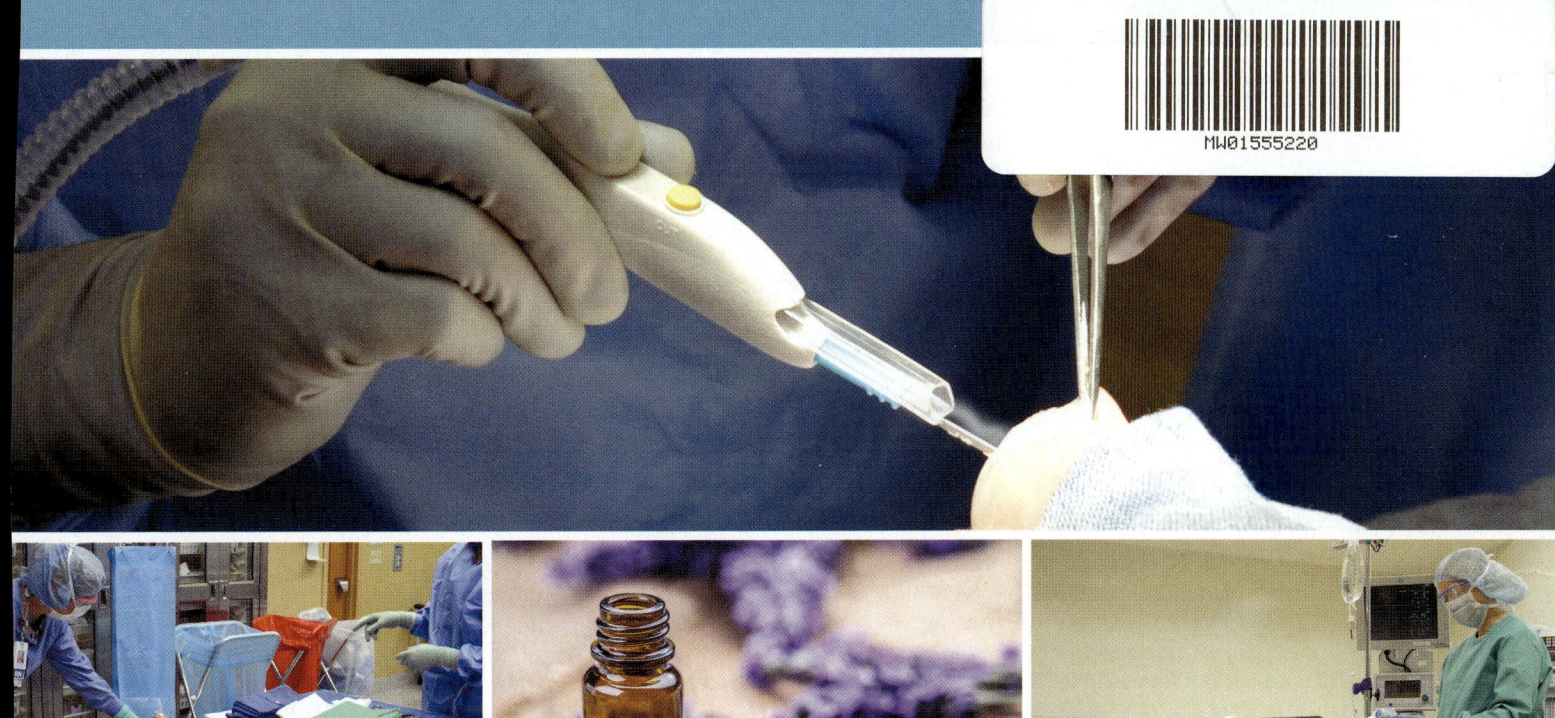

GUIDELINES FOR PERIOPERATIVE PRACTICE

2022 EDITION

Association of periOperative Registered Nurses

Editor-in-Chief
Erin Kyle, DNP, RN, CNOR, NEA-BC

Contributing Authors
Mary Alice Anderson, MSN, RN, CNOR
Byron Burlingame, MS, RN, CNOR
Julie A. Cahn, DNP, RN, CNOR, RN-BC, ACNS-BC, CNS-CP
Ramona Conner, MSN, RN, CNOR, FAAN
Jan Davidson, MSN, RN, CNOR, CASC
Karen deKay, MSN, RN, CNOR, CIC
Mary C. Fearon, MSN, RN, CNOR
Sharon Giarrizzo-Wilson, MS, RN-BC, CNOR
Esther M. Johnstone, DNP, RN, CNOR
Emily Jones, MSN, RN, CNOR, NPD-BC
Erin Kyle, DNP, RN, CNOR, NEA-BC
Terri Link, MPH, BSN, CNOR, CIC, FAPIC
Mary J. Ogg, MSN, RN, CNOR
Lisa Spruce, DNP, RN, CNS-CP, ACNS, ACNP, CNOR, FAAN
Cynthia Spry, MA, MS, RN, CNOR, CBSPDT
Sharon A. Van Wicklin, MSN, RN, CNOR, CRNFA(E), CPSN-R, PLNC, FAAN
Amber Wood, MSN, RN, CNOR, CIC, FAPIC

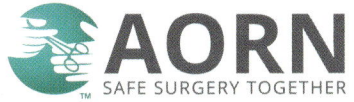

AORN
SAFE SURGERY TOGETHER

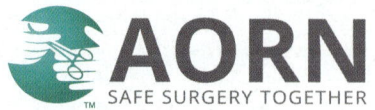

2170 South Parker Road, #400
Denver, CO 80231-5711
(800) 755-2676 | (303) 755-6300

Guidelines for Perioperative Practice, 2022 Edition
Copyright © 2022 AORN, Inc

CEO/Executive Director:
Linda Groah, MSN, RN, CNOR, NEA-BC, FAAN
Vice President of Nursing:
Renae Battié, MN, RN, CNOR
Director of Evidence-Based Perioperative Practice:
Lisa Spruce, DNP, RN, CNS-CP, ACNS, ACNP, CNOR, FAAN
Director of Publications & Product Strategy:
Richard L. Wohl, MFA, MBA

Senior Managing Editor:
Liz Cowperthwaite
Clinical Research Librarian:
Kristyn Beaty, MLS, BSN, RN, CNOR
Senior Manager, Creative Services:
Colleen Ladny
Graphic Designers: Keven Lewis,
Erynn McConnell
Illustrators: Kurt Jones, Colleen Ladny

AORN Mission, Vision, and Values

The Association of periOperative Registered Nurses (AORN) was founded in 1949 to establish a national community for operating room nurses who sought to share best practices for patients undergoing surgery. Today, we unite and empower perioperative nurses, health care organizations, and industry partners to support safe surgery for every patient, every time.

Mission: AORN defines, supports, and advocates for patient and staff safety through exemplary practice for each phase of perioperative nursing care using evidence-based guidelines, continuing education, and clinical practice resources.

Vision: AORN will provide indispensable evidence-based resources to establish the standards of excellence for each phase of perioperative nursing care to achieve optimal outcomes for every patient, every time.

Values:
- Diversity, Equity & Inclusiveness – honoring the contributions of all individuals
- Innovation – rewarding creativity, risk taking, leading-edge results
- Communication – respecting collaborative, open, and honest dialogue
- Quality – ensuring reliability, timeliness, and accountability
- Achievement – supporting growth and excellence

ISBN 978-0-939583-08-9   Printed in Canada

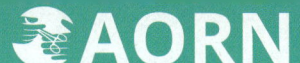
TABLE OF CONTENTS

Introduction

Guidelines for Perioperative Practice

REVISED *Documents appearing in print for the first time in 2022 and new/revised guidelines published electronically in 2021.*

SPECIAL FEATURES

Autologous Tissue Management

Complementary Care Interventions REVISED

Design and Maintenance

Electrosurgical Safety

SPECIAL FEATURES: CONTINUED

SPECIAL FEATURES: CONTINUED

Information Management

Instrument Cleaning

Laser Safety

Local Anesthesia

Medication Safety

Minimally Invasive Surgery

Moderate Sedation/Analgesia REVISED

Packaging Systems

Patient Skin Antisepsis REVISED

Pneumatic Tourniquets

Positioning the Patient

Product Evaluation

Radiation Safety REVISED

Retained Surgical Items REVISED

Safe Patient Handling and Movement

Sharps Safety

Specimen Management

Sterile Technique

AORN GUIDELINES FOR
PERIOPERATIVE PRACTICE,
2022 EDITION

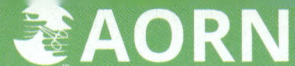
USING **THE AORN**
GUIDELINES FOR PERIOPERATIVE PRACTICE

AORN is committed to promoting excellence in perioperative nursing practice, advancing the profession, and supporting the professional perioperative registered nurse (RN). AORN promotes safe care for patients undergoing operative and other invasive procedures through the creation and maintenance of this collection of evidence-based perioperative guidelines. The descriptive and comprehensive guidelines in this collection reflect evidence-based practices for the perioperative RN in a range of topics that support both patient and worker safety. Each AORN guideline includes recommendations intended to optimize patient care that are informed by a systematic review of evidence and an assessment of the benefits and harms of alternative care options. The Preferred Reporting Items for Systematic Reviews and Meta-Analyses (PRISMA) is used to prepare transparent accounts of the systematic reviews that inform each guideline.

The guidelines are intended to be achievable and represent what is believed to be an optimal level of perioperative patient care and workplace safety. Each guideline contains recommendations that are broad statements to be used to guide the development of policies, procedures, and criteria for measuring individual competency in a variety of practice settings where operative and other invasive procedures are performed. These guidelines represent AORN's official position on questions regarding perioperative practice, and they have been approved by the AORN Guidelines Advisory Board.

Evidence-based practice is essential to improving patient care by promoting decisions based on the most recent, relevant evidence. The AORN guidelines are based on a comprehensive, systematic review of research and non-research evidence; the individual references are appraised and scored, and the recommendations are rated according to the strength and quality of the evidence supporting each recommendation. When adhering to the AORN Guidelines for Perioperative Practice, perioperative clinicians can be confident that they are following trustworthy guidelines developed in accordance with the principles set forth by the National Academy of Medicine.[1]

Perioperative practice specialists in the AORN Nursing Department serve as the lead authors of each guideline. the lead author facilitates guideline development through collaboration with a guideline development team that includes members of the AORN Guidelines Advisory Board, including a patient advocate, and Guideline Advisory Board liaisons representing the American Association of Nurse Anesthetists, the American College of Surgeons, the American Society of Anesthesiologists, the Association for Professionals in Infection Control and Epidemiology, the Healthcare Sterile Processing Association, the Society for Healthcare Epidemiology of America, and the Surgical Infection Society.

The AORN guideline development process is funded by AORN, Inc. Each guideline is posted for a 30-day public comment period at http://www.aorn.org, where members of the public, including scientific and clinical experts, organizations, agencies, and patients can review and comment on the guideline draft. The public comments are individually reviewed and reconciled by the guideline team members.

Each guideline is reviewed and updated on a 5-year cycle. Because only a portion of the guidelines are updated for publication in any given year, differences in format, content organization, and design may occur. Within the context of the guidelines, use of the word "should" indicates that a certain course of action is recommended. "Must" is used only to describe requirements mandated by government regulation. Use of "may" indicates that a course of action is permissible within the limits of the guideline, and "can" indicates possibility and capability.

Evidence Appraisal and Rating

Each guideline focuses on a specific question or topic. A clinical perioperative nurse research librarian employed by AORN conducts a systematic literature search to identify relevant literature. The Hierarchy of Evidence (Appendix A) is a visual depiction of the types of evidence used in the AORN Guidelines and demonstrates the strongest to the weakest types of evidence.

The lead author and an evidence appraiser independently evaluate and critically appraise the strength and quality of the evidence using the AORN Evidence Appraisal Tools (See Appendices B, C, and D). Each article or study is assigned a consensus appraisal score as agreed upon by the reviewers. Each appraisal score includes a Roman numeral (ie, I, II, III, IV, or V) and an alphabetical character (ie, A, B, or C). The Roman numeral represents the level of strength, and the alphabetical character represents the level of quality (eg, IIA). The appraisal scores of individual references are noted in brackets after each citation in the references section of the guideline as applicable.

After the evidence is individually appraised, the evidence supporting each recommendation is synthesized and rated as high-, moderate-, or low-quality using the AORN Evidence Rating Model (See Appendix E). The strength of the recommendation is rated based on the evidence rating, a benefit-harm assessment, and consideration of resource use. The recommendations in each guideline are given one of the following color-coded ratings:

- *[Regulatory Requirement]*
- *[Recommendation]*
- *[Conditional Recommendation]*
- *[No Recommendation]*

The recommendation strength rating is noted in brackets after each recommendation (See page xii).

DOCUMENT STRUCTURE

Topic Headings

Headings that represent the general subject of each section. The topic heading is in a bold font inside a colored bar and is identified by a number (eg, 1).

1. Product Selection and Use

Recommendations

Specific recommendations for treatment or action. Recommendations are identified by a number after the topic heading number (eg, 2.5). The recommendation statement is followed by a rationale detailing the evidence that supports the recommendation. The strength of each recommendation is rated using the AORN Evidence Rating Model and is noted in brackets after the recommendation statement (eg, *[Recommendation]*).

2.5 Perform cleaning activities in a methodical pattern that limits the transmission of micro-organisms.[21,81] *[Recommendation]*

Activities

Statements that describe the actions necessary to implement the recommendation. Activities are noted by a number following the topic heading number and the recommendation number (eg, 2.5.3). The strength of each activity is rated using the AORN Evidence Rating Model and is noted in brackets after the activity statement (eg, *[Conditional Recommendation]*).

2.5.3 The room may be cleaned in a clockwise or counter-clockwise direction in conjunction with clean-to-dirty and top-to-bottom methods.[21] *[Conditional Recommendation]*

Glossary

A list of definitions for terms used in the guideline with which the reader may be unfamiliar. Glossary terms are in a bold, underlined font in the text for easy identification. The definitions are located at the end of the guideline before the References.

A standardized product selection process assists in the selection of functional and reliable products that are safe, cost-effective, and **environmentally preferable** and that promote quality care, as well as decreases duplication or rapid obsolescence.[21,30]

Glossary

Environmentally preferable: Products or services that have lesser or reduced effect on human health and the environment compared to competing products or services that serve the same purpose.

References

A list of all references used in the guideline and the assigned appraisal scores. The appraisal score is noted in brackets after each citation.

References

1. Hess AS, Shardell M, Johnson JK, et al. A randomized controlled trial of enhanced cleaning to reduce contamination of healthcare worker gowns and gloves with multidrug-resistant bacteria. *Infect Control Hosp Epidemiol.* 2013;34(5):487-493. [IA]

DOCUMENT STRUCTURE: CONTINUED

Ambulatory Supplements

Each guideline is reviewed and vetted for applicability to ambulatory surgery centers, and supplemental information is provided related to recommendations that may have additional considerations unique to these perioperative practice settings. The Ambulatory Supplements are intended to be used as additional information for the perioperative RN practicing in a free-standing ambulatory surgery center or a physician office-based surgery center.

The (A) symbol in the text of a guideline indicates that there is additional information in the Ambulatory Supplement following the document. Relevant text from the guideline is repeated in the Supplement for easy reference and to give context to the ambulatory considerations. New text is denoted with the (A) symbol in the Supplement.

Pediatric Content

The (P) symbol in the text of a guideline indicates that the recommendation or supporting evidence is notably relevant to care of the pediatric patient.

7. Medical Gases

7.2.1 (A) Store an adequate emergency supply of oxygen at the facility to provide an uninterrupted supply for 1 day.[100]

The Ambulatory Supplement is an adjunct to the guideline on which it is based and is not intended to be a replacement for that document. Perioperative personnel who are developing and updating organizational policies and procedures should review and cite the full guideline.

1.1.3 Do not use disinfectants (eg, phenolics) to clean infant bassinets or incubators while these items are occupied.[8,21] If disinfectants (eg, phenolics) are used to terminally clean infant bassinets or incubators, prepare solutions in the correct concentrations per the manufacturer's IFU and rinse treated surfaces with water.[8,21] *[Recommendation]* (P)

AORN Guidelines and the PNDS

The Perioperative Nursing Data Set (PNDS) is the standardized nursing language developed and refined by AORN and recognized by the American Nurses Association to describe the nursing care, from preadmission to discharge, of patients undergoing operative or other invasive procedures.[2] The PNDS enables the perioperative registered nurse to document perioperative care in a standardized manner and allows the collection of reliable and valid comparable clinical data to evaluate the effectiveness of nurse-sensitive interventions and the relationship between these interventions and patient outcomes. The Guidelines for Perioperative Practice are the foundation of clinical knowledge from which the PNDS is derived.

The Guidelines for Perioperative Practice and the PNDS concepts are mapped to the clinical content within the AORN Syntegrity perioperative documentation solution for the electronic health record. The AORN Syntegrity solution provides standardized content for electronic perioperative nursing documentation. The PNDS is distributed only through an AORN Syntegrity license. To learn more about the AORN Syntegrity solution and implementation of the PNDS within the electronic health record, contact the AORN Syntegrity team via e-mail at syntegrity@aorn.org or visit http://www.aorn.org/syntegrity.

Implementation in Practice

Individual commitment, professional conscience, and the setting in which perioperative nursing is practiced should guide the RN in implementing these guidelines. Implementation of the guidelines in perioperative settings requires close examination of the organization's existing policies and procedures. This review may indicate that new or revised policies and procedures are needed. Although the guidelines are considered to represent the optimal level of practice, variations in practice settings and clinical situations may limit the degree to which each guideline can be implemented. AORN has created a comprehensive set of implementation tools to help health care organizations implement the guidelines. For more information, visit http://www.aorn.org.

References

1. Institute of Medicine. Field MJ, Lohr KN, eds. *Clinical Practice Guidelines: Directions for a New Program*. Washington, DC: National Academy Press; 1990:38.

2. Petersen C, ed. *Perioperative Nursing Data Set*. 3rd ed. Denver, CO: AORN, Inc; 2011.

AORN Hierarchy of Evidence

RESEARCH	**I**	SYSTEMATIC REVIEW – All studies RCTs RANDOMIZED CONTROLLED TRIAL (RCT)
	II	SYSTEMATIC REVIEW – All studies Quasi-Experimental or a combination of RCTs and Quasi-Experimental QUASI-EXPERIMENTAL
	III	SYSTEMATIC REVIEW – All studies Non-Experimental or a combination of RCTs, Quasi-Experimental, and Non-Experimental Any or all studies Qualitative NON-EXPERIMENTAL QUALITATIVE
NON-RESEARCH	**IV**	CLINICAL PRACTICE GUIDELINE CONSENSUS or POSITION STATEMENT
	V	LITERATURE REVIEW CASE REPORT EXPERT OPINION ORGANIZATIONAL EXPERIENCE

Copyright © AORN, Inc, 2022

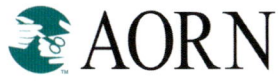 **AORN RESEARCH EVIDENCE APPRAISAL TOOL - STUDY**

DATE_____
REVIEWER_____
APPRAISAL SCORE _____

RW#	CITATION

Does this evidence address the perioperative practice question?
☐ Yes   ☐ No - Do not proceed with evidence appraisal.

Does this evidence have a major flaw?
☐ No   ☐ Yes - Determine level of evidence and score quality as C.
Provide explanation of flaw in comments.

LEVEL OF EVIDENCE

Is this a report of a single research study?
☐ Yes   ☐ No (If No, go to the AORN Research Evidence Appraisal Tool - Summary)

INTERVENTION/MANIPULATION The researcher performed an intervention with at least some of the participants (ie, there was some type of treatment being tested).		☐ Yes	☐ No
CONTROL/COMPARISON GROUP The researcher provided standard care or a comparison intervention that was different from the experimental intervention.		☐ Yes	☐ No
RANDOM ASSIGNMENT The researcher assigned participants to a control or treatment group on a random basis (ie, in a manner determined by chance).		☐ Yes	☐ No

YES to Intervention/Manipulation, Control/Comparison Group, and Random Assignment	☐ LEVEL I	Randomized Controlled Trial (RCT)
YES to Intervention/Manipulation or YES to Intervention/Manipulation, and Control/Comparison Group	☐ LEVEL II	Quasi-Experimental (eg, controlled trial, controlled trial without randomization, pre-test/post-test, time series)
NO to Intervention/Manipulation	☐ LEVEL III	Non-Experimental (eg, descriptive, comparative, observational, correlational, case-control, retrospective, cross-sectional)
	☐ LEVEL III	Qualitative (eg, interviews, surveys, focus groups)

ADDITIONAL COMMENTS:

QUALITY OF EVIDENCE	A HIGH	B GOOD	C LOW	NA
PURPOSE/BACKGROUND				
• Was the purpose of the study clearly defined?				�
• Were the research questions clear?				▣
• Did the researcher(s) identify what is known and not known about the research questions and how the study would address any gaps in knowledge?				▣
• Was the study approved by an institutional review board (IRB)?				
• Were the supporting references the most current available?				▣
• Were the supporting references relevant to the research question?				▣
RANDOMIZATION				
• Were the subjects randomly assigned to the Intervention and Control groups?				
• Were the subjects and providers blinded to the study group?		▣	▣	
CONTROL				
• Was the Control group clearly identified?				
• Was the Control group representative of the sample population?				
• Were the characteristics and/or demographics similar in both the Control and Intervention groups?				
• Were all groups treated equally, except for the Intervention group?				
• Were multiple settings used?				
• If multiple settings were used, were the settings similar?				
INTERVENTION(S)				
• Did the intervention support the research question?				
• Did the intervention(s) for each group contain sufficient details to allow replication?				
SAMPLE SIZE				
• Was an adequate description of sample size determination provided?				
• Was a power analysis performed?		▣	▣	
• If no power analysis was performed, did the sample size ensure confidence that the effect of the intervention was demonstrated?	▣			
• Was the inclusion/exclusion criteria for the study participants clear?				
• Were all study participants accounted for?				
DATA COLLECTION				
• Was the data collection process clearly described?				▣
• Were the methods of statistical analysis clearly described?				▣
• Was there a discussion of the instrument's validity?				
• Was the precision of each outcome supported with a measurement (eg, confidence interval) to show statistical significance, or lack thereof?				▣
• If surveys/questionnaires were used, was the response rate > 25%?				
RESULTS/CONCLUSIONS				
• If tables were presented, was the narrative consistent with the table content?				
• Were the outcomes of the study clearly explained?				▣
• Were the conclusions of the researcher(s) consistent with the results of the study?				
LIMITATIONS/FUTURE RESEARCH				
• Was the discussion of the limitations of the evidence accurate?				▣
BIAS				
• Did the researcher(s) implement methods to reduce distortion of the results of the study (eg, blinding)?				▣
• Has the effect of the intervention been over- or underestimated by the researcher(s)?				▣
VALIDITY				
• Were threats to validity controlled by the study design?				▣
GENERALIZABILITY				
• Are the results of the study transferrable or applicable to other settings or populations?				▣
FINAL QUALITY SCORE				

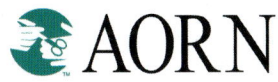 **AORN** **AORN RESEARCH EVIDENCE APPRAISAL TOOL - SUMMARY**

DATE_____
REVIEWER_____
APPRAISAL SCORE _____

RW#	CITATION

Does this evidence address the perioperative practice question?
☐ Yes ☐ No - Do not proceed with evidence appraisal.

Does this evidence have a major flaw?
☐ No ☐ Yes - Determine level of evidence and score quality as C.
Provide explanation of flaw in comments.

LEVEL OF EVIDENCE

Summary of multiple research studies? ☐ Yes ☐ No (If No, go to the AORN Research Evidence Appraisal Tool - Study)

Comprehensive search strategy and rigorous appraisal?
☐ Yes (Systematic Review) ☐ No (If No, go to the AORN Non-Research Appraisal Tool)

Results from studies combined and analyzed to generate new statistic or effect size (measure of strength of relationship between two variables)	☐ Yes – Systematic Review with Meta-Analysis ☐ No
Concepts from Qualitative studies analyzed and synthesized	☐ Yes – Systematic Review with Meta-Synthesis ☐ No
All studies are randomized controlled trials (RCTs)	☐ LEVEL I
All studies are Quasi-Experimental or a combination of RCTs and Quasi-Experimental	☐ LEVEL II
All studies are Non-Experimental or a combination of RCTs, Quasi-Experimental, and Non-Experimental	☐ LEVEL III
Any or all studies are Qualitative	☐ LEVEL III

ADDITIONAL COMMENTS:

Copyright © AORN, Inc, 2022

QUALITY OF EVIDENCE	A HIGH	B GOOD	C LOW	NA
PURPOSE/BACKGROUND				
• Was the purpose of the systematic review clearly defined?				▓
• Was the research question clear?				▓
• Did the researcher(s) identify what is known and not known about the research question and how the systematic review would address any gaps in knowledge?				▓
SEARCH				
• Was the search strategy reproducible?				▓
• Were the key search terms stated?				▓
• Were multiple databases searched and identified?				▓
• Was the inclusion/exclusion criteria described?				▓
• Was both published and unpublished literature identified and retrieved where possible?				▓
• Are the types of studies to be included in the review described?				▓
EVIDENCE REVIEW				
• Was there an explanation of the number of studies eliminated at each level of review?				▓
• Were the details of the included studies presented (design, sample, methods, results, outcomes, strengths, limitations)?				▓
• Were methods for appraising the strength of evidence (level and quality) rigorous?				▓
• Was the evidence reviewed and appraised by at least two members of the research team?				▓
• Were the supporting references the most current available?				▓
• Were the supporting references relevant to the research question?				▓
DATA COLLECTION				
• Were methods of statistical analysis described?				
• Were methods of retrieving data from the individual studies described?				
• Was the data extracted by at least two members of the research team?				
RESULTS/CONCLUSIONS				
• Were the conclusions of the researcher(s) consistent with the results of the studies and the overall strength of the evidence?				▓
• Was the strength of the phenomenon being studied quantified in a summary statistic (ie, effect size) that can be compared across the studies?		▓	▓	
LIMITATIONS/FUTURE RESEARCH				
• Were limitations of the review discussed?				▓
FINAL QUALITY SCORE				

AORN NON-RESEARCH EVIDENCE APPRAISAL TOOL

AORN

DATE_____
REVIEWER_____
APPRAISAL SCORE _____

RW#	CITATION

Does this evidence address the perioperative practice question?
☐ Yes   ☐ No - Do not proceed with evidence appraisal.

LEVEL OF EVIDENCE		
Systematically developed recommendations from recognized experts based on evidence or consensus opinion that guides members of a professional organization in decision-making related to practice or a particular issue of concern	☐ LEVEL IV	Clinical Practice Guideline Consensus or Position Statement
Summary of published literature on a topic of interest without a systematic appraisal of the strength and quality of the evidence	☐ LEVEL V	Literature Review
In-depth analysis of an individual, group, social unit, issue, or event	☐ LEVEL V	Case Report
Advice from an individual(s) with knowledge and expertise on a particular topic or issue	☐ LEVEL V	Expert Opinion
Initiative with a goal to improve the processes or outcome of care being delivered within a particular institution	☐ LEVEL V	Organizational Experience

ADDITIONAL COMMENTS:

QUALITY OF EVIDENCE	A HIGH	B GOOD	C LOW	NA
CLINICAL PRACTICE GUIDELINE/POSITION STATEMENT				
• Was the purpose of the guideline or position statement clearly stated?				
• Was the guideline or position statement developed, reviewed, or revised within the past five years?				
• Were stakeholders involved in the development of the guideline or position statement representative of the specialty?				
• Were the groups to which the recommendations apply and do not apply clearly defined?				
• Was the strategy for developing the guideline or position statement rigorous?				
• Was there a reproducible literature search or other systematic method used to search for evidence?				
• Was a rating scheme or grading method used to determine the quality and strength of the evidence included in the guideline or position statement?				
• Was there an objective description of the type of studies or the consensus process used to support the recommendations?				
• Were the recommendations of the author(s) unbiased and consistent with the literature reviewed?				
• Were the strengths and limitations of the body of evidence clearly described?				
• Were the supporting references the most current available?				
• Were the supporting references relevant to the recommendations?				
• Was the guideline or position statement subjected to a peer review process?				
LITERATURE REVIEW				
• Was the purpose of the literature review clearly stated?				
• Did the author(s) identify what is known and not known about the practice question and how the literature review will address any gaps in knowledge?				
• Were the supporting references the most current available?				
• Were the supporting references relevant to the subject being reviewed?				
• Did the author(s) provide a meaningful analysis and synthesis of the literature reviewed?				
• Were conclusions of the author(s) unbiased and consistent with the literature reviewed?				
• Were the findings of the literature review accurately summarized in tables or figures?				
• Were recommendations made for future practice or study?				
CASE REPORT				
• Was the purpose of the case report clearly stated?				
• Was the case report clearly presented?				
• Were the findings of the case report evidence-based?				
• Was follow-up sufficiently long and complete?				
• Was there a literature review?				
• Did the author(s) provide recommendations for practice?				
• Were the recommendations for practice clearly stated and linked to the findings of the case report?				
EXPERT OPINION				
• Has the individual published or presented on the topic?				
• Was the individual opinion evidence-based?				
• Was the individual opinion clearly stated?				
• Was the individual opinion unbiased and consistent with the evidence?				
ORGANIZATIONAL EXPERIENCE				
• Was the aim of the organizational project clearly stated and focused on assessing and improving current practice?				
• Was the methodology of the project adequately described?				
• Were process or outcome measures for the organizational project identified?				
• Were the results of the organizational project adequately described?				
• Were components of cost/benefit analysis described?				
• Were multiple sites involved?				
FINAL QUALITY SCORE				

AORN Evidence Rating Model

1. Evidence Rating

HIGH	MODERATE	LOW
IA or IB IIA or IIB	IIIA or IIIB	IC, IIC, or IIIC VA, VB, or VC
• Wide range of studies with no major limitations • Little variation between studies	• Few studies and some have limitations but not major flaws • Some variation between studies	• Studies have major flaws or there are no rigorous studies • Important variation between studies

2. Recommendation Rating

Evidence Rating

Benefit-Harm Assessment

Resource Use

↓

RECOMMENDATION

Regulatory Requirement

Recommendation

• Benefits clearly exceed harms
• Supported by high- to moderate-quality evidence
• May be based on low-quality evidence or expert opinion when
  - high-quality evidence is impossible to obtain
  - supported by a guideline, position statement, or consensus statement

Conditional Recommendation

• Benefits are likely to exceed harms
• May be supported by any level of evidence when
  - indicated for a specific patient population or clinical situation
  - impact of the intervention is difficult to separate from other simultaneously implemented interventions (eg, "bundled" practices)
  - benefit-harm assessment may change with further research or not be consistent
  - benefit is most likely if used as a supplemental measure

No Recommendation

• There is both a lack of evidence and an unclear balance between benefits and harms.

3. Implementation

Regulatory Requirement →

• Perioperative team members "must" implement the recommendation in accordance with regulatory requirements.

Recommendation →

• Perioperative team members "should" implement the recommendation, unless a clear and compelling rationale for an alternative approach is present.

Conditional Recommendation →

• Perioperative team members "may" implement the recommendation.
• The degree of implementation may vary depending on the benefit-harm assessment for the specific setting.

No Recommendation →

• Perioperative team members will need to evaluate whether or not to implement the practice issue.

AORN GRATEFULLY ACKNOWLEDGES THE WORK OF THE 2021-2022 GUIDELINES ADVISORY BOARD

Co-Chairs

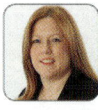
Susan Lynch, PhD, RN, CSSM, CNOR
Associate Director/Surgical Services
Penn Medicine - Chester County Hospital
Glen Mills, Pennsylvania
(Member 2019-2020, Chair 2020-2022)

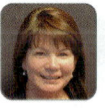
Mary C. Fearon, MSN, RN, CNOR
Service Line Director Neuroscience
Overlake Hospital Medical Center
Bellevue, Washington
(Member 2018-2021, Chair 2021-2022)

Members

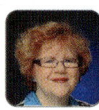
Linda C. Boley, MSN, BSN, RN, CNOR
Clinical Educator, Surgical Services
Norton Women's and Children's Hospital
Louisville, Kentucky
(2019-2022)

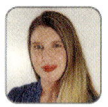
Crystal A. Bricker, MSN, RN, CNOR
Clinical Practice Partner, Perioperative Services
Advocate BroMenn Regional Medical Center
Bloomington, Illinois
(2019-2022)

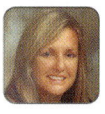
Michele J. Brunges, MSN, RNM, CNOR, CHSE
Director of Perioperative Services
University of Florida Health Shands Hospital
Gainesville, Florida
(2019-2022)

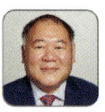
Bernard C. Camins, MD, MSc
Health System Infection Prevention Medical Director
Mount Sinai Medical Center
New York, New York
(Advisory Board Liaison 2016-2018,
Member 2018-2022)

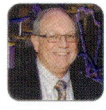
Rob J. Levin, MSN, RN, RRT, CNOR
OR Educator
Virtua Health Mt Holly
Mt Holly, New Jersey
(2020-2022)

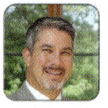
James Padilla, JD
Dean
Loras College
Dubuque, Iowa
(Patient Advocate, 2020-2022)

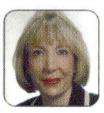
Donna A. Pritchard, MA, BSN, RN, NE-BC, CNOR
Director of Perioperative Services
Interfaith Medical Center
Brooklyn, New York
(Member 2017-2018, 2021-2022; Chair 2018-2021)

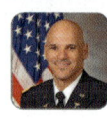
Jose Rodriguez, DNP, RN, CCNS, CNOR
Assistant Professor and Deputy Director
AG-CNS Program
Bethesda, Maryland
(2021-2022)

Advisory Board Liaisons

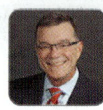
Craig S. Atkins, DNP, CRNA
American Association of Nurse Anesthesiology
(2019-2022)

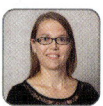
Shandra R. Day, MD
Society for Healthcare Epidemiology of America
(2020-2022)

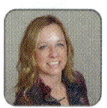
Cassie Dietrich, MD
American Society of Anesthesiologists
(2018-2022)

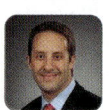
Jared M. Huston, MD
Surgical Infection Society
(2019-2022)

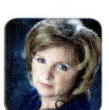
Sue G. Klacik, BS, CRCST, FCS
Healthcare Sterile Processing Association
(2017-2022)

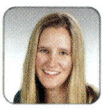
Sara Reese
Association for Professionals in Infection
Control and Epidemiology
(2020-2022)

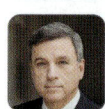
Juan A. Sanchez, MD, MPA, FACS, FACHE
American College of Surgeons
(2020-2022)

AORN Board Liaison

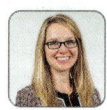
Brandy L. Miller, MHA, MSN, RN, CNOR
Director
Southwest Surgical Suites
Fort Wayne, Indiana
(2021-2022)

AUTOLOGOUS TISSUE MANAGEMENT

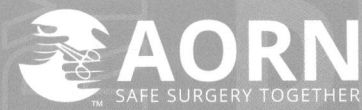

TABLE OF CONTENTS

MEDICAL ABBREVIATIONS & ACRONYMS

AATB – American Association of Tissue Banks
CDC – Centers for Disease Control and Prevention
CFR – Code of Federal Regulations
CHG – Chlorhexidine gluconate
CLIA-88 – Clinical Laboratory Improvement Amendments of 1988
DMEM – Dulbecco's modified Eagle's medium
EO – Ethylene oxide

FDA – US Food and Drug Administration
H₂O₂ – Hydrogen peroxide
IFU – Instructions for use
PSI – Pounds per square inch
RCT – Randomized controlled trial
RPMI – Roswell Park Memorial Institute
SSI – Surgical site infection
THA – Total hip arthroplasty

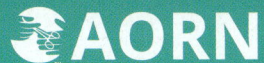
GUIDELINE FOR
AUTOLOGOUS TISSUE MANAGEMENT

The Guideline for Autologous Tissue Management was approved by the AORN Guidelines Advisory Board and became effective as of December 9, 2019. The recommendations in the guideline are intended to be achievable and represent what is believed to be an optimal level of practice. Policies and procedures will reflect variations in practice settings and/or clinical situations that determine the degree to which the guideline can be implemented. AORN recognizes the many diverse settings in which perioperative nurses practice; therefore, this guideline is adaptable to all areas where operative or other invasive procedures may be performed.

Purpose

This document provides guidance for preserving **autologous tissue**, including cranial bone flaps, parathyroid glands, skin, vessels (eg, veins, arteries), femoral heads, incus, and adipose tissue, in the perioperative setting. Guidance is also provided for team communication related to autologous tissue management; handling, packaging, labeling, storage, disposal, cleaning, transport, and documentation of autologous tissue; and policies and procedures for preservation and delayed **replantation** or **autotransplantation** of autologous tissue within the same facility.

Preserving and replanting autologous tissue may improve the patient's long-term outcomes. Some types of autologous tissue (eg, cranial bone flaps, parathyroid glands) are preserved because the patient's clinical symptoms (eg, swelling, hormone levels, infection) prevent the tissue from being replanted or autotransplanted during the same procedure in which it was removed. Other types of autologous tissue (eg, veins, skin, adipose tissue) are preserved because the tissue was harvested but was not all used during the original procedure and may be needed for a future procedure (eg, cardiovascular bypass graft, skin graft). In addition, the use of autologous tissue may be preferred over the use of **allograft** tissue or synthetic tissue implants in certain situations. Following good tissue practices described in 21 Code of Federal Regulations (CFR) Part 1271 Subpart D[1] and evidenced-based guidance for autologous tissue management may

- decrease the patient's risk for infection;
- decrease the risk for a packaging, labeling, or tissue identification error;
- decrease the risk to perioperative personnel of exposure to blood and other potentially infectious materials; and
- preserve the clinical viability of the tissue.

The following topics are outside the scope of this document:

- autologous tissue that is replanted into the patient during the same procedure in which it was removed (eg, tendons, ligaments, osteochondral grafts, fractional skin grafts, epidermal grafts);
- autologous blood products;
- autologous islet cell or stem cell transplantation;
- autologous cartilage used for staged microtia reconstruction procedures;
- autologous bone that is exposed to cryotherapy, radiation, or thermal therapy for eradication of cancer and replanted during the same procedure in which it was removed;
- tissue-engineered grafts grown from autologous cells;
- allograft organ or tissue transplantation;
- allograft fecal microbiota transplantation; and
- xenogeneic tissue (eg, bovine or porcine implants).

Refer to the AORN Guideline for Specimen Management[2] for information regarding surgical specimens and the AORN Guideline for Sterilization Packaging Systems[3] for recommendations on packaging systems for sterilization.

Evidence Review

A medical librarian with a perioperative background conducted a systematic search of the databases Ovid MEDLINE®, Ovid Embase®, EBSCO CINAHL®, and the Cochrane Database of Systematic Reviews. The search was limited to literature published in English from January 2014 through October 2018. At the time of the initial search, weekly alerts were created on the topics included in that search. Results from these alerts were provided to the lead author until February 2019. The lead author requested additional articles that either did not fit the original search criteria or were discovered during the evidence appraisal process. The lead author and the medical librarian also identified relevant guidelines from government agencies, professional organizations, and standards-setting bodies.

Search terms included *adipose aspirates, adipose tissue, autograft, bone flap, bone resorption, bone transplantation, cell culture techniques, cranial edema, craniotomy, cryopreservation, decompressive craniectomy, fat grafting, intercranial hypertension (surgery), internal mammary artery, internal mammary artery implantation, internal thoracic artery, mammary arteries, ossiculoplasty, parathyroid glands, pedicle flap, radial artery, renal artery, saphenous vein, skull (microbiology, cytology, surgery), sterilization (methods), sterilization and disinfection*

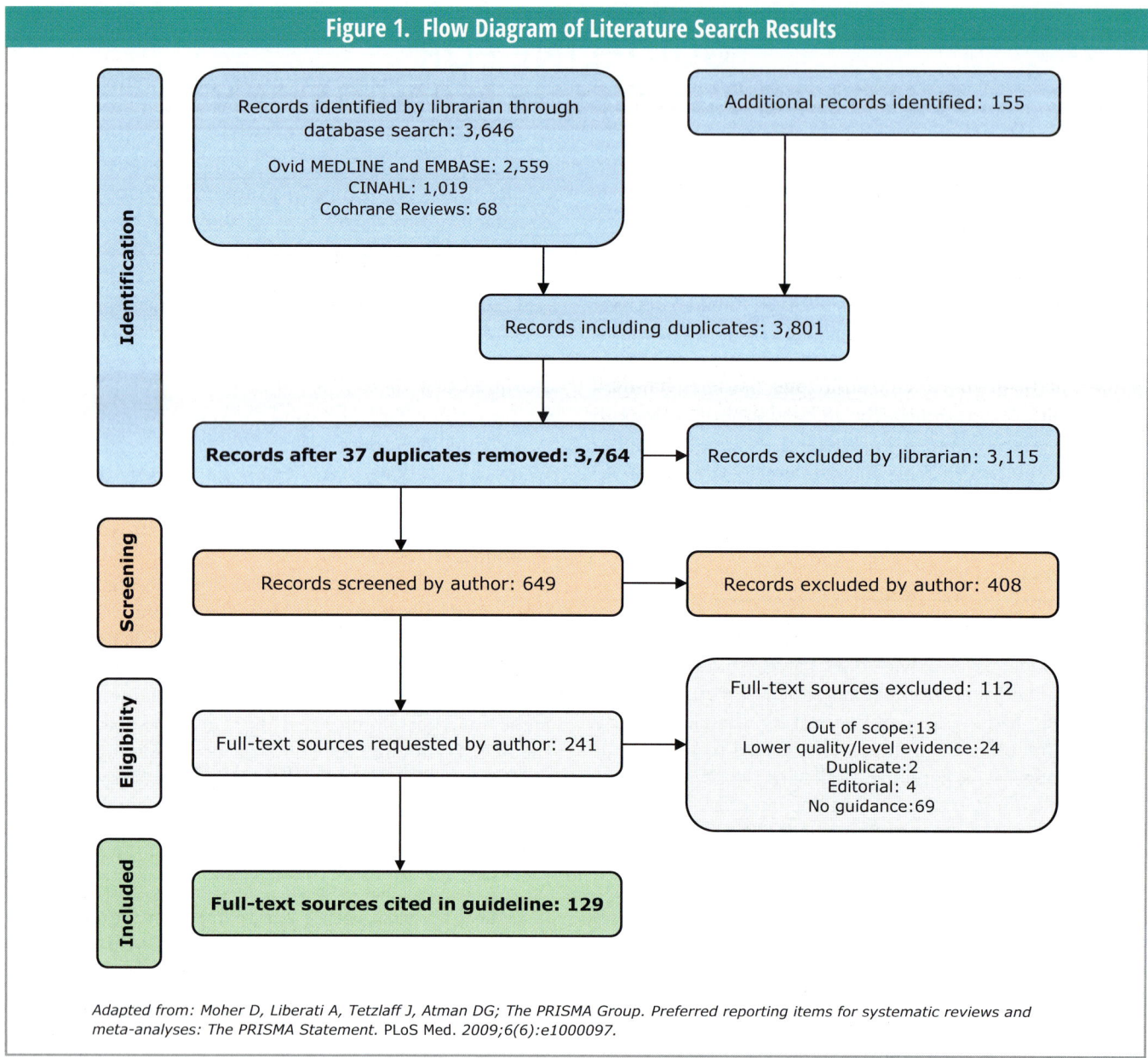

Figure 1. Flow Diagram of Literature Search Results

Identification

Records identified by librarian through database search: 3,646

Ovid MEDLINE and EMBASE: 2,559
CINAHL: 1,019
Cochrane Reviews: 68

Additional records identified: 155

Records including duplicates: 3,801

Records after 37 duplicates removed: 3,764

Records excluded by librarian: 3,115

Screening

Records screened by author: 649

Records excluded by author: 408

Eligibility

Full-text sources requested by author: 241

Full-text sources excluded: 112

Out of scope:13
Lower quality/level evidence:24
Duplicate:2
Editorial: 4
No guidance:69

Included

Full-text sources cited in guideline: 129

Adapted from: Moher D, Liberati A, Tetzlaff J, Atman DG; The PRISMA Group. Preferred reporting items for systematic reviews and meta-analyses: The PRISMA Statement. PLoS Med. 2009;6(6):e1000097.

(methods), surgical flaps, thoracic arteries, time factors, and *transplantation (autologous).*

Included were research and non-research literature in English, complete publications, and publications with dates within the time restriction when available. Excluded were non-peer-reviewed publications and older evidence within the time restriction when more recent evidence was available. Editorials, news items, and other brief items were excluded. Low-quality evidence was excluded when higher-quality evidence was available, and literature outside the time restriction was excluded when literature within the time restriction was available (Figure 1).

Articles identified in the search were provided to the project team for evaluation. The team consisted of the lead author and one evidence appraiser. The lead author and the evidence appraiser reviewed and critically appraised each article using the AORN Research or Non-Research Evidence Appraisal Tools as appropriate. A second appraiser was consulted if there was a disagreement between the lead author and the primary evidence appraiser. The literature was independently evaluated and appraised according to the strength and quality of the evidence. Each article was then assigned an appraisal score. The appraisal score is noted in brackets after each reference as applicable.

Each recommendation rating is based on a synthesis of the collective evidence, a benefit-harm assessment, and consideration of resource use. The strength of the recommendation was determined using the AORN Evidence Rating Model and the quality and consistency of the evidence supporting a recommendation. The recommendation strength rating is noted in brackets after each recommendation.

Note: The evidence summary table is available at http://www.aorn.org/evidencetables/.

Editor's note: MEDLINE is a registered trademark of the US National Library of Medicine's Medical Literature Analysis and Retrieval System, Bethesda, MD. Embase is a registered trademark of Elsevier B.V., Amsterdam, The Netherlands. CINAHL, Cumulative Index to Nursing and Allied Health Literature, is a registered trademark of EBSCO Industries, Birmingham, AL.

1. Tissue Establishment Registration

1.1 **Facilities in which autologous tissue is handled must register with the US Food and Drug Administration (FDA) as a tissue establishment unless the tissue is recovered, packaged, labeled, and stored in the original form for replantation or autotransplantation in the same patient at the same facility.** *[Regulatory Requirement]*

In 21 CFR 1271.15(b), the FDA provides an exception from registration as a tissue establishment as long as the autologous tissue is removed from and replanted or autotransplanted in the original form back into the same individual during the same surgical procedure.[1] In 2017, the FDA clarified that procedures involving the removal of and replantation or autotransplantation of the autologous tissue back into the same individual at the same facility are generally considered to be the same surgical procedure.[4] Surgical removal and subsequent replantation or autotransplantation of cranial bone flaps or portions of parathyroid tissue that occur a number of days apart may be considered the same surgical procedure under the 21 CFR 1271.15(b) exception. Processing steps for storage may include cleaning, rinsing, packaging, and labeling. However, the tissue must remain in its original form with no additional manufacturing steps (eg, sterilization, centrifuge for cell isolation).[4] The method used to store autologous tissue (eg, refrigeration, freezing, cryopreservation) does not, in itself, affect whether an establishment meets the same surgical procedure exception.

1.2 **Facilities must register with the FDA as a tissue establishment if autologous tissue handling includes manufacturing steps such as sterilization or other processing that changes the tissue from the original form.**[1,4] *[Regulatory Requirement]*

Registering with the FDA as a tissue establishment is required by 21 CFR 1271 when a facility manufactures tissue.[1] Manufacturing of tissue includes the steps involved in recovery, processing, storage, labeling, packaging, and distribution. Processing may include sterilization or other steps to inactivate or remove contaminants.[1] The FDA has clarified that the only processing steps that allow autologous tissue to stay in the original form are cleaning, rinsing, sizing, and shaping.[4] In general, use of only the specified processing steps allows facilities to use the exception in 21 CFR 1271.15(b) that eliminates the need for registration.[4]

1.3 **A facility that routinely distributes tissue to other facilities must register as a tissue establishment using the FDA's electronic Human Cell and Tissue Establishment Registration System and must comply with the applicable regulations in 21 CFR 1271.**[1] *[Regulatory Requirement]*

Under 21 CFR 1271.3(e), distribution of tissue from one facility to another is considered part of manufacturing and requires registration with the FDA as a tissue establishment.[1]

1.3.1 **A facility may not be required to register as a tissue establishment when tissue distribution is only for the purpose of burial or cremation.** *[Conditional Recommendation]*

Facilities that are asked to send tissue for burial or cremation are not required to register as a tissue establishment because the tissue is not intended for replantation or autotransplantation into a human recipient.[1]

2. Cranial Bone Flap

2.1 **Autologous cranial bone flaps may be frozen, cryopreserved, or stored in a subcutaneous pocket for replantation.** *[Conditional Recommendation]*

Moderate-quality evidence supports the preservation of autologous cranial bone by freezing, cryopreservation, and subcutaneous pocket storage.[5-10]

Corliss et al[5] conducted a systematic review of 48 studies that included 5,346 patients and compared cryopreservation and subcutaneous storage of autologous cranial bone flaps. The researchers found there was no significant difference between cryopreservation and subcutaneous storage for the outcomes of infection rates, bone resorption rates, or the need for revision procedures. The researchers concluded that both the cryopreservation and subcutaneous preservation methods for preserving autologous cranial bone flaps were safe and effective.

The evidence conflicts regarding the viability of bone after cryopreservation and the effect on patient outcomes (eg, resorption, infection). Some researchers have found that cranial bone flaps had some or complete viability after cryopreservation,[8,11-13] while others have reported limited or no viability after cryopreservation.[14-16] Only a few studies have investigated the outcomes of both bone viability and patient outcomes after cryopreservation.[8,11,16] However, because of variability in the study methodologies and the reported results, no conclusion can be drawn as to how cryopreservation affects viability or how cranial bone flap viability affects patient outcomes. Further research is needed.

The benefits of autologous bone flap preservation may exceed the harms. The benefits include no risk of immunoreactivity,[17] better insulation,[11] improved cosmetic appearance,[18-20] and reduced costs compared to use of synthetic cranial bone flap replacements.[7] The harms may include risks of

- reduced **osteoblast** viability after cryopreservation,[14,15]
- bone flap resorption compared to almost no risk of resorption with synthetic material use,[8,21-23]
- skin breakdown or necrosis when the **subgaleal** scalp area is used for preservation,[24] and
- bone formation in a subcutaneous pocket.[25]

In a nonexperimental study, Ernst et al[7] found a significant difference in cost between **cranioplasty** procedures involving autologous bone and procedures involving custom implants. The average cost of procedures involving autologous bone was $2,156.28 ± $1,144.60, whereas the average cost of procedures involving synthetic implants was $35,118.60 ± $2,067.51 (2017 dollars).

Conversely, Honeybul et al[26] conducted a randomized controlled trial (RCT) to compare patient outcomes and hospital costs for cranioplasty procedures (N = 64) and found that the use of titanium implants was associated with a reduction in reoperations and hospital costs compared with the use of autologous cranial bone flaps. However, the results were not statistically significant.

2.1.1 When an autologous cranial bone flap is stored in a subcutaneous pocket, provide the patient and the patient's designated caregiver(s) with instructions regarding the care of the surgical incision storage area. *[Recommendation]*

Providing patient education on care of the surgical wound area where the tissue is stored may help the patient understand how to help the area heal and prevent actions (eg, touching, rubbing, scratching) that might increase the risk of skin breakdown, bone formation in the subcutaneous pocket, or resorption or atrophy of the preserved tissue.

2.2 Determine a method for preparing cranial bone flaps for preservation, which may include

- preparing the bone for packaging as soon as a decision is made to preserve the bone,[27,28]

- removing blood[19,28,29] and excess soft tissue,[29,30]
- irrigating or immersing the bone in normal saline solution or a mixture of normal saline and antibiotics or povidone-iodine solution,[6,8,17,29-32]
- using low-linting sterile material to dry excess fluid from the bone,[6,28,29]
- wrapping the bone flap in sterile gauze,[32]
- using sterile technique and sealing the bone in at least two sterile bags[6,11,17,19,27-29,31,33] or a sterile container that can be sealed,
- packaging and labeling[11,27] the bone (See Recommendation 11),
- placing the packaged bone flap in a third sterile bag before handing it off the sterile field[6], and
- placing the bone in the tissue freezer as soon as possible.[11,27]

[Conditional Recommendation]

The benefits of preparing autologous cranial bone flaps for preservation are likely to exceed the harms. Wrapping the bone flap in sterile gauze may reduce the risk of the sharp edges of the bone flap puncturing the sterile bags. A potential harm of using nonradiopaque sterile gauze may be increased risk of a retained surgical item or foreign body reaction from contact with the fibers, although further research is needed.

No studies were found that specifically compared the effect of autologous cranial bone flap preparation on patient outcomes (eg, infection, resorption). However, several researchers reported how cranial bone flaps were prepared for storage as part of their study methodology. Bhaskar et al[17] reported a high level of variability in cranial bone flap preparation methods used in 25 major neurosurgical health care facilities in Australia. From a survey, the researchers found that in 52% of the facilities, cranial bone flaps were cryopreserved in a facility freezer, whereas in the remaining 48% of the facilities, cranial bone flaps were stored at a local **tissue bank**. Further research is needed to determine the effect of autologous bone flap preparation on patient outcomes.

2.2.1 Follow the manufacturer's instructions for use (IFU) when using a prepackaged cranial bone flap storage kit from a manufacturer or tissue establishment to freeze or cryopreserve cranial bone flaps. *[Recommendation]*

2.3 Determine the temperature range for freezing or cryopreserving autologous cranial bone flaps based on the anticipated length of storage, risk for microbial growth, and preservation of osteocyte viability. *[Recommendation]*

Moderate-quality evidence shows a wide variation in temperature ranges used for cryopreservation or freezing of autologous cranial bone flaps. In a systematic review of 48 studies, Corliss et al[5] reported that the storage temperatures for cranial bone flaps ranged from 8° C to -86° C (46.4° F to -122.8° F) with a mean temperature of -57° C (-70.6° F). Results of a survey of 25 major neurosurgical centers in Australia showed that bone flaps were cryopreserved at temperatures between -18° C to -83° C (-0.4° F to -117.4° F), with a mean of -62.1° C (-79.8° F).[17] The American Association of Tissue Banks (AATB) recommends that frozen or cryopreserved allograft musculoskeletal tissue be stored at temperatures between -20° C and -40° C (-4° F and -40° F) for temporary storage less than 6 months and -40° C (-40° F) or colder for storage durations longer than 6 months.[34] No studies comparing different temperature ranges were found, and further research is needed to determine the ideal temperature.

In a nonexperimental study, Tahir et al[27] investigated surgical site infection (SSI) rates associated with cranial bone flaps stored at -26° C (-14.8° F). The researchers found that only three patients (3.4%) who received the bone flaps developed an SSI. Two patients had superficial infections that resolved with oral antibiotics and the third patient required a second procedure for washout of the infection. No bone flap resorption was reported. The researchers concluded that storage at -26° C (-14.8° F) resulted in an acceptable rate of infection. Additionally, the researchers questioned the need to store autologous cranial bone flaps at deep freezer temperatures, stating that deep freezer storage temperatures may affect the viability of osteocytes and increase the risk of bone resorption. They recommended that cranial bone flaps be kept at a minimum temperature that prevents microbial growth, preserves osteocyte viability, and reduces the risk of bone resorption.

2.4   **Determine the maximum storage duration for frozen or cryopreserved cranial bone flaps based on the preservation method, temperature range, packaging method used, and patient-specific needs.**
[Recommendation]

There may also be patient-specific considerations (eg, chronic infections) that necessitate the storage of autologous cranial bone flaps for longer periods of time.

According to the AATB, the maximum storage period is determined by the type of tissue preserved, preservation method, temperature range, and packaging method used.[34] Moderate-quality evidence varies regarding the optimal length of storage time between **craniectomy** and cranioplasty procedures. The studies had high levels of variability in methodology[6,8,35-37] and, therefore, the study results cannot be compared for the purposes

of making a clinical practice recommendation for maximum storage duration. No studies were found that specifically compared the effects of varying lengths of storage durations on patient outcomes (eg, infection, resorption), and further research is needed (See Recommendation 12.5).

Several researchers reported the average or mean duration of storage in their results or study methodology. In a systematic review of 48 studies, Corliss et al[5] found that the mean storage duration for cryopreserved cranial bone flaps was 69.9 days. In a survey by Bhaskar et al[17] of 25 major neurosurgical facilities in Australia, the reported duration of cryopreservation storage was

- 6 months (16%),
- 9 months (4%),
- 2 years (8%),
- 5 years (56%),
- until the patient is deceased (4%), and
- not specified (12%).

Cheah et al[6] conducted a prospective study that compared the effect of cryopreservation and subcutaneous pocket storage methods on SSI rates. The bone flaps that were cryopreserved (n = 55) had a mean storage duration of 168 days; the shortest and longest storage durations were 25 days and 538 days, respectively. The infection rate was 5.45% (n = 3) in the cryopreservation group. The only variable associated with an increased infection rate was repeated cranioplasty procedures.

In a nonexperimental study, Wui et al[16] stated that cranial bone flaps were kept for 6 months then discarded due to concerns about the viability of bone after deep freezer preservation. Bhaskar et al[14] conducted a quasi-experimental study and concluded that replantation of cranial bone flaps after 6 months of storage should be discouraged unless there are exceptional circumstances.

There is also conflicting evidence on how storage duration of cryopreserved cranial bone flaps affects the risk of cranial bone flap resorption in children younger than 18 years of age. In a nonexperimental study, Piedra et al[37] found that children younger than 18 years were at a higher risk for bone flap resorption when the cranioplasty was performed after 6 weeks. Conversely, Bowers et al[38] conducted a nonexperimental study on pediatric patients younger than 16 years and did not find an association between the duration of the time in the freezer and bone flap resorption.

In a nonexperimental study, Chan et al[33] evaluated contamination rates by the duration of storage and size of 18 cranial bone flaps. Although the study sample was too small to reach statistical significance, the researchers concluded that longer storage durations for cranial bone flaps may increase the risk for contamination. Contaminated cranial bone flaps had been stored for a mean duration of 32.9 months ± 15.1 months, whereas bone flaps free of contamination had been stored for a shorter mean duration of 19.9 months ± 17.9 months. Additionally, the mean size of the infected bone flaps was considerably larger than the size of noninfected bone flaps. The infected bone flaps had a mean size of 117.7 cm² ± 44.96 cm² compared to uninfected bone flaps that had a mean size of 76.8 cm² ± 50.24 cm².

2.5 **No recommendation can be made regarding the use of cryoprotectants or storage solutions for cranial bone flaps that are cryopreserved.** *[No Recommendation]*

The balance between the benefits and harms of using cryoprotectants or storage solution is unclear. The benefits of cryoprotectants may include protection of the tissue while in deep frozen cryopreservation temperatures (eg, -80° C to -196° C [-112° F to -320.8° F]).[39] The harms may include incomplete removal of the cryoprotectant before reimplantation, which may increase the risk of exposing the patient to chemicals or solutions and potential loss of cell viability from intracellular ice formation or recrystallization.[39]

The following cryoprotectants and solutions were used in studies of cryopreservation of cranial bone flaps with varying results:

- dimethyl sulfoxide,[8]
- 20% glycerol solution,[40]
- povidone iodine,[41] and
- 100% ethanol.[42]

Several studies reported positive patient outcomes from cryopreservation of cranial bone flaps without cryoprotectants.[5,6,27,28] No studies were found that specifically compared the use of cryoprotectants versus no cryoprotectants on cell viability or patient outcomes.

2.6 **Determine a method for preparing frozen or cryopreserved cranial bone flaps for replantation, which may include**

- **retrieving the bone flap after the patient is in the OR and the surgeon has confirmed that it will be replanted**[29,32]**;**
- **thawing the bone flap in the sterile package at OR room temperature**[11,19,27,29,32,33]**;**
- **removing the bone flap from the packaging as close to the time of use as possible**[27]**;**
- **thawing the bone flap in warm solution**[41]**;**
- **wiping the bone flap of excess dust, soft tissue, and loose fragments**[8,27]**; and**
- **immersing, washing, or rinsing the bone flap in a solution (eg, normal saline solution, Ringer's solution, povidone iodine, a mixture**

of a solution and antibiotics or povidone iodine).[8,11,17,19,27,29-31] *[Conditional Recommendation]*

Although no studies were found that investigated the effect of cranial bone flap thawing and preparation methods on patient outcomes, several researchers reported thawing and preparation procedures in the description of their study methodology. Bhaskar et al[17] found that 68% of 25 major neurosurgical facilities surveyed in Australia did not have a specific procedure or instructions for thawing autologous cranial bone flaps.

2.7 **Cultures may be used to screen for microbial contamination of the cranial bone flap when clinically indicated.** *[Conditional Recommendation]*

The benefits of microbial culturing of the cranial bone flap when a patient presents with clinical signs and symptoms of infection may outweigh the harms. However, implementing routine cultures of cranial bone flaps prior to preservation may not provide an accurate indication of infection risk after a cranioplasty procedure.

Moderate-quality evidence varies on the use of culture results as a predictor of microbial contamination of cranial bone flaps and postoperative infection. In nonexperimental studies, Cheng et al[43] and Morton et al[36] found that bacteria on the cranial bone flap prior to preservation were different from the type of bacteria that cause SSIs.

Cheng et al[43] found no statistical association between positive or negative bone flap culture results and SSIs. This led the researchers to conclude that a negative culture result does not guarantee that there will be no infection, and conversely, a positive culture result is not predictive of a cranial bone flap infection. Cheng et al found that the use of cultures was not a cost-effective method for preventing infection. They recommended that cranial bone flap cultures only be performed in patients with a confirmed infection after craniectomy procedures.

Morton et al[36] also recommended against performing routine microbial cultures when there are no clinical indications of infection at the time of craniectomy since the results are not a useful predictor of cranioplasty infection rates. Additionally, they reported that routine discarding of the cranial bone flaps because of positive culture results led to an increased use of synthetic prostheses, which increased health care costs.

In a nonexperimental study, Cho et al[15] did not find bacterial growth on bone flaps (n = 47) that had been cryopreserved for an average of 83.2 months. In another nonexperimental study, Elwatidy et al[13] reported no microbial contamination of cranial bone flaps (n = 14) cryopreserved for a mean of 313 days. Conversely, Chan et al[33] found a 27.8% contamination rate for 18 cranial bone flaps that had been in cryopreservation and were removed for microbial culturing. Although the study sample was too small to reach statistical significance, the researchers concluded that cranial bone flaps that are larger in size and stored for longer durations may be more susceptible to contamination.[33]

In a nonexperimental study, Piitulainen et al[44] reported that any bone flap found to have a positive culture was discarded but also reported that of patients who had cranial bone flaps replanted (N = 20), 40% subsequently had the bone flap removed because of either infection (25%) or resorption (15%).

Herteleer et al[31] conducted a nonexperimental study comparing two protocols for bone flap preparation, one that included microbial culture screening and one that did not. In the culture screening protocol, cranial bone flaps with a positive culture were radiated and then cryopreserved again at -80° C (-112° F). Of the bone flaps that had microbial cultures taken, 36.8% (n = 14) were found to be contaminated and were radiated. It is unclear whether the bones were removed from sterile packaging for the radiation. The researchers reported that there were slightly lower complication rates for cranial bone flaps that had microbial cultures taken; however, the result was not statistically significant.

2.7.1 **Select the microbial culturing method (eg, swab, liquid, sponge) in collaboration with the surgeon(s), infection preventionist, and laboratory personnel.** [Recommendation]

Moderate-quality evidence exists on the effectiveness of different culturing methods.[45-47] Ronholdt and Bogdansky[45] conducted an RCT to compare two different culture swab products using the traditional method of swabbing. The method included swabbing the tissue in a "zig-zag" pattern to ensure that the greatest surface area of the allograft was swabbed. Both swab culturing systems tested exhibited low and variable microorganism recovery from allograft tissues. However, the researchers noted that moist swabs were more likely to capture and retain microorganisms than dry swabs.

In a nonexperimental study by Dennis et al[46] and a quasi-experimental study by Nguyen et al,[47] the researchers found that other methods of culturing (ie, liquid cultures, sponge cultures) had higher levels of efficacy than traditional methods of culture swabbing. Dennis et al[46] compared swabbing cultures to liquid cultures obtained by immersing the tissue in 4,000 mL of sterile normal saline solution for 10 minutes, shaking the tissue for 1 minute, then injecting 10 mL of the rinse solution into a culture medium. The results showed that the swab method detected only 20% of organisms while the liquid culture method detected 90%. Nguyen et al[47] found that a 4 cm x 8 cm sponge that was cut, moistened with 20 mL of sterile saline, and then rubbed on the tissue prior to placement in a specimen container inoculated with thioglycolate had a sensitivity and negative predictive value of 100%.

2.7.2 **When obtaining and performing cultures,**
- **collect the sample before the tissue is treated with antibiotics or cleansing agents,**
- **test for aerobic and anaerobic bacteria, and**
- **perform the test in a laboratory that is either certified under the Clinical Laboratory Improvement Amendments of 1988 (CLIA-88)[18] or another laboratory-accrediting organization that has deemed status for CLIA-88.[34]**

[Recommendation]

Using antibiotics or other cleansing agents before obtaining the culture may inhibit the detection of viable organisms and may produce a false-negative culture result. Using a certified laboratory for microbiologic culture testing is an AATB standard.[34]

2.7.3 **When the culture results are available, consult with the surgeon to determine whether the autograft may be placed on the sterile field.** [Recommendation]

2.7.4 **Provide education and competency verification for personnel who perform microbial tissue culturing.** [Recommendation]

Microbial culture results are important in determining effective and directed antibiotic therapy for prevention or treatment of patient infections. However, swab cultures may be prone to error as a result of variation in the way that the swab is manipulated. The ability of the swab to recover microorganisms is dependent on the ability to pick up viable microorganisms from the surface of the item being swabbed and to release those microorganisms from the swab into the culture medium.[45] The swab tip may be relatively small compared to the surface area of the autograft.[47] A small amount of bioburden reduces the potential for the swab to collect all microorganisms on the surface.[47] In addition, some microorganisms that are collected may become trapped in the matrix of the swab itself and thus not transferred to the culture medium and not detected.

2.8 **Determine a process for reducing the risk of dropping or contaminating a cranial bone flap, which may include**
- **stabilizing the bone flap during elevation, replantation, or drilling processes[49,50];**
- **holding a sterile container or sterile bag below the bone flap elevation and insertion site[50];**
- **designating an area on the sterile instrument table with a sterile towel, drilling tools, implants, and a toothed instrument (eg, Kocher forceps) or a radiopaque gauze sponge (eg, laparotomy sponge) for holding the bone flap steady while drilling[49];**
- **having the person who removed the bone flap place it on the instrument back table[50]; and**
- **transferring the bone flap in a container when moving it from the surgical incision site to the instrument table.**

[Conditional Recommendation]

Moderate-quality evidence indicates the rates of occurrence and reasons for dropped cranial bone flaps.[49,50] Two nonexperimental studies showed that occurrences of dropped cranial bone flaps are low, around 0.3%.[49,50] However, Jankowitz and Kondziolka[50] reported that 66% (n = 33) of neurosurgeons surveyed had experienced a dropped bone flap and that 83% (n = 45) would replant the bone flap after it was disinfected.[50] Bone flaps were dropped during the following events:
- bone flap elevation,[49,50]
- moving of the bone flap from the surgical site to the sterile table,[50]
- bone flap insertion,[49] and
- placement of implants in the bone flap on the sterile table.[49,50]

2.9 **In collaboration with the surgeon(s) and an infection preventionist, select a mechanical method (eg, scrubbing, low-pressure pulsatile lavage of 6 pounds per square inch [PSI] to 14 PSI, tissue bank decontamination) for decontaminating contaminated cranial bone flaps for replantation.**

[Recommendation]

Moderate-quality evidence shows that decontamination of bone has eliminated or reduced contamination[51-53] or infection rates,[49,50,54] especially when mechanical methods of decontamination (eg, scrubbing, low-pressure pulsatile lavage) were used.[52-56]

Cruz et al[54] found that when the contaminated bone was irrigated with 100 mL of any of the decontamination solutions used in the study (ie,

normal saline solution, povidone-iodine solution, cefazolin 1 g/L), there was a significant reduction in infection rates.

Bruce et al[52] found that soaking bone flaps for 5 or 10 minutes followed by mechanical scrubbing of the osteoarticular fragments with the bristles of a scrub brush resulted in no positive cultures regardless of which solution (ie, 0.9% normal saline solution, povidone iodine) was used for decontamination. However, when bulb syringe lavage was used, povidone iodine was effective in eliminating microbial contamination but normal saline solution was not.

Hirn et al[55] found a statistically significant reduction in contamination with the use of low-pressure pulsatile lavage with sterile saline solution compared to soaking in antibiotic solutions.

In two quasi-experimental studies, Bhandari et al[53,57] found that the use of low-pressure pulsatile lavage (14 PSI) was effective in removing bacteria from bone,[53] whereas the use of high-pressure pulsatile lavage (70 PSI) was correlated to bone damage and seeding of bacterial contamination into a bone fracture near the site of the lavage.[57] It is important to note that there is some disagreement in the literature about whether decontamination processes need to eliminate all potentially infectious material[58] or just reduce bacterial contamination to noninfectious levels.[50,54,55]

Four quasi-experimental studies evaluated the contamination levels of bone that had been on the floor for varying lengths of time, including 30 seconds, 1 minute, 5 minutes, or 60 minutes.[51,52,54,55] Two of the studies found that contamination from the OR floor did not lead to significant rates of microbial contamination[51] or infection[54] after the bone was decontaminated. Cruz et al[54] concluded that contact with the OR floor for 5 minutes did not correlate to levels of contamination that resulted in clinical infections. The researchers stated that contaminated bone flaps do not have to be discarded because decontamination through mechanical cleansing with any of the solutions used in the study would make the bone suitable for replantation.

Conversely, two of the studies reported higher levels of contamination from specimens that had been on the OR floor.[52,55] However, these two studies had important differences in methodology compared to the other studies on OR floor contamination, including the type of specimen used[52] and the length of time the specimen was on the floor.[55] Hirn et al[55] reported contamination rates of 55% and 73% depending on the swabbing method used on bone that had been rubbed on the OR floor and left there for 60 minutes.

Two studies that reviewed rates of dropped bone flaps and subsequent methods of decontamination found that there were no infections in the postoperative follow-up period,[49,50] which was as long as 20 to 44 months in one study.[49] In a nonexperimental study, Abdelfatah[49] found that 89.3% (n = 25) of the microbial cultures sent from the saline used during the initial rinse of the dropped cranial bone flaps were negative. In the remaining 10.7% (n = 3) of positive cultures, the patient's postoperative antibiotics were changed to cover the organisms identified in the culture.

The benefits of decontaminating contaminated cranial bone flaps that will be replanted exceed the harms. The benefits include reduction or elimination of potentially infectious material from the contaminated autologous bone flap, which may reduce the risk for infection. The harms associated with mechanical decontamination of contaminated cranial bone may include loss of cell viability.[56,59]

2.9.1 **The methods for decontaminating contaminated bone flaps may include**
- **a mechanical rinse with normal saline solution,[54]**
- **soaking in normal saline solution for 5 minutes followed by a 1-minute mechanical scrub with the bristles of a scrub brush and normal saline solution,[52]**
- **pulsatile lavage at low-pressure settings (eg, 6 PSI to 14 PSI) with normal saline solution,[53,55] and**
- **processing at a tissue bank.**

[Conditional Recommendation]

2.9.2 **No recommendation can be made for the use of antiseptic (eg, povidone iodine) or antibiotic additives in irrigation solution used during decontamination of cranial bone flaps.**

[No Recommendation]

It is unclear whether additional solutions are necessary for decontamination of contaminated cranial bone flaps when 0.9% normal saline solution is used with a mechanical method of decontamination.[53-55] Additionally, the effect of povidone iodine and antibiotics on cell viability[56,58,59] and the effectiveness of different solutions to decrease or eliminate microbial contamination of contaminated bone flaps[18,52,53,55,56,58] is unclear.[49,50,54]

Adding antiseptics or antibiotics to irrigation solution may be unnecessary and potentially harmful. Antiseptics and antibiotics may not have been validated for use in irrigation solutions and may therefore pose a risk to the patient. Antiseptic solutions are intended for external use and may be ineffective or toxic when used internally. Facility antimicrobial stewardship programs may provide additional guidance on the best use of antibiotics for prevention of infection. Additionally, manufacturer's IFU clarify the intended use of the product and how to use the product for maximum effectiveness. For instance, the IFU of some antiseptic agents may specify a dry time. See the AORN Guideline for Sterile Technique[60] for additional guidance on the use of items not labeled as sterile (eg, antiseptic solution) or not packaged for sterile delivery to the sterile field (eg, vancomycin powder).

There is low-quality evidence on the effects of different solutions on decontamination of bone,[18,52,53,55,56,58] infection rates,[49,50,54] and cell viability.[56,58,59] The evidence is limited because the researchers used varying methodologies and reported conflicting results.

Normal saline solution was used for bone decontamination in four quasi-experimental studies.[53-56] One study showed that a 100-mL normal saline solution rinse prevented infection of bone in an animal model.[54] The other three studies showed that use of normal saline solution with low-pressure pulsatile lavage (6 PSI and 14 PSI) was effective in eliminating[53] or reducing microbial contamination.[55,56] Bruce et al[52] found that a 5-minute or 10-minute saline soak followed by a mechanical scrub with the bristles of a scrub brush and saline solution resulted in no positive cultures from contaminated osteoarticular bone fragments.

Povidone iodine was used for bone decontamination in five quasi-experimental studies[52,54,56,58,59] and one nonexperimental study.[50] The use of a povidone-iodine solution rinse or irrigation was found to be effective for preventing infection[50,54] and microbial growth.[52] Yaman et al[58] found that povidone iodine can be used to effectively decontaminate bone without damaging the bone structure. Conversely, Kaysinger et al[59] found that the use of povidone-iodine solutions at concentrations typically found in the OR were **cytotoxic** to osteoblasts. Bhandari et al[56] found that povidone-iodine solution decreased the number of **osteoclasts** and impaired osteoblast function. In a quasi-experimental study, Lacey[61] found that the antibacterial effect of povidone iodine was inactivated in the presence of significant amounts of hemoglobin and whole blood.

Various antibiotics were used for bone decontamination in five quasi-experimental studies.[54-56,58,59] Cruz et al[54] found that rinsing bone flaps with 100 mL of cefazolin solution (1 g/L) prevented infection. Yaman et al[58] reported that immersion in cephazolin sodium, neomycin with polymyxin, or rifamycin effectively decontaminated bone without damaging the bone structure. However, they also found that only rifamycin was effective in eliminating all bacterial contamination.[58] Conversely, Hirn et al[55] concluded that cephalosporins and rifampicin should not be used in decontamination of bone but have applications in preoperative prophylaxis and treatment of severe infections, respectively.

There were also conflicting results about the use of bacitracin. One study found that bacitracin solution was safe for use on bone and osteoblasts,[59] but another study reported that exposure to 2 minutes of low-pressure pulsatile lavage using bacitracin resulted in a 70% decrease in cell density and decreased the number of osteoblasts.[56] Other solutions studied for their effects on decontamination of bone include liquid soap solution[56] and combinations of solutions used in succession (eg, normal saline followed by povidone iodine then antibiotic solution).[49,50,52,58]

2.9.3 **Do not use hydrogen peroxide (H_2O_2), chlorhexidine gluconate (CHG), or ethanol to decontaminate bone flaps.** *[Recommendation]*

There is an increased risk of patient harm from either ineffective decontamination[18,56,58] or cell toxicity[56,59] when H_2O_2, CHG, or ethanol are used for decontaminating bone.

Hydrogen peroxide solution was used for bone decontamination in three quasi-experimental studies and one experimental study. Jankowitz and Kondziolka[50] reported no incidents of infection in the follow-up period, which varied from 2 months to 176 months. However, this retrospective review of 14 dropped bone flaps only included one bone flap that was soaked in povidone iodine and then H_2O_2 solution. Two studies showed that H_2O_2 solution was either not effective for bacterial disinfection[58] or was not effective against all bacterial contamination used in the study.[18] Kaysinger et al[59] reported that concentrations of H_2O_2 typically used in the OR setting caused toxicity in bone.

Quasi-experimental studies have found CHG to be effective[52] and ineffective[56,58] for decontaminating contaminated bone grafts, and CHG has also been found to be toxic to bone cells, even at very low concentrations (ie, 1%).[56] Bhandari et al[56] found that ethanol was toxic to osteoblasts and that 2 minutes of exposure to low-pressure pulsatile lavage using ethanol decreased cell density.

2.9.4 **When decontaminating a contaminated cranial bone flap,**
- use a separate sterile field for decontamination of the flap[60];
- use interventions to prevent contamination of the sterile field during decontamination (eg, covering the main sterile field, covering the active hand piece of the pulsatile lavage)[60];
- change gown and gloves after decontamination is complete[60];
- change the wound classification to Class III, Contaminated[60]; and
- conduct a debriefing session with the team members involved to determine the root cause of the event and interventions to prevent another occurrence.

[Recommendation]

Creating and using a separate sterile field for decontamination of a cranial bone flap reduces the risk of contaminating the main sterile field. The use of pulsatile lavage can cause splash, splatter, and spray.[60] Interventions to minimize the effect of contaminated spray from the use of pulsatile lavage are detailed in the AORN Guideline for Sterile Technique.[60] Changing the gown and gloves after decontamination helps prevent the transfer of contaminants to the main sterile table.[60]

Replantation of a contaminated autograft constitutes a major break in sterile technique. According to the Centers for Disease Control and Prevention (CDC) surgical wound classification system, a surgical wound with a major break in sterile technique is classified as Class III, Contaminated.[62]

Debriefing with the perioperative team after an event has occurred may help prevent future incidents by examining underlying factors and system flaws that may have contributed to the event.

2.9.5 **Do not use sterilization to decontaminate cranial bone flaps.** *[Recommendation]*

Tissue sterilization is only allowed when a facility or health care organization is registered with the FDA as a tissue establishment **(See Recommendation 1.2).**[1]

The benefits of sterilizing cranial bone flaps for the purposes of decontamination do not outweigh the harms. The benefits include the potential for reduced microbial load,[18] but exposure to the OR floor may not be a significant source of contamination[51] and other methods of decontamination besides sterilization have been shown to be effective.[49,50,54] The harms include an increased risk for SSI.[16,42]

Moderate-quality evidence exists on steam sterilization as a method for decontaminating cranial bone flaps.[16,18,42] In a quasi-experimental study, Schültke et al[18] found that sterilization at 75° C (167° F) for 20 minutes was the only method that eradicated all the bacteria from cranial bone flap pieces that had been purposefully contaminated. However, Wui et al[16] found that sterilization after cryopreservation significantly increased the patient's risk for SSI. In a nonexperimental study, Matsuno et al[42] found a significantly higher rate of infection in patients for whom sterilized autologous bone or skull defect treated with polymethyl methacrylate was used during the cranioplasty procedure.

Sterilization was reported as a method for decontamination in two surveys on decontamination of dropped cranial bone flaps.[49,50] In both surveys, respondents reported soaking bone flaps in various solutions as the more prevalent method of decontamination. The total number of sterilized bone flaps between both surveys was 12. Neither study reported infections in the follow-up period, which in one survey was only 2 months. No information was provided on the sterilization parameters used.[49,50]

Yaman et al[58] reviewed the histological effects of steam sterilization on bone and found increased infiltration of lymphocytes, irregularity of blood vessels, and edema causing necrosis in the Haversian canals.

2.10 **No recommendation can be made regarding sterilization of cranial bone flaps for the purpose of preservation.** [No Recommendation]

Tissue sterilization is only allowed when a facility or health care organization is registered with the FDA as a tissue establishment (See Recommendation 1.2).[1]

Low-quality evidence varies on sterilization of cranial bone flaps as a preservation method.[23,63-66] All of the studies used different methodologies (eg, type of sterilization, preparation of the bone for sterilization, storage after sterilization, use of a second sterilization prior to replantation) and had varying results. The inconsistency between the study methodologies and the results prevent a clear understanding of the risks and benefits of sterilization as a method for preservation. The harms associated with sterilization of cranial bone flaps are bone flap resorption[23,64] and the potential for SSI after storage longer than 10 months.[66] Further research is needed.

Anto et al[63] and Mracek et al[64] conducted nonexperimental studies on the use of steam sterilization as a method of preservation. Anto et al[63] exposed cranial bone flaps to sterilization at 132° C (269.6° F) for 20 minutes then stored them at ambient temperatures in a cupboard. On the day of the scheduled cranioplasty, the cranial bone flaps were sterilized a second time. The researchers reported that complications occurred in 10 of the 72 patients (13.9%). Five patients had bone fracture or fragmentation, four patients had osteomyelitis, and one patient had bone resorption. The researchers concluded that the use of steam sterilization for bone flap preservation had good outcomes but required further study.

Conversely, Mracek et al[64] cleaned the bone flaps, boiled the flaps in distilled water for 30 minutes, and then sterilized the bone flaps at 121° C (249.8° F) for 20 minutes prior to storage in a refrigerator at 8° C (46.4° F). If the bone flap had been stored longer than 3 months, the bone flap was sterilized again prior to cranioplasty. The researchers reported that SSI occurred in 3.3% of patients (n = 5) and resorption occurred in 20% of patients (n = 22). They concluded that there was a low rate of SSI but a significant rate of bone resorption when this method was used.

A nonexperimental study by Jho et al[66] and quasi-experimental study by Missori et al[65] investigated ethylene oxide (EO) sterilization as a preservation method and found it to be safe and effective. Jho et al[66] reviewed the effect of EO sterilization and room temperature storage of cranial bone flaps on infection rates. Cranial bone flaps were replanted after an average of 4 months with a follow-up period averaging 14 months. The infection rate was 7.8% (n = 8). The researchers found that preservation beyond 10 months was significantly correlated to an increased risk for infection. This finding led the researchers to recommended that cranial bone flaps preserved after 10 months be discarded or sterilized a second time.

Missori et al[65] compared EO sterilization, steam sterilization at 121° C (249.8° F) for 45 minutes, and H_2O_2 gas plasma sterilization methods. Cranial bone flaps were replanted after a mean of 10 weeks with an average follow-up period for the EO sterilization group of 42 months. The infection rate was 2% (n = 1), with the only infection in the study occurring in the EO group. The researchers also described one case of partial bone resorption in a child from the EO sterilization group.

Neither study discussed precautions (eg, aeration time) used to mitigate any potential patient risks from EO sterilization. The harms of using EO sterilization methods are unknown. Ethylene oxide is a known human carcinogen, with a half-life of 69 to 149 days, that may damage the central nervous system.[67]

Kim et al[23] conducted a nonexperimental study of the infection and bone resorption rates for cranioplasty patients, using cranial bone flaps that had been sterilized with low-temperature H_2O_2 gas plasma as a preservation method compared to the use of polymethyl methacrylate used during the cranioplasty. The follow-up period was at least 1 year but averaged 15 months. To prepare the cranial bone flap for preservation, the bone flap was first cleaned of soft tissue then placed in a sterile drier at between 110° C and 120° C (230°F and 248° F) for 24 to 48 hours. Then the bone flap was placed in a low-temperature H_2O_2 gas plasma sterilizer at 70° C (158° F) for 75 minutes. After sterilization, the bone flap was placed in two layers of sterile bags and stored in a refrigerator at 8° C (46.4° F). Prior to replantation, the bone flap was sterilized a second time using the same method. The researchers found that use of the sterilized bone resulted in significant rates of bone flap resorption compared to the use of polymethyl methacrylate.

3. Parathyroid Tissue

3.1 **Parathyroid tissue may be cryopreserved and autotransplanted.** [*Conditional Recommendation*]

The benefits of parathyroid tissue cryopreservation are likely to exceed the harms. A benefit of cryopreserving autologous parathyroid tissue is having tissue available for patients who develop permanent hypoparathyroidism.[68-72] Permanent hypoparathyroidism is a serious condition that decreases quality of life[69] and increases risk of morbidity[69,73] but has limited treatment options.[69,74,75] Patients with permanent hypoparathyroidism can develop paresthesia[74] and adynamic bone disease[69,71,76] that requires lifelong serum monitoring and dependence on supplements.[72,74,75] The harms of cryopreserving parathyroid tissue include the potential for reduced cell viability,[70,73,77,78] risk of decreased graft success,[71] limited space at facilities that store cryopreserved tissue,[74] and increased cost.[69,74]

Low-quality evidence supports cryopreservation of parathyroid tissue.[68-75,77,78] The evidence is limited due to the small sample size of most of the available studies.[68,69,71-73,77,78] Although several studies have shown that cryopreservation of parathyroid tissue may reduce cell viability[70,73,77,78] or potentially decrease graft success,[71] the same studies still support its use with additional recommendations,[70,71,73,77,78] including autotransplantation of additional tissue[70,73] and tissue viability testing.[73,77,78] Researchers

in two studies recommended autotransplantation of additional amounts of parathyroid tissue to increase the probability of a functioning graft.[70,73]

Several studies discussed low rates of cryopreserved parathyroid tissue use and associated costs.[69,71,75] In a nonexperimental study, Cohen et al[71] reported that 448 parathyroid tissue samples from 436 patients were cryopreserved, but only 29 of the patients underwent autotransplantation procedures (6.6%). In a high-quality organizational experience article, Agarwal et al[75] stated that the cryopreservation rate of parathyroid tissue from more than 2,000 parathyroid procedures was 31% but that only 1.5% of samples were subsequently autotransplanted. In a nonexperimental study, Guerrero et al[74] noted that 501 specimens were cryopreserved from 149 patients during a 15-year period and that the facility was experiencing a surplus of cryopreserved parathyroid tissue at the storage facility. Conversely, Agarwal et al[75] stated that space and cost requirements were minimal. Guerrero et al[74] also stated that cryopreservation processing and storage uses multiple resources and is costly. Barreira et al[76] concurred that the special laboratory needed for cryopreservation may have high assembly and maintenance costs.

Because of the lifelong consequences of permanent hypoparathyroidism, Cohen et al[71] recommended cryopreservation of parathyroid tissue, regardless of the associated costs, as a treatment option for patients who do not respond to immediate autotransplantation. Agarwal et al[75] noted that parathyroid tissue cryopreservation, preparation, and storage fees have specific billing codes that can be used for facility reimbursement, but that patients at their facility are not billed beyond 2 years of storage.

3.2 Parathyroid tissue may be prepared in the OR for cryopreservation by

- placing the tissue in enough cold sterile 0.9% normal saline solution[69,71-75,78] or cold Roswell Park Memorial Institute (RPMI)-1640 medium[68,72] to cover the tissue;
- placing the specimen cup[74] on sterile ice[68,70,71] and covering it to prevent airborne contamination[60,79,80];
- dividing tissue into 1 x 1 x 1 mm or 2 x 2 x 2 mm pieces[68-75,77,78];
- sending a small portion of the specimen for a frozen section to confirm the tissue type, if requested by the surgeon[69,75,80];
- collecting 5 mL to 10 mL of the patient's blood into a tube with no additives to be sent with the tissue, if requested by the surgeon[71,75];

- transporting the prepared tissue as soon as possible[75] in an enclosed and labeled container (eg, specimen cup,[74] tuberculosis syringe,[75] cryovials[75]) within a biohazard-marked specimen bag on ice with required, completed, facility documentation[75] to an accredited clinical laboratory for cryopreservation[68,69,75,76,79,81]; and
- alerting the clinical laboratory when the tissue for cryopreservation is en route.

[Conditional Recommendation]

3.3 If temporary storage or transport of parathyroid tissue is necessary before cryopreservation, determine the method of preservation, temperature, and duration of storage. [Conditional Recommendation]

Some facilities may need to temporarily store[79] or transport parathyroid tissue before cryopreservation because the facility does not have personnel immediately available or does not have laboratory specializing in cryopreservation on site.[76] However, the ideal method of preserving parathyroid cell viability before cryopreservation is unknown because of limited and low-quality evidence on the subject.

In a quasi-experimental study, Barreira et al[76] compared the effects of refrigerated storage at 4° C (39.2° F) for different time intervals on the structural integrity of parathyroid tissue (N = 11). The parathyroid tissue was stored in a cell culture medium that included **Dulbecco's modified Eagle's medium** (DMEM), streptomycin 500 µg/mL, ampicillin 500 µg/mL, amphotericin B 3 mg/mL, and 25 mM of a buffering solution. Parathyroid tissue stored in the cell culture medium at 4° C (39.2° F) was found to be viable for as long as 12 hours. However, the researchers also found that all the samples had at least one structural change after 24 hours in refrigerated storage.

One quasi-experimental study[77] and two organizational experience articles[75,79] also described temporary storage of parathyroid tissue. Alvarez-Hernandez et al[77] stated that specimens were stored at 4° C (39.2° F) in RPMI medium for 16 to 20 hours prior to experimentation. Stotler et al[79] reported that part of the institutional process of parathyroid tissue preservation included either same-day cryopreservation or refrigerated storage overnight at 4° C (39.2° F). Agarwal et al[75] stated that specimens were occasionally placed in refrigerated storage between 2° C and 8° C (35.6° F and 46.4° F) if processing was delayed.

3.4 Determine the maximum storage duration for cryopreservation of parathyroid tissue based on tissue viability and patient-specific needs. [Recommendation]

The balance between the benefits and harms of storing cryopreserved parathyroid tissue longer than 24 months is unclear. A benefit of storing cryopreserved parathyroid tissue longer than 24 months is that a very small number of patients may develop delayed symptoms related to parathyroid hormone deficiency[69] and have limited treatment options.[75] Conversely, cryopreservation of parathyroid glands may affect the viability of the tissue or graft success rates. There may also be facility limitations including costs or storage availability.[74]

Low-quality evidence on the duration of cryopreserved parathyroid tissue in relation to cell viability[68,70,74,77,78] or patient outcomes[69,71,72,75,81,82] is limited due to small sample sizes, varying methodologies, and conflicting results. Four quasi-experimental[68,70,77,78] and four nonexperimental[69,71,72,74] studies supported a duration of cryopreservation between 6.66 months and less than 24 months. However, Schneider et al[69] reported that four of the 15 patients (26.6%) in a non-experimental study had autotransplant procedures more than 2 years after the initial procedure. Additionally, two case reports described positive patient outcomes (eg, elevated parathyroid hormone, reversed hypoparathyroidism) after 30 months and 36 months.[81,82] The author of an organizational experience article stated that the facility stored cryopreserved parathyroid tissue longer than 24 months due to the available space, low cost of storage, and the lack of treatment options for patients.[75]

Specific findings of the studies conflict. Two quasi-experimental studies found no significant difference between fresh parathyroid tissue and cryopreserved parathyroid tissue regardless of storage duration.[68,77] Three studies did not find a correlation between cell viability[70,78] or patient outcomes[72] and the duration of cryopreservation. Conversely, Cohen et al[71] found a significant difference between the cryopreservation storage duration of functional and nonfunctional grafts. The mean cryopreservation period was 7.9 months for functional grafts and 15.3 months for nonfunctional grafts.[71] The researchers concluded that the duration of cryopreservation was a significant predictor of graft failure.[71] Two studies stated that even though cryopreservation was not found to be detrimental to the tissue, the process of freezing or thawing may be.[70,72]

Guerrero et al[74] concluded that facilities would benefit from challenging the idea of storing cryopreserved parathyroid tissue indefinitely. They recommended that facilities establish a maximum period of preservation that balances the considerations of tissue viability, storage ability, and cost.

4. Skin

4.1 **Autologous skin may be preserved and auto-transplanted.** *[Conditional Recommendation]*

The benefits of storing autologous skin (eg, split-thickness skin grafts) for delayed autotransplantation may exceed the harms **(Figure 2)**. The benefits include minimizing the area of the donor site needed,[83] the potential elimination of a secondary donor site,[84] and cost efficiency.[83,85,86] The harms may include reduced graft success rates due to decreased skin viability over time[87-89] and risk for infection from contaminated skin grafts.[90,91]

Moderate-quality evidence indicates that preserved skin is viable, but the viability declines during the duration of storage.[87-89] Therefore, most of the available research on autologous skin seeks to determine which variables (eg, medium) may extend storage duration while optimizing graft success rates or some aspect of skin cell viability.[85-89,91,92] Five quasi-experimental studies[85-88,91] and four nonexperimental studies[83,84,89,90] compared the effect of tissue preservation on graft success rates or different aspects of skin cell viability. The evidence is limited by

- the small number of high-quality studies conducted on this practice issue,
- the small sample sizes of the studies,[83,84,86-89,91-93]
- missing information in the study methodology descriptions (eg, graft preparation, temperature, storage duration),[84,89,90,93]
- differences between the study methodology and how autologous skin is prepared in clinical practice (eg, not meshed, skin biopsies used),[83-87,93] and
- variable results in studies that investigated the same outcome (ie, graft success rates, skin viability).

Further research is needed to examine how skin viability after preservation affects the clinical outcomes of graft success rates in humans.

4.2 **No recommendation can be made regarding meshing skin prior to preservation.** *[No Recommendation]*

The balance between the benefits and harms of meshing the skin is unclear. Meshing the skin allows the skin graft to stretch and cover a larger area. Meshing the skin during the initial procedure when it is harvested may reduce time during a subsequent procedure. However, meshing the skin exposes it to mechanical trauma that may compromise cellular function,[88] which may affect clinical outcomes.

Moderate-quality evidence conflicts regarding meshing the skin prior to preservation. A quasi-experimental study that reviewed graft success rates of preserved and transplanted skin in an animal model found that the results for skin meshed before preservation were not significantly differ-

Figure 2. Split-Thickness and Full-Thickness Skin Grafts

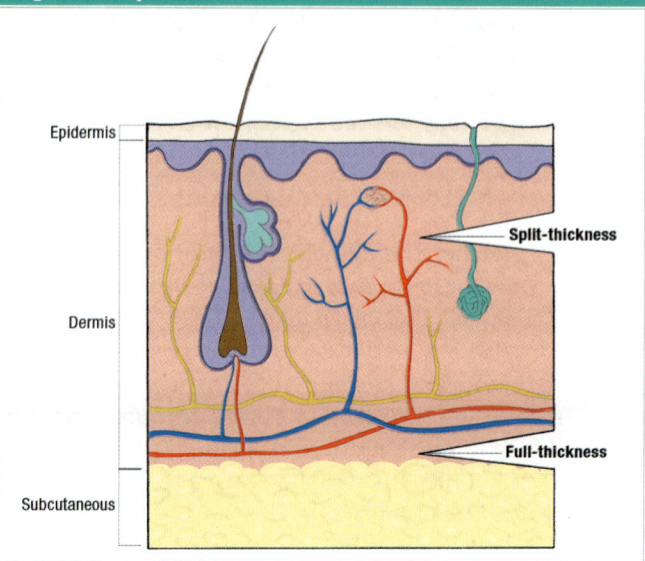

Epidermis
Dermis
Subcutaneous
Split-thickness
Full-thickness

A split-thickness skin graft includes the epidermis and part of the dermis. A full-thickness skin graft includes the epidermis and all of the dermis.

Illustration by Kurt Jones.

ent from those for nonmeshed skin.[92] Two quasi-experimental studies compared the effects of meshing split-thickness skin grafts on different aspects of skin cell viability after preservation.[88,91] Li et al[91] found decreases in cell viability of **meshed skin** over the duration of storage time. These findings led the researchers to recommend using meshed skin within 7 days of harvesting.

Sterne et al[88] found that meshed skin had initial swelling and pleomorphism that subsided by the 21st day of storage. However, the researchers suggested that after 3 weeks of preservation, the rates of successful skin grafts would be severely diminished. The study results also showed that meshed skin had more shrinkage and epidermal clefting, which predisposed the meshed skin to more deterioration than nonmeshed skin. The researchers recommended not meshing the skin and storing it in a roll.

No studies were found in which the results of graft success rates for skin meshed before and after preservation were compared. Further research is needed.

4.3 Determine a method of preparing the skin for preservation, which may include
- placing the epithelial side of the graft down[88] onto a sheet of **tulle gras**,[88,90]
- folding the graft in half dermis-to-dermis[83,88,90] then rolling it,[83,88]
- wrapping the graft in saline moistened gauze,[83,86-91] and
- placing the wrapped tissue into a sterile container.[88,91]

[Conditional Recommendation]

Low-quality evidence indicates that the viability of preserved skin was improved when the tissue was rolled during storage. In a quasi-experimental study, Sterne et al[88] reviewed the histological changes in split-thickness skin grafts from meshing and graft configuration during storage. The skin was stored either rolled or flat and wrapped in saline-soaked gauze sponges for a 4-week period. The researchers found that both rolled nonmeshed skin and rolled meshed skin had less shrinkage in the later weeks of storage and had less clefting between the dermis and epidermis than the skin that was stored flat. The researchers thought that rolling the skin might reduce moisture loss during the storage period. They concluded that the viability of the stored grafts was greatest when the grafts were stored as an unmeshed roll at 4° C (39.2° F) for fewer than 7 days. Further research is needed.

4.4 Preserve autologous skin by refrigeration at 4° C (39.2° F). [Recommendation]

The benefits of skin preservation exceed the potential for patient harm and have been found to be cost efficient.[85]

Moderate-quality evidence consistently shows that skin viability is preserved when autologous skin is stored at 4° C (39.2° F) for varying durations.[85-91] However, the evidence is limited because the methodology, medium used, storage duration, and conclusions were highly varied between studies. It is important to note that while stored skin remains viable for a period of time, at some point, the viability of the preserved skin diminishes.[87,88,90,91] Diminished skin viability may increase the rate of failed skin grafts in patients.[89] The AATB recommends that skin be preserved by refrigeration above freezing to 10° C (50° F) or by freezing or cryopreservation at -40° C (-40° F) or colder.[34]

In a nonexperimental study, Titley et al[90] investigated bacterial contamination and rates of graft success in eight patients and found that the skin of all eight patients was contaminated at the time of recovery. Interestingly, the researchers noted that except for *Acinetobacter* organisms, the other bacteria found in the study would not replicate in temperatures below 4° C (39.2° F).

4.5 In collaboration with the surgeon(s), an infection preventionist, and a pharmacist, determine which storage medium or solution will be used and if antibiotics will be added. [Recommendation]

4.5.1 Store skin in a storage medium or normal saline solution. [Recommendation]

The benefits of using a storage medium or solution, including retained pliability of the skin, exceed the harms, which may include loss of moisture.

High-quality evidence shows that normal saline solution was inferior to other storage media with which it was compared.[85-87,91] Storage media reported in studies to be superior to normal saline solution for preservation include

- RPMI-1640 medium,[86]
- RPMI-1640 medium with antibiotics,[87]
- DMEM,[91]
- DMEM/Ham F12 (DMEM/F12, 3:1 mixture),[91] and
- McCoy's 5A medium.[85]

However, most researchers also found that normal saline solution is the most commonly used solution[86-88,90,91] and that it demonstrated some preservation of skin viability for a period of time that was usually shorter than for other media.[85,87,91]

Furthermore, in their nonexperimental study, Knapik et al[89] discussed the common practice of using normal saline as a storage solution and that the corresponding patient outcomes (ie, graft success rates) may be clinically acceptable. The researchers questioned whether the use of more expensive storage media is of clinical interest.

4.5.2 Determine whether antibiotics will be added to storage media or solutions based on the patient's allergies, manufacturer's IFU, and the facility antibacterial stewardship program (if applicable). [Conditional Recommendation]

Moderate-quality evidence demonstrates that storage of skin in media with antibacterial properties may be useful.[90,91]

In a nonexperimental study, Titley et al[90] reviewed bacterial contamination rates of the skin at the moment of harvest and after 3 weeks of storage. Split-thickness skin grafts taken from patients were put on tulle gras and then wrapped in saline-moistened gauze prior to placement in a refrigerator. The preserved skin was grafted to 10 patients and data were available for eight patients. The researchers found that all eight skin grafts were contaminated at harvest with bacterial counts between 2.2×10^1 and 5.3×10^7 organisms per gram of skin and included seven different organisms. Of the eight grafts included in the study, three failed completely. The researchers found a significant correlation between lower numbers of organisms found on the skin at harvest and higher percentages of graft success rates. The researchers concluded that commonly used storage practices facilitate bacterial multiplication.

In a quasi-experimental study, Li et al[91] compared meshed split-thickness skin grafts from surgical burn patients. The grafts were stored in different storage solutions and reviewed for cell viability and microbial contamination over 28 days. The researchers found that storage in DMEM or DMEM/Ham F12 was better than storage in normal saline solution or Hartman's solution. They also found microbial contamination in 43.3% (n = 13) of the skin samples stored in antibiotic-free media compared with only 10% (n = 3) of the samples stored in media with antibiotics. The researchers concluded that use of storage solutions with antimicrobial agents may help minimize the risk of contamination, especially from skin recovered from burn patients that may be prone to higher levels of contamination.

4.5.3 **No recommendation can be made regarding changing storage solution or medium every 72 hours.** [*No Recommendation*]

No evidence was found on the effectiveness of changing storage solutions or media for preserved skin. The benefits of changing the solutions are unknown and the harms could include an increased risk of contaminating the skin.

4.6 **Determine the maximum storage duration for autologous split-thickness skin grafts.** [*Recommendation*]

Moderate-quality evidence suggests varying lengths of time that skin may be stored at 4° C (39.2° F).[85-91] The evidence is limited because the studies used different storage media and varying techniques for assessing the viability of preserved skin. The researchers reported findings of acceptable storage durations between 7 days and 4 weeks, which were conditional based on the methods used in the research.[85,88-91] Two of the studies did not report a cut-off point for when stored skin grafts may no longer be used.[86,87] In a quasi-experimental study, Boekema et al[87] concluded that it was not possible to determine a cut-off point when split-thickness skin grafts could no longer be used because the decline in skin viability was gradual. The researchers also concluded that more research is needed to correlate viability of preserved skin to graft success rates in patients.[87] The AATB recommends that refrigerated autologous skin not be stored for longer than 14 days.[34]

4.7 **Split-thickness skin grafts procured during free flap procedures may be stored on the patient's donor site for delayed autotransplantation.** [*Conditional Recommendation*]

The benefits of storing autologous split-thickness skin grafts at the donor site during free flap procedures are likely to exceed the harms. The benefits may include

- reduced surgical time,[83]
- elimination of a second procedure,[83,93]
- the ability to see the flap area during the immediate postoperative period,[83,93]
- increased flap survival rates,[93]
- no risk of a graft being placed on the wrong patient,[83,93]
- reduced size of the skin graft required,[83,93]
- decreased donor site morbidity,[83]
- improved healing of the unused skin graft left at the donor site,[83]
- decreased risk of scarring,[83]
- increased patient satisfaction,[83]
- elimination of biohazardous waste disposal,[93]
- cost efficiency,[83,93] and
- availability for all patients because refrigeration is unnecessary.[93]

The harms associated with storing autologous split-thickness skin grafts at the donor site include harvesting a larger split-thickness skin graft than is needed because it can be hard to estimate the size of graft needed. Additional high-quality research is needed to clarify the risks and confirm the benefits of storing split-thickness skin grafts at the donor site for delayed autotransplantation.

Low-quality evidence supports storage of the patient's autologous skin at the donor site for delayed autotransplantation over a free flap site.[83,93] One nonexperimental study[83] and one case report[93] discussed patient outcomes from storage of autologous skin at the donor site for delayed autotransplantation over the free flap site.

Ciudad et al[83] studied graft success rates from lymph node flap transfer procedures for grafts stored at the donor site in 10 patients. The bedside procedure to autotransplant the skin from the donor site to the recipient site was completed between the fourth and sixth postoperative day. The researchers reported that a single patient needed slightly more medication during the bedside graft transfer. There was a 100% flap survival rate and a 97% graft success rate. The researchers concluded that delayed skin grafting may reduce flap complications as well as decrease operative time and costs. A study limitation was that the researchers did not include patients with coagulopathy or diabetes mellitus.

Mardini et al[93] reviewed the clinical outcomes of initial free flap voice reconstruction procedures using skin grafts stored at the donor site in 10 patients. The bedside procedure was performed between 3 and 8 days after the initial procedure. The researchers stated that elevation of the stored graft was well tolerated. They reported 95% **engraftment** in all cases and that all the grafts healed completely during the 5- to 12-month follow-up period. The researchers concluded that storage of the skin autograft at the donor site for as long as 8 days was a reliable and cost-effective technique.[93]

5. Vessels

5.1 **Autologous vessels may be preserved and auto-transplanted.** *[Conditional Recommendation]*

The benefits of preserving autologous vessels are likely to exceed the harms. Preservation of remaining vessel segments results in the availability of autologous tissue during the initial recovery period when patients' vessels may occlude, requiring subsequent grafts.[94] Potential harms include occlusions in vascular grafts and subsequent graft failure.[94]

Moderate-quality evidence supports the preservation of autologous veins for delayed autotransplantation.[94-99] Two RCTs,[96,98] three quasi-experimental studies,[95,97,99] and one nonexperimental study[94] reviewed the effects of various storage solutions on veins or arteries for periods longer than several hours.

5.2 **Store vessels submerged in a buffered storage solution or tissue culture medium between 2° C and 8° C (35.6° F and 46.4° F) for no longer than 14 days.** *[Recommendation]*

Moderate-quality evidence addresses vessels stored at 4° C (39.2° F),[94-96,98] at a range from 0° C to 4° C (32° F to 39.2° F),[97] and at 21° C (69.8° F).[99] Additionally, the Organ Procurement and Transplantation Network states that extra vessels that come packaged separately with organs for transplant may be stored between 2° C to 8° C (35.6° F to 46.4° F) in an FDA-approved preservation solution and destroyed within 14 days of the recovery date of the organ.[100]

Two RCTs[96,98] and four quasi-experimental studies[94,95,97,99] reviewed the long-term effects of different storage solutions on vessels for preservation periods between 24 hours and 4 weeks. Several studies found that buffered solutions protect the endothelial cell lining[99] or maintain vessel function[94,96-99] better than other solutions studied. A secondary finding was that storage in normal saline solution had an adverse effect on the endothelial lining of the vessel[99] or did not preserve vessel function[94,96-99] compared to other solutions.

The specific period used for storage of vessels is dependent on the storage solution used. The evidence is limited due to the variability in the storage solutions studied, research methodologies,

and reported results. The AATB recommends packaging allograft vascular tissue in **isotonic** sterile solution (eg, tissue culture media) but not normal saline solution.[34] Buffered solutions and media found to preserve vessels include

- **TiProtec** solution for 4 days[94] and 7 to 14 days[96];
- tissue culture medium for up to 4 weeks[101];
- University of Wisconsin solution for 24 hours[98];
- GALA (glutathione, ascorbic acid, and L-arginine) solution for 24 hours[99]; and
- N-acetyl histidine–buffered, potassium chloride–enriched, amino acid–fortified solution augmented with iron chelators deferoxamine and LK 614 for 4 days.[97]

Harskamp et al[102] conducted an RCT involving 107 US facilities and 3,014 patients to compare intraoperative preservation solutions used on veins of patients undergoing coronary artery bypass graft procedures. The study revealed that the highest percentage of patients (44%) had veins stored in saline solution for intraoperative preservation. However, the study results showed that intraoperative vein preservation in buffered saline solution resulted in significantly lower vein graft failure rates at the 1-year follow-up period and improved but nonsignificant long-term clinical outcomes (ie, lower death rates, fewer cases of myocardial infarction, greater revascularization) than veins stored in saline or blood-based solutions.

However, contrary to other study findings, in a quasi-experimental study, Ebner et al[95] investigated the effects of storage in TiProtec solution at 4° C (39.2° F) for 2 hours and for 2 days and found that storage for 2 days or longer significantly impaired vessel tone development. Importantly, the study also found significant molecular alteration in the vessels after storage for 2 hours. This was a central finding because changes at the molecular level were evident before functional vessel changes, and alterations at the molecular level may affect graft function. The researchers concluded that further study is needed to understand the effects of these findings on graft success rate outcomes in patients.

5.2.1 **No recommendation can be made regarding changing storage solution or medium every 72 hours.** *[No Recommendation]*

No evidence was found on the effectiveness of changing storage solutions or media for preserved veins. The benefits of changing the solutions are unknown and the harms could include an increased risk of contaminating the vessels.

5.3 **No recommendation can be made regarding cryopreservation of vessels.** *[No Recommendation]*

The balance between the benefits and harms of preserving autologous vessels through cryopreservation is unclear. Vessels may be damaged by cryopreservation,[101,103] but vascular and cardiac patients who undergo multiple procedures may be more likely to have vessel disease that limits the number of vessels available for grafting[104] or may have vessels used during a previous procedure that could be cryopreserved for a future procedure as a method of longer-term storage than refrigeration.[104] The AATB recommends freezing or cryopreserving allograft vascular tissue at -100° C (-148° F) or colder.[34]

Low-quality evidence on cryopreservation of vessels includes one RCT,[101] one experimental study,[103] and one case report.[104] The evidence is limited because of considerable variability between study methodologies (eg, type of vessels used, tests used for comparison) and reported results. The researchers found that cryopreserved vessels had a significant decrease in lumen size,[101] a significant increase in vessel wall thickness,[101] and increased vessel stiffness as duration of storage increased.[103] Conversely, the studies also reported that vessels retained elastic properties and some contractility,[101] and that the mechanical properties of the vessels were similar before and after cryopreservation.[103]

Chang et al[103] reported that atherosclerotic areas of the cryopreserved arteries were more likely to have fragmentation. The authors of a case report on three patients who had greater saphenous vein grafts using autologous cryopreserved vein segments reported that no occlusions or aneurysmal dilations were found during the follow-up period.[104] No studies were found that examined the effect of using cryopreserved vessels on rates of successful grafts in patients. Further research is needed.

5.4 **No recommendation can be made regarding prewarming vessels before autotransplantation.** [*No Recommendation*]

The balance between the benefits and harms of vessel prewarming is unclear because there is no research on the subject.

No studies were found that compared prewarming processes for vessels that had been in cold storage. Three moderate-quality studies reported vessel prewarming processes used in the study methodology.[95-97] In all three studies, vessels were warmed to 37° C (98.6° F).[95-97] The vessels were placed in physiological saline solution[96] or phosphate-buffered saline solution[95] for warming. The prewarming process took place within 1 hour[97] and more than 1.5 hours.[96]

6. Femoral Head

6.1 **No recommendation can be made regarding freezing or cryopreserving the autologous femoral head.** [*No recommendation*]

No evidence was found on preservation of autologous femoral heads through cryopreservation or freezing. The benefits and risks of freezing or cryopreserving femoral heads are unknown. More research is needed.

6.2 **The patient's femoral head may be preserved within an iliac pocket.** [*Conditional Recommendation*]

The benefits of placing the femoral head from a total hip arthroplasty (THA) procedure into a newly created pocket in the patient's iliac area for preservation may exceed the harms. In a nonexperimental study, Shinar and Harris[105] reported that THA revision procedures were necessary in 60% of procedures using allograft tissue (n = 9 of 15) and 29% of procedures using autologous tissue (n = 16 of 55). Other sources agree that the use of autologous bone grafts is preferable to the use of allograft tissue.[106,107] The benefits include

- having autologous bone available for future use,[107] including if the patient moves out of the area[106];
- elimination of screening procedures, sterilization, risk of rejection,[106] storage facilities, and expenses associated with allograft bone use[107];
- cost effectiveness[106,107];
- minimal time needed for the pocket creation procedure[107]; and
- exposure of the iliac crest if additional autologous graft volume is needed.[106]

The harms may include

- infection, incisional hernia, or discomfort at the pocket site[107];
- morbidity of the pouch site[106];
- damage to the lateral cutaneous nerve of the thigh[106];
- potential preservation of a femoral head with malignancy[106]; and
- unnecessary storage of the femoral head if it is not used.

Low-quality evidence includes one organizational experience article[106] and one case report[107] that describe preservation of the femoral heads removed during THA procedures for use during future THA revision procedures. The femoral head was placed in an iliac pocket on the same side of the patient's body from which it was removed.[106,107] The pouch was subperiosteal[106] or extraperiosteal with iliacus muscle preservation.[107]

In an article by Hing et al,[106] patient selection criteria for femoral head preservation included a planned primary THA procedure for osteoarthritis and a previous THA procedure on the patient's other hip that had evidence of symptomatic loosening. The authors reported that the femoral head was cut in half and placed in the pocket with the cut surface closest to the iliac crest. Thirteen patients had the femoral head preserved in a pouch, and six of the patients had revision procedures using the preserved bone from 8 months to 8 years and 11 months after the preservation of the femoral head. The femoral head was morselized during the revision procedure and used as bone graft.

Hing et al[106] found that after preservation, the bone was viable and not contaminated. They also reported that postoperative mobilization was the same as for patients who had a conventional primary THA procedure performed. There was no morbidity at the implant site in any patient. Interestingly, the authors found that tissue viability appeared to be related to the distance of the cut surface to the ilium, with the cartilage and bone furthest from the ilium showing some signs of necrosis. They concluded that preservation of the femoral head is a viable option for specific patients; however, further study is needed.

A 2014 case report by Mohan et al[107] included patients having either partial hip arthroplasty or THA procedures but not patients with suspected joint infection. They reported that femoral heads from 17 patients were preserved within iliac pouches from 2008 to 2012 but none had been used. There were no complications at the pocket site except for discomfort in the initial postoperative period that resolved over a few weeks. The authors stated that younger patients may have increased risk for revisions in the future.[107] A regression analysis performed by Shinar and Harris[105] also showed that a younger age at the time of surgery was one factor correlated with the need for revision procedures.

6.2.1 **Preparation of the autologous femoral head may include**
- **rinsing thoroughly with sterile normal saline,**[107]
- **wiping the surface,**[107]
- **removing articular cartilage,**[107]
- **removing periosteum from the neck,**[107] **and**
- **dividing the bone in half.**[106]

[Conditional Recommendation]

In a case report, Mohan et al[107] discussed the preparation methods used for the femoral head prior to placement in the iliac pouch.

6.2.2 **Provide the patient and the patient's designated caregiver(s) with instructions regard-** ing the care of the surgical incision storage area for the autologous femoral head. *[Recommendation]*

Providing patient education on care of the surgical wound area where the tissue is preserved may help the patient understand how to help the area heal and prevent actions (eg, touching, rubbing, scratching) that might increase the risk of resorption, atrophy, or necrosis of the preserved tissue.

7. Incus

7.1 **No recommendation can be made regarding autologous incus preservation within the patient's body.** *[No Recommendation]*

The balance between the benefits and harms of preserving the autologous incus in a postauricular or posttragal pocket for staged ossicular chain reconstruction procedures is unclear. The benefits of storing the autologous incus within the patient between procedures may include elimination of the need for bone banking or tissue tracking[108] and cost effectiveness.[108] A limitation of storing the autologous incus inside of the patient between procedures is that the incus may resorb, atrophy, or fixate to surrounding tissue, therefore becoming unusable.[108] Additionally, between staged procedures, the patient's stapes superstructure may atrophy,[108] causing the surgeon to need a different implant type instead of the stored incus to reconstruct the ossicular chain.[109]

Low-quality evidence exists regarding the preservation of the autologous incus. Two nonexperimental studies[108,109] and one case report[110] support the preservation of the autologous incus in a postauricular pocket,[108] in the mastoid area,[109] or in a posttragal pocket.[110] Researchers considered the reconstructive surgery to be successful if the patient achieved an air-bone gap within 15 or 20 decibels.[108,109] Both nonexperimental studies reported acceptable postoperative air-bone gap rates of 78.9%[108] and 65%.[109] Reported resorption or atrophy rates of the preserved incus were 11.1%[108] and 4.1%.[109]

Faramarzi et al[108] asserted that in developing countries the cost of an allograft implant, synthetic incus, or bone bank preservation of the autologous incus may be prohibitive. The researchers concluded that the use of a postauricular pocket for preservation of the autologous incus may make ossicular chain reconstruction procedures more affordable.

Gyo et al[109] reported that after a follow-up period of between 5 and 9 years, 57% of patients still met the expected hearing outcomes. Both Faramarzi et al[108] and Gyo et al[109] concluded that preservation of the autologous incus in the postauricular area was safe and effective.

Fritsch and Moberly[110] preserved an incus for 8 months in the posterior tragus area. Upon removal, they found the incus to be intact with no absorption, and it was placed successfully during the second procedure. The authors stated that the tragal area had been used successfully in 16 procedures that included 14 incus bones and two malleus-head bones.

7.1.1 **Provide the patient and the patient's designated caregiver(s) with instructions regarding the care of the surgical incision storage area for the autologous incus.** [*Recommendation*]

Providing patient education on care of the surgical wound area where the tissue is preserved may help the patient understand how to help the area heal and prevent actions (eg, touching, rubbing, scratching) that might increase the risk of resorption or atrophy of the preserved tissue.

8. Adipose Tissue

8.1 **No recommendation can be made regarding the cryopreservation and delayed autotransplantation of cryopreserved adipose tissue.** [*No Recommendation*]

The balance between the benefits and harms of using cryopreserved adipose tissue for delayed autotransplantation is unclear. The benefits include reduced numbers of procedures to procure adipose tissue, thereby reducing procedure-related risks, postoperative pain, additional procedure time,[111] and costs.[112] Additional benefits include higher patient satisfaction rates compared to traditional adipose procurement and grafting methods.[112,113] The harms include the potential for partial or complete resorption of adipose tissue at the graft site, leading to graft failure.[114]

Low-quality evidence, including one quasi-experimental study,[111] two nonexperimental studies,[113,114] and one organizational experience article,[112] supports the use[111-113] and further research[111,113,114] of cryopreservation of adipose tissue for patient injection. The evidence is limited by the small number of studies on the topic, including limited high-quality studies done on patient outcomes, and the use of varied study methodologies.[111,113,114]

Because of the conflicting study methodologies, there is limited consistency in the reported outcomes and reported rates of resorption. Conti et al[114] found that 50% (n = 13) of the mice that received cryopreserved subcutaneous adipose injections in a study had limited resorption, and the other 50% had high levels of resorption after 1 week. Ibrahiem et al[112] found that only 8.65% (n = 9) of patient grafts had resorption. Ha et al[111] found the lowest resorption rate (13%) for adipose tissue that had been cryopreserved for less than 1 month and included added adipose tissue–derived stem cells in the injection.

Ma et al[113] reported a 0.6% complication rate (n = 1) from cryopreserved adipose autotransplantation, which was a case of lump formation on a patient's upper lip. Conversely, Ibrahiem et al[112] reported several cases of complications including nine infections, seven cases of formation of multiple tiny firm nodules that resolved spontaneously, three hematomas, and three cases of fat necrosis.

Injecting either smaller amounts of adipose tissue per graft[112] or smaller-sized pieces of adipose tissue per graft[113] may affect the graft success rate by improving the ability of the tissue to neovascularize. Other studies have suggested that stem cells were viable after cryopreservation[114] and that the addition of stem cells to adipose autotransplantation may be important because of the ability of the cells to differentiate into various cell types, thereby increasing the potential for regeneration and graft success.[111] Although some researchers performed part of the cryopreservation process in a laboratory,[111,114] the authors of one nonexperimental study and one organizational experience article performed all or portions of the process in the OR.[112,113]

One nonexperimental study[113] and one organizational experience article[112] reported positive patient satisfaction rates related to the use of delayed autotransplantation of cryopreserved adipose tissue.

9. Team Communication

9.1 **During the procedural briefing process, include a discussion of anticipated autologous tissue preservation, replantation, or autotransplantation.**[115] [*Recommendation*]

Including a discussion of anticipated preservation, replantation, or autotransplantation of autologous tissue during the briefing allows perioperative personnel to discuss tissue availability, the thawing process (if applicable), or preparation for tissue preservation.

9.2 **During the hand-over process between OR personnel, include a review of autologous tissue that is on the sterile field, is in the room, or has been sent for preservation.**[115,116] [*Recommendation*]

In a nonexperimental study of root causes of misplaced or dropped reconstructive free flaps, Wax et al[116] found that the durations of the procedures in which the incidents occurred were long enough that the personnel may have changed.

9.3 **During the procedural debrief, confirm the name of the autologous tissue and preservation method for tissue that has been or will be preserved.**[115] *[Recommendation]*

The benefits of confirming the name of the autologous tissue and the preservation method during the procedural debrief include clear identification of the autograft and the preservation method and the potential to reduce or eliminate errors related to tissue management.

10. Handling

10.1 **Implement measures to minimize the risk of contamination and cross contamination throughout the steps of tissue handling.** *[Recommendation]*

Minimizing the risk of contamination and cross contamination is important and is required in 21 CFR 1721 for facilities registered as tissue establishments when handling, recovering, processing, packaging, labeling, storing, and tracking tissue.[1]

10.1.1 **Transfer autologous tissue intended for preservation off the sterile field as soon as possible.** *[Recommendation]*

No studies comparing tissue contamination or integrity and the timing of tissue packaging were found. However, Hirn et al[55] stated that a method of minimizing bacterial contamination is to process and package tissue as soon as possible.

10.1.2 **Verify the patient and tissue information verbally with the surgeon using a read-back technique before transferring the tissue from the sterile field.** *[Recommendation]*

The benefits of using a read-back technique include a potential reduction in labeling or documentation errors and the prevention of patient or tissue misidentification.

A 2017 report from the ECRI Institute stated that the top two types of specimen errors involved mislabeled specimens and specimens with incomplete or missing labels.[117] The report also stated that most specimen errors occur in phases of specimen handling (eg, collection, ordering, handling, transport) that take place before the specimen's delivery to the laboratory.

In a nonexperimental study, Greenberg et al[118] investigated communication breakdowns from surgical malpractice claims and found that the majority of breakdowns were in verbal communication. The researchers suggested that one method to prevent the communication breakdown would be to read back the information to verify that it was received correctly.[118] AORN recommends using a read-back technique when transferring patient information.[115]

10.1.3 **Use standard precautions[119] and sterile technique[60] when transferring autologous tissue from the sterile field.** *[Recommendation]*

10.1.4 **Measures to prevent contamination of autologous tissue that is on the sterile field may include**
- **minimal handling of tissue,**
- **sterile glove changes before handling tissue, and**
- **containing or covering recovered tissue until a tissue disposition decision is made.**[60]

[Conditional Recommendation]

10.2 **Keep autologous tissue moist or in solution when it is on the sterile field. Do not place tissue on dry, absorbent surfaces or materials.** *[Recommendation]*

The benefits of keeping tissue moist or in solution include prevention of desiccation. The AATB recommends aseptically wrapping tissue in at least one moisture barrier.[34]

10.3 **Clearly label, sequester, and monitor autologous tissue that is kept on the sterile field.** *[Recommendation]*

The benefits of identifying, sequestering, and monitoring autologous tissue kept on the sterile field include reduced risk of the tissue being contaminated, compromised, or lost.

Wax et al[116] reviewed reasons for dropped free flaps and found 13 instances of free flaps that were dropped or misplaced (eg, wrapped in a sponge and discarded as waste) out of 8,382 reconstructive head and neck procedures performed at five institutions. The researchers reported that the root cause of the dropped or misplaced flaps was miscommunication in nine of the 13 instances (69.2%). In seven of the 13 incidents (53.8%), the flap had been wrapped in a sponge or towel and then discarded later during the procedure in a bucket off the sterile field. The study also reported that personnel in one facility wrapped the flap in a moist, countable sponge and then placed it in a clear plastic bag within a basin, with distinct labeling to facilitate tissue identification.

10.4 Before placing tissue on the sterile field, visually inspect the package or container for maintained sterility[60] and verbally verify the patient's autologous tissue information with the scrub person, including
- facility-approved patient identifiers,
- the name of the preserved tissue,
- the preservation solution (when applicable), and
- the expiration date (when applicable).

[Recommendation]

11. Packaging and Labeling

11.1 Package and label autologous tissue immediately after it is transferred from the sterile field. [Recommendation]

The benefits of containing and labeling autologous tissue immediately after transfer from the sterile field include preservation of tissue integrity (eg, moisture content) and prevention of contamination, damage, or loss. Correctly labeling the tissue may also help prevent mix-ups or transplantation of the tissue into an unintended recipient.

11.2 Packaging materials for autologous tissue must be leak proof and puncture resistant.[120] [Regulatory Requirement]

11.2.1 Packaging material should be designed to prevent contamination and the introduction, transmission, or spread of communicable diseases. [Recommendation]

Use of packaging material that meets these recommendations is required in 21 CFR 1271 for tissue establishments.[1]

11.3 Use autologous tissue packaging materials that
- are large enough to fit and protect the tissue,
- will maintain the integrity of the tissue during processing (eg, cryopreservation, thawing), and
- are validated to meet the anticipated temperature range (eg, -26° C [-14.8° F]) and duration of storage (eg, 5 years).

[Recommendation]

It is an AATB standard to use packaging materials that are validated to meet the anticipated storage conditions.[34] Use of packaging materials that will protect the tissue for the anticipated temperature range and duration of the storage prevents tissue compromise that may cause the tissue to become contaminated or unusable.

11.4 The autograft package must be labeled
- "For Autologous Use Only,"[1,34]
- "Not Evaluated for Infectious Substances" if infectious disease testing has not been performed,[1,34]
- with the biohazard legend if infectious disease testing was performed and any results were positive or if donor screening was performed and risk factors were identified,[1,34]
- "Warning: Reactive Test Results for (name of disease or agent)" when there is a reactive test result,[1] and
- with an expiration date (when available).[1,34]

[Regulatory Requirement]

Specific labeling practices are a regulatory requirement and part of good tissue practices.[1] See Recommendation 12.5 for information on determining expiration dates and maximum storage duration for tissue.

11.4.1 Clearly label autologous tissue with the
- unique patient identifiers (eg, patient's name and medical record number) as specified by the facility and
- tissue type and laterality (when applicable).[34]

[Recommendation]

Facilities registered as tissue establishments with the FDA are required to label tissue with a distinct identification code, a description of the tissue, and an expiration date if there is one.[1] Clear labeling with similar requirements is also an AATB standard.[34]

11.5 Facilities may use a bar-code labeling system for labeling when available. [Conditional Recommendation]

The benefits of using a bar-code labeling system may exceed the harms. The benefits of a bar-code labeling system may include improved accuracy in matching tissue to the recipient, fewer identification errors, and improved tissue tracking.[121,122] The harms may include increased facility costs. Labeling the autograft in a manner that minimizes the risk for errors is a regulatory requirement for good tissue practice[1] and an AATB standard.[34]

11.6 Evaluate labels to confirm that the material will remain affixed to the packaging of autologous tissue throughout processing (eg, cryopreservation) and the anticipated storage parameters (eg, temperature range and duration). [Recommendation]

The AATB recommends using labels designed to be firmly affixed to the container under the anticipated storage conditions for the length of use.[34]

11.7 Securely affix the label to both the inner and outer package or container. [Recommendation]

Use of both an internal and external label is recommended because the outer label may fall off or become unreadable during frozen storage (eg, smudged from condensation).

12. Storage, Disposal, and Cleaning

12.1 **Autologous tissue must be stored in a manner that prevents exposure of health care personnel to blood, body fluids, or other potentially infectious materials.**[120] *[Regulatory Requirement]*

12.2 **Store autologous tissue in a secured location.** *[Recommendation]*

Securing the storage area is a regulatory requirement for facilities registered with the FDA as tissue establishments.[1]

12.3 **Store autologous and allograft tissue separately.** *[Recommendation]*

The benefits of storing autologous and allograft tissue separately include reduced risk of misidentification of tissue types (eg, autologous, allograft).

No research comparing different storage configurations of autologous and allograft tissue was found. However, autologous tissue is not usually tested for contamination or communicable diseases, whereas allograft donors are screened and the tissue is tested.[34] Therefore, separating allograft and autologous tissue within a shared storage space (eg, different shelves of a freezer) may minimize the risk for cross contamination, contamination, or mix-ups.[34]

12.4 **Store autologous tissue at temperatures that**
- **are established in accordance with federal and state regulations,**
- **prevent contamination or degradation of the tissue, and**
- **are maintained and periodically reviewed to confirm that the temperatures are within acceptable limits.**
[Recommendation]

It is crucial to store autologous tissue at a temperature that maintains tissue integrity. Additionally, facilities registered with the FDA as tissue establishments are required to store tissue within acceptable temperature limits; however, acceptable temperature limits for each tissue type are not specified.[1]

12.5 **In collaboration with the surgeon(s) and an infection preventionist, determine the expiration date or a maximum storage duration for autologous tissue based on the**
- **tissue type,**

- preservation method (eg, refrigerated, frozen, cryopreserved),
- storage conditions (eg, temperature range),
- packaging type, and
- packaging expiration dates.
[Recommendation]

According to 21 CFR 1271.260(c), facilities registered with the FDA as tissue establishments must assign an expiration date to tissue based on specific factors (eg, type, preservation method, storage conditions, packaging) when appropriate.[1] The AATB recommendations for duration of preservation vary based on the tissue type.[34]

12.6 **On an established schedule, review the inventory of stored autografts for package integrity and identification of tissue that is nearing expiration or the maximum storage duration.** *[Recommendation]*

Periodic review provides an opportunity to look at packaging for compromised integrity and identify items nearing expiration or the maximum storage duration. Compromised tissue packages may be contaminated and using the tissue within a compromised package may increase the risk of infection. Comparing the preserved packages to the storage records during the autologous tissue inventory may help maintain accurate tissue tracking.

Cheah et al[6] discussed that the cranial bone flap freezer log in one facility was reviewed every 6 months to confirm the need for continued specimen storage. Bhaskar et al[17] found that 8% of 25 major neurosurgical facilities surveyed in Australia required periodic reviews of the stored bone flaps.

12.6.1 **Sequester any compromised tissue packages and determine, in collaboration with the surgeon and an infection preventionist, whether the tissue should be discarded.** *[Recommendation]*

Sequestering compromised tissue packages that are under investigation may reduce the risk of cross contamination with other stored tissue. Discussing the finding with an interdisciplinary team may help confirm whether the tissue needs to be discarded or if it can be decontaminated.

12.7 **In collaboration with the surgeon(s) and an infection preventionist, determine a process for managing tissue that is nearing the expiration date or the maximum storage duration for the packaging.** *[Recommendation]*

12.7.1 **The process for managing tissue that is nearing the expiration date or the maximum**

storage duration for the packaging may include

- reviewing the patient's status (eg, alive, deceased),
- assessing the condition of the tissue packaging,
- discussing tissue that is nearing expiration or the maximum storage duration with the patient's surgeon, and
- contacting the patient or patient's legal representative for release of tissue (eg, for burial or cremation) prior to disposal.

[Conditional Recommendation]

12.8 **Remove and discard autologous tissue by the expiration date or at the end of the maximum storage duration.** *[Recommendation]*

When an expiration date is specified by health care organization or facility policy for a specific tissue type, discarding the tissue by the expiration date is important to prevent the tissue from being used when it may have reduced viability and a decreased chance of graft success. The AATB recommends against using autologous tissue after the expiration date has passed.[34]

12.8.1 **Tissue must be disposed of as regulated waste in accordance with state and local regulations.** *[Regulatory Requirement]*

Regulated medical waste includes items that contain blood or other potentially infectious materials.[120] Hazardous waste disposal of human tissue may prevent exposure of health care personnel to blood, body fluids, or other potentially infectious materials. Local and state regulations related to disposal of human tissue vary.

12.9 **Regularly scheduled calibration checks must be performed on refrigerators and freezers used for storage of tissue[1] in accordance with the manufacturer's IFU.** *[Regulatory Requirement]*

12.9.1 **Maintenance, calibration, and other activities performed on refrigerators and freezers used for storage of tissue must be recorded, and the records must be readily available.[1]** *[Regulatory Requirement]*

12.10 **Equipment used to store tissue (ie, freezers, refrigerators, nitrogen tanks) should have**
- **continuous temperature monitoring,[34]**
- **daily temperature recording,**
- **an alarm,[34] and**
- **an emergency power source.[123,124]**

[Recommendation]

It is an accreditation standard to continuously monitor equipment, use a functioning alarm, and have a back-up plan for equipment used to store tissue.[123,124] The use of an alarm will alert personnel when the temperature is out of range.[34]

Two moderate-quality studies on autologous skin reviewed the effects of the type of refrigerator used (eg, domestic, monitored) on tissue preservation. In a quasi-experimental study, Sterne et al[88] hypothesized that use of domestic refrigerators might subject tissue to a wide range of temperature fluctuations. The researchers took a series of random temperature readings from an unmonitored refrigerator and found that the temperatures were higher and more variable than in the monitored refrigerator. The researchers stated that higher temperatures resulted from frequent door opening, the door being left open for a period of time, or items of warmer temperature being placed in the refrigerator and that refrigerator temperatures that are out of range may cause ice to form. Additionally, they reported that skin stored in the unmonitored domestic refrigerator displayed more severe clefting between the epidermis and the dermis than skin stored in the monitored refrigerator.

In an experimental study, Titley et al[90] tested the effectiveness of a domestic-style refrigerator by placing temperature probes on the top, middle, and bottom shelves. The researchers found that the mean temperatures were 9.8° C (49.6° F), 7.3° C (45.1° F), and 4° C (39.2° F) on the top, middle, and bottom shelves respectively. When the refrigerator was opened once during the monitoring period, the temperature on the top shelf reached 13.9° C (57° F). The researchers also found significant levels of contamination of tissue that was stored longer than 21 days in the domestic refrigerator. Based on the study findings, they concluded that strict temperature monitoring of refrigerators is necessary and that domestic-style refrigerators are not appropriate for tissue storage.

12.10.1 **The alarm system should**
- **sound in an area where an individual is always present to initiate corrective action or**
- **notify personnel who are available to respond.**

[Recommendation]

Rapid corrective action may be required to prevent compromise or degradation of tissue when storage equipment malfunctions or fails.

12.11 **Have a back-up plan for malfunctioning or broken equipment (eg, refrigerators, freezers,**

nitrogen tanks) that is used to store tissue. [Recommendation]

It is an accreditation standard to have a back-up plan for equipment used to store tissue.[123,124]

12.12 Establish a process for

- maintaining the temperature of stored tissue in the event of an equipment malfunction and
- responding to malfunctioning storage equipment when the facility is closed or the area where the tissue is stored is unoccupied.

[Recommendation]

Proactively creating a process for the possibility of equipment malfunction or failure may decrease the time spent responding to the event and reduce the possibility of tissue loss. The AATB recommends developing policies and procedures to designate alternative storage facilities and monitoring methods.[34] During process development, the AATB also recommends clarifying the temperature and time limits for emergency tissue transfer and the steps to take when the temperature or time limits have been exceeded.[34]

12.13 Clean, sanitize, and maintain equipment and devices used for storage of tissue on an established schedule. [Recommendation]

Cleaning, disinfecting, and maintaining equipment and devices used for tissue storage may prevent malfunctions, contamination, or cross contamination.[34] It is also a regulatory requirement for a facility registered with the FDA as a tissue establishment to establish procedures for cleaning and sanitation for the purposes of preventing the introduction, transmission, or spread of communicable diseases.[1]

12.13.1 Record cleaning and disinfection of equipment and devices used in tissue management, including the methods used, cleaning schedule, and personnel responsible. Maintain the records for 3 years. [Recommendation]

13. Transport

13.1 Tissue must be transported in a manner that

- prevents exposure of health care personnel to blood, body fluids, or other potentially infectious materials,[120]
- secures the confidentiality of protected patient information,[125-127] and
- is clearly labeled with the fluorescent orange or orange-red biohazard legend.[120]

[Regulatory Requirement]

13.2 Transport tissue in a manner that maintains tissue integrity (eg, temperature, sterility). [Recommendation]

13.3 In collaboration with the surgeon, an infection preventionist, and a risk manager, determine a method for preventing contamination or cross contamination of autologous tissue during unanticipated distribution from one facility to another. [Conditional Recommendation]

According to 21 CFR 1271.3(e), distribution of tissue from one facility to another is considered part of manufacturing and requires registration with the FDA as a tissue establishment.[1] However, the FDA has clarified that in limited circumstances, transfer of tissue for the medical needs of a specific patient may be acceptable.[4] The clarifying statement from the FDA specifically references distribution of cranial bone flaps and parathyroid tissue.[4]

13.4 An AATB-accredited tissue source facility may be contacted for assistance with packaging and shipping of autologous tissue to other facilities when the originating facility is not registered as a tissue establishment. [Conditional Recommendation]

Transferring tissue from one facility to another is considered distribution under 21 CFR 1271.[1] An AATB-accredited tissue source facility can offer expert assistance with packaging and shipping of autologous tissue.

14. Documentation

14.1 Maintain records for tracking of autologous tissue. [Recommendation]

Maintaining records for tracking of tissue is an accreditation standard,[128,129] an AATB recommendation,[34] and a regulatory requirement for facilities registered as tissue establishments.[1]

14.1.1 Records related to tissue must be maintained for 10 years after the tissue is dispensed or expired, whichever is longer.[1] [Regulatory Requirement]

14.2 Record the following information for autologous tissue:

- type of autologous tissue being preserved;
- date of recovery, procedure, and name of the surgeon;
- if the tissue was cultured and applicable results;
- date and time the autograft was placed in storage;
- identity of the person placing the autograft in storage;

- method of preservation;
- storage temperature;
- processing steps (eg, sterilization) performed (when applicable);
- method of decontamination (when applicable);
- solution(s) and medication(s) used in decontamination (when applicable);
- date and time the autograft was removed from storage;
- identity of the person removing the autograft from storage;
- date of subsequent use and the procedure (when applicable); and
- final disposition of the autograft (eg, replantation, autotransplantation, transfer to another facility, release to the patient or family, disposal).

[Recommendation]

Recording information is a regulatory requirement for good tissue practice[1] and an AATB standard.[34] Accurate recording of autologous tissue information is important for tissue tracking, quality monitoring, and investigations. The AATB recommends documenting the following in regard to autologous tissue recovery: patient identifiers (eg, name, medical record number, date of birth), tissue type, date and time of recovery, and the name of the physician recovering the tissue.[34]

15. Policies and Procedures

15.1 **Facilities must maintain procedures for autologous tissue that meet the core current good tissue practice requirements (eg, labeling, storage, records, tracking) for all steps performed in tissue management.**[1] *[Regulatory Requirement]*

Maintaining procedures for tissue management is a regulatory requirement according to 21 CFR 1271.180(a).[1] It is also a Joint Commission accreditation standard specific to autologous tissue to have policies and procedures that clarify tissue management practices including identifying, tracking, storing, handling, and adverse event management.[123,124] The AATB recommends that facilities maintain policies and procedures, including a written policy for discarding autologous tissue.[34]

Glossary

Allograft: A graft taken from a living or nonliving donor for transplantation to a different individual.

Autograft: Tissue recovered from an individual for implantation or transplantation exclusively on or in the same individual.

Autologous: Cells or tissues obtained from the same individual.

Autotransplantation: Transplantation of tissue from one site to another in the same individual.

Craniectomy: Surgical removal of a portion of the skull.

Cranioplasty: Surgical repair of a defect or deformity of the skull.

Cryopreservation: A process for freezing cells or tissue at very low temperatures.

Cryoprotectant: A chemical substance (eg, glycerol, dimethyl sulfoxide) used to protect biological tissue from damage caused by ice formation during the cryopreservation and thawing process.

Cytotoxic: A substance that is poisonous to living cells.

Dulbecco's modified Eagle's medium: A modified version of Eagle's minimum essential medium that contains iron, phenol red, four times the number of vitamins and amino acids, and two to four times more glucose.

Engraftment: A process that occurs when a piece of tissue (eg, skin) that has been surgically transplanted begins to function normally.

Isotonic: Having the same solute concentration as a reference solution.

McCoy's 5A medium: A sterile nutrient medium made up of amino acids, vitamins, minerals, antibiotics, and buffers.

Meshed skin: A skin graft with multiple cuts that allow it to be stretched to cover a larger area.

Osteoblasts: Large cells responsible for synthesis and mineralization of bone during bone formation and regeneration. Osteoblasts are the major cellular component of bone.

Osteoclasts: Large multinuclear bone cells that resorb bone tissue.

Pulsatile lavage: A method of delivering irrigation under pressure with pulsation. Used to remove microorganisms and debris from the surface of a wound.

Replantation: Replacing an organ or body part (eg, cranial bone flap) into its original site and reestablishing its circulation.

Storage medium: A physiologic solution that closely replicates conditions that help to preserve the viability of cells.

Subgaleal: The space between the skin and the skull.

TiProtec: A sterile, hypothermic solution enriched with potassium chloride and N-acetyl histidine used for long-term protection and storage of tissue.

Tissue bank: A facility that participates in procuring, processing, preserving, or storing human cells and tissue for transplantation.

Tissue establishment: A facility that manufacturers human cells, tissues, and cellular and tissue-based products (HCT/Ps) and must follow applicable requirements of 21 CFR 1271.

Tulle gras: A fine-meshed gauze impregnated with vegetable oil or soft paraffin.

References

1. 21 CFR 1271: Human cells, tissues, and cellular and tissue-based products. US Food and Drug Administration. https://www.accessdata.fda.gov/scripts/cdrh/cfdocs/cfcfr/CFRSearch.cfm?CFRPart=1271. Accessed August 29, 2019.

2. Guideline for specimen management. In: *Guidelines for Perioperative Practice.* Denver, CO: AORN, Inc; 2019:897-930. [IVA]

3. Guideline for sterilization packaging systems. In: *Guidelines for Perioperative Practice.* Denver, CO: AORN, Inc; 2019. [IVA]

4. Same surgical procedure exception under 21 CFR 1271.15(b): questions and answers regarding the scope of the exception. US Food and Drug Administration. https://www.fda.gov/regulatory-information/search-fda-guidance-documents/same-surgical-procedure-exception-under-21-cfr-127115b-questions-and-answers-regarding-scope. Published November 2017. Accessed August 29, 2019.

5. Corliss B, Gooldy T, Vaziri S, Kubilis P, Murad G, Fargen K. Complications after in vivo and ex vivo autologous bone flap storage for cranioplasty: a comparative analysis of the literature. *World Neurosurg.* 2016;96:510-515. [IIIA]

6. Cheah PP, Rosman AK, Cheang CK, Idris B. Autologous cranioplasty post-operative surgical site infection: does it matter if the bone flaps were stored and handled differently? *Malays J Med Sci.* 2017;24(6):68-74. [IIB]

7. Ernst G, Qeadan F, Carlson AP. Subcutaneous bone flap storage after emergency craniectomy: cost-effectiveness and rate of resorption. *J Neurosurg.* 2018;129(6):1604-1610. [IIIB]

8. Fan MC, Wang QL, Sun P, et al. Cryopreservation of autogous cranial bone flaps for cranioplasty: a large sample retrospective study. *World Neurosurg.* 2018;109:e853-e859. [IIIA]

9. Nobre MC, Veloso AT, Santiago CFG, et al. Bone flap conservation in the scalp after decompressive craniectomy. *World Neurosurg.* 2018;120:e269-e273. [IIIC]

10. Pasaoglu A, Kurtsoy A, Koc RK, et al. Cranioplasty with bone flaps preserved under the scalp. *Neurosurg Rev.* 1996;19(3):153-156. [IIIC]

11. Lu Y, Hui G, Liu F, Wang Z, Tang Y, Gao S. Survival and regeneration of deep-freeze preserved autologous cranial bones after cranioplasty. *Br J Neurosurg.* 2012;26(2):216-221. [IIIC]

12. Beez T, Sabel M, Ahmadi SA, Beseoglu K, Steiger H, Sabel M. Scanning electron microscopic surface analysis of cryoconserved skull bone after decompressive craniectomy. *Cell Tissue Bank.* 2014;15(1):85-88. [IIIC]

13. Elwatidy S, Elgamal E, Jamjoom Z, Habib H, Raddaoui E. Assessment of bone flap viability and sterility after long periods of preservation in the freezer. *Pan Arab J Neurosurg.* 2011;15(1):24-28. [IIIC]

14. Bhaskar IP, Yusheng L, Zheng M, Lee GY. Autogenous skull flaps stored frozen for more than 6 months: do they remain viable? *J Clin Neurosci.* 2011;18(12):1690-1693. [IIB]

15. Cho TG, Kang SH, Cho YJ, Choi HJ, Jeon JP, Yang JS. Osteoblast and bacterial culture from cryopreserved skull flap after craniectomy: laboratory study. *J Korean Neurosurg Soc.* 2017;60(4):397-403. [IIIC]

16. Wui SH, Kim KM, Ryu YJ, et al. The autoclaving of autologous bone is a risk factor for surgical site infection after cranioplasty. *World Neurosurg.* 2016;91:43-49. [IIIB]

17. Bhaskar IP, Zaw NN, Zheng M, Lee GYF. Bone flap storage following craniectomy: a survey of practices in major Australian neurosurgical centres. *ANZ J Surg.* 2011;81(3):137-141. [IIIC]

18. Schültke E, Hampl JA, Jatzwauk L, Krex D, Schackert G. An easy and safe method to store and disinfect explanted skull bone. *Acta Neurochir (Wien).* 1999;141(5):525-528. [IIB]

19. Iwama T, Yamada J, Imai S, Shinoda J, Funakoshi T, Sakai N. The use of frozen autogenous bone flaps in delayed cranioplasty revisited. *Neurosurgery.* 2003;52(3):591-596. [IIIB]

20. Shoakazemi A, Flannery T, McConnell RS. Long-term outcome of subcutaneously preserved autologous cranioplasty. *Neurosurgery.* 2009;65(3):505-510. [IIIB]

21. Spijker R, Ubbink DT, Becking AG, et al. Autologous bone is inferior to alloplastic cranioplasties: safety of autograft and allograft materials for cranioplasties: a systematic review. *World Neurosurg.* 2018;117:443-452. [IIIA]

22. Malcolm JG, Mahmooth Z, Rindler RS, et al. Autologous cranioplasty is associated with increased reoperation rate: a systematic review and meta-analysis. *World Neurosurg.* 2018;116:60-68. [IIIA]

23. Kim SH, Kang DS, Cheong JH, Kim JH, Song KY, Kong MH. Comparison of complications following cranioplasty using a sterilized autologous bone flap or polymethyl methacrylate. *Korean J Neurotrauma.* 2017;13(1):15-23. [IIIB]

24. Krishnan P, Bhattacharyya AK, Sil K, De R. Bone flap preservation after decompressive craniectomy—experience with 55 cases. *Neurol India.* 2006;54(3):291-292. [VC]

25. Wang WX, Jiang N, Wang JW, Kang X, Fu GH, Liu YL. Bone formation in subcutaneous pocket after bone flap preservation. *Clin Case Rep.* 2016;4(5):473-476. [VB]

26. Honeybul S, Morrison DA, Ho KM, Lind CRP, Geelhoed E. A randomised controlled trial comparing autologous cranioplasty with custom-made titanium cranioplasty: long-term follow-up. *Acta Neurochir.* 2018;160(5):885-891. [IB]

27. Tahir MZ, Shamim MS, Sobani ZA, Zafar SN, Qadeer M, Bari ME. Safety of untreated autologous cranioplasty after extracorporeal storage at -26 degree Celsius. *Br J Neurosurg.* 2013;27(4):479-482. [IIIB]

28. Daou B, Zanaty M, Chalouhi N, et al. Low incidence of bone flap resorption after native bone cranioplasty in adults. *World Neurosurg.* 2016;92:89-94. [IIIB]

29. Sundseth J, Sundseth A, Berg-Johnsen J, Sorteberg W, Lindegaard KF. Cranioplasty with autologous cryopreserved bone after decompressive craniectomy: complications and risk factors for developing surgical site infection. *Acta Neurochir (Wein).* 2014;156(4):805-811. [IIIB]

30. Cheng CH, Lee HC, Chen CC, Cho DY, Lin HL. Cryopreservation versus subcutaneous preservation of autologous bone flaps for cranioplasty: comparison of the surgical site infection and bone resorption rates. *Clin Neurol Neurosurg.* 2014;124:85-89. [IIIA]

31. Herteleer M, Ectors N, Duflou J, Van Calenbergh F. Complications of skull reconstruction after decompressive craniectomy. *Acta Chir Belg.* 2017;117(3):149-156. [IIIB]

32. Inamasu J, Kuramae T, Nakatsukasa M. Does difference in the storage method of bone flaps after decompressive craniectomy affect the incidence of surgical site infection after cranioplasty? Comparison between subcutaneous pocket and cryopreservation. *J Trauma.* 2010;68(1):183-187. [IIIB]

33. Chan DYC, Mok YT, Lam PK, et al. Cryostored autologous skull bone for cranioplasty? A study on cranial bone flaps' viability and microbial contamination after deep-frozen storage at -80°C. *J Clin Neurosci.* 2017;42:81-83. [IIIC]

34. *Standards for Tissue Banking.* 14th ed. McLean, VA: American Association of Tissue Banks; 2016. [IVC]

35. Schoekler B, Trummer M. Prediction parameters of bone flap resorption following cranioplasty with autologous bone. *Clin Neurol Neurosurg.* 2014;120:64-67. [IIIC]

36. Morton RP, Abecassis IJ, Hanson JF, et al. Predictors of infection after 754 cranioplasty operations and the value of intraoperative cultures for cryopreserved bone flaps. *J Neurosurg.* 2016;125(3):766-770. [IIIA]

37. Piedra MP, Thompson EM, Selden NR, Ragel BT, Guillaume DJ. Optimal timing of autologous cranioplasty after decompressive craniectomy in children. *J Neurosurg Pediatr.* 2012;10(4):268-272. [IIIB]

38. Bowers CA, Jay Riva-Cambrin, Hertzler DA, Walker ML. Risk factors and rates of bone flap resorption in pediatric patients after decompressive craniectomy for traumatic brain injury. *J Neurosurg Pediatr.* 2013;11(5):526-532. [IIIC]

39. Baust JM, Campbell LH, Harbell JW. Best practices for cryopreserving, thawing, recovering, and assessing cells. *In Vitro Cell Dev Biol Anim.* 2017;53(10):855-871. [VA]

40. Takeuchi H, Higashino Y, Hosoda T, et al. Long-term follow-up of cryopreservation with glycerol of autologous bone flaps for cranioplasty after decompressive craniectomy. *Acta Neurochir (Wien).* 2016;158(3):571-575. [IIIC]

41. Zhang J, Peng F, Liu Z, et al. Cranioplasty with autogenous bone flaps cryopreserved in povidone iodine: a long-term follow-up study. *J Neurosurg.* 2017;127(6):1449-1456. [IIIB]

42. Matsuno A, Tanaka H, Iwamuro H, et al. Analyses of the factors influencing bone graft infection after delayed cranioplasty. *Acta Neurochir (Wien).* 2006;148(5):535-540. [IIIB]

43. Cheng Y, Weng H, Yang J, Lee M, Wang T, Chang C. Factors affecting graft infection after cranioplasty. *J Clin Neurosci.* 2008;15(10):1115-1119. [IIIC]

44. Piitulainen JM, Kauko T, Aitasalo KMJ, Vuorinen V, Vallittu PK, Posti JP. Outcomes of cranioplasty with synthetic materials and autologous bone grafts. *World Neurosurg.* 2015;83(5):708-714. [IIIC]

45. Ronholdt CJ, Bogdansky S. The appropriateness of swab cultures for the release of human allograft tissue. *J Ind Microbiol Biotechnol.* 2005;32(8):349-354. [IB]

46. Dennis JA, Martinez OV, Landy DC, et al. A comparison of two microbial detection methods used in aseptic processing of musculoskeletal allograft tissues. *Cell Tissue Bank.* 2011;12(1):45-50. [IIIB]

47. Nguyen H, Morgan DAF, Cull S, Benkovich M, Forwood MR. Sponge swabs increase sensitivity of sterility testing of processed bone and tendon allografts. *J Ind Microbiol Biotechnol.* 2011;38(8):1127-1132. [IIB]

48. 42 CFR 493: Laboratory requirements. Government Publishing Office. https://www.govinfo.gov/app/details/CFR-2011-title42-vol5/CFR-2011-title42-vol5-part493. Published October 1, 2011. Accessed August 29, 2019.

49. Abdelfatah MA. Management of dropped skull flaps. *Turk Neurosurg.* 2017;27(6):912-916. [IIIC]

50. Jankowitz BT, Kondziolka DS. When the bone flap hits the floor. *Neurosurgery.* 2006;59(3):585-589. [IIIB]

51. Presnal BP, Kimbrough EE. What to do about a dropped bone graft. *Clin Orthop Relat Res.* 1993;296:310-311. [IIB]

52. Bruce B, Sheibani-Rad S, Appleyard D, et al. Are dropped osteoarticular bone fragments safely reimplantable in vivo? *J Bone Joint Surg Am.* 2011;93(5):430-438. [IIB]

53. Bhandari M, Schemitsch EH, Adili A, Lachowski RJ, Shaughnessy SG. High and low pressure pulsatile lavage of contaminated tibial fractures: an in vitro study of bacterial adherence and bone damage. *J Orthop Trauma.* 1999;13(8):526-533. [IIB]

54. Cruz NI, Cestero HJ, Cora ML. Management of contaminated bone grafts. *Plast Reconstr Surg.* 1981;68(3):411-414. [IIB]

55. Hirn M, Laitinen M, Pirkkalainen S, Vuento R. Cefuroxime, rifampicin and pulse lavage in decontamination of allograft bone. *J Hosp Infect.* 2004;56(3):198-201. [IIB]

56. Bhandari M, Adili A, Schemitsch EH. The efficacy of low-pressure lavage with different irrigating solutions to remove adherent bacteria from bone. *J Bone Joint Surg Am.* 2001;83(3):412-419. [IIB]

57. Bhandari M, Adili A, Lachowski RJ. High pressure pulsatile lavage of contaminated human tibiae: an in vitro study. *J Orthop Trauma.* 1998;12(7):479-484. [IIB]

58. Yaman F, Unlü G, Atilgan S, Celik Y, Ozekinci T, Yaldiz M. Microbiologic and histologic assessment of intentional bacterial contamination of bone grafts. *J Oral Maxillofac Surg.* 2007;65(8):1490-1494. [IIB]

59. Kaysinger KK, Nicholson NC, Ramp WK, Kellam JF. Toxic effects of wound irrigation solutions on cultured tibiae and osteoblasts. *J Orthop Trauma.* 1995;9(4):303-311. [IIB]

60. Guideline for sterile technique. In: *Guidelines for Perioperative Practice.* Denver, CO: AORN, Inc; 2019:931-972. [IVA]

61. Lacey RW. Antibacterial activity of povidone iodine towards non-sporing bacteria. *J Appl Bacteriol.* 1979;46(3):443-449. [IIB]

62. Surgical site infection (SSI) event. In: *National Healthcare Safety Network (NHSN) Patient Safety Component Manual.* Atlanta GA: National Healthcare Safety Network, Centers for Disease Control and Prevention; 2018.

63. Anto D, Manjooran RP, Aravindakshan R, Lakshman K, Morris R. Cranioplasty using autoclaved autologous skull bone flaps preserved at ambient temperature. *J Neurosci Rural Pract.* 2017;8(4):595-600. [IIIB]

64. Mracek J, Hommerova J, Mork J, Richtr P, Priban V. Complications of cranioplasty using a bone flap sterilised by

autoclaving following decompressive craniectomy. *Acta Neurochir (Wein)*. 2015;157(3):501-506. [IIIB]

65. Missori P, Marruzzo D, Paolini S, et al. Autologous skull bone flap sterilization after decompressive craniectomy: an update. *World Neurosurg*. 2016;90:478-483. [IIC]

66. Jho DH, Neckrysh S, Hardman J, Charbel FT, Amin-Hanjani S. Ethylene oxide gas sterilization: a simple technique for storing explanted skull bone: technical note. *J Neurosurg*. 2007;107(2):440-445. [IIIB]

67. Guideline for sterilization. In: *Guidelines for Perioperative Practice*. Denver, CO: AORN, Inc; 2019:973-1002. [IVA]

68. Herrera MF, Grant CS, van Heerden JA, Jacobsen D, Weaver A, Fitzpatrick LA. The effect of cryopreservation on cell viability and hormone secretion in human parathyroid tissue. *Surgery*. 1992;112(6):1096-1102. [IIC]

69. Schneider R, Ramaswamy A, Slater EP, Bartsch DK, Schlosser K. Cryopreservation of parathyroid tissue after parathyroid surgery for renal hyperparathyroidism: does it really make sense? *World J Surg*. 2012;36(11):2598-2604. [IIIB]

70. McHenry CR, Stenger DB, Calandro NK. The effect of cryopreservation on parathyroid cell viability and function. *Am J Surg*. 1997;174(5):481-484. [IIC]

71. Cohen MS, Dilley WG, Wells SA Jr, et al. Long-term functionality of cryopreserved parathyroid autografts: a 13-year prospective analysis. *Surgery*. 2005;138(6):1033-1040. [IIIB]

72. Saxe AW, Spiegel AM, Marx SJ, Brennan MF. Deferred parathyroid autografts with cryopreserved tissue after reoperative parathyroid surgery. *Arch Surg*. 1982;117(5):538-543. [IIIC]

73. Wagner PK, Rumpelt HJ, Krause U, Rothmund M. The effect of cryopreservation on hormone secretion in vitro and morphology of human parathyroid tissue. *Surgery*. 1986;99(3):257-264. [IIB]

74. Guerrero MA, Evans DB, Lee JE, et al. Viability of cryopreserved parathyroid tissue: when is continued storage versus disposal indicated? *World J Surg*. 2008;32(5):836-839. [IIIB]

75. Agarwal A, Waghray A, Gupta S, Sharma R, Milas M. Cryopreservation of parathyroid tissue: an illustrated technique using the Cleveland Clinic protocol. *J Am Coll Surg*. 2013;216(1):e1-e9. [VA]

76. Barreira CE, Cernea CR, Brandão LG, Custodio MR, Caldini ET, de Menezes Montenegro FL. Effects of time on ultrastructural integrity of parathyroid tissue before cryopreservation. *World J Surg*. 2011;35(11):2440-2444. [IIC]

77. Alvarez-Hernandez D, Gonzalez-Suarez I, Carrillo-Lopez N, Naves-Diaz M, Anguita-Velasco J, Cannata-Andia JB. Viability and functionality of fresh and cryopreserved human hyperplastic parathyroid tissue tested in vitro. *Am J Nephrol*. 2008;28(1):76-82. [IIC]

78. Brennan MF, Brown EM, Sears HF, Aurbach GD. Human parathyroid cryopreservation: in vitro testing of function by parathyroid hormone release. *Ann Surg*. 1978;187(1):87-90. [IIC]

79. Stotler BA, Reich-Slotky R, Schwartz J, et al. Quality monitoring of microbial contamination of cryopreserved parathyroid tissue. *Cell Tissue Bank*. 2011;12(2):111-116. [VB]

80. Monchik JM, Cotton TM. Technique for subcutaneous forearm transplantation of autologous parathyroid tissue. *Surgery*. 2017;161(5):1451-1452. [VB]

81. Leite AK, Junior CP, Arap SS, et al. Successful parathyroid tissue autograft after 3 years of cryopreservation: a case report. *Arq Bras Endocrinol Metabol*. 2014;58(3):313-316. [VB]

82. de Menezes Montenegro FL, Custodio MR, Arap SS, et al. Successful implant of long-term cryopreserved parathyroid glands after total parathyroidectomy. *Head Neck*. 2007;29(3):296-300. [VB]

83. Ciudad P, Date S, Orfaniotis G, et al. Delayed grafting for banked skin graft in lymph node flap transfer. *Int Wound J*. 2017;14(1):125-129. [IIIB]

84. Sheridan R, Mahe J, Walters P. Autologous skin banking. *Burns*. 1998;24(1):46-48. [IIIC]

85. DeBono R, Rao GS, Berry RB. The survival of human skin stored by refrigeration at 4 degrees C in McCoy's 5A medium: does oxygenation of the medium improve storage time? *Plast Reconstr Surg*. 1998;102(1):78-83. [IIB]

86. Turhan-Haktanır N, Dilek FH, Köken G, Demir Y, Yılmaz G. Evaluation of amniotic fluid as a skin graft storage media compared with RPMI and saline. *Burns*. 2011;37(4):652-655. [IIA]

87. Boekema BK, Boekestijn B, Breederveld RS. Evaluation of saline, RPMI and DMEM/F12 for storage of split-thickness skin grafts. *Burns*. 2015;41(4):848-852. [IIB]

88. Sterne GD, Titley OG, Christie JL. A qualitative histological assessment of various storage conditions on short term preservation of human split skin grafts. *Br J Plast Surg*. 2000;53(4):331-336. [IIC]

89. Knapik A, Kornmann K, Kerl K, et al. Practice of split-thickness skin graft storage and histological assessment of tissue quality. *J Plast Reconstr Aesthet Surg*. 2013;66(6):827-834. [IIIB]

90. Titley OG, Cooper M, Thomas A, Hancock K. Stored skin—stored trouble? *Br J Plast Surg*. 1994;47(1):24-29. [IIIB]

91. Li Z, Overend C, Maitz P, Kennedy P. Quality evaluation of meshed split-thickness skin grafts stored at 4°C in isotonic solutions and nutrient media by cell cultures. *Burns*. 2012;38(6):899-907. [IIA]

92. Rosenquist MD, Kealey GP, Lewis RW, Cram AE. A comparison of storage viability of nonmeshed and meshed skin at 4 degrees C. *J Burn Care Rehabil*. 1988;9(6):634-636. [IIB]

93. Mardini S, Agullo FJ, Salgado CJ, Rose V, Moran SL, Chen HC. Delayed skin grafting utilizing autologous banked tissue. *Ann Plast Surg*. 2009;63(3):311-313. [VB]

94. Wilbring M, Tugtekin SM, Zatschler B, et al. Preservation of endothelial vascular function of saphenous vein grafts after long-time storage with a recently developed potassium-chloride and N-acetylhistidine enriched storage solution. *Thorac Cardiovasc Surg*. 2013;61(8):656-662. [IIIB]

95. Ebner A, Poitz DM, Augstein A, Strasser RH, Deussen A. Functional, morphologic, and molecular characterization of cold storage injury. *J Vasc Surg*. 2012;56(1):189-198. [IIB]

96. Garbe S, Zatschler B, Muller B, et al. Preservation of human artery function following prolonged cold storage with a new solution. *J Vasc Surg*. 2011;53(4):1063-1070. [IB]

97. Zatschler B, Dieterich P, Muller B, Kasper M, Rauen U, Deussen A. Improved vessel preservation after 4 days of cold storage: experimental study in rat arteries. *J Vasc Surg.* 2009;50(2):397-406. [IIC]

98. Cavallari N, Abebe W, Hunter WJ 3rd, et al. University of Wisconsin solution effects on intimal proliferation in canine autogenous vein grafts. *J Surg Res.* 1995;59(4):433-440. [IB]

99. Thatte HS, Biswas KS, Najjar SF, et al. Multi-photon microscopic evaluation of saphenous vein endothelium and its preservation with a new solution, GALA. *Ann Thorac Surg.* 2003;75(4):1145-1152. [IIB]

100. Policy 16: Organ and extra vessel packaging, labeling, shipping, and storage. Organ Procurement and Transplantation Network. https://optn.transplant.hrsa.gov/media/1200/optn_policies.pdf. Effective August 15, 2019. Accessed August 29, 2019.

101. Molnar GF, Nemes A, Kekesi V, Monos E, Nadasy GL. Maintained geometry, elasticity and contractility of human saphenous vein segments stored in a complex tissue culture medium. *Eur J Vasc Endovasc Surg.* 2010;40(1):88-93. [IB]

102. Harskamp RE, Alexander JH, Schulte PJ, et al. Vein graft preservation solutions, patency, and outcomes after coronary artery bypass graft surgery: follow-up from the PREVENT IV randomized clinical trial. *JAMA Surg.* 2014;149(8):798-805. [IA]

103. Chang SK, Lau JW, Chui CK. Changes in mechanical, structural integrity and microbiological properties following cryopreservation of human cadaveric iliac arteries. *Ann Acad Med Singapore.* 2014;43(10):492-498. [IIB]

104. Coppi G, Ragazzi G, Cataldi V, Corvi V, Silingardi R. Cryopreserved autologous saphenous vein for staged treatment of bilateral popliteal aneurysms: report of three cases. *Ann Vasc Surg.* 2014;28(5):1322.e13-1322.e17. [VB]

105. Shinar AA, Harris WH. Bulk structural autogenous grafts and allografts for reconstruction of the acetabulum in total hip arthroplasty. Sixteen-year-average follow-up. *J Bone Joint Surg Am.* 1997;79(2):159-168. [IIIB]

106. Hing CB, Ball RY, Tucker JK. Autobanking of femoral heads for revision total hip replacement, a preliminary report of a new surgical technique. *Surgeon.* 2004;2(1):37-41. [VB]

107. Mohan MD, Sandeep RB, Roshan MW. Auto bone banking: innovative method for bone preservation. *J Orthop Case Rep.* 2014;4(4):16-18. [VB]

108. Faramarzi M, Roosta S, Dianat M. Outcome of incus interposition after preservation in soft tissue. *Iran J Otorhinolaryngol.* 2017;29(2):83-88. [IIIB]

109. Gyo K, Hato N, Shinomori Y, Hakuba N. Storage of the incus in the mastoid bowl for use as a columella in staged tympanoplasty. *Auris Nasus Larynx.* 2007;34(1):5-8. [IIIC]

110. Fritsch MH, Moberly AC. Tragal storage of autograft middle-ear ossicles. *Otolaryngol Head Neck Surg.* 2010;143(1):161-162. [VC]

111. Ha KY, Park H, Park SH, et al. The relationship of a combination of human adipose tissue-derived stem cells and frozen fat with the survival rate of transplanted fat. *Arch Plast Surg.* 2015;42(6):677-685. [IIB]

112. Ibrahiem SMS, Farouk A, Salem IL. Facial rejuvenation: serial fat graft transfer. *Alex J Med.* 2016;52(4):371-376. [VB]

113. Ma H, Fang YH, Lin CH, Perng CK, Tsai CH, Hsiao FY. Facial recontouring with autologous cryopreserved fat graft. *Formosan J Surg.* 2018;51(2):58-62. [IIIB]

114. Conti G, Jurga M, Benati D, et al. Cryopreserved subcutaneous adipose tissue for fat graft. *Aesthetic Plast Surg.* 2015;39(5):800-817. [IIIB]

115. Guideline for team communication. In: *Guidelines for Perioperative Practice.* Denver, CO: AORN, Inc; 2019:1061-1092. [IVA]

116. Wax MK, Futran ND, Rosenthal EL, Blackwell KE, Cannady S. Accidental dropping or misplacement of free flaps. *Laryngoscope.* 2015;125(8):1807-1810. [IIIB]

117. Ask HRC: Best practices for specimen handling. ECRI Institute. https://www.ecri.org/components/HRC/Pages/AskHRC072417.aspx. Published July 24, 2017. Accessed August 29, 2019. [VB]

118. Greenberg CC, Regenbogen SE, Studdert DM, et al. Patterns of communication breakdowns resulting in injury to surgical patients. *J Am Coll Surg.* 2007;204(4):533-540. [IIIB]

119. Guideline for transmission-based precautions. In: *Guidelines for Perioperative Practice.* Denver, CO: AORN, Inc; 2019. [IVA]

120. 29 CFR 1910.1030: Bloodborne pathogens. Occupational Safety and Health Administration. https://www.osha.gov/pls/oshaweb/owadisp.show_document?p_id=10051&p_table=STANDARDS. Accessed August 29, 2019.

121. Lost surgical specimens, lost opportunities. *PA PSRS Patient Saf Advis.* 2005;2(3):1-5. [VB]

122. Where do most lab errors occur? Not the lab. *ECRI PSO Monthly Brief.* June 2012. ECRI Institute. https://www.ecri.org/EmailResources/PSO_Monthly_Brief/2012/PSO_Brief_Jun12.pdf. Accessed August 29, 2019. [VB]

123. Program: Ambulatory. Transplant safety. TS.03.01.01: The organization uses standardized procedures for managing tissues. In: *Comprehensive Accreditation Manual.* E-dition ed. Oakbrook Terrace, IL: The Joint Commission; 2019.

124. Program: Hospital. Transplant safety. TS.03.01.01: The hospital uses standardized procedures for managing tissues. In: *Comprehensive Accreditation Manual.* E-dition ed. Oakbrook Terrace, IL: The Joint Commission; 2019.

125. Guideline for patient information management. In: *Guidelines for Perioperative Practice.* Denver, CO: AORN, Inc; 2019:371-400. [IVA]

126. 45 CFR parts 160 and 164: Modifications to the HIPAA privacy, security, enforcement, and breach notification rules under the health information technology for economic and clinical health act and the genetic information nondiscrimination act; other modifications to the HIPAA rules; final rule. *Fed Regist.* 2013;78(17):5566-5702.

127. Standards of perioperative nursing. In: *Guidelines for Perioperative Practice.* Denver, CO: AORN, Inc; 2015. [IVB]

128. Program: Hospital. Transplant safety. TS.03.02.01: The hospital traces all tissues bi-directionally. In: *Comprehensive Accreditation Manual.* E-dition ed. Oakbrook Terrace, IL: The Joint Commission; 2019.

129. Program: Ambulatory. Transplant safety. TS.03.02.01: The organization traces all tissues bi-directionally. In: *Comprehensive Accreditation Manual.* E-dition ed. Oakbrook Terrace, IL: The Joint Commission; 2019.

Guideline Development Group

Lead Author: Julie Cahn[1], DNP, RN, CNOR, RN-BC, ACNS-BC, CNS-CP, Perioperative Practice Specialist, AORN, Denver, Colorado

Methodologist: Amber Wood[2], MSN, RN, CNOR, CIC, FAPIC, Editor-in-Chief, *Guidelines for Perioperative Practice,* AORN, Denver, Colorado

Evidence Appraisers: Julie Cahn[1]; Janice Neil[3], PhD, CNE, RN, Associate Professor, East Carolina College of Nursing, Greenville, North Carolina; and Amber Wood[2]

Guidelines Advisory Board Members:

- Donna A. Pritchard[4], MA, BSN, RN, NE-BC, CNOR, Director of Perioperative Services, Interfaith Medical Center, Brooklyn, New York
- Bernard C. Camins[5], MD, MSc, Medical Director, Infection Prevention, Mount Sinai Health System, New York, New York
- Mary Fearon[6], MSN, RN, CNOR, Service Line Director Neuroscience, Overlake Medical Center, Sammamish, Washington
- Kate McGee[7], BSN, RN, CNOR, Staff Nurse, Aurora West Allis Medical Center, East Troy, Wisconsin
- Brenda G. Larkin[8], MS, ACNS-BC, CNS, CNOR, Clinical Nurse Specialist, Aurora Lakeland Medical Center, Lake Geneva, Wisconsin
- Vicki J. Barnett[9], MSN, RN, CNOR, Founder, VJB Perioperative Consulting, Northside Hospital, Atlanta, Georgia

External Review: Expert review comments were received from individual members of the American Association of Tissue Banks (AATB), American Association of Nurse Anesthetists (AANA), American College of Surgeons (ACS), Association for Professionals in Infection Control and Epidemiology (APIC), American Society of Anesthesiologists (ASA), International Association of Healthcare Central Service Materiel Management (IAHCSMM), and the Society for Healthcare Epidemiology of America (SHEA). Their responses were used to further refine and enhance this guideline; however, their responses do not imply endorsement. The draft was also open for a 30-day public comment period.

Financial Disclosure and Conflicts of Interest

This guideline was developed, edited, and approved by the AORN Guidelines Advisory Board without external funding being sought or obtained. The Guidelines Advisory Board was financially supported entirely by AORN and was developed without any involvement of industry.

Potential conflicts of interest for all Guidelines Advisory Board members were reviewed before the annual meeting and each monthly conference call. None of the members of the Guideline Development Group reported a potential conflict of interest.[1-9]

Publication History

Originally published in November 2014 in *Perioperative Standards and Recommended Practices* online.

Minor editing revisions made in November 2014 for publication in *Guidelines for Perioperative Practice,* 2015 edition.

Evidence ratings revised in *Guidelines for Perioperative Practice,* 2018 edition, to conform to the current AORN Evidence Rating Model.

Revised 2019 for online publication in *Guidelines for Perioperative Practice.*

Scheduled for review in 2024.

COMPLEMENTARY CARE

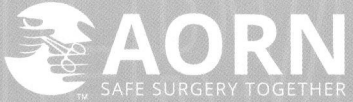

TABLE OF CONTENTS

[P] *indicates a recommendation or evidence relevant to pediatric care.*

MEDICAL ABBREVIATIONS & ACRONYMS

AANA – American Association of Nurse Anesthetists
AHNA – American Holistic Nurses Association
ASA – American Society of Anesthesiologists
BIS – Bispectral index
CAM – Complementary and alternative medicine
CPM – Continuous passive motion
ERAS – Enhanced Recovery After Surgery
FDA – US food and Drug Administration
GI – Gastrointestinal
ICC – Induction Compliance Checklist
ICU – Intensive care unit
IKDC – International Knee Documentation Committee Subjective Knee Form
INVR – Index of Nausea, Vomiting, and Retching
IU – International units
LOHS – Length of hospital stay
LOS – Length of stay
MRI – Magnetic resonance imaging

NIN – Noninvasive interactive neurostimulation
NSAID – Nonsteriodal anti-inflammatory drug
PACU – Postanesthesia care unit
PEMF – Postoperative pulsed electromagnetic field
PENS – Percutaneous electrical nerve stimulation
POD – Postoperative day
PDNV – Post-discharge nausea and vomiting
PONV – Postoperative nausea and vomiting
PT – Physical therapy
RCT – Randomized controlled trial
RN – Registered nurse
ROM – Range of motion
TCM – Traditional Chinese medicine
tDCS – Transcranial direct current stimulation
TENS – Transcutaneous electrical nerve stimulation
TKA – Total knee arthroplasty
VR – Virtual reality

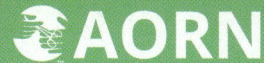
GUIDELINE FOR
COMPLEMENTARY CARE

The Guideline for Complementary Care was approved by the AORN Guidelines Advisory Board and became effective as of June 10, 2021. The recommendations in the guideline are intended to be achievable and represent what is believed to be an optimal level of practice. Policies and procedures will reflect variations in practice settings and/or clinical situations that determine the degree to which the guideline can be implemented. AORN recognizes the many diverse settings in which perioperative nurses practice; therefore, this guideline is adaptable to all areas where operative or other invasive procedures may be performed.

Purpose

This document provides guidance to perioperative registered nurses (RNs) for determining what **complementary** care interventions will be used in the organization and how to implement them in the perioperative setting. Optimal perioperative nursing practice promotes patient well-being, and implementing patient-centered complementary care interventions can improve the perioperative experience for patients, their families, and health care workers, as well as reduce health care costs. The perioperative experience begins when an operative or invasive procedure is scheduled and ends when the patient is released from follow-up surgical care. Patients can experience preoperative stress, intraoperative discomfort, and problems with postoperative healing, some of which can be addressed with complementary care interventions.

Assessing patients' individual values, health beliefs, and health experiences concerning physical, mental, emotional, spiritual, and environmental factors that can affect well-being and healing is essential when planning and implementing perioperative complementary care interventions. The use of complementary care has increased in many clinical areas, and an increasing number of researchers are studying perioperative outcomes that can be improved with complementary care interventions. As such, this guideline revision expands on the previous version, which was focused on reducing perioperative pain and anxiety, by including **holistic** methods for optimizing the overall health and well-being of perioperative patients through the use of a variety of complementary care interventions that can be implemented throughout the perioperative care plan.

The ability to provide complementary care interventions depends on several patient and organizational factors. Patient factors include the patient's acceptance and engagement, individual values, health beliefs, and experiences with health care. Organizational factors include the clinical experience, the education and competency of the perioperative team to provide complementary care interventions, and procedural and facility constraints. Considerations for cost and feasibility are also discussed in this guideline.

The variable nature of complementary care intervention studies (eg, implementation techniques, assessment, evaluation) limits the reliability and validity of the literature. Researchers have concluded that additional research studies are needed to confirm initial findings and conclusions because intervention techniques, outcomes, and settings have been inconsistent and limit generalizability.[1-10] Complementary care interventions may not be feasible or suitable for every patient; therefore, the perioperative RN plays an integral role in facilitating an optimal perioperative experience for the patient by individualizing complementary care based on the evidence-based practice recommendations in this guideline.

Researchers have examined current use of **complementary and alternative medicine** (CAM) and age-specific differences in use. In national surveys[11-14] conducted from 2012 to 2016, adults, **older adults**, and Hispanic respondents reported increased use of complementary care interventions. Clarke et al[13] found that use of dietary and herbal interventions was the most popular response. Ho et al[12] found that respondents born between 1946 and 1964 were more likely to use complementary care than other groups. Black et al[11] found that older pediatric patients were more likely to use complementary care interventions (eg, yoga). De Moura et al[14] found that younger pediatric patients were more likely to report postoperative pain and 42% of pediatric patients reported having preoperative anxiety. **P**

The recommendations and interventions described in this guideline are intended to complement **conventional treatment** and not intended to be alternatives to conventional surgical care[10] or **integrative treatments** for conditions, diseases, or illnesses. The National Institutes of Health defines complementary as an adjunct to conventional medicine and alternative as a replacement for conventional medicine.[10] Complementary and alternative medicine includes the use of natural products (eg, herbs, vitamins and minerals, probiotics, dietary supplements) and mind and body practices (eg, deep breathing, yoga, meditation, massage, homeopathy, relaxation, guided imagery). The definition of complementary care is expanding as new interventions continue to be the focus of study.

Figure 1. Flow Diagram of Literature Search Results

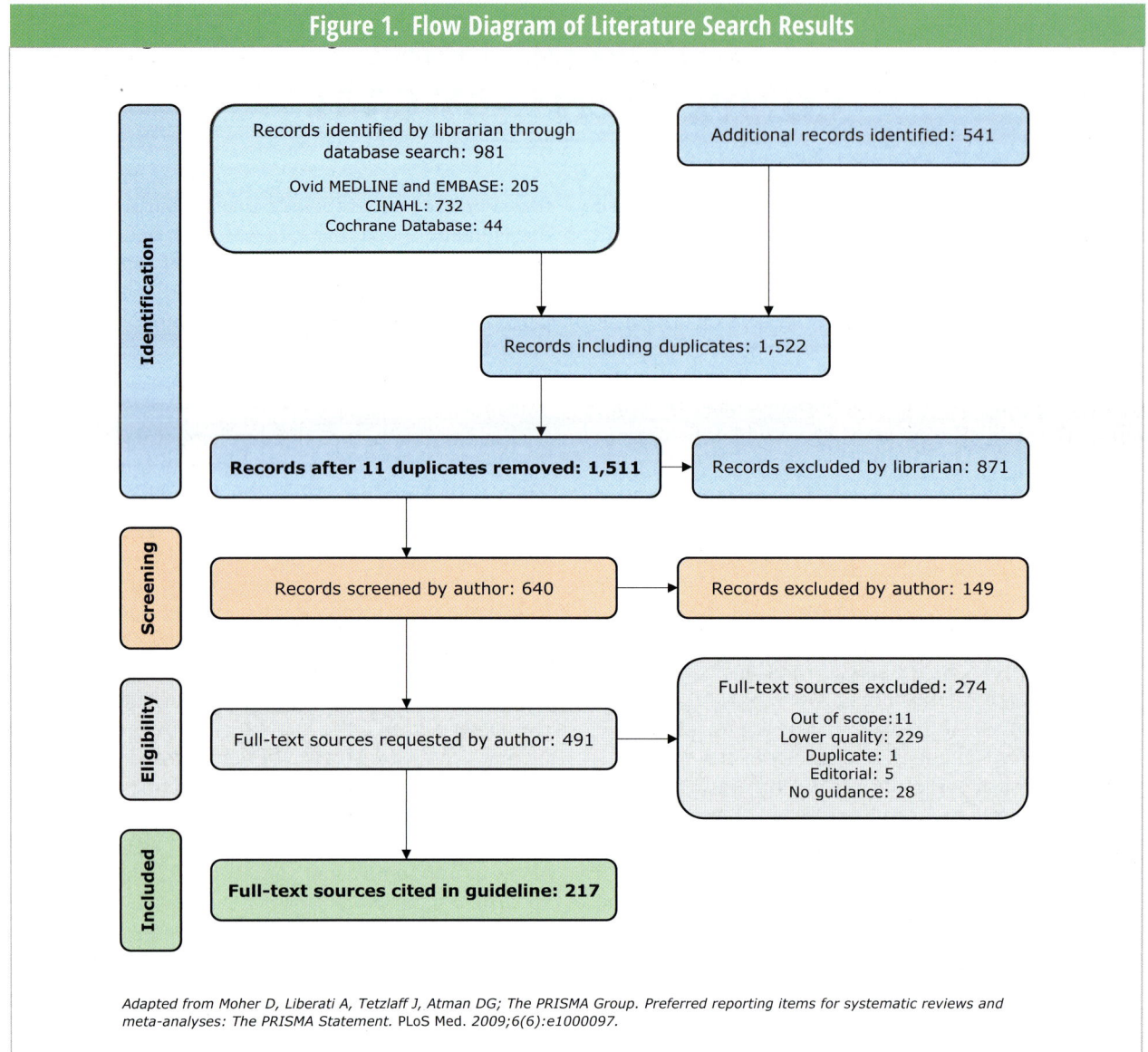

Adapted from Moher D, Liberati A, Tetzlaff J, Atman DG; The PRISMA Group. Preferred reporting items for systematic reviews and meta-analyses: The PRISMA Statement. PLoS Med. 2009;6(6):e1000097.

Topics outside the scope of this document are

- conventional medical treatment,
- nontraditional forms of conventional medicine prescribed by a licensed independent practitioner (eg, alternative medicine, functional medicine, integrative medicine),
- interventions that have limited use in the perioperative setting (eg, animal therapy, yoga),
- interventions that are implemented outside of the perioperative setting (eg, rehabilitation, physical therapy),
- interventions intended for the purpose of treating a condition or disease (eg, natural hormones, alternative medication, ERAS), and
- interventions to improve health care workers' well-being.

A discussion of **ERAS (Enhanced Recovery After Sugery)**[15] and other conventional medical care guidelines is outside the scope of this guideline, but many elements of ERAS can be found in these recommendations.

Evidence Review

A medical librarian with a perioperative background conducted a systematic search of the databases Ovid MEDLINE, Ovid Embase, EBSCO CINAHL, and the Cochrane Database of Systematic Reviews. The search was limited to literature published in English from January 2010 through April 2020. At the time of the initial search, weekly alerts were created on the topics included in that search. Results from these alerts were provided to the lead author until June 2020. The lead author requested additional articles that either did not fit the original search criteria or were discovered during the evidence appraisal process. The lead author and the medical librarian also identified relevant guidelines from government agencies, professional organizations, and standards-setting bodies.

Search terms included *acupressure, acupunctur*, adulterants, alternative analgesia, alternative medicine, alternative* therap*, anxiety, aromatherap*, audio visual distraction, ayurved*, bioelectromagnetics, biofield, biological field, bleeding, bruis*, carrier oil, chiropract*, chromatography, complementary care, complementary medicine, complementary therap*, conditioned aversion, contusions, cool cloths, cortisol, cough relief, deep breathing, diet therap*, discomfort, dislike smell, distress, electromagnetic fields, emotional distress, energy medicine, environmental trigger, essential oils, fear, flexibility, functional medicine, guided imagery, h*matoma, heart rate, heating pad, herbal medicine, herbal remedies, herbal*, holistic interventions, homeopath*, homeopathic medicine, hypnosis, hypnotherap*, ice, inflammation, integrative health, integrative medicine, LED lights, massage, muscle tension, nasal stuffiness, natural medicine, natural therap*, naturopath*, naturopathy, nausea, nonconventional therapy, nonpharmaceutical, nutrition*, operating room nurse, operating rooms, organic, osteopath*, PACU, pain tolerance, perioperative nursing, physiological stress, phytotherap*, pillows, positioning, postoperative, postoperative nausea and vomiting, postoperative pain, postoperative period, postoperative phase, preoperative, preoperative period, preoperative phase, purity, quality, range of motion, reflexolog*, safety data sheet, scent bias, scope of practice, sedative, skin irritation, stress, supplement, swelling, symptom relief, TENS, therapeutic touch, topical analgesic, traditional Chinese medicine, tranquility, undiluted, virtual reality, vitamin therapy, vomiting, and yoga.

Included were research and non-research literature in English, complete publications, and publications with dates within the time restriction when available. Excluded were non-peer-reviewed publications and older evidence within the time restriction when more recent evidence was available. Editorials, news items, and other brief items were excluded. Low-quality evidence was excluded when higher-quality evidence was available, and literature outside the time restriction was excluded when literature within the time restriction was available (Figure 1).

Articles identified in the search were provided to the project team for evaluation. The team consisted of the lead author and two evidence appraisers. The lead author divided the search results into topics and assigned members of the team to review and critically appraise each article using the AORN Research or Non-Research Evidence Appraisal Tools as indicated. The literature was independently evaluated and appraised according to the strength and quality of the evidence. Each article was then assigned an appraisal score. The appraisal score is noted in brackets after each reference as applicable.

Each recommendation rating is based on a synthesis of the collective evidence, a benefit-harm assessment, and consideration of resource use. The strength of the recommendation was determined using the AORN Evidence Rating Model and the quality and consistency of the evidence supporting a recommendation. The recommendation strength rating is noted in brackets after each recommendation.

Note: *The evidence summary table is available at http://www.aorn.org/evidencetables/.*

1. Selecting Interventions

1.1 Convene an interdisciplinary team to review, select, and evaluate complementary care interventions that will be used in the health care organization.[16] *[Recommendation]*

Using an interdisciplinary team approach can facilitate buy-in from perioperative team members and other health care personnel.[16]

1.1.1 The interdisciplinary team may include
- surgeons,
- anesthesia professionals,
- perioperative leaders,
- perioperative nurses (eg, preoperative RNs, RN circulators, postoperative RNs),
- perioperative team members (eg, scrub personnel, transporters/aides),
- quality improvement professionals,
- risk management and legal professionals,
- resource personnel (eg, registered dietitian, social workers, case managers), and
- other stakeholders identified by the organization.

[Conditional Recommendation]

Including representatives of all perioperative team members as well as other disciplines and departments facilitates safe and efficacious care when complementary care interventions involve multimodal techniques and settings for implementation. Many times, complementary care interventions can be performed preoperatively to positively influence postoperative outcomes, and this necessitates effective team communication, especially when adverse events are a concern. For instance, preoperative interventions are implemented through collaboration of multiple disciplines (eg, schedulers, preadmission personnel, preoperative RNs, intraoperative RNs, anesthesia professionals, surgeons, postoperative RNs); intraoperative interventions will necessitate collaboration from the OR team (eg, parental presence during induction); postoperative interventions will necessitate collaboration with other departments (eg, case managers scheduling follow ups). Some health care organizations have resources such as complementary care and alternative medicine practitioners and integrative medicine professionals who can be excellent resources during selection and planning of complementary care interventions in the perioperative setting.

1.2 Follow applicable local, state (eg, scope of practice[16]), and federal laws when defining and implementing complementary care interventions that will be used in the organization.[16] *[Regulatory Requirement]*

Some complementary care interventions require formal education, training, and licensure (eg, hypnosis, **biofield interventions**, massage, **reflexology**). An American Nurses Association position statement reflects the expanding role of nurses' practice based on education, evidence, and experience.[16] As informed decision makers, nurses can collaborate with patients and their families to implement complementary care interventions that they are suitably educated, trained, and competent to perform.[16]

1.3 When selecting complementary care interventions that may be used in the organization, review the
- patient population,
- types of procedures performed, and
- types of anesthesia administered.

[Conditional Recommendation]

Complementary care interventions are used in diverse populations and settings. Researchers study interventions in a specific population under controlled conditions. Interventions that have been studied and are believed to be beneficial for a specific population under specific conditions may be beneficial for other populations and conditions. The interdisciplinary team can weigh the benefits and harms of the intervention to determine whether it is generalizable to other patient populations, different procedures, or perioperative settings that were not studied.

1.4 When selecting individualized complementary care interventions, take into account information obtained from a comprehensive patient assessment (See Recommendation 2.1).[1,15,17-21] *[Recommendation]*

High-quality evidence[17-20] and guidelines[1,15,21] support using individualized (eg, age-specific[20]) complementary care that may increase patients' satisfaction with their care[22] and that may reduce negative perioperative outcomes.[20] Low-quality evidence supports regular assessment of the patient's preference and comfort with complementary care interventions.[23] Guidelines[1,15,21] emphasize that patient care should honor the patient's values, beliefs, and experiences, including a focus on healing the whole person's well-being and interrelationship with the environment[23] by integrating self-care, self-responsibility, spirituality, and reflection of life.[24]

An American Holistic Nurses Association (AHNA) position statement for the role of nurses in complementary and integrative health approaches includes several recommendations for collaborating on the plan of care with the patient (eg, preferences, family, culture, health beliefs, values) and integration steps (ie, identifying needs, finding providers, facilitating through education, coordinating, and evaluating effectiveness).[23]

1.5 Standardize protocols for implementing complementary care interventions.[1-9,15,25-27] *[Recommendation]*

Standardizing implementation protocols including education, assessments, interventions, and evaluations, can increase health care organizations' and nursing researchers' ability to implement evidence-based interventions[15] for patients who will receive the most benefit. Standardization of education and evaluations,[1,3,25] assessments,[1-3,9,26] and interventions[1,4-7,26,27] increases the feasibility for perioperative nurses to implement practice changes and for health care organizations to accurately assess efficacy and cost-effectiveness of each intervention.

1.5.1 Elements to standardize for complementary care interventions may include
- Intervention techniques,[1,4-7,26,27]
- outcome-specific assessments,[1-3,9,26]
- documentation,[28] and
- perioperative team education and competency evaluation.[1,3,25]

[Conditional Recommendation]

High-quality evidence supports standardization of complementary care in the perioperative setting.[4-9] Researchers have concluded that lack of standardized skills,[3] assessments,[3,9] and interventions,[4-8] have limited the study of complementary care interventions. The researchers agree that standardization could facilitate study of interventions and increase the reliability of their benefits in the perioperative setting.[1-9] Low-quality evidence[3] and guidelines[1,2] support standardization for optimal implementation of complementary care interventions in the perioperative setting.

1.5.2 Select and implement standardized and validated patient assessment[2] and evaluation[1,9,26] tools for complementary care interventions.[3] *[Recommendation]*

High-quality evidence supports using standardized assessment tools for baseline measurements[26] and standardized evaluation[9] tools for complementary care interventions. Several authors have concluded that using standardized assessment tools would increase the reliability of their conclusions and improve patient care.[3,9] The authors of one meta-analysis could not compare the efficacy of interventions because baseline assessments were not always included in the studies.[26] Low-quality evidence[3] and guidelines[1,2] support conducting a standardized assessment of the patient to facilitate gathering sufficient information for optimal perioperative care.

2. Patient Assessment

2.1

Before implementing complementary care interventions, assess the patient's

- **capability and willingness to participate in care[15];**
- **preference, tolerance, and willingness[29-31] to use complementary care interventions[13,32-34];**
- **understanding of and current use of complementary care interventions (eg, benefits, potential harms);**
- **developmental age, cognitive status (eg, delay, impairment) and understanding[20];**
- **mental state (eg, highly anxious, spiritual)[24];**
- **functional status;**
- **laboratory test results (eg, albumin as an indicator of nutritional status, cortisol as in indicator of stress response)[17-19,35];**
- **nutritional status (eg, malnourished)[17-19,35];**
- **current use of dietary and herbal supplements;**
- **understanding of potential drug-supplement interactions;**
- **history of postoperative nausea and vomiting (PONV); and**
- **risk for**
  - **falls when considering early ambulation,**
  - **pressure injury related to wearable devices,[36] and**
  - **surgical burns related to wearable devices when electrosurgery is used.[37]**

[Recommendation]

Assessing the patient's current use of complementary care practices and willingness to use complementary care interventions in the perioperative setting can facilitate creating the individualized plan of care.[29-31] Patients may already use complementary care interventions; however, patient surveys[29,30] and guidelines[31] report that few patients discuss their complementary or non-Western practices with their health care providers. Omitting this information in the assessment can be detrimental if the perioperative plan of care creates contraindications with the patient's complementary care practices. For example, many herbs can interfere with some anesthetics, increase adverse effects of the herbs or the conventional medicine, and increase the potential for perioperative adverse events.[31]

One national survey[12] found that the patient's biological sex may influence their choice about whether to use complementary care interventions and which they prefer to use.

Patients may be more willing to try complementary care interventions if they believe the interventions are beneficial. Patients who are interested in complementary care are likely to be more open to learning about and consenting to specific interventions. Patients who have used complementary care will have additional insight into what worked for them and can collaborate to reduce the time, money, and effort of implementing interventions that they have no interest in pursuing. Patients who are already using complementary care interventions may not be aware of suitable use, additional interventions, and potential synergistic or maladaptive interactions between their current interventions and the complementary care interventions proposed in the perioperative plan of care. Additional patient education may be required to promote safe perioperative care.[13,32-34]

Moderate-quality evidence supports identifying needs and risk factors related to perioperative care.[38] High-quality evidence[39] and guidelines[1,15,21] recommend assessing risk factors for PONV to determine the plan of care, including for whom and when each complementary care intervention may be used.

Low-quality evidence[29,30,40] and guidelines[31,41] support that many perioperative patients are unaware that dietary and herbal interventions can interact with their conventional medical plan of care, especially the consumption of herbs. Patients may not disclose this information if they perceive that their herbal supplementation is unrelated to their medical condition; however, herbal use may increase the patient's risk for adverse events and negative outcomes in the perioperative setting, regardless of the herbs indicated or desired intent. Sankar-Maharaj et al[40] found that patients who used cannabis preoperatively required active warming postoperatively.

In a survey of 526 patients at one facility, Levy et al[29] found that of 44% of patients who reported using dietary and herbal supplements, only 16.5% understood that these supplements could interact negatively with anesthesia or increase their risk for injury. The researchers concluded that perioperative management and health care workers' education about supplements should be emphasized to promote safe use.

The American Association of Nurse Anesthetists (AANA) recommends that anesthesia providers interview patients preoperatively and be aware of potential adverse effects, drug interactions, and complications associated with dietary and herbal interventions.[31] Though there is no official guidance, a patient education brochure from the AANA recommends that the patient discontinue taking herbal supplements at least 1 to 2 weeks before undergoing an operative or invasive procedure.[31] The AANA recommends requesting full disclosure of natural remedies and discussing the conventional surgical plan of care with patients and their families during the anesthesia preoperative visit.[31]

The American Society of Anesthesiologists (ASA) brochure on dietary and herbal interventions identifies that half of Americans take some herbal or dietary supplement.[41] These are not regulated by the US Food and Drug Administration (FDA), and some dietary and herbal interventions have been associated with prolonged anesthesia metabolism, increased bleeding, hypertension, interference with medications, and heart problems in some individuals. The brochure advises that patients should bring all supplement bottles to preoperative appointments because anesthesia professionals may recommend discontinuing use at least 2 weeks before an operative or invasive procedure.[41]

2.2 **Assess the patient's response to complementary care interventions and adjust as needed based on the patient's input and an evaluation of intended outcomes.**[28,42-46] *[Recommendation]*

Changes in the patient's condition may change the patient's response to complementary care interventions, resulting in a need for interventions to be modified or discontinued. The Institute of Medicine recommends evaluating CAM intervention implementation and efficacy.[28] Intervention methods may change in phases of care or depending on the patient's condition preferences, and potential interactions of the patient's current and desired complementary care interventions with the patient's individualized conventional surgical plan.

High-quality evidence supports that interventions may have synergistic effects in combination, though some effects may not be enhanced but diminished.[42-46] Perioperative RNs can help guide the patient to prioritize interventions that provide the most benefit and reduce conditions (eg, cost, time, mental energy) that may occur with additional interventions if one intervention has no effect or less effect than another.

Low-quality evidence supports regular assessment of the patient's desire for and the effectiveness and efficacy of complementary care interventions.[23]

In a qualitative study of perioperative nurses' perceptions of the preoperative assessment, Malley et al[38] organized the findings into four themes: understanding the patient's vulnerabilities, multi-dimensional communication, managing patients' expectations, and the nurses' role in compensating for gaps. The researchers concluded that the perioperative nurses' use of the preoperative assessment to identify the patients' needs and risk factors was associated with a positive perioperative care trajectory.

A position statement from the AHNA about the role of nurses in complementary and integrative health approaches recommends collaborating on the plan of care with the patient (eg, preferences, family, culture, health beliefs, values) and integration steps (ie, identifying needs, finding providers, facilitating through education, coordinating, and evaluating effectiveness).[23]

3. Planning Interventions

3.1 **Use individualized, multimodal complementary care interventions based on an assessment of the patient.**[1,12,15,17,19-21,28,46-62] *[Recommendation]* [P]

Clinical guidelines support individualized, multimodal interventions to improve desired outcomes.[1,15,21,28]

The Institute of Medicine CAM guidelines recommend an evaluation of the patient, history, physical examination, and conventional and other methods of diagnosis; documentation of medical options discussed, offered, tried, and refused; referral of treatment; risks and benefits; and extent of potential interference with other recommended or ongoing treatment.[28]

The ERAS guidelines are developed through a review of literature for multimodal conventional, CAM, and surgical techniques for specific patient populations to improve clinical and non-clinical outcomes.[15]

High-quality evidence also supports implementing individualized multimodal complementary care interventions together with conventional surgical care (eg, **essential oils** plus medications for PONV) to improve the patient's perioperative experience.[12,17,19,20,46-62] Specific patient populations may respond to complementary care interventions differently than others, and high-quality evidence supports additional research to determine the influence of age on complementary care intervention efficacy.[63]

Though there is limited research, evidence supports individualizing interventions based on patient factors, including

- age (eg, pediatric,[20,47,53-55,62] older adult[17,19,28,48,57-60]),
- nutrition status (eg, malnutrition),[49-51] and
- baseline anxiety scores.[46,52,56]

3.1.1

Complementary care interventions specific to reducing perioperative anxiety in pediatric patients may be used.[15,20,28,53,56,62] *[Conditional Recommendation]* **P**

High-quality evidence supports using complementary care interventions for pediatric patients.[20,53,56,62] Based on the limitations of their results, researchers found different levels of effectiveness and concluded that additional research can determine whether pediatric patients' ages are associated with the effectiveness of different interventions.[20,54,55] Guidelines also support age-suitable interventions, as pediatric populations may experience perioperative complementary care interventions differently than adult-only populations.[15,28]

In a systematic review of 33 trials and quasi-experimental studies, Bice and Wyatt[62] found four holistic comfort interventions (eg, music [2003-2007], n = 287; amusement and entertainment [1994-2015], n = 1,210; caregiver facilitation [2001-2013] n = 349], and a combination of interventions [2000-2015, n = 569]) that increased comfort for pediatric patients undergoing a variety of procedures (eg, venipuncture, port access, injections, burn wound care). A study criterion was that the patient sample must include children 4 to 7 years of age. The researchers concluded that various distraction techniques were beneficial for decreasing anxiety, distress, fear, and pain. The researchers suggested that future studies are needed to explore the children's experience of painful procedures, including those that are performed in the perioperative setting, to determine the benefits of each complementary care intervention.

In a randomized controlled trial (RCT), Liguori et al[53] provided 20 pediatric patients ages 6 to 11 years with a 6-minute video on a mobile app the night before their surgical procedures. The video depicted two surgeons dressed as clowns who gave a comical and informative tour of the operating room (OR) with the intention of reducing preoperative anxiety among the children who viewed it. Children who viewed the video had significantly lower anxiety scores before induction of general anesthesia compared to a control group that received standard care (n = 20). The researchers concluded that the mobile application–delivered video could substitute for education and tours delivered by health care workers to decrease costs. The researchers recommended that future studies control for age, sex, and history of previous surgery.

In an RCT, Kassai et al[56] gave pediatric patients ages 6 to 17 years a comic information leaflet before surgery (n = 54). The researchers found that compared to a group that received standard preoperative education (n = 57), anxiety was significantly lower in the intervention group. Patients with higher baseline anxiety scores had more significantly reduced anxiety, and the researchers concluded that these patients benefited more from the intervention.

In a quasi-experimental study that included 83 pediatric patients ages 9 to 18 years, Aytekin et al[20] found that tailoring the distraction technique (eg, games, music, cartoons, books) to the age group significantly decreased anxiety and separation anxiety in participants who received individualized interventions.

3.1.2

Complementary care interventions specific to older adult patients may be used.[15,17,19,28,48,57-60] *[Conditional Recommendation]*

High-quality evidence[17,19,48,58-60] supports specific interventions for the older adult patient including nutritional support,[57,59] acupoint for gastrointestinal (GI) functional recovery after GI procedures,[58] and cognitive health support.[48,60] Older adult patients are more at-risk for nutritional and cognitive deterioration, and perioperative complications. Nutrition status deficits among older adults can be improved with preoperative dietary supplementation for malnutrition[57,59] and electrical acupoint stimulation for GI functional recovery.[58] Music[48] and cognitive education and skills training[60] for older adult patients can significantly improve postoperative cognitive function.

Guidelines[15,28] also support age-specific interventions, as older adult patients may experience perioperative complementary care interventions differently than younger patients, including having an increased risk for adverse events (eg, medication interactions,[19] fractures[17,18]).

In a systematic review that included retrospective case series totaling 15 trials, the researchers found that preoperative nutrition status (eg, low serum albumin, more than 10% weight loss in the previous 6 months) was a significant indicator of postoperative outcome in older adult patients. The researchers concluded that older adult patients are subject to nutrition deterioration and complications and would benefit from dietary interventions.[57]

In an RCT, of 126 older adult patients with hip fractures, Myint et al[59] found oral liquid nutritional support significantly shortened length of stay (LOS) in the rehabilitation ward and decreased the infection rate. The researchers found that both the intervention and control groups had a decrease in body mass index, but the weight loss was less in the group that received oral liquid nutritional support (n = 65) compared with a group that received the standard hospital diet (n = 61). There were no changes in albumin level, functional status, or mobility. The researchers concluded there were nutritional benefits but no rehabilitation benefits to protein supplementation for older adult perioperative patients.

In an RCT conducted by Lili et al,[58] 40 older adult patients undergoing GI procedures were given electrical acupoint stimulation for 2 minutes every postoperative day (POD). The researchers found significant improvement in gastrin levels on POD 3 and 5, improved motilin levels on POD 3, shorter time to flatus, and a lower incidence of complications (eg, abdominal pain, distention, and diarrhea), as well as improved the electrocardiogram frequency and amplitude on POD 5. The researchers concluded that **acupuncture** stimulation promoted GI function recovery and could decrease complications efficiently and painlessly in older adult patients.

In an RCT conducted by Çetinkaya[48] in Turkey of 60 older adult patients undergoing total joint procedures, Turkish music was played for 20 minutes three times a day on the first, second, and third postoperative days. Patients' cognitive scores were significantly improved on POD 3 compared with POD 1. The researcher concluded that music prevented cognitive dysfunction, though the study sample was limited to patients in one facility and only one type of music was used.

In an RCT pilot, Kulason et al[60] found that providing 12 older adult postoperative patients with cognitive education and skills training (ie, **simple calculation and reading aloud** [SCRA]) drills 3 to 5 times a week for 30 minutes significantly improved the patients' motor function and quality of life. The researchers concluded that preoperative cognitive education and skills improved the cognitive and emotional state (eg, level of distress) of postoperative older adult patients.

In an RCT, Seidi et al[19] assigned patients to receive either one dose of 1 g of oral ginger (n = 40), two doses of 500 mg of oral ginger (n = 42), or a placebo (n = 40) before undergoing cataract procedures under general anesthesia. The researchers found significantly lower scores for nausea and vomiting for the participants who received two smaller doses. They concluded that oral ginger is safe and effective to reduce PONV, and two smaller doses may be more beneficial than one large dose. However, the researchers noted potential adverse effects in older adults and potential for adverse events with certain medications. They recommended that additional research include a longer preoperative consumption time to confirm the benefits of oral ginger.

In an RCT conducted by Bischoff-Ferrari et al,[17] older adult patients (65 years or older) with hip fractures were given extended postoperative physical therapy (PT) and either 2,000 international units (IU) or 800 IU of cholecalciferol per day (2,000 IU + standard PT [n = 42], 2,000 IU + extended PT [n = 44], 800 IU + standard PT [n = 44], 800 IU + extended PT [n = 43]). The researchers found a 25% reduction in falls and 39% reduction in hospital readmissions in both groups that received 2,000 IU. The patients who received 2,000 IU of cholecalciferol had a lower risk of hip fractures, lower vitamin D deficiency, and lower facility readmission rates that the patients who received 800 IU.

In an RCT, Chapuy et al[18] provided 1.2 g elemental calcium and 800 IU vitamin D3 (n = 1,634) compared to placebos (n = 1,636) to women ages 69 to 106 years who were living in nursing homes. The researchers found that calcium and vitamin D3 supplementation significantly lowered the incidence of hip and other nonvertebral fractures.

3.1.3

Plan complementary care interventions for patients who are identified as being highly anxious at the baseline measurement.[46,56] *[Recommendation]* **P**

High-quality evidence suggests that patients who are assessed as highly anxious receive greater benefit from complementary care interventions than those who are not identified as highly anxious in the preoperative assessment.[46,56]

In an RCT, Kassai et al[56] provided pediatric patients ages 6 to 17 years with a comic information leaflet before surgery (n = 54). The researchers found that compared to a group that received standard preoperative education (n = 57), anxiety was significantly lower in the intervention group. The researchers concluded that those with higher baseline anxiety scores had more significantly reduced anxiety and benefited more from the intervention.

In a quasi-nonequivalent controlled trial, Kim et al[46] evaluated the effects of intraprocedural handholding with or without sharing of verbal step-by-step information on the anxiety of patients undergoing percutaneous vertebroplasty under local anesthesia. Ninety-four patients received either standard care (n = 30), handholding (n = 30), or handholding and procedural information (n = 34) during their procedures. The researchers found a significant decrease in systolic blood pressure in the control group and significant decrease in anxiety among participants that received both handholding and verbal step-by-step information shared throughout the procedure. The researchers concluded that this study demonstrates the value of nursing care, specifically handholding, for anxious patients during a surgical intervention.

3.2 **In collaboration with the patient, plan complementary care interventions as early as possible after a surgical intervention is scheduled.**[1,21,23,38] *[Recommendation]*

Moderate-quality evidence supports that early assessment and collaboration with patients facilitates creating a complementary care plan that fits with the patient's needs, lifestyle, and perioperative plan of care by identifying the patient's physical, spiritual, or social needs.[23,38] Well-established complementary care interventions are associated with a positive effect on perioperative adverse outcomes (eg, PONV,[1,21] anxiety related to isolation, uncertainty about the procedure, pain or discomfort).

If there is limited preoperative time, some interventions may not be feasible, whereas delaying the assessment may prevent implementation of time-dependent interventions (eg, **prehabilitation**, massage, nutritional supplementation) or resource-heavy interventions (eg, stress diversion, music, aromatherapy, acupoint, massage).

In a qualitative study of perioperative nurses' perceptions of the preoperative assessment, Malley et al[38] organized the findings into four themes: understanding the patient's vulnerabilities, multidimensional communication, managing patients' expectations, and the nurses' role in compensating for gaps. The researchers concluded that perioperative nurses use the preoperative assessment to identify the patients' desires and risk factors associated with the perioperative care trajectory.

An AHNA position statement for the role of nurses in complementary and integrative health approaches includes recommendations for collaborating on the plan of care with the patient (eg, preferences, family, culture, health beliefs, values) and integration steps (ie, identifying needs, finding providers, facilitating through education, coordinating, and evaluating effectiveness).[23]

3.2.1 **Additional time may be scheduled for consultation**[28] **with practitioners in other disciplines,**[16] **to obtain any needed orders, and to implement the intervention in the indicated phase of care.** *[Conditional Recommendation]*

The time frame may extend months in advance of the planned procedure (ie, prehabilitation).

3.2.2 **Include the patient's priorities for surgical outcomes and expectations of complementary care interventions in the perioperative plan of care.**[3,28,64] *[Recommendation]*

Discussing priorities and expectations of complementary care interventions with the patient is essential when creating the perioperative plan of care. Moderate-quality evidence[3,64] and guidelines[28] support assessing expectations and priorities and educating patients on postoperative outcomes to promote realistic expectations and care plan goal setting.

Silva et al[64] conducted a survey in which patients reported high expectations for pain, thirst, and hunger discomfort. However, after their procedures, the patients reported that their discomfort regarding thirst, hunger, physical weakness, and coldness far surpassed their expectations.

In a survey of patients evaluating perception of nursing care, Fatma and Serife[3] established that an expectation for pain management and evaluating specific interventions for efficacy can improve the patient's experience and future experiences. The researchers suggested that perceived and actual patient needs, expectations, and responses to interventions may change for different events as well as throughout perioperative experiences and their lives.

3.3 **Obtain informed consent before implementing complementary care interventions.**[11-14] *[Recommendation]*

Complementary care interventions can have both benefits and potential harms to the patient, and these can be different for each patient. For this reason, a discussion of the benefits and potential harms is important as part of obtaining informed consent.

Moderate-quality evidence supports using a patient-centered approach when communicating the risks and benefits of complementary care interventions and when incorporating these interventions into the conventional surgical plan of care.[11-14] Based on national trends[11-14] and patient education[65] and preference,[12] nurses can suggest common interventions with which patients are more likely to have experience, that they may be willing to try, and that are likely to provide a benefit. Patients who are educated in complementary care intervention risks and benefits may be more willing to accept the interventions or decide which interventions would not improve their perioperative experience.

3.4 **Limit the intervention exposure (eg, music,[66] aromatherapy[67-69]) to the patient for whom it is intended.** [Recommendation] 🅿

Some interventions have the risk of affecting more than just the intended patient (eg, unwanted transfer of aromatherapy scent to other patients,[68] patient-selected music being heard by other patients, music contributing to noise in the care environment[66]). Restricting the exposure of interventions to only the intended patient preserves patients' autonomy for their care.

In a systematic review of 73 RCTs conducted between 1988 to 2013, Hole et al[66] evaluated research on perioperative music intervention benefits for postoperative pain, anxiety, use of analgesia, and patient satisfaction. The researchers found improvements in all of these outcomes and concluded that perioperative music interventions were beneficial. The researchers found that music was effective even when patients were under a general anesthetic. However, the benefits of allowing patients to choose the music and a suitable volume for music were unclear. Also unclear were conclusions about whether the use of headphones hindered communication between patients and perioperative health care workers and whether use of headphones alleviated imposing the music on the health care workers.

Aromatherapy delivery devices are meant to limit exposure of the aromatherapy intervention to a single user. High-quality evidence supports using aromatherapy delivery devices in perioperative settings to reduce PONV[68] and post-discharge nausea vomiting (PDNV).[67,69] Essential oil room-diffusers may pose challenges, and researchers in one study reported the difficulty of restricting aromatherapy interventions through a handheld device.[68] Creative methods may be required to restrict aromatherapy to its intended area.

Kiberd et al[68] found that a limitation of a pilot RCT of pediatric patients (N = 162) ages 4 to 16 years who used a handheld aromatherapy delivery device was that the researchers were unable to contain the aromatherapy intervention in a way that the control group was not also exposed to the aromatherapy. Even though research was limited by not having a true control group, the researchers did find that

there was a significant desire to continue use of the handheld aromatherapy delivery device among the intervention group.

In an RCT conducted by Stallings-Welden et al,[67] patients received a handheld aromatherapy delivery device after surgery (n = 108) versus standard care (n = 113). The aromatherapy used was a blend of pure essential oils including spearmint, peppermint, ginger, and lavender. There was no significant difference in PONV incidence, antiemetic dose, or patient satisfaction in the intervention group prior to patient discharge from the perioperative setting with the product for at-home use. However, the aromatherapy intervention was 100% effective in treating PDNV among the 11 patients who reported PDNV. The researchers concluded that identifying patients at risk for PONV and planning a holistic comfort approach to address PONV that included aromatherapy was beneficial.

A quasi-experimental study also supported use of aromatherapy delivery devices to reduce PONV. Lee and Shin[69] gave 60 patients either ginger essential oil or normal saline in a necklace delivery device in the postoperative setting. The researchers found significantly lower PONV measured by the Index of Nausea, Vomiting, and Retching (INVR) scale in the first 6 hours. The researchers concluded that even though there is no documented optimal delivery technique for aromatherapy, use of the necklaces decreased PONV, and the intervention was inexpensive and easy to administer

3.5 **When devices are used to deliver complementary care interventions (eg, headphones for music, a wristband for acupoint), follow the manufacturer's instructions for use.** [Conditional Recommendation]

3.6 **Establish a process for the care and cleaning of reusable devices.** [Recommendation]

3.7 **Encourage the patient's autonomy by having the patient select specific preferences related to each intervention (eg, music type,[43,70] stress diversion[71]) in each perioperative setting, when possible.** [Recommendation]

High-quality evidence supports encouraging patients' autonomy by allowing them to express a preference regarding complementary care interventions, when possible.[43,70,71]

In an RCT conducted by Nagata et al,[43] patients (N = 224) either listened to instrumental music, received aromatherapy, or both compared to a control group while undergoing colonography procedures (n = 56 in each group). The results for pain scores and vital signs were nonsignificant between the groups, though a significant number of patients asked to use the same intervention for the next screening. The researchers concluded that additional research including music chosen according to patient preference may be beneficial.

In an RCT that included 124 male patients undergoing flexible cystoscopy awake procedures, Zhang et al[70] compared an intervention with patient-selected music (n = 62) to standard care (n = 62). The researchers found heart rates, pain scores, and anxiety scores were significantly reduced in the intervention group.

3.8 **In collaboration with surgeons and anesthesia professionals, determine which dietary and herbal supplements should be discontinued before an operative or other invasive procedure, when they should be discontinued, and when the patient can resume taking dietary and herbal supplements after the procedure.[23,31,41,72]** *[Recommendation]*

Discontinuing use of dietary and herbal supplements preoperatively can mitigate the risk for adverse events. Low-quality evidence[72] and instructions from the AANA[31] include discontinuing supplements before procedures to reduce potential complications, though the recommended time frames vary.

Patients may not be aware of the interactions of their current practices with medications they may receive in the perioperative setting, and may not consider them relevant to disclose during the preoperative assessment. Perioperative nurses can facilitate open communication by delving into the patient's interests and background[23] and reviewing common complementary care practices and potential adverse events associated with them.

The AANA recommends that surgical patients discontinue herbal remedies 1 to 2 weeks before an operative or invasive procedure to reduce the risk for complications (eg, prolonged anesthesia metabolism, increased bleeding, hypertension, interference with medications, heart issues), inform their provider of historical or current use, and bring supplement containers to their appointments. The AANA also recommends that the patient tell their family members about their herbal supplement and medication use in case of an emergency when the patient cannot communicate this information.[31]

The ASA brochure on dietary and herbal interventions identifies that 50% of Americans take some herbal or dietary supplement. These are not regulated by the FDA, and some dietary and herbal interventions have been associated with prolonged anesthesia metabolism, increased bleeding, hypertension, interference with medications, and heart problems in some individuals. The brochure advises that patients should bring all supplement bottles to

preoperative appointments because anesthesia professionals may recommend discontinuing use at least 2 weeks before an operative or invasive procedure.[41]

In a case report that was included in a literature review, Pedroso et al[72] described one patient's chronic use of ginkgo biloba for a variety of conditions (ie, cognitive impairment, tinnitus, vertigo, asthma, allergies). The researchers found that these were an ill-founded use of the herb and that the patient required hospital admission for spontaneous cerebral bleeding attributed to chronic use of the herb, which improved after discontinuation.

4. Supportive Education Interventions

4.1 **Schedule time to provide patients with unrushed supportive education before the procedure[25,73] (eg, the night before surgery,[74,75] the morning of surgery[75,76]) and the opportunity to ask questions about the perioperative experience.** *[Recommendation]*

4.1.1 **Select and implement techniques for perioperative supportive education delivery that are tailored to the patient's age[77-80] and cognitive ability.[57]** *[Recommendation]* **P**

Moderate-quality evidence supports tailoring counseling based on the patient's age (eg, pediatric,[77-80] older adult[57]). Factors other than age can also affect understanding (eg, learning disabilities, cognitive disorders, distractors).

In a systematic review that included qualitative surveys, Perry et al[77] found that reducing preoperative anxiety in pediatric populations required age-specific teaching interventions, including the information that is shared, when and how it is shared, and who provides the information. They found that role-play or play therapy with dolls and toys was more efficacious for younger children, and OR tours, coloring books, or video games were more efficacious for school-aged children. They also found that patients between 3 and 6 years were less anxious when given interventions less than 7 days before the procedure, while patients older than 6 years needed interventions at least 5 days in advance and patients younger than 3 may not benefit from preoperative teaching interventions.

In an RCT, Rhodes et al[78] evaluated anxiety and patient satisfaction in 65 pediatric and young adult patients (ages 11 to 21 years) who received either standard care (n = 39) or standard care with the inclusion of 30 minutes of education (n = 26) before undergoing a posterior spinal fusion procedure to correct scoliosis. The researchers found that the education intervention did not lower anxiety as hypothesized, and the intervention group had significantly higher perioperative anxiety; however, both the patients' and caregivers' overall satisfaction was significantly higher. The researchers speculated that having more information increased the patients' perioperative anxiety but improved their postoperative expectations and experience, which could be associated with higher satisfaction as a result of the increased trust and stronger patient-family-caregiver relationship created by increased preoperative interaction.

In an RCT, Fernandes et al[79] assigned 125 pediatric patients ages 8 to 12 years to one of seven different preoperative education groups: education and entertainment via an education board (n = 15), video (n = 15), or booklet (n = 15); entertainment only via an education board (n = 15), video (n = 15), or booklet (n = 15); or a control group that received no materials (n = 35). The researchers found that regardless of the technique, receiving education significantly reduced the patients' anxiety compared to receiving entertainment alone. However, the was no difference in parental anxiety scores regardless of the child's intervention group. The researchers concluded that lower resource–intensive interventions could be beneficial, though they also recommended that additional studies include longer preoperative time frames and patients undergoing major inpatient procedures.

In an RCT of 42 pediatric patients ages 5 to 12 years, Batuman et al[80] found that preoperative information provided by video (n = 21) instead of verbally (n = 21) significantly lowered anxiety and postoperative maladaptive behaviors. The researchers concluded that future research should focus on comparing when the video is viewed and composition of video interventions.

4.1.2 **Deliver supportive education interventions in the patient's preferred language.**[81,82] *[Recommendation]*

High-quality evidence supports providing supportive education interventions in the patient's preferred language.[81,82]

In an RCT, West et al[81] found that when an instructional video in Spanish was used for patients whose preferred language was Spanish, they had significantly decreased anxiety scores and increased satisfaction. The researchers concluded that though there were no objective

measurements, videos provided in the patient's preferred language could be a beneficial substitution (eg, less cost, less time) when language interpreters are not available. The researchers of another RCT recommended that future studies regarding the efficacy of video education involve multiple languages.[82]

4.2 **Select and implement preoperative supportive education interventions for anxiety.** *[Recommendation]*

High-quality evidence supports providing patients with preoperative supportive education to decrease anxiety. Researchers found that compared to receiving no materials, receiving verbal,[83,84] written,[85] and audio-visual[81,82,86] materials designed to increase knowledge of the perioperative setting decreased patients' preoperative anxiety and could improve other clinical outcomes. Researchers also found improved cortisol levels with the use of structured verbal materials[84] and improved patient satisfaction with the use of structured verbal[83] and audio visual[86] materials.

In an RCT, Zhang et al[83] found that patients undergoing elective coronary artery bypass grafting who received 3 days of nurse-initiated preoperative structured education (n = 20) had significantly lower rates of complications and less anxiety than patients who were admitted only 1 day before surgery (n = 20). Patients in the intervention group had lower rates of postoperative lower-extremity edema, urinary retention, and constipation than those in the control group.

In an RCT, Amini et al[85] assigned patients undergoing elective hernia or cholecystectomy procedures to receive either preoperative verbal education (n = 20), education via a booklet (n = 20), or standard care (n = 20). There was a significant decrease in anxiety after the intervention in both interventional groups, and the researchers concluded that a well-designed booklet could decrease preoperative anxiety and reduce the resources required for in-person education. However, limitations include the pseudo-randomization in which patient groups were predictable to the researchers and that the results can be generalized only to patients undergoing hernia and cholecystectomy procedures.

In a RCT conducted by Bahrami et al[84] in Iran, patients undergoing elective gynecological procedures who participated in anxiety-reduction techniques (eg, deep breathing, distraction, repeating religious words) the night before their procedure (n = 30) had significantly lower serum cortisol levels on the morning of the procedure than those who received standard care (n = 30). However, no significant difference in vital signs was found between the intervention and control groups. The researchers concluded that individualized interventions to reduce patient anxiety may be included in the nursing plan of care.

In a pilot RCT, Tou et al[82] studied adult patients scheduled to undergo operative colorectal procedures (n = 16) who watched a 13-minute cartoon video step-by-step guide to colorectal surgery compared to a control group (n = 15). Fourteen (88%) of the patients in the intervention group reported that the video was helpful, and the researchers found a significant decrease in immediate and discharge anxiety in the group that watched the video compared to the control group. The researchers concluded that videos are beneficial and recommended that future studies involve videos for other procedures and in other languages.

In an RCT of 100 adults undergoing a variety of operative procedures (eg, upper abdominal surgery, lower abdominal surgery, other surgery [eg, thyroidectomy mastectomy, lower limb]) with either general or spinal anesthesia, Lin et al[86] had patients view an 8-minute video on perioperative anesthesia education (n = 50) or receive a verbal briefing by an anesthesia professional (n = 50) during their visit to the preoperative clinic for preanesthetic assessment. The video included information about the preoperative assessment, differences between general and spinal anesthesia, medication administration, and recovery management, whereas the verbal information included the process and protocols for anesthesia procedures. The researchers found no significant differences in opioid use in the immediate postoperative period and no difference in PONV incidence between the intervention and control groups. However, the patients in the video group had significantly lowered anxiety scores and increased patient satisfaction compared to those who received an 8-minute verbal briefing by an anesthesia professional.

In an RCT, West et al[81] found that an instructional video in Spanish for Spanish-speaking adults significantly decreased anxiety scores and increased patient satisfaction of the knowledge provided compared to patients whose immediate preoperative anesthesia evaluation was conducted through an interpreter. The researchers concluded that this interim study demonstrated that though the outcomes were subjective (ie, patient reported), and the patients' baseline literacy could influence the results, videos could be beneficial to supplement interpreter services in a cost-effective manner.

4.2.1 **Additional supportive education time (eg, the night before surgery,[74,75] the morning of**

surgery[75,76]) may be scheduled for patients with a high level of anxiety. *[Conditional Recommendation]*

Moderate-quality evidence[74-76] supports decreasing preoperative patient anxiety and improving the perioperative experience with additional preoperative visits from an OR health care worker (eg, perioperative nurse, surgical technician, nurse practitioner) based on when patients are admitted to the facility. Researchers have found

- decreased anxiety with additional visits on the night before[74,75] and morning of the procedure,[75,76]
- decreased complications with additional visits on the night before the procedure,[74] and
- improved quality of life scores with additional visits on the morning of the procedure.[76]

In an RCT, Sadati et al[74] assigned women undergoing laparoscopic cholecystectomy to receive either routine nursing care (n = 50) or two preoperative nursing visits that included patient education about the OR, anesthesia, the surgical procedure, and pre- and postoperative care (n = 50). The first visit occurred on the day before the procedure and the second occurred after transfer to the preoperative area. The researchers found no difference in anxiety scores between the groups on admission to the preoperative area; however, there was a significant decrease in anxiety just before patients entered the OR after the second nursing visit. Postoperative outcomes were also significantly better in the intervention group, including mean time to consciousness (ie, Aldrete score of 9), incidence of PONV, level of postoperative pain, duration of vital sign stabilization, and time to ambulation. The researchers concluded that additional nursing visits should be integrated into standard care for laparoscopic cholecystectomy patients.

In a quasi-experimental study conducted by Bagheri et al,[75] 70 adults undergoing elective hernia procedures in Iran received two preoperative visits from the same surgical technologist, first on the night before the procedure and again after transfer to the perioperative suite through anesthesia induction. The surgical technologist provided information about the surgeon, surgery, time of surgery, duration of surgery, OR setting, and duration of the immediate postoperative unit stay using simple and understandable language. Patients were given the opportunity to ask questions, and the surgical technologist reassured the patient that he would be present in the OR for the surgery.

Although the study was underpowered, the researchers found a significant decrease in the patients' anxiety scores and concluded that preoperative visitation could decrease anxiety for patients undergoing elective procedures.

In a quasi-experimental study conducted by Donker et al,[76] 214 older adults undergoing elective vascular procedures at one facility in the Netherlands received either standard care (ie, consultation by the surgeon alone [n = 81]) or additional education from a nurse practitioner involved with the operative procedures (n = 133). Both groups had a significant increase in quality of life scores and a decrease in anxiety scores, but no difference in depression scores. Researchers concluded that nurse practitioners could provide education as efficaciously as the surgeon. They also concluded that future studies should measure the effect of involving a nurse practitioner on patient satisfaction.

4.3 **When applicable, provide preoperative patient education for alcohol and smoking cessation.**[15,87]
[Recommendation]

ERAS guidelines[15] and an RCT[87] support cessation programs to reduce the potential for negative postoperative outcomes related to suboptimal preoperative patient conditions (eg, alcohol consumption, smoking.) Optimization for perioperative care guidelines, including ERAS,[15] may include minimizing or abstaining from alcohol and participating in smoking cessation programs, as these habits are known deterrents to incision healing.[15]

In an RCT, Lindstrom et al[87] assigned patients to receive either standard care (n = 54) or an 8-week smoking cessation program with 4 weeks before and 4 weeks after the procedure (n = 48). The researchers found a significant decrease in the complication rate (eg, requiring additional medical or surgical treatment) in the intervention group (21%) compared with the standard care group (41%). The researchers found a significant decrease in the overall complication rates 30 days post surgery in the intervention group, and they concluded that a 4-week preoperative program may be as effective as the 8-week program.[87]

4.4 **When applicable, provide information to patients about accessing postoperative support, including**
- postoperative support groups[88] and
- postoperative cognitive skills programs for older adult patients.[60]

[Conditional Recommendation]

High-quality evidence[60] supports postoperative cognitive skills training to improve older adult patients' mental and physical function and quality of life, and moderate-quality evidence[88] supports that patients sharing their experiences can increase coping postoperatively.

Increased coping skills may benefit all perioperative patients, especially those who undergo major procedures. Grouping patients in support groups according to procedure, age, and sex can increase participation and comradery among those who participate.[60,88] The potential barriers to implementing support groups include the challenge of scheduling multiple small groups, barriers to meeting in person (eg, geographic location) and limitations of online platforms, and challenges with buy-in resulting in the need for the support group to be participant-led and health care organization facilitated.

In an RCT pilot conducted by Kulason et al,[60] 12 older adult postoperative patients who received SCRA cognitive skills training had significantly improved motor function and quality of life scores. The researchers concluded that even with the study limitations (ie, performance bias and subjective motivation with a small sample and no placebo group), preoperative cognitive skills training can improve the cognitive and emotional state (ie, distress) of postoperative older adult patients.

In a nonrandomized case controlled trial, 34 of 67 women undergoing radiotherapy were included in a postoperative support group.[88] Emilsson et al[88] found a significant improvement in measures of coping; however, anxiety and depression measures were not significantly different between the groups. The researchers concluded that sharing the mutual experiences increased levels of coping resources, though future research of the long-term effects is needed for better understanding of the benefits.

4.5 **Information may be provided to the patient about how to prepare for operative and other invasive procedures, including**
- strength exercises to improve quality of life,[73]
- walking to improve cognitive recovery (eg, social function, emotional role[89]) and functional recovery (eg, increase walking capacity[89,90]), and
- a combination of activities (eg, walking, diet, relaxation skills).[91]

[Conditional Recommendation]

High-quality evidence[89-91] and guidelines[15] support the use of prehabilitation interventions to improve postoperative outcomes. Prehabilitation is mental or physical conditioning that the patient commits to completing before a scheduled procedure that is intended to improve outcomes during the postoperative recovery phase.

In an RCT, Gillis et al[91] assigned patients to receive either a combination of prehabilitation interventions (eg, exercise, diet, relaxation techniques) (n = 38) or standard postoperative rehabilitation (n = 39). The researchers found that at postoperative week 4, 50% of both groups were still below their preoperative functional exercise capacity baseline. After 8 weeks, the prehabilitation participants had significantly higher function on a 6-minute walking test compared to the rehabilitation group, who remained below their baseline. Though there were no differences in complications or LOS, the researchers found that there were clinically meaningful benefits to prehabilitation interventions.

In an RCT, 35 patients undergoing liver resection procedures participated in 4 weeks of high intensity cycle interval exercise before the scheduled procedure.[73] Dunne et al[73] found that the patients experienced preoperative improvements in oxygen and peak exercise levels and significant improvement of quality of life and overall mental health in the postoperative setting. The researchers concluded that prehabilitation interventions that include high-intensity exercise on the cycle improved the postoperative patient experience and that the additional time spent with patients and education provided to patients during prehabilitation interventions was also beneficial.

In an RCT conducted by Carli et al,[90] 112 patients received a structured exercise prehabilitation intervention (eg, strengthening [n = 58] compared with walking exercises [n = 54]) before undergoing a colorectal procedure. There was no difference in mean functional walking capacity between the groups before the prehabilitation intervention or at the first postoperative follow-up, however the walking capacity of the walking group was significantly improved compared to the strengthening group. The researchers concluded there was an unexpected benefit for patients in the walking intervention group though there was no baseline or control for at-home adherence. The researchers recommended assessing prehabilitation responders' characteristics to determine which patients would benefit most from the intervention.

In a quasi-experimental pilot study, Li et al[89] compared the outcomes of 42 patients who were assigned prehabilitation walking exercises with outcomes from a 45-patient cohort before prehabilitation was implemented. The researchers found significant improvement in walking in postoperative weeks 4 and 8 and recovery at week 8 for the prehabilitation group compared with the standard care cohort (81% versus 40%). The intervention group had significantly higher scores for social function, emotional role, and mental wellness. The researchers concluded that prehabilitation improved postoperative recovery.

4.6 **Provide the patient with information on the use of postoperative cold temperature interventions (eg, cryotherapy,[92-94] ice packs,[95] cold application plus aromatherapy[45]).** *[Conditional Recommendation]*

Some examples of postoperative cold temperature interventions include

- cryotherapy to decrease pain,[93,94,96] improve function,[93,96] improve temperature,[92,94] and decrease blood loss[93];
- ice packs to decrease pain and decrease opioid use[95]; or
- a combination (eg, cold application and lavender oil) to decrease pain and anxiety.[45]

High-quality evidence supports using cold therapy in the postoperative period,[45,92-96] although the authors of one systematic review found conflicting evidence of the benefits of cryotherapy interventions compared with the cost.[93] High-quality evidence also supports the use of cold therapy combined with other interventions (eg, lavender oil).[45]

In an RCT, Quinlan et al[95] compared targeted cold therapy of 1 L of ice to the lower back for 20 minutes (n = 74) with side-lying alone after spinal fusion procedures (n = 74). The researchers found both interventions decreased patients' pain, though there was a significant decrease in morphine-equivalent consumption and cumulative patient-controlled analgesia consumption from time point 7 to 12 hours in the group that received cold therapy. The researchers concluded that cold therapy is a beneficial adjunct to optimize pain management and reduce opioid consumption.

In a quasi-experimental study, Murata et al[92] compared 36 patients who received a cryotherapy icing system after undergoing spinal procedures (n = 16) to a control group (n = 20). The researchers found a significantly lower temperature of the wound and a positive correlation between the depth and temperature (ie, the deeper the wound the colder the temperature); however, cryotherapy had no effect on pain scores or bleeding outcomes. The researchers concluded that the benefits of cryotherapy are limited to decreasing the wound temperature.

Adie et al[93] performed a Cochrane review that included 12 trials (N = 809) in which cryotherapy was provided for 48 hours after total knee arthroplasty (TKA) procedures compared with standard care, the researchers found that cryotherapy had a significant but small benefit to reducing blood loss, decreasing pain scores at postoperative hour 48, and improved range of motion (ROM) at discharge. The researchers concluded that the results were not clinically significant, and the potential benefits could not justify the inconvenience and expense of the intervention.

In an RCT of 66 patients who underwent TKA procedures, Demoulin et al[94] investigated the effects of gaseous cryotherapy (n = 22) compared with standard cryotherapy (n = 22) or cold packs (n = 22). Gaseous cryotherapy significantly decreased wound temperature immediately in the postoperative setting and on POD 1. All groups reported an increase in pain immediately after the procedure, but pain scores in the standard cryotherapy group did not significantly increase. The researchers concluded that gaseous cryotherapy technology is not more beneficial than standard cryotherapy after TKA procedures.

In an RCT of 80 patients undergoing chest tube removal days after a coronary artery bypass grafting procedure, Hasanzadeh et al[45] compared three interventions, including cold application and lavender oil combined, cold application only, lavender oil only, and a control group (n = 20 in each group). The researchers found a significantly lower pain intensity and anxiety report for 15 minutes after chest tube removal in both groups in which cold interventions were applied. There was a significant decrease in anxiety in the combined intervention group compared to the group that received cold application alone, though the difference in pain scores was not significant between these groups.

5. Dietary and Herbal Interventions

5.1 **Provide information to the patient about dietary interventions that may affect perioperative outcomes, including**
- **the value of consulting with specialized personnel (eg, a registered dietitian, an herbologist) in the planning process[15];**
- **the benefits of following recommendations provided by specialized personnel[15] before and after an operative or other invasive procedure; and**
- **the benefits and risks (eg, potential for adverse interactions, bleeding risk) associated with dietary and herbal supplementation.**[15,17,18,29,35,49,97-101]

[Conditional Recommendation]

Guidelines support optimizing physical health during the perioperative period, including assessing nutritional status and using dietary and herbal interventions and glycemic control.[15] Several dietary and herbal interventions have been associated with improved perioperative outcomes that may outweigh the associated risks. Patients who are knowledgeable about risks and benefits can better discuss their current practices or potential implementation with their providers.

Fish Oil Supplementation

High-quality evidence supports preoperative and postoperative fish oil supplementation to improve postoperative outcomes[49,98,99] (eg, infection rate,[99] length of hospital stay [LOHS] and intensive care unit [ICU] stay[99]) without an associated increased risk of adverse events. However, the benefits were only studied in specific procedures (eg, abdominal,[99] esophagogastric[49]) and generalizability may be limited.

In a systematic review of 52 studies, Begtrup et al[98] found that fish oil supplementation reduced platelet aggregation but did not increase the risk for intraoperative bleeding or the postoperative blood transfusion rate. The researchers concluded that fish oil supplementation does not need to be discontinued before surgery.

In a meta-analysis that included 13 RCTs (N = 8,992), Chen et al[99] evaluated the effects of fish oil supplementation on the outcomes of adult patients who underwent abdominal procedures. The researchers found fish oil supplementation had a positive effect on LOHS, ICU LOS, and postoperative infection rates and no effect on mortality rates. The researchers concluded fish oil supplementation was a safe and effective way to improve clinical outcomes.

In an RCT, 195 patients received Omega-3 fatty acid enteral supplementation to improve their immunity compared with standard enteral nutrition before and after undergoing esophagogastric procedures.[49] Sultan et al[49] found a significantly higher Omega-3 concentration (ie, ratio of Omega 6 to Omega 3) in the intervention group. There was a significant increase in protein and energy consumption in the intervention group, as the volume needed to achieve target caloric and protein levels was lower and easier for patients to consume. Though there were no clinical or significant improvements in infection complications, ICU LOS, LOHS, morbidity, or mortality rate, the researchers concluded that patients who are malnourished or unable to consume enteral nutrition should supplement their dietary intake to optimize their postoperative healing.

Symbiotics

High-quality evidence supports that use of symbiotics[100] and probiotics[100,101] may decrease the patient's risk for developing sepsis. In a meta-analysis of

15 RCTs that included 1,201 patients undergoing GI procedures, the researchers found that probiotics and symbiotics significantly decreased the risk of sepsis.[101] In a meta-analysis conducted of 13 RCTs (including nine trials that were part of the previous meta-analysis[91]) (N = 962), symbiotics were found to be more beneficial than probiotics in reducing sepsis incidence.[100]

Vitamin D and Calcium

High-quality evidence[17,18] used to support clinical guidelines for orthopedic surgeons[35] indicates that postoperative vitamin D and calcium supplementation may decrease postoperative fracture complications in older adult nonoperative patients.

In an RCT, adult patients older than 65 years with hip fractures received extended physical therapy (n = 87) or standard physical therapy (n = 86) combined with either 2,000 IU (n = 86) or 800 IU of cholecalciferol per day (n = 87).[17] Bischoff-Ferrari et al[17] found a 25% reduction in falls and 39% reduction in readmissions in the groups that consumed 2,000 IU. The risk of facility readmission was lower for patients who received 2,000 IU of cholecalciferol.

In an RCT, Chapuy et al[18] provided either 1.2 g elemental calcium and 800 IU of vitamin D3 (n = 1,634) or placebos (n = 1,636) to female patients ages 69 to 106 years who were living in nursing homes. The researchers found that calcium and vitamin D3 supplementation lowered the incidence of nonvertebral and hip fractures.

Bleeding Risk

Low-quality evidence supports evaluating the patient's use of complementary practices and over-the-counter supplements for potential interactions with the surgical and anesthetic plans of care.[29,97] In a systematic review, Wang et al[30] evaluated the effects of dietary and herbal interventions on coagulation and bleeding among patients undergoing operative and other invasive procedures. The researchers found 11 common herbal medications (ie, echinacea, ephedra, garlic, ginger, ginkgo, ginseng, green tea, kava, saw palmetto, St John's wort, and valerian) and four supplements (ie, coenzyme Q10, glucosamine and chondroitin sulfate, fish oil, and vitamins) that may increase the risk for bleeding and cardiovascular instability.

In a cross-sectional cohort study, Levy et al[29] evaluated the effects of dietary supplements on general anesthesia and bleeding in surgery. The researchers found that patients who used sage as a dietary supplement had increased sedative toxicity and decreased blood level of anesthesia. The researchers also found that use of other dietary supplements had additional effects related to general anesthesia: chamomile prolonged sedation, green tea reduced anesthesia hypnotic effects, and lemon balm increased sedation. Several dietary supplements were identified as having effects on patient coagulation potential, including additive antiplatelets from Omega-3 fish oil, green tea, magnesium, rosemary, and flaxseed. Other platelet inhibitors were chamomile, ginger, and sage.

In a systematic review of nine trials including two observational studies, Marx et al[97] found that oral ginger reduced platelet aggregation in four of the studies. In these studies, varied delivery methods (eg, capsules, raw, powder, dried) and doses of ginger (eg, 10 g, 5 g, 625 mg four times a day, 1 g) or combinations with other medications (eg, nifedipine) decreased the ability of researchers to conclude whether one form of oral ginger had higher adverse associations with platelet aggregation. Evidence further conflicts as the remaining studies found no association with adverse events for varied routes (eg, capsules, raw, capsules with warfarin) and doses (eg, 4 g, 15 g, 3.6 g, 500 mg four times).

5.2 **Dietary and herbal interventions may be implemented for prevention of postoperative ileus complications.** *[Conditional Recommendation]*

Moderate-quality evidence,[102-104] and guidelines[15] support using dietary and herbal interventions to prevent postoperative ileus complications. Dietary and herbal supplement interventions that may prevent or reduce the incidence and severity of postoperative ileus complications include gum chewing (eg, LOHS, time to flatus, time to bowel movement)[102] and Dai-kenchu-to, a Japanese herbal medicine (eg, time to flatus,[103] health care organization costs, LOHS[104]).

Short et al[102] performed a Cochrane review of 81 RCTs (N = 9,072) in which patients received chewing gum to promote postoperative GI function versus a control group. Though the results were not statistically significant, the researchers found that gum chewing decreased time to flatus, slightly decreased the LOHS and time to bowel sounds, and improved postoperative healing after colorectal procedures.

In a quasi-experimental study patients received either 7.5 g of Dai-kenchu-to for 7 postoperative days (n = 15) or standard care (n = 15).[103] Yoshikawa et al[103] found that patients in the intervention group had a significantly shorter time to flatus and lower C-reactive protein on POD 3.

In a retrospective matched cohort study, Yasunaga et al[104] administered Dai-kenchu-to to 144 patients with adhesive small bowel obstruction. The researchers found that compared to a control group (n = 144), the intervention group had fewer requirements for long-tube decompression insertion as well as time to remove the tube and discharge the patient, which significantly lowered facility charges. Though the results were not adjusted for patient characteristics, the researchers concluded that Dai-kenchu-to was an effective intervention to decrease long-tube decompression requirements and associated costs.

5.3 **Postoperative interventions that can reduce thirst discomfort may be used in the postoperative phase of care.**[105-107] *[Conditional Recommendation]*

Moderate-quality evidence supports using interventions that may reduce a patient's thirst discomfort during postoperative recovery,[106,107] including menthol chewing gum[107] and oral care using menthol in normal saline swabs. Water interventions may include aromatherapy water, cold water, and menthol water.

In an RCT, Garcia et al[107] investigated the effects of menthol chewing gum (n = 51) versus standard care (n = 51) on thirst discomfort in the postoperative recovery area. The researchers found a significant decrease in the intensity and discomfort of postoperative thirst in the group that received menthol gum and concluded that the intervention was effective and safe.

In a quasi-experimental study, 60 patients received a menthol in normal saline oral care swab compared to standard oral care. Al Sebaee and Elhadary[105] found a significant decrease in thirst intensity and improvement in saliva and tongue health. The researchers concluded that adding menthol to the water used for oral care significantly improved postoperative recovery as part of an oral care bundle for patients recovering from abdominal procedures.

In a systematic literature review of 10 studies including one observational study, Garcia et al[106] found that frozen gauze, ice chips, cold water, menthol, chewing gum, acupressure, sipping liquids through a thin straw, and early oral fluids decreased thirst discomfort. Though they concluded that combining strategies can increase patient satisfaction, the researchers found that decreasing the temperature of the water was the most predominant and effective intervention to decrease thirst discomfort.

5.4 **Oral ginger may be used for postoperative nausea.**[1,19,21,108,109] *[Conditional Recommendation]*

High-quality evidence[19,108,109] and guidelines[1,21] support that ginger decreases postoperative nausea,[19,108,109] but conflict on differences in vomiting incidence[19,109] and administration (ie, dose, timing, and route).[19,108]

Tóth et al[108] performed a meta-analysis of 10 RCTs (N = 918) in which patients were given 100 mg to 1,500 mg of oral ginger. They found a significant decrease in nausea and vomiting severity, though PONV incidence and use of rescue medications were not statistically improved. The researchers concluded that underdosing may have contributed to nonsignificant results and that oral ginger is a safe and well-tolerated method for reducing PONV severity.

In an RCT of 100 patients undergoing cholelithiasis who received oral ginger, Soltani et al[109] found nausea severity was significantly lower at postoperative hours zero, 2, and 4, but the incidence of vomiting was only significantly lower at hour 16. The researchers concluded that oral ginger given 1 hour before surgery is an inexpensive, effective, and safe method to decrease PONV.

In another RCT, 122 patients received either one dose of 1 g or two doses of 500 mg of oral ginger or a placebo before undergoing cataract procedures under general anesthesia. Seidi et al[19] found significantly lower scores for nausea and vomiting with two smaller doses compared to one large dose or the placebo. The researchers concluded that oral ginger is a safe and effective intervention to reduce PONV, and two separate, smaller doses may be more beneficial than one larger dose. They recommended this intervention for older adult patients, for whom the risk of adverse events with antiemetic drug consumption is higher.

5.4.1 **Use oral ginger with caution in patients who are at risk for bleeding.**[97] *[Recommendation]*

Moderate-quality evidence found conflicting results on the potential adverse events (eg, bleeding risk associated with increased platelet aggregation) related to oral ginger use, depending on the dose.[97] Additional research is required to determine the optimal dose of oral ginger to avoid increasing platelet aggregation.

In a systematic review of nine trials including two observational studies, Marx et al[97] found oral ginger reduced platelet aggregation in four of the studies. In these studies, varied delivery methods (eg, capsules, raw, powder, dried) and doses of ginger (eg, 10 g, 5 g, 625 mg four times a day, 1 g) or combinations with other medications (eg, nifedipine) decreased the ability of researchers to conclude whether one form of oral ginger had higher adverse associations with platelet aggregation. Evidence further conflicts as the remaining studies found no association with adverse events for varied routes (eg, capsules, raw, capsules with warfarin) and doses (eg, 4 g, 15 g, 3.6 g, 500 mg four times).

5.5 Do not give patients essential oils for oral ingestion.[110] *[Regulatory Requirement]*

The FDA classifies essential oils as Generally Recognized as Safe as a regulated indirect additive for flavor, and they are not recognized as safe for any other indication.[110]

6. Music Interventions

6.1 Music interventions may be used in the perioperative environment.[66] *[Conditional Recommendation]*

In a high-quality systematic review of 73 RCTs conducted from 1988 to 2013, Hole et al[66] evaluated research on the benefits of perioperative music interventions for postoperative pain, anxiety, use of analgesia, and patient satisfaction. The researchers found improvements in all of these outcomes and concluded that perioperative music interventions were beneficial.

6.1.1 When music interventions will be used, determine
- **whether the music will be patient selected**[66,111,112] **or assigned,**[48,113]
- **what types of music will be used,**[27,48,55,66,111-117] **and**
- **what delivery mode will be used.**[113,114]

[Conditional Recommendation] **P**

High-quality evidence conflicts regarding using patient-selected music in the perioperative setting.[27,48,55,66,111-117] Researchers have found that patients desired to choose music based on their personal preferences[111,112] and, conversely, that a high percentage of patients requested to use again the same music genre that was assigned to them previously.[113] Other researchers found inconclusive evidence on whether music or music volume jeopardizes patient safety in the OR.[66]

Potential harms of music selection or volume can include negatively affecting the patient's response to anesthesia induction and emergence and volume at a level that introduces noise into the intraoperative environment and interrupts perioperative team communication.[66] Limitations to selecting a music intervention include the cost-effectiveness of using specific types of music (ie, **interactive music** interventions that require additional education and training)[27]; however, none of the researchers included a cost analysis in their studies.

In a systematic review of 73 RCTs, Hole et al[66] found a reduction in postoperative pain, anxiety, and use of analgesia and an increase in patient sat-

isfaction with the use of music interventions. However, the researchers concluded that allowing patients to choose the music and suitable volume were unclear limitations. It was also unclear whether the use of headphones created a risk of distracting patients from communicating with perioperative health care workers or a benefit of alleviating imposition of the music on the health care workers.

In an RCT, Palmer et al[114] assigned 207 female patients undergoing breast procedures to receive either patient-selected live music (eg, in-person guitar or keyboard) (n = 69), recorded music (n = 70), or usual preoperative area noises as a control in the preoperative setting (n = 68). In the OR, both music groups received therapist-selected intraoperative music and the control group received earmuffs. The researchers found a significant decrease in anxiety scores in the music groups, though the preoperative live music intervention resulted in a shorter recovery time, as indicated by discharge readiness. The researchers concluded that live music was more beneficial than recorded music; and preoperative music was safe and time efficacious to reduce anxiety.

In an RCT of 180 pediatric patients ages 3 to 15 years undergoing dental procedures, Ozkalayci et al[55] assigned participants to one of three groups: sound-isolating headphones with music, isolation headphones without music, or standard care (n = 60 in each group). The researchers found that there was a significantly prolonged recovery (ie, time to Aldrete discharge parameters) in the groups that did not receive a music intervention and concluded that use of a music intervention could decrease recovery time.

In an RCT conducted by Çetinkaya[48] in Turkey of 60 older adult patients undergoing total joint procedures, Turkish music was played for 20 minutes three times a day on the first, second, and third postoperative days. Cognitive scores significantly improved on POD 3 compared with POD 1. The researcher concluded that music prevented cognitive dysfunction, though the study sample was limited to patients in one facility and only one type of music was used.

In an RCT, Ko et al[115] found that patients undergoing colonoscopy without sedation (n = 138) had a significant decrease in anxiety when **Kern light music** was played intraoperatively. The researchers concluded it was a safe, convenient, and effective intervention.

In an RCT, Forooghy et al[112] compared patients who listened to 20 to 40 minutes of light instrumental music intraoperatively after local anesthesia was injected during percutaneous transluminal coronary angioplasty (n = 32) to a control group (n = 32). The researchers found a significant decrease in anxiety scores and a significant decrease in blood pressure immediately after the intervention and up to 30 minutes after the procedure and intervention were completed. Limitations included environmental noise and potential confounders related to patient's psychological or personality characteristics, attitudes, and beliefs. The researchers concluded that additional research is needed to determine the benefit of intraoperative light instrumental music.

In a pilot study of 34 patients undergoing colonoscopy procedures who received either muted headphones (n = 17) or listened to a loop of Bach music on headphones (n = 17) before and during their procedures, Martindale et al[113] found that anxiety scores decreased in both groups. However, all of the patients in the music group reported a desire to receive music for repeat procedures compared to 50% in the control group who said they would wear muted headphones again. Of interest, 64.7% of patients in the music group reported that they did not want to choose their own music, and the researchers concluded that any music genre may be beneficial to reduce anxiety.

In an RCT conducted with 98 patients, Weeks and Nilsson[116] found a significant postintervention reduction in anxiety and increase in well-being with use of a music intervention, regardless of whether music was provided by an audio pillow or loudspeaker during coronary angiographic procedures.

In an RCT conducted by Padmanabhan et al,[117] 100 patients in three groups preoperatively received either **binaural beat** music (n = 35), music without binaural tones (n = 34), or no intervention as a control group (n = 35). The researchers found a significant decrease in anxiety for both music groups and a significantly lower increase in anxiety in the binaural tones group compared to the control group. The researchers concluded that the potential to decrease acute preoperative anxiety warranted use of music interventions.

In a quasi-experimental study conducted by Hsu et al,[111] 49 older adults who had undergone TKA procedures completed 25 minutes of postoperative **continuous passive motion** (CPM) rehabilitation in the facility ward. Each patient performed CPM both with and without music during the course of 2 postoperative days. Patients reported significantly decreased pain and increased knee flexion angle when they listened to music during CPM rehabilitation. The researchers concluded that playing patient-selected music and decreasing environmental noise could improve the effectiveness of CPM rehabilitation.

6.2 Establish a process for the care and cleaning of reusable music delivery devices. [Recommendation]

6.3 Music intervention techniques may be used in all perioperative phases of care for anxiety and pain reduction for pediatric patients.[27,118] [Conditional Recommendation] P

High-quality evidence supports using music during all perioperative phases of care to decrease anxiety and pain in pediatric patients.[27,118]

In a systematic review and meta-analysis of 19 RCTs that included 1,513 pediatric patients ages 1 month to 18 years, Klassen et al[118] found a significant decrease in pain and anxiety when music was implemented in the perioperative setting. The researchers concluded that music was an effective adjunct to reduce pharmacologic requirements, pain, and anxiety.

In an RCT conducted to investigate an interactive music therapy intervention in pediatric patients ages 3 to 7 years, Kain et al[27] found that patients who received midazolam (n = 34) had significantly lower anxiety than patients in the music intervention group (n = 51) or control group (n = 38) on induction. The midazolam group had significantly lower anxiety even after the researchers controlled for the results for one music therapist whose group had significantly lower anxiety during preoperative parental separation and entrance to the OR. The researchers concluded that interactive music therapy may be helpful depending on the therapist, but not during anesthesia induction, and therefore, the intervention was not cost-effective.

6.4 Preoperative music interventions may be used for adult patients.[27,113,114,117,119] [Conditional Recommendation]

High-quality evidence supports the use of preoperative music interventions to improve vital signs[119] and decrease anxiety[113,114,117,119] and the length of time in the postanesthesia care unit (PACU).[114] Limitations of music interventions include the cost for a music therapist[114] and logistics for interactive music interventions.[27]

In a systematic review of 26 trials (N = 2,051 patients) that included quasi-experimental studies, Bradt et al[119] found that pre-recorded music in the preoperative setting decreased anxiety scores and had a small effect on patients' heart rate and diastolic blood pressure but not on systolic blood pressure, respiratory rate, or skin temperature. The researchers concluded that these results were consistent with the results of other Cochrane reviews that found preoperative music may decrease patient anxiety.

In a pilot study, Martindale et al[113] assigned 34 patients undergoing colonoscopy procedures to receive either muted headphones (n = 17) or to listen to a loop of Bach music (n = 17) before and during their procedures. During the study, anxiety scores decreased, and 100% of the patients in the music group reported a desire to receive music for repeat procedures compared to 50% in the control group that would wear muted headphones again. Limitations include the potential confounding factor of patient-controlled volume.

In an RCT conducted by Padmanabhan et al,[117] 104 patients received either binaural beat audios (n = 35), music without binaural tones (n = 34), or no intervention as a control group (n = 35). The researchers found a significant decrease in anxiety for both music groups and a significantly lower increase in anxiety in the group with the binaural beat audios. The researchers concluded that the potential to decrease acute preoperative anxiety warrants use of binaural tones.

In an RCT, Palmer et al[114] assigned 207 female patients undergoing breast procedures to listen to either patient-selected live music (ie, in-person guitar or keyboard) (n = 69), recorded music (n = 70), or usual preoperative area noises as a control in the preoperative setting (n = 68). The researchers found a significant decrease in anxiety with live music, resulting in a shorter recovery as indicated by discharge readiness. The researchers concluded that live music is safe and time efficacious, though determining the ideal timing of the intervention requires additional research.

6.5 **Intraoperative music interventions may be used.**[66,112,113,115,120-122] *[Conditional Recommendation]*

High-quality evidence supports that intraoperative music interventions may

- decrease analgesia use,[66,120]
- decrease anxiety,[66,112,113,115,120,121]
- decrease adrenaline and noradrenaline levels,[112,120,121]
- improve subjective coping,[122]
- improve vital signs,[112,120,121]
- increase patient satisfaction,[66,113,122] and
- decrease subjective stress.[121]

In a systematic review of 73 RCTs conducted between 1988 to 2013, Hole et al[66] found that use of a music intervention reduced postoperative pain, anxiety, and analgesia use and increased patient satisfaction. The researchers concluded that music interventions were effective in improving the studied outcomes and recommended the use of music in the perioperative setting.

In an RCT, Bashiri et al[120] evaluated music and anesthesia type for effects on patient anxiety scores. Group 1 received conscious sedation without music (n = 25), group 2 received conscious sedation with music (n = 33), group 3 received deep sedation without music (n = 55), and group 4 received deep sedation with music (n = 41). In each group that had a music intervention, the researchers found a decrease in anxiety and propofol use, increased patient satisfaction, and a desire to listen to music during future procedures. Heart rate and mean arterial pressure were also significantly lower during and after the procedure in the music groups. The researchers concluded that music interventions improved the comfort of patients undergoing procedures without general anesthesia.

In an RCT, Jiménez-Jiménez et al[121] provided either classical music (n = 20) or standard care (n = 20) to patients undergoing great saphenous vein stripping procedures. The researchers found significantly lower anxiety scores, lower serum adrenaline and noradrenaline levels, and improved vital signs in the group that listened to classical music. The researchers concluded that listening to the selected music reduced intraoperative anxiety.

In an RCT that included 26 women who underwent elective surgical abortions with either self-selected music and local anesthesia (n = 11) or local anesthesia alone (n = 13), Wu et al[122] found significantly better postoperative coping and less anxiety immediately after the procedure in the group that listened to music. The researchers concluded that music interventions as an adjunct to local anesthesia are associated with less postprocedure anxiety.

In a pilot study, Martindale et al[113] assigned 34 patients undergoing colonoscopy to either receive muted headphones (n = 17) or listen to a loop of Bach music (n = 17) before and during their procedures. Anxiety scores were reduced in both groups, and 100% of the patients in the music group reported a desire to receive music for repeat procedures compared to 50% in the control group who said they would wear muted headphones again. The researchers concluded that even though the music did not significantly reduce anxiety, pain scores, or medication doses (ie, midazolam, fentanyl), the patients expressed a clear preference to listen to music during future procedures.

In an RCT, Ko et al[115] found that 138 patients undergoing colonoscopy procedures without sedation had significantly decreased anxiety scores after listening to Kern light music. The researchers concluded it is a safe, convenient, and effective intervention.

In an RCT, Forooghy et al[112] compared patients who listened to 20 to 40 minutes of light instrumental music intraoperatively after receiving local anesthesia at the start of their percutaneous transluminal coronary angioplasty procedure (n = 32) to a control group (n = 32). The researchers found a significant decrease in postprocedure anxiety scores in the music group compared with the standard care group and concluded that music therapy is a safe, simple, inexpensive, and noninvasive nursing intervention that can significantly alleviate patient anxiety during coronary angioplasty.

6.6 **Postoperative music interventions may be used.**[48,66,111,123] *[Conditional Recommendation]*

High-quality evidence supports that using music therapy postoperatively for older adult patients may decrease their pain and cognitive decline.[48,66,123] Moderate-quality evidence supports postoperative use of music to decrease objective and subjective pain and anxiety outcomes and increase patient satisfaction.[111] Evidence conflicts on the ability of music to reduce analgesic consumption.[66,123]

Postoperative music interventions may

- decrease anxiety,[66]
- improve cognitive function,[48]
- improve physical function,[111]
- decrease pain,[66,111] and
- improve coping and stress.[123]

In a systematic review of 73 RCTs, Hole et al[66] found a reduction in postoperative pain, anxiety, and use of analgesia and an increase in patient satisfaction with the use of music interventions. The researchers concluded that allowing patients to choose the music and suitable volume were unclear limitations. It was also unclear whether the use of headphones created a risk of distracting patients from communicating with perioperative health care workers or a benefit of alleviating imposition of the music on the health care workers.

In an RCT of 163 patients, Easter et al[123] studied the effects of a music intervention on respiratory rate, oxygen saturation, and opioid consumption in the PACU after multiple outpatient procedures (eg, gastroenterology, ophthalmology, general, gynecology, neurology, oral, orthopedic, urology). The researchers found significantly lower respiratory rates with higher satisfaction in the music group (n = 111) compared to the control group (n = 102). There were no significant differences between the groups in oxygen saturation or opioid consumption in the PACU setting. The researchers concluded that music could be an alternative method to cope with postoperative pain.

In an RCT conducted by Çetinkaya[48] of 60 older adult patients undergoing total joint replacement procedures, Turkish music was played for 20 minutes three times a day on the first, second, and third postoperative days. Cognitive scores significantly improved on POD 3 compared with POD 1. The researcher concluded that music prevented cognitive dysfunction, though the study sample

was limited to patients in one facility and only one type of music was used.

In a quasi-experimental study conducted by Hsu et al,[111] 49 older adults who had undergone TKA procedures completed 25 minutes of postoperative CPM rehabilitation in the facility ward. Each patient performed CPM both with and without music during the course of 2 postoperative days. Patients reported significantly decreased pain and increased knee flexion angle when they listened to music during CPM rehabilitation. The researchers concluded that playing patient-selected music and decreasing environmental noise could improve the effectiveness of CPM rehabilitation.

7. Stress Diversion Interventions

7.1 **Select and implement perioperative stress diversion interventions based on the patient's age.**[20,53,54,56,71,124-140] *[Conditional Recommendation]* **P**

Types of stress diversion include

- preoperative humor,[53,56,132] play,[124] video,[71,125] and virtual reality (VR)[126-130] interventions;
- intraoperative distraction and a low stimulus environment[133,134];
- parental presence during emergence from anesthesia[135-137]; and
- postoperative patient visitation for both adult[139,140] and pediatric patients.[54,138]

High-quality evidence supports that preoperative stress diversion interventions can reduce anxiety,[53,56,71,124-131] including reducing the anxiety of the parents of pediatric patients.[20]

In a quasi-experimental study that included 83 pediatric patients ages 9 to 18 years, Aytekin et al[20] found that participating in distractions tailored to their age group (eg, games, music, cartoons, books) significantly decreased patients' anxiety and separation anxiety compared to patients in a control group. The researchers concluded that patients may benefit from different distraction methods geared toward developmental age.

7.2 **Preoperative humorous interventions may be used to decrease preoperative anxiety in pediatric patients.**[53,56,132] *[Conditional Recommendation]* **P**

High-quality evidence supports using humor (eg, costumes, toys, clowns, comical informational materials) to decrease preoperative anxiety in pediatric patients and their mothers.[53,56,132]

In an RCT, Kassai et al[56] gave a comic information leaflet to pediatric patients ages 6 to 17 years before surgery (n = 55). Anxiety scores were significantly decreased in the intervention group compared to a group that received standard care (n = 55). The researchers also found that those with a higher baseline anxiety scores benefited more from the intervention.

In an RCT, Liguori et al[53] provided pediatric patients ages 6 to 11 years with either a 6-minute video (ie, clown physicians giving a comical and informative tour of the OR) the night before the procedure (n = 20) or standard care (n = 20). Children who viewed the video, which was provided via an app, had significantly lower preoperative anxiety scores and significantly lower changes in anxiety before induction than those who did not view the video. The researchers concluded that the app could be used as a substitute when there is not enough time for health care workers to provide education and to decrease costs associated with staffing.

In a quasi-experimental study conducted by Berger et al,[132] 42 pediatric patients ages 4 to 17 years were distracted through humor, costumes, and toys while playing with their mothers. The researchers found significantly lower anxiety scores for the children on admission to the perioperative suite and significantly lower anxiety just before the procedure in both the children and their parents. The researchers concluded that costume and humor distraction was effective and improved the family perioperative experience.

7.2.1 | **Do not use clown humor interventions if the patient has an aversion to clowns.**[132] *[Recommendation]*

If the patient has an aversion to clowns, using this type of humor as a stress diversion intervention may negatively affect the patient's perioperative experience and may increase anxiety instead.[132]

7.2.2 | **Preoperative play interventions may be used to decrease preoperative anxiety in pediatric patients.**[124] *[Conditional Recommendation]* **P**

Moderate-quality evidence supports distracting pediatric patients preoperatively by providing a separate area dedicated to play.[124]

In an RCT, Hosseinpour and Memarzadeh[124] found that providing access to a preoperative playroom 30 minutes before a surgical procedure significantly decreased the anxiety scores for pediatric patients ages 2 to 6 years, compared with standard care.

7.3 | **Audio-video interventions may be used for preoperative anxiety reduction.**[71,125] *[Conditional Recommendation]* **P**

High-quality evidence[71,125] supports using videos to distract pediatric patients' and to reduce preoperative anxiety during high-anxiety preoperative peri-

ods, such as during transport to the OR[125] and during induction.[71,125] The benefits for pediatric patients could apply to other age groups.

In an RCT, Kerimoglu et al[125] assigned 96 pediatric patients ages 4 to 9 years to one of three groups: video glasses for distraction for 20 minutes, midazolam only, or video glasses for distraction combined with midazolam (n = 32 in each group). The interventions were implemented before transport and during anesthetic gas induction of general anesthesia. There was a significant decrease in anxiety during transport in the midazolam with video glasses group and significant increase in anxiety in the midazolam-only group, though the researchers did not find this to be clinically significant. The researchers concluded that the use of video glasses alone was not inferior to use of midazolam alone for decreasing preoperative anxiety. Limitations of the study include potential confounders that were not measured, such as **emergence delirium** and behavioral dysfunction.

In an RCT conducted by Mifflin et al[71] of 89 pediatric patients ages 2 to 10 years, patients streamed a video during induction (n = 42) or participated in traditional distraction methods (n = 47) including nonprocedural talk and game playing. The researchers found significantly lower anxiety scores and a significantly smaller increase in anxiety from the holding area to anesthesia induction time for those patients who watched the video. The researchers concluded that video distraction is useful, though future research should focus on confounding factors such as premedication with sedatives and parental presence during induction, as well as longer term effects of stress diversions used in recovery areas.

7.4 | **Virtual reality (eg, OR experience, gamification) audio-visual interventions may be used for preoperative anxiety reduction.**[126-130] *[Conditional Recommendation]* **P**

High-quality evidence supports that a short VR tour of the OR can decrease preoperative anxiety in both adult[126] and pediatric populations (ie, between 4 and 12 years of age).[126-130] Virtual reality gamification also significantly reduced patients' anxiety and improved induction compliance in one study; however, the cost of gamification (ie, adding gaming elements to non-game contexts) within VR interventions may not outweigh the benefits compared with general VR interventions.[129]

Evidence supports that VR interventions may benefit perioperative outcomes including decreased anxiety,[126-130] better induction compliance,[129,130] and increased patient satisfaction.[126] Evidence conflicts about effects on patient distress[126,127] and parental satisfaction.[127,130]

In an RCT, Bekelis et al[126] provided patients undergoing cranial and spinal procedures with a VR experience (n = 64) compared to a group that received standard care (n = 63). Patients were encouraged to watch the video as many times as desired and were given time for and encouraged to ask questions. After the intervention, the patients in the intervention group reported feeling more prepared and had higher satisfaction scores and lower stress even though they had a higher level of preoperative anxiety than the control group. The researchers concluded that an immersive OR environment experience with VR could minimize patients' preoperative stress.

In an RCT, Park et al[127] assigned 80 pediatric patients ages 4 to 10 years and their parents to one of two intervention groups. In the immersive mirroring intervention group (n = 40), patients watched a 4-minute VR tour via a headset while their parents watched the same 4-minute VR tour simultaneously on a separate monitor. In the second group, the patient watched the VR tour via headset, and the parents did not view the VR tour. Mirrored VR experiences significantly reduced the patients' preoperative anxiety and the parents' induction anxiety and increased parents' satisfaction. There was no difference in patient anxiety during anesthesia induction in either group, as measured by the **Induction Compliance Checklist** (ICC). The researchers concluded that having patients and their parents simultaneously watch an immersive VR tour was a feasible way to effectively reduce preoperative anxiety in pediatric patients and their parents.

In an RCT, Dehghan et al[128] assigned 40 pediatric patients ages 6 to 12 years to receive either 5 minutes of VR exposure to the OR or a control with or without a pretest (n = 10 in each group). The researchers found a significant decrease in anxiety among patients who received the VR intervention. The researchers concluded that distraction using VR decreased preoperative anxiety.

In an RCT of 69 pediatric patients ages 4 to 10 years, Ryu et al[130] found that a preoperative 4-minute VR tour of the OR (n = 35) versus standard care (n = 34) significantly lowered patients' preoperative anxiety scores and postoperative negative behaviors, as well as increasing their intraoperative ICC scores compared to the control group. The researchers concluded that VR could alleviate anxiety and increase induction compliance.

In another RCT conducted by Ryu et al[129] of 69 pediatric patients ages 4 to 10 years, the researchers found that 5 minutes of a VR gamification experience (n = 34) versus standard care (n = 35) did not have an effect on pediatric behaviors or parent satisfaction. However, preoperative anxiety and ICC scores were significantly decreased in participants in the intervention group, and the researchers concluded that the low cost and feasibility of a VR intervention can reduce pediatric anxiety.

7.5 **Stress diversion interventions may be used to reduce pain and distress in pediatric patients.**[133,134] *[Conditional Recommendation]* **P**

High-quality evidence supports the use of varied and multiple stress diversion interventions to reduce intraoperative pediatric pain and distress.[133,134] Types of stress diversion to reduce pain and distress include breathing exercises, cognitive behavioral therapy, distraction, information, hypnosis, memory alterations, positive suggestions,[133] and a low-stimulus environment.[134]

In an updated Cochrane review of pediatric pain and distress during needle procedures, Birnie et al[133] reviewed 20 new trials that included 5,550 pediatric patients and supported interventions such as distraction, cognitive behavioral therapy, hypnosis, increased information, breathing, positive suggestion, and memory alterations, as adjuncts to standard care.

In an RCT, Kain et al[134] assigned pediatric patients ages 2 to 7 years to receive either low sensory stimulus interventions including dim OR lights, soft background music, only one anesthesia professional, and no instrument noise from the sterile field (n = 33) or usual care (n = 37). The researchers found significantly lower anxiety scores for pediatric patients in the intervention group, lower anxiety scores for their parents, and significantly better cooperation with health care workers. The researchers concluded that manipulating the environment, including limiting loud noises, is a beneficial and low-cost intervention to reduce preoperative anxiety in pediatric patients.

7.6 **Parental presence during induction of general anesthesia for pediatric patients may be implemented, in collaboration with surgeons and anesthesia professionals, for anxiety reduction for both patients and their parents.**[135-137] *[Conditional Recommendation]* **P**

Moderate-quality evidence conflicts as to whether parental presence effectively reduces the parents' or pediatric patient's anxiety during anesthesia induction.[135-137] Educating perioperative team members and gaining their support for parental presence initiatives are critical for successful implementation. Without buy-in and understanding of the potential benefits, team members may be resistant or perceive the harms as outweighing the benefits. One potential roadblock may be the burden placed on the team to attend to the parent. Support for perioperative team members who facilitate parental presence may reduce the burden on the team and improve patient safety during critical phases of perioperative care. The team may also have concerns about the parent's attire because the parent's clothing may contaminate the perioperative area and increase the patient's risk for surgical site infection. Having the parent change into clean surgical attire may address this concern.

In a systematic review of RCTs of nonpharmacological interventions to assist during anesthesia induction in pediatric patients, Manyande et al[136] reviewed 28 trials (N = 2,681) and 17 interventions. They concluded that parental presence did not significantly reduce anxiety and additional studies are required to provide specific recommendations regarding other interventions, such as parental acupuncture, clown humor, playing videos of the patient's choice, low-sensory stimulation, and video game interventions.

In a quasi-experimental study, Chan and Molassiotis[137] provided 25 parents of pediatric patients ages 1 to 9 years with an education program, allowed them to be present during anesthesia induction, and allowed visitation with their children in the recovery area. The researchers found a significant decrease in parental anxiety and increase in patient satisfaction compared to parents in a control group (n = 25).

In 2014, Cagiran et al[135] surveyed 100 pediatric patients and their mothers and found that maternal anxiety was unrelated to the mother's level of education or socioeconomic status. However, the researchers found that maternal anxiety was reduced the most by increasing the mother's knowledge preoperatively (86%). Being present during transport and induction of anesthesia (37% and 46%, respectively) and speaking with other mothers (28%) were not as effective in lowering the mothers' preoperative anxiety. The researchers concluded that increasing the knowledge and experience with anesthesia processes reduced maternal anxiety.

7.7 **A procedure for patient visitation in the postanesthesia care unit may be implemented.**[54,138-140] *[Conditional Recommendation]* **P**

Health care organizations should weigh the benefits versus harms of including postoperative patient visitation when patient care and departmental conditions are suitable. Moderate-quality evidence supports family visits in the PACU to decrease patient anxiety and increase satisfaction for both the patient and family members.[54,138-140] Although guidelines support that family presence may benefit some patients, potential harms include an increased burden on health care workers and challenges with maintaining the privacy of other patients.

In an RCT, Burke et al[54] observed pediatric patients undergoing magnetic resonance imaging

(MRI) under general anesthesia for **emergence agitation** in the recovery area with parental presence (n = 45) versus parental absence (n = 43). Parents who were present reported earlier anxiety reduction than those who were not present; however, there was no significant difference in the children's agitation with parental presence.

In a quasi-experimental study, In et al[138] found that pediatric patients ages 3 to 6 years whose parent could be present while the patient was emerging from anesthesia (n = 46) had a significant decrease in emergence delirium compared to a control group (n = 47). Though the results at each time point were not statistically significant, the researchers concluded that the parental PACU visitation program could be beneficial.

Lower-quality evidence also supports family visitation. In an observational study, Wendler et al[140] found a significant decrease in patient anxiety and increase in family satisfaction when 5- to 10-minute supervised family visits during phase I recovery were provided for patients who underwent total joint procedures with spinal anesthesia.

In an organizational experience article, Pagnard and Sarver[139] reported that after familial presence was implemented (ie, one adult was allowed 5 minutes on the phone or in the PACU for patients requiring an overnight stay), there was an increase in family satisfaction and decrease in familial stress. Pre-intervention, 70% of the 29 PACU RNs were concerned that family visitation would increase their work stress; however, 94% were positive about the intervention at the end of the trial, and the researchers concluded that the intervention was beneficial to the patient and families without increasing the strain on health care workers.

8. Visualization Interventions

8.1 **Visualization interventions may be used in the perioperative environment.**[26,141-146] *[Conditional Recommendation]*

Types of visualization interventions include hypnosis,[26,141] **empathetic attention**,[142] guided imagery,[143,144] and relaxation recordings.[145,146]

8.1.1 **Hypnosis should only be performed by a certified hypnotherapist.** *[Recommendation]* **P**

Hypnosis implemented by an untrained individual has the potential to increase the risk for patient injury; facilitating this intervention with education and certification is recommended.[147,148]

Chandrasegaran[147] described a case in which the unintentional use of triggering suggestions (ie, verbiage used during hypnosis that causes adverse reactions to the patient during the intervention) increased the anxiety in a previously hypnosis-relaxed patient to the point where anesthesia induction could not occur and the procedure was cancelled. Trained professionals facilitate the optimal use of hypnosis interventions and lower the risk of adverse events.

In an expert opinion article, Kuttner[148] concluded that hypnosis was effective in reducing pain and anxiety in pediatric patients undergoing anesthesia procedures, but noted that training and supervised practice is required to practice hypnosis.

8.1.2 When hypnosis is used,
- individualize hypnotic scripts,[26]
- do not use hypnosis recordings, and
- evaluate the patient preoperatively for triggering words and do not use triggering suggestions when the patient is hypnotized.[147]

[Recommendation]

High-quality evidence supports individualizing hypnotherapy to provide the most effective intervention without potential negative effects.[26] Low-quality evidence supports individualizing hypnotic scripts to avoid using trigger words or phrases that could negatively affect patient care.[147] Researchers found that recorded hypnosis and **therapeutic suggestion** were not as effective as live hypnosis and may increase the risk of negative outcomes because the care is not individualized to avoid words that may trigger negative emotions based on the patient's life experiences.[26]

In a meta-analysis of 26 RCTs (N = 1,890), Kekecs et al[26] found that compared to therapeutic suggestion, hypnosis decreased anxiety and pain intensity but had no effect on analgesic use or nausea. The researchers concluded that live hypnosis could decrease anxiety and postoperative pain for minor surgeries, and more research is needed to understand the efficacy of therapeutic suggestion and recorded hypnosis interventions, which have the potential to include trigger words.

In a case report, Chandrasegaran[147] described hypnosis attempted to decrease the preoperative anxiety of a patient. The patient was successfully transported to the OR; however, during the hypnosis a trigger word was said that created higher anxiety in the patient and required cancelling the procedure. Preoperative hypnosis without the patient's trigger word was attempted later, which allowed for clinical management of the patient's claustrophobia and cold sensitivity during transport to the OR and allowed for a successful anesthesia induction and surgery. Later, the patient had no recollection of the transport and anesthesia induction in the OR, which increased her satisfaction with the procedure. The researchers noted that hypnosis should be individualized, as the previous hypnosis attempt with trigger words failed, and the researchers concluded that future studies should include hypnotic scripts, especially maintenance and termination scripts.

8.1.3 **Empathetic attention interventions may be used as an adjunct to hypnosis, but should not be used alone.**[142] *[Conditional Recommendation]*

In an RCT, Lang et al[142] assigned patients to receive either hypnosis (n = 82), empathetic attention without hypnosis (n = 66), or standard care (n = 70). Those who received self-hypnotic relaxation had significantly lower pain and anxiety scores and consumed fewer median drug units (eg, sedative and analgesic agents, 0.5 mg midazolam plus 25 µg fentanyl). Those in the empathetic attention–only group experienced significantly more adverse events. Because the adverse events were significant early in the study, the study was discontinued, and the researchers concluded that nonspecific support that does not provide the means to manage acute pain and anxiety may be more harmful than beneficial.

8.2 **Preoperative hypnosis interventions may be used.**[26,141] *[Conditional Recommendation]*

Preoperative hypnosis has been associated with
- avoiding unplanned conversion to general anesthesia,[141]
- decreasing intraoperative anesthesia medication demand,[141]
- decreasing postoperative fatigue and nausea/vomiting prophylaxis demand,[141] and
- decreasing preoperative anxiety.[26]

High-quality evidence conflicts as to whether preoperative hypnosis can reduce postoperative pain.[26,141]

In a meta-analysis of 26 RCTs (N = 1,890 patients), Kekecs et al[26] found that compared to therapeutic suggestion, hypnosis decreased anxiety and pain intensity but had no effect on analgesic use or nausea. The researchers concluded that live hypnosis could decrease anxiety and postoperative pain for minor surgeries.

In an RCT that included 150 female patients undergoing minor breast cancer surgeries, Amraoui et al[141] assigned patients to either an intervention group that received 15 minutes of preoperative hypnosis (n = 75) or a control group (n = 75). The intervention group had significantly increased pain scores and LOS in the recovery area, though pain was no different at discharge or at POD 30 follow-up compared to the control group. Patients who received hypnosis had significantly lower consumption of propofol and sufentanil but higher consumption of lidocaine, significantly higher use of noninvasive laryngeal masks for anesthesia, and significantly lower nausea and vomiting prophylaxis use. The researchers concluded that hypnosis did not reduce breast incision pain and that the lower intraoperative propofol use led to higher pain scores and longer recovery times, potentially related to emergence from hypnosis. However, the researchers found that the benefits of hypnosis (ie, less anesthesia drug consumption for airway management) may improve anesthesia outcomes and concluded that the use of perioperative patient hypnosis interventions was beneficial.

8.3 **Preoperative guided imagery interventions may be used for preoperative anxiety and postoperative pain reduction.**[143,144] *[Conditional Recommendation]* **P**

High-quality evidence supports using guided imagery for adult[144] and pediatric patients[143] to reduce anxiety,[144] preoperative anxiety,[143] and postoperative pain[143,144] and shorten length of PACU stay.[144]

In a meta-analysis of 21 studies conducted between 1995 and 2019 (N = 1,648) that included qualitative studies, Álvarez-Garcia and Yaban[143] found that guided imagery was effective in relieving preoperative state anxiety in pediatric patients and preoperative trait anxiety and postoperative pain in adult patients. The researchers concluded that the intervention was easy to implement, effective, and inexpensive.

In an RCT, Gonzales et al[144] assigned 44 adult participants to either listen to a 28-minute guided imagery recording (n = 22) or receive standard care (n = 22) before head and neck procedures. The intervention significantly decreased patients' anxiety and pain at 2 hours after surgery, with an almost significant decrease in recovery time in the PACU. The researchers concluded that guided imagery could be beneficial when there is a short preoperative period, such as for emergency procedures.

8.3.1 **Relaxation recordings with guided imagery interventions may be used for anxiety reduction.**[145,146] *[Conditional Recommendation]*

Low-quality evidence supports the use of relaxation recordings with guided imagery to decrease anxiety.[145,146]

In a quasi-experimental study, Lin[146] assigned a convenience sample of patients undergoing

total joint procedures to use a relaxation recording with guided imagery and breath work for 20 minutes preoperatively and on POD 3 (n = 45). The researcher found significantly lower severity of anxiety and difference in anxiety before and after the intervention and on POD 1 for the intervention group compared to a control group (n = 48). There was also a significant difference in systolic blood pressure, and the researcher concluded that relaxation therapy was effective.

Ko and Lin[145] conducted an observational study with a convenience sample of 80 patients who listened to a relaxation recording with deep breathing and guided imagery and meditation before surgery. The researchers found a significant improvement in respiratory rate, heart rate, systolic blood pressure, and anxiety after the intervention, and a significant decrease in anxiety when patients increased the time in the listening session. The researchers also found that female patients' anxiety scores changed significantly more than male patients' scores. The researchers determined they would include use of the relaxation recording as part of their standard care.

8.4 **Intraoperative hypnosis interventions**[149-151] **may be used to**
- **decrease emotional distress,**[149]
- **reduce medication consumption,**[149-151]
- **shorten operative time,**[149,150]
- **decrease pain,**[149,150]
- **improve physiological parameters,**[149,150] **and**
- **decrease recovery time (eg, length of PACU stay,**[149] **length of ICU stay).**[151]

[Conditional Recommendation]

High-quality evidence conflicts on the benefits of intraoperative hypnosis.[149-151]

In a meta-analysis of 34 RCTs (N = 2,597 patients), Tefikow et al[149] found that emotional distress, pain, medication consumption, physiological parameters, recovery, and operative time were clinically improved by hypnosis; however, the results were not statistically significant. The researchers concluded that a single session of hypnosis was as beneficial as multiple sessions for adults undergoing surgical or invasive procedures.

In an RCT, Lang et al[150] compared **self-hypnosis relaxation** (ie, hypnotic relaxation based on self-generated imagery) (n = 82) with structured attention (ie, an intervention with eight key components) (n = 80) and standard care (n = 79). The researchers found that the self-hypnotic relaxation technique significantly decreased pain, drug use, intraoperative hemodynamic instability, and procedure time compared to structured attention or standard care.

They concluded that the intervention was associated with lower opioid consumption, which positively affected oxygen saturation. The researchers concluded that hypnosis was beneficial.

In a quasi-experimental study of 143 consecutive patients who underwent transfemoral transcatheter aortic valve implantation under conscious sedation with either hypnotherapy (n = 36) or standard care (n = 107), Takahashi et al[151] found significantly decreased LOS in the ICU and lower consumption of propofol, remifentanil, and norepinephrine in the intraoperative phase in the hypnotherapy group. The researchers concluded that adjunctive hypnotherapy may facilitate perioperative care.

8.4.1   **Hypnosis interventions may be used for pediatric patients before anesthesia induction in the preoperative[152] or intraoperative area.[52,152]** *[Conditional Recommendation]* **P**

Evidence conflicts as to whether preinduction hypnosis in pediatric patients reduces postoperative anxiety and pain.[52,152]

In an RCT conducted by Duparc-Alegria et al,[152] pediatric patients ages 10 to 18 years who received a 5- to 10-minute preinduction personalized hypnosis imaginary journey (n = 59) had significantly reduced postoperative anxiety compared to patients who received standard care (n = 60). The researchers concluded that preoperative patient interviews conducted to personalize hypnosis imagery and practitioner education regarding hypnosis interventions may decrease postoperative anxiety.

In an RCT of 29 pediatric patients ages 5 to 12 years, Huet et al[52] found those who received hypnosis (n = 14) had significantly lowered anxiety and pain, and significantly more patients rated pain as "no pain" or "mild pain" than those in the control group (n = 15). Though this study was limited to pediatric patients undergoing dental procedures who had low baseline anxiety, the researchers concluded that hypnosis was beneficial.

9. Aromatherapy Interventions

9.1   **Aromatherapy interventions may be combined with other complementary care interventions to reduce pain[43] and nausea severity[44] and increase patient satisfaction.[43]** *[Conditional Recommendation]*

High-quality evidence supports combining citrus essential oil and music to reduce pain and increase patient satisfaction[43] and combining isopropyl alcohol and slow deep breathing to reduce nausea severity.[44]

In an RCT, Nagata et al[43] assigned 224 patients scheduled for screening colonography procedures into one of four groups (n = 56 in each group). The groups received either a combination of music and aromatherapy with citrus bergamia essential oil, the interventions separately, or standard care. Researchers found no significant difference in pain or satisfaction between the groups; however, there were a significant number of requests to use aromatherapy for the next colonography (ie, 67.3% in the group that received both interventions; 72.5% in the group that received aromatherapy alone). The researchers concluded that the intervention might be more beneficial if patients could select the music and aromatherapy scent.

In an RCT conducted by Cronin et al[44] that included female patients undergoing laparoscopic procedures, the patients who experienced nausea in the postoperative recovery setting were taught controlled breathing exercises to perform with (n = 41) or without (n = 41) isopropyl alcohol aromatherapy. The researchers found that nausea severity decreased significantly for both groups. Even though there were inconsistencies in the implementation and outcome evaluation (ie, a verbal scale difficult to use), the researchers concluded that breathing and isopropyl alcohol aromatherapy interventions are inexpensive, self-regulated, and low-risk methods to prevent or reduce PONV.

9.2   **Preoperative aromatherapy interventions may be used for patient anxiety and stress reduction.[153-157]** *[Conditional Recommendation]*

High-quality evidence supports using aromatherapy preoperatively to improve outcomes, including
- reduced self-reported anxiety (lavender[153,155]) and
- improved vital signs and cortisol levels (lavender,[154] lavender essential oil,[156,157] neroli oil[156]).

In an RCT, Trambert et al[153] sought to evaluate the effects of two essential oils on postoperative vital signs and anxiety in 87 women undergoing breast biopsy procedures. The researchers divided the participants into three groups that received either lavender-sandalwood aromatherapy (n = 30), orange-peppermint aromatherapy (n = 30), or a placebo (n = 27). The intervention was performed in the preoperative setting for an average of 64 minutes. The researchers found no postoperative changes in vital signs or anxiety in the orange-peppermint group but found a significant decrease in anxiety in the lavender-sandalwood group. They concluded that aromatherapy with lavender-sandalwood was beneficial.

In an RCT, Hosseini et al[154] compared patients who received two drops of lavender in distilled water for inhalation aromatherapy given the morning of surgery (n = 45) with a standard care control group (n = 45). The researchers found a significant decrease in anxiety scores and cortisol levels, as well as a significant correlation between cortisol levels and anxiety scores before and after the intervention. There was a significant improvement of vital signs in both groups, and the researchers found that 10.8% of anxiety changes and 69.9% of cortisol changes were correlated to the intervention in a post hoc analysis.

In an RCT that included 50 patients undergoing gastroscopy procedures, Hoya et al[157] diffused lavender essential oil and played a soothing recording of natural environmental images and sounds (n = 26) in the preoperative area. The intervention was compared with standard care (n = 24). The researchers found that neither the patients' self-reported anxiety nor systolic blood pressure increased significantly before gastroscopy in the intervention group and concluded that the intervention was effective in reducing preoperative anxiety.

In an RCT of 27 patients undergoing colonoscopy procedures, Hu et al[156] compared the effects of a sunflower oil placebo (n = 13) with neroli oil (eg, citrus aurantium, floral scent with citrus overtone) (n = 14) on procedural anxiety. The researchers found significantly lowered postprocedure systolic blood pressure in the intervention group, which also had a significantly higher preoperative systolic blood pressure. The researchers concluded that neroli oil may promote stress reduction and pain relief, though there were not significant improvements in anxiety or pain scores.

In a pilot observational study conducted by Januzel et al,[155] 30 women undergoing breast or axillary procedures received a lavender aromatherapy patch on the mid-sternal area in the preoperative setting, which was removed before transport to the OR. The average time worn was 58.1 minutes. Though there was no significant change in the patients' vital signs, the researchers found a significant decrease in preoperative anxiety scores after patients wore the patch for 15 minutes.

9.3 **Postoperative aromatherapy interventions may be used for anxiety, pain, and nausea reduction.**[1,9,21,158-161]
[Conditional Recommendation]

High-quality evidence[158-161] and guidelines[1,21] support the postoperative use and cost-effectiveness[9] of aromatherapy interventions to reduce anxiety[160] and pain.[159] High-quality evidence conflicts on the efficacy of aromatherapy interventions to reduce patients' experience of and incidence of PONV.[9,158]

In a systematic review of 60 RCTs (N = 1,326), Asay et al[9] concluded that aromatherapy (ie, peppermint; ginger oils; a combination of lavender, peppermint, ginger, and spearmint oils) is a cost-effective method to alleviate PONV and should be considered for use, even though the researchers found nonsignificant results.

In a Cochrane review of 11 RCTs and five controlled trials (N = 1,036), Hines et al[158] found that aromatherapy (eg, isopropyl alcohol, peppermint oil, ginger, combinations) significantly reduced the patients' requests for rescue antiemetics but was not effective in reducing the patient-reported severity of PONV. The use of isopropyl alcohol aromatherapy significantly decreased nausea by 50% during the study and also significantly reduced rescue antiemetic requirements but produced no difference in patient satisfaction. The researchers concluded that the aromatherapy interventions were beneficial.

Lane et al[161] conducted an RCT of 35 women who underwent cesarean delivery and received either peppermint spirits aromatherapy (n = 22), a placebo of colored water (n = 8), or standard care including antiemetic medication only (n = 5). The researchers found a significantly lower nausea score at 2 and 5 minutes postoperatively in the intervention group. The researchers concluded that aromatherapy was useful for decreasing nausea.

In an RCT, Olapour et al[159] assigned 30 women in labor to receive 5 minutes of lavender aromatherapy when they were dilated at 10 cm and again after the baby was delivered. The researchers found significantly lower pain at 4, 8, and 12 hours with a significant decrease in heart rate and an increase in patient satisfaction compared to a control group (n = 30). The researchers also found a significantly higher use of diclofenac in the control group. The researchers concluded that aromatherapy could be used as an adjunct but not treatment.

Braden et al[160] conducted an RCT to evaluate the effects of lavandin essential oil on preoperative anxiety. The researchers assigned 150 patients to one of three groups: one intervention group received lavandin essential oil in a cotton ball on the upper chest or shoulder of their gown as well as near the pedal pulse point, the second group received jojoba oil as a placebo in the same place, and the third group received standard care (n = 50 in each group). The researchers found that the placebo group reported significantly reduced anxiety; however, the intervention group had significantly higher anxiety at baseline, which may have confounded these results. The researchers concluded that use of lavandin essential oil for aromatherapy is a low-risk and cost-effective way to improve patient outcomes and satisfaction.

10. Acupoint Interventions

10.1 Acupoint interventions may be used in the perioperative environment.[4,7,8,39,47,58,69,162-187] *[Conditional Recommendation]*

10.1.1 Implementation considerations for acupoint interventions may include[162-164,184]
- selecting the delivery method for the specific intervention,[4,7,8,172,182,183]
- reviewing applicable regulations about scope of practice,[7,8,39,172]
- selecting delivery devices and settings,
- determining the length of the intervention, and
- recognizing precautions and warnings, such as
  - skin reactions[39,168,185] and
  - the need for forceful removal in the case of a wristband.[186]

[Conditional Recommendation] **P**

High-quality evidence[162-164] supports that use of acupoint interventions improves both adult and pediatric[164] patient outcomes, including PONV[162,163] and pain.[164]

In a 2015 Cochrane review, Lee et al[162] investigated 59 RCTs that included 7,667 patients, 727 of whom were pediatric patients, for the effect of PC6 (eg, Nei guan inner wrist) acupoint interventions on PONV. The researchers found that perioperative acupoint stimulation interventions (eg, acupressure, acupuncture, electrical acupoint stimulation) significantly decreased the incidence of PONV and patients' requests for antiemetics compared to patients who received sham acupoint stimulation. However, the intervention did not significantly decrease PONV.

The researchers also found that combining acupoint interventions with antiemetic drugs reduced the incidence of vomiting but not of nausea. In this Cochrane review, 14 trials reported adverse events related to acupuncture that were minor, transient, and self-limiting; these included skin irritation, blisters, redness, and pain where the intervention was applied to the patient's body. The researchers concluded that PC6 acupuncture stimulation efficacy was comparable to antiemetic drug use and that more high-quality trials are required to better understand the effects of PC6 acupoint interventions on PONV.[162]

In a systematic review of the efficacy of acupuncture on PONV that included an additional four reviews not included in the 2015 Cochrane review,[162] Yang et al[164] found that acupuncture in general may reduce PONV (N = 1,552 pediatric patients). The researchers concluded that additional high-quality research is warranted based on small sample sizes and methodology limitations of the RCTs included in the review.

Albooghobeish et al[163] conducted an RCT that included 63 patients undergoing strabismus procedures. Patients underwent 60 seconds of either laser acupuncture of acupoint P6 (n = 21) or of acupoints BL10, BL11, and GB34 (n = 21), compared with a control group that received acupuncture of a sham acupoint without laser (n = 21). The acupuncture was applied 15 minutes before anesthesia induction and 15 minutes after admission to the PACU. The researchers found no significant differences between the acupoint groups except that the incidence of emesis at postoperative hours 2 and 24 was reduced in the P6 acupoint intervention group. The researchers concluded that administering acupuncture to the P6 acupoint was more effective.

10.2 When wristbands are used for acupressure interventions, implement measures to prevent adverse events (eg, pressure injury related to intraoperative positioning, risk for burns when electrosurgery is used, skin reactions,[39,168,185] need for forceful removal[186]). *[Recommendation]*

High-quality evidence conflicts on the efficacy[39,186] and safety[168,185] of using wristbands to administer acupressure.

In a meta-analysis of RCTs that included 14 trials of 1,009 women undergoing breast procedures, Sun et al[168] concluded that non-needle stimulation may be used for PONV and that 30 minutes before induction to the end of the surgery seemed to be the most effective time frame. The researchers also concluded that the stimulation wristband was most likely to cause adverse reactions (eg, redness, swelling, tenderness, paresthesia).

Cooke et al[186] conducted a pilot RCT in 2015 in which 80 patients received a beaded acupoint wristband (n = 38) or a placebo wristband with no acupressure (n = 42). Researchers found that use of the wristband was well-tolerated, feasible, and justified. Rescue antiemetic consumption, PONV, and quality of recovery were significantly improved; however, the incidence of adverse events was also high (ie, six wristbands becoming tight, with one requiring forceful removal). The researchers recommended additional research with a larger sample size to prove efficacy of the wristbands.

In an RCT, Majholm and Møller[185] assigned 112 healthy, nonsmoking, female patients to receive either P6 acupressure or sham-point acupressure by a wristband before induction of anesthesia to a

24-hour follow-up interview. One-third of the patients had adverse skin reactions related to the wristband (eg, 40 reported redness, 17 reported swelling, 16 reported tenderness, four reported paresthesias), three of which were removed prematurely (ie, before 24 hours post surgery). The researchers concluded that the specific brand of acupressure wristband used was ineffective for perioperative patient outcomes.

In an RCT conducted by Oh and Kim,[39] 54 female patients who underwent gynecological procedures and wore a relief band postoperatively reported decreased PONV when educated and trained experts implemented postoperative electrical acupoint stimulation.

10.3 **Preoperative acupoint interventions (eg, acupressure, acupuncture, electrical acupoint stimulation) may be used.**[4,47,165,166,184,187] *[Conditional Recommendation]* Ⓟ

The use of preoperative acupoint interventions has been studied for a variety of outcomes and populations.[4,47,165 167,181,184,187] High-quality evidence supports the use of acupressure to reduce both preoperative patient anxiety[4,47,69,165-167] and preoperative parental anxiety.[47] High-quality evidence supports the use of bilateral acupressure before induction of anesthesia to decrease PONV and increase patient satisfaction.[184] High-quality evidence conflicts as to the benefits of placing auricular acupoint that remains in place during general anesthesia.[4,165,166] High-quality evidence supports using preoperative electrical stimulation to reduce postoperative complications (eg, abdominal pain, distention, duration of PACU stay, patient satisfaction, procedure acceptance).[167]

In an RCT, Acar et al[165] found that acupressure on relaxation points on the ear lowered bispectral index system (BIS) reactions, which suggests that the acupuncture intervention benefits are reduced by general anesthesia. Regardless of ear-point tape or needle use, relaxation points may be more beneficial than **traditional Chinese medicine** (TCM) points to reduce anxiety.[4,165]

In an RCT, Valiee et al[187] assigned 70 patients undergoing abdominal surgical procedures to receive either preoperative acupressure (ie, Yintang and Shenmen) or acupressure on two sham points (n = 35 in each group). The researchers found a significant decrease in anxiety scores and a significant decrease in both systolic and diastolic blood pressure after the intervention before surgery. The researchers concluded that acupressure on Yintang and Shenmen acupoints was clinically beneficial to reduce anxiety and blood pressure before abdominal surgery.

In an RCT, 100 patients classified as ASA physical status I and II who were undergoing major laparoscopic procedures received either sham-point (n = 50) or P6 (n = 50) acupressure stimulation bilaterally 30 to 60 minutes before general anesthesia induction.[184] White et al[184] found an overall significant decrease in vomiting from zero to 72 hours in the intervention group (12% versus 30% in the control group). The patients in the intervention group also reported significantly higher satisfaction and quality of postoperative recovery at 48 hours. There were no significant differences in recovery time or return to normal activity between the groups. The researchers concluded that acupressure to P6 combined with antiemetic drugs can reduce the incidence of vomiting among patients who have undergone major laparoscopic procedures.

In an RCT, Wu et al[166] compared acupuncture at four acupoints (ie, Baihui, Four God's Cleverness, Great Rush, Zu san li) (n = 17) to auricular acupuncture (ie, Shenmen) (n = 18) among patients undergoing ambulatory surgical procedures. The researchers found a significant reduction in anxiety scores in both groups but not between the groups. The researchers concluded that both auricular and body acupuncture treatment methods effectively decreased preoperative anxiety in patients.

In a pilot RCT, Wang et al[47] provided 61 parents (ie, one for each pediatric patient) with either 20 minutes of Yintang (n = 28) or sham-point (n = 33) acupuncture before their child's procedure. The researchers found significantly lower anxiety scores in the intervention group, but no significant difference in BIS, heart rate, and arterial blood pressure between the intervention and control groups. The researchers concluded that acupuncture may decrease the anxiety of parents of pediatric patients undergoing surgery.

In an RCT, Wang et al[4] compared responses to auricular acupuncture at different points. In this study, 91 adults with ASA physical status classification of I or II undergoing elective ambulatory surgery received auricular acupuncture at three points for 30 minutes at either TCM points (n = 31), relaxation points (n = 32), or sham/non-anxiety points (n = 27). The researchers found a significant decrease in anxiety scores with relaxation-point acupuncture and a nonsignificant but lower anxiety in the TCM group compared to the control group. The researchers concluded that a 1-minute application of this intervention using the relaxation acupoint technique produced significant improvement. The researchers noted that TCM acupuncture is typically individualized, which was not studied and potentially the reason why there were nonsignificant results for this group.

In an RCT, Chen et al[167] assigned patients with an ASA physical status classification of I or II to receive either 30 minutes of preoperative electrical stimulation on the Jiaji acupoint (n = 114) or a sham point (n = 115) before undergoing an elective colonoscopy procedure. The researchers found significantly lower abdominal pain, distention, and PACU LOS and higher patient satisfaction and acceptance of the procedure in the Jiaji acupoint intervention group. The researchers concluded that the intervention was an effective complementary resource.

10.3.1 **Acupoint interventions that are applied in the preoperative setting, remain in place during the operative or other invasive procedure, and are removed before the patient is transferred to the PACU may be used.**[168,169,181,182] *[Conditional Recommendation]* **P**

Acupuncture in adults[169] and pediatric patients,[181] acupoint stimulation wristbands in adults,[168] and electrical acupoint stimulation in adults[182] can improve nausea,[169,181] PONV,[168,181] and analgesic consumption.[182]

High-quality evidence supports using acupuncture to reduce nausea and PONV in pediatric patient populations,[168,169,181] though the varied techniques used in the studies limit the ability to generalize specific techniques to other patient populations. The evidence conflicts on whether electrical acupoint stimulation is beneficial;[168,181] one study showed no improvement in emergence agitation, length of PACU stay, or postoperative pain with electrical stimulation of acupoint H7 in pediatric patients.[181]

In a meta-analysis of RCTs that included 14 trials of 1,009 women undergoing breast procedures, Sun et al[168] concluded that non-needle stimulation may be used for PONV and that 30 minutes before induction to the end of the surgery seemed to be the most effective time frame. The researchers also concluded that the stimulation wristband was most likely to cause adverse reactions (eg, redness, swelling, tenderness, paresthesia).

In an RCT, Martin et al[169] assigned 161 pediatric patients ages 3 to 9 years to receive either bilateral P6 acupuncture and antiemetics (n = 86) or antiemetics only (n = 75). The researchers found significantly lower nausea in phase I and II recovery in the acupuncture group, but no difference was found at the final measurement (ie, 24 hours). The study was discontinued after interim analysis because the significant benefit of the intervention was evident. The researchers did not assess the potential effect of the duration of the intervention, which was placed and removed under anesthesia intraoperatively. Other limitations include that the quantity and frequency of the opioids used was not included.

In an RCT conducted by Nakamura et al,[181] pediatric patients ages 18 to 95 months received unilateral electrical acupoint stimulation of the H7 acupoint on the patient's right side at 1 Hz 50 mA throughout the procedure (n = 50) compared to a control group (n = 50). The researchers found no difference in pediatric anesthesia emergence delirium, emergence agitation, emergence agitation severity, PACU LOS, or postoperative pain between the intervention group and control groups; however, the study was underpowered, as the incidence of emergence anesthesia in the control group was low.

In an RCT conducted by Huang et al,[182] 80 adult patients in four groups of patients (n = 20 in each group) undergoing video-assisted thoracic surgical lobectomy procedures received different frequencies (ie, 2 Hz, 100 Hz, intermittent between 2 and 100 Hz, control at 0 Hz) of electrical acupoint stimulation on the same four acupoints (ie, Nei guan, Hegu, Lieque, Quchi) beginning 30 minutes before surgery, throughout the procedure, and during postoperative 30-minute sessions at 24 and 48 hours. The researchers found significantly lower opioid use and a decrease in intraoperative one-lung arterial oxygen partial pressure as well as lower PONV scores, a shorter time to extubation, and shorter PACU LOS when stimulation was set to intermittently change between 2 Hz and 100 Hz.

10.4 **Acupoint interventions may be used in the intraoperative phase of care.**[170,171] *[Conditional Recommendation]*

High-quality evidence supports the intraoperative use of electrical acupoint stimulation (ie, unilateral P6, bilateral P6) to reduce the incidence of PONV in women undergoing operative and other invasive procedures.[170,171] In contrast, other high-quality studies suggest that interoperative acupoint interventions are not effective and the costs may outweigh the benefits.[168,181]

In an RCT conducted by Carr et al,[170] 56 women received antiemetics either with (n = 26) or without (n = 27) P6 electrical acupoint stimulation intraoperatively during a laparoscopic cholecystectomy. The researchers found significantly lower PONV at PACU admission and at 30 and 60 minutes after PACU admission in patients who received acupuncture. The researchers concluded that the intervention was clinically meaningful but suggested that future research with larger sample sizes is needed.

In a RCT, El-Deeb and Ahmady[171] assigned 450 women undergoing elective cesarean delivery to receive either P6 bilateral electrical acupoint stimulation, placebo with a sham acupoint, or ondansetron only (n = 150 in each group) 30 minutes before spinal anesthesia. The researchers found a significantly lower incidence of nausea and vomiting during and 6 hours after surgery in both the electrical acupoint stimulation and ondansetron groups. Patients who received either acupoint stimulation or ondansetron also reported higher satisfaction than patients in the control group, although there was no significant difference in PONV incidence between postoperative hours 6 to 24. The researchers concluded that electrical acupoint stimulation was comparable to ondansetron for reducing PONV and could also improve patient satisfaction.

In a quasi-experimental pilot study, Wang et al[183] recruited 11 healthy volunteers to undergo S36 acupuncture (ie, anterior and inferior to the knee) during both awake and anesthetized MRI scans. The researchers found that patients' blood oxygen level dependent signals, a neurophysiological response to acupuncture stimulation, were lowered with concurrent use of propofol with general anesthesia. They concluded that additional research is needed to determine whether acupoint stimulation is beneficial with propofol use.

10.5 **Postoperative acupoint interventions may be used.**[7,8,39,58,172-180] *[Conditional Recommendation]* **P**

High-quality evidence supports that acupoint interventions result in a variety of improved outcomes[7,8,39,58,172-180]; however, high variability in study methodology and acupoint interventions was found in these studies.

In a meta-analysis of 14 RCTs (N = 1,653 patients), Chen et al[177] found significantly lower postoperative nausea, antiemetic rescue, dizziness, and pruritus with postoperative electrical acupoint stimulation used on various acupoints after patients underwent procedures with general anesthesia. The researchers concluded that postoperative electrical acupoint stimulation was effective in improving the studied outcomes and that future studies are needed to focus on the effect of spinal anesthesia and cultural biases on the efficacy of postoperative electrical acupoint stimulation.

In a systematic review of 12 trials (N = 1,025 patients), Cho et al[7] found that acupuncture after tonsillectomy significantly decreased pain scores at 4 hours and for the first 48 hours in both pediatric and adult patients (ages 1 to 80 years). Acupuncture also significantly reduced PONV without adverse effects. Analgesic requirements were significantly lower, and the researchers concluded that the intervention was beneficial.

In a systematic review and meta-analysis of 30 RCTs (N = 2,534 patients), Cheong et al[178] found that all acupoint interventions applied to the PC6 acupoint were effective; however, electrical acupoint stimulation with acupressure devices was more effective in reducing PONV than other methods. Electrical acupressure devices used for PONV prevention may be more costly upfront, though they can be reusable.

In an RCT, Yang et al[179] preoperatively assigned patients undergoing gynecological laparoscopic procedures under general anesthesia to receive either dexamethasone alone (n = 50), dexamethasone combined with electrical acupoint stimulation on the Nei guan acupoint at 1 mA/2 Hz (n = 50), or dexamethasone in combination with tropisetron (n = 53). The researchers did not investigate acupoint stimulation alone. The researchers found significantly lower PONV in patients who received acupressure in the first 24 hours compared to dexamethasone alone and nonsignificantly lower PONV in patients who received dexamethasone and tropisetron compared with dexamethasone alone. The researchers concluded that including acupuncture was more beneficial than dexamethasone alone, but had similar results to combining tropisetron with dexamethasone. Even though there was no assessment of patients' request for rescue medication during the first 24 hours, the researchers concluded that acupuncture is a beneficial intervention that can reduce the need for antiemetic medication.

In an RCT, Oh and Kim[39] postoperatively assigned 54 patients who had undergone gynecological procedures (eg, hysterectomy, ovarian cystectomy) to receive either a button wristband that put pressure on the Nei guan acupoint, a relief band with electrical acupoint stimulation to the Nei guan acupoint, or standard care (n = 18 in each group). The researchers concluded that the relief band reduced PONV in women undergoing gynecological procedures when an educated and trained researcher implemented the electrical acupoint stimulation.

In an RCT, Feng et al[173] assigned 150 patients undergoing TKA procedures who were identified as being at high-risk for PONV to receive either auricular acupressure (eg, Shenmen, Point Zero, Subcortex point) (n = 50), acupressure on a sham point (ie, tape with pellets 5 mm from the acupressure point) (n = 47), or a placebo (ie, tape without pellets) (n = 53) in the immediate postoperative period. The researchers found a significantly higher nausea incidence in the placebo group compared with either the acupressure group or the sham-point group. However, differences among all groups for episodes of emesis and recovery time were not significant. The researchers concluded that though nausea measurement is subjective, there was a significant decrease in nausea in the recovery area and at 24 hours post surgery in the acupressure intervention groups.

In an RCT, He et al[174] used **vaccaria seeds** to apply auricular acupressure including the Knee Joint, Shenmen, Subcortex, and Sympathesis points for 45 patients and to four non-acupuncture points for 45 patients undergoing TKA. The researchers found significantly lower pain scores on POD 3, 4, 5, and 7. There was also significantly lower analgesic consumption, fewer adverse events, and significantly higher scores on the Hospital for Special Surgery Knee Scoring System (eg, pain, function, ROM, muscle strength, flexion deformity, instability, subtractions), indicating higher function, at 2 weeks after surgery. The researchers concluded that the intervention was easy to apply, inexpensive, and safe to decrease pain and opioid use and facilitate early rehabilitation.

In an RCT conducted by Chang et al,[175] 62 patients undergoing TKA procedures received three sessions each of auricular acupressure (n = 31) or sham acupressure (ie, tape applied without acupressure) (n = 31) over 3 days. The researchers found a significant decrease in morphine consumption and significant increase in ROM on POD 3 for the intervention group compared with the sham group. They concluded that auricular acupressure interventions can reduce opioid analgesic consumption and improve passive ROM.

In an RCT conducted by Quinlan-Woodward et al,[8] 30 female patients with breast cancer received an average of 36 minutes of acupuncture (n = 15) compared to no acupuncture as a control (n = 15). Participants in the intervention group were significantly younger (mean difference 53.7 versus 62.5 years), and the researchers reported that differences in age may affect acceptance and efficacy of acupuncture. The researchers found a significant reduction in pain, anxiety, and nausea and an increase in coping on POD 1 and pain on POD 2 in the acupuncture group. They concluded that acupuncture could be used as a nonpharmacologic intervention, although further research is needed to determine a standard of care for the intervention.

In an RCT, Zhan and Tian[180] assigned 90 patients to receive either a transversus abdominis plane block with electrical acupoint stimulation (eg, 2 to 100 Hz at the Zusanli ST 36 and Nei guan acupoints), acupuncture (ie, at the Nei guan acupoint), or standard care after open abdominal procedures (n = 30 in each group). The researchers found pain scores decreased significantly at postoperative hours 24 and 48, with significantly lower adverse reactions and hemodynamic effects in the group that received

electrical acupoint stimulation. The researchers concluded that electrical acupoint stimulation is an ideal complementary postoperative analgesic strategy.

In an RCT, 18 female patients with cancer who were undergoing open gynecological procedures received either four treatments of acupuncture percutaneous electrical nerve stimulation (PENS) (ie, electrical acupoint stimulation, SP6 and SP8) (n = 9) or traditional acupuncture (ie, no electrical stimulation) at the same points (n = 9).[176] Gavronsky et al[176] found that pain relief was equivalent between the two groups; however, the patients in the PENS group had less pain from hours 24 to 48; at 48 hours there was no difference between the groups. Limitations include that the researchers did not measure opiate consumption, which could also affect bowel motility.

In an RCT, Lili et al[58] assigned patients age 60 years or older undergoing GI procedures to receive either electrical acupoint stimulation for 2 minutes every postoperative day through POD 5 (n = 20) or standard care (n = 20). The researchers found significant improvement for the intervention group in gastrin levels on POD 3 and 5 and motilin levels on POD 3, shorter time to flatus, and a lower incidence of complications (ie, abdominal pain, distention, diarrhea), as well as higher electrocardiogram frequency and amplitude on POD 5, which correlated with gastrin levels and contraction of GI muscles. The researchers concluded that acupuncture stimulation promoted GI function recovery and may decrease complications efficiently and painlessly in older adult patients.

11. Massage and Reflexology Interventions

11.1 **Massage and reflexology interventions may be used.**[188] *[Conditional Recommendation]*

Various massage (eg, general, hand, foot, back) and reflexology techniques are described in the literature, with no one technique determined to be superior.

A feasibility RCT conducted by Rosen et al[188] supports that massage interventions may decrease anxiety when used in both the preoperative and postoperative setting. Patients with cancer who were undergoing port placement received 20 minutes of massage (n = 40) or 20 minutes of structured attention (n = 20) pre- and postoperatively. The researchers found a significant decrease in anxiety in the massage intervention group after the first intervention and after adjusting for patients' baseline mean anxiety. There was also a significant decrease in pain after the procedure and on POD 1 in the massage intervention group.

11.2 Preoperative massage and reflexology interventions may be used.[189,190] [Conditional Recommendation]

High-quality evidence supports using preoperative massage to reduce pain,[189] stress,[189] and anxiety[189,190] for patients undergoing various procedures. Researchers found that compared to standard care, massage (ie, for older adults undergoing cardiovascular procedures)[190] and hand massage (ie, for women undergoing ambulatory procedures)[189] significantly decreased patients' preoperative anxiety.

In a pilot RCT, Wentworth et al[190] assigned 130 patients undergoing cardiovascular procedures (eg, radiofrequency ablation, angiogram, angiopercutaneous coronary intervention, permanent pacemaker, implantable cardioverter defibrillator) to receive either a preoperative massage (n = 64) or standard care (n = 66) for 20 to 30 minutes. The researchers found a significant decrease in pain, tension, and anxiety between the groups after adjusting for age, with a significant increase in patient satisfaction for those who received the massage. The researchers found that participants in the intervention group were significantly older (67.6 versus 59.7 years), which may influence the conclusions. A limitation of the study was that patients were not blinded to their intervention. The researchers recommended that future studies use a control match for the length of the massage and include objective outcomes.

In a quasi-experimental study, 86 female patients undergoing ambulatory procedures (eg, orthopedic, cataract, cystoscopy, colonoscopy) received preoperative hand massages performed with the room lights dimmed before attempted IV starts.[189] Brand et al[189] found that hand massages significantly lowered the patients' anxiety before surgery. They also found a significant decrease in anxiety and easier IV starts after massage. They concluded that the intervention was easy to implement and did not affect the flow or timing of the surgery. The researchers suggested that future studies evaluate vital signs and control for the patient's biological sex, family presence, and the scheduled procedure.

11.3 Intraoperative massage and reflexology interventions may be used for patients undergoing awake procedures.[5,46,191] [Conditional Recommendation]

The benefits of using intraoperative massage and reflexology interventions may outweigh the cost of implementation (eg, additional personnel, time, supplies). Intraoperative massage and reflexology interventions can reduce anxiety,[46,191] pain,[5] and vital signs.[46]

High-quality evidence indicates that intraoperative reflexology significantly lowers patients' anxiety and pain perception during varicose vein procedures.[5,46,191] Moderate-quality evidence indicates that general hand massage lowers patients' systolic blood pressure during percutaneous vertebroplasty procedures.[46] However, the evidence conflicts on whether massage significantly decreases pain and increases patient satisfaction.[46,191] Combining handholding with providing verbal step-by-step procedural information throughout the procedure was found to significantly lower anxiety for highly anxious patients but may not benefit all awake patients.[46]

In an RCT, Hudson et al[191] assigned 100 patients (ie, 83 women, 17 men) to receive either intraoperative hand reflexology (n = 50) or standard care (n = 50) during varicose vein procedures performed under local-only anesthesia. The researchers found significantly lower anxiety and shorter pain duration in patients who received the intervention compared to standard care; however, pain and patient satisfaction were not significantly improved.

In an RCT, Dolatian et al[5] assigned 120 women with low-risk pregnancies to one of three groups: 40 minutes of foot reflexology when the patient reached 4 cm to 5 cm cervical dilation during labor, emotional support, or standard care. The patients who received reflexology had significantly lower pain after the intervention, at 6 to 7 cm, and at 8 to 10 cm cervical dilation during labor, whereas emotional support did not significantly lower pain in the stages above 5-cm dilation. Although there was no standard massage technique, the researchers concluded that massage could benefit women in labor.

In a quasi-nonequivalent controlled trial conducted by Kim et al,[46] patients received handholding and information sharing (n = 30), handholding alone (n = 34), or standard care (n = 30) during percutaneous vertebroplasty procedures. The researchers found a significant decrease in systolic blood pressure in the control group, and a significant decrease in anxiety scores in both intervention groups. The researchers concluded that the intervention promotes the relationship between the patient and nurse (ie, qualitative patient responses included feeling supported and encouraged when provided with procedural information and handholding).

11.4 Postoperative massage and reflexology interventions may be used.[42,192-195] [Conditional Recommendation]

Postoperative massage and reflexology interventions can decrease anxiety,[42,192,194,195] decrease pain,[42,192,193] improve vital signs,[42] and increase patient satisfaction.[192]

High-quality evidence supports using massage techniques in the postoperative setting to improve the patient's response to pain and anxiety and to improve vital signs in the postoperative phase of care.[42,192-195] The researchers in these studies concluded that massage interventions can improve patient experiences; however, they also concluded that additional research is required to address limitations identified in these studies and understand generalizability among perioperative patients.[42,192-195]

Postoperative reflexology may reduce patients' anxiety; however, researchers report a lack of standardization in research methodologies, limiting the ability to generalize results to all patients in the postoperative setting.[194,195] Researchers have concluded that the benefits of massage may have been confounded with benefits of other complementary care interventions that were implemented simultaneously. For example, in one study, researchers found postoperative massage to be beneficial, but the intervention was combined with relaxation techniques.[42] In another study, the researchers had no control of the effects of the external environment during the intervention, which limited their ability to generalize findings about postoperative massage interventions.[192]

In an RCT conducted by Büyükyılmaz and Aştı,[42,30] patients participated in relaxation techniques (ie, breathing, exercises, and music for 30 minutes) and received a back massage (10 minutes lateral lying with lanolin oil) on POD 1 to 3 after total joint procedures. There was a significant decrease in pain intensity, anxiety, and vital signs for patients in the intervention group compared to patients in a control group (n = 30). Limitations of the study include that two interventions were studied without a way to measure the effects of each intervention independently. The researchers concluded that the combination of interventions was effective.

In a pilot RCT, Alameri et al[192] assigned 31 patients in the cardiac ICU after undergoing elective cardiac procedures to receive either a 10-minute foot massage (n = 16) or a 10-minute placebo hand massage (ie, handholding without massage technique) (n = 15). The researchers found a significant decrease in pain intensity and anxiety in the foot massage group compared to the placebo group. Even with a small sample size and potentially confounding variables, the researchers concluded that foot massage is a safe, inexpensive, nonpharmacological intervention that can reduce pain and anxiety.

In a quasi-experimental study, Ucuzal and Kanan[193] assigned patients undergoing breast procedures to receive either a foot massage (n = 35) or analgesics alone (n = 35). The researchers found a significant decrease in pain and improvement of blood pressure and heart rate in the foot massage intervention group but found no significant decrease in respiratory rate between the groups. The researchers found an increase in all the control group participants' vital signs except heart rate. They concluded that foot massages were effective in decreasing pain and that foot massage should be offered.

In an RCT conducted by Bagheri-Nesami et al,[194] 80 patients undergoing coronary artery bypass grafting were matched for age and biological sex then randomly assigned either left-foot 20-minute reflexology for POD 1 to 4 (n = 40) or a gentle 1-minute foot rub (n = 40). The researchers found a significant decrease in anxiety in the group that received reflexology. Variable intervention lengths were not controlled, which limited the researchers' conclusion that reflexology can reduce postoperative anxiety.

In an RCT conducted by Molavi Vardanjani et al,[195] male patients received either a 30-minute foot stimulation of three different reflexology points (n = 50) or a general foot massage (n = 50) on POD 1 after undergoing coronary angiography procedures. The researchers found a significant decrease in anxiety for both groups, with a significantly higher anxiety reduction in the reflexology group. The researchers found that reflexology significantly accounted for 7.5% of the patients' anxiety reduction. Even though the researchers reported a lack of methodological consistency, they recommended implementing two or more postoperative reflexology sessions.

11.5 **Individuals who are trained in specific massage and reflexology interventions may use these techniques.**[42,46,189,190,192,193,196] *[Conditional Recommendation]*

Having educated and trained personnel perform massage or reflexology interventions facilitates consistent knowledge and skills and may be regulated by the scope of practice according to local, state, and federal rules and regulations. This may include education, training, licensure, and certification.[196] If a state does not have reflexology-specific laws, personnel may be exempt or fall within the scope of massage laws.[196] Several researchers described the education and training of the personnel who performed the massage intervention, including certification[190,193] and training of research staff by a certified massage therapist.[42,46,189,192]

12. Electrical Stimulation Interventions

12.1 **Postoperative pulsed electromagnetic field (PEMF) interventions may be used.**[63,197-204] *[Conditional Recommendation]*

High-quality evidence supports the use of PEMF interventions to improve incision healing[198,201] and improve mental[197] and physical recovery.[63,197,199,200] However, the evidence conflicts on the benefits of PEMF interventions in reducing postoperative pain[198,201-204] and analgesic consumption.[198,202,203] Researchers in two studies found no improvement in pain reduction.[203,204] However, they suggested that using the patients' opposite side as their own control placebo potentially did not allow for the condition of both sides to be measured separately, if electrical stimulation transferred to the placebo side.[203,204]

In a meta-analysis, Akhter et al[63] included seven RCTs of 941 spinal fusion patients receiving postoperative electrical stimulus compared with a placebo. A postoperative PEMF intervention significantly increased the chances of a successful fusion by 2.5 times in this patient population. The researchers concluded there is moderate-quality support for using this intervention adjunctively for spinal fusion surgeries, and additional research is required to determine whether the patient's age and treatment effect outcomes, as well as measure the effect of the intervention on patient's pain and function.

In an RCT that was not included in the previously discussed meta-analysis,[63] Collarile et al[197] provided 30 patients who had undergone knee procedures with biophysical stimulation with a PEMF intervention for 4 hours every day for 60 days. Patients who received the intervention had a significant improvement in International Knee Documentation Committee Subjective Knee Form (IKDC) scores (ie, knee-specific patient reported outcome measures for subjective knee complaints affecting daily activities with varying score parameters) from 6 months to 60 months and a significant improvement at 60 months in disability and quality of life scores. The researchers also found a significant decrease in pain at 1, 2, and 60 months. They concluded that the PEMF intervention improved clinical outcomes.

In an RCT, Khooshideh et al[198] randomly assigned patients who underwent a cesarean delivery to either an intervention group that received a postoperative PEMF intervention (n = 36) or a control group (n = 36). The intervention group had significantly lower pain scores, fewer reports of severe pain at 24 hours, 1.9 times lower analgesic consumption, lower total doses of analgesics during POD 1 to 7, and significantly better incision healing at POD 7 than patients in the control group. The researchers concluded that lower amounts of exudate and edema increased patient satisfaction in addition to these benefits.

In an RCT, Osti et al[199] assigned patients to receive either a PEMF intervention (n = 32) or a pla-cebo (n = 34) after arthroscopic rotator cuff repair procedures. The researchers found that the intervention group had significant improvement in ROM scores and UCLA scores (ie, pain, function, active forward flexion, strength of forward flexion, patient satisfaction). The researchers concluded that the intervention was safe and reduced pain, analgesic consumption, and stiffness in short-term recovery. Limitations of the study methodology included a delay in providing the intervention (ie, it was not done immediately after surgery), no postoperative objective assessment of improvement (eg, MRI), and no cost analysis of the PEMF intervention.

In an RCT, Osti et al[200] assigned patients undergoing arthroscopic knee microfracture repair procedures to receive either a PEMF intervention (n = 34) or a placebo intervention (n = 34) 6 hours a day for 60 days. The researchers found significant improvement in both groups from baseline to 2 years and significant improvement in IKDC scores (eg, knee symptoms, function, sports activities) and Lysholm improvements (ie, 8 sections of common knee complaints for a total out of 100 points and a visual scale for pain related to each knee). At 5 years, a larger percentage of patients in the PEMF intervention group were still active at their preoperative level (82% compared to 68% in the placebo group). The study was limited by subjective outcomes to evaluate the quality of the repair. The researchers concluded that PEMF application can improve the effectiveness of microfracture repair in the long term.

In an RCT of patients undergoing dental molar extraction procedures, Stocchero et al[201] found significantly fewer incidents of dehiscence and decreased pain scores for patients who received a PEMF intervention (n = 38) compared with those who received a placebo (n = 38) and a control group (n = 38). The researchers also found a significant relationship between pain scores and the length of the intervention or medication (ie, NSAIDs). Though the difficulty of extraction and tooth sectioning may have confounded the results of this study, the researchers concluded that the PEMF intervention improved soft tissue healing and has the potential to be used for pain management in the future.

In an RCT of 32 patients undergoing breast reconstruction procedures, patients who received a PEMF intervention (n = 16) reported significantly lower pain at postoperative hours 6, 12, 24, 48, and 72 compared with a group that received the device but with no electromagnetic field initiated (n = 16).[202] Rhode et al[202] also found a significant decrease in overall narcotic use, interleukin-1b (ie, an inflammatory cytokine associated with pain hypersensitivity) concentration in wound exudate, and exudate volume at 24 hours in the intervention group. The researchers concluded that a PEMF intervention can positively affect the speed and quality of wound repair.

In an RCT of 49 healthy women who underwent elective cosmetic breast augmentation procedures, Svaerdborg et al[203] found no difference in pain scores or medication consumption through POD 7 when a PEMF device was placed intraoperatively to cover each breast implant incision immediately after skin closure and dressing application.

In an RCT of 11 patients undergoing oral surgical procedures, Menini et al[204] applied a PEMF device to both sides of the patient's face immediately after skin closure and dressing application but only activated the device on one cheek so the opposite side would act as a self-control. After 48 hours, there were no significant differences in swelling or pain scores, though the researchers concluded that the active benefits of the PEMF intervention may carry across to the other cheek related to their proximity. The researchers also did not account for the level of disease in each cheek and concluded that additional trials in more invasive surgeries should be studied.

12.2 **Transcutaneous electrical nerve stimulation (TENS) interventions may be used in the preoperative and postoperative periods for patients who have undergone thoracic[61,205] or total joint procedures.[96,206]** *[Conditional Recommendation]*

Outcomes improved by TENS interventions include decreased analgesic consumption, pain, and systolic blood pressure[61] when used preoperatively and decreased anxiety[206] and pain[96,205,206] and increased ROM[206] when used postoperatively.[205,206]

High-quality evidence supports the use of TENS to improve postoperative outcomes in several patient populations,[96,206] including patients undergoing thoracic[61,205] and TKA procedures.[206] Researchers in two RCTs found a significant decrease in pain after TENS was applied postoperatively for 30 minutes at 85 Hz/180 us pulse width,[61] for 20 minutes at 150 pps/150 us pulse duration,[206] and pre-procedurally at 80 Hz for 45 minutes.[61] Systolic blood pressure improved with diclofenac administration and TENS application after chest tube removal.[61]

In an RCT, 40 patients undergoing thoracic procedures received TENS (n = 20) compared with a control group (n = 20).[205] Erden and Senol Celik[205] found significantly lower pain and analgesic consumption in the intervention group and concluded that TENS was an easy and reliable analgesic method.

In an RCT conducted by Rakel et al,[206] patients who underwent TKA procedures received TENS 1 to 2 times per day (n = 122) compared with a placebo (n = 123) or standard care (n = 72). The researchers found significantly lower pain during active knee extension and fast walking and significantly lower anxiety and greater pain reduction during ROM exercises at 6 weeks in the intervention group. Patients in the TENS and placebo groups had significantly lower hyperalgesia compared with the control group. The researchers concluded that there was a placebo influence, and that the benefits of the intervention were reduced after 6 weeks. However, they also concluded that the patient's anxiety and pain reduction increased the overall benefit of using this intervention. Additional research may include potential tolerance buildup to the TENS effect and measurements for long-term results, general pain, and influence of ethnic diversity.

In an RCT, Chandra et al[61] compared patients who received diclofenac combined with 45 minutes of TENS while undergoing a pleurodesis procedure (n = 30) to a control group (n = 30). The researchers found significantly lower systolic blood pressure and pain scores at postoperative hours 4, 6, and 8 in the intervention group. The researchers also found that additional diclofenac dose requests were significantly lower in the intervention group. The researchers concluded that TENS may be used as an adjunct treatment to reduce postoperative pain.

12.3 **Postoperative brain stimulation interventions (eg, transcranial direct current stimulation [tDCS],[207] noninvasive interactive neurostimulation [NIN][208]) may be implemented after TKA procedures.** *[Conditional Recommendation]*

The benefits of postoperative brain stimulation may include increased ROM among patients who have undergone total hip and knee procedures[208] and decreased pain[208] and opioid analgesic consumption.[207]

High-quality evidence supports that using tDCS in TKA procedures decreases opioid use without increasing adverse events.[207] High-quality evidence also supports that the use of NIN after TKA procedures may decrease pain and increase ROM.[208]

In an RCT conducted by Borckardt et al,[207] patients undergoing TKA received standard care (n = 20) or 20 minutes of tDCS (ie, stimulation applied under the scalp dermis) in the PACU, 4 hours later, and in the morning and afternoon of POD 1, for 80 total minutes (n = 20). The researchers found significantly lower opioid use in the intervention group, though there was no subjective measurement of patients' mood or pain to confirm this outcome.

In an RCT, Nigam et al[208] assigned patients to receive either NIN (ie, TENS applied directly to the scalp only) (n = 28) or standard care (n = 30) after undergoing TKA procedures. The researchers found a significant decrease in pain and increase in ROM in the intervention group. There was a greater baseline ROM deficit in the intervention group, and the final difference was nonsignificant, indicating a larger increase in ROM is clinically significant. The researchers concluded that there was clear benefit of NIN, though limitations of the study include varied intervention lengths and the potential that NSAID consumption may have influenced study outcomes by further reducing swelling and pain results.

13. Biofield Interventions

13.1 Biofield interventions (eg, Reiki, healing touch therapy, therapeutic touch, energy field work) may be used in the perioperative environment.[6,209-214] *[Conditional Recommendation]*

The results of studies of perioperative patients indicate that the benefits of using biofield interventions may outweigh potential harms.[6,209-213] In one review of literature, the authors concluded that qigong (ie, regulation of breath rhythm and pattern, body movement and posture, meditation mind-body exercises) may aid in managing stress and emotion, strengthen respiratory muscles, reduce inflammation, and enhance the immune system in the older adult population,[214] and this intervention might also benefit perioperative patients.

Evidence indicates that there is low risk of patient harm when practitioners are trained and certified to perform biofield interventions.[6,209-214]

13.2 Reiki interventions may be used preoperatively and intraoperatively for anxiety and pain reduction.[6,209,210] *[Conditional Recommendation]*

High-quality evidence supports the use of Reiki interventions to reduce preoperative anxiety[209] and to reduce preoperative pain and pain on POD 1 to 3[6,209] in patients undergoing breast and joint procedures. Moderate-quality evidence is inconclusive about whether Reiki is associated with a reduction in intraoperative medication consumption[6,210] and decreased pain in the PACU.[6]

In a systematic review of 12 studies on the effect of Reiki interventions on pain and anxiety in patients undergoing noninvasive, invasive, and operative procedures, Thrane and Cohen[209] found there was a large effect size in anxiety reduction in patients undergoing breast biopsy procedures. The researchers concluded that Reiki may be effective in reducing patient pain and anxiety.

In an RCT pilot conducted by Notte et al,[6] patients undergoing TKA received either five Reiki sessions including 20 minutes of Reiki before surgery, 30 minutes in the PACU after their admission assessment, and 20 minutes on POD 1 to 3 (n = 23) or standard care (n = 20). The researchers found a significant decrease in preoperative pain and a significant decrease in pain on POD 1 to 3 in the Reiki group. Even with variations in the intervention that included the use of relaxing music during Reiki therapy and differences in Reiki technique, the researchers concluded that Reiki was beneficial.

In a quasi-experimental cohort comparison study, Bourque et al[210] evaluated the effect of Reiki delivered during colonoscopy on opioid consumption. Twenty-five patients received 10 minutes of Reiki during the procedure compared with 5 patients who received a placebo Reiki intervention and a control group that received standard care (n = 30). Although there was no significant difference in total meperidine administration, 16% of those patients who received Reiki received less than 50 mg of meperidine, whereas every patient in the control group received more than 50 mg. The researchers concluded that additional research is needed to determine the efficacy of Reiki interventions to reduce opioid consumption.

13.3 Perioperative healing touch interventions may be used.[211,215] *[Conditional Recommendation]*

High-quality evidence supports preoperative healing touch interventions as a method to reduce postoperative anxiety.[211,215]

In an RCT conducted by Goldberg et al,[211] women received magnetic clearing, a healing touch therapy intervention, 15 minutes before undergoing a breast biopsy procedure (n = 42) compared with a control group (n = 31). The researchers found a significant decrease in anxiety on POD 1 and trait anxiety post intervention compared to POD 1, as well as a significant decrease in scores for emotional and spiritual coping. Even though there is a potential bias related to studying the effect of only one healer in this study, the researchers concluded that the intervention may reduce anxiety.

In an RCT, MacIntyre et al[215] assigned patients undergoing coronary artery bypass grafting procedures to receive either healing touch from one of two certified healing touch providers (n = 99), a visit from a volunteer (n = 94), or standard care (n = 97). For the intervention groups, a certified healing touch provider or a volunteer visited each patient the day before and the day after surgery for 20 to 60 minutes and immediately before surgery for 60 to 90 minutes. Preoperative anxiety in both inpatients and outpatients and LOHS in outpatients were significantly reduced in the healing touch group. The researchers estimated that a $500,000 reduction in cost related to LOHS in this sample population offset the cost of hiring an experienced, certified healing touch provider. The researchers concluded that healing touch was a beneficial complementary intervention that warrants further research.

13.4 **Postoperative biofield interventions (eg, therapeutic touch,[212] energy field work[213]) may be used.** [Conditional Recommendation]

High-quality evidence supports using biofield interventions to reduce postoperative pain and increase participation with postoperative occupational therapy.[213] Moderate-quality evidence supports reduction of pain and improved biobehavioral stress markers with the use of therapeutic touch for patients who have undergone vascular procedures.[212]

In an RCT, McCormack[213] assigned 90 older adult postoperative patients to receive either energy field work for 10 minutes by a trained occupational therapy student, a metronome comparison (ie, an audible, rhythmic sound that can elicit a relaxation response), or standard care as a control (n = 30 in each group). The researchers found a significant decrease in pain and better participation with postoperative occupational therapy in the group that received energy field work. Though the study did not use a certified noncontact therapeutic touch practitioner, the researcher concluded that the intervention was beneficial.

In a quasi-experimental study, Bulette Coakley and Duffy[212] assigned 21 postoperative patients to either a group that received a **Krieger's therapeutic touch intervention** (n = 12) or a control group (n = 9). The researchers found significantly lower subjective pain as well as lower levels of cortisol and higher natural killer cells in the intervention group but determined that additional research is needed.

14. Education

14.1 **Health care organizations should design and implement complementary care intervention education for perioperative team members specific to perioperative complementary care interventions used in the organization.[9,25]** [Recommendation]

14.2 **Provide education, training, and supervised practice to personnel before implementing specific complementary care interventions (eg, interactive music therapy, hypnosis).[27,147,148]** [Recommendation] **P**

Low-quality evidence supports utilizing providers with suitable education, training, and supervised practice.[147,148]

Chandrasegaran[147] described that unintentional use of triggering suggestions during hypnosis to facilitate anesthesia induction in the OR increased anxiety in a previously hypnosis-relaxed patient. After hypnosis, as the patient was being wheeled into the OR, a member of the care team said "you are being wheeled [into the] OR now, but you don't have to worry, as you are in safe hands of doctors and nurses here, you can remain to be relaxed and enjoy your favorite safe place. If you feel cold, it is just the coldness of the operating room, which will be a signal for you to relax more and you could imagine hugging or wrapping yourself in a warm blanket."[147(p296)] At the mention of the OR and feeling cold, the patient began frowning and shivering and refused surgery. The anxiety induced by inadvertent use of the triggering suggestion was prohibitive to induction of general anesthesia and the procedure was cancelled. Trained professionals facilitate the optimal use of hypnosis interventions and lower the risk of adverse events related to triggering suggestions.

In an expert opinion article, Kuttner[148] described perianesthesia hypnosis techniques used for pediatric patients as either a patient-directed or a "magic glove" technique, and noted that education and supervised practice is required for both. For the patient-directed hypnosis technique, patients are invited to imagine that they are in their favorite place during the preoperative period and then can be reminded to visit their favorite place in the PACU. Health care workers are encouraged to gently touch the patient's shoulder when they recognize that the patient is experiencing discomfort in the hypnotic state. The magic glove is a quick technique to decrease perianesthesia pain and anxiety in which the patient is instructed to put on an imaginary glove that protects his or her hand (eg, the one in which IV insertion will be attempted). A hypnotic trance develops as the patient is guided to experience lower pain sensation in the gloved hand, including during the procedure. In the preoperative and postoperative setting, positive language and comfort-enhancing communication promotes hypnosis. The author concluded that though education is required, hypnosis promotes a positive experience for patients undergoing anesthetic procedures.

14.3 **Provide safety education and resources to health care workers who care for patients receiving complementary care interventions.[9,16,25,160]** [Recommendation]

High-quality evidence supports providing health care workers with education,[9,25] to develop and deliver efficient and safe complementary care interventions.[25] In a systematic review of the effect of aromatherapy on PONV, researchers concluded that inconsistent education led to inconsistent implementation and realized benefits of aromatherapy interventions.[9] In another systematic review regarding preoperative counseling, researchers concluded that health care workers' education should focus on developing and delivering complementary care interventions to substantiate the claims of an intervention's efficacy.[25] Braden et al[160] recommended that nurses collaborate with certified aromatherapists to develop safe protocols for the use of essential oils in their practice. The researchers concluded that to increase safety when using essential oils, the health care organization should provide education on suppliers, patch testing, plan of care application, safety data sheets, and fire safety.

Including members of the interdisciplinary team who will be involved in the care of patients receiving complementary care in the design and implementation of education facilitates interdisciplinary implementation of the interventions. For example, changes in dietary and herbal intervention timing parameters may confuse personnel and create unnecessary delays if nursing departments, preoperative nurses, and anesthesia providers are not all aware of the changes.[16]

14.4 Maintain records of health care personnel education and competency verification related to complementary care interventions that are used in the organization.[23,216,217] *[Recommendation]*

Many complementary care interventions can be implemented independently by nurses; however, the nature of the interventions requires collaboration with other caregivers and taking into account their interventions as well as the patients' current or desired lifestyle practices.[23,216,217]

14.5 Maintain records of current licensure and certification that are required for practitioners of certain complementary care interventions by local, state, and federal regulations.[23,216,217] *[Recommendation]*

Some complementary care interventions (eg, hypnosis, biofield interventions, aromatherapy, physical therapy, acupoint, massage, reflexology) may require education and certification in addition to nursing licensure and perioperative training for health care workers who care for perioperative patients.[23,216,217]

15. Policies and Procedures

15.1 Develop and review policies and procedures for complementary care interventions that will be used in the health care organization. Policies should include

- local, state, and federal regulations (eg, safety practices);
- required education, certification, or licensure for health care personnel implementing complementary care interventions;
- a method for obtaining informed consent for complementary care interventions;
- clinical documentation requirements (eg, informed consent, patient assessment, response to interventions);
- a method for obtaining orders, when required; and
- which tools will be used in the organization for assessment of patients receiving complementary care interventions.

[Recommendation]

Glossary

Acupuncture: Use of sharp, thin needles that are inserted at specific acupoints of the patient's body that are believed to positively adjust the body's energy flow.

Binaural beat: Use of an auditory phenomenon in which two tones of slightly different frequencies are played in separate ears simultaneously (usually via headphones) so the human brain perceives the creation of a new, third tone, whose frequency is equivalent to the difference between the two tones being played; the tone being perceived can alter brain waves through a process called entrainment, promoting specific states of mind.

Biofield: A complex endogenously generated sphere energy activity and information that surrounds a living system engaged in the generation, maintenance, and regulation of biological homeodynamics and physiological functions of the system it surrounds. The biofield is a massless field, not necessarily electromagnetic, that surrounds and permeates living bodies and affects the body.

Biofield (therapy) interventions: Noninvasive, practitioner-mediated therapies in which the biofield of both the practitioner and patient is used to stimulate a healing response (eg, healing touch, Johrei, Pranic healing, Reiki, qigong, therapeutic touch, non-contact therapeutic touch).

Complementary: Non-mainstream practice used together with conventional medicine.

Complementary and alternative medicine: Inclusion of complementary and alternative interventions in medical care.

Continuous passive motion: An exercise in which the affected foot is fixed in a track and the leg is moved toward and away from the body.

Conventional treatment: Treatment of symptoms and diseases by health care professionals using drugs, radiation, and surgery. Synonyms: Western medicine, allopathic, mainstream, orthodox, biomedicine.

Emergence agitation: Observable agitation in pediatric patients during anesthesia emergence. Synonym: emergence delirium.

Emergence delirium: Observable agitation in pediatric patients during anesthesia emergence. Synonym: emergence agitation.

Empathetic attention: Eight behaviors—matching verbal preference, adapting to nonverbal communication pattern, listening attentively, providing perception of control, swift response to requests, encouragement, avoiding negative language, and using emotionally neutral descriptors.

ERAS (Enhanced Recovery After Surgery): Pathways for a surgical specialty and facility culture created by interdisciplinary teams for evidence-based and patient-centered care; an integrated continuum from pre-hospital to home again to optimize patients' physiologic function, surgical stress response, and recovery.

Essential oils: Natural chemicals from the essence of certain plants whose scent is used for perfumes, food flavorings, medicine, and aromatherapy; usually distilled using steam or pressure.

Functional status: An evaluation of a person's ability to perform activities of daily living and fulfill personal roles through assessment of elements of the person's being. This assessment includes elements of the person's social support, living environment, mental and emotional state, physical health, economic situation, and use of assistive services.

Healing touch therapy: Energetic therapy to rebalance the energy field for healing of the body, mind, and spirit; the practitioner's hands may be placed on or above the client's body.

Holistic: Comprehension of the parts of something as intimately interconnected and explicable only by reference to the whole; treatment of the whole person, taking into account mental and social factors rather than just the symptoms of the disease.

Induction Compliance Checklist: An observational scale of compliance during induction of anesthesia, with higher scores indicating less compliance.

Integrative treatments: Conventional and complementary approaches used together in coordinated way between different providers and institutions; a holistic, patient-focused approach to treating the whole person.

Interactive music: An intervention developed that includes the use of different instruments and songs to promote the patient's emotional expression and physical release of preoperative anxiety.

Kern light music: Music by Kevin Kern, classified in the light music genre (eg, Western classical music).

Krieger's therapeutic touch: Therapeutic touch wherein the practitioner uses their health energy field to stimulate the patient's own immunological system to repattern itself.

Magnetic clearing: A healing touch technique that focuses on relaxation by releasing congested energy to reduce anger, fear, worry, tension, and anxiety.

Older adults: Persons ages 65 years or older. Further subdivided into

- Young old: ages 65 to 74 years;
- Middle old: ages 75 to 84 years;
- Old old: ages 85 years and older.

Postoperative nausea and vomiting: A common complication associated with perioperative surgical and anesthesia care.

Prehabilitation: The process of improving the functional capability of a patient before a surgical procedure so the patient can withstand any postoperative inactivity and associated decline.

Reflexology: A manual technique on specific reflex points on specific zones within main microcosms on the body (ie, feet, hands, and ears). This brings about psychological and physiological normalization of the total body.

Self-hypnosis relaxation: Hypnotic relaxation based on self-generated imagery.

Simple calculation and reading aloud: Simple arithmetic and reading cognitive skills training, used to improve mental capacity, especially for older adults after they have undergone general anesthesia.

Therapeutic suggestion: Suggestions given without hypnotic induction.

Traditional Chinese medicine: Practices in traditional Chinese medical care; non-Western medical care (eg, acupuncture, herbal supplementation, meditation).

Vaccaria seeds: Plant seeds that are used to stimulate acupressure, typically taped to auricular acupressure points to be worn for multiple days.

References

1. Gan TJ, Diemunsch P, Habib AS, et al. Consensus guidelines for the management of postoperative nausea and vomiting. *Anesth Analg.* 2014;118(1):85-113. [IVA]

2. Donoghue TJ. Herbal medications and anesthesia case management. *AANA J.* 2018;86(3):242-248 [VA]

3. Fatma A, Serife K. Experience of pain in patients undergoing abdominal surgery and nursing approaches to pain control. *Int J Caring Sci.* 2017;10(3):1456-1464. [IIIB]

4. Wang SM, Peloquin C, Kain ZN. The use of auricular acupuncture to reduce preoperative anxiety. *Anesth Analg.* 2001; 93(5):1178-1180. [IA]

5. Dolatian M, Hasanpour A, Montazeri S, Heshmat R, Alavi Majd H. The effect of reflexology on pain intensity and duration of labor on primiparas. *Iran Red Crescent Med J.* 2011;13(7):475-479. [IA]

6. Notte BB, Fazzini C, Mooney RA. Reiki's effect on patients with total knee arthroplasty: a pilot study. *Nursing.* 2016;46(2):17-23. [IB]

7. Cho HK, Park IJ, Jeong YM, Lee YJ, Hwang SH. Can perioperative acupuncture reduce the pain and vomiting experienced after tonsillectomy? A meta-analysis. *Laryngoscope*. 2016;126(3):608-615. [IA]

8. Quinlan-Woodward J, Gode A, Dusek JA, Reinstein AS, Johnson JR, Sendelbach S. Assessing the impact of acupuncture on pain, nausea, anxiety, and coping in women undergoing a mastectomy. *Oncol Nurs Forum*. 2016;43(6):725-732. [IA]

9. Asay K, Olson C, Donnelly J, Perlman E. The use of aromatherapy in postoperative nausea and vomiting: a systematic review. *J Perianesth Nurs*. 2019;34(3):502-516. [IA]

10. Complementary, alternative, or integrative health: what's in a name? National Center for Complementary and Integrative Health. https://www.nccih.nih.gov/health/complementary-alternative-or-integrative-health-whats-in-a-name. Accessed May 15, 2021. [VA]

11. Black LI, Clarke TC, Barnes PM, Stussman BJ, Nahin RL. Use of complementary health approaches among children aged 4-17 years in the United States: National Health Interview Survey, 2007-2012. *Natl Health Stat Report*. 2015;(78):1-19. [IIIA]

12. Ho TF, Rowland-Seymour A, Frankel ES, Li SQ, Mao JJ. Generational differences in complementary and alternative medicine (CAM) use in the context of chronic diseases and pain: baby boomers versus the silent generation. *J Am Board Fam Med*. 2014;27(4):465-473. [IIIA]

13. Clarke TC, Black LI, Stussman BJ, Barnes PM, Nahin RL. Trends in the use of complementary health approaches among adults: United States, 2002-2012. *Natl Health Stat Report*. 2015(79):1-16. [IIIA]

14. de Moura LA, Dias IMG, Pereira LV. Prevalence and factors associated with preoperative anxiety in children aged 5-12 years. *Rev Lat Am Enfermagem*. 2016;24:e2708. [IIIA]

15. ERAS society. https://erassociety.org/. Accessed May 15, 2021. [IVA]

16. Position statement: Care coordination and registered nurses' essential role. June 11, 2012. American Nurses Association. https://www.nursingworld.org/~4afbf2/globalassets/practiceandpolicy/health-policy/cnpe-care-coord-position-statement-final-draft-6-12-2012.pdf. Accessed May 15, 2021. [IVA]

17. Bischoff-Ferrari HA, Dawson-Hughes B, Platz A, et al. Effect of high-dosage cholecalciferol and extended physiotherapy on complications after hip fracture: a randomized controlled trial. *Arch Intern Med*. 2010;170(9):813-820. [IA]

18. Chapuy MC, Arlot ME, Duboeuf F, et al. Vitamin D3 and calcium to prevent hip fractures in elderly women. *N Engl J Med*. 1992;327(23):1637-1642. [IB]

19. Seidi J, Ebnerasooli S, Shahsawari S, Nzarian S. The influence of oral ginger before operation on nausea and vomiting after cataract surgery under general anesthesia: a double-blind placebo-controlled randomized clinical trial. *Electron Physician*. 2017;9(1):3508-3514. [IA]

20. 20. Aytekin A, Doru Ö, Kucukoglu S. The effects of distraction on preoperative anxiety level in children. *J Perianesth Nurs*. 2016;31(1):56-62. [IIA]

21. Hooper VD. SAMBA Consensus Guidelines for the Management of Postoperative Nausea and Vomiting: an executive summary for perianesthesia nurses. *J Perianesth Nurs*. 2015;30(5):377-382. [IVB]

22. Rajabpour S, Rayyani M, Mangolian Shahrbabaki P. The relationship between Iranian patients' perception of holistic care and satisfaction with nursing care. *BMC Nurs*. 2019;18:48. [IIIA]

23. Position Statement: Position on the Role of Nurses in the Practice of Complementary & Integrative Health Approaches (CIHA). June 2016. American Holistic Nurses Association. https://www.ahna.org/Portals/66/Docs/Committees/Corrected%20Position%20Statment%20on%20the%20Role%20of%20Nurses%20in%20the%20Practice%20of%20Complementary%20%20Integrative%20Health%20Approaches%20(CIHA)%202016.pdf?ver=HNA-u5c6jHUDiJCXgifuZg%3d%3d. Accessed May 15, 2021. [IVA]

24. Best M, Butow P, Olver I. Do patients want doctors to talk about spirituality? A systematic literature review. *Patient Educ Couns*. 2015;98(11):1320-1328. [VA]

25. Guo P. Preoperative education interventions to reduce anxiety and improve recovery among cardiac surgery patients: a review of randomised controlled trials. *J Clin Nurs*. 2015;24(1-2):34-46. [IA]

26. Kekecs Z, Nagy T, Varga K. The effectiveness of suggestive techniques in reducing postoperative side effects: a meta-analysis of randomized controlled trials. *Anesth Analg*. 2014;119(6):1407-1419. [IA]

27. Kain ZN, Caldwell-Andrews A, Krivutza DM, et al. Interactive music therapy as a treatment for preoperative anxiety in children: a randomized controlled trial. *Anesth Analg*. 2004;98(5):1260-1266. [IC]

28. Institute of Medicine (US). Committee on the Use of Complementary and Alternative Medicine by the American Public. Appendix E. Model guidelines for the use of complementary and alternative therapies in medical practice. In: *Complementary and Alternative Medicine in the United States*. Washington, DC: National Academies Press; 2005. [IVB]

29. Levy I, Attias S, Ben-Arye E, et al. Perioperative risks of dietary and herbal supplements. *World J Surg*. 2017;41(4):927-934. [IIIA]

30. Wang CZ, Moss J, Yuan CS. Commonly used dietary supplements on coagulation function during surgery. *Medicines (Basel)*. 2015;2(3):157-185. [IIIC]

31. Herbal products and your anesthesia. American Association of Nurse Anesthetists. https://www.aana.com/patients/herbal-products-and-your-anesthesia. Accessed May 15, 2021. [IVB]

32. Faith J, Thorburn S, Tippens KM. Examining the association between patient-centered communication and provider avoidance, CAM use, and CAM-use disclosure. *Altern Ther Health Med*. 2015;21(2):30-35. [IIIA]

33. Shere-Wolfe K, Tilburt JC, D'Adamo C, Berman B, Chesney MA. Infectious diseases physicians' attitudes and practices related to complementary and integrative medicine: results of a national survey. *Evid Based Complement Alternat Med*. 2013;2013:294381. [IIIA]

34. Kramlich D. Complementary health practitioners in the acute and critical care setting: nursing considerations. *Crit Care Nurse*. 2017;37(3):60-65. [VA]

35. Calcium and vitamin D: Moderate evidence supports use of supplemental vitamin D and calcium in patients following hip fracture surgery. American Academy of Orthopaedic Surgeons. http://www.orthoguidelines.org/guideline-detail?id=1287. Accessed May 15, 2021. [IVA]

36. Guideline for positioning the patient. In: *Guidelines for Perioperative Practice*. Denver, CO: AORN; 2021:643-718. [IVA]

37. Guideline for electrosurgical safety. In: *Guidelines for Perioperative Practice*. Denver, CO: AORN; 2021:83-108. [IVA]

38. Malley A, Kenner C, Kim T, Blakeney B. The role of the nurse and the preoperative assessment in patient transitions. *AORN J*. 2015;102(2):181.e1-181.e9. [IIIB]

39. Oh H, Kim BH. Comparing effects of two different types of Nei-Guan acupuncture stimulation devices in reducing postoperative nausea and vomiting. *J Perianesth Nurs*. 2017;32(3):177-187. [IA]

40. Sankar-Maharaj S, Chen D, Hariharan S. Postoperative shivering among cannabis users at a public hospital in Trinidad, West Indies. *J Perianesth Nurs*. 2018;33(1):37-44. [IIIB]

41. Herbal and dietary supplements and anesthesia. 2018. American Society of Anesthesiologists. https://www.asahq.org/madeforthismoment/wp-content/uploads/2018/10/ASA_Supplements-Anesthesia.pdf. Accessed May 15, 2021. [IVB]

42. Büyükyılmaz F, Aştı T. The effect of relaxation techniques and back massage on pain and anxiety in Turkish total hip or knee arthroplasty patients. *Pain Manag Nurs*. 2013;14(3):143-154. [IB]

43. Nagata K, Iida N, Kanazawa H, et al. Effect of listening to music and essential oil inhalation on patients undergoing screening CT colonography: a randomized controlled trial. *Eur J Radiol*. 2014;83(12):2172-2176. [IA]

44. Cronin SN, Odom-Forren J, Roberts H, Thomas M, Williams S, Wright MI. Effects of controlled breathing, with or without aromatherapy, in the treatment of postoperative nausea. *J Perianesth Nurs*. 2015;30(5):389-397. [IIB]

45. Hasanzadeh F, Kashouk NM, Amini S, et al. The effect of cold application and lavender oil inhalation in cardiac surgery patients undergoing chest tube removal. *EXCLI J*. 2016;15:64-74. [IA]

46. Kim BH, Kang HY, Choi EY. Effects of handholding and providing information on anxiety in patients undergoing percutaneous vertebroplasty. *J Clin Nurs*. 2015;24(23-24):3459-3468. [IIA]

47. Wang SM, Gaal D, Maranets I, Caldwell-Andrews A, Kain ZN. Acupressure and preoperative parental anxiety: a pilot study. *Anesth Analg*. 2005;101(3):666-669. [IB]

48. Çetinkaya F. Effect of listening to music on postoperative cognitive function in older adults after hip or knee surgery: a randomized controlled trial. *J Perianesth Nurs*. 2019;34(5):919-928. [IA]

49. Sultan J, Griffin SM, Di Franco F, et al. Randomized clinical trial of Omega-3 fatty acid-supplemented enteral nutrition versus standard enteral nutrition in patients undergoing oesophagogastric cancer surgery. *Br J Surg*. 2012;99(3):346-355. [IA]

50. Grode LB, Søgaard A. Improvement of nutritional care after colon surgery: the impact of early oral nutrition in the postanesthesia care unit. *J Perianesth Nurs*. 2014;29(4):266-274. [IB]

51. Fujita T, Daiko H, Nishimura M. Early enteral nutrition reduces the rate of life-threatening complications after thoracic esophagectomy in patients with esophageal cancer. *Eur Surg Res*. 2012;48(2):79-84. [IA]

52. Huet A, Lucas-Polomeni MM, Robert JC, Sixou JL, Wodey E. Hypnosis and dental anesthesia in children: a prospective controlled study. *Int J Clin Exp Hypn*. 2011;59(4):424-440. [IC]

53. Liguori S, Stacchini M, Ciofi D, Olivini N, Bisogni S, Festini F. Effectiveness of an app for reducing preoperative anxiety in children: a randomized clinical trial. *JAMA Pediatr*. 2016;170(8):e160533. [IA]

54. Burke CN, Voepel-Lewis T, Hadden S, et al. Parental presence on emergence: effect on postanesthesia agitation and parent satisfaction. *J Perianesth Nurs*. 2009;24(4):216-221. [IA]

55. Ozkalayci O, Araz C, Cehreli SB, Tirali RE, Kayhan Z. Effects of music on sedation depth and sedative use during pediatric dental procedures. *J Clin Anesth*. 2016;34:647-653. [IA]

56. Kassai B, Rabilloud M, Dantony E, et al. Introduction of a paediatric anaesthesia comic information leaflet reduced preoperative anxiety in children. *Br J Anaesth*. 2016;117(1):95-102. [IA]

57. van Stijn MF, Korkic-Halilovic I, Bakker MS, van der Ploeg T, van Leeuwen PA, Houdijk AP. Preoperative nutrition status and postoperative outcome in elderly general surgery patients: a systematic review. *JPEN J Parenter Enteral Nutr*. 2013;37(1):37-43. [IIIA]

58. Lili H, Lei X, Yan S, Fen G. Effect of electric acupoint stimulation on gastrointestinal hormones and motility among geriatric postoperative patients with gastrointestinal tumors. *J Tradit Chin Med*. 2016;36(4):450-455. [IB]

59. Myint MW, Wu J, Wong E, et al. Clinical benefits of oral nutritional supplementation for elderly hip fracture patients: a single blind randomised controlled trial. *Age Ageing*. 2013;42(1):39-45. [IA]

60. Kulason K, Nouchi R, Hoshikawa Y, Noda M, Okada Y, Kawashima R. The beneficial effects of cognitive training with simple calculation and reading aloud (SCRA) in the elderly postoperative population: a pilot randomized controlled trial. *Front Aging Neurosci*. 2018;10:68. [IB]

61. Chandra A, Dixit MB, Banavaliker JN, Thakur V., Ranjan R. Transcutaneous electrical nerve stimulation as an adjunct to non-steroidal anti-inflammatory medications for pain management during pleurodesis. *Anaesth Pain Intensive Care*. 2013;17(2):154-157. [IB]

62. Bice AA, Wyatt TH. Holistic comfort interventions for pediatric nursing procedures: a systematic review. *J Holist Nurs*. 2017;35(3):280-295. [IIA]

63. Akhter S, Qureshi AR, El-Khechen HA, et al. Efficacy of electrical stimulation for spinal fusion: a systematic review and meta-analysis of randomized controlled trials. *Sci Rep*. 2020;10(1):4568. [IA]

64. Silva RPJ, Rampazzo ARP, Nascimento LA, Fonesca LF. Discomfort patients expect and experience in the immediate postoperative period. *Rev Baiana Enferm*. 2018;32:e26070. [IIIB]

65. American College of Surgeons Statements on Principles. American College of Surgeons. https://www.facs.org/about-acs/

statements/stonprin. Updated April 12, 2016. Accessed May 15, 2021. [IVA]

66. Hole J, Hirsch M, Ball E, Meads C. Music as an aid for postoperative recovery in adults: a systematic review and meta-analysis. *Lancet.* 2015;386(10004):1659-1671. [IA]

67. Stallings-Welden LM, Doerner M, Ketchem EL, Benkert L, Alka S, Stallings JD. A comparison of aromatherapy to standard care for relief of PONV and PDNV in ambulatory surgical patients. *J Perianesth Nurs.* 2018;33(2):116-128. [IA]

68. Kiberd MB, Clarke SK, Chorney J, d'Eon B, Wright S. Aromatherapy for the treatment of PONV in children: a pilot RCT. *BMC Complement Altern Med.* 2016;16(1):450. [IB]

69. Lee YR, Shin HS. Effectiveness of ginger essential oil on postoperative nausea and vomiting in abdominal surgery patients. *J Altern Complement Med.* 2017;23(3):196-200. [IIB]

70. Zhang ZS, Wang XL, Xu CL, et al. Music reduces panic: an initial study of listening to preferred music improves male patient discomfort and anxiety during flexible cystoscopy. *J Endourol.* 2014;28(6):739-744. [IA]

71. Mifflin KA, Hackmann T, Chorney JM. Streamed video clips to reduce anxiety in children during inhaled induction of anesthesia. *Anesth Analg.* 2012;115(5):1162-1167. [IA]

72. Pedroso JL, Henriques Aquino CC, Escórcio Bezerra ML, et al. Ginkgo biloba and cerebral bleeding: a case report and critical review. *Neurologist.* 2011;17(2):89-90. [VA]

73. Dunne DF, Jack S, Jones RP, et al. Randomized clinical trial of prehabilitation before planned liver resection. *Br J Surg.* 2016;103(5):504-512. [IA]

74. Sadati L, Pazouki A, Mehdizadeh A, Shoar S, Tamannaie Z, Chaichian S. Effect of preoperative nursing visit on preoperative anxiety and postoperative complications in candidates for laparoscopic cholecystectomy: a randomized clinical trial. *Scand J Caring Sci.* 2013;27(4):994-998. [IC]

75. Bagheri H, Ebrahimi H, Abbasi A, Atashsokhan G, Salmani Z, Zamani M. Effect of preoperative visitation by operating room staff on preoperative anxiety in patients receiving elective hernia surgery. *J Perianesth Nurs.* 2019;34(2):272-280. [IIA]

76. Donker JM, de Vries J, de Lepper CC, et al. A novel finding: the effect of nurse practitioners on the relation to quality of life, anxiety, and depressive symptoms in vascular surgery. *Ann Vasc Surg.* 2014;28(3):644-650. [IIB]

77. Perry JN, Hooper VD, Masiongale J. Reduction of preoperative anxiety in pediatric surgery patients using age-appropriate teaching interventions. *J Perianesth Nurs.* 2012;27(2):69-81. [IIIA]

78. Rhodes L, Nash C, Moisan A, et al. Does preoperative orientation and education alleviate anxiety in posterior spinal fusion patients? A prospective, randomized study. *J Pediatr Orthop.* 2015;35(3):276-279. [IA]

79. Fernandes SC, Arriaga P, Esteves F. Providing preoperative information for children undergoing surgery: a randomized study testing different types of educational material to reduce children's preoperative worries. *Health Educ Res.* 2014;29(6):1058-1076. [IA]

80. Batuman A, Gulec E, Turktan M, Gunes Y, Ozcengiz D. Preoperative informational video reduces preoperative anxiety and postoperative negative behavioral changes in children. *Minerva Anestesiol.* 2016;82(5):534-542. [IA]

81. West AM, Bittner EA, Ortiz VE. The effects of preoperative, video-assisted anesthesia education in Spanish on Spanish-speaking patients' anxiety, knowledge, and satisfaction: a pilot study. *J Clin Anesth.* 2014;26(4):325-329. [IB]

82. Tou S, Tou W, Mah D, Karatassas A, Hewett P. Effect of preoperative two-dimensional animation information on perioperative anxiety and knowledge retention in patients undergoing bowel surgery: a randomized pilot study. *Colorectal Dis.* 2013;15(5):e256-e265. [IB]

83. Zhang CY, Jiang Y, Yin QY, Chen FJ, Ma LL, Wang LX. Impact of nurse-initiated preoperative education on postoperative anxiety symptoms and complications after coronary artery bypass grafting. *J Cardiovasc Nurs.* 2012;27(1):84-88. [IB]

84. Bahrami N, Soleimani MA, Sharifnia H, Shaigan H, Sheikhi MR, Mohammad-Rezaei Z. Effects of anxiety reduction training on physiological indices and serum cortisol levels before elective surgery. *Iran J Nurs Midwifery Res.* 2013;18(5):416-420. [IA]

85. Amini K, Alihossaini Z, Ghahremani Z. Randomized clinical trial comparison of the effect of verbal education and education booklet on preoperative anxiety. *J Perianesth Nurs.* 2019;34(2):289-296. [IA]

86. Lin SY, Huang HA, Lin SC, Huang YT, Wang KY, Shi HY. The effect of an anaesthetic patient information video on perioperative anxiety: a randomised study. *Eur J Anaesthesiol.* 2016;33(2):134-139. [IA]

87. Lindstrom D, Azodi OS, Wladis A, et al. Effects of a perioperative smoking cessation intervention on postoperative complications: a randomized trial. *Ann Surg.* 2008;248(5):739-745. [IA]

88. Emilsson S, Svensk AC, Tavelin B, Lindh J. Support group participation during the post-operative radiotherapy period increases levels of coping resources among women with breast cancer. *Eur J Cancer Care (Engl).* 2012;21(5):591-598. [IIA]

89. Li C, Carli F, Lee L, et al. Impact of a trimodal prehabilitation program on functional recovery after colorectal cancer surgery: a pilot study. *Surg Endosc.* 2013;27(4):1072-1082. [IIA]

90. Carli F, Charlebois P, Stein B, et al. Randomized clinical trial of prehabilitation in colorectal surgery. *Br J Surg.* 2010;97(8):1187-1197. [IA]

91. Gillis C, Li C, Lee L, et al. Prehabilitation versus rehabilitation: a randomized control trial in patients undergoing colorectal resection for cancer. *Anesthesiology.* 2014;121(5):937-947. [IA]

92. Murata K, Yoshimoto M, Takebayashi T, Ida K, Nakano K, Yamashita T. Effect of cryotherapy after spine surgery. *Asian Spine J.* 2014;8(6):753-758. [IIB]

93. Adie S, Kwan A, Naylor JM, Harris IA, Mittal R. Cryotherapy following total knee replacement. *Cochrane Database Syst Rev.* 2012(9):CD007911. [IIB]

94. Demoulin C, Brouwers M, Darot S, Gillet P, Crielaard JM, Vanderthommen M. Comparison of gaseous cryotherapy with

more traditional forms of cryotherapy following total knee arthroplasty. *Ann Phys Rehabil Med.* 2012;55(4):229-240. [IA]

95. Quinlan P, Davis J, Fields K, et al. Effects of localized cold therapy on pain in postoperative spinal fusion patients: a randomized control trial. *Orthop Nurs.* 2017;36(5):344-349. [IA]

96. Curry AL, Goehring MT, Bell J, Jette DU. Effect of physical therapy interventions in the acute care setting on function, activity, and participation after total knee arthroplasty: a systematic review. *J Acute Care Phys Ther.* 2018;9(3):1-14. [IIB]

97. Marx W, McKavanagh D, McCarthy AL, et al. The effect of ginger (Zingiber officinale) on platelet aggregation: a systematic literature review. *PLoS One.* 2015;10(10):e0141119. [IIIB]

98. Begtrup KM, Krag AE, Hvas AM. No impact of fish oil supplements on bleeding risk: a systematic review. *Dan Med J.* 2017;64(5):A5366. [IIA]

99. Chen B, Zhou Y, Yang P, Wan H, Wu X. Safety and efficacy of fish oil–enriched parenteral nutrition regimen on postoperative patients undergoing major abdominal surgery: a meta-analysis of randomized controlled trials. *JPEN J Parenter Enteral Nutr.* 2010;34(4):387-394. [IA]

100. Kinross JM, Markar S, Karthikesalingam A, et al. A meta-analysis of probiotic and synbiotic use in elective surgery: does nutrition modulation of the gut microbiome improve clinical outcome? *JPEN J Parenter Enteral Nutr.* 2013;37(2):243-253. [IA]

101. Arumugam S, Lau CSM, Chamberlain RS. Probiotics and synbiotics decrease postoperative sepsis in elective gastrointestinal surgical patients: a meta-analysis. *J Gastrointest Surg.* 2016;20(6):1123-1131. [IA]

102. Short V, Herbert G, Perry R, et al. Chewing gum for postoperative recovery of gastrointestinal function. *Cochrane Database Syst Rev.* 2015(2):CD006506. [IA]

103. Yoshikawa K, Shimada M, Nishioka M, et al. The effects of the Kampo medicine (Japanese herbal medicine) "Daikenchuto" on the surgical inflammatory response following laparoscopic colorectal resection. *Surg Today.* 2012;42(7):646-651. [IIB]

104. Yasunaga H, Miyata H, Horiguchi H, Kuwabara K, Hashimoto H, Matsuda S. Effect of the Japanese herbal Kampo medicine Dai-kenchu-to on postoperative adhesive small bowel obstruction requiring long-tube decompression: a propensity score analysis. *Evid Based Complement Alternat Med.* 2011;2011:264289. [IIIB]

105. Al Sebaee HA, Elhadary SM. Effectiveness of a care bundle on postoperative thirst relief and oral condition among patients undergoing abdominal surgeries. *IOSR J Nurs Health Sci.* 2017;6(5):82-90. [IIA]

106. Garcia AK, Fonseca LF, Aroni P, Galvão CM. Strategies for thirst relief: Integrative literature review. *Rev Bras Enferm.* 2016;69(6):1215-1222. [IIIA]

107. Garcia AKA, Furuya RK, Conchon MF, Rossetto EG, Dantas RAS, Fonseca LF. Menthol chewing gum on preoperative thirst management: randomized clinical trial. *Rev Lat Am Enfermagem.* 2019;27:e3180. [IA]

108. Tóth B, Lantos T, Hegyi P, et al. Ginger (Zingiber officinale): an alternative for the prevention of postoperative nausea and vomiting. A meta-analysis. *Phytomedicine.* 2018;50:8-18. [IA]

109. Soltani E, Jangjoo A, Afzal Aghaei M, Dalili A. Effects of preoperative administration of ginger (Zingiber officinale Roscoe) on postoperative nausea and vomiting after laparoscopic cholecystectomy. *J Tradit Complement Med.* 2017;8(3):387-390. [IA]

110. 21 CFR 501.22. Animal foods; labeling of spices, flavorings, colorings, and chemical preservatives. US Food and Drug Administration. https://www.ecfr.gov/cgi-bin/text-idx?SID=5f3a5f2bf61663047e77fc6506971be5&mc=true&node=pt21.6.501&rgn=div5#se21.6.501_122. Accessed May 17, 2021.

111. Hsu CC, Chen SR, Lee PH, Lin PC. The effect of music listening on pain, heart rate variability, and range of motion in older adults after total knee replacement. *Clin Nurs Res.* 2019;28(5):529-547. [IIA]

112. Foroughy M, Mottahedian Tabrizi E, Hajizadeh E, Pishgoo B. Effect of music therapy on patients' anxiety and hemodynamic parameters during coronary angioplasty: a randomized controlled trial. *Nurs Midwifery Stud.* 2015;4(2):e25800. [IA]

113. Martindale F, Mikocka-Walus AA, Walus BP, Keage H, Andrews JM. The effects of a designer music intervention on patients' anxiety, pain, and experience of colonoscopy: a short report on a pilot study. *Gastroenterol Nurs.* 2014;37(5):338-342. [IIA]

114. Palmer JB, Lane D, Mayo D, Schluchter M, Leeming R. Effects of music therapy on anesthesia requirements and anxiety in women undergoing ambulatory breast surgery for cancer diagnosis and treatment: a randomized controlled trial. *J Clin Oncol.* 2015;33(28):3162-3168. [IA]

115. Ko CH, Chen YY, Wu KT, et al. Effect of music on level of anxiety in patients undergoing colonoscopy without sedation. *J Chin Med Assoc.* 2017;80(3):154-160. [IA]

116. Weeks BP, Nilsson U. Music interventions in patients during coronary angiographic procedures: a randomized controlled study of the effect on patients' anxiety and well-being. *Eur J Cardiovasc Nurs.* 2011;10(2):88-93. [IC]

117. Padmanabhan R, Hildreth AJ, Laws D. A prospective, randomised, controlled study examining binaural beat audio and pre-operative anxiety in patients undergoing general anaesthesia for day case surgery. *Anaesthesia.* 2005;60(9):874-877. [IA]

118. Klassen JA, Liang Y, Tjosvold L, Klassen TP, Hartling L. Music for pain and anxiety in children undergoing medical procedures: a systematic review of randomized controlled trials. *Ambul Pediatr.* 2008;8(2):117-128. [IA]

119. Bradt J, Dileo C, Shim M. Music interventions for preoperative anxiety. *Cochrane Database Syst Rev.* 2013;(6):006908. [IIA]

120. Bashiri M, Akçalı D, Coşkun D, Cindoruk M, Dikmen A, Çifdalöz BU. Evaluation of pain and patient satisfaction by music therapy in patients with endoscopy/colonoscopy. *Turk J Gastroenterol.* 2018;29(5):574-579. [IA]

121. Jiménez-Jiménez M, García-Escalona A, Martín-López A, De Vera-Vera R, De Haro J. Intraoperative stress and anxiety reduction with music therapy: a controlled randomized clinical trial of efficacy and safety. *J Vasc Nurs.* 2013;31(3):101-106. [IA]

122. Wu J, Chaplin W, Amico J, et al. Music for surgical abortion care study: a randomized controlled pilot study. *Contraception.* 2012;85(5):496-502. [IC]

123. Easter B, DeBoer L, Settlemyer G, Starnes C, Marlowe V, Tart RC. The impact of music on the PACU patient's perception of discomfort. *J Perianesth Nurs.* 2010;25(2):79-87. [IA]

124. Hosseinpour M, Memarzadeh M. Use of a preoperative playroom to prepare children for surgery. *Eur J Pediatr Surg.* 2010;20(6):408-411. [IA]

125. Kerimoglu B, Neuman A, Paul J, Stefanov DG, Twersky R. Anesthesia induction using video glasses as a distraction tool for the management of preoperative anxiety in children. *Anesth Analg.* 2013;117(6):1373-1379. [IA]

126. Bekelis K, Calnan D, Simmons N, MacKenzie T, Kakoulides G. Effect of an immersive preoperative virtual reality experience on patient reported outcomes: a randomized controlled trial. *Ann Surg.* 2017;265(6):1068-1073. [IA]

127. Park JW, Nahm FS, Kim JH, Jeon YT, Ryu JH, Han SH. The effect of mirroring display of virtual reality tour of the operating theatre on preoperative anxiety: a randomized controlled trial. *IEEE J Biomed Health Inform.* 2019;23(6):2655-2660. [IA]

128. Dehghan F, Jalali R, Bashiri H. The effect of virtual reality technology on preoperative anxiety in children: a Solomon four-group randomized clinical trial. *Perioper Med (Lond).* 2019;8:5. [IA]

129. Ryu JH, Park JW, Nahm FS, et al. The effect of gamification through a virtual reality on preoperative anxiety in pediatric patients undergoing general anesthesia: a prospective, randomized, and controlled trial. *J Clin Med.* 2018;7(9):284. [IA]

130. Ryu JH, Park SJ, Park JW, et al. Randomized clinical trial of immersive virtual reality tour of the operating theatre in children before anaesthesia. *Br J Surg.* 2017;104(12):1628-1633. [IA]

131. Agostini F, Monti F, Neri E, Dellabartola S, de Pascalis L, Bozicevic L. Parental anxiety and stress before pediatric anesthesia: a pilot study on the effectiveness of preoperative clown intervention. *J Health Psychol.* 2014;19(5):587-601. [IA]

132. Berger J, Wilson D, Potts L, Polivka B. Wacky Wednesday: use of distraction through humor to reduce preoperative anxiety in children and their parents. *J Perianesth Nurs.* 2014;29(4):285-291. [IIB]

133. Birnie KA, Noel M, Chambers CT, Uman LS, Parker JA. Psychological interventions for needle-related procedural pain and distress in children and adolescents. *Cochrane Database Syst Rev.* 2018(10):CD005179. [IA]

134. Kain ZN, Wang SM, Mayes LC, Krivutza DM, Teague BA. Sensory stimuli and anxiety in children undergoing surgery: a randomized, controlled trial. *Anesth Analg.* 2001;92(4):897-903. [IA]

135. Cagiran E, Sergin D, Deniz MN, Tanattı B, Emiroglu N, Alper I. Effects of sociodemographic factors and maternal anxiety on preoperative anxiety in children. *J Int Med Res.* 2014;42(2):572-580. [IIIA]

136. Manyande A, Cyna AM, Yip P, Chooi C, Middleton P. Non-pharmacological interventions for assisting the induction of anaesthesia in children. *Cochrane Database Syst Rev.* 2015(7):CD006447. [IC]

137. Chan CS, Molassiotis A. The effects of an educational programme on the anxiety and satisfaction level of parents having parent present induction and visitation in a postanaesthesia care unit. *Pediatr Anaesth.* 2002;12(2):131-139. [IIA]

138. In WY, Kim YM, Kim HS, et al. The effect of a parental visitation program on emergence delirium among postoperative children in the PACU. *J Perianesth Nurs.* 2019;34(1):108-116. [IIB]

139. Pagnard E, Sarver W. Family visitation in the PACU: an evidence-based practice project. *J Perianesth Nurs.* 2019;34(3):600-605. [VA]

140. Wendler MC, Smith K, Ellenburg W, Gill R, Anderson L, Spiegel-Thayer K. "To see with my own eyes": experiences of family visits during phase 1 recovery. *J Perianesth Nurs.* 2017;32(1):45-57. [IIIA]

141. Amraoui J, Pouliquen C, Fraisse J, et al. Effects of a hypnosis session before general anesthesia on postoperative outcomes in patients who underwent minor breast cancer surgery: The HYPNOSEIN randomized clinical trial. *JAMA Netw Open.* 2018;1(4):e181164. [IB]

142. Lang EV, Berbaum KS, Pauker SG, et al. Beneficial effects of hypnosis and adverse effects of empathic attention during percutaneous tumor treatment: when being nice does not suffice. *J Vasc Interv Radiol.* 2008;19(6):897-905. [IA]

143. Álvarez-García C, Yaban ZŞ. The effects of preoperative guided imagery interventions on preoperative anxiety and postoperative pain: a meta-analysis. *Complement Ther Clin Pract.* 2020;38:101077. [IA]

144. Gonzales EA, Ledesma RJA, McAllister DJ, Perry SM, Dyer CA, Maye JP. Effects of guided imagery on postoperative outcomes in patients undergoing same-day surgical procedures: a randomized, single-blind study. *AANA J.* 2010;78(3):181-188. [IB]

145. Ko YL, Lin PC. The effect of using a relaxation tape on pulse, respiration, blood pressure and anxiety levels of surgical patients. *J Clin Nurs.* 2012;21(5-6):689-697. [IIIB]

146. Lin PC. An evaluation of the effectiveness of relaxation therapy for patients receiving joint replacement surgery. *J Clin Nurs.* 2012;21(5-6):601-608. [IIA]

147. Chandrasegaran A. Case study: clinical management of claustrophobia and cold sensitivity towards operating room environment with preoperative hypnosis. *Sleep Hypn.* 2018;20(4):294-298. [VB]

148. Kuttner L. Pediatric hypnosis: pre-, peri-, and post-anesthesia. *Pediatr Anesth.* 2012;22(6):573-577. [VB]

149. Tefikow S, Barth J, Maichrowitz S, Beelmann A, Strauss B, Rosendahl J. Efficacy of hypnosis in adults undergoing surgery or medical procedures: a meta-analysis of randomized controlled trials. *Clin Psychol Rev.* 2013;33(5):623-636. [IA]

150. Lang EV, Benotsch EG, Fick LJ, et al. Adjunctive non-pharmacological analgesia for invasive medical procedures: a randomised trial. *Lancet.* 2000;355(9214):1486-1490. [IA]

151. Takahashi M, Mouillet G, Khaled A, et al. Perioperative outcomes of adjunctive hypnotherapy compared with conscious sedation alone for patients undergoing transfemoral transcatheter aortic valve implantation. *Int Heart J.* 2020;61(1):60-66. [IIA]

152. Duparc-Alegria N, Tiberghien K, Abdoul H, Dahmani S, Alberti C, Thiollier AF. Assessment of a short hypnosis in a paediatric operating room in reducing postoperative pain and anxiety: a randomised study. *J Clin Nurs.* 2018;27(1-2):86-91. [IB]

153. Trambert R, Kowalski MO, Wu B, Mehta N, Friedman P. A randomized controlled trial provides evidence to support aromatherapy to minimize anxiety in women undergoing breast biopsy. *Worldviews Evid Based Nurs.* 2017;14(5):394-402. [IA]

154. Hosseini S, Heydari A, Vakili M, Moghadam S, Tazyky S. Effect of lavender essence inhalation on the level of anxiety and blood cortisol in candidates for open-heart surgery. *Iran J Nurs Midwifery Res.* 2016;21(4):397-401. [IA]

155. Jaruzel CB, Gregoski M, Mueller M, Faircloth A, Kelechi T. Aromatherapy for preoperative anxiety: a pilot study. *J Perianesth Nurs.* 2019;34(2):259-264. [IIA]

156. Hu PH, Peng YC, Lin YT, Chang CS, Ou MC. Aromatherapy for reducing colonoscopy related procedural anxiety and physiological parameters: a randomized controlled study. *Hepatogastroenterology.* 2010;57(102-103):1082-1086. [IC]

157. Hoya Y, Matsumura I, Fujita T, Yanaga K. The use of non-pharmacological interventions to reduce anxiety in patients undergoing gastroscopy in a setting with an optimal soothing environment. *Gastroenterol Nurs.* 2008;31(6):395-399. [IC]

158. Hines S, Steels E, Chang A, Gibbons K. Aromatherapy for treatment of postoperative nausea and vomiting. *Cochrane Database Syst Rev.* 2018;3(3):CD007598. [IIA]

159. Olapour A, Behaeen K, Akhondzadeh R, Soltani F, Al Sadat Razavi F, Bekhradi R. The effect of inhalation of aromatherapy blend containing lavender essential oil on cesarean postoperative pain. *Anesth Pain Med.* 2013;3(1):203-207. [IA]

160. Braden R, Reichow S, Halm MA. The use of the essential oil lavandin to reduce preoperative anxiety in surgical patients. *J Perianesth Nurs.* 2009;24(6):348-355. [IA]

161. Lane B, Cannella K, Bowen C, et al. Examination of the effectiveness of peppermint aromatherapy on nausea in women post C-section. *J Holist Nurs.* 2012;30(2):90-104. [IA]

162. Lee A, Chan SK, Fan LT. Stimulation of the wrist acupuncture point PC6 for preventing postoperative nausea and vomiting. *Cochrane Database Syst Rev.* 2015;(11):CD003281. [IA]

163. Albooghobeish M, Mohtadi A, Saidkhani V, et al. Comparative effects of the stimulation of BL10, BL11, and GB34 acupuncture points with P6 point using a low-level laser on the prevention of vomiting after strabismus surgery: a randomized, double-blind, controlled clinical trial. *Iran Red Crescent Med J.* 2019;21(2):e64713. [IA]

164. Yang C, Hao Z, Zhang LL, Guo Q. Efficacy and safety of acupuncture in children: an overview of systematic reviews. *Pediatr Res.* 2015;78(2):112-119. [IA]

165. Acar HV, Cuvas O, Ceyhan A, Dikmen B. Acupuncture on Yintang point decreases preoperative anxiety. *J Altern Complement Med.* 2013;19(5):420-424. [IA]

166. Wu S, Liang J, Zhu X, Liu X, Miao D. Comparing the treatment effectiveness of body acupuncture and auricular acupuncture in preoperative anxiety treatment. *J Res Med Sci.* 2011;16(1):39-42. [IC]

167. Chen Y, Wu W, Yao Y, Yang Y, Zhao Q, Qiu,L. Transcutaneous electric acupoint stimulation at Jiaji points reduce abdominal pain after colonoscopy: a randomized controlled trial. *Int J Clin Exp Med.* 2015;8(4):5972-5977. [IA]

168. Sun R, Dai W, Liu Y, et al. Non-needle acupoint stimulation for prevention of nausea and vomiting after breast surgery: a meta-analysis. *Medicine (Baltimore).* 2019;98(10):e14713. [IA]

169. Martin CS, Deverman SE, Norvell DC, Cusick JC, Kendrick A, Koh J. Randomized trial of acupuncture with antiemetics for reducing postoperative nausea in children. *Acta Anaesthesiol Scand.* 2018;63(3):292-297. [IA]

170. Carr KL, Johnson FE, Kenaan CA, Welton JM. Effects of P6 stimulation on postoperative nausea and vomiting in laparoscopic cholecystectomy patients. *J Perianesth Nurs.* 2015;30(2):143-150. [IB]

171. El-Deeb AM, Ahmady MS. Effect of acupuncture on nausea and/or vomiting during and after cesarean section in comparison with ondansetron. *J Anesth.* 2011;25(5):698-703. [IA]

172. Kwon JH, Shin Y, Juon HS. Effects of Nei-guan (P6) acupressure wristband: on nausea, vomiting, and retching in women after thyroidectomy. *Cancer Nurs.* 2016;39(1):61-66. [IIA]

173. Feng C, Popovic J, Kline R, et al. Auricular acupressure in the prevention of postoperative nausea and emesis: a randomized controlled trial. *Bull Hosp Jt Dis* (2013). 2017;75(2):114-118. [IA]

174. He BJ, Tong PJ, Li J, Jing HT, Yao XM. Auricular acupressure for analgesia in perioperative period of total knee arthroplasty. *Pain Med.* 2013;14(10):1608-1613. [IA]

175. Chang LH, Hsu CH, Jong GP, Ho S, Tsay SL, Lin KC. Auricular acupressure for managing postoperative pain and knee motion in patients with total knee replacement: a randomized sham control study. *Evid Based Complement Alternat Med.* 2012;2012:528452. [IA]

176. Gavronsky S, Koeniger-Donohue R, Steller J, Hawkins JW. Postoperative pain: acupuncture versus percutaneous electrical nerve stimulation. *Pain Manag Nurs.* 2012;13(3):150-156. [IB]

177. Chen J, Tu Q, Miao S, Zhou Z, Hu S. Transcutaneous electrical acupoint stimulation for preventing postoperative nausea and vomiting after general anesthesia: a meta-analysis of randomized controlled trials. *Int J Surg.* 2020;73:57-64. [IA]

178. Cheong KB, Zhang JP, Huang Y, Zhang ZJ. The effectiveness of acupuncture in prevention and treatment of postoperative nausea and vomiting—a systematic review and meta-analysis. *PLoS One.* 2013;8(12):e82474. [IA]

179. Yang XY, Xiao J, Chen YH, et al. Dexamethasone alone vs in combination with transcutaneous electrical acupoint stimulation or tropisetron for prevention of postoperative

nausea and vomiting in gynaecological patients undergoing laparoscopic surgery. *Br J Anaesth.* 2015;115(6):883-889. [IA]

180. Zhan W, Tian W. Addition of transcutaneous electric acupoint stimulation to transverse abdominis plane block for postoperative analgesia in abdominal surgery: a randomized controlled trial. *Eur J Integr Med.* 2020;35:101087. [IA]

181. Nakamura N, Mihara T, Hijikata T, Goto T, Ka K. Unilateral electrical stimulation of the heart 7 acupuncture point to prevent emergence agitation in children: a prospective, double-blinded, randomized clinical trial. *PLoS One.* 2018;13(10):e0204533. [IA]

182. Huang S, Peng W, Tian X, et al. Effects of transcutaneous electrical acupoint stimulation at different frequencies on perioperative anesthetic dosage, recovery, complications, and prognosis in video-assisted thoracic surgical lobectomy: a randomized, double-blinded, placebo-controlled trial. *J Anesth.* 2017;31(1):58-65. [IA]

183. Wang SM, Constable RT, Tokoglu FS, Weiss DA, Freyle D, Kain ZN. Acupuncture-induced blood oxygenation level-dependent signals in awake and anesthetized volunteers: a pilot study. *Anesth Analg.* 2007;105(2):499-506. [IIB]

184. White PF, Zhao M, Tang J, et al. Use of a disposable acupressure device as part of a multimodal antiemetic strategy for reducing postoperative nausea and vomiting. *Anesth Analg.* 2012;115(1):31-37. [IB]

185. Majholm B, Møller AM. Acupressure at acupoint P6 for prevention of postoperative nausea and vomiting: a randomised clinical trial. *Eur J Anaesthesiol.* 2011;28(6):412-419. [IA]

186. Cooke M, Rapchuk I, Doi SA, et al. Wrist acupressure for post-operative nausea and vomiting (WrAP): a pilot study. *Complement Ther Med.* 2015;23(3):372-380. [IA]

187. Valiee S, Bassampour SS, Nasrabadi AN, Pouresmaeil Z, Mehran A. Effect of acupressure on preoperative anxiety: a clinical trial. *J Perianesth Nurs.* 2012;27(4):259-266. [IB]

188. Rosen J, Lawrence R, Bouchard M, Doros G, Gardiner P, Saper R. Massage for perioperative pain and anxiety in placement of vascular access devices. *Adv Mind Body Med.* 2013;27(1):12-23. [IB]

189. Brand LR, Munroe DJ, Gavin J. The effect of hand massage on preoperative anxiety in ambulatory surgery patients. *AORN J.* 2013;97(6):708-717. [IIB]

190. Wentworth LJ, Briese LJ, Timimi FK, et al. Massage therapy reduces tension, anxiety, and pain in patients awaiting invasive cardiovascular procedures. *Prog Cardiovasc Nurs.* 2009;24(4):155-161. [IB]

191. Hudson BF, Davidson J, Whiteley MS. The impact of hand reflexology on pain, anxiety and satisfaction during minimally invasive surgery under local anaesthetic: a randomised controlled trial. *Int J Nurs Stud.* 2015;52(12):1789-1797. [IA]

192. Alameri R, Dean G, Castner J, Volpe E, Elghoneimy Y, Jungquist C. Efficacy of precise foot massage therapy on pain and anxiety following cardiac surgery: pilot study. *Pain Manag Nurs.* 2020;21(4):314-322. [IB]

193. Ucuzal M, Kanan N. Foot massage: effectiveness on postoperative pain in breast surgery patients. *Pain Manag Nurs.* 2014;15(2):458-465. [IIB]

194. Bagheri-Nesami M, Shorofi SA, Zargar N, Sohrabi M, Gholipour-Baradari A, Khalilian A. The effects of foot reflexology massage on anxiety in patients following coronary artery bypass graft surgery: a randomized controlled trial. *Complement Ther Clin Pract.* 2014;20(1):42-47. [IA]

195. Molavi Vardanjani M, Masoudi Alavi N, Razavi NS, Aghajani M, Azizi-Fini E, Vaghefi SM. A randomized-controlled trial examining the effects of reflexology on anxiety of patients undergoing coronary angiography. *Nurs Midwifery Stud.* 2013;2(3):3-9. [IA]

196. Laws Across the USA. Reflexology Association of America. https://reflexology-usa.org/wp-content/uploads/reflexology_laws_by_state2.pdf. Revised October 2013. Accessed May 17, 2021.

197. Collarile M, Sambri A, Lullini G, Cadossi M, Zorzi C. Biophysical stimulation improves clinical results of matrix-assisted autologous chondrocyte implantation in the treatment of chondral lesions of the knee. *Knee Surg Sports Traumatol Arthrosc.* 2018;26(4):1223-1229. [IA]

198. Khooshideh M, Latifi Rostami SS, Sheikh M, MD P, Ghorbani Yekta B, Shahriari A. Pulsed electromagnetic fields for postsurgical pain management in women undergoing cesarean section: a randomized, double-blind, placebo-controlled trial. *Clin J Pain.* 2017;33(2):142-147. [IA]

199. Osti L, Del Buono A, Maffulli N. Pulsed electromagnetic fields after rotator cuff repair: a randomized, controlled study. *Orthopedics.* 2015;38(3):e223-e228. [IA]

200. Osti L, Del Buono A, Maffulli N. Application of pulsed electromagnetic fields after microfractures to the knee: a mid-term study. *Int Orthop.* 2015;39(7):1289-1294. [IB]

201. Stocchero M, Gobbato L, De Biagi M, Bressan E, Sivolella S. Pulsed electromagnetic fields for postoperative pain: a randomized controlled clinical trial in patients undergoing mandibular third molar extraction. *Oral Surg Oral Med Oral Pathol Oral Radiol.* 2015;119(3):293-300. [IA]

202. Rohde CH, Taylor EM, Alonso A, Ascherman JA, Hardy KL, Pilla AA. Pulsed electromagnetic fields reduce postoperative interleukin-1[beta], pain, and inflammation: a double-blind, placebo-controlled study in TRAM flap breast reconstruction patients. *Plast Reconstr Surg.* 2015;135(5):808e-817e. [IB]

203. Svaerdborg M, Momsen OH, Damsgaard TE. Pulsed electromagnetic fields for postoperative pain treatment after breast augmentation: a double-blind, placebo-controlled study. *Aesthet Surg J.* 2016;36(6):NP199-NP201. [IB]

204. Menini M, Bevilacqua M, Setti P, Tealdo T, Pesce P, Pera P. Effects of pulsed electromagnetic fields on swelling and pain after implant surgery: a double-blind, randomized study. *Int J Oral Maxillofac Surg.* 2016;45(3):346-353. [IB]

205. Erden S, Senol Celik S. The effect of transcutaneous electrical nerve stimulation on post-thoracotomy pain. *Contemp Nurse.* 2015;51(2-3):163-170. [IA]

206. Rakel BA, Zimmerman BM, Geasland K, et al. Transcutaneous electrical nerve stimulation for the control of pain during rehabilitation after total knee arthroplasty: a randomized, blinded, placebo-controlled trial. *Pain.* 2014;155(12):2599-2611. [IA]

207. Borckardt JJ, Reeves ST, Robinson SM, et al. Transcranial direct current stimulation (tDCS) reduces postsurgical opioid

consumption in total knee arthroplasty (TKA). *Clin J Pain.* 2013;29(11):925-928. [IA]

208. Nigam AK, Taylor DM, Valeyeva Z. Non-invasive interactive neurostimulation (InterXTM) reduces acute pain in patients following total knee replacement surgery: a randomised, controlled trial. *J Orthop Surg Res.* 2011;6:45. [IA]

209. Thrane S, Cohen SM. Effect of Reiki therapy on pain and anxiety in adults: an in-depth literature review of randomized trials with effect size calculations. *Pain Manag Nurs.* 2014;15(4):897-908. [IA]

210. Bourque AL, Sullivan ME, Winter MR. Reiki as a pain management adjunct in screening colonoscopy. *Gastroenterol Nurs.* 2012;35(5):308-312. [IIC]

211. Goldberg DR, Wardell DW, Kilgarriff N, Williams B, Eichler D, Thomlinson P. An initial study using healing touch for women undergoing a breast biopsy. *J Holist Nurs.* 2016;34(2):123-134. [IA]

212. Bulette Coakley A, Duffy ME. The effect of therapeutic touch on postoperative patients. *J Holist Nurs.* 2010;28(3):193-200. [IIA]

213. McCormack GL. Using non-contact therapeutic touch to manage post-surgical pain in the elderly. *Occup Ther Int.* 2009;16(1):44-56. [IA]

214. Feng F, Tuchman S, Denninger JW, Fricchione GL, Yeung A. Qigong for the prevention, treatment, and rehabilitation of COVID-19 infection in older adults. *Am J Geriatr Psychiatry.* 2020;28(8):812-819. [VA]

215. MacIntyre B, Hamilton J, Fricke T, Ma W, Mehle S, Michel M. The efficacy of healing touch in coronary artery bypass surgery recovery: a randomized clinical trial. *Altern Ther Health Med.* 2008;14(4):24-32. [IA]

216. *AORN Position Statement on Patient Safety.* 2017. AORN, Inc. https://aorn.org/guidelines/clinical-resources/position-statements. Accessed May 17, 2021. [IVA]

217. *AORN Position Statement on a Healthy Perioperative Practice Environment.* 2015. AORN, Inc. https://aorn.org/guidelines/clinical-resources/position-statements. Accessed May 17, 2021. [IVA]

Guideline Development Group and Acknowledgments

Lead Author: Mary Alice Anderson[1], MSN, CNOR, RN, Perioperative Practice Specialist, AORN, Denver, Colorado
Contributing Author: Erin Kyle[2], DNP, RN, CNOR, NEA-BC, Editor-in-Chief, *Guidelines for Perioperative Practice,* AORN, Denver, Colorado
Methodologist: Erin Kyle[2]
Evidence Appraisers: Marie Bashaw[3], DNP, RN, NEA-BC, Professor and Director of Nursing, Wittenberg University, Springfield, Ohio; and Erin Kyle[2]

Guidelines Advisory Board Members:
- Susan Lynch[4], PhD, RN, CSSM, CNOR, Associate Director, Surgical Services, Penn Medicine-Chester County Hospital, West Chester, Pennsylvania
- Rob J. Levin[5], MSN, RN, FFT, CNOR, OR Educator Albert Einstein Medical Center, Philadelphia, Pennsylvania
- Elizabeth (Lizz) Pincus[6], MSN, RN, CNS-CP, CNOR, Clinical Nurse, Regional Medical Center of San Jose, California

External Review: Expert review comments were received from individual members of the American Association of Nurse Anesthetists (AANA), American College of Surgeons (ACS), Association for Professionals in Infection Control and Epidemiology (APIC), American Society of Anesthesiologists (ASA), International Association of Healthcare Central Service Materiel Management (IAHCSMM), the Society for Healthcare Epidemiology of America (SHEA), and the Surgical Infection Society (SIS). Their responses were used to further refine and enhance this guideline; however, their responses do not imply endorsement. The draft was also open for a 30-day public comment period.

Financial Disclosure and Conflicts of Interest

This guideline was developed, edited, and approved by the AORN Guidelines Advisory Board without external funding being sought or obtained. The Guidelines Advisory Board was financially supported entirely by AORN and was developed without any involvement of industry.

Potential conflicts of interest for all Guidelines Advisory Board members were reviewed before the annual meeting and each monthly conference call. None of the members of the Guideline Development Group reported a potential conflict of interest.[1-6]

Publication History

Originally published as Guideline for Complementary Care Interventions in *Guidelines for Perioperative Practice,* 2015 edition.

Evidence ratings revised in *Guidelines for Perioperative Practice,* 2018 edition, to conform to the current AORN Evidence Rating Model.

Evidence ratings revised and minor editorial changes made to conform to the current AORN Evidence Rating model, September 2019, for online publication in *Guidelines for Perioperative Practice.*

Revised June 2021 for online publication in *Guidelines for Perioperative Practice.*

Scheduled for review in 2026.

DESIGN AND MAINTENANCE

TABLE OF CONTENTS

🅿 *indicates a recommendation or evidence relevant to pediatric care.*

MEDICAL ABBREVIATIONS & ACRONYMS

ACH – Air changes per hour
HEPA – High-efficiency particulate air
HVAC – Heating, ventilation, and air conditioning
MRI – Magnetic resonance imaging

NFPA – National Fire Protection Association
OR – Operating room
PACU – Postanesthesia care unit
RN – Registered nurse

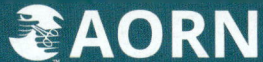
GUIDELINE FOR
DESIGN AND MAINTENANCE OF THE SURGICAL SUITE

The Guideline for Design and Maintenance of the Surgical Suite was approved by the AORN Guidelines Advisory Board and became effective August 1, 2018. It was presented as a proposed guideline for comments by members and others. The recommendations in the guideline are intended to be achievable and represent what is believed to be an optimal level of practice. Policies and procedures will reflect variations in practice settings and/or clinical situations that determine the degree to which the guideline can be implemented. AORN recognizes the many diverse settings in which perioperative nurses practice; therefore, this guideline is adaptable to all areas where operative or other invasive procedures may be performed.

Purpose

The physical design of the **surgical suite** should support safe patient care, efficient movement of patients and supplies, and workplace safety and security. The surgical suite includes the preoperative, intraoperative, and postoperative patient care areas and support areas, including central and satellite sterile processing areas, administrative areas, waiting areas, and locker rooms. This document provides guidance on the design of the surgical suite; security measures; safety measures during new construction or renovation; planning for utility service interruption; restoration of the surgical suite to full functionality after a utility failure; maintenance of structural surfaces; and design, monitoring, and maintenance of the heating, ventilation, and air conditioning (HVAC) system. The following topics are outside the scope of this document:

- use of portable/robotic ultraviolet light generators (See the AORN Guideline for Environmental Cleaning[1]);
- management of heater-cooler units (See the AORN Guideline for Sterile Technique[2]);
- accommodations for disabilities;
- interior design (eg, colors, furniture, cabinetry);
- control of surgical smoke (See the AORN Guideline for Surgical Smoke Safety[3]);
- security of information technology, including electronic health records (See the AORN Guideline for Patient Information Management[4]); and
- management of social media.

Evidence Review

A medical librarian conducted a systematic search of the databases Ovid MEDLINE®, EBSCO CINAHL®, Scopus®, and the Cochrane Database of Systematic Reviews. The search was limited to literature published in English from January 2012 through January 2018. At the time of the initial search, weekly alerts were created on the topics included in that search. Results from these alerts were provided to the lead author until January 2018. The lead author requested additional articles that either did not fit the original search criteria or were discovered during the evidence appraisal process. The lead author and the medical librarian also identified relevant guidelines from government agencies, professional organizations, and standards-setting bodies.

Search terms included *air conditioning, air filters, air microbiology, air pollutants (environmental), air pollution (indoor), airborne particles, anesthetics (inhalation), computer security, confidentiality, door openings/closings/swings, dust, electricity, energy conservation, environment (controlled), equipment contamination, equipment manufacturers, facility design and construction, fungi, gas scavengers, germicidal irradiation, green retrofit, Health Insurance Portability and Accountability Act, HIPAA, hospital design and construction, humidity, HVAC/unoccupied/night setback, illumination, laminar airflow, lighting, meaningful use, microbial colony count, mycoses, occupational exposure, operating room traffic patterns, particulate matter, power failure, privacy, restricted area, security measures, spores, traffic patterns/flow/deterrents, transition zone, ultraviolet germicidal irradiation, ultraviolet rays, unidirectional system, utility failure, vendors, violence, waste products,* and *workplace violence.*

Included were research and non-research literature in English, complete publications, and publications with dates within the time restriction when available. Exclusion criteria included documents deemed to be out of scope or not generalizable, duplicate articles, and older evidence within the time restriction when more recent evidence was available. Editorials, news items, and other brief items also were excluded. Evidence from non-peer-reviewed publications was excluded when evidence from peer-reviewed publications was available, and lower-quality evidence was excluded when higher-quality evidence was available **(Figure 1)**.

Articles identified in the search were provided to the project team for evaluation. The team consisted of the lead author and one evidence appraiser. The articles were reviewed and critically appraised using the AORN Research or Non-Research Evidence Appraisal Tools as appropriate. The literature was independently evaluated and appraised according to the strength and quality of the evidence. Each article was then assigned an appraisal score. The appraisal score is noted in brackets after each reference as applicable.

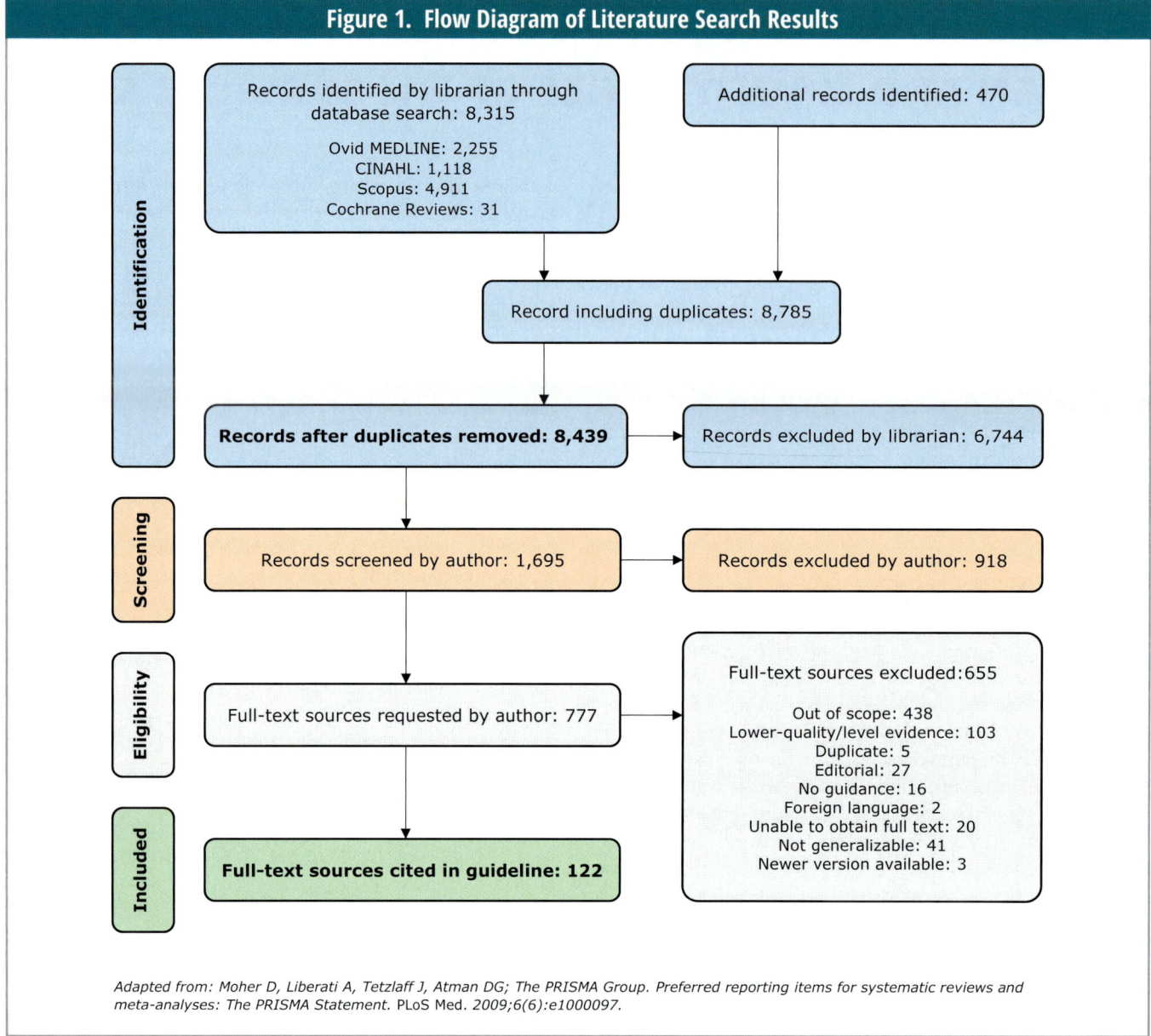

Figure 1. Flow Diagram of Literature Search Results

Records identified by librarian through database search: 8,315

Ovid MEDLINE: 2,255
CINAHL: 1,118
Scopus: 4,911
Cochrane Reviews: 31

Additional records identified: 470

Record including duplicates: 8,785

Records after duplicates removed: 8,439

Records excluded by librarian: 6,744

Records screened by author: 1,695

Records excluded by author: 918

Full-text sources requested by author: 777

Full-text sources excluded: 655

Out of scope: 438
Lower-quality/level evidence: 103
Duplicate: 5
Editorial: 27
No guidance: 16
Foreign language: 2
Unable to obtain full text: 20
Not generalizable: 41
Newer version available: 3

Full-text sources cited in guideline: 122

Identification · Screening · Eligibility · Included

Adapted from: Moher D, Liberati A, Tetzlaff J, Atman DG; The PRISMA Group. Preferred reporting items for systematic reviews and meta-analyses: The PRISMA Statement. PLoS Med. 2009;6(6):e1000097.

Each recommendation rating is based on a synthesis of the collective evidence, a benefit-harm assessment, and consideration of resource use. The strength of the recommendation was determined using the AORN Evidence Rating Model and the quality and consistency of the evidence supporting a recommendation. The recommendation strength rating is noted in brackets after each recommendation.

Note: The evidence summary table is available at http://www.aorn.org/evidencetables/.

Editor's note: MEDLINE is a registered trademark of the US National Library of Medicine's Medical Literature Analysis and Retrieval System, Bethesda, MD. Embase is a registered trademark of Elsevier B.V., Amsterdam, The Netherlands. CINAHL, Cumulative Index to Nursing and Allied Health Literature, is a registered trademark of EBSCO Industries, Birmingham, AL.

1. Interdisciplinary Team

1.1 Establish an **interdisciplinary team** with authority and responsibility to provide oversight of surgical suite construction or renovation projects. *[Recommendation]*

An interdisciplinary team can provide expertise on functional design, the functional needs of the users, infection prevention, sustainability, and regulatory requirements from a variety of viewpoints.[5-15]

In a case study, Guedon et al[16] described how an interdisciplinary team provided insights in the social and the organizational context of the facility. The authors concluded that the involvement of the interdisciplinary team helped in choosing the best technology to increase efficiency in the OR.

In a case report, Capolongo et al[17] described a participatory design process that included the use of a focus group for designing an emergency room, including choosing the color scheme. The authors determined that a participatory process allowed the users to understand the reasons for the color that was selected. The authors also stated that the members of the focus group can convey design decisions to their peers and to other key stakeholders. The authors recommended using a participatory design process, including a focus group, when designing a health care facility.

1.2 Include internal and external representatives on the interdisciplinary team. [*Recommendation*]

1.2.1 Include the following internal representatives of the health care organization on the team:
- perioperative registered nurses (RNs) with the responsibility and authority to represent the **perioperative team**;
- surgeons,
- anesthesia professionals,
- preoperative and postoperative nursing personnel,
- sterile processing personnel,
- environmental services personnel,
- surgical technologists,
- administrative personnel;
- infection preventionists; and
- representatives from other affected disciplines (eg, pharmacy, radiology, laboratory) as determined by the scope of the project.

[*Recommendation*]

Include the following external representatives:
- members of the design team (eg, architects, interior designers, engineers) and
- representatives of equipment manufacturers whose equipment requires provisions for structural support, space, and utilities.

[*Recommendation*]

Low-quality evidence and guidelines support the creation of an interdisciplinary team consisting of key stakeholders from some or all of the areas listed.[8,9,11,13,14,18-20] In an expert opinion article, Stichler[21] suggested hiring a consultant if the facility lacks the internal resources to assist with the management of any phase of the construction project.

1.2.2 The designated perioperative RN(s)
- provides input into the selection of equipment;
- provides input into the proposed flow of people, supplies, and equipment;
- provides input into space utilization;
- provides input for ergonomic safety;
- verifies the presence and integrity of construction barriers and infection pre-ven-tion measures (See Recommendation 10);
- participates in construction meetings;
- monitors the progress of the project by visual inspection;
- communicates to the perioperative team the progress of the project and information that will affect the daily functions of the surgical suite (eg, the presence of new barriers, additional cleaning required, noise and vibration that will be caused by the construction);
- collaborates with all stakeholders;
- collaborates with perioperative team members to resolve unanticipated problems as they arise during the construction process; and
- verifies that the components required (eg, surgical table, anesthesia machine, suction canister, back table) in an operating room (OR) are present in the simulated OR (See Recommendation 1.11).

[*Recommendation*]

In a systematic review of the literature, Stichler[22] concluded that RNs provide knowledge of the patient care environment and daily workflow processes and provide the clinical nurse's voice to help ensure the needs for safety, visual acuity, and efficiency to conserve energy are met. Devine et al[11] emphasized the importance of the perioperative RN being present to act as a liaison to keep peers informed.

1.3 The interdisciplinary team should participate in all phases of the project including scope development, budgeting, planning, design, construction, and **commissioning**. [*Recommendation*]

Experts agree that the interdisciplinary team should participate in all phases of the project.[13,14,23]

1.4 Create a functional program to include the
- scope and type of services to be provided;
- scope and type of anesthesia services to be provided;
- specialties to be served;
- procedures to be performed;
- type of patient care areas required (eg, preoperative, postoperative phase I and II);

- design and location of preoperative and post-operative patient care areas, such as
  - separate areas for preoperative, postoperative phase I, and postoperative phase II care;
  - separate areas for preoperative care and combined areas for postoperative phase I and postoperative phase II care;
  - separate areas for postoperative phase I care and combined areas for preoperative and postoperative phase II care; or
  - combined areas for preoperative, postoperative phase I, and postoperative phase II care;
- patient population (eg, patients of size, age, acuity levels);
- type of **patient care stations** for the preoperative and postoperative care areas (eg, **bay**, **cubicle**, **room**);
- projected volume of procedures;
- utility requirements;
- environmental (eg, HVAC) requirements;
- security requirements;
- communication requirements;
- storage requirements;
- technological requirements;
- sterile processing and supply movement requirements;
- location of support areas; and
- traffic patterns.

[Recommendation]

The functional program is a base for the design, communicates the owner's expectations for the project to the designers and others, and may be used as a supplemental construction document.[13,14]

| 1.4.1 | Determine the number of patient care stations in the preoperative and postoperative areas based on the number of ORs, anticipated volume, and scope of services.[13,14] *[Recommendation]*

1.5 Apply the design criteria established by the **authority having jurisdiction** when designing the surgical suite. *[Recommendation]*

State regulatory requirements may differ from the recommendations set forth in this guideline. This document references the most current guidelines and standards published by professional organizations.[13,14,24,25] These guidelines and standards are adopted in varying degrees by regulatory agencies.

| 1.5.1 | Perform a review of current design literature including federal, state, and local regulatory requirements and applicable construction guidelines (eg, Occupational Safety and Health Administration, Centers for Medicare & Medicaid Services, National Fire Protection Association [NFPA], Facility Guidelines Insti-

tute, American Society for Healthcare Engineering).[13,14,20,26-28] *[Recommendation]*

1.6 During the design phase, develop and implement a plan to minimize the impact on areas **adjacent** to the construction site (See Recommendation 10). *[Recommendation]*

1.7 Perform an ongoing safety assessment beginning early in the planning phase, continuing throughout the project, and ending at commissioning. *[Recommendation]*

| 1.7.1 | Include the following in the safety risk assessment:
- an infection control risk assessment;
- a patient handling and movement assessment (See the AORN Guideline for Safe Patient Handling and Movement[29]);
- a patient fall prevention assessment (See the AORN Guideline for Safe Patient Handling and Movement[29]);
- a medication safety assessment;
- a behavioral and mental health risk assessment;
- a security risk assessment; and
- factors that support a safe design and assist in creating the criteria for the selection of equipment, furnishings, finishes, surfaces, and HVAC systems.

[Recommendation]

Guidelines and low-quality evidence support completion of all or a portion of the items in this list.[8,13,14,20,30-32] The degree of detail expressed is dependent on the scope of the project and the population served.

1.8 Perform a security assessment, determine the zones of protection for each area, and determine security measures (See Recommendation 2.4.).[6,27,33] *[Recommendation]*

| 1.8.1 | Select security measures (eg, alarm systems, shatterproof glass, metal detectors, keyed or electronic door security systems [eg, digital, programmable, magstripe keycards and readers, contactless radio-frequency identification, cards or fobs with proximity readers, biometric systems that scan physical attributes (eg, fingerprints or retinas)], video surveillance, tracking systems, electronic identification access tracking systems, visitor logs) based on the security assessment.[6,27] *[Conditional Recommendation]*

In an expert opinion article, Yow[34] stated that video surveillance has positive and negative attributes. The positive attributes of a video system are that it may

- assist with improving the safety and security program,
- assist with preventing dishonest claims and false reports to law enforcement,
- assist with resolving all types of disputes,
- provide for real-time monitoring from internal or remote personal computers,
- provide for digital storage on network servers,
- provide visual evidence for internal and law enforcement investigations, and
- increase employee productivity.

Conversely, the negative attributes are that security cameras may

- lead to a decision not to provide additional physical security personnel because of over-reliance on the camera system,
- create a source for breach of patient privacy,
- lead to tampering with the cameras that can create an interruption of the video, and
- exceed the capacity of the information technology system.

1.9 Perform an environmental impact assessment of construction materials and design features during the planning phase. *[Recommendation]*

McGain and Naylor[35] completed a systematic review of the literature on hospital environmental sustainability and determined that there are instances in which the interests of patients and the environment coincide, but others where they conflict. The authors recommended more research be completed on the topic of sustainability. In a review of the literature, Beale and Kittredge[36] recommended incorporating sustainability into the design of a facility.

1.9.1 Assess the environmental impact by evaluating the projected water and energy consumption; the biodegradability and environmental toxicity of the building materials; and the ability to recycle, reuse, or renew building materials and construction debris. *[Recommendation]*

1.9.2 Environmental impact–reducing design features that may be included in the project are
- anesthetic gas reclamation systems,[37]
- LED surgical lamps,[37,38]
- closed fluid collection systems,[37,39]
- low flow water fixtures,
- bicycle racks and lockers,
- renewable energy sources,
- light switches that turn on and off automatically,

- heat pumps,
- a high-efficiency HVAC system,
- an HVAC setback strategy,
- surfaces and finishes that use low volatile organic compounds, and
- natural lighting.
[Conditional Recommendation]

1.10 Use energy consumption as a factor when purchasing products that use energy (eg, lighting, HVAC systems, water heaters). *[Recommendation]*

An energy-efficient device will decrease operating costs and may create lower amounts of emissions.[40] In an analysis of energy consumption, Ma et al[41] concluded that hospitals use more energy than schools and office buildings. The main factors that influence building energy consumption are the **building envelope**, lighting equipment, and air conditioning systems. The researchers recommended using energy-efficient lamps and air conditioning systems in addition to a building envelope with a low heat transfer coefficient to decrease the amount of energy used and therefore the carbon footprint.

1.10.1 Energy-saving methods (eg, energy audits, energy-saving lighting systems, alternative energy-generating systems) may be incorporated into the design of the perioperative care area. *[Conditional Recommendation]*

A case study illustrates the savings realized by one facility after low-energy-use devices were incorporated into the facility. The savings continued beyond the first year of service.[42] Completing an energy audit may assist with determining sources of energy waste (eg, lights and computers left on after personnel have gone home or the surgical procedures have been completed).[40]

1.11 During the surgical suite planning and design phase, use a simulated room or suite setup. *[Recommendation]*

Low-quality evidence supports use of a simulated room.[18,36,43,44] Mocked-up rooms are thought to assist with design because individual care providers (eg, physicians, nurses, ancillary staff members) are able to move through a simulation of their clinical practice areas and identify which layouts and configurations work best.[36] The team can also establish equipment and door placement, size of the rooms, and traffic and equipment flow patterns and visualize how the space will be used.

1.12 Develop and provide education for all key stakeholders on the use of new or remodeled spaces. *[Recommendation]*

1.12.1 Include the following in the education plan:
- emergency exits;
- location and use of electrical outlets, medical gas outlets, and other utilities;
- location of equipment and supplies; and
- movement of patients, personnel, supplies, and equipment through the facility.

[Recommendation]

2. Design Concepts

2.1 Use **evidence-based design** concepts in the design of the surgical suite. [Recommendation] **P**

Use of evidence-based design concepts has been reported to reduce infections, reduce stress on medical personnel, and improve patient healing.[8,45] Examples of evidence-based design concepts include integrated facility design, self-sufficiency design, and a human-centered design thinking process.

In a nonexperimental study, Pelly et al[5] described the impact of integrated facility design on the functionality of a pediatric ambulatory surgery center. An integrated facility design process is a process adapted from the Toyota 3P Program with a goal of accelerating development time and lowering start-up costs. The researchers compared the integrated facility design process to similar projects designed using traditional methods. They found that use of the integrated facility design process improved patient, family, and provider flow; reduced surgical and postanesthesia care unit (PACU) times; and reduced building space and change orders, leading to a savings of $30 million in the planned cost of the entire building.

The self-sufficiency design process permits the interdisciplinary design team to adapt the design and construction of new hospitals for optimal disaster functionality based on lessons learned from internal and external institutional experiences.[46]

The human-centered design thinking process supports the incorporation of an interdisciplinary team and the use of simulations.[15] Human-centered design thinking is defined as a process of creating solutions to complex problems for specific user groups, which focuses on needfinding, understanding, creating, thinking, and doing. Human-centered design thinking is a combination of creative thinking and critical thinking performed in an organized, replicable manner that enables personnel to express ideas; gain knowledge; make decisions; and improve products, services, or processes.

2.2 Divide the surgical suite into zones (ie, unrestricted, semi-restricted, restricted) based on the activities performed in each area; the access pathway; and the attire, HVAC, and surface requirements. [Recommendation]

2.2.1 The requirements for each zone include the following:
- All zones
  - have specific HVAC design requirements associated with the intended use of the space as described in *ANSI/ASHRAE/ASHE Standard 170-2017 Ventilation of Health Care Facilities*[13,14,24] and
  - have surfaces on floors, walls, ceilings, and cabinets that are durable, smooth, cleanable, and able to withstand cleaning practices.[13,14]
- Unrestricted zones
  - are accessible from the exterior of the building, other unrestricted areas, or semi-restricted areas and
  - do not require the wearing of surgical attire (ie, wearing of street clothes is permitted).
- Semi-restricted zones
  - are accessible from unrestricted, other semi-restricted, or restricted areas;
  - require the wearing of surgical attire[47];
  - have floors with no seams or sealed seams and a **cove base**;
  - have walls with no seams or sealed seams; and
  - have ceilings that are either **monolithic** or are drop-in ceiling tiles.
- Restricted zones
  - are accessible only from a semi-restricted area;
  - require the wearing of surgical attire[47] and masks in the presence of open sterile supplies[2];
  - have floors with no seams or sealed seams and a cove base;
  - have walls that are smooth with no seams or sealed seams; and
  - have ceilings that are monolithic or are drop-in gasketed ceiling tiles.

[Recommendation]

The HVAC, surgical attire, and traffic pattern requirements of the surgical suite are designed to be more stringent as one moves from unrestricted to restricted areas.[48] The progression of restrictions is intended to provide the cleanest environment in the restricted area.

Monolithic ceilings may assist in preventing dust and other contaminants from falling into the surgical wound or onto the sterile field. Ceilings require intermittent washing with harsh chemicals, which is facilitated by the surface being smooth.[13,14,48]

Surfaces that are durable, smooth, and cleanable allow for ease of cleaning and assist in preventing buildup of dirt and debris in crevices.[9,13,14]

2.2.2 **Separate the zones by signage indicating the attire required for entering the area and who is authorized to enter.** *[Recommendation]*

Signs provide a visual cue that alerts persons to the restrictions required for entry into each area. Doors provide a physical barrier to assist in maintaining control of the HVAC.

2.2.3 **Separate the unrestricted and semi-restricted areas by one or more visual cues (eg, doors, signage, floor or wall color change).** *[Recommendation]*

2.2.4 **Separate the restricted area from the semi-restricted area with a door.** *[Recommendation]*

2.3 **Assign the zones to the areas within the surgical suite as shown in Table 1.** *[Recommendation]*

2.4 **Determine the security zones for the surgical suite by the items stored in each location, and define the zones in the facility security plan (Table 2). The zones described in Recommendation 2.2. are not related to the security zones of protection.** *[Recommendation]*

The zones of protection recommended by the International Association for Healthcare Security and Safety include the following:

- "general areas accessible to the public at all times" have no restrictions regarding who enters or leaves the area and, depending on their locations in the building, may open to the exterior environment;
- "general areas restricted to the public during non-visiting hours, periods of lesser activity, or other periods of increased vulnerability" have time or situational restrictions as to when the public is admitted;
- "screened public areas" are accessible to only certain members of the public;
- "staff and accompanied public areas" may have a device on the doors (eg, card key entry, combination key pad) that permits entry only to those with permission to enter or those who are escorted by a person with permission to enter;
- "general staff-only areas" are accessible only to staff members and not the public; and

- "areas for designated staff with appropriate clearance" are accessible only to staff members with approved clearance.[6]

2.4.1 **Rooms in which biologicals or medical records are stored must be secured and accessible only to designated personnel with appropriate clearance.[49] [Regulatory Requirement]**

2.4.2 **Medications must be secured in a locked cabinet or a locked room.[49] [Regulatory Requirement]**

2.5 **Incorporate ergonomic design features in the design of the surgical suite that are based on the recommendations in the patient handling and movement assessment and the AORN Guideline for Safe Patient Handling and Movement.[29]** *[Recommendation]*

Ergonomic design principles include accommodations for handling patients of size; placement of electrical and gas outlets to prevent personnel from having to stretch, bend, or reach over the patient to access them; and measures to prevent slips, trips, and falls. Ergonomic accommodations may include structurally supported lifts, additional square footage for portable lift storage and operation, and increased structural supports (eg, hand rails, sinks, and commodes).[13,14,29,50,51]

In a systematic review, Stichler[22] concluded that the nursing workforce includes large numbers of aging nurses with physical and cognitive challenges that may result in injuries, and including ergonomic considerations in the design may help to decrease injuries for all nurses.

Thomas-Olsen et al[52] surveyed 29 perioperative staff members from a health system in Canada and found the reported number of injury claims due to patient handling decreased from five per year to fewer than one per year after the introduction of ceiling lifts in the OR.

2.6 **Design the HVAC system to meet the requirements associated with the intended use of the space.** *[Recommendation]*

The HVAC system assists with decreasing airborne microorganisms by filtering supplied air, diluting the contaminated air in the OR, and preventing entry of contaminated air from the areas outside the OR.[23] The pressure differentials between areas assists in preventing back-flow of air from contaminated areas within the suite or the facility.[23]

The rate of air changes per hour (ACH) in an OR is supported in a descriptive study by Gormley and Wagner.[53] The researchers measured the number of airborne particles in 30 simulated surgeries at 15 ACH, 20 ACH, and 25 ACH at the patient location, on

Table 1. Surgical Suite Zones[1,2]

Area	Zone
Preoperative patient care area Postoperative patient care area	Unrestricted*
Corridor leading from unrestricted area to restricted area Sterile processing clean and decontamination room or area** Satellite sterile processing area	Semi-restricted
Operating room	Restricted
Clean equipment and supply storage room Satellite laboratory Satellite pharmacy Specimen holding area Clean and soiled workrooms Supply breakout area/room Clean linen storage area Soiled linen storage area Environmental services room Garbage storage/holding area	Unrestricted* when access is obtained from a semi-restricted area and an unrestricted area or from an unrestricted area only - or - Semi-restricted when access is obtained from a semi-restricted area only
Locker rooms Waiting rooms Information systems control room Patient waiting rooms Administrative areas (eg, offices, reception areas, business offices) Medical records storage area Nurse station Multipurpose rooms	Unrestricted*

* Any unrestricted area can be a semi-restricted area if the area or room is located within a semi-restricted area.
** AAMI defines these areas as restricted.[3]

References

1. *Facility Guidelines Institute, US Department of Health and Human Services, American Society for Healthcare Engineering.* Guidelines for Design and Construction of Hospitals. *Chicago, IL: American Society for Healthcare Engineering of the American Hospital Association; 2018.*
2. *Facility Guidelines Institute, US Department of Health and Human Services, American Society for Healthcare Engineering.* Guidelines for Design and Construction of Outpatient Facilities. *Chicago, IL: American Society for Healthcare Engineering of the American Hospital Association; 2018.*
3. ANSI/AAMI ST79:2017 Comprehensive Guide to Steam Sterilization and Sterility Assurance in Health Care Facilities. *Arlington, VA: Association for the Advancement of Medical Instrumentation; 2017.*

the back table, and by an air return vent. The researchers found there were fewer particles at 20 ACH than at 15 ACH, and there was not an appreciable difference between 20 ACH and 25 ACH. The researchers recommended that the air change rate be 20 ACH.

Wan et al[54] conducted a nonexperimental study in which they sampled the particulate matter in the air 33 times in each of five different types of ORs. The ORs had either 20 ACH or 15 ACH. The researchers found a lower level of particulate matter in the ORs with the 20 ACH and recommended that this rate be used.

2.6.1 Use the HVAC design parameters for each area, as described in Table 3, for the design of a new or remodeled system, unless other

parameters are required by state or local regulations.[13,14] *[Recommendation]*

The design parameters provide a guide for the interdisciplinary team to use when selecting the HVAC system equipment and may be different from the operational values **(See Recommendation 12).**

2.7 In the design for the surgical suite, include the number of electrical outlets, the number of gas ports; and presence or absence of a waste anesthesia line and a nurse call system as associated with the intended use of the space **(Table 4).** *[Recommendation]*

2.7.1 Provide instrument air, via an outlet or portable tank, in all areas in which air is required

Table 2. Security Zones

Area	Zone
Interior of nurse station Clean workroom Soiled workroom Space for storing clean linen Space for storing dirty linen Storage for patient belongings Equipment and supply storage Multipurpose rooms Locker rooms Specimen management area Equipment storage rooms Satellite laboratory	General staff-only areas
Facilities for patient bathing	Screened public areas
Operating rooms Corridors leading to ORs from unrestricted areas Administrative areas/offices Preoperative patient care stations Postoperative patient care stations Phase I Postoperative patient care stations Phase II	Staff and accompanied public areas
Information systems control room Satellite pharmacy Medication storage and preparation area	Areas for designated staff with appropriate clearance

Note: The security zones may differ based on the care delivery model. If the care delivery model requires the area to be a closet, such as a supply closet, the doors to the closet should be accessible to staff members only.

for powering medical devices unrelated to human respiration, drying medical devices, powering air driven booms and pendants, and similar applications.[13,14,27] *[Recommendation]*

2.8 The surgical suite must be designed with electrical safeguards in place as described in *NFPA 70: National Electrical Code*[28]; *NFPA 99: Health Care Facilities Code Handbook*[27]; *Guidelines for Design and Construction of Hospitals*[13]; *Guidelines for Design and Construction of Outpatient Facilities*[14]; and local, state, and national regulations.[55] *[Regulatory Requirement]*

2.8.1 Determine whether the OR floor will be frequently flooded when a patient is present, making the room a "wet location." *[Recommendation]*

The NFPA defines locations where the floor is frequently flooded as a wet location. If it is determined that the room is a wet location, the room requires either an isolated power system or ground-fault circuit interrupters.[27,28]

2.9 Design the surgical suite with multiple lighting options appropriate to the tasks to be performed in the area.[56] (See Recommendation 4.12. for lighting of the sterile field). *[Recommendation]*

Stichler[22] performed a systematic literature review and concluded that multiple lighting options in patient rooms and in nurses' work areas provided the appropriate amount of light required to meet the needs of the patient and caregiver.

Dianat et al[57] conducted a nonexperimental study to evaluate the effect of lighting conditions in a hospital setting on employee satisfaction, job performance, safety, and health, and to find the most appropriate methods of improving lighting in this setting. The researchers surveyed 208 employees regarding the lighting conditions (eg, lighting characteristics and lighting disturbances) in the facility and the influence of lighting conditions on subjective assessments of employee satisfaction, job performance, safety, and health. There were also questions on potential improvements to the lighting conditions. The survey consisted of constructs for measuring

- satisfaction (2 items: satisfaction with general lighting condition and task visibility),
- job performance (2 items: decreased performance due to low light levels and lighting disturbances),
- safety (2 items: falls or slips due to light levels and lighting disturbances), and
- health (4 items: eye tiredness due to low light levels and lighting disturbances as well as the need to change posture for better viewing of the

Table 3. Heating, Ventilating, and Air Conditioning Design Parameters[1-4]

Area*	Minimum Total Air Changes per Hour	Minimum Total Outdoor Air Changes	Design Temperature ° F (° C)	Design Relative Humidity	Pressure Relationship to Adjacent Areas
Operating room	20	4	68° - 75° (20° - 24°)	20% - 60%[5]	Positive
Sterile processing clean workroom	4	2	68° - 73° (20° - 23°)	Maximum 60%	Positive
Sterile processing decontamination room	6	2	60° - 73° (16° - 23°)	NR	Negative
Clean workroom	4	2	NR	NR	Positive
Soiled workroom	10	2	NR	NR	Negative
Sterile storage room	4	2	Maximum 75° (24°)	Maximum 60%	Positive
Gastrointestinal endoscopy procedure room	6	2	68° - 73° (20° - 23°)	20% - 60%	NR
Endoscope cleaning room	10	2	NR	NR	Negative
Postanesthesia care unit	6	2	70° - 75° (21° - 24°)	20% - 60%	NR
Procedure room	15	3	70° - 75° (21° - 24°)	20% - 60%	Positive

* For areas not listed, consult the *ANSI/ASHRAE/ASHE Standard 170-2017 Ventilation of Health Care Facilities.*[1] This is a dynamic document and the most current edition or addendum should be consulted at the time of design.

NR = No recommendation

References

1. ANSI/ASHRAE/ASHE Standard 170-2017: Ventilation of Health Care Facilities. *New York, NY: American Society of Heating, Refrigerating and Air-Conditioning Engineers; 2017.*
2. *Facility Guidelines Institute, US Department of Health and Human Services, American Society for Healthcare Engineering.* Guidelines for Design and Construction of Hospitals. *Chicago, IL: American Society for Healthcare Engineering of the American Hospital Association; 2018.*
3. *Facility Guidelines Institute, US Department of Health and Human Services, American Society for Healthcare Engineering.* Guidelines for Design and Construction of Outpatient Facilities. *Chicago, IL: American Society for Healthcare Engineering of the American Hospital Association; 2018.*
4. *Berrios-Torres SI, Umscheid CA, Bratzler DW, et al. Centers for Disease Control and Prevention Guideline for the Prevention of Surgical Site Infection, 2017. JAMA Surg. 2017;152(8):784-791.*
5. State Operations Manual Appendix I: Survey Procedures for Life Safety Code Surveys. *Rev 159; 2016. https://www.cms.gov/Regulations-and-Guidance/Guidance/Manuals/downloads/som107ap_i_lsc.pdf. Accessed June 7, 2018.*

objects or working items due to low light levels and lighting disturbances).

The researchers found that 56% of the respondents reported eye tiredness related to the inadequate lighting conditions, 48% stated they had to change position to be able to see better, and 14% stated inadequate lighting increased the risk for slips or falls. The researchers concluded that light levels and light disturbances, such as unwanted shadows, were correlated with job performance.

2.9.1 Design the surgical suite lighting system to provide
- light for monitoring the patient and performance of other patient care tasks,
- dimmable lighting, and
- low operating and maintenance costs.

[Recommendation]

2.10 Select cabinets and countertops in the surgical suite that are made of nonabsorbent materials

Table 4. Minimum Utility Requirements[1-4]

Items*	Number per Operating Room	Number per Patient Station in Phase I PACU	Number per Patient Station in Phase II PACU	Number per Procedure Room	Number per Preprocedure Room	Number per Endoscopy Procedure Room	Number per Sterile Processing Decontamination Room	Number per Sterile Processing Clean Room	Number per Endoscopy Processing Room
Electrical outlets	36	8	4	12	NR	12	NR	NR	NR
Suction ports	5 (1ª,3ᵇ)	3 (1)	1	2	NR	3	NR	NR	e
Oxygen ports	2 (1)	2 (1)	1 (0)	2	0	1ᵈ	NR	NR	NR
Medical air ports	1 (1ᵇ)	1	NR	1	NR	NR	NR	NR	NR
Instrument air ports	1	NR	NR	NR	NR	NR	1ᵈ	ᵈ ᵉ	ᵈ ᵉ (1)
Waste anesthesia lines	1 (ᶜ)	NR	NR	NR	NR	NR	NR	NR	NR
Staff assist stations	1	1	1	1	1	NR (1)	NR	NR	NR (1)
Nurse call systems	NR	NR	Optional (1)	NR	1	NR	NR	NR	NR
Emergency call stations	1	1	1	1	1	NR	NR	NR	NR

PACU = Postanesthesia care unit; NR = No recommendation

* Numbers of items are the same for inpatient and outpatient facilities except where noted.
( ) = Outpatient facility information
ª = 255 sq ft ambulatory OR
ᵇ = 270 sq ft ambulatory OR
ᶜ = Waste anesthesia gas disposal is required when giving inhalation anesthesia.
ᵈ = Portable equipment in lieu of a piped gas system may be used.
ᵉ = Vacuum and/or instrument air is required if needed for the cleaning methods used.

References

1. *Facility Guidelines Institute, US Department of Health and Human Services, American Society for Healthcare Engineering.* Guidelines for Design and Construction of Hospitals. *Chicago, IL: American Society for Healthcare Engineering of the American Hospital Association; 2018.*
2. *Facility Guidelines Institute, US Department of Health and Human Services, American Society for Healthcare Engineering.* Guidelines for Design and Construction of Outpatient Facilities. *Chicago, IL: American Society for Healthcare Engineering of the American Hospital Association; 2018.*
3. NFPA 99: Health Care Facilities Code Handbook. *Quincy, MA: National Fire Protection Association; 2018.*
4. NFPA 70: National Electrical Code. *Quincy, MA: National Fire Protection Association; 2017.*

(eg, laminate, stainless steel, glass)[13,14] and free of seams, including edge seams. *[Recommendation]*

2.11 Select wall materials for the surgical suite that are made of an impact-resistant material.[9,48] *[Recommendation]*

When a wall surface is breached, a potential source of contamination is created.

2.11.1 Conduct an assessment to determine which walls and what amount of the walls should be covered with the impact-resistant material. *[Recommendation]*

2.12 Self-disinfecting surfaces (eg, copper, silver, antimicrobial surfactant, quaternary ammonium salt) may be used in the surgical suite. *[Conditional Recommendation]*

In a quasi-experimental study, Hinsa-Leasure et al[58] measured the bacterial concentration on 18 different high-touch objects in a 47-bed hospital. The experimental group contained copper alloys and the control group contained no copper. The researchers found the bacterial concentration on the objects containing the copper alloy was significantly lower than on the objects that did not contain the copper. The researchers concluded that copper alloy components should be used in health care facilities.

Karpanen et al[59] conducted a nonexperimental study on a surgical ward in which they measured microbial counts on 14 high-touch items made of a copper alloy. These counts were then compared to counts taken from the same items that did not contain the copper alloy. The researchers found lower counts on all of the items that contained the copper. They concluded that the use of copper in combination with optimal infection prevention strategies may reduce the risk to patients of acquiring an infection in a health care setting.

In a systematic review of the literature, O'Gorman and Humphreys[60] concluded that more research is needed before they could recommend widespread implementation of copper surfaces. Weber and Rutala[61] and Barzoloski-O'Connor[30] reached the same conclusion in reviews of the literature.

Further research is needed to determine the areas that should be covered in a self-disinfecting material and what self-disinfecting material is the most effective.

3. Preoperative Area

3.1 Use evidence-based design concepts in the planning and design of the **preoperative area**. *[Recommendation]*

3.2 Include the following in the preoperative area design:
- patient care stations,
- a **medication safety zone**,
- **hand washing stations**,
- provisions for storing patients' belongings,
- bathrooms for patients and personnel, and
- other support areas (See Recommendation 7).
[Recommendation]

3.2.1 Design hand washing stations to be located in every toilet room and patient care room. In patient care areas with more than one patient care station, include one hand washing station for every four or fewer patient care stations. If the number of patient care stations is not divisible by four, include one hand washing station for any fraction up to one (eg, if five, six, or seven patient care stations are present, two hand washing stations would be needed).[13,14] *[Recommendation]*

3.2.2 These areas may be shared with intraoperative or postoperative areas as defined in the functional program.[13,14] *[Conditional Recommendation]*

3.3 Determine the number of preoperative patient care stations and support areas based on the functional program (See Recommendation 1). *[Recommendation]*

3.4 Perform a risk/cost/benefit analysis to determine whether preoperative and postoperative care will be administered in the same area or different areas. *[Recommendation]*

3.4.1 If preoperative and postoperative care will be administered in the same area, design the area to meet the requirements of the area with the more stringent criteria.[13,14] *[Recommendation]*

4. Operating Rooms

4.1 Use evidence-based design concepts in the planning and design of the **intraoperative area.** *[Recommendation]*

Use of evidence-based design, such as human-centered OR design, may assist in decreasing the number of flow disruptions per procedure. In a nonexperimental study, Palmer et al[62] identified 1,080 flow disruptions by the entire perioperative team during 10 cardiac procedures. The researchers concluded that 33% of the disruptions were related to OR layout and design. They recommended this information be used in future design projects to decrease threats to patient safety caused by flow disruptions.

4.2 Design operating rooms to be of sufficient size to accommodate the number of anticipated personnel and amount of fixed and mobile equipment.[9,13,14,48] *[Recommendation]*

4.3 When determining the size and floor plan of the OR, divide the area into four zones: sterile field, circulation pathway, movable equipment zone, and anesthesia zone.[13,14] *[Recommendation]*
- The sterile field zone includes the OR bed, a clear area on each side for personnel and outstretched patient arm rests, and clearance at the foot of the OR bed for personnel and equipment.
- The circulation pathway zone includes the back table, other sterile equipment, and personnel in sterile attire. This space should accommodate the movement of two people in sterile attire and allow them to meet and pass each other without touching each other or nonsterile surfaces. The circulation pathway should include all four sides of the OR bed and should provide sufficient space for personnel to perform patient care tasks; pass between the sterile field and the wall during the procedure; and pass

between the anesthesia professional(s), anesthesia equipment, and the wall.

- The movable equipment zone includes the equipment not needed in close proximity to the sterile zone (eg, garbage cans, case cart).
- The anesthesia zone includes sufficient space for the anesthesia professional to perform patient care tasks and space for anesthesia equipment and supplies.

4.4 Use the following dimensions of the zones in a 400 sq ft (37.2 m²) inpatient or outpatient OR[13,14]:

- The sterile field clear area: 3 ft (0.91 m) on each side and at the foot of the OR bed, gurney, or procedural chair on which the patient is placed. The traditional OR bed measures 3 ft × 7 ft (0.91 m × 2.13 m).
- The circulation pathway: 3 ft (0.91 m) on both sides and 2 ft (0.61 m) at the foot of the sterile field.
- The movable equipment zone: 2 ft 6 inches (0.762 m) on each side and 2 ft (0.61 m) at the foot of the OR bed.
- The anesthesia zone: 6-ft × 8-ft (1.83-m × 2.44-m) space at the head of the OR bed. After the patient has been anesthetized, the 2 ft (0.61 m) closest to the wall becomes a portion of the circulation pathway.

[Recommendation]

4.5 Use the following dimensions of the zones in a 255 sq ft (23.69 m²) outpatient OR, in which no anesthetics will be administered using an anesthesia machine and supply cart[14]:

- The sterile field clear area: 3 ft (0.91 m) on each side and at the head and foot of the OR bed, gurney, or procedural chair on which the patient is placed. The traditional OR bed measures 3 ft × 7 ft (0.91 m × 2.13 m).
- The combined circulation pathway and mobile equipment zone measures 3 ft (0.91 m) on each side and 2 ft (0.61 m) at the head and foot of the sterile field.

[Recommendation]

4.6 Use the following dimensions of the zones in a 270 sq ft (25.08 m²) outpatient OR in which anesthetics will be administered using an anesthesia machine and supply cart[14]:

- The sterile field clear area: 3 ft (0.91 m) on each side and at the foot of the OR bed, gurney, or procedural chair on which the patient is placed. The traditional OR bed measures 3 ft × 7 ft (0.91 m × 2.31 m).
- The combined circulation pathway and mobile equipment zone measures 3 ft (0.91 m) on each side and 2 ft (0.61 m) at the foot of the sterile field.

- The anesthesia work zone measures 6 ft × 8 ft (1.83 m × 2.44 m) at the head of the OR bed, gurney, or procedural chair on which the patient is placed.

[Recommendation]

4.7 Include space for documentation in each OR.[13,14] *[Recommendation]*

4.7.1 The documentation area may be fixed or mobile.[13,14] If fixed, orient the area so the RN circulator can face the patient while documenting. *[Conditional Recommendation]*

4.8 Design a hand scrub area to be located outside each OR and adjacent to the door from the semi-restricted corridor.[13,14] *[Recommendation]*

4.8.1 The hand scrub area may be shared between two ORs if located adjacent the door of each OR.[13,14] *[Conditional Recommendation]*

4.9 Design the OR to have a positive pressure gradient to all surrounding areas including supply storage areas (eg, sterile core, central core) that are **directly accessible** to the OR.[13,14] *[Recommendation]*

Keeping the OR at a positive pressure is supported by a case report that describes an investigation following a polymicrobial outbreak that caused 22 sternal surgical site infections. The investigation identified a negative pressure gradient to the substerile room as an environmental component that was not within the recommended settings and was thought to be a causative factors in the outbreak.[63]

4.9.1 When the storage room (eg, sterile core, central core) is directly accessible to the OR, the storage room should be pressured negative to the OR but positive to the semi-restricted corridor and other directly accessible areas. *[Recommendation]*

4.10 Waste anesthesia gas disposal systems must be installed in any location where anesthesia gases are administered[13,14,64] and in compliance with *NFPA 99: Health Care Facilities Code Handbook*[27] or other regulations if more stringent. *[Regulatory Requirement]*

4.10.1 A waste anesthesia gas disposal system may be an active or passive system.[64] *[Conditional Recommendation]*

An active system is a vacuum system and a passive system is a non-recirculating HVAC system for removal of waste anesthesia gases.[64]

4.10.2 A waste anesthesia gas disposal system may include a scavenging or recycling system. *[Conditional Recommendation]*

Expert opinion articles suggest that a scavenging or a recycling system decreases the amount of waste anesthesia gas released into the atmosphere, which is thought to assist with decreasing the carbon footprint.[65,66] Further research is needed to determine the feasibility and the benefits of using a scavenging or a recycling system.

4.11 Perform a risk/benefit/cost analysis during the planning phase to determine whether a ventilation setback strategy, for periods when the OR is unoccupied, should be incorporated into the HVAC system. *[Recommendation]*

Guidelines support the use of a ventilation setback strategy.[13,14,23] In a nonexperimental study, Wang et al[67] measured the temperature and humidity in an unoccupied OR when the air changes were set at 20 ACH, 10 ACH, and 5 ACH. The researchers found the humidity and temperature stayed in the acceptable ranges with the decreased ACH rates. They concluded that the ACH may be safely decreased to 5 ACH when the OR is unoccupied. Wang et al[68] reached the same conclusions in a nonexperimental study involving 10 ORs.

Thiel et al[69] performed a nonexperimental study to review the energy used for a vaginal, an abdominal, a laparoscopic, and a robotic hysterectomy. They found that 70% of the energy was used by the HVAC system, and laparoscopic and robotic procedures used less lighting energy than vaginal or abdominal procedures. The researchers recommended using a ventilation setback to decrease the energy used by the HVAC system when the OR is unoccupied.

Aydin Çakir et al[70] illustrated the need for continuous air changes and air filtration in a nonexperimental study. The researchers measured the air microbial counts before and after a disinfection process 54 times for Hospital 1 and 42 times for Hospital 2 during a 3-month period. In Hospital 1, the counts were lower during each test, but in Hospital 2, the counts were higher after the disinfection process but not during the remainder of the counts. The researchers determined that the counts were higher in that test because the HVAC and air filtering system had been turned off.

4.11.1 Include the following in the risk/benefit/cost analysis:
- actual or projected usage of the setback system,
- applicable local building code requirements,
- existing ventilation system design, and
- energy savings.

[Recommendation]

4.11.2 Use a ventilation setback strategy that
- maintains the temperature and humidity settings within the design parameters for the intraoperative area (See Recommendation 2.6.1),
- maintains the positive-pressure relationship of the OR to the adjacent area, and
- provides a mechanism to restore the system to normal operation.[23,71]

[Recommendation]

4.12 Perform a risk/benefit/cost analysis during the planning phase when selecting the surgical field lighting by assessing the
- required ceiling support system,
- amount of interference with other ceiling-mounted equipment,
- ability to focus and control the spot size,
- amount of heat generated,
- time and effort required for lamp replacement,
- color and temperature of the light,
- amount of shadow produced,
- ease of cleaning,
- type of lighting (eg, LED),
- amount of interference with airflow,
- amount of energy for movement and focusing, and
- ability to control settings at the sterile field.

[Recommendation]

Lighting in the OR that is comfortable, safe, and provides optimal visibility and color recognition provides a satisfactory visual environment and meets the requirements of the OR personnel.[56] Surgical lights may produce high amounts of radiant heat that may cause damage to exposed tissues and discomfort to the surgical team.[72] The color of light produced can change the color and appearance of the skin and other tissue.[72,73] Shadows may be produced by equipment that blocks the light. Lights require frequent cleaning to protect against infections caused by dust.[73]

An observational study of 46 hours of surgery revealed that high forces were required to move the lights and an interruption was caused by adjustment of the lights, which at times required assistance from the RN circulator.[74] Comparisons of surgical lights found that amounts of force required to move the lights and degrees of interruption caused by light adjustment varied among lights made by different manufacturers.[38,75]

Incidents of patient burns from surgical lights have been reported when multiple light heads were aimed at one small area and operating at or near maximum power.[76]

4.13 Do not place sinks or drains in the OR. *[Recommendation]*

Sinks and the drains associated with them have been linked to infections in patients. In a nonexperimental study, Zhou et al[77] examined the link between patients infected with *Pseudomonas aeruginosa* and the presence of *P aeruginosa* in sink drain traps. The researchers found 46 of 244 samples from the sink drain traps contained *P aeruginosa*, and the strain found in the trap matched the strain found in 11 of the 17 infection cases. Bédard et al[78] conducted a post-outbreak investigation and discovered *Pseudomonas* in 24 of 28 drains. The researchers in both studies concluded that sinks contribute to the incidence of *P aeruginosa* infections.

5. Hybrid OR

5.1 Use evidence-based design concepts in the planning and design of the **hybrid OR**. *[Recommendation]*

5.2 Perform a risk/benefit/cost analysis during the planning phase to determine whether a hybrid OR will be a part of the surgical suite by
- identifying the specialties that will use the hybrid OR,
- identifying what type of imaging system will be used,
- determining whether the OR bed is compatible with the imaging system,
- identifying the type of procedures (eg, traditional open procedures, interventional procedures, diagnostic nonsurgical procedures, a combination of the procedure types) that will be performed in the hybrid OR, and
- determining the required safety precautions (eg, for radiation, magnetic resonance imaging [MRI]).

[Recommendation]

Low-quality evidence supports making all or some of these determinations when defining the need for and the equipment to be placed in a hybrid OR.[18,43,79-81]

5.3 Design the hybrid OR to include an imaging system control area, procedure area, and imaging system component room.[13] *[Recommendation]*

5.3.1 The control area
- should be sized to meet manufacturers' specifications;
- may be shared between multiple ORs;
- contains walls, windows, and a door that may be removed if the control room serves only one room and the room is built, main-

tained, and controlled in the same way as the OR.[13]

[Recommendation]

5.3.2 The system component room may be shared between multiple hybrid rooms and should not be accessible from the OR, but can be accessible from either the semi-restricted or unrestricted area.[13] *[Conditional Recommendation]*

5.4 Design the hybrid OR to
- comply with all the requirements of the non-hybrid OR (See Recommendations 2.6.1 and 2.7),
- be sized to accommodate the equipment to be used based on the manufacturers' specifications,
- have hazard protection based on the type and amount of protection required for the type of system used (eg, MRI, radiation),
- have signage indicating the types of precautions required based on the type of imaging equipment present, and
- be placed in an area **readily accessible** to both the surgical and radiology suites.

[Recommendation]

Guidelines and low-quality evidence support inclusion of all or a portion of these items.[7,13,18,43,79-83]

Locating the hybrid OR close to both the surgery and radiology departments is thought to increase patient safety because when there is an emergency, there is better access to emergency equipment and appropriate personnel. Location of the hybrid OR in an area with little noise and vibration assists with decreasing the potential for low-quality images.[79]

6. Postoperative Areas

6.1 Use evidence-based design concepts in the planning and design of the postoperative areas (ie, PACU Phase I and II). *[Recommendation]*

6.2 Include the following in the postoperative area design:
- patient care stations,
- a medication safety zone,
- hand washing stations,
- provisions for storing patients' belongings,
- bathrooms for patients and personnel,
- a nourishment area for patients in Phase II recovery,
- ice-making equipment, and
- other support areas (See Recommendation 7).[13,14]

[Recommendation]

6.2.1 These areas may be shared with the preoperative and intraoperative areas as defined in the functional program (See Recommendation 1).[13,14] [Conditional Recommendation]

6.2.2 Design hand washing stations to be located in every toilet room and patient care room. In patient care areas with more than one patient care station (eg, PACU Phase I), include one hand washing station for every four or fewer patient care stations. If the number of patient care stations is not divisible by four, include one hand washing station for any fraction up to one (eg, if five, six, or seven patient care stations are present, two hand washing stations should be installed).[13,14] [Recommendation]

6.3 Determine the number of the postoperative areas based on the functional program (See Recommendation 1). [Recommendation]

6.4 Perform a risk/cost/benefit analysis to determine whether the preoperative and postoperative care will be administered in the same area or different areas. [Recommendation]

6.4.1 If preoperative and postoperative care will be administered in the same area, design the area to meet the requirements of the area with the more stringent criteria.[13,14] [Recommendation]

6.5 Include the following in the nourishment area or room design:
- a hand washing station,
- a work counter,
- a refrigerator,
- a microwave,
- storage cabinets,
- a garbage container, and
- provisions and space for temporary storage of food service implements and unused and soiled meal trays if meal trays are provided.[13,14] [Recommendation]

7. Support Areas

7.1 Use evidence-based design concepts in the planning and design of the surgical suite support areas. [Recommendation]

7.2 Include the following in the surgical suite support area design:
- locker rooms;
- the nurse station;
- clean equipment storage areas, which may be combined with or separate from clean or sterile supply storage areas, and a clean linen storage area;
- a soiled workroom, which may be combined with or separate from a garbage storage/holding area, and a soiled linen storage area;
- an environmental services room;
- a **supply breakout area/room**;
- a sterile processing department; and
- administrative areas (eg, reception area, business offices).

[Recommendation]

7.3 The surgical suite support areas may include
- an information systems control room,
- medical records storage areas,
- multipurpose rooms,
- patient waiting rooms,
- specimen holding areas,
- a satellite sterile processing area,
- a satellite laboratory, and
- a satellite pharmacy.

[Conditional Recommendation]

7.4 Support areas may be shared between the preoperative, intraoperative, and postoperative areas; be dedicated to only one or two of the areas; or be shared with other departments in the facility unless otherwise designated and defined in the functional program (See Recommendation 1).[13,14] [Conditional Recommendation]

7.5 Determine the size, number, and location of the surgical suite support areas based on the functional program (See Recommendation 1). [Recommendation]

7.6 Design the support areas, including clean equipment and supply storage areas and work spaces (eg, cabinet countertops, tables), to be located adjacent to the patient care areas. [Recommendation]

Ley-Chavez et al[84] conducted a nonexperimental study on the effect that location of support areas has on walking distances and time spent waiting for elevators. The study involved the escorts who transported patients with limited mobility to more than 200 locations within a cancer hospital consisting of 3 million sq ft on 18 floors. The researchers determined that after relocation of support areas closer to the patient care areas, the escorts walked a total of 4,740 fewer miles per year and spent a total of 842 fewer hours waiting for elevators.

7.7 Design locker rooms to be in a location that is readily accessible to the surgical suite. Locker rooms may be shared with all areas in the facility.[13,14] *[Recommendation]*

7.8 Include work surfaces with a hand washing station(s) in or adjacent to the nurse station.[13,14] *[Recommendation]*

7.8.1 The nurse station may be combined with or include reception areas. *[Conditional Recommendation]*

7.9 The surgical suite equipment and supply storage areas may house both sterile and clean supplies and clean equipment. *[Conditional Recommendation]*

7.9.1 If clean and sterile supplies are stored in the same room, follow the HVAC requirements for the sterile storage room (See Recommendation 2.6.1). *[Recommendation]*

7.9.2 Determine the size of equipment and supply storage areas based on the size of the equipment and supplies to be stored in the area.[13,14,48] Use a room that is of sufficient size to allow for easy access to all equipment and supplies, allow for orderly storage, and support the use of safe ergonomic practices. *[Recommendation]*

An observational study in cardiovascular ORs and the associated surgical suites at five different facilities identified the lack of storage areas as a safety hazard that resulted in restricted hallways and caused difficulty during transfer of patients into and out of the OR. Lack of horizontal work spaces led to items being stored in a disorderly fashion, being difficult to locate, and falling on the floor.[85] An inadequate amount of storage space can lead to cluttered hallways and ORs.[9]

7.9.3 Position the bottom shelf of an open shelving unit to be 8 to 10 inches off the floor and the top shelf to allow 18 inches between the top of the product stored on the top shelf and the sprinkler head above it.[86] *[Recommendation]*

The distance between the bottom shelf and the floor is to allow for cleaning of the floor without contaminating the supplies stored on the bottom shelf. The distance between the product stored on the top shelf and the sprinkler head permits proper functioning of the sprinkler head.[86]

7.10 Include the following in the soiled workroom design:
- a hand washing station,
- a flushing-rim clinical service sink with a bedpan-rinsing device (ie, hopper) or equivalent flushing-rim fixture,
- an eyewash station,
- a work counter,
- space for separate containers for waste and soiled linen, and
- electrical and plumbing connections per manufacturer requirements and space for the docking station(s) when a fluid management system is used.[13,14]

[Recommendation]

7.10.1 The soiled workroom may be the decontamination room or a holding room for dirty linen and garbage. *[Conditional Recommendation]*

7.11 The clean linen storage area may be a room or an area within a room, such as a closet, or an area dedicated to a cart for clean linen within the clean workroom or equipment supply room. *[Conditional Recommendation]*

7.12 Design a supply breakout area/room to be located adjacent to the semi-restricted area of the surgical suite or within the supply processing department.[13,14,25] *[Recommendation]*

Items should be removed from external shipping containers and web-edged (ie, corrugated) boxes because dust, debris, and insects may enter the container or boxes during shipment, and the containers or boxes can carry contaminants into the semi-restricted area.[25]

8. Sterile Processing Areas

8.1 Use evidence-based design concepts in the planning and design of the sterile processing areas. *[Recommendation]*

8.2 When designing the sterile processing department or area, determine the
- anticipated volume of work based on the departments to be served;
- type of distribution system (eg, vertical, horizontal, case cart, exchange cart, par level, requisition);
- equipment required (eg, sterilizers, washer-disinfectors, washer-decontaminators, single- or multi-chamber tunnel washers, cart washers, ultrasonic cleaners, automated endoscope processors, detergent management system);

- utilities required (eg, steam supply, water purification, instrument air);
- space and equipment requirements for processing reusable textiles (eg, receiving, transporting, collecting, storing);
- storage requirements (eg, patient care equipment, packaging material supplies, sterilization process, indicators, case carts, sterilizer carts);
- space for receipt and return of loaned instruments and devices;
- space and equipment requirements for management of infectious waste, hazardous waste, and recyclable materials;
- support areas if not shared with other portions of the surgical suite; and
- traffic patterns.[25]

[Recommendation]

8.3 Design the sterile processing area to be a two-room configuration except when the sterilization equipment is limited to a table-top or similar-sized sterilizer(s).[13,14] [Recommendation]

8.4 In a two-room sterile processing configuration, include a decontamination room and a clean workroom that are separated by
- a wall with a door,
- a pass-through window, or
- a built-in washer-disinfector or washer-sterilizer with the dirty side opening in the decontamination room and the clean side opening in the clean workroom.[13,14,25]

[Recommendation]

8.4.1 Include the following in the decontamination room design:
- a washer-sterilizer or washer-decontaminator;
- an ultrasonic cleaner;
- a case cart washer, if case carts are used;
- a dirty case cart storage area, if case carts are used;
- a work counter(s);
- a hand washing station;
- three decontamination sinks or one sink with three divisions;
- a flushing-rim clinical sink or equivalent fixture unless alternative methods for disposal of bio-waste are provided;
- space for waste and soiled linen receptacle(s);
- a fixed or mobile documentation area;
- storage for decontamination supplies and personal protective equipment;
- space for donning and doffing personal protective equipment;

- space and equipment for inspection of items (eg magnification, borescope, laparoscopic insulation tester); and
- an eyewash station if required by the safety risk assessment.[13,14,25]

[Recommendation]

8.4.2 Include the following in the clean workroom design:
- a sterilizer,
- a work counter(s) with space to accommodate the volume of equipment assembly for the procedures performed in the facility and the expected staffing levels,
- a hand washing station,
- an eyewash station if required by the safety risk assessment,
- storage space for instrument inventory,
- storage space for sterilization and packaging supplies,
- space for cooling racks after sterilization, and
- a mobile or fixed documentation area.[13,14]

[Recommendation]

8.4.3 Include the following in the clean workroom design when required by the functional program (See Recommendation 1):
- a low-temperature sterilizer,
- a cooling area for the sterilization cart,
- sterile storage, and
- space for case cart storage.[13,14,25]

[Recommendation]

8.4.4 In a one-room sterile processing area, include
- a partial wall or partition at least 4 ft high and the width of the counter or
- a distance of 4 ft between the instrument-washing sink and the area where the instruments are prepared for sterilization.[13,14,25]

[Recommendation]

8.5 Provide functionally equivalent space in the building design for decontamination and sterilization of surgical instruments in all locations where sterilization processes are performed (eg, satellite sterile processing areas).[13,14] [Recommendation]

9. Procedure Rooms

9.1 Use evidence-based design concepts in the planning and design of **procedure rooms**. [Recommendation]

9.2 The surgical suite may include a procedure room. [Conditional Recommendation]

9.2.1 Perform a risk/benefit/cost analysis during the planning phase to determine whether a procedure room will be included in the surgical suite, and assess
- what specialties will use the procedure room and
- what types of procedures will be performed in the procedure room (eg, pain clinic, dental procedures, flexible endoscopy).[13,14]
[Recommendation]

9.3 Design procedure rooms to be 130 sq ft unless inhalation anesthesia will be administered, in which case the room should be 160 sq ft.[13,14]
[Recommendation]

9.4 The procedure room may have either a fixed or mobile work surface. [Conditional Recommendation]

9.5 Design a hand washing station to be provided in the procedure room unless a hand scrub station is directly accessible, in which case the hand washing station may be omitted. [Recommendation]

10. Environmental Contamination

10.1 Establish, maintain, and monitor measures for preventing environmental contamination when renovation or new construction occurs in close proximity to an occupied health care facility.
[Recommendation]

In a nonexperimental study, Loschi et al[87] assessed the effectiveness of mechanical preventive measures on the incidence of invasive pulmonary aspergillosis in neutropenic patients during a hospital renovation. The researchers found no increase in the incidence of invasive pulmonary aspergillosis in neutropenic patients and attributed this to multiple factors that they recommended be performed during all construction projects, including monitoring by the interdisciplinary team and the team making changes in the barriers as needed.

10.2 Create a plan for infection control and maintaining internal air quality.[88] [Recommendation]

10.2.1 Include interventions to control or mitigate
- dust generation,
- dust from entering occupied (or completed) areas of the facility,
- dust from entering the existing or finished HVAC system,
- generation of aerosols from contaminated water sources,
- debris buildup,

- alterations in ambient interior temperature and humidity levels, and
- mold and bacteria growth.
[Recommendation]

Low-quality evidence and guidelines support containing the by-products of demolition and construction.[8,32,88,89] The dust may contain asbestos or fungal contaminants.[87,88] In a nonexperimental study, Scarlett et al[90] found asbestos in 16 of 26 hospitals. The asbestos was found mainly in the thermal system insulation. The researchers concluded that an asbestos containment policy is needed during demolition and construction.

10.3 Establish the frequency and designate the person or persons responsible for construction site and infection control barrier monitoring.
[Recommendation]

A systematic review of the literature supports surveillance of the construction site to ensure compliance with recommended infection prevention interventions.[31]

10.4 Implement safety and infection control measures, including
- utilization of a dust collection system, such as during finishing of gypsum wallboard partitions;
- creation of barriers applicable to the type of construction occurring;
- maintenance of barrier integrity;
- creation of special construction-related traffic pathways, entrances, and exits; and
- use of negative pressure and high-efficiency particulate air (HEPA) filters on the construction side of the barrier.
[Recommendation]

Experts recommend adherence to these measures.[31,32,88,89,91] In a case report, Semchuk[92] found that following these measures resulted in fewer materials being rejected from the site, minimal shrinkage of gypsum wallboard and flooring installations, a clean and neat site, and easy turnover after completion.

10.4.1 Use high-efficiency particulate air filters to filter the incoming air when construction is occurring outside of the building.[32,88,89]
[Recommendation]

High-efficiency particulate air filters have been shown to decrease the particulate count in the air after filtration. In a nonexperimental study, Brace et al[93] measured particle counts in the air inside an OR and outside of the building. The researchers found the fine particle count was lower in the OR ($0.43/cm^3$) than outside the building (14.53/cm³). They attributed the difference to the use of HEPA filters to filter the incoming air.

Brun et al[94] conducted a nonexperimental study to measure the levels of fungi in the air in two hospitals, one without HEPA filtered air and one with HEPA filtered air in the patient rooms. The researchers found a lower concentration of fungi in the patient rooms in the facility with the HEPA filter. The researchers concluded that the presence of HEPA filters reduced the amount of fungi present.

Case reports by Saliou et al[95] and Barreiros et al[96] describe the fungal concentration in the air as being less in areas with HEPA filtration than in areas without filtration. The authors also state the amount of fungi found in the air outside of the hospital during demolition in close proximity to the building was greater than that in the building, because of the presence of the HEPA filters.[47]

10.4.2 **Place barriers (eg, solid fiberboard or sheet-rock walls, sealed plastic walls) between the construction site and the surgical suite and maintain them at all times.**[88,89] *[Recommendation]*

Nguyen et al[63] described eight cases of sternal infections caused by *Gordonia* that occurred during construction in which no physical barriers were placed between the ORs and the construction areas. The absence of the barriers was thought to be a causative factor in the outbreak.

In a nonexperimental study, Loschi et al[87] assessed the effectiveness of mechanical preventive measures on the incidence of invasive pulmonary aspergillosis in neutropenic patients during a hospital renovation. The researchers found no increase in the incidence of invasive pulmonary aspergillosis and attributed this to multiple factors that they recommended be performed during all construction projects, including the use of preventive measures. This study does not involve the OR, but the principles apply to all locations. More research is needed regarding the effect of preventive measures taken during renovation and construction on surgical site infection rates.

10.4.3 **Develop, communicate, and implement traffic plans for construction personnel and movement of supplies, equipment, and debris.** *[Recommendation]*

Loschi et al[87] assessed the effectiveness of mechanical preventive measures on the incidence of invasive pulmonary aspergillosis in neutropenic patients during a hospital renova-

tion. They found no increase in the incidence and attributed this to multiple factors that they recommended be performed during all construction projects, including rerouting traffic away from the construction site.

Establishing construction traffic routes assists with minimizing disruptions in care; maximizing safety; and preventing transmission of infectious agents to patients, personnel, and visitors.[30]

11. Utility Failures

11.1 **Create and implement a plan for managing and restoring the utilities and repairing damage to the surgical suite after failure of an internal or external utility.** *[Recommendation]*

Utility disruptions occur because of natural and man-made disasters and structural failure (eg, breaking of a water line in the building, HVAC system breakdown). The utility system includes internal components (eg, medical air compressors, medical vacuum pump, emergency generator, chiller, boiler) and external components (eg, electricity, internet, water, sewer).

The Centers for Disease Control and Prevention states that creating a utility failure remediation plan assists in preparing a facility for a utility failure.[97]

11.2 **In the utility failure plan, include protocols to be followed during a failure of the**
- **electrical power,**
- **emergency back-up power,**
- **gas delivery system,**
- **boilers/steam system,**
- **water system,**[98]
- **plumbing system,**
- **sewage system,**
- **medical gas delivery system,**
- **vacuum system,**
- **communication system, and**
- **HVAC system.**

[Recommendation]

Klinger et al[99] conducted a systematic literature search on the health effects of power outages and determined that all utilities can be lost at the same time, such as when caused by an electrical outage, or can be lost independently of each other. The loss of electrical power alone can lead to a loss in lighting, HVAC systems, clean water, sewage disposal, food and medication storage, life support devices and technologies, safety mechanisms, and transportation including elevators. The authors recommended that plans be created for handling extended outages and for educating health care workers about what resources are available during emergencies.

11.2.1 Include the following in the utility failure plan:
- measures to be performed in preparation for, during, and after any utility failure;
- critical services to remain operational during a utility outage[98];
- utility conservation steps to be taken;
- essential personnel and their roles and responsibilities based on the type of failure[100]; and
- sources for medical supplies and back-up utilities.[100]

[Recommendation]

11.3 Perform a damage assessment of the surgical suite after any utility failure, to determine the potential effects on both the patients and caregivers. *[Recommendation]*

The assessment is completed to determine whether there is damage and the extent of damage to equipment, supplies, and the facility.[101]

11.3.1 Assess for the
- level of contamination and the contaminating agent (eg, clear water, gray water, black water, no water, presence of mold) if applicable,[89]
- environmental cleanliness (eg, presence of dirt, debris, condensation on surfaces including walls and flooring),
- integrity of clean and sterile supplies (eg, presence of condensation on package surfaces, signs of water damage),
- functionality of the power supply (eg, fully restored, emergency generator in use),
- availability of water (eg, water pressure, water quality, steam supply) and other utilities,
- functionality of the HVAC system, and
- functionality of all fixed and mobile equipment.[89]

[Recommendation]

11.3.2 Based on the assessment, measures to be taken immediately may include
- rescheduling or redirecting procedures to areas of the surgical suite where the utilities are functioning within accepted parameters,
- delaying elective procedures,
- limiting surgical procedures to emergency procedures only,
- closing the affected OR(s), or
- taking no action.

[Conditional Recommendation]

11.3.3 Based on the assessment, measures that should be taken to restore the surgical suite to full functionality after any utility restoration may include
- terminally cleaning when there is evidence of contamination on surfaces or the event type increases the risk of contamination[1];
- reprocessing or discarding any supplies with packaging that may have been compromised[102];
- inventorying discarded, damaged supplies for insurance claim purposes and to assist with obtaining replacements;
- determining whether fixed or mobile medical equipment is salvageable;
- confirming functionality of the HVAC system[89,103];
- confirming functionality of the water system[97,102]; and
- confirming the quality of steam.

[Conditional Recommendation]

Low-quality evidence and the ANSI/AAMI ST79 guideline support performing one or more of the listed interventions when restoring an OR to full functionality.[25,101]

11.4 The utility failure plan may include the temporary use of mobile health care facilities including support services. *[Conditional Recommendation]*

Mobile facilities can allow the continuation of services during renovation or after a disaster. In a nonexperimental study, Boubour et al[104] validated for use a mobile sterile processing unit made from a shipping container. Sterilization was successfully achieved in 61 trials using four indicators of sterilization efficacy, including autoclave tape, an indicator strip, a biological indicator, and time and temperature.

11.5 Following a utility failure, determine whether to use a mobile health care facility and support services by performing a risk/benefit/cost analysis that includes
- patient flow,
- infection control measures,
- fire prevention measures,
- security measures,
- utilities connections,
- connections for communication systems,
- maintenance,
- requirements for linking corridors,
- emergency exits,
- interdepartmental pathways, and
- patient accommodations.

[Recommendation]

11.6 In the power failure portion of the plan, include interventions to be performed for various types of power system failures (eg, normal power system failure with or without emergency power system operating, partial power system failure with or without emergency system operating). [Recommendation]

11.6.1 List the following in the power failure protocol:
- the essential equipment that should be connected to the outlets powered by the emergency generator[105] and
- the life-sustaining medical equipment that has battery backup.
[Recommendation]

11.6.2 Develop a plan for temporary measures to use during a power failure, including
- working flashlights in every OR and available in or on every anesthesia machine or supply cart,
- manual monitoring equipment (eg, blood pressure cuff, stethoscope),
- long extension cords,
- battery-operated communication devices,
- mechanisms for gaining access into medication dispensing equipment, and
- paper documentation forms/records.
[Recommendation]

11.6.3 Batteries should be
- labeled with the expiration date,
- checked monthly for expiration, and
- replaced as needed.[106]
[Recommendation]

11.7 In the communications system failure portion of the plan, include a list of interventions to be performed in preparation for a communications system failure, including
- creating a detailed perioperative team contact list that includes multiple methods for contacting the personnel,
- designating preset meeting places and evacuation destinations in case of an inability to communicate, and
- determining alternative methods of communication (eg, web page updates, answering machine messages, texting, paper documentation).[100]
[Recommendation]

11.8 In the HVAC system failure portion of the plan, include guidelines for inspection of the HVAC system if compromised[107] and a method of reporting a variance in HVAC system parameters. [Recommendation]

11.9 Establish and determine intervals for education and competency verification activities for its personnel related to utility failure,[99] including
- which life-sustaining medical equipment has battery backup[28,105,108];
- the locations of alternate sources of lighting, power, and supplies for use when the normal power is interrupted, including
  - charged transport monitors,
  - manual monitoring devices (eg, blood pressure cuff, stethoscope),
  - flashlights,
  - the utility failure emergency procedures manual,
  - back-up resources for documentation and for supplies that are secured in devices that require power to open,
  - long extension cords, and
  - nonelectrical powered communication devices[105,108,109]; and
- interventions to perform during
  - various types of power system failure (eg, normal power system failure with or without the emergency power system operating, partial power system failure with or without the emergency system operating),[110,111]
  - gas service interruptions,
  - boiler/steam system failures,
  - water service interruptions,
  - sewage system interruptions,
  - medical gas service interruptions,
  - vacuum service interruptions,
  - communication system interruptions, and
  - HVAC system interruptions.
[Recommendation]

12. Surface and HVAC Maintenance

12.1 Create and implement a systematic process for monitoring and maintaining structural surfaces and HVAC system performance. [Recommendation]

Heating, ventilation, and air conditioning systems control room air quality, temperature, humidity, and air pressure of the room in comparison to the surrounding areas. The HVAC system reduces the amount of environmental contamination (eg, microbial-laden skin squames, dust, lint) in the surgical suite by carrying airborne contaminants away from the sterile field and removing them through the return duct vents located at the periphery of the room. The restricted areas are intended to be the cleanest; therefore, the HVAC requirements for the restricted areas are the most stringent.[112]

12.2 Maintain the integrity of structural surfaces (eg, doors, floors, walls, ceilings, cabinets) and have surfaces repaired when damaged. *[Recommendation]*

12.2.1 Report damage to floors, walls, ceilings, cabinets, and other structural surfaces according to the health care organization's policy. *[Recommendation]*

Damaged structural surfaces may create a reservoir for the collection of dirt and debris that cannot be removed during cleaning. Damage to floor surfaces may create a trip or fall hazard.

12.2.2 Determine repair priorities based on an assessment that determines the potential for the damage to result in an adverse outcome. *[Recommendation]*

12.3 Maintain the operational values for HVAC settings at either the settings described in **Recommendation 2.6.1** or the settings that applied at the time of design or the most recent renovation of the HVAC system and as stated in the state or local regulations.[113] *[Recommendation]*

12.4 Develop a method for reporting a variance in HVAC system parameters. *[Recommendation]*

12.4.1 Establish a reporting system that enables two-way conversation between perioperative personnel and plant operations personnel. *[Recommendation]*

12.5 Personnel who identify an unintentional variance in the predetermined HVAC system parameters should report the variance according to the health care organization's policy and procedures. *[Recommendation]*

Rapid communication between affected and responsible personnel can help facilitate resolution of the variance.

12.6 Designated perioperative team members in collaboration with the interdisciplinary team should perform a risk assessment of the surgical suite if a variance in the parameters of the HVAC system occurs. *[Recommendation]*

The literature search for this guideline did not reveal any evidence of clinical significance related to the acceptable degree of variance in the HVAC system design parameters. Further research is warranted.

The effect of the HVAC system parameters falling out of range is variable. A small variance for a short period of time may not be of clinical concern, whereas a large variance for a longer period may have clinical significance.

12.6.1 Based on the risk assessment, corrective measures may include
- rescheduling or redirecting procedures to areas of the surgical suite where the HVAC system is functioning within accepted parameters,
- delaying elective procedures,
- limiting surgical procedures to emergency procedures only,
- closing the affected OR(s), or
- taking no action.

[Conditional Recommendation]

12.6.2 Based on the risk assessment, measures taken to restore the surgical suite to full functionality after the HVAC system variance has been corrected may include
- terminally cleaning when there is evidence of contamination on surfaces[1];
- reprocessing or discarding any supplies with packaging that may have been compromised[102]; and
- inventorying discarded, damaged supplies for insurance claim purposes and to assist with obtaining replacements.

[Conditional Recommendation]

12.7 Create and implement a systematic process for monitoring HVAC system equipment and a mechanism for resolving unintentional variances. *[Recommendation]*

12.7.1 The HVAC system functionality must be monitored and maintained within accepted standards of practice.[49,114] *[Regulatory Requirement]*

12.8 The temperature may be intentionally adjusted based on the individual needs of the patient and occupant comfort. *[Conditional Recommendation]* **P**

Adjusting the temperature up or down may assist with preventing or inducing hypothermia as applicable.[115]

12.9 If a ventilation setback system is installed, create a protocol for restoring the HVAC system before an emergency or scheduled procedure begins. The protocol should
- include actions to be taken to activate and deactivate the system,
- designate who is responsible for activating and deactivating the system, and
- describe when the system is to be activated and deactivated.

[Recommendation]

The evidence is inconclusive regarding a time for the HVAC system to return to normal operating conditions after deactivation of the setback system. In a nonexperimental study, Traversari et al[116] examined the number of airborne particles in the OR during normal operating conditions and when the HVAC system was turned off, and determined how long it took to return to normal conditions after the HVAC system was turned back on. The researchers determined that a 30-minute period was required after restarting the HVAC system to return the air to the levels achieved during normal operating conditions. In a nonexperimental study, Dettenkofer et al[117] made the same recommendation for a 30-minute period between deactivating the setback system and beginning surgical activity. A limitation of both studies is that no HVAC settings are provided for the setback system. Guidelines from the Working Party of the British Hospital Infection Society recommend waiting 15 minutes after deactivating the setback system before the patient enters the OR.[23]

12.10 **In consultation with the HVAC design engineer and plant operations personnel, determine the frequency for filter changes and establish a mechanism for maintaining the system.** *[Recommendation]*

A properly functioning HVAC system minimizes the risk of contaminating the sterile field and is an essential component in surgical site infection prevention.[48]

Gniadek and Macura[118] conducted a nonexperimental study in a Polish hospital to measure the amount of *Aspergillus* in 50 air samples. The spores found were large enough to be removed by a HEPA air filtration system. The researchers concluded that the air filtering system requires regular maintenance, including filter changes.

An investigation of an outbreak of postoperative shoulder arthritis caused by *Propionibacterium acnes* infection (ie, four cases within 1 month) revealed that the HVAC system was not functioning properly. After repair of the system and increased environmental cleaning, no additional cases were reported.[119]

12.11 **Do not use free-standing fans, portable humidifiers, air conditioners, and dehumidifiers.** *[Recommendation]*

These devices all contain a fan that when running can disrupt the planned airflow within the room and may transfer unwanted particles from the floor to the surgical site. Humidifiers and dehumidifiers contain standing water that may be a source for *Legionella,* as reported in a case study by Yiallouros et al.[120]

Vladut et al[121] conducted a nonexperimental study that demonstrated the increased mixing of the room air and the alterations to the air pattern that were created when a portable air conditioner was used. This disruption in the airflow pattern could cause contaminants from the floor to become airborne, leading to potential contamination of the surgical site.

In a nonexperimental study, Casha et al[122] measured the average particle counts (eg, 0.5 micrometers, 5 micrometers) and the bacterial counts in an empty OR, an OR with 10 people present, and the same OR 1 hour later during the performance of a simulated thoracic surgical procedure. The counts were made with the fan off and the fan on. The counts of particles of 0.5 micrometers in the empty OR decreased (from 267,496 to 244,377) after the fan was turned on but the particles of 5 micrometers and the bacterial counts expressed as colony-forming units per 1,000 L increased (from 824 to 906 and 10 to 13, respectively) after the fan was turned on. In the initial test with 10 staff members present, there was an increase in all three of the criteria, but after 1 hour, the bacterial counts remained the same and particle counts decreased. No changes in the particle counts and the bacterial counts were of statistical significance. The researchers concluded that when the "bladeless fan" was used, the clean room conditions of the OR (ie, ISO Class 7/8) were maintained. A limitation of this study is that there is no description of where the fan was located and what direction the airflow was aimed.

12.12 **Do not place equipment and supplies in front of return air ducts.** *[Recommendation]*

An unobstructed airflow out of the room is required to maintain the correct pressure gradient within the room.

Glossary

Adjacent: Located next to but not necessarily connected to the identified area or room.

Authority having jurisdiction: An individual or organization designated by a state or government agency to enforce building codes or other regulations related to construction projects.

Bay: A space intended for human occupancy with one hard wall and three soft walls (eg, cubicle curtains, portable privacy screens).

Building envelope: All of the outer shell, including the exterior walls, floor, and roof, of a building that assists with maintaining a dry, heated, or cooled indoor environment and facilitates its climate control.

Commissioning: A quality process used to achieve, validate, and document that facilities and component infrastructure systems are planned, constructed, installed, tested, and capable of being operated and maintained in conformity with the design intent or performance expectations.

Cove base: Molding or trim used to create a curved right-angle transition from the wall to the floor.

Cubicle: A space intended for human occupancy with three full- or partial-height hard walls and one soft wall (eg, cubicle curtains, portable privacy screens).

Directly accessible: Connected to the identified room through a doorway, pass through, or other opening that does not require going through an intervening room or public space.

Evidence-based design: A process used by architects, interior designers, and facility managers in the planning, design, and construction of health care facilities. Individuals using evidence-based design make decisions based on the best information available from research, project evaluations, and evidence gathered from client operations. An evidence-based design is intended to result in improvements to an organization's outcomes, economic performance, productivity, and customer satisfaction.

Hand washing station: An area that includes a sink with a faucet that can be operated without using the hands and contains cleansing agents and a means for drying the hands.

Hybrid OR: An operating room designed with imaging technologies (eg, 3-D angiography, computed tomography, magnetic resonance imaging, positron-emission tomography, intravascular ultrasound) to support surgical procedures that require multiple care providers with varied expertise to provide patient care in one location.

Interdisciplinary team: A group of experts from different fields who work in a coordinated fashion toward a common goal.

Intraoperative area: The portion of the surgical suite that includes the operating room, interventional radiology room, hybrid operating room, and the semi-restricted corridors connecting the unrestricted area to the restricted area.

Medication safety zone: A critical area where medications are prescribed, orders are entered into a computer or transcribed onto paper documents, or medications are prepared or administered.

Monolithic: A surface constructed to be free of fissures, cracks, and crevices.

Patient care station: A designated space for individual patient care; may be defined as rooms, cubicles, or bays.

Perioperative team: An interdisciplinary group inclusive of all who act together to achieve a common goal before, during, and after an operative or other invasive procedure.

Preoperative area: The portion of the surgical suite in which preoperative care takes place. May include admission areas, waiting rooms, and patient care stations in which care is administered before the patient enters the intraoperative area.

Procedure room: A room designated for the performance of patient care that requires high-level disinfection or sterile instruments and some environmental controls but is not required to be performed with the environmental controls of an operating room.

Readily accessible: Available on the same floor or in the same building as the identified area or room.

Room: A space that has a door and is enclosed by four hard walls.

Supply breakout area/room: An area or room where items are removed from external shipping cartons before being taken into the semi-restricted area.

Surgical suite: An area or areas of the building containing the preoperative, intraoperative, and postoperative patient care areas and provisions for support areas.

References

1. Guideline for environmental cleaning. In: *Guidelines for Perioperative Practice.* Denver, CO: AORN Inc; 2018:7-28. [IVA]

2. Guideline for sterile technique. In: *Guidelines for Perioperative Practice.* Denver, CO: AORN Inc; 2018:75-104. [IVA]

3. Guideline for surgical smoke safety. In: *Guidelines for Perioperative Practice.* Denver, CO: AORN Inc; 2018:469-498. [IVA]

4. Guideline for patient information management. In: *Guidelines for Perioperative Practice.* Denver, CO: AORN Inc; 2018:573-598. [IVA]

5. Pelly N, Zeallear B, Reed M, Martin L. Utilizing integrated facility design to improve the quality of a pediatric ambulatory surgery center. *Paediatr Anaesth.* 2013;23(7):634-638. [IIIB]

6. *Security Design Guidelines for Healthcare Facilities.* Glendale Heights, IL: International Association for Healthcare Security & Safety (IAHSS); 2016. [IVC]

7. Sabnis R, Ganesamoni R, Mishra S, Sinha L, Desai MR. Concept and design engineering: endourology operating room. *Curr Opin Urol.* 2013;23(2):152-157. [VB]

8. Clair JD, Colatrella S. Opening Pandora's (tool) box: health care construction and associated risk for nosocomial infection. *Infect Disorder Drug Targets.* 2013;13(3):177-183. [VC]

9. Al-Benna S. Infection control in operating theatres. *J Perioper Pract.* 2012;22(10):318-322. [VB]

10. Spagnolo AM, Ottria G, Amicizia D, Perdelli F, Cristina ML. Operating theatre quality and prevention of surgical site infections. *J Prev Med Hyg.* 2013;54(3):131-137. [VA]

11. Devine DA, Wenger B, Krugman M, et al. Part 1: Evidence-based facility design using Transforming Care at the Bedside principles. *J Nurs Adm.* 2015;45(2):74-83. [VA]

12. Krugman M, Sanders C, Kinney LJ. Part 2: Evaluation and outcomes of an evidence-based facility design project. *J Nurs Adm.* 2015;45(2):84-92. [VB]

13. Facility Guidelines Institute, US Department of Health and Human Services, American Society for Healthcare Engineering. *Guidelines for Design and Construction of Hospitals.* Chicago, IL: American Society for Healthcare Engineering of the American Hospital Association; 2018. [IVC]

14. Facility Guidelines Institute, US Department of Health and Human Services, American Society for Healthcare Engineering.

Guidelines for Design and Construction of Outpatient Facilities. Chicago, IL: American Society for Healthcare Engineering of the American Hospital Association; 2018. [IVC]

15. Criscitelli T, Goodwin W. Applying human-centered design thinking to enhance safety in the OR. *AORN J.* 2017;105(4):408-412. [VC]

16. Guedon ACP, Wauben LSGL, de Korne DF, Overvelde M, Dankelman J, van den Dobbelsteen JJ. A RFID specific participatory design approach to support design and implementation of real-time location systems in the operating room. *J Med Syst.* 2015;39(1):168. [VB]

17. Capolongo S, Bellini E, Nachiero D, Rebecchi A, Buffoli M. Soft qualities in healthcare. Method and tools for soft qualities design in hospitals' built environments. *Ann Ig.* 2014;26(4):391-399. [VB]

18. Schaadt J, Landau B. Hybrid OR 101: a primer for the or nurse. *AORN J.* 2013;97(1):81-100. [VC]

19. Baker JD. The Orwellian nature of radio-frequency identification in the perioperative setting. *AORN J.* 2016;104(4):281-284. [VB]

20. Olmsted RN. Prevention by design: construction and renovation of health care facilities for patient safety and infection prevention. *Infect Dis Clin North Am.* 2016;30(3):713-728. [VA]

21. Stichler JF. Using consultants in the design, construction, and occupancy of new healthcare facilities. *J Nurs Adm.* 2015;45(11):537-539. [VB]

22. Stichler JF. Healthy work environments for the ageing nursing workforce. *J Nurs Manag.* 2013;21(7):956-963. [IIIB]

23. Hoffman PN, Williams J, Stacey A, et al. Microbiological commissioning and monitoring of operating theatre suites. *J Hosp Infect.* 2002;52(1):1-28. [IVB]

24. *ANSI/ASHRAE/ASHE Addendum H to ANSI/ASHRAE/ASHE Standard 170-2017: Ventilation of Health Care Facilities.* New York, NY: American Society of Heating, Refrigerating and Air-Conditioning Engineers; 2017. [IVC]

25. *ANSI/AAMI ST79:2017 Comprehensive Guide to Steam Sterilization and Sterility Assurance in Health Care Facilities.* Arlington, VA: Association for the Advancement of Medical Instrumentation; 2017. [IVB]

26. *NFPA 101: Life Safety Code.* Quincy, MA: National Fire Protection Association; 2018. [IVC]

27. *NFPA 99: Health Care Facilities Code Handbook.* Quincy, MA: National Fire Protection Association; 2018. [IVC]

28. *NFPA 70: National Electrical Code.* Quincy, MA: National Fire Protection Association; 2017. [IVC]

29. Guideline for safe patient handling and movement. In: *Guidelines for Perioperative Practice.* Denver, CO: AORN, Inc; 2018:e1-e48. [IVA]

30. Barzoloski-O'Connor B. Preventing infections during construction in the perioperative area. *OR Nurse.* 2013;7(1):10-12. [VC]

31. Kanamori H, Rutala WA, Sickbert-Bennett EE, Weber DJ. Review of fungal outbreaks and infection prevention in healthcare settings during construction and renovation. *Clin Infect Dis.* 2015;61(3):433-444. [IIIB]

32. Chang CC, Ananda-Rajah M, Belcastro A, et al. Consensus guidelines for implementation of quality processes to prevent invasive fungal disease and enhanced surveillance measures during hospital building works, 2014. *Intern Med J.* 2014;44(12):1389-1397. [IVC]

33. Smith TA. Secure design. *Health Facil Manage.* 2012;25(9):55-58. [VC]

34. Yow JA. The electronic security partnership of safety/security and information systems departments. *J Healthc Prot Manage.* 2012;28(1):108-111. [VC]

35. McGain F, Naylor C. Environmental sustainability in hospitals—a systematic review and research agenda. *J Health Serv Res Policy.* 2014;19(4):245-252. [IIIB]

36. Beale C, Kittredge FD Jr. Current trends in health facility planning, design, and construction. *Front Health Serv Manage.* 2014;31(1):3-17. [VC]

37. Kagoma Y, Stall N, Rubinstein E, Naudie D. People, planet and profits: the case for greening operating rooms. *CMAJ.* 2012;184(17):1905-1911. [VB]

38. Surgical lights: an illuminating look at the LED marketplace. *Health Devices.* 2010;39(11):390-402. [VB]

39. Horn M, Patel N, MacLellan M, Millard N. Traditional canister-based open waste management system versus closed system: hazardous exposure prevention and operating theatre staff satisfaction. *ACORN J.* 2015;28(1):18-22. [IIIB]

40. Finding ways to go green. *Can Nurse.* 2013;109(2):8-9. [VC]

41. Ma H, Du N, Yu S, et al. Analysis of typical public building energy consumption in northern China. *Energy Build.* 2017;136:139-150. [IIIC]

42. Whitson BA. The 50 percent solution to reducing energy costs. *Healthc Financ Manage.* 2012;66(11):132-138. [VC]

43. Kaneko TD, Michael J. Use of the hybrid operating room in cardiovascular medicine. *Circulation.* 2014;130(11):910-917. [VB]

44. Holmdahl T, Lanbeck P. Design for the post-antibiotic era: experiences from a new building for infectious diseases in Malmö, Sweden. *Health Environ Res Design J.* 2013;6(4):24-52. [VB]

45. Alfonsi E, Capolongo S, Buffoli M. Evidence based design and healthcare: an unconventional approach to hospital design. *Ann Ig.* 2014;26(2):137-143. [VA]

46. Brands CK, Hernandez RG, Stenberg A, et al. Complete self-sufficiency planning: designing and building disaster-ready hospitals. *South Med J.* 2013;106(1):63-68. [VB]

47. Guideline for surgical attire. In: *Guidelines for Perioperative Practice.* Denver, CO: AORN Inc; 2018:105-128. [IVA]

48. Allo MD, Tedesco M. Operating room management: operative suite considerations, infection control. *Surg Clin North Am.* 2005;85(6):1291-1297, xii. [VC]

49. *State Operations Manual Appendix A: Survey Protocol, Regulations and Interpretive Guidelines for Hospitals.* Rev 176; 2017. Centers for Medicare & Medicaid Services. https://www.cms.gov/Regulations-and-Guidance/Guidance/Manuals/downloads/som107ap_a_hospitals.pdf. Accessed June 7, 2018.

50. *Safe Patient Handling and Mobility: Interprofessional National Standards.* Silver Spring, MD: American Nurses Association: 2013. [IVB]

51. Cohen MH; 2010 Health Guidelines Revision Committee Specialty Subcommittee on Patient Movement. *Patient Handling and Movement Assessments: A White Paper.* Dallas, TX: Facility Guidelines Institute; 2010. [VA]

52. Thomas-Olson L, Gee M, Harrison D, Helal N. Evaluating the use of ceiling lifts in the operating room. *ORNAC J.* 2015;33(1):13-28. [IIIC]

53. Gormley T, Wagner J. Studying airflow in the OR: measuring the environmental quality indicators in a dynamic hospital operating room setting. *Health Facil Manage.* January 9, 2018. https://www.hfmmagazine.com/articles/3246-studying-airflow-in-the-or?utm_medium=email&utm_source=newsletter&utm_campaign=hfminsider&utm_content=20180116&eid=333111138&bid=1972574. Accessed June 6, 2018. [IIIC]

54. Wan G, Chung F, Tang C. Long-term surveillance of air quality in medical center operating rooms. *Am J Infect Control.* 2011;39(4):302-308. [IIIB]

55. Chapter IV. Subchapter G. Part 482. Conditions of Participation for Hospitals. Electronic Code of Federal Regulations. https://www.ecfr.gov/cgi-bin/text-idx?rgn=div5;node=42:5.0.1.1.1;cc=ecfr#se42.5.482_142. Accessed June 7, 2018.

56. *Lighting for Hospitals and Health Care Facilities.* New York, NY: Illuminating Engineering Society of North America; 2006. [IVC]

57. Dianat I, Sedghi A, Bagherzade J, Jafarabadi MA, Stedmon AW. Objective and subjective assessments of lighting in a hospital setting: implications for health, safety and performance. *Ergonomics.* 2013;56(10):1535-1545. [IIIA]

58. Hinsa-Leasure SM, Nartey Q, Vaverka J, Schmidt MG. Copper alloy surfaces sustain terminal cleaning levels in a rural hospital. *Am J Infect Control.* 2016;44(11):e195-e203. [IIC]

59. Karpanen TJ, Casey AL, Lambert PA, et al. The antimicrobial efficacy of copper alloy furnishing in the clinical environment: a crossover study. *Infect Control Hosp Epidemiol.* 2012;33(1):3-9. [IIIB]

60. O'Gorman J, Humphreys H. Application of copper to prevent and control infection: where are we now? *J Hosp Infect.* 2012;81(4):217-223. [IIIB]

61. Weber DJ, Rutala WA. Self-disinfecting surfaces: review of current methodologies and future prospects. *Am J Infect Control.* 2013;41(5 Suppl):S31-S35. [VB]

62. Palmer G 2nd, Abernathy JH 3rd, Swinton G, et al. Realizing improved patient care through human-centered operating room design: a human factors methodology for observing flow disruptions in the cardiothoracic operating room. *Anesthesiology.* 2013;119(5):1066-1077. [IIIB]

63. Nguyen DB, Gupta N, Abou-Daoud A, et al. A polymicrobial outbreak of surgical site infections following cardiac surgery at a community hospital in Florida, 2011-2012. *Am J Infect Control.* 2014;42(4):432-435. [VB]

64. Anesthetic gases: guidelines for workplace exposures. Occupational Safety and Health Administration. https://www.osha.gov/dts/osta/anestheticgases/index.html. Accessed June 7, 2018. [IVB]

65. Yasny JS, White J. Environmental implications of anesthetic gases. *Anesth Prog.* 2012;59(4):154-158. [VB]

66. Bosenberg M. Anaesthetic gases: environmental impact and alternatives. *South Afr J Anaesth Analg.* 2011;17(5):345-348. [VC]

67. Wang F, Hung J, Chen Y, Hsu C. Performance evaluation for operation rooms by numerical simulation and field measurement. *Int J Vent.* 2017;16(3):189-199. [IIIC]

68. Wang F, Lee M, Chang T, Hsu C. Evaluation of indoor environment parameters and energy-efficient HVAC system for an unoccupied operating room. In: *Indoor Air 2014—13th International Conference on Indoor Air Quality and Climate.* Santa Cruz, CA: International Society of Indoor Air Quality and Climate; 2014:769-776. [IIIB]

69. Thiel CL, Eckelman M, Guido R, et al. Environmental impacts of surgical procedures: life cycle assessment of hysterectomy in the United States. *Environ Sci Technol.* 2015;49(3):1779-1786. [IIIA]

70. Aydin Çakir N, Ucar FB, Haliki Uztan A, Corbaci C, Akpinar O. Determination and comparison of microbial loads in atmospheres of two hospitals in Izmir, Turkey. *Ann Agric Environ Med.* 2013;20(1):106-110. [IIIB]

71. *Operating Room HVAC Setback Strategies.* Chicago, IL: American Society for Healthcare Engineering; 2011. [VB]

72. Cockram A. Correct lighting of hospital buildings. 1976. *Health Estate.* 2007;61(4):21-23. [VC]

73. Verrinder J. Use of right lighting levels essential. *Health Estate.* 2007;61(6):31-32. [VC]

74. Knulst AJ, Mooijweer R, Jansen FW, Stassen LP, Dankelman J. Indicating shortcomings in surgical lighting systems. *Minim Invasive Ther Allied Technol.* 2011;20(5):267-275. [VC]

75. Baillie J. Stars of the theatre show true colours. *Health Estate.* 2012;66(1):31-36. [VC]

76. ECRI Institute. Hazard report. Overlap of surgical lighthead beams may present burn risk. *Health Devices.* 2009;38(10):341-342. [IVC]

77. Zhou Z, Hu B, Gao X, Bao R, Chen M, Li H. Sources of sporadic *Pseudomonas aeruginosa* colonizations/infections in surgical ICUs: association with contaminated sink trap. *J Infect Chemother.* 2016;22(7):450-455. [IIIC]

78. Bédard E, Laferrière C, Charron D, et al. Post-outbreak investigation of *Pseudomonas aeruginosa* faucet contamination by quantitative polymerase chain reaction and environmental factors affecting positivity. *Infect Control Hospital Epidemiol.* 2015;36(11):1337-1343. [IIIC]

79. Eder SP, Register JL. 10 management considerations for implementing an endovascular hybrid OR. *AORN J.* 2014;100(3):260-270. [VB]

80. Guideline for minimally invasive surgery. In: *Guidelines for Perioperative Practice.* Denver, CO: AORN Inc; 2018:611-640. [IVA]

81. Expert Panel on MR Safety; Kanal E, Barkovich AJ, Bell, C, et al. ACR guidance document on MR safe practices: 2013. *J Magn Reson Imaging.* 2013;37(3):501-530. [IVB]

82. Cowperthwaite L, Fearon MC. Guideline implementation: minimally invasive surgery, part 2—hybrid ORs. *AORN J.* 2017;106(2):145-153. [VC]

83. Childs S, Bruch P. Successful management of risk in the hybrid OR. *AORN J.* 2015;101(2):223-237. [VB]

84. Ley-Chavez A, Hmar-Lagroun T, Douglas-Ntagha P, Cumbo CL. Layout improvement study to reduce staff walking distance in a large health care facility: how to not walk an extra 4740 miles. *Qual Manag Health Care.* 2016;25(3):134-140. [VB]

85. Gurses AP, Kim G, Martinez EA, et al. Identifying and categorising patient safety hazards in cardiovascular operating rooms using an interdisciplinary approach: a multisite study. *BMJ Qual Saf.* 2012;21(10):810-818. [IIIA]

86. *NFPA 13: Standard for the Installation of Sprinkler Systems.* Quincy, MA: National Fire Protection Association; 2016:488. [IVC]

87. Loschi M, Thill C, Gray C, et al. Invasive aspergillosis in neutropenic patients during hospital renovation: effectiveness of mechanical preventive measures in a prospective cohort of 438 patients. *Mycopathologia.* 2015;179(5-6):337-345. [IIIB]

88. Lee L. Clean construction: infection control during building and renovation projects. *Health Facil Manage.* 2010;23(4):36-8; quiz 39. [VB]

89. Apisarnthanarak A, Mundy LM, Khawcharoenporn T, Mayhall CG. Hospital infection prevention and control issues relevant to extensive floods. *Infect Control Hosp Epidemiol.* 2013;34(2):200-206. [VA]

90. Scarlett HP, Postlethwait E, Delzell E, Sathiakumar N, Oestenstad RK. Asbestos in public hospitals: are employees at risk? *J Environ Health.* 2012;74(6):22-26. [IIIB]

91. Boix-Palop L, Nicolás C, Xercavins M, et al. *Bacillus* species pseudo-outbreak: construction works and collateral damage. *J Hosp Infect.* 2017;95(1):118-122. [VB]

92. Semchuk P. Breathing easy during building projects. *Health Estate.* 2015;69(2):17-20. [VC]

93. Brace MD, Stevens E, Taylor SM, et al. "The air that we breathe": Assessment of laser and electrosurgical dissection devices on operating theater air quality. *J Otolaryngol Head Neck Surg.* 2014;43(1):39-57. [IIIB]

94. Brun CP, Miron D, Silla LMR, Pasqualotto AC. Fungal spore concentrations in two haematopoietic stem cell transplantation (HSCT) units containing distinct air control systems. *Epidemiol Infect.* 2013;141(4):875-879. [IIIB]

95. Saliou P, Uguen M, Le Bars H, Le Clech L, Baron R. Fungal outbreaks and infection prevention during demolition: influence of high-efficiency particulate air filtration. *Clin Infect Dis.* 2016;62(7):950-951. [VC]

96. Barreiros G, Akiti T, Magalhães ACG, Nouér SA, Nucci M. Effect of the implosion and demolition of a hospital building on the concentration of fungi in the air. *Mycoses.* 2015;58(12):707-713. [VB]

97. Healthcare water system repair and recovery following a boil water alert or disruption of water supply. Centers for Disease Control and Prevention. https://www.cdc.gov/disasters/watersystemrepair.html. Accessed June 7, 2018. [IVC]

98. Centers for Disease Control and Prevention, American Water Works Association, eds. *Emergency Water Supply Planning Guide for Hospitals and Health Care Facilities.* Atlanta, GA: US Department of Health and Human Services; 2012. [IVC]

99. Klinger C, Landeg O, Murray V. Power outages, extreme events and health: a systematic review of the literature from 2011-2012. *Plos Curr.* 2014;6. [IIIB]

100. Working without technology: how hospitals and healthcare organizations can manage communication failure. Public Health Emergency. http://www.phe.gov/Preparedness/planning/cip/Documents/workingwithouttechnology.pdf. Accessed June 7, 2018. [VC]

101. Mitchell L, Anderle D, Nastally K, Sarver T, Hafner-Burton T, Owens S. Lessons learned from hurricane Ike. *AORN J.* 2009;89(6):1073-1078. [VB]

102. Remediation and infection control considerations for reopening healthcare facilities closed due to extensive water and wind damage. Centers for Disease Control and Prevention. https://www.cdc.gov/disasters/reopen_healthfacilities.html. Accessed June 7, 2018. [IVC]

103. Storm, flood, and hurricane response. Centers for Disease Control and Prevention. https://www.cdc.gov/niosh/topics/emres/cleaning-flood-hvac.html. Accessed June 7, 2018. [IVC]

104. Boubour J, Jenson K, Richter H, Yarbrough J, Oden ZM, Schuler DA. A shipping container-based sterile processing unit for low resources settings. *Plos One.* 2016;11(3):e0149624. [IIIC]

105. Carpenter T, Robinson ST. Case reports: response to a partial power failure in the operating room. *Anesth Analg.* 2010;110(6):1644-1646. [VA]

106. National Fire Protection Association, American National Standards Institute. *NFPA 110: Standard for Emergency and Standby Power Systems.* Quincy, MA: National Fire Protection Association; 2016. [IVC]

107. NIOSH alert: preventing occupational respiratory disease from exposures caused by dampness in office buildings, schools, and other nonindustrial buildings. November 2012. Centers for Disease Control and Prevention. https://www.cdc.gov/niosh/docs/2013-102/default.html. Accessed June 7, 2018. [VA]

108. Eichhorn JH, Hessel EA 2nd. Electrical power failure in the operating room: a neglected topic in anesthesia safety. *Anesth Analg.* 2010;110(6):1519-1521. [VB]

109. The Joint Commission. Preventing adverse events caused by emergency electrical power system failures. Sentinel Event Alert. September 6, 2006;37. https://www.jointcommission.org/sentinel_event_alert_issue_37_preventing_adverse_events_caused_by_emergency_electrical_power_system_failures/. Accessed June 7, 2018. [VC]

110. Stymiest DL. Power up: best practices for hospital power system reliability. Advice for planning, design, installation, inspection, maintenance and more. *Health Facil Manage.* 2016;29(3):25-29. [VC]

111. Stymiest DL. After the storm. expanding the concept of emergency power reliability. *Health Facil Manage.* 2013;26(1):21-24. [VC]

112. American Society of Heating, Refrigerating and Air-Conditioning Engineers. Infection control. In: *HVAC Design Manual for Hospitals and Clinics.* Atlanta, GA: American Society of Heating, Refrigerating and Air-Conditioning Engineers, Inc (ASHRAE); 2013:19-34. [IVC]

113. Berrios-Torres SI, Umscheid CA, Bratzler DW, et al. Centers for Disease Control and Prevention Guideline for the Prevention of Surgical Site Infection, 2017. *JAMA Surg.* 2017;152(8):784-791. [IVB]

114. *State Operations Manual Appendix L—Guidance for Surveyors: Ambulatory Surgical Centers.* Rev 137; 2015. Centers for Medicare & Medicaid Services. https://www.cms.gov/Regulations-and-Guidance/Guidance/Manuals/downloads/som107ap_l_ambulatory.pdf. Accessed June 7, 2018.

115. Guideline for prevention of unplanned patient hypothermia. In: *Guidelines for Perioperative Practice.* Denver, CO: AORN Inc; 2018:549-572. [IVA]

116. Traversari AA, Bottenheft C, van Heumen SP, Goedhart CA, Vos MC. Effect of switching off unidirectional downflow systems of operating theaters during prolonged inactivity on the period before the operating theater can safely be used. *Am J Infect Control.* 2017;45(2):139-144. [IIB]

117. Dettenkofer M, Scherrer M, Hoch V, et al. Shutting down operating theater ventilation when the theater is not in use: infection control and environmental aspects. *Infect Control Hosp Epidemiol.* 2003;24(8):596-600. [IIIB]

118. Gniadek A, Macura AB. Air-conditioning vs. presence of pathogenic fungi in hospital operating theatre environment. *Wiad Parazytol.* 2011;57(2):103-106. [IIIB]

119. Berthelot P, Carricajo A, Aubert G, Akhavan H, Gazielly D, Lucht F. Outbreak of postoperative shoulder arthritis due to *Propionibacterium acnes* infection in nondebilitated patients. *Infect Control Hosp Epidemiol.* 2006;27(9):987-990. [VB]

120. Yiallouros PK, Papadouri T, Karaoli C, et al. First outbreak of nosocomial *Legionella* infection in term neonates caused by a cold mist ultrasonic humidifier. *Clin Infect Dis.* 2013;57(1):48-56. [VB]

121. Vladut G, Sbirna LS, Sbirna S, Codresi C, Martin L. CFD simulation of the airflow pattern within a three-bed hospital room with or without a portable air conditioner in use. In: *2014 18th International Conference on System Theory, Control and Computing, ICSTCC.* Piscataway, NJ: IEEE; 2014:243-248. [IIIB]

122. Casha AR. Manche A, Camilleri L, Gauci M, Grima, JN, Borg MA. A novel method of personnel cooling in an operating theatre environment. *Interact Cardiovasc Thorac Surg.* 2014;19(4):687-689. [IIIB]

Acknowledgments

Lead Author

Byron Burlingame, MS, BSN, RN, CNOR
Senior Perioperative Nursing Specialist
AORN Nursing Department
Denver, Colorado

Contributing Author

Ramona Conner, MSN, RN, CNOR, FAAN
Editor in Chief, Guidelines for Perioperative Practice
AORN Nursing Department
Denver, Colorado

The authors and AORN thank Brenda G. Larkin, MS, ACNS-BC, CNS, CNOR, Clinical Nurse Specialist, Aurora Lakeland Medical Center, Lake Geneva, Wisconsin; Dawn Yost, MSN, BSDH, RN, RDH, CNOR, CSSM, Manager of Training & Development, Surgical Services, WVU Medicine-Ruby Memorial Hospital, Morgantown, West Virginia; Jennifer L. Butterfield, MBA, RN, CNOR, CASC, Administrator/CEO, Lakes Surgery Center, West Bloomfield, Michigan; Gerald McDonnell, PhD, BSc, Senior Director, Johnson & Johnson Family of Companies, Raritan, New Jersey; Susan Ruwe, MSN, RN, CPHQ, CIC, Senior Infection Preventionist, Carlie Foundation Hospital, Urbana, Illinois; and Janice A. Neil, PhD, RN, CNE, Full Time Faculty School of Nursing, East Carolina University, Winterville, North Carolina, for their assistance in developing this guideline.

Publication History

Originally published May 2014 as Guideline for a Safe Environment of Care, Part 2, in *Perioperative Standards and Recommended Practices* online.

Minor editing revisions made in November 2014 for publication in *Guidelines for Perioperative Practice,* 2015 edition.

Minor revisions to functional area terminology and recommendations for facility temperatures made in October 2016 for publication in *Guidelines for Perioperative Practice,* 2017 edition.

Revised August 2018 for publication in *Guidelines for Perioperative Practice* online.

Evidence ratings revised and minor editorial changes made to conform to the current AORN Evidence Rating model, September 2019, for publication in *Guidelines for Perioperative Practice* online.

ELECTROSURGICAL SAFETY

TABLE OF CONTENTS

🅿 *indicates a recommendation or evidence relevant to pediatric care.*

MEDICAL ABBREVIATIONS & ACRONYMS

ESU – Electrosurgical unit
AEC – Argon-enhanced coagulation
EMI – Electromagnetic interference
IED – Implanted electromechanical device
MAUDE – Manufacturer and User Facility Device Experience

SSEP – Somatosensory evoked potentials
IFU – Instructions for use
FDA – US Food and Drug Administration
CIED – Cardiac implanted electronic device
ID – Identification

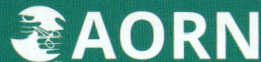
GUIDELINE FOR
ELECTROSURGICAL SAFETY

The Guideline for Electrosurgical Safety was approved by the AORN Guidelines Advisory Board and became effective as of July 29, 2020. The recommendations in the guideline are intended to be achievable and represent what is believed to be an optimal level of practice. Policies and procedures will reflect variations in practice settings and/or clinical situations that determine the degree to which the guideline can be implemented. AORN recognizes the many diverse settings in which perioperative nurses practice; therefore, this guideline is adaptable to all areas where operative or other invasive procedures may be performed.

Purpose

This document provides guidance to the perioperative team for the safe use of electrosurgical units (ESUs), **electrocautery** devices, and argon-enhanced coagulators.

An ESU includes a generator, an electrical cord and plug, and accessories. The accessories include the active electrode with tip(s), **dispersive electrode**, foot switch with cord (if applicable), adapters, and connectors.[1] The electrosurgical generator performs three functions. First, it converts the low-frequency alternating **current** received from the electrical circuit in the wall, which is at 60 Hertz, to approximately 500,000 Hertz (ie, **radio frequency**). The second function enables adjustment of the power setting. The third function controls the proportion of time over which a waveform is produced (ie, the **duty cycle**). These waveforms are known as *cut,* which is heating of the cellular water that leads to the cell bursting; *coagulation,* which causes a temperature rise in the cells leading to cellular dehydration and shrinkage; and *blend,* which is a modulated form of cut that results in an output with a higher voltage than cut at the same power setting.[1,2] The radio-frequency energy produced is transferred to the patient by various modalities, including monopolar, bipolar, advanced bipolar, bipolar ligating-cutting, and tripolar (ie, plasma knife) devices and **argon-enhanced coagulation** (AEC). These modalities are used to cut, coagulate, dissect, ablate, and shrink tissue.

The monopolar modality transfers the energy to the patient through an active electrode that usually has only a single tip. The intended current flow is from the generator through the active electrode cord to the active electrode tip, through the patient to the dispersive electrode, and then through the dispersive electrode cord back to the generator. The monopolar modality requires both an active and a dispersive electrode.[1,2]

The bipolar modality has a two-tip electrode that transfers the energy to the patient. The **current pathway** for this device goes from the generator through the cord to one tip of the forceps, through the tissue between the tips to the other tip, and then back to the generator. The current flows only through the tissue that is between the forceps tips. The only accessory required is the active electrode and the associated cord. **Bipolar electrosurgery** can be used as an alternative to **monopolar electrosurgery** when devices or implants would be in the current pathway between the monopolar active and dispersive electrodes.[1,2]

The advanced bipolar modality uses bipolar electrosurgery with a computer-controlled tissue feedback response system to sense tissue impedance. This allows for the continuous adjustment of the voltage and current generated by the unit. Continuous adjustment permits use of the lowest possible power setting that will achieve the desired tissue effect. The advanced bipolar modality does not require a dispersive electrode and requires less voltage. The energy flows only through the tissue that is between the forceps tips.[1,2] Some of the devices also have a cutting mechanism, allowing for cutting and coagulating of tissue between the forceps tips.[3]

The **tripolar device** has a tripolar tip consisting of a central pole and an outer pole on either side. The current flows from the center pole to the outer poles, creating a corona of energy that makes a blade-like incision. The primary current alternates with a second current that passes from one of the outer poles to the other, resulting in simultaneous cutting and coagulation.[1,3]

Argon-enhanced coagulation, also known as argon beam coagulation, is radio-frequency coagulation from an electrosurgical generator that delivers monopolar current through a flow of ionized argon gas. The risks related to this modality are similar to those for monopolar electrosurgery with the addition of the risk for gas emboli.[4]

The electrical current used by the ESU consistently flows on a pathway from the wall, through the device, to the accessories, through tissue, through the accessories, back to the device, and to the wall. Most adverse events associated with **electrosurgery** are related to the current trying to flow back to ground.[1,3] The majority of adverse events that result from the use of electrosurgery or electrocautery are burns. Burns may be caused by **direct application** that results in **thermal spread** beyond the intended target tissue, **insulation failure**, **antenna coupling**, **direct coupling**, **capacitive coupling**, **residual heat**, or **inadvertent activation** and may be described as **alternate site injuries.**[1,5-12] Adverse events have been reported to occur during various procedures and with all surgical approaches.[13-29] Burns may occur anywhere the tip of the active electrode is placed, under the dispersive electrode, inside the body during laparoscopic procedures, or at trocar sites.[1,5-12] Other types of adverse events include electrical shocks, **electromagnetic interference** (EMI), and fires.[1]

Electrical shocks do not often involve the patient because they occur off the sterile field; if strong enough, however, a shock can cause injury to a person in contact with the device or the electrical cord. A shock may result in a burn, another type of injury, or no injury.[1]

Electromagnetic interference may cause oversensing, cause a function reset, or stop the functioning of an implanted electromechanical device (IED) and could also damage a lead or the pulse generator itself.[30,31] In a retrospective study of 1,398 patients undergoing cardiac pacemaker generator replacement or upgrade surgery, Lin et al[32] found that four patients (0.3%) developed output failure or an inappropriate low pacing rate during use of electrosurgery. The researchers also reviewed the Manufacturer and User Facility Device Experience (MAUDE) database for events or patient injuries related to pacemaker malfunction and found 37 cases of pacemaker malfunction related to the use of electrosurgery. The adverse events included the pacemaker resorting to the backup pacing mode (32.4%), loss of output or capture function (59.5%), inappropriate low pacing rate (5.4%), and ventricular fibrillation (2.7%). The dates of review of the MAUDE database were not included in the report. Other authors have also reported on situations in which EMI during the use of electrosurgery led to complications, including ventricular tachycardia,[33] ventricular fibrillation,[28,34,35] and inappropriate defibrillation that occurred when an implantable cardioverter defibrillator sensed EMI from an electrosurgical active electrode as ventricular fibrillation.[36-38]

The active electrode is the most common ignition source in OR fires.[1] A fire may or may not result in patient burns.

Electrosurgical accessories, including the active and dispersive electrodes, have been implicated as the cause of injuries.[3,15,20,39,40] Overbey et al[16] reviewed reports to the MAUDE database from January 1, 1994, to December 31, 2013, and found 3,553 injuries and 178 deaths related to energy-generating devices. The energy-generating devices were classified as monopolar instruments (n = 1,670; 44.8%), radio-frequency/microwave **ablation** devices (n = 728, 19.5%), **advanced bipolar devices** (n = 538, 14.4%), ultrasonic devices (n = 350, 9.3%), bipolar instruments (n = 270, 7.2%), plasma beam monopolar devices (n = 163, 4.4%), and other (n = 12, 0.3%). The incidents involved thermal burns (n = 2,353, 63.1%), hemorrhage (n = 642, 17.2%), mechanical failure (n = 442, 11.8%), and fire (n = 294, 7.9%). The authors concluded that the risk for injury from surgical energy-generating devices is significant and warrants further research and education.

A limitation of the evidence is that randomized controlled trials related to electrosurgical injury prevention may expose patients to harm and, as such, would not be ethical. A limited number of other types of studies have contributed valuable knowledge to the field. However, interpretation of these studies is limited by the nature of this type of research, which can only show association among study variables and cannot determine causation. Because of a lack of research on interventions to prevent injury from the use of ESUs, much of the available evidence is based on generally accepted practices and expert opinion.

The following subjects are outside the scope of this guideline:
- general fire safety (See the AORN Guideline for a Safe Environment of Care)[41];
- surgical smoke safety (See the AORN Guideline for Surgical Smoke Safety)[42];
- selection of endoscopic distention fluid (See the AORN Guideline for Minimally Invasive Surgery)[43];
- procedure-related decisions (eg, the amount of time the tissue is exposed to the active electrode);
- therapeutic diathermy;
- use of electrical dental equipment (eg, battery-operated curing lights, ultrasonic baths, ultrasonic scalers, electric pulp testers, electric toothbrushes); and
- selection of electrosurgical devices.

Evidence Review

A medical librarian with a perioperative background conducted a systematic search of the databases Ovid MEDLINE®, Ovid Embase®, EBSCO CINAHL®, and the Cochrane Database of Systematic Reviews. The search was limited to literature published in English from January 2009 through June 2019. At the time of the initial search, weekly alerts were created on the topics included in that search. Results from these alerts were provided to the lead author until August 2019. The lead author requested additional articles that either did not fit the original search criteria or were discovered during the evidence appraisal process. The lead author and the medical librarian also identified relevant guidelines from government agencies, professional organizations, and standards-setting bodies.

Search terms included *ablation techniques, access control, accident prevention, accidental activation, airway fires, argon beam coagulation, argon plasma coagulation, artificial pacemaker, bipolar, burns, burns (electric), capacitive coupling, cauterization, cautery, device failure, device safety, diathermy, durable medical equipment, electric power supplies, electric wiring, electrical equipment and supplies, electrical power supplies, electrocautery, electrocoagulation, electrodes (implanted), electrosurgery, endocavitary fulguration, endometrial ablation techniques, energy device, equipment and supplies (hospital), equipment contamination, equipment defects, equipment failure, equipment failure analysis, equipment hazard, equipment malfunction, equipment safety, eye protective devices, fire extinguisher, fire management, fire safety, fires, grounding, high-intensity focused*

Figure 1. Flow Diagram of Literature Search Results

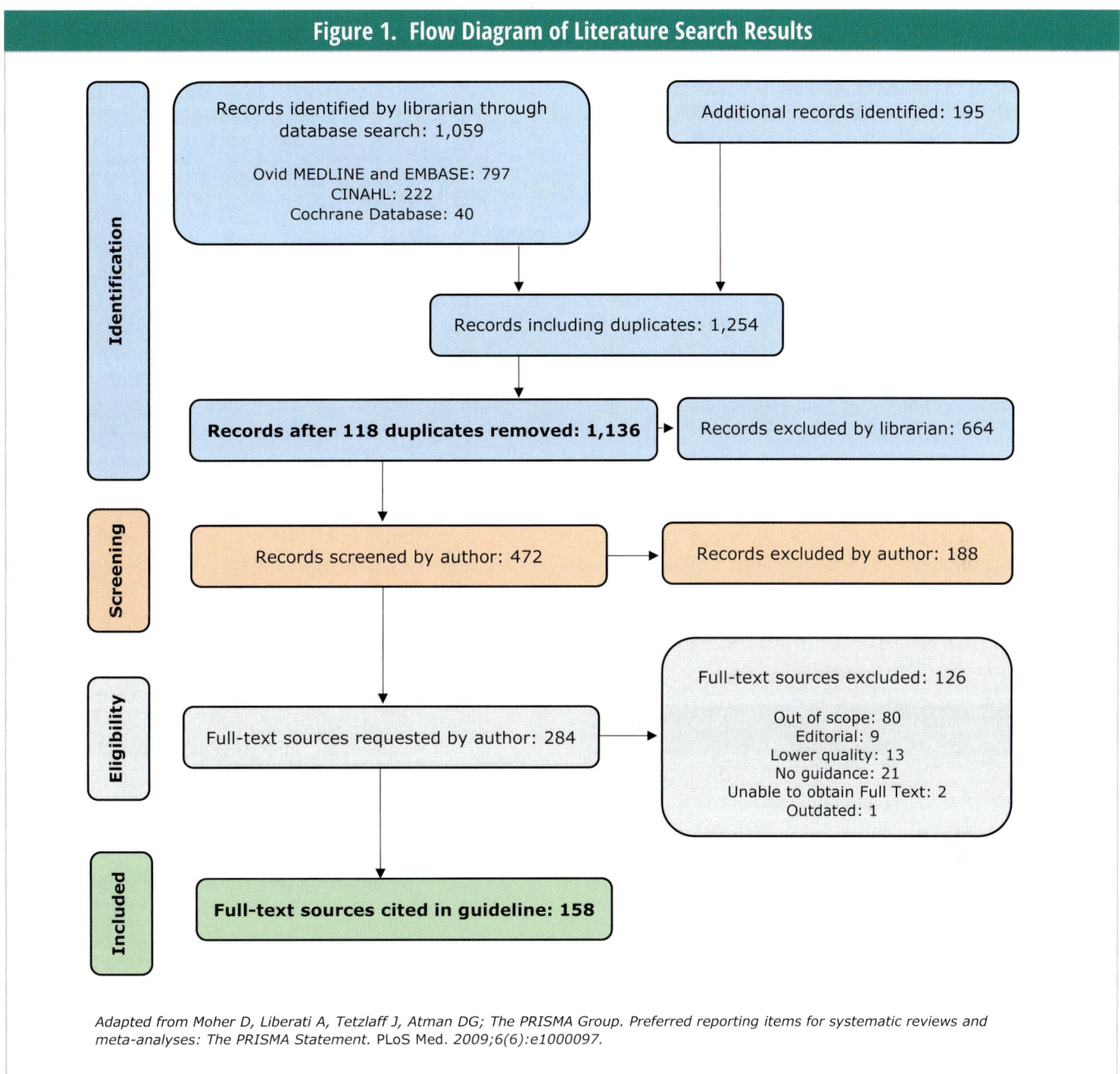

Records identified by librarian through database search: 1,059

Ovid MEDLINE and EMBASE: 797
CINAHL: 222
Cochrane Database: 40

Additional records identified: 195

Identification

Records including duplicates: 1,254

Records after 118 duplicates removed: 1,136

Records excluded by librarian: 664

Screening

Records screened by author: 472

Records excluded by author: 188

Eligibility

Full-text sources requested by author: 284

Full-text sources excluded: 126

Out of scope: 80
Editorial: 9
Lower quality: 13
No guidance: 21
Unable to obtain Full Text: 2
Outdated: 1

Included

Full-text sources cited in guideline: 158

Adapted from Moher D, Liberati A, Tetzlaff J, Atman DG; The PRISMA Group. Preferred reporting items for systematic reviews and meta-analyses: The PRISMA Statement. PLoS Med. 2009;6(6):e1000097.

ultrasound ablation, hospital incident reporting, hospital risk reporting, implantable electronic devices, implanted electrode, ligation, medical device safety, misdirection, nurses, occupational exposure, occupational hazards, occupational injuries, occupational safety, occupational-related injuries, pacemaker (artificial), patient safety, perioperative nursing, personal protective equipment, postoperative complications, power sources, power sources and settings, power supplies, protective clothing, protective devices, radiofrequency ablation, risk management, safety, shared airway procedures, shared airway safety, surgical diathermy, surgical equipment, surgical equipment and supplies, surgical fires, thermocoagulation, ultrasonic surgery, ultrasonic surgical procedures, and ultrasonic therapy.

Included were research and non-research literature in English, complete publications, and publications with dates

within the time restriction when available. Historical studies also were included. Excluded were non-peer-reviewed publications and older evidence within the time restriction when more recent evidence was available. Editorials, news items, conference proceedings, and poster abstracts were excluded. Low-quality evidence was excluded when higher-quality evidence was available, and literature outside the time restriction was excluded when literature within the time restriction was available. After evaluating the literature, the project team decided to exclude ultrasonic devices because they are not electrosurgical devices **(Figure 1)**.

Articles identified in the search were provided to the project team for evaluation. The team consisted of the lead author and one evidence appraiser. The lead author and the evidence appraiser reviewed and critically appraised each article using the AORN Research or Non-Research Evidence Appraisal Tools as appropriate. A second appraiser was consulted in the event of a disagreement between the lead author and the primary evidence appraiser. The literature was independently evaluated and appraised according to the strength and quality of the evidence. Each article was then assigned an appraisal score. The appraisal score is noted in brackets after each reference, as applicable.

Each recommendation rating is based on a synthesis of the collective evidence, a benefit-harm assessment, and consideration of resource use. The strength of the recommendation was determined using the AORN Evidence Rating Model and the quality and consistency of the evidence supporting a recommendation. The recommendation strength rating is noted in brackets after each recommendation.

Note: The evidence summary table is available at http:// www.aorn.org/evidencetables/.

Editor's note: MEDLINE is a registered trademark of the US National Library of Medicine's Medical Literature Analysis and Retrieval System, Bethesda, MD. Embase is a registered trademark of Elsevier B.V., Amsterdam, The Netherlands. CINAHL, Cumulative Index to Nursing and Allied Health Literature, is a registered trademark of EBSCO Industries, Birmingham, AL.

1. Injury Prevention

1.1 **Assess the patient preoperatively for the presence of foreign bodies (eg, IED, jewelry, prosthetic implants).** *[Recommendation]*

Assessment will help to determine the presence of items that will create the need to take actions to prevent injury.

1.2 **Place patient monitoring electrodes (eg, electrocardiogram, oximetry, fetal) as far as possible from the surgical site.**[44] *[Recommendation]*

Placing electrodes as far as possible from the surgical site decreases the risk for a burn at the electrode site.[44]

1.3 **Use alternate technologies (eg, bipolar, ultrasonic) instead of monopolar electrosurgery when neuromonitoring electrodes (eg, somatosensory evoked potentials [SSEP]) are present (See also 5. Implanted Electronic Devices).**[45] *[Recommendation]*

The findings of a laboratory study conducted by Townsend et al[45] support the use of alternate technologies. The researchers examined the temperature of the surface of a porcine tissue model onto which a neuromuscular monitoring lead was placed. They found an insignificant increase in the temperature at the neuromonitoring site with the use of an advanced bipolar device ($0.2° C \pm 0.4° C$ [$0.4° F \pm$

$0.7° F$]) and an ultrasonic device ($0° C \pm 0.3° C$ [$0° F \pm 0.5° F$]) compared to the temperature increase with the use of a monopolar ESU ($39° C \pm 13° C$ [$70° F \pm 23° F$]) or an argon beam generator ($34° C \pm 15° C$ [$61° F \pm 27° F$]). The researchers recommended using alternative technologies when neuromonitoring electrodes are used.

1.4 **During the use of monopolar devices, prevent contact between the patient and metal objects.**[44,46-48] *[Recommendation]*

Alternate site burns may occur because the electricity seeks an alternate pathway to ground, from the patient's skin to the metal object, instead of flowing to the dispersive electrode.[44,46-48] Low-quality evidence indicates that the risk for alternate site burns related to the phenomenon of stray current leakage has been almost eliminated by technological improvements in ESUs.[49,50]

A clinical guideline supports preventing contact between the patient and metal objects (eg, OR beds, stirrups, positioning devices, safety strap buckles) to prevent alternate site burns.[51]

1.5 **Remove all metal jewelry that will be between the active and dispersive electrodes.**[25,49,50,52] *[Recommendation]*

Metal jewelry, including body piercings, **subdermal implants**, and **transdermal** or **microdermal implants**, some of which may not be removable, presents a risk for thermal injury at the location where the jewelry touches the skin. The injury is caused by the heating of the metal as the electrical current moves through it.[52]

Nguyen et al[53] conducted a bench study to examine the effect of monopolar radio-frequency energy on the temperature of bovine myocardial tissue surrounding implanted metal objects. The objects consisted of insulated and noninsulated esophageal temperature probes, copper wire, a defibrillator lead, and a circular mapping catheter. The researchers applied radio-frequency energy to the tissue at 30 W using an ablation catheter. They found the temperature in the tissue surrounding the objects was elevated by a mean of $5.8° C$ to $8.9° C$ ($10.4° F$ to $16° F$) when the objects were between the active and dispersive electrodes and at a distance of 1 mm from the site of the active electrode. The researchers concluded that a significant rise in myocardial tissue temperature occurs when radio-frequency ablation is performed near metal items.

In contrast, the results of a quasi-experimental study conducted by Sheldon et al[54] did not support the need to remove microdermal implants. The researchers measured the skin temperature at microdermal implant sites located between the active and dispersive electrodes on swine skin. The dispersive electrode was placed 2 cm below an implant made of surgical stainless steel. The simulated surgical site was 2 cm above the implant. The researchers set the monopolar electrocautery at 30 W coagulation and administered it continuously for 30 seconds. They used thermal imaging to measure the surface skin temperature and assessed the tissue using gross examination and a histological evaluation.

The researchers found the skin temperature at the surgical site rose 27.7° C (49.9° F), and at the implant site the temperature was elevated 1.6° C (2.9° F). The researchers also measured the temperature at a control site on the contralateral side. The temperature increase at the subdermal site was 2° C (3.6° F) when the energy was applied on the contralateral site, which was not a significant difference. The researchers found no thermal injury on the tissue in close proximity to the subdermal implant site. They concluded that subdermal implants do not have to be removed even when in close proximity to the active electrode.[54]

1.5.1 When jewelry cannot be removed,
- notify the surgeon,
- consider using alternate technologies if jewelry is in the current pathway,[25,49,50,52]
- provide education to the patient regarding potential adverse events and document the education provided,
- assess all jewelry sites postoperatively for any evidence of burns, and
- document preoperative and postoperative assessment of jewelry sites.
[Recommendation]

1.6 Follow the manufacturer's written instructions for use (IFU) for all ESU components.[46] [Recommendation]

1.7 Perform the following fire prevention interventions when using an electrosurgical device:
- use technologies other than monopolar (eg, bipolar devices, coblation technology, non-energy-applying instruments) during surgical procedures on anatomical structures that present special fire hazards (eg, bowel, trachea)[12,19,23,26,55-59];
- use moist radiopaque sponges near the ignition source[12-14,19,21,57,60,61];
- remove alcohol-soaked sponges or other application devices from the sterile field[14,18,22,62-65]; and
- allow alcohol-based solutions to dry and fumes to dissipate before using any type of electrosurgical active electrodes.[14,18,22,62-65]
[Recommendation]

Low-quality evidence[12-14,17,19,21-23,26,55-58,60-65] and a clinical guideline[66] identify electrosurgical devices as an ignition source and support performing these interventions. For more information, see the fire prevention recommendations in the AORN Guideline for a Safe Environment of Care.[41]

Matt and Cottee[56] conducted a descriptive laboratory study in which they placed a bipolar radio-frequency ablation device in direct contact with flammable materials found in the OR: alcohol, four individual salt packets dissolved in alcohol, two pumps of ethanol-based foam hand sanitizer, saline-dampened gauze, plastic packaging filled with 5 mL of saline, and a 4.0 endotracheal tube with 100% oxygen flowing through the tube. The researchers found that the bipolar radio-frequency ablation device did not ignite the various materials even when set at the highest settings (ie, 9 ablation, 5 coagulation). They concluded that the tested bipolar radio-frequency ablation device did not produce an adequate amount of heat to serve as an ignition source at the surgical site, and therefore decreased the potential for fire.

In a laboratory study, Roy and Smith[55] compared the time to ignition of a chicken carcass (as a human tissue surrogate) when using a standard monopolar device at 15 W coagulate mode versus a bipolar radio-frequency ablation wand set at 9, 7, and 3 in the ablate mode. The researchers inserted an endotracheal tube into the gut of the chicken, with 100% oxygen flowing through the tube. Contact between the chicken and the device was made near the end of the endotracheal tube. Ignition occurred after 25 to 80 seconds during use of the monopolar device, and no ignition occurred during use of the bipolar device. The researchers concluded that use of a bipolar radio-frequency ablation device eliminates the risk for fire during open cavity surgery.

1.8 Perform the following fire prevention interventions when using an electrocautery device:
- use radiopaque sponges moistened with non-flammable liquid near the ignition source,[67]
- apply the protective cap when the cautery is not in use,[68] and
- remove the wire loop and batteries from the electrocautery device before discarding it.[59,68]
[Recommendation]

An electrocautery device has been identified as an ignition source.[68]

In a non-experimental study, Axelrod et al[67] tested the flammability of plastic tubing, an OR cap, paper tape, dry and moist cotton gauze, a paper gown, dry and moist cotton towels, a plastic drape, and a cellulose eye spear. The researchers found all the items except the moist towel and moist cotton gauze would ignite, melt, or char when touched with an electrocautery device at 1.5 or 3.0 volts. The researchers recommended using moist sponges near the site of electrocautery use.

1.9 When patient or personnel injuries or equipment failures occur during the use of an electrosurgical generator or accessories,

- **remove the electrosurgical generator and accessories from service;**
- **retain all accessories and packaging if possible[69]; and**
- **report the adverse event details, including device identification and maintenance and service information, according to the health care organization's policy and procedures.** *[Recommendation]*

A clinical guideline supports removing malfunctioning ESUs from service.[51] Retaining the generator, accessories, and packaging can facilitate a complete incident investigation.[69]

1.9.1 The health care organization must report to the US Food and Drug Administration (FDA) and the manufacturer when a medical device is suspected of having contributed to a death, or only to the FDA if the medical device manufacturer is unknown.[70] *[Regulatory Requirement]*

The FDA provides specific guidance for mandatory reporting.[70]

1.9.2 The health care organization or personnel may report ESU malfunctions to the FDA.[70] *[Conditional Recommendation]*

The FDA provides specific guidance for voluntary reporting.[70]

1.9.3 The health care organization must report to other regulatory bodies as defined by state or local regulations. *[Regulatory Requirement]*

2. ESU Generator

2.1 Keep safety and warning alarms and activation indicators on the generator operational, audible, and visible at all times.[1,44,69] *[Recommendation]*

Safety and warning alarms alert the operator to potential equipment failure. The indicators and alarms immediately alert the perioperative team when the active electrode is activated.[1,69]

2.2 Select the lowest power setting on the electrosurgical generator that achieves the desired result.[45,71,72] *[Recommendation]*

High-quality evidence supports that using the lowest power setting needed to achieve the desired result reduces

- damage from capacitive coupling,[71]
- the amount of undesirable tissue effect (ie, depth of tissue debridement plus depth of chondrocyte death in underlying cartilage),[73]
- the size of the ablation area,[74]
- the depth and area of injury,[75]
- the amount and depth of cell death,[76]
- damage from antenna coupling,[72]
- the temperature of the skin under a neuromuscular and an electrocardiogram lead,[45]
- thermal spread,[77] and
- development of esophageal ulcerations.[78]

These studies were quasi-experimental, and all of the studies except one[78] were conducted in laboratory settings using animal tissue.[45,71-77]

Lower-quality evidence also showed that using the lowest power setting needed to achieve the desired effect reduced the incidence of

- thermal spread,[79,80]
- antenna coupling,[81]
- thermal injury,[82]
- hemorrhage,[83] and
- EMI.[84,85]

These studies were nonexperimental, and all of the studies except one[83] were conducted in laboratory settings using animal tissue.[79-82,84,85]

Clinical guidelines also support use of the lowest effective power setting.[59,86] However, the findings of a nonexperimental study by Metzner et al[87] conflict with those of the previous studies. The researchers assigned 30 patients undergoing pulmonary vein isolation with an endoscopic ablation system to one of three groups:

- in Group 1 (n = 10), ablation was performed at power settings of 5.5 W and 7.0 W;
- in Group 2 (n = 10), ablation was performed at power settings of 7.0 W and 8.5 W; and
- in Group 3 (n = 10), ablation was performed at power settings of 8.5 W and 10.0 W.

Pulmonary vein isolation was successfully performed in each of the groups (ie, 69% in Group 1, 73% in Group 2, 90% in Group 3). One patient in each of Groups 2 and 3 developed esophageal thermal lesions; none were reported in Group 1. The researchers concluded that higher energy settings increase efficacy and are safe to use. They also stated that the study was small and further research should be conducted before final conclusions are drawn.[87]

2.2.1 Confirm the power settings on the electrosurgical generator with the operator before activation.[51] *[Recommendation]*

Clinical guidelines support confirming the power settings before activation.[51,86]

2.2.2 If the operator repeatedly requests an increase in power, confirm the integrity of the entire circuit including the generator and all accessories.[69,88,89] *[Recommendation]*

A nonintact circuit, such as a loss of adhesion between the dispersive electrode and the patient, may cause ineffective coagulation and cutting, resulting in a request by the user for an increase in power.[88]

2.3 Mount the electrosurgical generator securely to a tip-resistant cart or shelf.[51] *[Recommendation]*

A clinical guideline supports mounting the generator on a tip-resistant cart or shelf to help prevent the unit from falling to the floor and possibly causing injury to the patient or personnel.[51]

2.4 Do not place items including equipment or containers of liquids on the electrosurgical generator.[69,90,91] *[Recommendation]*

Use of the generator as a table may create a fire hazard or cause malfunctioning of the equipment placed on top of the generator.[69,90] Putting containers of liquids on the generator may increase the potential of an unintentional activation, a device failure, or an electrical hazard resulting from liquids entering the electrosurgical generator.[69,91]

A clinical guideline advises against putting containers of liquids on the generator.[51]

2.5 Qualified personnel (eg, a biomedical engineering services representative) must perform periodic monitoring, inspection, testing, and maintenance on the electrosurgical generator.[92,93] *[Regulatory Requirement]*

The Centers for Medicare & Medicaid Services requires that equipment be inspected, tested, and maintained.[92,93]

2.5.1 Document inspection and maintenance according to the health care organization's policy. *[Recommendation]*

2.6 Document the following in the patient's medical record in a manner consistent with the health care organization's policies and procedures:
- electrosurgical generator identification (eg, serial or biomedical number),
- location of dispersive electrode placement, and
- the patient's skin condition before application and after removal of the dispersive electrode.[94]

[Recommendation]

2.7 Follow the electrosurgical generator and accessory manufacturers' IFU when multiple ESUs are used simultaneously.[69] *[Recommendation]*

A clinical guideline recommends following the manufacturers' IFU.[59]

2.7.1 Label accessories to correspond with the generator to which they are attached.[95] *[Recommendation]*

Labeling individual generators and accessories to match helps identify which ESU requires adjustment or, during a move by the operator from one side of the table to the other, which operator is using which unit.[95]

2.7.2 Use one single-use dispersive electrode for each generator when multiple generators are used and
- place the dispersive electrodes as close as possible to the surgical site,
- do not overlap the dispersive electrodes, and
- place the dispersive electrodes equidistant from the surgical site when it is a single site.[39]

[Recommendation]

Equidistant placement results in the equal distribution of the electrical current.[39]

3. ESU Accessories

3.1 Use accessories that are compatible with the generator as specified in the manufacturers' IFU. *[Recommendation]*

A clinical guideline supports using only compatible accessories.[86]

3.2 Place the cords that connect the monopolar active electrode and the dispersive electrode to the generator as far as possible from or perpendicular to other cords (eg, cardiac and neuromuscular monitoring cords, light cords, second electrosurgery cords, camera cord).[45,72,81,96-98] *[Recommendation]*

High-quality evidence supports placing these cords as far as possible from or perpendicular to other cords.[45,98]

Robinson et al[98] conducted a randomized controlled trial that included 84 patients undergoing laparoscopic cholecystectomy. The researchers measured the amount of thermal injury at the skin adjacent to the umbilical trocar site in control group procedures (n = 42) during which active electrodes and camera cords were oriented parallel and located in close proximity and in experimental group procedures (n = 42) during which the cords were separated. The researchers found that thermal injury was significantly less in the experimental group than in the control group (31% versus 57%). They concluded that cords should be separated and not oriented parallel or located in close proximity.

Townsend et al[45] used a porcine model to examine the temperature of the surface of the tissue where a neuromuscular and an electrocardiogram lead were attached. The items were tested with an ESU power setting at 30 W and 15 W and cords placed close to or 15 cm away from the electrodes. The researchers noted a significant decrease in the temperature when the lower power setting was used and when the cords were not in close proximity. Based on these findings, they recommended setting the power as low as possible and placing the wires as far from the electrodes as possible.

Lower-quality evidence also supports placing cords that connect the monopolar active or dispersive electrode to the generator as far as possible from or perpendicular to other cords.[72,81,96,97]

Jones et al[81] illustrated antenna coupling in a laboratory study. The researchers measured the tissue temperature in a bovine liver using an L-hook device as the active electrode and an unlit 10-mm laparoscope as the instrument receiving the energy. The researchers compared the temperature at the end of the scope when the cords were parallel and bundled to the temperature when the cords were completely separated. They found the increase was greater when the cords were bundled than when the cords were separated (38.2° C [68.8° F] versus 15.7° C [28.3° F]). The researchers recommended separating the camera and light cords and the wires leading from the generator to the active electrode. Robinson et al[72] found similar results and drew the same conclusion in a descriptive laboratory study using bovine muscle tissue.

In a non-experimental laboratory study, Townsend et al[97] measured the temperature at the end of a 10-mm 30-degree laparoscopic telescope and a Maryland laparoscopic grasper after activating a monopolar L-hook placed 4 cm away during simulated four-port laparoscopic procedures on porcine liver tissue. The ESU was activated 10 times with the monopolar generator set at 30 W coagulation mode. The researchers found a significant increase in temperature when the active electrode and the telescope cord were in close proximity compared to when the cords were separated at the end of the telescope, which has a cord, but not at the end of the Maryland grasper. Townsend et al[96] achieved similar results when the dispersive electrode cord was in close proximity to the camera cord compared to when they were separated.

3.3 Secure electrosurgical accessory cords to the sterile drapes
- with a non-piercing plastic or other nonconductive device, and
- in a manner that does not crush or damage the cord or compromise the sterile field.[69]

[Recommendation]

Plastic devices do not conduct electricity if there is leakage. Use of a non-piercing device decreases the potential for sterile field contamination that could be caused by holes made in the drapes. Crushing or damaging a cord may create a place at which the current can escape from the cord, creating a fire on the drapes or causing the device to malfunction.[69]

3.4 Track the number of uses of reusable accessories (eg, cords, handles, shafts), and handle an accessory per the manufacturer's IFU when the maximum number of uses has been reached. *[Recommendation]*

Manufacturers' IFU contain instructions on the maximum number of sterilization cycles for which integrity testing has been performed.[86]

3.5 Visually inspect electrosurgical accessories for damage (eg, insulation breakage) before and after use and, if reusable, during reprocessing.[8,20,24,29,48,69,87,99-101] *[Recommendation]*

Inspection helps to identify malfunctioning accessories (eg, active electrode internal wires, electrode insulation, sheaths) that have caused procedure delays (eg, while replacement equipment is obtained), injury to personnel or patients, or ignition of surgical drapes or clinicians' gowns.[8,29,48,69,87,100,101] Refer to the AORN Guideline for Care and Cleaning of Surgical Instruments[102] for more detailed recommendations for instrument inspection.

Munro[82] conducted a laboratory comparative study to identify mechanisms of thermal injury to a patient's lower genital tract during radio-frequency resectoscopic surgery. The researcher used a tissue model to represent the uterus and created defects in the insulation on the electrode. He found injuries resulting from capacitive coupling occurred when the insulation was damaged.

Montero et al[103] examined 165 reusable laparoscopic instruments for breaks in insulation and found 19% of the instruments had insulation failure. The researchers recommended that surgeons be made aware of the many insulation failures that can occur and adopt practices to decrease the potential for complications related to insulation failure.

Clinical guidelines also support inspecting accessories.[51,59,86]

3.5.1 Use an active electrode insulation integrity tester while preparing active electrodes for packaging during processing.[104,105] [Recommendation]

Moderate-quality evidence[104,105] and a clinical guideline[59] support the use of an active electrode insulation integrity tester.

In a descriptive study, Tixier et al[105] inspected and tested 489 instruments for insulation failure. The researchers found 24.1% of the instruments failed a visual inspection and 37.2% failed with the use of an active electrode insulation integrity tester. Failure occurred in a median location in 50.4% of the laparoscopic instruments and in a distal location in 40.4% of the non-laparoscopic instruments.

In another descriptive study, Espada et al[104] tested 78 robotic and 298 laparoscopic instruments at 20 W and 2.64 kV in phase A and tested 60 robotic and 308 laparoscopic instruments at 20 W/1 kV and 20 W/4.2 kV in phase B. In phase A, the researchers found insulation failures in 80% of the robotic instruments and 36% of the laparoscopic instruments. In phase B, they detected failures in 81.7% of the robotic instruments and 19.5% of the laparoscopic instruments. The researchers recommended routine testing of laparoscopic and robotic instruments for insulation failure.

3.5.2 If an insulation failure is identified during processing, sterile processing personnel should remove the damaged device from service.[86] [Recommendation]

3.6 An interdisciplinary team that includes members of the perioperative and sterile processing teams should determine a standardized communication strategy and actions to perform when an insulation failure is found during processing. [Recommendation]

3.6.1 Include the following:
- the communication pathway between sterile processing and surgical personnel,
- physician notification,
- device handling, and
- documentation according to facility policy and procedure.

[Recommendation]

3.7 The electrosurgical generator foot pedal activation switch should be activated exclusively by the person in control of the active electrode.[60,69] [Recommendation]

Activation of the active electrode exclusively by the operator helps prevent unintentional activation of the device, minimizing the potential for patient and personnel injury.[60,69]

Clinical guidelines support activation of the active electrode exclusively by the operator.[51,59]

3.8 Place a fluid-resistant cover over the foot pedal when there is potential for fluid spills. [Recommendation]

Covering the foot pedal with a fluid-resistant cover helps keep the foot pedal dry, therefore decreasing the potential for an electrical shock or a mechanical malfunction.

Clinical guidelines support use of a fluid-resistant cover on the foot pedal.[59,86]

3.9 When using an active electrode,
- connect the cord directly into a designated receptacle on the electrosurgical generator[59,106];
- place the electrode in a clean, dry, nonconductive safety holster when it is not in use[1,29,59,60,63,64,69,91]; and
- use only adaptors approved by the manufacturers of the ESU and the accessory.

[Recommendation]

A clinical guideline supports performing the listed interventions.[86]

Use of a nonconductive safety holster helps prevent the active electrode from falling off the sterile field and from unintentional activation.[1,29,59,63,91]

3.10 Do not activate the active electrode until it is in close proximity to the surface if fulgurating, or in contact with the target tissue if cutting or coagulating.[1,8,40,47,48,107] [Recommendation]

Activation of the active electrode only when it is in close proximity to or in contact with the target tissue helps prevent alternate site burns.[1,8,40,48,107]

Makedonov and Lee[47] used a computer-generated model to determine the potential for an alternate site burn. They found that an alternate site burn would occur under following conditions:
- 20 seconds of continuous ESU activation,
- activation of the ESU without contact between the active electrode and the patient,
- a small alternate return site contact area of 1 cm^2, and
- the use of a high-power (ie, 200-W) cut mode.

The researchers concluded that to prevent alternate site burns, the active electrode should not be activated prior to contact with the patient.

A clinical guideline supports not activating the active electrode except when it is in close proximity to the target tissue.[59]

3.11 When using an active electrode tip,
- use the tip according to the manufacturer's IFU;

- firmly seat the tip into the hand piece with no gaps between the tip insulation and the hand piece[107];
- clean the tip
  - whenever there is visible **eschar** present,
  - away from the incision,
  - with a sponge moistened with sterile water or with an instrument wipe for nonstick-coated electrosurgical tips, and
  - with an abrasive electrode cleaning pad for noncoated electrodes[29,52,69,106]; and
- do not alter (eg, bend) the tip unless this is permitted by the manufacturer's IFU. *[Recommendation]*

Cleaning the tip decreases the amount of resistance; therefore the active electrode requires less power.[29,52]

3.11.1 **An anti-stick phospholipid solution may be used to decrease eschar buildup.**[108,109] *[Conditional Recommendation]* **P**

High-quality evidence[108,109] supports use of an anti-stick phospholipid solution to reduce surgical time.

In a randomized controlled trial, Baker and Ramadan[108] measured the differences in the number of hand backs (ie, the number of times the electrode tip needed to be handed back to the scrub person for cleaning) and the length of surgery between pediatric adenoidectomy procedures in which an anti-stick phospholipid solution was (n = 31) or was not (n = 30) applied to the electrosurgery suction tip. The researchers found a 1-minute 45-second decrease in the length of the procedure and a mean decrease of three hand backs per procedure with use of the anti-stick solution. Roy et al[109] found similar results in a randomized controlled trial of 50 patients undergoing rhytidectomy with use of a bipolar electrosurgical electrode.

3.12 **Assess the patient's skin before surgery in the vicinity of the potential dispersive electrode application site and after surgery at the point of contact with the dispersive electrode.** *[Recommendation]*

Preoperative and postoperative assessments are necessary to evaluate the patient's skin for injuries at the dispersive electrode site.

A clinical guideline supports performing a skin assessment.[59]

3.13 **Use a single-use dispersive electrode according to the manufacturer's IFU.**[49] *[Recommendation]*

3.13.1 **Select the single-use dispersive electrode size based on the patient's weight, as described in** the manufacturer's IFU (eg, neonate, infant, pediatric, adult).[20,25,39,44,69] *[Recommendation]* **P**

3.13.2 **Confirm that the manufacturer's beyond-use date has not expired before opening the single-use dispersive electrode, and do not use it if the beyond-use date has passed.** *[Recommendation]*

3.13.3 **Open single-use dispersive electrode packaging immediately before the electrode is needed.**[49] *[Recommendation]*

Opening the single-use dispersive electrode immediately before use helps decrease the potential for drying of the dispersive electrode's adhesive and conductive gel.[49]

A clinical guideline recommends not opening the package until the electrode is needed.[51]

3.13.4 **Check the single-use dispersive electrode for flaws, damage, discoloration, lack of adhesiveness, and dryness before application, and do not use the electrode if any of these conditions are present.**[49] *[Recommendation]*

Using a single-use dispersive electrode that has any of these problems increases the potential for patient injury, especially at the dispersive electrode site.[49]

A clinical guideline supports checking the dispersive electrode for the issues listed.[86]

3.14 **When placing a single-use dispersive electrode on the patient,**
- place the electrode
  - after final patient positioning[69];
  - close to the surgical site[25,38,49,69,110,111];
  - on clean, dry skin[20,69];
  - over a large, well-perfused muscle mass[25,38,44,49,69,110];
  - on the surgical side when indicated (eg, left or right shoulder, hip, kidney)[25,49,110];
  - to avoid any metal or monitoring leads between the dispersive and active electrodes[49,110,111];
  - away from a warming device[111]; and
  - so that it is in uniform contact with the patient's skin[2,20,40,44,49,112];
- do not place the electrode
  - over a bony prominence or potential pressure point[20,25,38,44,49,69,110];
  - over scar tissue[20,25,38,40,44,49,69];
  - over an implant containing metal components[25,38,44,49,69];
  - over skin folds[38];
  - on areas with dense hair[20,38,49,69];

- on areas where pooling of prep solutions may occur[20,44,46];
- where the cord could cause a pressure injury; or
- on areas distal to tourniquets[69];
- do not reposition or reapply the electrode[49]; and
- do not alter (eg, cut, fold) the electrode.

[Recommendation]

Clinical guidelines support implementing the criteria listed.[51,59,86]

A lack of good contact between the skin and the dispersive electrode can result in patient injuries.[10] Skin burns have been reported at the dispersive electrode site.[2,39,47,48,88,89,112,113]

Nguyen et al[53] conducted a bench study to examine the effect of monopolar radio-frequency energy on the temperature of bovine myocardial tissue surrounding implanted metal objects. The researchers found the temperature was elevated in the tissue surrounding the objects by a mean of 5.8° C to 8.9° C (10.4° F to 16° F) when the objects were between the active and dispersive electrodes and at a distance of 1 mm from the site of the active electrode. The researchers concluded that the dispersive electrode should be placed in a location with no metal objects between it and the active electrode.

3.15 Check the single-use dispersive electrode for uniform contact if the patient has been moved or repositioned or if any tension has been applied to the dispersive electrode cord.[49,88,112] *[Recommendation]*

Injuries have been reported that resulted from inadequate adhesion of the dispersive electrode.[49,88,112]

3.15.1 Perform corrective measures if inadequate contact between the single-use dispersive electrode and the patient occurs, including
- removing oil, lotion, moisture, or prep solution[86,88];
- removing excessive hair[86,88]; and
- applying a new single-use dispersive electrode to the same or a different site.[49,86]

[Recommendation]

Performing these interventions assists with obtaining adequate adhesion of the dispersive electrode.[49,88,112]

3.16 When using a dual-foil, single-use dispersive electrode, use a generator with <u>return-electrode contact quality monitoring</u>.[2,25,29,48,49,114] *[Recommendation]*

Return-electrode contact quality monitoring confirms that there is adequate contact between the return electrode and the patient and inhibits the output of the ESU if the dispersive electrode contact area is too small. An audible alarm or visual indicator alerts the user to a misconnection.[2,25,48,49,114]

A clinical guideline supports using a dual single-use dispersive electrode with a generator that has return-electrode contact quality monitoring.[86]

3.17 When using a reusable dispersive electrode cable,
- securely connect the cable to the electrode,
- cover the gel-free connecting lugs or tabs with the attachment clip, and
- inspect the cable for wear and replace it when worn.[49,86]

[Recommendation]

Connecting the cable to the electrode in this fashion helps prevent a patient burn related to the electrical current traveling from the exposed lugs or tabs to the patient.[49]

3.18 When using and storing a reusable dispersive electrode, follow the manufacturer's IFU.[86] *[Recommendation]*

3.18.1 Select the size based on the patient's weight, as described in the manufacturer's IFU (eg, neonate, infant, pediatric, adult).[86] *[Recommendation]* **P**

3.18.2 Confirm the manufacturer's beyond-use date has not passed prior to application, and do not use the electrode if the beyond-use date has passed.[86] *[Recommendation]*

3.18.3 Use the reusable dispersive electrode with minimal or no material between the electrode and the patient. *[Recommendation]*

3.18.4 Check the reusable dispersive electrode for tears or breaks in the surface material before and after use, and do not use the electrode if damage is present.[46,86] *[Recommendation]*

3.18.5 Clean and disinfect the reusable dispersive electrode with a health care facility–approved and Environmental Protection Agency–registered agent between uses in accordance with the manufacturer's IFU. *[Recommendation]*

3.18.6 Inspect the reusable, dispersive electrode cables for integrity before use, and replace the cables if damaged.[46] *[Recommendation]*

3.19 When high current (eg, ablation) is used for a prolonged period and there are no specific manufacturer's instructions, either a second single-use dispersive electrode or a reusable dispersive electrode may be used.[112,113] *[Conditional Recommendation]*

Using a second single-use dispersive electrode site helps increase the dispersive area, therefore decreasing the potential for a burn when high-current, long-activation-time procedures are performed.[112,113] Reusable dispersive electrodes cover a large dispersive area.

4. Minimally Invasive Surgery

4.1 Use conductive trocar systems when using electrosurgery during minimally invasive surgery.[1,20,24,46,48,99] *[Recommendation]*

Conductive trocar cannulas provide a means for the electrosurgical current to flow safely between the cannula and the abdominal wall. This reduces high-density current concentration and heating of non-target tissue, therefore decreasing the potential for injury related to capacitive coupling.[1,24,46,99]

Clinical guidelines support the use of conductive trocar systems.[59,86]

4.2 Prevent contact between the monopolar active electrode and other conductive instruments or materials.[1,29,40,69,115] *[Recommendation]*

Preventing contact between the monopolar active electrode and other conductive instruments or materials helps decrease the potential for a burn related to direct coupling.[1,29,40,69,115]

A clinical guideline supports preventing contact.[86]

4.3 Use an **active electrode monitoring** and shielding device.[116-118] *[Recommendation]*

Moderate-quality evidence[116-118] and clinical guidelines[59,86] support using an active electrode monitoring and shielding device.

In a laboratory study, Martin et al[116] measured the amount of energy transferred via capacitive coupling to determine whether the use of active electrode monitoring equipment decreased the amount of energy that escapes from a laparoscopic active electrode with insulation defects during laparoscopic surgery. The researchers used porcine tissue as a substitute for human tissue. They found that the use of the active electrode monitoring equipment decreased the number of tissue burns and the amount of energy transferred via capacitive coupling.

Guzman et al[117] reviewed 192,794 patients' records and found that 694 patients had experienced an accidental puncture or laceration during laparoscopic abdominal procedures. The researchers recommended using an active electrode monitoring and shielding device to decrease the incidence of adverse events.

Mendez-Probst et al[118] conducted a descriptive laboratory study to identify the amount of current leakage in 37 robotic instruments with visually intact insulation. Stray currents were found from 100% of the instruments with a mean leakage of 4.1 W. The researchers recommended adoption of an active electrode monitoring technology program.

5. Implanted Electronic Devices

5.1 When use of electrosurgery is possible for a patient with an IED, the anesthesia professional and the perioperative RN should consult with the team managing the IED preoperatively to define interventions necessary for safe management of the device during the intraoperative and postoperative phases of care.[30,31,51] *[Recommendation]* **P**

Preoperatively consulting with the team managing the IED helps the perioperative team obtain directions for caring for the patient.[25,30,31,37,38,44,51,111,119-132] Team members that the anesthesia professional and the perioperative RN may contact are listed below for specific devices:

- Pacemaker—cardiologist, electrophysiology team, health care industry representative
- Cochlear implant—implanting surgeon, health care industry representative
- Neurostimulator device—implanting surgeon, neurologist, health care industry representative
- Implanted infusion pump—implanting surgeon, physician responsible for managing care, health care industry representative

5.2 In an emergent situation when the team managing the IED cannot be contacted, the anesthesia professional and the preoperative RN or the RN circulator should consult with the implant manufacturer to determine interventions to perform for safe use of electrosurgery.[31,37,133] *[Recommendation]*

Many IED manufacturers have a 24-hour hotline available to assist in caring for a patient with an IED.[37] Clinical guidelines support contacting the manufacturer.[31,59,133]

5.2.1 Provide the following information to the team managing the device or the IED manufacturer's representative:

- the patient's level of dependence on the IED;
- the availability of a person competent to perform reprogramming if applicable;

- the scheduled procedure, including the site;
- whether cardioversion or defibrillation is anticipated;
- the intraoperative patient position;
- the potential for EMI based on the type of electrosurgical device to be used (eg, radio-frequency ablation, monopolar, bipolar);
- other potential sources of EMI (eg, shivering, nerve stimulators, large tidal volumes, extracorporeal shockwave lithotripsy);
- the location of the generator;
- the procedure room location (eg, OR, interventional radiology); and
- the postprocedure patient disposition (eg, outpatient, inpatient).[30,122,124]

[Recommendation]

Clinical guidelines support providing this information.[30,31,133,134] Obtaining this information will help the team managing the patient with an IED to determine the interventions to be performed during the perioperative period.[30,122,124]

The surgical site may determine the actions required. For example, if the site is 15 cm away from the generator and the dispersive electrode is placed so the generator is not in the pathway between the active and dispersive electrode, then no interventions beyond monitoring may be required.[134]

5.2.2 A chest x-ray may be performed if identification of a cardiac implanted electronic device (CIED) is not possible.[120,128] *[Conditional Recommendation]*

Performing a chest x-ray helps confirm the device lead placement and identify the device. The device identification is visible on a chest x-ray.[120,128]

5.3 Create an interdisciplinary team to develop and implement a clinical support tool that contains interventions to perform for a patient with an IED, for use when the team managing the IED or the manufacturer cannot be contacted. *[Recommendation]*

A clinical support tool can provide instructions for caring for the patient with an IED in an emergency situation or when the necessary people are not available to provide direction.

5.3.1 Include the following personnel on an interdisciplinary team responsible for developing the clinical support tool:
- perioperative RNs,
- scrub personnel,

- anesthesia professionals,
- surgeons who implant and manage IEDs,
- representatives from IED manufacturers, and
- other stakeholders.

[Recommendation]

Having a diverse team helps cover all aspects of patient care.

5.3.2 The IED clinical support tool should contain interventions specific to each IED (eg, reprogramming, removal of external parts, use of alternatives to monopolar electrosurgery, when to inactivate the device). *[Recommendation]*

5.3.3 Determine the applicable intervention based on the following IED information:
- type of implanted device;
- patient's level of dependence and severity of symptoms if the device is turned off;
- location of the device and leads (eg, within or outside the path between the active and dispersive electrodes);
- device manufacturer and model;
- clinical indication for the device;
- date of the last device interrogation or evaluation;
- battery life;
- device function; and
- device settings.

Obtain the following additional information when the patient has a CIED:
- lead polarity (eg, unipolar or bipolar),
- need for programming,
- response to a magnet,
- presence of an alert status on the generator or on the lead, and
- the last pacing threshold.[30,122,124]

[Recommendation]

Clinical guidelines support using the listed information when determining interventions to be performed for the patient with a CIED.[30,31,133] Gathering the listed information helps the team determine the necessary interventions to perform on the patient with an IED.[37,49,119-125,127,129,130,135,136] The information may be available from the patient assessment, the patient's caregivers, the implant identification (ID) card carried by the patient, and the medical record.

5.4 Perform the following interventions when a patient has an IED:
- inactivate or reprogram the IED if it is safe to do so[25,31,124,131,132,136,137];
- place the dispersive electrode as close as possible to the surgical site, but as far as possible

from the device's generator and leads[49,124,125,131,132,136,137];

- place the active electrode cord away from the pulse generator[25,131];
- verify that the implanted device and leads are not between the active electrode and the dispersive electrode[49,124,125,131];
- activate the ESU for the shortest amount of time possible[25,49,124,131,132,136];
- use the lowest effective power settings[124,131]; and
- use alternative technology (eg, electrocautery, bipolar forceps, ultrasonic technology, a **ferromagnetic surgical system**) instead of monopolar electrosurgery when possible.[25,49,124,125,132,136,137]

[Recommendation] **P**

Low-quality evidence[25,49,124,125,131,132,136-140] and clinical guidelines[30,31,59,134] support performing the listed interventions to decrease the risk of adverse events in patients with IEDs.

Bipolar electrosurgery does not produce EMI unless the forceps come into direct contact with the CIED.[86] Short activation bursts and a low power setting are beneficial because the amount of EMI produced is directly proportional to the amount of time of activation and the power setting.[132] The greater the distance between the generator and the active and dispersive electrode, the smaller the amount of EMI.[132]

In a nonexperimental study, Friedman et al[141] reviewed the records of 103 patients who had surgery after cardioverter defibrillator implantation. The researchers found no EMI with the use of bipolar technology but 11 cases of EMI with the use of monopolar technology. The researchers also found no cases of EMI when the surgical site and the dispersive electrode site were both below the hips. The researchers concluded that EMI does not occur when bipolar technology is used or when the surgical site and the dispersive electrode site are below the hip joint.

In a cadaveric study, Jeyakumar et al[142] assessed whether changes to an implanted cochlear device occurred during the use of monopolar electrosurgery and if there were changes in the intracochlear temperature. The researchers found no changes in the device, and the temperature of the cochlear device did not increase after 30 minutes of electrosurgical energy delivered at 30 W into the oral cavity. The researchers concluded that no damage or temperature increase occurred, but further study is required before changing existing practice.

5.5 **Perform the following interventions when a patient presents with a CIED:**

- place a magnet over the pacemaker to reprogram the device when indicated,[2,25,36-38,49,119,121,122,124,126,128,129,135,140,143,144]
- use an electrocardiogram system that has five or more leads,[30,37,127,140]
- use a beat-to-beat indicator (eg, arterial line, pulse oximeter),[2,37,120-122,126,129,143]
- have temporary pacing equipment and an external defibrillator immediately available,[25,31,36,37,49,121]
- have a magnet immediately available if the pacemaker will respond to a magnet and one is not used for reprogramming[2,124,140], and
- use continuous cardiac monitoring whenever the CIED has been reprogrammed.[2,25,35,44,49,69,120,122,123,126,128,129,135,144]

[Recommendation]

Low-quality evidence[2,25,33,35-38,44,49,52,69,120-125,127-130,136,140,141,144,145] and clinical guidelines[30,31,51,133,134] support performing the listed precautions to decrease the risk of adverse events in a patient with a CIED.

Use of a magnet is not always indicated because the response of a pacemaker is based on the model, age, and manufacturer of the device. In addition, use of a magnet on a pacemaker with a low battery may lead to device failure because the power of the battery may become rapidly exhausted.[25,37,49,119,121,126,135] Use of a magnet on a pacemaker will switch it to an asynchronous mode and inactivate the rate response feature. Use of a magnet on an implantable cardioverter defibrillator inactivates the anti-tachycardia features and does not alter the pacing mode.[134]

Pacemakers may incorrectly interpret the electrical signals from an electrosurgical device, leading to a misfiring or failure to fire that can result in arrhythmia, such as ventricular fibrillation or ventricular tachycardia.[49]

The tolerance for EMI is different for different types of pacemakers (unipolar, bipolar) and different makes and models of pacemakers.[37]

Use of a five-lead electrocardiogram configuration provides multiple leads to view in case one lead is obscured or difficult to interpret because of EMI.[37]

Electromagnetic interference is unlikely with a CIED generator implanted in the thoracic area when the procedure is below the umbilicus and the return electrode is placed on the lower body (thigh or gluteal area).[31,140]

Using a beat-to-beat indicator provides a signal for the pulse in case the electrocardiogram is obscured or difficult to interpret because of EMI.[2,37]

Moderate-quality evidence shows that EMI affects pacemakers.[32,84,85,145]

Lin et al[32] found four patients (0.3% of 1,398 patient records reviewed) who developed output failure or an inappropriate low pacing rate during use of electrosurgery. The patients were undergoing pacemaker generator replacement or upgrade surgeries. The researchers also reviewed the MAUDE database for events or patient injuries related to pacemaker malfunction and found 37 cases of pacemaker malfunction related to the use of electrosurgery. The adverse events included the pacemaker resorting to the backup pacing mode (32.4%), loss of output/capture (59.5%), inappropriate low pacing rate (5.4%), and ventricular fibrillation (2.7%). The dates of review of the MAUDE database were not included in the report. The researchers concluded that certain pacemaker models may exhibit loss of pacing or inappropriate low pacing rate during the use of monopolar electrosurgery during pacemaker replacement or upgrade surgery.

Paniccia et al[145] measured the average maximum EMI that occurred during activations of various surgical energy-based devices on a cardiac device implanted in a pig. The researchers found the mean EMI transferred to the implanted cardiac device varied for each device:

- 0.1 mV for a traditional bipolar device at 30 W,
- 0.004 mV for an advanced bipolar device,
- 0.1 mV for ultrasonic shears,
- 0.5 mV for a monopolar device at 30 W coagulation,
- 0.92 mV for a monopolar device at 30 W blend,
- 0.21 mV for a monopolar device without a dispersive electrode,
- 3.48 mV for a plasma energy-generating device, and
- 2.58 mV for an argon beam coagulator.

The researchers concluded that bipolar and ultrasonic devices are useful for decreasing the EMI on implanted cardiac defibrillators.

Govekar et al[85] conducted a laboratory study to determine whether the location of the dispersive electrode affected the functionality of a pacemaker in the heart of a pig. The dispersive electrode was placed on the right gluteus, left gluteus, right shoulder, and left shoulder. The ESU was set at a power of 30 W in the coagulate mode. The active electrode was activated for 5 seconds at a distance of 7.5 cm from the pacemaker generator. The researchers found more beats were dropped (1.5 versus 0.2) when the current vector traveled from the active electrode to the dispersive electrode through the pacemaker or through the leads. The researchers concluded that the dispersive electrode should be located such that the current vector does not pass through the pacemaker or the leads.

In a laboratory study, Robinson et al[84] examined the effect of monopolar electrosurgery devices on CIEDs implanted in pigs. The researchers measured the amount of EMI present after they changed the orientation of the active electrode cord from across the chest wall to coming from the feet, which changed the current vector so it did not flow across the CIED. The researchers found significantly less EMI when the orientation of the active electrode was from the feet and the current vector avoided the CIED. They concluded that the active electrode cord should be placed at the greatest distance possible from the CIED generator, and the CIED generator should not be in the pathway of the current from the active electrode to the dispersive electrode.

5.6 **Take the following precautions for a patient with an existing cochlear implant:**

- **remove all external components,**
- **do not use electrosurgical devices including bipolar devices within 2 cm to 3 cm of the implant generator electrodes,**[25,123,146,147]
- **use only bipolar electrosurgery above the clavicles,**[147] **and**
- **monopolar electrosurgery may be used below the clavicles if the dispersive electrode is also below the clavicles.**[147]

[Recommendation] **P**

Keeping the recommended distance from the device and removing external parts reduces the risk of accidental activation or damage to the device.[25,123,146,147]

5.7 **Decrease the amplitude to the lowest level and then inactivate deep brain stimulators, sacral nerve stimulators, spinal cord stimulators, vagal nerve stimulators, or gastric pacemakers, if this is advised by the manufacturer and can be tolerated by the patient.**[124,125,137] *[Recommendation]*

Low-quality evidence[124,125,137] and a clinical guideline[30] support inactivating the device to prevent inadvertent stimulation and decreasing the amplitude to decrease the amount of stimulation if the device is accidently turned on.

5.8 **Consult with the team managing the implant to determine postoperative interventions as soon as possible after surgery.**[30] *[Recommendation]*

Consultation allows the team managing the implant to confirm functioning of the implant or to restart the implant if it has been inactivated.[37,121,124-126,128,132,135,139]

Clinical guidelines support postoperative contact with the team managing the implant.[30,31]

5.9 **Provide education and postoperative instructions to patients and their caregivers on the effects of electrosurgery on IEDs.**[148] *[Recommendation]* **P**

Frampton and Mitchell[148] conducted a survey of 50 adults with cochlear implants and the parents of 50 children with cochlear implants to determine their knowledge of the risks for complications when a cochlear implant is present and electrosurgery is used during head and neck procedures. The researchers found that 86% of the adult patients possessed an implant ID card, and 71% carried it with them. Seventy-seven percent stated that if surgery were required, they would show their implant ID card and discuss the issue of electrosurgery with the physician.

Eighty-four percent of the parents reported that the child possessed an ID card; 8% of parents ensured the child carried the card at all times, and 12% reported that they carried the card for the child. Seventy-six percent of the parents believed that surgeons would be unaware of the electrosurgical restrictions, but none of the 12% of parents whose children had undergone surgery had brought the issue to the surgeon's attention. The researchers concluded that cochlear implant recipients should receive education about the risks of complications that could occur when electrosurgery is used for patients with cochlear implants.[148]

6. Argon-Enhanced Coagulation

6.1 **Follow all safety precautions for monopolar electrosurgery during use of AEC technology in addition to safety precautions described in the AEC manufacturer's IFU.**[38,49,149] *[Recommendation]*

The use of monopolar electrosurgery precautions is recommended for AEC because AEC is monopolar electrosurgery delivered while surrounded by argon gas.[38,49,149]

A clinical guideline supports following monopolar electrosurgery precautions when using AEC.[59]

6.1.1 **Use the lowest possible gas flow rate to achieve the desired tissue effect.**[4,150] *[Recommendation]*

Lower gas flow rates help prevent gas emboli.[4,150]

A clinical guideline supports use of the lowest flow rate possible.[59]

6.2 **Provide education and verify competency of personnel on recognition of the signs and symptoms of gas emboli and treatment measures.**[4,151-153] *[Recommendation]*

There have been reports of gas embolism when AEC is used.[4,151-153]

7. Education

7.1 **Provide education and verify competency regarding precautions to be taken during use of**

an ESU, as applicable to the person's job responsibilities.[48,69,117,146,154,155] *[Recommendation]* **P**

Providing education to personnel on all aspects of electrosurgery gives them information needed to avoid hazards associated with electrosurgery.[48,69]

Feldman et al[155] conducted a pretest-posttest study of 48 surgeons and 27 residents to determine the participants' knowledge of use of electrosurgical devices. On the pretest, the median percent of correct answers was 59% in the surgeon group and 55% in the resident group. After the groups received the education, a median of 90% correct was achieved on the posttest. The researchers concluded that there was a knowledge gap and education was required.

Frampton et al[146] surveyed 35 head and neck surgeons to assess the surgeons' knowledge of safety considerations when using electrosurgery in the presence of a cochlear implant. Seventy-seven percent of the respondents did not know about the published guidelines covering the use of electrosurgery in the patient with a cochlear implant, and 11% thought it was safe to use monopolar electrosurgery for this group of patients. The researchers concluded that surgeons need education on the safety guidelines regarding the use of electrosurgery when the patient has a cochlear implant.

Ahrens et al[154] conducted a survey of 17 shoulder surgeons and eight residents in the United Kingdom to determine the physicians' knowledge of possible locations for pacemaker lead placement and knowledge of the type of electrosurgery to use in the presence of a pacemaker lead. The researchers found that 65% of the surgeons and 70% of the residents knew that the cephalic vein may be used for the route of the pacemaker electrode. When asked what type of electrosurgery to use on the cephalic vein in the presence of a pacemaker, four surgeons reported they would use monopolar electrosurgery, 12 surgeons and six residents reported they would use bipolar electrosurgery, and one surgeon and two residents reported they would not use electrosurgery in the presence of a pacemaker. The researchers concluded that surgeons and residents need education on the proper use of electrosurgery and techniques used in other medical specialities (eg, the path the cardiologist uses to run the pacemaker leads).

Guzman et al[117] reviewed 192,794 records of patients who underwent laparoscopic abdominal procedures and found 694 patients had experienced an accidental puncture or laceration. They recommended physician education to decrease adverse events.

No study of other perioperative team member education was found in the literature search; therefore, further research is needed.

7.1.1 Include the following in education and competency verification:
- principles of electrosurgery;
- risks to patients and personnel;
- measures to minimize the risks from increased thermal spread, insulation failure, antenna coupling, direct coupling, capacitive coupling, residual heat, or inadvertent activation;
- precautions that must be taken when caring for patients with IEDs;
- steps for operation, care, and handling of the generator and accessories before, during, and after use that are in alignment with the manufacturers' IFU;
- the potential for electrosurgical-induced artefactual changes in patient monitoring devices (eg, cardiac, electroencephalogram, capnography, bispectral index);
- documentation in the patient's record;
- reporting methods if an adverse event occurs;
- equipment manufacturers' IFU and warnings; and
- instrumentation preparation, inspection, and sterilization processes.

[Recommendation]

Low-quality evidence[1,24,46,50,156-158] and a clinical guideline[86] support including the listed subjects in education.

Glossary

Ablation: A form of treatment that uses electrical energy, heat, cold, alcohol, or other modalities to destroy a small section of damaged tissue.

Active electrode monitoring: A dynamic process of searching for insulation failures and capacitive coupling during monopolar surgery. If the monitor detects an unsafe level of stray energy, it signals the generator to deactivate.

Advanced bipolar device: A bipolar electrosurgery unit that uses a computer-controlled tissue feedback response system to sense tissue impedance, allowing for the continuous adjustment of the voltage and current generated by the unit. This allows the lowest possible power setting to achieve the desired tissue effect.

Alternate site injuries: Injuries caused by an electrosurgical device that occur away from the dispersive electrode site.

Antenna coupling: Radio-frequency energy emitted by a monopolar active electrode and transferred without direct contact through conductive materials (eg, neuromuscular, cardiac monitoring electrode wires).

Argon-enhanced coagulation: Radio-frequency coagulation from an electrosurgical generator that is capable of delivering monopolar current through a flow of ionized argon gas.

Bipolar electrosurgery: Electrosurgery in which current flows between two tips of a bipolar forceps that are positioned around tissue to create a surgical effect. Current passes from the active electrode of one tip of the forceps through the patient's tissue to the other dispersive electrode tip of the forceps, thus completing the circuit without entering another part of the patient's body.

Capacitive coupling: Transfer of electrical current from the active electrode through intact insulation to adjacent conductive items (eg, tissue, trocars).

Current: A movement of electrons analogous to the flow of a stream of water.

Current pathway: The route taken by the current when traveling from the active to the dispersive electrode. Generally, it is the shortest route and a straight line.

Direct application: Intentional application to the surgical site.

Direct coupling: The contact of an energized active electrode tip with another metal instrument or object within the surgical field.

Dispersive electrode: The accessory that directs electrical current flow from the patient back to the electrosurgical generator. Often called the patient plate, return electrode, inactive electrode, or grounding pad. Synonym: passive electrode.

Duty cycle: The duration of electrosurgical generator activation.

Electrocautery: A surgical device, often battery powered, that is used to cauterize blood vessels. No electrodes are used. The current flows through the wire at the end of the application device and not through the patient. Cauterization is produced by heat.

Electromagnetic interference: The disruption of operation of an electronic device (eg, pacemaker, cochlear implant) when it is in the vicinity of an electromagnetic field in the radio-frequency spectrum that is caused by another electronic device (eg, electrosurgery unit).

Electrosurgery: The cutting and coagulation of body tissue with a high-frequency (ie, radio-frequency) current. The current is passed through the body or the tissue and between two poles. Heat is generated in the tissue through which the current passes.

Electrosurgical accessories: The active electrode with tip(s), dispersive electrode, adapters, and connectors to attach these devices to the electrosurgery generator.

Eschar: Charred tissue residue.

Ferromagnetic surgical system: An electrocautery device in which the electricity travels through a closed loop and produces heat by excitation of the ferromagnetic coating on the loop.

Inadvertent activation: An unintentional activation of the active electrode.

Insulation failure: Damage to the insulation of the active electrode that provides an alternate pathway for the current to leave that electrode as it completes the circuit to the dispersive electrode.

Microdermal implant: A form of body modification that has the appearance of a transdermal implant and is composed of two components: an anchor, which is implanted beneath the skin, and a piece protruding from (or flush with) the surface of the surrounding skin that is used to secure exchangeable jewelry. A microdermal implant is usually foot shaped and is inserted with a needle or a punch.

Monopolar electrosurgery: Electrosurgery in which only the active electrode is in the surgical wound, and the electrical current is directed through the patient's body, received by the dispersive electrode, and transferred back to the generator, completing the monopolar circuit.

Radio frequency: Radio waves used to conduct therapeutic procedures. The specific frequency, dosage, and intensity used vary depending on the desired effects which include heating, electrical stimulation, or ablation of tissues.

Residual heat: The heat that remains in the tip of the electrosurgical or electrocautery device after inactivation and before it has had a chance to cool.

Return-electrode contact quality monitoring: A dynamic monitoring circuit measuring impedance of the dispersive return electrode. If the dispersive electrode becomes compromised, the circuit inhibits the electrosurgical unit's output.

Subdermal implant: A body modification that is placed under the skin, creating a raised design.

Thermal spread: The distance that the heat travels from the activated electrosurgical device tip. Thermal spread is determined by the temperature of the active electrode tip, the amount of time the device is activated, the thermal mass of the device, and the thermal conductivity of the tissue.

Transdermal implant: a form of body modification consisting of an object (ie, anchor) placed partially below and partially above the skin. The jewelry attached to the anchor may be interchangeable. The implanted portion of the transdermal implant is flat and circular and is inserted with a dermal punch.

Tripolar device: An electrosurgical device with a tripolar tip consisting of a central pole and an outer pole on either side. The current flows from the center pole to the outer poles, creating a corona of energy that makes a blade-like incision. The current alternates with a second current that passes from one of the outer poles to the other, resulting in simultaneous cutting and coagulating.

References

1. Jones DB, Brunt LM, Feldman LS, Mikami DJ, Robinson TN, Jones SB. Safe energy use in the operating room. *Curr Probl Surg.* 2015;52(11):447-468. [VA]

2. Suchanek S, Grega T, Zavoral M. The role of equipment in endoscopic complications. *Best Pract Res Clin Gastroenterol.* 2016;30(5):667-678. [VB]

3. Law KS, Abbott JA, Lyons SD. Energy sources for gynecologic laparoscopic surgery: a review of the literature. *Obstet Gynecol Surv.* 2014;69(12):763-776. [VA]

4. Sankaranarayanan G, Resapu RR, Jones DB, Schwaitzberg S, De S. Common uses and cited complications of energy in surgery. *Surg Endosc.* 2013;27(9):3056-3072. [VA]

5. Hannah J. Probable postpolypectomy thermal burn: a case study. *Gastroenterol Nurs.* 2018;41(3):244-247. [VC]

6. Humes DJ, Ahmed I, Lobo DN. The pedicle effect and direct coupling: delayed thermal injuries to the bile duct after laparoscopic cholecystectomy. *Arch Surg.* 2010;145(1):96-98. [VC]

7. Sapienza P, Venturini L, Cigna E, Sterpetti AV, Biacchi D, di Marzo L. Deep gluteal grounding pad burn after abdominal aortic aneurysm repair. *Ann Ital Chir.* 2015;86(ePub). [VB]

8. Cormier B, Nezhat F, Sternchos J, Sonoda Y, Leitao MM Jr. Electrocautery-associated vascular injury during robotic-assisted surgery. *Obstet Gynecol.* 2012;120(2 Pt 2):491-493. [VB]

9. Cassaro S. Delayed manifestations of laparoscopic bowel injury. *Am Surg.* 2015;81(5):478-482. [VA]

10. Saaiq M, Zaib S, Ahmad S. Electrocautery burns: experience with three cases and review of literature. *Ann Burns Fire Disasters.* 2012;25(4):203-206. [VB]

11. Huffman SD, Huffman NP, Lewandowski RJ, Brown DB. Radiofrequency ablation complicated by skin burn. *Semin Intervent Radiol.* 2011;28(2):179-182. [VC]

12. Bansal A, Bhama JK, Varga JM, Toyoda Y. Airway fire during double-lung transplantation. *Interact Cardiovasc Thorac Surg.* 2013;17(6):1059-1060. [VC]

13. Hudson DW, Guidry OF, Abernathy JH 3rd, Ehrenwerth J. Case 4–2012. Intrathoracic fire during coronary artery bypass graft surgery. *J Cardiothorac Vasc Anesth.* 2012;26(3):520-521. [VC]

14. Herman MA, Laudanski K, Berger J. Surgical fire during organ procurement. *Internet J Anesthesiol.* 2009;19(1). [VC]

15. Kim MS, Lee JH, Lee DH, Lee YU, Jung TE. Electrocautery-ignited surgical field fire caused by a high oxygen level during tracheostomy. *Korean J Thorac Cardiovasc Surg.* 2014;47(5):491-493. [VC]

16. Overbey DM, Townsend NT, Chapman BC, et al. Surgical energy-based device injuries and fatalities reported to the Food and Drug Administration. *J Am Coll Surg.* 2015;221(1):197-205. [VA]

17. Mehta SP, Bhananker SM, Posner KL, Domino KB. Operating room fires: a closed claims analysis. *Anesthesiology.* 2013;118(5):1133-1139. [VB]

18. Chung SH, Lee HH, Kim TH, Kim JS. A patient who was burned in the operative field: a case report. *Ulus Travma Acil Cerrahi Derg.* 2012;18(3):274-276. [VC]

19. Haith LR Jr, Santavasi W, Shapiro TK, et al. Burn center management of operating room fire injuries. *J Burn Care Res.* 2012;33(5):649-653. [VC]

20. Alkatout I, Schollmeyer T, Hawaldar NA, Sharma N, Mettler L. Principles and safety measures of electrosurgery in laparoscopy. *JSLS.* 2012;16(1):130-139. [VC]

21. Moskowitz M. Fire in the operating room during open heart surgery: a case report. *AANA J.* 2009;77(4):261-264. [VA]

22. Chae SB, Kim WK, Yoo CJ, Park CW. Fires and burns occurring in an electrocautery after skin preparation with alcohol during a neurosurgery. *J Korean Neurosurg Soc.* 2014;55(4):230-233. [VC]

23. Lee JY, Park CB, Cho EJ, et al. Airway fire injury during rigid bronchoscopy in a patient with a silicon stent—a case report. *Korean J Anesth.* 2012;62(2):184-187. [VC]

24. Liu Q, Sun XB. Indirect electrical injuries from capacitive coupling: a rarely mentioned electrosurgical complication in monopolar laparoscopy. *Acta Obstet Gynecol Scand.* 2013;92(2):238-241. [VC]

25. Messenger D, Carter F, Francis N. Electrosurgery and energized dissection. *Surgery (Oxford).* 2014;32(3):126-130. [VB]

26. Mumith A, Thuraisingham J, Gurunathan-Mani S. Ignition of free gas in the peritoneal cavity: an explosive complication. *Case Rep Surg.* 2013;2013:746430. [VC]

27. Abu-Rafea B, Vilos GA, Al-Obeed O, AlSheikh A, Vilos AG, Al-Mandeel H. Monopolar electrosurgery through single-port laparoscopy: a potential hidden hazard for bowel burns. *J Minim Invasive Gynecol.* 2011;18(6):734-740. [IIIB]

28. Gunaruwan P, Barlow M. Diathermy-induced ventricular fibrillation with Riata high-voltage lead insulation failure. *Europace.* 2013;15(4):473. [VC]

29. Recommendations to reduce surgical fires and related patient injury: FDA Safety Communication. US Food and Drug Administration. https://www.fda.gov/medical-devices/safety-communications/recommendations-reduce-surgical-fires-and-related-patient-injury-fda-safety-communication. Updated July 18, 2018. Accessed March 30, 2020. [VB]

30. Healey JS, Merchant R, Simpson C, et al. Society Position Statement: Canadian Cardiovascular Society/Canadian Anesthesiologists' Society/Canadian Heart Rhythm Society joint position statement on the perioperative management of patients with implanted pacemakers, defibrillators, and neurostimulating devices. *Can J Anesth.* 2012;59(4):394-407. [IVB]

31. Crossley GH, Poole JE, Rozner MA, et al. The Heart Rhythm Society (HRS)/American Society of Anesthesiologists (ASA) Expert Consensus Statement on the perioperative management of patients with implantable defibrillators, pacemakers and arrhythmia monitors: facilities and patient management. *Heart Rhythm.* 2011;8(7):1114-1154. [IVA]

32. Lin Y, Melby DP, Krishnan B, Adabag S, Tholakanahalli V, Li JM. Frequency of pacemaker malfunction associated with monopolar electrosurgery during pulse generator replacement or upgrade surgery. *J Interv Card Electrophysiol.* 2017;49(2):205-209. [IIIB]

33. Goel AK, Korotkin S, Walsh D, Bess M, Frawley S. Monomorphic ventricular tachycardia caused by electrocautery during pacemaker generator change in a patient with normal left ventricular function. *Pacing Clin Electrophysiol.* 2009;32(7):957-958. [VC]

34. Cassagneau R, Hanninen M, Yee R. Electrocautery-induced ventricular fibrillation during routine implantable cardioverter-defibrillator generator replacement. *Europace.* 2014;16(3):319. [VC]

35. Russo V, Rago A, Di Meo F, et al. Ventricular fibrillation induced by coagulating mode bipolar electrocautery during pacemaker implantation in Myotonic Dystrophy type 1 patient. *Acta Myol.* 2014;33(3):149-151. [VB]

36. Mohammed I, Ratib K, Creamer J. An unusual intracardiac electrogram showing cause for false electrical discharge from an ICD. *BMJ Case Rep.* 2013;2013. [VC]

37. Castillo JG, Silvay G, Viles-González J. Perioperative assessment of patients with cardiac implantable electronic devices. *Mt Sinai J Med.* 2012;79(1):25-33. [VB]

38. King C. Endoscopic electrosurgery—an overview. *Gastrointest Nurs.* 2011;9(4):28-33. [VB]

39. Fonseca AZ, Santin S, Gomes LG, Waisberg J, Ribeiro MA Jr. Complications of radiofrequency ablation of hepatic tumors: frequency and risk factors. *World J Hepatol.* 2014;6(3):107-113. [VB]

40. Munro MG. Complications of hysteroscopic and uterine resectoscopic surgery. *Obstet Gynecol Clin North Am.* 2010;37(3):399-425. [VB]

41. Guideline for a safe environment of care. In: *Guidelines for Perioperative Practice.* Denver, CO: AORN, Inc; 2020:115-150. [IVA]

42. Guideline for surgical smoke safety. In: *Guidelines for Perioperative Practice.* Denver, CO: AORN, Inc; 2020:1007-1038. [IVA]

43. Guideline for minimally invasive surgery. In: *Guidelines for Perioperative Practice.* Denver, CO: AORN, Inc; 2020:482-514. [IVA]

44. Bisinotto FMB, Dezena RA, Martins LB, Galvão MC, Sobrinho JM, Calçado MS. Burns related to electrosurgery—report of two cases. *Rev Bras Anestesiol.* 2017;67(5):527-534. [VC]

45. Townsend NT, Jones EL, Paniccia A, Vandervelde J, McHenry JR, Robinson TN. Antenna coupling explains unintended thermal injury caused by common operating room monitoring devices. *Surg Laparosc Endosc Percutan Tech.* 2015;25(2):111-113. [IIB]

46. Demirçin S, Aslan F, Karagöz YM, Atılgan M. Medicolegal aspects of surgical diathermy burns: a case report and review of the literature. *Rom J Leg Med.* 2013;21(3):173-176. [VB]

47. Makedonov I, Lee J. An evaluation of potential for alternate return site burns due to capacitive coupling between active electrode and ground while using electrosurgery units. *J Clin Eng.* 2011;36(1):29-31. [IIIC]

48. O'Riley M. Electrosurgery in perioperative practice. *J Periop Pract.* 2010;20(9):329-333. [VC]

49. Nelson G, Morris ML. Electrosurgery in the gastrointestinal suite: knowledge is power. *Gastroenterol Nurs.* 2015;38(6):430-439. [VA]

50. Vilos GA, Rajakumar C. Electrosurgical generators and monopolar and bipolar electrosurgery. *J Minim Invasive Gynecol.* 2013;20(3):279-287. [VA]

51. Rey JF, Beilenhoff U, Neumann CS, Dumonceau JM; European Society of Gastrointestinal Endoscopy (ESGE). European Society of Gastrointestinal Endoscopy (ESGE) guideline: the use of electrosurgical units. *Endoscopy.* 2010;42(9):764-772. [IVC]

52. Gould J. Overview of electrosurgery. UptoDate. https://www.uptodate.com/contents/overview-of-electrosurgery. Updated January 7, 2019. Accessed March 30, 2020. [VB]

53. Nguyen DT, Barham W, Zheng L, Dinegar S, Tzou WS, Sauer WH. Effect of radiofrequency energy delivery in proximity to metallic medical device components. *Heart Rhythm.* 2015;12(10):2162-2169. [IIIB]

54. Sheldon RR, Loughren MJ, Marenco CW, et al. Microdermal implants show no effect on surrounding tissue during surgery with electrocautery. *J Surg Res.* 2019;241:72-77. [IIB]

55. Roy S, Smith LP. Device-related risk of fire in oropharyngeal surgery: a mechanical model. *Am J Otolaryngol.* 2010;31(5):356-359. [IIIC]

56. Matt BH, Cottee LA. Reducing risk of fire in the operating room using coblation technology. *Otolaryngol Head Neck Surg.* 2010;143(3):454-455. [IIIC]

57. González CEM, Fernández VO. Case report: airway burn. *Colombian Journal of Anesthesiology.* 2013;41(3):226-228. [VB]

58. Roy S, Smith LP. Preventing and managing operating room fires in otolaryngology-head and neck surgery. *Otolaryngol Clin North Am.* 2019;52(1):163-171. [VA]

59. *AST Standards of Practice for Use of Electrosurgery.* Littleton, CO: Association of Surgical Technologists; 2012. [IVC]

60. Dennis E. Decreasing airway fires. *OR Nurse 2012.* 2012;6(2):37-40. [VB]

61. Partanen E, Koljonen V, Salonen A, Bäck LJ, Vuola J. A patient with intraoral fire during tonsillectomy. *J Craniofac Surg.* 2014;25(5):1822-1824. [VA]

62. Smędra A, Meissner E, Barzdo M, et al. Iatrogenic burns of the neckline in a patient with tetraparesis during tracheotomy. *J Forensic Sci.* 2017;62(1):250-253. [VC]

63. Vo A, Bengezi O. Third-degree burns caused by ignition of chlorhexidine: a case report and systematic review of the literature. *Plast Surg.* 2014;22(4):264-266. [VA]

64. Seifert PC, Peterson E, Graham K. Crisis management of fire in the OR. *AORN J.* 2015;101(2):250-263. [VA]

65. Khatiwada S, Bhattarai B, Acharya R, Chettri ST, Dhital D, Rahman TR. Surgical site fire: a case of evil spirit or lapsed communication? *Nepal Med Coll J.* 2011;13(2):140-141. [VA]

66. Apfelbaum JL, Caplan RA, Barker SJ, et al. Practice advisory for the prevention and management of operating room fires: an updated report by the American Society of Anesthesiologists Task Force on Operating Room Fires. *Anesthesiology.* 2013;118(2):271-290. [IVA]

67. Axelrod EH, Kusnetz AB, Rosenberg MK. Operating room fires initiated by hot wire cautery. *Anesthesiology.* 1993;79(5):1123-1126. [IIIB]

68. Fire caused by improper disposal of a battery-powered electrocautery pen. *Health Devices.* 2013;42(10):346. [VC]

69. Potty AG, Khan W, Tailor HD. Diathermy in perioperative practice. *J Perioper Pract.* 2010;20(11):402-405. [VB]

70. Medical Device Reporting (MDR): How to report medical device problems. US Food and Drug Administration. https://www.fda.gov/medical-devices/medical-device-safety/medical-device-reporting-mdr-how-report-medical-device-problems. Updated July 8, 2019. Accessed March 30, 2020.

71. Robinson TN, Pavlovsky KR, Looney H, Stiegmann GV, McGreevy FT. Surgeon-controlled factors that reduce monopolar electrosurgery capacitive coupling during laparoscopy. *Surg Laparosc Endosc Percutan Tech.* 2010;20(5):317-320. [IIA]

72. Robinson TN, Barnes KS, Govekar HR, Stiegmann GV, Dunn CL, McGreevy FT. Antenna coupling—a novel mechanism of radiofrequency electrosurgery complication: practical implications. *Ann Surg.* 2012;256(2):213-218. [IIB]

73. Mitchell ME, Kidd D, Lotto ML, et al. Determination of factors influencing tissue effect of thermal chondroplasty: an ex vivo investigation. *Arthroscopy.* 2006;22(4):351-355. [IIB]

74. Itoi T, Isayama H, Sofuni A, et al. Evaluation of effects of a novel endoscopically applied radiofrequency ablation biliary catheter using an ex-vivo pig liver. *J Hepatobiliary Pancreat Sci.* 2012;19(5):543-547. [IIB]

75. Goulet CJ, Disario JA, Emerson L, Hilden K, Holubkov R, Fang JC. In vivo evaluation of argon plasma coagulation in a porcine model. *Gastrointest Endosc.* 2007;65(3):457-462. [IIB]

76. Huang Y, Zhang Y, Ding X, Liu S, Sun T. Working conditions of bipolar radiofrequency on human articular cartilage repair following thermal injury during arthroscopy. *Chin Med J (Engl).* 2014;127(22):3881-3886. [IIB]

77. Sutton PA, Awad S, Perkins AC, Lobo DN. Comparison of lateral thermal spread using monopolar and bipolar diathermy, the Harmonic Scalpel and the Ligasure. *Br J Surg.* 2010;97(3):428-433. [IIB]

78. Martinek M, Bencsik G, Aichinger J, et al. Esophageal damage during radiofrequency ablation of atrial fibrillation: impact of energy settings, lesion sets, and esophageal visualization. *J Cardiovasc Electrophysiol.* 2009;20(7):726-733. [IIB]

79. Brzeziński J, Kałużna-Markowska K, Naze M, Stróżyk G, Dedecjus M. Comparison of lateral thermal spread using monopolar and bipolar diathermy, and the bipolar vessel sealing system ThermoStapler™ during thyroidectomy. *Pol Przegl Chir.* 2011;83(7):355-360. [IIIB]

80. Hefermehl LJ, Largo RA, Hermanns T, Poyet C, Sulser T, Eberli D. Lateral temperature spread of monopolar, bipolar and ultrasonic instruments for robot-assisted laparoscopic surgery. *BJU Int.* 2014;114(2):245-252. [IIIB]

81. Jones EL, Robinson TN, McHenry JR, et al. Radiofrequency energy antenna coupling to common laparoscopic instruments: practical implications. *Surg Endosc.* 2012;26(11):3053-3057. [IIIB]

82. Munro MG. Mechanisms of thermal injury to the lower genital tract with radiofrequency resectoscopic surgery. *J Minim Invasive Gynecol.* 2006;13(1):36-42. Erratum in: *J Minim Invasive Gynecol.* 2007;14(2):268. [IIIB]

83. Lowe D, Cromwell DA, Lewsey JD, et al. Diathermy power settings as a risk factor for hemorrhage after tonsillectomy. *Otolaryngol Head Neck Surg.* 2009;140(1):23-28. [IIIA]

84. Robinson TN, Varosy PD, Guillaume G, et al. Effect of radiofrequency energy emitted from monopolar "Bovie" instruments on cardiac implantable electronic devices. *J Am Coll Surg.* 2014;219(3):399-406. [IIIB]

85. Govekar HR, Robinson TN, Varosy PD, et al. Effect of monopolar radiofrequency energy on pacemaker function. *Surg Endosc.* 2012;26(10):2784-2788. [IIIC]

86. *CSA Z387-2019. Safe Use of Electrosurgical Medical Devices and Systems in Health Care.* Toronto, ON: CSA Group; 2019. [IVC]

87. Metzner A, Wissner E, Schoonderwoerd B, et al. The influence of varying energy settings on efficacy and safety of endoscopic pulmonary vein isolation. *Heart Rhythm.* 2012;9(9):1380-1385. [IIIB]

88. Sabzi F, Niazi M, Ahmadi A. Rare case-series of electrocautery burn following off-pump coronary artery bypass grafting. *J Inj Violence Res.* 2014;6(1):44-49. [VB]

89. Sanders SM, Krowka S, Giacobbe A, Bisson LJ. Third-degree burn from a grounding pad during arthroscopy. *Arthroscopy.* 2009;25(10):1193-1197. [VB]

90. Gil Franco F, Bailard N. Peripheral nerve stimulator response triggered by proximity to electrosurgical unit. *Anesth Analg.* 2012;114(5):1142-1143. [VC]

91. Guglielmi CL, Flowers J, Dagi TF, et al. Empowering providers to eliminate surgical fires. *AORN J.* 2014;100(4):412-428. [VB]

92. *State Operations Manual Appendix L: Guidance for Surveyors: Ambulatory Surgical Centers.* Rev. 200, 02-21-20. Centers for Medicare & Medicaid Services. https://www.cms.gov/media/423701. Accessed March 31, 2020.

93. *State Operations Manual Appendix A: Survey Protocol, Regulations and Interpretive Guidelines for Hospitals.* Rev. 200, 02-21-20. Centers for Medicare & Medicaid Services. https://www.cms.gov/media/423601. Accessed March 31, 2020.

94. Guideline for patient information management. In: *Guidelines for Perioperative Practice.* Denver, CO: AORN, Inc; 2020:357-386. [IVA]

95. Hachach-Haram N, Saour S, Alamouti R, Constantinides J, Mohanna PN. Labelling of diathermy consoles when multiple systems are used: should this be part of the WHO checklist? *BMJ Qual Saf.* 2013;22(9):775-776. [VB]

96. Townsend NT, Nadlonek NA, Jones EL, et al. Unintended stray energy from monopolar instruments: beware the dispersive electrode cord. *Surg Endosc.* 2016;30(4):1333-1336. [IIIC]

97. Townsend NT, Jones EL, Overbey D, Dunne B, McHenry J, Robinson TN. Single-incision laparoscopic surgery increases the risk of unintentional thermal injury from the monopolar "Bovie" instrument in comparison with traditional laparoscopy. *Surg Endosc.* 2017;31(8):3146-3151. [IIIC]

98. Robinson TN, Jones EL, Dunn CL, et al. Separating the laparoscopic camera cord from the monopolar "Bovie" cord reduces unintended thermal injury from antenna coupling: a randomized controlled trial. *Ann Surg.* 2015;261(6):1056-1060. [IA]

99. Brill AI. Electrosurgery: principles and practice to reduce risk and maximize efficacy. *Obstet Gynecol Clin North Am.* 2011;38(4):687-702. [VB]

100. Shah AJ, Janes R, Holliday J, Thakur R. Radiofrequency transseptal catheter electrode fracture. *Pacing Clin Electrophysiol.* 2010;33(6):e57-e58. [VB]

101. Hazard report. Internal wire breakage in reusable electrosurgical active electrode cables may cause sparking and surgical fires. *Health Devices.* 2009;38(7):228-229. [VB]

102. Guideline for cleaning and care of surgical instruments. In: *Guidelines for Perioperative Practice.* Denver, CO: AORN, Inc; 2020:387-426. [IVA]

103. Montero PN, Robinson TN, Weaver JS, Stiegmann GV. Insulation failure in laparoscopic instruments. *Surg Endosc.* 2010;24(2):462-465. [IIIB]

104. Espada M, Munoz R, Noble BN, Magrina JF. Insulation failure in robotic and laparoscopic instrumentation: a prospective evaluation. *Am J Obstet Gynecol.* 2011;205(2):121.e1-121.e5. [IIIB]

105. Tixier F, Garçon M, Rochefort F, Corvaisier S. Insulation failure in electrosurgery instrumentation: a prospective evaluation. *Surg Endosc.* 2016;30(11):4995-5001. [IIIA]

106. Alternate-site burns from improperly seated or damaged electrosurgical pencil active electrodes. *Health Devices.* 2012;41(10):334. [VC]

107. Lowry TR, Workman JR. Avoiding oral burns during electrocautery tonsillectomy. *Ear Nose Throat J.* 2009;88(2):790-792. [VC]

108. Baker JC, Ramadan HH. The effects of an antistick phospholipid solution on pediatric electrocautery adenoidectomy. *Ear Nose Throat J.* 2012;91(1):E20-E23. [IA]

109. Roy S, Buckingham H, Buckingham E. The effects of an antistick phospholipid solution on bipolar electrocautery efficacy in rhytidectomy. *Am J Cosmet Surg.* 2017;34(3):156-160. [IB]

110. Sanders A, Andras L, Lehman A, Bridges N, Skaggs DL. Dermal discolorations and burns at neuromonitoring electrodes in pediatric spine surgery. *Spine (Phila PA 1976).* 2017;42(1):20-24. [VA]

111. Gallagher K, Dhinsa B, Miles J. Electrosurgery. *Surgery.* 2011;29(2):70-72. [VB]

112. Ertuğrul İ, Karagöz T, Aykan HH. A rare complication of radiofrequency ablation: skin burn. *Cardiol Young.* 2015;25(7):1385-1386. [VC]

113. Dhillon PS, Gonna H, Li A, Wong T, Ward DE. Skin burns associated with radiofrequency catheter ablation of cardiac arrhythmias. *Pacing Clin Electrophysiol.* 2013;36(6):764-767. [VC]

114. Odell RC. Surgical complications specific to monopolar electrosurgical energy: engineering changes that have made electrosurgery safer. *J Minim Invasive Gynecol.* 2013;20(3):288-298. [VB]

115. Talati RK, Dein EJ, Huri G, McFarland EG. Cutaneous burn caused by radiofrequency ablation probe during shoulder arthroscopy. *Am J Orthop (Belle Mead NJ).* 2015;44(2):E58-E60. [VA]

116. Martin KE, Moore CM, Tucker R, Fuchshuber P, Robinson T. Quantifying inadvertent thermal bowel injury from the monopolar instrument. *Surg Endosc.* 2016;30(11):4776-4784. [IIIB]

117. Guzman C, Forrester JA, Fuchshuber PR, Eakin JL. Estimating the incidence of stray energy burns during laparoscopic surgery based on two statewide databases and

retrospective rates: an opportunity to improve patient safety. *Surg Technol Int.* 2019;34:30-34. [IIIA]

118. Mendez-Probst CE, Vilos G, Fuller A, et al. Stray electrical currents in laparoscopic instruments used in da Vinci® robot-assisted surgery: an in vitro study. *J Endourol.* 2011;25(9):1513-1517. [IIIB]

119. Schulman PM, Rozner MA. Case report: use caution when applying magnets to pacemakers or defibrillators for surgery. *Anesth Analg.* 2013;117(2):422-427. [VA]

120. Ubee SS, Kasi VS, Bello D, Manikandan R. Implications of pacemakers and implantable cardioverter defibrillators in urological practice. *J Urol.* 2011;186(4):1198-1205. [VA]

121. Peter NM, Ribes P, Khooshabeh R. Cardiac pacemakers and electrocautery in ophthalmic surgery. *Orbit.* 2012;31(6):408-411. [VC]

122. Stone ME, Salter B, Fischer A. Perioperative management of patients with cardiac implantable electronic devices. *Br J Anaesth.* 2011;107(Suppl 1):i16-i26. [VA]

123. Voutsalath MA, Bichakjian CK, Pelosi F, Blum D, Johnson TM, Farrehi PM. Electrosurgery and implantable electronic devices: review and implications for office-based procedures. *Dermatol Surg.* 2011;37(7):889-899. [VA]

124. Howe N, Cherpelis B. Obtaining rapid and effective hemostasis: part II. electrosurgery in patients with implantable cardiac devices. *J Am Acad Dermatol.* 2013;69(5):677.e1-677.e9. [VC]

125. Venkatraghavan L, Chinnapa V, Peng P, Brull R. Noncardiac implantable electrical devices: brief review and implications for anesthesiologists. *Can J Anaesth.* 2009;56(4):320-326. [VA]

126. Navaratnam M, Dubin A. Pediatric pacemakers and ICDs: how to optimize perioperative care. *Paediatr Anaesth.* 2011;21(5):512-521. [VB]

127. García Bracamonte B, Rodriguez J, Casado R, Vanaclocha F. Electrosurgery in patients with implantable electronic cardiac devices (pacemakers and defibrillators). *Actas Dermosifiliogr.* 2013;104(2):128-132. [VB]

128. Chia PL, Foo D. A practical approach to perioperative management of cardiac implantable electronic devices. *Singapore Med J.* 2015;56(10):538-541. [VB]

129. Stone ME, Apinis A. Current perioperative management of the patient with a cardiac rhythm management device. *Semin Cardiothorac Vasc Anesth.* 2009;13(1):31-43. [VB]

130. Pavlović S, Milasinović G, Zivković M. Approach to patients with implanted pacemaker and scheduled surgical or diagnostic procedure. *Acta Chir Iugosl.* 2011;58(2):25-29. [VC]

131. Tom J. Management of patients with cardiovascular implantable electronic devices in dental, oral, and maxillofacial surgery. *Anesth Prog.* 2016;63(2):95-104. [VB]

132. Kumar A, Dhillon SS, Patel S, Grube M, Noheria A. Management of cardiac implantable electronic devices during interventional pulmonology procedures. *J Thorac Dis.* 2017;9(Suppl 10):S1059-S1068. [VA]

133. Practice advisory for the perioperative management of patients with cardiac implantable electronic devices: pacemakers and implantable cardioverter–defibrillators 2020: an updated report by the American Society of Anesthesiologists Task Force on Perioperative Management of Patients with Cardiac Implantable Electronic Devices. *Anesthesiology.* 2020;132(2):225-252. [IVA]

134. Sticherling C, Menafoglio A, Burri H, et al. Recommendations for the peri-operative management of patients with cardiac implantable electronic devices. *Kardiovaskulare Medizin.* 2016;19(1):13-18. [IVC]

135. Rozner MA. Perioperative care of the patient with a cardiac pacemaker or ICD. *Revista Mexicana de Anestesiologia.* 2009;32(Suppl 1):S190-S197. [VB]

136. Ramos JA, Brull SJ. Perioperative management of multiple noncardiac implantable electronic devices. *A A Case Rep.* 2015;5(11):189-191. [VA]

137. Harned ME, Gish B, Zuelzer A, Grider JS. Anesthetic considerations and perioperative management of spinal cord stimulators: literature review and initial recommendations. *Pain Physician.* 2017;20(4):319-329. [VA]

138. Hammwöhner M, Stachowitz J, Willich T, Goette A. Induction of ventricular tachycardia during radiofrequency ablation via pulmonary vein ablation catheter in a patient with an implanted pacemaker. *Europace.* 2012;14(2):298-299. [VC]

139. Wong TS, Abu Bakar J, Chee KH, et al. Posterior spinal fusion in a scoliotic patient with congenital heart block treated with pacemaker: an intraoperative technical difficulty. *Spine.* 2019;44(4):E252-E257. [VC]

140. Beinart R, Nazarian S. Effects of external electrical and magnetic fields on pacemakers and defibrillators: from engineering principles to clinical practice. *Circulation.* 2013;128(25):2799-2809. [VA]

141. Friedman H, Higgins JV, Ryan JD, Konecny T, Asirvatham SJ, Cha YM. Predictors of intraoperative electrosurgery-induced implantable cardioverter defibrillator (ICD) detection. *J Interv Card Electrophysiol.* 2017;48(1):21-26. [IIIB]

142. Jeyakumar A, Wilson M, Sorrel JE, et al. Monopolar cautery and adverse effects on cochlear implants. *JAMA Otolaryngol Head Neck Surg.* 2013;139(7):694-697. [IIIB]

143. Misiri J, Kusumoto F, Goldschlager N. Electromagnetic interference and implanted cardiac devices: the medical environment (part II). *Clin Cardiol.* 2012;35(6):321-328. [VA]

144. Santini L, Forleo GB, Santini M. Implantable devices in the electromagnetic environment. *J Arrhythm.* 2013;29(6):325-333. [VB]

145. Paniccia A, Rozner M, Jones EL, et al. Electromagnetic interference caused by common surgical energy-based devices on an implanted cardiac defibrillator. *Am J Surg.* 2014;208(6):932-936. [IIIB]

146. Frampton SJ, Ismail-Koch H, Mitchell TE. How safe is diathermy in patients with cochlear implants? *Ann R Coll Surg Engl.* 2012;94(8):585-587. [IIIB]

147. Behan J, Higgins S, Wysong A. Safety of cochlear implants in electrosurgery: a systematic review of the literature. *Dermatol Surg.* 2017;43(6):775-783. [VA]

148. Frampton SJ, Mitchell TE. Surgical safety issues relating to the use of diathermy in patients with cochlear implants:

the patient's perspective. *Cochlear Implants Int.* 2014;15(1):48-52. [IIIB]

149. Law SC, Wong JC, Cheung HY, Chung CC, Li MK. Colonic injury from electric arcing: a significant complication of argon plasma coagulation. *Hong Kong Med J.* 2009;15(3):227-229. [VC]

150. Sachdeva A, Pickering EM, Lee HJ. From electrocautery, balloon dilatation, neodymium-doped:yttrium-aluminum-garnet (Nd:YAG) laser to argon plasma coagulation and cryotherapy. *J Thorac Dis.* 2015;7(Suppl 4):S363-S379. [VB]

151. Mendelson BJ, Feldman JM, Addante RA. Argon embolus from argon beam coagulator. *J Clin Anesth.* 2017;42:86-87. [VB]

152. Shaw Y, Yoneda KY, Chan AL. Cerebral gas embolism from bronchoscopic argon plasma coagulation: a case report. *Respiration.* 2012;83(3):267-270. [VA]

153. Sutton C, Abbott J. History of power sources in endoscopic surgery. *J Minim Invasive Gynecol.* 2013;20(3):271-278. [VB]

154. Ahrens PM, Siddiqui NA, Rakhit RD. Pacemaker placement and shoulder surgery: is there a risk? *Ann R Coll Surg Engl.* 2012;94(1):39-42. [IIIC]

155. Feldman LS, Fuchshuber P, Jones DB, Mischna J, Schwaitzberg SD; FUSE (Fundamental Use of Surgical Energy™) Task Force. Surgeons don't know what they don't know about the safe use of energy in surgery. *Surg Endosc.* 2012;26(10):2735-2739. [IIIB]

156. AlNomair N, Nazarian R, Marmur E. Complications in lasers, lights, and radiofrequency devices. *Facial Plast Surg.* 2012;28(3):340-346. [VB]

157. Brown J, Blank K. Minimally invasive endometrial ablation device complications and use outside of the manufacturers' instructions. *Obstet Gynecol.* 2012;120(4):865-870 [VC]

158. Surve R, Madhusudan S, Sriganesh K. Electrocautery interference with intraoperative capnography during neurosurgery. *J Clin Monit Comput.* 2014;28(4):429-430. [VB]

Guideline Development Group

Lead Author: Byron L. Burlingame[1], MS, BSN, RN, CNOR, Senior Perioperative Practice Specialist, AORN, Denver, Colorado

Contributing Author: Erin Kyle[2], DNP, RN, CNOR, NEA-BC, Editor-in-Chief, Guidelines for Perioperative Practice, AORN, Denver, Colorado

Methodologist: Amber Wood[3], MSN, RN, CNOR, CIC, FAPIC, Editor-in-Chief, Guidelines for Perioperative Practice, AORN, Denver, Colorado

Evidence Appraisers: Byron L. Burlingame[1] and Janice Neil[4], PhD, CNE, RN, Associate Professor, East Carolina College of Nursing, Greenville, North Carolina

Guidelines Advisory Board Members:
- Donna A. Pritchard[5], MA, BSN, RN, NE-BC, CNOR, Director of Perioperative Services, Interfaith Medical Center, Brooklyn, New York
- Vangie V. Dennis[6], BSN, RN, CNOR, CMLSO, Executive Director Perioperative Services, Wellstar Health System Cobb Hospital, Duluth, Georgia
- Brenda G. Larkin[7], MS, ACNS-BC, CNS, CNOR, Clinical Nurse Specialist, Aurora Lakeland Medical Center, Lake Geneva, Wisconsin
- Kate McGee[8], BSN, RN, CNOR, Staff Nurse, Aurora West Allis Medical Center, East Troy, Wisconsin[8]
- Darlene B. Murdock[9], BSN, BA, RN, CNOR, Clinical Staff Nurse IV, Memorial Herman Texas Medical Center, Houston
- Elizabeth (Lizz) Pincus[10], MSN, RN, CNS-CP, CNOR, Clinical Nurse, Regional Medical Center of San Jose, California

Guidelines Advisory Board Liaison:
- Susan G. Klacik[11], BS, CRCST, FCS, Clinical Educator, International Association of Healthcare Central Service Materiel Management (IAHCSMM), Chicago, Illinois

External Review: Expert review comments were received from individual members of the American Association of Nurse Anesthetists (AANA), American College of Surgeons (ACS), Association for Professionals in Infection Control and Epidemiology (APIC), American Society of Anesthesiologists (ASA), International Association of Healthcare Central Service Materiel Management (IAHCSMM), Practice Greenhealth, and the Society for Healthcare Epidemiology of America (SHEA). Their responses were used to further refine and enhance this guideline; however, their responses do not imply endorsement. The draft was also open for a 30-day public comment period.

Financial Disclosure and Conflicts of Interest

This guideline was developed, edited, and approved by the AORN Guidelines Advisory Board without external funding being sought or obtained. The Guidelines Advisory Board was entirely supported financially by the AORN and was developed without any involvement of industry.

Potential conflicts of interest for all Guidelines Advisory Board members were reviewed before the annual meeting and each monthly conference call. The advisory board concluded that individuals with potential conflicts that may arise could remain on the advisory board if they had occurred if they agreed to recuse themselves from related discussion. None of the members of the Guideline Development Group reported a potential conflict of interest during the development of this guideline.[1-11]

Publication History

Originally published March 1985, *AORN Journal* as Recommended Practices: Electrosurgery. Revised April 1991; revised July 1993.

Revised November 1997; published January 1998, *AORN Journal* as Recommended Practices for Electrosurgery. Reformatted July 2000.

Revised November 2003; published February 2004, *AORN Journal.*

Revised November 2004; published in *Standards, Recommended Practices, and Guidelines,* 2005 edition. Reprinted March 2005, *AORN Journal.*

Revised July 2009 for online publication in *Perioperative Standards and Recommended Practices.*

Minor editing revisions made in November 2009 for publication in *Perioperative Standards and Recommended Practices,* 2010 edition.

Editorial revisions made July 2012. Recommendation X was revised and approved by the Recommended Practices Advisory Board. Reformatted September 2012 for publication in *Perioperative Standards and Recommended Practices,* 2013 edition.

Minor editing revisions made in November 2014 for publication as *Guideline for Electrosurgery in Guidelines for Perioperative Practice,* 2015 edition.

Revised and combined with the Guideline for Laser Safety, as Guideline for Safe Use of Energy-Generating Devices, September 2016, for online publication in *Guidelines for Perioperative Practice.*

Evidence ratings revised and minor editorial changes made to conform to the current AORN Evidence Rating model, September 2019, for online publication in *Guidelines for Perioperative Practice.*

Revised July 2020 for publication in *Guidelines for Perioperative Practice* online.

Scheduled for review in 2024.

ENVIRONMENT
OF CARE

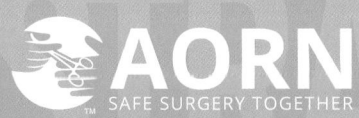

TABLE OF CONTENTS

Ⓐ *indicates additional information is available in the Ambulatory Supplement.*

MEDICAL ABBREVIATIONS & ACRONYMS

dBA – Decibels A-scale
ESU – Electrosurgical unit
FDA – US Food and Drug Administration
IFU – Instructions for use
IgE – Immunoglobulin E
MAUDE – Manufacturer and User Facility Device Experience
MMA – Methyl methacrylate

NFPA – National Fire Protection Association
NIOSH – National Institute for Occupational Safety and Health
OR – Operating room
ppm – Parts per million
RN – Registered nurse
SDS – Safety data sheet

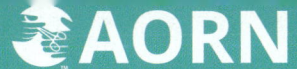

GUIDELINE FOR
SAFE ENVIRONMENT OF CARE

The Guideline for a Safe Environment of Care was approved by the AORN Guidelines Advisory Board and became effective October 1, 2018. It was presented as a proposed guideline for comments by members and others. The recommendations in the guideline are intended to be achievable and represent what is believed to be an optimal level of practice. Policies and procedures will reflect variations in practice settings and/or clinical situations that determine the degree to which the guideline can be implemented. AORN recognizes the many diverse settings in which perioperative nurses practice; therefore, this guideline is adaptable to all areas where operative or other invasive procedures may be performed.

Purpose

This document provides guidance for maintaining a safe environment of care for patients and perioperative personnel. The recommendations include information on
- **clinical** and **alert alarms**,
- **noise** and **distractions**,
- occupational injuries (eg, slips, trips, and falls),
- fire safety,
- electrical equipment,
- blanket and fluid warming cabinets,
- medical gas cylinders,
- waste anesthesia gases,
- **latex allergy**,
- hazardous chemicals, and
- hazardous waste.

The following topics are outside the scope of this document:
- chemotherapeutic agents (See the AORN Guideline for Medication Safety[1]);
- heating, ventilation, and air conditioning (See the AORN Guideline for Design and Maintenance of the Surgical Suite[2]);
- lifting equipment and moving patients (See the AORN Guideline for Safe Patient Handling and Movement[3]);
- patient injuries related to incorrect tubing connections (See the AORN Guideline for Medication Safety[1]);
- personnel injuries related to exposure to bloodborne pathogens (See the AORN Guideline for Transmission-Based Precautions[4]);
- product evaluation (See the AORN Guideline for Medical Device and Product Evaluation[5]);
- radiation (See the AORN Guideline for Radiation Safety[6]); and
- surgical smoke (See the AORN Guideline for Surgical Smoke Safety[7]).

Evidence Review

A medical librarian conducted a systematic literature search of the databases Ovid MEDLINE®, EBSCO CINAHL®, Scopus®, and the Cochrane Database of Systematic Reviews. The search was limited to literature published in English from 2012 through March 2018. At the time of the initial search, weekly alerts were created on the topics included in the search. Results from these alerts were provided to the lead author until April 2018. The lead author also requested additional articles that did not fit the original search criteria or were discovered during the appraisal process.

Search terms included *abortion spontaneous, activation indicators, airway fires, alarm fatigue, alert alarms, blanket warmer, bone cements, burns, clinical alarms, combustion, control of noise and distractions, dermatitis (allergic contact), electrical equipment, electrical equipment and supplies, ethylene oxide, fire, fire blanket, fire extinguisher, fire extinguishing equipment, fire prevention, fire safety, fire triangle, firefighting equipment and supplies, formalin, glutaraldehyde, hazardous substances, hazardous waste, hazardous waste disposal, latex, latex hypersensitivity, methyl methacrylate, methylmethacrylate, miscarriage, noise, occupational diseases, protective clothing, scalding, smoke alarms, solution warmer, surgical fires, teratogens, thermal injuries, warming techniques, waste products,* and *Zimmer bone cement.*

Included were research and non-research literature in English, complete publications, and publication dates within the time restriction when available. Excluded were non-peer-reviewed publications and older evidence within the time restriction when more recent evidence was available. Editorials, news items, and other brief items were excluded. Low-quality evidence was excluded when higher-quality evidence was available, and literature outside the time restriction was excluded when literature within the time restriction was available (Figure 1).

Articles identified in the search were provided to the project team for evaluation. The team consisted of the lead author and one evidence appraiser. The lead author divided the search results into topics, and both members of the team reviewed and critically appraised each article using the AORN Research or Non-Research Evidence Appraisal Tools as appropriate. The literature was independently evaluated and appraised according to the strength and quality of the evidence. Each article was then assigned an appraisal score. The appraisal score is noted in brackets after each reference, as applicable.

Each recommendation rating is based on a synthesis of the collective evidence, a benefit-harm assessment, and consideration of resource use. The strength of the recommendation was determined using the AORN

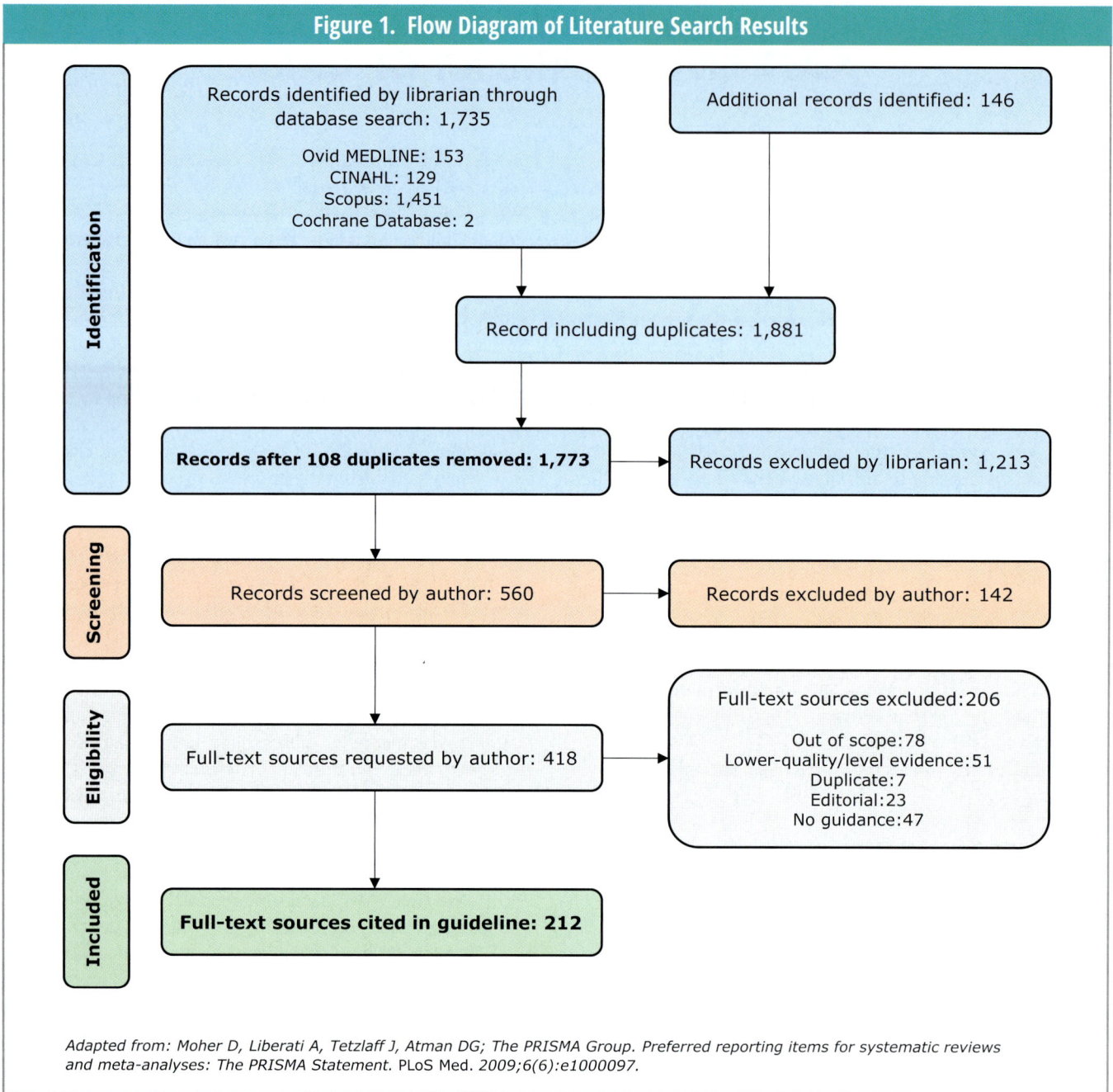

Figure 1. Flow Diagram of Literature Search Results

Adapted from: Moher D, Liberati A, Tetzlaff J, Atman DG; The PRISMA Group. Preferred reporting items for systematic reviews and meta-analyses: The PRISMA Statement. PLoS Med. 2009;6(6):e1000097.

Evidence Rating Model and the quality and consistency of the evidence supporting a recommendation. The recommendation strength rating is noted in brackets after each recommendation.

Note: The evidence summary table is available at http://www.aorn.org/evidencetables/.

Editor's note: MEDLINE is a registered trademark of the US National Library of Medicine's Medical Literature Analysis and Retrieval System, Bethesda, MD. CINAHL, Cumulative Index to 11211Nursing and Allied Health Literature, is a registered trademark of EBSCO Industries, Birmingham, AL. Scopus is a registered trademark of Elsevier B.V., Amsterdam, The Netherlands.

1. Clinical and Alert Alarms

1.1 **Take precautions to mitigate hazards associated with non-functioning clinical and alert alarms.** *[Recommendation]*

Patients have experienced injuries and near misses because alarms were turned off or inaudible. The reported causes of injuries and near misses include disabled alarm systems (eg, blood bank refrigerators, code blue alarms, electrosurgical unit [ESU] alarms, ethylene oxide level alarms, fire alarms, water treatment alarms), distractions, and failure of personnel to hear or to act on clinical alarms.[8]

1.2 Test clinical and alert alarms according to organizational policy and procedures. [Recommendation]

Periodic testing assists with maintaining a working system.[9,10]

1.3 Collaborate with clinical engineering personnel to conduct an inventory of clinical and alert alarms. [Recommendation]

Completing an inventory assists with identifying the pieces of equipment that have alarms, maintaining an accurate alarm inventory, and tracking testing.[11]

1.3.1 In the alarm inventory, include all devices and systems in the facility with alarms, including

- anesthesia equipment;
- refrigerators, freezers, or warmers designated for patient use;
- carbon dioxide insufflators;
- ESUs;
- infusion pumps;
- pneumatic tourniquets;
- patient monitoring devices (eg, cardiac monitors, oximeters);
- security systems;
- medical gas system; and
- sequential compression devices.

[Recommendation]

1.4 Test clinical and alert alarms on initial setup.[12] [Recommendation]

1.5 Set clinical and alert alarms to be sufficiently loud to allow them to be heard above competing noise, and reduce noise so that alarms can be heard. [Recommendation]

Noise makes it difficult to hear and differentiate among alarms.[9,10] In a study that evaluated the sound levels in the OR, researchers found that in 25 consecutive elective cardiac procedures, an anesthesia alarm sounded an average of once every 1.2 minutes.[13]

1.6 Communicate changes in clinical alarm default parameters (eg, volume, high or low limits) verbally and visually during changes of personnel. [Recommendation]

Communicating changes to alarm settings prepares oncoming personnel to respond appropriately.[14]

1.6.1 A clearly distinguishable visual cue, such as a posted sign, may be used to indicate the change in the default. [Conditional Recommendation]

1.7 Establish and implement a process for responding to alert alarms when perioperative personnel are not present. [Recommendation]

There may be systems within the perioperative suite that contain critical supplies that must be maintained under set conditions (eg, blood bank refrigerator, bone freezer), and the perioperative suite may not be staffed 24 hours per day. If no one hears and responds to the alarm, critical supplies could be damaged.

1.7.1 Have the alert alarm sound at a location in the building that is staffed 24 hours a day or connect the alarm to a remote location. [Recommendation]

2. Noise and Distractions

2.1 Minimize noise and distractions. [Recommendation]

In the perioperative setting, noise and distractions are created by equipment and personnel.[15-19] Noises created by equipment include clinical and alert alarms; heating, ventilating, and air conditioning systems; telephones and other communication devices; and tools related to the provision of surgical procedures (eg, equipment, powered instruments, ESUs, smoke evacuators, suction devices, ventilators).[15] Noises created by personnel include conversation; doors opening and closing, overhead pages, and music. Some noise is unavoidable in the perioperative environment, but certain noise levels can be controlled.

Moderate-quality evidence indicates that noise in the perioperative setting can interfere with verbal communication.[15-20] The Joint Commission has identified failures in communication as a leading cause of medical errors and negative patient outcomes.[21]

In a literature review, Katz[16] found that the noisiest periods during a surgical procedure were at the beginning and the end of surgery when surgical equipment is being prepared or disassembled. This coincides with the induction and patient's emergence from anesthesia. Equipment-related noise has been measured to be as high as 120 decibels A-Scale (dBA) and is caused by suction apparatus, anesthetic monitors, alarms, clanging and dropping of equipment, movement of equipment, and hammers. Personnel-related noise can reach levels of 78 dBA and includes conversation and other staff-related activities.

In one investigation, the National Institute for Occupational Safety and Health (NIOSH) measured noise levels in 18 ORs and found that the noise levels were the highest in the orthopedic and neurosurgery rooms. The levels were higher the closer the person was to the source of the sound (eg, higher for the people in the sterile field compared to the registered nurse [RN] circulator). The authors concluded that noise protection was not required because the noise levels were below the NIOSH-recommended criterion level of 85 dBA. The NIOSH criterion level describes the level of noise exposure that can be safely tolerated during an 8-hour shift without ear protection. There were peak levels that exceeded 90 dBA but that lasted for only short periods of time. The researchers concluded that the levels were high enough to potentially cause interference with understanding of the spoken word.[22]

In a systematic review, Mentis et al[18] found that distractions caused by movement and non-case-related conversation occurred most frequently, but the most severe distractions were equipment and procedure related. They also found that surgeons perceived that distractions in the operating room (OR) negatively affected surgical performance. The surgeons perceived the greatest amount of disruption was caused by equipment and procedural distractions. The researchers concluded that controlling distractions is important to successful patient outcomes and suggested creating OR policies and procedures to reduce equipment and procedural distractions.

Antoniadis et al[19] conducted a nonexperimental research study to identify **interruption** events in the OR. The researchers found there are interruption sources extrinsic to surgical procedures, such as people entering or exiting the OR and beeper and phone calls, and factors intrinsic to surgical procedures, such as interruptions caused by equipment failures, distractions from the work environment, and procedural problems. The researchers concluded that there are considerable distractions and interruptions in the OR that interfere with the work of the perioperative team and that the intrinsic factors caused more intense interference in the functioning of the OR team.

Keller et al[23] conducted a nonexperimental research study to investigate the effect of noise peaks on surgical teams' communication during 109 abdominal surgeries. The results of the study demonstrated that high noise peaks reduced the frequency of patient-related communication but not patient-irrelevant communication. The researchers concluded that the results support the need for developing noise-reducing programs in the OR.

Way et al[17] conducted a prospective study to investigate the effects of OR-simulated listening conditions on auditory processing in surgeons with normal hearing. The participants were asked to repeat the last word of a short sentence under four different conditions. The 50 short sentences were stated in a quiet setting, with filtered noise, with filtered noise plus OR noise, and with filtered noise plus OR noise and music. The results demonstrated that auditory performance decreased with each increase in the level of noise. The researchers recommended that ambient noise levels be decreased to avoid possible miscommunications.

2.2 **Implement measures to minimize noise created by personnel, including**
- **limiting nonessential conversations,**[20,24-27]
- **controlling the tone and volume of essential conversations,**[24] **and**
- **limiting the number of personnel in the OR.**[25]

[Recommendation]

Low-quality evidence supports implementing these measures to minimize noise and decrease the potential for distractions caused by the noise.[20,24-27]

2.3 **Implement measures to minimize noise generated by equipment and devices including**
- **portable communication devices (eg, pagers, smart phones, cell phones, wireless communication systems, hand held two-way radio transceivers [eg, walkie-talkies]),**
- **fixed communication devices (eg, overhead paging systems, intercoms, telephones),**
- **electronic music devices (eg, radios, CD players, digital audio players), and**
- **medical equipment and devices (eg, radiology equipment, the waste management system, smoke evacuators, powered surgical instruments, monitors, clinical and alert alarms, metal instruments).**

[Recommendation]

Cheriyan et al[15] measured the effect of intraoperative noise on intraoperative communication during percutaneous nephrolithotomy with ambient noise (53.49 dBA), with equipment in use (78.79 dBA), and with equipment and music (81.78 dBA). The surgeon spoke 20 different medical words or phrases five times, and responses from the first assistant, anesthesiologist, and circulating nurse were recorded. The correct response rates decreased with each increase in the amount of noise (97%, 81%, 56% when percutaneous nephrolithotomy equipment was in use, and 90%, 48%, 13% after music was added for the first assistant, anesthesiologist, and circulating nurse, respectively). The researchers concluded that noise pollution decreased effective intraoperative communication.

2.3.1 **When portable communication devices are present in the OR,**
- **place them on vibrate or silent mode,**
- **turn them off unless directly needed for job performance, or**
- **leave them at a common location outside of the OR.**

[Recommendation]

2.3.2 Use fixed communication devices
- only for essential communications,
- at the lowest volume possible, and
- for essential communication instead of opening the door and entering the OR.[24] *[Recommendation]*

The use of fixed communication devices is preferred to opening the door because opening the door causes a greater distraction and affects the airflow within the surgical suite.[28]

2.3.3 Set the volume of electronic music devices to be low enough to allow communication among team members.[15-17,24,25,29,30] *[Recommendation]*

Shambo et al[29] performed a review of the literature on music in the OR. The authors concluded that music contributes to the overall stress of the environment, interferes with communication, decreases the ability to accomplish tasks safely, and creates a safety threat to patients and personnel. The authors recommended that if music is played in the OR, it should be done judiciously and with the consent of all stakeholders.

2.4 Minimize distractions (eg, non-patient-care related noises, door openings, and conversation) during critical phases of the surgical procedure.[26,27] *[Recommendation]*

Critical phases of the surgical procedure are described as events in routine surgery during which there is a high risk of an adverse occurrence.[24,27,31,32] The critical phases of surgery include
- surgical briefings,[24,27]
- the surgical time out,[24,27,31,32]
- anesthesia induction,[24,25,27,31,32]
- emergence from anesthesia,[24,25,27,31,32]
- surgical counts,[24,27,31,32]
- crucial portions of the procedure (eg, delicate dissection, aneurysm clipping, anastomosis, implant sizing), and
- surgical specimen management.[27]

Implementing measures to limit distractions during these critical phases may promote a safer environment of care for patients and perioperative personnel.[27] Limiting the distractions during critical phases of the surgical procedure is supported in moderate-quality evidence that applies the use of the aviation concept referred to as the "**sterile cockpit** rule" to the OR.[27,31-34]

In response to complaints from anesthesia professionals about the high level of noise and distractions during critical phases of anesthesia induction and emergence, Hogan and Harvey[25] performed a quality improvement project at two community hospitals. The authors measured noise levels in the OR during anesthesia induction and the patient's emergence from anesthesia. The noise levels were measured before and after implementation of an educational inservice program about noise reduction strategies provided to all perioperative personnel. The authors found the sound levels were significantly lower during the induction and emergence phases of anesthesia at both hospitals after implementation of the educational inservice program. The authors concluded that reducing and controlling noise levels during critical phases of anesthesia may minimize annoyance, distraction, and stress for personnel.

In a nonexperimental research study, Ginsberg et al[35] measured noise levels in the cardiac OR during 23 cardiac surgeries performed with the patient under general anesthesia. The researchers found that at each anesthesia critical phase (ie, induction, emergence, termination of extracorporeal circulation, drape removal, transport), noise levels were louder than the levels at room setup, surgical skin incision, and 1 hour into the surgery. The researchers concluded that noise in the OR is louder during the critical phases of anesthesia and suggested that activities may be controlled by personnel during these critical phases.

Jenkins et al[34] conducted a nonexperimental research study in an obstetric OR setting in the United Kingdom. The researchers observed women undergoing cesarean deliveries under regional spinal-epidural anesthesia and identified three phases of anesthesia that are similar to critical phases of the surgical procedure: the period from when the anesthetist begins preparation of medications and equipment until the removal of the needle from the patient's back, the period when the patient is in the supine position, and the delivery of the infant's head. The researchers measured the noise levels with a sound level meter. The results indicated that the highest ambient noise levels, the highest rate of incidental noisy events, and the highest rate of nonclinical conversations occurred during the delivery of the infant's head. The researchers recommended turning off music and limiting nonessential or case-irrelevant conversations during critical phases in the obstetric OR to improve patient safety.

3. Slips, Trips, and Falls

3.1 Take precautions to mitigate the risk of occupational injuries associated with slips, trips, and falls. *[Recommendation]*

Occupational injuries can impair a perioperative employee's ability to do his or her job, increase work-related compensation claims, diminish the ability of the employee to care for patients, cause lost workdays, and reduce productivity.[36] In 2011,

NIOSH reported that the second most common cause of work-related injuries was slips, trips, and falls.[36] In 2015, Gomaa et al[37] reported rates of falls in 61 participating health care facilities. There were 382 work-related falls reported in the OR, which was the highest of all areas reporting.

3.2 Establish and implement a slip, trip, and fall prevention program. [Recommendation]

Low-quality evidence supports a slip, trip, and fall prevention program.[36-38] Research conducted by NIOSH demonstrated that implementing a prevention program led to a reduction of slip-, trip-, and fall-related workers' compensation claims.[37]

3.2.1 Perform an assessment of the environmental hazards and review of injury data within the health care organization. [Recommendation]

An assessment serves to identify factors that contribute to risk of slips, trips, and falls. Analysis of a slip, trip, and fall risk assessment can assist in reducing occupational slip, trip, and fall hazards in the perioperative setting.[36,37,39-42]

3.2.2 Include the following strategies for minimizing slips, trips, and falls:

- arranging equipment and supplies to provide unobstructed pathways,[38]
- cleaning up spills or debris as soon as possible,[36,38,39,41,42]
- covering electrical cables that are on the floor with a facility-approved floor cord covering,[38]
- reducing clutter and electrical cables on the floor,
- providing adequate lighting,[36,38,39]
- posting signs warning of wet floor hazards,[38] and
- wearing slip-resistant shoes.[36]

[Recommendation]

Perioperative personnel are at the greatest risk for occupational slips, trips, and falls associated with exposure to spills, body fluids, and slippery walking surfaces.[36]

4. Fire Safety

4.1 Identify potential hazards associated with fire safety and establish safe practices for communication, prevention, suppression, and evacuation. [Recommendation]

In a perioperative setting, a fire may occur and cause injury to both the patient and personnel because all three elements of the fire triangle (ie, fuel, oxidizer, ignition source) are present (Figure

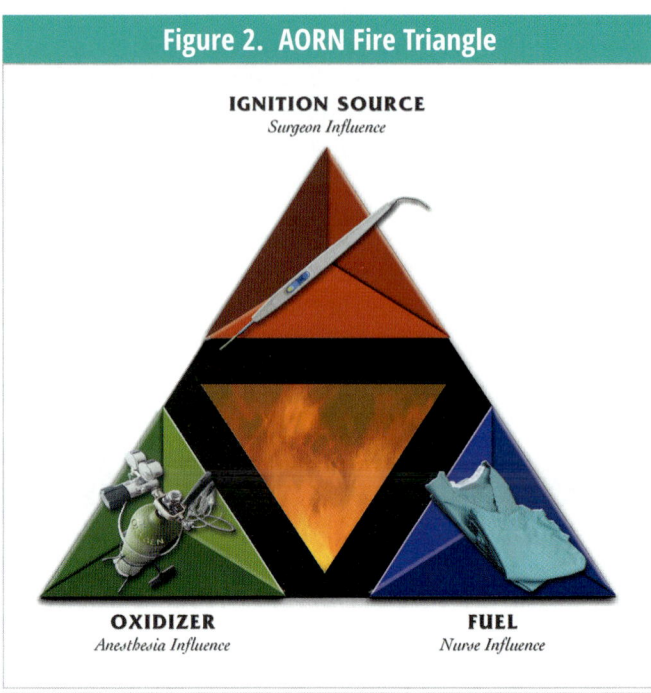

Figure 2. AORN Fire Triangle

IGNITION SOURCE
Surgeon Influence

OXIDIZER
Anesthesia Influence

FUEL
Nurse Influence

The AORN Fire Triangle illustrates the three elements necessary for a fire and the members of the perioperative team who frequently influence the element.

2).[43-51] The most common sites of fires that occur on a patient are the head, face, neck, or upper chest (44%).[45-47,49,52-58] Twenty-one percent of fires occur in the patient's airway. Fires have been reported during various types of procedures including blepharoplasty,[53,54] coronary bypass grafting,[59] colectomy,[60,61] laparoscopic cholecystectomy,[62,63] otolaryngology,[52,55-57,64] thoracotomy,[52] and tracheostomy.[47,55,64,65] Patient outcomes have included burns,[43,44,46,47,53,55,65,66] disfigurement,[43,47,53] severe injury,[51,60,67-70] extended medical care,[47] and death.[43,47,50,51,67-72] A majority (59.1%[53]) of surgical fires occur in the hospital setting.[44,46,49-53,58-60,62,65,69,73-81] Thirty percent of surgical fires occur in ambulatory surgery centers, and 10.8% occur in office procedure rooms.[53,65,80] Five incidents of surgical fires have been reported in obstetric ORs during cesarean deliveries.[44,82] All five women sustained second- or third-degree burns.

4.2 Have an interdisciplinary team composed of key stakeholders within the organization develop a written fire prevention and management plan. [Recommendation]

4.2.1 Perioperative RNs should have an active role in writing the fire prevention and management plan.[43,58,75,83,84] [Recommendation]

4.2.2 Include the following in the written fire prevention and management plan:

- perioperative team members' roles,[43,47,48,80,84]
- communication procedures,[53,61,65,69,75,78,80,84-88]

- methods of prevention,[43,48,51,61,62,65,81]
- processes for safely managing different fire scenarios,[43,48,51,59,61,62,80]
- alarm activation procedures,[48,71,79,80,83]
- methods to extinguish a fire,[48,61,62,81,83]
- preferred routes and levels of evacuation,[43,86,89,90]
- a description of the facility's fire prevention algorithm,[48]
- the required content for and frequency of fire safety education, and
- the frequency of and procedures for fire drills.[43,48,71,86,90-93]

[Recommendation]

4.3 Preoperatively, the RN circulator should complete a fire prevention assessment in collaboration with the perioperative team and communicate the results to the perioperative team during the standardized briefing process (See the AORN Guideline for Team Communication).[94] [Recommendation]

Moderate-quality evidence supports the use of a fire prevention assessment to identify causative factors for fires and interventions for prevention of surgical fires.[31,33,56,58,59,65,73,78,80-82,88]

4.3.1 Identify the following in the fire prevention assessment:

- ignition sources that are present (See Recommendation 4.6),[43,45-47,50,51,53-60,62,66,67,71,73-75,77,80,82,88,95,96]
- fuels that are present (See Recommendation 4.7),[43,47,56,67,73,77,80,88] and
- the potential for the presence of an oxygen-enriched environment (See Recommendation 4.8).[45-47,49-51,53-56,58,59,62,65,69,73,74,77,80,82,88,95,96] [Recommendation]

The assessment identifies which of the three components of the fire triangle are present (eg, ignition, fuel, oxidizer).[43,44,46-53,59-61,65-67,69,74,75,77,80-82,78,84,88,95,96]

4.4 Based on the results of the fire prevention assessment, implement the necessary interventions as described in the facility fire prevention protocol. [Recommendation]

4.4.1 Include preventive measures as described in Recommendations 4.6, 4.7, and 4.8 as interventions in the fire prevention protocol. [Recommendation]

4.5 Use ignition sources (eg, active electrosurgical electrodes, drills, heated probes, lasers, electrocautery devices, fiber-optic light cords, retractors) according to manufacturers' instructions for use (IFU) and applicable professional guidelines.[43,97,98] [Recommendation]

Manufacturers' written IFU and labels include fire safety information, such as the laser resistance of the endotracheal tube and methods of disposal for equipment (eg, battery packs).

There is a large body of moderate-quality evidence on ignition sources typically present in the OR.[43,46-48,50,53,65,75,77,80-82,88] Electrosurgical units and lasers can be ignition sources, especially when they are used in the presence of oxidizers, flammable solutions, or volatile or combustible chemicals or liquids. A fiber-optic light cable can be an ignition source if it is connected to the working element and allowed to contact drapes, sponges, or other fuel sources. The most common ignition source is the ESU, which contributes to 90% of surgical fires.[50,53,56,65,67,73,81,95]

4.5.1 Use sterile saline to cool devices that create heat during use (eg, burrs, drills, saw blades).[43,53,60,81,83,99] [Recommendation]

4.6 Prevent contact between fuels (eg, alcohol-based skin antiseptic agents, collodion, drapes, endotracheal tubes, gowns) and ignition sources. [Recommendation]

Preventing contact between fuels and ignition sources breaks the fire triangle, thereby preventing fire.[44,48,61,67,83,96] Many potential fuels will not burn in ambient air but will burn in an oxygen-enriched environment.[99,100] Fuels are present in every procedure and include the drapes and the patient's body (eg, gastrointestinal gases, hair, tissue[43,47,50,55,60,65,74,77,80,81,84,88]). The most common fuel source associated with surgical fires is surgical drapes, which contribute to 81% of surgical fires.[45,47]

Sibia et al[50] reported an incident of a surgical fire associated with the use of methyl methacrylate (ie, the fuel) and an ESU (ie, the ignition source) during a total knee arthroplasty. The use of the ESU near the bone cement ignited a fire in the surgical field. The burned bone cement was removed and the artificial joint was implanted with new cement. The patient did not sustain any injuries. The authors recommended appropriate selection and use of bone cement and proper assessment of set time (ie, time needed for final solidification and shaping of the applied cement). The authors' further recommended avoiding use of the ESU during the pick-up time (ie, the minimum time required for putty to increase in viscosity) because the risk for vapor ignition by an ESU is highest during the pick-up time.

4.6.1 Before use of a skin antiseptic, determine the flammable or combustible rating of the skin antiseptic agent by reviewing the applicable safety data sheet (SDS). [Recommendation]

Skin antiseptic solutions can be rated as "combustible" or "flammable" on the SDS. A solution with a rating of "combustible" has a flash point higher than 100° F (37.8° C). A rating of "flammable" indicates a solution that has a flash point lower than 100° F (37.8° C). A combustible solution will burn, but requires a higher temperature for ignition.[101]

4.6.2 **Prevent pooling or soaking of flammable skin antiseptic agents by**
- **using reusable or disposable sterile towels to absorb drips and excess solution during application,**
- **removing materials that are saturated with the skin antiseptic agent before draping the patient, and**
- **moving flammable antiseptic solution–soaked materials away from ignition sources.**[43,44,48,51,53,75,78,82,85,100,102]

[Recommendation]

4.6.3 **Allow flammable skin antiseptic agents to dry completely before sterile drapes are applied.** [Recommendation]

The National Fire Protection Association (NFPA)[100] states that allowing flammable skin antiseptic agents to dry completely before applying drapes helps to prevent the accumulation of volatile fumes beneath the drapes. The volatile fumes are flammable and may ignite without a connection between the ignition source and the antiseptic agent.[43,44,51,62,80,82,88,100,102]

4.6.4 **For surgical procedures that involve the head or neck, use a water-soluble gel to cover the patient's facial hair and use water-based eye lubricants.** [Recommendation]

The patient's hair is a fuel source[43,45,50,51,53,65, 75,77,80,81,84] and covering hair with water-soluble gel decreases the risk of combustion.[99] Eye lubricants that are not water based may be a fuel source.

4.6.5 **Local and state fire regulations must be followed regarding the storage of flammable liquids (eg, acetone, alcohol, alcohol-based skin antiseptic solutions, collodion, hand sanitizer) and the location of dispensers.**[93] [Regulatory Requirement]

4.7 **Use oxidizers (eg, nitrous oxide, oxygen) with caution near any ignition or fuel sources.** [Recommendation]

An environment is oxygen enriched when the oxygen concentration is greater than 21% by volume.[43,45,46,53,55,77] In an oxygen-enriched environment, the temperature and energy required for fuels to ignite is lower than that for ambient or medical air.[44,53,77] Nitrous oxide is considered an oxidizer and requires the same precautions that are used with oxygen.[43,44,50,51,53,55,65,74,77,80,88]

4.7.1 **The anesthesia professional should verify that the anesthesia circuit is free of leaks.** [Recommendation]

Leaks in the anesthesia circuit can increase the oxygen concentration under the drapes, creating an oxygen-enriched environment that increases the risk for fire. The anesthesia circuit includes the endotracheal tube, the seal between the tube and the patient's airway, the bag reservoir, and the tubing that leads from the anesthesia machine to the endotracheal tube.[43,49,52,56,57,59]

Hudson et al[59] reported the case of an intrathoracic fire that occurred as a result of an air leak that caused 100% oxygen to spill into the operative field. When the surgeon used the ESU, the laparotomy sponge in the patient's chest caught on fire. The authors recommended notifying the surgeon immediately if any circuit leak is detected and stopping the use of the electrocautery or other ignition source.

4.7.2 **When an open gas delivery system is used and the surgical procedure is above the xiphoid, take the following steps:**
- **The surgeon should notify the anesthesia professional prior to using an ignition source in the area of the face, head, or neck.**
- **The anesthesia professional should stop or reduce the delivery of supplemental oxygen to the minimum required to avoid hypoxia.**
- **After waiting a few minutes, the anesthesia professional should inform the surgeon that it is okay to activate the ignition source.**
- **The anesthesia professional should evacuate accumulated anesthetic gas before an ignition source is used in or near an oxygen-enriched environment.**

[Recommendation]

The evacuation of anesthetic gases will assist with removing excess oxidizing agents to create an atmosphere that is closer to ambient air.[43,56]

4.7.3 **Use the lowest possible oxygen concentration or flow that provides adequate patient oxygen saturation for a patient who requires supplemental oxygen.**[43,53,55,65] [Recommendation]

4.7.4 A laryngeal mask airway or an endotracheal tube may be used when the patient requires supplementary oxygen greater than 30% and when clinically indicated.[43,81] *[Conditional Recommendation]*

Use of a laryngeal mask airway or an endotracheal tube decreases the risk for fire by decreasing the oxygen concentration under the drapes and in the patient's upper airway.[43,81]

4.7.5 Minimize the potential of airway fires during surgical procedures involving the airway by placing wet radiopaque sponges or throat packs in the back of the patient's throat and inflating endotracheal tube cuffs with tinted solutions. *[Recommendation]*

Placing wet radiopaque sponges in the back of the patient's throat assists with decreasing or preventing oxygen leaks from the endotracheal tube.[43,46,52] Inflating endotracheal tube cuffs with solutions helps increase the temperature required for the endotracheal tube cuff to rupture after being in contact with the ignition source. The tinting of the solution provides a visual indicator of cuff rupture.[43]

4.7.6 When open source oxygen is used, place drapes over the patient's head in a manner that allows the oxygen to flow freely and prevents accumulation under the drapes.[43,45,57,65,103] *[Recommendation]*

4.7.7 During surgical procedures on anatomical structures that present special fire hazards (eg, bowel, trachea), take additional precautions (eg, using a scalpel rather than an electrosurgical active electrode to create the incision). *[Recommendation]*

Hydrogen and methane, which are flammable gases, may be present in the bowel and ignite when they are exposed to an ignition source, such as an active electrosurgical electrode. An oxygen-enriched environment may be present within the trachea because of the presence of anesthesia gases.[43,50,60,74,77,80,81,84]

4.8 Follow the health care organization's policies for communication, suppression, and evacuation procedures in the event of a fire. *[Recommendation]*

Following established procedures assists in protecting patients and perioperative personnel from injury or may decrease the severity of sustained injuries.[43,53,56,61,65,66,69,75,84-86,78,88]

4.8.1 The person who discovers the fire should alert the perioperative team members to the presence of the fire. *[Recommendation]*

The presence of a fire may be indicated by flames, smoke, or sounds consistent with a fire or explosion. Alerting the team allows team members to carry out their responsibilities and decreases the risks of injury to the patient and personnel.[43]

4.8.2 Use water, normal saline, or another safe method of smothering to extinguish a fire, if it can be accomplished safely. *[Recommendation]*

Extinguishing a fire as soon as possible decreases the risk of injury to the patient and personnel.[43,53,60,81,83]

4.8.3 In the event of an airway fire, remove the endotracheal tube immediately; stop flow of all airway gases; remove sponges and any other flammable material from the airway if present; and pour saline into the airway. These steps should be taken in collaboration with the anesthesia professional. *[Recommendation]*

Removing the endotracheal tube removes the source of the fuel, and normal saline cools burned tissue.[43,50,52,84]

4.8.4 In the event of a non-airway fire, the anesthesia professional should immediately stop the flow of all airway gases, and the perioperative team should simultaneously remove the fuel source from the patient and extinguish the fire.[43,65,73] *[Recommendation]*

4.8.5 After the fuel source has been removed from the patient, reestablish ventilation, assess the patient, and report the findings to the surgeon.[43] *[Recommendation]*

4.8.6 After extinguishing the fire, follow the required procedures for reporting and save all items that were involved in the fire.[43] *[Recommendation]*

Saving all items that are involved in the fire is necessary to provide evidence for an investigation. The investigation may be performed by the quality or risk management department personnel but also may involve the local fire department.[43]

4.8.7 Evacuate the OR according to the health care organization's fire plan if perioperative team members are unable to extinguish the fire. *[Recommendation]*

Evacuation protects the patient and perioperative team members from injury from the byproducts of the fire or the fire itself.[43]

4.9 **Disconnect equipment that emits unanticipated smoke, whether in use or not, from the electrical current source. Move the equipment and all of the accessories in use to a safe area, if this can be done safely.** [Recommendation]

Smoke suggests the presence of fire, and equipment may be an ignition source for nearby items. Disconnecting the piece of equipment from the electrical current source and moving the equipment out of the OR decreases the risk to the patient and perioperative team members in that room.[104]

4.9.1 **Evacuate the room immediately if the equipment cannot be removed safely.** [Recommendation]

4.10 **Place fire extinguishers in locations as required by the authority having jurisdiction.**[104] [Recommendation]

4.10.1 **Select fire extinguishers according to standards established by the NFPA 10**[104] **and the authority having jurisdiction. Factors that assist in determining the correct type of fire extinguishers include the**
- **presence of electrical equipment,**[104]
- **hazards that are present and may create adverse chemical reactions with the extinguishing agent,**[104]
- **maintenance requirements,**[93]
- **potential fire size,**[104]
- **physical abilities of the potential users,**[55,80,104]
- **ease of use,**[104] **and**
- **types of fuels that are present.**[104]

[Recommendation]

The NFPA 10[104] recommends that either a water mist or carbon dioxide fire extinguisher be used in the OR. Water mist extinguishers are rated Class 2A:C. Carbon dioxide extinguishers are rated Class B (eg, flammable liquids, alcohol, grease, oil) and Class C (eg, electrical equipment), but also may be used for Class A (eg, wood, cloth, paper) fires.

4.10.2 **Regularly inspect, test, and maintain fire extinguishing equipment and supplies.**[48,104] [Recommendation]

4.10.3 **Do not use fire extinguishers as a first line of defense in a fire.** [Recommendation]

Extinguishing a fire using noncombustible and nonflammable solutions from the back table or a smothering technique can be faster than obtaining a fire extinguisher.[99]

4.10.4 **All perioperative personnel should know the location of medical gas control valves, be able to identify the areas that the valves control, and have the ability to turn the control valves off in the event of a fire.** [Recommendation]

Removing the oxidizer by turning off the medical gas supply assists with breaking the fire triangle.[43]

4.11 **Do not store equipment (eg, case carts, patient beds, stretchers, supply carts) in locations that block access to fire pull alarms, medical gas control valves, or electrical panels.**[48,93] [Recommendation]

4.12 **Do not use fire blankets in an OR.** [Recommendation]

Fire blankets may trap fire next to or under the patient and cause more harm. Fire blankets are made of wool and can burn in an oxygen-enriched environment. During application of a fire blanket, instruments may be dislodged, causing injury to the patient. Usage can lead to wound contamination or spread the fire.[48,55]

4.13 **In collaboration with local authorities, establish evacuation routes for the perioperative environment that are guided by the NFPA regulations.**[93] [Recommendation]

4.13.1 **Provide education to personnel and emergency responders regarding how to implement the evacuation plan.**[43,89,90] [Recommendation]

4.13.2 **Clearly display evacuation routes in multiple locations throughout the health care facility.**[43] [Recommendation]

4.13.3 **The evacuation destination should be the closest safe location where patient care can be continued.**[43] [Recommendation]

4.14 **Provide education and competency verification activities for perioperative team members, according to their roles, on the following topics:**
- **the elements of a fire triangle;**
- **use of the perioperative fire prevention assessment**[80];
- **the locations of fire extinguishers**[43,80];
- **use of fire extinguishers and other fire-fighting equipment**[43,80];
- **evacuation routes**[80];
- **medical gas panel locations and operation, including how to turn them off in an emergency**[43,80];

- the location of shut-off controls for and procedures for turning off electrical systems[80];
- the location of fire alarm pull stations[80];
- how and when to activate the fire safety and evacuation plan[43,80]; and
- the roles and responsibilities of each perioperative team member in various fire scenarios.[43,47,80,81] *[Recommendation]*

The literature supports perioperative education and training that includes fire safety protocols, preparing for surgical fires, and participating in mock fire drills. Fire safety training prepares the perioperative team to respond quickly and appropriately in the event of a fire.[43,48,65,80]

4.14.1 **Hold fire drills periodically as required by the local authority having jurisdiction.** *[Recommendation]*

The NFPA 101[93] recommends that fire drills be held at least quarterly on each shift. The NFPA 99[100] recommends holding fire drills that include evacuation annually or as determined by the relevant building code. The local authority having jurisdiction may not have adopted the most current NFPA guidelines and therefore may be following the earlier edition.[43,93,100]

5. Electrical Equipment

5.1 **Take precautions to mitigate the risk for injury associated with the use of electrical equipment.** *[Recommendation]*

Injuries to patients, personnel, or visitors may occur from medical equipment that has frayed cords, from damaged outlets, or from extension cords.[100]

5.2 **Inspect all electrical equipment, including all loaned equipment, for damage periodically and before each use.** *[Recommendation]*

Damaged electrical equipment and power cords can cause unsafe conditions. Power cords are frequently subject to damage from daily use.[100]

Fires related to improper cleaning or malfunctions of booms and other equipment have been reported.[21] The ECRI Institute[105] reported that one of the top 10 health technology hazards for 2017 was equipment device failures caused by use of improper cleaning products and practices. Improper cleaning practices may create the potential for equipment malfunction and can result in damage to power supplies, electronics, and motors.

5.2.1 **Check power cords for fraying and examine the strain relief and plugs for damage.**[100] *[Recommendation]*

5.2.2 **Remove equipment that is found to be in disrepair, including the electrical cord, immediately from service.** *[Recommendation]*

Using equipment that is in a state of disrepair can create unsafe conditions.[100]

5.3 **Use device cords that are secured and have the appropriate characteristics for the intended use, including adequate length.** *[Recommendation]*

Cords that do not lie flat create the risk of tripping or accidental unplugging of the equipment.[106,107] A cord may cause damage to the machine if it does not meet the necessary electrical characteristics (eg, grounding resistance, power cord ampacity, correct polarization).[100] Adequate length of device cords from the device to the electrical outlet decreases the risk of tripping or accidental unplugging of the equipment.[40,100]

5.3.1 **Do not change device cords unless the replacement cord meets the electrical characteristic of the original cord.** *[Recommendation]*

Changing the device cord may nullify the device warranty. The cord may cause damage to the equipment if the electrical characteristics do not match the characteristics of the original cord.[100]

5.3.2 **Secure cords in a safe manner with an electrically safe device as defined by the NFPA.**[100] *[Recommendation]*

Safely securing cords helps prevent trips and falls.[40] Using an electrically safe device to secure cords decreases the potential for an electrical shock.[100]

5.3.3 **Use an extension cord only if it has the correct electrical characteristics.** *[Recommendation]*

Incorrect electrical characteristics can cause damage to the equipment and overheating of the cord.[48,100]

5.3.4 **Mount multiple outlet connections to a movable equipment assembly (eg, cart, table, pedestal, boom), provided that the cord and the connection have the capacity to allow the total number of amps required to pass through the cord without creating unsafe conditions. Calculate the total number of amps by adding together the amps required by each piece of equipment.** *[Recommendation]*

The use of a multiple outlet connection allows for multiple pieces of equipment to be plugged in to one connection so only one cord is on the floor instead of one cord for each piece of equipment.[100]

5.4 Label all electrical equipment charger adaptor cords with the name of the piece of equipment to which they belong. [Recommendation]

Equipment has been reported to overheat and malfunction when incorrect charger adaptor cords are used.[108]

6. Warming Cabinets

6.1 Take precautions to reduce the risk for thermal injuries related to warming solutions, blankets, and linens in blanket and solution-warming cabinets. [Recommendation]

The danger of burns from heated solutions, blankets, or linens is increased in the perioperative setting because patients may be unconscious or sedated and not able to feel an increase in temperature or communicate discomfort. Even when solutions and blankets do not feel warm to the touch, heat continues to build in these items and can be transferred to the patient.[109]

Injuries to the patient can result from irrigation solution being warmed to high temperatures. In one report, a patient experienced full-thickness skin burns and joint damage from irrigation solutions that were warmed in a cabinet in which the temperature ranged from 100.4° F (38° C) on the top shelf to 118.4° F (48° C) on the bottom shelf.[110]

6.2 Store solutions, blankets, and linens in separate warming cabinets or in cabinets with separate compartments that have independent temperature controls. [Recommendation]

Using separate temperature-controlled warming cabinets allows for better temperature control compared to single compartment cabinets. Separate compartments with separate controls allow for each compartment to be set to an individual temperature and for accurate regulation of both cabinets. Fluids cannot be warmed to the same temperature as blankets because fluids attain a higher temperature and retain the temperature longer, presenting a greater risk for thermal injury.[109]

6.2.1 Label warming cabinets to identify items that may be placed within the cabinet and the maximum permissible temperature settings. If the cabinet has separate compartments, label each compartment.[109] [Recommendation]

6.3 Set, maintain, and monitor warming cabinet temperatures according to organizational policy. [Recommendation]

Monitoring the temperature of warming cabinets is necessary to verify that temperature settings are maintained within specified limits.[109] A malfunctioning cabinet can cause temperature variation.[110]

6.3.1 Equip warming cabinets with an alarm mechanism that will alert personnel to an equipment failure. [Recommendation]

The equipment alarm will notify personnel so that corrective action can be taken in a timely manner.

6.3.2 Take precautions when a warming cabinet malfunctions, including
- removing the cabinet from service;
- labeling the cabinet as out of order;
- removing all solutions, blankets, and patient linens from the warmer;
- not using blankets if they are overheated until the temperatures are within the acceptable range;
- following the fluid manufacturers' written IFU to determine the usability of solutions; and
- reporting the malfunction to the facility clinical engineering department for repair and maintenance.

[Recommendation]

6.3.3 Rotate warming cabinet contents on a first-in, first-out basis. [Recommendation]

6.4 Provide the number of warming cabinets that is sufficient to support the anticipated need for warmed items. [Recommendation]

Perioperative personnel have been reported to use unsafe means, such as autoclaves or microwaves, to warm blankets.[111] When the supply of warm blankets is not sufficient, staff members may increase the temperature of the warmer, which can cause overheating of the blankets and potentially lead to burns.[109,112]

6.5 Have an interdisciplinary team conduct a risk assessment to establish and implement a maximum temperature limit for blanket-warming cabinets based on evidence and the cabinet manufacturer's IFU. [Recommendation]

The evidence conflicts about the optimal temperature for blanket-warming cabinets. The ECRI Institute investigated multiple cases of patient burns at hospitals during a 10-year period. Three patients at three different hospitals sustained burns from blankets heated in warming cabinets set to higher than 130° F (54.4° C).[113] The patients received rolled or folded blankets and were sedated or anesthetized.

Sutton et al[114] conducted a quasi-experimental study at a 384-bed metropolitan medical center to examine blanket thermal behavior and the blanket temperature preference of postoperative patients. The intervention group (n = 76) received blankets warmed to 155° F (68° C), whereas the control group (n = 110) received blankets warmed to 110° F (43° C). The researchers found the intervention group had higher skin temperatures and more thermal comfort throughout the 10 minutes of data collection. The researchers concluded blankets warmed to 150° F (66° C) are safe to use, and patients experienced a higher thermal comfort level. The limitations of this study are that participants were awake postoperative patients and that the study did not address the risk for potential thermal injuries ranging from minor skin irritation to partial- or full-thickness burns from the increased temperature setting when blankets are folded or rolled against the skin of semiconscious patients.

Kelly et al[115] conducted a randomized descriptive comparative study at a large urban hospital to determine the time-dependent cooling of cotton blankets after their removal from warming cabinets at two temperatures. The participants (N = 20) received one or two blankets warmed in 130° F (54° C) or 200° F (93° C) cabinets. The researchers found no skin temperature approached levels that cause epidermal damage. They recommended warming cotton blankets in cabinets set at 200° F (93° C) or less to improve thermal comfort without compromising patient safety.

In a similar randomized descriptive comparative study, Kelly et al[116] measured skin temperature and thermal comfort in healthy volunteers before and after the application of rolled and folded dry cotton blankets that were warmed in cabinets at 130° F (54° C) or 200° F (93° C). Study participants (N = 20) received each type of blanket at each of the warmed temperatures. The folded blanket was applied to the volunteer's back and the rolled blanket was applied to the neck. Skin temperatures from blankets warmed to 200° F (93° C) were greater than those from blankets warmed to 130° F (54° C). There was no evidence of skin temperature elevated high enough or long enough to cause dermal injury.

The limitations of these studies include having only awake, healthy, volunteer participants and small sample sizes.

6.6 Follow the solution manufacturers' IFU regarding the maximum temperature and length of time solutions should remain in the warming cabinet or compartment and for usability after removal. [Recommendation]

Solution manufacturers' recommendations for maximum temperature setting, time limit that solutions may remain in the warming device, and solution use after removal vary. Manufacturers' settings may be determined by the stability of the container and the solution.[109]

6.6.1 When solutions are placed in warming cabinets, label them with the date of insertion or the date the solutions should be removed from the warmer. [Recommendation]

Labeling identifies when a solution has reached its maximum shelf life and prevents overheating related to being left in the warmer too long.

6.6.2 Measure the temperatures of solutions on the sterile field before administration. [Recommendation]

Burns have been associated with the administration of overheated solutions. Huang et al[110] reported the case of a patient undergoing a routine knee arthroscopy who sustained full-thickness skin burns from 2 L arthroscopic fluid irrigation that was warmed in a fluid-heating cabinet. The fluid-heating cabinet temperature was measured to range from 38.5° C (101.3° F) at the top to 48.5° C (119.3° F) at the bottom of the warming cabinet. The patient required debridement of soft tissues, a gastrocnemius muscle flap, and split thickness skin grafting. The damage to his joint required a joint fusion with an external fixator. On postoperative day 48, the patient was discharged to a rehabilitation facility. The authors suggest that the temperature of any warmed arthroscopic irrigation fluid should be measured before and during its use because the warming cabinet may have temperature variations despite having an external monitor.

6.6.3 Warm solutions intended for IV administration using technology designed for this purpose. [Recommendation]

The temperature of solutions warmed in warming cabinets will vary depending on the design of the cabinet, load configuration, and the elapsed time from the removal of the solution from the cabinet to administration of the solution to the patient.[109,117] Using technology designed specifically to warm IV solutions provides accurate and consistent fluid temperature.

6.7 Do not warm skin antiseptic agents unless this is allowed in the manufacturer's IFU. [Recommendation]

Heating may alter the chemical composition and effectiveness of the skin antiseptic.

7. Medical Gases

7.1 Take precautions to mitigate risks associated with handling, storage, and use of compressed medical gas cylinders and liquid oxygen containers. *[Recommendation]*

The US Food and Drug Administration (FDA) has received reports of patient deaths and injuries related to connection errors in medical gas systems.[118]

7.2 Determine storage conditions for medical gases by the volume stored in a location, the need for immediate use, and regulatory requirements. *[Recommendation]*

The NFPA and regulatory agencies have determined the various medical gas storage condition requirements and are responsible for enforcement.[100]

7.2.1 Store an adequate emergency supply of oxygen at the facility to provide an uninterrupted supply for 1 day.[100] *[Recommendation]* **A**

7.2.2 Medical gases must be stored in secured locations and separately from industrial gases. *[Regulatory Requirement]*

The FDA considers compressed medical gases to be drugs for dispensing by prescription only.[100,119,120]

7.2.3 The combined volume of medical gas cylinders not considered to be for immediate patient use should not exceed 3,000 cu ft per **smoke compartment**. *[Recommendation]*

Cylinders on patient gurneys are considered to be in use or for immediate patient use. Cylinders and carts directly associated with a specific patient are considered to be in use. Cylinder and carts not directly associated with a specific patient for 30 minutes or more are considered not in use or in storage.[100]

7.2.4 Store medical gas cylinders that are not intended for immediate use indoors and
- in a room with a minimum 1-hour fire resistance rating,
- in a holder or storage rack with a chain-like securing device, and
- away from heat sources.

[Recommendation]

Securing cylinders with a chain-like securing device or in a rack prevents the cylinders from falling over.[100]

7.2.5 Do not store medical gas cylinders in an egress hallway.[100] *[Recommendation]*

7.2.6 Keep empty medical gas cylinders segregated from full cylinders. *[Recommendation]*

Segregating empty cylinders from full ones minimizes the risk of connecting to an empty cylinder and delaying administration of vital gases to the patient.[100]

7.3 Transport medical gas cylinders secured in a carrier that is designed to prevent the cylinder from tipping or being dropped or damaged. *[Recommendation]*

Transporting a cylinder without using an appropriate carrier increases the potential for damage to the cylinder and causing sudden release of the compressed gas, which can cause propulsion of the cylinder and subsequent injury.[100]

7.4 Secure medical gas cylinders used during patient transport to the transport cart or bed in holders designed for this purpose. *[Recommendation]*

Holders minimize the risk of the cylinder falling, which can cause propulsion of the cylinder and subsequent injury. Many transport carts are available with built-in holders.[100]

7.5 Check gas cylinders before use for the appropriate label, pin-index safety system connector, and color coding. *[Recommendation]*

The color of the cylinder, written labels, and a unique pin-index safety system connector are used to clearly identify the medical gas contained within a medical gas cylinder.[100]

The pin-index safety system connector for different medical gases prevents connecting the wrong gas to the delivery system.[121] The Compressed Gas Association has approved standardized colors for identification of different medical gases (eg, green indicates oxygen).[100,122] Serious injuries and deaths have resulted from the use of an incorrectly identified medical gas.[118]

7.6 Do not alter the fittings on medical gas cylinders and hoses.[100] *[Recommendation]*

Serious injuries and deaths have resulted from altering of the pin-index safety system, thereby permitting delivery of an incorrect gas into the medical gas administration system.[118,123]

7.6.1 If the fitting does not connect easily, recheck the label on the gas cylinder or hose to verify that it is correct.[100,123] *[Recommendation]*

7.6.2   If the label is correct, return the cylinder to the distributor for examination.[100] *[Recommendation]*

7.6.3   If the label is incorrect, replace the cylinder with a correctly labeled gas cylinder.[100] *[Recommendation]*

7.7   Use only approved regulators or other flow control devices.[100,123] *[Recommendation]*

7.7.1   Inspect the regulator, gasket, and washers before use.[123] *[Recommendation]*

7.7.2   Tighten the regulator with a T-handle until it is firmly in place. *[Recommendation]*

7.8   Take precautions during use of medical gas cylinder valves. *[Recommendation]*

Improper use of a medical gas cylinder valve can result in contamination of the gas and leakage of the contents into the environment.[100]

7.8.1   When a cylinder valve is opened, release a small amount of gas before attaching the regulator. *[Recommendation]*

Opening the valve removes any dust that may have accumulated.[100,123]

7.8.2   Open the valve slowly to determine whether there is a leak, and close the valve quickly if a leak is found. *[Recommendation]*

7.8.3   Open compressed medical gas tank valves fully during use.[100] *[Recommendation]*

7.8.4   Close the valves on medical gas cylinders properly to avoid leakage during storage. *[Recommendation]* **Ⓐ**

7.9   Liquid oxygen containers must be handled, filled, stored, and transported according to state and federal regulations and manufacturers' written instructions and labeling.[100] *[Regulatory Requirement]*

7.9.1   Store liquid oxygen containers
- outside of the building in a cool, dry place or
- inside the building as long as the containers
  - are secured to prevent them from tipping over,
  - do not interfere with foot traffic,
  - are not exposed to open flames or high-temperature devices, and
  - are not subject to damage from falling devices.[100]

[Recommendation]

8. Waste Anesthesia Gases

8.1   Take precautions to mitigate hazards related to waste anesthesia gases. *[Recommendation]*

The adverse health effects of exposure to trace amounts of waste anesthesia gases is currently unknown. The International Agency for Research on Cancer classifies volatile anesthetics as group 3, which is defined as not classifiable as to its carcinogenicity to humans.[124] A literature review revealed that the effects of waste anesthesia gases are disputed and the acceptable occupational levels vary by country.[125] A NIOSH report shows inconsistencies in the literature regarding the effects of waste anesthesia gases, confirms the means of exposure, and provides guidance for reducing exposures.[126] All anesthesia machines have the potential to leak, which increases the level of waste anesthesia gases in the ambient air.[127]

A study of 15,317 live births between 1990 and 2000 to 9,433 mothers who were exposed to waste anesthesia gases consisting of halothane, isoflurane, sevoflurane, and nitrous oxide revealed a potential exposure-response relationship between gas exposure and the development of congenital anomalies in the children, although the study did not establish a causal link. Results suggest the anomalies may correlate with the type of waste anesthesia gas to which the mother was exposed.[128]

A report of two cases from 2008 suggests a potential relationship between personnel exposure to high nitrous oxide concentrations and persistent cognitive deficits.[129]

A study in Poland involving 55 female nurses and 29 male anesthesiologists showed a link between waste nitrous oxide and DNA damage. If the concentration of nitrous oxide exceeded the occupational exposure level of 180 mg/m^3, the genetic injury was aggravated. In contrast, the researchers found no significant correlation between the DNA damage score and exposure to sevoflurane and isoflurane.[130]

A British study revealed a link between lower vitamin B$_{12}$ metabolism and levels of nitrous oxide greater than the recommended occupational exposure level, but no link existed if the level was less than the occupational exposure level.[131]

Baysal et al[132] examined 30 OR personnel and 30 non-OR personnel for DNA damage. The OR personnel had been exposed to a complex mixture of halothane, isoflurane, sevoflurane, nitrous oxide, and desflurane. The researchers found a correlation between levels of waste anesthesia gases and DNA damage. They also found a correlation between DNA damage and an increased oxidative stress index and total oxidative status.

Rozgaj et al[133] measured DNA damage in 50 OR personnel (ie, anesthesiologists, technicians, nurses) and 50 non-OR personnel in a facility in Croatia. A gas scavenging system was in use at the facility. The researchers found the presence of DNA damage in all participants who had been exposed to sevoflurane, isoflurane and nitrous oxide. Similar results were found in a study by Chandrasekhar et al[134] that took place in India and involved a group of 45 OR personnel who had been exposed to waste anesthesia gases and 45 non-exposed health care workers. The OR personnel had been exposed to a mixture of halothane, isoflurane, sevoflurane, sodium pentothal, nitrous oxide, desflurane, and enflurane.

A descriptive study in Turkey revealed that a group of anesthesiologists who were exposed to higher than the NIOSH-acceptable levels of waste anesthesia gases (ie, sevoflurane and nitrous oxide) experienced higher levels of sister chromatid exchanges (ie, DNA mutation) compared to internists who did not work in the OR, and the levels dropped after a 2-month absence from the OR. These ORs did not have scavenging systems or low-leakage anesthesia machines, and no preventive maintenance had been performed.[135]

8.2 Establish a waste anesthesia gas management program to be in compliance with the NIOSH recommendations. *[Recommendation]*

The NIOSH standard for nitrous oxide exposure levels is no more than 25 parts per million (ppm) during an 8-hour period and no more than 2 ppm of any halogenated anesthetic agent in 1 continuous hour.[136]

8.2.1 In the waste anesthesia gas management program, define the engineering controls, work practice controls, administrative controls, personal protective equipment and monitoring requirements for each type of anesthesia being used. *[Recommendation]*

One study showed various types of leaks were present during anesthesia administration.[137] Higher levels of waste anesthesia gases related to the use of uncuffed endotracheal tubes and during induction with a mask were reported in a review of the literature.[138] Researchers who compared four different administration techniques found that variance in the level of waste anesthesia gases was related to the administration technique.[139]

8.3 Anesthesia delivery systems located throughout the facility must be in proper working order and maintained on a regularly scheduled basis, consistent with the manufacturer's written instructions and organizational policy and procedures.[127,136] *[Regulatory Requirement]*

A report summarizing the results of one facility's testing of 24 anesthesia machine revealed differing high- and low-level leaks at the time of testing. One group of machines had leaks primarily at the absorbent canister bases. The remainder of the machines had leaks in other locations.[140] It is required by OSHA and recommended by NIOSH that a program for routine inspection and maintenance of all anesthesia machines be in place.[127,136]

9. Latex-Safe Environment

9.1 Develop and implement a protocol to establish a natural rubber latex–safe environment. *[Recommendation]*

Natural rubber latex has been identified as a common cause of anaphylaxis during surgical and interventional procedures.[141-143] There is a large body of moderate-quality evidence that establishes that frequent exposure to natural rubber latex is an occupational risk factor for development of latex sensitivity,[144-151] latex allergy,[144-155] and anaphylaxis[144-146,149,150,152-155] among health care workers (eg, RNs, clinical support personnel, housekeepers, physicians, physiotherapists, technicians).[144-146,148-153,155] An observational study performed at two facilities in Wisconsin found that health care providers are exposed to latex antigens from airborne sources, and the use of powder-free latex gloves reduces the risk of sensitization.[156]

Perioperative health care personnel and patients are at high risk for developing latex sensitivity, latex allergy, and anaphylaxis from exposure to latex.[144-155,157] Routes of exposure to natural rubber latex identified in the literature include

- direct external contact (eg, natural rubber latex gloves, face masks, blood pressure cuff tubing)[144,146-155,157];
- airborne sources that can affect the mucous membranes of the eyes, nose, trachea, bronchi and bronchioles, and oropharynx[144-153];
- particles that are swallowed after entering the nasopharynx or oropharynx[144-147,150-154];
- direct contact of the mucous membranes with indwelling natural rubber latex devices such as catheters[144,147,148,151,152,154,157];
- internal patient exposure from health care provider use of natural rubber latex gloves during surgical procedures[144,146-151,153,157]; and
- internally placed natural rubber latex devices, such as wound drains.[144,148,149,154,155,158]

Reactions to latex can include dermal or cutaneous symptoms such as contact dermatitis,[144-147,149-152,155,157] eczema,[145,149,151,153] redness or itching,[144,147-149,153,157] and urticaria[144-147,149-151,155] and respiratory or non-cutaneous symptoms such as anaphylaxis,[144,145,149-155,157] asthma,[144-146,149-151,153] red and itchy eyes,[144,148-151,153] and rhinitis.[144-151,153] The quality of life for those allergic to latex is improved by avoiding latex.[144-151,153-155] The symptoms of a reaction may resolve quickly after the source of the latex protein has been removed, but the immunoglobulin E (IgE)—a class of antibody that indicates continued sensitivity—remains in the body for at least 5 years.

9.2 Purchase products made from alternatives to natural rubber latex, if available. *[Recommendation]*

9.2.1 Maintain a list of supplies for products that contain natural rubber latex and alternatives that do not contain natural rubber latex.[144,151,157-159] *[Recommendation]*

The American Latex Allergy Association[159] and the Spina Bifida Association of America[158] maintain an electronic listing of products that contain latex and alternatives that do not contain latex.

9.3 Assess all patients preoperatively for latex sensitivity risk factors. *[Recommendation]*

Early recognition of risk factors for sensitivity and implementation of a latex-safety protocol can prevent the progression of anaphylaxis.[144,154,155] Anaphylaxis to latex usually presents during the maintenance phase of anesthesia.[154,157] **Latex sensitization** reportedly occurs in 17% to 25% of health care workers, and in 27% of patients with spina bifida,[149,152] and more frequently in patients with a history of multiple surgical procedures than those who have fewer procedures.[154]

9.3.1 Include the following risk factors for latex sensitivity in the preoperative assessment:
- a history of long-term bladder care[144,152];
- a history of spina bifida, spinal cord trauma, and urogenital abnormalities in children[144,152,154];
- a history of multiple surgical procedures[144,146-152,154];
- occupational exposure to latex, such as work in health care[144-155,160];
- food allergies (eg, avocado, banana, kiwi, chestnuts, raw potato)[144,149-152,154];
- a history of frequent gynecological examinations, obstetric procedures, or contact with latex-containing contraceptives (ie, diaphragms, condoms)[144,160]; and
- a history of symptoms of
  o asthma,[144-146,149-151,153,161]
  o dermatitis,[144-147,149-152,155,157]
  o eczema,[144,145,149,151,153]
  o contact dermatitis, especially of the hands,[144-147,149-152,155,157]
  o contact urticaria,[144-147,149-151,155]
  o hay fever,[146,149,153,161] and
  o rhinitis.[144-146,149,151,153,161]

[Recommendation]

9.4 Implement latex precautions for patients with latex sensitivity or allergy.[144,146-148,150-155,157] *[Recommendation]*

Latex precautions in health care settings have helped reduce the risk to patients and have led to a decline in latex-triggered anaphylaxis.[150,152,154]

9.4.1 Identify patients with a sensitivity or allergy to latex with a wristband[154,157] or bracelet[144,152,157] and on the patient's medical record. *[Recommendation]*

These interventions provide multiple visual cues for health care team members and promote patient safety.[144,154]

9.4.2 During care of a patient with latex sensitivity who requires surgery or another invasive procedure in an environment that is not latex-safe,
- remove all products containing natural rubber latex from the room the evening before the procedure, except those that are sealed or contained[144,154];
- avoid using products containing natural rubber latex during terminal cleaning of the room the evening before the procedure[144,154];
- schedule an elective surgery as the first procedure of the day[144,154];
- restrict traffic and equipment in the OR before and during the procedure[154]; and
- when no alternative to a product containing natural rubber latex is available, provide a barrier between the latex-containing products and the patient's skin.

[Recommendation]

In a literature review, Worth and Sheikh[154] found that removing latex-containing products from the room the evening before a procedure and using latex-free products during terminal cleaning may reduce the release of latex particles. Scheduling an elective procedure as the first procedure of the day provides time for room air to be completely exchanged after terminal cleaning.[144,154]

9.4.3 Post signs stating "latex allergy" before the start of the procedure on all doors leading into the OR where the procedure will be performed.[154,157,160] *[Recommendation]*

9.4.4 After surgery, transfer the patient to a latex-safe care area, if one is available.[144] *[Recommendation]*

9.5 Include latex sensitivity in all hand-over communications during the transfer of patient care.[144,154,157] *[Recommendation]*

Communication failures during the transfer of information are common in the perioperative setting, and failure to communicate a patient's latex sensitivity or allergy could compromise the patient's safety.[94,162]

The Pennsylvania Patient Safety Authority 2018 report[157] indicates that perioperative settings are high-risk areas where latex exposures and near misses continue to occur. The report also states that urinary catheters made of latex accounted for more exposures than latex gloves. The Pennsylvania Patient Safety Authority recommends sharing information about a patient's allergy to latex during hand-over communication to prevent latex exposures.

9.6 Wear low-protein, powder-free, natural rubber latex gloves[144,145,147,149,151,152,154,160] or gloves labeled as "not made with natural rubber latex."[144,151,157,160] *[Recommendation]*

Moderate-quality evidence is clear that health care personnel are susceptible to developing latex allergies when they are exposed to latex gloves and glove powder.[144-155] Use of low-protein, powder-free natural rubber latex gloves or latex-free gloves can minimize latex exposure and the risk of reactions in both health care workers and patients.[144-147,149,151,152,154,160] Studies have shown that using low-protein, powder-free, natural rubber latex gloves or latex-free gloves significantly reduces natural rubber latex aeroallergens in the environment, as well as sensitivity and asthma in health care workers.[144-147,149,151,152,154,160]

Phaswana and Naidoo[148] conducted a nonexperimental study to evaluate the prevalence of latex sensitization and latex allergy among 510 health care workers who used either lightly powdered latex gloves (exposed) or hypoallergenic powder-free gloves (unexposed) in a hospital setting in South Africa. The participants completed a questionnaire and underwent skin-prick testing. The researchers found the overall prevalence of latex sensitization and latex allergy to be 5.9% (n = 29) and 4.6% (n = 23), respectively. The prevalence of latex sensitization was higher among the exposed group (7.1%) than the unexposed group (3.1%) and was higher among those who were exposed and had an employment duration of less than 10 years. The researchers indicated the

elimination of powdered latex gloves has reduced the concentration of aeroallergens in the OR as evidenced by the low prevalence of latex allergy in the study population. The researchers concluded that despite the availability of powder-free hypoallergenic gloves, health care workers exhibited latex sensitivity and latex allergy symptoms, and these continue to be an important occupational hazard for health care workers.

9.6.1 For patients with latex sensitivity or allergy, perioperative personnel wearing gloves made of natural rubber latex should remove the gloves, wash their hands, and don gloves that are not made of natural rubber latex before entering the room. *[Recommendation]*

Natural rubber latex proteins on gloves bind to the glove powder (eg, cornstarch powder) and release allergens into the air when gloves are removed.[144,147,148,151,152,154,155,160]

10. Chemicals

10.1 Take precautions to mitigate the risks associated with the use of chemicals in the perioperative setting. *[Recommendation]*

Improper handling of chemicals can result in injury to health care workers and patients. Injuries may result from exposure of any portion of the body, including the integumentary, reproductive, or respiratory systems.[163-176]

Casey et al[174] conducted a cross-sectional research study to evaluate use of environmental disinfectant products among 163 health care workers in Morgantown, West Virginia. The air quality was measured in the breathing zones of the environmental health care workers while they performed their regular cleaning duties. The air quality samples were analyzed for the three chemicals found in the environmental disinfectants: hydrogen peroxide, peracetic acid, and acetic acid. The researchers found that the air quality measurements were well below the OSHA permissible exposure limits. However, they found higher levels of chemical in the labor and delivery department. This was a result of short-term patient stays that required consecutive terminal cleaning, quick turnaround times, and frequent admissions.

In addition, the researchers compared health care workers who used disinfectants and those who did not use disinfectants who reported asthma-like symptoms, eye irritation, and nasal problems in a survey. The researchers observed an increase in work-related asthma-like symptoms, eye irritation, and nasal problems after use of the disinfectant. They did not find a significant difference in the prevalence of asthma between health care workers who did or did not use disinfectants. However, the researchers concluded that the use of environmental products that contain acetic acid, hydrogen peroxide, and peracetic acid may result in adverse health effects among health care workers exposed to these products.

10.2 The health care organization must follow the most stringent federal, state, or local regulations for chemical handling and disposal.[163,177] *[Regulatory Requirement]*

State and local requirements may be more stringent than federal regulations. The most stringent regulations take precedence over less-restrictive regulations.

10.3 For every potentially hazardous chemical, an SDS must be readily accessible to employees either electronically or in print within the practice setting.[163] *[Regulatory Requirement]*

Safety data sheets include information on hazard identification; recommendations for precautions or special handling; signs and symptoms of toxic exposure; first aid treatments for exposure; and other information, including pictograms and signal words (eg, danger, warning).[163,178]

10.4 A chemical hazard risk assessment for all chemicals within the facility must be performed annually using the SDS and the manufacturer's IFU for each chemical.[163,178] Include the following in the assessment:
- chemical identification and properties,[163]
- information on the composition or list of ingredients of each chemical,[163]
- disposal requirements,[163]
- exposure control measures,[163]
- first aid measures,[163]
- fire safety measures,[163]
- handling and storage requirements,[163]
- hazard identification,[163]
- PPE measures,[163,179]
- reproductive toxicity (eg, risk of spontaneous abortion),[163,176]
- whether a chemical that has less risk of causing and injury can be used, and
- whether a chemical that is present is no longer being used and therefore should be discarded.

[Regulatory Requirement]

The risk assessment helps determine the precautions to take and provides information for developing an action plan in the event of spills or exposures.

10.5 All chemicals must be handled according to their respective SDS and the manufacturer's IFU, including
- disinfectants and sterilants (eg, glutaraldehyde, ortho-phthalaldehyde, ethylene oxide, hydrogen peroxide, peracetic acid),[165,180,181]
- tissue preservatives (eg, formalin),[164] and
- antiseptic agents (eg, hand hygiene products, surgical prep solutions, alcohol).[93,182,183]

[Regulatory Requirement]

10.6 An emergency spill plan must be developed for chemicals listed in the chemical hazard risk assessment, if required by regulation. *[Regulatory Requirement]*

Some chemicals may not require an emergency spill plan, or the requirement may be based on the volume of the chemical spilled (eg, formaldehyde, glutaraldehyde). A written emergency spill plan for each chemical identified in the chemical hazard risk assessment is an OSHA requirement.[177]

10.7 Chemicals must be stored according to
- federal, state, and local regulations[163,180];
- SDS information[163,180];
- manufacturers' IFU[163,180]; and
- flammability and combustibility.[163,180]

[Regulatory Requirement]

10.8 The health care organization must provide PPE for employees who handle chemicals in the workplace.[179] *[Regulatory Requirement]*

Personal protective equipment is defined as any clothing or other equipment that protects a person from exposure to chemicals. It may include gloves, aprons, chemical splash goggles, and impervious clothing.[179] Scrub clothes and lab coats worn by health care workers are not considered PPE because they are not impervious.[184]

10.8.1 Perioperative personnel must wear PPE during exposure and handling of hazardous chemicals.[179] *[Regulatory Requirement]*

10.9 The health care organization must develop a respiratory protection plan for each chemical listed in the chemical hazard risk assessment.[185] *[Regulatory Requirement]*

Use of respiratory protection including local exhaust ventilation (eg, hoods) or general ventilation above a designated number of air changes per hour is an OSHA[185] requirement. Respirators are required as a portion of the respiratory protection plan for certain chemicals and when the appropriate ventilation cannot be provided.

10.10 Eyewash stations, either plumbed or self-contained, must be provided where chemicals that are hazardous to the eyes are located.[186] *[Regulatory Requirement]*

10.10.1 Plumbed eyewash stations should deliver warm water (ie, 60° F to 100° F [16° C to 38° C]) at a rate of 1.5 L/minute.[186] *[Recommendation]*

10.10.2 Plumbed eyewash stations should be flushed weekly.[186] *[Recommendation]*

Weekly flushing removes stagnant water, which may contain microbial contamination, from the system.[186]

10.10.3 Eyewash stations should be located so that travel time is no greater than 10 seconds from the location of chemical use or storage, or should be immediately available if the chemical is caustic or is a strong acid.[186] *[Recommendation]*

10.10.4 All eyewash stations must be inspected on an annual basis or when a concern is reported.[186] *[Regulatory Requirement]*

10.11 Health care organizations must provide education to employees about the hazardous chemicals in the workplace.[163] *[Regulatory Requirement]*

10.12 Safe practices must be established and implemented for the use of methyl methacrylate (MMA) as required by federal, state, and local regulation.[187,188] *[Regulatory Requirement]*

Bone cement is a combination of MMA monomer, which is a liquid, and beads of polymethyl methacrylate or a polymethyl methacrylate-based polymer.[189] The liquid portion of MMA can be absorbed through the skin and respiratory tract and by ingestion and may cause irritation to the area exposed.[188,190] The OSHA permissible exposure limit for MMA is 100 ppm or a time-weighted average of 410 mg/m³.[187,188]

Karnwal et al[168] reported that some studies suggest MMA can cause birth defects in pregnant animals exposed to extremely high levels. It is not known whether MMA can affect pregnancy in humans and further research is warranted.

10.12.1 The health care organization must provide PPE for employees who handle MMA. *[Regulatory Requirement]*

The use of PPE reduces the risk of handling MMA and exposure of perioperative personnel.[179]

10.12.2 Perioperative personnel must wear eye protection when mixing and inserting MMA bone cement.[179,188] *[Regulatory Requirement]*

Methyl methacrylate fumes may irritate the eyes.[168,188,190,191]

10.12.3 Do not allow mixed cement to come in contact with gloves until it has reached the dough stage. Wear a second pair of gloves made of the material recommended in the MMA manufacturer's IFU and then discard them after contact with the cement. *[Recommendation]*

Methyl methacrylate can penetrate many plastic and latex compounds and can be absorbed through the skin, leading to contact dermatitis. The liquid portion of MMA can be absorbed through the skin and respiratory tract and by ingestion and may cause irritation to the area exposed.[188,190]

Ponce et al[169] reported the case of an orthopedic perioperative RN who developed an occupational allergic contact dermatitis of his hands after handling MMA for knee replacements. The RN experienced blistering, edema, erythema, and cracking of the fingertips and sides of the second, third, and fourth fingers of the right hand and the fourth finger of the left hand. The authors indicated that surgical gloves may not provide protection, as acrylates can penetrate rubber; MMA is capable of easily dissolving plastic and synthetic rubber compounds. Despite wearing two pairs of rubber or nitrile gloves, the orthopedic RN continued to develop erythema and itching and small vesicles formed on his fingertips.

10.12.4 Use a closed system when mixing MMA.[190,191] *[Recommendation]*

Closed mixing systems help reduce exposure to MMA. Closed mixing systems, with or without a vacuum, release less MMA vapor into the breathing zone of the surgical team compared with open mixing systems.[190,192]

Jelecevic et al[191] conducted a nonexperimental study to evaluate the use of two commonly used vacuum mixing systems for effectiveness in preventing MMA vapor release in a simulated laboratory and OR environment. The researchers identified three main causes of MMA vapor leakage into the environment during use of vacuum mixing systems for bone cements in orthopedic procedures. The first occurs during filling of the cartridge with the MMA liquid, the second occurs during mixing of the bone cement, and the third occurs during evacuation of the bone cement out of the mixing cartridge and handling of the cement as the reaction progresses.

However, the researchers concluded that vacuum mixing systems can significantly reduce MMA vapor concentrations in the OR compared to the traditional open hand mixing, thus reducing occupational exposures.

Downes et al[171] conducted a literature review that included studies on occupational exposure to MMA and the risk to pregnant or lactating women. The researchers indicated the risk of exposure to high levels of MMA in the OR is minimal, and the potential risk of adverse effects in pregnant and lactating personnel in the orthopedic OR is low. They suggested that use of a vacuum mixer and personal hood protectant system may help reduce the risk of occupational exposure to MMA.

10.12.5 **Do not leave discarded bone cement in contact with the patient's skin.** *[Recommendation]*

Methyl methacrylate is a known liquid monomer, is a mild skin irritant, and may induce skin sensitization.[188,190]

During the curing process, the cement releases heat and has been shown to cause burns to the patient's skin during total hip arthroplasty.[193]

10.12.6 **In the event MMA liquid is spilled,**
- **ventilate the spill area until the odor has dissipated,**[190]
- **remove all sources of ignition,**[163,190]
- **wear PPE during cleanup as required by the manufacturer's IFU or SDS,**[163,178,179]
- **isolate the spill area,**[163]
- **cover the MMA with an activated charcoal absorbent,**[178] **and**
- **dispose of the MMA waste product in a hazardous waste container.**[163,194]

[Recommendation]

10.12.7 **Methyl methacrylate monomer is hazardous waste and must be disposed of according to federal, state, and local requirements.**[190] *[Regulatory Requirement]*

10.13 **The health care organization must establish and implement safe handling practices for glutaraldehyde as required by federal, state, and local regulation.**[163,177] *[Regulatory Requirement]*

Glutaraldehyde-based agents are used to disinfect heat-sensitive medical equipment that cannot be steam sterilized. High-level disinfection using glutaraldehyde-based products may occur in a variety of locations, including sterile processing, surgery, endoscopy, and respiratory therapy departments.

Glutaraldehyde is a transparent, oily liquid with a pungent odor. The NIOSH recommended exposure limit with an up to 10-hour time-weighted average limit at the ceiling is 0.2 ppm (0.8 mg/m³) and the American Conference of Governmental Industrial Hygienists threshold limit value at the ceiling is 0.05 ppm (0.02 mg/m³).[195,196]

Personnel can be exposed to glutaraldehyde through inhalation or skin contact[197] while performing many activities, including
- activating and pouring glutaraldehyde solution into or out of a cleaning container system (eg, a soaking basin in manual disinfecting operations or a reservoir in automated processors);
- opening the cleaning container system to immerse instruments to be disinfected;
- agitating glutaraldehyde solution;
- handling soaked instruments;
- removing instruments from the container system;
- rinsing the channels of instruments containing residual glutaraldehyde solution;
- flushing out instrument parts with a syringe;
- drying instrument interiors with compressed air;
- disposing of "spent" glutaraldehyde solutions to the sanitary sewer; and
- performing maintenance procedures, such as filter or hose changes on automated processors that have not been pre-rinsed with water.[198]

Exposure to glutaraldehyde may result in throat and lung irritation, asthma and difficulty breathing, dermatitis, nasal irritation, sneezing, wheezing, burning eyes, and conjunctivitis.[197] The level of exposure depends on the dose, duration, and work being done.[198] Continuous exposure to glutaraldehyde for longer than 1 hour has been shown to increase the risk of a spontaneous abortion according to one study.[176]

Walters et al[170] conducted a nonexperimental study to evaluate the causes and trends of occupational asthma among health care workers between 1991 and 2011. There were 182 cases of occupational asthma, with the majority of cases occurring in the nursing, OR, endoscopy, and radiology personnel. The most frequent causes of occupational asthma were exposure to glutaraldehyde and cleaning products. The researchers concluded that continuing efforts are required to reduce the number of occupational asthma cases among health care workers.

Lawson et al[176] conducted a descriptive research study that included 7,482 pregnant nurses, of whom 775 experienced a spontaneous abortion at less than 20 weeks of pregnancy. The researchers concluded that nurses who were exposed to sterilizing agents (eg, ethylene oxide, formaldehyde, glutaraldehyde) during pregnancy had a two-fold increased risk of late spontaneous abortion.

10.13.1 **Use alternatives for glutaraldehyde for disinfection if any are listed in the device IFU.**[197] *[Recommendation]*

Alternative methods of high-level disinfection or sterilization that are less toxic to humans and the environment than glutaraldehyde are available.[180,181]

10.13.2 **Use a closed automated system if possible.**[197] *[Recommendation]*

10.13.3 **Use a local exhaust ventilation system or use a room that has a minimum air change rate of 7 to 15 air changes per hour.**[197] *[Recommendation]*

10.13.4 **Containers that contain glutaraldehyde solutions should**
- **be covered and sealed when not in use,**
- **only be opened for insertion or removal of the device to be soaked,**
- **be sized for the item to be soaked, and**
- **have close-fitting lids.**[197]

[Recommendation]

10.13.5 **When disposing of glutaraldehyde, use a pump to transfer the solution from the container to the drain.**[197] *[Recommendation]*

10.13.6 **Limit the number of people working in areas where glutaraldehyde is present.**[197] *[Recommendation]*

10.13.7 **Clean up glutaraldehyde spills immediately.**[197] *[Recommendation]*

10.14 **Safe practices must be established and implemented for use of formaldehyde as required by federal, state, and local regulation.**[164] *[Regulatory Requirement]*

Formaldehyde, the active ingredient in formalin, is a known carcinogen and may cause an increased risk of spontaneous abortion.[176] Formaldehyde may cause acute and chronic health conditions through inhalation, ingestion, and exposure to the skin or eyes. The reaction is based on the amount of exposure.
- Ingestion of a 10% to 40% solution may lead to severe irritation and inflammation of the mouth, throat, and stomach and possible loss of consciousness and death. Ingestion of 0.03% to 0.04% solutions may cause discomfort in the stomach and pharynx.
- Inhalation may lead to irritation of the eyes, nose, and throat (0.5 ppm to 2.0 ppm); tearing of the eyes (3 ppm to 5 ppm); difficulty in breathing, burning of the nose and throat, cough, and heavy tearing of the eyes (10 ppm to 20 ppm); severe respiratory tract injury leading to pulmonary edema and pneumonitis (25 ppm to 30 ppm); and death (at a concentration of > 100 ppm).
- Skin contact may lead to severe skin irritation and sensitization, white discoloration, smarting, drying, cracking, and scaling. Prolonged and repeated contact can result in numbness and a hardening or tanning of the skin.
- Eye contact can result in injuries ranging from transient discomfort to severe, permanent corneal clouding and loss of vision. The severity of the injury is related to the concentration and whether the eyes were flushed with water immediately after the accident.[164]

Berton and Di Novi[166] conducted a nonexperimental study that included 171 interviews and 156 observations to quantify respiratory issues among hospital workers exposed to formaldehyde. The researchers found that exposure to formalin produced respiratory symptoms.

10.14.1 **Locations where formaldehyde is used must**
- **be free of ignition sources,**[164]
- **have posted signs warning of formaldehyde use,**[164] **and**
- **have ventilation systems with adequate capacity to maintain levels below the permissible exposure limits (ie, 8-hour total weighted average of 0.75 ppm; 15-minute, short-term exposure limit of 2.0 ppm).**[164]

[Regulatory Requirement]

Formaldehyde is a combustible liquid. The permissible exposure limits are set by OSHA and individual states.[164]

10.14.2 **Formaldehyde must not be stored in the OR unless the ventilation system is adequate to keep levels within the recommended exposure limits.**[164] *[Regulatory Requirement]*

10.14.3 **Personnel handling formaldehyde must wear proper PPE including gloves, impervious clothes, aprons, chemical splash goggles, and respiratory protection based on the potential for exposure.**[164] *[Regulatory Requirement]*

Latex gloves provide no protection against formaldehyde. Butyl and nitrile gloves provide 8 hours of protection, and polyethylene gloves provide 4 hours of protection. Respiratory protection (eg, respirators, ventilation hoods) is required if the levels of formalin in the area are greater than 100 ppm.[164]

10.14.4 Medical surveillance must be provided if workers are exposed to levels of formaldehyde above the permissible exposure limits.[164] *[Regulatory Requirement]*

Per OSHA requirements, formaldehyde levels should not exceed the 8-hour total weighted average of 0.75 ppm or the 15-minute, short-term exposure limit of 2.0 ppm.[164]

10.14.5 Health care organizations must monitor levels of formaldehyde
- when the agent is introduced into the space where it will be stored or used,[164]
- if there is a change in processes or practices involving formaldehyde,[164]
- periodically after introduction,[164]
- after a change in processes or practices (unless permission has been granted by the regulatory agency having jurisdiction to stop monitoring after two consecutive measurements that were taken at least 7 days apart showed the levels were below the recognized safe limits),[164,199] and
- when an employee reports symptoms of respiratory or dermal exposure.[164,181,199]

[Regulatory Requirement]

10.14.6 Facilities may provide specimen containers pre-filled with formalin. *[Conditional Recommendation]*

Providing specimen containers that are pre-filled reduces the need for perioperative personnel to transfer formalin into the specimen container, which reduces the risk of splash exposures.

11. Hazardous Waste

11.1 Take precautions to avoid hazards associated with handling waste. *[Recommendation]*

The types of precautions taken when handling wastes are based on the US Environmental Protection Agency classifications (eg, hazardous, nonhazardous). Hazardous waste is further classified by the Environmental Protection Agency as listed waste, characteristic waste, universal waste, and mixed waste. Medical waste is considered nonhazardous waste and disposal may or may not be regulated.[200]

11.2 The health care organization must follow the most stringent federal, state, or local regulations that govern the disposal of hazardous and nonhazardous waste.[194] *[Regulatory Requirement]*

Legal requirements vary by state and local jurisdiction. The most stringent requirement supersedes others.[194]

11.2.1 The appropriate regulatory body should be consulted for the applicable definition of medical waste (ie, regulated, nonregulated), which may include specific requirements (eg, volume of body fluids, type of waste exposed to human body fluids) to classify the item as regulated medical waste.[194] *[Recommendation]*

11.3 Waste that is classified as hazardous must be placed in hazardous waste containers at the point of use.[194] *[Regulatory Requirement]*

This action alerts handlers to take precautions during disposal.

11.3.1 The waste container must be labeled with the type of waste it contains (eg, red bags indicate regulated medical waste, yellow bags indicate hazardous waste such as waste contaminated by chemotherapy agents).[194] *[Regulatory Requirement]*

11.3.2 The waste container must protect personnel handling the container against exposure to the contents (eg, a container used to dispose of sharps must be puncture resistant, the container for hazardous liquids must be fracture resistant, the lid of the waste container must seal).[194] *[Regulatory Requirement]*

11.3.3 Batteries that contain cadmium, lead, or silver must be disposed of as hazardous waste.[194,201] *[Regulatory Requirement]*

11.3.4 Any product that contains mercury must be disposed of as a hazardous waste.[194,201] *[Regulatory Requirement]*

11.3.5 Flammable liquids (eg, alcohol, benzoin, collodion, formalin, MMA monomer, silver nitrate) are considered characteristic wastes and must be contained and placed into a hazardous waste receptacle for disposal.[194] *[Regulatory Requirement]*

These chemicals pose fire and environmental hazards if they are discarded into the regular waste stream.

11.4 Medications must be disposed of in accordance with guidelines from the state or regulatory body[1] and in consultation with the health care organization's pharmacist. *[Regulatory Requirement]*

Regulations that cover medication disposal vary between states and locality. The category of waste, which dictates the method of disposal, may vary based on the volume of waste and other conditions.[200]

11.5 The health care organization must provide education and competency verification activities for perioperative personnel who work with chemicals and other potentially hazardous agents in the workplace. Education should include safe handling practices, a description of potential hazards, exposure prevention practices, and spill management procedures.[163,201,202] *[Regulatory Requirement]*

12. Quality

12.1 Participate in a variety of quality assurance and performance improvement activities that are consistent with the health care organization's plan to improve understanding of and compliance with the principles and processes of maintaining a safe environment of care. *[Recommendation]*

Quality assurance and performance improvement programs can facilitate the identification of problem areas and assist personnel in evaluating and improving the quality of patient care and the presence of environmental safety hazards and formulating plans for corrective actions. These programs provide data that may be used to determine whether an individual organization is within benchmark goals, and if not, to identify areas that may require corrective action. A quality management program provides a mechanism to evaluate effectiveness of processes and compliance with maintaining a safe environment of care.

12.2 An interdisciplinary team that includes representatives from all disciplines of the perioperative team should establish and implement a quality management plan that includes guidance for

- collecting and analyzing information about adverse outcomes associated with the environment of care (eg, latex allergy) as a part of the organization-wide performance improvement program that addresses adverse events and near misses;
- monitoring actual and potential risks in each care area on a regular basis (eg, at least monthly environment of care rounds by a team that includes clinicians, administrators, and support personnel);
- monitoring and reporting incidents of equipment malfunction that lead to patient harm as outlined in the Safe Medical Devices Act of 1990[203];

- monitoring and reporting incidents of alarm malfunction and events related to the inability of the team members to respond to alarms[9,10,204];
- conducting scheduled "walk around" safety rounds to test clinical and alert alarms and to observe staff members' responses to the alarms;
- monitoring compliance with requirements for safe handling of chemicals and hazardous wastes in the workplace;
- developing processes to regularly inspect, test, and maintain fire extinguishing equipment and supplies;
- critiquing fire drill performance by a team that includes representatives from all disciplines of the perioperative department to identify deficiencies and opportunities for improvement; and
- reporting work-related health problems, such as by using the E-OSHA 300 log.[205]

[Recommendation]

Collecting data to monitor and improve safety, patient care, treatment, and services is a regulatory and accreditation requirement for both hospitals and ambulatory settings.[206-210]

12.2.1 Include the following in the quality assurance and performance improvement program for maintaining a safe environment of care:
- review and evaluation of safety data,
- verification of compliance with the health care organization safety policies,
- identification of needed corrective action,
- implementation of a corrective action plan, and
- evaluation of results.

[Recommendation]

Reviewing and evaluating quality assurance and performance improvement activities facilitates identification of safety hazards and facilitates development of risk reduction strategies to promote a safe environment of care.[58]

12.3 Participate in quality assurance and performance improvement activities related to maintaining a safe environment of care to
- identify safety hazards,
- take appropriate corrective actions, and
- report hazards according to organizational policy.

[Recommendation]

12.4 Report and document near misses and adverse events according to the health care organization's policy and review for potential opportunities for improvement. *[Recommendation]*

Reports of near misses and adverse events can be used to identify actions that may prevent similar occurrences and reveal opportunities for improvement.

12.5 **Submit reports regarding device malfunction that led to serious injury or death to MedWatch: The FDA Safety Information and Adverse Event Reporting Program.**[211] *[Recommendation]*

The FDA uses medical device reports to monitor device performance, detect potential device-related safety issues, and contribute to risk-benefit assessments of suspected device-associated deaths, serious injuries, or malfunction.[211] The Manufacturer and User Facility Device Experience (MAUDE) database houses reports submitted to the FDA by mandatory reporters (ie, manufacturers, importers, device user facilities) and voluntary reporters (ie, health care professionals, patients, consumers).[212]

Mandatory reporters are required to submit reports when they become aware of information that reasonably suggests that one of their marketed devices may have caused or contributed to a death or serious injury or has malfunctioned and that the malfunction of the device would be likely to cause or contribute to a death or serious injury if the malfunction were to recur.[211] Voluntary reporters are required to submit reports when they become aware of information that reasonably suggests a device may have caused or contributed to a death or serious injury of a patient.[211]

Glossary

Alert alarm: An alarm connected to a system such as a medical gas system, blood bank refrigerator, or fire alarm. Alarms can be audible, visual, or a combination of both.

Clinical alarm: An alarm for alerting caregivers to patient-related situations that have varying degrees of urgency. Alarms can be audible, visual, or a combination of both.

Distraction: An event that causes a diversion of attention or concentration during performance of a task.

Interruption: An unplanned or unexpected event that results in discontinuation of a task.

Latex allergy: An IgE-mediated (ie, immunologic) reaction to the proteins present in natural rubber latex that comes from the milky fluid of the Brazilian rubber tree.

Latex-safe environment: An environment in which every reasonable effort has been made to remove high-allergen and airborne latex sources from coming into direct contact with affected individuals. The airborne latex protein load should be less than 0.6 ng/m³.

Latex sensitization: A hypersensitivity reaction (Type 4) to the allergens that include rubber additives, accelerators, and natural latex.

Noise: Any undesired sound that interferes with normal hearing.

Smoke compartment: A space within a building enclosed by smoke barriers on all sides, including the top and bottom.

Strain relief: An electrical cable design that allows the cable to move without cracking or breaking away from the plug or connector that connects to an electrical outlet or a hardware device. The strain relief is typically a series of ridges at the point where the cabling meets the connector or plug that allows flexibility in the cable without putting stress on that vulnerable point in the cord.

Sterile cockpit: An environment in which personnel refrain from nonessential activities to minimize distractions during important tasks.

References

1. Guideline for medication safety. In: *Guidelines for Perioperative Practice.* Denver, CO: AORN, Inc; 2018:295-330. [IVA]

2. Guideline for design and maintenance of the surgical suite. In: *Guidelines for Perioperative Practice.* Denver, CO: AORN, Inc; 2018:e49-e76. [IVA]

3. Guideline for safe patient handling and movement. In: *Guidelines for Perioperative Practice.* Denver, CO: AORN, Inc; 2018:e1-e48. [IVA]

4. Guideline for prevention of transmissible infections. In: *Guidelines for Perioperative Practice.* Denver, CO: AORN, Inc; 2018:499-534. [IVA]

5. Guideline for medical device and product evaluation. In: *Guidelines for Perioperative Practice.* Denver, CO: AORN, Inc; 2018:183-190. [IVA]

6. Guideline for radiation safety. In: *Guidelines for Perioperative Practice.* Denver, CO: AORN, Inc; 2018:331-366. [IVA]

7. Guideline for surgical smoke safety. In: *Guidelines for Perioperative Practice.* Denver, CO: AORN, Inc; 2018:469-498. [IVA]

8. Cram N. Medical device alarm fatigue: a systems engineering perspective. *J Clin Eng.* 2015;40(4):189-194. [VC]

9. Clinical Alarms Task Force. Impact of clinical alarms on patient safety: a report from the American College of Clinical Engineering Healthcare Technology Foundation. *J Clin Eng.* 2007;32(1):22-33. [VB]

10. *A Siren Call to Act: Priority Issues from the Medical Device Alarms Summit.* Arlington, VA: Association for the Advancement of Medical Instrumentation; 2011. [IVB]

11. Criscitelli T. Alarm management: promoting safety and establishing guidelines. *AORN J.* 2016;103(5):518-521. [VB]

12. 2008 ASA recommendations for pre-anesthesia checkout procedures. American Society of Anesthesiologists. https://www.asahq.org/resources/clinical-information/2008-asa-recommendations-for-pre-anesthesia-checkout. Accessed August 21, 2018. [IVB]

13. Schmid F, Goepfert MS, Kuhnt D, et al. The wolf is crying in the operating room: patient monitor and anesthesia workstation alarming patterns during cardiac surgery. *Anesth Analg.* 2011;112(1):78-83. [IIIB]

14. Brown JC, Anglin-Regal P. Patient safety focus. Clinical alarm management: a team effort. *Biomed Instrum Technol.* 2008;42(2):142-144. [VA]

15. Cheriyan S, Mowery H, Ruckle D, et al. The impact of operating room noise upon communication during percutaneous nephrostolithotomy. *J Endourol.* 2016;30(10):1062-1066. [IIIB]

16. Katz JD. Noise in the operating room. *Anesthesiology.* 2014;121(4):894-898. [VB]

17. Way TJ, Long A, Weihing J, et al. Effect of noise on auditory processing in the operating room. *J Am Coll Surg.* 2013;216(5):933-938. [IIIC]

18. Mentis HM, Chellali A, Manser K, al e. A systematic review of the effect of distraction on surgeon performance: directions for operating room policy and surgical training. *Surg Endosc.* 2015;30:1713-1724. [IIIA]

19. Antoniadis S, Passauer-Baierl S, Baschnegger H, Weigl M. Identification and interference of intraoperative distractions and interruptions in operating rooms. *J Surg Res.* 2014; 188(1):21-29. [IIIB]

20. Plaxton H. Communication, noise, and distractions in the operating room: the impact on patients and strategies to improve outcomes. *ORNAC J.* 2017;35(2):13-22. [VB]

21. Sentinel event data - event type by year (1995- Q2-2016). The Joint Commission. https://www.jointcommission.org/se_data_event_type_by_year_/. Published August 1, 2016. Accessed August 21, 2018. [VB]

22. Chen L, Brueck SE, Niemeier MT. Evaluation of potential noise exposures in hospital operating rooms. *AORN J.* 2012;96(4):412-418. [IIIB]

23. Keller S, Tschan F, Beldi G, Kurmann A, Candinas D, Semmer NK. Noise peaks influence communication in the operating room. An observational study. *Ergonomics.* 2016; 59(12):1541-1552. [IIIA]

24. Ford DA. Speaking up to reduce noise in the OR. *AORN J.* 2015;102(1):85-89. [VB]

25. Hogan LJ, Harvey RL. Creating a culture of safety by reducing noise levels in the OR. *AORN J.* 2015;102(4):410.e1-410. e7. [IIB]

26. *AORN Position Statement on Managing Distractions and Noise during Perioperative Patient Care.* AORN, Inc. http://www.aorn.org/guidelines/clinical-resources/position-statements. Revised 2014. Accessed August 21, 2018. [IVB]

27. Wright MI. Implementing no interruption zones in the perioperative environment. *AORN J.* 2016;104(6):536-540. [VB]

28. Panahi P, Stroh M, Casper DS, Parvizi J, Austin MS. Operating room traffic is a major concern during total joint arthroplasty. *Clin Orthop.* 2012;470(10):2690-2694. [IIIB]

29. Shambo L, Umadhay T, Pedoto A. Music in the operating room: is it a safety hazard? *AANA J.* 2015;83(1):42-48. [IIIA]

30. Weldon S, Korkiakangas T, Bezemer J, Kneebone R. Music and communication in the operating theatre. *J Adv Nurs.* 2015;71(12):2763-2774. [IIIA]

31. Gibbs J, Smith P. A pathway to clinician-led culture change in the operating theatre. *J Perioper Pract.* 2016;26(6): 134-137. [VC]

32. Clark GJ. Strategies for preventing distractions and interruptions in the OR. *AORN J.* 2013;97(6):702-707. [VB]

33. Yoong W, Khin A, Ramlal N, Loabile B, Forman S. Interruptions and distractions in the gynaecological operating theatre: irritating or dangerous? *Ergonomics.* 2015;58(8):1314-1319. [IIIB]

34. Jenkins A, Wilkinson JV, Akeroyd MA, Broom MA. Distractions during critical phases of anaesthesia for caesarean section: an observational study. *Anaesthesia.* 2015;70(5):543-548. [IIIB]

35. Ginsberg SH, Pantin E, Kraidin J, Solina A, Panjwani S, Yang G. Noise levels in modern operating rooms during surgery. *J Cardiothorac Vasc Anesth.* 2013;27(3):528-530. [IIIB]

36. Bell J, Collins JW, Dalsey E, Sublet V. *Slip, Trip, and Fall Prevention for Healthcare Workers.* DHHS (NIOSH) Publication Number 2011-123; 2010. Centers for Disease Control and Prevention. https://www.cdc.gov/niosh/docs/2011-123/pdfs/2011-123.pdf. Accessed August 21, 2018. [IVB]

37. Gomaa AE, Tapp LC, Luckhaupt SE, et al. Occupational traumatic injuries among workers in health care facilities—United States, 2012-2014. *MMWR Morb Mortal Wkly Rep.* 2015;64(15):405-410. [VA]

38. Brogmus G, Leone W, Butler L, Hernandez E. Best practices in OR suite layout and equipment choices to reduce slips, trips, and falls. *AORN J.* 2007;86(3):384-394. [IVB]

39. Bell JL, Collins JW, Wolf L, et al. Evaluation of a comprehensive slip, trip and fall prevention programme for hospital employees. *Ergonomics.* 2008;51(12):1906-1925. [IIB]

40. Chang WR, Leclercq S, Lockhart TE, Haslam R. State of science: occupational slips, trips and falls on the same level. *Ergonomics.* 2016;59(7):861-883. [VA]

41. Hamel KD. Identifying same-level slip and fall hazards in the workplace. *Occup Health Saf.* 2014;83(11):52-53. [VB]

42. Leclercq S, Cuny-Guerrier A, Gaudez C, Aublet-Cuvelier A. Similarities between work related musculoskeletal disorders and slips, trips and falls. *Ergonomics.* 2015;58(10):1624-1636. [VB]

43. Apfelbaum JL, Caplan RA, Connis RT, et al. Practice advisory for the prevention and management of operating room fires: an updated report by the American Society of Anesthesiologists Task Force on Operating Room Fires. *Anesthesiology.* 2013;118(2):271-290. [IVA]

44. Bonnet A, Devienne M, De Broucker V, Duquennoy-Martinot V, Guerreschi P. Operating room fire: should we mistrust alcoholic antiseptics? *Ann Chir Plast Esthet.* 2015;60(4): 255-261. [VB]

45. Culp WC Jr, Kimbrough BA, Luna S. Flammability of surgical drapes and materials in varying concentrations of oxygen. *Anesthesiology.* 2013;119(4):770-776. [IIIB]

46. Engel SJ, Patel NK, Morrison CM, et al. Operating room fires: part II. Optimizing safety. *Plast Reconstr Surg.* 2012;130(3):681-689. [IIB]

47. Fisher M. Prevention of surgical fires: a certification course for healthcare providers. *AANA J.* 2015;83(4):271-274. [IIC]

48. Flowers J. Fire safety in procedural areas. *J Radiol Nurs.* 2012;31(1):13-19. [VB]

49. Huddleston S, Hamadani S, Phillips ME, Fleming JC. Fire risk during ophthalmic plastic surgery. *Ophthalmology.* 2013;120(6):1309. [IIB]

50. Sibia US, Connors K, Dyckman S, et al. Potential operating room fire hazard of bone cement. *Am J Orthop.* 2016;45(7):E512-E514. [VC]

51. Tao JP, Hirabayashi KE, Kim BT, Zhu FA, Joseph JM, Nunery W. The efficacy of a midfacial seal drape in reducing oculofacial surgical field fire risk. *Ophthal Plast Reconstr Surg.* 2013;29(2):109-112. [IIB]

52. Bansal A, Bhama JK, Varga JM, Toyoda Y. Airway fire during double-lung transplantation. *Interact Cardiovasc Thorac Surg.* 2013;17(6):1059-1060. [VB]

53. Connor MA, Menke AM, Vrcek I, Shore JW. Operating room fires in periocular surgery. *Int Ophthalmol.* 2017:1-9. [IIIB]

54. De Almeida CED, Curi EF, Brezinscki R, De Freitas RC. Fire in the surgical center. *Rev Bras Anestesiol.* 2012;62(3):432-438. [VB]

55. Haith LR, Santavasi W, Shapiro TK, et al. Burn center management of operating room fire injuries. *J Burn Care Res.* 2012;33(5):649-653. [VB]

56. Hempel S, Maggard-Gibbons M, Nguyen DK, et al. Wrong-site surgery, retained surgical items, and surgical fires a systematic review of surgical never events. *JAMA Surg.* 2015;150(8):796-805. [IIIA]

57. Vancleave AM, Jones JE, James D, Saxen MA, Sanders BJ, Walker LA. Factors involved in dental surgery fires: a review of the literature. *Anesth Prog.* 2014;61(1):21-25. [VA]

58. Steelman VM, Graling PR, Perkhounkova Y. Priority patient safety issues identified by perioperative nurses. *AORN J.* 2013;97(4):402-418. [IIIA]

59. Hudson DW, Guidry OF, Abernathy JH 3rd, Ehrenwerth J. Case 4—2012: intrathoracic fire during coronary artery bypass graft surgery. *J Cardiothorac Vasc Anesth.* 2012;26(3):520-521. [VB]

60. Raghavan K, Lagisetty KH, Butler KL, Cahalane MJ, Gupta A, Odom SR. Intraoperative fires during emergent colon surgery. *Am Surg.* 2015;81(2):E82-E83. [VB]

61. Di Pasquale L, Ferneini EM. Fire safety for the oral and maxillofacial surgeon and surgical staff. *Oral Maxillofac Surg Clin North Am.* 2017;29(2):179-187. [VB]

62. Chung K, Lee S, Oh S, Choi J, Cho H. Thermal burn injury associated with a forced-air warming device. *Korean J Anesthesiol.* 2012;62(4):391-392. [VB]

63. Lalla RK, Koteswara CM. Fire in the operating room due to equipment failure. *J Anaesthesiol Clin Pharmacol.* 2013;29(1):141. [VC]

64. ElBardissi AW, Sundt TM. Human factors and operating room safety. *Surg Clin North Am.* 2012;92(1):21-35. [VB]

65. Mehta SP, Bhananker SM, Posner KL, Domino KB. Operating room fires: a closed claims analysis. *Anesthesiology.* 2013;118(5):1133-1139. [IIIB]

66. Preventing surgical fires. *Bull Am Coll Surg.* 2013;98(8):65-66. [VC]

67. Culp WC Jr, Kimbrough BA, Luna S, Maguddayao AJ. Operating room fire prevention: creating an electrosurgical unit fire safety device. *Ann Surg.* 2014;260(2):214-217. [IIB]

68. Fuchshuber P, Jones S, Jones D, Feldman LS, Schwaitzberg S, Rozner MA. Ensuring safety in the operating room: the "Fundamental Use of Surgical Energy" (FUSE) program. *Int Anesthesiol Clin.* 2013;51(4):65-80. [VA]

69. Kung TA, Kong SW, Aliu O, Azizi J, Kai S, Cederna PS. Effects of vacuum suctioning and strategic drape tenting on oxygen concentration in a simulated surgical field. *J Clin Anesth.* 2016;28:56-61. [IB]

70. Fuchshuber PR, Robinson TN, Feldman LS, Jones DB, Schwaitzberg SD. The SAGES FUSE program: bridging a patient safety gap. *Bull Am Coll Surg.* 2014;99(9):18-27. [VB]

71. Holla R, Darshan B, Unnikrishnan B, et al. Fire safety measures: awareness and perception of health care professionals in coastal Karnataka. *Indian J Public Health Res Dev.* 2016;7(3):246-249. [IIIB]

72. Cvach M, Rothwell KJ, Cullen AM, Nayden MG, Cvach N, Pham JC. Effect of altering alarm settings: a randomized controlled study. *Biomed Instrum Technol.* 2015;49(3):214-222. [IB]

73. Arefiev K, Warycha M, Whiting D, Alam M. Flammability of topical preparations and surgical dressings in cutaneous and laser surgery: a controlled simulation study. *J Am Acad Dermatol.* 2012;67(4):700-705. [IIIA]

74. Chowdhury K. Fires in Indian hospitals: root cause analysis and recommendations for their prevention. *J Clin Anesth.* 2014;26(5):414-424. [VC]

75. Jones EL, Overbey DM, Chapman BC, et al. Operating room fires and surgical skin preparation. *J Am Coll Surg.* 2017;225(1):160-165. [IIIB]

76. Michaels JPS, MacDonald P. Ignition of eyelash extensions during routine minor eyelid surgery. *Ophthal Plast Reconstr Surg.* 2014;30(3):e61-e62. [VB]

77. Rapp C, Gaines R. Fire in the operating room: a previously unreported ignition source. *Am J Orthop.* 2012;41(8):378-379. [VB]

78. Rocos B, Donaldson LJ. Alcohol skin preparation causes surgical fires. *Ann R Coll Surg Engl.* 2012;94(2):87-89. [IIIB]

79. Schroeder RT. Using best practices to respond to an OR fire. *AORN J.* 2013;97(6):605-606. [VB]

80. Seifert PC, Peterson E, Graham K. Crisis management of fire in the OR. *AORN J.* 2015;101(2):250-263. [VA]

81. Stewart MW, Bartley GB. Fires in the operating room: prepare and prevent. *Ophthalmology.* 2015;122(3):445-447. [VB]

82. Wolf O, Weissman O, Harats M, et al. Birth wind and fire: raising awareness to operating room fires during delivery. *J Matern Fetal Neonatal Med.* 2013;26(13):1303-1305. [VC]

83. Kaye AD, Kolinsky D, Urman RD. Management of a fire in the operating room. *J Anesth.* 2014;28(2):279-287. [VA]

84. Gibbs VC. Thinking in three's: changing surgical patient safety practices in the complex modern operating room. *World J Gastroenterol.* 2012;18(46):6712-6719. [VC]

85. Poore SO, Sillah NM, Mahajan AY, Gutowski KA. Patient safety in the operating room: II. intraoperative and postoperative. *Plast Reconstr Surg.* 2012;130(5):1048-1058. [VB]

86. Porteous J. Evacuating an OR is a complex process: who does what? *ORNAC J.* 2013;31(1):15, 17-19, 30-32 passim. [VC]

87. Joint Commission on Accreditation of Healthcare. Maintaining fire equipment and building features. A deep dive into EC.02.03.05. *Jt Comm Perspect.* 2013;33(12):12-15. [VC]

88. Spratt D, Cowles CE, Berguer R, et al. Workplace safety equals patient safety. *AORN J.* 2012;96(3):235-244. [VB]

89. Bongiovanni I, Leo E, Ritrovato M, Santoro A, Derrico P. Implementation of best practices for emergency response and recovery at a large hospital: a fire emergency case study. *Saf Sci.* 2017;96:121-131. [VB]

90. Silva JF, Almeida JE, Rossetti RJF, Coelho AL. A serious game for EVAcuation training. In: *Book of Proceedings. IEEE 2nd International Conference on Serious Games and Applications for Health (SeGAH 2013).* Vilamoura Algarve, Portugal: IEEE; 2013. [IIIC]

91. Prosper D. Boosting fire drill participation in hospital settings. *J Healthc Prot Manage.* 2015;31(1):23-30. [VB]

92. Fire alarm led to center evacuation. *Same Day Surg.* 2012:83-84. [VC]

93. *NFPA 101: Life Safety Code.* Quincy, MA: National Fire Protection Association; 2018. [IVB]

94. Guideline for team communication. In: *Guidelines for Perioperative Practice.* Denver, CO: AORN, Inc; 2018:745-772. [IVA]

95. Culp WC, Kimbrough BA, Luna S, Maguddayao AJ. Mitigating operating room fires: development of a carbon dioxide fire prevention device. *Anesth Analg.* 2014;118(4):772-775. [IIIB]

96. Van Cleave AM, Jones JE, McGlothlin JD, Saxen MA, Sanders BJ, Vinson LA. The effect of intraoral suction on oxygen-enriched surgical environments: a mechanism for reducing the risk of surgical fires. *Anesth Prog.* 2014;61(4):155-161. [IIIB]

97. Guideline for safe use of energy-generating devices. In: *Guidelines for Perioperative Practice.* Denver, CO: AORN, Inc; 2018:129-156. [IVA]

98. Feldman LS, Fuchshuber PR, Jones DB. *The SAGES Manual on the Fundamental Use of Surgical Energy (FUSE).* New York, NY: Springer; 2012. [IVC]

99. ECRI Institute. New clinical guide to surgical fire prevention. Patients can catch fire—here's how to keep them safer. *Health Devices.* 2009;38(10):314-332. [VA]

100. Bielen RP, Lathrop JK; National Fire Protection Association. *NFPA 99: Health Care Facilities Code Handbook.* Quincy, MA: National Fire Protection Association; 2018. [IVB]

101. *NFPA 30: Flammable and Combustible Liquids Code.* Quincy, MA: National Fire Protection Association; 2018. [IVB]

102. Kim JB, Jung HJ, Im KS. Operating room fire using an alcohol-based skin preparation but without electrocautery. *Can J Anesth.* 2013;60(4):413-414. [VC]

103. Chapp K, Lange L. Warming blanket head drapes and trapped anesthetic gases: understanding the fire risk. *AORN J.* 2011;93(6):749-760. [IIIA]

104. *NFPA 10: Standard for Portable Fire Extinguishers.* Quincy, MA: National Fire Protection Association; 2018. [IVB]

105. Executive brief: top 10 health technology hazards for 2017. ECRI Institute. https://www.ecri.org/Resources/White papers_and_reports/Haz17.pdf. Accessed August 21, 2018. [VC]

106. Cappell MS. Accidental occupational injuries to endoscopy personnel in a high-volume endoscopy suite during the last decade: mechanisms, workplace hazards, and proposed remediation. *Dig Dis Sci.* 2011;56(2):479-487. [VB]

107. Cappell MS. Injury to endoscopic personnel from tripping over exposed cords, wires, and tubing in the endoscopy suite: a preventable cause of potentially severe workplace injury. *Dig Dis Sci.* 2010;55(4):947-951. [VB]

108. Hargrove M, Aherne T. Possible fire hazard caused by mismatching electrical chargers with the incorrect device within the operating room. *J Extra Corpor Technol.* 2007;39(3):199-200. [VC]

109. ECRI Institute. Warming cabinets. *Operating Room Risk Management.* 2017. [VC]

110. Huang S, Gateley D, Moss AL. Accidental burn injury during knee arthroscopy. *Arthroscopy.* 2007;23(12):1363.e1-1363.e3. [VC]

111. Bujdoso PJ. Blanket warming: comfort and safety. *AORN J.* 2009;89(4):717-722. [VB]

112. Guideline for prevention of unplanned patient hypothermia. In: *Guidelines for Perioperative Practice.* Denver, CO: AORN; Inc; 2018:549-572. [IVA]

113. ECRI institute continues to recommend maximum temperature setting of 130 degrees Fahrenheit for blanket warming cabinets. ECRI Institute. https://www.ecri.org/com ponents/PSOCore/Pages/PSMU040114_ecri.aspx. Published April 1, 2014. Accessed August 21, 2018. [VC]

114. Sutton LT, Baker FS, Faile NJ, Tavakoli A. A quasi-experimental study examining the safety profile and comfort provided by two different blanket temperatures. *J Perianesth Nurs.* 2012;27(3):181-192. [IIB]

115. Kelly PA, Cooper SK, Krogh ML, et al. Thermal comfort and safety of cotton blankets warmed at 130°F and 200°F. *J Perianesth Nurs.* 2013;28(6):337-346. [IIC]

116. Kelly PA, Morse EC, Swanfeldt JV, et al. Safety of rolled and folded cotton blankets warmed in 130°F and 200°F cabinets. *J Perianesth Nurs.* 2017;32(6):600-608. [IIC]

117. Limiting temperature settings on blanket and solution warming cabinets can prevent patient burns. *Health Devices.* 2005;34(5):168-171. [VC]

118. US Department of Health and Human Services, Food and Drug Administration, Center for Drug Evaluation and Research. Guidance for Hospitals, Nursing Homes, and Other Health Care Facilities. https://www.fda.gov/downloads/drugs/guidance complianceregulatoryinformation/guidances/ucm070285.pdf. Published 2001. Accessed August 21, 2018.

119. US Department of Health and Human Services, Food and Drug Administration. Medical gas containers and closures; current good manufacturing practice requirements. *Fed Regist.* 2006;71(68):18039-18053.

120. Compressed medical gases guideline. US Food and Drug Administration. https://www.fda.gov/drugs/guidancecom plianceregulatoryinformation/guidances/ucm124716.htm. Revised 1989. Accessed August 21, 2018.

121. ISO 407:2004. Small medical gas cylinders—pin-index yoke-type valve connections. International Organization for Standardization. http://www.iso.org/iso/catalogue_detail .htm?csnumber=40148. Accessed August 21, 2018. [IVB]

122. *Standard Color Marking of Compressed Gas Cylinders Intended for Medical Use.* 4th ed. Chantilly, VA: Compressed Gas Association; 2004. [IVB]

123. ECRI. Compressed gases. *Healthcare Risk Control.* 2007; 3(Environmental Issues 17.1). [VB]

124. Anesthetics, volatile. IARC monographs on the evaluation of carcinogenic risks to humans. Overall evaluations of carcinogenicity: An updating of IARC Monographs volumes 1 to 42. Supplement 7 (1987). International Agency for Research on Cancer. https://monographs.iarc.fr/iarc-monographs-on-the-evaluation-of-carcinogenic-risks-to-humans-80/. Accessed August 21, 2018. [IVC]

125. Oliveira CR. Occupational exposure to anesthetic gases residue. *Rev Bras Anestesiol.* 2009;59(1):110-124. [VC]

126. Waste anesthetic gases: occupational hazards in hospitals. DHHS (NIOSH) Publication No 2007-151. National Institute for Occupational Safety and Health. https://www.cdc.gov/niosh/docs/2007-151/default.html. Published September 2007. Accessed August 21, 2018. [IVB]

127. Anesthetic gases: guidelines for workplace exposures. Occupational Safety and Health Administration. https://www.osha.gov/dts/osta/anestheticgases/index.html. Published 1999. Revised 2000. Accessed August 21, 2018. [IVB]

128. Teschke K, Abanto Z, Arbour L, et al. Exposure to anesthetic gases and congenital anomalies in offspring of female registered nurses. *Am J Ind Med.* 2011;54(2):118-127. [IIIB]

129. Dreyfus E, Tramoni E, Lehucher-Michel MP. Persistent cognitive functioning deficits in operating rooms: two cases. *Int Arch Occup Environ Health.* 2008;82(1):125-130. [VC]

130. Wronska-Nofer T, Palus J, Krajewski W, et al. DNA damage induced by nitrous oxide: study in medical personnel of operating rooms. *Mutat Res.* 2009;666(1-2):39-43. [IIIB]

131. Krajewski W, Kucharska M, Pilacik B, et al. Impaired vitamin B12 metabolic status in healthcare workers occupationally exposed to nitrous oxide. *Br J Anaesth.* 2007;99(6):812-818. [IIIB]

132. Baysal Z, Cengiz M, Ozgonul A, Cakir M, Celik H, Kocyigit A. Oxidative status and DNA damage in operating room personnel. *Clin Biochem.* 2009;42(3):189-193. [IIIB]

133. Rozgaj R, Kasuba V, Brozovic G, Jazbec A. Genotoxic effects of anaesthetics in operating theatre personnel evaluated by the comet assay and micronucleus test. *Int J Hyg Environ Health.* 2009;212(1):11-17. [IIIB]

134. Chandrasekhar M, Rekhadevi PV, Sailaja N, et al. Evaluation of genetic damage in operating room personnel exposed to anaesthetic gases. *Mutagenesis.* 2006;21(4):249-254. [IIIB]

135. Eroglu A, Celep F, Erciyes N. A comparison of sister chromatid exchanges in lymphocytes of anesthesiologists to nonanesthesiologists in the same hospital. *Anesth Analg.* 2006;102(5):1573-1577. [IIIB]

136. Criteria for a recommended standard: occupational exposure to waste anesthetic gases and vapors. NIOSH Publication Number 77-140. National Institute for Occupational Safety and Health. https://www.cdc.gov/niosh/docs/77-140/default.html. Published March 1977. Accessed August 21, 2018. [IVB]

137. Sartini M, Ottria G, Dallera M, Spagnolo AM, Cristina ML. Nitrous oxide pollution in operating theatres in relation to the type of leakage and the number of efficacious air exchanges per hour. *J Prev Med Hyg.* 2006;47(4):155-159. [IIIB]

138. Irwin MG, Trinh T, Yao CL. Occupational exposure to anaesthetic gases: a role for TIVA. *Expert Opin Drug Saf.* 2009;8(4):473-483. [VA]

139. Barberio JC, Bolt JD, Austin PN, Craig WJ. Pollution of ambient air by volatile anesthetics: a comparison of 4 anesthetic management techniques. *AANA J.* 2006;74(2):121-125. [IVA]

140. Smith FD. Management of exposure to waste anesthetic gases. *AORN J.* 2010;91(4):482-494. [VA]

141. Mertes PM, Lambert M, Gueant-Rodriguez RM, et al. Perioperative anaphylaxis. *Immunol Allergy Clin North Am.* 2009;29(3):429-451. [VB]

142. Heitz JW, Bader SO. An evidence-based approach to medication preparation for the surgical patient at risk for latex allergy: is it time to stop being stopper poppers? *J Clin Anesth.* 2010;22(6):477-483. [VC]

143. Pollart SM, Warniment C, Mori T. Latex allergy. *Am Fam Physician.* 2009;80(12):1413-1418. [VB]

144. Latex allergy management guidelines. 2014. American Association of Nurse Anesthetists. https://www.aana.com/docs/default-source/practice-aana-com-web-documents-(all)/latex-allergy-management.pdf?sfvrsn=9c0049b1_2. Accessed August 21, 2018. [IVB]

145. Boonchai W, Sirikudta W, Iamtharachai P, Kasemsarn P. Latex glove-related symptoms among health care workers: a self-report questionnaire-based survey. *Dermatitis.* 2014;25(3):135-139. [IIB]

146. Larese Filon F, Bochdanovits L, Capuzzo C, Cerchi R, Rui F. Ten years incidence of natural rubber latex sensitization and symptoms in a prospective cohort of health care workers using non-powdered latex gloves 2000-2009. *Int Arch Occup Environ Health.* 2014;87(5):463-469. [IIA]

147. Liu Q, He X, Liang K, et al. Prevalence and risk factors for latex glove allergy among female clinical nurses: a multicenter questionnaire study in China. *Int J Occup Environ Health.* 2013;19(1):29-34. [IIB]

148. Phaswana SM, Naidoo S. The prevalence of latex sensitization and allergy and associated risk factors among healthcare workers using hypoallergenic latex gloves at King Edward VIII Hospital, KwaZulu-Natal South Africa: a cross-sectional study. *BMJ Open.* 2013;3(12):e002900. [IA]

149. Supapvanich C, Povey AC, Vocht FD. Latex sensitization and risk factors in female nurses in Thai governmental hospitals. *Int J Occup Med Environ Health.* 2014;27(1):93-103. [IIIB]

150. Wang ML, Kelly KJ, Klancnik M, Petsonk EL. Self-reported hand symptoms: a role in monitoring health care workers for latex sensitization? *Ann Allergy Asthma Immunol.* 2012;109(5):314-318. [IIB]

151. Köse S, Mandiracioglu A, Tatar B, Gül S, Erdem M. Prevalence of latex allergy among healthcare workers in Izmir (Turkey). *Cent Eur J Public Health.* 2014;22(4):262-265. [IIIA]

152. Risenga SM, Shivambu GP, Rakgole MP, et al. Latex allergy and its clinical features among healthcare workers at Mankweng Hospital, Limpopo Province, South Africa. *S Afr Med J.* 2013;103(6):390-394. [IIC]

153. Supapvanich C, Povey AC, de Vocht F. Respiratory and dermal symptoms in Thai nurses using latex products. *Occup Med (Lond).* 2013;63(6):425-428. [IIIA]

154. Worth A, Sheikh A. Prevention of anaphylaxis in healthcare settings. *Expert Rev Clin Immunol.* 2013;9(9):855-869. [VA]

155. Al-Niaimi F, Chiang YZ, Chiang YN, Williams J. Latex allergy: assessment of knowledge, appropriate use of gloves and prevention practice among hospital healthcare workers. *Clin Exp Dermatol.* 2013;38(1):77-80. [IIIB]

156. Kelly KJ, Wang ML, Klancnik M, Petsonk EL. Prevention of IgE sensitization to latex in health care workers after reduction of antigen exposures. *J Occup Environ Med.* 2011;53(8):934-940. [IIIC]

157. Liberatore K. Latex: a lingering and lurking safety risk. *Penn Patient Saf Advis.* 2018;15(1). [VB]

158. Latex in the hospital environment. Spina Bifida Association. https://spinabifidaassociation.org/wp-content/uploads/2015/07/latex-in-the-hospital-environment-eng.pdf. Updated 2015. Accessed August 21, 2018. [VC]

159. Medical products. American Latex Allergy Association. http://latexallergyresources.org/medical-products. Accessed August 21, 2018.

160. Bigat Z, Kayacan N, Ertugrul F, Karsli B. Latex allergy on anaesthesiologist and anaesthesia managements: are the health workers high risk patients? *J Pak Med Assoc.* 2014;64(4):453-456. [VB]

161. Gentili A, Lima M, Ricci G, et al. Perioperative treatment of latex-allergic children. *J Patient Saf.* 2007;3(3):166-172. [IIIB]

162. Nagpal K, Arora S, Vats A, et al. Failures in communication and information transfer across the surgical care pathway: interview study. *BMJ Qual Saf.* 2012;21(10):843-849. [IIIB]

163. 29 CFR §1910.1200. Hazard communication: toxic and hazardous substances. US Government Publishing Office. https://www.gpo.gov/fdsys/pkg/CFR-2014-title29-vol6/pdf/CFR-2014-title29-vol6-sec1910-1200.pdf. Accessed August 21, 2018.

164. 29 CFR §1910.1048: Formaldehyde. US Government Publishing Office. https://www.gpo.gov/fdsys/granule/CFR-2016-title29-vol6/CFR-2016-title29-vol6-sec1910-1048/content-detail.html. Accessed August 21, 2018.

165. 29 CFR §1910.1047: Ethylene oxide. US Government Publishing Office. https://www.gpo.gov/fdsys/granule/CFR-2010-title29-vol6/CFR-2010-title29-vol6-sec1910-1047. Accessed August 21, 2018.

166. Berton F, Di Novi C. Occupational hazards of hospital personnel: assessment of a safe alternative to formaldehyde. *J Occup Health.* 2012;54(1):74-78. [IB]

167. Davies T. Health problems have come in wake of contact with chemicals. *Nurs Stand.* 2016;30(39):30-31. [VC]

168. Karnwal A, Lippmann M, Kakazu C. Bone cement implantation syndrome affecting operating room personnel. *Br J Anaesth.* 2015;115(3):478. [VB]

169. Ponce V, Muñoz-Bellido F, González A, Gracia M, Moreno A, Macías E. Occupational contact dermatitis to methacrylates in an orthopaedic operating room nurse. *J Investig Allergol Clin Immunol.* 2013;23(4):286. [VC]

170. Walters GI, Moore VC, McGrath EE, Burge PS, Henneberger PK. Agents and trends in health care workers' occupational asthma. *Occup Med (Lond).* 2013;63(7):513-516. [IIIB]

171. Downes J, Rauk PN, Vanheest AE. Occupational hazards for pregnant or lactating women in the orthopaedic operating room. *J Am Acad Orthop Surg.* 2014;22(5):326-332. [VA]

172. Olsen F, Kotyra M, Houltz E, Ricksten SE. Bone cement implantation syndrome in cemented hemiarthroplasty for femoral neck fracture: incidence, risk factors, and effect on outcome. *Br J Anaesth.* 2014;113(5):800-806. [IIIB]

173. *Ethylene Oxide (EtO): Evidence of Carcinogenicity.* Atlanta, GA: US Department of Health & Human Services: Centers for Disease Control and Prevention, The National Institute for Occupational Safety and Health (NIOSH); 2014. [IVB]

174. Casey ML, Hawley B, Edwards N, Cox-Ganser J, Cummings KJ. Health problems and disinfectant product exposure among staff at a large multispecialty hospital. *Am J Infect Control.* 2017;45(10):1133-1138. [IIIB]

175. Reducing ethylene oxide use. US Environmental Protection Agency. http://www.glrppr.org/docs/r5-eto-factsheet-revised-feb2018.pdf. Accessed August 21, 2018.

176. Lawson CC, Rocheleau CM, Whelan EA, et al. Occupational exposures among nurses and risk of spontaneous abortion. *Am J Obstet Gynecol.* 2012;206(4):327.e1-327.e8. [IIIB]

177. 29 CFR §1910.120. Hazardous waste operations and emergency response. US Government Publishing Office. https://www.gpo.gov/fdsys/pkg/CFR-2009-title29-vol5/pdf/CFR-2009-title29-vol5-sec1910-120.pdf. Accessed August 21, 2018.

178. Healthcare wide hazards: hazardous chemicals. Occupational Safety and Health Administration. https://www.osha.gov/SLTC/etools/hospital/hazards/hazchem/haz.html. Accessed August 21, 2018. [VC]

179. 29 CFR §1910.132. General requirements. US Government Publishing Office. https://www.gpo.gov/fdsys/pkg/CFR-2009-title29-vol5/pdf/CFR-2009-title29-vol5-sec1910-120.pdf. Accessed August 21, 2018.

180. Guideline for high-level disinfection. In: *Guidelines for Perioperative Practice.* Denver, CO: AORN, Inc; 2018:883-906. [IVA]

181. Guideline for sterilization. In: *Guidelines for Perioperative Practice.* Denver, CO: AORN, Inc; 2018:957-984. [IVA]

182. Guideline for preoperative patient skin antisepsis. In: *Guidelines for Perioperative Practice.* Denver, CO: AORN, Inc; 2018:51-74. [IVA]

183. Guideline for hand hygiene. In: *Guidelines for Perioperative Practice.* Denver, CO: AORN, Inc; 201829-50:29-50. [IVA]

184. Guideline for surgical attire. In: *Guidelines for Perioperative Practice.* Denver, CO: AORN, Inc; 2018:105-128. [IVA]

185. 29 CFR §1910.134. Respiratory protection. US Government Publishing Office. https://www.govinfo.gov/app/details/CFR-2018-title29-vol5/CFR-2018-title29-vol5-sec1910-134/context. Accessed August 21, 2018.

186. *American National Standard for Emergency Eyewash and Shower Equipment.* Arlington, VA: International Safety Equipment Association (ISEA); 2014:22. [IVC]

187. International chemical safety cards: methyl methacrylate. Centers for Disease Control and Prevention. http://www.cdc.gov/niosh/ipcsneng/neng0300.html. Updated July 1, 2014. Accessed August 21, 2018. [IVB]

188. Methyl methacrylate. Occupational Safety and Health Administration. https://www.osha.gov/chemicaldata/chemResult.html?RecNo=712. Accessed September 20, 2017.

189. Methyl methacrylate. In: *IARC Monographs on the Evaluation of Carcinogenic Risks to Humans.* Vol 60. Lyon, France: World Health Organization: International Agency for Research on Cancer; 1994. [VC]

190. Medical devices; reclassification of polymethylmethacrylate (PMMA) bone cement. Final rule. *Fed Regist.* 2002; 67(137):46852-46855.

191. Jelecevic J, Maidanjuk S, Leithner A, Loewe K, Kuehn KD. Methyl methacrylate levels in orthopedic surgery: comparison of two conventional vacuum mixing systems. *Ann Occup Hyg.* 2014;58(4):493-500. [IIIB]

192. Ungers LJ, Vendrely TG, Barnes CL. Control of methyl methacrylate during the preparation of orthopedic bone cements. *J Occup Environ Hyg.* 2007;4(4):272-280. [IIIB]

193. Burston B, Yates P, Bannister G. Cement burn of the skin during hip replacement. *Ann R Coll Surg Engl.* 2007;89(2):151-152. [VC]

194. 40 CFR §260: Hazardous waste system: General. US Government Publishing Office. https://www.gpo.gov/fdsys/pkg/CFR-2017-title40-vol28/xml/CFR-2017-title40-vol28-part260.xml. Accessed August 23, 2018.

195. Glutaraldehyde. OSHA Occupational Chemical Database. https://www.osha.gov/chemicaldata/chemResult.html?recNo=123. Updated 2018. Accessed August 21, 2018.

196. *Glutaraldehyde: TLV Chemical Substances.* 7th ed. Cincinnati, OH: American Conference of Governmental Industrial Hygienists (ACGIH); 2015. [IVB]

197. Smith DR, Wang R. Glutaraldehyde exposure and its occupational impact in the health care environment. *Environ Health Prev Med.* 2005;11(1):3-10. [VB]

198. *Best Practices for the Safe Use of Glutaraldehyde in Health Care.* Washington, DC: Occupational Safety and Health Administration; 2006.

199. Sampling strategy and analytical methods for formaldehyde. Occupational Safety and Health Administration. https://www.osha.gov/pls/oshaweb/owadisp.show_document?p_table=standards&p_id=10077. Accessed August 21, 2018.

200. Hazardous waste. US Environmental Protection Agency. https://www.epa.gov/hw. Accessed August 21, 2018.

201. 40 CFR §266: Standards for the management of specific hazardous wastes and specific types of hazardous waste management facilities. US Government Publishing Office. https://www.gpo.gov/fdsys/granule/CFR-2012-title40-vol28/CFR-2012-title40-vol28-part266. Accessed August 21, 2018.

202. 29 CFR Appendix D to §1910.1200: Definition of "trade secret" (mandatory). US Government Publishing Office. https://www.gpo.gov/fdsys/granule/CFR-2000-title29-vol6/CFR-2000-title29-vol6-sec1910-1200-appD/content-detail.html. Accessed August 21, 2018.

203. *Safe Medical Devices Act of 1990 and the Medical Device Amendments of 1992.* HHS Publication FDA 93-4243. Washington, DC: US Department of Health and Human Services, Public Health Service/Food and Drug Administration, Center for Devices and Radiological Health; 1993.

204. Phillips J. Clinical alarms: complexity and common sense. *Crit Care Nurs Clin North Am.* 2006;18(2):145-156. [VB]

205. Randall SB, Pories WJ, Pearson A, Drake DJ. Expanded Occupational Safety and Health Administration 300 log as metric for bariatric patient-handling staff injuries. *Surg Obes Relat Dis.* 2009;5(4):463-468. [IIIA]

206. 42 CFR §482: Conditions of participation for hospitals. US Government Publishing Office https://www.gpo.gov/fdsys/granule/CFR-2011-title42-vol5/CFR-2011-title42-vol5-part482. Accessed August 21, 2018.

207. 42 CFR §416: Ambulatory surgical services. US Government Publishing Office. https://www.gpo.gov/fdsys/granule/CFR-2011-title42-vol3/CFR-2011-title42-vol3-part416. Accessed August 21, 2018.

208. *State Operations Manual Appendix A—Survey Protocol, Regulations and Interpretive Guidelines for Hospitals.* Rev 137; 2105. Centers for Medicare & Medicaid Services. https://www.cms.gov/Regulations-and-Guidance/Guidance/Manuals/downloads/som107ap_a_hospitals.pdf. Accessed August 21, 2018.

209. *State Operations Manual Appendix L—Guidance for Surveyors: Ambulatory Surgical Centers.* Rev 137; 2015. Centers for Medicare & Medicaid Services. https://www.cms.gov/Regulations-and-Guidance/Guidance/Manuals/Downloads/som107ap_l_ambulatory.pdf. Accessed August 21, 2018.

210. Quality management and improvement. In: *Accreditation Handbook for Ambulatory Health Care.* Skokie, IL: Accreditation Association for Ambulatory Health Care, Inc; 2016:46-50.

211. MedWatch: The FDA Safety Information and Adverse Event Reporting Program. http://www.fda.gov/Safety/MedWatch/default.htm. Accessed August 21, 2018.

212. MAUDE—Manufacturer and User Facility Device Experience. https://www.accessdata.fda.gov/scripts/cdrh/cfdocs/cfMAUDE/search.CFM. Updated July 31, 2018. Accessed August 21, 2018.

Acknowledgments

Lead Author
Esther M. Johnstone, DNP, RN, CNOR
Perioperative Practice Specialist
AORN Nursing Department
Denver, Colorado

Co-Author
Byron L. Burlingame, MS, RN, BSN, CNOR
Senior Perioperative Practice Specialist
AORN Nursing Department
Denver, Colorado

Contributing Author
Ramona L. Conner, MSN, RN, CNOR, FAAN
Editor-in-Chief, Guidelines for Perioperative Practice
AORN Nursing Department
Denver, Colorado

The authors and AORN thank Janice Neil, PhD, CNE, RN, Associate Professor, East Carolina College of Nursing, Greenville, North

Carolina; Donna A. Pritchard, MA, BSN, RN, NE-BC, CNOR, Director of Perioperative Services, Interfaith Medical Center, Brooklyn, New York; Gerald McDonnell, PhD, BSc, Johnson & Johnson Family of Companies, Raritan, New Jersey; Sue G. Klacik, BS, CRCST, FCS, President, Klacik Consulting, Canfield, Ohio; Jay Bowers, BSN, RN, CNOR, Clinical Coordinator for Trauma, General Surgery, Bariatric, Pediatric and Surgical Oncology, West Virginia University Hospitals, Morgantown; Brenda G. Larkin, MS, ACNS-BC, CNS, CNOR, Clinical Nurse Specialist, Aurora Lakeland Medical Center, Lake Geneva, Wisconsin; Julie K. Moyle, MSN, RN, Member Engagement Manager, Centura – Avista Adventist Hospital, Golden, Colorado; Darlene Murdock, BSN, BA, RN, CNOR, Clinical Staff Nurse IV, Memorial Hermann TMC, Missouri City, Texas; Jane Flowers, MSN, RN, CNOR, NEA-BC, CRCST, Sterile Processing Manager, University of Maryland Shore Regional Health, Easton, Maryland; and Amber Wood, MSN, RN, CNOR, CIC, FAPIC, Senior Perioperative Practice Specialist, AORN, Denver, Colorado, for their assistance in developing this guideline.

Publication History

Originally published February 1988, *AORN Journal,* as "Recommended practices for safe care through identification of potential hazards in the surgical environment." Revised March 1992.

Revised November 1995; published March 1996, *AORN Journal.* Reformatted July 2000.

Revised; published March 2003, *AORN Journal.*

Revised 2007; published in *Perioperative Standards and Recommended Practices,* 2008 edition, as "Recommended practices for a safe environment of care."

Revised November 2009 for online publication in *Perioperative Standards and Recommended Practices.*

Minor editing revisions made in November 2010 for publication in *Perioperative Standards and Recommended Practices,* 2011 edition.

Revised and reformatted December 2012 for online publication in *Perioperative Standards and Recommended Practices.*

Evidence ratings revised 2013 to conform to the AORN Evidence Rating Model.

Minor editing revisions made in November 2014 for publication in *Guidelines for Perioperative Practice,* 2015 edition.

Evidence ratings revised in *Guidelines for Perioperative Practice,* 2018 edition, to conform to the current AORN Evidence Rating Model.

Revised October 2018 for publication in *Guidelines for Perioperative Practice* online.

Evidence ratings revised and minor editorial changes made to conform to the current AORN Evidence Rating model, September 2019, for publication in *Guidelines for Perioperative Practice* online.

AMBULATORY SUPPLEMENT:
A SAFE ENVIRONMENT OF CARE

7. Medical Gases

7.2.1 **Store an adequate emergency supply of oxygen at the facility to provide an uninterrupted supply for 1 day.**[A1]

Ⓐ Oxygen delivery may only be available on certain days, and emergency supplies may be unavailable.

Ⓐ An alarm system should indicate oxygen reserve status and 1-day supply.[A2-A4]

Ⓐ Oxygen supply levels should be verified daily when the facility is open for business.[A2,A3]

Ⓐ Surgical procedures should not be started until a sufficient oxygen supply is confirmed.

7.8.4 **Close the valves on medical gas cylinders properly to avoid leakage during storage.**

Ⓐ Gas cylinder valves and oxygen delivery unit valves (eg, anesthesia machines, flow meters) should be checked at the close of every business day to confirm they are in the off position.

Ⓐ A cylinder valve or delivery unit valve left open overnight or over the weekend may deplete the facility's entire oxygen supply.

Ambulatory Recommendation

Ⓐ **Develop policies and procedures for the provision of a safe environment of care, review them annually, revised them as necessary, and make them readily available in the practice setting.**

Include the following in policies and procedures:
- the minimum oxygen supply level to be maintained,[A4]
- oxygen storage capabilities,[A4]
- the oxygen procurement process,[A4]
- processes for verifying the daily oxygen supply,[A2,A3] and

- processes for checking gas cylinder valves and oxygen delivery unit valves (eg, anesthesia machines, flow meters) at the close of every business day to confirm they are in the off position.

References

A1. Bielen RP, Lathrop JK. *Health Care Facilities Code Handbook.* Quincy, MA: National Fire Protection Association; 2018.

A2. EC.02.05.09: The organization inspects, tests, and maintains medical gas and vacuum systems. In: *Comprehensive Accreditation Manual for Ambulatory Care.* Oakbrook Terrace, IL: Joint Commission; 2018.

A3. Anesthesia care services. In: *2018 Accreditation Handbook for Ambulatory Health Care.* Skokie, IL: Accreditation Association for Ambulatory Health Care; 2018:87.

A4. *NFPA 99: Health Care Facilities Code.* Quincy, MA: National Fire Protection Association; 2018.

Acknowledgments

Lead Author, Ambulatory Supplement
Jan Davidson, MSN, RN, CNOR, CASC
Director, Ambulatory Surgery Division
AORN, Inc
Denver, Colorado

Publication History

Originally published in *Perioperative Standards and Recommended Practices,* 2014 edition.

Revised January 2016 for publication in *Guidelines for Perioperative Practice,* 2016 edition.

Revised October 2018 for online publication in *Guidelines for Perioperative Practice.*

Minor editorial changes made to conform to revised guideline format, September 2019, for publication in *Guidelines for Perioperative Practice* online.

AORN GUIDELINES FOR
PERIOPERATIVE PRACTICE,
2022 EDITION

ENVIRONMENTAL CLEANING

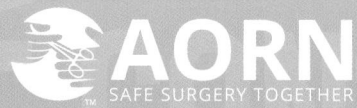

TABLE OF CONTENTS

🅿 *indicates a recommendation or evidence relevant to pediatric care.*

MEDICAL ABBREVIATIONS & ACRONYMS

ATP – Adenosine triphosphate
CDC – Centers for Disease Control and Prevention
CJD – Creutzfeldt-Jakob disease
EPA – Environmental Protection Agency
FIFRA – Federal Insecticide, Fungicide, and Rodenticide Act
FMUV – Focused multivector ultraviolet
HAI – Health care–associated infection
ICU – Intensive care unit
IDSA – Infectious Diseases Society of America
IFU – Instructions for use

IV – Intravenous
MDRO – Multidrug-resistant organism
MRSA – Methicillin-resistant *Staphylococcus aureus*
NaOH – Sodium hydroxide
OR – Operating room
PPE – Personal protective equipment
RVA – Remote video auditing
SHEA – Society for Healthcare Epidemiology of America
SSI – Surgical site infection
VRE – Vancomycin-resistant enterococci

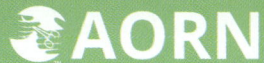

GUIDELINE FOR
ENVIRONMENTAL CLEANING

The Guideline for Environmental Cleaning was approved by the AORN Guidelines Advisory Board and became effective as of January 13, 2020. The recommendations in the guideline are intended to be achievable and represent what is believed to be an optimal level of practice. Policies and procedures will reflect variations in practice settings and/or clinical situations that determine the degree to which the guideline can be implemented. AORN recognizes the many diverse settings in which perioperative nurses practice; therefore, this guideline is adaptable to all areas where operative or other invasive procedures may be performed.

Purpose

This document provides guidance on the selection and use of cleaning products, cleaning procedures, personnel education and competency verification, and monitoring cleanliness through performance improvement processes. All perioperative team members have a responsibility to provide a **clean** and safe environment for patients. Perioperative and environmental services leaders can cultivate an environment in which perioperative and environmental services personnel work collaboratively to accomplish cleanliness in a culture of safety and mutual support.

Researchers have shown that cleaning practices in the operating room (OR) are not always thorough or consistent with the policies of the health care organization.[1-3] Jefferson et al[3] observed a mean cleaning rate of 25% for objects monitored in the OR setting in six acute care hospitals. Munoz-Price et al[1] observed cleaning in 43 ORs of a large urban hospital and found only 50% of the surfaces were being cleaned. In both studies, fluorescent gel markers were used to measure cleanliness. These findings demonstrate that some ORs may not be as clean as previously thought,[1] although the literature has not defined the concept of cleanliness.

In a literature review, Ibrahimi et al[4] stated that the amount of bacteria present in the operative site is one of the most important factors associated with surgical site infection (SSI) development, although the minimum number of bacteria that causes an infection varies depending on the qualities of the organism, the host, and the procedure performed. The review authors also found that **fomites** near the surgical field may harbor bacteria. These fomites may serve as a reservoir for wound contamination through either direct contact with the patient's skin or by personnel contact with the fomite and subsequent skin-to-skin or glove-to-skin contact with the patient.

A high risk for pathogen transmission exists in the perioperative setting because of multiple contacts between perioperative team members, patients, and environmental surfaces.[5-7] Cleaning and disinfecting the environment is a basic infection prevention principle used to reduce the likelihood that exogenous sources will contribute to health care–associated infections (HAIs).[8,9] Operating room environmental surfaces and equipment can become contaminated with pathogens that cause SSIs, particularly if cleaning is suboptimal, and pathogens can then be transmitted to the hands of perioperative team members. Thus, thorough cleaning and **disinfection** of **high-touch objects** as part of a comprehensive **environmental cleaning** and disinfection program that includes hand hygiene are essential in preventing the spread of potentially pathogenic microorganisms.[1]

In a prospective multifacility observational study, Loftus et al[10] followed patients undergoing general anesthesia (N = 548) to identify which bacterial reservoir was associated with transmission events from intravenous (IV) tubing three-way stopcocks. The researchers sampled three bacterial reservoirs: providers' hands, the patient's axillae and nasopharynx, and two high-touch sites on the anesthesia machine. All three reservoirs contributed to transmission, although 64% of stopcock contamination was traced to the anesthesia machine. The researchers also linked the bacterial reservoirs to 30-day postoperative infections. Loftus et al[11] conducted a subset analysis of the previous study[10] and found that gram-negative organisms caused 85% of the HAIs, with the source most often being the anesthesia machine. In two additional analyses[12,13] of the original data,[10] researchers examined the transmission of *Staphylococcus aureus* and found that two strains were frequently transmitted in the anesthesia work area and were highly transmissible, virulent, and drug resistant.

Other studies have identified microorganisms that contribute to environmental contamination of surfaces in the OR, including staphylococcal species,[1,5,14,15] *Corynebacterium* species,[14] *Micrococcus* species,[6,14] *Bacillus* species,[6,14] *Klebsiella pneumoniae*,[1,16] *Pseudomonas* species,[1,6] *Acinetobacter* species,[1] *Enterococcus* species,[1,17] and *Escherichia coli*.[1]

Environmental cleaning and disinfection includes considerations for a safe environment of care, transmission-based precautions, and hand hygiene. Although these topics are mentioned briefly where applicable (eg, standard precautions), they are addressed in other AORN guidelines,[18-20] and broader discussions are outside the scope of this document. Laundering of textiles and evaluation of self-disinfecting surfaces are also outside the scope of these recommendations.

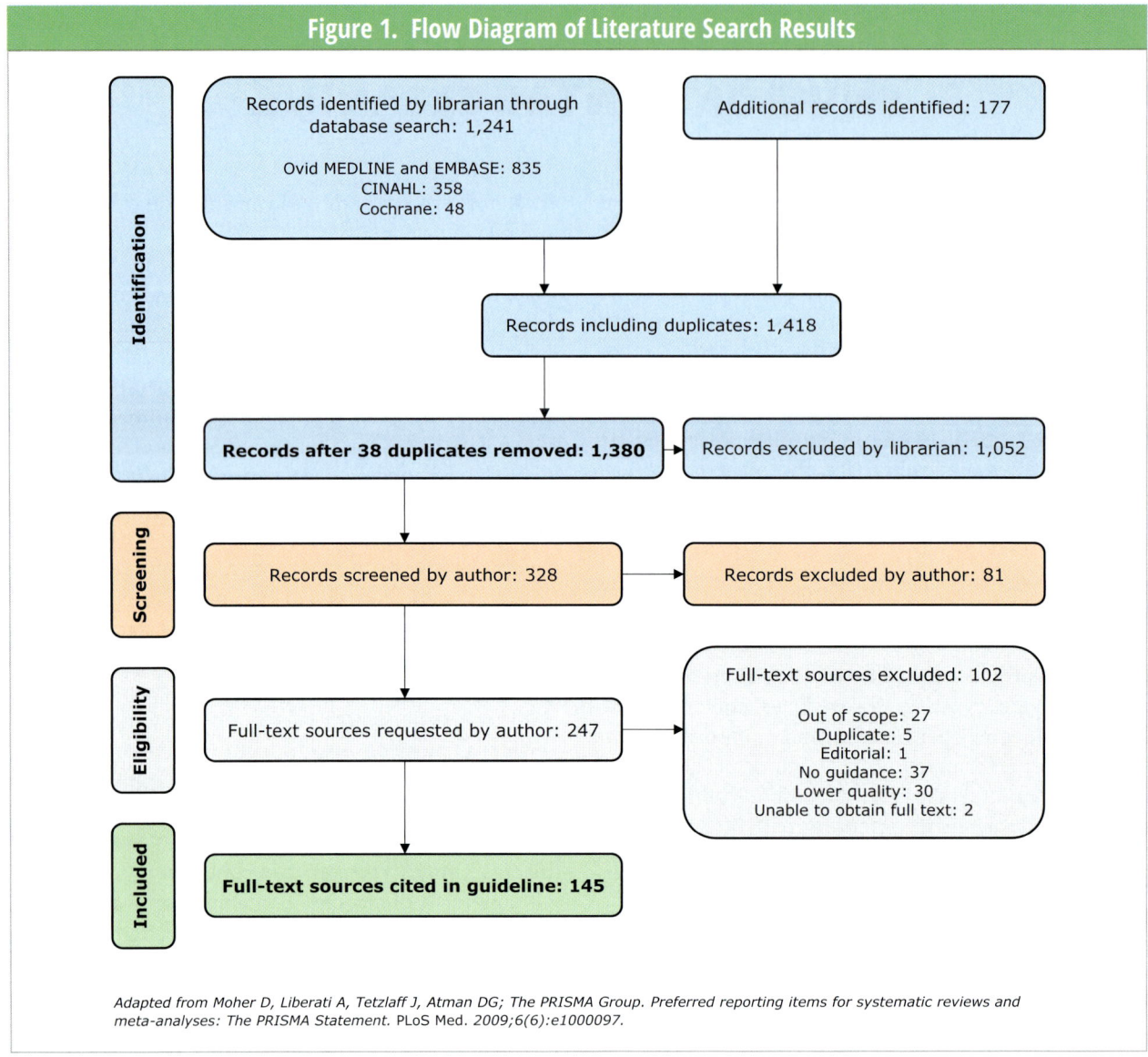

Figure 1. Flow Diagram of Literature Search Results

Adapted from Moher D, Liberati A, Tetzlaff J, Atman DG; The PRISMA Group. Preferred reporting items for systematic reviews and meta-analyses: The PRISMA Statement. PLoS Med. 2009;6(6):e1000097.

Evidence Review

A medical librarian with a perioperative background conducted a systematic search of the databases Ovid MEDLINE®, Ovid Embase®, EBSCO CINAHL®, and the Cochrane Database of Systematic Reviews. The search was limited to literature published in English from January 2013 through November 2018. At the time of the initial search, weekly alerts were created on the topics included in that search. Results from these alerts were provided to the lead author until May 2019. The lead author requested additional articles that either did not fit the original search criteria or were discovered during the evidence appraisal process. The lead author and the medical librarian also identified relevant guidelines from government agencies, professional organizations, and standards-setting bodies.

Search terms included *adenosine triphosphate, air sampling, ambulatory surgery center/facilit*, ants, aspergill*, auto scrubber, bacterial count, bacterial load, bedding and linens, beds, biolumi-nescence detection, bleach, body fluids, central processing, central service department, central supply (hospital), checklist, cleaning program/regimen/schedule/standard/policies/guideline/protocol/routine, cleaning zone, cleansing agents, cloths, cockroaches, colony count (microbial), contact surface, contact time, Creutzfeldt-Jakob disease/syndrome, cross infection, curtains, decontamination, decontamination (hazardous materials), detergents, diphtheria, disease reservoirs, disease transmission (infectious), disinfectants, disinfection, dust, dwell time, enhanced environmental cleaning, environmental microbiology/monitoring/cleaning/services/surface, fleas, flies, fluid waste management, fluorescent light, fomites, gram-negative bacteria, gram-positive bacteria, green cleaning, healthcare associated infection, heater-cooler, high-touch objects/surfaces, hospital housekeeping, hospital laundry service, housekeeping department, housekeeping (hospital), hydrogen peroxide, ice machine, infection control, insects, keyboard covers, laundry, laundry department, laundry service (hospital), lice, luminescent measurements, mattresses, microbial colony count, microfib*, mites, mouse, nosocomial infection, occupational health/exposure/*

injuries/safety, operating room tables, operating rooms/suites/ theat*, ozone, patient monitors/transfer board, pest control/management, phenols, Phthiraptera, previous patient, prior patient/ room occupant, quaternary ammonium compounds/disinfectant, room contamination, scrub sink, silver, Siphonaptera, sodium hypochlorite, solvents, sterile processing/supply, sterilization and disinfection, sticky mat, storage areas, subacute spongiform encephalopathy, surgical wound infection, surgical wound infection, surgicenters, tacky mat, terminal cleaning/disinfection/ decontamination, textiles, ultraviolet light, ultra-violet light, ultraviolet rays, vermin, viruses, visual inspection, waste disposal (fluid), and wet time.

Included were research and non-research literature in English, complete publications, and publications with dates within the time restriction when available. Historical studies were also included. Excluded were non-peer-reviewed publications and older evidence within the time restriction when more recent evidence was available. Editorials, news items, and other brief items were excluded. Low-quality evidence was excluded when higher-quality evidence was available, and literature outside the time restriction was excluded when literature within the time restriction was available (Figure 1).

Articles identified in the search were provided to the project team for evaluation. The team consisted of the lead author and one evidence appraiser. The lead author and the evidence appraiser reviewed and critically appraised each article using the AORN Research or Non-Research Evidence Appraisal Tools as appropriate. A second appraiser was consulted if there was a disagreement between the lead author and the primary evidence appraiser. The literature was independently evaluated and appraised according to the strength and quality of the evidence. Each article was then assigned an appraisal score. The appraisal score is noted in brackets after each reference as applicable.

Each recommendation rating is based on a synthesis of the collective evidence, a benefit-harm assessment, and consideration of resource use. The strength of the recommendation was determined using the AORN Evidence Rating Model and the quality and consistency of the evidence supporting a recommendation. The recommendation strength rating is noted in brackets after each recommendation.

Note: *The evidence summary table is available at http:// www.aorn.org/evidencetables/.*

Editor's note: *MEDLINE is a registered trademark of the US National Library of Medicine's Medical Literature Analysis and Retrieval System, Bethesda, MD. CINAHL, Cumulative Index to Nursing and Allied Health Literature, is a registered trademark of EBSCO Industries, Birmingham, AL. Scopus is a registered trademark of Elsevier, B.V., Amsterdam, The Netherlands.*

1. Product Selection and Use

1.1 Have an interdisciplinary team select disinfectants for use in the perioperative setting based on the following factors:
- Environmental Protection Agency (EPA) registration and hospital-grade rating[8,21];
- targeted microorganisms[8,22-24];
- contact times[8,22,25,26];
- manufacturers' instructions for use (IFU)[8,21,23];
- compatibility with surfaces, cleaning materials, and equipment[8,21,24,26];
- patient population (eg, neonatal)[8,21];
- cost[8,21,22,24,26];
- safety[8,21,26-29]; and
- effect on the environment.[21]

[Recommendation]

A standardized product selection process assists in the selection of functional and reliable products that are safe, cost-effective, and environmentally preferable and that promote quality care, as well as decreases duplication or rapid obsolescence.[21,30] For further guidance on pre-purchase evaluation, see the AORN Guideline for Medical Device and Product Evaluation.[30]

The Centers for Disease Control and Prevention (CDC) recommends that EPA-registered disinfectants be used in health care settings.[8]

1.1.1 Do not use high-level disinfectants or liquid chemical sterilants to clean and disinfect environmental surfaces or noncritical devices.[8,26] [Recommendation]

These chemicals are not intended for use on environmental surfaces and are not labeled for use as low- or intermediate-level disinfectants. Potential harms include chemical safety hazards for personnel and patients and damage to surfaces or equipment, which could create a reservoir for pathogens.

1.1.2 Do not use alcohol (ie, ethyl alcohol 60%– 90%, isopropyl alcohol 60%–90%) to disinfect large environmental surfaces (eg, tables, OR bed).[8] [Recommendation]

The risk for fire is a potential harm of using alcohol to disinfect environmental surfaces in the OR because of the oxygenated environment and presence of ignition sources. Furthermore, alcohol (eg, isopropyl alcohol 70%) is an antiseptic and is not an EPA-registered disinfectant.

1.1.3 Do not use disinfectants (eg, phenolics) to clean infant bassinets or incubators while these items are occupied.[8,21] If disinfectants (eg, phenolics) are used to terminally clean infant bassinets or incubators, prepare solutions in the correct concentrations per the manufacturer's IFU and rinse treated surfaces with water.[8,21] *[Recommendation]* **P**

Hyperbilirubinemia in newborns has been linked to poor ventilation and cleaning of incubators and other nursery surfaces with inadequately diluted phenolic solutions.[8]

1.2 Cleaning chemicals must be prepared, handled, used, stored, and disposed of in accordance with manufacturers' IFU and local, state, and federal regulations.[8,23,25,31] *[Regulatory Requirement]*

The users of EPA-registered disinfectants are required to follow the manufacturers' IFU in accordance with the Federal Insecticide, Fungicide, and Rodenticide Act (FIFRA), and noncompliance can be punishable by law.[25] Microbial contamination of disinfectants has been reported with improper dilution of the disinfectant.[8,25]

1.2.1 If the cleaning chemical is removed from the original container, the secondary container must immediately be labeled with the chemical name, concentration, and expiration date.[31] *[Regulatory Requirement]*

1.2.2 If there are no disposal restrictions from regulatory bodies, cleaning chemicals may be discarded along with copious amounts of cold utility water into a drain connected to a sanitary sewer.[26] *[Conditional Recommendation]*

1.3 Safety data sheets must be available and reviewed for each cleaning chemical used in the perioperative setting.[31] *[Regulatory Requirement]*

1.4 Conduct an annual chemical hazard risk assessment of all cleaning chemicals in use.[26,31] *[Recommendation]*

Assessing chemical hazards annually provides a mechanism for reviewing updated chemical safety data from the manufacturers and for identifying new, safer products that become available. For further guidance see the AORN Guideline for a Safe Environment of Care.[18]

1.5 Before applying a disinfectant, remove visible soil (eg, dust, debris) from the surface.[21,25] *[Recommendation]*

The presence of visible soil, dirt, and organic material inhibits the process of disinfection by preventing the disinfectant from interacting with the surface.[21,26]

1.6 Do not use a spray bottle to apply disinfectants to environmental surfaces in the perioperative practice setting.[8] *[Recommendation]*

Disinfectants that are sprayed produce more aerosols than solutions that are poured or ready-to-use wipes.[8] If the cleaning solution is contaminated, the spray mechanism may provide a route for airborne transmission of disease.[8] Aerosols generated may contaminate the surgical wound, sterile supplies, or the sterile field, or may cause respiratory symptoms (acute or chronic) in personnel and patients.

1.6.1 Disinfectants may be applied by a cloth or poured onto environmental surfaces in a manner that prevents splashing.[21] *[Conditional Recommendation]*

1.7 Apply the disinfectant for the contact time required on the product label for the targeted microorganism (eg, bacteria, viruses, *Clostridioides difficile* [formerly called *Clostridium difficile*]).[21,25] If the IFU require that the surface remain wet for the duration of the contact time, reapply the disinfectant as needed. *[Recommendation]*

The contact time required for disinfection varies by the type of microorganism and disinfectant. The manufacturer determines the amount of contact time needed to kill various types of microorganisms, and this is listed on the product label. If the disinfectant does not remain in contact with the microorganism for the full contact time, disinfection may not be achieved.[22,32]

Hong et al[32] conducted a nonexperimental study to evaluate the bactericidal efficacy of accelerated hydrogen peroxide, quaternary ammonium compounds, and sodium hypochlorite liquid disinfectants against *S aureus* and *Pseudomonas aeruginosa* on hard nonporous surfaces at six different contact times and eight different concentrations. The researchers found that deviation from label contact time or concentrations significantly reduced the disinfectants' efficacy.

In a quasi-experimental study, West et al[33] tested six types of disinfectant towelettes at 10 different contact times (ie, 30 seconds, 1 minute, 2 minutes, 3 minutes, 4 minutes, 5 minutes, 10 minutes, 20 minutes, 30 minutes, 60 minutes) to determine whether contact time and dry time influenced bactericidal efficacy against *S aureus*. The researchers found significant differences in the time it took the disinfectants to dry completely. Extending the recommended contact time or dry time beyond 30 seconds did not enhance disinfection; the log reductions at 30 seconds were not significantly different from those at 60 minutes. Towelette composition (eg, inactive ingredients, alcohol presence, disinfectant concentration) was also a significant variable in bactericidal efficacy.

Rutala et al[34] conducted a quasi-experimental study to test common health care disinfectants (ie, quaternary ammonium compound, phenolic, sodium hypochlorite) against *S aureus, Escherichia coli, P aeruginosa,* and *Salmonella choleraesuis* at 30 seconds and 5 minutes. The researchers found that the maximum log reduction was achieved in 30 seconds and was identical to the log reduction at 5 minutes.

West et al[35] conducted a nonexperimental comparative study to test the efficacy of 10 different disinfectant wipes over a 1-, 2-, 4-, and 8-ft square surface area. In this study, the wipes that dried out first reduced the amount of *Staphylococcus* and *Pseudomonas* species better than wipes that stayed wet longer. As the surface area increased, less disinfectant was applied by the wipes.

Regardless of the research findings, using a contact time that differs from the EPA-registered product label is considered off-label use, and as such the user assumes liability for any injuries and is potentially subject to enforcement action under FIFRA.[25]

1.8 **Have an interdisciplinary team select cleaning materials, tools, and equipment based on the following factors:**
- **surface composition of the items to be cleaned,**[21,36]
- **manufacturers' IFU for cleaning materials and equipment,**[21]
- **compatibility with detergents and disinfectants,**[21,37]
- **durability and life cycle,**[21,22,36]
- **cost,**[21]
- **personnel ergonomics and safety,**[21] **and**
- **effect on the environment.**[21]

[Recommendation]

A standardized product selection process assists in the selection of functional and reliable products that are safe, cost-effective, and environmentally preferable and that promote quality care, as well as decreases duplication or rapid obsolescence.[21,30] Effective cleaning and disinfection is accomplished when the correct tools and equipment are paired with the correct chemical solutions.[21]

In a quasi-experimental study, Gonzalez et al[36] tested five types of disinfectant wipes on anesthesia machine surfaces and simulated smooth and ridged knobs. The researchers found that device design and the texture of the cleaning cloth affected bacterial removal.

1.8.1 **Use low-linting cleaning materials (eg, mop heads, cloths).**[38,39] *[Recommendation]*

Excess lint can be deposited onto surfaces in the perioperative environment where it can be aerosolized and carried to the surgical wound or sterile supplies.

1.8.2 **Determine whether to select reusable or single-use cleaning materials (eg, mop heads, cloths) based on the following factors:**
- **laundering processes,**
- **laundry turnaround time,**
- **size of the areas to be cleaned,**
- **frequency of cleaning,**
- **cost,**
- **effect on the environment, and**
- **storage space.**[8,21,40]

[Recommendation]

1.8.3 **Microfiber cleaning materials may be used.**[21,38,39]

[Conditional Recommendation]

In a comparative study, Rutala et al[38] reported that microfiber mopping systems were more effective than cotton string mops at microbial removal (95% and 68% respectively) and that microbial removal with microfiber was equally effective with and without use of a disinfectant. Diab-Elschahawi et al[39] found in a comparative study that although microfiber cloths were best for decontamination, cotton was most effective after multiple launderings. However, the laundering methods used to process the microfiber cloths in this study were at a higher temperature than that recommended by the CDC, which may have altered their effectiveness.

In another nonexperimental study, Sifuentes et al[41] evaluated the effect of laundering and cleaning practices at 10 facilities on microbial load of both cotton and microfiber towels. The researchers found that regardless of the laundering method (ie, central, in-house laundering), microfiber towels had significantly greater microbial contamination than cotton towels.

Trajtman et al[42] conducted a quasi-experimental study to evaluate the removal and transfer of *C difficile* spores from moistened ceramic surfaces using both cotton and microfiber cloths on a simulated cleaning apparatus. The cotton cloths transferred spores between wet surfaces significantly more often than the microfiber cloths, and the microfiber cloths released significantly fewer spores onto the clean surface than cotton cloths.

Additional research is needed to determine the most effective material for cleaning and disinfecting environmental surfaces in perioperative areas.[24]

1.8.4 **Do not use a broom with bristles to sweep the floor in the semi-restricted and restricted areas.** [Recommendation]

Brooms with bristles are difficult to clean and may harbor pathogens that can be aerosolized during sweeping.

1.9 **Dedicate cleaning materials, tools, and equipment for use only in restricted and semi-restricted areas.**[21] [Recommendation]

The wheels on cleaning carts and equipment can transfer soil and microorganisms from areas outside the restricted and semi-restricted areas. Dedicated equipment may prevent cross contamination of the OR from other patient care areas.[21]

1.10 **Before storage and reuse, disassemble cleaning equipment according to the manufacturers' IFU, then clean, disinfect with an EPA-registered disinfectant, and dry the equipment.**[8] [Recommendation]

Cleaning the equipment prevents the growth of microorganisms during storage and prevents subsequent contamination of the perioperative area.[8]

1.11 **Room decontamination systems (ie, ultraviolet light,**[43-56] **hydrogen peroxide**[57-63]**) may be evaluated as an adjunct to manual cleaning procedures.**[64] [Conditional Recommendation]

The benefits of using room decontamination systems as an adjunct to cleaning procedures are likely to exceed the harms. The benefits may include reduction of contamination on environmental surfaces in the OR that could lead to transmission and patient infection. However, further research is needed to determine the clinical benefit for prevention of SSIs and other HAIs. Further research is also needed to evaluate the potential harms of using these devices in the OR, including their effect on sterile supplies and environmental parameters (eg, temperature, humidity). Additionally, decontamination devices have not been regulated and a variety of testing protocols are being used, making the need for standardized testing and product registration essential.[65] The effectiveness of the device may also vary by the technology used and product configuration. Furthermore, the cost-benefit analysis and the availability of resources needed to implement these systems will depend on the benefit-harm assessment in the local setting.

A systematic review by Leas et al[24] and a literature review by Weber et al[66] describe advantages and disadvantages of ultraviolet and hydrogen peroxide systems. An advantage of both systems is the ability to consistently eliminate residual contamination. However, neither system will physically remove organic or inorganic material. Ultraviolet light systems are dependent on distance and orientation of items to be disinfected and require shorter delivery time than hydrogen peroxide systems. Disinfecting an entire room with a hydrogen peroxide system requires sealing of air vents. However, hydrogen peroxide systems may have a greater sporicidal efficacy than ultraviolet systems. More studies are needed to determine the effect of hydrogen peroxide and ultraviolet systems on patient outcomes.

In a systematic review with meta-analysis, Marra et al[67] evaluated the use of hydrogen peroxide and ultraviolet light systems for reduction of HAIs caused by multidrug-resistant organisms (MDROs). Their analysis of 13 ultraviolet light system studies found a significant reduction in both *C difficile* and vancomycin-resistant enterococci (VRE) infections with use of these systems. The researchers concluded that further research is needed to evaluate hydrogen peroxide systems, although they found two studies that showed these systems also reduced VRE infections.

In another systematic review, Cobb[68] compared methicillin-resistant *S aureus* (MRSA) log reduction by ultraviolet light to log reduction by hydrogen peroxide vapor. Cobb's analysis of 12 studies on ultraviolet light and eight studies on hydrogen peroxide vapor found a significant reduction of MRSA on nonporous surfaces from both treatments. The researchers stated that a limitation of the review was their inability to control for other factors that may have influenced the reduction of MRSA on surfaces, such as the presence of soil and the dosage or intensity of the room decontamination systems.

Because of limited data, the Infectious Diseases Society of America (IDSA) and the Society for Healthcare Epidemiology of America (SHEA)[69] do not recommend the use of automated sporicidal terminal disinfection as a component of *C difficile* infection prevention.

Ultraviolet Light Systems

High-quality evidence is available regarding the use of ultraviolet light–emitting systems as adjunct technology to cleaning for the following outcomes:

- MDRO reduction on surfaces of patient rooms,[43,45,70-74] simulated patient rooms,[44,47,49] and the OR[53-56];
- MDRO transmission to subsequently admitted patients[48,50,52];
- SSI rates[51]; and
- time required to use the system.[56,70]

Five quasi-experimental studies[43-46,49] and one prospective cluster-randomized crossover trial[48] evaluated continuous ultraviolet light systems, with cycle times ranging from 20 to 83.7 minutes. The researchers found that continuous ultraviolet light systems significantly lowered the incidence of patient infections caused by MRSA, VRE and *C difficile*[48] and reduced environmental contamination by vegetative bacteria,[43] VRE,[45,46] *C difficile*,[43-46] *Acinetobacter* species,[45,49] MRSA,[46] *S aureus*,[49] and *Enterococcus faecalis.*[49]

Eleven quasi-experimental studies evaluated **pulsed xenon ultraviolet light systems**, with cycle times ranging from 8 to 20 minutes.[47,50-54,70-74] The researchers found that the pulsed xenon ultraviolet light systems

- significantly decreased SSI rates for Class I (clean) procedures,[51]
- significantly lowered hospital-acquired *C difficile* rates[50,73,74] and VRE rates,[73]
- reduced patient acquisition of VRE,[52]
- significantly reduced contamination of high-touch surfaces in the OR 54 and patient rooms,[70-72]
- decreased the labor burden,[47]
- were practical for daily disinfection of surfaces,[47] and
- may contribute to efficacy and efficiency of standard between-patient cleaning procedures in the OR when used on a 2-minute cycle.[53]

Two quasi-experimental studies evaluated the use of focused multivector ultraviolet (FMUV) light systems in the OR, with cycle times of 90 seconds.[55,56] The researchers found that the FMUV systems significantly reduced microbial contamination of the OR bed, back table, and electrosurgical unit[55] and that there was no significant difference in cleaning time when using FMUV with manual cleaning compared to manual cleaning alone.[56]

Hydrogen Peroxide Systems
High-quality evidence is available regarding the use of hydrogen peroxide systems as adjunct technology to discharge cleaning for the outcome of MDRO reduction on surfaces in patient rooms,[57,59,61,62] simulated patient rooms,[58,60] and a simulated OR.[63]

Two studies evaluated dry-mist hydrogen peroxide, with cycle times ranging from 18 to 52 minutes.[57,58] In a prospective randomized study conducted at two hospitals in France, Barbut et al[57] found that a hydrogen peroxide mist system was significantly more effective than 0.5% sodium hypochlorite solution in eradicating *C difficile* spores in patient rooms. Bartels et al[58] conducted a quasi-experimental study in a simulated setting and found that a dry-mist hydrogen peroxide and silver ion vapor decreased environmental contamination in intensive care unit (ICU) settings as an adjunct to **terminal cleaning** procedures.

Five quasi-experimental studies evaluated hydrogen peroxide vapor, with cycle times ranging from 1.5 to 3 hours.[59-63] The researchers found that use of hydrogen peroxide vapor as an adjunct to

other cleaning procedures reduced the rate of *C difficile* infections,[59] patient acquisition of MDROs,[62] and surface contamination with VRE,[60] MRSA,[61] and multidrug-resistant *Acinetobacter baumannii.*[63] In a simulated OR, Lemmen et al[63] did not identify any visual damage or alteration of surfaces after three applications of hydrogen peroxide vapor.

2. Cleaning Procedures

2.1 **Have an interdisciplinary team determine cleaning procedures and frequencies based on the type of surfaces and tasks to be performed.**[75,76] *[Recommendation]*

Involvement of an interdisciplinary team (eg, perioperative nursing, sterile processing, environmental services, infection prevention, anesthesia) allows input from personnel who perform environmental cleaning in perioperative areas and from personnel with expertise beyond clinical end-users (eg, infection prevention personnel). As part of a bundled approach to implementing best practices for environmental cleaning, Havill[76] recommended that cleaning procedures be developed by an interdisciplinary team.

Operational guidelines for cleaning frequency in the perioperative setting were identified as a gap in the literature based on the evidence review.

2.2 **Identify high-touch objects and surfaces to be cleaned and disinfected.**[5,6,8,15,77] *[Recommendation]*

Contamination of environmental surfaces that are touched frequently creates a risk for hands to acquire pathogens that could be transmitted to patients.[5-7,64,78] Moderate-quality evidence indicates that high-touch objects in the OR are more contaminated than low-touch objects and supports more frequent disinfection of high-touch objects.[5,7,15]

In a two-part descriptive study, Link et al[7] observed 43 surgical procedures and recorded the number of times a surface was touched by unsterile surgical team members' hands during patient care. The five surfaces touched most frequently were the anesthesia computer mouse, OR bed, nurse computer mouse, OR door, and anesthesia cart. The researchers found that a low-touch surface on the top of the OR light dome was less contaminated than the high-touch surfaces, except for the OR bed.

In a nonexperimental study, Alexander et al[5] collected 517 cultures from a variety of surfaces in 33 ORs. The researchers found that surfaces disinfected routinely (eg, back table, work station) had lower levels of bacteria than surfaces that came in contact with a higher number of OR personnel and that were not disinfected as often (eg, computer mouse, telephone).

Additionally, they found that vertical surfaces had fewer bacteria than horizontal surfaces.

As part of a nonexperimental study, Dallolio et al[15] cultured 10 high-touch surfaces (eg, anesthesia cart, OR bed and remote, vitals monitor, instrument table) in 10 ORs before the first scheduled surgery of the day and then again after completion of disinfection between procedures. The surfaces that exceeded the established limits for bacterial growth were an anesthesia computer touch screen, surgical lights, internal door opening buttons, and an intercom.

2.2.1 When cleaning high-touch objects, clean the frequently touched areas of the item (eg, control panel, switches, knobs, work area, handles).[8] [Recommendation]

In a nonexperimental study, Richard and Bowen[78] tested 13 surfaces in six orthopedic ORs before the first surgery of the day and found that items with buttons or controls (eg, tourniquet machine, electrosurgical unit, patient warming device, keyboards) and patient positioning devices were the items with the highest bioburden.

2.3 Determine the frequency and extent of cleaning required when areas are not occupied (eg, unused rooms, weekends).[8,64] [Recommendation]

The presence of personnel generates dust from shedding skin squames, which can harbor bacteria.[8,64] However, further evidence is needed to determine ideal terminal cleaning frequencies and the extent of cleaning and disinfection required in unoccupied perioperative areas.

2.4 Assign responsibility for cleaning perioperative areas and equipment to competent personnel.[21,64,79] [Recommendation]

Assigning cleaning responsibilities is an important component of defining cleaning procedures. After responsibility is determined, appropriate training programs, communication, and standardization can be implemented.[21,79] In a literature review, Dancer[64] discussed the importance of assigning cleaning responsibilities to reduce the number of items that personnel forget to clean.

When cleaning the OR between procedures, having personnel assigned to designated cleaning areas may prevent cross contamination between dirty and clean surfaces and may improve efficiency during turnovers. In an organizational experience to increase compliance with between-patient cleaning, Pederson et al[80] introduced a "pit crew" method to assign personnel specific tasks. Overall compliance with the cleaning protocol between procedures increased from 79% to 93%.

2.5 Perform cleaning activities in a methodical pattern that limits the transmission of microorganisms.[21,81] [Recommendation]

Cleaning an area in a methodical pattern establishes a routine for cleaning so that items are not missed during the cleaning process.[21] The method for cleaning may limit the transmission of microorganisms and reduce the risk of cross contamination of environmental surfaces.[81]

In an observational study, Bergen et al[81] evaluated the spread of bacteria on surfaces when cleaning with microfiber cloths moistened with sterile water and a detergent in a 16-side method and found that although bacterial counts of *E faecalis* and *Bacillus cereus* were lower after cleaning, the bacteria from contaminated surfaces were spread to clean surfaces. Additional research is needed to determine optimal cleaning methods for the perioperative setting and to evaluate the risk for microbial transmission across environmental surfaces during cleaning activities.

2.5.1 When cleaning with the same cleaning material (eg, cloth, wipe, mop head), progress from clean to dirty areas.[21,81] [Recommendation]

Cleaning the least soiled areas before moving to the most soiled areas diminishes the likelihood of spreading contaminants from dirtier areas to cleaner surfaces.[21]

2.5.2 When cleaning and damp dusting, progress from top to bottom.[21] [Recommendation]

During cleaning of high areas, dust, debris, and contaminated cleaning solutions may contaminate lower areas. If low areas are cleaned first, these areas could potentially be recontaminated with debris from the higher areas.[21]

2.5.3 The room may be cleaned in a clockwise or counter-clockwise direction in conjunction with clean-to-dirty and top-to-bottom methods.[21] [Conditional Recommendation]

Using the same sequence each time provides consistency and lowers the chance of missing items that need to be cleaned.

2.6 Do not return used cleaning materials (eg, mop heads, cloths) to the cleaning solution container.[8,21] [Recommendation]

Used cleaning materials are considered contaminated and returning them to the cleaning solution container contaminates the solution.

2.7 Change reusable cleaning materials after each use. Discard disposable cleaning materials after each use according to the manufacturer's IFU.[8] *[Recommendation]*

Using a dirty mop or cloth on a clean area or to clean for multiple patients may increase the risk of cross contamination. Discarding disposable material in non-designated areas (eg, toilets) can lead to clogging of pipes or sewer systems.

2.8 **Always consider floors in the perioperative practice setting to be contaminated.**[8,25,82,83] *[Recommendation]*

Even in the best scenario, the floor is essentially contaminated as soon as it is cleaned because of air contaminants settling on the floor after mopping and new contaminants being introduced by air currents or traffic.[25] In a nonexperimental study, Andersen et al[82] investigated the reduction of bacterial contamination of the floor using various cleaning methods and found that even with the best results, the floor and air was contaminated after use of each method.

Deshpande et al[83] conducted a nonexperimental study to evaluate floor contamination in patient rooms at five hospitals, either while the patient occupied the room or after terminal cleaning. The researchers found that floors were contaminated both during admission and after discharge. *C difficile* was the pathogen most frequently isolated from the floors, although MRSA and VRE were recovered significantly more often from *C difficile* isolation room floors.

2.8.1 **Consider items that contact the floor for any amount of time to be contaminated.**[1,83] *[Recommendation]*

In a quasi-experimental study, Munoz-Price et al[1] found that the OR floor was a potential reservoir for microorganisms because of inadvertent contamination of items during routine patient care. When patient care items (eg, IV tubing, safety straps) inadvertently touched the floor, the items were potentially contaminated by the floor and could transmit pathogens to the patient if they were not disinfected before contact with the patient.

Deshpande et al[83] conducted a point prevalence survey of 100 occupied isolation and non-isolation rooms at five hospitals to determine the number of patient care objects that touched the floor and the potential for those objects to transfer pathogens. When an item fell to the floor, if possible, the researcher picked it up with gloved or ungloved hands, depending on the patient's isolation status. Ungloved hands were cultured before and after item retrieval, and gloved hands were cultured only after item retrieval. Forty-one patient rooms had one or more items come into contact with the floor. Thirty-one hand or glove cultures were collected of which six grew MRSA, two grew VRE, and one grew *C difficile*.

2.8.2 **Clean and disinfect noncritical items (eg, safety straps, positioning devices) per the manufacturer's instructions after these items contact the floor.**[8,25] *[Recommendation]*

2.9 **Mop floors with damp or wet mops. Do not dust the floor with a dry mop in semi-restricted and restricted areas.**[8,82] *[Recommendation]*

In an observational study, Andersen et al[82] found that wet and moist mopping using a detergent was most effective in reducing organic soil on floors. Although all methods of mopping in the study increased bacterial counts in the air just after mopping, wet methods of mopping produced fewer aerosols than dry methods.

2.9.1 **When mopping, progress from the cleanest to dirtiest areas of the floor.**[21] *[Recommendation]*

The center of the room, where most of the patient care occurs, is most likely to have higher levels of contamination.

2.10 **After each patient use, clean and disinfect reusable noncritical, nonporous surfaces such as mattress covers, pneumatic tourniquets, blood pressure cuffs, and other patient equipment according to the manufacturers' instructions.**[8] *[Recommendation]*

The CDC recommends low- or intermediate-level disinfection of noncritical patient care items.[8]

2.10.1 **Clean and disinfect patient transport vehicles including the straps, handles, side rails, and attachments after each patient use.**[8] *[Recommendation]*

2.10.2 **Discard single-use items after each patient use.**[21] *[Recommendation]*

2.11 **Apply a protective barrier covering to noncritical equipment surfaces if the surface cannot withstand disinfection or is difficult to clean (eg, computer keyboards, foot pedals, touchscreen computer monitors).**[8,84] *[Recommendation]*

Protecting surfaces that cannot withstand disinfection, in accordance with the equipment manufacturer's instructions for cleaning, provides a mechanism to prevent surfaces from becoming a reservoir for microorganisms. Equipment that is difficult to clean may harbor pathogens in crevices that are not easy to disinfect. Using a barrier covering may prevent contamination of these areas and other areas that are difficult to reach.[8,84]

2.11.1 If a protective barrier covering is used, remove or clean and disinfect the cover per the manufacturer's IFU after each patient use.[8,84,85] *[Recommendation]*

The use of a protective barrier covering does not replace the need to clean the item. In a prospective interventional study, Das et al[85] evaluated the bacterial contamination of keyboards with and without protective covers. After 6 months of use, the researchers found that 96% of all the keyboards were positive for both nonpathogenic and potentially pathogenic bacteria (eg, *S aureus*, *Streptococcus* species, gram-negative rods). However, the amount of potentially pathogenic bacteria was higher on covered keyboards than on uncovered keyboards. The researchers theorized that the covered keyboards may not have been cleaned as often.

2.11.2 Clean noncritical medical equipment that cannot be covered and cannot withstand disinfection (eg, robots, imaging system components) in accordance with the equipment manufacturers' IFU.[8] *[Recommendation]*

Computers and other sensitive electronic devices are likely to become contaminated and may be difficult to clean. Electronic components may be damaged by cleaning chemicals.

2.12 Clean and disinfect equipment that is stored outside the surgical suite before bringing it into the semi-restricted area. *[Recommendation]*

The benefits of cleaning equipment before it is brought to the semi-restricted area include removal of any dust or microorganisms that may contaminate the semi-restricted environment.

2.13 Before cleaning, inspect mattresses and padded positioning device surfaces (eg, OR beds, arm boards, patient transport carts) for any moisture, stains, or damage.[8,86] *[Recommendation]*

Nonintact surfaces may become reservoirs for microorganisms and may harbor pathogens. Regular inspection for visible signs of compromise or wear, such as tears, cracks, pinholes or stains, facilitates prompt replacement and prevention of cross contamination resulting from underlying surface exposure.[86]

2.13.1 Remove and replace damaged or worn mattress coverings according to facility policy and the manufacturer's instructions.[8,86] *[Recommendation]*

The CDC does not recommend using patches for tears or holes in mattress coverings because the patches do not provide an impermeable surface.[8]

2.13.2 Avoid penetration of the mattress by needles and other sharp items.[8] *[Recommendation]*

Inadvertent puncture of a mattress cover provides a reservoir for blood and body fluids to enter the mattress.

3. Waste and Laundry

3.1 Standard precautions must be followed when cleaning, to prevent contact with blood, body fluids, or other potentially infectious materials.[19,75] *[Regulatory Requirement]*

All body fluids except sweat (eg, semen, vaginal secretions, cerebrospinal fluid, synovial fluid, pleural fluid, pericardial fluid, peritoneal fluid, amniotic fluid, saliva) are potentially infectious.[75]

3.1.1 Personal protective equipment (PPE) must be worn during handling of contaminated items or cleaning of contaminated surfaces, to reduce the risk of exposure to blood, body fluids, and other potentially infectious materials.[8,75] *[Regulatory Requirement]*

3.1.2 Gloves must be worn when it is reasonably anticipated that there may be contact with blood, body fluids, or other potentially infectious materials during handling or touching of contaminated items or surfaces.[75] *[Regulatory Requirement]*

3.1.3 Masks, eye protection, and face shields must be worn whenever contact with splashes, spray, splatter, or droplets of blood, body fluids, or other potentially infectious materials is anticipated.[75] *[Regulatory Requirement]*

3.1.4 Wear respiratory protection (ie, an N95 respirator, a powered air-purifying respirator) if cleaning procedures are expected to generate infectious aerosols.[8,19] *[Recommendation]*

3.1.5 Perform hand hygiene after PPE is removed and as soon as possible after hands are soiled.[20] *[Recommendation]*

3.2 When visible soiling by blood, body fluids, or other potentially infectious materials appears on surfaces or equipment, the area must be cleaned and disinfected immediately or as soon as feasible.[8,75] *[Regulatory Requirement]*

Soil on environmental surfaces increases the risk of cross contamination and is more difficult to remove the longer it remains on the surface. Critical patient care activities occurring at the same time as contamination may necessitate delay in removal.

3.3 Take the following steps when cleaning a spill of blood or body fluids:

1. Apply an EPA-registered disinfectant that is effective against bloodborne pathogens (eg, human immunodeficiency virus, hepatitis B virus) to the spill.[25]

2. Soak up the spill with an absorbent material (eg, lint-free towel, absorbent gel) and discard it.[8,21,25,75]

3. Clean and disinfect the surface.[25]

[Recommendation]

Applying an EPA-registered disinfectant to a spill of blood or body fluids inactivates bloodborne viruses and minimizes the risk for infection to personnel during cleanup.[75]

3.3.1 When an EPA-registered disinfectant is not available, a freshly diluted sodium hypochlorite solution may be used:

- for a small spill (< 10 mL), apply a 1:100 dilution (525-615 ppm available chlorine) to the spill before cleaning;

- for a large spill (> 10 mL), apply a 1:10 dilution (5,000 ppm to 6,150 ppm available chlorine) to the spill before cleaning and then use a 1:100 dilution to disinfect the surface.[25]

[Conditional Recommendation]

Environmental Protection Agency–registered disinfectants are preferred because they are reviewed for safety and microbial efficacy. However, the CDC recommends use of sodium hypochlorite solutions when EPA-registered products are not available.[25]

3.4 Items that would release blood, body fluids, or other potentially infectious materials in a liquid or semi-liquid state if compressed and items that are caked with dried blood, body fluids, or other potentially infectious materials must be placed in closable, leak-proof containers or bags that are color coded, labeled, or tagged for easy identification as biohazardous waste.[75] *[Regulatory Requirement]*

Leak-proof containers prevent exposure of personnel to blood, body fluids, and other potentially infectious materials and prevent contamination of the environment. Color coding or labeling alert personnel and others to the presence of items potentially contaminated with infectious microorganisms, prevent

exposure of personnel to infectious waste, and prevent contamination of the environment.[75]

3.4.1 Manage waste generated during care of patients on transmission-based precautions in accordance with standard waste management procedures per local, state, and federal regulations.[8,19,87] *[Recommendation]*

3.5 Containers or bags containing **regulated medical waste** must be transported in closed, impervious containers according to state and federal regulations.[8,75] *[Regulatory Requirement]*

3.6 Regulated waste must be stored in a ventilated area that is inaccessible to pests until it is transported for treatment and disposal according to state and federal regulations.[8] *[Regulatory Requirement]*

3.7 Contaminated liquid waste must be disposed of according to state and federal regulations (eg, pouring the liquid down a sanitary sewer, adding a solidifying powder to the liquid, using a medical liquid waste disposal system).[8,75] *[Regulatory Requirement]*

A well-ventilated area and large amounts of water are necessary to prevent inadvertent exposure of health care workers when pouring liquids into the sanitary sewer.[88]

In a nonexperimental study, Horn et al[89] found that when compared to an open suction cannister system, a closed system was a less hazardous and more efficient way to dispose of fluid waste.

3.8 Immediately or as soon as possible after use, contaminated sharps (eg, needles, blades, sharp disposable instruments) must be discarded in a closeable, puncture-resistant container that is leak proof on its sides and bottom and is labeled or color coded.[8,75] *[Regulatory Requirement]*

3.8.1 Sharps containers must not be overfilled.[75] *[Regulatory Requirement]*

An overfilled container increases the risk for injury each time additional items are added and makes proper closure of the container difficult.

3.8.2 Broken glassware must not be touched with hands.[75] Use mechanical means, such as forceps, tongs, or a dustpan to handle broken glass. *[Regulatory Requirement]*

Handling broken glassware with hands increases the potential for a sharps injury.

3.9 Laundry contaminated with blood, body fluids, or other potentially infectious materials must be handled as little as possible.[8,75] *[Regulatory Requirement]*

Handling contaminated laundry with a minimum of agitation avoids contamination of air, surfaces, and personnel.[8]

3.9.1 Contaminated laundry must be placed in labeled or color coded containers or bags at the location where it was used.[8,75] *[Regulatory Requirement]*

3.9.2 Contaminated laundry that is wet and may soak or leak through the container or bag must be placed and transported in closed containers or bags that prevent soak-through or leakage of fluids to the exterior.[8,75] *[Regulatory Requirement]*

4. OR and Procedure Rooms

4.1 Damp dust all horizontal surfaces (eg, furniture, surgical lights, booms, equipment) before the first scheduled surgical or other invasive procedure of the day.[8,64] *[Recommendation]*

Dust is known to contain human skin and hair, fabric fibers, pollens, mold, fungi, insect parts, glove powder, and paper fibers, among other components.[8,18] Airborne particles range from 0.001 micrometers to several hundred micrometers. In settings with dry conditions, gram-positive cocci (eg, coagulase-negative *Staphylococcus* species) found in dust may persist; in settings with surfaces that are moist and soiled, the growth of gram-negative bacilli may persist.[8]

4.1.1 Complete damp dusting before case carts, supplies, and equipment are brought into the room.[21] *[Recommendation]*

4.1.2 Use a clean, low-linting cloth moistened with a disinfectant to damp dust.[21] *[Recommendation]*

4.2 Operating and procedure rooms must be cleaned and disinfected after each patient procedure (Figure 2).[90-93] *[Regulatory Requirement]*

4.2.1 Do not begin environmental cleaning, including trash and contaminated laundry removal, until the patient has left the OR or procedure room.[8,21] *[Recommendation]*

Environmental surfaces may be recontaminated if cleaning begins while the patient is still occupying the room. Increased room traffic and movement for cleaning activities may generate unnecessary noise and be a distraction from patient care activities, including emergence from anesthesia.

4.2.2 Remove trash and used linen from the room[21] (See Recommendation 3). *[Recommendation]*

4.2.3 Clean and disinfect all items used during patient care, including
- anesthesia carts, including the top and drawer handles[7,21,84,94,95];
- anesthesia equipment (eg, IV poles, IV pumps)[21,84];
- anesthesia machines, including dials, knobs, and valves[3,84,94-96];
- patient monitors, including cables[43];
- OR beds[1,7,8,21];
- reusable table straps[21];
- OR bed attachments (eg, arm boards, stirrups, head rests)[1,21];
- positioning devices (eg, viscoelastic polymer rolls, vacuum pack positioning devices, socket attachments)[78];
- patient transfer devices (eg, roll boards)[16];
- overhead procedure lights[1,3,15,21];
- tables and Mayo stands[1,5,21,78]; and
- mobile and fixed equipment (eg, sitting or standing stools, suction regulators, pneumatic tourniquets, imaging viewers, viewing monitors, radiology equipment, electrosurgical units, microscopes, robots, lasers).[3,21,78]

[Recommendation]

The anesthesia work area, consisting of the anesthesia machine, anesthesia cart, IV poles, IV pumps, and monitoring equipment, contains irregular, complex surfaces that encounter frequent hand contact. Failing to clean these surfaces properly can lead to cross transmission of potential pathogens.[84] Moderate-quality evidence supports cleaning of the anesthesia machine and cart after patient care.[36,95,96]

4.2.4 Clean and disinfect the floor with a mop after each surgical or invasive procedure when visibly soiled or potentially soiled by blood or body fluids (eg, splash, splatter, dropped item).[1,8,21,38,82] *[Recommendation]*

4.2.5 Spot clean and disinfect the walls after each surgical or invasive procedure when visibly soiled.[8] *[Recommendation]*

4.3 Performing terminal cleaning or closing the OR after a contaminated or dirty/infected procedure (ie, Class III, Class IV) is not necessary.[14,97-99] If the patient is infected or colonized with an

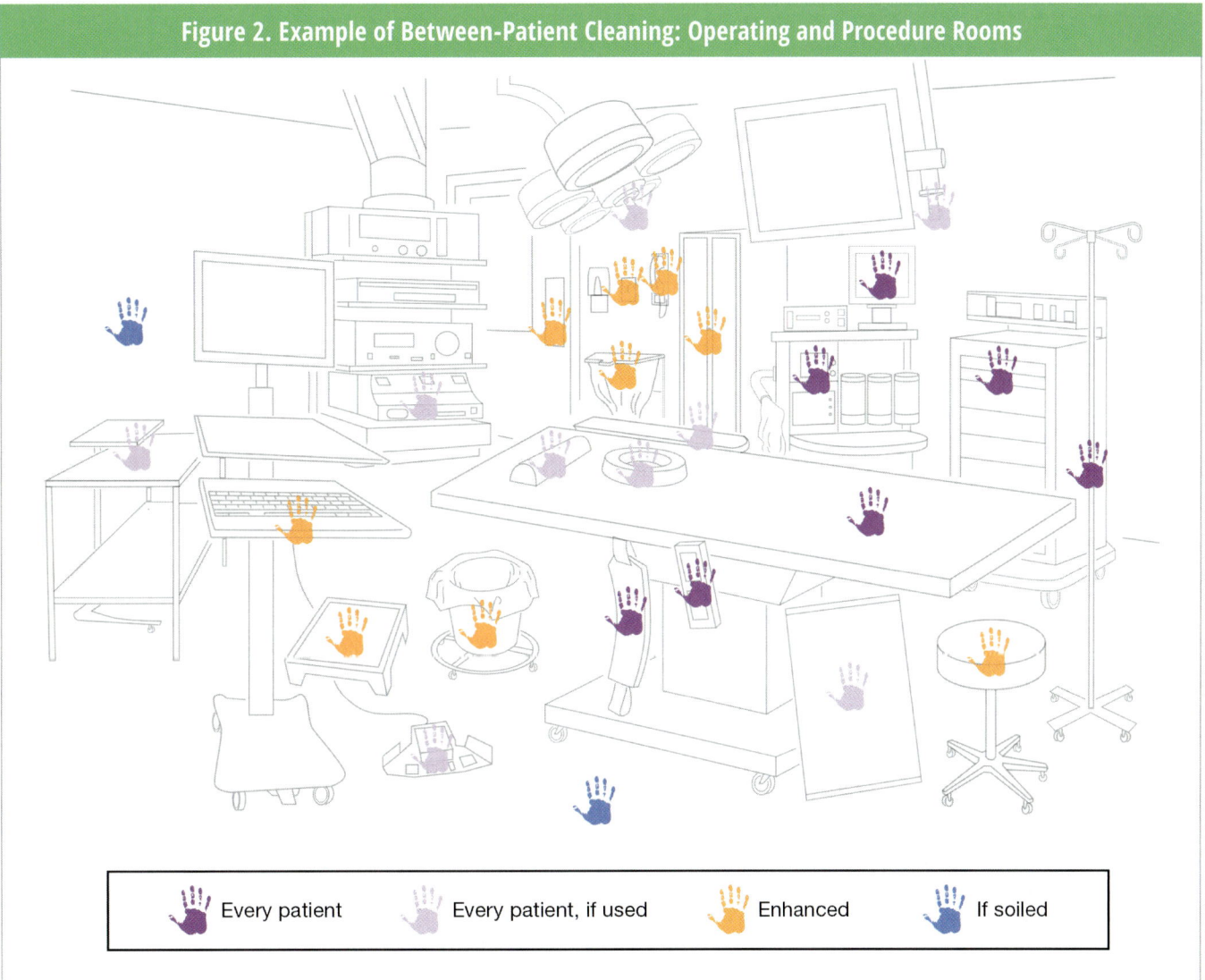

Figure 2. Example of Between-Patient Cleaning: Operating and Procedure Rooms

Every patient   Every patient, if used   Enhanced   If soiled

MDRO, implement enhanced environmental cleaning procedures (see Recommendation 8.1). [Recommendation]

The CDC and moderate-quality evidence support not performing terminal cleaning or closing the OR after surgery on a patient with an infected wound.[14,97-99]

In a retrospective controlled study in a large Canadian hospital, Abolghasemian et al[98] evaluated the incidence of HAIs in 83 patients who had an arthroplasty procedure in an OR in which the previous patient had a known infection. The researchers found that an infection was no more likely to occur in a patient whose surgery followed that of a patient with an infection than that of a patient without an infection. Of note, between-patient cleaning was completed using diluted 7% chlorhexidine solution, which is not an EPA-registered disinfectant, and neither unilateral ultraclean air flow nor orthopedic surgical space suits were used.

Balkissoon et al[14] conducted a prospective correlational study at an academic medical center in the United States to evaluate microbial surface contamination after standard between-patient cleaning following 14 surgeries on patients with infections and 16 surgeries on patients without infections. The surgeries were open procedures in multiple surgical specialties. The researchers did not find significant differences in bacterial contamination of high-touch surfaces in the OR between the two groups. The researchers concluded that standard between-patient cleaning reduced surface contamination to a minimum regardless of the infection status of the previous patient, and therefore the need for additional cleaning after a contaminated or dirty/infected procedure is not necessary.

In an exploratory prospective observational study at a German university hospital, Harnoss et al[99] evaluated the microbial room air concentration, as well as microbial sedimentation at 0.5 m and 1.5 m from the sterile field for 16 general surgeries on

Figure 3. Example of Between-Patient Cleaning: Preoperative and Postoperative Areas

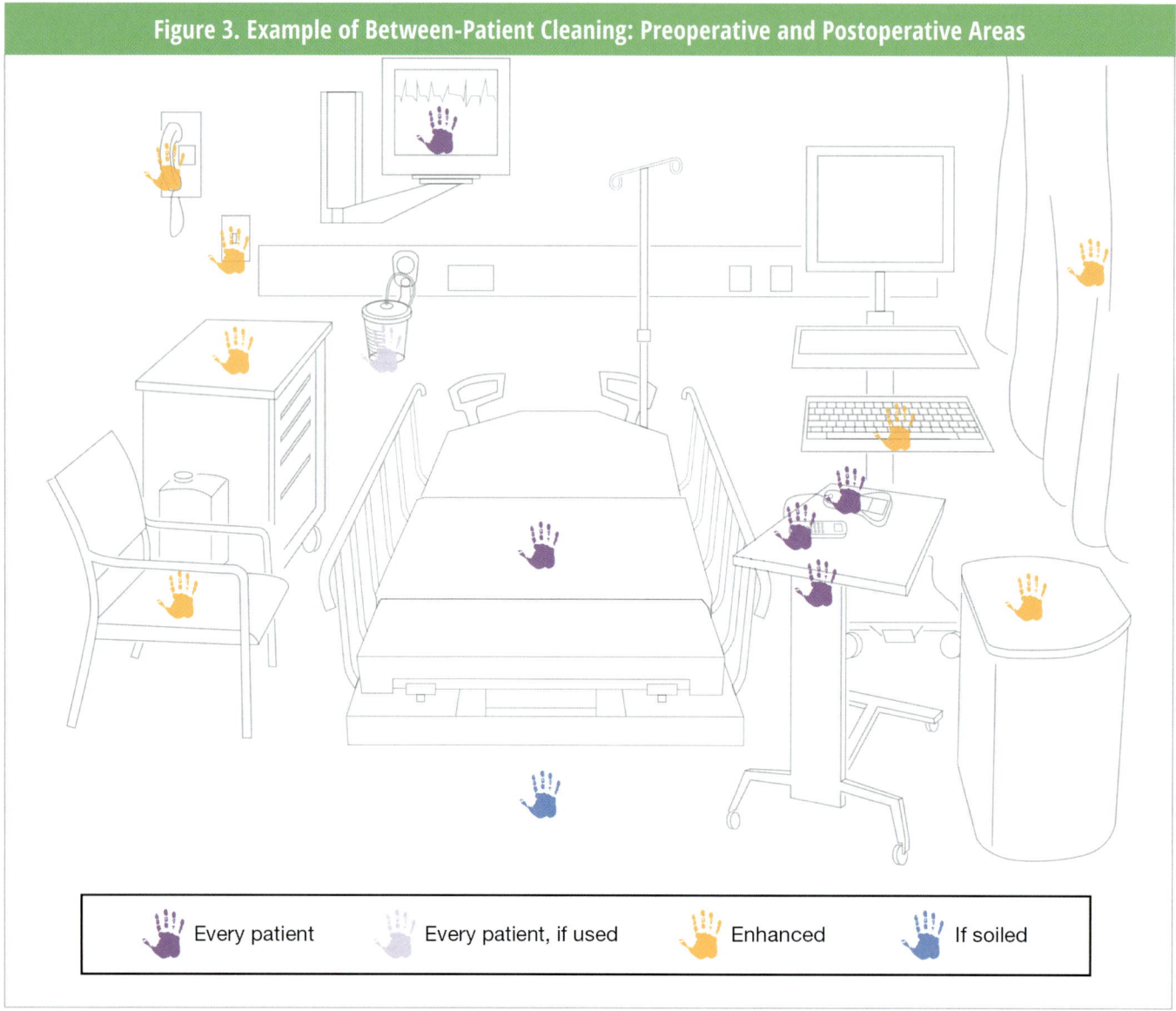

Every patient		Every patient, if used	Enhanced	If soiled

patients with infections and 14 general surgeries on patients without infections. Air samples were taken at the start of the procedure, every 30 minutes during the procedure, at the procedure end, and 30 minutes after the procedure. Microbial sedimentation was measured before the procedure and at the end of the procedure. No significant differences were found in microbial concentration of air or sedimentation between the surgeries, leading the researchers to conclude that procedures for patients with and without infections do not need to be spatially separated. However, one limitation was that the type of ventilation was not described.

4.4 Terminally clean operating and procedure rooms each day the rooms are used. *[Recommendation]*

4.4.1 Clean and disinfect the exposed surfaces, including wheels and casters, of all items, including

- anesthesia carts, including the top and drawer handles[7,21,84,94,95];
- anesthesia equipment (eg, IV poles, IV pumps)[21,84];
- anesthesia machines, including dials, knobs, and valves[3,84,94-96];
- patient monitors, including cables[43];
- OR beds[1,7,8,21];
- reusable table straps[21];
- OR bed attachments (eg, arm boards, stirrups, head rests)[1,21];
- positioning devices (eg, viscoelastic polymer rolls, vacuum pack positioning devices, socket attachments)[78];
- patient transfer devices (eg, roll boards)[16];
- overhead procedure lights[1,3,15,21,100];
- tables and Mayo stands[1,5,21,78];
- mobile and fixed equipment (eg, suction regulators, pneumatic tourniquets, imaging

viewers, viewing monitors, radiology equipment, electrosurgical units, microscopes, robots, lasers)[3,21,78];

- storage cabinets, supply carts, and furniture[3,21];
- light switches[3,21];
- door handles and push plates[3,7,21];
- telephones and mobile communication devices[5,15,21];
- computer accessories (eg, keyboards, mouse, touch screen)[5,7,78];
- chairs, stools, and step stools[21]; and
- trash and linen receptacles.[3,8,21]

[Recommendation]

4.4.2 Clean and disinfect the entire floor, including areas under the OR bed and mobile equipment,[21] using either a wet vacuum or mop.[8] *[Recommendation]*

5. Preoperative and Postoperative Areas

5.1 Preoperative and postoperative patient care areas must be cleaned after each patient has left the area **(Figure 3)**.[8,21,90,91] *[Regulatory Requirement]*

5.1.1 Clean and disinfect items that are used during patient care, including

- patient monitors,[43,79]
- infusion pumps and IV poles,[79,101]
- patient beds or stretchers,[43,44,77,102,103]
- over-bed tables,[2,40,43,44,77,79,102-107]
- television remote controls,[44,102,103] and
- call lights.[2,77,79,104,105,107]

[Recommendation]

5.1.2 Clean and disinfect mobile and fixed equipment (eg, suction regulators, medical gas regulators, imaging viewers, radiology equipment, warming equipment) that is used during patient care.[3,21] *[Recommendation]*

5.1.3 Clean and disinfect the floor with a mop when visibly soiled or potentially soiled by blood or body fluids (eg, splash, splatter, dropped item).[1,8,21,38,82] *[Recommendation]*

5.1.4 Spot clean and disinfect the walls when visibly soiled.[8] *[Recommendation]*

5.2 Terminally clean the preoperative and postoperative patient care areas each day the areas are used. *[Recommendation]*

5.2.1 Clean and disinfect the exposed surfaces, including wheels and casters, of all items in the area, including

- patient monitors[43,79];
- patient beds or stretchers[43,44,77,79,101-103,107];
- over-bed tables[2,43,44,77,79,102-105];
- television remote controls[44,102,103];
- call lights[2,77,79,104,105];
- mobile and fixed equipment (eg, suction regulators, medical gas regulators, imaging viewers, radiology equipment, warming equipment)[3,21];
- storage cabinets, supply carts, and furniture[3,21];
- light switches[3,21];
- door handles and push plates[3,21];
- telephones and mobile communication devices[21];
- computer accessories (eg, keyboard, mouse, touch screen)[1,69];
- chairs, stools, and step stools[21]; and
- trash and linen receptacles.[8,21]

[Recommendation]

5.2.2 Clean and disinfect the entire floor, including areas under mobile equipment,[21] using either a wet vacuum or mop.[8] *[Recommendation]*

6. Sterile Processing Areas

6.1 Damp dust all horizontal surfaces in the sterilization packaging area (eg, countertops, workstations) at least daily.[108] *[Recommendation]*

Dust or debris on surfaces can be aerosolized onto instruments being prepared for sterilization or onto sterilized items. Daily damp dusting helps to minimize the opportunity for dust dispersal.

6.1.1 Use a clean, low-linting cloth moistened with a disinfectant to damp dust.[21] *[Recommendation]*

6.2 Terminally clean sterile processing areas each day the areas are used.[108] *[Recommendation]*

Sterile processing personnel conduct critical processes, such as decontaminating, assembling, and sterilizing surgical instrumentation, in support of operating and invasive procedure rooms. As such, the recommendations for terminal cleaning apply in sterile processing areas as in areas where surgical and other invasive procedures are performed. Furthermore, sterile processing areas where decontamination occurs have some of the highest risks for environmental contamination of all perioperative areas. Environmental cleaning in sterile processing areas is critical for reducing the risk of disease transmission from reservoirs of blood-borne pathogens and microorganisms in the decontamination environment.

The Association for the Advancement of Medical Instrumentation recommends that floors and horizontal work surfaces in sterile processing areas be cleaned daily.[108]

6.3 Clean and disinfect the clean work areas, such as the packaging area and sterile storage area, before the dirty work areas, such as the decontamination area, to reduce the possibility of contaminating the clean areas.[108] *[Recommendation]*

6.4 When feasible, avoid terminal cleaning when personnel are actively decontaminating instruments. *[Recommendation]*

Aerosolization and dispersal of contaminated water can occur during instrument decontamination. If cleaning of surfaces and floors is occurring at same time, there is potential for cross transmission of pathogens.

6.5 Clean and disinfect all work surfaces and high-touch objects in the clean work areas and decontamination areas using a clean, low-linting cloth.[108] *[Recommendation]*

6.6 Remove trash from receptacles in sterile processing areas at least daily and when they are full.[108] *[Recommendation]*

6.7 Clean and disinfect all floors in sterile processing areas each day the areas are used.[108] *[Recommendation]*

7. Scheduled Cleaning

7.1 Determine a cleaning schedule (eg, weekly, monthly) for areas and equipment that are not terminally cleaned, including
- clean and soiled storage areas;
- sterile storage areas;
- shelving, drawers, and storage bins;
- corridors, including stairwells and elevators;
- walls and ceilings;
- privacy curtains;
- pneumatic tubes and carriers;
- sterilizers and loading carts;
- sterilizer service access rooms;
- lounges, waiting rooms, locker rooms, bathrooms, offices; and
- environmental services closets.[8,21]

[Recommendation]

Areas and equipment that are not cleaned according to a schedule may be missed during rou-tine cleaning procedures and become environmental reservoirs for dust, debris, and microorganisms.

7.2 Clean ventilation ducts, including air vents and grilles, and change their filters on a routine basis according to the manufacturers' IFU.[8] *[Recommendation]*

Clean ventilation ducts and filters support optimal performance of the ventilation system.

7.3 Clean and disinfect linen chutes on a routine basis.[8] *[Recommendation]*

Linen chutes become contaminated by dirt and debris with use.

7.4 Clean and disinfect all refrigerators and ice machines on a routine basis according to the manufacturers' IFU.[8] *[Recommendation]*

Refrigerators and ice machines become contaminated with use.

7.5 Clean and disinfect sinks, including eye wash stations, on a routine basis.[8] *[Recommendation]*

8. Special Pathogens

8.1 Implement enhanced environmental cleaning procedures following the care of patients who are known or suspected to be infected or colonized with MDROs, including
- MRSA,
- VRE,
- vancomycin-intermediate *Enterococcus* species,
- vancomycin-resistant *S aureus,*
- vancomycin-intermediate *S aureus,*
- carbapenem-resistant *Enterobacteriaceae,*
- multidrug-resistant *Acinetobacter* species,
- *Candida auris,*[109]
- extended spectrum beta-lactamase-producing organisms, and
- *Klebsiella pneumoniae* carbapenemase-producing organisms.[48,87,101,110-114]

[Recommendation]

Decreasing environmental contamination on high-touch surfaces may decrease the risk of MDRO transmission. Moderate-quality evidence supports enhanced environmental cleaning of high-touch surfaces following the care of patients who are infected or colonized with MDROs.[101,111,113,114] A limitation of this evidence is that the researchers did not use an objective method to identify high-touch objects, such as measuring the frequency of touch or contamination level of the surfaces. Furthermore, these studies were performed in the inpatient setting and further research is needed to evaluate enhanced environmental cleaning in the perioperative setting.

In a multi-center stepped-wedge trial, Mitchell et al[114] evaluated the effect of a cleaning bundle that emphasized daily cleaning of high-touch surfaces, a consistent cleaning sequence, and compliance with product manufacturers' instructions on the incidence of health care–associated *S aureus* bacteremia, *C difficile* infection, and VRE infection. The intervention resulted in a significant reduction in VRE infections, but not other infection types. The researchers proposed that use of bundle to reduce VRE would lead to decreased length of stay and antimicrobial resistance treatment cost and also eliminate bacteria similar to VRE.

In a randomized controlled trial, Hess et al[101] evaluated enhanced cleaning procedures in an ICU setting and found that intense cleaning of patient rooms contaminated with identified MRSA or multidrug-resistant *A baumannii* did not significantly decrease contamination of health care workers' gowns and gloves. However, in an observational study, Morgan et al[113] found that environmental contamination was the main determinant of transmission of MDROs to health care workers' clothing, gloves, and gowns. In a quasi-experimental study, Datta et al[111] found that enhanced cleaning significantly reduced MRSA and VRE contamination and decreased the risk of MRSA transmission from the room's previous occupant.

The CDC recommends meticulous cleaning and disinfection of both patient rooms and mobile equipment to reduce the risk of transmission of *C auris*.[109]

8.1.1 **Clean and disinfect all items touched during patient care, including**
- **storage cabinets, supply carts, and furniture**[3,21]**;**
- **light switches**[3,21]**;**
- **door handles and push plates**[3,21,87]**;**
- **telephones and mobile communication devices**[21,87]**;**
- **computer accessories (eg, keyboard, mouse, touch screen)**[1,87]**;**
- **chairs, stools, and step stools**[21]**;**
- **trash and linen receptacles**[21]**; and**
- **privacy curtains in the perioperative patient care areas.**[115,116]

[Recommendation]

8.1.2 **In addition to standard precautions, wear a gown and gloves when performing enhanced environmental cleaning procedures.**[8,19] *[Recommendation]*

8.2 **Following the care of patients diagnosed with or suspected of infection with *C difficile*, use an** EPA-registered disinfectant that is effective against *C difficile* spores when cleaning.[8,19,25] *[Recommendation]*

C difficile presents unique challenges for environmental cleaning. In its spore form, *C difficile* can survive for long periods, up to 5 months, on environmental surfaces. *C difficile* spores also are resistant to several cleaning chemicals (eg, alcohols, phenols, quaternary ammonium compounds).[69] Selection of a cleaning chemical that is effective against *C difficile* spores and removal of the spores from environmental surfaces are important when disinfecting a surface contaminated with *C difficile*.[69,77]

8.2.1 **An interdisciplinary team that includes an infection preventionist may determine whether a nonsporicidal disinfectant will be used in a nonoutbreak situation.**[69] *[Conditional Recommendation]*

In a review of the literature, McDonald et al[69] found minimal evidence to support the use of sporicidal disinfectant in a nonoutbreak setting. Therefore, IDSA and SHEA[69] recommend daily and terminal cleaning with sporicidal disinfectant in the inpatient setting only during outbreaks or sustained high rates of *C difficile* infections and for reoccurrence of infections in the same patient room.

8.3 **Following the care of patients diagnosed with or suspected of infection or colonization with *C auris*, use an EPA-registered disinfectant that is effective against *C difficile* spores.**[109] *[Recommendation]*

Some disinfectants may not be effective against *C auris*. Until further information is available, the CDC recommends using an EPA-registered disinfectant that is effective against *C difficile* spores.[109]

However, Rutala et al[117] recently conducted a quasi-experimental study to evaluate the efficacy of disinfectants against *C auris* inoculated onto stainless steel discs. The researchers found that several commonly used disinfectants (eg, phenolic, 1.4% hydrogen peroxide, alcohol-quaternary ammonium compound) were as effective against *C auris* as chlorine-based products, which are primarily used as disinfectants for *C difficile* spores.

8.4 **Restrict room access following the care of a patient diagnosed with or suspected of infection with an airborne transmissible disease (eg, tuberculosis) and following aerosolization activities (eg, intubation, extubation, cough-generating activities) of a patient diagnosed with or suspected of infection with a droplet transmissible disease (eg, influenza) until adequate time has passed for air exchanges per hour to remove 99% of airborne particles from**

the air (eg, 15 air exchanges per hour for 28 minutes to remove 99.9% of airborne contaminants).[8,19,118] *[Recommendation]*

Patients and personnel entering a room that has transmissible disease particles in the air are at risk for contracting the disease.[19]

8.4.1 If entering the room before a complete air exchange occurs, wear respiratory protection (eg, an N95 respirator) to perform environmental cleaning.[8,118] *[Recommendation]*

8.5 Use special cleaning procedures for environmental contamination with high-risk tissue (ie, brain, spinal cord, eye tissue, pituitary tissue) from a patient who is diagnosed with or suspected of having Creutzfeldt-Jakob disease (CJD). If the environment is not contaminated with high-risk tissue, follow routine cleaning procedures.[8,119] *[Recommendation]*

Currently, no EPA-registered disinfectants claim to inactivate prions on environmental surfaces.[119] When the environment is contaminated with tissue that has a high risk of containing prions, the causative infectious agent in CJD, extraordinary cleaning procedures are necessary in accordance with recommendations from the CDC and SHEA.[8,119]

8.5.1 Before the operative or invasive procedure begins, remove unnecessary equipment and cover work surfaces with a disposable, impervious material that can be removed and decontaminated after the procedure if contaminated with high-risk tissue.[8,119] *[Recommendation]*

Covering environmental surfaces (eg, anesthesia cart, prep stand) minimizes contamination of the environment.

8.5.2 When linens are not contaminated with high-risk tissue, follow routine laundering processes.[119] *[Recommendation]*

8.5.3 Clean noncritical environmental surfaces contaminated with high-risk tissue with a detergent and then decontaminate with a solution of either sodium hypochlorite (1:5 to 1:10 dilution with 10,000 ppm to 20,000 ppm available chlorine) or sodium hydroxide (1N NaOH), depending on surface compatibility.[8,119] *[Recommendation]*

No transmissions of prion diseases from environmental surfaces have been reported; however, it remains prudent to eliminate highly infectious material from OR surfaces that will be contacted during subsequent surgeries.[8,119]

8.5.4 Perform cleaning and disinfection of surfaces contaminated with high-risk tissues in the following order:

1. Remove the gross tissue from the surface.
2. Clean the area with a detergent solution.
3. Apply the disinfectant solution for a contact time of 30 minutes to 1 hour.
4. Use an absorbent material to soak up the solution.
5. Discard the cleaning material in an appropriate waste container.
6. Rinse the treated surface thoroughly with water.[8,119]

[Recommendation]

8.5.5 Use standard cleaning procedures to disinfect surfaces that are not contaminated with high-risk tissue.[119] *[Recommendation]*

8.5.6 Manage regulated medical waste generated during patient care, including waste that was contaminated by high-risk tissue and has been decontaminated, in accordance with standard waste management procedures per local, state, and federal regulations.[8] *[Recommendation]*

No epidemiological evidence has linked CJD transmission to waste disposal practices.[8]

9. Environmental Contamination

9.1 Implement cleaning and disinfection procedures for construction, renovation, repair, demolition, and disaster remediation.[8] *[Recommendation]*

According to the CDC, cleaning and disinfection measures during internal and external construction projects reduce contamination of environmental air and surfaces from dust and potential pathogens, such as *Aspergillus* and *Bacillus,* and are key elements of an infection prevention program.[8] Several reports have linked environmental air and surface contamination from construction projects to outbreaks of infection in health care settings.[120-123] However, in a literature review of construction-related fungal case reports from 1974 to 2014, Kanamori et al[124] found a decline in the number of reported cases, which the authors thought could be a result of guidelines and policies on infection prevention and control during construction.

9.1.1 Determine the cleaning and disinfection procedures and frequencies based on the infection control risk assessment. *[Recommendation]*

An interdisciplinary team that includes an infection preventionist performs an infection control risk assessment before starting any construction project.[8,125,126]

9.1.2 **Perform cleaning and disinfection of environmental surfaces to remove dust and debris.**[8,123,125] **If dust is contaminating areas outside of the construction barriers, assess the barriers to determine their effectiveness and reestablish the barriers.** *[Recommendation]*

While investigating an outbreak of deep bacterial eye infections, Gibb et al[123] reported that fine dust from a construction project was found on horizontal surfaces in the OR. After the ORs were cleaned of dust and reopened, no additional eye infections were reported during the surveillance period.

9.1.3 **Perform terminal cleaning before equipment and supplies are placed in the area where the construction, renovation, repair, demolition, or disaster remediation has been completed.**[8] *[Recommendation]*

9.2 **If flooding or a water-related emergency occurs, including sewage intrusion, inspect the area for water damage and implement a cleaning and disinfection process.**[8] *[Recommendation]*

9.2.1 **When surfaces remain in good repair, allow them to dry for 72 hours and perform terminal cleaning.**[8] *[Recommendation]*

9.2.2 **When surfaces are damaged or cannot dry within 72 hours, perform remediation to replace the surface with new materials after the facility engineer determines that the underlying structure is dry.**[8] *[Recommendation]*

9.3 **Perform terminal cleaning of affected areas when condensation is observed on surfaces.**[8] *[Recommendation]*

Condensation can contain debris or infectious organisms and can contaminate surfaces where sterile supplies are placed or serve as a cross-contamination source.

9.4 **When contamination of the incoming air occurs, perform terminal cleaning of the affected areas, including ventilation ducts, air vents, and grilles, and change air filters after the source of the contamination is identified and contained.**[8,120] *[Recommendation]*

10. Pests

10.1 **Take measures to prevent pest infestation of the perioperative environment, including removing food, containing biological waste, and keeping windows and doors closed.**[8] *[Recommendation]*

Pests may cause disease and microorganism transmission by serving as a vector.[8,127-130] Insects in health care settings have been shown to carry more pathogens than insects in residential settings. Pathogens isolated from insects in health care settings also have been shown to have antibiotic resistance.[8,129]

10.2 **If preventive measures fail to eliminate the cause of the infestation, consult a credentialed pest control specialist.**[8] *[Recommendation]*

Identification of the species, life cycle, diet, and virulence potential can aid in determining necessary actions.[131] A credentialed pest control specialist trained in integrated pest management uses this information to select the most economical actions with the least possible hazard to the environment and personnel.[21,132]

10.2.1 **Terminally clean the area after an infestation is resolved.**[8] *[Recommendation]*

The presence of open sterile supplies, patients' compromised tissue integrity, and mixing of medications in perioperative areas necessitates the removal of any residue from the environment.[131]

11. Education

11.1 **Provide education and complete competency verification activities related to the principles and processes of environmental cleaning.** *[Recommendation]*

Moderate-quality evidence supports educating personnel on the principles and processes of environmental cleaning.[24,94,114,133] In a systematic review, Leas et al[24] found 23 studies that included education as a key component to improve environmental cleaning.

Before implementing a cleaning bundle in a quasi-experimental study, Mitchell et al[114] allotted 2 weeks at each facility for facilitators to deliver multiple education sessions to environmental services personnel on cleaning procedures, roles and responsibilities, and the relationship of cleaning to HAI reduction. One component of the education was identification of frequent touch points in the patient care environment, which led to an increased cleaning compliance during the course of the study.

Hota et al[133] conducted a quasi-experimental study and found that surface contamination with

VRE was related to a failure to clean rather than failure of a product or cleaning procedure. Cleaning thoroughness and site contamination improved significantly after implementation of an education program for housekeeping personnel.

In a prospective cohort study, Goebel et al[94] found a significant decrease in post-procedure contamination after providing education to housekeeping personnel that was specific to anesthesia workspace cleaning. After two education sessions that included demonstrations and hands-on sessions, the housekeeping personnel completed post-procedure cleaning for 100 orthopedic surgeries. Another 100 post-procedure room cleanings were performed by nurse anesthetists, who normally cleaned the area as part of their job. The housekeeping group took less time to clean and had a 67% reduction in bacterial load compared to the nurse anesthetist group. Additionally, no patients in the rooms cleaned by housekeeping personnel developed HAIs, but six patients in the rooms cleaned by the nurse anesthetists developed HAIs.

In an organizational experience report, Armellino et al[134] found that standardized checklists, competency verification, and education were necessary for improving cleaning compliance. A baseline audit of facility cleaning practices revealed large variability in processes. On further exploration, the researchers discovered that competency verification occurred shortly after hire but was sporadically validated thereafter. Consequently, the organization developed sequenced protocols, reeducated personnel, and implemented an ongoing competency verification process.

In a literature review, Dancer[64] found that cleaning education was often no more than a "perfunctory introduction to the cleaning process" and that a lack of understanding of the basic microbiologic principles underlying cleaning processes can allow potential reservoirs of pathogens in the environment to go unrecognized. Dancer further described the consequences of limited training in environmental cleaning, such as improper maintenance of cleaning equipment, inappropriate use of cleaning chemicals, and exposing patients to contaminated surfaces.

11.1.1   Incorporate topics for education and competency verification related to the principles and processes of environmental cleaning, including

- basic principles of microbiology[21,64,126];
- signs and labels or color coding required for contaminated items[75];
- the modes of transmission of bloodborne pathogens and the employer's exposure control plan[75];

- the use and limitation of methods for reducing the exposure (eg, engineering controls, work practices, PPE)[21,75];
- the hepatitis B vaccine, its efficacy and safety, the method of administration, and the benefits of vaccination[75];
- location and use of eye wash stations[18];
- types, proper selection, proper use, location, removal, handling, decontamination, and disposal of PPE[19,21,23,75];
- location of safety data sheets[18];
- identification and handling of hazardous chemicals[18];
- hazardous and medical waste disposal[18,21];
- review of the organization's policies and procedures[126];
- selection of cleaning chemicals, materials, and equipment based on the intended use and compatibility with surfaces[126]; and
- reading and interpreting the disinfectant product labels, including contact times.[26]

[Recommendation]

11.1.2   **Trained observers may use knowledge assessment tools to verify competence.** *[Conditional Requirement]*

In a literature review, Kak et al[135] concluded that competence is best measured through evaluation of performance by experts or trained observers. To provide accurate evaluations, assessors must be trained but the length of training depends on the expertise of the assessor, what is to be assessed, and the instrument to be used. Other methods to evaluate competency include objective structured examinations, interviews, or simulations.[126,135]

11.1.3   **Develop educational materials appropriate in content, vocabulary level, literacy, and language for the target personnel.**[24,75,79] *[Recommendation]*

11.1.4   **Provide education when new disinfectants, equipment, or processes are introduced.**[23] *[Recommendation]*

11.2   **Personnel at risk for occupational exposure to blood, body fluids, or other potentially infectious materials must receive training before assignment to tasks where occupational exposure may occur, at least annually, and when changes to procedures or tasks effect occupational exposure risk.**[75] *[Regulatory Requirement]*

The Occupational Safety and Health Administration requires employers to provide training on the

Bloodborne Pathogens standard during working hours at no cost to employees.[75]

11.3 Provide education that addresses human factors related to the principles and processes of environmental cleaning.[24,136,137] *[Recommendation]*

Human factors include the interpersonal and social aspects of the perioperative environment (eg, coordination of activities, teamwork, collaboration, communication).[24] Effectively implementing the principles and processes of environmental cleaning requires that perioperative and environmental services personnel demonstrate not only procedural knowledge and technical proficiency but also the ability to anticipate needs, coordinate multiple activities, work collaboratively with other team members, and communicate effectively.

Matlow et al[136] conducted focus groups and administered questionnaires to evaluate ICU environmental service workers' attitudes and beliefs and intent about their jobs and found that the environmental services workers' attitudes and beliefs may affect intent and effectiveness of their cleaning practices.

Mitchell et al[137] conducted a cross-sectional survey of 923 environmental services personnel before and after implementation of a cleaning bundle, which included optimizing product use, cleaning technique, staff training, auditing with feedback, and communication. The survey focused on knowledge, reported practices, attitudes, roles, and perceived organizational support. A high level of knowledge and role importance was noted by participants both before and after the survey. However, the perception of lack of organizational support and investment in cleaning resources did not change during the course of the study, which led the researchers to conclude that the attitudes of personnel may be determinants of cleaning performance and to recommend taking human factors into consideration when developing interventions for cleaning improvement.

12. Quality

12.1 Perform process monitoring as part of an overall environmental cleaning program, including
- **compliance with regulatory standards**[90,91];
- **a review of products and manufacturers' IFU**[8];
- **monitoring cleaning and disinfection practices**[23,69]; and
- **reporting and investigation of adverse events (eg, outbreaks, product issues, corrective actions, evaluation).**[23]

[Recommendation]

12.2 Establish a process for evaluating cleaning thoroughness.[1,107,133] *[Recommendation]*

High-quality evidence supports the importance of cleaning thoroughness.[1,107,133] In a prospective study conducted at a large teaching hospital, Munoz et al[1] used fluorescent markers and cultures of environmental surfaces to evaluate cleaning thoroughness in the OR. The researchers found that improvement in thoroughness of cleaning practices in the OR significantly decreased surface contamination with potentially pathogenic organisms.

Hota et al[133] conducted a quasi-experimental study and found that surface contamination with VRE was related to a failure to clean rather than failure of a product or cleaning procedure. Cleaning thoroughness and site contamination improved significantly after implementation of an education program for environmental services personnel.

In an interrupted times series study to introduce a new method of daily patient room cleaning using disposable disinfectant wipes at a large tertiary hospital, Alfa et al[107] used fluorescent markers to monitor cleaning practices for high-touch surfaces. The researchers found that when there was an 80% or greater compliance with fluorescent marker removal, there was significant reduction in *C difficile*, MRSA, and VRE infection rates.

12.3 Measure cleaning practices using qualitative methods[2,3,48,80,103-105,114,134,138] (eg, visual observation of cleaning process, visual inspection of cleanliness, fluorescent marking) and quantitative methods[5,14,15,55,78,102,106,116,139-143] (eg, cultures, adenosine triphosphate [ATP] monitoring). *[Recommendation]*

Environmental monitoring programs allow health care organizations to provide measurable, objective data on the cleanliness of the environment. Data generated by measurement of cleaning practices provide complementary information that can be used to drive process improvement activities, encourage compliance with established cleaning protocols, educate personnel, and verify personnel competency.

In a systematic review of monitoring methods, Leas et al[24] found few studies that compared one method against another, no randomized controlled trials, and inconsistent benchmarks for cleanliness. The researchers concluded that more studies are needed to compare methods, determine validated consensus benchmarks, and correlate cleanliness measurements with clinical outcomes (eg, patient colonization, infection).

The CDC tool kit Options for Evaluating Environmental Cleaning describes an interdisciplinary approach to implementing a comprehensive environmental monitoring program that is specific to the level of monitoring desired by the health care organization.[79]

Qualitative Measures

Moderate-quality evidence is available regarding the use of qualitative fluorescent marking methods for assessing environmental cleanliness.[3,103-105,114] The researchers found that fluorescent marking

- improved thoroughness of daily terminal cleaning in the OR[3];
- led to significant improvements in ICU room cleaning[104];
- improved cleaning of high-touch objects in the patient's immediate environment[105];
- improved inpatient room cleaning as part of a bundled approach[114]; and
- was useful for determining the frequency of high-touch surface cleaning during terminal cleaning, although it was not as reliable for detecting surface contamination levels as quantitative measures.[103]

Low-quality evidence is available regarding the use of qualitative remote video auditing (RVA) methods for assessing environmental cleanliness.[80,134] Two organizations reported using RVA with independent observers to improve cleaning in ORs.[80,134]

Before beginning RVA for a 17-room OR, Pederson et al[80] developed explicit standards and audit tools for between-patient and terminal cleaning. Shortly after introduction of the standards, audit tools, and RVA, compliance for between-patient cleaning was 79% and compliance for terminal cleaning was 67%. However, after introduction of a "pit crew" concept, in which personnel were assigned specific tasks before beginning between-patient cleaning, compliance rose to 93%. As a result of the low compliance score for terminal cleaning, remedial training and re-education of environmental services personnel was initiated, leading to a 94% compliance score. A secondary measure of the RVA intervention was reduction of SSIs, which decreased by 10% compared to the previous year.[80]

Armellino et al[134] used RVA to improve and maintain compliance with terminal cleaning in the ORs of two facilities. Before beginning RVA, the terminal cleaning process was placed into sequential steps and used to develop an audit tool. After the first week of RVA, Facility 1 reported 52% compliance with protocol and Facility 2 had 33% compliance. However, after 3 months of continuous daily feedback to personnel and reporting of findings to perioperative and organizational administration, Facility 1 increased compliance to 98% and Facility 2 increased to 88%. Twelve months later when RVA was used again to evaluate practices, Facility 1 had 97.8% and Facility 2 had 99.7% compliance.

For the most objective approach to monitoring, the CDC recommends using an independent observer who is not part of the environmental services department, such as an infection preventionist or a health care epidemiologist.[79]

Quantitative Measures

Moderate-quality evidence is available regarding the use of quantitative culturing for assessing environmental cleanliness.[5,15,106] The researchers found that culturing methods

- identified the specific type of bacteria or fungi on the surface,[14,116,143]
- determined the density of organisms on a surface,[5,55]
- identified surface contamination on a contact culture plate that was not found by ATP methods,[106]
- were a cost-effective method for identifying environmental contamination,[5]
- used contact culture plates on flat surfaces,[15] and
- used culture swabs on irregular surfaces.[15]

Moderate-quality evidence is available regarding the use of ATP methods for assessing environmental cleanliness.[78,102,106,140-142] The researchers found that ATP monitoring

- identified suboptimal cleaning practices[102];
- improved cleaning of high-touch objects when implemented with an education and feedback program[102];
- identified areas that may need additional cleaning[78];
- could have detected nonviable debris[141,142];
- reached surface areas that contact culture plates could not[142];
- was a good method to evaluate high-touch sites that may have bacterial contamination[106];
- was a quick and objective method for assessing hospital cleanliness, but thresholds appeared to be poorly standardized[140]; and
- was limited in its' ability to detect bacterial spores.[144]

12.3.1 **Multiple qualitative and quantitative methods may be used to assess environmental cleaning practices.**[103] *[Conditional Recommendation]*

Using multiple qualitative and quantitative methods provides a comprehensive assessment of cleaning practices. In a prospective observational study, Boyce et al[103] found that although fluorescent marking was useful for determining cleaning frequency, this method was not as reliable for detecting surface contamination levels as were quantitative measures.

12.3.2 **Provide feedback of assessment findings to personnel and leaders.**[2,24,102,104,107,134] *[Recommendation]*

Measurement and feedback improve cleaning thoroughness. Moderate-quality evidence supports the sharing of monitored data, along with follow-up education to improve cleaning compliance.[2,24,102,104,107,134]

In a systematic review, Leas et al[24] found that in addition to organizational culture and leadership, standardization of processes and feedback to personnel were key to improving. cleaning practices.

Boyce et al[102] reported in a prospective intervention study conducted at a university-affiliated community teaching hospital that use of an ATP assay showed suboptimal cleaning practices, and implementation of an education and feedback program improved cleanliness of high-touch objects in patient rooms. The researchers found that the instant results of the ATP assay were useful in improving cleaning practice.

Carling et al[2] conducted a quasi-experimental study in 36 acute care hospitals and found that cleaning can be significantly improved with a combined approach of a highly objective targeting method, repeat performance feedback to environmental services personnel, and administrative interventions. In another quasi-experimental study, Carling et al[104] found that repeated performance feedback to environmental services personnel as part of an objective fluorescent targeting method led to significant improvements in ICU room cleaning.

Alfa et al[107] also conducted a quasi-experimental study and found a significant reduction in HAIs after implementing a clearly defined cleaning protocol, use of an effective disinfectant, and monitoring of compliance with same-day feedback.

Mitchell et al[137] administered a cross sectional survey to environmental services personnel and found that they desired feedback but felt feedback on a regular basis was lacking.

As part of organizational improvement project, Armellino et al[134] conducted a 3-month feedback period to provide daily results of OR terminal cleaning audits to appropriate personnel, along with remedial education. The researchers found that combined monitoring program with feedback resulted in sustained improvement in terminal cleaning.

12.4 Record completion of terminal and scheduled cleaning procedures on a checklist or log.[24,126] *[Recommendation]*

Checklists that outline the health care organization's cleaning procedures guide cleaning personnel in performing terminal and scheduled cleaning procedures so that items are not missed. A checklist or log also facilitates communication between perioperative team members and environmental services personnel that the environment is safe and clean for patients.

As part of a systematic review, Leas et al[24] identified checklists as a means to standardize procedures and support adherence to best practices. In a multisociety expert opinion document,[126] the authors recommended creating a checklist to ensure all surfaces are cleaned and disinfected as part of a bundled approach for a successful cleaning program.

12.4.1 The cleaning checklist may be designed for the specific setting and workflow of the area and modified when there is a change in equipment or workflow.[114,145] *[Conditional Recommendation]*

New technologies or changes in workflow or standards of practice may require modification of a checklist or log.[145] To avoid checklist fatigue, Burian et al[145] recommended that a checklist be designed for a specific setting and the workflow that occurs in that area. When conducting a quasi-experimental study, Mitchell et al[114] allowed for customization of a cleaning bundle by each of the 11 facilities, to take into context the facility's existing cleaning products and schedules.

Glossary

Clean: The absence of visible dust, soil, debris, or blood.

Contact time: The specific length of time a disinfectant must remain in contact with a microorganism to achieve disinfection. Synonyms: dwell time, kill time.

Disinfection: A process that kills pathogenic and other microorganisms by physical or chemical means.

Enhanced environmental cleaning: Cleaning of surfaces that extends beyond routine cleaning and is performed following the care of a patient who is infected or colonized with a multidrug-resistant organism.

Environmental cleaning: The process of cleaning, disinfecting, and monitoring for cleanliness.

Environmentally preferable: Products or services that have lesser or reduced effect on human health and the environment compared to competing products or services that serve the same purpose.

Focused multivector ultraviolet light system: An ultraviolet light delivery system that uses modular panels and reflectors to create a target zone that allows UV-C light to contact item surfaces from many directions.

Fomite: An inanimate object that, when contaminated with a viable pathogen (eg, bacterium, virus), can transfer the pathogen to a host.

High-touch object: A frequently touched item or surface.

Continuous ultraviolet system: An ultraviolet light delivery system that delivers UV-C light in a constant-on mode for a set time. Low pressure mercury lamps are most often used for UV-C delivery.

Pulsed xenon ultraviolet system: An ultraviolet light delivery system that uses a xenon lamp to produce intense pulses of UV-C light.

Regulated medical waste: Liquid or semi-liquid blood or other potentially infectious materials, contaminated items that would release blood or other potentially infectious materials in a liquid or semi-liquid state if compressed, items that are caked with dried blood or other potentially infectious materials and are capable of releasing these materials during handling, contaminated sharps, and pathological and microbiological wastes containing blood or other potentially infectious materials.

Scheduled cleaning: Periodic cleaning (eg, weekly, monthly) of areas and equipment that are not cleaned daily or after every use.

Surgical suite: An area or areas of the building containing the preoperative, intraoperative, and postoperative patient care areas and provisions for support areas.

Terminal cleaning: Thorough environmental cleaning that is performed at the end of each day the room or area is used.

Utility water: Water obtained directly from a faucet that has not been purified, distilled, or otherwise treated. Synonym: tap water.

References

1. Munoz-Price LS, Birnbach DJ, Lubarsky DA, et al. Decreasing operating room environmental pathogen contamination through improved cleaning practice. *Infect Control Hosp Epidemiol.* 2012;33(9):897-904. [IIA]

2. Carling PC, Parry MM, Rupp ME, et al. Improving cleaning of the environment surrounding patients in 36 acute care hospitals. *Infect Control Hosp Epidemiol.* 2008;29(11):1035-1041. [IIA]

3. Jefferson J, Whelan R, Dick B, Carling P. A novel technique for identifying opportunities to improve environmental hygiene in the operating room. *AORN J.* 2011;93(3):358-364. [IIIB]

4. Ibrahimi OA, Sharon V, Eisen DB. Surgical-site infections and routes of bacterial transfer: which ones are most plausible? *Dermatol Surg.* 2011;37(12):1709-1720. [VB]

5. Alexander JW, Van Sweringen H, Vanoss K, Hooker EA, Edwards MJ. Surveillance of bacterial colonization in operating rooms. *Surg Infect (Larchmt).* 2013;14(4):345-351. [IIIB]

6. Yezli S, Barbut F, Otter JA. Surface contamination in operating rooms: a risk for transmission of pathogens? *Surg Infect (Larchmt).* 2014;15(6):694-699. [VB]

7. Link T, Kleiner C, Mancuso MP, Dziadkowiec O, Halverson-Carpenter K. Determining high touch areas in the operating room with levels of contamination. *Am J Infect Control.* 2016;44(11):1350-1355. [IIIA]

8. Sehulster L, Chinn RY, Arduino MJ, et al. *Guidelines for Environmental Infection Control in Health-Care Facilities. Recommendations of CDC and the Healthcare Infection Control Practices Advisory Committee (HICPAC).* Chicago, IL: American Society for Healthcare Engineering/American Hospital Association; 2004. https://www.cdc.gov/infectioncontrol/pdf/guidelines/environmental-guidelines-P.pdf. Updated July 2019. Accessed September 11, 2019. [IVA]

9. Armellino D. Minimizing sources of airborne, aerosolized, and contact contaminants in the OR environment. *AORN J.* 2017;106(6):494-501. [VA]

10. Loftus RW, Brown JR, Koff MD, et al. Multiple reservoirs contribute to intraoperative bacterial transmission. *Anesth Analg.* 2012;114(6):1236. [IIIA]

11. Loftus RW, Brown JR, Patel HM, et al. Transmission dynamics of gram-negative bacterial pathogens in the anesthesia work area. *Anesth Analg.* 2015;120(4):819-826. [IIIB]

12. Loftus RW, Koff Brown JR, Patel HM, et al. The epidemiology of *Staphylococcus aureus* transmission in the anesthesia work area. *Anesth Analg.* 2015;120(4):807-818. [IIIB]

13. Loftus RW, Dexter F, Robinson ADM. High-risk *Staphylococcus aureus* transmission in the operating room: a call for widespread improvements in perioperative hand hygiene and patient decolonization practices. *Am J Infect Control.* 2018;46(10):1134-1141. [IIIA]

14. Balkissoon R, Nayfeh T, Adams KL, Belkoff SM, Riedel S, Mears SC. Microbial surface contamination after standard operating room cleaning practices following surgical treatment of infection. *Orthopedics.* 2014;37(4):e339-e344. [IIIB]

15. Dallolio L, Raggi A, Sanna T, et al. Surveillance of environmental and procedural measures of infection control in the operating theatre setting. *Int J Environ Res Public Health.* 2018;15(1):E46. [IIIB]

16. van 't Veen A, van der Zee A, Nelson J, Speelberg B, Kluytmans JA, Buiting AG. Outbreak of infection with a multiresistant *Klebsiella pneumoniae* strain associated with contaminated roll boards in operating rooms. *J Clin Microbiol.* 2005;43(10):4961-4967. [VB]

17. Loftus RW, Koff Brown JR, Patel HM, et al. The dynamics of enterococcus transmission from bacterial reservoirs commonly encountered by anesthesia providers. *Anesth Analg.* 2015;120(4):827-836. [IIIB]

18. Guideline for a safe environment of care. In: *Guidelines for Perioperative Practice.* Denver, CO: AORN, Inc; 2019:137-172. [IVA]

19. Guideline for transmission-based precautions. In: *Guidelines for Perioperative Practice.* Denver, CO: AORN, Inc; 2019:1093-1122. [IVA]

20. Guideline for hand hygiene. In: *Guidelines for Perioperative Practice.* Denver, CO: AORN, Inc; 2019:289-314. [IVA]

21. Association for the Healthcare Environment, American Hospital Association, American Society for Healthcare

Environmental Services. *Practice Guidance for Healthcare Environmental Cleaning: The Essential Resource for Environmental Cleaning and Disinfection.* Chicago, IL: Association for the Healthcare Environment of the American Hospital Association; 2012. [IVC]

22. Rutala WA, Weber DJ. Selection of the ideal disinfectant. *Infect Control Hosp Epidemiol.* 2014;35(7):855-865. [VA]

23. Healthcare Infection Control Practices Advisory Committee, ed. *Core Infection Prevention and Control Practices for Safe Healthcare Delivery in All Settings—Recommendations of the Healthcare Infection Control Practices Advisory Committee (HICPAC).* Atlanta, GA: Centers for Disease Control and Prevention; 2017. [IVA]

24. Leas BF, Sullivan N, Han JH, Pegues DA, Kaczmarek JL, Umscheid CA, eds. *Environmental Cleaning for the Prevention of Healthcare-Associated Infections* [Technical brief no. 22 (prepared by the ECRI Institute – Penn Medicine Evidence-Based Practice Center under contract no. 290-2012-00011-I). AHRQ publication no. 15-EHC020-EF]. Rockville, MD: Agency for Healthcare Research and Quality; 2015. [IIIA]

25. Rutala WA, Weber DJ; Healthcare Infection Control Practices Advisory Committee. *Guideline for Disinfection and Sterilization in Healthcare Facilities, 2008.* Update May 2019. Atlanta, GA: Centers for Disease Control and Prevention; 2008. [IVA]

26. *ANSI/AAMI TIR68:2018. Low and Intermediate-Level Disinfection in Healthcare Settings for Medical Devices and Patient Care Equipment and Sterile Processing Environmental Surfaces.* Arlington, VA: AAMI; 2018. [VA]

27. Arif AA, Delclos GL. Association between cleaning-related chemicals and work-related asthma and asthma symptoms among healthcare professionals. *Occup Environ Med.* 2012;69(1):35-40. [IIIB]

28. Casey ML, Hawley B, Edwards N, Cox-Ganser JM, Cummings KJ. Health problems and disinfectant product exposure among staff at a large multispecialty hospital. *Am J Infect Control.* 2017;45(10):1133-1138. [IIIB]

29. Su FC, Friesen MC, Stefaniak AB, et al. Exposures to volatile organic compounds among healthcare workers: modeling the effects of cleaning tasks and product use. *Ann Work Expo Health.* 2018;62(7):852-870. [IIIB]

30. Guideline for medical device and product evaluation. In: *Guidelines for Perioperative Practice.* Denver, CO: AORN, Inc; 2019:715-724. [IVA]

31. 29 CFR 1910.1200: Hazard communication. Occupational Safety and Health Administration. https://www.osha.gov/pls/oshaweb/owadisp.show_document?p_id=10099&p_table=STANDARDS. Accessed September 12, 2019.

32. Hong Y, Teska PJ, Oliver HF. Effects of contact time and concentration on bactericidal efficacy of 3 disinfectants on hard nonporous surfaces. *Am J Infect Control.* 2017;45(11):1284-1285. [IIIB]

33. West AM, Teska PJ, Oliver HF. There is no additional bactericidal efficacy of environmental protection agency–registered disinfectant towelettes after surface drying or beyond label contact time. *Am J Infect Control.* 2019;47(1):27-32. [IIB]

34. Rutala WA, Barbee SL, Aguiar NC, Sobsey MD, Weber DJ. Antimicrobial activity of home disinfectants and natural products against potential human pathogens. *Infect Control Hosp Epidemiol.* 2000;21(1):33-38. [IIB]

35. West AM, Nkemngong CA, Voorn MG, et al. Surface area wiped, product type, and target strain impact bactericidal efficacy of ready-to-use disinfectant towelettes. *Antimicrob Resist Infection Control.* 2018;7:122. [IIIB]

36. Gonzalez EA, Nandy P, Lucas AD, Hitchins VM. Ability of cleaning-disinfecting wipes to remove bacteria from medical device surfaces. *Am J Infect Control.* 2015;43(12):1331-1335. [IIC]

37. Engelbrecht K, Ambrose D, Sifuentes L, Gerba C, Weart I, Koenig D. Decreased activity of commercially available disinfectants containing quaternary ammonium compounds when exposed to cotton towels. *Am J Infect Control.* 2013;41(10):908-911. [IIIB]

38. Rutala WA, Gergen MF, Weber DJ. Microbiologic evaluation of microfiber mops for surface disinfection. *Am J Infect Control.* 2007;35(9):569-573. [IIB]

39. Diab-Elschahawi M, Assadian O, Blacky A, et al. Evaluation of the decontamination efficacy of new and reprocessed microfiber cleaning cloth compared with other commonly used cleaning cloths in the hospital. *Am J Infect Control.* 2010;38(4):289-292. [IIB]

40. Wiemken TL, Curran DR, Pacholski EB, et al. The value of ready-to-use disinfectant wipes: compliance, employee time, and costs. *Am J Infect Control.* 2014;42(3):329-330. [IIB]

41. Sifuentes LY, Gerba CP, Weart I, Engelbrecht K, Koenig DW. Microbial contamination of hospital reusable cleaning towels. *Am J Infect Control.* 2013;41(10):912-915. [IIIB]

42. Trajtman AN, Manickam K, Alfa MJ. Microfiber cloths reduce the transfer of *Clostridium difficile* spores to environmental surfaces compared with cotton cloths. *Am J Infect Control.* 2015;43(7):686-689. [IIC]

43. Rutala WA, Gergen MF, Weber DJ. Room decontamination with UV radiation. *Infect Control Hosp Epidemiol.* 2010;31(10):1025-1029. [IIB]

44. Boyce JM, Havill NL, Moore BA. Terminal decontamination of patient rooms using an automated mobile UV light unit. *Infect Control Hosp Epidemiol.* 2011;32(8):737-742. [IIB]

45. Anderson DJ, Gergen MF, Smathers E, et al. Decontamination of targeted pathogens from patient rooms using an automated ultraviolet-C-emitting device. *Infect Control Hosp Epidemiol.* 2013;34(5):466-471. [IIB]

46. Nerandzic MM, Cadnum JL, Pultz MJ, Donskey CJ. Evaluation of an automated ultraviolet radiation device for decontamination of *Clostridium difficile* and other healthcare-associated pathogens in hospital rooms. *BMC Infect Dis.* 2010;10:197. [IIB]

47. Umezawa K, Asai S, Inokuchi S, Miyachi H. A comparative study of the bactericidal activity and daily disinfection housekeeping surfaces by a new portable pulsed UV radiation device. *Curr Microbiol.* 2012;64(6):581-587. [IIA]

48. Anderson DJ, Chen LF, Weber DJ, et al. Enhanced terminal room disinfection and acquisition and infection caused by multidrug-resistant organisms and *Clostridium difficile* (the benefits of enhanced terminal room disinfection study): a

cluster-randomised, multicentre, crossover study. *Lancet.* 2017;389(10071):805-814. [IA]

49. Nottingham M, Peterson G, Doern C, et al. Ultraviolet-C light as a means of disinfecting anesthesia workstations. *Am J Infect Control.* 2017;45(9):1011-1013. [IIC]

50. Levin J, Riley LS, Parrish C, English D, Ahn S. The effect of portable pulsed xenon ultraviolet light after terminal cleaning on hospital-associated *Clostridium difficile* infection in a community hospital. *Am J Infect Control.* 2013;41(8):746-748. [IIB]

51. Catalanotti A, Abbe D, Simmons S, Stibich M. Influence of pulsed-xenon ultraviolet light-based environmental disinfection on surgical site infections. *Am J Infect Control.* 2016;44(6):e99-e101. [IIC]

52. Sampathkumar P, Folkert C, Barth JE, et al. A trial of pulsed xenon ultraviolet disinfection to reduce *Clostridioides difficile* infection. *Am J Infect Control.* 2019;47(4):406-408. [IIA]

53. El Haddad L, Ghantoji SS, Stibich M, et al. Evaluation of a pulsed xenon ultraviolet disinfection system to decrease bacterial contamination in operating rooms. *BMC Infect Dis.* 2017;17(1):672. [IIB]

54. Simmons S Jr, Dale C, Holt J, Passey DG, Stibich M. Environmental effectiveness of pulsed-xenon light in the operating room. *Am J Infect Control.* 2018;46(9):1003-1008. [IIB]

55. Armellino D, Walsh TJ, Petraitis V, Kowalski W. Assessment of focused multivector ultraviolet disinfection with shadowless delivery using 5-point multisided sampling of patient care equipment without manual-chemical disinfection. *Am J Infect Control.* 2019;47(4):409-414. [IIB]

56. Armellino D, Walsh TJ, Petraitis V, Kowalski W. Assessing the feasibility of a focused multivector ultraviolet system between surgery cases with a parallel protocol for enhanced disinfection capabilities. *Am J Infect Control.* 2019;47(8):1006-1008. [IIB]

57. Barbut F, Menuet D, Verachten M, Girou E. Comparison of the efficacy of a hydrogen peroxide dry-mist disinfection system and sodium hypochlorite solution for eradication of *Clostridium difficile* spores. *Infect Control Hosp Epidemiol.* 2009;30(6):507-514. [IB]

58. Bartels MD, Kristoffersen K, Slotsbjerg T, Rohde SM, Lundgren B, Westh H. Environmental meticillin-resistant *Staphylococcus aureus* (MRSA) disinfection using dry-mist-generated hydrogen peroxide. *J Hosp Infect.* 2008;70(1):35-41. [IIB]

59. Boyce JM, Havill NL, Otter JA, et al. Impact of hydrogen peroxide vapor room decontamination on *Clostridium difficile* environmental contamination and transmission in a healthcare setting. *Infect Control Hosp Epidemiol.* 2008;29(8):723-729. [IIB]

60. Chan HT, White P, Sheorey H, Cocks J, Waters MJ. Evaluation of the biological efficacy of hydrogen peroxide vapour decontamination in wards of an Australian hospital. *J Hosp Infect.* 2011;79(2):125-128. [IIB]

61. Manian FA, Griesenauer S, Senkel D, et al. Isolation of *Acinetobacter baumannii* complex and methicillin-resistant *Staphylococcus aureus* from hospital rooms following terminal cleaning and disinfection: can we do better? *Infect Control Hosp Epidemiol.* 2011;32(7):667-672. [IIB]

62. Passaretti CL, Otter JA, Reich NG, et al. An evaluation of environmental decontamination with hydrogen peroxide vapor for reducing the risk of patient acquisition of multidrug-resistant organisms. *Clin Infect Dis.* 2013;56(1):27-35. [IIA]

63. Lemmen S, Scheithauer S, Häfner H, Yezli S, Mohr M, Otter JA. Evaluation of hydrogen peroxide vapor for the inactivation of nosocomial pathogens on porous and nonporous surfaces. *Am J Infect Control.* 2015;43(1):82-85. [IIB]

64. Dancer SJ. Hospital cleaning in the 21st century. *Eur J Clinical Microbiol Infect Dis.* 2011;30(12):1473-1481. [VA]

65. Donskey CJ. Decontamination devices in health care facilities: practical issues and emerging applications. *Am J Infect Control.* 2019;47S:A23-A28. [VA]

66. Weber DJ, Rutala WA, Anderson DJ, Chen LF, Sickbert-Bennett E, Boyce JM. Effectiveness of ultraviolet devices and hydrogen peroxide systems for terminal room decontamination: focus on clinical trials. *Am J Infect Control.* 2016;44(5):e77-e84. [VB]

67. Marra AR, Schweizer ML, Edmond MB. No-touch disinfection methods to decrease multidrug-resistant organism infections: a systematic review and meta-analysis. *Infect Control Hosp Epidemiol.* 2018;39(1):20-31. [IIIA]

68. Cobb TC. Methicillin-resistant *Staphylococcus aureus* decontamination: is ultraviolet radiation more effective than vapor-phase hydrogen peroxide? *Rev Med Microbiol.* 2017;28(2):69-74. [IIIB]

69. McDonald LC, Gerding DN, Johnson S, et al. Clinical practice guidelines for *Clostridium difficile* infection in adults and children: 2017 update by the Infectious Diseases Society of America (IDSA) and Society for Healthcare Epidemiology of America (SHEA). *Clin Infect Dis.* 2018;66(7):e1-e48. [IVA]

70. Hosein I, Madeloso R, Nagaratnam W, Villamaria F, Stock E, Jinadatha C. Evaluation of a pulsed xenon ultraviolet light device for isolation room disinfection in a United Kingdom hospital. *Am J Infect Control.* 2016;44(9):e157-e161. [IIB]

71. Jinadatha C, Villamaria FC, Restrepo MI, et al. Is the pulsed xenon ultraviolet light no-touch disinfection system effective on methicillin-resistant *Staphylococcus aureus* in the absence of manual cleaning? *Am J Infect Control.* 2015;43(8):878-881. [IIC]

72. Zeber JE, Pfeiffer C, Baddley JW, et al. Effect of pulsed xenon ultraviolet room disinfection devices on microbial counts for methicillin-resistant *Staphylococcus aureus* and aerobic bacterial colonies. *Am J Infect Control.* 2018;46(6):668-673. [IIB]

73. Vianna PG, Dale CR Jr, Simmons S, Stibich M, Licitra CM. Impact of pulsed xenon ultraviolet light on hospital-acquired infection rates in a community hospital. *Am J Infect Control.* 2016;44(3):299-303. [IIB]

74. Nagaraja A, Visintainer P, Haas JP, Menz J, Wormser GP, Montecalvo MA. *Clostridium difficile* infections before and during use of ultraviolet disinfection. *Am J Infect Control.* 2015;43(9):940-945. [IIA]

75. 29 CFR 1910.1030: Bloodborne pathogens. Occupational Safety and Health Administration. https://www.osha.gov/pls/oshaweb/owadisp.show_document?p_id=10051&p_table=STANDARDS. Accessed September 12, 2019.

76. Havill NL. Best practices in disinfection of noncritical surfaces in the health care setting: creating a bundle for success. *Am J Infect Control.* 2013;41(5 Suppl):S26-S30. [VB]

77. Dancer SJ. The role of environmental cleaning in the control of hospital-acquired infection. *J Hosp Infect.* 2009;73(4):378-385. [VB]

78. Richard RD, Bowen TR. What orthopaedic operating room surfaces are contaminated with bioburden? A study using the ATP bioluminescence assay. *Clin Orthop.* 2017;475(7):1819-1824. [IIIC]

79. Guh A, Carling P; Environmental Evaluation Workgroup. *Options for Evaluating Environmental Cleaning Toolkit.* Centers for Disease Control and Prevention; 2010. https://www.cdc.gov/hai/toolkits/evaluating-environmental-cleaning.html. Accessed September 12, 2019. [VB]

80. Pedersen A, Getty Ritter E, Beaton M, Gibbons D. Remote video auditing in the surgical setting. *AORN J.* 2017;105(2):159-169. [VA]

81. Bergen LK, Meyer M, Hog M, Rubenhagen B, Andersen LP. Spread of bacteria on surfaces when cleaning with microfibre cloths. *J Hosp Infect.* 2009;71(2):132-137. [IIIB]

82. Andersen BM, Rasch M, Kvist J, et al. Floor cleaning: effect on bacteria and organic materials in hospital rooms. *J Hosp Infect.* 2009;71(1):57-65. [IIIB]

83. Deshpande A, Cadnum JL, Fertelli D, et al. Are hospital floors an underappreciated reservoir for transmission of health care-associated pathogens? *Am J Infect Control.* 2017;45(3):336-338. [IIIB]

84. Munoz-Price LS, Bowdle A, Johnston BL, et al. Infection prevention in the operating room anesthesia work area. *Infect Control Hosp Epidemiol.* 2018; December 11:1-17. Epub ahead of print. [IVA]

85. Das A, Conti J, Hanrahan J, Kaelber DC. Comparison of keyboard colonization before and after use in an inpatient setting and the effect of keyboard covers. *Am J Infect Control.* 2018;46(4):474-476. [IIB]

86. *2019 Top 10 Health Technology Hazards; Executive Brief.* Plymouth Meeting, PA: ECRI Institute; 2018. [VB]

87. Siegel JD, Rhinehart E, Jackson M, Chiarello L; Health Care Infection Control Practices Advisory Committee. 2007 guideline for isolation precautions: preventing transmission of infectious agents in health care settings. *Am J Infect Control.* 2007;35(10 Suppl 2):S65-S164. [IVA]

88. *ANSI/AAMI TIR67:2018. Promoting Safe Practices Pertaining to the Use of Sterilant and Disinfectant Chemicals in Health Care Facilities.* Arlington, VA: Association for the Advancement of Medical Instrumentation; 2018. [VA]

89. Horn M, Patel N, MacLellan DM, Millard N. Traditional canister-based open waste management system versus closed system: hazardous exposure prevention and operating theatre staff satisfaction. *ORNAC J.* 2016;34(2):36-50. [IIIC]

90. 42 CFR 416: Ambulatory surgical services. Government Publishing Office. https://www.govinfo.gov/app/details/CFR-2011-title42-vol3/CFR-2011-title42-vol3-part416. Accessed September 12, 2019.

91. 42 CFR 482: Conditions of participation for hospitals. Government Publishing Office. https://www.govinfo.gov/app/details/CFR-2011-title42-vol5/CFR-2011-title42-vol5-part482. Accessed September 12, 2019.

92. *State Operations Manual Appendix A: Survey Protocol, Regulations and Interpretive Guidelines for Hospitals.* Rev. 183; 2018. Centers for Medicare & Medicaid Services. https://www.cms.gov/Regulations-and-Guidance/Guidance/Manuals/downloads/som107ap_a_hospitals.pdf. Accessed September 12, 2019.

93. *State Operations Manual Appendix L: Guidance for Surveyors: Ambulatory Surgical Centers.* Rev. 137; 2015. Centers for Medicare & Medicaid Services. https://www.cms.gov/Regulations-and-Guidance/Guidance/Manuals/Downloads/som107ap_l_ambulatory.pdf. Accessed September 12, 2019.

94. Goebel U, Gebele N, Ebner W, et al. Bacterial contamination of the anesthesia workplace and efficiency of routine cleaning procedures: a prospective cohort study. *Anesth Analg.* 2016;122(5):1444-1447. [IIIB]

95. Clark C, Taenzer A, Charette K, Whitty M. Decreasing contamination of the anesthesia environment. *Am J Infect Control.* 2014;42(11):1223-1225. [IIB]

96. Birnbach DJ, Rosen LF, Fitzpatrick M, Carling P, Munoz-Price LS. The use of a novel technology to study dynamics of pathogen transmission in the operating room. *Anesth Analg.* 2015;120(4):844-847. [IIIC]

97. Berrios-Torres SI, Umscheid CA, Bratzler DW, et al; Healthcare Infection Control Practices Advisory Committee. Centers for Disease Control and Prevention Guideline for the Prevention of Surgical Site Infection; 2017. *JAMA Surg.* 2017;152(8):784-791. [IVA]

98. Abolghasemian M, Sternheim A, Shakib A, Safir OA, Backstein D. Is arthroplasty immediately after an infected case a risk factor for infection? *Clin Orthop.* 2013;471(7):2253-2258. [IIB]

99. Harnoss JC, Assadian O, Diener MK, et al. Microbial load in septic and aseptic procedure rooms. *Dtsch Arztebl Int.* 2017;114(27-28):465-475. [IIIC]

100. Kalava A, Midha M, Kurnutala LN, SchianodiCola J, Yarmush JM. How clean are the overhead lights in operating rooms? *Am J Infect Control.* 2013;41(4):387-388. [VB]

101. Hess AS, Shardell M, Johnson JK, et al. A randomized controlled trial of enhanced cleaning to reduce contamination of healthcare worker gowns and gloves with multidrug-resistant bacteria. *Infect Control Hosp Epidemiol.* 2013;34(5):487-493. [IA]

102. Boyce JM, Havill NL, Dumigan DG, Golebiewski M, Balogun O, Rizvani R. Monitoring the effectiveness of hospital cleaning practices by use of an adenosine triphosphate bioluminescence assay. *Infect Control Hosp Epidemiol.* 2009;30(7):678-684. [IIB]

103. Boyce JM, Havill NL, Havill HL, Mangione E, Dumigan DG, Moore BA. Comparison of fluorescent marker systems with 2 quantitative methods of assessing terminal cleaning practices. *Infect Control Hosp Epidemiol.* 2011;32(12):1187-1193. [IIIA]

104. Carling PC, Parry MF, Bruno-Murtha LA, Dick B. Improving environmental hygiene in 27 intensive care units

to decrease multidrug-resistant bacterial transmission. *Crit Care Med.* 2010;38(4):1054-1059. [IIA]

105. Carling PC, Parry MF, Von Beheren SM; Healthcare Environmental Hygiene Study G. Identifying opportunities to enhance environmental cleaning in 23 acute care hospitals. *Infect Control Hosp Epidemiol.* 2008;29(1):1-7. [IIIB]

106. Watanabe R, Shimoda T, Yano R, et al. Visualization of hospital cleanliness in three Japanese hospitals with a tendency toward long-term care. *BMC Res Notes.* 2014;7:121. [IIIA]

107. Alfa MJ, Lo E, Olson N, MacRae M, Buelow-Smith L. Use of a daily disinfectant cleaner instead of a daily cleaner reduced hospital-acquired infection rates. *Am J Infect Control.* 2015;43(2):141-146. [IIB]

108. *ANSI/AAMI ST79:2010 & A1:2010 & A2:2011 & A3:2012: Comprehensive Guide to Steam Sterilization and Sterility Assurance in Health Care Facilities.* Arlington, VA: Association for the Advancement of Medical Instrumentation; 2012:250-254. [IVC]

109. *Candida auris.* Infection prevention and control: environmental disinfection. Centers for Disease Control and Prevention. https://www.cdc.gov/fungal/candida-auris/c-auris-infection-control.html#disinfection. Accessed September 12, 2019.

110. Siegel JD, Rhinehart E, Jackson M, Chiarello L; Healthcare Infection Control Practices Advisory Committee. *Management of Multidrug-Resistant Organisms in Healthcare Settings.* Atlanta, GA: Centers for Disease Control and Prevention; 2006. [IVA]

111. Datta R, Platt R, Yokoe DS, Huang SS. Environmental cleaning intervention and risk of acquiring multidrug-resistant organisms from prior room occupants. *Arch Intern Med.* 2011;171(6):491-494. [IIB]

112. Landman D, Babu E, Shah N, et al. Transmission of carbapenem-resistant pathogens in New York City hospitals: progress and frustration. *J Antimicrob Chemother.* 2012;67(6):1427-1431. [IIIA]

113. Morgan DJ, Rogawski E, Thom KA, et al. Transfer of multidrug-resistant bacteria to healthcare workers' gloves and gowns after patient contact increases with environmental contamination. *Crit Care Med.* 2012;40(4):1045-1051. [IIIA]

114. Mitchell BG, Hall L, White N, et al. An environmental cleaning bundle and health-care-associated infections in hospitals (REACH): a multicentre, randomised trial. *Lancet Infect Dis.* 2019;19(4):410-418. [IIB]

115. Ohl M, Schweizer M, Graham M, Heilmann K, Boyken L, Diekema D. Hospital privacy curtains are frequently and rapidly contaminated with potentially pathogenic bacteria. *Am J Infect Control.* 2012;40(10):904-906. [IIIB]

116. Shek K, Patidar R, Kohja Z, et al. Rate of contamination of hospital privacy curtains in a burns/plastic ward: a longitudinal study. *Am J Infect Control.* 2018;46(9):1019-1021. [IIIB]

117. Rutala WA, Kanamori H, Gergen MF, Sickbert-Bennett E, Weber DJ. Susceptibility of *Candida auris* and *Candida albicans* to 21 germicides used in healthcare facilities. *Infect Control Hosp Epidemiol.* 2019;40(3):380-382. [IIB]

118. Jensen PA, Lambert LA, Iademarco MF, Ridzon R; CDC. Guidelines for preventing the transmission of *Mycobacterium tuberculosis* in health-care settings, 2005. *MMWR Recomm Rep.* 2005;54(RR-17):1-141. [IVA]

119. Rutala WA, Weber DJ; Society for Healthcare Epidemiology of America. Guideline for disinfection and sterilization of prion-contaminated medical instruments. *Infect Control Hosp Epidemiol.* 2010;31(2):107-117. [IVA]

120. Balm MN, Jureen R, Teo C, et al. Hot and steamy: outbreak of *Bacillus cereus* in Singapore associated with construction work and laundry practices. *J Hosp Infect.* 2012;81(4):224-230. [VA]

121. Campbell JR, Hulten K, Baker CJ. Cluster of *Bacillus* species bacteremia cases in neonates during a hospital construction project. *Infect Control Hosp Epidemiol.* 2011;32(10):1035-1038. [VA]

122. Fournel I, Sautour M, Lafon I, et al. Airborne *Aspergillus* contamination during hospital construction works: efficacy of protective measures. *Am J Infect Control.* 2010;38(3):189-194. [IIIB]

123. Gibb AP, Fleck BW, Kempton-Smith L. A cluster of deep bacterial infections following eye surgery associated with construction dust. *J Hosp Infect.* 2006;63(2):197-200. [VB]

124. Kanamori H, Rutala WA, Sickbert-Bennett EE, Weber DJ. Review of fungal outbreaks and infection prevention in healthcare settings during construction and renovation. *Clin Infect Dis.* 2015;61(3):433-444. [VA]

125. Olmsted RN. Prevention by design: construction and renovation of health care facilities for patient safety and infection prevention. *Infect Dis Clin North Am.* 2016;30(3):713-728. [VB]

126. The Health Research & Educational Trust of the American Hospital Association, American Society for Health Care Engineering, Association for Professionals in Infection Control and Epidemiology, Society of Hospital Medicine, University of Michigan. *Using the Health Care Physical Environment to Prevent and Control Infection.* Chicago, IL: The American Society for Health Care Engineering of the American Hospital Association; 2015. [VB]

127. Faulde M, Spiesberger M. Role of the moth fly *Clogmia albipunctata (Diptera: Psychodinae)* as a mechanical vector of bacterial pathogens in German hospitals. *J Hosp Infect.* 2013;83(1):51-60. [IIIB]

128. Munoz-Price LS, Safdar N, Beier JC, Doggett SL. Bed bugs in healthcare settings. *Infect Control Hosp Epidemiol.* 2012;33(11):1137-1142. [VB]

129. Abdolmaleki Z, Mashak Z, Safarpoor Dehkordi F. Phenotypic and genotypic characterization of antibiotic resistance in the methicillin-resistant *Staphylococcus aureus* strains isolated from hospital cockroaches. *Antimicrob Resist Infect Control.* 2019;8(1):54. [IIIB]

130. Schulz-Stübner S, Danner K, Hauer T, Tabori E. *Psychodidae* (drain fly) infestation in an operating room. *Infect Control Hosp Epidemiol.* 2015;36(3):366-367. [VA]

131. Schouest JM, Heinrich L, Nicholas B, Drach F. Fly rounds: validation and pilot of a novel epidemiologic tool to guide infection control response to an infestation of *Sarcophagidae* flies in a community hospital's perioperative department. *Am J Infect Control.* 2017;45(9):e91-e93. [VB]

132. *Joint Statement on Bed Bug Control in the United States from the U.S. Centers For Disease Control And Prevention (CDC) and the U.S. Environmental Protection Agency (EPA).* Atlanta, GA: Centers for Disease Control and Prevention, US Environmental Protection Agency; 2010. [VA]

133. Hota B, Blom DW, Lyle EA, Weinstein RA, Hayden MK. Interventional evaluation of environmental contamination by vancomycin-resistant enterococci: failure of personnel, product, or procedure? *J Hosp Infect.* 2009;71(2):123-131. [IIB]

134. Armellino D, Dowling O, Newman SB, et al. Remote video auditing to verify OR cleaning: a quality improvement project. *AORN J.* 2018;108(6):634-642. [VA]

135. Kak N, Burkhalter B, Cooper M. *Measuring the Competence of Healthcare Providers.* Operations Research Issue Paper 2(1). Bethesda, MD: US Agency for International Development (USAID), Quality Assurance (QA) Project; 2001. [VA]

136. Matlow AG, Wray R, Richardson SE. Attitudes and beliefs, not just knowledge, influence the effectiveness of environmental cleaning by environmental service workers. *Am J Infect Control.* 2012;40(3):260-262. [IIIC]

137. Mitchell BG, White N, Farrington A, et al. Changes in knowledge and attitudes of hospital environmental services staff: the researching effective approaches to cleaning in hospitals (REACH) study. *Am J Infect Control.* 2018;46(9):980-985. [IIIA]

138. Knelson LP, Ramadanovic GK, Chen LF, et al. Self-monitoring by environmental services may not accurately measure thoroughness of hospital room cleaning. *Infect Control Hosp Epidemiol.* 2017;38(11):1371-1373. [IIIA]

139. Havill NL, Havill HL, Mangione E, Dumigan DG, Boyce JM. Cleanliness of portable medical equipment disinfected by nursing staff. *Am J Infect Control.* 2011;39(7):602-604. [IIIB]

140. Amodio E, Dino C. Use of ATP bioluminescence for assessing the cleanliness of hospital surfaces: a review of the published literature (1990–2012). *J Infect Public Health.* 2014;7(2):92-98. [VA]

141. Saito Y, Yasuhara H, Murakoshi S, Komatsu T, Fukatsu K, Uetera Y. Time-dependent influence on assessment of contaminated environmental surfaces in operating rooms. *Am J Infect Control.* 2015;43(9):951-955. [IIIB]

142. Ellis O, Godwin H, David M, Morse DJ, Humphries R, Uslan DZ. How to better monitor and clean irregular surfaces in operating rooms: insights gained by using both ATP luminescence and RODAC assays. *Am J Infect Control.* 2018;46(8):906-912. [IIIB]

143. Alfonso-Sanchez JL, Martinez IM, Martín-Moreno JM, González RS, Botía F. Analyzing the risk factors influencing surgical site infections: the site of environmental factors. *Can J Surg.* 2017;60(3):155-161. [IIIA]

144. Gibbs SG, Sayles H, Colbert EM, Hewlett A, Chaika O, Smith PW. Evaluation of the relationship between the adenosine triphosphate (ATP) bioluminescence assay and the presence of *Bacillus anthracis* spores and vegetative cells. *Int J Environ Res Public Health.* 2014;11(6):5708-5719. [IIIB]

145. Burian BK, Clebone A, Dismukes K, Ruskin KJ. More than a tick box: medical checklist development, design, and use. *Anesth Analg.* 2018;126(1):223-232. [VA]

Guideline Development Group

Lead Author: Karen deKay[1], MSN, RN, CNOR, CIC, Perioperative Practice Specialist, AORN, Denver, Colorado

Methodologist: Amber Wood[2], MSN, RN, CNOR, CIC, FAPIC, Editor-in-Chief, Guidelines for Perioperative Practice, AORN, Denver, Colorado

Evidence Appraisers: Karen deKay[1]; Janice Neil[3], PhD, CNE, RN, Associate Professor, East Carolina College of Nursing, Greenville, North Carolina; and Amber Wood[2]

Guidelines Advisory Board Members:
- Bernard C. Camins[4], MD, MSc, Medical Director, Infection Prevention, Mount Sinai Health System, New York, New York
- Crystal A. Bricker[5], MSN, RN, CNOR, Clinical Practice Partner, Perioperative Services, Advocate Health Care, Normal, Illinois
- Elizabeth (Lizz) Pincus[6], MSN, RN, CNS-CP, CNOR, Clinical Nurse, Regional Medical Center of San Jose, San Jose, California
- Stephen Balog[7], MSN, RN, CNOR, Staff Nurse, Hilton Head Hospital, Hilton Head Island, South Carolina
- Nakeisha M. Archer[8], MBA, RN, NE-BC, CNOR, Director Perioperative Services, Texas Children's Hospital Membership, Missouri City, Texas
- William (Bill) Duffy[9], RN, MJ, CNOR, FAAN, Director of Health Systems Management Program, Loyola University of Chicago, Illinois

Guidelines Advisory Board Liaisons:
- Jennifer Hanrahan[10], DO, Medical Director of Infection Prevention, Metrohealth Medical Center, Cleveland, Ohio
- Susan Ruwe[11], MSN, RN, CPHQ, CIC, Senior Infection Preventionist, Carle Foundation Hospital, Argenta, Illinois
- Susan G. Klacik[12], BS, CRCST, FCS, Clinical Educator, International Association of Healthcare Central Service Materiel Management (IAHCSMM), Chicago, Illinois

External Review: Expert review comments were received from individual members of the American Association of Nurse Anesthetists (AANA), American College of Surgeons (ACS), Association for Professionals in Infection Control and Epidemiology (APIC), American Society of Anesthesiologists (ASA), International Association of Healthcare Central Service Materiel Management (IAHCSMM), the Society for Healthcare Epidemiology of America (SHEA), and the Surgical Infection Society (SIS). Their responses were used to further refine and enhance this guideline; however, their responses do not imply endorsement. The draft was also open for a 30-day public comment period.

Financial Disclosure and Conflicts of Interest

This guideline was developed, edited, and approved by the AORN Guidelines Advisory Board without external funding being sought or obtained. The Guidelines Advisory Board was financially supported entirely by AORN and was developed without any involvement of industry.

Potential conflicts of interest for all Guidelines Advisory Board members were reviewed before the annual meeting and each monthly conference call. Ten members of the Guideline Development Group reported no potential conflict of interest.[1-8,11-12] Two members[9,10] disclosed potential conflicts of interest. After review and discussion of these disclosures, the advisory board concluded that individuals with potential conflicts could remain on the advisory board if they reminded the advisory board of potential conflicts before any related discussion and recused themselves from a related discussion if requested.

Publication History

Originally published June 1975, *AORN Journal,* as "Recommended practices for sanitation in the surgical practice setting."

Format revised March 1978; March 1982; July 1982. Revised April 1984; November 1988; December 1992.

Revised June 1996; published October 1996, *AORN Journal.* Reformatted July 2000.

Revised; published December 2002, *AORN Journal.*

Revised 2007; published in *Perioperative Standards and Recommended Practices,* 2008 edition.

Minor editing revisions made to omit PNDS codes; reformatted September 2012 for publication in *Perioperative Standards and Recommended Practices,* 2013 edition.

Revised September 2013 for online publication in *Perioperative Standards and Recommended Practices.*

Minor editing revisions made in November 2014 for publication in *Guidelines for Perioperative Practice,* 2015 edition.

Evidence ratings revised in *Guidelines for Perioperative Practice,* 2018 edition, to conform to the current AORN Evidence Rating Model.

Revised 2019 for publication in *Guidelines for Perioperative Practice,* 2020 edition.

Scheduled for review in 2025.

FLEXIBLE ENDOSCOPES

AORN
SAFE SURGERY TOGETHER

TABLE OF CONTENTS

MEDICAL ABBREVIATIONS & ACRONYMS

AAMI – Association for the Advancement of Medical Instrumentation
AGEA – Australian Gastrointestinal Endoscopy Association
ANSI – American National Standards Institute
APIC – Association for Professionals in Infection Control and Epidemiology
ASGE – American Society for Gastrointestinal Endoscopy
ASHRAE – American Society of Heating, Refrigerating and Air-Conditioning Engineers
ATP – Adenosine triphosphate
AUD – Australian dollars
β – Beta
CDC – Centers for Disease Control and Prevention
CFU – Colony-forming units
CJD – Creutzfeldt-Jakob disease
CRKP – Carbapenemase-resistant *Klebsiella pneumoniae*
ED – Emergency department
EGD – Esophagogastroduodenoscopy
EPA – Environmental Protection Agency
ERCP – Endoscopic retrograde cholangiopancreatography
ESGE – European Society of Gastrointestinal Endoscopy
ESGENA – European Society of Gastroenterology and Endoscopy Nurses and Associates
EU – Endotoxin unit
FDA – US Food and Drug Administration
FGI – Facility Guidelines Institute
GENCA – Gastroenterological Nurses College of Australia

GESA – Gastroenterological Society of Australia
HEPA – High-efficiency particulate air
HLD – High-level disinfection
HSV – Herpes simplex virus
HVAC – Heating, ventilation, and air conditioning
ICU – Intensive care unit
IFU – Instructions for use
ILD – Intermediate-level disinfection
IRPA – Imipenem-resistant *Pseudomonas aeruginosa*
ISEA – International Safety Equipment Association
MAUDE – Manufacturer and User Facility Device Experience
MDR-TB – Multidrug-resistant *Mycobacterium tuberculosis*
MERV – Minimum efficiency reporting value
NDM-1 – New Delhi metallo-β-lactamase-1
OSHA – Occupational Safety and Health Administration
PAS – Portable anteroom system
PFU – Plaque-forming units
PPE – Personal protective equipment
RLU – Relative light units
SEM – Scanning electron microscopy
SFERD – Steering Group for Flexible Endoscope Cleaning and Disinfection
SGNA – Society of Gastroenterology Nurses and Associates
SHEA – Society for Healthcare Epidemiology of America
TSE – Transmissible spongiform encephalopathy
vCJD – Variant Creutzfeldt-Jakob disease
VIM – Verona integron-encoded metallo-β-lactamase

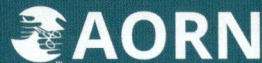
GUIDELINE FOR
PROCESSING FLEXIBLE ENDOSCOPES

The Guideline for Processing Flexible Endoscopes was approved by the AORN Guidelines Advisory Board and became effective February 1, 2016. It was presented as a proposed guideline for comments by members and others. The recommendations in the guideline are intended to be achievable and represent what is believed to be an optimal level of practice. Policies and procedures will reflect variations in practice settings and/or clinical situations that determine the degree to which the guideline can be implemented. AORN recognizes the many diverse settings in which perioperative nurses practice; therefore, this guideline is adaptable to all areas where operative or other invasive procedures may be performed.

Purpose

This document provides guidance to perioperative, endoscopy, and sterile processing personnel for processing all types of reusable flexible endoscopes and accessories. Recommendations are provided for design and construction of the **endoscopy suite** as well as for controlling and maintaining the environment to support processing activities. Guidance is provided for maintaining records of processing for traceability and for quality assurance measures related to processing flexible endoscopes and accessories.

Patients have a right to undergo endoscopic procedures in a safe, clean environment where personnel adhere to consistent, evidence-based practices for processing every flexible endoscope every time care is provided. It is essential that the risk of patient-to-patient transmission of infection via flexible endoscopes be minimized as much as is reasonably possible.

Infections related to endoscopy procedures may be caused by endogenous microorganisms that colonize the mucosal surfaces of the gastrointestinal or respiratory tract and gain access to the bloodstream or other sterile tissues as a consequence of the procedure.[1] Endogenous infections include infections such as cholangitis that may occur after endoscopic procedures of the biliary tract or pneumonia that may occur after endoscopic procedures of the respiratory tract.[1]

Infections related to endoscopy procedures may also be caused by exogenous microorganisms that are transmitted from previous patients or from the inanimate environment by contaminated endoscopes or accessories.[1] The US Food and Drug Administration (FDA) has identified two recurrent themes as contributing to persistent bronchoscope contamination and transmission of exogenous infection:

- a failure to meticulously follow the manufacturer's written instructions for processing and

- the continued use of bronchoscopes despite issues with integrity, maintenance, and mechanical problems.[2]

If flexible endoscopes are not correctly processed, exposure to body fluids and tissue remnants from previous patients may result in the transmission of pathogens to large numbers of subsequent patients.[3] In a systematic search of the literature to clarify the epidemiology of *Klebsiella* species in endoscopy-associated outbreaks, Gastmeier and Vonberg[4] found that insufficient processing was the main reason for subsequent pathogen transmission. The authors concluded that strict adherence to guidelines for processing flexible endoscopes in combination with alertness to the potential for pathogen transmission after endoscopy procedures was required, and that additional studies were needed to determine the true risk of pathogen transmission via flexible endoscopes.

Because of the many different types of flexible endoscopes and the differences in flexible endoscope construction, not all steps discussed in this guideline (eg, leak testing) will apply to all endoscopes; however, some steps (eg, manual cleaning) will apply to all flexible endoscopes. The European Society of Gastrointestinal Endoscopy (ESGE) has proposed a classification of endoscope families[5] based on similar characteristics, including the number, construction, and purpose of the different endoscope channels and their clinical applications.

- Group 1 endoscopes are typically intended for use in the gastrointestinal tract. This group includes endoscopes that have air/water channels, have an instrument/suction channel, and may have an additional instrument or waterjet channel. Examples of Group 1 endoscopes are gastroscopes, colonoscopes, and duodenoscopes with an encapsulated elevator channel.

- Group 2 endoscopes are also intended for use in the gastrointestinal tract. This group includes endoscopes that have air/water channels, have an instrument/suction channel, and may have an additional instrument channel. Group 2 endoscopes also may have an elevator channel and up to two control channels for balloon functions. Examples of Group 2 endoscopes are duodenoscopes with an open elevator channel, echoendoscopes used for endoscopic ultrasound, and enteroscopes.

- Group 3 endoscopes are used in bronchoscopy, otorhinolaryngology applications, gynecology, and urology. This group includes endoscopes with only one channel system for biopsy, irrigation, and suction or endoscopes without any channel. Examples of Group 3 endoscopes are bronchoscopes, cystoscopes, laryngoscopes, and nasendoscopes.

In addition to following the guidance provided in this document, it is critically important for individuals who are responsible for processing Group 1, 2, or 3 flexible endoscopes to follow the manufacturer's instructions for use (IFU) and the IFU for all products and equipment used for processing flexible endoscopes. Processing flexible endoscopes is a complex cycle of multiple steps that includes point-of-use precleaning, transporting, leak testing, cleaning, inspecting, **high-level disinfection** (HLD) or liquid chemical sterilization, packaging and **sterilization**, storage, and use **(Figure 1)**.

The complex design of flexible endoscopes increases the efficiency and effectiveness of endoscopic procedures; however, it creates enormous challenges for effective processing.[3] Some parts of the endoscope may be difficult or impossible to access, and effective cleaning of all areas of flexible duodenoscopes may not be possible.[6]

Although single-use devices may meet the quality of reusable endoscopic devices and may provide an option for reducing the risk for transmission of infection,[7-10] a discussion of the potential benefits of single-use flexible endoscopes is outside the scope of this guideline. The use of airborne, contact, or droplet precautions, the various chemicals used as **high-level disinfectants** or **liquid chemical sterilants**, the methods used for HLD or low-temperature sterilization, the methods for determining water quality used for processing flexible endoscopes and accessories, the protocols for microbiological surveillance of flexible endoscopes, the management of processing failures, sharps and medication safety, and the ergonomic injuries associated with the endoscopy environment are also outside of the scope of this guideline.

A full discussion of the design and construction of endoscopy suites in hospitals and outpatient facilities, the design of ventilation systems for controlling personnel exposure limits to chemicals used in the endoscopy suite, and the performance and use requirements for eyewash and shower equipment are outside of the scope of this document. However, because the design of the endoscopy suite and the procedures performed in the facility affect the processing of flexible endoscopes, some recommendations have been provided relative to **procedure rooms** and other elements of the endoscopy suite

Evidence Review

A medical librarian conducted a systematic search of the databases Ovid MEDLINE®, EBSCO CINAHL®, and Scopus® as well as of the Ovid Cochrane Database of Systematic Reviews. Search results were limited to literature published in English from 1994 through 2014. At the time of the initial search, the librarian established weekly alerts on the search topics and until October 2015, presented relevant results to the lead author. The author and the librarian also identified relevant guidelines and guidance from government agencies, professional organizations, and standards-setting bodies. During the development of this guideline, the author requested supplementary searches for topics not included in the original search as well as articles and other sources that were discovered during the evidence-appraisal process.

Search terms included the subject headings *endoscopes, disinfection, decontamination, sterilization, disinfectants, detergents, biofilms, infection control, cross-infection, equipment contamination, occupational exposure, protective clothing,* and *hypersensitivity.* Subject headings and key words for specific types of endoscopes, bacteria, disinfectants, and protective devices also were included, as were headings and terms related to the concepts of endoscope storage, methods of reprocessing, disinfection monitoring, infection transmission, disposable and reusable equipment, occupational allergies and injuries, and air pollution and ventilation. Complete search strategies are available upon request.

Excluded were non-peer-reviewed or retracted publications and evidence specific to the mechanism of action or health hazards associated with specific high-level disinfectants or liquid chemical sterilants, rigid endoscopic instrumentation, endoscopic medical treatment protocols, techniques, patient management, or functional design of flexible endoscopes.

In total, 1,257 research and non-research sources of evidence were identified for possible inclusion, and of these, 418 were cited in the guideline **(Figure 2)**.

Articles identified by the search were provided to the lead author and an evidence appraiser. The lead author and the evidence appraiser reviewed and critically appraised each article using the AORN Research or Non-Research Evidence

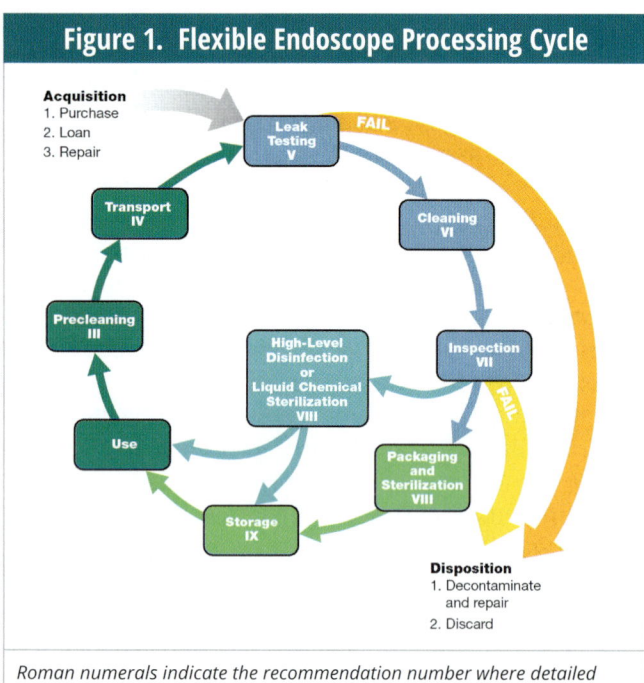

Figure 1. Flexible Endoscope Processing Cycle

Roman numerals indicate the recommendation number where detailed guidance is provided.

Figure 2. Flow Diagram of Literature Search Results

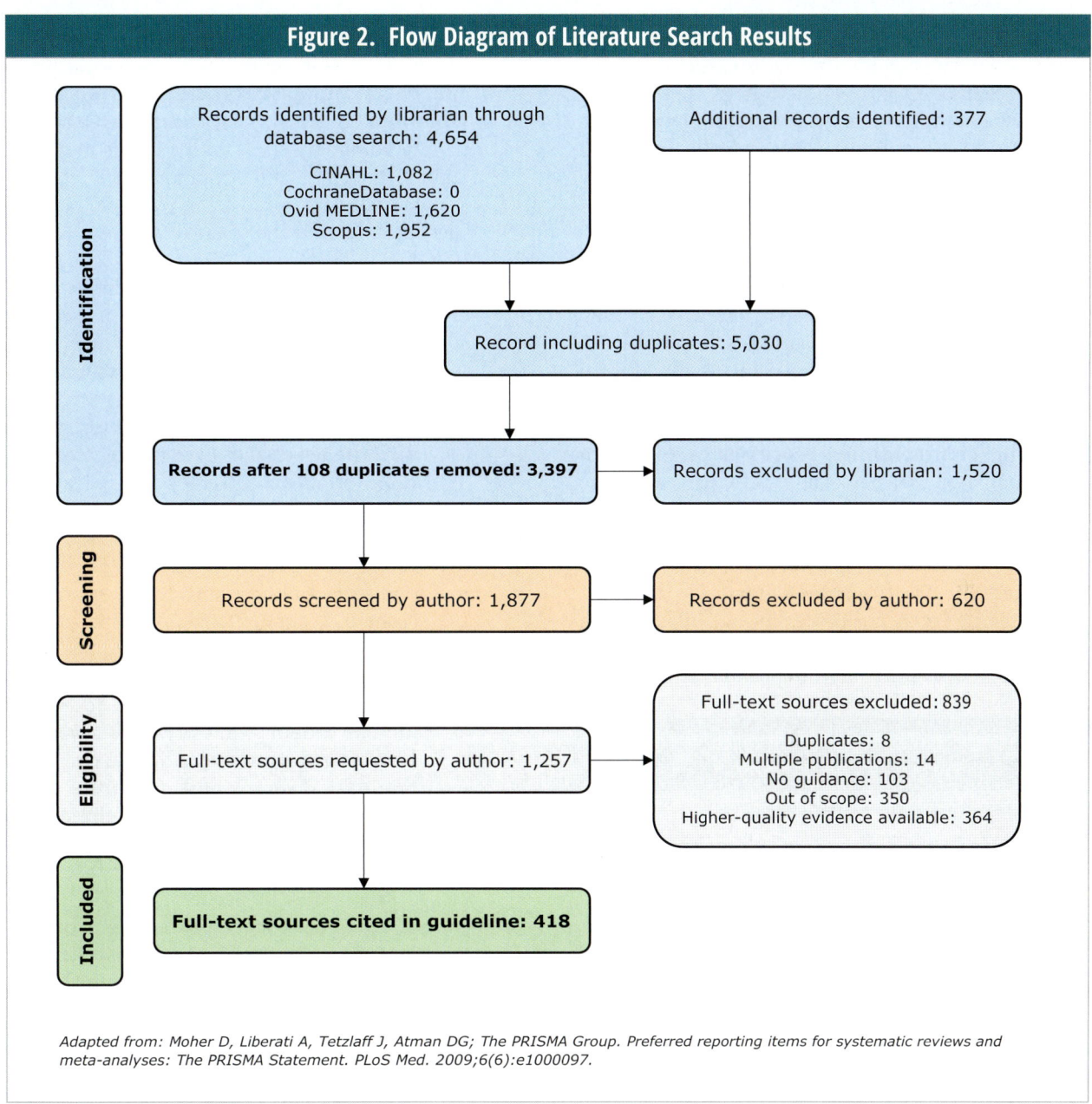

Records identified by librarian through database search: 4,654

CINAHL: 1,082
CochraneDatabase: 0
Ovid MEDLINE: 1,620
Scopus: 1,952

Additional records identified: 377

Identification

Record including duplicates: 5,030

Records after 108 duplicates removed: 3,397

Records excluded by librarian: 1,520

Screening

Records screened by author: 1,877

Records excluded by author: 620

Eligibility

Full-text sources requested by author: 1,257

Full-text sources excluded: 839

Duplicates: 8
Multiple publications: 14
No guidance: 103
Out of scope: 350
Higher-quality evidence available: 364

Included

Full-text sources cited in guideline: 418

Adapted from: Moher D, Liberati A, Tetzlaff J, Atman DG; The PRISMA Group. Preferred reporting items for systematic reviews and meta-analyses: The PRISMA Statement. PLoS Med. 2009;6(6):e1000097.

Appraisal Tools as appropriate. The literature was independently evaluated and appraised according to the strength and quality of the evidence. Each article was then assigned an appraisal score. The appraisal score is noted in brackets after each reference as applicable.

Each recommendation rating is based on a synthesis of the collective evidence, a benefit-harm assessment, and consideration of resource use. The strength of the recommendation was determined using the AORN Evidence Rating Model and the quality and consistency of the evidence supporting a recommendation. The recommendation strength rating is noted in brackets after each recommendation.

Note: *The evidence summary table is available at http://www.aorn.org/evidencetables/.*

Editor's note: MEDLINE is a registered trademark of the US National Library of Medicine's Medical Literature Analysis and Retrieval System, Bethesda, MD. CINAHL, Cumulative Index to Nursing and Allied Health Literature, is a registered trademark of EBSCO Industries, Birmingham, AL. Scopus is a registered trademark of Elsevier B.V., Amsterdam, The Netherlands.

1. Processing Area

1.1 Process flexible endoscopes in an area designed and constructed to support processing activities.[1,11-19] *[Recommendation]*

The endoscopy suite consists of a minimum of three functional areas: procedure room(s), **processing room**(s), and **patient care area**(s).[11] The design of the endoscopy suite, and the procedures performed in the facility affect processing of flexible endoscopes.

Low-quality evidence and several clinical practice guidelines support processing flexible endoscopes in an area designed and constructed for processing activities.[1,11-19]

The benefits are that construction and design to support processing activities may improve efficiency, help to reduce the risk of cross contamination, and provide a safe work environment. Refer to the Facility Guidelines Institute (FGI) *Guidelines for Design and Construction of Hospitals and Outpatient Facilities*[11] for additional guidance.

1.2 **Except for precleaning processes performed at the point of use, perform endoscope processing in a room where only processing activities are performed and that is physically separated from locations where patient care activities are performed.[12,14,16-18,20-22]** *[Recommendation]*

Limiting endoscope processing activities to designated processing rooms may help prevent contamination of procedure rooms and patient care areas.[22]

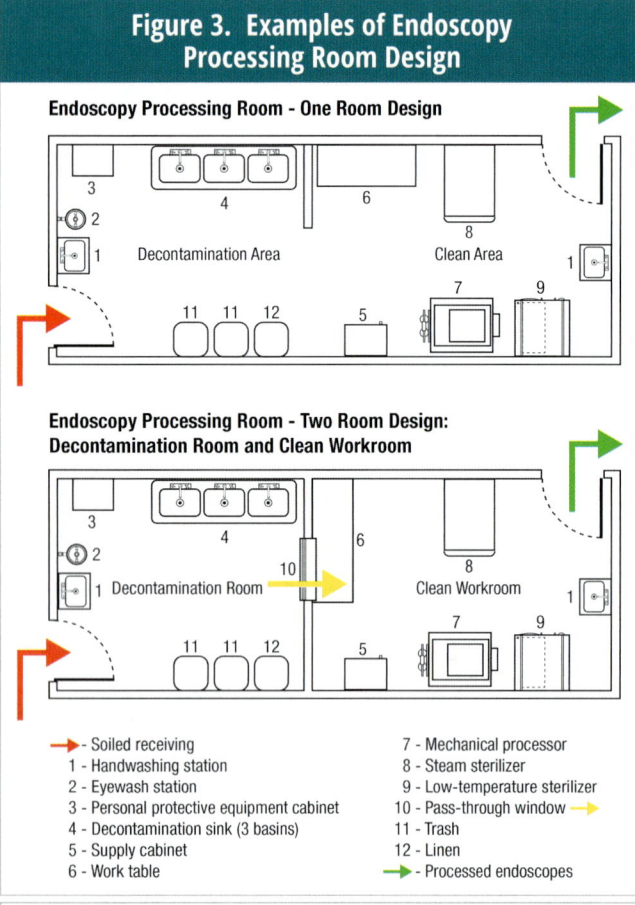

Figure 3. Examples of Endoscopy Processing Room Design

Endoscopy Processing Room - One Room Design

Decontamination Area — Clean Area

Endoscopy Processing Room - Two Room Design: Decontamination Room and Clean Workroom

Decontamination Room — Clean Workroom

→ - Soiled receiving
1 - Handwashing station
2 - Eyewash station
3 - Personal protective equipment cabinet
4 - Decontamination sink (3 basins)
5 - Supply cabinet
6 - Work table
7 - Mechanical processor
8 - Steam sterilizer
9 - Low-temperature sterilizer
10 - Pass-through window →
11 - Trash
12 - Linen
→ - Processed endoscopes

Note: *These examples are conceptual illustrations of one- and two-room design, equipment placement, and traffic flow. They are not intended to represent complete schematic designs.*

1.3 **Endoscope processing may occur in a single endoscopy processing room[14] or in two separate rooms (ie, decontamination room, clean workroom) as shown in Figure 3.[11]** *[Conditional Recommendation]*

The minimum standard for design and construction of hospitals and outpatient care facilities is a single endoscopy processing room containing both decontamination and clean areas.[23]

1.3.1 **During the infection control risk assessment, a multidisciplinary team that includes infection preventionists, endoscopy and perioperative RNs, sterile processing personnel, endoscopists, and other involved personnel should determine the potential harms compared with the benefits of performing decontamination and clean activities in separate rooms.** *[Recommendation]*

Having separate decontamination and clean rooms may avoid the risk of cross contamination from multiple individuals performing both clean and contaminated processing activities in a single area.[23,24]

1.3.2 **The endoscopy processing room should include a door[11] that provides access to and from the decontamination area or decontamination room[12] and a separate door that provides access to and from the clean area or clean workroom.[25]** *[Recommendation]*
- **Automatic sliding doors or foot-operated doors may be used.[21]**
- **When endoscope processing activities will occur in two separate rooms, either a door or a pass-through window may be used as access from the decontamination room to the clean workroom.[12,26]**

[Conditional Recommendation]

Doors to the decontamination area and clean area help contain contaminants within the processing room and help prevent cross contamination.[25] Automatic sliding doors and foot-operated doors facilitate hands-free movement of flexible endoscopes and other items to and from the endoscopy processing room.

1.3.3 **An endoscopy processing room with a one-room design should provide**
- **a minimum of 3 ft (0.9 m) between the decontamination area and the clean work area[11,14] and**
- **either a separating wall or a barrier that extends a minimum of 4 ft (1.2 m) above the sink rim to separate soiled work areas from clean work areas.[14,23]**

[Recommendation]

Cross contamination can result when soiled items are placed in close proximity to clean items or are placed on surfaces upon which clean items are later placed. Separation of the decontamination area from the clean area minimizes the potential for contamination of clean and processed flexible endoscopes.[12,13,16,22,23,27]

Hota et al[28] demonstrated that contaminated water droplets had the ability to travel a distance of 39.4 inches (1 m). There is no evidence to indicate that contaminated water droplets from endoscope cleaning activities would be dispersed farther than 39.4 inches (1 m). It is unlikely that microorganisms would be disseminated by air over longer distances because they would be contained within water droplets.[23]

Separating soiled and clean work areas by a distance of at least 3 ft (0.9 m) aligns with current recommendations from the Centers for Disease Control and Prevention (CDC) that patients who require droplet precautions should be placed at least 3 ft from other patients.[29]

Having a wall or physical barrier for separation of the decontamination area provides protection and minimizes the potential for contamination of clean and processed flexible endoscopes.

1.4 **The endoscopy processing room should be designed to facilitate a unidirectional workflow from the decontamination area or decontamination room to the clean area or clean workroom and then to clean storage in a separate location.[1,11-15,17,18,20,25,30]** *[Recommendation]*

A unidirectional flow improves efficiency and helps to contain contaminants within the decontamination area or decontamination room.[11,12,17,18,25,30]

1.5 **Heating, ventilation, and air conditioning (HVAC) systems for the endoscopy suite should be designed in compliance with state and local building codes and other guidelines as set forth by the FGI and American Society of Heating, Refrigerating and Air-Conditioning Engineers (ASHRAE).[11,15,31]** *[Recommendation]*

Heating, ventilation, and air conditioning systems control the air quality, temperature, humidity, and air pressure of the room in comparison to the surrounding areas.[32] The HVAC system is intended to reduce the amount of environmental contamination (eg, microbial-laden skin squames, dust, lint) in the endoscopy suite.[31,32]

1.5.1 Heating, ventilation, and air conditioning systems in the endoscopy suite should be constructed and designed to meet the parameters shown in Table 1. *[Recommendation]*

The minimum HVAC values are for new construction or major renovations. They are not intended to be used as values for operating older facilities built when lesser standards were in place.

1.5.2 **Maintain the minimum number of air changes in the endoscopy suite, including the percentage of outdoor air, within the HVAC design parameters at the rate that was applicable at the time of design or of the most recent renovation of the HVAC system.[32]** *[Recommendation]*

Filtered air minimizes the recirculation of indoor contaminants within the area.[32]

1.5.3 **The incoming air should be sequentially filtered through two filters. The first filter should be rated as 7 MERV (ie, minimum efficiency reporting value) and the second should be rated as 14 MERV.[11,32]** *[Recommendation]*

The incoming air requires continuous filtration because dust and airborne fungi are present at all times.[32]

Minimum efficiency reporting values measure the effectiveness of the air filters on a scale from 1 to 16.[31] The higher the MERV rating on a filter, the fewer the dust particles and other contaminants that can pass through it.[31]

1.5.4 **Maintain the airflow direction (ie, pressure relationship of one area to adjacent areas) for the endoscopy suite within the HVAC parameters.[32] When endoscope processing activities will occur in two rooms, the pressure relationship should be**
- **negative in the decontamination room[33] and**
- **positive in the clean workroom.[33]**
[Recommendation]

There is no recommendation for the pressure relationship when endoscope processing activities will occur in a single room.[33,34]

The direction of the airflow from one room to the adjacent area is engineered to minimize the flow of contaminants from dirty to clean areas.[31] Negative pressure in the decontamination room helps prevent contaminants from flexible endoscopes and other items being processed from reaching surrounding environments.[26] Positive pressure in the clean workroom helps prevent contaminants from surrounding environments from reaching the clean room.[26]

1.5.5 **Bronchoscopy procedure rooms should be designed to be under negative pressure to the surrounding areas.[11,32,35,36]** *[Recommendation]*

Table 1. HVAC Design Parameters for Endoscopy Suites				
Functional Area	Minimum Total Air Changes Per Hour	Settings for Airflow Patterns (Pressure)	Humidity	Temperature
Endoscopy processing room - One-room design	10	NR	Maximum 60%	60° F to 73° F (16° C to 23° C)
Endoscopy processing room - Two-room design				
Decontamination room	10	Negative	Maximum 60%	60° F to 73° F (16° C to 23° C)
Clean workroom	10	Negative	Maximum 60%[1]	68° F to 73° F (20° C to 23° C)
Clean/sterile storage room	4	Positive	Maximum 60%	< 75° F (< 24° C)
Endoscopy procedure room	6	NR	Maximum 60%	68° F to 73° F (20° C to 23° C)
Bronchoscopy procedure room	12	Negative	NR	68° F to 73° F (20° C to 23° C)
Sterilizer service access room	10	Negative	NR[2]	NR[2]
Environmental services closet	10	Negative	NR	NR

NR = No recommendation
[1] Check the manufacturer's instructions for use, for storage requirements (eg, reusable linens, chemical indicators, biological indicators)
[2] Check sterilizer manufacturer's specifications

Note: The terminology and parameters noted above represent the consensus of a joint heating, ventilation, and air-conditioning (HVAC) task force brought together on April 29, 2015 in Annapolis, Maryland, for the purpose of harmonizing the conflicting and sometimes unclear HVAC standards and guidelines established by a variety of professional organizations. The task force included representatives from the American Society of Heating, Refrigerating, and Air-Conditioning Engineers (ASHRAE), the American Society for Healthcare Engineering (ASHE), the Association for the Advancement of Medical Instrumentation (AAMI), the Association of periOperative Registered Nurses (AORN), the Facility Guidelines Institute (FGI), and other sterile processing experts and consultants.

1.5.6 For patients who require airborne precautions when a negative pressure room is not available, a portable, industrial grade high-efficiency particulate air (HEPA) filter or portable anteroom system (PAS)-HEPA combination unit may be used to supplement air cleaning.[32,35] *[Conditional Recommendation]*

Use of an airborne infection isolation room; negative pressure room; or portable, industrial grade HEPA filter or PAS-HEPA combination unit helps prevent the spread of airborne pathogens, particularly tuberculosis, rubeola, and varicella zoster, and is recommended during procedures that can generate infectious aerosols (eg, bronchoscopy).[29,36] The reader can refer to the Healthcare Infection Control Practices Advisory Committee "Guideline for isolation precautions: preventing transmission of infectious agents in healthcare settings"[29] and the AORN Guideline for Prevention of Transmissible Infections[35] for additional guidance.

1.5.7 Ventilation within the endoscopy suite must be controlled to meet personnel limits for chemical exposure as required by local, state, and federal Occupational Safety and Health Administration (OSHA) regulations[37,38] and should be accomplished in accordance with industry standards[11,31] and professional guidelines.[18,22,39-46] *[Regulatory Requirement]*

1.6 Structural surfaces (eg, doors, floors, walls, ceilings, cabinets, shelves, work surfaces), furniture (eg, tables), and equipment in the endoscopy processing room, procedure rooms, and patient care areas should be smooth and made of materials that are water resistant, stain resistant, and able to withstand frequent cleaning.[11-13,21] *[Recommendation]*

Structural surfaces that are smooth and able to withstand frequent cleaning ease the cleaning process. A clean environment will reduce the number of microorganisms present.

1.6.1 Ceiling surfaces in the endoscopy processing room, procedure rooms, and patient care areas should not be composed of perforated, serrated, cut, or highly textured tiles.[11] *[Recommendation]*

Perforated, serrated, cut, and highly textured ceiling tiles may create a reservoir for the collection of dirt and debris that cannot be removed during cleaning.

1.6.2 Pipes and other fixtures above work areas in the endoscopy suite should be enclosed and tightly sealed.[11,12] *[Recommendation]*

Providing tight seals and enclosing pipes and other fixtures above work areas helps prevent contamination from dust, condensation, and other potential sources of contamination.[12]

1.6.3 Floor surfaces in endoscopy processing rooms, procedure rooms, and patient care areas should be **monolithic**.[11] Junctions between floors and walls should have an integral **coved wall base** that is carried up the wall a minimum of 6 inches (152 mm) and is tightly sealed to the wall.[11,13] *[Recommendation]*

Seams, joints, or crevices may harbor microorganisms.[12]

1.6.4 Maintain the integrity of surfaces within the endoscopy suite and have damaged surfaces repaired.[32] *[Recommendation]*

Damaged surfaces may shed particles into the environment[12] and may create a reservoir for the collection of dirt and debris that cannot be removed during cleaning.[32] Damage to floor surfaces may create a trip or fall hazard.[32]

1.7 Lighting in the endoscopy suite should be designed in compliance with state and local building codes and other guidelines as set forth by the Illuminating Engineering Society of North America.[47] *[Recommendation]*

Well-designed lighting facilitates visual inspection of flexible endoscopes and other tasks performed in the endoscopy suite.

1.7.1 Lighting should be designed to provide good visibility for personnel to perform necessary tasks and should be adjustable.[47] *[Recommendation]*

Although a very high illuminance capability may be required for some tasks, too much light can be uncomfortable. Adjustable lighting improves comfort by allowing personnel to increase or decrease the lighting level as needed to perform the task.[47]

1.8 **Hand washing stations** in the endoscopy suite must be readily accessible[48] and should be provided in the decontamination room and the clean workroom.[11,21] When endoscope processing activities will occur in a single room, a hand washing station should be provided in the decontamination area.[11] *[Regulatory Requirement]*

Providing readily accessible hand washing stations is a regulatory requirement.[48] Hand washing stations that are easy to access facilitate hand washing and may improve hand hygiene compli-

ance.[17] Hand hygiene is required after removal of personal protective equipment (PPE).[35,48]

1.9 A minimum of two **decontamination sinks** (or one sink with two divisions) should be provided in the endoscopy processing room.[12,13]

- When two decontamination sinks (or one sink with two divisions) are provided, designate one sink (or division) for leak testing and manual cleaning, and the other for rinsing.[12]
- Three decontamination sinks (or one sink with three divisions) may be provided in the endoscopy processing room.[12] When three decontamination sinks (or one sink with three divisions) are provided, designate one sink (or division) for leak testing, the second for manual cleaning, and the third for rinsing.[12,13]

[Recommendation]

Sinks are required for functions such as leak testing, cleaning, and rinsing of flexible endoscopes and other items being processed. Separate sinks or divisions facilitate endoscope processing and may help prevent cross contamination.

Silva et al[49] reported a **pseudo-outbreak** of *Pseudomonas aeruginosa* and *Serratia marcescens* involving 41 patients who underwent bronchoscopy procedures in a 380-bed private hospital in Sao Paulo, Brazil, between December 1994 and October 1996. As part of the investigation, the investigators reviewed and observed endoscopy processing procedures. They found that in addition to other inadequacies in the processing procedures, the same sink was used for both washing and rinsing the bronchoscopes. The pseudo-outbreak resolved with improved processing procedures that included separate sinks for washing and rinsing of the endoscopes.

1.9.1 Use decontamination sinks that are deep enough to allow complete submersion of the endoscope and large enough to allow the endoscope to be positioned in the sink without tight coiling.[12,13,15,22,25] *[Recommendation]*

Complete submersion of the endoscope minimizes aerosolization during cleaning.[12] Tight coiling of the endoscope may damage the light bundles, internal channels, tubes, or angulation wires.[12]

1.10 **Instrument air** should be provided in the endoscopy processing room.[50,51] *[Recommendation]*

Compressed air facilitates flushing and drying of channels and lumens.[12] Clean, filtered air is required for drying lumens and small channels without introducing contaminants into the clean device.

1.11 Eyewash stations, either plumbed or self-contained, must be provided within the endoscopy suite where chemicals that are hazardous to the eyes are located.[52] *[Regulatory Requirement]*

It is a regulatory requirement that emergency eyewash stations or showers be immediately accessible in locations where the eyes or body of any person may be exposed to injurious corrosive materials.[52]

Plumbed eyewash stations are connected to a continual source of water that is safe to drink.[53] Self-contained eyewash stations are stand-alone devices that contain flushing fluid.[53]

Many chemicals are eye irritants. Eyewash stations are necessary to provide flushing fluid when the safety data sheet identifies the chemical as a hazard and recommends immediate flushing of the eyes as an emergency first aid measure.

1.11.1 Eyewash stations should be located
- in a well-lit area identified with a highly visible sign positioned within the area served by the eyewash station,[53]
- so that travel time is no greater than 10 seconds from the location of chemical use or storage,[53] and
- on the same level as the hazard, with the path of travel free of obstructions (eg, doors) that may inhibit immediate use of an eyewash station.[53]

[Recommendation]

1.11.2 Eyewash stations should be positioned with the flushing fluid nozzles not less than 33 inches (83.8 cm) and not more than 45 inches (114.3 cm) from the surface on which the person using the eyewash station stands and a minimum of 6 inches (15.2 cm) from the wall or the nearest obstruction.[53] *[Recommendation]*

1.11.3 Eyewash stations should not be installed in a location that requires flushing of the eyes in the decontamination sink. *[Recommendation]*

Splashing from the decontamination sink could potentially contaminate the eyes of personnel using the sink.

1.11.4 Once activated, eyewash stations should be capable of delivering tepid (60° F to 100° F [16° C to 38° C]) flushing fluid to both eyes simultaneously at not less than 0.4 gallons (1.5 L) per minute for 15 minutes at a velocity low enough to be noninjurious to the user and without requiring the use of the operator's hands.[53] *[Recommendation]*

Refer to the current *ANSI/International Safety Equipment Association (ISEA) American National Standard for Emergency Eyewash and Shower Equipment*[53] for additional guidance.

2. Room Control and Maintenance

2.1 Process flexible endoscopes in an area that is controlled and maintained to support processing activities.[1,11-19,24] *[Recommendation]*

Low-quality evidence and several clinical practice guidelines support processing flexible endoscopes in an area where activities such as temperature, humidity, environmental cleaning, **surgical attire**, traffic patterns, and security are managed in accordance with specific policies and procedures that promote processing activities.[1,11-19,24]

The benefits are that this may improve efficiency, maintain functionality of flexible endoscopes and other medical devices, help to reduce the risk of cross contamination, and provide a safe work environment.

The limitations of the evidence are that no research studies have investigated the link between patient outcomes and flexible endoscopes processed in a controlled area.[30]

2.2 Create and implement a systematic process for establishing and monitoring performance of the HVAC system in the endoscopy suite.[27,32] *[Conditional Recommendation]*

Monitoring performance of the HVAC systems helps ensure that the desired HVAC parameters are being achieved and maintained.

2.2.1 Maintain relative humidity within the HVAC design parameters for endoscopy suites.[32] *[Recommendation]*

The effect of relative humidity on bacterial, fungal, and viral growth is inconclusive. Additional research is warranted to determine optimal relative humidity levels for control of environmental contamination.[32]

2.2.2 Adjust the room temperature in the endoscopy suite based on the needs of the patient and the comfort of personnel.[32] *[Conditional Recommendation]*

Maintaining comfort and normothermia of patients in procedure rooms or patient care areas may require that room temperature be adjusted outside of the recommended range. Temperature settings in nonclinical areas may also need to be adjusted to provide comfortable temperatures for personnel based on the activities being performed (eg, a lower temperature may be required in the decontamination area where PPE may be worn for long periods of time).[12]

2.2.3 **Report unintentional variances in the predetermined HVAC system parameters in the endoscopy suite according to the health care organization's policy and procedure.**[32] *[Conditional Recommendation]*

Rapid communication between affected and responsible personnel can help facilitate resolution of the variance.[32]

2.2.4 **Designate personnel from the health care organization to perform a risk assessment if a variance in the parameters of the HVAC system occurs.**[32] *[Conditional Recommendation]*

The effect of the HVAC system parameters falling out of range is variable. A small variance for a short period of time may not be of clinical concern, whereas a large variance for a longer period may have clinical significance.[32]

2.2.5 **Based on the risk assessment, take corrective measures that may include**

- **terminal cleaning of surfaces when there is evidence of contamination on surfaces;**
- **reprocessing or discarding any supplies with packaging that may have been compromised;**
- **inventorying discarded, damaged supplies to obtain replacements; and**
- **modifying or updating the HVAC system.**[32]

[Conditional Recommendation]

2.3 **Implement hand hygiene practices in the endoscopy suite in accordance with the AORN Guideline for Hand Hygiene.**[54] *[Recommendation]*

Hand hygiene has been recognized as a primary method of decreasing health care–associated infections.[54] Health care–associated infections can result in untoward outcomes such as escalated cost of care, increased rates of morbidity and mortality, and longer lengths of stay, as well as the pain and suffering a patient may experience.[54]

Because of a severe outbreak of *Klebsiella pneumoniae*-producing extended-spectrum beta (β)-lactamase that occurred in 16 patients undergoing endoscopic retrograde cholangiopancreatography (ERCP) procedures in a hospital in France between December 2008 and August 2009, Aumeran et al[55] observed the duodenoscope processing procedures. They found a lack of personnel compliance with recommended hand hygiene practices, and they concluded that

the hands of personnel may have been a source or vehicle for transmission of the outbreak strain.

2.3.1 **Do not use hand washing sinks to clean flexible endoscopes.**[12,20,22] *[Recommendation]*

Cleaning endoscopes in hand washing sinks could contaminate the sink, faucet, and hands of personnel subsequently washed in the same sink.[12]

2.3.2 **Do not use decontamination sinks for hand washing.**[12] *[Recommendation]*

Hand washing in the decontamination sinks could contaminate the endoscope or other items subsequently washed in the same sink.[12]

2.4 **Follow processes and procedures for environmental cleaning in the endoscopy suite in accordance with the AORN Guideline for Environmental Cleaning.**[56] *[Recommendation]*

A clean environment will minimize the exposure risk of health care personnel and patients to potentially infectious microorganisms.[56]

2.5 **Wear clean surgical attire and head coverings in the processing room and procedure rooms of the endoscopy suite.** *[Recommendation]*

Surgical attire is worn to provide a high level of cleanliness and hygiene within the endoscopy environment and to promote patient and worker safety.[57] Head coverings contain hair and minimize microbial dispersal.[57]

2.6 **Personnel working in the endoscopy suite must wear PPE.** *[Regulatory Requirement]*

It is a regulatory requirement that PPE be worn whenever splashes, spray, spatter, or droplets of blood, body fluids, or other potentially infectious materials may be generated and eye, nose, or mouth contamination can be reasonably anticipated.[48] Employers are required to ensure that employees are protected when exposed to eye or face hazards from liquid chemicals.[59]

2.6.1 **Wear personal protective equipment in accordance with the AORN Guideline for Prevention of Transmissible Infections,**[35] **the AORN Guideline for Surgical Attire,**[57] **and the AORN Guideline for Cleaning and Care of Surgical Instruments.**[58] *[Recommendation]*

2.6.2 **When working in the endoscopy processing room and handling contaminated flexible endoscopes, wear PPE that includes**

- **surgical masks in combination with eye protection devices, such as goggles, glasses** with solid side shields, or chin-length face shields;

- fluid-resistant gowns;
- general purpose utility gloves with cuffs that extend beyond the cuff of the gown; and
- fluid-resistant shoe covers.

[Recommendation]

Contaminated flexible endoscopes are a potential source of transmissible pathogens.[58] Personal protective equipment helps to protect processing and procedural personnel from exposure to blood, body fluids, and other potentially infectious materials.[58]

Surgical masks in combination with eye protection devices can protect the wearer's face, eyes, nose, and mouth from exposure to hazardous chemicals as well as pathogenic microorganisms, body fluids, and other potentially infectious materials.[57] The mucous membranes of the nose, mouth, and eyes may act as portals of entry to infectious agents.[60] In addition to the risk for injury from a direct splash to the eye, there is also a risk of developing conjunctivitis or a systemic infection.[60] Skin may also act as a portal when its integrity is compromised by trauma or disease.[60]

Kaye[61] reported an unusual complication of inoculation in the eye by effluent from the open biopsy port of a flexible esophagoscope. The patient was diagnosed with herpetic esophagitis. After esophageal brushings and biopsies had been obtained, the endoscopist attempted air inflation and a jet of fluid was directed from the patient's esophagus into the endoscopist's right eye, which was immediately flushed with copious amounts of water. One week later, the endoscopist noted an itchy papule beneath the right eyelid that developed into multiple conjunctival vesicles. Conjunctival cultures were positive for herpes simplex virus (HSV). The endoscopist subsequently developed a sore throat (also culture-positive for HSV), neck stiffness, lymphadenopathy, and splenomegaly that resolved within a week. The conjunctival HSV reappeared approximately two weeks later and resolved without further recurrence. The author concluded that although this was a rare event, it is conceivable that diseases such as tuberculosis and hepatitis could be transmitted in a similar way. The author recommended that endoscopists keep their faces away from the biopsy port and seal it as soon as the forceps have been withdrawn. In all likelihood, the splashing of fluid into the endoscopist's eye would have been prevented by the use of protective eyewear.

Fluid-resistant gowns can prevent transfer of microorganisms from contaminated items to skin.[58]

General purpose utility gloves can minimize the potential for punctures, nicks, and cuts, and exposure of the hands and forearms to blood, body fluids, and other potentially infectious materials.[58] Wearing utility gloves with cuffs that extend beyond the cuff of the gown helps provide protection from fluids during cleaning of flexible endoscopes and other items in the decontamination sink.[58]

Fluid-resistant shoe covers can protect shoes from splashes, splatters, and spills.[58]

2.6.3 **Perform hand hygiene after removal of PPE.[29]**
[Recommendation]

The CDC recommends performing hand hygiene after removal of PPE.[29] Hands may become contaminated when removing PPE. Damage to PPE in the form of tears, punctures, and abrasions may occur and be undetected, exposing the wearer to microbial contamination and bloodborne pathogens.[60]

2.6.4 **Reusable PPE must be decontaminated and the integrity of the PPE verified between uses.[48] Reusable PPE must be discarded if there are signs of deterioration or its ability to function as a barrier has been compromised.[48]**
[Regulatory Requirement]

Decontaminating reusable PPE and verifying its integrity between uses is a regulatory requirement.[48] Reusable gloves, gowns, aprons, and protective eyewear or face shields may become contaminated and their integrity compromised during use.

2.7 **Personnel working in the endoscopy suite should be immunized against vaccine-preventable diseases in accordance with the AORN Guideline for Prevention of Transmissible Infections.[35]** [Recommendation]

Personnel may come into contact with patients or infectious material from patients that may put them at risk for exposure and possible transmission of vaccine-preventable diseases.[35]

2.8 **Implement traffic patterns within the endoscopy suite that facilitate movement of patients, personnel, equipment, and supplies into, through, and out of defined areas within the endoscopy suite.**
[Recommendation]

Effective traffic patterns support safe patient care, workplace safety, and security.[32]

2.8.1 **Keep the processing room doors closed except during the entry and exit of personnel.** *[Recommendation]*

Keeping the doors closed helps prevent contaminated particles from entering or leaving the room and maintains the pressure differential required for decontamination rooms. Keeping the door closed also assists with venting contaminated room air out of the building, minimizing contamination of adjacent areas.[32]

2.9 **Designate personnel from the health care organization to develop a security plan for the endoscopy suite in consultation with security personnel or law enforcement representatives.[32] [Conditional Recommendation]**

Including the endoscopy suite in the facility-wide plan takes into consideration the unique security risks created by the presence of high-value equipment, medications, and supplies and the variable hours during which the suite may be unoccupied.[32] Security personnel and law enforcement representatives have expertise in identifying security risks and in prevention and mitigation tactics.[32]

2.9.1 **Select security measures based on a risk assessment; these may include the use of devices (eg, alarm systems, video surveillance, shatterproof glass) or controls (eg, locked doors, tracking systems, visitor logs).[32] [Conditional Recommendation]**

Security measures provide for the safety of patients, personnel, and visitors.[32]

2.10 **Implement processes and procedures for purchasing, evaluating, and selecting flexible endoscopes, accessories, equipment, and other items and products related to the use and processing of flexible endoscopes in accordance with the AORN Guideline for Product Selection.[62] [Recommendation]**

Patient and worker safety, quality, and cost containment are primary concerns of endoscopy personnel as they participate in evaluating and selecting medical devices and products for use in endoscopy settings.[62]

2.10.1 **Use endoscopes, accessories, and equipment that have manufacturer-validated IFU.** *[Recommendation]*

Manufacturers of reusable devices cleared by the FDA provide validated cleaning and processing instructions and guidance on how to process devices between uses. Items cannot be assumed to be correctly processed unless the manufacturer's IFU are derived from **validation** testing and the instructions have been followed.[58]

Validation by the manufacturer provides objective evidence that the requirements for the specific intended use of the product or device can be consistently fulfilled.[63-65]

2.10.2 **When performing prepurchase evaluation of flexible endoscopes, accessories, and equipment,**
- **ensure that the facility has the capability to comply with the manufacturer's IFU,**
- **confirm that the manufacturer's IFU can be replicated, and**
- **verify compatibility with other relevant manufacturers' IFU.**

[Recommendation]

Manufacturers' IFU vary widely. Some devices or items may have unique requirements that may not be achievable within the facility.

2.10.3 **Obtain endoscope accessories and devices specified by the endoscope or mechanical processor manufacturer for cleaning and processing at the time of endoscope purchase and use these in accordance with the IFU.[58]** *[Recommendation]*

Using accessories and devices that are designed and manufactured to the endoscope or mechanical processor manufacturer's specifications helps ensure the endoscope can be used effectively and facilitates performance of cleaning and processing procedures.[58]

2.11 **Implement processes and procedures for managing new, loaned, and repaired endoscopes, accessories, and equipment in the endoscopy suite in accordance with the AORN Guideline for Cleaning and Care of Surgical Instruments.[58]** *[Recommendation]*

Adhering to the AORN guideline will help ensure successful management of new, loaned, or repaired items.

2.12 **Flexible endoscopes and endoscope accessories should be cleaned and processed by individuals who have received education and completed competency verification activities related to endoscope processing.[15,66] [Recommendation]**

Moderate-quality evidence shows that ensuring flexible endoscopes and endoscope accessories are processed by individuals whose primary duties are to clean and process flexible endoscopes minimizes variability and improves processing effectiveness.[67,68] Having individuals who have received education and demonstrated competency process flexible endoscopes and accessories helps reduce the risk for errors and cross contamination.[66,69] Individuals whose primary duties are to clean and process flexible endoscopes bring a specialized level of knowledge to the processing procedure that may include

- an improved understanding of the health and safety issues that can arise when endoscopes are not correctly processed,[69]
- an in-depth knowledge of the structure and operation of the endoscopes they are responsible for processing,[69]
- an in-depth knowledge of the structure and operation of the mechanical processors they are using for processing,[69] and
- a desire for additional education related to processing of flexible endoscopes and accessories that may improve the quality and standard of processing.[69]

A dedicated team of individuals responsible for processing flexible endoscopes may also allow endoscopy nurses to focus on clinical responsibilities.[69]

Kolmos et al[70] reported a pseudo-outbreak of *P aeruginosa* in eight consecutive HIV-infected patients undergoing bronchoscopy in Denmark. None of the patients developed signs of respiratory tract infection that could be ascribed to the organism. The investigators found the source to be *P aeruginosa* contamination in the suction channels of two bronchoscopes. Due to the lack of a dedicated processing person, the nurses, who were inexperienced with processing procedures for flexible bronchoscopes, were not manually cleaning the endoscopes. Further, the mechanical processor was not working correctly, so the bronchoscopes were being manually soaked in glutaraldehyde in a location other than the endoscopy processing room. Interviews with the nurses confirmed that the suction channels had not been cleaned for many weeks before the pseudo-outbreak. When the channels were inspected, there were deposits of organic material in both bronchoscopes. The contaminated bronchoscopes were effectively cleaned and processed, and this stopped the outbreak. The investigators recommended having dedicated personnel process flexible bronchoscopes.

Ensuring flexible endoscopes and endoscope accessories are processed by individuals whose primary duties are to clean and process flexible endoscopes may also reduce repair costs and extend the life of the endoscope.[67,68]

McGill et al[71] conducted a nonexperimental study to ascertain the durability of flexible cystoscopes in relation to their use in the outpatient setting. The researchers prospectively investigated cystoscope processing and repair costs for six new cystoscopes from July 1, 2008, through August 31, 2009, and com-

pared these data with retrospective data from the previous eight months. During the prospective study period, the flexible cystoscopes were only processed by urology nursing personnel skilled in processes for handling and maintaining flexible cystoscopes. The researchers found there was a 43.9% decrease in repair costs and mechanical failure when the nurses processed the endoscopes.

To investigate the causes and costs of flexible ureteroscope damage and to develop recommendations to limit damage, Sooriakumaran et al[72] analyzed repair costs and damage to 35 ureteroscopes sent for repair during a 1-year period. The researchers found that the majority (72%) of the damages occurred during the cleaning and processing phase rather than during procedural use. The researchers suggested that having a skilled, dedicated team clean and process the ureteroscopes could help prevent damage and reduce costs.

In an effort to reduce costs and damage to flexible ureteroscopes, Semins et al[73] studied the effect and analyzed the cost per use of having dedicated urology personnel clean and process all ureteroscopes rather than the facility processing personnel who cleaned and processed all other facility items. Between April 2007 and March 2008, when the urology team processed the ureteroscopes, 11 ureteroscopes were processed 478 times. The average number of uses per ureteroscope before repair was necessary was 28.1. The average repair cost per use was $120.63 ($134.33 in 2015 US dollars). During the previous year, when the processing was performed by facility personnel, the average number of uses per ureteroscope before repair was necessary was only 10.8. The average repair cost per use was $418.19 ($465.69 in 2015 US dollars). The authors concluded that having a skilled and dedicated team process ureteroscopes was an effective measure to reduce repair costs and processing-related damage to flexible ureteroscopes.

McDougall et al[74] conducted a quasi-experimental study to determine whether the technique used to clean flexible ureteroscopes or the number of persons handling the endoscope during the cleaning process influenced function or number of repairs. The researchers used a new, flexible ureteroscope for each of two 30-day study periods. During the first study period, the endoscope was leak tested, cleaned, and processed by the endourology support team. During the second study period, the endoscope was leak tested, cleaned, and processed by the surgeon. The researchers found that the function and durability of the endoscope was not affected by the technique used to clean it or the number of people involved in cleaning and processing the endoscope. The function and durability of the endoscope was found to be affected by the demands of the surgical procedure and the technique of the surgeon.

2.12.1 **Process flexible endoscopes in the same manner in all processing locations.** *[Recommendation]*

Smith[75] reported two cases of septicemia caused by *P aeruginosa* following ERCP procedures. The investigators found that the accessory instruments used through the endoscope were cleaned with chlorhexidine gluconate and soaked in glutaraldehyde for 1 hour. After soaking, they were rinsed with **utility water**, and the lumens of the endoscope were flushed using single-use syringes. The accessory instruments were then placed into their original shipping containers while still wet and were stored in a cupboard. The syringes were stored in a wet condition and reused. The investigators sampled the syringes and found them to be culture-positive for the same strain of *P aeruginosa* that was found in the septic patients. The bacteria had been introduced into the patients' biliary tract on endoscopy instruments contaminated after disinfection by the syringes used for flushing the endoscope channels. The endoscopes were being processed at multiple sites, with processing personnel following different processing procedures at different sites.

In a case control study of an outbreak of multidrug-resistant *P aeruginosa*, Machida et al[76] found a relationship between the infections and contaminated bronchoscopes. Between June and August 2007, isolates from five patients in the intensive care unit (ICU) and emergency department (ED) of a 1,076-bed university hospital were culture-positive for multidrug-resistant *P aeruginosa*. All of the patients had undergone bronchoscopy procedures in the ICU or ED. The organism was not found in any of the bronchoscopes in use at the hospital; however, the investigators found that the bronchoscopes used in the ICU and the ED were processed differently from other hospital endoscopes.

The researchers retrospectively reviewed medical records from 2006 and found 11 additional patients with multidrug-resistant *P aeruginosa*. The review showed that these patients also had bronchoscopy procedures in the ICU or ED. Processing procedures were reviewed and showed poor compliance with hospital procedures for processing the endoscopes. The manual cleaning step was often skipped when the endoscopes were processed in the ICU or ED. The outbreak ended when effective cleaning and high-level disinfecting processes were established in all processing areas.[78]

2.12.2 **Provide sufficient time and numbers of personnel to permit thorough cleaning and processing of flexible endoscopes.**[58,77,78] *[Recommendation]*

Time constraints and insufficient numbers of endoscope-processing team members may create a disincentive for personnel to adhere to recommended cleaning and processing procedures.[58]

2.12.3 **Schedule endoscopy procedures to allow sufficient time for cleaning and processing of flexible endoscopes.**[78] *[Recommendation]*

Time constraints may create a disincentive for personnel to adhere to recommended cleaning and processing procedures.[58]

2.12.4 **Maintain an inventory of flexible endoscopes and accessories sufficient to meet the anticipated demand.**[58,77,78] *[Recommendation]*

Having an adequate inventory provides sufficient time for personnel to follow correct cleaning and processing procedures.[58,78]

2.12.5 **A multidisciplinary team that includes endoscopy personnel, RNs from departments where bedside endoscopy procedures are performed, infection preventionists, risk managers, endoscopy processing personnel, endoscopists, and other involved personnel should establish policies and procedures requiring that flexible endoscopes used for procedures performed at the bedside or outside of normal operating hours be processed in the same manner as endoscopes used during normal operating hours.** *[Recommendation]*

Flexible endoscopes are complex and costly devices that require multiple processing steps. Having skilled, dedicated personnel process flexible endoscopes for emergency procedures performed outside of normal operating hours helps ensure that the endoscopes have been processed correctly and are safe to use.[68]

Bou et al[79] conducted a cohort study to identify risk factors for infection following an outbreak of *P aeruginosa* infections in the 27-bed ICU of a community hospital in Spain during July 2003. The investigators identified 17 case patients with 25 *P aeruginosa* infections that included respiratory tract infections (n = 21), a bloodstream infection (n = 1), a urinary tract infection (n = 1), a pressure ulcer (n = 1), and a surgical site infection (n = 1). Ten of the 17 case patients had undergone bronchoscopy procedures in the ICU during a weekend. A review of the weekend processing procedures showed major deviations from hospital policies. Adequate cleaning and HLD were not performed. The weekend procedure involved rinsing the bronchoscope with povidone iodine and placing the bronchoscope into its storage case without drying. The bronchoscope was then transported to the endoscopy unit where it was stored in a drawer until its next use. On weekdays, the bronchoscope was either manually or mechanically cleaned and high-level disinfected without a sterile water rinse, alcohol flush, or purging with air. Notably, the manufacturer's IFU were not being followed in the ICU or the endoscopy unit. The researchers concluded that education of processing personnel was necessary to ensure processing was carried out in accordance with published guidelines in all areas of the hospital and during all hours processing procedures were performed.

Srinivasan et al[80] conducted a survey among 46 practicing bronchoscopists to assess their knowledge of recommended guidelines and processing procedures. The survey was distributed to participants in two bronchoscopy courses attended by pulmonologists from the United States. The results of the survey showed that 65% of the bronchoscopists (n = 30) were not familiar with bronchoscope processing guidelines and 39% (n = 18) did not know what processing procedures were used in their own facilities.

To audit processing of flexible endoscopes used during procedures performed outside of normal operating hours, Radford et al[81] conducted a telephone survey of 104 ear, nose, and throat units in England. On-call clinicians from 72 units (69%) agreed to participate. The researchers found that the on-call clinician processed the flexible endoscope in 60 units (83%); however, the on-call clinician had only received education and hands-on instruction on processing procedures in 27 units (38%). In addition, clinicians in 19 units (26%) followed inadequate processing procedures, and clinicians in 16 units (22%) were unsure of the correct processing method. In one case, the clinician admitted to not cleaning the endoscope between procedures. In 35 units (49%), the endoscope was stored in an unsterile carrying case. In seven units (10%), the on-call clinician did not know how the endoscope was stored. The researchers concluded there was an urgent need for compliance with effective processing procedures for flexible endoscopes used for emergent endoscopy procedures performed outside of normal operating hours.

3. Point-of-Use Treatment

3.1 **Preclean flexible endoscopes and accessories at the point of use.** *[Recommendation]*

Low-quality evidence supports precleaning of flexible endoscopes at the point of use as a mechanism for moistening, diluting, softening, and removing organic soils (eg, blood, feces, respiratory secretions) and reducing the formation of **biofilm**. If organic soil and biofilm are not removed completely, the subsequent HLD or sterilization process might not be effective.[82] The need for precleaning at the point of use is emphasized in numerous clinical practice guidelines.[12,13,15-22,27,44,45,83-85]

The benefits of precleaning flexible endoscopes at the point of use are that it eases[86] and improves[87] the cleaning process and helps reduce the formation of biofilm, which can interfere with HLD or sterilization.[82]

3.2 **Preclean flexible endoscopes and accessories at the point of use as soon as possible after the endoscope is removed from the patient (or the procedure is completed) and before organic material has dried on the surface or in the channels of the endoscope.**[12,13,18-22,27,44,45,83-85,88] *[Recommendation]*

The presence of dried organic material makes cleaning difficult.[85,89] When using an enzymatic cleaner, dried organic material has to be rehydrated in order for the **enzymes** to be effective.[90]

In a quasi-experimental laboratory study, Merritt et al[86] evaluated the effects of 12 different cleaning solutions on four microorganisms known to adhere to polystyrene and medical implant materials (ie, *Staphylococcus epidermidis, Candida albicans, Escherichia coli, P aeruginosa*). The results of the study showed that allowing **bioburden** to dry on surfaces made cleaning very difficult. The researchers recommended that microorganisms, protein, or other materials not be allowed to dry on flexible endoscopes before cleaning.

Biofilm is difficult to remove and may begin to form within minutes after the procedure is completed.[82,85] In an expert opinion article discussing biofilm development on the surfaces of medical devices and the role of biofilm in device processing, Roberts[82] explained that the formation of biofilm begins when a layer of organic material is deposited on the surface of a medical device **(Figure 4)**. Colonizing microorganisms subsequently become attached to this foundational layer. At this point,

Figure 4. Biofilm Formation[1,2]

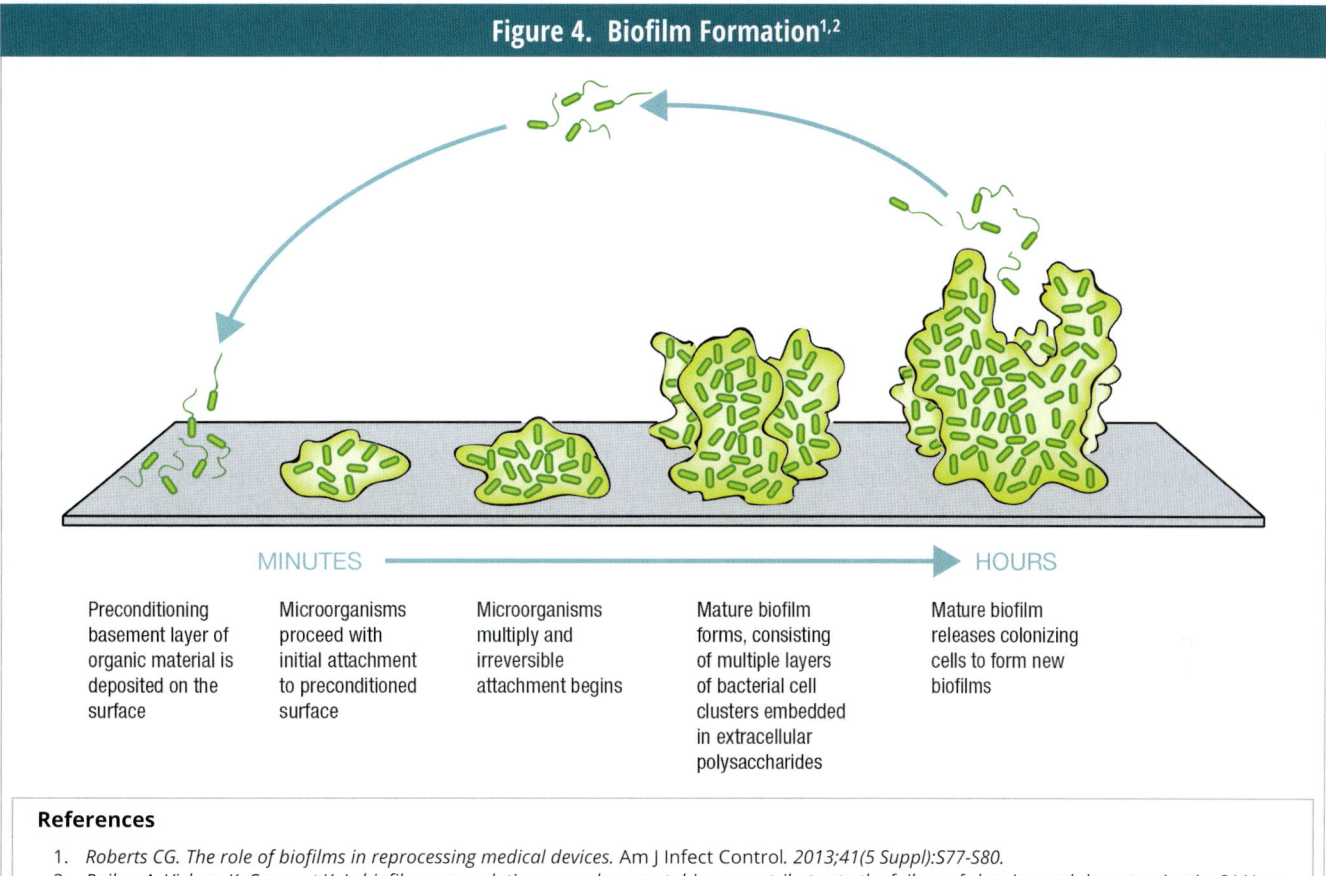

MINUTES ———————————————→ HOURS

Preconditioning basement layer of organic material is deposited on the surface

Microorganisms proceed with initial attachment to preconditioned surface

Microorganisms multiply and irreversible attachment begins

Mature biofilm forms, consisting of multiple layers of bacterial cell clusters embedded in extracellular polysaccharides

Mature biofilm releases colonizing cells to form new biofilms

References

1. Roberts CG. The role of biofilms in reprocessing medical devices. Am J Infect Control. 2013;41(5 Suppl):S77-S80.
2. Pajkos A, Vickery K, Crossart Y. Is biofilm accumulation on endoscope tubing a contributor to the failure of cleaning and decontamination? J Hosp Infect. 2004;58(3):224-229.

the microorganisms are loosely attached and can be removed by cleaning.[91]

Nearly irreversible attachment occurs as the microorganisms begin to multiply and form a mature biofilm.[91,92] A mature biofilm consists of layers of bacterial cell clusters embedded in towers of **polysaccharides** secreted by the microorganisms into their environment.[91-94] Microorganisms within a mature biofilm are protected by the secreted extracellular substances and may not be easily penetrated or killed by antibiotics, HLD, or sterilization.[82,93-96] This protective mechanism may be related to physical, genetic, or physiological characteristics of the bacteria or their ability to produce neutralizing enzymes.[45] The mature biofilm releases colonizing cells to form new biofilms on other surfaces of the device.[82,94]

Certain conditions are necessary for biofilm formation, including

- the presence of colonizing microorganisms,
- sufficient nutrients,
- acceptable temperature conditions for growth, and
- time required for the formation of biofilm.[82]

Some microorganisms undergo cell division every 20 to 30 minutes; however, it may take several hours for a mature biofilm to form.[82] The time frame within which the cleaning of flexible endoscopes or other reusable medical devices occurs is therefore a key factor in the prevention of biofilm formation and buildup.[82] Performing precleaning and the remaining processing steps within an hour after a procedure may prevent formation of a mature biofilm even under conditions favorable to rapid biofilm development.[82]

Biofilm can form on the inner surface of endoscope channels and is especially prone to form when these inner channels become scratched or damaged.[93] Herrmann et al[87] performed microscopic examinations of the inner surfaces of the suction and biopsy channels of new flexible endoscopes. They found that the channels were only partially smooth and contained small indentations and irregularities where biofilm could form and be retained even after cleaning. They noted that the formation of biofilm in the small indentations and irregularities was even more likely to occur if the endoscope was not cleaned immediately after use.

Effective precleaning processes may help to prevent patient infection. Naas et al[97] reported an outbreak of carbapenemase-producing *Klebsiella pneumoniae* transmitted via a flexible endoscope. Retrospective analysis showed that 17 patients from five regional hospitals in France had undergone endoscopy with the same gastroscope. Of the 17 patients, six were colonized and two developed infections. A review of the endoscope processing procedures revealed that one potential explanation for the contamination was that the precleaning of the endoscope had been delayed for 24 hours, allowing organic material to dry on the device.

3.3 Perform precleaning in accordance with the endoscope manufacturer's IFU. *[Recommendation]*

There are multiple types of flexible endoscopes, and recommended precleaning processes may vary among manufacturers.

Variations from the manufacturer's IFU may result in insufficient cleaning or in processing failure.

3.3.1 Perform precleaning by
- **preparing a fresh solution of a cleaning product with properties recommended by the manufacturer**[12,15];
- **washing the exterior surfaces of the endoscope with a soft, lint-free cloth or sponge saturated with the cleaning solution**[12,13,15,19,21,27,44,83-85,89];
- **suctioning the cleaning solution through the suction and biopsy channels**[12,13,15,19,21,44,85,89];
- **placing the distal end of the endoscope in the cleaning solution and suctioning the solution through the endoscope**[12,15,21];
- **flushing the air, water, and other channels of the endoscope alternately with the cleaning solution and air,**[12,15,16,17,21,83] **finishing with air**[13,85,89];
- **visually inspecting the endoscope for damage**[12,19]; **and**
- **discarding the cleaning solution and cleaning cloth or sponge after use.**[13,15,83]

[Recommendation]

Using a fresh solution for each new cleaning process may help prevent cross contamination of flexible endoscopes.[98] Recommended cleaning solutions vary among endoscope manufacturers. Manufacturers have validated products with specific properties for effective cleaning of their devices.[90]

Washing the external surfaces of the endoscope and flushing the internal channels helps moisten, dilute, soften, and remove organic soils.

Suctioning all channels and cleaning the distal end assists with removing gross soil. Alternating cleaning solution with air may be more effective in loosening and removing organic soils. Finishing with air may help prevent excess fluid from remaining in the channels.[13]

Visually inspecting the endoscope after precleaning helps detect obvious damage to the endoscope.

The cleaning solution and cleaning cloth or sponge may support bacterial growth if stored or reused.[45,99]

3.4 When the precleaning process will be delayed (eg, an endoscope is used for intubation and remains in the procedure room for potential reuse), wipe the external surfaces with a soft, lint-free cloth or sponge saturated with utility or sterile water and suction water through the channels.[85] *[Recommendation]*

Wiping the external surfaces and suctioning water through the channels of the endoscope may help prevent organic soils from drying, reducing bacterial adherence and the risk of biofilm formation until precleaning with a cleaning solution can be accomplished.

Microorganisms readily adhere to surfaces and begin forming biofilm.[82] Biofilm that has formed in lumens is difficult to remove. If not removed, biofilm may reduce the efficacy of subsequent disinfection or sterilization.[45]

Shimono et al[100] reported an outbreak of *P aeruginosa* infections that occurred following thoracic surgery in seven patients. The authors determined that one cause of the outbreak was dried organic material in the bronchoscope that occurred when the bronchoscope was reused several times during the surgeries without any cleaning or flushing between uses.

4. Transport to the Processing Area

4.1 After precleaning at the point of use, transport contaminated flexible endoscopes and accessories to the endoscopy processing room. *[Recommendation]*

Low-quality evidence and several clinical practice guidelines support transporting flexible endoscopes from the procedure room to the endoscopy processing room.[12,13,16,17,21,44,84,101]

The benefit of transporting flexible endoscopes to designated decontamination areas is that this may help prevent contamination of procedure rooms and patient care areas and also limits the number of areas where chemicals are used for cleaning and disinfection.[22]

4.2 Transport contaminated flexible endoscopes and accessories to the endoscopy processing room as soon as possible after use. *[Recommendation]*

Transporting the contaminated endoscope as soon as possible facilitates the ability to expeditiously

Figure 5. Biohazard Legend

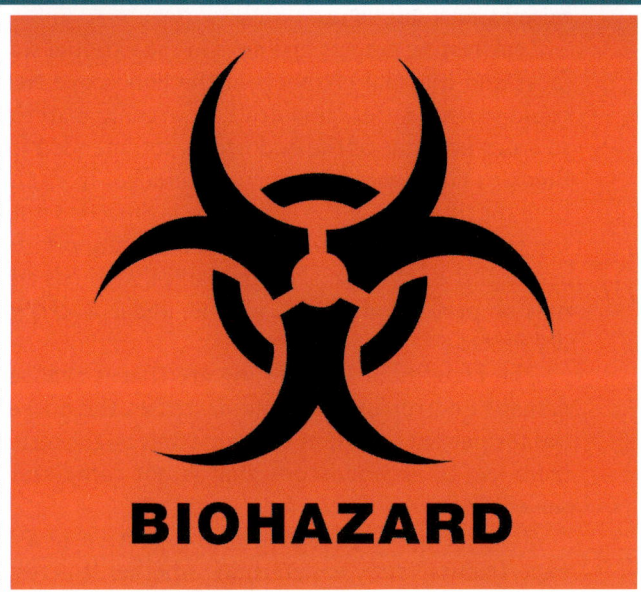

initiate the cleaning process and helps prevent organic material from drying on the surface or in the lumens, which facilitates cleaning.[69,86,87]

4.3 Keep endoscopes and accessories wet or damp but not submerged in liquid during transport. *[Recommendation]*

Keeping the endoscope and accessories wet helps dilute, soften, and ease removal of organic soils. Allowing organic material to dry on the surface and in the channels of the endoscope makes the cleaning process difficult.[15,24,86]

Submerging the endoscope in liquid during transport may increase the risk of spillage and could lead to fluid invasion if the endoscope has an unknown leak.

4.4 Contaminated endoscopes and accessories must be transported to the decontamination area in a closed container or closed transport cart.[48] The container or cart must be

- leak proof,[13,48]
- puncture resistant,[48] and
- large enough to contain all contents.[48,84]

[Regulatory Requirement]

Transporting items in leak-proof, puncture-resistant containers and in a manner that prevents exposing personnel to blood, body fluids, and other potentially infectious materials is a regulatory requirement.[48]

4.4.1 Use a container that is of sufficient size to accommodate the endoscope when the endoscope is coiled in large loops.[12,16] *[Recommendation]*

Using containers of sufficient size to fully contain the endoscope and allow loose coiling helps prevent damage to the endoscope.[16,84,102]

In a nonexperimental study to assess the costs of flexible ureterorenoscopy, Collins et al[103] found there was significant damage to a new ureteroscope that produced a crescent-shaped defect in the field of vision after only 12 procedures. The defect was determined to be the result of coiling the ureteroscope too tightly in the cleaning tray.

4.4.2 The transport cart or container must be labeled with a fluorescent orange or orange-red label containing a **biohazard** legend (Figure 5).[48] Biohazard labels must be securely affixed so as to prevent separation from the contents.[48] *[Regulatory Requirement]*

Labeling containers of biohazardous material is a regulatory requirement[48] and communicates to others that the contents may be biohazardous.

4.4.3 Transport flexible endoscopes in a horizontal position and not suspended.[102] *[Recommendation]*

Fluid may leak from the contaminated endoscope if the endoscope is transported vertically. When suspended, the endoscope may become damaged because of compression on dependent components.[102]

4.4.4 Transport endoscope accessories with the endoscope[13] but in a separate container.[12,101,102] *[Recommendation]*

Keeping the accessories with the endoscope helps prevent them from being lost or misplaced[13] and supports traceability of the endoscope and accessories as a single unit. Placing the accessories in a separate container helps prevent damage to the endoscope and accessories.[12,101,102]

4.5 Process endoscopes and endoscope accessories as soon as possible after transport to the endoscopy processing room or within the manufacturer's recommended time to processing. *[Recommendation]*

Performing processing steps within 1 hour after a procedure may help prevent formation of biofilm.[15,82]

4.5.1 When it is not possible to initiate the cleaning process within the endoscope manufacturer's recommended time to cleaning, follow the manufacturer's IFU for delayed processing.[12,16] *[Recommendation]*

4.5.2 Do not leave flexible endoscopes soaking in enzymatic cleaning solutions beyond the endoscope manufacturer's designated contact time unless this is recommended in the manufacturer's IFU for delayed processing. *[Recommendation]*

Alfa and Howie[104] demonstrated the ability of microorganisms to replicate in enzymatic cleaning solutions when held at room temperature (77° F [25° C]). Soaking endoscopes in enzymatic cleaning solutions beyond the manufacturer's designated contact time may increase the potential for microbial contamination, biofilm formation, ineffective disinfection or sterilization, and moisture damage to the endoscope.[99]

4.5.3 Develop and implement a procedure for recording the times that the procedure is completed and cleaning is initiated. *[Conditional Recommendation]*

A process for recording the times that the procedure ended and cleaning was initiated enables processing personnel to ascertain how long the endoscope has been awaiting processing, to establish priority order, and to determine whether routine processing within the manufacturer's recommended time to cleaning is achievable, and if not, to implement the manufacturer's procedures for delayed processing.

4.6 After each use, mechanically clean transport carts or containers used for flexible endoscopes and thermally disinfect or chemically disinfect them with a compatible Environmental Protection Agency (EPA)-registered hospital-grade disinfectant.[69] *[Recommendation]*

Cleaning and disinfecting transport carts and containers after each use helps prevent cross contamination that could occur if clean items were placed on contaminated transport carts.[69] Disinfectants that are incompatible with the cart or container surface may cause damage to the cart or container and may be ineffective when applied to the incompatible surface.

5. Leak Testing

5.1 Leak test flexible endoscopes that are designed to be leak tested after each use, after any event that may have damaged the endoscope, and before use of a newly purchased, repaired, or loaned endoscope. *[Recommendation]*

Not every endoscope requires leak testing.

Low-quality evidence and several clinical practice guidelines support leak testing as a method to help ensure the endoscope has not been compromised and is safe to use.[1,12,13,15-17,19,21,44,83-85,89,93,105,106]

Leak testing detects openings in the external surfaces and internal channels of the endoscope that could permit water, chemicals, or organic material to enter portions of the endoscope not intended for fluids.[106] These materials may accumulate from the time the integrity of the endoscope is breached until the time the leak is identified. Leak testing may be accomplished by manual or mechanical methods and may be performed using a wet (ie, under water) or dry process.[65]

The benefits of leak testing are that it reduces damage and repair costs and decreases the potential for patient infection or injury that might result from use of an endoscope that is not completely sealed.[85,89,107]

Khan et al[108] conducted a prospective quasi-experimental study to determine whether leak testing flexible ureteroscopes after ureterorenoscopy and laser fragmentation of renal calculi procedures reduced damage and repair costs. The new ureteroscope used for the Group 1 procedures (n = 95) was not leak tested after each procedure. The new ureteroscope used for the Group 2 procedures (n = 98) was leak tested after each procedure. Both groups were comparable for surgeon's years of experience, stone location, size and number of stones, access sheath usage, and duration of lasering. During the study period, October 2010 to March 2011, there were seven repairs costing $46,264.40 in Group 1 ($49,322.39 in 2015 US dollars) and three repairs costing $9,952.80 in Group 2 ($10,610.66 in 2015 US dollars). The researchers concluded that leak testing of flexible ureteroscopes significantly reduced the costs of maintenance and repair by promoting early recognition of damage, allowing for earlier repair, and preventing further use of a damaged ureteroscope.

In an effort to determine the longevity of flexible ureteroscopes used in the urology department of a London hospital, Bultitude et al[101] analyzed data for the number of procedures and repairs required for each of four new ureteroscopes used during 375 procedures. The results showed that on average, each ureteroscope was used 94 times, required two repairs, and was used for 36 procedures between each repair. To extend the life of the ureteroscope and help prevent unnecessary repairs, the authors recommended having dedicated personnel process the endoscopes, transporting endoscopes separately from the rest of the supplies and equipment, and performing a leak test after every procedure in order to detect and repair minor problems before they become major problems.

Leak testing may decrease the risk for an infection transmitted by a flexible endoscope. Ramsey et al[109] reported an outbreak of *Mycobacterium tuberculosis* transmitted from a patient with active tuberculosis to at least two patients via a contaminated bronchoscope. Examination of the bronchoscope revealed a small leak in the external sheath of the bronchoscope tip. The hole had not been discovered previously because leak testing was not routinely performed after bronchoscope use. The hole allowed the *M tuberculosis* from the index case to be delivered directly to the distal airways of subsequent patients.

Cêtre et al[110] identified 117 bronchoalveolar lavage samples contaminated with *Enterobacteriaceae* during three consecutive outbreaks among 418 patients between March 2001 and October 2001 in a 700-bed hospital in France. The source of the contamination was found to be a loose port of the biopsy channel of two of the seven bronchoscopes used in the endoscopy suite. The bronchoscopes were subsequently recalled by the manufacturer due to a potential design flaw. The researchers speculated that leak testing performed after each procedure might have allowed for much earlier detection of the problem.

In a report that illustrates the importance of leak testing in preventing patient injury, Krishna et al[111] described two cases of caustic mucosal injury of the larynx from exposure to glutaraldehyde retained in a damaged endoscope channel. The same laryngoscope was used for both patients. After examination, the laryngoscope was found to have retained glutaraldehyde because of an undetected perforation in the lining of the working channel. Both patients required inpatient admission with airway monitoring, and one patient required admission to the ICU. After treatment with antibiotics and steroids, the patients recovered with no further problems. The authors did not state whether leak testing was included in the processing of the laryngoscope in question; however, they concluded that leak testing was an important and necessary aspect of processing to determine whether the instrument channel had been damaged and to confirm the integrity of the laryngoscope.

5.2 **Perform leak testing before manual cleaning and before the endoscope is placed into cleaning solutions.**[1,12,13,16,84,89] *[Recommendation]*

Performing leak testing before cleaning verifies the integrity of the endoscope and helps prevent damage that might occur during the cleaning process if the endoscope has been compromised.

The addition of cleaning solution to the water used for leak testing may discolor the water or introduce bubbles, limiting the ability of the person performing the leak test to see the entire endoscope or bubbles from the endoscope that indicate leaks.[16,107] Leaks may also go undetected because bubbles from leaks may be assumed to be bubbles from the cleaning solution.[107]

5.3 **Perform leak testing in accordance with the endoscope and leak-testing equipment manufacturers' IFU.**[12,13,15-17,44,85] *[Recommendation]*

There are multiple types of endoscopes and leak-testing equipment. Steps to complete leak testing may vary among manufacturers.

5.3.1 Perform leak testing by
- **removing all port covers and function valves;**
- **pressurizing the endoscope to the recommended pressure**[12,13,16,21,83,84,107]**;**
- **placing the endoscope in a loose configuration**[12,13,16,21,83,107]**;**
- **manipulating all moving parts, including the elevator and angulating the bending section of the distal end**[12,13,16,84,107]**;**
- **actuating video switches; and**
- **maintaining pressure and inspection for a minimum of 30 seconds.**[12]

[Recommendation]

Underpressurizing may allow a leak to go undiscovered; overpressurizing may stress seals and cause damage to the endoscope.[107]

Tight coiling of the endoscope may hide leaks;[12] loose coiling helps remove structural impediments and improves visibility.[107]

Angulating the bending section of the distal end exposes the surfaces to maximum extension and helps reveal leaks.[12,107]

Maintaining pressure and inspection for a minimum of 30 seconds may help reveal small leaks. Evidence for leak testing time is based on expert opinion. The AAMI[12] recommends 30 seconds. Thomas[107] recommended 90 seconds in order to help detect leaks that may not be detected immediately.

5.4 **When an endoscope fails a leak test, remove it from service and have it repaired or replaced (See Recommendation 7.5.1).**[12,13,83-85] *[Recommendation]*

Removing the endoscope from service will prevent further damage to the endoscope[84] and will prevent the damaged endoscope from being used.

6. Manual Cleaning

6.1 **After leak testing and before high-level disinfection or sterilization, manually clean flexible endoscopes.** [*Recommendation*]

Low-quality evidence and clinical practice guidelines indicate that cleaning is the most important step in the processing of flexible endoscopes.[18,22,85,93,112-114] Because of the body cavities they enter, some flexible endoscopes acquire high levels of microbial contamination.[45,112,113] Some flexible endoscopes contain multiple channels and ports that can easily collect organic material.[45,93] The environment in which flexible endoscopes are used provides optimal conditions for contamination and growth of biofilm.[93] When inadequately cleaned, contaminated endoscopes may be vectors of normal bacterial flora as well as pathogenic bacteria.[115,116] When endoscopes are effectively cleaned, bioburden is reduced to a level that does not present a challenge to subsequent disinfection or sterilization.[46,112,114,117]

In a landmark study, Chu et al[113] investigated and compared the bioburden levels on the exterior surfaces of the insertion tube and in the suction channels of colonoscopes immediately after use and after manual cleaning. The colonoscopes were collected from a free-standing endoscopy center and a hospital. Ten colonoscopes were sampled immediately after use, and 10 colonoscopes were sampled immediately after manual cleaning. The results of this randomized controlled trial showed that immediately after use, the level of bioburden on the exterior surfaces of the insertion tubes ranged from 1.2×10^4 to 1.5×10^6 **colony-forming units** (CFU) per device. The level of bioburden in the suction channels ranged from 1.3×10^7 to 2.0×10^{10} CFU per device. After manual cleaning, the level of bioburden on the exterior surfaces of the insertion tube decreased to a range of 8.2×10^2 to 9.5×10^4 CFU per device, establishing that manual cleaning achieved a mean reduction of greater than 1 log. The level of bioburden in the suction channels decreased to a range of 1.3×10^3 to 4.3×10^5 CFU per device, establishing that manual cleaning achieved a mean reduction of 5.5 logs. The 4-log difference can be attributed to the fact that the suction channel is the working channel of the device through which suction occurs and accessories are inserted into the intended locations, so this lumen is exposed to a greater volume of intestinal material.

If endoscopes are not adequately cleaned, the disinfection or sterilization process can fail and increase the possibility for transmission of infectious microorganisms from one patient to another.[112,114,116,117] Some disinfectants are inactivated in the presence of organic material.[1,16]

In a quasi-experimental laboratory study to demonstrate the effectiveness of a high-level disinfectant (ie, orthophalaldehyde), Alfa and Sitter[115] sampled 10 bronchoscopes, 10 gastroscopes, and 10 colonoscopes immediately after use. They found the level of bioburden for the bronchoscopes was 6.4×10^5 CFU/mL^{-1}, the level of bioburden for the gastroscopes was 1.7×10^5 CFU/mL^{-1}, and the level of bioburden for the colonoscopes was 5.2×10^5 CFU/mL^{-1}. The researchers noted that the average load of microorganisms was higher for the gastroscopes than for the bronchoscopes, reflecting the higher number of bacteria in the gastrointestinal tract compared with the respiratory tract, and was likewise higher for the colonoscopes than for the gastroscopes due to the higher concentration of microorganisms in the colon compared with the upper gastrointestinal tract or the bronchi. The endoscopes were cleaned and disinfected, and the residual microbial load was monitored by sampling the suction channels. The researchers found that the cleaning process alone removed up to 10^3 organisms, leaving fewer organisms for the disinfectant to kill. The cleaning and disinfection procedure achieved more than a 5-$\log_{10}$ reduction in bacterial load. The researchers emphasized the need to combine effective cleaning with the high-level disinfectant to ensure maximum efficacy of the disinfectant.

Cleaning is a process that uses friction, cleaning solution, and water to remove organic and inorganic debris to the extent necessary for further processing or for the intended use.[12,58,89,93,112,117] Cleaning removes rather than kills microorganisms. The effectiveness of the cleaning process can vary based on a number of factors including the type of device being cleaned, the design of the device being cleaned, the person performing the cleaning, the amount of time spent cleaning, and the site where the device is cleaned.[112] Routine cleaning procedures may not effectively remove biofilm from endoscope channels. Biofilm remaining in the lumen of an endoscope may prevent effective HLD or sterilization.[92,115]

In a quasi-experimental laboratory study, Pajkos et al[92] assessed 13 biopsy channels and 12 air channels removed from 13 endoscopes that had been sent to an endoscope processing center in Sydney, Australia. The endoscopes were of various ages from 13 different hospitals, and no information was provided to the researchers as to the reason for servicing or how frequently the endoscopes had been used. The researchers used scanning electron microscopy (SEM) to examine the endoscope channels for the presence of biofilm. The SEM showed that biofilm was present on five of the 13 biopsy channels and on all 12 of the air channel samples. In addition, the researchers found surface defects that included cracks, grooves, and pits in many of the channels. The researchers concluded that cleaning had not removed all biofilm from any of the channels, and they noted that the presence of biofilm could lead to failure of the HLD process by inactivating or preventing penetration of the disinfectant.

Alfa and Howie[104] investigated whether the repeated exposure to high levels of microorganisms and the wet and dry conditions that occur during the use and processing of flexible endoscopes could lead to an accumulation of organic material in endoscope channels, and whether this biofilm buildup presented a greater challenge to remove than traditional biofilm that forms when a surface is exposed to microorganisms and continually bathed in fluid. The results of the study showed that the biofilm buildup facilitated high levels of organism survival and reduced the efficacy of the two high-level disinfectants evaluated during the study (ie, glutaraldehyde, accelerated hydrogen peroxide). The researchers theorized that these results provided an explanation for the persistence of residual levels of biofilm remaining in endoscope channels even when the endoscopes were correctly processed. As flexible endoscopes are repeatedly used and processed, the load of bioburden increases, reducing the efficacy of the high-level disinfectant and increasing the risk for pathogen transmission.

The benefits of manual cleaning are that it removes visible soil and reduces the amount of microbial contamination and biofilm formation on and in the endoscope.[16,83,84] If microbial contamination and biofilm are not removed completely, the surface under the bioburden may not be disinfected or sterilized.[16,22,83,84,104,112,114,116] Manual cleaning helps ensure effective HLD or sterilization and may protect patients from exposure to contaminated endoscopes that could result in transmissible infections.[114,118]

6.2 **Perform manual cleaning as soon as possible after leak testing.** *[Recommendation]*

Initiating the cleaning process as soon as possible after leak testing helps prevent the formation of biofilm.[82,83] Biofilm is difficult to remove and may begin to form within minutes after the procedure is completed.[82] If biofilm is present on or in the endoscope, the subsequent HLD or sterilization process may not be effective.[82,95,96]

6.3 **Perform manual cleaning in accordance with the endoscope manufacturer's IFU.** *[Recommendation]*

There are multiple types of endoscopes. Steps to complete cleaning may vary among manufacturers. Adherence to the manufacturer's IFU may minimize the risk for infection.[6]

6.4 **Use the type of water recommended by the endoscope manufacturer for manual cleaning.** *[Recommendation]*

Recommendations for the type of water to be used for manual cleaning may vary among endoscope manufacturers. Utility water is often adequate for precleaning, manual cleaning, and rinsing; however, water quality is affected by the presence of dissolved minerals, solids, chlorides, and other impurities and by its acidity and alkalinity.[119] The **pH** level of the water affects the performance of cleaning solutions.[119] Untreated water quality fluctuates over time, varies with geographic location and season, and can affect the outcome of cleaning actions.[119]

6.5 **Use the cleaning solution recommended by the endoscope manufacturer for manual cleaning.** *[Recommendation]*

There are multiple types of endoscopes. Recommended cleaning solutions may vary among manufacturers. Following the endoscope manufacturer's IFU decreases the possibility of selecting and using cleaning solutions that may damage the endoscope.

The chemical actions of cleaning solutions vary and are intended for different applications. The pH and rinsability of cleaning products also vary. Some cleaning solutions target specific types of bioburden (eg, protein, lipids); others are intended for general purpose cleaning.[90] General purpose cleaners function primarily as **surfactants**.[65,120]

Enzymatic cleaners contain one or a combination of enzymes to help break down organic material and facilitate its removal.[65,90,120,121] Enzymes are specific in terms of the soils they remove. Protease enzymes target proteins.[120,121] Amylase enzymes target carbohydrates, starches, and sugars.[90,120-122] Lipase enzymes break down fats and oils.[90,120-122] Cellulase enzymes break down cellulose.[90] Enzymatic cleaners attempt to remove biofilm by decomposing the extracellular polysaccharides surrounding and protecting the embedded microorganism.[95] Because the diversity of extracellular polysaccharides in the biofilm is unique to the microorganism, a mixture of enzymes may be needed for sufficient degradation of bacterial biofilm.[91]

Enzymatic cleaners are effective at room temperature (ie, 68° F to 72° F [20° C to 22° C]) but function more effectively at warmer temperatures.[19,69,89,120] A temperature that is too hot (ie, ≥ 140° F [≥ 60° C]) denatures proteins and may negate the desired enzymatic activity.[69,120]

Enzymatic cleaners are often recommended for cleaning flexible endoscopes and other medical devices because they help remove proteins, lipids, and carbohydrates by breaking down large molecules into smaller, water-soluble molecules that are easily rinsed away after cleaning[83,122]; however, the collective evidence conflicts regarding the benefits of using enzymatic cleaning solutions compared with nonenzymatic cleaners that may contain disinfectants or other chemicals to enhance cleaning and reduce viable bioburden.[91,95,123] Decontamination is a physical or chemical process that removes or reduces the number of microorganisms or infectious agents and renders reusable medical devices safe for use, handling, or disposal.[12,45,58] Decontamination requires a microbicidal process after cleaning.[12,58] Microbicidal cleaning solutions do not eliminate the need for HLD or sterilization, but they may reduce the risk of exposure to biohazardous substances for processing personnel.[22,120]

In a quasi-experimental laboratory study, Merritt et al[86] evaluated the effects of 12 different cleaning products, including enzymatic and nonenzymatic cleaning solutions, on organisms known to adhere to polystyrene and medical implant materials (ie, *S epidermidis, C albicans, E coli, P aeruginosa*). The results of the study showed that the enzymatic cleaners were effective at cleaning contaminated surfaces and removed all of the microorganisms while the solutions without enzymes were no more effective than utility water.

In a quasi-experimental laboratory study conducted to determine the effectiveness of five enzymatic and nine nonenzymatic cleaners on *E coli* biofilm, Henoun Loukili et al[123] found that of the six products with the highest effectiveness scores (ie, mean percent activity of detergent > 70%), three were enzymatic cleaners and three were nonenzymatic cleaners. The three enzymatic cleaners had the highest scores (ie, 92%, 90%, 89%). The researchers concluded that enzymatic cleaners were not more effective than nonenzymatic cleaners. A major limitation of the study was that the enzymatic solutions were used at room temperature (ie, 68° F to 77° F [20° C to 25° C]), which may not have been in accordance with the manufacturers' recommendations and may have affected overall performance. Another limitation was that the biofilm was prepared on a glass surface that is not representative of the materials used in many medical devices, including flexible endoscopes.

In a study to compare the effectiveness of enzymatic and nonenzymatic cleaners on *E coli* biofilm on the inner surface of gastroscopes, Fang et al[124] randomly and equally assigned 15 Teflon® tubes coated with biofilm to one of three groups:

- Group 1 tubes were treated with a 1-minute wash with water, followed by a 3-minute wash with enzymatic cleaner, followed by a 1-minute wash with water.
- Group 2 tubes were treated with a 1-minute wash with water, followed by a 3-minute wash with nonenzymatic cleaner, followed by a 1-minute wash with water.
- Group 3 tubes were treated with a 1-minute wash with water, followed by a 3-minute wash with sterile distilled water, followed by a 1-minute wash with water.

The researchers found that although none of the cleaning solutions completely eliminated the biofilm, there was a 2.39-$\log_{10}$ CFU per tube reduction of bacterial burden in the nonenzymatic group compared with a 0.23-$\log_{10}$ CFU per tube reduction of bacterial burden in the enzymatic group. The researchers concluded that the nonenzymatic cleaners were more effective than the enzymatic cleaners. A limitation of this study was the use of only one bacterial biofilm. Another limitation was that the enzymatic cleaner was noted to be most effective at a temperature higher than room temperature (ie, 68° F [20° C]), but was used at 59° F (15° C). The researchers believed this temperature was more representative of the temperature at which enzymatic cleaning solutions are often used in actual practice.

In a study to evaluate the effects of various cleaning products and contact times on the removal of biofilm from flexible endoscopes, Ren et al[95] randomly and equally assigned 60 Teflon tubes coated with E coli biofilm to one of four groups:

- Group 1 tubes were treated with enzymatic cleaner 1.
- Group 2 tubes were treated with enzymatic cleaner 2.
- Group 3 tubes were treated with a nonenzymatic cleaner.
- Group 4 tubes were treated with sterile water for injection.

The researchers found a statistically significant difference between the amount of residual biofilm in the enzymatic groups (Group 1 = 4.61 ± 0.52 CFU/cm²; Group 2 = 4.67 ± 0.59 CFU/cm²) compared with the nonenzymatic group (1.29 ± 0.13 CFU/cm²). Both enzymatic and nonenzymatic cleaners demonstrated the ability to remove biofilm; however, the amount of biofilm removal was greater with the nonenzymatic cleaner. A limitation of this study was the use of only one bacterial biofilm, although the researchers noted that *E coli* is a major component of normal intestinal flora and source of bacterial contamination of gastrointestinal endoscopes.[95]

In a quasi-experimental laboratory study, Vickery et al[125] tested the efficacy of four enzymatic cleaning solutions and one nonenzymatic cleaning product on Teflon and polyvinyl chloride tubes coated with *E coli* biofilm. The researchers found that the nonenzymatic cleaner resulted in a 4.7-$\log_{10}$ CFU/cm^2 reduction in biofilm bacteria, while the most effective enzymatic cleaner resulted in only a 1.57-$\log_{10}$ CFU/cm^2 reduction. Notably, the nonenzymatic cleaner used in the study was a quaternary ammonium disinfectant and for this reason would be expected to have a greater bacterial **log reduction** compared with cleaning solutions that are not microbicidal.[126]

Alfa and Jackson[121] conducted a quasi-experimental laboratory study to evaluate the cleaning and bactericidal effectiveness of a hydrogen peroxide-based nonenzymatic cleaner compared with two enzymatic cleaners. Test organisms (*Enterococcus faecalis, Salmonella choleraesuis, Staphylococcus aureus, P aeruginosa*) were suspended in artificial test soil on polyvinyl chloride carriers and then exposed to the cleaning solutions. The nonenzymatic cleaner demonstrated a 5-$\log_{10}$ CFU per carrier reduction in microbial load, even in the presence of a dried organic challenge of *E faecalis* and *S aureus*. The researchers found that none of the enzymatic cleaners achieved this level of log reduction.

Marion et al[127] recommended an approach for removing biofilm that involved the use of detachment-promoting cleaners in endoscope channels and automated washer-disinfectors. The researchers contaminated the operating channel of three new endoscopes with biofilm developed from human serum inoculated with a bacterial culture of *P aeruginosa, S epidermidis, Enterobacter cloacae,* and *K pneumoniae*. One endoscope was left untreated; two endoscopes were treated with different detachment-promoting cleaners. The treated endoscopes underwent a static brushing procedure that involved immersing the endoscope in the selected cleaner and brushing the contaminated operating channel for 1 minute using the manufacturer's recommended cleaning brush, simulating a manual cleaning process. The treated endoscopes also underwent a dynamic flushing procedure that involved the use of a peristaltic pump to circulate the cleaner through the operating channel, simulating a mechanical cleaning process. The researchers examined the internal surfaces of the operating channel using SEM and found that the biofilm was completely removed by the detachment-promoting cleaners.

Perret-Vivancos et al[128] reported the case of a highly contaminated colonoscope that was effectively treated with a combination of biofilm detachment-promoting agents. The treatment included application of a multienzymatic solution designed to digest the foundation where the biofilm was anchored, followed by an enriched detergent solution designed to detach the biofilm as a single unit. After the first treatment, the authors found there was a decrease in the contamination level but the biofilm was not completely eliminated. A second identical treatment was applied and showed a significant reduction in the amount of biofilm. After a third treatment, the biofilm was almost totally removed.

The authors speculated that using these detachment-promoting cleaners could represent an approach to biofilm control that might improve the efficacy of cleaning and reduce the risk of transmitting infections. In addition, these cleaners have the potential to reduce costs by allowing for salvage of endoscopes contaminated with biofilm or as a preventive mechanism to avoid accumulation of biofilm in endoscope channels.[128] Further research is warranted.

6.5.1 **If the manufacturer's recommended cleaning solution is not available, contact the endoscope manufacturer for recommendations for other cleaning solutions that may be used.** [*Recommendation*]

6.5.2 **Use a freshly prepared cleaning solution to perform manual cleaning.**[12,13,15,16,27,69,83,84,89,98] **Change cleaning solutions before they become cloudy or discolored, and before there are visible particulates in the solution.** [*Recommendation*]

Using a freshly prepared solution for each new cleaning process helps prevent cross contamination.[12,13,15,16,27,69,83,84,89,98] Cleaning solutions are not microbicidal and may support bacterial growth if stored or reused beyond their expiration date.[45,65,84,99,129] Repeated use of cleaning solutions decreases the amount of active ingredients in the solution and reduces cleaning efficacy. Residual contaminants in cleaning solutions could increase the potential for cross contamination.[96] Bioburden is deposited in the cleaning solution during the cleaning process. Changing the cleaning solution minimizes bioburden.

In a nonexperimental study to investigate biofilm on endoscope channels, Ren-Pei et al[96] collected 66 endoscope suction and biopsy channels and 13 water and air channels from 66 endoscopy centers in hospitals throughout

China. They used SEM to examine biofilm on the inner surface of the channels. A total of 36 suction and biopsy channels (54.5%) and 10 water and air channels (76.9%) were found to have biofilm.

After examining the endoscope channels, the researchers sent a questionnaire to each of the 66 endoscopy centers to explore the correlation between endoscope processing procedures and the amount of biofilm in the endoscope channels. They divided the responses (N = 66) into hospitals without biofilm on endoscopes (Group A; n = 30), and hospitals with biofilm on endoscopes (Group B; n = 36). The researchers found that the proportion of reuse of enzymatic cleaning solutions in Group A was 60% (18 of 30), whereas in Group B the proportion was 91.6% (33 of 36) and in some cases, the cleaning solution was reused more than four times. The researchers concluded that the formation of biofilm on the endoscope channels could be related to reuse of cleaning solutions.[96]

6.5.3 **Do not add products to the cleaning solution unless this is recommended by the manufacturer.** [Recommendation]

Adding products that are not recommended by the manufacturer could cause a chemical reaction that could damage the endoscope or render the cleaning solution ineffective.[83]

6.5.4 **Follow the cleaning solution manufacturer's IFU for**
- **water quality, hardness, and pH**[58,119];
- **concentration and dilution**[19,20,58,65,83,98];
- **water temperature**[20,58,83,120];
- **contact time**[16,58,65,83,84,98,120];
- **conditions of storage**[58]; and
- **use life** and **shelf life**.[58,69,98]

[Recommendation]

Deviations from the manufacturer's IFU may render the cleaning product ineffective.[129]

Water quality, including hardness, and pH can alter the effectiveness of cleaning solutions.[25,90,119] The enzymes used in enzymatic cleaners may be most effective at a neutral pH and may be inactivated by a high or low pH.[98]

Using the product in the concentration recommended by the manufacturer helps ensure consistent and accurate cleaning chemistry.[77] A weak solution may not effectively break down proteins and other organic material; a strong solution may produce an increased number of bubbles, creating air pockets that prohibit surface contact of the cleaning chemical with the endoscope.[122,129] Undiluted or under-diluted

enzymatic cleaning solutions are difficult to remove and may lead to residual cleaning solutions and proteinaceous material in the endoscope that provide a foundation for biofilm formation and lead to processing failures.

If the water temperature is not warm enough, the cleaning product may not mix with the water as intended,[122,129] and the enzymes may not be able to effectively dissolve and remove organic soil.[25] If the temperature is too hot, it may cause coagulation of proteins and fix proteinaceous soil to the endoscope.[25]

Contact of the cleaning solution with all surfaces of the endoscope for the minimum contact time is necessary for effective cleaning.[16,120,121]

Enzymes used in enzymatic cleaners can lose their effectiveness over time.[83,90,98] The cleaning solution may be ineffective if used beyond the defined period of useful life or the expiration date.

Hutchisson and LeBlanc[98] conducted a quasi-experimental study to demonstrate the need to follow the manufacturer's IFU when using enzymatic cleaning solutions. The researchers tested five colonoscopes used during procedures at a Texas hospital after precleaning at the point of use, and then manually cleaned them using a low-sudsing enzymatic cleaner in the following formulations:
- Endoscope 1: 1 oz of low-sudsing enzymatic cleaner in 1 gallon of water followed by a water rinse.
- Endoscope 2: 2 oz of low-sudsing enzymatic cleaner in 1 gallon of water followed by a water rinse.
- Endoscope 3: 4 oz of low-sudsing enzymatic cleaner in 1 gallon of water followed by a water rinse.
- Endoscope 4: 1 oz of low-sudsing enzymatic cleaner in 1 gallon of water with no rinse.
- Endoscope 5: undiluted low-sudsing enzymatic cleaner followed by a water rinse.

The manufacturer's IFU called for 1 oz of enzymatic cleaner in 1 gallon of water.

After manual cleaning, the colonoscopes were mechanically processed, rinsed, and disinfected with orthophalaldehyde. They were hung vertically to dry without an alcohol flush. An absorbent white cloth was placed on the floor of the endoscope cabinet to catch effluent dripping from the distal tips of the endoscopes. Orthophalaldehyde reacts with residual bioburden to form dark stains. The researchers observed no staining of proteinaceous material with Endoscope 1 that had been cleaned with correctly diluted cleaning solution followed by a water rinse. The researchers observed some staining with Endoscope 4 that had been cleaned with correctly diluted cleaning solution but not rinsed. They observed significant staining with Endoscopes 2, 3, and 5 that were cleaned with underdiluted and nondiluted cleaning solution and then rinsed.[98]

The results of the study demonstrated that when endoscopes were cleaned using incorrect dilutions of cleaning solutions, small amounts of residual proteinaceous material were left on the interior and exterior surfaces of the endoscope. There could be a buildup of this residual material over time, which raises concerns about cleaning effectiveness as well as the potential negative effect of residual buildup on the optimal functioning and life of the endoscope.[98]

6.5.5 **An automated titration unit may be used to concentrate cleaning products at a consistent ratio.**[58] *[Conditional Recommendation]*

The concentration of the solution can vary when it is mixed manually. Using a titration unit can aid in accurate measurement of the chemical during preparation of the cleaning solution and help personnel to consistently obtain the recommended concentration of the cleaning product.[58]

6.5.6 **Change cleaning solutions when the temperature of the solution does not meet the temperature specified in the manufacturer's IFU.**[77] *[Recommendation]*

Cleaning solutions may not be effective when used at temperatures outside of the manufacturer-specified parameters.

6.5.7 **A digital temperature measuring device may be used to monitor the temperature of the cleaning solution.** *[Conditional Recommendation]*

6.6 **Completely submerge the endoscope in the cleaning solution during the cleaning process.**[12,13,16,20,22,65,84,85,89] **Detach removable parts (eg, valves, buttons, caps) from the endoscope and submerge if recommended by the endoscope manufacturer's IFU.**[85] *[Recommendation]*

Cleaning the endoscope under the surface of the solution helps prevent splashing of the contaminated solution and reduces the potential for aerosolization and exposure to biohazardous substances.[16] Detaching removable parts and completely submerging the endoscope and removable parts helps ensure contact between the cleaning solution and all surfaces of the endoscope.[65]

Figure 6. Anatomy of an Endoscope

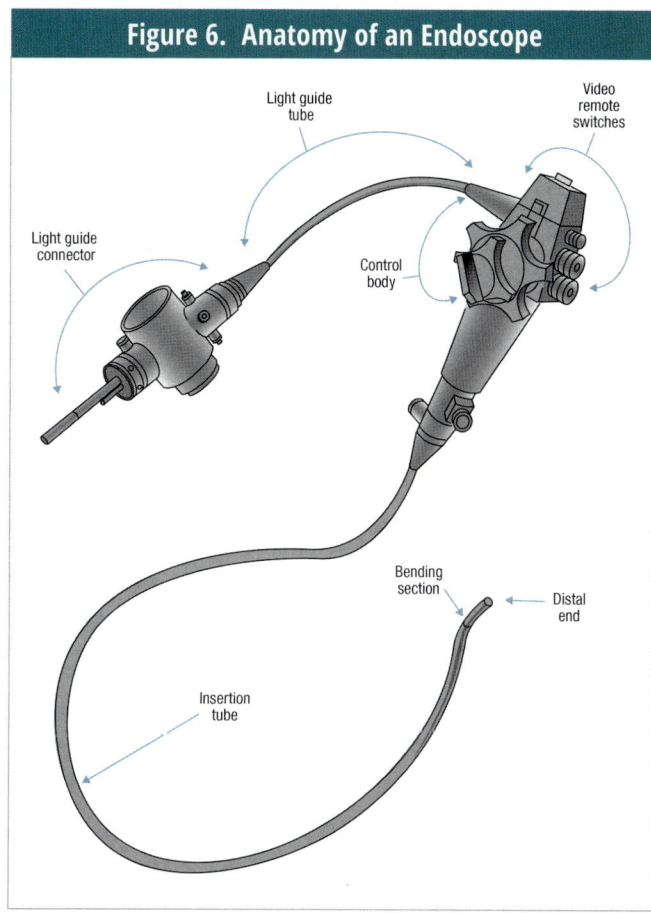

6.7 **Clean all exterior surfaces of the endoscope (Figure 6) with a soft, lint-free cloth or sponge saturated with the cleaning solution.**[1,12,13,15,16,18,19,22,27,65,83,84,89,105] *[Recommendation]*

Washing the external surfaces of the endoscope helps remove organic material that remains after precleaning.

6.8 **Clean all accessible channels and the distal end of the endoscope with a cleaning brush of the length, width, and material recommended by the endoscope manufacturer.**[1,13,15,18,19,22,45,65,83,85,89,105,129] **Manually actuate the endoscope valves while cleaning.**[12,19,22] *[Recommendation]*

Clinical practice guidelines recommend thorough and careful brushing of the accessible endoscope channels **(Figure 7)** with a correctly-sized brush as a method of dislodging and removing organic material and biofilm.[1,18,45] Cleaning the distal end helps ensure there is no debris or tissue lodged in or around the water nozzle and suction biopsy channel.[85] The presence and buildup of organic material in the lumens of endoscopes can have significant implications, including toxic reactions, device damage, inadequate disinfection or sterilization, increased risk of biofilm development, and the potential transmission of infection.[130,131]

Figure 7. Endoscope Channels

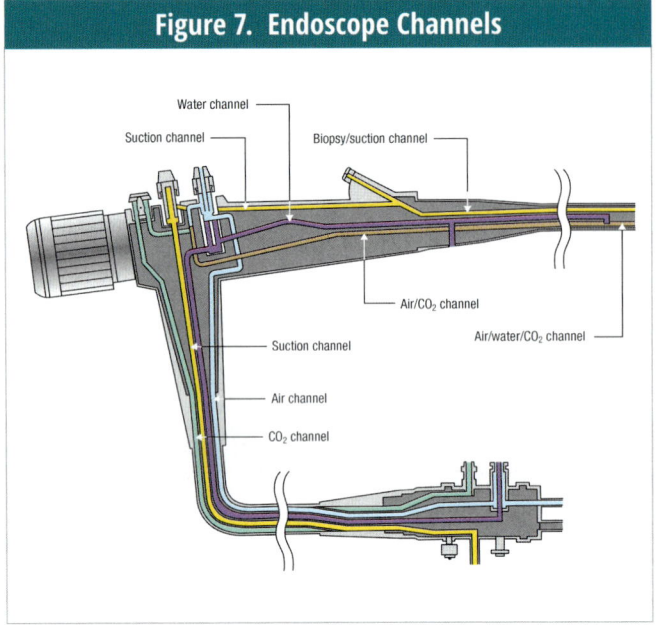

Figure 7. Endoscope Channels

Using the correct-size brush increases contact between the brush and the walls of the endoscope channels and maximizes the amount of soil removed.[19,129] If the brush is too small, it will not make contact with the organic material or channel walls.[129] If the brush is too large, it may get lodged in the channel and cause damage to the internal channels, or the bristles may be deflected upward, only swiping the sides of the channel and not effectively removing organic material or contacting the channel walls.[129] Some endoscopes will require the use of two different brush sizes for effective cleaning.[129]

Manually actuating the valves during cleaning helps ensure brushing of all internal parts.[12,19]

Pineau and De Philippe[132] assessed 206 samples from flexible endoscopes (ie, 87 colonoscopes, 93 gastroscopes, 26 bronchoscopes) from four different hospitals in France for levels of bioburden. In this nonexperimental study, the researchers compared samples that had been collected

- after point-of-use precleaning (n = 30);
- after point-of-use precleaning and manual brushing of channels (n = 34);
- after point-of-use precleaning, manual brushing of channels, and double washing and rinsing in a mechanical processor (n = 111); and
- after point-of-use precleaning, manual brushing of channels, double washing and rinsing in a mechanical processor, and HLD in a mechanical processor (n = 31).

The researchers found that brushing significantly reduced the contamination present in the endoscope channels after point-of-use precleaning. Brushing endoscope channels reduced the number of viable bacteria by at least 2.5-$\log_{10}$/cm². The researchers concluded that brushing was important for reducing contamination remaining in endoscopes after point-of-use precleaning.

In a quasi-experimental laboratory study, Dietze et al[133] investigated the influence of design on the efficacy of manual cleaning of endoscope channels. The researchers tested two duodenoscopes and two gastroscopes. The air channels of one duodenoscope (A) and one gastroscope (B) were freely accessible and able to be flushed and brushed. The air channels of the other duodenoscope (C) and the other gastroscope (D) were only able to be flushed. The researchers contaminated the air channels of all four endoscopes with blood containing *Enterococcus faecium* as a test organism. They implemented manual cleaning by flushing and brushing for endoscopes A and B and flushing only for endoscopes C and D and then calculated the recovery rates.

The researchers found that the rate of microorganisms recovered after flushing alone was between 4.8×10^5 CFU/180 mL and 5.8×10^5 CFU/180 mL. The rate of microorganisms recovered after flushing and brushing was between 1.6×10^7 CFU/180 mL and 2.3×10^7 CFU/180 mL. This indicated that the cleaning rate for flushing alone was only 2.6% of the cleaning rate obtained by flushing and brushing.[133]

In a quasi-experimental study, Ishino et al[134] alternately assigned endoscopes used for upper gastrointestinal examinations into Group A (n = 20), where the air and water channels were brushed three times with a sterile, correctly sized brush, and Group B (n = 22), where the air and water channels were not brushed. The researchers examined the endoscope channels using a protein-staining dye and found no residual protein in the air channels of either Group A or Group B endoscopes. The water channels of the Group A endoscopes also had no residual protein; however, one water channel from the Group B endoscopes did have residual protein. The researchers concluded that the proteinaceous material remaining in the water channel of the non-brushed endoscope was likely organic debris, and unless removed by brushing, this material could become fixed on the inner surface of the endoscope channels and become a potential source of infection.

Bajolet et al[118] reported transmission of an extended-spectrum β-lactamase-producing *P aeruginosa* in four patients who underwent esophagogastroduodenoscopy (EGD) procedures with the same gastroscope between May 2011 and August 2011. The gastroscope had been purchased in January 2011. Microbiological sampling before its first use showed negative results. Observation of the endoscope processing procedures during the investigation identified cleaning failures that included inadequate brushing and flushing of the channels and the use of a single-diameter cleaning brush for all gastrointestinal endoscopes. The investigators concluded that the lack of sufficient cleaning and the use of an incorrectly sized brush may have supported the development of a persistent biofilm that contributed to patient-to-patient transmission of a serious infection.

Agerton et al[135] reported a case of transmission of multidrug-resistant *M tuberculosis* (MDR-TB) caused by a contaminated bronchoscope. Five patients from a South Carolina community who were family members or close friends were diagnosed with tuberculosis. Three additional patients were hospitalized in the same facility as one of the five patients diagnosed with tuberculosis. These three patients had bronchoscopy procedures performed with the same bronchoscope in the same hospital within 17 days of the tuberculosis patient. As a result of the contaminated bronchoscope, two patients had false-positive MDR-TB cultures from specimens obtained during their bronchoscopy procedures, and one patient developed and died from MDR-TB. A review of the processing procedures for bronchoscopes revealed that leak-testing equipment was available but never used, manual cleaning time averaged less than 3 minutes, and a cleaning brush was passed through the endoscope only one time.

6.8.1 **Clean and brush the elevator mechanism and the recesses surrounding it with a cleaning brush of the length, width, and material recommended by the endoscope manufacturer.**[1,6,13,15,22,45,65,83,85,89,129] **Raise and lower the elevator throughout the manual cleaning process.**[6,85] *[Recommendation]*

Some duodenoscopes have a movable elevator channel at the distal end **(Figure 8)** that allows the accessory instrument to access the pancreatic and biliary ducts.[6] The complex design of the duodenoscope improves the efficiency and effectiveness of ERCP procedures; however, some parts of the endoscope may be extremely difficult to access, and this creates challenges for cleaning.[6] In fact, effective cleaning of all areas of the duodenoscope may not be possible.[6] The moving parts of the elevator mechanisms contain microscopic crevices that may not be reachable with a brush.[6] Residual body fluids and organic material may remain in these crevices after cleaning and disinfection.[6] If this fluid or material contains microbial contamination, subsequent patients may be exposed to serious infections.[6,136,137] Although the risk of infection transmission associated with these complex devices cannot

Figure 8. Distal End of Flexible Endoscope and Duodenoscope

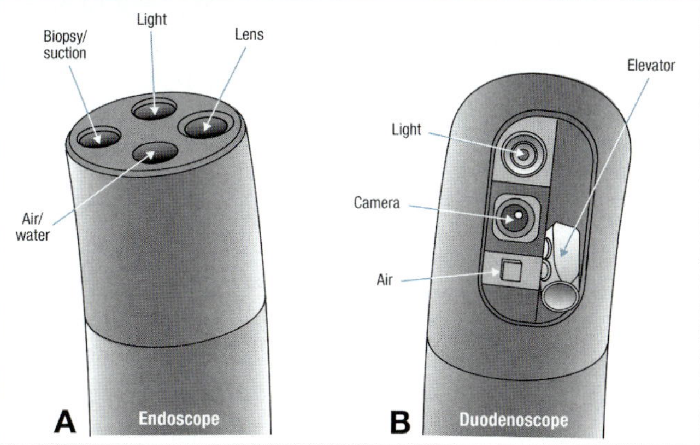

A — Endoscope

B — Duodenoscope

be completely eliminated, the benefits of treatment outweigh the risks in appropriately selected patients.[138]

Raising and lowering the elevator during the cleaning process helps ensure that no organic material is lodged in the moveable mechanism and allows for more effective brushing of all surfaces, including the base of the elevator apparatus.[6,85,139]

Alrabaa et al[136] reported seven cases of carbapenemase-producing *K pneumoniae* in patients from two tertiary hospitals in South Florida between June 2008 and January 2009. All seven patients had ERCP procedures at the same outpatient endoscopy center within 60 days before the outbreak. Six patients had undergone procedures with a common endoscope.[140] The endoscope was examined and found to have residual organic material under the elevator that cultured positive for carbapenemase-producing *E coli*, *Pseudomonas*, and *Serratia* species.[140] The investigators observed processing procedures at the endoscopy center and found the cleaning procedure for the duodenoscopes was inadequate. The manufacturer's IFU that required cleaning with a brush the complex terminal part of the endoscope that contains the elevator were not followed, and bioburden remained under the elevator of the endoscope after the cleaning process was completed. The investigators concluded that processing duodenoscopes was more complex than processing traditional endoscopes, and additional steps were required to ensure effective decontamination.[140]

The CDC[141] reported an outbreak of New Delhi metallo-β-lactamase-1 (NDM-1)-producing *E coli* involving 28 colonized and 10 infected patients. All 38 patients were exposed while undergoing

ERCP in a Chicago hospital between January 2013 and September 2013. After manual cleaning and mechanical processing, the terminal section of a side-viewing duodenoscope used for five of the case patients remained culture-positive for NDM-1-producing *E coli* and carbapenemase-producing *K pneumoniae,* despite no obvious lapses in protocol. Although cultured from the same endoscope, no colonization or infections were identified from this second strain of carbapenem-resistant *Enterobacteriaceae.* The CDC observed that the design of ERCP endoscopes makes them particularly challenging to clean and disinfect. In an independent inspection of the hospital's procedures, the Centers for Medicare & Medicaid Services reported that the hospital was using unapproved cleaning solutions and brushes and failed to process the endoscopes as recommended by the manufacturer.[142,143]

Wendorf et al[137] described an outbreak of AmpC-producing *E coli* at a medical center in Seattle between November 2012 and August 2013. Thirty-two patients who had undergone ERCP procedures were found to harbor one of two genetically similar strains of the organism.[144,145] The investigators found no violations of the recommended processing procedures. During the investigation, the endoscope manufacturer observed personnel manually cleaning and inspecting the endoscopes and concluded that the cleaning process was not only consistent with manufacturer guidelines, it was above the industry standard. Even after implementing procedures that included enhanced manual cleaning, the investigators found that gastrointestinal bacteria continued to be recovered from the endoscope elevator channels.[137]

Nine endoscopes, which included the eight endoscopes in use during the outbreak plus an additional endoscope, were evaluated by the manufacturer. The manufacturer found that all of the endoscopes (whether in need of repair or not) harbored pathogenic bacteria in the elevator channel and continued to have positive cultures even after repair. Notably, three of the endoscopes had passed leak tests at the hospital but failed the manufacturer's leak test, and seven endoscopes were determined to have at least one critical defect. The investigators concluded that obscure mechanical defects in combination with the difficulty of cleaning the elevator channel facilitated the transmission of the infection.

Kola et al[146] reported an outbreak of carbapenemase-resistant *K pneumoniae* (CRKP)

associated with a contaminated duodenoscope in a German university hospital. Between December 2012 and January 2013, CRKP was cultured from 12 patients staying on four different wards. Molecular typing confirmed the close relation between all 12 isolates. Six of the patients were from the same ward; they were immediately transferred to separate rooms and placed on contact precautions. The remaining six patients had all undergone ERCP procedures with the same duodenoscope. Culturing the duodenoscope did not recover CRKP.

The investigators reviewed processing procedures for the duodenoscope and could not find deviations from the manufacturer's IFU; however, they did obtain positive cultures for *Enterococci,* which they suggested was indicative of insufficient cleaning. The duodenoscope was sent to the manufacturer who found a defective distal cap. The outbreak ended when the duodenoscope was removed from service. The investigators concluded that the processing procedures may not have been sufficient in every case because of the complex physical design of the distal end of the duodenoscope.[146]

Verfaillie et al[147] reported a large outbreak of Verona integron-encoded metallo-β-lactamase (VIM)-2-producing *P aeruginosa* linked to the use of a duodenoscope with a sealed elevator channel intended to obviate the need for special cleaning measures. Between January 2012 and April 2012, 30 patients were identified with a VIM-2-positive *P aeruginosa;* 22 of these patients had undergone ERCP with the same duodenoscope. The investigators confirmed that the strain in all 22 cases was identical to the strain that was cultured from the recess under the forceps elevator of the duodenoscope. Dismantling the distal end of the duodenoscope revealed that the sealed elevator channel design may have hampered effective cleaning. The outbreak resolved when the endoscope was withdrawn from clinical use.

6.8.2 **Use a clean brush for each endoscope cleaning. Visually inspect brushes and other items used to clean endoscope channels before use; if the integrity of the brush or other cleaning item is in question, do not use it.[89]** *[Recommendation]*

Using a clean brush for each cleaning of the endoscope helps prevent cross contamination. Verifying the brush is intact and safe to use (ie, the protective tip is present, the coiling is braided, all bristles are present, the delivery tube is not kinked) assists with effective cleaning and helps prevent damage to the endoscope.[129]

Behnia et al[148] reported a pseudo-outbreak of and *Acinetobacter baumannii* in six patients in a community hospital in Augusta, Georgia. The source was traced to a contaminated bronchoscope that had been used in two ICUs at the same hospital. The investigators reviewed the processing procedures for the bronchoscope and found that brushes intended for single-use were being shared between several different bronchoscopes and were not discarded after each use.

6.8.3 **Brush the accessible channels of the endoscope multiple times until no debris appears on the brush.**[12,13,15,16,20,21,27,45,65,83,85,89] **Remove debris from the brush before the brush is retracted back through the channel and after each pass by swirling the brush in the cleaning solution and rinsing it.**[13,15,16,65,83,85,89] *[Recommendation]*

Cleaning and rinsing the cleaning brush after each pass removes visible debris and helps prevent it from being redeposited in the endoscope channel.[12,13]

6.8.4 **New technologies for brush design and lumen cleaning may be used when compatible with the endoscope.** *[Conditional Recommendation]*

There is discussion in the literature regarding the need for enhanced brush design to improve cleaning efficacy, decrease brushing time and effort, and reduce the potential for exposure of processing personnel to biohazardous material.

In a quasi-experimental laboratory study to evaluate protein deposits and removal in the channels of flexible endoscopes, Hervé and Keevil[130] took 8-inch (20-cm) sections of new endoscope biopsy and air and water channels and contaminated them with artificial test soil. An enzymatic cleaner and single-use endoscope brushes were used to clean the soiled channel sections by inserting the brush head at one end of the channel section and pushing it out the other end. This brushing maneuver was repeated several times. The channel sections were then flushed with deionized water and purged with air. After cleaning, dye was injected into the lumen, which was then rinsed with deionized water and purged with air. The channel sections were examined with an episcopic differential contrast/epifluorescence microscope.

The researchers found that brushing the channels did not remove proteinaceous residues because endoscope channels **adsorb** pro-

teins as a thin film on the internal surfaces. Brushing did have some beneficial effect; however, brushing also appeared to increase microcontamination. The researchers suggested that because **prions** represent the proteinaceous contamination most resistant to decontamination, this inability to completely remove proteinaceous contamination could be problematic in countries with a population at risk for **variant Creutzfeldt-Jakob disease** (vCJD); however, the risk of transmission was unclear. They posited that the cleaning outcome could be improved with better brush design.[130]

New technologies for brush design and lumen cleaning may be more effective and less damaging to the internal lumens of flexible endoscopes. Charlton[149] compared the cleaning efficacy of a lumen-cleaning device to three lumen-cleaning brushes (ie, triple-headed brush, single-use brush, reusable brush). The lumen-cleaning device had elastomer discs designed to make contact with the internal walls of the endoscope channels and wipe soil from the surface as it is pulled through the channel. In this nonexperimental laboratory study, the researchers applied simulated blood soil to the lumens of two different-sized endoscope channels (ie, 2.8 mm, 5.0 mm) that had been removed from used endoscopes during servicing. The lumen-cleaning device was passed through the soiled lumens one time. The lumen-cleaning brushes were pushed down and then pulled up through the lumen three times. The researchers found there was very little residual soil in the lumen cleaned with the lumen-cleaning device and substantial quantities of soil in the lumens cleaned with the lumen-cleaning brushes. The lumen-cleaning device removed significantly more soil (92%) compared with the lumen-cleaning brushes (52% to 65%).

The researchers noted that multiple passes with a brush was more time-consuming than a single pass with the lumen-cleaning device. They suggested that the lumen-cleaning device was safer to use than a brush because the lumen-cleaning device emerged only once from the contaminated channel compared with the cleaning motion for brushing that requires the brush to emerge multiple times from the contaminated channel. As the tip of the brush emerges from the lumen, the bristles have the potential to flick soil into the environment, onto other parts of the endoscope, or onto other instruments, increasing the risk for cross contamination and the potential for biohazardous spray and splatter. Brushes may also increase the formation of biofilm by causing surface abrasion or grooves in the channel wall. Notably, this study was funded by the manufacturer of the lumen-cleaning device.[149]

Charlton[150] conducted a second nonexperimental study in a clinical setting to compare the lumen-cleaning device used in the previous laboratory study to reusable lumen-cleaning brushes. The study was completed during a four-day period in an endoscopy clinic of a major hospital in Sydney, Australia. Immediately after the endoscope was removed from the patient, a sterile saline solution was flushed down the biopsy channel of the endoscope and submitted for microbiological sampling. The endoscope was cleaned using either one pass of the lumen-cleaning device (n = 26), or three passes (ie, pushed down and then pulled up through the lumen) of the reusable cleaning brush (n = 27), and a second microbiological sample was submitted.

The researchers found no significant difference between the effectiveness of the lumen-cleaning device compared with the reusable lumen-cleaning brushes. The lumen-cleaning devices reduced CFU by $3.302\text{-log}_{10}/\text{cm}^2$. The reusable lumen-cleaning brushes reduced CFU by $3.003\text{-log}_{10}/\text{cm}^2$. The researchers concluded that one pass of the lumen-cleaning device was as effective as three passes of the reusable lumen-cleaning brushes. Notably, this study was funded by the manufacturer of the lumen-cleaning device.[150]

A report of a study prepared by Highpower Validation Testing & Lab Services[151] detailed the methods used to evaluate and compare the cleaning efficacy of a unique microfiber endoscopic channel brush and the endoscope manufacturer's recommended cleaning brush. The researchers extracted the endoscope cleaning channels, inoculated them with artificial test soil containing blood and protein, allowed the soil to dry for 24 hours, and compared the effectiveness of the brushes in removing the soil. The results showed that the microfiber channel brush removed 99.98% of the soil (ie, a 4-log reduction). The manufacturer's recommended cleaning brush removed 93.35% of the soil (ie, a 1.2-log reduction). Notably, this study was funded by the manufacturer of the microfiber endoscopic channel brush. Further research is warranted.

6.9 **Flush the channels of the endoscope with cleaning solution.**[12,15-17,19-21,27,89] **A cleaning adapter or auto-**

matic flushing system may be used when compatible with the endoscope.[12] *[Recommendation]*

Flushing all internal channels helps dislodge and remove organic material and biofilm and exposes these surfaces to the cleaning solution.[27] Cleaning adapters and automatic flushing systems facilitates opening of the ports and cleaning of the channels.[1]

6.10 **Flush the exterior surfaces and internal channels of the endoscope and rinse them with utility water until all cleaning solution and residual debris is removed.**[12,13,15-17,20,27,83-85,89] *[Recommendation]*

Thorough flushing of the channels and rinsing of the endoscope with utility water helps remove residual debris and cleaning solutions and prevents dilution of the high-level disinfectant or liquid chemical sterilant.[13,16,65,89,90] If not adequately rinsed, enzymatic cleaning solutions may contribute to protein buildup within the endoscope channels.[131]

6.11 **Dry the exterior surfaces of the endoscope with a soft, lint-free cloth or sponge and purge all channels with instrument air.**[12,13,15,16,84,89] *[Recommendation]*

Moisture remaining on the surface or in the endoscope lumens may dilute the high-level disinfectant or interfere with the sterilization process, potentially reducing its effectiveness.[13,16,84] Hydrogen peroxide vapor and hydrogen peroxide gas plasma sterilization cycles may abort in the presence of excess moisture.[40] Ethylene oxide combines with water to form ethylene glycol (ie, antifreeze), which is toxic and not removed during aeration.[41]

6.12 **Clean, brush, rinse, and high-level disinfect or sterilize reusable parts (eg, valves, buttons, port covers, tubing, water bottles), accessories (eg, forceps), and cleaning implements (eg, brushes, channel cleaning adapters).**[1,12,13,17-21,27,44,83,89,152,153] *[Recommendation]*

Effective processing of reusable endoscope parts and accessories is necessary for safe and successful treatment of patients.[120,152,154] Reusable brushes that are not decontaminated can cause contaminants to be transferred from one device to another.[58]

The FDA[155] has received reports that, in the absence of a valve to prevent backflow, patient fluids such as blood and stool can travel through the auxiliary water channel and into the water inlet and irrigation system; however, there have been no reports of infection directly attributed to backflow. The FDA recommends that the following be processed or replaced after each patient use:
- any device directly connected to the auxiliary water inlet (up to and including the distal valve in the fluid pathway),[155]

- the one-way valve in the auxiliary water channel of an endoscope with an internal one-way valve,[155] and

- any device directly connected to the biopsy channel (up to and including the distal one-way valve in the fluid path).[155]

The Department of Veterans Affairs[156] reported an incident involving a patient who underwent a colonoscopy procedure. During the procedure, the endoscopy team noticed blood in the tubing of the auxiliary water system used for irrigation during procedures. The equipment was taken out of service and an investigation was initiated. The investigators found that a required one-way valve had not been used during the procedure, the tubings had been incorrectly connected, and the tubings were not being disinfected or discarded according to the manufacturer's IFU. Notably, both connectors were the same color and roughly the same size and shape. The investigators were unable to determine when or why the switch occurred. Likewise, they were unable to determine how long the required one-way valve had not been in use.

6.12.1 | **High-level disinfect or sterilize water and irrigation bottles at least daily.**[22,44,45,93,153] **There should be no residual water or moisture remaining in the water-bottle assembly.**[153,157] *[Recommendation]*

Water bottles consist of the water container, cap, and tubing used for insufflation of air and lens washing.[153] Irrigation bottles consist of the water container, tubing, and accessories used to flush water through the endoscope.[153]

Water and irrigation bottles can be a source of endoscope contamination[22]; however, the optimal frequency for replacing, disinfecting, or sterilizing them has not been established and warrants further research.[44] Residual water remaining in the water-bottle assembly may support bacterial growth.

6.12.2 | **Use sterile water to fill water and irrigation bottles.**[1,22,44,45,93,153] *[Recommendation]*

The collective evidence conflicts regarding the need for sterile water in the water and irrigation bottles, and further research is warranted. The American Society for Gastrointestinal Endoscopy (ASGE) recommends using utility water in irrigation bottles because the rates of bacterial contamination are similar with the use of utility water and sterile water and neither has been associated with clinical infections.[30] This conflicts with the recommendation for using sterile water provided in the "Multisociety guideline on processing flexible gastrointestinal endoscopes."[44] Using sterile water is also recommended by some professional organizations to help prevent contamination from organisms in utility water[1,22,44,45,153]; however, there is a small amount of evidence that indicates this may not be necessary.[158-160]

In a two-phase quasi-experimental study to determine whether the endoscope water source holds potential for transmission of infection, Puterbaugh et al[158] compared utility water in clean water bottles (Phase 1; n = 303) with sterile water in sterile water bottles (Phase 2; n = 106). The researchers took cultures of the water in the bottles before starting and after completing the day's procedures. The researchers found that 29 (9.6%) of the samples from Phase 1 were positive for normal flora found in city water. Four of the samples from Phase 2 (3.8%) were positive for similar bacteria. They concluded that the use of utility water in clean water bottles carried no greater risk than using sterile water in sterile water bottles.

Wilcox et al[159] conducted a quasi-experimental study in a university teaching hospital to determine whether there was a need for sterile water in the water bottles used during endoscopy procedures. During a 12-week period, the water bottles were sterilized weekly and then filled with either sterile or utility water. At the end of each week, the remaining water in the bottles was cultured. During the study period, 437 procedures were performed and 36 cultures were submitted. Nine of the cultures were positive, including three cultures from bottles where sterile water had been used. The bacterial isolates included *Flavobacterium* species (n = 5), *Acinetobacter* species (n = 4), *Pseudomonas* species (n = 2), and *Stenotrophomonas maltophilia* (n = 1). Colony counts ranged from 900/mL to more than 10,000/mL. No patient developed infections from any of the organisms recovered. The researchers concluded that the use of utility water compared with sterile water may be reasonable and may also reduce costs.

In response to this study, Patton et al[161] countered that utility water contains minerals that can leave deposits on flexible endoscopes and in the channels of the endoscope. The mineral deposits could lead to a costly repair or a need to replace the endoscope. The author estimated repair costs at $1,000 to $5,500 ($1,470.59 to $8,088.24 in 2015 US dollars) and noted that the cost of a 1,000 mL bottle of sterile water was $2.38 ($3.50 in 2015 US dollars); therefore, several cases of sterile water were less expensive than a single repair. The author concluded that using sterile water would not only decrease the risk of transmission of pathogenic organisms, it would also decrease the need for repair or replacement of the endoscope.

In an expert opinion piece, Rockey[160] debated the need for sterile water in water bottles, stating there was no evidence to support the concern that using utility water could damage the endoscope and contending that it would take years for mineral deposits to form. If mineral deposits were to form on the internal channels of the endoscope, they would likely be washed away by the force of the fluid flushed through the channels during mechanical processing. The author further stated that using sterile water is necessary when entering sterile body cavities, but should not be necessary when entering portions of the gastrointestinal tract that are not sterile since utility water is acceptable for drinking. Likewise, utility water is used in other body systems without complication (eg, oxygen humidification).

6.12.3 **Process insulated electrosurgical devices used during endoscopic procedures in accordance with the AORN Guideline for Cleaning and Care of Surgical Instruments[58] and handle them in accordance with the AORN Guideline for Electrosurgery.[162]** *[Recommendation]*

6.13 **Single-use parts, accessories, and cleaning implements may be used when compatible with the endoscope.** *[Conditional Recommendation]*

The intricate design and configuration of certain components and accessories used with flexible endoscopes represent a significant challenge to cleaning.[154] Using single-use products may be helpful in reducing the risk of cross contamination from reusable products.[18,27,120] Using single-use brushes may help ensure that a clean brush is used each time.[58]

Parente[154] conducted a nonexperimental study to evaluate the difficulty with manual cleaning and disinfection of endoscopic biopsy port valves. The researchers collected 15 reusable biopsy port valves from three endoscopy centers across the United States. The valves had been reprocessed and were deemed to be clean, disinfected, and ready for use. The biopsy port valves were examined using brightfield microscopy and then further studied to identify potential sources of contamination using Fourier transform infrared spectroscopy. The researchers found that eight of the 15 valves (53.3%) exhibited some form of debris or potential contamination. Testing confirmed the debris to be proteinaceous material. The researchers also found

that many of the valves were damaged, increasing the potential for leakage and providing reservoirs for bacterial colonization. At least one valve came from each of the three facilities. The researchers concluded that single-use biopsy port valves provided a higher degree of patient safety.

6.13.1 **Discard single-use parts, accessories, and cleaning implements after use and do not reprocess them.[1,13,15,22,27,45,83]** *[Recommendation]*

Wilson et al[163] reported a pseudo-outbreak of *Aureobasidium* species found in 10 broncheoalveolar lavage fluid cultures taken from nine patients between June 1998 and August 1998. Based on the clinical and laboratory data, there did not appear to be a true infection in any of the patients; however, all of the patients had their bronchoscopy procedures performed in the same outpatient bronchoscopy suite. The investigators observed the processing procedures and found that single-use plastic stopcocks were routinely being reused. The stopcocks were attached to sterile syringes containing sterile water used for the broncheoalveolar lavage. After each use, the stopcocks were manually washed and placed into a mechanical processor. Notably, the manufacturer of the mechanical processor did not recommend disinfecting the stopcocks in this manner.

After HLD, the stopcocks were stored in a sterile, plastic container with a screw top. At the time of the investigation, the container held approximately 20 stopcocks. There was no record of how many times each stopcock was being reused. Culture of the stopcocks yielded heavy growth of *Aurebasidium* species. The practice of reusing the single-use stopcocks was discontinued.[163]

7. Visual Inspection

7.1 **Visually inspect flexible endoscopes, accessories, and associated equipment for cleanliness, integrity, and function before use, during the procedure, after the procedure, after cleaning, and before disinfection or sterilization.** *[Recommendation]*

Clinical practice guidelines support visual inspection of endoscopes, accessories, and equipment after cleaning and throughout use and processing as a method to help identify residual organic material and defective items in need of repair.[1,12,13,21,58,65,90]

The benefits are that visual inspection and evaluation provide an opportunity to identify and remove from service soiled or defective items that might put patients at risk for infection or injury until these items are cleaned or repaired.[24,58]

7.2 **Before use, visually inspect and process all new, repaired, refurbished, and loaned endoscopes, accessories, or other equipment according to the manufacturer's IFU.** *[Recommendation]*

It is not possible to verify how all new, repaired, refurbished, or loaned equipment and devices have been handled, cleaned, inspected, or processed before receipt in the facility. Failure to correctly clean, inspect, or process an item may lead to transmission of pathogenic microorganisms from a contaminated device and create a risk for patient injury or infection.

Visually inspecting endoscopes, accessories, and equipment upon receipt and before processing can help verify there are no obvious defects and may prevent damaged or malfunctioning endoscopes from being used on patients.

7.3 **Visually inspect and evaluate endoscopes, accessories, and equipment for**
- **cleanliness,**[12,13,21,58,65]
- **missing parts,**[1,58]
- **clarity of lenses,**[58,106]
- **integrity of seals and gaskets,**[58,106]
- **moisture,**[58]
- **physical or chemical damage,**[106] **and**
- **function.**[12,13,21,58,65,106]

[Recommendation]

Visual inspection and evaluation help detect the presence of residual soil and identify items in need of repair.

7.4 **Use lighted magnification to inspect endoscopes and accessories for cleanliness and damage.**[12,13,65] *[Recommendation]*

An endoscope that appears clean may harbor debris that cannot be seen without magnification. Lighted magnification may increase the ability to identify residual soil or damage.

7.4.1 **Internal channels of flexible endoscopes may be inspected using an endoscopic camera or borescope.** *[Conditional Recommendation]*

Endoscopic cameras and borescopes penetrate the lumen and allow for improved visual inspection.[12,58]

7.5 **Remove defective endoscopes, accessories, and equipment from service and have the items repaired or replaced.**[1,13,58] *[Recommendation]*

Identification of defective endoscopes, accessories, and equipment and removal from service

reduces the risk of a defective item being used and helps prevent further damage from use.[84]

7.5.1 **Medical equipment being sent for repair must be decontaminated to the fullest extent possible and a biohazard label attached before transportation.**[48] *[Regulatory Requirement]*

Decontaminating and labeling medical equipment before transport is a regulatory requirement and communicates to others which portions of the device being transported are contaminated.[48]

Incorrectly preparing the item being sent for repair may further damage the item and expose personnel handling the item to contaminants.

The manufacturer or service representative may provide recommendations that align with regulatory requirements for safe processes to follow for return or repair of the endoscope.[85]

8. HLD or Sterilization

8.1 **After manual cleaning and inspection, high-level disinfect or sterilize flexible endoscopes and endoscope accessories.**[45] *[Recommendation]*

The Spaulding classification system, developed by Earl Spaulding in 1968, classifies items as critical, semicritical, or noncritical.[117] The level of processing required (ie, sterilization, HLD, **intermediate-level disinfection** [ILD], low-level disinfection) is based on the nature of the item that requires processing and the manner in which the item is to be used.[117] The classification system has been used by infection preventionists and others for more than 47 years.[164]

According to the Spaulding classification, devices that enter sterile tissue or the vascular system are considered critical items.[117] When critical items, such as biopsy forceps, are contaminated with microorganisms, the risk of infection transmission is substantial.[117] Therefore, Spaulding et al[117] recommended that critical items be processed by sterilization. Sterilization eliminates all microbial life, including pathogenic and nonpathogenic microorganisms and bacterial spores.[117] Notably, sterilization is a validated process used to render a product free from all forms of viable microorganisms.[155] Liquid chemical sterilization may not convey the same sterility assurance as sterilization using thermal or other low-temperature sterilization methods.[155]

Items such as flexible endoscopes that come in contact with nonintact skin or mucous membranes, are considered to be semicritical.[117] Mucous membranes provide a barrier to common bacterial spores, but not to organisms such as tubercle bacilli and viruses.[117] Therefore, Spaulding et al[117] recommended

Table 2. Spaulding Classification Modification for Critical Items[1-3]		
Classification	**Disinfection Level**	**Effectiveness**
Critical Items that directly or **secondarily (ie, via a muscous membrane)** enter sterile tissue or vascular system **(eg, bronchoscope, cystoscope, duodenoscope)**. Sterile tissue and the vascular are at a high risk of infection if contaminated with microorganisms.	**Sterilization** Use saturated steam if possible. Use ethylene oxide, dry heat, ozone, low-temperature hydrogen peroxide gas, or liquid chemical sterilization for heat-sensitive items.	Sterilization eliminates all microbial life, including pathogenic and nonpathogenic microorganisms and bacterial spores.

References

1. *Spaulding EH, Lawrence CA, Block SS, Reddish GF, Chemical disinfection of medical and surgical materials. In: Lawrence CA, Block SS, Reddish GF, eds. Disinfection, Sterilization, and Preservation. Philadelphia, PA: Lea & Febiger; 1968:517-531.*
2. *Rutala WA. Weber DJ; the Healthcare Infection Control Practices Advisory Committee (HICPAC). Guideline for Disinfection and Sterilization in Healthcare Facilities, 2008. Atlanta, GA: Centers for Disease Control and Prevention; 2008.*
3. *Rutala WA. ERCP Scopes: A Need to Shift from Disinfection to Sterilization? Meeting of the FDA Gastroenterology and Urology Devices Panel of the Medical Devices Advisory Committee [transcript]. Annapolis, MD: Free State Reporting, Inc; May 14, 2015.*

that semicritical items be processed by sterilization, or at a minimum, by HLD. High-level disinfection eliminates all pathogenic microorganisms except for small numbers of bacterial spores.[46,117]

8.2 **A multidisciplinary team that includes infection preventionists, endoscopy and perioperative RNs, sterile processing personnel, endoscopists, and other involved personnel should conduct a risk assessment to determine whether items that secondarily enter sterile tissue or the vascular system (ie, via a mucous membrane) should be sterile.** *[Recommendation]*

At a meeting of the Gastroenterology-Urology Devices Panel convened by the FDA in May 2015 to seek expert scientific and clinical opinion related to reprocessing of duodenoscopes and other flexible endoscopes, Rutala proposed a modification of the Spaulding system wherein items that secondarily enter sterile tissue or the vascular system are considered to be critical items **(Table 2)**.[165] Devices secondarily entering sterile tissue would include devices that enter sterile tissue by way of a mucous membrane, such as a bronchoscope, a cystoscope, or a duodenoscope.[165] For example, a bronchoscope enters the bronchi through the mouth or nose, a cystoscope enters the bladder through the urethra, and a duodenoscope enters the bile or pancreatic ducts through the mouth. Requiring sterilization of items that secondarily enter sterile tissue or the vascular system may help prevent patient infection.

There are challenges to implementing the current Spaulding classification system when processing complex, heat-sensitive devices such as flexible endoscopes.[120] Because of the heavy microbial load that may be present on some flexible endoscopes and the difficulty in cleaning and disinfecting long, narrow channels, current HLD processes may not

be adequate to ensure flexible endoscopes are safe for use on patients.[166]

The Spaulding classification does not address how to process semicritical items used in conjunction with critical items.[120] Although flexible endoscopes are categorized as semicritical, the accessory devices used in combination with flexible endoscopes may be critical items because they enter sterile tissue or the vascular system.[120] These critical items are passed through an endoscope categorized as semicritical, which requires a minimum of HLD rather than sterilization.[120] Endoscopic accessories may emerge from the distal end of the endoscope and contact the mucosal surface of the bowel, bladder, or esophagus before they are used for the procedure. In addition, the Spaulding classification does not address the need for inactivating certain types of infectious agents, such as prions.[120] Thus, there are concerns about whether semicritical items should be sterilized rather than high-level disinfected.[165,167]

Incidents of reduced susceptibility to aldehyde disinfectants and high-level disinfectant failure also have been reported.[164,168,169] Tschudin-Sutter et al[168] detected *P aeruginosa* in 23 of 73 routine samples (32%) obtained from endoscopes during November 2009, and in 29 of 99 investigational samples (29%) obtained between November 4, and December 7, 2009. The investigators observed endoscope processing procedures and found no lapses; however, they noted that the drying time on the mechanical processor had been reduced from 10 minutes to 5 minutes to expedite turnaround time.

Environmental samples were obtained, and *P aeruginosa* was detected in the rinsing water and in the drain of one of the mechanical processors. The pathogen could not be detected in the water pipes or in any of the cleaning solutions or disinfectants used for processing the endoscopes. Infectious disease specialists reviewed medical records and detected six patients with lower respiratory tract and bloodstream infections possibly caused by the pseudo-outbreak strain. The investigators found that the glutaraldehyde-based disinfectant demonstrated no activity against the microorganism when used in the recommended concentration and at the recommended temperature. They concluded the *P aeruginosa* was resistant to the glutaraldehyde disinfectant.[168]

In a quasi-experimental study to investigate the potential for bacterial resistance in mechanical processors using aldehyde disinfectants, Fisher et al[169] randomly sampled three mechanical processors in the United States using aldehydes for HLD of flexible endoscopes. The researchers found bacterial contamination after disinfection in all of the mechanical processors and found that some mycobacteria isolates demonstrated significant resistance to glutaraldehyde and orthophalaldehyde disinfectants. The researchers concluded that bacteria can survive aldehyde-based HLD and may pose a cross contamination risk to patients.

In some outbreaks and pseudo-outbreaks, resolution was only achieved when the endoscope was sterilized by ethylene oxide.[166,170-172] Epstein et al[170] conducted a case control study to identify the source and interrupt transmission of NDM-producing carbapenem-resistant *E coli* in a tertiary care hospital in northeastern Illinois. The investigators identified 39 case patients from January 2013 through December 2013, of whom 35 had undergone ERCP procedures in the same hospital. No lapses in duodenoscope processing were identified; however, NDM-producing *E coli* that shared a 92% genetic similarity to all case patients was recovered from a processed duodenoscope. After the investigators changed from using from HLD with orthophalaldehyde to sterilization with ethylene oxide, the duodenoscopes were culture-negative and no additional case patients were identified.

Between October and December 2010, Chang et al[173] identified ertapenem-resistant *E cloacae* in the urine cultures of 15 patients who had undergone ureteroscopy with the same ureteroscope. The investigators did not find any breaches in the processing procedures. The endoscope was culture-positive for the ertapenem-resistant *E cloacae*. The ureteroscope was meticulously cleaned and high-level disinfected for an additional 5 minutes beyond the manufacturer's recommended HLD time. The ureteroscope was sampled, and the results were again culture-positive. The ureteroscope was sterilized with ethylene oxide, sampled, and found to be culture-negative.

Smith et al[174] questioned current processing guidelines for duodenoscopes in a report describing transmission of carbapenem-resistant *Enterobacteriaceae*. Between May and November 2013, three patients at a Wisconsin medical center were identified as having NDM-1 carbapenem-resistant *E coli* after undergoing ERCP procedures with the same duodenoscope. The investigators observed the processing procedures and found no lapses. They sampled the duodenoscope and found it was culture-negative; however, the evidence was sufficiently strong to implicate the duodenoscope as the mode of transmission. The duodenoscope was sterilized with ethylene oxide and no additional infections were diagnosed. The researchers noted that for procedures in which duodenoscopes were used, there may be a risk of transmission of infection despite HLD.

Müller et al[175] described infections of multidrug-resistant *P aeruginosa* in two patients who had undergone ERCP procedures with the same duodenoscope for which sterilization by ethylene oxide did not eliminate the organism. The endoscope was quarantined and sampled and found to be culture-positive for the same strain of *P aeruginosa* as the infected patients. The endoscope was manually cleaned, soaked in 2% glutaraldehyde for 10 hours, sampled, and again found to be culture-positive. The duodenoscope was then sterilized with ethylene oxide, sampled, and once again found to be culture-positive. The endoscope was returned to the manufacturer for replacement of all internal channels. The investigators concluded that constant vigilance related to processes for cleaning and HLD was needed to ensure safe and effective processing of endoscopes.

Notably, many facilities do not have the capability of performing ethylene oxide sterilization. Sterilization and aeration using ethylene oxide may take 12 to 15 hours or more.[166] Penetration of ethylene oxide into long, narrow lumens is a concern, and flexible endoscopes may not have been validated by the manufacturer for sterilization with ethylene oxide.[120]

In a quasi-experimental laboratory study, Alfa et al[176] assessed the effect of serum and salt on the performance of two 100% ethylene oxide sterilizers, two ion plasma sterilizers, a vaporized hydrogen peroxide sterilizer, and a 12/88 ethylene oxide sterilizer. The researchers inoculated test carriers with *E coli*, *E faecalis*, *P aeruginosa*, *Mycobacterium chelonae*, *Bacillus stearothermophilus* spores, *Bacillus subtilis* spores, and *Bacillus circulans* spores; subjected them to sterilization; and calculated the residual bacterial load. The inoculum was prepared with and without 10% serum and 0.65% salt. The researchers found that all of the sterilizers effected a 6-log reduction of the bacterial inoculum; however, none of the sterilizers could effect a 6-log reduction in the presence of 10% serum and 0.65% salt. The researchers commented that the inability of sterilizers to reliably eliminate microorganisms in narrow channels in the presence of serum and salt raises concerns about the practice of using ethylene oxide sterilization as a mechanism for controlling outbreaks related to contaminated flexible endoscopes. Bile salts are the major organic component in bile whose function is to emulsify fats and facilitate intestinal absorption.[177]

In a second, similar study, Alfa et al[178] compared the ability of a liquid chemical sterilant and ethylene oxide to sterilize long, narrow lumens. The researchers found that the liquid chemical sterilant achieved a 6-log reduction in bacterial load compared with a 2.5- to 6-log reduction for ethylene oxide. The researchers noted that residual salt appeared to be a major problem for ethylene oxide sterilization, and this raised questions about the practice of using ethylene oxide to sterilize flexible endoscopes used in procedures where there might be residual protein, serum, blood, or salt remaining in the lumen. These data support the need to ensure effective cleaning of narrow lumens before initiating any HLD or sterilization method.

In a quasi-experimental study to assess cleaning and sterilization efficacy in narrow-lumened devices using artificial test soil and to assess the use of artificial test soil as a worst-case organic challenge to the microbial killing efficacy of various sterilization methods, Alfa et al[179] inoculated the biopsy channel of a flexible endoscope with artificial test soil containing 108 CFU/mL of *Geobacillus stearothermophilus*, *M chelonae*, and *E faecalis*. Suboptimal cleaning (ie, no brushing, no immersion, only flushing) was compared to optimal manual cleaning (ie, brushing, flushing, immersion) for organic soil removal. The sterilization efficacy of pre-vacuum steam, 100% ethylene oxide, and peracetic acid was evaluated in the presence of this organic challenge. The researchers found that suboptimal cleaning resulted in less than 99% removal of hemoglobin, carbohydrate, and **endotoxin**, whereas optimal cleaning resulted in greater than 99% removal. The survival of *G stearothermophilus* and *E faecalis* in lumens after sterilization suggested that high residual soil loads affect the efficacy of the sterilization process.

8.3 After manual cleaning and inspection and when compatible with the endoscope manufacturer's IFU, either mechanically clean and mechanically process flexible endoscopes and accessories by exposure to a high-level disinfectant or a liquid chemical sterilant or mechanically clean and sterilize flexible endoscopes and accessories. *[Recommendation]*

Mechanical processing includes mechanical cleaning, mechanical HLD or sterilization, and mechanical rinsing. Moderate-quality evidence shows that mechanical processing improves cleaning effectiveness, increases efficiency, minimizes personnel exposure to biohazardous materials, and can be more successfully monitored for quality and consistency.[1,12,15,16,18,22,45,83,85,93,114,122,180-183]

Although mechanical processing is more effective than manual processing, recommendations from professional organizations supporting mechanical processing are inconsistent. Some experts[93,105,120,182] and clinical practice guidelines[13,17-22,122] recommend using only mechanical processing, while other experts[89] and clinical practice guidelines[15,16,27,44,83,84] support the use of manual methods.

Unless the manufacturer of the mechanical processor has validated the processor to exclude manual cleaning, mechanical processing does not eliminate the need for manual cleaning.[122] The sequence of manual cleaning followed by mechanical cleaning most effectively removes bioburden and helps prevent the buildup of dead microorganisms that may occur when incompletely cleaned devices are subjected to HLD or sterilization.[120] The physical force of the water pressure used by mechanical processors to flush endoscope channels allows the bioburden to be physically lifted and removed by the flow of fluid.[120,182,184]

In a quasi-experimental study to evaluate the effectiveness of five methods of HLD for removal of biofilm in endoscopes, Balsamo et al[185] used Teflon tubes to simulate the channels of flexible endoscopes. The researchers contaminated the tubes with *P aeruginosa* biofilm and subjected them to one of five processing methods:

- manual processing using 2% glutaraldehyde,
- mechanical processing using 2% glutaraldehyde,
- manual processing using 0.09% to 0.15% active peracetic acid,
- mechanical processing using 35% peracetic acid, or
- mechanical processing using acidic electrolytic water.

The researchers found that none of the processing methods completely removed the biofilm. Mechanical processing using 2% glutaraldehyde or 35% peracetic acid were the most effective in removing the biofilm. The biofilm remained attached to 35.7% of the sample segments (15 of 42) and was completely removed in 26% of the sample segments (11 of 42). There was a statistically significant difference between manual and mechanical processing methods.

Ubhayawardana et al[182] conducted a nonexperimental study to evaluate the effectiveness of manual processing for removal of bioburden from side-view endoscopes used for ERCP procedures in a tertiary referral endotherapy unit in Sri Lanka. The researchers obtained samples from 102 different flexible side-view endoscopes before and after processing and then tested them for microbial growth. The researchers found that despite strict adherence to recommended processing protocols, the average culture-positive rates from the endoscope tips was 90% (92 of 102) before processing and 21% (21 of 102) after processing. The culture-positive rate from the working channel after processing was 10% (10 of 102). Notably, manual processing was completed in the procedure room, and this may have contributed to the high culture-positive rate. *Klebsiella* and *Candida* species were the most common microorganisms found. The results of this study suggest that processing of the endoscope tip was less effective than processing of the working channels. The researchers concluded that there was a high culture-positive rate after manual processing of side-view endoscopes.

Some mechanical processors also provide a thermal or chemical decontamination process that removes or reduces the number of microorganisms or infectious agents and renders reusable medical devices safe for use, handling, or disposal.[12,45,58,90]

In addition to improved cleaning and decontamination, mechanical processors may also provide improved rinsing of disinfectants and reduce the potential for patient injury associated with residual disinfectants remaining in the endoscope. In a non-experimental laboratory study, Farina et al[186] determined residual levels of glutaraldehyde in two gastroscopes and two colonoscopes following manual and automatic disinfection procedures. The researchers found that residual glutaraldehyde levels were much higher after manual disinfection (< 0.2 to 159.5 mg/L) than after mechanical disinfection (< 0.2 to 6.3 mg/L).

Mechanical processors may reduce the risk of cross contamination from one load to another by allowing for single-use cleaning and disinfecting solutions.[122]

Using mechanical processors reduces the potential for breaches in recommended processing protocols associated with human error and noncompliance.[67,122,139,182] Audits have shown that personnel do not consistently adhere to guidelines for processing, and this has led to outbreaks of infection.[15,45] Procedures for manual processing of flexible endoscopes may be inadequate or inconsistent and may vary significantly from one health care facility to another, as well as within the same facility.[89,180]

Studies from the United States[80,181,187-189] and other countries[131,190-207] have demonstrated varying degrees of compliance with recommended processing procedures.

Ofstead et al[181] conducted a prospective multisite observational study to evaluate procedures, employee perceptions, and occupational health issues related to processing flexible endoscopes. The researchers collected data from two gastroenterology specialty centers, two multispecialty hospitals, and one outpatient surgery center from five geographically diverse regions in the United States. The researchers found that when performing manual processing, personnel performed all required steps for only one of 69 endoscopes processed (1.4%). When performing mechanical processing, personnel performed all required steps for 86 of 114 endoscopes processed (75.4%). Steps commonly omitted during manual processing included brushing, forced-air drying, and flushing with 70% isopropyl alcohol. The only step routinely omitted during mechanical processing was the final external drying of the endoscope after removal from the processor.

In an examination of the peer-reviewed and non-peer-reviewed literature to identify lapses in processing flexible endoscopes reported in North America from 2005 to 2012, Dirlam Langlay et al[187] found that lapses occurred in various types of facilities and in all major steps of processing. Lapses included failing to

- comply with established guidelines,
- preclean endoscopes before processing,
- correctly contain contaminated endoscopes,
- adequately brush endoscope channels,
- adequately clean the elevator channel of duodenoscopes,
- perform adequate HLD,
- correctly program mechanical processors,
- report malfunctioning mechanical processors, and
- document processing personnel competency.

These lapses may have resulted in patient exposure to potentially contaminated gastrointestinal endoscopes.

In a study to determine common practices for endoscope processing at regional endoscopy centers, Moses and Lee[188] sent anonymous questionnaires to 367 members of the Society of Gastroenterology Nurses and Associates (SGNA) in Pennsylvania, Delaware, Virginia, Maryland, and the District of Columbia. The survey was completed by 230 members (63%), the majority of whom (59%; n = 136) practiced in hospital-based endoscopy units performing more than 3,000 procedures a year. The results of the study showed wide variation in the manual cleaning process. Only 70% (n = 161) suctioned cleaning solution through the endoscope channels and also brushed channels and valves. There was variation in the number of times the channels were brushed, with the majority (37%; n = 85) brushing three to five times. In 6% of the units (n = 14), manual cleaning was the only processing step, and 18% (n = 42) reported omitting manual cleaning before mechanical processing.

Surveyors from the Centers for Medicare & Medicaid Services[189] assessed adherence to infection control practices in 68 ambulatory surgery centers in three states (ie, 32 in Maryland, 16 in North Carolina, 20 in Oklahoma). The surveyors assessed compliance with hand hygiene, injection safety and medication handling, equipment processing, environmental cleaning, and handling of blood glucose monitoring equipment. They found that overall, 46 (67.6%) of the surgery centers had at least one lapse in infection control, and 12 (17.6%) had identified lapses in three or more infection control categories. Errors in processing included failing to adequately clean instruments before sterilization or HLD (four of 60; 6.7%); failing to use chemical or biologic indicators in sterilizer loads (two of 55; 3.6%); failing to prepare, test, or replace high-level disinfectants (eight of 48; 16.7%); failing to document HLD or sterilization (two of 66; 3%); failing to store sterilized or disinfected equipment in a clean area (one of 65; 1.5%); and reprocessing single-use devices (four of 10; 40%).

Although mechanical processors provide many advantages compared with manual processing, there are some disadvantages. Mechanical processors require preventive maintenance to ensure safe and effective operation.[122,180] The use of contaminated or defective mechanical processors for cleaning, disinfecting, or rinsing can result in inadequate processing[22,122,183] that has been associated with outbreaks of endoscopy-related infections and **pseudo-infections**[100,208-219] and patient injury.[220,221] In addition, the presence of biofilm has been detected in mechanical processors.[208,209]

An Endoscope Task Force was established to review endoscope processing incidents in England from 2003 to 2004 and to make recommendations to prevent recurrences. The task force found there were a total of 18 incidents. Eight of the incidents (44%) involved failures to adequately clean endoscope channels. Seven incidents (39%) involved problems with mechanical processors. In one incident, a pump had failed and, due to the lack of a functional alarm system, the failure to irrigate endoscopes with cleaning solution and disinfectant was not being signaled. Another incident involved a malfunction in which the cleaning solution was frothing excessively. The cause was identified as a faulty valve; however, processing personnel had removed the pressure sensors and alarm systems from the machine to stop the signal when it was incorrectly deemed that there was nothing wrong.

An additional incident involved an incorrect adaptor. Three incidents involved the incorrect use of cleaning solutions.[222]

Vanhems et al[223,224] described the possible transmission of pathogens to 236 persons exposed to an endoscope processed in a defective mechanical processor in a gastrointestinal endoscopy unit. In March 2002, a nurse from the digestive diseases unit questioned the "tactile sensation" of the gastrointestinal endoscopes after they had been mechanically processed. The manufacturer was contacted and determined that the pump for injecting disinfectants into the biopsy channels was malfunctioning and the alarm system designed to detect such a flaw was also malfunctioning. The endoscopes had not been disinfected, and patients had potentially been exposed to contaminants. Notably, the endoscopes had been manually cleaned before being placed into the mechanical processor. A total of 197 (83.5%) patients found to be at risk for infection completed follow-up. No acute infection was observed. The investigators noted that the problem was identified because of the subjective perception of an experienced nurse.

The time required for mechanical processing may be longer[180] or shorter[225] than the time required for manual processing, and costs may be increased[180] or offset by financial gains as a result of increased productivity.[226] The consistency of mechanical processing also may minimize the potential for damage and the need for repairs.[67]

Alfa et al[225] compared the efficacy of the cleaning phase of a mechanical processor with optimal manual cleaning in a quasi-experimental laboratory study. A bronchoscope, gastroscope, and colonoscope were each inoculated with artificial test soil containing *P aeruginosa* and *E faecalis* and then allowed to dry for 1 hour. The endoscopes were either manually cleaned following the endoscope manufacturer's IFU or mechanically processed following the IFU for the processor. The results showed a greater than 90% reduction in soil levels for both manual and mechanical cleaning. Manual cleaning was slightly better for exterior surfaces, and mechanical cleaning was slightly better for removal of microorganisms from the channels. The researchers noted that manual cleaning time varied between 15 to 25 minutes per endoscope, depending on the type of endoscope being cleaned. This was substantially longer than the 6 to 7 minutes of cleaning time required for mechanical cleaning of endoscopes.

Forte and Shum[227] used a time and motion study to compare the costs of personnel resources and consumable supplies associated with mechanical processors that do and do not require manual cleaning before processing. For 3 days, the researchers timed and observed two technicians who performed all endoscope processing activities. The researchers found that the total time to process endoscopes was significantly shorter when the technicians used the processor that did not require manual cleaning. The difference in median time to process was 12.6 minutes per colonoscope, 6.31 minutes per gastroscope, and 5.66 minutes per bronchoscope. The amount of time saved per day was 6.2 hours. The researchers determined that the cost of consumable supplies was slightly higher per processing with use of the processor that did not require manual cleaning ($8.91 [$9.50 in 2015 US dollars]) compared with use of the processor that did require manual cleaning ($8.31 [$8.86 in 2015 US dollars]).

Funk and Reaven[226] used data from peer-reviewed published literature and country-specific market research to compare manual processing to mechanical processing relative to productivity, need for endoscope repair, and infection transmission in India, China, and Russia. The researchers found that conversion to mechanical processing had a positive effect on financial performance, paying back the capital investment within 14 months in China and within seven months in Russia. In India, the additional revenue generated by the change to mechanical processing offset nearly all of the operating costs.

8.3.1 **After precleaning and leak testing, and when directed by the mechanical processor manufacturer's IFU, mechanical processing may be accomplished without manual cleaning.** [Conditional Recommendation]

The mechanical processor manufacturer has validated the processes required for effective processing without manual cleaning.[90]

In a quasi-experimental laboratory study to assess the efficacy of a mechanical processor that did not require manual cleaning before use, Alfa et al[228] evaluated patient-used duodenoscopes (n = 15), bronchoscopes (n = 10), colonoscopes (n = 15), and gastroscopes (n = 15). The endoscopes had been precleaned at the point of use and mechanically processed without additional manual cleaning before processing. All endoscope channels and two external surface sites were sampled to determine residual organic and microbial load. The results of the study showed that 99.7% of lumens and 98.8% of surfaces met or surpassed the predetermined cleaning endpoints for protein (< 6.4 µg/cm^2) and bioburden (< 4-log$_{10}$ viable bacteria/cm^2) residuals.

The researchers also conducted simulated use testing by inoculating the channels and

two surface sites of bronchoscopes (n = 3), colonoscopes (n = 3), and duodenoscopes (n = 3) with artificial test soil containing 108 CFU/mL of *E faecalis, P aeruginosa,* and *C albicans.* The endoscopes were allowed to dry for 1 hour before sampling. The results showed that 100% of both lumens and surface sites met or surpassed the cleaning end points for protein and bioburden residuals.[228]

8.4 **Perform mechanical processing in accordance with the endoscope manufacturer's IFU and the mechanical processor manufacturer's IFU.**[17] [Recommendation]

There are multiple types of flexible endoscopes and mechanical processors. Instructions for use may vary among manufacturers. Even slight deviations from the recommended protocols can lead to the survival of microorganisms and an increased risk for infection.[225] Kressel and Kidd[208] reported a pseudo-outbreak of *M chelonae* and *Methylobacterium mesophilicum* caused by a contaminated mechanical processor in an academic medical center between July 1998 and October 1998. An unusual number of fungal cultures obtained during bronchoscopy procedures (26 of 131; 20%) grew *M chelonae.* The 26 cultures came from 22 patients; however, none of the patients had clinical evidence of pulmonary mycobacterial infection.

The investigators sampled the bronchoscopes, the mechanical processors, and the glutaraldehyde from the mechanical processors, and obtained positive results for *M chelonae.* They discovered that because of time constraints, employees had modified the connections required for the alcohol flush, rendering it inadequate. As a result, the mechanical processors became contaminated with biofilm that could not be removed. The processors then contaminated the bronchoscopes. The outbreak ended when the facility purchased a new mechanical processor.[208]

8.4.1 **Verify compatibility between the endoscope and the mechanical processor before processing.**[1,16,18,27,44] [Recommendation]

Compatibility between the endoscope and the mechanical processor is necessary to ensure effective processing of the endoscope and to prevent patient infection.[180]

Larson et al[219] investigated a potential outbreak of tuberculosis in a community hospital in New York in October 2000. Three patients had bronchoscopy specimen cultures that were positive for *M tuberculosis;* however, only one patient had clinical signs and symptoms consistent with tuberculosis. The three culture-positive specimens of *M tuberculosis* were obtained within

9 days of each other from the same bronchoscope. A review of the processing procedures showed that the mechanical processor was not approved for use with the bronchoscope by the bronchoscope manufacturer.

8.4.2 **Position flexible endoscopes and accessories within the mechanical processor in a manner that ensures contact of the processing solutions with all surfaces of the endoscope.** *[Recommendation]*

Contact of all surfaces of the endoscope with processing solutions is necessary to achieve effective processing.

The complexity of flexible endoscopes and the variety of processing equipment available make it essential to follow the manufacturers' IFU to achieve optimal processing.

In a nonexperimental study to determine whether the noncritical portions of a flexible laryngoscope could harbor microorganisms, Bhatt et al[229] randomly sampled six flexible laryngoscopes from the eye piece and handle immediately before use and after subsequent HLD wherein only the shaft of the endoscope was immersed in the high-level disinfectant. The researchers found there was bacterial growth in 41% (seven of 17) of samples. The results of the study demonstrate that despite HLD of the endoscope shaft, the noncritical portions of the endoscope can harbor microorganisms, and complete submersion of the endoscope is necessary to achieve complete processing.

8.4.3 **Verify that all connectors between the endoscope and the mechanical processor are connected correctly.**[13,20,44,69] *[Recommendation]*

Correct connections are necessary to ensure exposure of all surfaces of the endoscope to the processing solutions.[20,44]

Mechanical processors may require that endoscope channels be fitted with flow restrictors or tubing connectors to regulate fluid outflow.[225] The restrictors and tubing direct fluids into specific channels, thereby ensuring perfusion of the channels with necessary fluid flow dynamics.[225] Because of the complexity of the channels and their internal connections, it is critical that the correct connection tubing and flow restrictors be used to achieve adequate flow dynamics.[225] Flow restrictors and tubing connectors are often specific to the make and model of the flexible endoscope.[225]

The CDC[212] reported three clusters of culture-positive bronchoscopy specimens obtained from patients at local health care facilities in New York between 1996 and 1998. The first cluster involved five patients at a health care facility whose bronchial specimens yielded *M tuberculosis* with the same genetic pattern, suggestive of a common source. Samples taken from the bronchoscopes used during the procedures were negative. The investigators identified an inconsistency between the processing procedures recommended in the manufacturer's IFU and those followed by processing personnel. The biopsy port cap was not replaced before the bronchoscope was placed into the mechanical processor, and this led to a 50% reduction in flow and a 25% reduction in pressure, resulting in processing failure.

The second cluster involved bronchial specimens that were culture-positive for *Mycobacterium avium-intracellulare* from seven patients who had all undergone bronchoscopy with the same bronchoscope. The investigators found that the bronchoscope was being processed in a mechanical processor using the connectors provided by the bronchoscope manufacturer rather than the connectors recommended by the mechanical processor manufacturer.[212]

The third cluster involved 18 patients at a health care facility who had bronchial specimens that grew imipenem-resistant *P aeruginosa* (IRPA). None of the patients had IRPA isolated from sputum samples obtained before bronchoscopy, and all but one isolate had identical genetic patterns. The investigators found that the bronchoscopes were not being connected to the mechanical processor in accordance with the mechanical processor manufacturer's IFU.[212] The investigators concluded that there was a need for processing personnel to review and adhere to manufacturer's IFU and ensure correct connections between the endoscope and the mechanical processor.

Sorin et al[230] reported 18 isolates of IRPA from 18 patients who underwent bronchoscopy procedures during a 3-month period immediately after implementation of a new mechanical processor. Three patients demonstrated clinical signs and symptoms of infection and were treated with antibiotics. A representative of the mechanical processor manufacturer noted several incorrect connections from the bronchoscope to the processor. The investigators concluded that the incorrect connections led to an insufficient flow of the chemical sterilant through the bronchoscope lumen, resulting in incomplete processing of the bronchoscope.

8.4.4 Monitor mechanical processing cycles to verify they are completed as programmed. If a mechanical processing cycle is interrupted, repeat the entire cycle.[16,17,20,21,44,83] *[Recommendation]*

Monitoring mechanical processing cycles helps ensure processing parameters have been achieved. Effective processing cannot be assured when the cycle has been interrupted.[16,44,83]

8.5 Use **critical water** to perform mechanical processing of flexible endoscopes.[119] *[Recommendation]*

Critical water meets the following parameters:
- hardness: < 1 mg/L calcium carbonate,[119]
- pH: 5 to 7,[119]
- chloride: < 1 mg/L,[119]
- bacteria: < 10 CFU/mL,[119] and
- endotoxin: < 10 endotoxin units (EU)/mL.[119]

Water quality is affected by the presence of dissolved minerals, solids, chlorides, and other impurities and by its acidity and alkalinity.[119] Untreated water quality fluctuates over time, varies with geographic location and season, and can affect the outcome of cleaning actions.[119]

Hard water can decrease the effectiveness of cleaning solutions and disinfectants, and can also adversely affect the performance of mechanical processors.[119] Deposits can form on medical devices that may prevent microorganisms and organic material from being removed during cleaning.[119] Hard water may be incompatible with some high-level disinfectants and liquid chemical sterilants.[119]

Water with pH levels that are acidic or alkaline may affect the performance of cleaning solutions (especially enzymatic cleaning solutions), disinfectants, or sterilants.[119]

Controlling bacterial and endotoxin levels in water used for processing flexible endoscopes helps reduce the risk for patient infection.[119]

8.6 Use cleaning, disinfectant, and sterilant solutions and chemicals recommended by the endoscope manufacturer and the mechanical processor manufacturer.[13,18,20,22,44,45,46,83,84] *[Recommendation]*

There are multiple types of endoscopes and mechanical processors. Recommended cleaning and disinfectant or sterilant solutions may vary among manufacturers.

The chemical actions of cleaning, disinfectant, and sterilant solutions vary and are intended for different applications. Following the manufacturers' IFU decreases the possibility of selecting and using solutions that may damage the endoscope or mechanical processor.[44,45]

8.6.1 Use chemicals and solutions in the mechanical processor at the concentration, volume, temperature, and contact time recommended by the mechanical processor manufacturer.[13,18-20,40,43,44,69]
- If recommended by the mechanical processor manufacturer, use a test strip or other FDA-cleared testing device specific for the disinfectant and minimum effective concentration of the active ingredient for monitoring solution potency.[1,40,43]
- If a solution falls below its minimum effective concentration, discard it, even if the designated expiration date has not been reached.[40,43]

[Recommendation]

Some mechanical processors may require the use of a test strip or device to verify efficacy of the high-level disinfectant or liquid chemical sterilant used for processing.[40] The concentration of a high-level disinfectant or liquid chemical sterilant will decrease with dilution by water, the presence of organic material, evaporation of the solution, and exposure of the solution to light.[40] Checking the concentration of the high-level disinfectant or liquid chemical sterilant before use reduces the risk of inadequate processing.[40] High-level disinfection solution potency cannot be guaranteed when the solution falls below the minimum effective concentration. Incorrect dilution, volume, temperature, or contact time may result in a processing failure.[40,69,93,131]

8.6.2 Chemicals and solutions used for cleaning and processing flexible endoscopes and endoscope accessories must be handled in accordance with local, state, and federal regulations and the manufacturer's IFU.[38]
- The safety data sheets must be readily accessible to employees within the workplace.[38]
- Chemical spill kits must be stored in close proximity to areas where chemicals or other hazardous materials are stored.[38]

[Regulatory Requirement]

Cleaning products, high-level disinfectants, and liquid chemical sterilants can be hazardous to the individuals who are using them. It is a regulatory requirement that employers have a program to ensure that information about the identification, hazards, composition, safe handling practices, and emergency control measures of a chemical is readily available to employees.[38] When employees have information about the chemicals being used, they can take steps to reduce exposure, establish safe work practices, and implement first aid measures when necessary. Chemical spill kits enable prompt response by providing items that may be required in the cleanup of spills, leaks, or other discharges of hazardous materials.

8.6.3 **Do not use the following products for processing flexible endoscopes:**
- **skin antiseptics**,[1]
- **hypochlorites**,[1,45]
- **phenolics**,[1,45] and
- **quaternary ammonium compounds**.[1,45]

[Recommendation]

Skin antiseptics (eg, povidone iodine, chlorhexidine gluconate) are not formulated as disinfectants.[1] Hypochlorites (eg, bleach) are corrosive and may be inactivated by organic material.[1,45] Phenolics (eg, ortho-benzyl-para-chlorophenol) may cause tissue irritation and injury to mucous membranes.[1,45] Quaternary ammonium compounds (eg, benzalkonium chloride) do not provide adequate disinfection of flexible endoscopes.[1,45]

Esteban et al[231] reported a pseudo-outbreak of 15 *Aeromonas hydrophila* isolates from colon biopsies between January 1998 and May 1998. The investigators found that the endoscopes had been manually cleaned with an enzymatic cleaning solution and rinsed with utility water and then placed into a quaternary ammonium solution for 20 minutes. The pseudo-outbreak ended when the quaternary ammonium solution was replaced with 2% glutaraldehyde for HLD.

8.7 **Following disinfection, mechanically rinse and flush the endoscope and endoscope channels with critical or sterile water.**[1,15,19,20,22,44,83,89,93] **Rinse endoscope accessories and removable parts with critical or sterile water.** *[Recommendation]*

Thorough rinsing and flushing with critical water helps prevent patient injury associated with disinfectant or sterilant retained in the endoscope.[1,45,186,232-240] Utility water may contain microorganisms and endotoxins that can be deposited on the endoscope during the final rinse.[1,119] Tissue contaminated with endotoxins can cause severe inflammation.[119] Outbreaks of endoscopy-related infections and pseudo-infections have been linked to rinsing flexible endoscopes with utility water.[49,93,241] Using critical or sterile water reduces the potential for introducing microbes into the endoscope.[65]

Farina et al[186] conducted a nonexperimental study to determine residual levels of 2% glutaraldehyde in flexible endoscopes after manual and mechanical HLD. In a total of 92 measurements taken after manual HLD (n = 24) and mechanical HLD (n = 68) for two gastroscopes and two colono-scopes, the researchers found that residual levels of glutaraldehyde were higher and more variable after manual HLD (< 0.2 mg/mL to 159.5 mg/mL) than after mechanical HLD (< 0.2 mg/mL to 6.3 mg/mL). The researchers concluded that residual 2% glutaraldehyde levels (especially after manual disinfection) could be high enough to be toxic and a cause of colitis or proctitis following endoscopy.

In an attempt to reduce processing time, Kim and Baek[233] changed from using 2% glutaraldehyde to process flexible endoscopes in their endoscopy unit to using a peracetic acid compound. After the change, the researchers observed a series of 12 patients who experienced **colonic mucosal pseudolipomatosis**. The protocol for mechanical disinfection included a 60-second rinse cycle. The researchers reviewed the processing records and found that the colonic pseudolipomatosis occurred only when one of six nurses was on duty. The nurse sometimes rinsed the endoscopes for only 10 seconds and at other times omitted the mechanical rinsing cycle, opting to manually rinse the endoscopes under running water. No more cases occurred after the 60-second rinse cycle was reinstated. The researchers noted that this case highlighted the importance of completing all processing steps and following the manufacturer's IFU when using mechanical processors.

Wendleboe et al[242] investigated an outbreak of seven *P aeruginosa* infections associated with outpatient cystoscopy performed by a urologist in New Mexico from January to April 2007. The investigators found multiple breaches in processing procedures including rinsing of the cystoscope in unsterile water after processing. Specifically, sterile water was placed in a container and replaced every 2 weeks or when it began to smell. The outbreak resolved when improved procedures for processing flexible cystoscopes were implemented.

8.8 **A multidisciplinary team that includes infection preventionists, endoscopy and perioperative RNs, endoscopy processing personnel, endoscopists, and other involved personnel should conduct a risk assessment to determine whether endoscope lumens should be flushed with 70% to 90% ethyl or isopropyl alcohol.** *[Recommendation]*

Flushing endoscope lumens with alcohol may not be necessary if the endoscope is effectively dried.[243] Because of the fixative properties of alcohol, this practice is not recommended in some countries.[18-20,22,69,93]

Alfa and Sitter[243] conducted a prospective, quantitative assessment of the effect of drying on the bacterial load in duodenoscopes used for ERCP procedures. The researchers sampled 42 duodenoscopes that had been manually cleaned and then mechanically processed at 2, 24, and 48 hours after disinfection. They found that 21 duodenoscopes (50%) were contaminated. There was visible moisture remaining in the suction channel even though processing personnel had followed the mechanical processor manufacturer's IFU. The bacterial counts ranged from 1×10^1 CFU/mL^{-1} to 1×10^7 CFU/mL^{-1}. The researchers added 10 minutes of drying time to 19 of the 21 contaminated duodenoscopes, either by purging the lumens of the endoscopes with instrument air or by adding 10 minutes of drying time in the mechanical processor. The results showed that there were no microorganisms detected after the additional drying time. The researchers concluded that the additional 10 minutes of drying time prevented bacterial growth in the endoscopes and eliminated the need for an alcohol flush.

Many clinical practice guidelines[1,15,16,19,44-46,83] and experts in the field[89,93,244] recommend manual or mechanical flushing of endoscope lumens with alcohol because it facilitates drying of the endoscope lumens by binding with residual water and enhancing evaporation.[1,16,65] Alcohol prevents colonization and transmission of waterborne bacteria.[46,65,89] Some mechanical processors automatically flush the endoscope with 70% isopropyl alcohol, others do not.

Wang et al[245] reported a pseudo-infection of *M chelonae* involving 25 patients with 25 positive isolates (ie, 18 bronchial, one soft tissue, one plural, five corneal) between September 1992 and December 1992. The investigators found the suction channels of four different bronchoscopes to be the sources of contamination and noted that the processing procedure did not include flushing the suction channels with 70% isopropyl alcohol. The bronchoscope processing procedures were modified to include flushing the endoscope lumens with 70% isopropyl alcohol after mechanical processing, and no further episodes of cross contamination or infection occurred.

In a quasi-experimental study to analyze whether flushing endoscope lumens with 70% ethyl alcohol after processing reduced the risk of microbiological contamination, Gavalda et al[246] sampled 18 different bronchoscopes after processing. The samples were collected on a monthly basis during a 4-year period. Nine of the bronchoscopes were processed manually, and nine were processed mechanically. A total of 620 samples was obtained. The researchers found that 564 samples (91%) tested negative, and 56 samples (9%) tested positive, of which two (3.3%) contained pathogenic microorganisms. Only one positive sample (0.6%) was detected among the 167 samples from endoscopes flushed with alcohol after disinfection. The researchers recommended flushing broncho-scope channels with 70% ethyl alcohol after each disinfection cycle.

8.9 **After mechanical processing, dry the exterior surfaces of the endoscope with a soft, lint-free cloth or sponge.**[15,16,22,83,89]
- **Dry the endoscope channels by purging with instrument air or using a mechanical processor drying system.**[1,15,16,19,22,44-46,83,89,131,244]
- **Dry removable parts and endoscope accessories.**[16]
[Recommendation]

Some mechanical processors have drying systems, others do not.

Effectively drying the internal and external surfaces of the endoscope is as important as effective cleaning and disinfection or sterilization.[244] The long, narrow channels of the endoscope make it difficult to verify thorough drying.[157] Any moisture remaining on the exterior and interior surfaces of the endoscope can facilitate microbial growth and biofilm formation during storage.[19,46,65,93,131] Because bacteria can double in population every 20 to 30 minutes, an inadequately dried endoscope contaminated with only one or two viable bacteria can, after 8 hours of storage, be contaminated with tens of thousands of bacteria.[247] These multiplying bacteria could pose a risk for infection.[247]

In a nonexperimental study to mimic disinfection and drying of biofilm in contaminated endoscopes, Kovaleva et al[248] prepared single species biofilm (ie, *C albicans*, *Candida parapsilosis*, *P aeruginosa*, or *S maltophilia*) and dual species biofilm (ie, *C parapsilosis* with *P aeruginosa* or *C parapsilosis* with *S maltophilia*) in sterile tissue culture plates and treated the single and dual strains with 1% peracetic acid. The culture plates were incubated at 122° F (50° C) for 2 hours to mimic the drying process, and then sealed and incubated at room temperature (ie, 68° F to 72° F [20° C to 22° C]), for 1, 3, and 5 days to mimic the storage process. The researchers found that there was no biofilm regrowth when the drying process was applied, but regrowth of all biofilms occurred when the drying process was not implemented. The researchers concluded that thorough drying was an important factor in the maintenance of bacteria-free endoscopes.

In a nonexperimental study, Ren-Pei et al[96] investigated biofilm on endoscope channels. The researchers collected 66 endoscope suction and biopsy channels and 13 water and air channels from 66 endoscopy centers in hospitals throughout China and used SEM to examine biofilm on the inner surface of the channels. A total of 36 suction and biopsy channels (54.5%) and 10 water and air channels (76.9%) were found to have biofilm.

After examining the endoscope channels, the researchers sent a questionnaire to each of the 66 endoscopy centers to explore the correlation between endoscope processing procedures and the amount of biofilm found in the endoscope channels. They divided the responses (N = 66) into hospitals without biofilm on endoscopes (Group A; n = 30), and hospitals with biofilm on endoscopes (Group B; n = 36). The researchers found that the proportion of endoscopy centers using an alcohol flush and compressed air drying in Group A was 76.6% (23 of 30) compared with 38.9% (14 of 36) in Group B. The researchers concluded that the formation of biofilm on the endoscope channels could be related to inadequate drying.[96]

Purging the endoscope channels with instrument air or using a mechanical drying system facilitates drying without introducing contaminants into the clean device, removes residual alcohol, and reduces the likelihood of contamination of the endoscope by waterborne pathogens and the transmission of pathogens that may result in patient infection.[1,22,44,45,89,99,157]

Bajolet et al[118] reported transmission of an extended-spectrum β-lactamase-producing *P aeruginosa* in four patients who underwent an EGD procedure with the same gastroscope between May and August 2011. The gastroscope had been purchased in January 2011. Microbiological sampling before its first use showed negative results. The investigators observed processing procedures and found the endoscopes were still wet at the end of the cleaning process and were not adequately dried before storage. They concluded that the moist environment in the channels of the endoscope had supported development of a persistent biofilm that contributed to transmission of a serious infection.

Hagan et al[249] reported a pseudo-infection of *Rhodotorula rubra* related to a contaminated bronchoscope in a Kansas City medical center. Between October and November 1992, bronchoscopy specimens from 11 patients yielded growth of *R rubra*. The outbreak ended when investigators initiated changes to the processing procedures that included adding an alcohol flush and purging the lumens of the bronchoscope with air for 3 minutes.

Carbonne et al[250] reported an outbreak of *K pneumoniae* carbapenemase-producing *K pneumoniae* type 2 that was detected in two hospitals in France during September 2009. Of the 13 patients, seven had been examined with the same duodenoscope that had been used to examine the source patient. The investigators found that the cleaning and disinfection processes were consistent with French national guidelines; however, the drying process was not optimal. The procedures were revised to include a systematic drying step after each disinfection cycle, and no additional cases were identified.

Because of a severe outbreak of *K pneumoniae* producing extended-spectrum β-lactamase that occurred in 16 patients undergoing ERCP procedures in a hospital in France between December 2008 and August 2009, Aumeran et al[55] observed the duodenoscope processing procedures. They found that the duodenoscopes were not fully dried before they were stored. The investigators hypothesized that bacteria were introduced into the channels of the duodenoscope during the procedures, and despite repeated cleaning and disinfection, the contamination persisted because the moisture remaining in the endoscope channels created conditions favorable to the persistence and growth of the involved organism. The infection was transmitted to 12 patients. Implementing adequate drying of the endoscopes and ensuring that the elevator channel was dry before storage led to an abrupt termination of the outbreak.

8.10 **A multidisciplinary team that includes infection preventionists, endoscopy and perioperative RNs, endoscopy processing personnel, endoscopists, and other involved personnel should conduct a risk assessment to determine the potential harms compared with the benefits of initiating one or more enhanced methods for processing duodenoscopes.[138]** *[Recommendation]*

Initiating enhanced processing methods for duodenoscopes may decrease the potential for pathogenic microorganisms to remain on the endoscope after processing.[138,165,251] Before processing, gastrointestinal endoscopes carry a microbial load of approximately 10^7 to 10^{10} (ie, 10,000,000 to 10,000,000,000) organisms.[112,113,115,252] Cleaning results in a 2-log to 6-log reduction.[253,254] High-level disinfection results in a 4-log to 6-log reduction.[254]

Theoretically, if a flexible endoscope carried a microbial load of 10^{10}, and cleaning reduced the microbial load by 2-log (10^{-2}), followed by HLD that resulted in a 4-log reduction (10^{-4}), the device would still have a 4-log (10^4) microbial load after processing (ie, 10,000 microorganisms). Repeat HLD or sterilization would increase the margin of safety and further decrease the number of pathogenic microorganisms remaining on the endoscope.[165,251]

The **sterility assurance level** for sterile items is 10^{-6}.[77] A 6-log reduction theoretically reduces a population of 1 million microorganisms to zero.[77]

8.10.1 Enhanced methods for processing flexible duodenoscopes may include implementing HLD followed by
- endoscope quarantine until the duodenoscope is culture-negative,[138,165,251]
- a liquid chemical sterilant processing system,[138,165,251]

- a second HLD,[138,165,251]
- ethylene oxide sterilization,[138,165,251] or
- FDA-cleared low-temperature sterilization.[165,251]

[Conditional Recommendation]

Culturing duodenoscopes after every processing cycle and quarantining the endoscope until culture results are known may be an effective method for assessing processing effectiveness.

Ross et al[144] implemented a process for quarantining flexible duodenoscopes following an outbreak of multidrug-resistant *E coli* that occurred in a Seattle medical center between November 2012 and August 2013. Thirty-two patients were found to harbor one of two genetically similar strains of the organism. All of the patients had undergone ERCP procedures. The investigators were unable to find any lapses in HLD or infection control procedures. The genetic strain of *E coli* was identified by culture on four of eight duodenoscopes, three of which required critical repairs despite a lack of noticeable malfunction. Twenty new duodenoscopes were purchased to implement the quarantine process.

After mechanical processing performed in accordance with the manufacturer's IFU, cultures were taken of the duodenoscope, mechanical processing was repeated after culturing, and the duodenoscope was hung vertically in a storage cabinet with passive airflow for 48 hours. If the culture report was negative, the endoscope was released for use. If bacterial pathogens were identified, the duodenoscope was reprocessed, cultured, and quarantined for an additional 48 hours and only released if the cultures were negative. During a 1-year period, a total of 1,524 cultures were collected from the duodenoscopes, of which 200 (13.1%) were positive for bacterial growth. The majority, 171 (85.5%) grew common skin flora and nonpathogenic organisms. The remaining 29 (14.5%) were positive for pathogenic bacterial growth. In two cases, the duodenoscopes required more than one repeat cycle of HLD in order to be culture-negative. The two endoscopes were returned to the manufacturer for inspection, and one had to be taken out of service. The investigators concluded that the quarantine process was successful in ending the outbreak of duodenoscope-related infections.

Because some duodenoscopes may have persistent microbial contamination despite HLD, repeat HLD or sterilization may provide a greater margin of safety.[138] Using a liquid chemical sterilant system after HLD may provide a greater margin of safety and may be effective for heat-sensitive devices such as flexible endoscopes; however, because this process may require rinsing with unsterile water after sterilization, the endoscope may not remain completely free of all viable microorganisms.[138]

Ethylene oxide sterilization following HLD may also provide a greater margin of safety, and may be effective for heat-sensitive devices such as flexible endoscopes; however, it can fail in the presence of organic material, it is costly and not accessible to all health care facilities, and it may affect the material and mechanical properties of the duodenoscope.[138]

Performing HLD followed by HLD, liquid chemical sterilization, low-temperature sterilization, or ethylene oxide sterilization has not been validated by the endoscope, mechanical processor, or sterilizer manufacturers, and further research is warranted.

8.11 **Implement processes and procedures for packaging and sterilizing flexible endoscopes and endoscope accessories in accordance with the AORN Guideline for Selection and Use of Packaging Systems for Sterilization[255] and the AORN Guideline for Sterilization.[256]** *[Recommendation]*

Sterilization provides the highest level of assurance that processed items are free of viable microbes.[45]

Packaging systems permit sterilization of the contents within the package, protect the integrity of the sterilized contents, prevent contamination of the contents until the package is opened for use, and permit the aseptic delivery of the contents.[255]

8.11.1 **Sterilize endoscopic accessories (eg, biopsy forceps) that enter sterile tissue or the vascular system.[27,44,256]** *[Recommendation]*

Devices that enter sterile tissue or the vascular system are considered critical items.[117]

8.12 **Implement precautions to minimize the risk for transmission of prion diseases from flexible endoscopes and endoscope accessories in accordance with the AORN Guideline for Cleaning and Care of Surgical Instruments.[58]** *[Recommendation]*

Prions are a unique class of infectious proteins that cause fatal neurological diseases.[257] Examples of prion diseases are Gerstmann-Sträussler-Scheinker syndrome, fatal familial insomnia syndrome, and Creutzfeldt-Jakob disease (CJD).[257] Creutzfeldt-Jakob disease is a rare and ultimately fatal degenerative disease that belongs to a group of neurological disorders known as **transmissible spongiform encephalopathies** (TSEs).[20] Variant Creutzfeldt-Jakob disease is acquired from cattle with bovine spongiform encephalopathy, or "mad cow disease."[46,167,257,258]

There are concerns about the potential for endoscopic transmission of prions and other TSEs, including CJD, and vCJD.[46,122] For an endoscope to act as a vehicle for transmission of prions, contact with infective tissue is required.[46,257]

Table 3. Recommendations for Processing Flexible Endoscopes Used with High-Risk Patients

Type of Patient	Type of Tissue	Method of Processing
High-risk: • Patients with known prion disease • Patients with familial history of CJD, Gerstmann-Straüssler-Scheinker syndrome, or familial insomnia syndrome • Patients with a known mutation in the PrP (prion protein) gene (involved in familial transmissible spongiform encephalopathies [TSEs]) • Patients with a history of dura mater transplantation • Patients with electroencephalograph findings or laboratory evidence suggesting of TSE (eg, markers of neuronal injury such as 14-3-3 protein) • Patients with a known history of cadaver-derived pituitary hormone injection	High-risk: • brain (including dura mater) • spinal cord • posterior eye (including retina or optic nerve) • pituitary gland	Discard
	Low-risk: • cerebrospinal fluid • kidney • liver • spleen • lung • placenta • olfactory epithelium • lymph nodes	No recommendation (Unresolved issue) • Conduct a risk assessment with a multidisciplinary team to determine whether to process or discard • Discard neurosurgical endoscopes with central nervous system contact
	No-risk: • peripheral nerve • intestine • bone marrow • blood • leukocytes • serum • thyroid gland • adrenal gland • heart • skeletal muscle • adipose tissue • gingiva • prostate • testis • tears • saliva • sputum • urine • feces • semen • vaginal secretions • milk • sweat	Process in accordance with the AORN Guideline for Cleaning and Care of Surgical Instruments

References

1. *Rutala WA, Weber DJ; Society for Healthcare Epidemiology of America. Guideline for disinfection and sterilization of prion-contaminated medical instruments.* Infect Control Hosp Epidemiol. *2010;31(2):107-117*
2. *Guideline for cleaning and care of surgical instruments. In:* Guidelines for Perioperative Practice. *Denver, CO: AORN, Inc; 2015:615-650.*

In CJD, the prions accumulate in the central nervous system and are transmitted by exposure to infectious brain, pituitary, or eye tissue. Because flexible endoscopes do not come in contact with brain, pituitary, or eye tissue, endoscopic transmission of CJD or other TSEs is unlikely.[46,257]

In vCJD, the prions accumulate in both central nervous system and lymphoid tissue.[167,258] Patients with vCJD have infectivity detectable in the appendix, spleen, tonsils, thymus, and lymph nodes.[20,46,93,167,257,258] The prions responsible for vCJD are found in abundance in the Peyer patches located in the terminal ileum.[20,167] Aggregates of lymphoid prions are also found in the large intes-tine and the stomach.[167] Transmission of vCJD via a flexible gastrointestinal endoscope is therefore theoretically possible because of the lymphatic distribution of prions. The risk for transmission is greater during invasive interventional procedures (eg, biopsy, polypectomy, mucosal resection, sphincterotomy) than during noninterventional procedures[20,258]; however, there have been no reports of such transmission described in the literature.[93,167,258]

8.12.1 Process flexible endoscopes and accessories used during endoscopy procedures on high-risk patients as shown in Table 3. [Recommendation]

Prions are highly resistant to conventional physical and chemical disinfection and sterilization and can remain infectious for years.[46,167,257,258]

Methods for processing instruments contaminated with prions are unsuitable for semicritical, heat-labile devices such as flexible endoscopes.[20,257] Current recommendations for processing instruments exposed to prions include decontamination with concentrated sodium hydroxide (ie, lye) or sodium hypochlorite (ie, bleach), which are corrosive to flexible endoscopes, followed by prolonged steam sterilization, which most flexible endoscopes cannot tolerate.[93,257] Dry heat, glutaraldehyde, and ethylene oxide are not effective disinfection or sterilization methods for flexible endoscopes contaminated with prions.[20,93,258] Aldehyde disinfectants (eg, glutaraldehyde, orthophalaldehyde) may anchor prion proteins within endoscope channels and also render them more difficult to remove. For this reason, aldehyde disinfectants are not recommended for HLD in some countries.[20,167,258] Further research is warranted relative to the use of cleaning chemistries and low-temperature sterilization technologies for inactivating prions.[257]

Discarding the endoscope and accessories after use on high-risk tissue from high-risk patients ensures the endoscope and accessories will not be used on subsequent patients and eliminates the risk of inadequate prion inactivation or patient-to-patient transmission of prion disease.

There is no recommendation for processing critical or semicritical devices contaminated with low-risk tissue from high-risk patients. Although low-risk tissue has been found to transmit CJD, this has been demonstrated only when low-risk tissue has been inoculated into the brain of a susceptible animal.[257]

Flexible endoscopes contaminated with no-risk tissue do not present a risk for prion transmission.

8.13 **A multidisciplinary team that includes infection preventionists, endoscopy and perioperative RNs, endoscopy processing personnel, endoscopists, and other involved personnel should conduct a risk assessment to determine whether single-use endoscope sheaths will be used with compatible flexible endoscopes, and if used, whether, and under what circumstances the endoscope will be disinfected using ILD or HLD.** *[Recommendation]*

Flexible endoscopes contact mucous membranes and are considered semicritical items requiring a minimum of HLD[117,259]; however, high-quality evidence shows that when compatible with the sheath, and used in accordance with the sheath manufacturer's IFU, flexible endoscopes may be effectively processed using 70% isopropyl alcohol (an ILD)[45] rather than HLD, and processing time is reduced.[83,89,260-264]

In a quasi-experimental study to compare the efficacy of various high-level disinfectants against mycobacteria when used in combination with manual cleaning, Foliente et al[253] found that 70% isopropyl alcohol was as effective against mycobacteria as two high-level disinfectants. The researchers inoculated five colonoscopes and five duodenoscopes with *M chelonae*. Each endoscope was manually cleaned, and then exposed to one of two high-level disinfectants (ie, 2% glutaraldehyde, 7.5% hydrogen peroxide), 70% isopropyl alcohol, a liquid chemical sterilant (ie, 0.2% peracetic acid), or ethylene oxide sterilization. The researchers sampled the endoscopes after inoculation, manual cleaning, and disinfection or sterilization. The results showed the average number of microorganisms recovered after inoculation was 9.4×10^6 CFU. After manual cleaning, the average number of microorganisms was 9.9×10^3 CFU, reflecting a 3-log reduction. The researchers found no mycobacteria after exposure to ethylene oxide or 0.2% peracetic acid. The average number of microorganisms after exposure to 70% alcohol was 19 CFU/endoscope and after exposure to the high-level disinfectants was 13 CFU/endoscope for 2% glutaraldehyde and 40 CFU/endoscope for 7.5% hydrogen peroxide.

Sheaths reduce but do not eliminate the risk of contamination and do not eliminate the need for manual cleaning of the endoscope after use.[89] The endoscope may also be contaminated by the soiled hands or gloves of personnel during application or removal of the sheath.[89] The sheath may be breached or may break or tear during use,[89] potentially exposing the patient to a flexible endoscope processed by ILD rather than HLD. Sheath failure may not be obvious.[259]

Lawrentschuk and Chamberlain[260] described their experience of using a flexible cystoscope with a single-use endoscope sheath designed to function as a microbial barrier on 200 consecutive patients. The authors found that using the single-use sheath eliminated the need for HLD or sterilization, thus saving time and minimizing personnel exposure to hazardous chemicals. Notably, the sheath failed in 5% of procedures. The authors noted that using the sheath reduced contact of the cystoscope with body fluids and chemicals, and this reduced contact could theoretically prolong the life of the endoscope.

In a nonexperimental study to evaluate the use of endoscope sheaths as barriers to viruses on flexible ear, nose, and throat endoscopes, Baker et al[261] challenged the sheaths by applying laser-drilled holes (2 μg to 30 μg) and inoculating the sheaths with suspensions of **bacteriophage** (1.0 × 10⁸ **plaque-forming units** (PFU)/mL). The sheath and the endoscope were sampled to recover any virus particles that had penetrated through the holes in the sheath. The researchers found that up to 500 virus particles could pass through the 30 μg holes, indicating a very low viral passage. The researchers concluded that meticulous cleaning of the endoscope followed by ILD provided an instrument that was safe to use on patients.

Elackattu et al[262] conducted a quasi-experimental study to evaluate the number of microorganisms on patient-used flexible nasopharyngolaryngoscopes with and without endoscope sheaths. The researchers took samples from multiple sites on 100 flexible nasopharyngolaryngoscopes. The endoscopes were assigned to either the sheath group (n = 50) or the HLD group (n = 50). Samples were taken from the handle of the endoscopes and the lower third of the insertion shaft of the endoscopes before and after use. The results showed that one in 50 endoscope insertion shafts was culture-positive after disinfection in the sheath group and there was no growth in the HLD group. There were four positive cultures of handles in the HLD group after disinfection and one positive culture of a handle in the sheath group. The sheath method averaged 89 seconds to process, whereas the HLD method averaged 14 minutes. The researchers concluded that using the endoscope sheath reduced processing time and was a safe method for preventing transmission of infection from one patient to the next. Notably, this study was funded by a grant from the sheath manufacturer.

In a randomized controlled trial to investigate the function and processing of flexible gastroscopes, Mayinger et al[263] compared the performance of 50 sheathed with 50 unsheathed gastroscopes using a 10-point **analog rating scale**. The researchers recorded processing times, took samples before and after use and processing, and examined the endoscope sheaths for leaks or tears. The researchers found no leaks or tears in any of the endoscope sheaths. Microbial contamination was found in 10% (five of 50) of the unsheathed endoscopes processed by HLD and in 16% (eight of 50) of the sheathed endoscopes. The processing time for the sheathed system was significantly shorter at 8.9 minutes compared with 48.4 minutes for processing by HLD. Based on the results of the analog rating scale, the endoscopists preferred the unsheathed endoscope, while the processing personnel preferred the sheathed endoscope for its ease of processing.

Alvarado et al[264] conducted a randomized controlled trial to determine whether sheathed nasopharyngoscopes could provide reliable protection against bacterial contamination and obviate the need for HLD. The researchers obtained baseline samples at three time periods from the control heads and insertion shafts of three nasopharyngoscopes used in 100 clinical examinations. The samples were obtained

- before application of the sheath and the procedure;
- immediately after the procedure and removal of the sheath; and
- after point-of-use precleaning, disinfection with 70% isopropyl alcohol, and drying.

The researchers found no bacteria on any of the endoscopes after processing. No sheath showed loss of barrier integrity during leak testing. The researchers concluded that after following point-of-use precleaning, disinfection with 70% isopropyl alcohol, and drying processes, the endoscopes were safe to use. This study was funded by a grant from the sheath manufacturer.[264]

In an evaluation to measure image clarity, ease of use, and handling performance of a flexible bronchoscope and single-use sheath, Colt et al[265] measured the performance using a linear rating scale of 1 (poor) to 5 (excellent) after use on 24 patients at three tertiary care centers. The mean performance ratings were > 4.0 for image clarity, illumination, lack of fogging, distal tip angulation, and ease of transnasal passage. All other ratings were > 3.0, with the lowest for handling comfort. The authors concluded that the single-use sheath had the potential to reduce bronchoscope downtime by eliminating the need for HLD between procedures. This study was supported in part by the sheath manufacturer.

Using endoscope sheaths may potentially extend the life of the endoscope[83,89,260,266]; however, sheaths increase the diameter of the endoscope and this may lead to patient discomfort.[266,267] Securely fitted sheaths may also cause damage to the delicate tip of the endoscope when the sheath is removed.[266]

In a nonexperimental study to evaluate bacterial contamination of flexible cystoscopes protected by single-use sheaths, Jorgensen et al[267] leak tested 100 cystoscopes and then sampled the cystoscopes after removal of the sheath and after ILD. The researchers found that all samples had less than 5 CFU per sample. The researchers concluded that processing flexible cystoscopes using ILD was an acceptable alternative to HLD, provided there was a low risk for pathogen transmission. Using the sheath reduced processing time between 4 and 31 minutes per procedure. The researchers noted that using the sheaths resulted in some reduced visualization for the urologist and increased discomfort for the patient.

Street et al[266] audited the costs of disinfection practices in a UK hospital between July 2003 and January 2004 and found that endoscope sheaths had damaged two flexible laryngoscopes with repair costs totaling $15,551.77 (£10,252 [$19,735.77 and £13,029.32 in 2015]). The cause of the damage in one instance was determined to be the sheath being incorrectly fitted, and in the other, the sheath being left on the endoscope overnight. The lining of each flexible endoscope was torn about 2 cm from the tip. Sheaths tightly grip the tip of the flexible endoscope and can shear off the lining of the tip when removed. The authors also opined that the use of sheaths increased patient discomfort and the likelihood of trauma to the nasal mucosa because of the increased diameter of the endoscope, which they calculated to be a 12% increase.

8.13.1 **Discard single-use endoscope sheaths after each use.** *[Recommendation]*

Discarding the endoscope sheath after use helps ensure it is not used on subsequent patients. Brake et al[207] conducted a survey of 171 otolaryngologists to compare practices in Canada for disinfection of flexible nasopharyngoscopes. The researchers found that 36.4% of otolaryngologists who used endoscope sheaths were unsure whether the sheaths were to be discarded after use, and 18.2% believed that sheaths were intended to be used multiple times. Only 63.6% always cleaned the nasopharyngoscopes between sheath uses, and 9.1% did not know how often the endoscopes were cleaned between uses. The researchers did not disclose how many of the otolaryngologists who responded to the survey used endoscope sheaths.

8.13.2 **If processing by ILD is approved by the multidisciplinary team, visually inspect the endoscope and single-use endoscope sheath after each use.**[83] *[Recommendation]*

Inspection of the endoscope sheath confirms the integrity of the sheath and may determine the subsequent level of processing (ie, HLD or ILD).[83]

8.13.3 **If the sheath is intact, disinfect the endoscope by**
- washing all external surfaces with a soft, lint-free cloth or sponge saturated with the endoscope manufacturer's recommended cleaning solution[1,12,13,15,16,18,19,22,27,65,83,84,89,105];

- rinsing the exterior surfaces of the endoscope with utility water until all cleaning solution and residual debris is removed[12,13,15-17,20,27,83-85,89];
- wiping the external surfaces of the endoscope with 70% isopropyl alcohol[83]; and
- drying the external surfaces of the endoscope with a soft, lint-free cloth or sponge.[83]

[Conditional Recommendation]

The manufacturer has validated the sheath to be impermeable to penetration by microorganisms and has validated that sheath application and removal can be accomplished without contamination of the endoscope. The barrier properties of the sheath have been validated, and a minimum of ILD is required before application of a new sheath.[268]

8.13.4 **If the endoscope sheath is torn or any portion of the endoscope appears soiled or wet, clean and process the endoscope by HLD or sterilization.**[83] *[Recommendation]*

If the endoscope has been contaminated due to a torn sheath, processing by ILD may not be sufficient to prevent patient-to-patient transmission of pathogenic microorganisms, and HLD is required.[89]

8.13.5 **If an endoscope is to be used without the sheath for a subsequent patient, process the endoscope by HLD or sterilization, even though the sheath appears intact and the endoscope was processed by ILD.**[12] *[Recommendation]*

8.13.6 **If the endoscope is only used with a single-use sheath, the multidisciplinary team, should conduct a risk assessment to establish intervals for leak testing, inspection, and HLD or sterilization.** *[Recommendation]*

8.14 A multidisciplinary team that includes infection preventionists, endoscopy and perioperative RNs, endoscopy processing personnel, endoscopists, and other involved personnel should conduct a risk assessment to determine whether chlorine dioxide wipes may be used for disinfection of non-channeled flexible endoscopes when compatible with the endoscope and used in accordance with the disinfectant manufacturer's IFU. *[Recommendation]*

Chlorine dioxide wipes incorporate a three-step process for cleaning and disinfecting non-channeled flexible endoscopes that includes cleaning, disinfection, and rinsing; however, chlorine dioxide has not been cleared by the FDA as a high-level disinfectant for processing reusable medical equipment.[269]

Non-channeled flexible endoscopes can become contaminated with mucous, debris, microorganisms, and blood during use.[270] Non-channeled flexible endoscopes contact mucous membranes and are considered semicritical items requiring a minimum of HLD.[117]

Bhattacharyya and Kepnes[271] conducted a quasi-experimental study to determine whether HLD rendered non-channeled flexible laryngoscopes free of nonviral infectious microorganisms. The researchers sampled six laryngoscopes after HLD at the beginning, middle, and end of two clinical workdays (n = 36), and after contamination with saliva on two additional days (n = 12). The researchers recovered only one positive culture (2.1%) for mold species. No cultures were positive for bacteria. The researchers concluded that HLD was effective and provided a flexible laryngoscope that was safe for patient use.

Protocols for processing non-channeled flexible endoscopes are derived from protocols for processing channeled flexible endoscopes, which carry a much higher bioload after use and have different design properties than non-channeled endoscopes.[272,273] Other technologies may be effective for processing non-channeled endoscopes.

In a quasi-experimental study to compare various methods for processing non-channeled flexible laryngoscopes, Liming et al[274] applied eight different processes to patient-used endoscopes, sampled the endoscopes after processing, and compared the results. The methods applied included a

- 30-second wash with utility water,
- 30-second scrub with antimicrobial soap,
- 30-second wipe with 70% isopropyl alcohol,
- 30-second scrub with antimicrobial soap followed by a 30-second wipe with 70% isopropyl alcohol,
- 30-second wipe with a germicidal cloth,
- 12-minute soak in orthophalaldehyde,
- 15-minute soak in orthophalaldehyde, and
- 20-minute soak in orthophalaldehyde.

The researchers found that each of the methods used was statistically efficacious in removing bacterial contamination and equally as effective as HLD. The researchers concluded that fast, cost-effective practices were acceptable for processing non-channeled flexible endoscopes.

In a quasi-experimental study to determine the efficacy of various cleaning and disinfecting methods in reducing bacterial and fungal loads on flexible fiberoptic laryngoscopes, Chang et al[272] contaminated clean endoscopes with *S aureus* and *C albicans*. The researchers exposed the contaminated endoscopes to

- 20-, 15-, 10-, and 5-minute soaks in orthophalaldehyde after precleaning in an enzymatic cleaning solution;
- 20-, 15-, 10-, and 5-minute soaks in orthophalaldehyde without precleaning in an enzymatic cleaning solution;

- a 5-minute soak in enzymatic cleaning solution;
- a 30-second wipe with antibacterial soap and water;
- a 30-second wipe with 70% isopropyl alcohol;
- a 30-second wipe with antibacterial soap followed by a 30-second wipe with 70% isopropyl alcohol; and
- a 30-second wipe with a germicidal cloth.

All exposures were followed by a 30-second rinse with utility water. The results showed that all exposures except the 5-minute soak in enzymatic cleaning solution were successful in completely eliminating the *S aureus* and *C albicans* from the contaminated endoscopes. The researchers concluded that short and simple cleaning and disinfecting protocols for non-channeled endoscopes were acceptable without sacrificing efficacy and patient safety.

In a nonexperimental study to evaluate the efficacy of chlorine dioxide wipes for disinfection of flexible nasendoscopes, Tzanidakis et al[273] randomly sampled the handles and distal tips of 31 endoscopes from a number of otolaryngology outpatient clinics. The samples were taken immediately before and after use on patients and immediately after cleaning. The researchers found that none of the samples were culture-positive after disinfection with the chlorine dioxide wipes. Three of the samples from the handles of the nasendoscope were positive for *S aureus* before use on the patient, demonstrating the potential for contamination of the area of the nasendoscope that is handled during transport that occurs after cleaning and before use. The researchers concluded that the chlorine dioxide wipes provided a safe and effective alternative to mechanical processing but recommended that personnel perform hand hygiene and don gloves before handling flexible endoscopes.

Javed et al[270] conducted a survey of 200 ear, nose, and throat outpatient departments in the United Kingdom to investigate practices for disinfection of flexible nasal endoscopes. The response to the survey was 61% (n = 121). The researchers found that the preferred method for disinfection of nasal endoscopes was chlorine dioxide wipes (58%; n = 70); however, mechanical processors were also used (34%; n = 41), as were flexible sheaths (7%; n = 8). The vast majority of respondents (65%; n = 79) performed precleaning at the point of use with an enzymatic cleaning solution. Notably, the researchers found the use of 2% glutaraldehyde as a high-level disinfectant was rare (0.8%; n = 1).

The use of chlorine dioxide wipes may be more costly than mechanical processing[270] but less costly than use of single-use endoscope sheaths.[266] Phua et al[275] evaluated the efficacy and cost-effectiveness of chlorine dioxide wipes compared with mechanical processing for processing flexible nasendoscopes. The researchers contaminated clean nasendoscopes with *S epidermidis,* exposed them to disinfection using either chlorine dioxide wipes (n = 50) or mechanical processing (n = 50), and then sampled the endoscopes. The researchers used *S epidermidis* as the test organism because it is representative of the normal flora found in the nasopharynx and larynx. The samples showed *S epidermidis* in 2% of samples (one of 50) from the chlorine dioxide group and 28% of samples (14 of 50) from the mechanical processor group. The researchers estimated costs over a 10-year period and determined that even with the expense of installation and maintenance, the mechanical processor would be less costly than the chlorine dioxide wipes and would provide an annual cost savings of approximately $25,355.82 (£16,715 [$26,467.45 in 2015 US dollars and £17,473.49 in 2015 British pounds]).

Street et al[266] audited the costs of disinfection practices in a UK hospital between July 2003 and January 2004. After determining that the cost of single-use sheaths averaged $6079.94 (£4008 [$7715.66 in 2015 US dollars and £5093.79 in 2015 British pounds]) per month, the authors introduced the use of chlorine dioxide wipes and achieved a monthly cost savings of $4770.81 (£3145 [$6054.33 in 2015 US dollars and £3997 in 2015 British pounds]).

9. Endoscope Storage

9.1 **Store flexible endoscopes and endoscope accessories in a manner that minimizes contamination and protects the device or item from damage.**[1,12,13,16,44,45,65,83] *[Recommendation]*

Several guidelines recommend effective storage of flexible endoscopes and endoscope accessories as a means of helping to ensure devices are safe for patient use.[1,12,13,16,44,45,83] The benefits of effective storage are that it helps protect the endoscopes and endoscope accessories from damage and reduces contamination.[1,12,13,16,44,45,83] Some evidence is limited due to inconsistency in outcome measures, small sample sizes,[276-282] and lack of a control.[283-287] There is no consensus regarding maximum safe storage times.[1,12,13,15,16,18-22,27,44,83]

9.2 **Store flexible endoscopes in cabinets that are situated in a secure location in the clean workroom of the endoscopy processing room in a two-room design or in a separate clean area close to, but not within, the endoscopy procedure room.**[65,288] *[Recommendation]*

Situating the storage cabinet in a secure location helps protect inventories of flexible endoscopes

and supplies that are vulnerable to misappropriation.[69,288] Locating the storage cabinet in the clean workroom or in a clean area outside of the procedure room helps prevent contamination of processed endoscopes.[69]

9.2.1 **Use storage cabinets that have doors**[23] **and are located at least 3 ft (0.9 m) from any sink.**[23] *[Recommendation]*

Ensuring storage cabinets have doors and are separated from sinks by at least 3 ft (0.9 m) provides protection and reduces the potential for processed flexible endoscopes to be contaminated by water droplets.[12,13,16,22,23,27]

9.3 **Store flexible endoscopes in accordance with the endoscope and storage cabinet manufacturers' IFU.** *[Recommendation]*

Following the manufacturers' IFU helps ensure safe and effective storage of endoscopes.

9.3.1 **Store flexible endoscopes in a drying cabinet.**[15,18,27,69] *[Recommendation]*

Optimal storage of flexible endoscopes facilitates drying, decreases the potential for contamination, and provides protection from environmental contaminants.[69,85,288]

A wide variety of storage cabinets are available.[20] Drying cabinets include a drying system that circulates HEPA-filtered air through the cabinet while filtered air under pressure is forced through the endoscope channels.[69,276,278] The internal and external surfaces of the endoscope are continuously dried, suppressing bacterial growth.[12,20,69,276,277] Studies related to the efficacy of drying cabinets compared with other methods of storage showed that drying cabinets effectively limited bacterial proliferation during storage.[276-278,283]

In a quasi-experimental study to determine whether bacterial growth occurred in flexible endoscopes during a 72-hour storage period in a drying cabinet, Foxcroft et al[276] processed 55 endoscopes, sampled the endoscopes, stored 40 of the endoscopes in a drying cabinet designed for horizontal storage of the endoscopes, and placed 15 of the endoscopes in an open storage cabinet in the endoscopy unit designed for vertical storage of the endoscopes. Each endoscope in the drying cabinet was connected individually to the HEPA-filtered air source. The cabinet was opened eight times daily to simulate normal use. At the end of the 72-hour storage period, the endoscopes were removed and sampled.

The researchers found that of a total of 64 samples collected from the endoscopes stored in the drying cabinet, only one sample (taken immediately after processing) showed bacterial growth (1 CFU coagulase-negative *Staphylococcus*). The researchers theorized this was likely the result of laboratory contamination since no other cultures from the endoscope were positive. Of the 44 samples collected from the endoscopes stored in the open cabinet, only one sample (taken immediately after processing) showed bacterial growth (1 CFU *Streptococcus*, 1 CFU *Propionbacterium*). The researchers also placed culture plates in the storage cabinets to evaluate and compare environmental contaminants within the cabinets. They found that the culture plates from the drying cabinet had significantly fewer organisms detected than the culture plates placed in the open cabinet. The researchers concluded that a 72-hour storage time did not result in increased bacterial counts in any of the stored endoscopes.[276]

Grandval et al[283] evaluated the microbial levels of endoscopes after clinical use and processing, followed by 72 hours of storage in

- a drying cabinet designed for horizontal storage of the endoscopes (Group 1; n = 41 [colonoscopes = 13; gastroscopes = 21; duodenoscopes = 7]),
- a dedicated storage cabinet designed for vertical storage of the endoscopes without daily disinfection (Group 2; n = 41 [colonoscopes = 17; gastroscopes = 17; duodenoscopes = 7]), and
- a dedicated storage cabinet designed for vertical storage of the endoscopes with daily disinfection (Group 3; n = 41 [colonoscopes = 20; gastroscopes = 15; duodenoscopes = 6]).

The researchers found that 100% of the Group 1 endoscopes had a contamination level consistent with the preset target level (< 5 CFU/endoscope), and 56% of these (n = 23) were completely free of contamination. Of the Group 2 and 3 endoscopes, 88% (n = 36) had a contamination level consistent with the preset target level. Of the Group 2 endoscopes, 41% (n = 17) were completely free of contamination, and of the Group 3 endoscopes, 61% (n = 25) were completely free of contamination. The researchers concluded that the use of a drying cabinet was the most effective method for maintaining microbial loads within the preset target level.[283]

In a quasi-experimental study of the efficacy of a drying cabinet, Pineau et al[277] artificially contaminated one colonoscope, one gastroscope, and one enteroscope with *P aeruginosa*;

stored them first inside and then outside of a drying cabinet designed for vertical storage of the endoscopes; and then sampled the endoscopes at 12, 24, 28, and 72 hours. The results showed that when the endoscopes were stored in the drying cabinet, microbial contamination levels were lower than the number of bacteria initially introduced. The researchers theorized that the level would continue to decrease considerably thereafter. For endoscopes stored outside of the drying cabinet, microbial levels were stable or increased. These data demonstrated the advantages of drying cabinets in limiting bacterial proliferation in the internal channels of endoscopes during storage.

Wardle[278] conducted a quasi-experimental study to determine whether gastroscopes and colonoscopes stored in a drying cabinet designed for vertical storage of the endoscopes grew microorganisms in the channels within 72 hours. The researcher evaluated the microbial levels of two gastroscopes and six colonoscopes after clinical use and processing followed by 72 hours of storage in a drying cabinet. The results showed there was no microbial growth in any of the endoscopes. The researcher concluded that flexible endoscopes could be stored in the drying cabinet and used without reprocessing for up to 72 hours but speculated that because of the effectiveness of the cabinet, the endoscopes could be safely used after storage for up to 1 week.

9.3.2 | **If a drying cabinet is not available, store flexible endoscopes in a closed cabinet with HEPA-filtered air that provides positive pressure and allows air circulation around the flexible endoscopes.**[1,13,19,27,65,85] *[Conditional Recommendation]*

Ventilation promotes continued drying of the endoscope. Using HEPA-filtered air may help prevent bacterial growth in the endoscope. Positive pressure may help prevent contamination of stored endoscopes.

9.3.3 | **Do not store flexible endoscopes in the original shipment cases.**[12,15,27,45,65,83,84] *[Recommendation]*

The cases are difficult to clean, may be contaminated,[45] and are designed for shipping only.[65]

9.4 | **Store flexible endoscopes that have been mechanically processed in a cabinet that is either**
- **designed and intended by the cabinet manufacturer for horizontal storage of flexible endoscopes or**

- of sufficient height, width, and depth to allow flexible endoscopes to hang vertically, without coiling and without touching the bottom of the cabinet.[1,12,13,15-20,27,44,45,65,85,93]

[Recommendation]

Some drying cabinets are designed by the manufacturer for horizontal storage of flexible endoscopes. Using a cabinet of sufficient height, depth, and width helps prevent damage that might occur from one endoscope hitting another.[16] Hanging flexible endoscopes vertically helps prevent coiling or kinking of the endoscope.[12,17,65]

9.5 Store flexible endoscopes with all valves open[22] and removable parts detached but stored with the endoscope.[1,13,15,16,18-20,22,27,44,83,85] *[Recommendation]*

Leaving valves open and removable parts detached facilitates drying of the endoscope.[85] Insufficient drying creates an environment conducive to microbial growth and promotes the formation of biofilm.[82] Storing removable parts with the endoscope helps prevent loss and facilitates traceability.[13,22]

Alfa et al[131] surveyed 37 hospitals across Canada and collected samples from the biopsy channel of duodenoscopes to assess processing practices and evaluate levels of bioburden in patient-ready duodenoscopes. The researchers found that 43% of centers (n = 16) were compliant with national processing guidelines. All of the samples with low levels of organisms (< 200 CFU/mL) had gram-positive organisms, whereas the samples with more than 200 CFU/mL had predominantly gram-negative organisms. *S maltophilia* was the most common organism (ie, in six of eight samples). The researchers suggested that this was likely caused by growth of water-related organisms resulting from removable parts being left on the endoscope during storage.

9.6 Identify flexible endoscopes that are processed and ready for use with a distinct visual cue.[12,17,19,45,65,83] *[Recommendation]*

Identifying endoscopes that are ready for use and distinguishing them from unprocessed endoscopes may help prevent use of a contaminated endoscope.[12,65]

After identifying two incidents in which used, contaminated flexible endoscopes were returned to the clean storage area without HLD, Nomides et al[289] created a visual cue that would readily identify endoscopes that had been processed and were ready for patient use. Infection prevention and sterile processing team members worked with a manufacturer to develop a green locking tie that was applied to the endoscopes after processing. The tie prevented the endoscope from being used until removal by the user.[289]

Personnel who processed flexible endoscopes were educated about the new system and the use of locking ties was implemented in all areas where endoscopes were processed. Endoscopes with the locking tie were readily identified as processed and ready for patient use. If there was no tie on the endoscope, it was processed and a tie was applied before storage. After implementation of this system, 94% of the endoscopy suites were compliant, and no additional incidents of using contaminated endoscopes were identified. The authors concluded that the use of a distinct, visual cue was an effective way to identify processed endoscopes and improve patient safety.

9.7 Visually inspect flexible endoscopes and storage cabinets for cleanliness before endoscopes are placed into or removed from storage.[13]

- If there is any evidence of contamination of the endoscope (eg, soil, moisture), reprocess the endoscope before use.[13]
- If there is any evidence of contamination of the cabinet (eg, wet spots, soil, fecal odor), remove and reprocess all endoscopes in the cabinet and clean the cabinet.

[Recommendation]

Reprocessing endoscopes that could be contaminated helps ensure they are safe for use. Visible soil in the storage cabinet may indicate that one or more of the stored endoscopes is contaminated. Soil in the cabinet may contaminate endoscopes stored in the cabinet.[13]

9.8 Wear clean, low-protein, powder-free, natural rubber latex gloves or latex-free gloves when handling processed flexible endoscopes and when transporting them to and from the storage cabinet. *[Recommendation]*

Sterile gloves are not required for handling processed flexible endoscopes unless the endoscope is intended to be placed on a sterile field.

Wearing clean gloves may lessen contamination of processed flexible endoscopes by the hands of personnel.[69] Using low-protein, powder-free natural rubber latex gloves or latex-free gloves can minimize latex exposure and the risk of reactions in both health care workers and patients.[42] Studies related to storage of flexible endoscopes have confirmed endoscope contamination from the hands of personnel and environmental surfaces.[279-282,284,286,287]

Muscarella[290] described the case of a processed endoscope randomly selected from an endoscope storage cabinet for surveillance purposes that yielded positive growth for both patient-borne and environmental bacteria. To investigate the potential for disease transmission, a second colonoscope was sampled immediately after use (ie, the positive control), and a third colonoscope that had been sterilized with ethylene oxide was also

Table 4. Recommendations from Professional Organizations for Flexible Endoscope Storage Time

Professional organization	Storage time
American College of Chest Physicians[27] American Associates for Bronchology	No recommendation
American Urological Association[83] Society of Urologic Nurses and Associates	7 to 10 days
American Society for Gastrointestinal Endoscopy[44]	10 to 14 days
Association for the Advancement of Medical Instrumentation[12]	Based on risk assessment
Association for Professionals in Infection Control[1]	No recommendation
Association of periOperative Registered Nurses	Based on risk assessment
British Society of Gastroenterology[20]	Up to 1 month per cabinet manufacturer
British Thoracic Society[18]	Per manufacturer
Department of Health: United Kingdom[51]	3 hours unless stored in a way validated to extend usable storage life or in a sterile package
Dutch Nurses Association: Division Gastroenterology and Hepatology[21] Sterilization Association of the Netherlands Dutch Society of Experts on Sterile Medical Devices Dutch Society for Infection Prevention and Control in the Health Care Setting	Up to 1 month in a drying or dust-free storage cabinet
European Society of Gastrointestinal Endoscopy[22] European Society of Gastroenterology and Endoscopy Nurses and Associates	Based on risk assessment
Gastroenterological Society of Australia[15] Gastroenterological Nurses College of Australia	72 hours • bronchoscopes (intubating) • colonoscopes • endoscopic ultrasound (radial) • enteroscopes (stored with continuous airflow) • gastroscopes 12 hours • bronchoscopes • duodenoscopes • endoscopic ultrasound (linear) • enteroscopes (stored hanging vertically)
Health Service Executive United Kingdom[13]	72 hours
Society of Gastroenterology Nurses and Associates[16]	7 days when processed and stored according to professional guidelines and manufacturer's instructions
World Gastroenterology Organisation[19] World Endoscopy Organization	No recommendation

sampled (ie, the negative control). Environmental surfaces were sampled, as were the hands and fingernails of personnel who handled the endoscopes. The investigator found that the bacteria from the insertion tube of the negative control and contaminated colonoscope yielded *S aureus* identical to the strain cultured from the fingernails of a newly hired team member. These results suggested that the team member's hands and fingernails were the source of the bacteria and con-

tamination of the colonoscope after processing. The investigator recommended that personnel wear clean gloves when handling processed endoscopes to prevent contamination of endoscopes before they are used on patients.

9.9 A multidisciplinary team that includes infection preventionists, endoscopy and perioperative RNs, endoscopy processing personnel, endoscopists, and other involved personnel should establish a

policy to determine the maximum storage time that processed flexible endoscopes are considered safe to use without reprocessing. *[Recommendation]*

The collective evidence regarding the maximum safe storage time for processed endoscopes is inconclusive. Recommendations from professional organizations for maximum storage times for flexible endoscopes are not in agreement; recommended storage times range from 3 hours to 1 month **(Table 4)**.

There is limited evidence to definitively establish the length of time that processed flexible endoscopes remain safe for use during storage. Studies have shown that when correctly processed, flexible endoscopes may be safe to use for 48 hours to 56 days after processing.[279,280,282,284-287] There are benefits to reducing unnecessary processing that include reduced processing costs (eg, personnel, processing supplies), reduced wear and tear on the endoscope and processing equipment, and lower replacement and repair costs.[280,286] Safe storage times may be affected by factors unique to the facility including the type of endoscopes processed and stored, processing effectiveness (eg, level of residual contamination), storage conditions (eg, restricted access, drying cabinet, HEPA-filtered air), compliance with manufacturers' IFU (ie, endoscope, mechanical processor, storage cabinet), frequency of use, and patient population.[22]

In a nonexperimental study to evaluate the survival of aerobic bacteria and fungi in gastrointestinal endoscopes that were processed after routine procedures and stored in an endoscope cabinet over the weekends, Alfa et al[285] tested all channels from 20 flexible gastrointestinal endoscopes (ie, five gastroscopes, nine colonoscopes, six duodenoscopes) used at an endoscopy clinic. The endoscopes were sampled for the presence of bacteria and fungi every Monday morning during a 7-month period. Bacteria and fungi were detected in 50.1% (n = 192) of the 383 channels tested. Of the 141 endoscopes tested, 14.1% (n = 20) had detectable microbial growth in at least one channel. The researchers concluded that with correct processing and drying, flexible endoscopes were safe to use for 48 to 72 hours after processing.

Osborne et al[284] conducted a prospective, observational study to determine a safe shelf life for flexible endoscopes in a four-suite gastroenterology unit. All flexible endoscopes in active clinical use (ie, 23 endoscopes) during a 3-week period were sampled before storage and when removed from storage (N = 194). The median shelf life ranged from 5.27 hours to 165.35 hours. The researchers found that 15.5% of samples were culture-positive (n = 30); however, only 0.5% were positive for pathogenic microorganisms (n = 1). The researchers concluded

that when processed and stored correctly, the endoscopes were safe to use for at least 120 hours.

Rejchrt et al[279] evaluated the bacterial load of gastroscopes, duodenoscopes, and colonoscopes stored in a dust-proof cabinet for 5 days. After clinical use, the endoscopes were cleaned at the point of use, manually cleaned, mechanically processed without an alcohol flush, sampled, and then stored hanging vertically in the cabinet. The researchers sampled the endoscopes for aerobic and anaerobic bacteria, including bacterial spores, and for *Candida* species after 5 days of storage. The results showed that all endoscopes were culture-negative after processing. A total of 135 samples were obtained after storage, four of which were positive for normal skin flora (*Corynebacterium pseudodiphtheriae, S epidermidis*). Notably, these samples were taken from the external surface of the endoscopes. All of the samples from the internal channels of the endoscopes were negative.

In a second phase of the study, 10 endoscopes were mechanically processed and stored in a dust-proof cabinet for 5 days and then sampled. All 10 samples were culture-negative. The researchers concluded that when correctly processed and stored, flexible endoscopes were safe to use for up to 5 days without reprocessing.[279]

Riley et al[287] conducted a nonexperimental, simulated study to establish an acceptable duration of storage before reprocessing for flexible colonoscopes processed with a liquid chemical sterilant. The researchers artificially contaminated all channels of a colonoscope with *S aureus, P aeruginosa,* and *B subtilis.* The endoscope was manually cleaned, sampled, processed, and stored by hanging vertically in a ventilated endoscope storage cabinet. The endoscope was sampled five times after 24 hours of storage and five times after 168 hours of storage. The results showed no growth at 24 hours. At 168 hours, there was no bacterial growth on four of five occasions (80%) and sparse growth (< 5 CFU/mL) of two non-test organisms (ie, coagulase-negative *Staphylococcus* [skin flora], *Micrococcus* species [skin and environmental flora]). The researchers theorized that the presence of the organisms was not a result of inadequate processing but of contamination during testing procedures or storage. The researchers concluded that when correctly processed and stored, flexible endoscopes were safe to use for a period of 7 days before reprocessing.

In a multiphase study to assess the microbiological load of endoscopes after HLD, Vergis et al[280] evaluated four duodenoscopes and three colonoscopes. In Phase 1, the endoscopes were sampled daily after HLD for a period of 2 weeks. This process was repeated in Phase 2. In Phase 3, the endoscopes were sampled daily after HLD for a period of 7 days. The researchers found that in Phase 1, six of 70 samples (8.6%) were culture-positive. No cultures were positive in Phase 2. In Phase 3, one endoscope had a positive culture for *S epidermidis*, a low-virulence skin organism. The researchers concluded that with correct processing and storage, flexible endoscopes were safe to use for a period of at least 7 days and possibly up to 14 days before reprocessing.

Brock et al[286] conducted a prospective, observational study to demonstrate whether flexible endoscopes were safe to use after storage for as long as 21 days before reprocessing. The researchers tested four duodenoscopes, two gastroscopes, and four colonoscopes. Immediately after use, the endoscopes were precleaned at the point of use, leak tested, manually cleaned, mechanically processed, flushed with alcohol, dried, sampled, and stored in a dust-free endoscope storage cabinet until removed for sampling at 7, 14, and 21 days. Notably, the cabinet was also used for storing endoscopes in active clinical use and was left open during the day but closed at night for security.

The results showed there were 33 positive cultures from 28 of the 96 sites tested, resulting in a 29.2% overall contamination rate. Of the culture-positive samples, 29 were typical skin or environmental contaminants, and thus clinically insignificant. Four potential pathogens were sampled that included *Enterococcus, C parapsilosis,* alpha-hemolytic *Streptococcus,* and *Aureobasidium pullulans;* however, the researchers theorized they were likely clinically insignificant as each was only recovered at one time point at one site and all grew in low concentrations. There were no true pathogenic isolates. The researchers concluded that correctly processed and stored flexible endoscopes were safe to use for a period of 21 days before reprocessing.[286]

Saliou and Baron[291] responded that the level of bacterial colonization in the study might have been underestimated by the researchers' use of sterile water for culture sampling. Brock et al[291] responded that the sampling methods they used were acceptable and were recommended by professional organizations such as ESGE, the CDC, and the Gastroenterological Society of Australia.

In a quasi-experimental study to examine bacterial growth in colonoscopes after various storage times, Ingram et al[282] sampled four new colonoscopes for anaerobic and aerobic bacteria after processing and after storage for 3, 5, 7, 14, 21, 28, 42, and 56 days. The colonoscopes were stored vertically in an open-air storage area. The results showed that none of the endoscopes were culture-positive after 3, 5, or 7 days of storage. After 14 days of storage, one of the endoscopes had fewer than

2 CFU of *S epidermidis* and *Staphylococcus hominis,* both common skin flora. The only other microbial growth was ≤ 1 CFU of *S epidermidis* noted in one of the endoscopes after 42 days of storage. None of the endoscopes had bacterial growth at 56 days. The researchers concluded that when correctly processed and stored, the period of time for which flexible endoscopes were considered safe to use before reprocessing could be extended to 56 days; however, further research examining viral and fungal growth on stored endoscopes was warranted.

Schmelzer et al[292] conducted a systematic review to evaluate the evidence related to endoscope storage time and included 10 studies that measured the length of endoscope storage time and microbial growth. They concluded that flexible endoscopes were safe to use for a period of 7 days before reprocessing; however, the acceptable length of storage was dependent on effective processing, thorough drying, controlled storage, and microbiological surveillance.

9.9.1 **The multidisciplinary team should establish a policy for removing and reprocessing the endoscope before use if the maximum storage time has been exceeded.** *[Recommendation]*

9.10 **Clean and disinfect storage cabinets used for flexible endoscopes with an EPA-registered hospital-grade disinfectant when visibly soiled and on a regular (eg, daily, weekly) basis.**[13,15,16,65] *[Recommendation]*

Visible soil in the storage cabinet may contaminate endoscopes stored in the cabinet.[13] Areas and equipment that are not cleaned according to a schedule may be missed during routine cleaning procedures and become environmental reservoirs for dust, debris, and microorganisms.

9.10.1 **A multidisciplinary team that includes infection preventionists, endoscopy and perioperative RNs, endoscopy processing personnel, endoscopists, and other involved personnel should establish a policy to determine the cleaning frequency of the storage cabinet.** *[Recommendation]*

Facilities with high volumes of endoscopy procedures will require more frequent cleaning of the storage cabinet.

9.11 **Store sterilized items (eg, biopsy forceps) in a sterile storage area and in accordance with the AORN Guideline for Sterilization.**[256] *[Recommendation]*

Limiting exposure to moisture, dust, or excessive handling decreases potential contamination of sterilized items.[77,256]

10. Processing Records

10.1 **The health care organization should maintain records of flexible endoscope processing and procedures.** *[Recommendation]*

Records provide data for the identification of trends and demonstration of compliance with regulatory requirements and accreditation agency standards.

Highly reliable data collection is necessary to demonstrate the health care organization's progress toward quality care outcomes.[293] Effective management and collection of health care information that accurately reflects the patient's care, treatment, and services is a regulatory requirement[294-297] and an accreditation agency standard for both hospitals[298,299] and ambulatory settings.[299-306]

10.2 **Include the following in records related to flexible endoscope processing:**
- **date**[12,13,15,83] **and time**[12,13,83];
- **identity of the endoscope and endoscope accessories**[12,13,15,20,83,84];
- **method and verification of cleaning and results of cleaning verification testing**[13,15,83,84];
- **number or identifier of the mechanical processor or sterilizer and results of process efficacy testing**[3,12,13,15,20,83,84];
- **identity of the person(s) performing the processing**[3,12,13,83];
- **lot numbers of processing solutions**[12,15];
- **disposition of defective items or equipment**[3]; **and**
- **maintenance of water systems, endoscopes and endoscope accessories, and processing equipment.**[3,12,15,83]

[Recommendation]

Records of flexible endoscope processing enable traceability in the event of a processing failure.[13,20,69,77,84] Records of endoscopes, mechanical processors or sterilizers, and processing solutions provide a source of evidence for review during investigation of clinical issues, including infections and pseudo-infections.[44] Records of water systems, endoscopes and accessories, and processing equipment maintenance provide evidence of maintenance,[69] compliance with manufacturers' IFU, and information that may be useful in determining the need for repair or replacement. Records of repairs may help to identify trends in endoscopes and processing equipment damage and help to define practices that may reduce damage.

10.3 **Include the following in records related to flexible endoscope procedures:**
- **date**[3,12,15,84] **and time,**[3,12,84]
- **identity of the patient,**[3,12,13,15,20,44,84]
- **procedure,**[3,12,44,84]
- **identity of the licensed independent practitioner performing the procedure,**[12,84] **and**
- **identity of the endoscope and endoscope accessories used during the procedure.**[3,12,13,15,18,20,44,69,84]

[Recommendation]

Records of endoscopy procedures enable traceability in the event of a processing failure.[13,18,20,69,77,84]

10.4 **Maintain records for a time period specified by the health care organization.**[77] *[Conditional Recommendation]*

11. Education

11.1 **Personnel with responsibility for processing flexible endoscopes should receive initial and ongoing education and complete competency verification activities related to processing flexible endoscopes.** *[Recommendation]*

Initial and ongoing education of endoscopy personnel facilitates the development of knowledge, skills, and attitudes that affect safe patient care. It is the responsibility of the health care organization to provide initial and ongoing education and to verify the competency of its personnel[307]; however, the primary responsibility for maintaining ongoing competency remains with the individual.[308]

Competency verification activities provide a mechanism for competency documentation and help verify that personnel processing flexible endoscopes and accessories understand the principles and processes necessary for effective processing and reducing the risk of infection from flexible endoscopes and mechanical processors.

Ongoing development of knowledge and skills and documentation of personnel participation is a regulatory requirement[294-297] and an accreditation agency standard for both hospitals[309,310] and ambulatory settings.[310-316]

11.2 **The health care organization should establish education and competency verification activities for its personnel and determine intervals for education and competency verification related to processing flexible endoscopes and accessories.** *[Conditional Recommendation]*

Education and competency verification needs and intervals are unique to the facility and to its personnel and processes.

To determine whether deficiencies existed in the processing of contaminated flexible sigmoidoscopes in family practice and internal medicine offices and whether education of office personnel resulted in a correction of identified deficiencies, Jackson and Ball[317] conducted a prospective review of processing before and after an educational course. A total of 25 persons from 19 offices (ie, 14 family practice, five internal medicine) attended one of three separate educational sessions. The course included both didactic and hands-on instruction. The instructor was a certified gastroenterology RN with infection prevention experience.

The researchers reviewed standards published by the SGNA, the Association for Professionals in Infection Control and Epidemiology (APIC), the ASGE, and the CDC, and selected 17 common standards as those most critical to effective endoscope processing. All of the participants completed a questionnaire based on the 17 standards before the course and again 2 months after the course. The researchers found that before the educational course, the 19 offices had between four and 11 deficiencies per office, with an average of 6.8 deficiencies per office. After the educational course, deficiencies ranged from zero to eight, with an average of 0.9 deficiencies per office. The researchers concluded that before the educational course, personnel from the family practice and internal medicine offices were insufficiently educated to perform flexible endoscope processing and that endoscopes were not being processed in accordance with standards. However, after the educational course, personnel processed the endoscopes according to the standards.

Lunn et al[318] reported their experience with endoscope repairs before and after implementing an educational program designed to improve handling of flexible endoscopes and equipment. The authors retrospectively reviewed the cost of endoscope repair in the 3 years preceding and in the 5 years following an educational program that included both didactic and hands-on components. The authors found that the cost of repairs during the 3 years before the educational program averaged $42 per procedure ($62.18 in 2015 US dollars). After the educational program, the repair costs dropped dramatically to $8 per procedure ($10.63 in 2015 US dollars). These reduced costs were realized despite an average 10% increase in the number of procedures being performed each year. The authors concluded that an educational program was effective in decreasing the costs of endoscope and equipment repairs.

11.3 Include the following in education and competency verification activities related to processing flexible endoscopes and accessories:
- **controlling and maintaining an environment that supports processing actions**[1,12,19,44];

- **precleaning at the point of use**[3,12,17,19,44,69,84,85];
- **transporting**[3,12,17,19,44,69,84,85];
- **leak testing**[3,12,17,19,44,69,84,85];
- **manual cleaning**[3,12,17,19,44,69,84,85];
- **inspecting**[3,12,17,19,44,69,84,85];
- **HLD, liquid chemical sterilization, packaging and sterilization**[3,12,17,19,44,69,84,85];
- **storage**[12];
- **maintaining records of processing and procedures for traceability**[12]; and
- **quality assurance measures.**[2,3]
[Recommendation]

Providing education and verifying competency helps reduce the risk of processing errors.[66]

11.4 Provide education and competency verification activities to personnel before new flexible endoscopes, accessories, cleaning and processing solutions, equipment, or procedures are introduced. *[Recommendation]*

Receiving education and completing competency verification activities before new endoscopes, accessories, cleaning and processing solutions, equipment, or procedures are introduced helps ensure safe practices in the endoscopy suite.

12. Policies and Procedures

12.1 Develop policies and procedures for processing flexible endoscopes, review them periodically, revise as necessary, and make them readily available in the practice setting in which they are used. *[Recommendation]*

Policies and procedures assist in the development of patient safety, quality assessment, and performance improvement activities. Policies and procedures also serve as operational guidelines used to minimize patients' risk for injury or complications, standardize practice, direct personnel, and establish continuous performance improvement programs. Policies and procedures establish authority, responsibility, and accountability within the practice setting.

Having policies and procedures that guide and support patient care, treatment, and services is a regulatory requirement[294-297] and an accreditation agency standard for both hospitals[319,320] and ambulatory settings.[312,320-326]

12.2 Address the following in policies and procedures related to processing flexible endoscopes:
- **controlling and maintaining an environment that supports processing actions**[30];
- **precleaning at the point of use**[12];

- transporting[12];
- leak testing[12];
- manual cleaning[12];
- inspecting[12];
- HLD, liquid chemical sterilization, packaging, and sterilization[12];
- storage[12];
- maintaining records of processing and procedures for traceability[12]; and
- quality assurance measures.[2,3]

[Recommendation]

Effective processing of flexible endoscopes and accessories begins with clear and detailed policies and procedures.

12.3 **Make the manufacturers' IFU readily available and monitor that personnel responsible for processing flexible endoscopes are following the IFUs. Review the manufacturer's IFU periodically, and align processing practices to comply with the most current IFU. [Recommendation]**

Instructions for use identify the validated processes necessary to achieve effective processing.[77] Manufacturers may make modifications to their IFU when new technology becomes available, when regulatory requirements change, or when modifications are made to a device.

12.4 **Develop policies and procedures for managing loaned endoscopes, accessories, and equipment in accordance with the AORN Guideline for Cleaning and Care of Surgical Instruments.[58] [Recommendation]**

The systematic management of loaned instrumentation reduces loss and helps ensure effective processing through increased collaboration, communication, and accountability.[58]

13. Quality

13.1 **The health care organization's quality management program should evaluate processing of flexible endoscopes. [Recommendation]**

Quality assurance and performance improvement programs can facilitate the identification of problem areas and assist personnel in evaluating and improving the quality of patient care and formulating plans for corrective action. These programs provide data that may be used to determine whether an individual organization is within **benchmark** goals, and if not, to identify areas that may require corrective action. A quality management program provides a mechanism to evaluate effectiveness of processes, compliance with manufacturer's IFU, endoscopy processing policies and procedures, and function of equipment.

Collecting data to monitor and improve patient care, treatment, and services is a regulatory requirement[294-297] and an accreditation agency standard for both hospitals[327-334] and ambulatory settings.[332-345]

13.2 **Include the following in the quality assurance and performance improvement program for processing flexible endoscopes:**
- **periodically reviewing and evaluating processing activities to verify compliance or to identify the need for improvement,**
- **identifying corrective actions directed toward improvement priorities, and**
- **taking additional actions when improvement is not achieved or sustained.**

[Recommendation]

Reviewing and evaluating quality assurance and performance improvement activities may identify failure points that contribute to errors in processing flexible endoscopes and help define actions for improvement and increased competency.[85] Taking corrective actions may improve patient safety by enhancing understanding of the principles of and compliance with best practices for processing flexible endoscopes.

Evans[346] described a quality improvement initiative undertaken to improve processing of flexible cystoscopes following anecdotal reports of an increased incidence of urinary tract infections after cystoscopy procedures. The author first conducted a literature search to determine best practices for processing flexible cystoscopes. She reviewed the manufacturer's IFU to ensure cystoscopes were being processed in a manner consistent with the IFU, conducted a gap analysis to identify problematic areas, and developed a plan to address them. She then shadowed clinical personnel for 2 days and conducted interviews to ensure that personnel understood and adhered to best practices for effective processing. The author developed a process improvement tool to audit compliance, and provided remediation on an ongoing basis as needed. The quality improvement process was successful in improving processing of flexible cystoscopes and enhancing patient safety.

13.3 **Personnel participating in endoscopy procedures or responsible for processing flexible endoscopes and accessories should participate in ongoing quality assurance and performance improvement activities related to processing flexible endoscopes by identifying processes that are important for**
- **monitoring quality,**
- **developing strategies for compliance,**
- **establishing benchmarks to evaluate quality indicators,**

- collecting data related to the levels of performance and quality indicators,
- evaluating practice based on the cumulative data collected,
- taking action to improve compliance, and
- assessing the effectiveness of the actions taken. [Recommendation]

Participating in ongoing quality assurance and performance improvement activities is a primary responsibility of endoscopy personnel engaged in practice.[307]

13.4 The health care organization should monitor compliance with the use of PPE in the endoscopy suite. [Recommendation]

Moderate-quality evidence shows there are lapses in compliance with the use of PPE.[190,347,348]

In a survey commissioned by the Disinfection Management Committee of the Korean Society of Gastrointestinal Endoscopy, Park et al[190] assessed compliance of 100 nurses and nursing assistants from the endoscopy units of eight secondary or tertiary Korean hospitals with Korean national guidelines for processing flexible endoscopes. The researchers found that the activity with the lowest compliance was wearing protective eyewear, with only 32% of respondents complying; 72% complied with wearing surgical masks, and 80% complied with wearing gloves. The researchers concluded that education combined with periodic surveillance could improve compliance.

Angtuaco et al[347] conducted a survey of 250 gastroenterologists and gastrointestinal endoscopy nurses from the American Board of Internal Medicine and the SGNA to determine and compare compliance with standard precautions and the use of PPE. A total of 77 gastroenterologists and 157 gastrointestinal endoscopy nurses responded to the survey. The results of the survey showed that

- 32% of the gastroenterologists (n = 25) and 50% of the nurses (n = 79) washed their hands before and after contact with patients,
- 5% of the gastroenterologists (n = 4) and 30% of the nurses (n = 47) wore gloves during patient contact,
- 14% of the gastroenterologists (n = 11) and 21% of the nurses (n = 33) wore face shields during procedures, and
- 29% of the gastroenterologists (n = 22) and 46% of the nurses (n = 72) wore protective gowns during procedures.

When asked to provide an assessment of their own compliance with standard precautions and use of PPE, 45% of gastroenterologists (n = 35) and 60% of nurses (n = 94) reported that they always complied. The researchers concluded that compliance

with standard precautions for both groups was low, but was greater for the nurses than for the gastroenterologists.[347]

In a survey of 300 randomly selected gastrointestinal endoscopy units in Spain to assess compliance with occupational risk prevention measures, Baudet et al[348] received responses from 196 units (65%). The researchers found that personnel in

- 19% of the units (n = 38) wore protective eyewear,
- 99% of the units (n = 195) wore gloves,
- 46% of the units (n = 90) wore masks, and
- 21% of the units (n = 42) wore protective gowns.

The researchers concluded that compliance with occupational risk prevention measures in Spain was lacking and improvement was needed.

13.5 A multidisciplinary team that includes facility engineers, endoscopy processing personnel, infection preventionists, and other involved personnel should establish a policy to determine processes for monitoring and auditing facility water quality to ensure compliance with requirements for endoscope processing as specified in the endoscope, processing equipment, and processing products manufacturers' IFU. Assess water quality and water filtration systems at established intervals[119,213,214,216,247,349-358] and after major maintenance to the water supply system.[359] [Recommendation]

Water quality varies seasonably and after water-source maintenance. Periodic testing can indicate whether the chemical combination used to condition the water used for endoscope processing requires adjusting.[119] Water-quality checks measure objective performance criteria (eg, pH, hardness) that have a direct effect on the outcomes.[119] The quality of the water is a consideration when determining the necessary level of filtration.[119,215,353,354,357,359-362] The need for repairs or modifications to the water treatment system can be identified from a water-quality check.[119] Monitoring water quality also assists in determining the performance of the filters and whether replacement is necessary.[353,356,358] Failing to regularly replace filters may result in bacterial growth on the filter and contamination of the water supply.[354,356] Contamination of the water supply may increase the patient's risk for infection. Monitoring water quality provides an opportunity for controlling exposure of the endoscope to waterborne contamination and subsequent exposure of patients to potential pathogens.[214,358,361,363]

Quality processes can be enhanced by audits that are conducted on a regular basis.[119,358,362] Regular monitoring and auditing of water quality may help prevent incidents related to contaminated water,[247,349,350,352,353,362,364] including infection[365] and pseudo-infection.[213-216,356,357,359,360]

Rossetti et al[357] reported 16 isolates of *Mycobacterium gordonae* from 267 patients undergoing bronchoscopy procedures. This finding was significant because in the previous 7 years, only one isolate of *M gordonae* was found among 1,368 patients. The investigators found there had been a failure in water filter replacement and water system maintenance. Replacement of the water filters and restoration of periodic assessment of water quality ended the pseudo-infections.

Rosengarten et al[215] reported a cluster of *Burkholderia cepacia* pseudo-infections associated with a contaminated mechanical processor in a bronchoscopy unit. Bronchoalveolar lavage samples obtained from three patients on three consecutive days grew organisms identified as *B cepacia* on culture; however, there were no clinical manifestations of infection in any of the patients. All of the patients had been examined with the same bronchoscope. Examination of the mechanical processor revealed that the 0.2-μm bacteria-retentive filter on the water supply line was missing, and this missing filter was the probable cause of the cluster of pseudo-infections. The mechanical processor was thoroughly cleaned and disinfected, and the missing filter was replaced. Subsequent samples were negative for *B cepacia.* The investigators concluded that a failure to follow the manufacturer's IFU by not installing the 0.2-μm filter had enabled bacteria to enter the mechanical processor and contaminate it and the bronchoscopes.

Chroneou et al[213] described a pseudo-outbreak of *M chelonae* in bronchoalveolar lavage fluid that was traced to a contaminated mechanical processor. The investigators obtained environmental samples from 17 different components of the processor, from the brushes used to clean the bronchoscopes, and from the utility water used to rinse the bronchoscopes. The investigators found the source of the outbreak was a filtration system malfunction that occurred because of a failure to change the water filters on schedule. It was not clear who had the responsibility for changing the filters at the scheduled time. Developing a process to ensure the water filters were changed on a monthly basis and assigning this responsibility to biomedical personnel eliminated the pseudo-outbreak strain.

13.6 **A multidisciplinary team that includes facility engineers, endoscopy processing personnel, infection preventionists, and other involved personnel should collaborate with manufacturer service personnel to determine schedules for preventive maintenance of flexible endoscopes,** mechanical processors, and other equipment (eg, the drying cabinet) used for processing flexible endoscopes. *[Recommendation]*

A regular program of preventative maintenance helps identify and mitigate potential risks.[22] Mechanical processors that are not maintained or functioning correctly may cause processing failures of flexible endoscopes and increase the risk for transmission of infection.[209,218,367] Schlenz and French[209] reported an outbreak of multidrug-resistant *P aeruginosa* infection involving 11 patients, eight of whom had undergone bronchoscopy procedures with two of three facility bronchoscopes that had been processed in a malfunctioning mechanical processor. There were no maintenance records, and no maintenance had been performed on the processor since its purchase 1 year previously. The tubing, filter, and pump system had to be replaced before the processor was free of *Pseudomonas* species. The bronchoscopes had likewise not been maintained and required replacement parts. The investigators concluded that regular, controlled, professional maintenance of mechanical processors and bronchoscopes was necessary for safe, effective processing of flexible endoscopes.

In a study to monitor the quality of gastrointestinal endoscope processing, Chiu et al[367] randomly sampled flexible endoscopes immediately after completion of mechanical processing. During the study, the researchers found that the endoscopes processed in one particular mechanical processor were culture-positive in spite of manual cleaning and mechanical processing. The service representative discovered that a relief valve from the mechanical processor was damaged and loose. After the valve was replaced, subsequent cultures were negative. The researchers recommended that mechanical processors undergo preventive maintenance at least every 3 to 6 months.

Méan et al[218] reported an incident involving 72 patients who underwent endoscopy procedures. The endoscopes used during the procedures were mechanically processed in a malfunctioning mechanical processor. The malfunction was reported by a nurse who became alarmed when the processor printed a validation ticket even though there was no cleaning solution in the mechanical processor. The processing failure was caused by a malfunction of the sensor whose function was to control the level of cleaning solution in the processor. An undetermined number of cleaning cycles had been skipped; however, the manual cleaning and HLD cycles were completed correctly. The investigators concluded that this incident highlighted the importance of regular preventive maintenance for mechanical processors.

Regular maintenance and replacement of endoscope lumens contaminated with biofilm may help to prevent transmission of infection.[368] In some cases, outbreaks of infection[136,217,365,369,370] and pseudo-infection[368] transmitted via flexible endoscopes were only stopped when the scope was sent to the manufacturer for repair and replacement of the lumen.[368]

DiazGranados et al[371] reported a cluster of 12 patients with respiratory cultures positive for *P aeruginosa*, 11 of whom had undergone bronchoscopy with the same bronchoscope. Processing procedures were reviewed by the infection prevention team and found to be acceptable. Despite appropriate processing, *P aeruginosa* was recovered from the bronchoscope. The investigators found that the bronchoscope had been in use for 16 months, and during that time, regular visual inspections and leak testing had been performed. The bronchoscope had been submitted to the manufacturer for repair three times but not for preventive maintenance, and the last repair was performed 8 months before the pseudo-outbreak. The bronchoscope was sent to the manufacturer who found multiple defects including kinking of the forceps channel tube, damage to the bending section sheath cover, pinching of the insertion tube, and peeling of the light-guide tube coating. The investigators concluded that regular preventive maintenance inspections were necessary to prevent similar occurrences.

Corne et al[368] investigated an outbreak of *P aeruginosa* infections (n = 9) and pseudo-infections (n = 7). Inspection of the internal channels of the involved bronchoscopes revealed large surface defects in the internal channels. The researchers theorized the defects were caused by biopsy forceps. The breaches in the internal channels prevented effective cleaning and processing of the endoscopes even though processing personnel adhered to the manufacturer's IFU. The outbreaks were controlled when the manufacturer replaced the inner channels of the bronchoscopes and the facility began using single-use biopsy forceps. The investigators concluded that the outbreaks emphasized the need to establish maintenance procedures for detecting damage to the internal channels of flexible bronchoscopes.

Qiu et al[369] investigated a duodenoscope that was manually cleaned and mechanically processed multiple times but continued to be culture-positive for *P aeruginosa*. The duodenoscope was sent to the manufacturer, who replaced the internal lumens of the device. Thereafter, the duodenoscope was culture-negative.

Zweigner et al[217] reported an outbreak of carbapenem-resistant *K pneumoniae* involving eight patients. A review of the processing procedures did not identify any deviations from the manufacturer's IFU. The outbreak ended when the bronchoscopes associated with the infections (n = 2) were submitted to the manufacturer who found defects in the internal channels of both endoscopes. The investigators concluded that the outbreak underlined the importance of regular preventive maintenance for flexible endoscopes.

In a CDC Epidemic Intelligence Service[370] investigation to review a duodenoscope-associated cluster of carbapenem-resistant *Bacteriaceae* infections in which no breaches in processing or device defects were identified to explain transmission, the investigators returned all duodenoscopes with positive cultures (n = 8) to the manufacturer for assessment. Only one duodenoscope was returned because it was not functioning correctly. The remaining seven duodenoscopes were returned as part of the investigation and had no obvious defects or functional issues. They had undergone and passed leak tests after each use and were functioning without any noticeable problems.

The manufacturer identified critical repair issues in all eight duodenoscopes that included cracks, leak test failures, frayed bending sections, and other issues related to biopsy forceps passage (eg, breaches in the biopsy channel). Notably, there was no preventive maintenance schedule recommended by the manufacturer. The investigators concluded that the lack of preventive maintenance was concerning. A process for the manufacturer to regularly inspect and service duodenoscopes was established that included random selection of duodenoscopes that were then sent to the manufacturer at predetermined intervals.[370]

Damage may occur with repetitive use of endoscopes that suggests a need for limiting the duration a reusable device is used.[372] Lee et al[372] conducted a quasi-experimental study to compare differences in surface alterations between not-aged and simulated-aged samples of endoscope materials. The researchers inoculated the samples with *E coli*, *P aeruginosa*, and *Mycobacterium terrae* artificial test soil, and then exposed the endoscope materials to identical processing conditions. The researchers found significantly more abrasions, cracks, and holes in the aged samples. They concluded that surface alterations on the samples of the endoscope material increased during repetitive use and processing. The possibility of accumulation of microorganisms and organic substances increased accordingly, and this also increased the risk of infection transmission.

13.6.1 Align the schedule for preventive maintenance with the manufacturer's IFU.[13,21,58,366] *[Recommendation]*

13.6.2 Base the frequency of preventive maintenance on variables that are unique to the facility.[366] *[Conditional Recommendation]*

Variables unique to the facility, such as the type of endoscopes that are used, the amount of use of the endoscopes, the type of damage that occurs to the endoscope, the thoroughness of the cleaning processes, the implements that are used to clean the endoscopes, the type of water used in the facility, and other factors may affect the need to increase or decrease the frequency of preventative maintenance.

13.6.3 Test mechanical processors for performance on installation; at regular, established intervals (eg, daily, weekly); after major repairs; and after changes in programmed parameters (eg, temperature, cycle time).[21,58] *[Recommendation]*

Testing the function of mechanical processors confirms the equipment is operating correctly. Effective processing is dependent on correctly functioning equipment.

13.6.4 Have qualified individuals perform preventive maintenance.[21,22,85] *[Recommendation]*

Preventive maintenance requires special skills and knowledge that includes systematic inspection, testing, measurement, adjustment, detection, parts replacement, and correction of device or equipment malfunction either before it occurs or before it develops into major failure. Having qualified personnel perform preventive maintenance increases the probability that repair and service will be performed correctly.[58]

13.7 Verify manual cleaning of flexible endoscopes using cleaning verification tests when new endoscopes are purchased and at established intervals (eg, after each use, daily). *[Recommendation]*

Moderate-quality evidence shows that manual cleaning is a learned skill subject to human error.[373] Cleaning verification tests are used to verify the ability of the cleaning process to remove, or reduce to an acceptable level, the organic soil and microbial contamination that occurs during use of a reusable device.[77,374] Cleaning verification tests include **adenosine triphosphate** (ATP) and chemical **reagent** tests for detecting clinically relevant soils (eg, protein, carbohydrate). Periodic verification of cleaning effectiveness may help reduce errors in manual cleaning and improve effectiveness.[90,183,373]

No single method of cleaning verification has been established as a standard for assessing the outcome of endoscope processing.[45]

Efficacy of cleaning has traditionally been evaluated visually; however, visual inspection alone, even with magnification, is not sufficient to determine cleanliness of complex devices such as flexible endoscopes.[12,90,374,375] Visual inspection is subjective. Infectious microorganisms are not visible to the naked eye. It is also not possible to visually inspect the lumens of flexible endoscopes.[12,90,374] Residual soil may remain and prevent effective subsequent HLD or sterilization.[375]

There is a need for rapid testing methods to detect residual soil and verify the adequacy of manual cleaning.[376] Although no studies have been conducted linking clinical outcomes with using monitors for cleaning verification,[377] auditing the manual cleaning of flexible endoscopes provides an objective method for verifying cleanliness and helps ensure that insufficiently cleaned flexible endoscopes are recleaned before HLD or sterilization.[90,183,377,378]

Alfa et al[252] conducted a quasi-experimental study to determine the type and amount of soil found in various types of flexible endoscopes before and after cleaning. The researchers' intent was that the determination of expected soil levels would help establish parameters for worst-case soil cleaning efficacy benchmarks. The researchers assessed suction channels from 10 bronchoscopes, 10 duodenoscopes, and 10 colonoscopes immediately after use for levels of bilirubin, hemoglobin, protein, sodium ion, carbohydrate, endotoxin, and viable bacteria. An additional set of endoscope suction channels (ie, 10 bronchoscopes, 10 duodenoscopes, 10 colonoscopes) were evaluated for the same components after manual cleaning but before mechanical processing for subsequent clinical use. The researchers found the worst-case soil levels in the suction channels were

- protein: 115 $\mu g/cm^2$,
- sodium ion: 7.4 micromole/cm^2,
- hemoglobin: 85 $\mu g/cm^2$,
- bilirubin: 299 nanomole/cm^2,
- carbohydrate: 29.1 $\mu g/cm^2$,
- endotoxin: 9852 EU/cm^2, and
- bacteria: 7.1-$\log_{10}$ CFU/cm^2.

After cleaning, the levels of protein, endotoxin, and sodium ion were reduced five- to ten-fold. Carbohydrate and bilirubin were reduced to undetectable levels. The average load of viable bacteria was reduced from between 3-$\log_{10}$ to 5-$\log_{10}$ CFU/cm^2. Residual hemoglobin was only detectable in bronchoscopes. The researchers concluded the data demonstrated that cleaning reduced or eliminated many components of organic soil, but a substantial amount of viable bacteria and protein may still remain on the endoscope.[252]

In a study to evaluate contamination of patient-used endoscopes using visual inspection and rapid cleaning verification tests and to determine which testing instruments and methods could be used for quality improvement initiatives related to flexible endoscope processing, Visrodia et al[375] sampled endoscopes used for gastrointestinal procedures after precleaning at the point of use and after manual cleaning. During 37 examinations of 12 endoscopes, the researchers visually inspected 121 endoscope components and conducted 249 rapid cleaning verification tests. The researchers found that regardless of whether there was visible soil on the endoscope after precleaning at the point of use, all endoscopes had high levels of ATP and detectable blood or protein. Although there was no visible soil on any of the endoscopes after manual cleaning, 82% had at least one positive cleaning verification test. The researchers concluded that relying solely on visual inspection after manual cleaning and before HLD was insufficient to ensure processing effectiveness. The researchers theorized that using more than one cleaning verification testing method may be necessary to ensure contamination is consistently detected before endoscopes are processed and used on patients.

In a quasi-experimental study to determine whether colonoscope and gastroscope contamination that occurred during clinical use persisted despite processing in accordance with US guidelines, Ofstead et al[379] performed microbiological cultures and rapid cleaning verification tests for ATP, protein, hemoglobin, and carbohydrate residue during 60 examinations of 15 endoscopes (ie, two new and 13 patient-used [ie, seven colonoscopes, six esophagogastroduodenoscopes without elevator channels]). Benchmarks were set at ATP < 200 relative light units (RLU), protein 120 µg/mL, carbohydrate 210 µg/mL, and hemoglobin 0.25 µg/mL. The researchers assessed endoscope contamination immediately after point-of-use precleaning, manual cleaning, HLD, and overnight storage. The researchers found that

- after point-of-use precleaning, 13 of 13 endoscopes (100%) had detectable protein, hemoglobin, and ATP, and 12 of 13 (92%) harbored viable microorganisms;
- after manual cleaning, 12 of 13 endoscopes (92%) had protein or ATP exceeding the benchmarks and six endoscopes (46%) had at least one positive culture;
- after HLD, eight of 11 endoscopes (73%) were positive for contamination exceeding benchmarks,

and viable microorganisms were found on seven endoscopes (64%); and

- after overnight storage, nine of 11 endoscopes (82%) were positive, and one of 11 (9%) harbored microorganisms.

Viable microorganisms were recovered from patient-ready endoscopes after all processing steps including HLD. The researchers concluded that despite processing in accordance with US guidelines, viable microorganisms persisted on patient-used flexible endoscopes, and this suggested that current guidelines might not be sufficient to ensure successful processing. The results of the study also suggested that rapid cleaning verification tests were valid and reliable and that it might be beneficial to test for both protein and ATP because one was often present without the other. Assessing the efficacy of manual cleaning using rapid cleaning verification tests allowed processing personnel to be immediately informed when test results exceeded established benchmarks. Endoscopes could then be recleaned before HLD or sterilization.[379]

Hansen et al[380] compared ATP testing with microbiological culturing by examining 108 flexible endoscopes (ie, 40 gastroscopes, eight duodenoscopes, 42 bronchoscopes, 18 colonoscopes) after processing. Benchmarks for positive ATP were set at < 30 RLU and < 100 RLU based on the manufacturer's IFU. The researchers considered all microbiological growth to be positive, regardless of the species or number of CFU. The researchers found that 26% of the endoscopes had bacterial growth (n = 28 [ie, nine gastroscopes, one duodenoscope, 13 bronchoscopes, five colonoscopes]). Using < 30 RLU as the benchmark, 62% of the endoscopes were positive for ATP (n = 67 [ie, 25 gastroscopes, six duodenoscopes, 24 bronchoscopes, 12 colonoscopes]). Using < 100 RLU as the benchmark, 19% were positive for ATP (n = 21; [ie, seven gastroscopes, one duodenoscope, eight bronchoscopes, five colonoscopes]). The researchers concluded that it was beneficial to implement ATP testing as a method to identify ineffective cleaning of flexible endoscopes and the need for recleaning before HLD or sterilization.

13.7.1 **A multidisciplinary team that includes infection preventionists, endoscopists, endoscopy processing personnel, and other involved personnel should establish the type of cleaning verification test to be performed.** *[Recommendation]*

There are a number of tests that can be used to assess cleaning efficacy.[90,373,378,381] Chemical tests involve the use of a reagent and observing for a color change that indicates the presence of organic markers such as protein or blood.[90,373,381]

In a dual phase (ie, simulated-use, in-use) study to validate the use of an audit tool composed of reagent test strips in 43 endoscopy clinics across Canada, Alfa et al[381] collected samples from 30 patient-used endoscopes (ie, 10 colonoscopes, 10 duodenoscopes, 10 gastroscopes) and tested them for residual protein, carbohydrate, and hemoglobin using the audit tool test strips. The test strips had three reagent pads designed to rapidly detect organic residuals of protein, carbohydrate, and hemoglobin after manual cleaning. The researchers confirmed that the audit tool flagged endoscopes with residual protein, hemoglobin, or carbohydrate.[373] In the second phase of the study, the researchers sent prototype testing kits to 44 endoscopy clinics in 23 health care facilities across Canada and conducted a survey to obtain feedback from processing personnel using a 5 point analog rating scale. The results of the survey showed that processing personnel valued the audit tool and thought it was important for confirming the adequacy of manual cleaning. Respondents also thought the test was easy to use, that it should be used on some endoscopes daily, and that it should be part of the quality assurance program for the endoscopy unit.[381]

Quantitative tests provide a measurement against which cleaning results can be compared.[90] Adenosine triphosphate bioluminescence is an example of a quantitative test.[378] The item to be tested is swabbed to collect ATP, the swab is inserted into a reaction tube, and the ATP on the swab reacts with the chemicals in the reaction tube.[58] The reaction tube is then inserted into a hand-held luminometer that converts the ATP released from microorganisms or human cells into a light signal, which is measured in RLU.[58]

Obee et al[374] conducted a nonexperimental study to compare the efficacy of endoscope processing using microbiological surveillance and ATP bioluminescence. Following visual observation of manual cleaning, the researchers sampled eight different areas on 63 gastrointestinal endoscopes (N = 504) before, during, and after processing. The benchmarks for positive results were set at ATP > 500 RLU and microbiological culture ≥ 3 CFU per sample. The researchers found that a total of 32 cultures (6.3%) and 95 ATP tests (18.8%) were positive; however, after processing, only three cultures (0.6%) and one ATP test (0.2%) were positive. The researchers concluded that ATP provided a rapid means of assessing the efficacy of manual cleaning before HLD.

In a prospective study carried out in a gastrohepatology unit to evaluate using ATP bioluminescence to verify manual cleaning of flexible endoscopes, Fernando et al[382] obtained samples from the lumens of endoscopes and tested the endoscopes using ATP in 120 endoscopic procedures. The samples were obtained before the procedure, after the procedure, after manual cleaning, and after mechanical processing. The ATP benchmark was set at < 100 RLU. If the after-processing benchmark was exceeded, the endoscope was reprocessed and retested.

The researchers found the average RLU reading before the procedure was 48 RLU. After the procedure, the average reading was 124,052 RLU. After manual cleaning the average reading was 1,423 RLU, and after mechanical processing, the average reading was 144 RLU. The corresponding culture results before the procedure were all negative. After the procedure, only four cultures were negative. After manual cleaning, 26 cultures were negative, and after mechanical processing, all cultures were negative. Twenty-one (18%) of the post-mechanical processing cultures were initially positive; however, after reprocessing, the cultures were negative. The researchers concluded that ATP testing had the potential to play an important role in verifying that flexible endoscopes had been effectively processed and were safe to use. They posited that because the results were available so rapidly, the test could be easily performed before every procedure.[382]

In a nonexperimental study to evaluate ATP, microbial load, and protein as potential indicators of gastrointestinal endoscope cleanliness, Fushimi et al[383] sampled exterior surfaces and interior suction/accessory channels of 12 endoscopes used in 41 patients. The researchers found that before cleaning, the ATP levels were 10,417 RLU from the exterior surfaces and 30,281 RLU from the channels. After cleaning, these values decreased to 82 RLU and 104 RLU, respectively. Before cleaning, the microbial load was 5,143 CFU per sample exterior and 95,827 CFU per sample channels. After cleaning, the microbial load was 1 CFU per sample exterior and 104 CFU per sample channels. Before cleaning, the protein level was 36 μg per sample channels; after cleaning, the level was 20 μg per sample. There was a significant change in ATP and microbial load; however, the decrease in protein levels was not significant. The researchers concluded that ATP measurement provided a reliable, rapid, and practical assessment of endoscope cleanliness for routine monitoring in the clinical setting.

In a quasi-experimental, three-phase study, Sciortino et al[384] investigated and evaluated the use of a portable luminometer system for detecting contamination after cleaning and HLD of flexible endoscopes. In Phase 1, the researchers conducted a microbiological analysis of 15 endoscopes (ie, five processed, one cleaned, nine contaminated). The researchers found that the five processed endoscopes were culture-negative. The other 10 endoscopes were culture-positive. Notably, the internal channel of one of the culture-positive endoscopes was visibly contaminated with feces, yet had been cleaned but not disinfected for patient use.

In Phase 2, the researchers examined 31 endoscopes and tested them before cleaning, after cleaning, after HLD, and after storage at 1- to 2-week intervals. The researchers found that of the 31 endoscopes tested, eight (25.8%) were sterile (0 RLU; < 1 CFU), 12 (38.7%) were clean (< 5,000 RLU; < 50 CFU), and 11 (35.5%) were contaminated (> 5,000 RLU; > 50 CFU).[384]

In Phase 3, the researchers tested 63 endoscopes that had been processed and stored for reuse. The results showed that none of the endoscopes were sterile, 10 (15.9%) were clean, and 53 (84.1%) were contaminated.[384]

The researchers found that the storage room was moist and humid, and there was an open window 16 ft from the storage cabinet. The researchers observed there were disadvantages of ATP testing that included a lack of specificity for certain pathogenic microorganisms. In addition, the swab did not reach into crevices and could not be used deep inside internal channels without potential damage to the endoscope. Regardless, the researchers concluded that application of the ATP test was beneficial because it enabled monitoring of processing problems that could be addressed and immediately corrected.[384]

In response to a study by Visrodia et al[375] that supported the use of rapid cleaning verification tests, Whiteley et al[385] criticized ATP systems because of the lack of correlation between ATP and specific pathogens of concern and because of the measurement variability between commercially branded devices. In reply, Visrodia et al[386] countered that their research[375] had shown that flexible endoscopes with and without visually apparent organic soil had high levels of blood, protein, and ATP. The intent of their study was to identify methods for rapidly evaluating the effectiveness of manual cleaning in the clinical setting. The ATP testing system provided a numerical result reflecting the amount of ATP present, and these data can assist in quality monitoring of flexible endoscope processing and help ensure the adequacy of manual cleaning before mechanical processing.

There are quantitative tests that can be used for cleaning verification testing of other residual soils, including

- protein,
- carbohydrate,
- hemoglobin,
- endotoxin,
- lipid,
- sodium ion,
- bioburden, and
- total organic carbon.[90]

Quantitative testing can be used as part of a quality monitoring program to observe for trends and to monitor performance of a manual or a mechanical process.[58] Readings that trend lower indicate effective cleaning, whereas readings that trend higher may indicate a need for improved manual cleaning processes.[58] Further research is warranted.

13.7.2 **The multidisciplinary team should establish the benchmarks for the cleaning verification tests to be performed.** *[Recommendation]*

Standards for clinically significant levels of residual soil remaining after cleaning are lacking,[90] and this lack of widely accepted residual soil benchmarks has limited the implementation of rapid cleaning verification testing.[373,377,378,387]

Manufacturers may establish quantitative benchmarks for cleaning verification tests to measure manual cleaning of flexible endoscopes.[58] Endoscopes not meeting this reference point after manual cleaning require recleaning before HLD or sterilization.[58] However, variability has been identified as a concern in the use of hand-held ATP monitors, and this variability is greatest at the boundary between acceptable and unacceptable cleanliness verification.[388] Variability may also lead to poor repeatability.[388] The RLU reading scale has not been quantified against a known standard and therefore cannot be calibrated, diminishing interbrand compatibility.[388] An additional concern is the risk for random error, which may be undetectable in single monitoring samples.[388]

Whiteley et al[388] investigated the reliability of ATP bioluminometers and documented precision and variability measurements using known and quantitative standard methods. The researchers subjected four commercially branded ATP bioluminometers to known quantities of various bacteria in suspension cultures. The researchers found that the variability of commercial ATP bioluminometers was unacceptably high. They concluded that the advantages of the ATP rapid response test were undermined by the imprecision of the instrument.

However, studies have demonstrated the adequacy of an ATP benchmark of < 200 RLU for ATP[252,378,387] for both manual[387] and pump-assisted manual cleaning.[389] In a simulated-use, quasi-experimental study to validate the use of ATP for monitoring manual cleaning of flexible endoscopes, Alfa et al[387] contaminated all channels of a duodenoscope with artificial test soil containing 106 CFU of *P aeruginosa* and *E faecalis*. Residual levels of ATP, protein, hemoglobin, and bioburden were calculated from an uncleaned, partially cleaned, and fully cleaned duodenoscope. The benchmarks for clean were set at ATP < 200 RLU, protein < 6.4 mg/cm^2, hemoglobin < 2.2 mg/cm^2, and bioburden < 4-log$_{10}$ CFU/cm^2. The researchers found that the benchmarks for protein, hemoglobin, and bioburden were met if ATP < 200 RLU was achieved. The researchers concluded that effectively cleaned flexible endoscopes would have < 200 RLU of ATP.

In a quasi-experimental study to determine whether the published benchmarks[252,378,387] for protein (< 6.4 µg/cm^2), bioburden (< 4-log$_{10}$ CFU/cm^2), and ATP (< 200 RLU) were relevant for pump-assisted manual cleaning, Alfa et al[389] sampled the suction biopsy channel of patient-used endoscopes after precleaning at the point of use (ie, 10 colonoscopes, 10 duodenoscopes, 10 gastroscopes) and after pump-assisted manual cleaning (ie, 20 colonoscopes, 20 duodenoscopes, 20 gastroscopes) and then tested them for protein, bioburden, and ATP levels. The researchers found that after pump-assisted manual cleaning, 25% of gastroscopes (n = 5) exceeded the ATP benchmark, whereas all duodenoscopes (n = 20) and colonoscopes (n = 20) were below the benchmark level. The protein and bioburden residuals were also consistently lower than existing benchmarks after pump-assisted cleaning. The researchers concluded that the benchmark for protein could be low-

ered to < 2 µg/cm^2, and the benchmark for bioburden could be lowered to < 2-log$_{10}$ CFU/cm^2, for pump-assisted manual cleaning; however, the ATP benchmark of < 200 RLU was still adequate.

13.7.3

The multidisciplinary team should evaluate the need to implement protocols for cleaning verification testing of flexible duodenoscopes with elevator channels. [*Recommendation*]

Duodenoscopes with elevator channels pose a particular challenge for cleaning because of the design of the intricate distal end that provides access to the pancreatic and bile ducts. Even in cases where processing personnel performed all required processing steps, multidrug-resistant microorganisms have been transmitted to patients via flexible endoscopes, resulting in colonization, infection, or death.[137,170,171]

Alfa et al[378] conducted a quasi-experimental study to verify that the ATP benchmark of < 200 RLU was achievable in a busy endoscopy clinic. The researchers sampled all channels from patient-used colonoscopes (n = 20) and duodenoscopes (n = 20) after manual cleaning and tested them for residual ATP. Benchmarks for achieving adequate cleaning were set at ATP < 200 RLU, protein < 6.4 µg/cm^2, and bioburden < 4-log$_{10}$ CFU/cm^2. The researchers found that 96% (115 of 120) of manually cleaned endoscopes met the ATP benchmark of < 200 RLU. All 120 endoscopes tested had protein and bioburden levels lower than the benchmark levels. The researchers recommended the use of ATP testing after manual cleaning as an audit tool to confirm adequacy of cleaning. Notably, the five endoscopes that exceeded benchmark levels were duodenoscopes with elevator channels. The researchers suggested these data indicated that the elevator channel required additional monitoring to verify cleaning adequacy.

Bommarito et al[390] tested three types of flexible endoscopes (ie, 30 duodenoscopes, 116 gastroscopes, 129 colonoscopes) with ATP at five different hospitals, and determined the number of cleaning failures using < 200 RLU as the benchmark. The researchers observed that the failure rates in the manual cleaning step was highest for duodenoscopes (33%; n = 10) and gastroscopes (24%; n = 28), and lowest for colonoscopes (3%; n = 4). The researchers suggested that a more rigorous protocol was needed for manual cleaning of upper gastrointestinal endoscopes, and cleaning verification testing helped ensure cleaning effectiveness.

13.8 **A multidisciplinary team that includes infection preventionists, endoscopists, endoscopy processing personnel, microbiologists, laboratory personnel, risk managers, and other involved personnel should evaluate the need to implement a program for regular microbiologic surveillance cultures of flexible endoscopes and mechanical processors.** *[Recommendation]*

The collective evidence regarding the need for routine microbiological surveillance cultures is inconclusive. Routine microbiological surveillance culturing of flexible endoscopes after processing, during storage, or before use has not been advised in current US guidelines. The CDC,[45] APIC,[1] and the "Multisociety guideline on reprocessing flexible endoscopes"[44] representing ASGE, the Society for Healthcare Epidemiology of America (SHEA), AORN, and APIC do not recommend routine microbiologic sampling of flexible endoscopes except when focused microbiologic testing is indicated as a result of clinical or epidemiologic findings that suggest endoscopy-related transmission of infection.

A program of regular microbiological surveillance culturing of flexible endoscopes and mechanical processors is advised in the processing guidelines of several international organizations, including the combined Gastroenterological Society of Australia (GESA), Gastroenterological Nurses College of Australia (GENCA), and Australian Gastrointestinal Endoscopy Association (AGEA)[15]; the combined ESGE and European Society of Gastroenterology and Endoscopy Nurses and Associates (ESGENA) committee[391]; and the Steering Group for Flexible Endoscope Cleaning and Disinfection (SFERD).[21] However, there are variances among the recommendations.

Routine surveillance microbiological culturing is supported in the literature as an effective method for monitoring the effectiveness and quality of processing, reinforcing best practices, evaluating the effectiveness of corrective interventions, and detecting endoscopes requiring service.[93,183,281,367,392-400]

Chiu et al[401] assessed the effectiveness of mechanical processing of double-balloon enteroscopes by collecting and analyzing samples before and after processing of oral and anal route enteroscopes. Before processing, the positive culture rate was 83.9% (26 of 31) for the oral route enteroscopes, and 100% (26 of 26) for the anal route enteroscopes. After processing, the positive culture rate was 12.9% (four of 31) for the oral route enteroscopes, and 19.2% (five of 26) for the anal route enteroscopes. The researchers concluded that surveillance culture monitoring was an effective method for assessing the effectiveness of HLD of double-balloon enteroscopes.

In a nonexperimental study to evaluate the quality of gastrointestinal endoscope processing and the advantages of microbiological culture surveillance of flexible endoscopes, Saviuc et al[393] conducted a retrospective analysis of the results of endoscope sampling performed from October 1, 2006, to December 31, 2014, in a gastrointestinal unit of a French teaching hospital equipped with 89 flexible endoscopes and three mechanical processors. The compliance rate was defined as the proportion of results that met target (< 5 CFU and absence of indicator microorganisms) and alert (≤ 5 to ≤ 25 CFU and absence of indicator microorganisms). Indicator microorganisms included *Enterobacteriaceae, Pseudomonas, S maltophilia, S aureus, Acinetobacter,* and *Candida.* A total of 846 samples were taken, and the researchers found the overall compliance rate was 86% (n = 728). A total of 14% (n = 118) samples carried indicator microorganisms. The researchers concluded that microbiological surveillance was indispensable for monitoring processing, reinforcing good practices, and detecting endoscopes in need of service.

Bisset et al[402] monitored patient-ready endoscopes during an 80-week period to determine the efficacy of decontamination procedures in a busy endoscopy center. The researchers sampled the internal surface of the endoscopes from 1,376 upper gastrointestinal procedures and 987 lower gastrointestinal procedures after mechanical processing. The researchers found that gastroscopes (1.8%; n = 25) and colonoscopes (1.9%; n = 19) were equally likely to grow bacteria, with all numbers of bacteria < 10 organisms/mL. A change in procedure to processing endoscopes with the buttons attached to the endoscope resulted in a cluster of culture-positive results. No clinically untoward consequences were observed, but the researchers concluded that cultures after changes in protocols were necessary to confirm that the change in protocol did not alter processing effectiveness.

Routine microbiological surveillance may also help to identify the source of contamination and rectify processing methods to prevent transmission of infection.[367,394,398,400] Tunuguntla and Sullivan[394] performed 300 cultures at 3- to 6-month intervals on 12 flexible endoscopes between 1994 and 2003. In 1995, they found that all but two endoscopes were culture-positive for *Pseudomonas* species ranging from 1,000 CFU/mL to 7,000 CFU/mL. The culture-positive endoscopes were reprocessed and recultured, but again were culture-positive for *Pseudomonas* with CFU ranging from 20,000 CFU/mL to 75,000 CFU/mL. The authors then investigated the water source and mechanical processors and found that one of the processors was culture-positive for 50,000 CFU/mL of *Pseudomonas* due to a contaminated water source. The contaminated mechanical processor was replaced and the water source was changed, resulting in negative cultures. The authors theorized that these deficiencies in processing might have led to patient infection and would not have been detected except for routine culture surveillance.

Microbiological sampling of rinse water used during mechanical processing may reduce the risk of patient infection or pseudo-infection from waterborne bacteria.[247]

In a literature review to determine the need for microbiological culturing of rinse water used in mechanical processors, Muscarella[247] discussed the regulatory requirement[403,404] and recommendations[45,77,256] for validating the sterilization process using biological indicators to ensure that conditions for sterilization have been achieved and the similar need for verifying that utility water passed through water filtration systems, such as those connected to mechanical processors used for flexible endoscopes, is cultured. The filtered water used to rinse the endoscope may be labeled "sterile" or "bacteria free"; however, there is no way to know whether the rinse water actually meets this claim if it is not routinely sampled. Routine sampling of the rinse water may also provide information about the effectiveness of the water filtration system.

Endoscopes are complex devices. There may be debris and bacterial growth in inaccessible portions of the endoscope. Viruses such as hepatitis B and C and HIV cannot be cultured using standard methods.[138] Commonly used disinfectants may inhibit cultures. There may be false-positive results from contaminated equipment or skin. A negative culture does not guarantee that the scope has been adequately processed. Surveillance cultures of processed endoscopes have not been validated by correlating viable counts on an endoscope with infection after an endoscopic procedure.[44,45] Notably, the false-positive rate, the false-negative rate, and the limits of detection also have not been established.[138] The sensitivity of routine cultures may be unreliable for detecting the organisms associated with outbreaks.

Between May and November 2013, three patients at a Wisconsin medical center were identified as having NDM-1 carbapenem-resistant *E coli* after undergoing ERCP procedures with the same duodenoscope. Smith et al[174] observed the endoscope processing procedures and found no lapses. The investigators obtained three cultures from the duodenoscope: one sonication culture, one brush culture with the elevator channel open, and one brush culture with the elevator channel closed. Despite these measures, the duodenoscope was culture-negative;

however, the evidence was sufficiently strong to implicate the duodenoscope as the mode of transmission. The investigators concluded that it was questionable whether routine surveillance cultures would have led to an earlier identification of endoscope colonization since the NDM-1-producing *E coli* was not able to be isolated from the implicated duodenoscope.

Kola et al[146] reported an outbreak of CRKP in a German university hospital associated with a contaminated duodenoscope. Between December 2012 and January 2013, CRKP was cultured from 12 patients staying on four different wards. Molecular typing confirmed the close relation between all 12 isolates. Six of the patients were from the same ward; they were immediately transferred to separate rooms and placed on contact precautions. The remaining six patients had all undergone ERCP procedures using the same duodenoscope. Culturing of the duodenoscope did not recover CRKP. The investigators reviewed processing procedures for the duodenoscope and could find no deviations from the manufacturer's IFU; however, they did obtain positive cultures for *Enterococci*, which they suggested was indicative of insufficient cleaning. The investigators concluded that although culturing of the duodenoscope did not recover CRKP, it did not exclude it as the vehicle of transmission. They theorized that flushing the channels with normal saline may not have been sensitive enough to reveal the contamination, particularly after the endoscope had been processed several times before sampling, as it was in this case.

Fraser et al[405] conducted a case-control study following an outbreak of multidrug-resistant *P aeruginosa* sepsis in five patients who underwent ERCP procedures with the same duodenoscope. The endoscope, which was on loan from the manufacturer, had been processed and cultured with negative results 1 month earlier before being put into clinical use. The investigators concluded that the organism that caused the outbreak had most likely been transmitted from patient to patient by the loaned endoscope. In an attempt to prevent such an outbreak, endoscopes at the facility had been cultured quarterly before the outbreak; however, the outbreak occurred despite a negative surveillance culture of the implicated endoscope. The investigators suggested that routine cultures were not helpful in preventing the outbreak and were therefore of no benefit. They theorized that the endoscopist's awareness of the potential for opportunistic infection following ERCP procedures was more valuable than routine endoscope surveillance cultures.

The use of surveillance cultures is confounded by the delay in feedback and the frequent isolation of nonpathogenic organisms resulting from environmental contamination.[44,93] The need to quarantine flexible endoscopes until the culture results have been obtained may not allow for rapid reuse of the tested endoscope and could also lead to delays in patient care.[138]

Microbiological culturing is resource-intensive, and requires additional expenditures for microbiological testing and time for personnel to collect and process samples.[138,367,406] Culturing for bacterial load is impractical for many endoscopy centers that may not have access to microbiology laboratories.[138] Implementing a recommendation for routine surveillance cultures may require that some facilities outsource culture testing to qualified microbiologists. This could be quite costly, and it might also be difficult for facilities to find a laboratory that is willing to perform the necessary culture testing. Outsourcing surveillance culturing to environmental or contract laboratories may also lead to uncertainty in interpretation of results.[138]

Gillespie et al[407] reviewed microbiological testing conducted between January 1, 2002, and December 31, 2006, at two health campuses in Southern Australia in which, together, more than 3,500 endoscopic procedures were performed annually. Bronchoscopes, duodenoscopes, and mechanical processors were microbiologically sampled every 4 weeks. Gastroscopes and colonoscopes were cultured every 3 months. Positive cultures were investigated and followed up by the endoscopy and infection prevention teams. Costs for processing team members to sample the endoscopes were calculated at weekend pay rates because the samples were obtained outside of normal operating hours. Time to sample was calculated at 22 minutes per sample and $10.54 ($AUD 15) per hour. During the 5-year period, 2,374 microbiological tests were undertaken. The annual cost of microbiological testing was $14,109.55 ($AUD 20,080). The total cost of testing over 5 years was $70,547.75 ($AUD 100,400). In 2015, this would equate to a sampling cost of $12.53 ($AUD 17.83) per hour, an annual cost of $83,885.55 ($AUD 119,369.14), and a 5-year cost of $419,427.75 ($AUD 596,845.70).

13.8.1 **The multidisciplinary team should establish the methods and frequencies for microbiological surveillance culturing of flexible endoscopes and mechanical processors.** *[Recommendation]*

Standards for performing microbiological cultures, including the frequency of testing and the interpretation of results have not been determined.[44,45,93,183,367,399] A protocol for culturing and a sampling method has not yet been validated.[93,399] Different techniques may be required for different portions of the endoscope. For example, a swab-rinse technique may be recommended for sampling exterior surfaces and the distal opening of the suction/biopsy channel port.[93] A flush/brush/flush technique with rinsing through the channels using a sterile fluid and sterile cleaning brush to obtain samples through the biopsy port may be recommended for sampling the interior surface of the endoscope channels.[93] A flush technique may be recommended when brushing the channel lumens is not possible.[93]

Anterograde sampling, where the last-rinse water from the endoscope is collected inside the mechanical processor at the distal end of the endoscope, or retrograde sampling, where the suction/biopsy channel and the air/water channel are each manually flushed with sterile fluid from the distal to the proximal end, may be recommended.[93] Collection of microbiological samples requires the use of sterile technique and this may be difficult when culturing a long, flexible instrument.[407] It may be necessary to have more than one person perform the collection to prevent contamination. Developing effective standardized procedures for obtaining the cultures, as well as the actions to be implemented based on the results of the cultures, is challenging.

In a 5-year (ie, February 2006 to January 2011) prospective quasi-experimental study to assess the effectiveness of HLD by comparing cultured samples from biopsy channels of gastrointestinal endoscopes and the internal surfaces of mechanical processors, Chiu et al[392] collected rinse samples from 420 biopsy channels (ie, 300 gastroscopes, 120 colonoscopes) and swab samples from mechanical processors and examined them for the presence of aerobic and anaerobic bacteria and mycobacteria. The researchers found the number of culture-positive samples obtained from the biopsy channels (13.6%; 57 of 420) was significantly higher than that obtained from the mechanical processors (1.7%; seven of 420). In addition, the number of culture-positive samples obtained from the biopsy channels of gastroscopes (10.7%; 32 of 300) and colonoscopes (20.8%; 25 of 120) was significantly higher than those obtained from the mechanical processors used for HLD of gastroscopes (2.0%; six of 300) and the mechanical processors used for HLD of colonoscopes (0.8%; one of 120).

The researchers concluded that culturing rinse samples from biopsy channels provided a better indication of the effectiveness of HLD of gastrointestinal endoscopes than culturing swab samples from the inner surfaces of mechanical processors. They recommended using rinse samples for performing regular surveillance monitoring of flexible endoscopes. Lu et al[408] described the same study but concluded that swab culturing was also a useful method for monitoring the contamination level of the mechanical processor and the effectiveness of the HLD process.[392]

Because of a severe outbreak of *K pneumoniae* producing extended-spectrum β-lactamase that occurred in 16 patients undergoing ERCP procedures in a hospital in France between December 2008 and August 2009, Aumeran et al[55] observed duodenoscope processing procedures. They found that the duodenoscopes were not fully dried before they were stored. The investigators hypothesized that bacteria were introduced into the channels of the duodenoscope during the procedures, and despite repeated cleaning and disinfection, the contamination persisted because the moisture remaining in the endoscope channels created conditions favorable to the persistence and growth of the involved organism. The infection was transmitted to 12 patients. Surveillance cultures of the endoscopes were repeatedly negative during the outbreak, but the epidemic strain was finally isolated by flushing and brushing the duodenoscope channels.

In an expert opinion piece, Muscarella[409] discussed the limitations of surveillance culturing demonstrated by the Aumeran report[55] and the false-negative result that erroneously confirmed the endoscope was safe for patient use. Only when the sampling technique was modified to include brushing of the endoscope's suction channel in addition to flushing it was the effectiveness of sampling sufficient to culture the outbreak strain. Recovery of bacteria from a sampled channel confirms that the sampling technique effectively recovered microorganisms from the endoscope (ie, a true positive result), whereas non-recovery does not necessarily confirm effective processing.

Recommendations regarding the frequency of surveillance conflict. The ESGE-ESGENA[391] recommends periodic microbiological surveillance of endoscopes, mechanical processors, and the water used in endoscopy concurrently, at intervals no greater than 3 months.[44] The GESA and the GENCA[15] recommend sampling of mechanical processors, duodenoscopes, bronchoscopes, and ultrasound instruments at 4-week intervals, and sampling of all other gastrointestinal endo-

scopes at 3-month intervals. The SFERD[21] recommends microbial testing of water following installation of mechanical processors or water treatment systems, and additionally recommends quarterly testing and testing following incidents or after process-altering repairs. The SFERD recommends annual microbiological culturing of endoscopes and mechanical processors as well as supplemental culturing of loaned endoscopes and culturing of endoscopes and mechanical processors following repair, outbreak, or when deemed necessary by supervisory personnel.

13.8.2

The multidisciplinary team should establish benchmarks for microbial levels in flexible endoscope channels and mechanical processors. [Recommendation]

Correlations with patients' clinical outcomes is preferred for validation of benchmarks for microbial levels in flexible endoscope channels; however, this type of validation is difficult to perform. The introduction of low-virulence microorganisms to the gastrointestinal tract does not necessarily mean that the patient will have clinical symptoms or develop an infection.

In a nonexperimental study to define a realistic benchmark for residual microbial levels that could be achieved 99% of the time in a routine clinical setting, Alfa et al[285] tested all channels of 20 flexible gastrointestinal endoscopes (ie, five gastroscopes, nine colonoscopes, six duodenoscopes) used at an endoscopy clinic. The endoscopes were sampled for the presence of bacteria and fungi every Monday morning during a 7-month period. Bacteria and fungi were detected in 5.7% (n = 22) of the 383 channels tested. Of the 141 endoscopes tested, 14.1% (n = 20) had detectable microbial growth in at least one channel. The samples from only two channels grew > 100 CFU/mL of bacteria. The researchers recommended that < 100 CFU/mL be used as a clinically relevant benchmark for the number of bacteria detected from processed endoscopes.

13.8.3

The multidisciplinary team should evaluate the need to implement a program for regular microbiological culturing of duodenoscopes.[138] [Recommendation]

Routine or periodic surveillance culturing may help to assess the adequacy of duodenoscope processing and identify duodenoscopes with persistent contamination despite processing in accordance with the manufacturer's IFU.[138,410]

The ECRI recommends performing baseline cultures on all duodenoscope channels and elevator mechanisms using a media specific for carbapenem-resistant *Enterobacteriaceae* followed by regular surveillance culturing for carbapenem-resistant *Enterobacteriaceae* as well as quarantining cultured duodenoscopes until negative results are received. The ECRI further recommends that if current resources will not allow for culturing each duodenoscope after each use, weekly culturing may be considered. If cultures are positive, the ECRI recommends reprocessing and repeat culturing, and if the repeat culture is positive, permanently removing the endoscope from service or sending it back to the manufacturer for additional assessment.[411]

The CDC has provided interim guidance for performing culture surveillance for bacterial contamination of duodenoscopes or other endoscopes that have an elevator mechanism (eg, endoscopic ultrasound) after processing.[410,412,413] The CDC guidance is intended to supplement and not replace or modify manufacturer recommended processing procedures.[410] The interim protocol provided by the CDC may change as new information becomes available.[410]

13.8.4 Consider duodenoscopes with positive cultures of ≤ 10 CFU of **low-concern organisms** in the context of typical culture results at the facility.[410] *[Conditional Recommendation]*

Small numbers (< 10 CFU) of low-concern organisms (ie, organisms less often associated with disease and potentially a result of contamination of cultures during collection), such as coagulase-negative staphylococci (excluding *Staphylococcus lugdunensis*, *Bacillus* species, and diphtheroids) might occasionally be detected. Levels of low-concern organisms can vary depending on the processing procedures in the facility.[410]

13.8.5 Take duodenoscopes with positive cultures of any quantity of **high-concern organisms** out of service and initiate corrective actions that may include

- quarantining the duodenoscope, reprocessing it, and repeating post-processing cultures until it is culture-negative[410];
- reviewing the manufacturer's IFU to ensure compliance with processing procedures[410];
- notifying infection prevention and other relevant personnel to initiate corrective actions, as necessary[410];
- following the manufacturer's IFU for having the duodenoscope evaluated for defects[410]; or

- reviewing positive cultures among affected patients to determine whether other clusters of pathogens could have been transmitted.[410]

[Recommendation]

Positive cultures of organisms of high concern (ie, organisms more often associated with disease), such as gram-negative bacteria (eg, *E coli*, *K pneumoniae*, *Enterobacteriaceae*, *P aeruginosa*), *S aureus*, and *Enterococcus* necessitate corrective actions.[410]

13.8.6 If a cluster of suspected or confirmed endoscopy-related infections is identified, the infection preventionist should initiate an investigation in consultation with a health care epidemiologist and the multidisciplinary team.[3,12,17]

[Recommendation]

Initiating an investigation helps determine possible routes of infection and end further transmission.

Weber and Rutala[416] proposed a 15-step sequential approach to assist health care facilities in evaluating and managing potential failures of processing semicritical and critical items that includes

1. confirming failure of processing;
2. immediately removing from service any potentially incorrectly processed semicritical or critical item;
3. not using a questionable mechanical processor until correct functioning has been restored;
4. informing key stakeholders;
5. conducting a thorough evaluation to determine the cause of the processing failure;
6. preparing a list of potentially exposed patients;
7. assessing whether the processing failure increased the patients' risk for infection;
8. informing an expanded list of stakeholders of the processing failure;
9. developing a hypothesis for the processing failure and initiating corrective action;
10. developing a method to assess potential adverse patient events;
11. considering notifying appropriate state and federal authorities;
12. considering patient notification;
13. if patients are notified, considering whether they require medical evaluation for possible postexposure therapy with anti-infectives or additional follow-up to detect infection and offering it, if warranted;
14. developing a detailed plan to prevent similar failures in the future; and
15. performing an after-action report.

Refer to the ASGE guideline for reprocessing failure[414] and other relevant documents[66,223,224,415-417] for additional guidance.

13.8.7 **If a breach in protocol for endoscope processing is recognized, the infection preventionist, epidemiologist, and multidisciplinary team should perform an assessment and investigation to determine whether patient notification is required, and if so, how patients will be notified and followed.[17,78]** *[Recommendation]*

Health care facilities have an ethical obligation to inform affected patients in a timely manner when a significant breach in processing occurs.[414] Prompt notification allows patients to take precautions to minimize the risk of transmitting the infection to others and allows for early serologic testing.[414] Where a breach in processing has been determined to pose a negligible patient risk, health care providers have to consider the ethical issue of a patient's right to know compared with the potential for causing unnecessary patient distress in a situation where the risk for infection may be very small.[414-416] Reporting a processing-related outbreak may also cause patients to avoid potential life-saving endoscopic procedures because of an unwarranted fear of infection.[414]

13.9 **Report and document adverse events according to the health care organization's policy and procedure and review these events for potential opportunities for improvement.** *[Conditional Recommendation]*

Reports of adverse events and near misses can be used to identify actions that may prevent similar occurrences and reveal opportunities for improvement.

13.9.1 **Investigate near misses (ie, unplanned events that do not result in injury) and take corrective action to prevent serious adverse events.** *[Recommendation]*

13.9.2 **Submit reports regarding device malfunction leading to serious injury or death to MedWatch: The FDA Safety Information and Adverse Event Reporting Program.[418]** *[Recommendation]*

The FDA uses medical device reports to monitor device performance, detect potential device-related safety issues, and contribute to risk-benefit assessments of suspected device-associated deaths, serious injuries, or malfunction. The MAUDE (ie, Manufacturer and User Facility Device Experience) database houses reports submitted to the FDA by mandatory reporters (ie, manufacturers, importers, device user facilities) and voluntary reporters (ie, health care professionals, patients, consumers).[418]

Mandatory reporters are required to submit reports when they become aware of information that reasonably suggests that one of their marketed devices may have caused or contributed to a death or serious injury or has malfunctioned and that the malfunction of the device would be likely to cause or contribute to a death or serious injury if the malfunction were to recur.[418] Voluntary reporters are required to submit reports when they become aware of information that reasonably suggests a device may have caused or contributed to a death or serious injury of a patient.[418]

Editor's note: Teflon is a registered trademark of the Chemours Co, Wilmington, DE.

Glossary

Adenosine triphosphate: A substance present in all living cells that provides energy for many metabolic processes and is involved in making ribonucleic acid.

Adsorb: The adhesion by gases, solutes, or liquids in an extremely thin layer of molecules to the surfaces of solid bodies or liquids with which they come in contact.

Analog rating scale: An instrument for measuring subjective phenomena in which a subject selects from a gradient of alternatives arranged in linear fashion.

Bacteriophage: A virus that lives within a bacterium, replicating itself and eventually destroying the bacterial cell.

Benchmark: A standard or point of reference against which things may be compared or measured.

Bioburden: The degree of microbial load; the number of viable organisms contaminating an object.

Biofilm: A thin layer of microorganisms adhering to the surface of a structure, which may be organic or inorganic, together with the polysaccharides that they secrete.

Biohazard: A biological or chemical substance that is dangerous to human beings and the environment.

Borescope: A device used to inspect the inside of an instrument through a small opening or lumen of the instrument.

Colonic mucosal pseudolipomatosis: A rare, benign complication of a colonoscopy involving a characteristic white, slightly elevated lesion usually preceded by an effervescent release of molecular oxygen.

Colony-forming unit: A measure of the number of viable bacterial cells in a sample.

Coved wall base: Molding or trim used to create a curved transition from the wall to the floor.

Critical water: Water that is extensively treated to remove microorganisms and other materials.

Decontamination: The process of removing pathogenic microorganisms from objects so they are safe to handle, use, or discard.

Decontamination sink: A sink located in the decontamination room or endoscopy processing room that is used for endoscope processing tasks, such as leak testing, cleaning, and rinsing of flexible endoscopes and other reusable items.

Drying cabinet: A medical device designed for storage of flexible endoscopes that circulates continuous filtered air through each endoscope channel and within the cabinet.

Endoscopy suite: A facility or unit within a facility designed for care of the patient undergoing procedures requiring the use of an endoscope. The suite includes waiting rooms, offices, lounges, endoscopy procedure rooms, other patient care areas, and endoscopy processing rooms.

Endotoxin: A toxic substance present in the outer membrane of gram-negative bacteria that is released from the cell when it disintegrates.

Enzymes: Proteins that act as catalysts to bring about specific biochemical reactions.

Hand washing station: An area that includes a sink, a hands-free faucet, cleansing solutions, and a means for drying the hands.

High-concern organisms: Organisms often associated with disease, such as gram-negative bacteria (eg, *Escherichia coli, Klebsiella pneumoniae, Enterobacteriaceae, Pseudomonas aeruginosa*), *Staphylococcus aureus,* and *Enterococcus.* Positive cultures of organisms of high concern require corrective action.

High-level disinfectant: A germicide that inactivates all microbial pathogens, except bacterial endospores.

High-level disinfection: Processes that kill all microbial pathogens, but not necessarily all bacterial spores.

Hypochlorites: Oxidizing agents composed of chlorine and oxygen.

Infection control risk assessment: A documented process to proactively identify and plan safe design elements, including consideration of long-range infection prevention; identify and plan for internal and external building areas and sites that will be affected during construction/renovation; identify potential risk for transmission of airborne and waterborne biological contaminants during construction and/or renovation and commissioning; and develop infection control risk mitigation recommendations to be considered.

Instrument air: A medical gas that falls under the general requirements for medical gases as defined by the *NFPA 99: Health Care Facilities Code,* is not respired, is compliant with the *ANSI/ISA S-7.0.01: Quality Standard for Instrument Air,* and is filtered to 0.01 micron, free of liquids and hydrocarbon vapors, and dry to a dew point of –40° F (–40° C).

Intermediate-level disinfection: A process that destroys all vegetative bacteria, including tubercle bacilli, lipid and some nonlipid viruses, and fungi, but not bacterial spores.

Liquid chemical sterilant: A chemical that has been validated to provide microbial kill adequate to obtain clearance by the US Food and Drug Administration for a sterilization label claim.

Log reduction: A 10-fold reduction in the number of live bacteria. A 1-log reduction would reduce 100 bacteria to 10.

Low-concern organisms: Organisms less often associated with disease and potentially a result of contamination of cultures during collection, such as coagulase-negative staphylococci. Levels of low-concern organisms can vary depending on the processing procedures in the facility.

Mechanical processor: A device that mechanically cleans, rinses, and exposes flexible endoscopes and accessories to a high-level disinfectant or liquid chemical sterilant.

Minimum efficiency reporting value (MERV): A measure of the effectiveness of air filters on a rating scale of 1 to 16. The higher the MERV rating, the more effective the filter.

Monolithic: A single-piece surface with no seams or joints unless the surface joints are chemically or heat welded.

Patient care area: An area used for the provision of patient care (eg, monitoring, evaluation, treatments).

pH: A numeric scale used to specify the acidity or alkalinity of an aqueous solution. Solutions with a pH lower than 7 (ie, the pH of water) are acidic and solutions with a pH higher than 7 are alkaline or basic.

Phenolics: Germicides derived from carbolic acid.

Plaque-forming unit: A measure of the number of particles capable of forming plaques per unit volume, such as virus particles.

Polysaccharide: A carbohydrate consisting of bonded sugar molecules.

Prions: A unique class of infectious proteins that cause fatal neurological diseases and are resistant to disinfection and sterilization.

Procedure room: A room designated for the performance of procedures that do not require a restricted environment but may require the use of sterile instruments or supplies.

Processing room: A room dedicated to cleaning, decontaminating, inspecting, and preparing surgical instruments and other medical devices (eg, flexible endoscopes) for high-level disinfection or sterilization.

Pseudo-infection: Laboratory evidence of the presence of pathogenic microorganisms in the absence of infection.

Pseudo-outbreak: An episode of false increased disease incidence due to enhanced surveillance (eg, microbiological culturing) or other factors (eg, laboratory contamination, false positive test).

Quaternary ammonium compounds: Disinfectants derived from ammonium in which the nitrogen atom is attached to four organic groups.

Reagent: A substance that is used to test for the presence of another substance by causing a chemical reaction.

Shelf life: The period of time during which a stored product remains effective, useful, or suitable for use.

Skin antiseptics: Products with antimicrobial activity that are applied to the skin to reduce the number of microbial flora.

Sterility assurance level (SAL): The probability of a single viable microorganism remaining on an item after sterilization. A SAL of 10^{-6} means there is less than or equal to one chance in 1 million that a single viable microorganism is present on a sterilized item.

Sterilization: Processes by which all microbial life, including pathogenic and nonpathogenic microorganisms and spores, are killed.

Surfactant: A substance that reduces the surface tension of a liquid in which it is dissolved.

Surgical attire: Nonsterile apparel designated for the perioperative practice setting that includes two-piece pantsuits, scrub dresses, cover jackets, head coverings, shoes, masks, and protective eyewear.

Transmissible spongiform encephalopathies: Fatal prion diseases that affect the brain and nervous system. The development of tiny holes in the brain causes it to appear like a sponge, hence the term *spongiform*.

Use life: The defined period for safe use of a product after the container is opened.

Utility water: Water obtained directly from a faucet that has not been purified, distilled, or otherwise treated. Synonym: tap water.

Validation: Confirmation by examination and provision of objective evidence, performed by the manufacturer, that the particular requirements for a specific intended use can be consistently fulfilled.

Variant Creutzfeldt-Jakob disease: A fatal degenerative neurological disease caused by a prion. The human form of bovine spongiform encephalopathy (ie, mad cow disease).

References

1. Alvarado CJ, Reichelderfer M. APIC guideline for infection prevention and control in flexible endoscopy. Association for Professionals in Infection Control. *Am J Infect Control.* 2000;28(2):138-155. [IVB]

2. Infections associated with reprocessed flexible bronchoscopes: FDA safety communication. US Food and Drug Administration. http://www.fda.gov/MedicalDevices/Safety/AlertsandNotices/ucm462949.htm. Accessed December 9, 2015. [VA]

3. Preventing cross-contamination in endoscope processing: FDA safety communication. US Food and Drug Administration. http://www.fda.gov/MedicalDevices/Safety/AlertsandNotices/ucm190273.htm. Accessed December 9, 2015. [VB]

4. Gastmeier P, Vonberg RP. *Klebsiella spp.* in endoscopy-associated infections: we may only be seeing the tip of the iceberg. *Infection.* 2014;42(1):15-21. [VA]

5. Kampf B, Makowski T, Weiss H, et al. ESGE newsletter. Definition of "endoscope families" as used in EN ISO 15883-4. *Endoscopy.* 2013;45(2):156-157. [VB]

6. Design of endoscopic retrograde cholangiopancreatography (ERCP) duodenoscopes may impede effective cleaning: FDA safety communication. US Food and Drug Administration.

http://www.fda.gov/MedicalDevices/Safety/AlertsandNotices/ucm434871.htm. Accessed December 9, 2015. [VA]

7. Boylu U, Oommen M, Thomas R, Lee BR. In vitro comparison of a disposable flexible ureteroscope and conventional flexible ureteroscopes. *J Urol.* 2009;182(5):2347-2351. [IIIB]

8. Piepho T, Werner C, Noppens RR. Evaluation of the novel, single-use, flexible aScope for tracheal intubation in the simulated difficult airway and first clinical experiences. *Anaesthesia.* 2010;65(8):820-825. [VB]

9. Pujol E, Lopez AM, Valero R. Use of the Ambu® aScope in 10 patients with predicted difficult intubation. *Anaesthesia.* 2010;65(10):1037-1040. [VB]

10. Tvede MF, Kristensen MS, Nyhus-Andreasen M. A cost analysis of reusable and disposable flexible optical scopes for intubation. *Acta Anaesthesiol Scand.* 2012;56(5):577-584. [VB]

11. *Guidelines for Design and Construction of Hospitals and Outpatient Facilities.* Chicago, IL: Facility Guidelines Institute; 2014. [IVC]

12. *ANSI/AAMI ST91:2015 Flexible and Semi-rigid Endoscope Processing in Health Care Facilities.* Arlington, VA: Association for the Advancement of Medical Instrumentation; 2015. [IVC]

13. Health Service Executive Advisory Group. *HSE Standards and Recommended Practices for Endoscope Reprocessing Units.* Tipperary, Ireland: HSE; 2012. [IVB]

14. CLARIFICATION: requirements for an endoscopy equipment processing room. *Jt Comm Perspect.* 2012;32(3):13-14. [VA]

15. *Infection Control in Endoscopy.* 3rd ed. Victoria, Australia: Gastroenterological Society of Australia and the Gastroenterological Nurses College of Australia; 2010. [IVB]

16. Society of Gastroenterology Nurses and Associates. Standards of infection control in reprocessing of flexible gastrointestinal endoscopes. *Gastroenterol Nurs.* 2013;36(4):293-303. [IVB]

17. Hookey L, Armstrong D, Enns R, Matlow A, Singh H, Love J. Summary of guidelines for infection prevention and control for flexible gastrointestinal endoscopy. *Can J Gastroenterol.* 2013;27(6):347-350. [VA]

18. Du Rand IA, Blaikley J, Booton R, et al. British Thoracic Society guideline for diagnostic flexible bronchoscopy in adults. *Thorax.* 2013;68(Suppl 1):i1-i44. [IVA]

19. World Gastroenterology Organisation/World Endoscopy Organization. *Endoscope Disinfection—A Resource-Sensitive Approach.* World Endoscopy Organisation. http://www.worldendo.org/assets/downloads/pdf/guidelines/wgo_weo_endoscope_disinfection.pdf. Accessed December 9, 2015. [IVC]

20. Guidance on decontamination of equipment for gastrointestinal endoscopy. 2014. British Society of Gastroenterology. http://www.bsg.org.uk/clinical-guidance/general/guidelines-for-decontamination-of-equipment-for-gastrointestinal-endoscopy.html. Accessed December 9, 2015. [IVA]

21. *Professional Standard Handbook Cleaning and Disinfection Flexible Endoscopes.* Version 3.1 ed. The Netherlands: Steering Group for Flexible Endoscope Cleaning and Disinfection; 2014. [IVB]

22. Beilenhoff U, Neumann CS, Rey JF, et al. ESGE-ESGENA Guideline: cleaning and disinfection in gastrointestinal endoscopy. *Endoscopy.* 2008;40(11):939-957. [IVC]

23. *Formal Interpretations: Guidelines for Design and Construction of Hospitals and Outpatient Facilities, 2014.* Facility Guidelines Institute. http://fgiguidelines.org/pdfs/FGI-interps_2014 Guidelines_141222.pdf. Accessed December 9, 2015. [VA]

24. *Choice Framework for local Policy and Procedures 01-06—Decontamination of flexible endoscopes: Policy and management.* 2013. UK Department of Health. https://www.gov.uk/government/uploads/system/uploads/attachment_data/file/192522/Decontamination_of_flexible_endoscopes.pdf. Accessed December 9, 2015. [IVB]

25. *Choice Framework for local Policy and Procedures 01-06 - Decontamination of flexible endoscopes: Design and installation.* 2013. UK Department of Health. https://www.gov.uk/government/uploads/system/uploads/attachment_data/file/148560/CFPP_01-06_Design_and_installation_Final.pdf. Accessed December 9, 2015. [IVB]

26. Burlingame BL. Airflow in endoscope cleaning rooms [Clinical Issues]. *AORN J.* 2013;98(5):541-542. [VA]

27. Mehta AC, Prakash UBS, Garland R, et al. American College of Chest Physicians and American Association for Bronchoscopy Concensus Statement: Prevention of flexible bronchoscopy-associated infection. *Chest.* 2005;128(3):1742-1755. [IVC]

28. Hota S, Hirji Z, Stockton K, et al. Outbreak of multidrug-resistant *Pseudomonas aeruginosa* colonization and infection secondary to imperfect intensive care unit room design. *Infect Control Hosp Epidemiol.* 2009;30(1):25-33. [VB]

29. Siegel JD, Rhinehart E, Jackson M, Chiarello L; Healthcare Infection Control Practices Advisory Committee. 2007 Guideline for Isolation Precautions: Preventing Transmission of Infectious Agents in Healthcare Settings. *Am J Infect Control.* 2007;35(10 Suppl 2):S65-S164. [IVA]

30. ASGE Ensuring Safety in the Gastrointestinal Endoscopy Unit Task Force; Calderwood AH, Chapman FJ, et al. Guidelines for safety in the gastrointestinal endoscopy unit. *Gastrointest Endosc.* 2014;79(3):363-372. [IVB]

31. Overview of health care HVAC systems. In: *HVAC Design Manual for Hospitals and Clinics.* 2nd ed. Atlanta, GA: American Society of Heating, Refrigerating and Air-Conditioning Engineers; 2013. [IVC]

32. Guideline for a safe environment of care, part 2. In: *Guidelines for Perioperative Practice.* Denver, CO: AORN, Inc; 2015:265-290. [IVA]

33. Table 7.1: Design parameters. In: *ANSI/ASHRAE/ASHE 170-2013: Ventilation of Health Care Facilities.* Atlanta, GA: American Society of Heating, Refrigerating and Air-Conditioning Engineers; 2013. [IVC]

34. *Interpretation IC 170-2013-4 of ANSI/ASHRAE/ASHE Standard 170-2013 Ventilation of Health Care Facilities.* Atlanta, GA: American Society of Heating, Refrigerating and Air-Conditioning Engineers; January 27, 2015. [IVC]

35. Guideline for prevention of transmissible infections. In: *Guidelines for Perioperative Practice.* Denver, CO: AORN, Inc; 2015:419-454. [IVA]

36. Tan HL, Lo PLC, Eng CTP. Bronchoscopy during SARS: perspectives from a non-SARS designated hospital. *J Bronchol.* 2006;13(4):223-225. [VB]

37. Occupational Safety and Health Act of 1970 (Public Law 91-596, December 29, 1970, as amended through January 1, 2004). Occupational Safety and Health Administration. https://www.osha.gov/pls/oshaweb/owadisp.show_document?p_table=OSHACT&p_id=2743. Accessed December 9, 2015.

38. 29 CFR 1910.1200: Hazard Communication. 2011. Occupational Safety and Health Administration. https://www.osha.gov/pls/oshaweb/owadisp.show_document?p_table=standards&p_id=10099. Accessed December 9, 2015.

39. *Industrial Ventilation: A Manual of Recommended Practice for Design.* Cincinnati, OH: ACGIH; 2013. [IVC]

40. *ANSI/AAMI ST58: Chemical Sterilization and High-level Disinfection in Health Care Facilities.* Arlington, VA: Association for the Advancement of Medical Instrumentation; 2013. [IVC]

41. *ANSI/AAMI ST41: Ethylene Oxide Sterilization in Health Care Facilities: Safety and Effectiveness.* Arlington, VA: Association for the Advancement of Medical Instrumentation; 2012. [IVC]

42. Guideline for a safe environment of care, part 1. In: *Guidelines for Perioperative Practice.* Denver, CO: AORN, Inc; 2015:239-264. [IVA]

43. Guideline for high-level disinfection. In: *Guidelines for Perioperative Practice.* Denver, CO: AORN, Inc; 2015:601-614. [IVB]

44. ASGE Quality Assurance In Endoscopy Committee; Petersen BT, Chennat J, et al. Multisociety guideline on reprocessing flexible gastrointestinal endoscopes: 2011. *Gastrointest Endosc.* 2011;73(6):1075-1084. [IVA]

45. Rutala WA. Weber DJ; the Healthcare Infection Control Practices Advisory Committee (HICPAC). *Guideline for Disinfection and Sterilization in Healthcare Facilities, 2008.* Atlanta, GA: Centers for Disease Control and Prevention; 2008. [IVA]

46. SGNA Practice Committee 2013-14. Guideline for use of high-level disinfectants and sterilants for reprocessing flexible gastrointestinal endoscopes. *Gastroenterol Nurs.* 2015;38(1):70-80. [IVB]

47. *ANSI/IESNA RP-29-06: Lighting for Hospitals and Health Care Facilities.* RP-29-06 ed. New York, NY: Illuminating Engineering Society of North America; 2006. [IVC]

48. 29 CFR §1910.1030: Bloodborne Pathogens. Occupational Safety and Health Administration. http://www.osha.gov/pls/oshaweb/owadisp.show_document?p_table=STANDARDS&p_id=10051. Accessed December 9, 2015.

49. Silva CV, Magalhaes VD, Pereira CR, Kawagoe JY, Ikura C, Ganc AJ. Pseudo-outbreak of *Pseudomonas aeruginosa* and *Serratia marcescens* related to bronchoscopes. *Infect Control Hosp Epidemiol.* 2003;24(3):195-197. [VC]

50. NFPA 99: Health Care Facilities Code Handbook. Quincy, MA: National Fire Protection Association; 2015. [IVC]

51. *ANSI/ISA S7.0.01-1996 Quality Standard Instrument Air.* Research Triangle Park, NC: Instrument Society of America; 1996. [IVC]

52. 29 CFR 1910.151: Medical and First Aid. Occupational Safety and Health Administration. https://www.osha.gov/pls/oshaweb/owadisp.show_document?p_table=STANDARDS&p_id=9806. Accessed December 9, 2015.

53. American National Standards Institute/International Safety Equipment Association. *American National Standard for*

Emergency Eyewash and Shower Equipment. Arlington, VA: International Safety Equipment Association; 2009. [IVC]

54. Guideline for hand hygiene. In: *Guidelines for Perioperative Practice.* Denver, CO: AORN, Inc; 2015:31-42. [IVB]

55. Aumeran C, Poincloux L, Souweine B, et al. Multidrug-resistant *Klebsiella pneumoniae* outbreak after endoscopic retrograde cholangiopancreatography. *Endoscopy.* 2010;42(11):895-899. [VA]

56. Guideline for environmental cleaning. In: *Guidelines for Perioperative Practice.* Denver, CO: AORN, Inc; 2015:9-30. [IVA]

57. Guideline for surgical attire. In: *Guidelines for Perioperative Practice.* Denver, CO: AORN, Inc; 2015:97-120. [IVA]

58. Guideline for cleaning and care of surgical instruments. In: *Guidelines for Perioperative Practice.* Denver, CO: AORN, Inc; 2015:615-650. [IVA]

59. 29 CFR 1910.133: Eye and Face Protection. Occupational Safety and Health Administration. https://www.osha.gov/pls/oshaweb/owadisp.show_document?p_table=STANDARDS&p_id=9778. Accessed December 9, 2015.

60. ASGE Technology Committee; Pedrosa MC, Farraye FA, et al. Minimizing occupational hazards in endoscopy: personal protective equipment, radiation safety, and ergonomics. *Gastrointest Endosc.* 2010;72(2):227-235. [VB]

61. Kaye MD. Herpetic conjunctivitis as an unusual occupational hazard (endoscopists' eye). *Gastrointest Endosc.* 1974;21(2):69-70. [VB]

62. Guideline for product selection. In: *Guidelines for Perioperative Practice.* Denver, CO: AORN, Inc; 2015:179-186. [IVB]

63. 21 CFR Chapter 1. Subchapter H: Medical Devices. 2015. US Food and Drug Administration. https://www.accessdata.fda.gov/scripts/cdrh/cfdocs/cfCFR/CFRSearch.cfm?CFRPart=820. Accessed December 9, 2015.

64. *Reprocessing Medical Devices in Health Care Settings: Validation Methods and Labeling Guidance for Industry and Food and Drug Administration Staff.* Silver Spring, MD: US Food and Drug Administration; 2015.

65. Rudy SF, Adams J, Waddington C. Implementing the SOHN-endorsed AORN guidelines for reprocessing reusable upper airway endoscopes. *ORL Head Neck Nurs.* 2012;30(1):6-15. [VB]

66. Weber DJ. Managing and preventing exposure events from inappropriately reprocessed endoscopes. *Infect Control Hosp Epidemiol.* 2012;33(7):657-660. [VA]

67. Statham MM, Willging JP. Automated high-level disinfection of nonchanneled flexible endoscopes: duty cycles and endoscope repair. *Laryngoscope.* 2010;120(10):1946-1949. [IIIB]

68. Hutson P. Staffing the endoscopy department: what is the appropriate skill mix? *Gastrointest Nurs.* 2011;9(1):28-33. [VB]

69. Choice Framework for local Policy and Procedures 01-06—Decontamination of flexible endoscopes: Operational management. 2013. UK Department of Health. https://www.gov.uk/government/uploads/system/uploads/attachment_data/file/148559/CFPP_01-06_Operational_mgmt_Final.pdf. Accessed December 9, 2015. [IVB]

70. Kolmos HJ, Lerche A, Kristoffersen K, Rosdahl VT. Pseudo-outbreak of *Pseudomonas aeruginosa* in HIV-infected patients undergoing fiberoptic bronchoscopy. *Scand J Infect Dis.* 1994;26(6):653-657. [VC]

71. McGill JJ, Schaeffer AJ, Gonzalez CM. Durability of flexible cystoscopes in the outpatient setting. *Urology.* 2013;81(5):932-937. [IIIB]

72. Sooriakumaran P, Kaba R, Andrews HO, Buchholz NP. Evaluation of the mechanisms of damage to flexible ureteroscopes and suggestions for ureteroscope preservation. *Asian J Androl.* 2005;7(4):433-438. [IIIB]

73. Semins MJ, George S, Allaf ME, Matlaga BR. Ureteroscope cleaning and sterilization by the urology operating room team: the effect on repair costs. *J Endourol.* 2009;23(6):903-905. [VB]

74. McDougall EM, Alberts G, Deal KJ, Nagy JM 3rd. Does the cleaning technique influence the durability of the <9F flexible ureteroscope? *J Endourol.* 2001;15(6):615-618. [IIC]

75. Smith F. *Pseudomonas* infection. *Nurs Times.* 1994;90 (46):55-56. [VB]

76. Machida H, Seki M, Yoshioka N, et al. Correlation between outbreaks of multidrug-resistant *Pseudomonas aeruginosa* infection and use of bronchoscopes suggested by epidemiological analysis. *Biol Pharm Bull.* 2014;37(1):26-30. [IIIB]

77. *ANSI/AAMI ST79: Comprehensive Guide to Steam Sterilization and Sterility Assurance in Health Care Facilities.* Arlington, VA: Association for the Advancement of Medical Instrumentation; 2013. [IVC]

78. Centers for Disease Control and Prevention. *Immediate Need for Healthcare Facilities to Review Procedures for Cleaning, Disinfecting, and Sterilizing Reusable Medical Devices.* Health Alert Network. September 11, 2015. http://stacks.cdc.gov/view/cdc/34153. Accessed December 9, 2015. [VB]

79. Bou R, Aguilar A, Perpinan J, et al. Nosocomial outbreak of *Pseudomonas aeruginosa* infections related to a flexible bronchoscope. *J Hosp Infect.* 2006;64(2):129-135. [IIIB]

80. Srinivasan A, Wolfenden LL, Song X, Perl TM, Haponik EF. Bronchoscope reprocessing and infection prevention and control: bronchoscopy-specific guidelines are needed. *Chest.* 2004;125(1):307-314. [IIIB]

81. Radford PD, Unadkat SN, Rollin M, Tolley NS. Disinfection of flexible fibre-optic endoscopes out-of-hours: confidential telephone survey of ENT units in England—10 years on. *J Laryngol Otol.* 2013;127(5):489-493. [IIIC]

82. Roberts CG. The role of biofilms in reprocessing medical devices. *Am J Infect Control.* 2013;41(5 Suppl):S77-S80. [VA]

83. Joint AUA/SUNA white paper on reprocessing of flexible cystoscopes. *J Urol.* 2010;184(6):2241-2245. [VC]

84. Cavaliere M, Iemma M. Guidelines for reprocessing non-lumened heat-sensitive ear/nose/throat endoscopes. *Laryngoscope.* 2012;122(8):1708-1718. [VB]

85. Lind N, Ninemeier JD, Bird BT; International Association of Healthcare Central Service Materiel Management. *Central Service Technical Manual.* Chicago, IL: International Association of Healthcare Central Service Materiel Management; 2007. [IVC]

86. Merritt K, Hitchins VM, Brown SA. Safety and cleaning of medical materials and devices. *J Biomed Mater Res.* 2000;53(2):131-136. [IIB]

87. Herrmann IF, Heeg P, Matteja B, et al. Silent risks and hidden dangers in endoscopy: what to do? *Acta Endoscopica.* 2008;38(5):493-502. [IIIC]

88. Alfa MJ. Medical-device reprocessing. *Infect Control Hosp Epidemiol.* 2000;21(8):496-498. [VA]

89. Muscarella LF. Prevention of disease transmission during flexible laryngoscopy. *Am J Infect Control.* 2007;35(8):536-544. [VA]

90. *TIR 30: A Compendium of Processes, Materials, Test Methods, and Acceptance Criteria for Cleaning Reusable Medical Devices.* Arlington, VA: Association for the Advancement of Medical Instrumentation; 2011. [IVC]

91. Johansen C, Falholt P, Gram L. Enzymatic removal and disinfection of bacterial biofilms. *Appl Environ Microbiol.* 1997;63(9):3724-3728. [IIIC]

92. Pajkos A, Vickery K, Cossart Y. Is biofilm accumulation on endoscope tubing a contributor to the failure of cleaning and decontamination? *J Hosp Infect.* 2004;58(3):224-229. [IIC]

93. Kovaleva J, Peters FT, van der Mei HC, Degener JE. Transmission of infection by flexible gastrointestinal endoscopy and bronchoscopy. *Clin Microbiol Rev.* 2013;26(2):231-254. [VA]

94. Costerton JW, Stewart PS, Greenberg EP. Bacterial biofilms: a common cause of persistent infections. *Science.* 1999;284(5418):1318-1322. [VB]

95. Ren W, Sheng X, Huang X, Zhi F, Cai W. Evaluation of detergents and contact time on biofilm removal from flexible endoscopes. *Am J Infect Control.* 2013;41(9):e89-e92. [IB]

96. Ren-Pei W, Hui-Jun X, Ke Q, Dong W, Xing N, Zhao-Shen L. Correlation between the growth of bacterial biofilm in flexible endoscopes and endoscope reprocessing methods. *Am J Infect Control.* 2014;42(11):1203-1206. [IIIB]

97. Naas T, Cuzon G, Babics A, et al. Endoscopy-associated transmission of carbapenem-resistant *Klebsiella pneumoniae* producing KPC-2 beta-lactamase. *J Antimicrob Chemother.* 2010;65(6):1305-1306. [VB]

98. Hutchisson B, LeBlanc C. The truth and consequences of enzymatic detergents. *Gastroenterol Nurs.* 2005;28(5):372-376. [IIB]

99. Alfa MJ. Can biofilm prevent high level disinfection? *J GENCA.* 2006;16(1):23-24. [VA]

100. Shimono N, Takuma T, Tsuchimochi N, et al. An outbreak of *Pseudomonas aeruginosa* infections following thoracic surgeries occurring via the contamination of bronchoscopes and an automatic endoscope reprocessor. *J Infect Chemother.* 2008;14(6):418-423. [VB]

101. Bultitude MF, Dasgupta P, Tiptaft RC, Glass JM. Prolonging the life of the flexible ureterorenoscope. *Int J Clin Pract.* 2004;58(8):756-757. [VB]

102. Thomas LA. Transporting the endoscope. *Gastroenterol Nurs.* 2005;28(2):145-146. [VB]

103. Collins JW, Keeley FX Jr, Timoney A. Cost analysis of flexible ureterorenoscopy. *BJU Int.* 2004;93(7):1023-1026. [IIIC]

104. Alfa MJ, Howie R. Modeling microbial survival in buildup biofilm for complex medical devices. *BMC Infect Dis.* 2009;9:56. [IIB]

105. Yanaihara H, Hamasuna R, Takahashi S, et al. Current controversial issues in the decontamination process for urological endoscopes. *Int J Urol.* 2012;19(1):5-6. [VB]

106. Endoscope inspections fraught with challenges. *Healthc Purchasing News.* 2013;37(11):16-18. [VB]

107. Thomas LA. Essentials for endoscopic equipment. Leak testing. *Gastroenterol Nurs.* 2005;28(5):430-432. [VB]

108. Khan F, Mukhtar S, Marsh H, et al. Evaluation of the pressure leak test in increasing the lifespan of flexible ureteroscopes. *Int J Clin Pract.* 2013;67(10):1040-1043. [IIB]

109. Ramsey AH, Oemig TV, Davis JP, Massey JP, Torok TJ. An outbreak of bronchoscopy-related *Mycobacterium tuberculosis* infections due to lack of bronchoscope leak testing. *Chest.* 2002;121(3):976-981. [VC]

110. Cetre JC, Nicolle MC, Salord H, et al. Outbreaks of contaminated broncho-alveolar lavage related to intrinsically defective bronchoscopes. *J Hosp Infect.* 2005;61(1):39-45. [IIIB]

111. Krishna PD, Statham MM, Rosen CA. Acute glutaraldehyde mucosal injury of the upper aerodigestive tract due to damage to the working channel of an endoscope. *Ann Otol Rhinol Laryngol.* 2010;119(3):150-154. [VB]

112. Chu NS, Favero M. The microbial flora of the gastrointestinal tract and the cleaning of flexible endoscopes. *Gastrointest Endosc Clin N Am.* 2000;10(2):233-244. [VA]

113. Chu NS, McAlister D, Antonoplos PA. Natural bioburden levels detected on flexible gastrointestinal endoscopes after clinical use and manual cleaning. *Gastrointest Endosc.* 1998;48(2):137-142. [IC]

114. Kampf G, Fliss PM, Martiny H. Is peracetic acid suitable for the cleaning step of reprocessing flexible endoscopes? *World J Gastrointest Endosc.* 2014;6(9):390-406. [VA]

115. Alfa MJ, Sitter DL. In-hospital evaluation of orthophthalaldehyde as a high level disinfectant for flexible endoscopes. *J Hosp Infect.* 1994;26(1):15-26. [IIB]

116. Weber DJ, Rutala WA. Lessons from outbreaks associated with bronchoscopy. *Infect Control Hosp Epidemiol.* 2001;22(7):403-408. [VA]

117. Spaulding EH, Lawrence CA, Block SS, Reddish GF. Chemical disinfection of medical and surgical materials. In: Lawrence CA, Block SS, Reddish GF, eds. *Disinfection, Sterilization, and Preservation.* Philadelphia, PA: Lea & Febiger; 1968:517-531. [VA]

118. Bajolet O, Ciocan D, Vallet C, et al. Gastroscopy-associated transmission of extended-spectrum beta-lactamase-producing *Pseudomonas aeruginosa. J Hosp Infect.* 2013;83(4):341-343. [VA]

119. *Technical Information Report 34: Water for the Reprocessing of Medical Devices.* Atlanta, GA: Association for the Advancement of Medical Instrumentation; 2014. [IVC]

120. Alfa MJ. Methodology of reprocessing reusable accessories. *Gastrointest Endosc Clin N Am.* 2000;10(2):361-378. [VA]

121. Alfa MJ, Jackson M. A new hydrogen peroxide-based medical-device detergent with germicidal properties: comparison with enzymatic cleaners. *Am J Infect Control.* 2001; 29(3):168-177. [IIB]

122. Rey JF, Kruse A, Neumann C; ESGE (European Society of Gastrointestinal Endoscopy); ESGENA (European Society of Gastrointestinal Endoscopy Nurses and Associates). ESGE/ ESGENA technical note on cleaning and disinfection. *Endoscopy.* 2003;35(10):869-877. [VB]

123. Henoun Loukili N, Zink E, Grandadam S, Bientz M, Meunier O. Effectiveness of detergent-disinfecting agents on *Escherichia coli* 54127 biofilm. *J Hosp Infect.* 2004;57(2):175-178. [IIC]

124. Fang Y, Shen Z, Li L, et al. A study of the efficacy of bacterial biofilm cleanout for gastrointestinal endoscopes. *World J Gastroenterol.* 2010;16(8):1019-1024. [IB]

125. Vickery K, Pajkos A, Cossart Y. Removal of biofilm from endoscopes: evaluation of detergent efficiency. *Am J Infect Control.* 2004;32(3):170-176. [IIB]

126. Sava A. Biofilm digestion: more confusion than answers. *Am J Infect Control.* 2005;33(10):614. [VB]

127. Marion K, Freney J, James G, Bergeron E, Renaud FN, Costerton JW. Using an efficient biofilm detaching agent: an essential step for the improvement of endoscope reprocessing protocols. *J Hosp Infect.* 2006;64(2):136-142. [IIB]

128. Perret-Vivancos C, Marion K, Renaud FN, Freney J. Efficient removal of attached biofilm in a naturally contaminated colonoscope using detachment-promoting agents. *J Hosp Infect.* 2008;68(3):277-278. [VB]

129. Thomas LA. Essentials for endoscopic equipment. Manual cleaning. *Gastroenterol Nurs.* 2005;28(6):512-513. [VB]

130. Herve R, Keevil CW. Current limitations about the cleaning of luminal endoscopes. *J Hosp Infect.* 2013;83(1):22-29. [IIC]

131. Alfa MJ, Olson N, Degagne P, Jackson M. A survey of reprocessing methods, residual viable bioburden, and soil levels in patient-ready endoscopic retrograde choliangiopancreatography duodenoscopes used in Canadian centers. *Infect Control Hosp Epidemiol.* 2002;23(4):198-206. [IIIA]

132. Pineau L, De Philippe E. Evaluation of endoscope cleanliness after reprocessing: a clinical-use study. *Zentralsterilisation.* 2013;21(1):15-27. [IIIB]

133. Dietze B, Kircheis U, Schwarz I, Martiny H. Freely accessible endoscope channels improve efficacy of cleaning. *Endoscopy.* 2001;33(6):523-528. [IIB]

134. Ishino Y, Ido K, Koiwai H, Sugano K. Pitfalls in endoscope reprocessing: brushing of air and water channels is mandatory for high-level disinfection. *Gastrointest Endosc.* 2001;53(2):165-168. [IIB]

135. Agerton T, Valway S, Gore B, et al. Transmission of a highly drug-resistant strain (strain W1) of *Mycobacterium tuberculosis.* Community outbreak and nosocomial transmission via a contaminated bronchoscope. *JAMA.* 1997;278(13):1073-1077. [VA]

136. Alrabaa SF, Nguyen P, Sanderson R, et al. Early identification and control of carbapenemase-producing *Klebsiella pneumoniae,* originating from contaminated endoscopic equipment. *Am J Infect Control.* 2013;41(6):562-564. [VA]

137. Wendorf KA, Kay M, Baliga C, et al. Endoscopic retrograde cholangiopancreatography-associated AmpC *Escherichia coli* outbreak. *Infect Control Hosp Epidemiol.* 2015;36(6):634-642. [IIIA]

138. Supplemental measures to enhance duodenoscope reprocessing: FDA safety communication. US Food and Drug Administration. http://www.fda.gov/MedicalDevices/Safety/Alerts andNotices/ucm454766.htm. Accessed December 9, 2015. [VA]

139. Edmiston CE Jr, Spencer M. Endoscope reprocessing in 2014: why is the margin of safety so small? *AORN J.* 2014;100(6): 609-615. [VA]

140. An outbreak of carbapenem-resistant *Klebsiella pneumoniae* infections associated with endoscopic retrograde cholangiopancreatography (ERCP) procedures at a hospital. *Am J Infect Control.* 2010;38(5):e141. [VB]

141. Notes from the field: New Delhi metallo-β-lactamase–producing *Escherichia coli* associated with endoscopic retrograde cholangiopancreatography—Illinois, 2013. *Morb Mortal Weekly Rep.* 2014;62(51):1051. [VA]

142. Advocate Lutheran General Hospital. Report No. 8196. January 16, 2014. Association of Health Care Journalists. http://www.hospitalinspections.org/report/8196. Accessed December 9, 2015.

143. Muscarella LF. Risk of transmission of carbapenem-resistant *Enterobacteriaceae* and related "superbugs" during gastrointestinal endoscopy. *World J Gastrointest Endosc.* 2014;6(10):457-474. [VA]

144. Ross AS, Baliga C, Verma P, Duchin J, Gluck M. A quarantine process for the resolution of duodenoscope-associated transmission of multidrug-resistant *Escherichia coli. Gastrointest Endosc.* 2015;82(3):477-483. [VA]

145. *Meeting of the FDA Gastroenterology and Urology Devices Panel of the Medical Devices Advisory Committee* [transcript]. Annapolis, MD: Free State Reporting, Inc; May 14, 2015. [VA]

146. Kola A, Piening B, Pape UF, et al. An outbreak of carbapenem-resistant OXA-48-producing *Klebsiella pneumonia* associated to duodenoscopy. *Antimicrob Resist Infect Control.* 2015;4:8-015-0049-4. eCollection 2015. [VA]

147. Verfaillie CJ, Bruno MJ, F Voor In 't Holt A, et al. Withdrawal of a novel-design duodenoscope ends outbreak of a VIM-2-producing *Pseudomonas aeruginosa. Endoscopy.* 2015;47(6):493-502. [VA]

148. Behnia MM, Amurao K, Clemons V, Lantz G. Pseudo-outbreak of and *Acinetobacter baumannii* by a contaminated bronchoscope in an intensive care unit. *Tanaffos.* 2010;9(3):44-49. [VB]

149. Charlton TS. A comparison of the efficacy of lumen-cleaning devices for flexible gastrointestinal endoscopes. *Aust Infect Control.* 2007;12(3):81. [IIIC]

150. Charlton TS. A comparison of two devices for the manual cleaning of flexible gastrointestinal endoscopes in a clinical setting. *Aust Infect Control.* 2007;12(4):130-130, 132, 134, passim. [IIIB]

151. *Final report: Comparative Brush Study of the Cygnus Medical Dragon Tail Cleaning Brush and the Olympus Single Use Combination Cleaning Brush Protein Analysis.* Study No. 1504-244. Rochester, NY: HIGHPOWER Validation Testing & Lab Services; 2015. [IIB]

152. Society of Gastroenterology Nurses and Associates. Reprocessing of endoscopic accessories and valves. *Gastroenterol Nurs.* 2013;36(4):291-292. [IVB]

153. Society of Gastroenterology Nurses and Associates. *Position Statement on Reprocessing of Water Bottles Used During Endoscopy.* Updated 2011. http://www.ascquality.org/Library/endoscopereprocessingtoolkit/SGNA%20Water%20Bottle%20Reprocessing.pdf. Accessed December 9, 2015. [IVB]

154. Parente DM. Could biopsy port valves be a source for potential flexible endoscope contamination? *Infect Control Today.* 2007;11(5). [IIIC]

155. Liquid chemical sterilization. US Food and Drug Administration. http://www.fda.gov/MedicalDevices/Productsand MedicalProcedures/GeneralHospitalDevicesandSupplies/ ucm208018.htm. Accessed December 9, 2015.

156. Veterans Affairs Office of Inspector General. *Use and Reprocessing of Flexible Fiberoptic Endoscopes at VA Medical Facilities.* Report No. 09-01784-146. Washington, DC: Department of Veterans Affairs; 2009. [VA]

157. Muscarella LF. Disinfecting endoscopes immediately before the first patient of the day. *AORN J.* 2001;73(6):1159-1163. [VA]

158. Puterbaugh M, Barde C, Van Enk R. Endoscopy water source: tap or sterile water? *Gastroenterol Nurs.* 1997;20(6):203-206. [IIC]

159. Wilcox CM, Waites K, Brookings ES. Use of sterile compared with tap water in gastrointestinal endoscopic procedures. *Am J Infect Control.* 1996;24(5):407-410. [IIC]

160. Rockey DC. Endoscopy: dollars and sense. *Gastroenterology.* 1995;108(6):1957. [VB]

161. Patton RF, Wilcox CM, Blakely J. Benefits of sterile water use in an endoscopic laboratory [4] (multiple letters). *Am J Infect Control.* 1998;26(3):366-367. [VC]

162. Guideline for electrosurgery. In: *Guidelines for Perioperative Practice.* Denver, CO: AORN, Inc; 2015:121-138. [IVB]

163. Wilson SJ, Everts RJ, Kirkland KB, Sexton DJ. A pseudo-outbreak of *Aureobasidium* species lower respiratory tract infections caused by reuse of single-use stopcocks during bronchoscopy. *Infect Control Hosp Epidemiol.* 2000;21(7):470-472. [VB]

164. Rutala WA, Weber DJ. New developments in reprocessing semicritical items. *Am J Infect Control.* 2013;41(5 Suppl):S60-S66. [VA]

165. *Meeting of the FDA Gastroenterology and Urology Devices Panel of the Medical Devices Advisory Committee* [transcript]. Annapolis, MD: Free State Reporting, Inc; May 15, 2015. [VA]

166. Rutala WA, Weber DJ. Gastrointestinal endoscopes: a need to shift from disinfection to sterilization? *JAMA.* 2014; 312(14):1405-1406. [VA]

167. Puzey A. Managing the risks of prion disease transmission through flexible endoscopy. *Gastrointest Nurs.* 2010; 8(2):18-25. [VA]

168. Tschudin-Sutter S, Frei R, Kampf G, et al. Emergence of glutaraldehyde-resistant *Pseudomonas aeruginosa. Infect Control Hosp Epidemiol.* 2011;32(12):1173-1178. [VA]

169. Fisher CW, Fiorello A, Shaffer D, Jackson M, McDonnell GE. Aldehyde-resistant mycobacteria bacteria associated with the use of endoscope reprocessing systems. *Am J Infect Control.* 2012;40(9):880-882. [IIC]

170. Epstein L, Hunter JC, Arwady MA, et al. New Delhi metallo-beta-lactamase-producing carbapenem-resistant *Escherichia coli* associated with exposure to duodenoscopes. *JAMA.* 2014;312(14):1447-1455. [IIIA]

171. McCool S, Clarke L, Querry A, et al. Carbapenem-resistant *Enterobacteriaceae* (CRE) *Klebsiella pneumonia* (KP) Cluster Analysis Associated with GI Scopes with Elevator Channel [poster]. 2013. Infectious Diseases Society of America. https:// idsa.confex.com/idsa/2013/webprogram/Handout/id1798/ POSTER188_1619.pdf. Accessed December 9, 2015. [VA]

172. Campagnaro RL, Teichtahl H, Dwyer B. A pseudoepidemic of *Mycobacterium chelonae*: contamination of a bronchoscope and autocleaner. *Aust New Zealand J Med.* 1994;24(6):693-695. [VB]

173. Chang CL, Su LH, Lu CM, Tai FT, Huang YC, Chang KK. Outbreak of ertapenem-resistant *Enterobacter cloacae* urinary tract infections due to a contaminated ureteroscope. *J Hosp Infect.* 2013;85(2):118-124. [IIIB]

174. Smith ZL, Oh YS, Saeian K, et al. Transmission of carbapenem-resistant *Enterobacteriaceae* during ERCP: time to revisit the current reprocessing guidelines. *Gastrointest Endosc.* 2015;81(4):1041-1045. [VA]

175. Müller S, Maguilnilk I, Konkewicz LR, Barth AL, Kuchenbecker RS. Biofilm in duodenoscope: hospital infection by pan-resistant *Aeruginosa pseudomonas* related to endoscopic retrograde cholangiopancreatography (ERCP). *J GENCA.* 2010; 20(1):13-14. [VC]

176. Alfa MJ, DeGagne P, Olson N, Puchalski T. Comparison of ion plasma, vaporized hydrogen peroxide, and 100% ethylene oxide sterilizers to the 12/88 ethylene oxide gas sterilizer. *Infect Control Hosp Epidemiol.* 1996;17(2):92-100. [IIB]

177. Boyer JL. Bile formation and secretion. *Compr Physiol.* 2013;3(3):1035-1078. [VA]

178. Alfa MJ, DeGagne P, Olson N, Hizon R. Comparison of liquid chemical sterilization with peracetic acid and ethylene oxide sterilization for long narrow lumens. *Am J Infect Control.* 1998;26(5):469-477. [IIB]

179. Alfa MJ, DeGagne P, Olson N. Validation of ATS as an appropriate test soil to assess cleaning and sterilization efficacy in narrow lumened medical devices such as flexible endoscopes. *Zentralsterilisation.* 2005;13(6):387-402. [IIB]

180. Muscarella LF. Automatic flexible endoscope reprocessors. *Gastrointest Endosc Clin N Am.* 2000;10(2):245-257. [VA]

181. Ofstead CL, Wetzler HP, Snyder AK, Horton RA. Endoscope reprocessing methods: a prospective study on the impact of human factors and automation. *Gastroenterol Nurs.* 2010;33(4):304-311. [IIIA]

182. Ubhayawardana DL, Kottahachchi J, Weerasekera MM, Wanigasooriya IW, Fernando SS, De Silva M. Residual bioburden in reprocessed side-view endoscopes used for endoscopic retrograde cholangiopancreatography (ERCP). *Endosc Int Open.* 2013;1(1):12-16. [IIIB]

183. Kenters N, Huijskens EG, Meier C, Voss A. Infectious diseases linked to cross-contamination of flexible endoscopes. *Endosc Int Open.* 2015;3(4):E259-E265. [VA]

184. Vickery K, Ngo QD, Zou J, Cossart YE. The effect of multiple cycles of contamination, detergent washing, and disinfection on the development of biofilm in endoscope tubing. *Am J Infect Control.* 2009;37(6):470-475. [IIB]

185. Balsamo AC, Graziano KU, Schneider RP, Antunes Junior M, Lacerda RA. Removing biofilm from an endoscopic: evaluation of disinfection methods currently used. *Rev Esc Enferm USP.* 2012;46(Spec): 91-98. [IIB]

186. Farina A, Fievet MH, Plassart F, Menet MC, Thuillier A. Residual glutaraldehyde levels in fiberoptic endoscopes: measurement and implications for patient toxicity. *J Hosp Infect.* 1999;43(4):293-297. [IIIC]

187. Dirlam Langlay AM, Ofstead CL, Mueller NJ, Tosh PK, Baron TH, Wetzler HP. Reported gastrointestinal endoscope reprocessing lapses: the tip of the iceberg. *Am J Infect Control.* 2013;41(12):1188-1194. [VA]

188. Moses FM, Lee JS. Current GI endoscope disinfection and QA practices. *Dig Dis Sci.* 2004;49(11-12):1791-1797. [IIIB]

189. Schaefer MK, Jhung M, Dahl M, et al. Infection control assessment of ambulatory surgical centers. *JAMA.* 2010;303(22):2273-2279. [IIIA]

190. Park JB, Yang JN, Lim YJ, et al. Survey of endoscope reprocessing in Korea. *Clin Endosc.* 2015;48(1):39-47. [IIIB]

191. Przytulski K, Reguła J. Disinfection of endoscopes and sterilization of accessories for gastrointestinal endoscopy in Polish units—analysis of the questionnaire. *Gastroenterol Pol.* 2004;11(3):241-243. [IIIC]

192. Yamada G, Takahashi H, Abe S. A survey of bronchoscope reprocessing procedure in Japan [2]. *J Bronchol.* 2005;12(3):184-185. [IIIC]

193. Zhang X, Kong J, Tang P, ct al. Currcnt status of clcaning and disinfection for gastrointestinal endoscopy in China: a survey of 122 endoscopy units. *Dig Liver Dis.* 2011;43(4):305-308. [IIIB]

194. Akamatsu T, Tabata K, Hironga M, Kawakami H, Uyeda M. Transmission of *Helicobacter pylori* infection via flexible fiberoptic endoscopy. *Am J Infect Control.* 1996;24(5):396-401. [IIIB]

195. Ahuja V, Tandon RK. Survey of gastrointestinal endoscope disinfection and accessory reprocessing practices in the Asia-Pacific region. *J Gastroenterol Hepatol.* 2000;15(Suppl):G78-G81. [IIIB]

196. Barbosa JM, Souza AC, Tipple AF, Pimenta FC, Leao LS, Silva SR. Endoscope reprocessing using glutaraldehyde in endoscopy services of Goiania, Brazil: a realidade em servicos de endoscopia de Goiania, GO. *Arq Gastroenterol.* 2010;47(3):219-224. [IIIB]

197. Fratila O, Tantau M. Cleaning and disinfection in gastrointestinal endoscopy: current status in Romania. *J Gastrointest Liver Dis.* 2006;15(1):89-93. [IIIC]

198. Heudorf U, Exner M. German guidelines for reprocessing endoscopes and endoscopic accessories: guideline compliance in Frankfurt/Main, Germany. *J Hosp Infect.* 2006;64(1):69-75. [IIIC]

199. Honeybourne D, Neumann CS. An audit of bronchoscopy practice in the United Kingdom: a survey of adherence to national guidelines. *Thorax.* 1997;52(8):709-713. [IIIC]

200. Lubbe DE, Fagan JJ. South African survey on disinfection techniques for the flexible nasopharyngoscope. *J Laryngol Otol.* 2003;117(10):811-814. [IIIC]

201. Orsi GB, Filocamo A, Di Stefano L, Tittobello A. Italian National Survey of Digestive Endoscopy Disinfection Procedures. *Endoscopy.* 1997;29(8):732-738. [IIIC]

202. Soares JB, Goncalves R, Banhudo A, Pedrosa J. Reprocessing practice in digestive endoscopy units of district hospitals: results of a Portuguese National Survey. *Eur J Gastroenterol Hepatol.* 2011;23(11):1064-1068. [IIIB]

203. Spinzi G, Fasoli R, Centenaro R, Minoli G; SIED Lombardia Working Group. Reprocessing in digestive endoscopy units in Lombardy: results of a regional survey. *Dig Liver Dis.* 2008;40(11):890-896. [IIIB]

204. Ribeiro MM, de Oliveira AC, Ribeiro SM, Watanabe E, de Resende Stoianoff MA, Ferreira JA. Effectiveness of flexible gastrointestinal endoscope reprocessing. *Infect Control Hosp Epidemiol.* 2013;34(3):309-312. [IIIB]

205. Lakhani R, Smithard A, Bleach N. How clean is your scope? A completed audit cycle of the disinfection of nasendoscopes. *Ann R Coll Surg Engl.* 2010;92(7):587-590. [IIB]

206. Banfield GK, Hinton AE. A national survey of disinfection techniques for flexible nasen*doscopes* in UK ENT out-patient departments. *J Laryngol Otol.* 2000;114(3):202-204. [IIIC]

207. Brake MK, Lee BS, Savoury L, et al. Survey of nasopharyngoscope decontamination methods in Canada. *J Otolaryngol Head Neck Surg.* 2010;39(6):714-722. [IIIB]

208. Kressel AB, Kidd F. Pseudo-outbreak of *Mycobacterium chelonae* and *Methylobacterium mesophilicum* caused by contamination of an automated endoscopy washer. *Infect Control Hosp Epidemiol.* 2001;22(7):414-418. [VB]

209. Schelenz S, French G. An outbreak of multidrug-resistant *Pseudomonas aeruginosa* infection associated with contamination of bronchoscopes and an endoscope washer-disinfector. *J Hosp Infect.* 2000;46(1):23-30. [VB]

210. Blanc DS, Parret T, Janin B, Raselli P, Francioli P. Nosocomial infections and pseudoinfections from contaminated bronchoscopes: two-year follow up using molecular markers. *Infect Control Hosp Epidemiol.* 1997;18(2):134-136. [IIIB]

211. Maloney S, Welbel S, Daves B, et al. *Mycobacterium abscessus* pseudoinfection traced to an automated endoscope washer: utility of epidemiologic and laboratory investigation. *J Infect Dis.* 1994;169(5):1166-1169. [IIIB]

212. Centers for Disease Control and Prevention (CDC). Bronchoscopy-related infections and pseudoinfections—New York, 1996 and 1998. *MMWR Morb Mortal Wkly Rep.* 1999;48(26):557-560. [VA]

213. Chroneou A, Zimmerman SK, Cook S, et al. Molecular typing of *Mycobacterium chelonae* isolates from a pseudo-outbreak involving an automated bronchoscope washer. *Infect Control Hosp Epidemiol.* 2008;29(11):1088-1090. [VC]

214. Gillespie TG, Hogg L, Budge E, Duncan A, Coia JE. *Mycobacterium chelonae* isolated from rinse water within an endoscope washer-disinfector. *J Hosp Infect.* 2000;45(4):332-334. [VC]

215. Rosengarten D, Block C, Hidalgo-Grass C, et al. Cluster of pseudoinfections with Burkholderia cepacia associated with a contaminated washer-disinfector in a bronchoscopy unit. *Infect Control Hosp Epidemiol.* 2010;31(7):769-771. [VA]

216. Ramirez J, Ahmed Z, Gutierrez CN, Byrd RP Jr, Roy TM, Sarubbi FA. Impact of atypical mycobacterial contamination of bronchoscopy on patient care: report of an outbreak and review of the literature. *Infect Dis Clin Pract (Baltim Md).* 1998;7(6):281-285. [VC]

217. Zweigner J, Gastmeier P, Kola A, Klefisch F-R, Schweizer C, Hummel M. A carbapenem-resistant *Klebsiella pneumoniae* outbreak following bronchoscopy. *Am J Infect Control.* 2014;42(8):936-937. [VB]

218. Mean M, Mallaret MR, Bichard P, Shum J, Zarski JP. Gastrointestinal endoscopes cleaned without detergent substance following an automated endoscope washer/disinfector dysfunction. *Gastroenterol Clin Biol.* 2006;30(5):665-668. [VC]

219. Larson JL, Lambert L, Stricof RL, Driscoll J, McGarry MA, Ridzon R. Potential nosocomial exposure to *Mycobacterium tuberculosis* from a bronchoscope. *Infect Control Hosp Epidemiol.* 2003;24(11):825-830. [VA]

220. Kara M, Turan I, Polat Z, Dogru T, Bagci S. Chemical colitis caused by peracetic acid or hydrogen peroxide: a challenging dilemma. *Endoscopy.* 2010;42(Suppl 2):E3-E4. [VC]

221. Cammarota G, Cesaro P, Cazzato A, et al. Hydrogen peroxide-related colitis (previously known as "pseudolipomatosis"): a series of cases occurring in an epidemic pattern. *Endoscopy.* 2007;39(10):916-919. [VC]

222. Gamble HP, Duckworth GJ, Ridgway GL. Endoscope decontamination incidents in England 2003-2004. *J Hosp Infect.* 2007;67(4):350-354. [VB]

223. Vanhems P, Gayet-Ageron A, Ponchon T, et al. Follow-up and management of patients exposed to a flawed automated endoscope washer-disinfector in a digestive diseases unit. *Infect Control Hosp Epidemiol.* 2006;27(1):89-92. [VB]

224. Vanhems P, Gayet-Ageron A, Ponchon T, et al. Erratum: Follow-up and management of patients exposed to a flawed automated endoscope washer-disinfector in a digestive diseases unit (Infection Control and Hospital Epidemiology [January 2006] 27 [89-91]). *Infect Control Hosp Epidemiol.* 2006;27(4):431.

225. Alfa MJ, Olson N, DeGagne P. Automated washing with the Reliance Endoscope Processing System and its equivalence to optimal manual cleaning. *Am J Infect Control.* 2006;34(9):561-570. [IIB]

226. Funk SE, Reaven NL. High-level endoscope disinfection processes in emerging economies: financial impact of manual process versus automated endoscope reprocessing. *J Hosp Infect.* 2014;86(4):250-254. [IIIC]

227. Forte L, Shum C. Comparative cost-efficiency of the EVOTECH endoscope cleaner and reprocessor versus manual cleaning plus automated endoscope reprocessing in a real-world Canadian hospital endoscopy setting. *BMC Gastroenterology.* 2011;11:105. [IIIB]

228. Alfa MJ, DeGagne P, Olson N, Fatima I. EVOTECH endoscope cleaner and reprocessor (ECR) simulated-use and clinical-use evaluation of cleaning efficacy. *BMC Infect Dis.* 2010;10:200. [IIA]

229. Bhatt JM, Peterson EM, Verma SP. Microbiological sampling of the forgotten components of a flexible fiberoptic laryngoscope: what lessons can we learn? *Otolaryngol Head Neck Surg.* 2014;150(2):235-236. [IIIC]

230. Sorin M, Segal-Maurer S, Mariano N, Urban C, Combest A, Rahal JJ. Nosocomial transmission of imipenem-resistant *Pseudomonas aeruginosa* following bronchoscopy associated with improper connection to the Steris System 1 processor. *Infect Control Hosp Epidemiol.* 2001;22(7):409-413. [IIIB]

231. Esteban J, Gadea I, Fernandez-Roblas R, et al. Pseudo-outbreak of Aeromonas hydrophila isolates related to endoscopy. *J Hosp Infect.* 1999;41(4):313-316. [VC]

232. West AB, Kuan SF, Bennick M, Lagarde S. Glutaraldehyde colitis following endoscopy: clinical and pathological features and investigation of an outbreak. *Gastroenterology.* 1995;108(4):1250-1255. [VC]

233. Kim SJ, Baek IH. Colonic mucosal pseudolipomatosis: disinfectant colitis? *Gastroenterol Nurs.* 2012;35(3):208-213. [IIIB]

234. Rozen P, Somjen GJ, Baratz M, Kimel R, Arber N, Gilat T. Endoscope-induced colitis: description, probable cause by glutaraldehyde, and prevention. *Gastrointest Endosc.* 1994;40(5):547-553. [VC]

235. Tsai MS, Chiu HH, Li JH. Education and imaging. Gastrointestinal: glutaraldehyde proctocolitis. *J Gastroenterol Hepatol.* 2008;23(9):1460. [VC]

236. Yen HH, Chen YY. Glutaraldehyde colitis. *Endoscopy.* 2006;38(Suppl 2):E98. [VB]

237. Mohamad MZ, Koh KS, Chong VH. Gluteraldehyde-induced colitis: a rare cause of lower gastrointestinal bleeding. *Am J Emerg Med.* 2014;32(6):685.e1-685.e2. [VC]

238. Mee AS, Bower M. Risk factors for pancreatitis [2]. *Gut.* 1997;40(2):289. [VC]

239. Stein BL, Lamoureux E, Miller M, Vasilevsky CA, Julien L, Gordon PH. Glutaraldehyde-induced colitis. *Can J Surg.* 2001;44(2):113-116. [VC]

240. Caprilli R, Viscido A, Frieri G, Latella G. Acute colitis following colonoscopy. *Endoscopy.* 1998;30(4):428-431. [VC]

241. Bennett SN, Peterson DE, Johnson DR, Hall WN, Robinson-Dunn B, Dietrich S. Bronchoscopy-associated *Mycobacterium* xenopi pseudoinfections. *Am J Respir Crit Care Med.* 1994;150(1):245-250. [IIIA]

242. Wendelboe AM, Baumbach J, Blossom DB, Frank P, Srinivasan A, Sewell CM. Outbreak of cystoscopy related infections with *Pseudomonas aeruginosa*: New Mexico, 2007. *J Urol.* 2008;180(2):588-592. [IIIB]

243. Alfa MJ, Sitter DL. In-hospital evaluation of contamination of duodenoscopes: a quantitative assessment of the effect of drying. *J Hosp Infect.* 1991;19(2):89-98. [IIIA]

244. Muscarella LF. Inconsistencies in endoscope-reprocessing and infection-control guidelines: the importance of endoscope drying. *Am J Gastroenterol.* 2006;101(9):2147-2154. [VA]

245. Wang HC, Liaw YS, Yang PC, Kuo SH, Luh KT. A pseudo-epidemic of *Mycobacterium chelonae* infection caused by contamination of a fibreoptic bronchoscope suction channel. *Eur Respir J.* 1995;8(8):1259-1262. [IIIC]

246. Gavalda L, Olmo AR, Hernandez R, et al. Microbiological monitoring of flexible bronchoscopes after high-level disinfection and flushing channels with alcohol: results and costs. *Respir Med.* 2015;109(8):1079-1085. [IIB]

247. Muscarella LF. Application of environmental sampling to flexible endoscope reprocessing: the importance of monitoring the rinse water. *Infect Control Hosp Epidemiol.* 2002;23(5):285-289. [VA]

248. Kovaleva J, Degener JE, van der Mei HC. Mimicking disinfection and drying of biofilms in contaminated endoscopes. *J Hosp Infect.* 2010;76(4):345-350. [IIIB]

249. Hagan ME, Klotz SA, Bartholomew W, Potter L, Nelson M. A pseudoepidemic of *Rhodotorula rubra*: a marker for microbial contamination of the bronchoscope. *Infect Control Hosp Epidemiol.* 1995;16(12):727-728. [VC]

250. Carbonne A, Thiolet JM, Fournier S, et al. Control of a multi-hospital outbreak of KPC-producing *Klebsiella pneumoniae* type 2 in France, September to October 2009. *Euro Surveill.* 2010;15(48):pii:19734. [VA]

251. Rutala WA, Weber DJ. ERCP scopes: what can we do to prevent infections? *Infect Control Hosp Epidemiol.* 2015;36(6):643-648. [VA]

252. Alfa MJ, Degagne P, Olson N. Worst-case soiling levels for patient-used flexible endoscopes before and after cleaning. *Am J Infect Control.* 1999;27(5):392-401. [IIA]

253. Foliente RL, Kovacs BJ, Aprecio RM, Bains HJ, Kettering JD, Chen YK. Efficacy of high-level disinfectants for reprocessing GI endoscopes in simulated-use testing. *Gastrointest Endosc.* 2001;53(4):456-462. [IIC]

254. Rutala WA, Weber DJ. FDA labeling requirements for disinfection of endoscopes: a counterpoint. *Infect Control Hosp Epidemiol.* 1995;16(4):231-235. [VB]

255. Guideline for selection and use of packaging systems for sterilization. In: *Guidelines for Perioperative Practice.* Denver, CO: AORN, Inc; 2015:651-664. [IVA]

256. Guideline for sterilization. In: *Guidelines for Perioperative Practice.* Denver, Co: AORN, Inc; 2015:665-692. [IVA]

257. Rutala WA, Weber DJ; Society for Healthcare Epidemiology of America. Guideline for disinfection and sterilization of prion-contaminated medical instruments. *Infect Control Hosp Epidemiol.* 2010;31(2):107-117. [IVA]

258. Widmer A. Prions and endoscopy: an unresolved problem. *Zentralsterilisation.* 2004;12(Suppl 1):70-77. [VB]

259. Cooke RP, Goddard SV. Endoscopes and protective sheaths. *J Hosp Infect.* 2002;52(2):153-154. [VC]

260. Lawrentschuk N, Chamberlain M. Sterile disposable sheath system for flexible cystoscopes. *Urology.* 2005;66(6):1310-1313. [VC]

261. Baker KH, Chaput MP, Clavet CR, Varney GW, To TM, Lytle CD. Evaluation of endoscope sheaths as viral barriers. *Laryngoscope.* 1999;109(4):636-639. [IIIC]

262. Elackattu A, Zoccoli M, Spiegel JH, Grundfast KM. A comparison of two methods for preventing cross-contamination when using flexible fiberoptic endoscopes in an otolaryngology clinic: disposable sterile sheaths versus immersion in germicidal liquid. *Laryngoscope.* 2010;120(12):2410-2416. [IIB]

263. Mayinger B, Strenkert M, Hochberger J, Martus P, Kunz B, Hahn EG. Disposable-sheath, flexible gastroscope system versus standard gastroscopes: a prospective, randomized trial. *Gastrointest Endosc.* 1999;50(4):461-467. [IB]

264. Alvarado CJ, Anderson AG, Maki DG. Microbiologic assessment of disposable sterile endoscopic sheaths to replace high-level disinfection in reprocessing: a prospective clinical trial with nasopharygoscopes. *Am J Infect Control.* 2009;37(5):408-413. [IA]

265. Colt HG, Beamis JJ, Harrell JH, Mathur PM. Novel flexible bronchoscope and single-use disposable-sheath endoscope system. A preliminary technology evaluation. *Chest.* 2000;118(1):183-187. [VB]

266. Street I, Hamann J, Harries M. Audit of nasendoscope disinfection practice. *Surgeon.* 2006;4(1):11-13. [VC]

267. Jorgensen PH, Slotsbjerg T, Westh H, Buitenhuis V, Hermann GG. A microbiological evaluation of level of disinfection for flexible cystoscopes protected by disposable endosheaths. *BMC Urol.* 2013;13:46. [IIIB]

268. Guidance for manufacturers seeking marketing clearance of ear, nose, and throat endoscope sheaths used as protective barriers: guidance for industry. US Food and Drug Administration. http://www.fda.gov/RegulatoryInformation/Guidances/ucm073746.htm. Accessed December 9, 2015.

269. FDA-cleared sterilants and high level disinfectants with general claims for processing reusable medical and dental devices—March 2015. http://www.fda.gov/MedicalDevices/DeviceRegulationandGuidance/ReprocessingofReusableMedicalDevices/ucm437347.htm. Accessed December 9, 2015.

270. Javed F, Sood S, Banfield G. Decontamination methods for flexible nasal endoscopes. *Br J Nurs.* 2014;23(15):850-852. [IIIB]

271. Bhattacharyya N, Kepnes LJ. The effectiveness of immersion disinfection for flexible fiberoptic laryngoscopes. *Otolaryngol Head Neck Surg.* 2004;130(6):681-685. [IIB]

272. Chang D, Florea A, Rowe M, Seiberling KA. Disinfection of flexible fiberoptic laryngoscopes after in vitro contamination with *Staphylococcus aureus* and *Candida albicans*. *Arch Otolaryngol Head Neck Surg.* 2012;138(2):119-121. [IIB]

273. Tzanidakis K, Choudhury N, Bhat S, Weerasinghe A, Marais J. Evaluation of disinfection of flexible nasendoscopes using Tristel wipes: a prospective single blind study. *Ann R Coll Surg Engl.* 2012;94(3):185-188. [IIIB]

274. Liming B, Funnell I, Jones A, Demons S, Marshall K, Harsha W. An evaluation of varying protocols for high-level disinfection of flexible fiberoptic laryngoscopes. *Laryngoscope.* 2014;124(11):2498-2501. [IIB]

275. Phua CQ, Mahalingappa Y, Karagama Y. Sequential cohort study comparing chlorine dioxide wipes with automated washing for decontamination of flexible nasendoscopes. *J Laryngol Otol.* 2012;126(8):809-814. [IIB]

276. Foxcroft L, Monaghan W, Faoagali J. Controlled study of the Lancer FD8 drying/storage cabinet for endoscopes. *J GENCA.* 2008;18(2):5-11. [IIB]

277. Pineau L, Villard E, Duc DL, Marchetti B. Endoscope drying/storage cabinet: interest and efficacy. *J Hosp Infect.* 2008;68(1):59-65. [IIC]

278. Wardle B. Endoscope storage cabinets. *J GENCA.* 2007;17(3):5. [IIC]

279. Rejchrt S, Cermak P, Pavlatova L, McKova E, Bures J. Bacteriologic testing of endoscopes after high-level disinfection. *Gastrointest Endosc.* 2004;60(1):76-78. [IIC]

280. Vergis AS, Thomson D, Pieroni P, Dhalla S. Reprocessing flexible gastrointestinal endoscopes after a period of disuse: is it necessary? *Endoscopy.* 2007;39(8):737-739. [IIB]

281. Marino M, Grieco G, Moscato U, et al. Is reprocessing after disuse a safety procedure for bronchoscopy?: a cross-sectional study in a teaching hospital in Rome. *Gastroenterol Nurs.* 2012;35(5):324-330. [IIB]

282. Ingram J, Gaines P, Kite R, Morgan M, Spurling S, Winsett RP. Evaluation of medically significant bacteria in

colonoscopes after 8 weeks of shelf life in open air storage. *Gastroenterol Nurs.* 2013;36(2):106-111. [IIB]

283. Grandval P, Hautefeuille G, Marchetti B, Pineau L, Laugier R. Evaluation of a storage cabinet for heat-sensitive endoscopes in a clinical setting. *J Hosp Infect.* 2013;84(1):71-76. [IIIB]

284. Osborne S, Reynolds S, George N, Lindemayer F, Gill A, Chalmers M. Challenging endoscopy reprocessing guidelines: a prospective study investigating the safe shelf life of flexible endoscopes in a tertiary gastroenterology unit. *Endoscopy.* 2007;39(9):825-830. [IIIB]

285. Alfa MJ, Sepehri S, Olson N, Wald A. Establishing a clinically relevant bioburden benchmark: a quality indicator for adequate reprocessing and storage of flexible gastrointestinal endoscopes. *Am J Infect Control.* 2012;40(3):233-236. [IIIB]

286. Brock AS, Steed LL, Freeman J, Garry B, Malpas P, Cotton P. Endoscope storage time: assessment of microbial colonization up to 21 days after reprocessing. *Gastrointest Endosc.* 2015;81(5):1150-1154. [IIIB]

287. Riley R, Beanland C, Bos H. Establishing the shelf life of flexible colonoscopes. *Gastroenterol Nurs.* 2002;25(3):114-119. [IIIB]

288. Thomas LA. Essentials for endoscopic equipment. Recommended care and handling of flexible endoscopes: endoscope storage. *Gastroenterol Nurs.* 2005;28(1):45-46. [VB]

289. Nomides N, Sweeney J, Sturm L, et al. Ready for patient use? Implementing a visual cue for high level disinfected endoscopes. *Am J Infect Control.* 2014;42:S40-S41. [VA]

290. Muscarella LF. The study of a contaminated colonoscope. *Clin Gastroenterol Hepatol.* 2010;8(7):577-580.e1. [VA]

291. Saliou P, Baron R. Method for assessing the microbial contamination of GI endoscopes. *Gastrointest Endosc.* 2015;82(3):582. [VA]

292. Schmelzer M, Daniels G, Hough H. Safe storage time for reprocessed flexible endoscopes: a systematic review. *JBI Database System Rev Implement Rep.* 2015;13(9):187-243. [IIIC]

293. Guideline for health care information management. In: *Guidelines for Perioperative Practice.* Denver, CO: AORN, Inc; 2015:491-512. [IVB]

294. *State Operations Manual Appendix A—Survey Protocol, Regulations and Interpretive Guidelines for Hospitals.* Rev. 105. Washington, DC: Department of Health and Human Services, Centers for Medicare & Medicaid Services. 2014.

295. *State Operations Manual Appendix L—Guidance for Surveyors: Ambulatory Surgical Centers.* Rev. 99. Washington, DC: Department of Health and Human Services, Centers for Medicare & Medicaid Services. 2014.

296. 42 CFR 482. Conditions of participation for hospitals. 2013. US Government Publishing Office. https://www.gpo.gov/fdsys/granule/CFR-2011-title42-vol5/CFR-2011-title42-vol5-part482/content-detail.html. Accessed December 10, 2015.

297. 42 CFR 416: Ambulatory surgical services. 2013. US Government Publishing Office. https://www.gpo.gov/fdsys/granule/CFR-2011-title42-vol3/CFR-2011-title42-vol3-part416. Accessed December 10, 2015.

298. RC.01.01.01: The hospital maintains complete and accurate medical records for each individual patient. In: *Hospital Accreditation Standards.* 2014 ed. Oakbrook Terrace, IL: Joint Commission Resources; 2014.

299. MS.16 Medical record maintenance. In: *NIAHO Interpretive Guidelines and Surveyor Guidance.* 10.1 ed. Milford, OH: DNV Healthcare Inc; 2012:29.

300. RC.01.01.01: The organization maintains complete and accurate clinical records. In: *Standards for Ambulatory Care 2014: Standards, Elements of Performance, Scoring, Accreditation Policies.* Oakbrook Terrace, IL: Joint Commission Resources; 2014.

301. Clinical records and health information. In: *2014 Accreditation Handbook for Ambulatory Health Care.* Skokie, IL: Accreditation Association for Ambulatory Health Care; 2014:37-39.

302. Medical records: pre-operative medical record. In: *Regular Standards and Checklist for Accreditation of Ambulatory Surgery Facilities.* Version 14 ed. Gurnee, IL: American Association for Accreditation of Ambulatory Surgery Facilities; 2014:59-60.

303. Medical records: operating room records. In: *Regular Standards and Checklist for Accreditation of Ambulatory Surgery Facilities.* Version 14 ed. Gurnee, IL: American Association for Accreditation of Ambulatory Surgery Facilities; 2014:62-64.

304. Medical records: general. In: *Regular Standards and Checklist for Accreditation of Ambulatory Surgery Facilities.* Version 14 ed. Gurnee, IL: American Association for Accreditation of Ambulatory Surgery Facilities; 2014:58-59.

305. Medical records: general. In: *Procedural Standards and Checklist for Accreditation of Ambulatory Surgery Facilities.* Version 3 ed. Gurnee, IL: American Association for Accreditation of Ambulatory Surgery Facilities; 2011:60-61.

306. Medical records: procedure room records. In: *Procedural Standards and Checklist for Accreditation of Ambulatory Surgery Facilities.* Version 3 ed. Gurnee, IL: American Association for Accreditation of Ambulatory Surgery Facilities; 2011:64-66.

307. Standards of perioperative nursing practice. In: *Guidelines for Perioperative Practice.* Denver, CO: AORN, Inc; 2015:693-708. [IVB]

308. Jordan C, Thomas MB, Evans ML, Green A. Public policy on competency: how will nursing address this complex issue? *J Contin Educ Nurs.* 2008;39(2):86-91. [VA]

309. HR.01.05.03: Staff participate in ongoing education and training. In: *Comprehensive Accreditation Manual: CAMH for Hospitals.* 2014 ed. Oakbrook Terrace, IL: Joint Commission Resources; 2014.

310. MS.10 Continuing education. In: *NIAHO Interpretive Guidelines and Surveyor Guidance.* 10.1 ed. Milford, OH: DNV Healthcare Inc; 2012:24.

311. HR.01.05.03: Staff participate in ongoing education and training. In: *Comprehensive Accreditation Manual: CAMAC for Ambulatory Care.* 2014 ed. Oakbrook Terrace, IL: Joint Commission Resources; 2014.

312. Governance. In: *2014 Accreditation Handbook for Ambulatory Health Care.* Skokie, IL: Accreditation Association for Ambulatory Health Care; 2014:19-26.

313. Personnel: personnel records; individual personnel files. In: *Regular Standards and Checklist for Accreditation of Ambulatory Surgery Facilities.* Version 14 ed. Gurnee, IL: American Association for Accreditation of Ambulatory Surgery Facilities; 2014:75-76.

314. Personnel: knowledge, skill & CME training. In: *Regular Standards and Checklist for Accreditation of Ambulatory Surgery*

Facilities. Version 14 ed. Gurnee, IL: American Association for Accreditation of Ambulatory Surgery Facilities; 2014:77-78.

315. Personnel: personnel safety. In: *Procedural Standards and Checklist for Accreditation of Ambulatory Surgery Facilities.* Version 3 ed. Gurnee, IL: American Association for Accreditation of Ambulatory Surgery Facilities; 2011:79-80.

316. Personnel: knowledge, skill & CME training. In: *Procedural Standards and Checklist for Accreditation of Ambulatory Surgery Facilities.* Version 3 ed. Gurnee, IL: American Association for Accreditation of Ambulatory Surgery Facilities; 2011:79.

317. Jackson FW, Ball MD. Correction of deficiencies in flexible fiberoptic sigmoidoscope cleaning and disinfection technique in family practice and internal medicine offices. *Arch Fam Med.* 1997;6(6):578-582. [IIC]

318. Lunn W, Garland R, Gryniuk L, Smith L, Feller-Kopman D, Ernst A. Reducing maintenance and repair costs in an interventional pulmonology program. *Chest.* 2005;127(4):1382-1387. [VB]

319. LD.04.01.07: The hospital has policies and procedures that guide and support patient care, treatment, and services. In: *Hospital Accreditation Standards.* 2014 ed. Oakbrook Terrace, IL: Joint Commission Resources; 2014.

320. SS.1: Organization. In: *NIAHO Interpretive Guidelines and Surveyor Guidance.* 10.1 ed. Milford, OH: DNV Healthcare Inc; 2012:70-71.

321. LD.04.01.07: The organization has policies and procedures that guide and support patient care, treatment, or services. In: *Standards for Ambulatory Care 2014: Standards, Elements of performance, Scoring, Accreditation policies.* Oakbrook Terrace, IL: Joint Commission Resources; 2014.

322. Personnel: personnel safety. In: *Regular Standards and Checklist for Accreditation of Ambulatory Surgery Facilities.* Version 14 ed. Gurnee, IL: American Association for Accreditation of Ambulatory Surgery Facilities; 2014:79.

323. Personnel: personnel records. In: *Procedural Standards and Checklist for Accreditation of Ambulatory Surgery Facilities.* Version 3 ed. Gurnee, IL: American Association for Accreditation of Ambulatory Surgery Facilities; 2011:77-79.

324. 200.35: High Level Disinfection of Endoscopes. In: *Regular Standards and Checklist for Accreditation of Ambulatory Surgery Facilities.* Gurnee, IL: American Association for Accreditation of Ambulatory Surgery Facilities; 2014:28.

325. 200.40: Instrument Processing. In: *Regular Standards and Checklist for Accreditation of Ambulatory Surgery Facilities.* Gurnee, IL: American Association for Accreditation of Ambulatory Surgery Facilities; 2014:28.

326. 200.30: Procedures—Sterilization. In: *Procedural Standards and Checklist for Accreditation of Ambulatory Surgery Facilities.* Gurnee, IL: American Association for Accreditation of Ambulatory Surgery Facilities; 2011:34-36.

327. PI.03.01.01: The hospital improves performance on an ongoing basis. In: *Hospital Accreditation Standards.* 2014 ed. Oakbrook Terrace, IL: Joint Commission Resources; 2014.

328. IC.02.01.01: The hospital implements its infection prevention and control plan. In: *Comprehensive Accreditation Manual for Hospitals e-dition.* Washington, DC: The Joint Commission; August 2014.

329. IC.02.02.01: The hospital reduces the risk of infections associated with medical equipment, devices, and supplies. In: *Comprehensive Accreditation Manual for Hospitals e-dition.* Washington, DC: The Joint Commission; August 2014.

330. IC.03.01.01: The hospital evaluates the effectiveness of its infection prevention and control plan. In: *Comprehensive Accreditation Manual for Hospitals e-dition.* Washington, DC: The Joint Commission; August 2014.

331. EC.02.04.03: The hospital inspects, tests, and maintains medical equipment. In: *Hospital Accreditation Standards.* 2015 ed. Oakbrook Terrace, IL: Joint Commission Resources; 2015.

332. Quality management system. In: NIAHO Interpretive Guidelines and Surveyor Guidance. 10.1 ed. Milford, OH: DNV Healthcare Inc; 2012:10-16.

333. Infection prevention and control. In: *NIAHO Accreditation Requirements Interpretive Guidelines & Surveyor Guidance.* 10.1 ed. Milford, OH: DNV Healthcare; 2012.

334. Physical environment. PE.1 Facility. In: *NIAHO Accreditation Requirements Interpretive Guidelines & Surveyor Guidance Revision.* 10.1 ed. Milford, OH: DNV Healthcare; 2012.

335. PI.03.01.01: The organization improves performance. In: *Standards for Ambulatory Care 2014: Standards, Elements of Performance, Scoring, Accreditation Policies.* Oakbrook Terrace, IL: Joint Commission Resources; 2014.

336. IC.02.01.01: The organization implements infection prevention and control activities. In: *Comprehensive Accreditation Manual for Ambulatory Care e-dition.* Washington, DC: The Joint Commission; August 2014.

337. IC.02.02.01: The organization reduces the risk of infections associated with medical equipment, devices, and supplies. In: *Comprehensive Accreditation Manual for Ambulatory Care e-dition.* Washington, DC: The Joint Commission; August 2014.

338. IC.03.01.01: The organization evaluates the effectiveness of its infection prevention and control activities. In: *Comprehensive Accreditation Manual for Ambulatory Care e-dition.* Washington, DC: The Joint Commission; August 2014.

339. EC.02.04.03: The organization inspects, tests, and maintains medical equipment. In: *Ambulatory Accreditation Standards.* 2015 ed. Oakbrook Terrace, IL: Joint Commission Resources; 2015.

340. Quality managment and improvement. In: *Accreditation Handbook for Ambulatory Health Care.* Skokie, IL: Accreditation Association for Ambulatory Health Care; 2014:32-36.

341. Infection prevention and control and safety. In: *Accreditation Handbook for Ambulatory Health Care.* Skokie, IL: Accreditation Association for Ambulatory Health Care; 2014:40-43.

342. Faciliites and environment. In: *Accreditation Handbook for Ambulatory Health Care.* Skokie, IL: Accreditation Association for Ambulatory Health Care; 2014:44-45.

343. Quality assessment/quality improvement: quality improvement. In: *Regular Standards and Checklist for Accreditation of Ambulatory Surgery Facilities.* Version 14 ed. Gurnee, IL: American Association for Accreditation of Ambulatory Surgery Facilities; 2014:65.

344. Quality assessment/quality improvement: unanticipated operative sequelae. In: *Regular Standards and Checklist for Accreditation of Ambulatory Surgery Facilities.* Version 14 ed.

Gurnee, IL: American Association for Accreditation of Ambulatory Surgery Facilities; 2014:68-70.

345. Operating room policy, environment, and procedures: equipment. In: *Regular Standards and Checklist for Accreditation of Ambulatory Surgery Facilities.* Version 14 ed. Gurnee, IL: American Association for Accreditation of Ambulatory Surgery Facilities; 2014:45.

346. Evans P. Cystoscope reprocessing safety: one practice's experience. *AAACN Viewpoint.* 2014;36(2):10-11. [VB]

347. Angtuaco TL, Oprescu FG, Lal SK, et al. Universal precautions guideline: self-reported compliance by gastroenterologists and gastrointestinal endoscopy nurses—a decade's lack of progress. *Am J Gastroenterol.* 2003;98(11):2420-2423. [IIIC]

348. Baudet JS, Martín JM, Sánchez del Rio A, Aguirre-Jaime A. Occupational risk prevention in endoscopy units: a pending issue. *Rev Esp Enferm Dig.* 2011;103(2):83-88. [IIIB]

349. Joint Working Group of the Hospital Infection Society (HIS) and the Public Health Laboratory Service (PHLS). Rinse water for heat labile endoscopy equipment. *J Hosp Infect.* 2002;51(1):7-16. [IVA]

350. Kovaleva J, Degener JE, van der Mei HC. Methylobacterium and its role in health care-associated infection. *J Clin Microbiol.* 2014;52(5):1317-1321. [VA]

351. Phillips G, McEwan H, Butler J. Quality of water in washer-disinfectors. *J Hosp Infect.* 1995;31(2):152-154. [VC]

352. Marek A, Smith A, Peat M, et al. Endoscopy supply water and final rinse testing: five years of experience. *J Hosp Infect.* 2014;88(4):207-212. [VA]

353. Cooke RP. Hazards of water. *J Hosp Infect.* 2004;57(4):290-293. [VB]

354. Cooke RP, Whymant-Morris A, Umasankar RS, Goddard SV. Bacteria-free water for automatic washer-disinfectors: an impossible dream? *J Hosp Infect.* 1998;39(1):63-65. [IIIC]

355. Curtis B, Cooke RPD, Whymant-Morris A, Umasankar RS, Goddard SV. Testing water quality for automatic washer-disinfectors (multiple letters) [5]. *J Hosp Infect.* 1999;42(1):74-76. [VB]

356. Falkinham JO 3rd. Hospital water filters as a source of *Mycobacterium* avium complex. *J Med Microbiol.* 2010;59(Pt 10): 1198-1202. [VC]

357. Rossetti R, Lencioni P, Innocenti F, Tortoli E. Pseudoepidemic from *Mycobacterium gordonae* due to a contaminated automatic bronchoscope washing machine. *Am J Infect Control.* 2002;30(3):196-197. [VB]

358. Khalsa K, Smith A, Morrison P, et al. Contamination of a purified water system by *Aspergillus fumigatus* in a new endoscopy reprocessing unit. *Am J Infect Control.* 2014;42(12):1337-1339. [VB]

359. Mitchell DH, Hicks LJ, Chiew R, Montanaro JC, Chen SC. Pseudoepidemic of *Legionella pneumophila* serogroup 6 associated with contaminated bronchoscopes. *J Hosp Infect.* 1997;37(1):19-23. [VB]

360. Kiely JL, Sheehan S, Cryan B, Bredin CP. Isolation of *Mycobacterium chelonae* in a bronchoscopy unit and its subsequent eradication. *Tuber Lung Dis.* 1995;76(2):163-167. [VC]

361. Phillips L. Identification and resolution of contamination causes found in flexible endoscopes. *Gastroenterol Nurs.* 1997;20(1):9-11. [VC]

362. Hubner NO, Assadian O, Poldrack R, et al. Endowashers: an overlooked risk for possible post-endoscopic infections. *GMS Krankenhhyg Interdiszip.* 2011;6(1):o13. [IIB]

363. Robertson P, Smith A, Mead A, et al. Risk-assessment-based approach to patients exposed to endoscopes contaminated with *Pseudomonas* spp. *J Hosp Infect.* 2015;90(1):66-69. [VB]

364. Phillips G, McEwan H, McKay I, Crowe G, McBeath J. Black pigmented fungi in the water pipe-work supplying endoscope washer disinfectors. *J Hosp Infect.* 1998;40(3):250-251. [VC]

365. Imbert G, Seccia Y, La Scola B. *Methylobacterium* sp. bacteraemia due to a contaminated endoscope. *J Hosp Infect.* 2005; 61(3):268-270. [VC]

366. *Choice Framework for local Policy and Procedures 01-06—Decontamination of flexible endoscopes: Validation and verification.* 2013. UK Department of Health. https://www.gov.uk/government/uploads/system/uploads/attachment_data/file/148562/CFPP_01-06_Validation_Final.pdf. Accessed December 10, 2015. [IVB]

367. Chiu KW, Fong TV, Wu KL, et al. Surveillance culture of endoscope to monitor the quality of high-level disinfection of gastrointestinal reprocessing. *Hepatogastroenterology.* 2010;57(99-100):531-534. [IIC]

368. Corne P, Godreuil S, Jean-Pierre H, et al. Unusual implication of biopsy forceps in outbreaks of *Pseudomonas aeruginosa* infections and pseudo-infections related to bronchoscopy. *J Hosp Infect.* 2005;61(1):20-26. [VB]

369. Qiu L, Zhou Z, Liu Q, Ni Y, Zhao F, Cheng H. Investigating the failure of repeated standard cleaning and disinfection of a *Pseudomonas aeruginosa*-infected pancreatic and biliary endoscope. *Am J Infect Control.* 2015;43(8):e43-e46. [VB]

370. Hunter J, Epstein L. Epi-Aid trip report: cluster of plasmid-mediated AmpC-producing carbapenem-resistant *Enterobacteriaceae* (CRE)—Washington, 2014. Atlanta, GA: Department of Health and Human Services, Centers for Disease Control and Prevention; 2014. [VA]

371. DiazGranados CA, Jones MY, Kongphet-Tran T, et al. Outbreak of *Pseudomonas aeruginosa* infection associated with contamination of a flexible bronchoscope. *Infect Control Hosp Epidemiol.* 2009;30(6):550-555. [IIIA]

372. Lee DH, Kim DB, Kim HY, et al. Increasing potential risks of contamination from repetitive use of endoscope. *Am J Infect Control.* 2015;43(5):e13-e17. [IIB]

373. ASGE Technology Committee; Komanduri S, Abu Dayyeh BK, et al. Technologies for monitoring the quality of endoscope reprocessing. *Gastrointest Endosc.* 2014;80(3):369-373. [VB]

374. Obee PC, Griffith CJ, Cooper RA, Cooke RP, Bennion NE, Lewis M. Real-time monitoring in managing the decontamination of flexible gastrointestinal endoscopes. *Am J Infect Control.* 2005;33(4):202-206. [IIIB]

375. Visrodia KH, Ofstead CL, Yellin HL, Wetzler HP, Tosh PK, Baron TH. The use of rapid indicators for the detection of organic residues on clinically used gastrointestinal endoscopes with and without visually apparent debris. *Infect Control Hosp Epidemiol.* 2014;35(8):987-994. [IIB]

376. Petersen BT. Monitoring of endoscope reprocessing: accumulating data but best practices remain undefined. *Infect Control Hosp Epidemiol.* 2014;35(8):995-997. [VA]

377. Alfa MJ. Monitoring and improving the effectiveness of cleaning medical and surgical devices. *Am J Infect Control.* 2013;41(5 Suppl):S56-S59. [VA]

378. Alfa MJ, Fatima I, Olson N. The adenosine triphosphate test is a rapid and reliable audit tool to assess manual cleaning adequacy of flexible endoscope channels. *Am J Infect Control.* 2013;41(3):249-253. [IIA]

379. Ofstead CL, Wetzler HP, Doyle EM, et al. Persistent contamination on colonoscopes and gastroscopes detected by biologic cultures and rapid indicators despite reprocessing performed in accordance with guidelines. *Am J Infect Control.* 2015;43(8):794-801. [IIB]

380. Hansen D, Benner D, Hilgenhoner M, Leisebein T, Brauksiepe A, Popp W. ATP measurement as method to monitor the quality of reprocessing flexible endoscopes. *Ger Med Sci.* 2004;2:o04. [IIIB]

381. Alfa MJ, Olson N, Degagne P, Simner PJ. Development and validation of rapid use scope test strips to determine the efficacy of manual cleaning for flexible endoscope channels. *Am J Infect Control.* 2012;40(9):860-865. [IIIA]

382. Fernando G, Collignon P, Beckingham W. ATP bioluminescence to validate the decontamination process of gastrointestinal endoscopes. *Healthc Infect.* 2014;19(2):59-64. [IIA]

383. Fushimi R, Takashina M, Yoshikawa H, et al. Comparison of adenosine triphosphate, microbiological load, and residual protein as indicators for assessing the cleanliness of flexible gastrointestinal endoscopes. *Am J Infect Control.* 2013;41(2):161-164. [IIIB]

384. Sciortino CV Jr, Xia EL, Mozee A. Assessment of a novel approach to evaluate the outcome of endoscope reprocessing. *Infect Control Hosp Epidemiol.* 2004;25(4):284-290. [IIC]

385. Whiteley GS, Derry C, Glasbey T. Sampling plans for use of rapid adenosine triphosphate (ATP) monitoring must overcome variability or suffer statistical invalidity. *Infect Control Hosp Epidemiol.* 2015;36(2):236-237. [VA]

386. Visrodia KH, Ofstead CL, Wetzler HP, Tosh PK, Baron TH. Reply to Whiteley et al. *Infect Control Hosp Epidemiol.* 2015;36(2):237-238. [VA]

387. Alfa MJ, Fatima I, Olson N. Validation of adenosine triphosphate to audit manual cleaning of flexible endoscope channels. *Am J Infect Control.* 2013;41(3):245-248. [IIB]

388. Whiteley GS, Derry C, Glasbey T, Fahey P. The perennial problem of variability in adenosine triphosphate (ATP) tests for hygiene monitoring within healthcare settings. *Infect Control Hosp Epidemiol.* 2015;36(6):658-663. [IIIA]

389. Alfa MJ, Olson N, Murray BL. Comparison of clinically relevant benchmarks and channel sampling methods used to assess manual cleaning compliance for flexible gastrointestinal endoscopes. *Am J Infect Control.* 2014;42(1):e1-e5. [IIA]

390. Bommarito M, Thornhill GA, Morse DJ. A multi-site field study evaluating the effectiveness of manual cleaning of flexible endoscopes with an ATP detection system. *Am J Infect Control.* 2013;41(6 Suppl):S24. [IIIC]

391. Beilenhoff U, Neumann CS, Rey JF, et al. ESGE-ESGENA guideline for quality assurance in reprocessing: microbiological surveillance testing in endoscopy. *Endoscopy.* 2007;39(2):175-181. [IVC]

392. Chiu KW, Tsai MC, Wu KL, Chiu YC, Lin MT, Hu TH. Surveillance cultures of samples obtained from biopsy channels and automated endoscope reprocessors after high-level disinfection of gastrointestinal endoscopes. *BMC Gastroenterol.* 2012;12:120. [IIA]

393. Saviuc P, Picot-Gueraud R, Shum Cheong Sing J, et al. Evaluation of the quality of reprocessing of gastrointestinal endoscopes. *Infect Control Hosp Epidemiol.* 2015;36(9):1017-1023. [IIIA]

394. Tunuguntla A, Sullivan MJ. Monitoring quality of flexible endoscope disinfection by microbiologic surveillance cultures. *Tenn Med.* 2004;97(10):453-456. [VB]

395. Merighi A, Contato E, Scagliarini R, et al. Quality improvement in gastrointestinal endoscopy: microbiologic surveillance of disinfection. *Gastrointest Endosc.* 1996;43(5):457-462. [VC]

396. Moses FM, Lee J. Surveillance cultures to monitor quality of gastrointestinal endoscope reprocessing. *Am J Gastroenterol.* 2003;98(1):77-81. [VA]

397. Bretthauer M, Jorgensen A, Kristiansen BE, Hofstad B, Hoff G. Quality control in colorectal cancer screening: systematic microbiological investigation of endoscopes used in the NORCCAP (Norwegian Colorectal Cancer Prevention) trial. *BMC Gastroenterol.* 2003;3:15. [IIIA]

398. Buss AJ, Been MH, Borgers RP, et al. Endoscope disinfection and its pitfalls—requirement for retrograde surveillance cultures. *Endoscopy.* 2008;40(4):327-332. [VA]

399. Hong KH, Lim YJ. Recent update of gastrointestinal endoscope reprocessing. *Clin Endosc.* 2013;46(3):267-273. [VA]

400. Kovaleva J, Meessen NE, Peters FT, et al. Is bacteriologic surveillance in endoscope reprocessing stringent enough? *Endoscopy.* 2009;41(10):913-916. [VA]

401. Chiu KW, Lu LS, Wu KL, et al. Surveillance culture monitoring of double-balloon enteroscopy reprocessing with high-level disinfection. *Eur J Clin Invest.* 2012;42(4):427-431. [IIIC]

402. Bisset L, Cossart YE, Selby W, et al. A prospective study of the efficacy of routine decontamination for gastrointestinal endoscopes and the risk factors for failure. *Am J Infect Control.* 2006;34(5):274-280. [IIIA]

403. Infection Control Devices Branch Division of General and Restorative Devices Office of Device Evaluation Center for Devices and Radiological Health Food and Drug Administration. *Guidance on Premarket Notification [510(k)] Submissions for Sterilizers Intended for Use in Health Care Facilities.* March 1993. US Food and Drug Administration. http://www.fda.gov/downloads/medicaldevices/deviceregulationandguidance/guidancedocuments/ucm081341.pdf. Accessed December 10, 2015.

404. *Addendum to: Guidance on Premarket Notification [510(k)] Submissions for Sterilizers Intended for Use in Health Care Facilities.* September 19, 1995. US Food and Drug Administration. http://www.fda.gov/RegulatoryInformation/Guidances/ucm080300.htm. Accessed December 10, 2015.

405. Fraser TG, Reiner S, Malczynski M, Yarnold PR, Warren J, Noskin GA. Multidrug-resistant *Pseudomonas aeruginosa* cholangitis after endoscopic retrograde cholangiopancreatography:

failure of routine endoscope cultures to prevent an outbreak. *Infect Control Hosp Epidemiol.* 2004;25(10):856-859. [IIIC]

406. Nelson DB. Recent advances in epidemiology and prevention of gastrointestinal endoscopy related infections. *Curr Opin Infect Dis.* 2005;18(4):326-330. [VB]

407. Gillespie EE, Kotsanas D, Stuart RL. Microbiological monitoring of endoscopes: 5-year review. *J Gastroenterol Hepatol.* 2008;23(7 Pt 1):1069-1074. [IIIB]

408. Lu LS, Wu KL, Chiu YC, Lin MT, Hu TH, Chiu KW. Swab culture monitoring of automated endoscope reprocessors after high-level disinfection. *World J Gastroenterol.* 2012;18(14):1660-1663. [IIIA]

409. Muscarella LF. Investigation and prevention of infectious outbreaks during endoscopic retrograde cholangiopancreatography. *Endoscopy.* 2010;42(11):957-959. [VA]

410. Interim duodenoscope surveillance protocol. Centers for Disease Control and Prevention. http://www.cdc.gov/hai/organisms/cre/cre-duodenoscope-surveillance-protocol.html. Accessed December 10, 2015. [VA]

411. *H0245 01: ECRI Institute Recommends Culturing Duodenoscopes as a Key Step to Reducing CRE Infections [Hazard Report].* Plymouth Meeting, PA: ECRI Institute. March 3, 2015. [VA]

412. Interim duodenoscope sampling method. Centers for Disease Control and Prevention. http://www.cdc.gov/hai/settings/lab/lab-duodenoscope-sampling.html. Accessed December 10, 2015. [VB]

413. Interim duodenoscope culture method. Centers for Disease Control and Prevention. http://www.cdc.gov/hai/settings/lab/lab-duodenoscope-culture-method.html. Accessed December 10, 2015. [VB]

414. Banerjee S, Nelson DB, Dominitz JA, et al. Reprocessing failure. *Gastrointest Endosc.* 2007;66(5):869-871. [IVA]

415. Patel PR, Srinivasan A, Perz JF. Developing a broader approach to management of infection control breaches in health care settings. *Am J Infect Control.* 2008;36(10):685-690. [VA]

416. Weber DJ, Rutala WA. Assessing the risk of disease transmission to patients when there is a failure to follow recommended disinfection and sterilization guidelines. *Am J Infect Control.* 2013;41(5):S67-S71. [VA]

417. Holodniy M, Oda G, Schirmer PL, et al. Results from a large-scale epidemiologic look-back investigation of improperly reprocessed endoscopy equipment. *Infect Control Hosp Epidemiol.* 2012;33(7):649-656. [IIIA]

418. MAUDE—Manufacturer and User Facility Device Experience. https://www.accessdata.fda.gov/scripts/cdrh/cfdocs/cfmaude/search.cfm. Accessed December 9, 2015.

Acknowledgments

Lead Author

Sharon A. Van Wicklin, MSN, RN, CNOR, CRNFA(E), CPSN-R, PLNC
Senior Perioperative Practice Specialist
AORN Nursing Department
Denver, Colorado

Contributing Authors
Ramona Conner, MSN, RN, CNOR
Editor-in-Chief, Guidelines for Perioperative Practice
AORN Nursing Department
Denver, Colorado

Cynthia Spry, MA, MS, RN, CNOR(E), CSPDT
Independent Consultant
New York, New York

The authors and AORN thank Marie A. Bashaw, DNP, RN, NEA-BC, CNOR, Assistant Professor, Wright State University College of Nursing and Health, Dayton, Ohio; Cori L. Ofstead, MSPH, President and CEO, Ofstead & Associates, Inc, St Paul, Minnesota; John E. Eiland, RN, MS, Senior Research Associate, Ofstead & Associates, Inc, St Paul, Minnesota; Judith Goldberg, DBA, MSN, RN, CNOR, CSSM, CHL, CRCST, Director, Patient Care Services, Perioperative and Procedural Services, Lawrence + Memorial Hospital, New London, Connecticut; Sheryl P. Eder, MSN, RN, CNOR CRCST, Director, Sterile Processing Department, LeeSar Regional Service Center, Fort Myers, Florida; Angela Hewitt, MD, MS, Associate Professor, Division of Infectious Diseases, Associate Medical Director, Department of Infection Control and Epidemiology, Associate Medical Director, Nebraska Biocontainment Unit, Director, Infectious Diseases Outpatient Clinics, University of Nebraska Medical Center, Omaha; Heather A. Hohenberger, BSN, RN, CIC, CNOR, CPHQ, Quality Improvement Consultant, Perioperative Services, Indiana University Health, Indianapolis; and Donna Ford, MSN, RN-BC, CNOR, CRCST, Nursing Education Specialist, Mayo Clinic, Rochester, Minnesota, for their assistance in developing this guideline.

Publication History

Originally published February 1993, *AORN Journal.*

Revised November 1997; published January 1998. Reformatted July 2000.

Revised November 2002; published in *Standards, Recommended Practices, and Guidelines,* 2003 edition.

Reprinted February 2003, *AORN Journal.*

Revised November 2008; published in *Perioperative Standards and Recommended Practices,* 2009 edition.

Reformatted September 2012 for publication in *Perioperative Standards and Recommended Practices,* 2013 edition.

Minor editing revisions made in November 2014 for publication as Guideline for Cleaning and Processing Flexible Endoscopes and Endoscope Accessories in *Guidelines for Perioperative Practice,* 2015 edition.

Revised February 2016 for publication in *Guidelines for Perioperative Practice,* 2016 edition.

Evidence ratings revised and minor editorial changes made to conform to the current AORN Evidence Rating model, September 2019, for publication in *Guidelines for Perioperative Practice* online.

HAND HYGIENE

AORN
SAFE SURGERY TOGETHER

TABLE OF CONTENTS

MEDICAL ABBREVIATIONS & ACRONYMS

AANA – American Association of Nurse Anesthetists
AST – Association of Surgical Technologists
CDC – Centers for Disease Control and Prevention
CFU – Colony-forming units
CHG – Chlorhexidine gluconate
FDA – US Food and Drug Administration
FGI – Facility Guidelines Institute
IDSA – Infectious Diseases Society of America
NICE – National Institute for Health and Care Excellence

OR – Operating room
RCT – Randomized controlled trial
RN – Registered nurse
SHEA – Society for Healthcare Epidemiology of America
SSI – Surgical site infection
TFM – Tentative Final Monograph
UV – Ultraviolet
WHO - World Health Organization

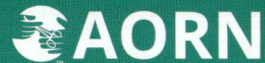
GUIDELINE FOR
HAND HYGIENE

The Guideline for Hand Hygiene was approved by the AORN Guidelines Advisory Board and became effective September 1, 2016. It was presented as a proposed guideline for comments by members and others. The recommendations in the guideline are intended to be achievable and represent what is believed to be an optimal level of practice. Policies and procedures will reflect variations in practice settings and/or clinical situations that determine the degree to which the guideline can be implemented. AORN recognizes the many diverse settings in which perioperative nurses practice; therefore, this guideline is adaptable to all areas where operative or other invasive procedures may be performed.

Purpose

This document provides guidance for **hand hygiene** and **surgical hand antisepsis** in the perioperative setting. Hand hygiene is widely recognized as a primary method to prevent health care-associated infections and the transmission of pathogens in the health care setting.[1] Health care-associated infections can result in untoward patient outcomes, such as morbidity and mortality, pain and suffering, longer lengths of hospital stay, delayed wound healing, increased use of antibiotics, and higher costs of care.[2] Thus, prevention of health care-associated infections is a priority for all health care personnel. Hand hygiene and surgical hand antisepsis are effective and cost-efficient ways to prevent and control infections in the perioperative setting.

Normal skin flora on the hands include transient and resident microorganisms. Transient flora are microorganisms that colonize the superficial layers of the skin. Perioperative team members acquire these microorganisms while caring for patients and when coming into contact with contaminated environmental surfaces. Transient microorganisms are easier to remove by hand hygiene than are resident microorganisms, which are seated in the deeper layers of the skin. Skin and nail condition and the presence of jewelry contribute to the number of transient microorganisms on the hands.

The goal of surgical hand antisepsis is to remove soil and transient microorganisms from the hands of perioperative team members and suppress the growth of resident microorganisms for the duration of the surgical procedure to reduce the risk that the patient will develop a surgical site infection (SSI).[3] Safe and effective **surgical hand antiseptics** rapidly and persistently remove transient microorganisms and suppress the growth of resident microorganisms with minimal skin and tissue irritation.[2]

The perioperative registered nurse (RN) plays a crucial role in developing and implementing protocols for hand hygiene and surgical hand antisepsis in the perioperative setting, including involvement in the selection of surgical hand antiseptics and hand hygiene products. This guideline provides perioperative RNs and other perioperative team members with evidence-based practice guidance for hand hygiene and surgical hand antisepsis to promote patient and personnel safety and reduce the risk for health care-associated infections, especially SSIs.

Hand hygiene in health care settings other than the perioperative setting is outside the scope of this document.

Evidence Review

A medical librarian conducted a systematic search of the databases Ovid MEDLINE®, EBSCO CINAHL®, Scopus®, and the Cochrane Database of Systematic Reviews. The search was limited to literature published in English from January 2010 through September 2015. Between September 2015 and February 2016, the results of alerts established at the time of the initial search were assessed, and the lead author requested additional articles that either did not fit the original search criteria or were discovered during the evidence appraisal process. Finally, the lead author and the medical librarian identified relevant guidelines from government agencies, professional organizations, and standards-setting bodies.

The search was limited to the concept of hand hygiene in the perioperative setting. Hand hygiene search terms included the subject headings *handwashing* and *hand disinfection*, supplemented by the keywords *hand washing, handwashing, hand hygiene, hand antisepsis, hand contamination,* and *hand decontamination*. Search terms related to the perioperative setting included the subject headings *operating rooms, surgicenters, anesthesia, perioperative care, perioperative period, perioperative nursing,* and *operating room personnel* and keywords such as *operating theater, surgical suite, operating suite,* and *perioperative setting*. To retrieve additional relevant articles, the keywords *surgical, preoperative, preoperative, presurgical,* and *pre-surgical* were combined with the keywords *hand antisepsis, wash, scrub, rub,* and *hand preparation*. Subject headings and keywords for cross contamination and infection, fingernails and jewelry, skin irritation and inflammation, and specific antiseptic agents and products also were included.

Inclusion criteria were research and non-research literature in English, complete publications, and publication dates within the time restriction unless none were available. Excluded were non-peer-reviewed publications and

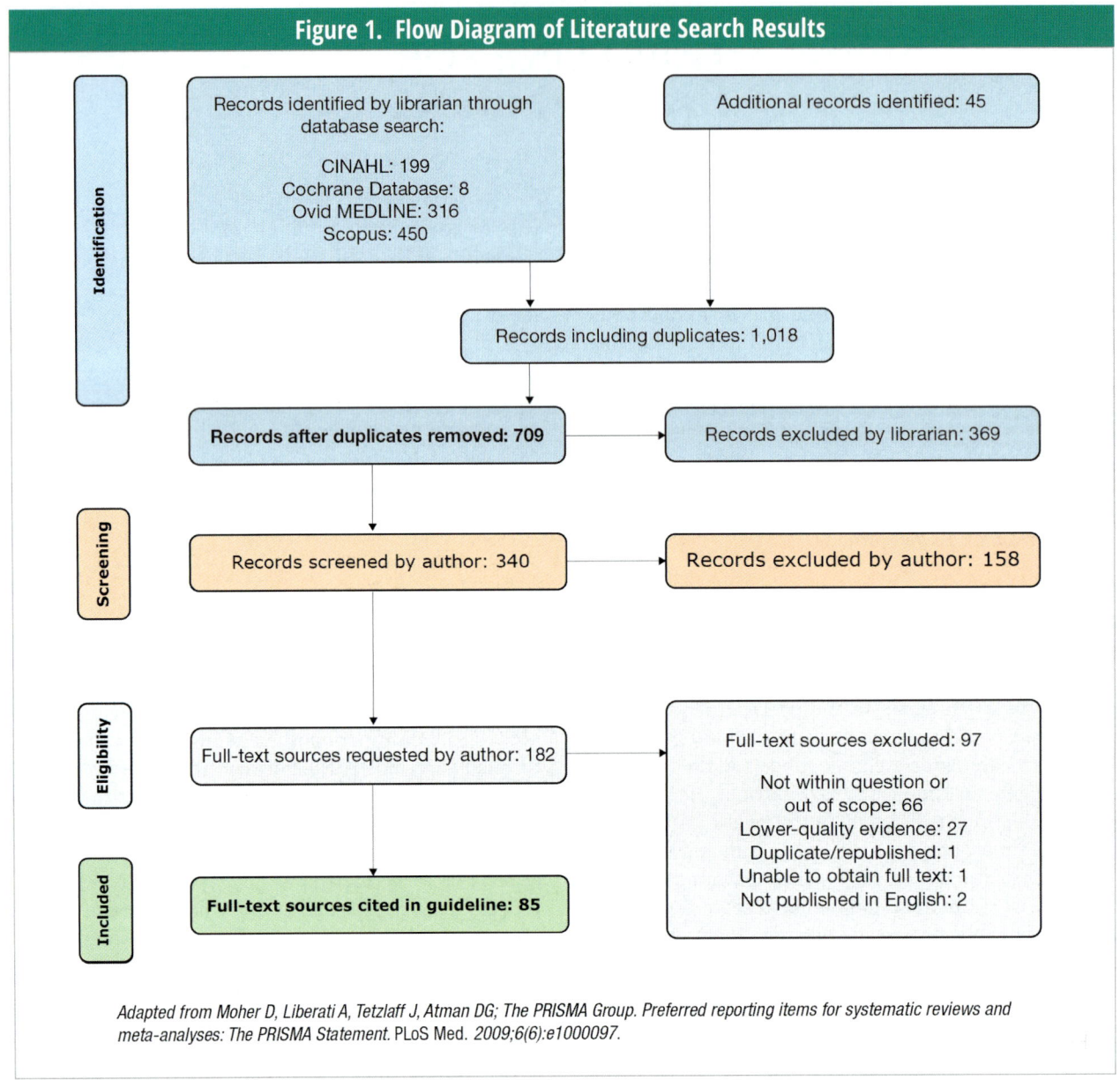

Figure 1. Flow Diagram of Literature Search Results

Records identified by librarian through database search:

CINAHL: 199
Cochrane Database: 8
Ovid MEDLINE: 316
Scopus: 450

Additional records identified: 45

Records including duplicates: 1,018

Records after duplicates removed: 709

Records excluded by librarian: 369

Records screened by author: 340

Records excluded by author: 158

Full-text sources requested by author: 182

Full-text sources excluded: 97

Not within question or out of scope: 66
Lower-quality evidence: 27
Duplicate/republished: 1
Unable to obtain full text: 1
Not published in English: 2

Full-text sources cited in guideline: 85

Identification

Screening

Eligibility

Included

Adapted from Moher D, Liberati A, Tetzlaff J, Atman DG; The PRISMA Group. Preferred reporting items for systematic reviews and meta-analyses: The PRISMA Statement. PLoS Med. 2009;6(6):e1000097.

literature on hand hygiene in patient care settings other than the perioperative setting. Editorials, news, and brief items were excluded. Low-quality evidence was excluded when higher-quality evidence was available, and literature outside the time restriction was excluded when literature within the time restriction was available (Figure 1).

Articles identified in the search were provided to the project team for evaluation. The team consisted of the lead author and two evidence appraisers. The lead author divided the search results into topics and assigned members of the team to review and critically appraise each article using the AORN Research or Non-Research Evidence Appraisal Tools as appropriate. The literature was independently evaluated and appraised according to the strength and quality of the evidence. Each article was then assigned an appraisal score. The appraisal score is noted in brackets after each reference as applicable.

Each recommendation rating is based on a synthesis of the collective evidence, a benefit-harm assessment, and consideration of resource use. The strength of the recommendation was determined using the AORN Evidence Rating Model and the quality and consistency of the evidence supporting a recommendation. The recommendation strength rating is noted in brackets after each recommendation.

Note: The evidence summary table is available at http://www.aorn.org/evidencetables/.

Editor's note: MEDLINE is a registered trademark of the US National Library of Medicine's Medical Literature Analysis and Retrieval System, Bethesda, MD. CINAHL, Cumulative Index to Nursing and Allied Health Literature, is a registered trademark of EBSCO Industries, Birmingham, AL. Scopus is a registered trademark of Elsevier B.V., Amsterdam, The Netherlands.

1. Fingernail and Hand Condition

1.1 **All perioperative team members should maintain healthy fingernail and hand skin condition.** *[Recommendation]*

Moderate-quality evidence and guidance from professional organizations[1,3-5] indicate that having unhealthy skin or fingernails may impede the removal of microorganisms from the hands during hand hygiene.

Hand hygiene is critical for preventing the transmission of microorganisms from the hands of perioperative team members to the patient and the environment. Transmission to the patient of microorganisms that are harbored in unhealthy skin or fingernails may result in the patient developing a health care–associated infection.

1.2 **Maintain short, natural fingernails. Keep fingernail tips no longer than 2 mm (0.08 inch).**[6,7] *[Recommendation]*

Moderate-quality evidence and guidance from professional organizations support that health care personnel should maintain their fingernails at a short length.[1,3,4,6-10] The most recent research found in the evidence review supports maintaining fingernails at a length no longer than 2 mm (**Figure 2**).[6,7] Benefits of maintaining short nails include reducing the risk of harboring potential pathogens under fingernails. In addition, the harms of having long nails may include puncturing gloves,[1,3,9] limiting the effectiveness of hand hygiene,[3,8] or injuring patients during patient handling.

Historical studies cited by the Centers for Disease Control and Prevention (CDC)[4] and the World Health Organization (WHO)[3] have found that the areas under the fingernails can harbor high concentrations of bacteria (eg, coagulase-negative staphylococci, gram-negative rods [*Pseudomonas*], *Corynebacteria*) and yeasts, which can remain present even after careful hand hygiene or surgical hand antisepsis. Based on this evidence, in 2002, the CDC[4] recommended keeping natural nail length shorter than 0.25 inches. In 2009, the WHO[3] also recommended that health care personnel who have direct contact with patients keep natural nails short, with tips shorter than 0.25 inches or 0.5 cm. Rather than providing a specific recommendation on fingernail length, the Association of Surgical Technologists (AST)[9] recommended in 2008 that fingernail length not extend beyond the fingertips due to the risk for glove puncture.

More recent research has indicated that the 6 mm (0.25 inch) recommendation for length of the fingernail is too long. In 2008, Rupp et al[7] conducted a

Figure 2. Measuring Fingernail Tip Length

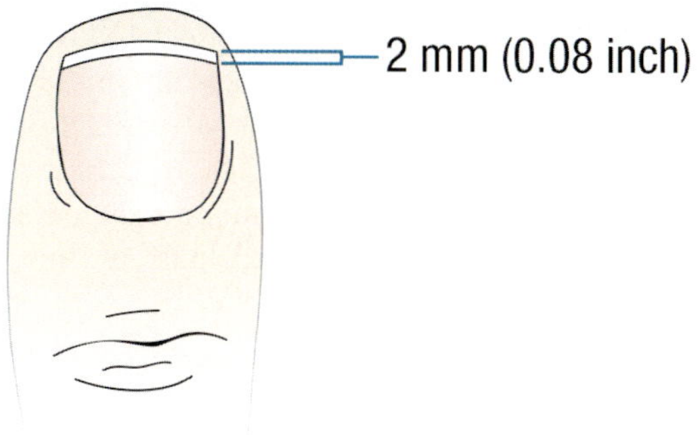

2 mm (0.08 inch)

prospective controlled cross-over trial to introduce **alcohol-based hand rubs** in two medical-surgical intensive care units at a tertiary care teaching hospital. This study was designed to investigate whether the introduction of an alcohol-based hand rub improved hand hygiene compliance, affected patient outcomes, or altered the microbial flora on the hands of health care personnel. The researchers used a modified glove juice method to culture the hands of personnel (N = 174) and found that fingernail length longer than 2 mm (0.08 inches) was significantly associated with a higher number of microorganisms compared with fingernail lengths shorter than 2 mm.

Fagernes and Lingaas[6] evaluated the microflora on the hands of 465 Norwegian health care personnel by using the **glove juice method** in a 2011 observational study. The researchers found that fingernails longer than 2 mm were significantly associated with the prevalence of *Staphylococcus aureus.* Thus, they recommended that the fingernails of health care personnel be no longer than 2 mm.

In a prospective observational study with an educational intervention, Hautemaniere et al[8] evaluated factors associated with hand hygiene effectiveness for 3,067 hospital personnel in France. The researchers evaluated hand hygiene before and after an educational intervention, which consisted of a 30-minute session to teach best practices for use of alcohol-based hand rub. Evaluation of hand hygiene effectiveness was determined using a validated technique of observation of rubbing time (limit 30 seconds), adherence to the application method protocol, and evaluation by visual criteria. The evaluation of visual criteria was assessed by applying fluorescent alcohol-based hand rub and using ultraviolet light to evaluate the percentage of hand coverage. In this study, having long nails was associated with ineffective hand rub use by the evaluation criteria. However, the researchers did not describe the nail length that was used to classify nails as long in this study.

1.3 **Do not wear artificial fingernails or extenders in the perioperative setting.**[1,3-5,9] *[Recommendation]*

Artificial nails have been associated with hand contamination and epidemiologically implicated in outbreaks caused by gram-negative bacteria and yeasts.[1,3,4] Based on this historical evidence, professional organizations recommend that personnel who have direct contact with patients not wear artificial nails or extenders.[1,3-5,9]

Clinical trials of artificial nails may expose patients to harm and thus may not be ethical. Further research is needed to determine whether the length of the fingernail or the artificial nail itself poses a risk for the transmission of microorganisms.[3,4]

1.4 **Have a multidisciplinary team that includes perioperative RNs, physicians, and infection preventionists determine whether fingernail polish may be worn in the perioperative setting.**[3] *[Conditional Recommendation]*

Low-quality evidence is inconclusive regarding the effect of fingernail polish on hand hygiene. Professional organizations provide differing opinions on the wearing of nail polish based on the inconclusive evidence. For example, the WHO[3] recommends that health care facilities develop policies on the wearing of nail polish by health care personnel. The CDC does not make any recommendation on the wearing of nail polish, although the CDC guideline for hand hygiene discusses the evidence on nail polish.[4] The National Institute for Health and Care Excellence (NICE)[5] guidelines in the United Kingdom recommend that the operating team remove nail polish before surgeries because of the lack of evidence on the effect of nail polish on hand contamination. The AST[9] recommends that nail polish be freshly applied and free of chips if the health care facility allows nail polish to be worn.

Arrowsmith and Taylor[11] conducted a systematic review with meta-analysis of one small randomized controlled trial (RCT) published in 1994. The RCT compared the bacterial counts measured in colony-forming units (CFU) on the hands of perioperative nurses (N = 102) with and without nail polish before and after surgical hand antisepsis. In the study, the participants had either unpolished nails (n = 34), freshly applied nail polish that was less than 2 days old (n = 34), or old nail polish that was either obviously chipped or more than 4 days old (n = 34). The researchers found a significantly higher median number of CFU after surgical hand antisepsis in the group wearing old or chipped nail polish compared with the groups with unpolished nails or freshly applied nail polish. However, in the meta-analysis of this RCT, Arrowsmith and Taylor[11] did not find significant differences in the mean CFU between any of the study groups.

A limitation of the RCT is that the data were skewed because of a contaminated sample in the freshly applied nail polish group before surgical hand antisepsis. Thus, the researchers used the median CFU values rather than the mean CFU values to test for statistical significance. Although the median values showed a statistically significant difference in CFU in the old or chipped nail polish group after surgical hand antisepsis, the mean values did not show any difference. Arrowsmith and Taylor[11] describe as a limitation of this RCT that it was underpowered to detect clinically important differences in colonization. Limitations of Arrowsmith and Taylor's systematic review are that the review and meta-analysis was limited to one RCT and the median CFU values were not included in the analysis.

In their observational study, Fagernes and Lingaas[6] cultured the hands of 465 Norwegian health care personnel. They recorded the presence of nail polish for each study participant as either no polish present (n = 377), intact polish (n = 35), or chipped polish (n = 51), or nail polish status was not registered (n = 2). Previous studies of nail polish sampled only the fingernails for culturing, whereas this study cultured the whole hand using the glove juice method. The researchers found no effect of nail polish status on the bacterial count for the whole hand. A limitation of this study is that there was no power analysis to determine whether the sample size was sufficient to determine an effect of nail polish on hand colonization.

A limitation of the evidence on nail polish is that the quality of the research is low. Further research is needed to determine whether wearing nail polish affects hand contamination or patient outcomes, including the rate of SSI.

Although evidence is lacking to determine any harms of wearing nail polish, the potential harms could include nail polish hindering the effectiveness of hand hygiene, transmission to a patient of pathogens harbored in chipped or old nail polish, or chipped polish becoming deposited in the sterile field or wound.

1.4.1 **Determine whether ultraviolet (UV)-cured nail polish (eg, gel, Shellac®) may be worn in the perioperative setting.**[1] *[Conditional Recommendation]*

The evidence review found no research to support or refute wearing UV-cured nail polish. The Society for Healthcare Epidemiology of America (SHEA)/Infectious Diseases Society of America (IDSA) hand hygiene practice recommendations[1] also cite a lack of evidence-based guidance on wearing UV-cured nails and nail enhancements in the patient care setting. A conservative approach recommended by SHEA/IDSA[1] is for the health care organization to consider UV-cured nails as artificial and to not allow health care personnel to wear this type of polish in high-risk areas, such as the operating room (OR). Research is needed to determine whether UV-cured nail polish affects the performance of hand hygiene and the microflora on the hands of health care personnel.

Whether UV-cured nail polish carries the same risk of harboring pathogens or transmission of infection to patients as artificial nails is unknown. The harms of wearing UV-cured nail polish may include damage to the natural fingernail and harboring of pathogens in the gaps created as the nail and cuticle grow.

1.5 **Take measures to prevent hand dermatitis.**[3]
[Recommendation]

High-quality evidence indicates that hand dermatitis may have a negative effect on hand hygiene.[3,12] According to the WHO,[3] damage to the skin may change skin flora and has been associated with more frequent colonization by staphylococci and gram-negative bacilli.

Personnel with hand dermatitis and eczema are less likely to perform hand hygiene.[12] In an RCT conducted by van der Meer et al,[12] personnel in 48 departments of a hospital in the Netherlands were randomly assigned by department to either a control group or a group that participated in an educational intervention to prevent hand eczema. Participants (N = 1,649) self-reported hand eczema and preventive behavior. The researchers found that 12 months after the baseline report, the intervention group was significantly more likely to report hand eczema, less hand washing, more frequent moisturizer use, and more use of cotton undergloves. The researchers suggested that increased awareness of hand eczema symptoms may have led to the increased reporting of hand eczema in the intervention group.

The limitations of the evidence are that research has not confirmed the effect of dermatitis on hand hygiene or the effect of prevention strategies on the development of hand dermatitis.

Having hand dermatitis may result in hand colonization with pathogens, less hand washing, and increased risk for infection of both patients and perioperative team members. The benefits of preventing hand dermatitis outweigh the harms. Benefits of using hand dermatitis preventative measures may include preventing skin damage and promoting optimal hand hygiene.

1.5.1 **Use moisturizing skin care products approved by the health care organization.**[1,3,4,13]
[Recommendation]

High-quality evidence and guidance from professional organizations support the use of moisturizing skin care products to maintain healthy skin condition.[1,3,4,13] Further research is needed to determine the effect of hand lotion use on bacterial colonization (**See Recommendation 5.5** for guidance on selection of skin care products).

The WHO[3] recommends that health care personnel use moisturizing skin care products after hand cleansing to minimize irritant contact dermatitis caused by hand hygiene. The CDC[4] and the SHEA/IDSA[1] also encourage the use of lotion by health care personnel as a strategy to prevent and manage hand hygiene-related irritant contact dermatitis.

Harnoss et al[13] conducted a survey of 16,000 German surgeons and received 1,433 responses (response rate 11%). Although 50% of the respondents reported having experienced skin irritation or discomfort, only 5% reported that they used skin protection or skin care products at the beginning of their shifts. Ten percent of the surgeons refused to use skin care products because of concern that the product would reduce the antimicrobial efficacy of the surgical hand rub. A limitation of this survey is the risk of participation bias by respondents who may have had a personal interest in hand hygiene or skin disorders.

Following the survey, Harnoss et al[13] conducted an experimental crossover study (N = 26) using European Norm standards for testing to determine the effect of skin protection and skin care products on surgical hand antisepsis and glove microperforations after 3 hours of glove wear at rest. After using the skin care products three times daily for 8 days, the participants in the intervention group (n = 13) had significantly higher skin moisture with no significant changes in surgical hand rub effectiveness or glove microperforations than the group that did not use any skin care products (n = 13). Although the study did not find a statistically significant rate of glove microperforations, the group with no skin care product use had a higher perforation rate (23.1%) than the group that used skin care products (7.7%), which may indicate that having dry hands increases the microperforation rate. However, this study was not designed to examine the correlation of dry skin to glove microperforation, so further research is needed to evaluate this relationship.

In the interpretation of this study, Harnoss et al[13] cautioned readers to assess the compatibility of skin care products with hand hygiene products during the product selection process.

In an observational study, Fagernes and Lingaas[6] cultured the hands of 465 Norwegian health care personnel using the glove juice method. For each study participant, the minutes between application of hand lotion and hand culturing were recorded. The researchers found that 10 health care personnel used hand lotion within 5 minutes before sampling, and this was significantly associated with the presence of *Staphylococcus aureus*. The researchers postulated that use of hand lotion may increase the efficiency of the skin to acquire staphylococci or may cause better recovery in culturing methods during sampling due to surface-active ingredients or that the findings might be a result of statistical chance. However, the researchers cited a historical report of increased hand bacterial counts after hand lotion use, which supported their findings. A limitation of this study is that there was no power analysis to determine whether the sample size was sufficient to determine the effect of hand lotion on hand colonization.

1.5.2   **Completely dry hands before donning gloves.**[3] *[Recommendation]*

The WHO[3] recommends that health care personnel allow their hands to dry completely before donning gloves after either hand washing or use of an alcohol-based hand rub because of an increased risk for skin irritation from wearing gloves on wet hands.

1.5.3   **Control water temperature for hand hygiene between 70° F and 80° F (21.1° C and 26.7° C).**[14] *[Recommendation]*

The Facility Guidelines Institute (FGI)[14] recommends controlling water temperature at **hand washing stations** between 70° F and 80° F (21.1° C and 26.7° C). Water temperatures higher than 80° F (26.7° C) are conducive to the growth of *Legionella* bacteria.[14]

The WHO,[3] the CDC,[4] and the SHEA/IDSA[1] recommend avoiding hand washing in hot water because repeated exposure to hot water can irritate the skin and may lead to dermatitis or bacterial colonization. As an alternative, the SHEA/IDSA[1] recommends using either warm or cold water for hand washing due to a lack of evidence that either water temperature is superior. Notably, these professional organizations do not define temperature ranges for hot, warm, and cold water. Further research is needed to determine the effect of water temperature on hand dermatitis and bacterial colonization.

1.5.4   **In the absence of visible soil, disinfect hands with an alcohol-based hand rub rather than washing with soap and water.**[1,3] *[Recommendation]*

The WHO[3] and the SHEA/IDSA[1] recommend promoting the use of alcohol-based hand rub for routine hand hygiene over hand washing with soap and water because alcohol-based hand rubs are well tolerated and associated with less irritant contact dermatitis.

1.5.5   **Cotton glove liners may be worn under nonsterile gloves. Sterile cotton glove liners may be worn under sterile gloves.**[1] *[Conditional Recommendation]*

The SHEA/IDSA[1] recommends use of cotton glove liners for individuals with irritant contact dermatitis to maintain healthy skin condition when extended use of gloves is anticipated.

1.5.6   **Discard single-use cotton glove liners after each use. Reprocess reusable cotton glove liners in accordance with the manufacturer's instructions for use.** *[Recommendation]*

1.5.7   **Provide education to perioperative team members on the recognition and prevention of hand dermatitis.**[1,3,12] *[Recommendation]*

The WHO[3] and the SHEA/IDSA[1] recommend educating health care personnel on hand care practices to prevent irritant contact dermatitis and other skin damage from hand hygiene practices.

van der Meer et al[12] studied use of an educational intervention to prevent hand eczema in the Netherlands. The multifaceted intervention included education, participatory work groups, and role models. The study found that the educational intervention was effective in influencing personnel to implement evidence-based hand eczema preventative measures, including more frequent moisturizer use and more use of cotton undergloves in the intervention group. Further research is needed to determine the effect of education on the prevalence of hand eczema in health care personnel.

1.6   Restrict the activities of health care personnel with dermatitis, infections, exudative lesions, and nonintact skin when these activities pose a risk for transmission of infection to patients and other health care providers.[15] Follow state, federal, and professional guidelines and strategies to determine the need for work restrictions for health care personnel with bloodborne infections.[16,17] *[Recommendation]*

Perioperative team members with breaks in skin integrity or infections of the nails, hands, or arms may be at risk for acquiring infections or transmitting infection to patients (See the AORN Guideline for Prevention of Transmissible Infections[15] for additional guidance).

2. Jewelry

2.1 **Do not wear jewelry (eg, rings, watches, bracelets) on the hands or wrists in patient care areas.**[3,5,6,8,9,18] *[Recommendation]*

Wearing jewelry may impede the removal of microorganisms from the hands during hand hygiene.[1,3-5]

Moderate-quality evidence and guidance from professional organizations support perioperative team members removing rings, watches, and bracelets before caring for patients in the perioperative setting.[3,5,6,8,9] Wearing jewelry on the hands and wrists has been associated with increased bacterial counts on the hands[6] and ineffective use of alcohol-based hand rubs.[8] Transmission to the patient of microorganisms that are harbored on jewelry worn by perioperative team members may result in the patient developing a health care–associated infection.

Several professional organizations have provided guidance on the wearing of jewelry in the health care setting. The WHO[3] strongly discourages the wearing of rings or other jewelry in the health care setting and recommends that all rings or jewelry be removed in the OR. The WHO[3] recognizes that religious and cultural attitudes may strongly condition health care workers' attitudes toward removing their wedding rings. Thus, the WHO[3] advises that for these individuals, wearing a simple wedding band may be acceptable except in a high-risk setting such as the OR. The NICE[5] guidelines recommend that the operating team remove hand jewelry before surgeries as a measure to decrease the risk for SSI. The AST[9] recommends that all jewelry including rings, bracelets, and watches be removed before surgical hand antisepsis is performed. The AORN Guideline for Surgical Attire[18] recommends that jewelry that cannot be contained within the surgical attire not be worn in the semi-restricted or restricted areas. The CDC[4] makes no recommendation for the wearing of rings in health care settings, designating the issue as unresolved due to the lack of evidence to determine whether wearing rings results in increased transmission of pathogens.

Although a systematic review by Arrowsmith and Taylor[11] did not find any RCTs to evaluate the effect of wearing rings on the effectiveness of surgical hand antisepsis or SSI rates, other types of evidence were found in the evidence review for this guideline.

Fagernes and Lingaas[6] evaluated the microflora on the hands of 465 Norwegian health care personnel by using the glove juice method and found that wearing a wristwatch (n = 79) was significantly associated with a higher total bacteria count on hands than not wearing a watch (n = 121). Wristwatch status was not recorded for 265 study participants. The study also found that wearing one ring (n = 192) increased the rate of colonization with Enterobacteriaceae. However, there was insufficient statistical power to detect a significant difference between wearing of a single decorative ring (n = 50) or wearing of multiple rings (n = 10).

Fagernes and Lingaas[6] also found that wearing rings was associated with a higher total number of bacteria on hands. However, they found that study participants wearing rings were more likely to also wear watches. Because of this confounding factor, the researchers did not use these data in statistical analysis. Based on their findings, they recommended that health care personnel not wear finger rings or watches.

The study conducted by Hautemaniere et al,[8] as described in **Recommendation 1.2**, also evaluated the wearing of jewelry on hand hygiene effectiveness. This study found that wearing a watch, bracelet, and rings other than a wedding ring was significantly associated with ineffective hand rub use by the evaluation criteria. Wearing a wedding ring was not independently associated with hand hygiene ineffectiveness in this study. Notably, the researchers did not describe characteristics of a wedding ring, such as the band type or stone setting. However, they discussed that even though wedding rings had a strong symbolic and sentimental value to the health care personnel, some personnel became aware of the importance of removing their rings because the alcohol solution did not penetrate under the ring, and thus the ring could harbor microorganisms.

A limitation of the evidence is that research has not confirmed the risk of direct transmission of microorganisms to the patient from health care personnel wearing jewelry or watches on the hands or wrists. Further research is needed to determine the effectiveness of hand hygiene in the presence of jewelry on the hands and wrists of health care personnel.

3. Hand Hygiene

3.1 **Perioperative team members should perform hand hygiene.**[1,3,4] *[Recommendation]*

Moderate-quality evidence and guidance from professional organizations support that hand hygiene reduces the incidence of health care–associated infections.[1,3,4]

Observational research studies have demonstrated that IV stopcocks become contaminated with bacteria in the perioperative setting.[19,20] Loftus et al[21] found that IV stopcock contamination is significantly associated with patient mortality and 30-day postoperative infections. Although the source remains unclear, potential sources of IV stopcock contamination include the patient, the environment, and the hands of anesthesia professionals.

A limitation of the evidence is that current hand hygiene guidelines have not taken into account the rapid pace and task density associated with the administration of anesthesia in the perioperative setting.[22-26] Further research is needed to establish hand hygiene protocols that are feasible for anesthesia professionals and do not compromise patient safety.

Another limitation of the evidence is that research has not established the clinical benefit of performing hand hygiene prior to donning gloves for patient contact that is not associated with a clean or sterile task.[1] Some evidence suggests that glove boxes may be contaminated by the hands of health care personnel retrieving gloves, which may be an indication for performing hand hygiene before donning gloves or for the need for a solution to reduce box contamination during glove dispensing.[1] Further research is also needed to determine the benefits of performing hand hygiene before donning gloves for patient contact.[1]

The benefits of performing hand hygiene outweigh the harms. Benefits include removal of soil and transient microorganisms from the hands of perioperative team members, possibly reducing occupational exposure and the risk for the patient to develop a health care–associated infection.

3.2 Perform hand hygiene
- **before and after patient contact,**[1,3,4,19,22,23,27-29]
- **before performing a clean or sterile task,**[3]
- **after risk for blood or body fluid exposure,**[1,3,4]
- **after contact with patient surroundings,**[1,3,4]
- **when hands are visibly soiled**[1,3,4]
- **before and after eating,**[4] and
- **after using the restroom.**[3,4]

[Recommendation]

The WHO[3] and the CDC[4] recommend performing hand hygiene before and after patient contact, before performing a clean or sterile task, after risk for blood or body fluid exposure, after contact with patient surroundings, and any time hands are visibly dirty or soiled. **Table 1** provides examples of hand hygiene indications in the perioperative setting.

3.2.1 **Perform hand hygiene before and after patient contact, including**

- **performing a physical exam,**[27,29,30]
- **marking the site,**[27]
- **transferring or positioning the patient,**[27,30]
- **assessing an invasive device (eg, vascular catheter [peripheral, arterial, central], urinary catheter),**[27] and
- **assessing wound dressing.**[27]

[Recommendation]

3.2.2 **Perform hand hygiene before a clean or sterile task, including**

- **inserting an invasive device (eg, vascular catheter**[31] **[peripheral,**[29,30,32-34] **arterial,**[30] **central**[22,23,32]**], urinary catheter**[35]**)**[1,3,4,10,27,36]**;**
- **accessing a vascular device (eg, port,**[10] **stopcock,**[19-21] **IV tubing**[23,27,33,36]**)**[31]**;**
- **moving from a contaminated body site (eg, perineum) to a clean body site (eg, face) on the same patient**[1,3,4]**;**
- **administering or preparing medication, including delivery of medications to the sterile field and preparation of IV fluids**[1,3,27,30,33,36]**;**
- **performing neuraxial procedures (eg, epidural, spinal, lumbar puncture, spinal tap, epidural blood patch, epidural lysis of adhesions, intrathecal chemotherapy, lumbar or spinal drainage catheters, spinal cord simulation trials)**[10,23,27,32,37,38]**;**
- **administering regional anesthesia**[30,32,38]**;**
- **performing phlebotomy**[30]**;**
- **opening sterile supplies**[27,30,33,36]**; and**
- **performing patient skin antisepsis.**[27]

[Recommendation]

3.2.3 **Perform hand hygiene after risk for blood or body fluid exposure, including**

- **removing personal protective equipment (eg, gloves, mask)**[1,3,4,10,22,23]**;**
- **having contact with blood, body fluids, excretions, mucous membranes, nonintact skin, or wound dressings**[1,3,4]**;**
- **inserting or assessing an invasive device (ie, vascular catheter [peripheral, arterial, central], urinary catheter)**[27,30,32]**;**
- **performing airway manipulation (ie, intubation, suctioning)**[27,29,30,32,33,36] **as patient safety allows**[10,23,25]**;**
- **handling used sponges**[27,33]**;**
- **handling specimens**[27]**;**
- **draining urinary catheter bags, colostomy bags, or other drains**[27,33]**; and**
- **removing surgical drapes.**[27,33]

[Recommendation]

3.2.4 **Perform hand hygiene after contact with patient surroundings, including**

Table 1. Examples of Hand Hygiene Indications in the Perioperative Setting

Hand Hygiene Indications	Perioperative Examples
Before and after patient contact[1,3,4,19,22,23,27-29]	• Performing a physical exam[27,29,30] • Marking the site[27] • Transferring or positioning the patient[27,30] • Assessing an invasive device (eg, vascular catheter [peripheral, arterial, central], urinary catheter)[27] • Assessing wound dressing[27]
Before performing a clean or sterile task[3]	• Inserting an invasive device (eg, vascular catheter [peripheral, arterial, central], urinary catheter)[1,3,4,10,22,23,27,29-36] • Accessing a vascular device (eg, port, stopcock, IV tubing)[10,19-21,23,27,31,33,36] • Moving from a contaminated body site (eg, perineum) to a clean body site (eg, face) on the same patient[1,3,4] • Administering or preparing medication, including delivery of medications to the sterile field and preparation of IV fluids[1,3,27,30,33,36] • Performing neuraxial procedures (eg, epidural, spinal, lumbar puncture, spinal tap, epidural blood patch, epidural lysis of adhesions, intrathecal chemotherapy, lumbar or spinal drainage catheters, spinal cord simulation trials)[10,23,27,32,37,38] • Administering regional anesthesia[30,32,38] • Performing phlebotomy[30] • Opening sterile supplies[27,30,33,36] • Performing patient skin antisepsis[27]
After risk for blood or body fluid exposure[1,3,4]	• Removing personal protective equipment (eg, gloves, mask)[1,3,4,10,22,23] • Having contact with blood, body fluids, excretions, mucous membranes, non-intact skin, or wound dressings[1,3,4] • Inserting or accessing an invasive device (ie, vascular catheter [peripheral, arterial, central], urinary catheter)[27,30,32] • Performing airway manipulation (ie, intubation, suctioning) as patient safety allows[10,23,25,27,29,30,32,33,36] • Counting used sponges[27,33] • Handling specimens[27] • Draining urinary catheter bags, colostomy bags, or other drains[27,33] • Removing surgical drapes[27,33]
After contact with patient surroundings[1,3,4]	• Inanimate surfaces and objects, including medical equipment, in the immediate vicinity of the patient[1,3,4] • OR bed controls[29] • Patient bed and linens[34] • The floor or items that have come in contact with the floor[23,30,39]
Other	• Before and after assembling items for sterilization • When hands are visibly dirty or soiled[1,3,4] • Before and after eating[4] • After using the restroom[3,4]

Note: *The reference numbers in this table correspond to the numbers in the reference list at the end of the guideline.*

- inanimate surfaces and objects, including medical equipment, in the immediate vicinity of the patient[1,3,4];
- OR bed controls[29];
- patient bed and linens[34]; and
- the floor or items that have come in contact with the floor.[23,30,39]

[Recommendation]

3.2.5 **When gloves are worn and hand hygiene is indicated, remove the gloves to perform hand hygiene.**[3,4] *[Recommendation]*

The use of gloves does not replace the need for hand hygiene.[3,4]

3.2.6 **Performing a single act of hand hygiene may fulfill multiple indications (eg, opening multiple sterile items sequentially).**[3] *[Conditional Recommendation]*

Multiple indications for hand hygiene may arise simultaneously that create a single opportunity to perform hand hygiene.[3]

3.3 **In the event that performing hand hygiene would put the patient's safety at risk, weigh the risks and benefits of delaying hand hygiene.** *[Recommendation]*

The benefits of performing hand hygiene may not outweigh the harms, depending on the clinical situation. Benefits include reducing the risk for the patient developing a health care–associated infection. The harms may include patient injury or delaying necessary, possibly life-saving interventions, such as ventilation.

3.3.1 **The anesthesia professional may wear two pairs of gloves (ie, double glove), remove the contaminated outer gloves after airway manipulation, and continue patient care until the patient's status allows for removal of the inner gloves and performance of hand hygiene.**[10,40,41] *[Conditional Recommendation]*

The American Association of Nurse Anesthetists (AANA)[10] recommends that anesthesia professionals double glove during airway manipulation. The AANA[10] recommends maintaining patient oxygenation by ventilating immediately after airway manipulation, auscultating breath sounds, and confirming end-tidal carbon dioxide. Removing gloves to perform hand hygiene immediately after airway management may jeopardize patient safety. As an alternative, the AANA[10] recommends that anesthesia professionals don two pairs of gloves before airway manipulation, remove the outer gloves after the airway device is inserted, and perform hand hygiene when the patient is stable.

Birnbach et al[40] conducted an RCT to assess contamination of the OR surfaces during simulated laryngoscopy and intubation by anesthesiology residents (N = 22). The intervention group members (n = 11) wore two pairs of gloves and removed the outer pair of gloves after intubation, whereas the control group members (n = 11) each wore a single pair of gloves. The study found that the group wearing two pairs of gloves during intubation and removing the outer gloves immediately after intubation contaminated significantly fewer surfaces, as measured by fluorescent marking gel.

In a similar RCT with anesthesiology residents in simulations (N = 45), Birnbach et al[41] compared the level of OR surface contamination after single gloving (n = 15), double gloving with the outer gloves removed (n = 15), and double gloving with the outer gloves used to cover the laryngoscope (n = 15). The study found that both double-gloving techniques were associated with significantly less contamination than single gloving. Use of the outer pair as a sheath for the laryngoscope immediately after intubation was associated with the least contamination of the IV hub, patient, and intraoperative environment.

3.4 **Perform hand washing with soap and water**
- **after being exposed to blood or body fluids,**[3,4]
- **after using the restroom,**[3,4]
- **when hands are visibly soiled,**[1,3,4] **and**
- **when caring for patients with spore-forming organisms (eg,** *Clostridium difficile, Bacillus anthracis***) or norovirus.**[1,3,4]

[Recommendation]

Performing hand hygiene with an alcohol-based hand rub may not be effective when hands are visibly or potentially soiled with organic matter, such as blood and body fluids. Also, spores may be removed from the hands more effectively with soap and water than with an alcohol-based hand rub.[1,3,4]

3.4.1 **Perform a standardized hand washing protocol using soap and water in the following order:**
1. **Remove jewelry from hands and wrists (eg, rings, watches, bracelets).**[3,4]
2. **Adjust water for a comfortable temperature, avoiding hot water.**[3]
3. **Wet hands thoroughly with water.**[3,4]
4. **Apply the amount of soap needed to cover all surfaces of the hands.**[3,4]
5. **Rub hands together vigorously covering all surfaces of the hands and fingers for at least 15 seconds.**[4]
6. **Rinse with water to remove all soap.**[3,4]
7. **Dry hands thoroughly with a disposable paper towel.**[3,4]
8. **When hand-free controls are not available on the sink, use a clean paper towel to turn off the water.**[4]

[Recommendation]

3.5 **When hands are not visibly soiled or dirty, perform hand hygiene using an alcohol-based hand rub according to the manufacturer's instructions for use.**[3,4] *[Recommendation]*

The WHO[3] and the CDC[4] recommend performing hand hygiene with an alcohol-based hand rub when hands are not visibly soiled or dirty.

3.5.1 **Perform a standardized hand hygiene protocol using an alcohol-based hand rub in the following order:**
1. **Remove jewelry from hands and wrists (eg, rings, watches, bracelets).**[3,4]
2. **Apply the amount of alcohol-based hand rub recommended by the manufacturer to cover all surfaces of the hands.**[3,4]
3. **Rub hands together, covering all surfaces of the hands and fingers until dry.**[3,4]

[Recommendation]

3.6 Place hand washing stations in convenient locations as determined in an infection control risk assessment and in accordance with federal, state, and local regulatory requirements and applicable construction guidelines. *[Recommendation]*

The FGI[14] has established the minimum number and locations for hand washing stations. The FGI recommends conducting an infection control risk assessment to evaluate the convenience of hand washing station locations for clinical use and to further identify locations that will enhance accessibility to hand hygiene products.

3.6.1 For areas with multiple patient care stations, include at least one hand washing station for every four patient care stations. Position the hand washing station to be approximately an equal distance between the furthest stations.[14] *[Recommendation]*

3.6.2 Sinks designated for hand hygiene should only be used for hand hygiene. *[Recommendation]*

Performing activities other than hand washing or surgical hand antisepsis could contaminate the sink, faucet, or hands of personnel subsequently using the sink.

3.7 Select hand washing station sinks with controls that can be operated without using hands, including single-lever or wrist blade devices and electronic sensor controls. When the operation of the scrub sink is dependent on the building electrical service, connect the controls to the essential electrical system.[14] *[Recommendation]*

Hands-free sinks reduce the risk of cross contamination after hand hygiene is performed.

3.8 Provide paper towel dispensers at hand washing stations that dispense paper towels without the need to touch the dispenser.[14] *[Recommendation]*

3.9 Place alcohol-based hand rub product dispensers (eg, wall-mounted, table-top) in convenient locations as determined by the infection control risk assessment and in accordance with federal, state, and local regulatory requirements.[1,3,4] *[Recommendation]*

The infection control risk assessment identifies locations that will enhance accessibility to hand hygiene products and evaluates the convenience of locations for clinical use.

Professional organizations support placement of alcohol-based hand rub products at the point of use.[1,3,4] The WHO[3] recommends that hand hygiene product dispensers be as close as possible, ideally within arm's reach, to where patient contact is tak-

ing place, to avoid personnel having to leave the care or treatment zone. The CDC[4] and the SHEA/IDSA[1] recommend having alcohol-based hand rub products available at the patient's bedside and in other convenient locations to promote hand hygiene adherence by personnel who perform a high volume of patient care.

3.9.1 Dispenser placement and storage of flammable alcohol-based hand hygiene products must be in compliance with local, state, and federal regulations.[42-44] *[Regulatory Requirement]*

The Centers for Medicare & Medicaid Services[42,45] states in §482.41(c)(2) that "facilities, supplies, and equipment must be maintained to ensure an acceptable level of safety and quality," including storage in compliance with fire codes. The National Fire Protection Association[44] makes recommendations for storage of flammable solutions.

3.9.2 Alcohol-based hand hygiene product dispensers should

- be at least 4 ft apart;
- hold a maximum of 1.2 L in rooms, corridors, and areas open to corridors;
- not be placed above an ignition source (eg, electrical outlet, switch) or within 1 inch of the ignition source; and
- not total more than 10 gallons (37.8 L) outside of a storage cabinet in a single smoke compartment.[44]

[Recommendation]

3.10 Health care organizations may permit use of personal dispensers of alcohol-based hand hygiene products.[3,4] *[Conditional Recommendation]*

Low-quality evidence and guidance from professional organizations support use of personal dispensers of alcohol-based hand hygiene product in the perioperative setting.[3,4,23,46-48]

The CDC[4] recommends having alcohol-based hand rub available at the patient's bedside and in other convenient locations, including in individual containers carried by health care workers, to promote hand hygiene adherence by personnel who perform a high volume of patient care.

The WHO[3] supports use of personal hand hygiene product containers when combined with wall-mounted dispensing systems to increase access to hand hygiene products at the point of care. However, the WHO[3] discusses the limitations of using personal hand hygiene products in the clinical setting:

- Many of the personal dispensers are not transparent and may be found to be empty when needed.

- The amount of hand rub may be so small (10 mL to 20 mL) that several containers per person are needed each day.
- The personal dispensers may not be cost-effective, and maintaining the dispenser supply may be challenging if dependent on a single manufacturer.
- Using disposable dispensers may have a negative impact on the environment.
- The external surface of the bottle may become contaminated, although this may be considered to be negligible because of the excess spillage of the disinfectant and the overall short time until replacement.

Several experts support the use of personal hand hygiene dispensers in the perioperative setting, especially to increase access to hand hygiene products for anesthesia professionals.[23,46,47] In an RCT conducted at a tertiary care and Level 1 trauma center, Koff et al[48] examined the effect of personal hand hygiene product dispenser use by anesthesia professionals (N = 111) on hourly hand decontamination events, contamination of the anesthesia work area and IV tubing, and health care–associated infection rates. As a reminder to the anesthesia professional, the personal dispenser sounded an audible alarm every 6 minutes if no product had been dispensed. Wall-mounted and table-top dispensers were also available in the clinical setting. Use of the personal dispenser was associated with significantly more hourly hand decontamination events, less IV tubing contamination, and lower health care–associated infection rates. A limitation of this study was that a standardized system was not used for health care–associated infection surveillance.

3.11 **Verify hand hygiene product dispenser function in accordance with the manufacturer's instructions each time a new refill is installed.**[44] *[Recommendation]*

3.12 **Make hand washing stations and products accessible to patients and visitors in unrestricted areas (eg, waiting room, preoperative area, postoperative area) unless contraindicated for a specific patient population or individual patient.** *[Recommendation]*

Providing opportunities to perform hand hygiene engages the patient and visitors in the mission of the perioperative team to prevent the patient from developing a health care–associated infection and may reduce the contamination of the patient's environment.

The SHEA/IDSA[1] recommends conducting a point-of-care risk assessment to guide placement of dispensers. Based on the risk assessment, the health care organization may decide to provide patients and visitors with nontoxic hand hygiene products because cognitively impaired, behavioral health, or substance abuse patients may be injured by ingestion of alcohol-based hand rub.

The WHO[3] also recommends careful consideration for placement of dispensers in areas with patients who are likely to ingest the product, such as disoriented elderly patients, psychiatric patients, young children, or patients with alcohol dependence.

3.13 **Provide education and competency verification activities that address performance of hand hygiene in accordance with the product manufacturer's instructions and the health care organization's policies and procedures.**[1,3,4] *[Recommendation]*

Lack of knowledge, experience, and education are factors associated with low hand hygiene compliance.[3] Moderate-quality evidence and guidance from professional organizations support educating health care personnel on hand hygiene indications and performance as part of a multifaceted hand hygiene program (eg, education, training, observation, feedback).[1,3,4,8,28,29,33,34,36,49-54]

Gould et al[49] conducted a systematic review to evaluate the success of strategies to improve hand hygiene compliance. The researchers found that using multiple strategies for education and training, such as engaging personnel in planning and social marketing strategies, may be helpful for improving hand hygiene compliance. However, the quality of the evidence was insufficient to allow for drawing a firm conclusion, and further research is needed to evaluate the effectiveness of educational interventions in increasing hand hygiene compliance.

Several studies have found low compliance with hand hygiene protocols in the perioperative setting[28,32-34,50,54] and knowledge deficits among perioperative team members.[29,36,51,52] In an organizational experience report from Brazil, Santos et al[50] found a significant improvement in hand hygiene rates in an endoscopy unit after a hand hygiene education intervention that included task-oriented training and live demonstrations.

In an organizational report from Australia, Bellaard-Smith and Gillespie[33] found a significant improvement in hand hygiene compliance after they implemented multiple hand hygiene strategies in the operating suite, including education about the WHO five moments of hand hygiene specific to the perioperative setting, appropriate glove use, correct hand hygiene technique, and hand care.

Jericho et al[54] investigated two interventions to improve hand hygiene compliance in the perioperative setting: use of educational posters and including hand hygiene in the time-out process. The researchers found that compliance with using an alcohol-based hand foam was significantly improved after educational posters were placed in strategic locations and hand hygiene was included in the time-out process.

Elkaradawy et al[51] studied the effect of a hand hygiene educational intervention for anesthesia professionals and found a significant reduction in bacterial contamination of the anesthesia machine and the hands of personnel after the intervention.

Some researchers have suggested that use of a fluorescent indicator is an effective hand hygiene education intervention to enhance active participation.[8,53] Pan et al[53] assessed the thoroughness of health care personnel hand hygiene by using a fluorescent substance to simulate hand contamination. The personnel (N = 388) then performed hand hygiene with soap and water, and the researchers used an ultraviolet light detector to identify missed areas where the fluorescent substance remained after the hand wash. The researchers found that the most missed areas of the hand were the nails. The researchers recommended using fluorescent products as part of a "seeing is believing" hand hygiene campaign to encourage active participation.

Hautemaniere et al[8] used a fluorescent alcohol-based hand rub solution to assess thoroughness of hand coverage by using an ultraviolet light to identify any missed areas of the hand that were not covered by the solution. The study found that health care personnel (N = 3,067) significantly improved compliance with a hand hygiene protocol after an educational intervention.

The limitations of the evidence are that the quality of evidence for educational interventions is low, and research has not confirmed the most effective and sustainable education methods to improve hand hygiene compliance. Further research is needed to determine the most effective method to educate health care personnel regarding activities that can result in hand contamination during patient care.[3]

3.13.1 | **Provide education and competency verification when new hand hygiene products or processes are introduced.** [Recommendation]

4. Surgical Hand Antisepsis

4.1 | **Perform surgical hand antisepsis before donning sterile gowns and gloves for operative and other invasive procedures.**[1,3,4,9,55] [Recommendation]

Surgical hand antisepsis is the primary line of defense to protect the patient from pathogens on the hands of perioperative team members, whereas sterile surgical gloves are the secondary line of defense.[55] Due to the risk for glove failure,[56] the per-

formance of surgical hand antisepsis is critical for the prevention of SSIs.[3,4,55]

The limitation of the evidence is that due to low quality, the available research has not confirmed the effect of surgical hand antisepsis on the development of SSIs.[2] Although research has demonstrated that surgical hand antisepsis reduces the number of bacteria on the hands of health care personnel, a systematic review by Tanner et al[2] found that the evidence is unclear about how the number of bacteria correlates to the likelihood of a patient developing an SSI. However, further research to confirm this correlation is not ethical to conduct in clinical trials because it may expose patients to harm.[3]

There is indirect historical evidence that supports the correlation of bacteria on the hands of health care personnel with patient infection. For example, historical evidence has shown that bacteria on the hands of surgeons can cause wound infections if introduced to the sterile field during surgery.[4] Older studies have also shown that bacteria multiply rapidly under surgical gloves when hands are washed with non-antimicrobial soap[4] and that switching to the use of a non-antimicrobial surgical scrub was implicated in an outbreak of SSIs.[3]

The benefits of surgical hand antisepsis outweigh the harms. Benefits include reduction of transient and resident microorganisms on the hands of perioperative team members, which may lower the risk of the patient developing an SSI.[2]

4.2 | **Perform surgical hand antisepsis using a surgical hand rub according to the manufacturer's instructions for use.** [Recommendation]

The evidence review found no literature related to application technique. Antiseptic manufacturers' instructions for use convey important safety and efficacy instructions to the user. Failure to adhere to the manufacturer's instructions for use may result in harm or ineffectiveness of the surgical hand antiseptic.

4.2.1 | **Perform a standardized surgical hand antisepsis protocol using a surgical hand rub in the following order:**
1. **Remove jewelry from hands and wrists (eg, rings, watches, bracelets).**[3,4]
2. **Don a surgical mask.**[3,56]
3. **If hands are visibly soiled, wash hands with soap and water.**[3,4]
4. **Remove debris from underneath fingernails using a disposable nail cleaner under running water.**[3,4]
5. **Dry hands and arms thoroughly**[3,4] **with a disposable paper towel.**

6. Apply the surgical hand rub product to the hands and arms according to the manufacturer's instructions for use (eg, amount, method, time).[3,4]

7. Allow hands and arms to dry completely[3,4] before using sterile technique to don a surgical gown and gloves.[56]

[Recommendation]

4.3 Perform surgical hand antisepsis using a surgical hand scrub according to the manufacturer's instructions for use. [Recommendation]

The evidence review found no literature related to application technique, including sequence of scrubbing, alternating between arms, and the need to scrub above the elbow. Antiseptic manufacturers' instructions for use convey important safety and efficacy instructions to the user. Failure to adhere to the manufacturer's instructions for use may result in harm or ineffectiveness of the surgical hand antiseptic.

4.3.1 Perform a standardized surgical hand antisepsis protocol using a surgical hand scrub in the following order:

1. Remove jewelry from hands and wrists (eg, rings, watches, bracelets).[3,4]

2. Don a surgical mask.[3,56]

3. If hands are visibly soiled, wash hands with soap and water.[3,4]

4. Remove debris from underneath fingernails using a disposable nail cleaner under running water.[3,4]

5. Apply the amount of surgical hand scrub product recommended by the manufacturer to the hands and forearms using a soft, nonabrasive sponge.

6. Visualize each finger, hand, and arm as having four sides. Wash all four sides effectively, keeping the hands elevated.[3]

7. Scrub for length of time recommended by the manufacturer.[4] The scrub should be timed to allow adequate product contact with skin.[3]

8. For water conservation, turn off water when it is not in use, if possible.

9. Avoid splashing surgical attire.[3]

10. Discard sponges, if used.

11. Rinse hands and arms under running water in one direction from fingertips to elbows.[3]

12. Hold hands higher than elbows and away from surgical attire.

13. In the OR or procedure room, dry hands and arms with a sterile towel using sterile technique before donning a surgical gown and gloves.[3,56]

[Recommendation]

4.3.2 Do not perform the surgical hand scrub using a brush.[3,4,57-59] [Recommendation]

Scrubbing with a brush may damage skin and increase the amount of bacteria shedding from the hands.[4] Several studies have shown that use of a brush is not necessary to reduce the number of bacteria on the hands.[3,4,57-59]

4.4 Install a hand scrub sink in the semi-restricted area near the entrance to the OR or procedure room.[14] One hand scrub sink with two scrub positions may serve two operating or procedure rooms if located next to the entrance to each room.[14] [Recommendation]

The FGI[14] recommends that hand scrub facilities be located near the entrance of each cesarean delivery, trauma, operating, interventional imaging procedure, and procedure room in hospitals, outpatient facilities, and office-based surgery settings.

4.5 Install hand scrub sinks that have foot, knee, or electronic sensor controls.[14] When the operation of the scrub sink is dependent on the building electrical service, connect the controls to the essential electrical system.[14] [Recommendation]

Operating the scrub sink with hands-free controls allows perioperative team members to maintain sterile technique during surgical hand antisepsis. The FGI[14] recommends that hand scrub sinks have foot, knee, or electronic sensor controls.

4.6 Provide education and competency verification activities that address performance of surgical hand antisepsis in accordance with the product manufacturer's instructions for use. [Recommendation]

Two studies found that misuse of a surgical hand rub product may have contributed to an increase in SSI rates and that peer education in a skills lab may increase compliance with a surgical hand antisepsis protocol.[60,61]

Haessler et al[60] described an investigation of an SSI cluster at an academic, Level 1 trauma, tertiary care medical center. As part of the investigation, direct observations of surgical hand antisepsis, including scrub and alcohol rub products, were performed. Observers noted inadequate pre-washing when required (eg, for soiled hands), lack of use of a nail pick, and incorrect application of the alcohol surgical hand rub product. Interviews revealed that the surgeons lacked understanding about correct alcohol rub product usage. After the product being misused was removed and the surgeons received education on proper surgical hand antisepsis technique, the SSI rate returned to a level at or below the medical center's historical rates.

In a pilot study, Fichtner et al[61] studied the effect of a skills lab on the surgical hand scrubbing compliance of fourth year medical students (N = 161) in Germany. Students randomly assigned to the intervention group underwent a 45-minute standardized peer training session of practical competencies on surgical hand scrubbing according to the European standard EN1500. Compliance was measured by hand coverage with a fluorescent surgical hand scrub antiseptic. The researchers found that the intervention group (n = 80) had significantly better hand coverage than the control group (n = 81), which received training after the test.

> **4.6.1** **Provide education and competency verification when new surgical hand antiseptic products or processes are introduced.** [Recommendation]

5. Product Evaluation

5.1 **A multidisciplinary team should select hand hygiene products to be used in the perioperative setting following an analysis of product effectiveness, user acceptance, and cost.**[3] [Recommendation]

The WHO[3] recommends that a multidisciplinary team evaluate the antimicrobial efficacy, user acceptance, and cost during the selection of hand hygiene products.

5.2 **The multidisciplinary team should include the infection prevention committee or designated authority with specialized knowledge in infection prevention. Committee representatives should include perioperative RNs and other perioperative team members.** [Recommendation]

Members of the infection prevention committee have specialized knowledge in the selection of hand hygiene products.

5.3 **Develop a mechanism for product evaluation and selection of hand hygiene products.**[62] [Recommendation]

Developing a mechanism for hand hygiene product selection provides a structured process for product evaluation by the health care organization.

5.4 **Evaluate the safety and efficacy of hand hygiene products.**[3,4] [Recommendation]

The WHO[3] and the CDC[4] recommend evaluating the safety and efficacy of hand hygiene products during the product selection process.

In a systematic review, Tanner et al[2] found that no one surgical hand antiseptic was more effective than another for preventing SSI. The evidence involving surgical hand antiseptic efficacy conflicts. Some research indicates that alcohol-based antisep-

tics may be more effective for reducing bacterial counts on hands than aqueous-based solutions.[2,63-67] However, some studies have found that aqueous-based solutions are as effective as alcohol-based antiseptics for reducing bacterial counts.[68,69] Some of these studies indicated a preference for alcohol-based antiseptics because of efficiency and user acceptance.[70,71]

High-quality evidence on the effectiveness of chlorhexidine gluconate (CHG) in surgical hand antiseptics also conflicts. Research indicates that aqueous CHG scrubs may reduce bacterial counts on hands more effectively than aqueous povidone iodine.[2,72] With regard to alcohol-based CHG products, some research indicates that alcohol combined with CHG is superior to other alcohol-based surgical hand antiseptics.[67,73] However, some researchers found that other alcohol-based antiseptics were equally or more effective than the alcohol-and-CHG combination surgical hand antiseptics.[74,75]

Tanner et al[2] found the available evidence on surgical hand antisepsis to be of low quality. Another limitation of some evidence, as described in a laboratory study by Kampf et al,[76] is that studies assessing the efficacy of CHG without using neutralizing agents in the culture sampling fluid may be flawed by overestimating efficacy.

With a gap in the evidence to guide practice, decisions about which surgical hand antiseptic to select for use in the practice setting are complex. This is an unresolved issue that warrants additional research. A variety of products may be necessary to meet the needs of various perioperative team members with skin sensitivities and allergies. Input from a multidisciplinary team with diverse experience and knowledge of hand antiseptics is helpful during review of research, clinical guidelines, and literature from the product manufacturers.

> **5.4.1** **Select products for hand hygiene and surgical hand antisepsis that meet US Food and Drug Administration (FDA) requirements.**[77] [Recommendation]

The FDA approval process includes evaluation of product efficacy and safety. For efficacy, the FDA requires surgical hand antiseptic products to be fast acting (ie, within 1 minute), broad spectrum, and persistent (ie, no return to baseline flora count at 6 hours post application).[77,78] Health care hand wash or rub products must reduce the bacteria on the hands within 5 minutes.[77,78] The FDA approval process also includes evaluating the safety of hand hygiene and surgical hand antiseptics by reviewing human safety studies (eg, maximal use trials), nonclinical safety studies (eg, developmental and reproductive toxicity studies, carcinogenicity studies), data to characterize hormonal effects, and data to evaluate the development of antimicrobial resistance.[77,78]

The FDA currently categorizes active ingredients in the 1994 Tentative Final Monograph (TFM) for hand antiseptic products as either Category I, II, or III.[77]

- Category I means that the product is generally recognized as safe and effective;
- Category II means that the product is not generally recognized as safe and effective; and
- Category III means that available data is insufficient to classify the product as safe and effective, and additional testing is required.

Due to the availability of advanced understanding in safety and efficacy testing methods, however, in a 2015 proposed rule to finalize the TFM by 2018, the FDA requested additional scientific evidence from manufacturers to evaluate whether the ingredients in certain antiseptic products are safe and effective.[78] Thus, the proposed rule categorizes all the antiseptics as IIISE, until the FDA has received all requested safety and efficacy data for each antiseptic. While the FDA gathers scientific evidence from the manufacturers, they recommend that health care personnel continue to use health care antiseptics to maintain a standard of care to prevent patient infection.[79]

The proposed rule also recommended changes to the FDA clinical simulation testing efficacy requirements for health care personnel hand wash or rub and surgical hand scrub or rub.[78] **Table 2** provides a summary of the TFM and proposed rule clinical simulation testing protocols and efficacy requirements.

A limitation of using FDA testing requirements as a tool for evaluating product safety and efficacy is that the FDA testing protocols are based on simulation with volunteers in the laboratory setting. The laboratory protocols may not accurately reflect actual use of hand wash and surgical hand scrub or rub products in the clinical setting.[3,4] Further research is needed to determine the generalizability of these studies and protocols to the clinical setting.

5.4.2 Non-antimicrobial and <u>antimicrobial soaps</u> may be selected for evaluation. *[Conditional Recommendation]*

The CDC[4] and the SHEA/IDSA[1] recommend using either non-antimicrobial or antimicrobial soaps in the health care setting.

5.4.3 Do not select soaps containing triclosan for evaluation.[1] *[Recommendation]*

The SHEA/IDSA[1] recommends avoiding use of soaps containing the antiseptic triclosan in the health care setting due to an assessment of benefits and harms. Evidence is lacking to establish clinical benefit from use of triclosan compared to other antiseptics. The harms of triclosan may include environmental contamination and the potential for development of bacterial resistance.[1] Further research is needed to assess the benefits and harms of triclosan use in the perioperative setting.

5.5 Evaluate the compatibility of hand hygiene products with skin care products (eg, lotions, moisturizers) and types of gloves used at the facility.[3,4] *[Recommendation]*

The WHO[3] and the CDC[4] recommend reviewing information from the manufacturer regarding any known interactions between products used to clean hands, skin care products, and gloves. Oil-containing lotions have been associated with altered integrity of latex rubber gloves, reduced persistent effects of hand antiseptics, and bacterial contamination of the lotion.[3,4]

5.6 Evaluate the cost of hand hygiene products, but cost should not be the primary factor for selection.[3,4] *[Recommendation]*

The WHO[3] and the CDC[4] recommend evaluating cost during the selection of hand hygiene products. However, both organizations emphasize the importance of product effectiveness and user acceptance over cost.

5.7 Conduct end-user evaluations to determine acceptability of the hand hygiene and skin care products to perioperative team members.[1,3,4] *[Recommendation]*

Acceptability of hand hygiene products is a key factor that influences health care personnel compliance with hand hygiene.[1,3,4] The WHO,[3] the CDC,[4] and the SHEA/IDSA[1] recommend involving health care personnel in the choice of hand hygiene and skin care products.

5.7.1 Determine the time frame and season for end-user evaluation of hand hygiene products. When more than one product is evaluated, establish a mechanism for a time period between product evaluations.[3] *[Recommendation]*

The WHO[3] recommends end-user evaluation for at least 2 to 3 weeks, although a fast-track method has also been validated. When more than one product is being evaluated, the WHO[3] recommends either a period of routine product

Table 2. US Food and Drug Administration Clinical Simulation Testing Protocol[1,2]			
Product	**Testing Method**	**1994 Tentative Final Monograph**	**Proposed Rule**
Hand wash or rub	**ASTM E-1174** • Artificial contamination with *Serratia marcescens* and *Escherichia coli* • Test solution applied to hands and lower 1/3 of forearms for 30 seconds and rinsed with water • Sterile loose fitting gloves donned and secured at wrist, 75 mL of eluent added and kneaded for 1 minute, and eluate cultured for bacteria	**1st wash** • 2 $\log_{10}$ reduction, each hand, within 5 minutes **10th wash** • 3 $\log_{10}$ reduction, each hand, within 5 minutes	**Single wash or rub** • 2.5 $\log_{10}$ reduction, each hand, within 5 minutes
Surgical hand scrub or rub	**ASTM E-1115** • No artificial contamination, resident skin flora • Volunteer cleans under fingernails with nail stick, clips fingernails, and removes all jewelry from the hands and arms • Hands and lower 2/3 of forearms rinsed with water for 30 seconds, washed with non-antimicrobial soap for 30 seconds, and rinsed with water for 30 seconds • Test solution is applied per manufacturer's instructions • Sterile loose fitting gloves donned and secured at wrist, 75 mL of eluent added and kneaded for 1 minute, and eluate cultured for bacteria	**1st wash, Day 1** • 1 $\log_{10}$ reduction, each hand, within 1 minute • Does not exceed baseline at 6 hours **Day 2** • 2 $\log_{10}$ reduction, each hand, within 1 minute **Last wash, Day 5** • 3 $\log_{10}$ reduction, each hand, within 1 minute	**Single wash or rub** • 2 $\log_{10}$ reduction, each hand, within 1 minute • Does not exceed baseline at 6 hours

References
1. *US Food and Drug Administration. Tentative final monograph for healthcare antiseptic drug products proposed rule. Fed Regist. 1994;59(116): 31402-31452.*
2. *CFR part 310 safety and effectiveness of health care antiseptics; topical antimicrobial drug products for over-the-counter human use; proposed amendment of the tentative final monograph; reopening of administrative record; proposed rule. Fed Regist. 2015;80(84):25166-25205.*

use or a 2-day period between product evaluations when feasible.

The WHO[3] recommends avoiding the testing of new hand hygiene products during seasons of low humidity because health care personnel may have more skin reactions in this weather and the results of the end-user evaluation could be affected by this seasonal variation. In a European field study, Girard et al[80] investigated factors that influenced the testing of alcohol-based hand rubs and found that test periods during colder seasons were significantly associated with skin reactions.

5.7.2 **Include the following in end-user evaluations:**
- **skin tolerance,**
- **skin reactions,**
- **ease of use (eg, volume, dry time),**
- **feel (eg, consistency, texture),**
- **color, and**
- **fragrance.**[3,4]

[Recommendation]

As part of the end-user evaluations, the WHO[3] and the CDC[4] recommend that skin tolerance, skin reactions, ease of use, and the aesthetic preferences (ie, fragrance, color, texture)

of health care personnel be considered in the selection of hand hygiene products.

5.7.3 **Include patients in end-user evaluations of hand hygiene products.**[3] *[Recommendation]*

The WHO[3] recommends that the patient's aesthetic preferences (ie, fragrance, color, texture, ease of use) be considered in the selection of hand hygiene products. Patients may be especially sensitive to the fragrance of hand hygiene products.[3]

5.7.4 **The multidisciplinary team should review written end-user evaluations.** *[Recommendation]*

Written questionnaires or evaluations provide the multidisciplinary team with data to assess acceptability to end-users.

5.8 **Evaluate hand hygiene product dispensers (eg, wall-mounted, table-top, personal) for adequate, reliable function and delivery of the recommended product volume.**[3,4] *[Recommendation]*

The WHO[3] and the CDC[4] recommend evaluating hand hygiene product dispensers for adequate and reliable function in the delivery of hand hygiene products.

5.8.1 The multidisciplinary team may evaluate automated wall-mounted dispensers.[3] *[Conditional Recommendation]*

Moderate-quality evidence is inconclusive regarding the benefits of automated wall-mounted dispensers. The theoretical benefit of automated wall-mounted dispensers is that they can be used without being touched and potentially contaminating the hands of the perioperative team member.[3] The German and Austrian Society for Hospital Hygiene[81] requires that hand hygiene dispensers be triggered without using hands, operated either by a sensor or an elbow.

In an observational study, Assadian et al[82] cultured 17 hand sanitizer dispensers in a 12-bed intensive care unit at an urban teaching hospital. The dispensers were disinfected on a daily basis. This study found that all dispensers were contaminated with bacteria, both from common skin flora and gram-negative bacteria, and that contamination was greatest on the lever. The results of this study implicate hand sanitizer dispensers as potential reservoirs for bacteria in the health care environment. The researchers recommended cleaning the dispensers to reduce contamination and suggested that automated or pedal-operated dispensers may reduce the risk of dispenser contamination. A limitation of this study is that it was not designed to evaluate the effect of disinfection on contamination. Another limitation is that the small sample size may limit the generalizability of the study findings.

The WHO[3] discusses that the downside to automated wall-mounted dispensers is that they have a higher chance for malfunction and are more expensive to maintain than non-automated dispensers.

Further research is needed to determine the effect of contaminated dispensers on hand hygiene effectiveness, the best method for preventing contamination of hand hygiene product dispensers, and the optimal method for dispensing hand hygiene products.

5.8.2 Use dispensers of alcohol-based hand hygiene products that
- do not release products except when the dispenser is activated,
- only activate when an object is placed within 4 inches of the sensor,
- only activate once when an object is left in place in the activation zone,
- do not dispense more product than the amount recommended by the manufacturer for hand hygiene, and
- are designed to prevent accidental or malicious activation of the dispenser.[44]

[Recommendation]

6. Quality

6.1 Participate in a variety of quality assurance and performance improvement activities that are consistent with the facility or health care organization plan to improve understanding and compliance with the principles and processes of hand hygiene. *[Recommendation]*

Quality assurance and performance improvement programs assist in evaluating and improving the quality of patient care and formulating plans for corrective action. These programs provide data that may be used to determine whether an individual organization is within benchmark goals and, if not, to identify areas that may require corrective action.

6.2 Identify barriers for performing hand hygiene in the perioperative setting and address these through interventions to improve hand hygiene compliance.[1] *[Recommendation]*

Identifying barriers to hand hygiene allows the health care organization to develop relevant interventions to improve hand hygiene compliance.[1] The SHEA/IDSA[1] recommends identifying unit-specific barriers and creating interventions specific to the unit's needs.

6.3 Monitor adherence to policies and procedures for hand hygiene as part of quality assurance and process improvement initiatives.[1,3,4] *[Recommendation]*

Professional organizations recommend monitoring health care personnel adherence to recommended hand hygiene practices.[1,3,4] According to the WHO,[3] monitoring hand hygiene adherence as a performance indicator serves several functions including system monitoring, incentive for performance improvement, outbreak investigation, and infrastructure design.

6.3.1 Measure hand hygiene in the perioperative setting by direct observation.[1,3,4,83] *[Recommendation]*

The SHEA/IDSA[83] recommends performing direct observation audits of hand hygiene in the perioperative setting as a strategy to prevent SSIs. The authors of several studies and organizational experience reports monitored hand hygiene compliance in the perioperative setting using direct observation.[24,25,28,30,32-34,36,50,52,54,84]

Limitations of direct observation are the risk for selection and observer bias[3] and that the method is subject to the Hawthorne effect.[1] Direct observation audits are performed by a human observer, either in person or by video recording, which can be labor intensive. Video observations may be beneficial in the perioperative setting due to the high number of hand hygiene indications and numerous perioperative team members. However, video observations may also compromise patient privacy.[1]

Rowlands et al[26] used video observations of anesthesia professionals to evaluate hand hygiene compliance with WHO criteria. Three perioperative team members (ie, an anesthesiologist, an anesthesiology resident, and a perioperative RN) reviewed the videos independently. The researchers found that hand hygiene compliance in the anesthesia work area was low and that compliance with current hand hygiene guidelines was not feasible. A limitation of the study was that the perioperative team being observed was aware of the recording, which could have biased the observations by creating a Hawthorne effect.

6.3.2 **Other measures to evaluate hand hygiene practices may include product usage or automated monitoring.**[1,3,4] *[Conditional Recommendation]*

Measuring product usage, such as of alcohol-based hand rub products, provides an indicator of overall hand hygiene activity.[3] However, this method does not reliably measure hand hygiene based on opportunities,[1,3] and the CDC-recommended measurement of product volume usage per 1,000 patient-days[4] is not a perioperative indicator of patient volume. This evidence review found no literature to support or refute the use of product usage measurement as a hand hygiene indicator in the perioperative setting.

Automated hand hygiene monitoring is an emerging technology that may detect hand hygiene opportunities within the patient encounter.[1,3] The evidence review found no literature to support or refute the use of automated hand hygiene monitoring systems in the perioperative setting.

6.3.3 **Provide feedback on hand hygiene performance to perioperative team members.**[1,3,4] *[Recommendation]*

Professional organizations[1,3,4] recommend providing health care personnel with performance feedback when monitoring adherence to hand hygiene practices.

6.4 **Encourage patients and visitors to remind perioperative team members to perform hand hygiene before care.**[1,3,4,85] *[Recommendation]*

Moderate-quality evidence and guidance from professional organizations support encouraging patients and their family members to remind health care personnel to clean their hands before care episodes.[1,3,4,85] The WHO[3] recommends a structured approach to incorporating patient engagement into the hand hygiene promotion strategy, including developing ownership and shared responsibility for the program at the health care organization, reviewing existing empowerment programs, and developing the program based on organization-specific factors such as culture, program implementation, and evaluation.

The WHO[3] conducted a global survey of patient experiences with hand hygiene (N = 459) and found that 29% of respondents had asked health care personnel to wash their hands, and 25% reported receiving a negative response to the request. The survey found that patients were more likely to feel comfortable reminding health care personnel to wash their hands when encouraged by health care personnel. Patients with direct experience of a health care–associated infection were more likely to question the health care personnel.

In another patient survey, Ottum et al[85] surveyed 200 patient respondents (response rate 94.78%) about their comfort in reminding health care personnel to perform hand hygiene. The study found that 99.5% of patients surveyed believed that personnel were supposed to wash their hands before and after care and that 90.5% believed in reminding health care personnel to wash their hands only if they forgot. However, only 14% of patients reported having asked personnel to wash their hands, with 64% comfortable reminding nurses and 54% comfortable reminding physicians. Patients who had worked in health care were significantly more likely to be comfortable asking personnel to wash their hands than patients who had not worked in health care. The implications of these findings are that the baseline beliefs of the patients about the importance of hand hygiene were universally high, which suggests that more education would be unlikely to empower their participation further. Thus, the researchers recommended focusing interventions on making patients more comfortable with asking health care personnel to wash their hands.

Editor's note: Shellac is a registered trademark of Creative Nail Design, Inc, San Diego, CA.

Glossary

Alcohol-based hand rub: An alcohol-containing preparation (eg, liquid, gel, foam) designed for application to the hands to inactivate microorganisms and temporarily suppress their growth.

Antimicrobial soap: Soap containing an antiseptic at a concentration sufficient to inactivate microorganisms and temporarily suppress their growth.

Artificial nails: Substances or devices applied or added to the natural nails to augment or enhance the wearer's own nails. They include, but are not limited to, bonding, extensions, tips, wraps, gel and acrylic overlays, and tapes.

Eluent: A solvent used for separating material from a surface.

Glove juice method: A method for culturing the hands that involves donning a sterile glove, instilling an eluent solution into the glove, securing the glove at the wrist, kneading the gloved hand in a standardized manner for 60 seconds, and extracting the eluent fluid (glove juice) for culture.

Hand hygiene: Any activities related to hand condition and cleansing.

Hand washing station: An area that includes a sink, a hands-free faucet, cleansing solutions, and a means for drying the hands.

Invasive procedure: The surgical entry into tissues, cavities, or organs or the repair of major trauma injuries.

Surgical hand antisepsis: Hand wash or hand rub using a surgical hand antiseptic, performed preoperatively by the surgical team to remove transient flora and reduce resident skin flora.

Surgical hand antiseptic: A product that is a broad-spectrum, fast-acting, and nonirritating preparation containing an antimicrobial ingredient designed to significantly reduce the number of microorganisms on intact skin. Surgical hand antiseptic agents demonstrate both persistent and cumulative activity.

Ultraviolet-cured nail polish: Nail polish created by polymerization of a methacrylate or acrylate that hardens when exposed to ultraviolet (UVA) light.

References

1. Ellingson K, Haas JP, Aiello AE, et al. Strategies to prevent healthcare-associated infections through hand hygiene. *Infect Control Hosp Epidemiol.* 2014;35(8):937-960. [IVA]

2. Tanner J, Dumville JC, Norman G, Fortnam M. Surgical hand antisepsis to reduce surgical site infection. *Cochrane Database Syst Rev.* 2016;1:CD004288. [IB]

3. *WHO Guidelines on Hand Hygiene in Health Care.* Geneva, Switzerland: World Health Organization; 2009. [IVA]

4. Boyce JM, Pittet D; Healthcare Infection Control Practices Advisory Committee. Society for Healthcare Epidemiology of America. Association for Professionals in Infection Control. Infectious Diseases Society of America. Hand Hygiene Task Force. Guideline for Hand Hygiene in Health-Care Settings: recommendations of the Healthcare Infection Control Practices Advisory Committee and the HICPAC/SHEA/APIC/IDSA Hand Hygiene Task Force. *Infect Control Hosp Epidemiol.* 2002;23(12 Suppl):S3-S40. [IVA]

5. *Surgical Site Infection: Evidence Update June 2013* [Evidence Update 43]. Manchester, United Kingdom: National Institute for Health and Care Excellence; 2013. [IVA]

6. Fagernes M, Lingaas E. Factors interfering with the microflora on hands: a regression analysis of samples from 465 healthcare workers. *J Adv Nurs.* 2011;67(2):297-307. [IIIB]

7. Rupp ME, Fitzgerald T, Puumala S, et al. Prospective, controlled, cross-over trial of alcohol-based hand gel in critical care units. *Infect Control Hosp Epidemiol.* 2008;29(1):8-15. [IIB]

8. Hautemaniere A, Cunat L, Diguio N, et al. Factors determining poor practice in alcoholic gel hand rub technique in hospital workers. *J Infect Public Health.* 2010;3(1):25-34. [IIB]

9. *AST Standards of Practice for Surgical Attire, Surgical Scrub, Hand Hygiene and Hand Washing.* April 13, 2008. Association of Surgical Technologists. http://www.ast.org/uploadedFiles/Main_Site/Content/About_Us/Standard_Surgical_Attire_Surgical_Scrub.pdf. Accessed June 27, 2016. [IVC]

10. *Infection Prevention and Control Guidelines for Anesthesia Care.* 2015. American Association of Nurse Anesthetists. http://www.aana.com/resources2/professionalpractice/Pages/Infection-Prevention-and-Control-Guidelines-for-Anesthesia-Care.aspx. Accessed June 27, 2016. [IVB]

11. Arrowsmith VA, Taylor R. Removal of nail polish and finger rings to prevent surgical infection. *Cochrane Database Syst Rev.* 2014;8:CD003325. [IC]

12. Van Der Meer EWC, Boot CRL, Van Der Gulden JWJ, et al. Hands4U: The effects of a multifaceted implementation strategy on hand eczema prevalence in a healthcare setting. Results of a randomized controlled trial. *Contact Derm.* 2015;72(5):312-324. [IB]

13. Harnoss JC, Brune L, Ansorg J, Heidecke C-D, Assadian O, Kramer A. Practice of skin protection and skin care among German surgeons and influence on the efficacy of surgical hand disinfection and surgical glove perforation. *BMC Infect Dis.* 2014;14:315. [IB]

14. Facility Guidelines Institute, US Department of Health and Human Services, American Society for Healthcare Engineering. *Guidelines for Design and Construction of Hospitals and Outpatient Facilities.* Chicago, IL: American Society for Healthcare Engineering of the American Hospital Association; 2014. [IVC]

15. Guideline for prevention of transmissible infections. In: *Guidelines for Perioperative Practice.* Denver, CO: AORN, Inc; 2016:471-506. [IVA]

16. Bolyard EA, Tablan OC, Williams WW, Pearson ML, Shapiro CN, Deitchmann SD. Guideline for infection control in healthcare personnel, 1998. Hospital Infection Control Practices Advisory Committee. *Infect Control Hosp Epidemiol.* 1998;19(6):407-463. [IVA]

17. Henderson DK, Dembry L, Fishman NO, et al. SHEA guideline for management of healthcare workers who are

infected with hepatitis B virus, hepatitis C virus, and/or human immunodeficiency virus. *Infect Control Hosp Epidemiol.* 2010;31(3):203-232. [IVA]

18. Guideline for surgical attire. In: *Guidelines for Perioperative Practice.* Denver, CO: AORN, Inc; 2016:95-118. [IVA]

19. Loftus RW, Muffly MK, Brown JR, et al. Hand contamination of anesthesia providers is an important risk factor for intraoperative bacterial transmission. *Anesth Analg.* 2011;112(1):98-105. [IIIA]

20. Mermel LA, Bert A, Chapin KC, LeBlanc L. Intraoperative stopcock and manifold colonization of newly inserted peripheral intravenous catheters. *Infect Control Hosp Epidemiol.* 2014;35(9):1187-1189. [IIIB]

21. Loftus RW, Brown JR, Koff MD, et al. Multiple reservoirs contribute to intraoperative bacterial transmission. *Anesth Analg.* 2012;114(6):1236-1248. [IIIA]

22. Cosgrove MS. Infection control in the operating room. *Crit Care Nurs Clin North Am.* 2015;27(1):79-87. [VB]

23. Munoz-Price LS, Birnbach DJ. Hand hygiene and anesthesiology. *Int Anesthesiol Clin.* 2013;51(1):79-92. [VA]

24. Munoz-Price LS, Lubarsky DA, Arheart KL, et al. Interactions between anesthesiologists and the environment while providing anesthesia care in the operating room. *Am J Infect Control.* 2013;41(10):922-924. [VA]

25. Munoz-Price LS, Riley B, Banks S, et al. Frequency of interactions and hand disinfections among anesthesiologists while providing anesthesia care in the operating room: induction versus maintenance. *Infect Control Hosp Epidemiol.* 2014;35(8):1056-1059. [IIIB]

26. Rowlands J, Yeager MP, Beach M, Patel HM, Huysman BC, Loftus RW. Video observation to map hand contact and bacterial transmission in operating rooms. *Am J Infect Control.* 2014;42(7):698-701. [IIIA]

27. Allen G. Hand hygiene and the surgical team. *Perioper Nurs Clin.* 2010;5(4):411-418. [VA]

28. Krediet AC, Kalkman CJ, Bonten MJ, Gigengack ACM, Barach P. Hand-hygiene practices in the operating theatre: an observational study. *Br J Anaesth.* 2011;107(4):553-558. [IIIB]

29. Fernandez PG, Loftus RW, Dodds TM, et al. Hand hygiene knowledge and perceptions among anesthesia providers. *Anesth Analg.* 2015;120(4):837-843. [IIIA]

30. Biddle C, Shah J. Quantification of anesthesia providers' hand hygiene in a busy metropolitan operating room: what would Semmelweis think? *Am J Infect Control.* 2012;40(8):756-759. [IIIB]

31. O'Grady NP, Alexander M, Burns LA, et al. Guidelines for the prevention of intravascular catheter-related infections. *Am J Infect Control.* 2011;39(4 Suppl 1):S1-S34. [IVA]

32. Sahni N, Biswal M, Gandhi K, Yaddanapudi S. Quantification of hand hygiene compliance in anesthesia providers at a tertiary care center in northern India. *Am J Infect Control.* 2015;43(10):1134-1136. [VB]

33. Bellaard-Smith ER, Gillespie EE. Implementing hand hygiene strategies in the operating suite. *Healthc Infect.* 2012;17(1):33-37. [VA]

34. Megeus V, Nilsson K, Karlsson J, Eriksson BI, Andersson AE. Hand hygiene and aseptic techniques during routine

anesthetic care—observations in the operating room. *Antimicrob Resist Infect Control.* 2015;4(1):5. [IIIB]

35. Gould CV, Umscheid CA, Agarwal RK, Kuntz G, Pegues DA; Healthcare Infection Control Practices Advisory Committee. Guideline for prevention of catheter-associated urinary tract infections 2009. *Infect Control Hosp Epidemiol.* 2010;31(4):319-326. [IVA]

36. Andersson AE, Bergh I, Karlsson J, Eriksson BI, Nilsson K. The application of evidence-based measures to reduce surgical site infections during orthopedic surgery—report of a single-center experience in Sweden. *Patient Saf Surg.* 2012; 6(1):11. [IIIB]

37. American Society of Anesthesiologists Task Force on Infectious Complications Associated with Neuraxial Techniques. Practice advisory for the prevention, diagnosis, and management of infectious complications associated with neuraxial techniques: a report by the American Society of Anesthesiologists Task Force on Infectious Complications Associated with Neuraxial Techniques. *Anesthesiology.* 2010;112(3):530-545. [IVB]

38. Jochum D, Iohom G, Bouaziz H. Asepsis in regional anesthesia. *Int Anesthesiol Clin.* 2010;48(4):35-44. [VB]

39. Guideline for environmental cleaning. In: *Guidelines for Perioperative Practice.* Denver, CO: AORN, Inc; 2016:7-28. [IVA]

40. Birnbach DJ, Rosen LF, Fitzpatrick M, Carling P, Arheart KL, Munoz-Price LS. Double gloves: a randomized trial to evaluate a simple strategy to reduce contamination in the operating room. *Anesth Analg.* 2015;120(4):848-852. [IB]

41. Birnbach DJ, Rosen LF, Fitzpatrick M, Carling P, Arheart KL, Munoz-Price LS. A new approach to pathogen containment in the operating room: sheathing the laryngoscope after intubation. *Anesth Analg.* 2015;121(5):1209-1214. [IB]

42. *State Operations Manual Appendix A—Survey Protocol, Regulations and Interpretive Guidelines for Hospitals.* Rev 151; 2015. Centers for Medicare & Medicaid Services. https://www.cms.gov/Regulations-and-Guidance/Guidance/Manuals/downloads/som107ap_a_hospitals.pdf. Accessed June 27, 2016.

43. Guideline for a safe environment of care, part 1. In: *Guidelines for Perioperative Practice.* Denver, CO: AORN, Inc; 2016:237-262. [IVA]

44. *NFPA 101: Life Safety Code.* Quincy, MA: National Fire Protection Association; 2015.[IVC]

45. *State Operations Manual Appendix L—Guidance for Surveyors: Ambulatory Surgical Centers.* Rev 137; 2015. Centers for Medicare & Medicaid Services. https://www.cms.gov/Regulations-and-Guidance/Guidance/Manuals/downloads/som107ap_l_ambulatory.pdf. Accessed June 27, 2016.

46. Petty WC. Closing the hand hygiene gap in the postanesthesia care unit: a body-worn alcohol-based dispenser. *J Perianesth Nurs.* 2013;28(2):87-97. [VB]

47. Loftus RW, Koff MD, Birnbach DJ. The dynamics and implications of bacterial transmission events arising from the anesthesia work area. *Anesth Analg.* 2015;120(4):853-860. [VA]

48. Koff MD, Loftus RW, Burchman CC, et al. Reduction in intraoperative bacterial contamination of peripheral

intravenous tubing through the use of a novel device. *Anesthesiology.* 2009;110(5):978-985. [IB]

49. Gould DJ, Moralejo D, Drey N, Chudleigh JH. Interventions to improve hand hygiene compliance in patient care. *Cochrane Database Syst Rev.* 2010;9:CD005186. [IIC]

50. Santos LX, Souza Dias MB, Borrasca VL, et al. Improving hand hygiene adherence in an endoscopy unit. *Endoscopy.* 2013;45(6):421-425. [VA]

51. Elkaradawy SA, Helaly GF, Abdel Wahab MM. Effect of an infection control educational programme on anaesthetists' attitude and anaesthetic field bacterial contamination. *Egypt J Anaesth.* 2012;28(2):149-156. [IIA]

52. Swenne CL, Alexandrén K. Surgical team members' compliance with and knowledge of basic hand hygiene guidelines and intraoperative hygiene. *J Infect Prev.* 2012;13(4):114-119. [IIIB]

53. Pan S-C, Chen E, Tien K-L, et al. Assessing the thoroughness of hand hygiene: "Seeing is believing." *Am J Infect Control.* 2014;42(7):799-801. [IIA]

54. Jericho BG, Kalin AM, Schwartz DE. Improving hand hygiene compliance by incorporating it into the verification process in the operating room. *Internet J Anesthesiol.* 2013;32(3):2. [VA]

55. Adams AB. Surgical hand antisepsis: where we have been and where we are today. *Perioper Nurs Clin.* 2010;5(4):443-448. [VB]

56. Guideline for sterile technique. In: *Guidelines for Perioperative Practice.* Denver, CO: AORN, Inc; 2016:65-94. [IVA]

57. Abdelatiff DA, El-Haiyk KS, Ghobashi NH, El-Qudaa RF, El-Sabouni RS. Comparing of using sterile brush during surgical scrubbing versus brushless for surgical team in operating room. *Life Sci J.* 2014;11(1):387-393. [IC]

58. da Cunha ÉR, Matos FGOA, da Silva AM, de Araújo EAC, Ferreira KASL, Graziano KU. The efficacy of three hand asepsis techniques using chlorhexidine gluconate (CHG 2%). *Rev Esc Enferm USP.* 2011;45(6):1440-1445. [IIB]

59. Okgün Alcan A, Demir Korkmaz F. Comparison of the efficiency of nail pick and brush used for nail cleaning during surgical scrub on reducing bacterial counts. *Am J Infect Control.* 2012;40(9):826-829. [IB]

60. Haessler S, Connelly NR, Kanter G, et al. A surgical site infection cluster: the process and outcome of an investigation—the impact of an alcohol-based surgical antisepsis product and human behavior. *Anesth Analg.* 2010;110(4):1044-1048. [VB]

61. Fichtner A, Haupt E, Karwath T, Wullenk K, Pöhlmann C, Jatzwauk L. A single standardized practical training for surgical scrubbing according to EN1500: effect quantification, value of the standardized method and comparison with clinical reference groups. *GMS Z Med Ausbild.* 2013;30(2):Doc24. [IC]

62. Guideline for product selection. In: *Guidelines for Perioperative Practice.* Denver, CO: AORN, Inc; 2016:177-184. [IVB]

63. Barbadoro P, Martini E, Savini S, et al. Invivo comparative efficacy of three surgical hand preparation agents in reducing bacterial count. *J Hosp Infect.* 2014;86(1):64-67. [IIC]

64. Shen N-J, Pan S-C, Sheng W-H, et al. Comparative antimicrobial efficacy of alcohol-based hand rub and conventional surgical scrub in a medical center. *J Microbiol Immunol Infect.* 2015;48(3):322-328. [IIIB]

65. Lai KW, Foo TL, Low W, Naidu G. Surgical hand antisepsis—a pilot study comparing povidone iodine hand scrub and alcohol-based chlorhexidine gluconate hand rub. *Ann Acad Med Singapore.* 2012;41(1):12-16. [IIC]

66. Chen S-H, Chou C-Y, Huang J-C, Tang Y-F, Kuo Y-R, Chien L-Y. Antibacterial effects on dry-fast and traditional water-based surgical scrubbing methods: a two-time points experimental study. *Nurs Health Sci.* 2014;16(2):179-185. [IIB]

67. Hamed Mahmoud M, Morad Asaad A, Ansar Qureshi M. Hand rubbing and scrubbing in relation to microbial count among surgical team members in a Saudi hospital. *Life Sci J.* 2013;10(3):198-205. [IIB]

68. Ghorbani A, Shahrokhi A, Soltani Z, Molapour A, Shafikhani M. Comparison of surgical hand scrub and alcohol surgical hand rub on reducing hand microbial burden. *J Perioper Pract.* 2012;22(2):67-70. [IC]

69. Howard JD, Jowett C, Faoagali J, McKenzie B. New method for assessing hand disinfection shows that pre-operative alcohol/chlorhexidine rub is as effective as a traditional surgical scrub. *J Hosp Infect.* 2014;88(2):78-83. [IIB]

70. Chen C-F, Han C-L, Kan C-P, Chen S-G, Hung PW. Effect of surgical site infections with waterless and traditional hand scrubbing protocols on bacterial growth. *Am J Infect Control.* 2012;40(4):e15-e17. [IIC]

71. Weight CJ, Lee MC, Palmer JS. Avagard hand antisepsis vs. traditional scrub in 3600 pediatric urologic procedures. *Urology.* 2010;76(1):15-17. [IIC]

72. Jarral OA, McCormack DJ, Ibrahim S, Shipolini AR. Should surgeons scrub with chlorhexidine or iodine prior to surgery? *Interact Cardiovasc Thorac Surg.* 2011;12(6):1017-1021. [IIIB]

73. Olson LKM, Morse DJ, Duley C, Savell BK. Prospective, randomized in vivo comparison of a dual-active waterless antiseptic versus two alcohol-only waterless antiseptics for surgical hand antisepsis. *Am J Infect Control.* 2012;40(2):155-159. [IIA]

74. Macinga DR, Edmonds SL, Campbell E, McCormack RR. Comparative efficacy of alcohol-based surgical scrubs: the importance of formulation. *AORN J.* 2014;100(6):641-650. [IB]

75. Cargill DI, Roche ED, Van Der Kar CA, et al. Development of a health care personnel handwash with 6-hour persistence. *Am J Infect Control.* 2011;39(3):226-234. [IIA]

76. Kampf G, Reichel M, Hollingsworth A, Bashir M. Efficacy of surgical hand scrub products based on chlorhexidine is largely overestimated without neutralizing agents in the sampling fluid. *Am J Infect Control.* 2013;41(1):e1-e5. [IIB]

77. US Food and Drug Administration. Tentative final monograph for healthcare antiseptic drug products proposed rule. *Fed Regist.* 1994;59(116):31402-31452.

78. 21 CFR Part 310. Safety and effectiveness of health care antiseptics; topical antimicrobial drug products for over-the-counter human use; proposed amendment of the tentative final monograph; reopening of administrative record; proposed rule. *Fed Regist.* 2015;80(84):25166-25205.

79. Q&A for consumers: health care antiseptics. US Food and Drug Administration. http://www.fda.gov/Drugs/DrugSafety/InformationbyDrugClass/ucm445063.htm. Accessed June 27, 2016.

80. Girard R, Carre E, Mermet V, et al. Factors influencing field testing of alcohol-based hand rubs. *Infect Control Hosp Epidemiol.* 2015;36(3):302-310. [IIIB]

81. Eiref SD, Leitman IM, Riley W. Hand sanitizer dispensers and associated hospital-acquired infections: friend or fomite? *Surg Infect.* 2012;13(3):137-140. [IIIB]

82. Assadian O, Kramer A, Christiansen B, et al. Recommendations and requirements for soap and hand rub dispensers in healthcare facilities. *GMS Krankenhhyg interdiszip.* 2012;7(1):Doc03. [IVC]

83. Anderson DJ, Podgorny K, Berrios-Torres SI, et al. Strategies to prevent surgical site infections in acute care hospitals: 2014 update. *Infect Control Hosp Epidemiol.* 2014;35(6):605-627. [IVA]

84. Homa K, Kirkland KB. Determining next steps in a hand hygiene improvement initiative by examining variation in hand hygiene compliance rates. *Qual Manage Health Care.* 2011;20(2):116-121. [VB]

85. Ottum A, Sethi AK, Jacobs EA, Zerbel S, Gaines ME, Safdar N. Do patients feel comfortable asking healthcare workers to wash their hands? *Infect Control Hosp Epidemiol.* 2012;33(12):1283-1284. [IIIB]

Acknowledgments

Lead Author
Amber Wood, MSN, RN, CNOR, CIC
Senior Perioperative Practice Specialist
AORN Nursing Department
Denver, Colorado

Contributing Author
Ramona L. Conner, MSN, RN, CNOR
Editor-in-Chief, Guidelines for Perioperative Practice
AORN Nursing Department
Denver, Colorado

The authors and AORN thank Rodney W. Hicks, PhD, RN, FNP-BC, FAANP, Professor, Western University of Health Sciences, Pomona, California; Bernard C. Camins, MD, MSc, Associate Professor of Medicine Division of Infectious Diseases, University of Alabama at Birmingham Healthcare Epidemiologist, UAB Health System Medical Director, UAB Hospital Employee Health and UA HSF Employee Health, Birmingham; Barbara L. Nalley, MSN, CRNP, CNOR, Manager, Anne Arundel Medical Group, Annapolis, Maryland; Heather A. Hohenberger, BSN, RN, CIC, CNOR, CPHQ, Quality Improvement Consultant, Perioperative Services, Indiana University Health, Indianapolis; Jocelyn M. Chalquist, BSN, RN, CNOR, Surgical Services Educator, Aurora Medical Center-Kenosha, Wisconsin; Lisa Spruce, DNP, RN, CNS-CP, ACNS, ACNP, CNOR, FAAN, Director of Evidence-based Perioperative Practice, AORN Nursing Department, Denver, Colorado; Mary C. Fearon, MSN, RN, CNOR, Perioperative Practice Specialist, AORN Nursing Department, Denver, Colorado; Jay Bowers, BSN, RN, CNOR, TNCC, Clinical Educator, WVU Health Care, Morgantown, West Virginia; Missi Merlino, MHA, RN-BC, CNOR, Staff Nurse II, Baylor Scott & White Health, Temple, Texas; Nathalie Walker, MBA, RN, CNOR, Member of the Louisiana Nursing Supply and Demand Commission, a subcommittee of the Health Works Commission of Louisiana, Metairie; and Sandy Albright, MSHM, BSN, RN, CNOR, Clinical Consultant, Cardinal Health, Dublin, Ohio, for their assistance in developing this guideline.

Publication History

Originally published May 1976, *AORN Journal*, as "Recommended practices for surgical hand scrubs."

Revised March 1978, July 1982, May 1984, October 1990. Published as proposed recommended practices August 1994.

Revised November 1998; published April 1999, *AORN Journal.* Reformatted July 2000.

Revised November 2003; published in *Standards, Recommended Practices, and Guidelines,* 2004 edition. Reprinted February 2004, *AORN Journal.*

Revised March 2009 for online publication in *Perioperative Standards and Recommended Practices.* Revised July 2009 for online publication in *Perioperative Standards and Recommended Practices.*

Minor editing revisions made in October 2009 for publication in *Perioperative Standards and Recommended Practices,* 2010 edition.

Reformatted September 2012 for publication in *Perioperative Standards and Recommended Practices,* 2013 edition.

Minor editing revisions made in November 2014 for publication in *Guidelines for Perioperative Practice,* 2015 edition, as Guideline for Hand Hygiene.

Revised September 2016 for online publication in *Guidelines for Perioperative Practice.*

Evidence ratings revised and minor editorial changes made to conform to the current AORN Evidence Rating model, September 2019, for online publication in *Guidelines for Perioperative Practice.*

AORN GUIDELINES FOR
PERIOPERATIVE PRACTICE,
2022 EDITION

HIGH-LEVEL DISINFECTION

AORN
SAFE SURGERY TOGETHER

TABLE OF CONTENTS

MEDICAL ABBREVIATIONS & ACRONYMS

CDC – Centers for Disease Control and Prevention
CFU – Colony-forming units
FDA – US Food and Drug Administration
FIFRA - Federal Insecticide, Fungicide, and
    Rodenticide Act
HLD – High-level disinfectant

HPV – Human papillomavirus
IFU – Instructions for use
MEC – Minimum effective concentration
MRC – Minimum recommended concentration
PPE – Personal protective equipment
SDS – Safety data sheet

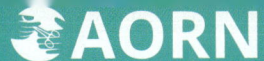
GUIDELINE FOR
MANUAL CHEMICAL HIGH-LEVEL DISINFECTION

The Guideline for Manual Chemical High-Level Disinfection was approved by the AORN Guidelines Advisory Board and became effective January 15, 2018. It was presented as a proposed guideline for comments by members and others. The recommendations in the guideline are intended to be achievable and represent what is believed to be an optimal level of practice. Policies and procedures will reflect variations in practice settings and/or clinical situations that determine the degree to which the guideline can be implemented. AORN recognizes the many diverse settings in which perioperative nurses practice; therefore, this guideline is adaptable to all areas where operative or other invasive procedures may be performed.

Purpose

High-level disinfection is a process that deactivates all types of microorganisms with the exception of bacterial spores and prions.[1] The purpose of this document is to provide guidance to health care personnel for

- performing safe and effective manual chemical high-level disinfection of reusable **semicritical items** and
- preventing patient and health care worker injury associated with the handling and use of liquid chemical high-level disinfectants (HLDs).

The Spaulding classification system defines reusable medical items as critical, semicritical, or noncritical.[2] The level of processing required (ie, sterilization; high-, intermediate-, or low-level disinfection) is based on the manner in which the item is to be used.[2] Items that contact mucous membranes (eg, endocavity ultrasound probes) or nonintact skin are considered to be semicritical.[2] Spaulding[2] recommended that semicritical items be processed by sterilization or, at a minimum, by high-level disinfection.

Failure to correctly perform high-level disinfection can lead to transmission of pathogens via contaminated medical or surgical devices.[3,4] The vast majority of patient infections and exposures related to processing medical or surgical devices have involved high-level disinfection of reusable semicritical items.[3] In a recent safety report, The Joint Commission[5] noted that processes for high-level disinfection of equipment and devices are frequently found to be inadequate, especially in ambulatory care centers and decentralized locations in hospitals. Breaches in the performance of high-level disinfection can result in outbreaks of viral or bacterial organisms.[5]

High-level disinfectants are harmful to human tissue and the environment.[6] Health hazards associated with the use of HLDs vary from minor irritation of mucous membranes to more serious injury (eg, chemical burns).[1] Health care organizations are responsible for informing health care workers about chemical hazards in the workplace and for implementing measures to reduce personnel exposure and mitigate identified hazards.[7] Implementing safe processes for handling and using chemical HLDs is essential for preventing injury to both patients and personnel.[6]

Guidance for the following topics is outside of the scope of this document:

- processing critical items for sterilization;
- processing semicritical items using thermal high-level disinfection (ie, pasteurization);
- processing flexible endoscopes and accessories and other semicritical items using mechanical (ie, automated) processes for high-level disinfection or liquid chemical sterilization (See the AORN Guideline for Processing Flexible Endoscopes[8]);
- processing endocavity ultrasound probes and other semicritical items using nebulized hydrogen peroxide mist;
- processing semicritical items potentially contaminated with prions;
- processing noncritical items for intermediate- or low-level disinfection;
- assessing risk and notifying patients regarding high-level disinfection failures; and
- using specific HLDs.

Evidence Review

A medical librarian conducted a systematic literature search of the Ovid MEDLINE®, CINAHL®, and Scopus® databases and the Cochrane Database of Systematic Reviews for meta-analyses, randomized and nonrandomized trials and studies, and systematic and nonsystematic reviews. The initial search was conducted in August 2014, and an additional search was performed in December 2016. In each search, the results were limited to literature published in English in the 5 years prior to the search date. The medical librarian established continuing alerts on the topics covered in this guideline and provided relevant results to the lead author. During the development of this guideline, the author requested supplementary searches for topics not included in the original search as well as articles and other sources that were discovered during the evidence-appraisal process. The lead author and the medical librarian also identified and obtained relevant guidelines from government agencies, standards-setting bodies, and other professional organizations.

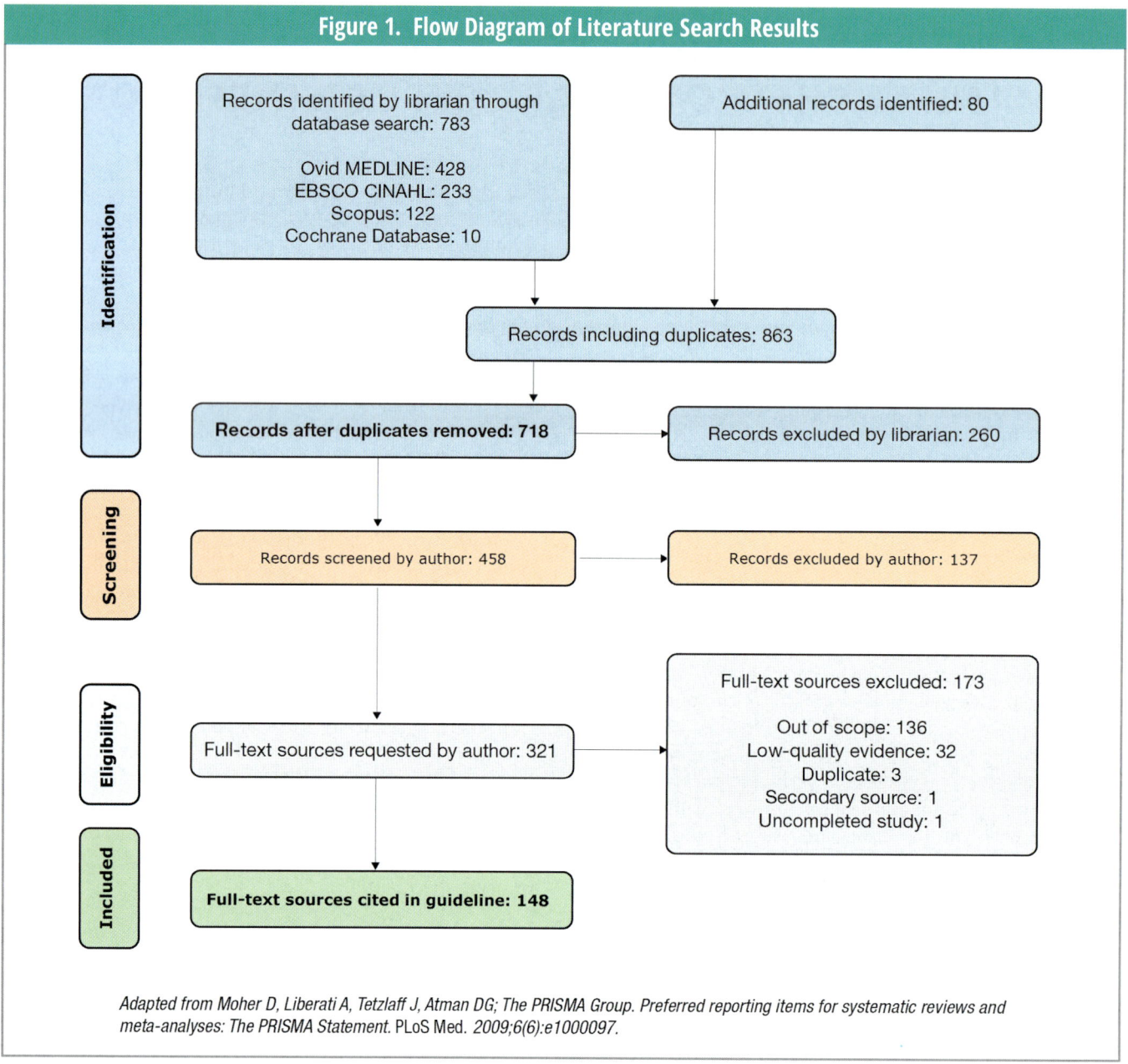

Figure 1. Flow Diagram of Literature Search Results

Records identified by librarian through database search: 783

Ovid MEDLINE: 428
EBSCO CINAHL: 233
Scopus: 122
Cochrane Database: 10

Additional records identified: 80

Identification

Records including duplicates: 863

Records after duplicates removed: 718

Records excluded by librarian: 260

Screening

Records screened by author: 458

Records excluded by author: 137

Eligibility

Full-text sources requested by author: 321

Full-text sources excluded: 173

Out of scope: 136
Low-quality evidence: 32
Duplicate: 3
Secondary source: 1
Uncompleted study: 1

Included

Full-text sources cited in guideline: 148

Adapted from Moher D, Liberati A, Tetzlaff J, Atman DG; The PRISMA Group. Preferred reporting items for systematic reviews and meta-analyses: The PRISMA Statement. PLoS Med. 2009;6(6):e1000097.

Search terms included *high-level disinfection, semi-critical item or device, automated endoscope reprocessor, Spaulding schema or criteria, peracetic acid, hydrogen peroxide, glutaraldehyde, ortho-phthalaldehyde, thermal or heat disinfection, pasteurization, medical device washer, equipment contamination or reuse, anesthesia equipment, disease transmission, cross-infection, biofilm, bacteria, microbial, spores, fungus, prion, Creutzfeldt-Jacob syndrome, Klebsiella, Pseudomonas aeruginosa, carbapenemase-producing Enterobacteriaceae, Staphylococcus aureus, Pseudomonas putida, Mycobacterium massiliense, storage, shelf life, cabinet, transport, protective clothing, eye protective devices, occupational disease or exposure, hypersensitivity, health personnel, medical waste disposal, waste management,* and *documentation.* Subject headings and key words for specific types of endoscopes also were included.

Included were research and non-research literature in English, complete publications, and publication dates within the time restriction when available. Excluded were non-peer-reviewed publications, older evidence within the time restriction when more recent evidence was available, and research and non-research evidence related to thermal high-level disinfection, specific disinfectants, workplace safety and occupational illness not related to high-level disinfection, sterile processing activities not associated with high-level disinfection, environmental and surface disinfection, and high-level disinfection of single-use devices. Editorials, news items, and other brief items were excluded. Low-quality evidence was excluded when higher-quality evidence was available, and literature outside the time restriction was excluded when literature within the time restriction was available. In total, 321 research and non-research sources of evidence were identified for possible inclusion, and of these, 148 are cited in the guideline (Figure 1).

Articles identified in the search were provided to the project team for evaluation. The team consisted of the lead author and one evidence appraiser. The lead author and the evidence appraiser critically appraised each reference using the AORN Research or Non-Research Evidence Appraisal Tools as appropriate. The literature was independently evaluated and appraised according to the strength and quality of the evidence. Each reference was then assigned an appraisal score. The appraisal score is noted in brackets after each reference, as applicable.

Each recommendation rating is based on a synthesis of the collective evidence, a benefit-harm assessment, and consideration of resource use. The strength of the recommendation was determined using the AORN Evidence Rating Model and the quality and consistency of the evidence supporting a recommendation. The recommendation strength rating is noted in brackets after each recommendation.

Note: The evidence summary table is available at http://www.aorn.org/evidencetables/.

Editor's note: MEDLINE is a registered trademark of the US National Library of Medicine's Medical Literature Analysis and Retrieval System, Bethesda, MD. CINAHL, Cumulative Index to Nursing and Allied Health Literature, is a registered trademark of EBSCO Industries, Birmingham, AL. Scopus is a registered trademark of Elsevier B.V., Amsterdam, The Netherlands.

1. Criteria for Manual High-Level Disinfection

1.1 **Reusable semicritical items may be processed using manual methods when manual chemical high-level disinfection is the only processing method recommended by the manufacturer.** *[Recommendation]*

Some reusable semicritical items cannot be sterilized or mechanically processed.

1.2 **The health care organization should appoint an interdisciplinary team of key stakeholders to conduct a risk assessment to identify reusable semicritical items used within the facility that may be processed by manual chemical high-level disinfection when recommended by the device manufacturer.** *[Recommendation]*

Having an interdisciplinary team conduct a risk assessment allows for a comprehensive, holistic review of the organization's needs by individuals with a range of relevant knowledge and skills and a variety of perspectives.

1.3 **Sterilize reusable semicritical items that are manufacturer-validated for sterilization, if possible.** *[Recommendation]*

Reusable semicritical items processed by high-level disinfection present a greater risk of disease transmission than items processed by sterilization.[3] Sterilization eliminates all microbial life, including pathogenic and nonpathogenic microorganisms and bacterial spores.[2] Correctly sterilized and handled items are rarely associated with patient infection[9]; however, some sterilization methods can affect the material and mechanical properties of the item. Sterilization may not be possible for all reusable semicritical devices in all health care facilities.

1.4 **Conduct a risk assessment to determine whether each semicritical item that secondarily enters sterile tissue or the vascular system (ie, via a mucous membrane) should be sterile.** *[Recommendation]*

Sterilization provides the greatest margin of safety and assurance that the item is safe for use.[3,10] Because of the heavy microbial load that may be present on some semicritical items (eg, flexible gastrointestinal endoscopes) and the difficulty of cleaning and disinfecting items with lumens and long, narrow channels, current high-level disinfection processes may not be adequate to ensure all items that enter sterile tissue via a mucous membrane are safe for use on patients.[11]

High-level disinfection may not effectively eliminate some viruses, bacteria, mycobacteria, and protozoa.[12] There have been reports of increased resistance profiles in some bacteria (including mycobacteria) to glutaraldehyde-based HLDs. Lorena et al[13] and Duarte et al[14] reported on an outbreak of postoperative infections due to *Mycobacterium massiliense* BRA100 involving 197 patients. All the involved hospitals (N = 63) were using 2% glutaraldehyde for high-level disinfection of endoscopic instruments unable to tolerate steam sterilization. The outbreak resolved when use of the glutaraldehyde-based HLD was discontinued.

Tschudin-Sutter et al[15] detected *Pseudomonas aeruginosa* in 23 of 73 routine samples obtained from endoscopes and in 29 of 99 subsequent samples obtained from the endoscopes. The investigators found that the glutaraldehyde-based HLD used for disinfection of the endoscopes demonstrated no activity against *P aeruginosa* when used at the manufacturer's recommended concentration and temperature. They concluded the *P aeruginosa* was resistant to the glutaraldehyde-based disinfectant.

Some HLDs may not be effective against certain types of viral pathogens.[12] Meyers et al[16] conducted a nonexperimental laboratory study of the susceptibility of infectious human papillomavirus (HPV) type 16 to commonly used clinical disinfectants (N = 11), including glutaraldehyde and ortho-phthalaldehyde.

The researchers found that both glutaraldehyde and ortho-phthalaldehyde did not demonstrate any significant reduction of infectivity of the virus. Because HLDs are commonly used to disinfect vaginal and rectal endocavity ultrasound probes, further research is warranted, and when possible, sterilization may be the preferred method for processing these and other semicritical items.[10]

1.5 **Mechanically process reusable semicritical items that are manufacturer-validated for high-level disinfection or liquid chemical sterilization using automated methods.**[8] *[Recommendation]*

Moderate-quality evidence shows that using automated methods (ie, mechanical processing) for high-level disinfection or sterilization of reusable semicritical items improves cleaning effectiveness, increases efficiency, and minimizes personnel exposure to hazardous substances (eg, chemical, biological).[1,17,18] Mechanical processors contain the disinfection process, reducing worker exposure to HLDs.[19-24] Mechanical processing methods can also be more successfully monitored for quality and consistency than manual methods of high-level disinfection.[1,17,18]

Ubhayawardana et al[18] conducted a nonexperimental study in the endotherapy unit of a university teaching hospital in Sri Lanka to evaluate the quality of manual processes for high-level disinfection of flexible side-view endoscopes. The researchers collected and analyzed 102 samples obtained from the tip and working channel of the endoscopes after manual chemical high-level disinfection. The results of the study showed that 20% (n = 21) of tips and 9% (n = 10) of channels were culture-positive. The researchers concluded that using mechanical processing methods for high-level disinfection increased processing effectiveness, reduced bioburden, and decreased human variability.

1.6 **Process endocavity ultrasound probes by high-level disinfection or sterilization.**[1,3,25-34] *[Recommendation]*

Endocavity ultrasound probes are introduced into a variety of body orifices (eg, vagina, rectum, trachea).[25] These probes contact mucosal tissue and are therefore classified as semicritical devices that require cleaning and a minimum of high-level disinfection.[2,25] The Centers for Disease Control and Prevention (CDC)[1] and the American Institute of Ultrasound Medicine[26] recommend that endocavity probes, used with or without a sheath or cover, be processed with high-level disinfection at a minimum.

Moderate-quality evidence shows that endocavity ultrasound probes present a high risk of contamination with pathogenic microorganisms after ultrasound procedures and that disinfection by methods other than high-level disinfection or sterilization may

not be sufficient to eliminate the organisms even when a sheath or cover is used.[27-31,35]

Westerway et al[27] conducted a blinded prospective study in the ultrasound unit of a private clinic and public hospital in Australia. They collected and analyzed a total of 129 samples from transvaginal and transabdominal ultrasound probes. The samples from the probes were collected after use (transvaginal: n = 28; transabdominal: n = 32), after low-level disinfection (transvaginal: n = 26; transabdominal: n = 32), and after high-level disinfection (transvaginal: n = 9; transabdominal: n = 2). The researchers found that although a sheath or cover was used with all of the probes, 60% (n = 19) of the transabdominal and 14% (n = 4) of the transvaginal probes showed bacterial contamination after use. Contaminating pathogenic species on the transabdominal probes included *Staphylococcus haemolyticus* and *Staphylococcus warneri.* After low-level disinfection, 3% (n = 1) of the transabdominal probes and 4% (n = 1) of the transvaginal probes remained contaminated. No contaminating bacteria were detected on any of the probes after high-level disinfection.

Inadequately disinfected endocavity probes also increase the risk for transmission of HIV, hepatitis B virus, hepatitis C virus, *Neisseria gonorrhea, Chlamydia trachomatis, Trichomonas vanginalis,* and HPV.[28] In a random probability distribution computer simulation performed to produce hypothetical cohorts for a population of 4 million annual ultrasound examinations in France, Leroy et al[29] estimated the number of patients infected by HIV, herpes simplex virus, hepatitis B virus, hepatitis C virus, HPV, cytomegalovirus, and *C trachomatis.* The simulation showed that despite the use of a sheathed probe and low-level disinfection, the probability of infection from a contaminated probe ranged from 1% to 6%, depending on the pathogen. For cases of HIV, this would result in approximately 60 infected patients per year. The researchers recommended using high-level disinfection for vaginal and rectal endocavity ultrasound probes.

Casalegno et al[30] conducted a prospective study in two phases in the gynecology department of a university hospital in France. In the first phase, the researchers collected and analyzed 217 samples from endocavity ultrasound probes after these were used for patient examination. In the second phase, the researchers collected and analyzed 200 samples before the probe was used for patient examination. Despite the use of sheathed probes, human DNA was detected in 36 (18%) of the post-examination samples, and 61 (28%) of the pre-examination samples. Seven post-examination samples (3.5%) were HPV positive, and six pre-examination samples (2.8%) were HPV positive, with four samples (2%) positive for high-risk HPV.

The researchers recommended replacing the current method of processing (ie, low-level disinfection with quaternary ammonium compound wipes) with a more stringent high-level disinfection process.

In a prospective study conducted in a French radiology center, M'Zali et al[31] collected and analyzed a total of 300 samples from endocavity ultrasound probes for HPV (n = 100), *C trachomatis* (n = 100), and commensal or environmental bacteria (n = 100). The samples were collected after disinfection of the probes with wipes impregnated with a quaternary ammonium compound and chlorhexidine. The researchers found HPV on 13% of the samples (n = 13), *C trachomatis* on 20% of the samples (n = 20), and commensal or environmental bacterial flora on 86% of the samples (n = 86). The researchers concluded that endocavity ultrasound probes remained contaminated after low-level disinfection.

Notably, not all HLDs may be effective against all pathogens that could potentially be found on endocavity ultrasound probes. Ryndock et al[35] conducted a nonexperimental study to compare the efficacy of immersion in a liquid chemical HLD (ie, ortho-phthalaldehyde) and exposure to nebulized hydrogen peroxide mist against HPV type 16 and HPV type 18 on endocavity ultrasound probes. The researchers found the liquid chemical HLD had only minimal efficacy against HPV. The HPV type 16 was highly resistant to the ortho-phthalaldehyde, demonstrating only a $0.52 \log_{10}$ reduction in viral infectivity. The HPV type 18 was also highly resistant to the ortho-phthalaldehyde, demonstrating only a $0.39 \log_{10}$ reduction in viral activity. The nebulized hydrogen peroxide mist method showed greater than $5 \log_{10}$ reductions for both HPV type 16 and HPV type 18.

2. Selection of High-Level Disinfectants (HLDs)

2.1 **The interdisciplinary team should select HLDs that will be used within the health care organization.** *[Recommendation]*

It is the responsibility of the health care organization to select HLDs using a systematic evaluation process that includes compliance with federal, state, and local regulations and a review of product safety, effectiveness, materials compatibility, and cost-effectiveness[36] (See the AORN Guideline for Medical Device and Product Evaluation[37]).

2.2 **Select a US Food and Drug Administration (FDA)-cleared HLD for high-level disinfection of reusable semicritical items.** *[Recommendation]*

The FDA regulates HLDs used to process medical devices and surgical instruments.[38] Notably, the FDA uses the term *liquid chemical sterilant* in conjunction with the term *high-level disinfectant* based on the position that, given sufficient time, many HLDs are also indicated for use as liquid chemical sterilants.[38,39] Refer to the "FDA-cleared sterilants and high-level disinfectants with general claims for processing reusable medical and dental devices"[38] for additional information.

2.3 **Select the HLD based on a risk assessment of the potential health hazards associated with the disinfectant.**[40] *[Recommendation]*

Health hazards associated with exposure to HLDs can be serious. Reported reactions have included
- headache,[20,23]
- ocular irritation and conjunctivitis,[20,23]
- nasal membrane irritation and rhinitis,[20]
- cough,[20]
- skin staining,[22,41]
- contact dermatitis,[20,24,42-45]
- occupational asthma,[20,24,45-51] and
- allergic reactions including anaphylaxis.[22,52,53]

Input from a variety of stakeholders can assist health care organizations with decisions related to potential health hazards and selection of HLDs for use in the facility.[54]

Rideout et al[54] surveyed personnel from 51 acute care hospitals in Canada to gather information about the decision-making process for selection of HLDs. The researchers found the decision about which HLD to use generally involved more than one person or personnel from more than one department. Members of the team selecting HLDs for use in the facility most frequently included personnel performing high-level disinfection and personnel from occupational health, infection prevention, and regional health departments. The researchers also found the greatest concern of team members selecting HLDs was protecting the health of individuals using the HLDs.

2.4 **Assess compatibility of the HLD and the HLD manufacturer's instructions for use (IFU) with existing semicritical items and current processes, products, and equipment used for high-level disinfection within the facility.** *[Recommendation]*

Having an interdisciplinary team evaluate compatibility requirements helps ensure that the new HLD will be compatible with existing products and processes, or if not compatible, helps clarify the need for additional items or equipment necessary for use of the HLD being evaluated.

3. HLD Storage Locations

3.1 Determine the locations where HLDs will be stored within the health care organization. [Recommendation]

Confining HLDs to designated storage locations may help to mitigate the risk for spills and exposure of personnel.

3.2 High-level disinfectants must be stored in accordance with
- safety data sheet (SDS) information;
- the manufacturer's IFU; and
- federal, state, and local regulations[7] (eg, requirements for storage of flammable or combustible items, patient and personnel safety requirements).

[Regulatory Requirement]

Safe and compliant storage of HLDs reduces the potential for exposure and injury to patients and personnel.

3.3 Store high-level disinfectants in a secure location.[36] [Recommendation]

Storing HLDs in secure locations may help prevent accidental damage to the HLD containers and unauthorized removal or use of HLDs.[36]

3.4 Store high-level disinfectants within the manufacturer's recommended temperature range.[36] [Recommendation]

Manufacturers' IFU recommend product storage at specified temperatures.

3.5 Store activated HLDs in covered containers[20] with tight-fitting lids.[19,24] [Recommendation]

Keeping containers tightly closed helps prevent spills; reduces the potential for personnel exposure to vapors; and decreases evaporation of the HLD, which could lead to a change in HLD concentration.[36]

3.5.1 Clearly label containers of activated HLDs with the contents and **reuse-life** dates.[36] [Recommendation]

Labeling containers of activated HLDs communicates to others the contents and period of time the HLD solution may be used.

3.5.2 If it is necessary to transport activated HLDs from one designated location to another, transport them in closed containers with tight-fitting lids[19,21] that are clearly labeled with the contents.[36] [Recommendation]

Transporting HLDs in closed containers with tight-fitting lids reduces the potential for spills.[19] Labeling containers communicates the contents to others.

4. Disinfection Areas

4.1 Perform manual chemical high-level disinfection in areas controlled and maintained to support processing activities. [Recommendation]

Performing manual chemical high-level disinfection in locations that are controlled and maintained to support high-level disinfection processes minimizes contamination of the environment, reduces the risk for cross contamination, decreases personnel exposure to hazardous chemicals, improves efficiency, and enhances process control and monitoring (See the AORN Guideline for Processing Flexible Endoscopes[8]).

4.2 Determine the locations where manual chemical high-level disinfection will occur within the health care organization. [Recommendation]

Confining manual chemical high-level disinfection to locations determined by an interdisciplinary team may help reduce the risk for patient and personnel exposure.

4.3 Perform high-level disinfection in an area where access is limited to authorized personnel.[19] [Recommendation]

Confining high-level disinfection processes reduces the potential for exposure of unauthorized personnel.[19,21,36]

4.3.1 Warning signs may be posted at the entrance to the disinfection area.[19] [Conditional Recommendation]

Warning signs may reduce the potential for exposure by preventing unauthorized personnel from entering the area.[19,36]

4.4 Perform manual chemical high-level disinfection in a designated area that is separate from locations where patient care activities are performed.[1] [Recommendation]

Performing high-level disinfection in designated areas helps prevent contamination of patient care areas and reduces the potential for adverse exposure effects on patients.[36] Local exhaust and ventilation systems used in areas where high-level disinfection is performed might not be recommended for areas where patient care activities are carried out.[36]

4.5 Perform high-level disinfection in a designated clean area that is separate from the decontamination area. *[Recommendation]*

Separating the clean area from the area where devices are cleaned and prepared for high-level disinfection reduces the risk of device contamination that might occur when both clean and contaminated processing activities are performed in a single area.[36] Droplets and aerosols created during cleaning of soiled instruments or other items can cause cross contamination of nearby clean items or surfaces.[55]

4.5.1 If the clean and decontamination areas are located within the same room, the area where high-level disinfection will occur should be separated from the decontamination area by
- a minimum of 3 ft (0.9 m)[56] and
- a separating wall or a barrier that extends a minimum of 4 ft (1.2 m) above the sink rim.[57]

[Recommendation]

Hota et al[58] demonstrated that contaminated water droplets had the ability to travel a distance of 1 m (39 inches). Based on the results of this report, the Facility Guidelines Institute determined it is unlikely that microorganisms from a decontamination area would be disseminated by air over distances longer than 1 m because they would be contained within water droplets.[57] Separating decontamination and clean work areas by a distance of at least 3 ft aligns with current recommendations from the CDC that patients who require droplet precautions are separated by at least 3 ft from other patients.[59] Having a wall or physical barrier for separation of the decontamination area provides protection and minimizes the potential for contamination of items that have been processed by high-level disinfection.

4.6 Design the workflow for high-level disinfection processes to facilitate a unidirectional flow that prevents recontamination of the item during or after completion of the disinfection process.[56,60] *[Recommendation]*

A unidirectional flow improves efficiency and helps contain contaminants within the decontamination area.[56,60]

4.7 Perform high-level disinfection in an area with sufficient space to permit freedom of movement of personnel during the disinfection process.[19,61] *[Recommendation]*

Crowded work spaces may increase the potential for spills.[19]

4.8 Do not perform high-level disinfection in areas near potential sources of contamination.[36] *[Recommendation]*

Performing high-level disinfection in areas near scrub sinks, hoppers, waste or linen containers, or other potential sources of contamination increases the potential for cross contamination.[36]

4.9 Do not perform high-level disinfection in high-traffic areas.[36] *[Recommendation]*

Performing high-level disinfection in high-traffic areas increases the potential for spills and cross contamination.[36]

5. Preparation of Items for Disinfection

5.1 Prepare reusable semicritical items to be processed by high-level disinfection according to the device manufacturer's IFU. *[Recommendation]*

The device manufacturer is responsible for ensuring the device can be effectively cleaned and for providing validated cleaning instructions.[36] Preparing the device for high-level disinfection by effective cleaning, rinsing, **purging**, and drying is a critical step necessary to reduce bioburden and moisture to a level that does not present a challenge to subsequent high-level disinfection.

5.2 If precleaning is recommended by the device manufacturer, preclean the device in accordance with the device manufacturer's IFU. *[Recommendation]*

Precleaning recommendations and procedures vary among manufacturers. Deviations from the manufacturer's IFU may result in insufficient cleaning of the item or high-level disinfection failure.[8]

5.2.1 Preclean at the point of use. *[Recommendation]*

Precleaning at the point of use assists with moistening, diluting, softening, and removing organic soils and reducing the formation of biofilm that might prevent effective high-level disinfection.[1,8,55,62]

5.3 After precleaning at the point of use or after use, personnel must transport contaminated items to be prepared for high-level disinfection in a closed container or closed transport cart.[63] *[Regulatory Requirement]*

Transporting items to the decontamination area in a manner that prevents exposing personnel to blood, body fluids, and other potentially infectious materials is a regulatory requirement.[63]

5.3.1 The container or cart must be
- leak proof,
- puncture resistant,
- large enough to contain all contents, and
- labeled with a fluorescent orange or orange red label containing a biohazard legend.[63]

[Regulatory Requirement]

Securing and labeling containers of biohazardous material is a regulatory requirement and communicates to others that the contents may be biohazardous.[63]

5.3.2 Keep semicritical items wet or damp, but not submerged in liquid during transport. *[Recommendation]*

Keeping the items wet helps dilute, soften, and ease removal of organic soils.[64] Dried organic materials and debris can make the item more difficult to clean and potentially lead to the formation of biofilm.[64] Submerging the device in liquid during transport may increase the risk of spillage and could lead to fluid invasion if the device has an unknown leak.

5.4 After transport of items to the decontamination area, leak test items designed to be leak tested in accordance with the device and leak-testing equipment manufacturers' IFU.[8] *[Recommendation]*

Not every device requires leak testing. Leak testing helps detect breaches in the integrity of the device being tested.[60] Leak testing also helps reduce damage and repair costs and decreases the potential for patient infection or injury that might result from use of a device that is not completely sealed.

5.5 After transport of items to the decontamination area or after leak testing, clean the items in accordance with the device manufacturers' IFU.[8,55] *[Recommendation]*

Clinical practice guidelines and low-quality evidence show that cleaning is essential to successful high-level disinfection because HLDs are inactivated by or less effective in the presence of organic material.[1,4,6,26,33,34,65] There have been reports of endocavity ultrasound probes or portions of endocavity ultrasound probes not being cleaned or being inadequately cleaned before disinfection, leading to residual contamination remaining on the device.[32,66,67] Reducing the level of microbial contamination on the item is necessary when performing high-level disinfection because there is a lower margin of safety (ie, a reduced ability to inactivate high levels of bacteria) compared with sterilization.[68] Effective cleaning can reduce bioburden to a level that does not inhibit high-level disinfection.[6]

Some HLDs may fix organic soil and blood to the surface of the item being disinfected.[69] Effective cleaning and removal of fixed soils before manual chemical high-level disinfection is necessary for successful high-level disinfection.[69] In a nonexperimental laboratory study, Kampf et al[69] found that exposure to disinfectants and liquid chemical sterilants led to variable amounts of blood fixation on the surface of surgical instruments processed by high-level disinfection. The glutaraldehyde-based disinfectants showed blood fixation between 77% and 100%. The peracetic acid-based disinfectants showed fixation rates between 19% and 78%. The researchers concluded that effective cleaning before disinfection was essential for effective high-level disinfection or liquid chemical sterilization.

5.6 After cleaning, rinse the item and flush any lumens or channels with utility water in accordance with the device manufacturer's IFU.[8] *[Recommendation]*

Thorough rinsing and flushing helps dislodge and remove residual debris and cleaning solutions.[70] If not adequately rinsed, enzymatic cleaning solutions may contribute to protein buildup within device channels.[70] Unless prohibited by the device manufacturer's IFU, using utility water is acceptable during the cleaning process. In some cases, a final rinse with water treated to remove organic and inorganic substances may be recommended by the device manufacturer to prevent staining and help ensure effective high-level disinfection or sterilization.

5.7 After rinsing, remove visible moisture from the external surfaces of the device using a clean, lint-free cloth.[8,60] *[Recommendation]*

Water remaining on the surface of the device can dilute the HLD.[36] If sufficiently diluted, the concentration of the active ingredients in the HLD can be reduced to a level that is too low to effectively eliminate certain microorganisms within the recommended exposure time.[36]

5.7.1 Purge device lumens with instrument air in accordance with the device manufacturer's IFU.[8,60] *[Recommendation]*

Water remaining in the lumens of devices can dilute the HLD.[36]

5.8 After removing visible moisture and purging, inspect the item for cleanliness, damage, and function.[8,9,55,60,71-73] *[Recommendation]*

Inspection helps identify residual soil or organic material that might put patients at risk for infection and allows soiled items to be removed from service until they are sufficiently cleaned.[9,71,73] Inspection also identifies damaged and defective items and allows them to be removed from service until repaired or replaced.[72]

5.8.1 **Inspect items using lighted magnification.**[8,55,60] *[Recommendation]*

An item that appears clean may harbor debris that cannot be seen without magnification.[8,55] Lighted magnification may increase the ability of personnel to identify soiled or damaged items.[8,55]

5.8.2 **Internal channels and lumens may be inspected using an endoscopic camera or a borescope.**[8,55] *[Conditional Recommendation]*

Endoscopic cameras and borescopes penetrate the lumen and allow for improved inspection.[8] Retained organic material in lumens can lead to patient injury.[9,73]

5.8.3 **Reclean soiled items.**[71] *[Recommendation]*

Residual soil remaining on the item can prevent effective high-level disinfection.[1,4,6,26,33,34,65]

5.8.4 **Remove damaged or defective items from service and have them repaired or replaced.**[55,60] *[Recommendation]*

Using damaged or defective instruments or devices can cause or contribute to patient injury.[72]

6. Preparation and Use of HLDs

6.1 **Personnel must prepare and use HLDs in accordance with the disinfectant and device manufacturers' IFU.**[74] *[Regulatory Requirement]*

Label claims, contraindications for use, and requirements for effective high-level disinfection are unique to each HLD. Failing to follow the manufacturer's IFU can jeopardize the effectiveness of the disinfection process or the performance of the device.[36] In the United States, HLDs are regulated under the Federal Insecticide, Fungicide, and Rodenticide Act (FIFRA).[74,75] Under FIFRA, any substance or mixture of substances intended to prevent, destroy, repel, or mitigate any pest (including microorganisms, but excluding those in or on living humans or animals) is required to be registered before sale or distribution.[74,75]

The device manufacturer is responsible for registering the device, ensuring the device can be effectively disinfected, and providing validated instructions for high-level disinfection.[36] Users of products registered under FIFRA are required to follow the manufacturer's IFU.[74,75] Failure to follow the manufacturer's IFU is considered a misuse of the product and is potentially subject to enforcement action under FIFRA.[74,75]

6.2 **Monitor processes for manual chemical high-level disinfection and the use of HLDs within the health care organization.** *[Recommendation]*

Oversight of high-level disinfection processes by an interdisciplinary team supports safe use of HLDs and implementation of work practices that will reduce occupational and patient exposure to HLDs.[36] Reducing the risk of patient infection associated with inadequate disinfection or sterilization of medical devices is a regulatory requirement[76-79] and an accreditation agency standard for both hospitals[80,81] and ambulatory settings.[81-84]

6.3 **Before performing high-level disinfection, verify compatibility of the HLD with the item to be processed by high-level disinfection.**[6,26] *[Recommendation]*

Using an HLD that is not compatible with the item may void the device warranty.[6] Not all HLDs are safe for use with all endocavity ultrasound probes.[26] Incompatibility between a device and a disinfectant may result in changes in appearance, integrity, and performance of the device.[3,6] Materials such as metals, alloys, and plastics and their polymers can be adversely affected by exposure to certain chemicals.[36] Some materials might become brittle and crack.[36] Others (eg, polymeric adhesives) might dissolve. Still others might swell or become distorted.[36] Any of these effects could cause the device to malfunction or fail.[36]

6.4 **Use activated HLDs at the concentration recommended by the disinfectant manufacturer.**[36,85] *[Recommendation]*

The **minimum recommended concentration** (MRC) or **minimum effective concentration** (MEC) and reuse-life date are established by the manufacturer.[6] Using the HLD at the recommended concentration reduces the potential for inadequate disinfection.[36]

Howie et al[86] conducted a quasi-experimental laboratory study to determine the efficacy of optimal and suboptimal concentrations of two HLDs—glutaraldehyde and activated hydrogen peroxide—for inactivating enveloped and non-enveloped viruses, bacteria, yeast, and mycobacteria. The researchers found that when used at the manufacturer's recommended concentration, 2.6% glutaraldehyde inactivated all test organisms except a specific *Mycobacterium chelonae* strain. When used at the manufacturer's recommended concentration, 7% activated hydrogen peroxide inactivated all test organisms, including *M chelonae*. A substantial number and variety of microorganisms survived exposure when the disinfectants were diluted. The researchers noted that these findings underscore the importance of and need for quality assurance monitoring of the HLD concentration before each use because HLDs can be used for multiple days. Dilution, evaporation, chemical breakdown, neutralization from accumulated proteins, or other actions that may limit the biocidal activity can occur before the reuse-life date of the HLD has been reached.

6.4.1 Use a test strip or other FDA-cleared testing device specific to the disinfectant and the active ingredient in the disinfectant before each use of the HLD solution.[6,36,85] *[Recommendation]*

Solution test strips are used to determine whether the concentration of the active ingredient in the HLD is above or below the MRC or MEC.[36] The concentration of the active ingredient in an HLD solution decreases with dilution by water, the presence of organic or inorganic soil, time, evaporation of the solution, and exposure of the solution to light.[6,36] High-level disinfectant solution potency cannot be guaranteed when the solution concentration falls below the MRC or MEC.[36,87]

6.4.2 Use and store test strips or testing devices in accordance with the test strip or testing device manufacturer's IFU.[36,85] *[Recommendation]*

6.4.3 Perform efficacy testing of the test strip or testing device as recommended by the test strip or testing device manufacturer's IFU.[6,36] *[Recommendation]*

Test strips can deteriorate and become less accurate over time.[6]

6.4.4 If the test strip or testing device indicates the concentration of the active ingredient is inadequate, discard the solution, even if the designated reuse-life date has not been reached.[6,36] *[Recommendation]*

6.5 Use activated HLDs at the temperature recommended by the disinfectant manufacturer.[36,85,87] *[Recommendation]*

6.5.1 Verify the temperature of the HLD solution before each use with a thermometer calibrated within the applicable range. *[Recommendation]*

Monitoring the solution temperature helps ensure effectiveness of the HLD and confirms the HLD is being used at the manufacturer's recommended temperature.[36]

6.5.2 Verify the accuracy of thermometers used to measure temperature of the HLD solution at established intervals. *[Recommendation]*

Verifying accuracy of thermometers helps ensure correct temperature measurement.

6.6 Use activated HLDs at the volume recommended by the disinfectant manufacturer.[36] *[Recommendation]*

Using the HLD at the recommended volume helps ensure complete immersion and contact with all surfaces of the device.[36]

6.6.1 If it is necessary to add activated HLD solution to an existing container of activated HLD solution (eg, the solution has evaporated, there is insufficient volume of solution to immerse the device),
- consult the HLD manufacturer's IFU to verify adding activated solution is an acceptable practice,
- test the activated HLD solution after the additional solution has been added to verify MRC or MEC, and
- do not use the activated HLD solution beyond the original solution container's reuse-life date.

[Recommendation]

6.7 Use the type of soaking container recommended by the HLD manufacturer. *[Recommendation]*

Using the type of container recommended by the manufacturer helps ensure there is no interaction between the container and the active or inert ingredients in the HLD.[36]

6.7.1 Use a soaking container that is large enough to contain the volume of solution recommended by the HLD manufacturer while reducing the surface contact area to the smallest amount possible.[19] *[Recommendation]*

Using the smallest container possible that holds the HLD manufacturer's recommended volume of solution helps reduce the amount of HLD that is used and decreases the potential for exposure and spills.

6.8 Discard activated HLDs on or before the manufacturer's recommended reuse-life date, even if the concentration of the ingredients is at or above the MRC or MEC.[36] *[Recommendation]*

Following the manufacturer's IFU for the period of time the disinfectant can be used may help prevent use of an ineffective HLD solution.

6.9 **Inspect the HLD solution before use.[36] Discard the HLD solution if precipitates are present or if the solution appears cloudy.[36]** *[Recommendation]*

Inspection before use may help prevent use of a contaminated HLD solution. The presence of precipitates or a cloudy solution may indicate the solution has been contaminated.[36]

6.10 **Handle the HLD solution in a manner that minimizes agitation of the solution and personnel exposure.[19]** *[Recommendation]*

Reducing solution agitation helps decrease exposure levels.[19] Solution agitation may be increased during tasks such as

- activating and pouring HLD solutions into or out of soaking containers,
- opening the soaking container,
- immersing items to be disinfected,
- handling soaked items,
- removing items from the soaking container, and
- disposing of HLD solutions into the sanitary sewer.[19]

6.11 **Disassemble the item to be processed by high-level disinfection according to the manufacturer's IFU.[1,88]** *[Recommendation]*

Disassembling the item helps ensure all surfaces are exposed to the disinfectant. Rutala et al[88] conducted a nonexperimental laboratory study to investigate the effectiveness of high-level disinfection of a probe used in ultrasound-guided prostate biopsy. The researchers inoculated the interior lumen of the biopsy needle guide, the outside surface of the biopsy needle guide, and the interior lumen of the ultrasound probe with 107 colony-forming units (CFU) of *P aeruginosa*. After inoculation, the researchers immersed the probe in an HLD for the manufacturer's recommended contact time and then assessed the probe for microbial contamination. They found that disinfection (defined by the researchers as a reduction in bacterial load greater than 7 $\log_{10}$ CFU) could only be achieved if the needle guide was removed from the probe. When the needle guide was left in the probe during immersion, disinfection was not achieved (ie, the reduction in bacterial load was only 1 $\log_{10}$ CFU). The disinfection failure occurred because the microorganisms that contaminated the surfaces of the probe lumen and outside surfaces of the needle guide were not exposed to the HLD and were able to survive the disinfection process. The researchers recommended disassembling the device before high-level disinfection. However, some items cannot be disassembled or are designed by the device manufacturer to remain assembled during high-level disinfection or sterilization.

6.12 **Immerse the item to be disinfected in the HLD solution.[1]** *[Recommendation]*

Complete immersion helps ensure all surfaces of the device are in contact with the HLD. It is not possible to ensure that all surfaces of an incompletely immersed item (eg, an item that floats on the surface of the disinfectant solution) will be effectively processed by high-level disinfection.[1]

Some cryosurgical probes are not fully immersible.[1,3] Manufacturers of endocavity ultrasound transducers may advise against submersion of the transducer handle because only the head portion of an ultrasound transducer contacts the patient's mucous membranes[25] and because the handle is not fully sealed.[32] The handle does not directly contact the patient, but it does contact the gloved hands of the technician during positioning of the probe and is therefore in need of high-level disinfection due to potential contamination from mucous membrane secretions.[25]

In a prospective cross-sectional study conducted at an ultrasound clinic and public hospital in Australia, Ngu et al[32] collected samples from 152 transducer handles that were cleaned and dried after routine use. The researchers randomly separated the transducers into two study groups. In the first group (n = 77), the transducer head was processed by high-level disinfection using 2.4% glutaraldehyde, but the handle was not disinfected (per usual practice). In the second group (n = 75), both the transducer head and handle were disinfected using a nebulized hydrogen peroxide mist. The researchers found that residual bacteria, including pathogenic bacteria, persisted on 80.5% (n = 62) of the handles that were not disinfected. Bacterial contamination on the handles that were disinfected was significantly lower at 5.3% (n = 4). The researchers concluded that ultrasound transducer handles could become contaminated with clinically significant organisms if they were not completely immersed or were processed using a method that did not disinfect the handle.

6.12.1 **If a portion of the device cannot be immersed in the HLD,**
- **immerse the portion of the device that can be immersed, and**
- **disinfect the portion of the device that cannot be immersed in accordance with the device manufacturer's IFU.[1,3]**

[Recommendation]

6.12.2 **For items that cannot be immersed in the HLD,**
- **replace the items with fully immersible items or**
- **process the items by high-level disinfection using the device manufacturer's**

validated methods that do not involve immersion in a liquid HLD.[1,3] [Recommendation]

High-level disinfection of the entire device reduces the potential for cross contamination and transmission of infection.[25] Methods found to be acceptable for high-level disinfection of both the endocavity probe head and handle include ultraviolet C light[89,90] or nebulized hydrogen peroxide mist.[3,10,33,91-93]

6.13 **Flush and completely fill lumens and ports with the HLD solution while the item is immersed.[94]** [Recommendation]

Eliminating air bubbles and flushing and filling lumens and ports with the HLD solution helps ensure that all surfaces of the item are exposed to the disinfectant. Rutala et al[94] conducted a nonexperimental laboratory study of channeled cystoscopes to examine the effectiveness of immersion compared with immersion and perfusion of the channel with the HLD. The researchers inoculated the channel of a flexible cystoscope with a suspension of test organisms (ie, vancomycin-resistant *Enterobacteriaceae*, carbapenem-resistant *Enterobacteriaceae*, *Klebsiella pneumoniae*), allowed the cystoscope to dry, and then immersed the cystoscope in an HLD for the manufacturer's recommended contact time. They found that high-level disinfection (defined by the researchers as a reduction in bacterial load greater than 7 $\log_{10}$ CFU) did not occur unless the cystoscope channel was actively perfused with the HLD while the device was completely submerged. Failure to fully perfuse the channel achieved only minimal reduction in bacterial contamination; however, complete inactivation (ie, a reduction equal to 8 $\log_{10}$ CFU) was achieved when the channel was actively perfused.

6.13.1 **Actuate moving parts while the item is immersed in the HLD solution.** [Recommendation]

Actuating moving parts helps ensure that all surfaces of the item are exposed to the disinfectant.

6.14 **Immerse the item to be disinfected in the HLD solution for the full duration of the disinfectant manufacturer's recommended contact time.[1,26,85]** [Recommendation]

Immersion for the full duration of the recommended contact time helps ensure that all surfaces of the item are exposed to the disinfectant and that any microorganisms on the device are completely inactivated.

6.14.1 **If there is a discrepancy between the disinfectant and device manufacturers' recom-**

mended contact times, immerse the device for the longer of the recommended contact times.** [Recommendation]

Using the longer recommended contact time may provide a margin of safety and help ensure the device is adequately disinfected.

6.14.2 **Use a timing device to verify the exposure time.** [Recommendation]

Using a timing device helps ensure the item was exposed to the HLD for the full duration of the HLD manufacturer's recommended contact time.

6.15 **Place the HLD soaking tray as close as possible to the rinsing sinks or containers.[19]** [Recommendation]

Locating the rinsing sinks or soaking containers in close proximity to the HLD soaking tray minimizes the potential for dripping HLDs onto other surfaces.[19]

6.16 **After high-level disinfection, thoroughly rinse and flush the item as described in the device manufacturer's IFU.[6,26]** [Recommendation]

Moderate-quality evidence and clinical practice guidelines show that thorough rinsing and flushing helps prevent patient injury associated with HLD remaining on the device.[6,52,53,95,96] High-level disinfectants not completely rinsed from the device can injure mucous membranes.[6] There have been reports of serious patient injury including toxic anterior segment syndrome,[95] anaphylaxis,[52,53] and bowel injury[96,97] associated with inadequate rinsing of medical devices and surgical instruments processed by high-level disinfection. Thorough rinsing reduces the potential for patient exposure to the disinfectant chemical.[6] Thorough rinsing also decreases the potential for HLDs to be absorbed into and subsequently released from the device.[52,53]

6.16.1 **Rinse the device with critical or sterile water.** [Recommendation]

Using **critical water** or sterile water reduces the potential for introducing microorganisms onto the disinfected device. Some manufacturers recommend rinsing with utility water; however, utility water may contain microorganisms and **endotoxins** that can be deposited on the item during the rinsing process.[98] Tissue contaminated with endotoxins can experience severe inflammation.[98]

Gillespie et al[99] reported an outbreak of *P aeruginosa* in four patients who underwent transrectal ultrasound-guided prostate biopsy. The authors concluded that rinsing the biopsy needle guide, a device intended for use on the sterile field, with utility water was a cause of the outbreak.

6.16.2 If not defined in the HLD manufacturer's IFU, establish the frequency for changing rinse water and rinsing containers. At a minimum, change the rinse water and rinsing containers daily. *[Conditional Recommendation]*

Some HLD manufacturer's do not specify how often the rinse water and rinsing containers are to be changed. In that case, the frequency of changing rinse water and rinsing containers is best determined by an interdisciplinary team because the number and type of devices undergoing high-level disinfection is unique to the facility.

Wendelboe et al[100] investigated an outbreak of seven *P aeruginosa* infections associated with outpatient cystoscopy performed by a urologist in New Mexico from January to April 2007. The investigators found multiple breaches in processing procedures, including rinsing of the cystoscope in unsterile water after high-level disinfection. Specifically, sterile water was placed in a rinsing container and replaced every 2 weeks or when it began to smell. The outbreak was resolved when improved procedures for processing flexible cystoscopes were implemented.

6.17 When removing the device from the HLD and when rinsing the device, handle it in a controlled manner that prevents the disinfected item from coming into contact with the soaking or rinsing containers. *[Recommendation]*

Handling the device in a controlled manner prevents contamination of the device by unintended contact with surfaces or items.

6.18 After rinsing, if the device will be stored for future use,
- dry the external surfaces of the device with a clean, lint-free cloth and
- dry device lumens with instrument air.[1,6]

[Recommendation]

Moisture remaining on the external or internal surfaces of the device can facilitate microbial growth during storage.[1,6,70] Clean, filtered air is required for drying lumens and small channels without introducing contaminants into the clean device.

6.19 If the device will be placed on a sterile field, rinse, dry, contain, transport and place the device on the sterile field using sterile technique.[1,3] *[Recommendation]*

Using sterile technique is necessary to maintain a sterile field (See the AORN Guideline for Sterile Technique).[101] Notably, a sterile field ceases to be sterile when a device that has not been sterilized is placed upon it.

6.19.1 The device may be covered with a sterile sheath or drape (eg, camera drape).[1,3] *[Conditional Recommendation]*

Covering the device with a sterile sheath or drape may help to maintain a sterile field and reduce the risk of patient infection.[1,3]

7. Transport and Storage

7.1 Protect reusable semicritical items that have been processed by high-level disinfection from contamination until the item is delivered to the point of use.[1] *[Recommendation]*

Protecting disinfected items is necessary to prevent contamination.

7.2 Transport items that are processed by high-level disinfection immediately before use to the point of use using aseptic technique.[36] *[Recommendation]*

Using aseptic technique during transport to the point of use helps prevent contamination of the device.

7.3 Transport and store items that are processed by high-level disinfection and stored before use in accordance with the device manufacturer's IFU and in a manner that protects the device from damage or contamination. *[Recommendation]*

Correct storage and protection of items that have been processed by high-level disinfection may reduce the potential for contamination of processed devices.

7.3.1 Clearly identify devices that have been processed by high-level disinfection and will be stored before use with a distinct visual cue as processed and ready for use.[1] *[Recommendation]*

Identifying items that have been processed by high-level disinfection and are ready for use may help to prevent use of a contaminated device.[1]

7.3.2 If the item will be stored in a cabinet or other storage device, follow the storage cabinet or storage device manufacturer's IFU. *[Recommendation]*

Following the storage cabinet manufacturer's IFU may prevent contamination of the item being stored in the cabinet and reduce the risk of patient infection. Stigt et al[102] reported a **pseudo-outbreak** of *Stenotrophomonas maltophilia* in the cultures of bronchial aspirations obtained from three patients via two different bronchoscopes. The pseudo-outbreak was caused by inadequate disinfection of ultrasound endoscopes. The contaminated ultrasound endoscopes subsequently contaminated bronchoscopes stored in the same drying cabinet via the connecting tubes in the cabinet. The authors found the humidity of the air being blown through the channels in the drying cabinet was higher than that recommended by the drying cabinet manufacturer. Excessively humidified air led to inadequate drying that promoted the outgrowth of residential microorganisms in the inadequately disinfected ultrasound endoscopes.

7.3.3 Visually inspect storage cabinets and disinfected devices for cleanliness before the item is placed into or removed from storage.[60]
- If there is any evidence of contamination of the disinfected device (eg, soil, moisture), reprocess the item before use.[60]
- If there is any evidence of contamination of the storage cabinet (eg, wet spots, soil, odor), remove and reprocess all items in the cabinet and clean the cabinet.[60]

[Recommendation]

Visible soil in the storage cabinet may indicate that one or more of the stored items is contaminated. Soil in the cabinet could also contaminate other items stored in the cabinet.[60] Reprocessing items that might be contaminated helps ensure they are safe for use.

7.3.4 Wear clean, latex-safe gloves when handling items that have been processed by high-level disinfection and when transporting them to and from the storage cabinet. *[Recommendation]*

Wearing gloves may lessen the risk of contamination of processed items by the hands of personnel. Using latex-safe gloves can minimize latex exposure and the risk of reactions in both health care workers and patients.[103] Sterile gloves are not required for handling processed items unless they are intended to be placed on a sterile field.

8. Safe Environment

8.1 The health care organization must provide a safe environment for personnel who handle or use HLDs.[7] *[Regulatory Requirement]*

High-level disinfectants are harmful to human tissue and the environment; therefore, implementing safe processes for handling and use is essential for the safety of patients and personnel.[6] It is a regulatory requirement that employers have a program to ensure that information about the identification, hazards, and composition of chemicals and safe handling practices and emergency control measures for chemicals is communicated and readily available to personnel.[7]

8.2 The health care organization must develop a written hazard communication program for all chemicals used within the facility.[7] *[Regulatory Requirement]*

It is a regulatory requirement that employers provide their employees with information about the hazards of all chemicals used in the workplace.[7]

8.2.1 The hazard communication program must include a list of the hazardous chemicals present in the facility and information about
- the specific hazards of each chemical,
- the SDS, and
- how the chemicals will be labeled.[7]

[Regulatory Requirement]

8.2.2 Safety data sheets for each chemical used in the facility must be readily accessible to personnel within the workplace.[7] *[Regulatory Requirement]*

Safety data sheets provide information about the chemical hazards; safety precautions for handling, storing, and transporting the chemical; signs and symptoms of toxic exposure; and first aid treatments after exposure. Providing personnel with information about the chemicals being used in the workplace is a regulatory requirement[7] that allows personnel to implement procedures to reduce exposure, establish safe work practices, and apply first aid measures when necessary.

8.3 The health care organization must develop a chemical spill control and cleanup plan.[7] *[Regulatory Requirement]*

Developing a chemical spill control and cleanup plan is a regulatory requirement[7] that promotes a rapid, efficient, and effective response to chemical spills.[36]

8.3.1 Include the following in the spill control plan:
- designate the individuals responsible for managing spill cleanup,
- include the HLD manufacturer's recommendations for emergency response and cleanup procedures,
- specify the location of spill control supplies and required personal protective equipment (PPE),

- **delineate respiratory protection requirements for HLDs,**
- **identify methods for preventing the dispersal of HLDs to other areas of the facility through the general ventilation system,**
- **describe evacuation procedures for nonessential personnel,**
- **outline medical treatment plans for exposed individuals,**
- **explain site-specific reporting requirements, and**
- **define education and competency verification requirements for personnel.**[19]

[Recommendation]

Effective management of chemical spills reduces the amount of vapor dispersed into the air and the potential for contact with skin, eyes, and mucous membranes.[6]

8.3.2 **Store chemical spill kits in close proximity to areas where HLDs and other hazardous materials are stored or used.**[19] *[Recommendation]*

Readily accessible chemical spill kits enable a prompt response by providing items that may be required in the cleanup of spills, leaks, or other discharges of hazardous materials.

8.4 **The health care organization must provide single-action eyewash stations, either plumbed or self-contained, in areas where HLDs that are hazardous to the eyes are located.**[104] *[Regulatory Requirement]*

It is a regulatory requirement that emergency eyewash stations or showers be immediately accessible in locations where the eyes or body of any person may be exposed to injurious corrosive materials.[104] Many HLDs are eye irritants. Eyewash stations are necessary to provide flushing fluid when the SDS identifies the chemical as a hazard and recommends immediate flushing of the eyes as an emergency first aid measure.[21] Refer to the *American National Standard for Emergency Eyewash and Shower Equipment*[105] for additional guidance.

8.5 **The health care organization must control and maintain ventilation in areas where HLDs will be handled or used, to meet limits for chemical exposure of personnel as required by federal, state, and local regulations.**[7,106] *[Regulatory Requirement]*

Ventilation control and maintenance of ventilation systems should be accomplished in accordance with industry standards[56,107] and professional guidelines.[1,6,36,108-110]

Controlling ventilation systems to provide adequate ventilation dilutes vapor and reduces personnel exposure to HLD fumes.[20,23,24] Maintaining ventilation systems helps ensure correct and continued functioning.[6]

8.5.1 **Rooms where manual chemical high-level disinfection is performed should have a minimum of 10 air changes per hour.**[19,21,36,56,107] *[Recommendation]*

8.5.2 **Install additional ventilation (eg, local exhaust ventilation) necessary to control personnel exposure within the threshold limit values at the point of release of HLD vapors.**[19,36] **Local exhaust ventilation systems for high-level disinfection processes may include a**
- **local exhaust hood (eg, laboratory fume hood) or**
- **self-contained, freestanding, recirculating exhaust ventilation system (eg, ductless fume hood).**[19]

[Recommendation]

Local exhaust ventilation captures and removes vapor at the source before it can escape into the general work environment.[19,21,36] Local exhaust hoods capture HLD vapor and conduct it into the exhaust system (via the hood) where it is transported through a duct system and discharged to the outside.[19,36] Ductless fume hoods have ventilated enclosures that draw air out of the hood, pass it through an air-cleaning filter, and discharge the cleaned air back into the work area.[19,36] Local exhaust ventilation is not required for all HLDs.

8.5.3 **Enclosed work stations may be used.** *[Conditional Recommendation]*

Enclosed work stations help manage air flow and reduce exposure to HLD fumes. Work stations also provide an enclosed area for soaking trays that helps protect personnel from splashes and spills.[19]

8.5.4 **Keep doors closed in areas where high-level disinfection is performed.**[19] *[Recommendation]*

Keeping doors closed helps maintain air pressure differentials to surrounding areas.[19]

8.6 **Monitor exposure levels in areas where HLDs are handled or used if there is a potential for chemical vapors to be dispersed into the air in amounts that may be hazardous to health care personnel.**[19,36] *[Recommendation]*

Health care organizations have a responsibility to minimize health care worker exposure to chemical vapors.[36] Monitoring exposure levels helps ensure a safe work environment and enables monitoring results to be compared with recommended threshold limit values for HLDs.[19] Monitoring is not required for all HLDs. The reader can refer to the American Conference of Governmental Industrial Hygienists[111] and the Occupational Safety and Health Administration Occupational Chemical Database[112] for information regarding permissible exposure limits and validated sampling methods for HLDs.

8.6.1 When exposure monitoring is required, at a minimum, evaluate exposure levels

- after initial use of the HLD[19];
- whenever there is a significant change in protocol, work practices, or caseload[19];
- after major heating, ventilation, or air conditioning equipment repairs or disruptions[6,19]; and
- when personnel have concerns about or symptoms of overexposure.[19]

[Recommendation]

8.7 Use HLD transfer pumps or safety nozzles whenever possible.[19,21] *[Recommendation]*

Transfer pumps reduce personnel exposure by containing the release of HLD vapor within a closed system during transfer of HLDs from one container to another.[19] Safety nozzles reduce the potential for splashing when HLD solutions are poured.[19]

8.8 The health care organization must develop and implement a written respiratory protection program for required respirator use.[113] *[Regulatory Requirement]*

Respirators are required as part of the respiratory protection program for certain chemicals if the limits for chemical exposure of personnel cannot be achieved by using engineering controls (eg, local exhaust ventilation) or when using engineering controls is not feasible.[113]

8.9 The health care organization must ensure that personnel handling HLDs or performing high-level disinfection wear PPE.[63,114-116] *[Regulatory Requirement]*

Employers are required to ensure that employees are protected when exposed to eye or face hazards from liquid chemicals, bloodborne pathogens or other potentially infectious material, or mechanical irritants capable of causing injury or impairment through absorption, inhalation, or physical contact.[1,20,63,114-116]

In a retrospective review of health care personnel seen for injuries related to chemical exposures at a University of North Carolina hospital between 2003 and 2012, Weber et al[24] found that splashes to mucous membranes were reported by 30 health care personnel, with 19 splashes to the eye; however, 33 personnel reported exposure events in which no injury occurred because they were wearing PPE.

8.9.1 During manual chemical high-level disinfection, wear personal protective equipment including

- masks,
- protective eyewear (eg, goggles),
- **chemical-resistant gloves** recommended by the glove and disinfectant manufacturers for use with the HLD,[36] and
- additional PPE as recommended by the SDS (eg, respirators, impervious gowns, aprons).

[Recommendation]

The specific PPE worn for each task depends on the potential for and the anticipated length of exposure[1] (See the AORN Guideline for Prevention of Transmissible Infections,[117] the AORN Guideline for Surgical Attire,[118] and the AORN Guideline for Cleaning and Care of Surgical Instruments[55]). Personnel handling or using HLDs are vulnerable to injury from a direct chemical splash.[24] Surgical masks in combination with eye protection devices protect the wearer's eyes, nose, face, and mouth from exposure to hazardous chemicals. Goggles or safety glasses are necessary whenever there is a potential for a chemical to contact the eyes.[21,114] Eye glasses or contact lenses do not provide sufficient protection from chemical splashes.[6]

Skin may also act as a portal of entry. Employers are required to ensure workers' hands are protected from exposure to potential skin absorption of substances such as chemical HLDs.[116] Chemical resistance and glove permeability vary among glove manufacturers. Polyvinyl chloride, neoprene, and latex examination gloves may not provide adequate skin protection from HLDs.[19] Additional PPE may be needed based on the task and the recommendations of the SDS.

8.9.2 Wear gloves that are fitted at the wrist and long enough to provide protection of the forearm or clothing from splashes or seepage.[6,21,36] *[Recommendation]*

Wearing close-fitting, elbow-length gloves or protective sleeves provides protection of the hands and forearms.[19]

8.9.3 Inspect gloves for integrity after donning, before contact with the HLD, and throughout use.[101] *[Recommendation]*

Careful inspection of glove integrity after donning and before contact with the HLD may reveal holes and defects in the unused product that may have occurred during the manufacturing or donning process and could allow for the passage of the HLD through the glove to the hands of personnel. Careful inspection of glove integrity throughout use may prevent unnoticed glove perforation that may present an increased risk for direct contact with the HLD.

8.9.4 **Perform hand hygiene after removal of PPE.**[59] *[Recommendation]*

The CDC recommends performing hand hygiene after removal of PPE.[59] Hands may become contaminated when removing PPE. Damage to PPE in the form of tears, punctures, and abrasions may occur and be undetected, exposing the wearer to chemical hazards.

8.9.5 **Reusable PPE must be**
- **verified for integrity before each use,**
- **decontaminated after each use, and**
- **discarded if there are signs of deterioration or if its ability to function as a barrier has been compromised.**[63]

[Regulatory Requirement]

8.10 **The health care organization must dispose of HLDs in accordance with federal, state, and local regulations.**[119-121] *[Regulatory Requirement]*

The US Environmental Protection Agency regulates the treatment, storage, and disposal of hazardous chemical wastes under the Resource Conservation and Recovery Act.[119,120] States are permitted to administer their own hazardous waste program providing they enact laws that are at least as stringent as the federal laws.[121] State regulations are often more restrictive than federal regulations.[122] Local governments also have laws and regulations pertaining to the disposal of hazardous materials.[123]

8.10.1 **If there are no disposal restrictions, activated HLDs may be disposed of, along with copious amounts of cold water, into a drain connected to the sanitary sewer system.**[19,21,36] *[Conditional Recommendation]*

Some local regulations may prohibit disposal of HLDs into the sewer system or may require neutralization before disposal.[19]

8.10.2 **When recommended by the disinfectant manufacturer, add a neutralizer to the activated HLD before disposal.** *[Recommendation]*

High-level disinfectant vapors may increase when the solution is poured out of a soaking container. Adding a neutralizer may reduce exposure levels.

8.10.3 **Do not dispose of activated HLDs, including neutralized HLDs, into septic systems.**[19,36] *[Recommendation]*

Disposing of HLDs in a septic system can disrupt the biodegradation process by killing beneficial microorganisms.[19,36]

8.10.4 **When discarding activated HLD into a sink, use a sink that is**
- **close to the area where the HLD is stored and**
- **large enough to accommodate the volume of HLD being discarded.**[36]

[Recommendation]

Discarding the HLD into a sink that is in close proximity and of sufficient size reduces the potential for spills.

8.10.5 **When the HLD is discarded from a reusable soaking container, clean and dry the soaking container before reuse.** *[Recommendation]*

Cleaning and drying soaking containers that have been used to store HLDs reduces the potential for cross contamination and helps ensure that residual HLD has been removed from the container.

8.10.6 **Dispose of empty HLD containers in accordance with the disinfectant manufacturer's IFU.**[19,36] *[Recommendation]*

Disposing of empty HLD containers in accordance with the disinfectant manufacturer's IFU may prevent accidental chemical exposure or inappropriate use of containers.[36]

9. Processing Records

9.1 **Maintain records of manual chemical high-level disinfection processes.** *[Recommendation]*

Records provide data for the identification of trends and demonstration of compliance with regulatory requirements and accreditation agency standards. Highly reliable data collection is necessary to demonstrate the health care organization's progress toward quality care outcomes.[124] Effective management and collection of health care information that accurately reflects the patient's care, treatment, and services is a regulatory requirement[76-79] and an accreditation agency standard for both hospitals[125,126] and ambulatory settings.[126-130]

9.2 **Include the following information in records related to manual chemical high-level disinfection:**
- **date and time of high-level disinfection**[36]**;**
- **HLD solution lot number**[36]**;**
- **HLD solution shelf-life date**[36]**;**

347

- HLD solution **activation** date[36];
- HLD solution reuse-life date[36];
- results of solution test strip testing, if applicable[36];
- results of MRC or MEC testing, if applicable[36];
- HLD solution temperature[36];
- HLD solution exposure time[36];
- quantity and description of the device or item[36];
- unique device identification number, if available[36];
- identity of the person performing high-level disinfection[36];
- identity of the patient on whom the device was used, if possible[36]; and
- identity of the physician and procedure where the device was used, if possible.[36]

[Recommendation]

Maintaining records of manual chemical high-level disinfection helps ensure that parameters for correct high-level disinfection have been met,[85] enables retrieval of HLD solutions in the event of a recall, and establishes traceability and accountability.

9.3 Maintain records of manual chemical high-level disinfection for a time period specified by the health care organization. *[Recommendation]*

10. Education

10.1 Provide initial and ongoing education and competency verification activities related to manual chemical high-level disinfection for personnel who are handling and using chemical HLDs.[5,6,21,36] *[Recommendation]*

Initial and ongoing education of perioperative personnel facilitates the development of knowledge, skills, and attitudes that affect safe patient care. It is the responsibility of the health care organization to provide initial and ongoing education and to verify the competency of its personnel; however, the primary responsibility for maintaining ongoing competency remains with the individual.

Competency verification activities provide a mechanism for competency documentation and help verify that personnel understand the principles and processes necessary for safe and effective manual chemical high-level disinfection. Having competent personnel perform manual chemical high-level disinfection increases the likelihood that personnel will adhere to best practices and reduces the potential for exposure and adverse events to both patients and personnel.[36] Advances and developments in high-level disinfection processes, the emergence of new diseases and microorganisms, the increasing complexity of medical devices, and the responsibility for implementing safe and effective processing of reusable semicritical devices underscore the need for health care organizations to ensure that manual chemical high-level disinfection is performed by educated and competent personnel.[36] Ongoing development of knowledge and skills and documentation of personnel participation is a regulatory requirement[76-79] and an accreditation agency standard for both hospitals[131,132] and ambulatory settings.[132-135]

10.2 The health care organization must provide education about the written hazard communication program for personnel who use, handle, or may be exposed to HLDs.[7,103] *[Regulatory Requirement]*

Personnel who have received education and completed competency verification activities related to the plan may have a greater understanding of how to reduce potential adverse effects associated with exposure to hazardous chemicals.

10.2.1 Education related to the hazard communication program must include

- an explanation of the SDS and chemical labeling system, and how to obtain and use this hazard information;
- methods and observations that may be used to detect the presence or release of all chemicals used in the workplace;
- the physical and health hazards of all chemicals used in the workplace; and
- the measures personnel can take to protect themselves, including specific procedures the organization has implemented to protect personnel from exposure to chemicals used in the workplace (eg, emergency procedures, PPE).[7]

[Regulatory Requirement]

Henn et al[136] surveyed 4,657 members of professional practice organizations representing RNs, technologists/technicians, dental professionals, respiratory therapists, and others who reported handling HLDs in the previous 7 days. The results showed that 44% of the respondents did not always wear protective gowns, 42% did not always wear eye and face protection, and 9% did not always wear gloves. The most frequent explanation provided for not wearing PPE was that "exposure was minimal," even though 12% of the respondents reported direct skin contact with an HLD in the previous 7 days. The researchers noted the results of the survey indicated the respondents did not fully recognize the hazards and potential adverse health effects of HLD exposure and the need for PPE.

10.3 Establish education and competency verification activities for personnel and determine intervals for education and competency verification related to manual chemical high-level disinfection. *[Recommendation]*

Manual chemical high-level disinfection is a complex process requiring performance by educated and competent personnel.[85] The Joint Commission has identified sufficient education and competency verification of personnel performing high-level disinfection processes as one of the areas most frequently needing improvement in health care facilities.[85]

Education and competency verification needs and intervals are unique to the facility and to its personnel and processes. Educational and skill mastery needs will vary among personnel and may also vary among organizational processing sites.[137,138] Some personnel will require greater levels of remediation and reinforcement.[139]

10.3.1 Verify that the personnel responsible for providing education and competency verification to individuals who perform manual chemical disinfection are sufficiently educated and competent to do so.[5,85] *[Recommendation]*

10.4 Include the following in education and competency verification activities related to manual chemical high-level disinfection:
- information about devices and disinfectants approved by the interdisciplinary team for manual chemical high-level disinfection;
- procedures for safe and effective preparation and use of chemical HLDs,[20,21,110]
- elements of a safe environment for personnel who are performing manual chemical high-level disinfection, including the location and use of
  o SDS,
  o eyewash stations,
  o chemical spill kits, and
  o PPE;[1,21,110]
- requirements for maintaining records of manual chemical high-level disinfection;
- quality assurance measures for manual chemical high-level disinfection; and
- processes for reporting adverse events and occupational exposure incidents related to manual chemical high-level disinfection. *[Recommendation]*

11. Policies and Procedures

11.1 Develop policies and procedures for manual chemical high-level disinfection that are reviewed periodically, revised as necessary, and readily available in the practice setting in which they are used. *[Recommendation]*

Policies and procedures assist in the development of patient safety, quality assessment, and performance improvement activities. Policies and procedures also serve as operational guidelines used to minimize patients' risk for injury or complications, standardize practice, direct personnel, and support continuous performance improvement programs. Policies and procedures establish authority, responsibility, and accountability within the practice setting. Having policies and procedures that guide and support patient care, treatment, and services is a regulatory requirement[76-79] and an accreditation agency standard for both hospitals[81,140] and ambulatory settings.[81,134,141,142]

11.2 Include the following in policies and procedures related to manual chemical high-level disinfection:
- devices and disinfectants approved by the interdisciplinary team for manual chemical high-level disinfection,
- procedures for safe and effective preparation and use of chemical HLDs,[21,143]
- elements of a safe environment for personnel who are performing manual chemical high-level disinfection,
- maintaining records of manual chemical high-level disinfection,
- quality assurance measures for manual chemical high-level disinfection, and
- processes for reporting adverse events related to manual chemical high-level disinfection. *[Recommendation]*

11.3 The manufacturers' IFU for all components of the high-level disinfection process (eg, device, equipment, supplies, HLD solutions) should be readily available to and followed by personnel responsible for manual chemical high-level disinfection.[5] *[Recommendation]*

Instructions for use identify the manufacturers' validated processes and procedures necessary to achieve effective manual chemical high-level disinfection.

11.3.1 Review the device and HLD manufacturers' IFU at established intervals and verify that manual chemical high-level disinfection practices are in compliance with the most current IFUs.[110] *[Recommendation]*

Manufacturers may make modifications to their IFUs when new technology becomes available, when regulatory requirements change, or when modifications are made to their product.

12. Quality

12.1 **The health care organization's quality management program should evaluate manual chemical high-level disinfection processes.**[5] *[Recommendation]*

Quality assurance and performance improvement programs can facilitate the identification of problem areas and assist personnel in evaluating and improving the quality of patient care and formulating plans for corrective action. These programs provide data that may be used to determine whether an individual organization is within benchmark goals, and if not, to identify areas that may require corrective action. A quality management program provides a mechanism to evaluate effectiveness of manual chemical high-level disinfection processes, compliance with manufacturer's IFU, and equipment function. Collecting data to monitor and improve patient care, treatment, and services is a regulatory requirement[76-79] and an accreditation agency standard for both hospitals[144,145] and ambulatory settings.[145-148]

12.2 **Include the following in the quality assurance and performance management program for manual chemical high-level disinfection:**
- **periodically reviewing and evaluating manual chemical high-level disinfection to verify compliance with or to identify the need for improvement with established processes for manual chemical high-level disinfection,**
- **identifying corrective actions directed toward improvement priorities, and**
- **taking additional actions when improvement is not achieved or sustained.**

[Recommendation]

Reviewing and evaluating quality assurance and performance improvement activities may identify failure points that contribute to errors in manual chemical high-level disinfection and help define actions for improvement. Monitoring compliance with established safe practices can increase workplace safety and help reduce personnel exposure to HLDs. Taking corrective actions may improve patient safety by verifying that personnel understand the principles of and comply with best practices for manual chemical high-level disinfection.

Nayebzadeh[23] conducted a nonexperimental study to investigate the effects of work practices and work-related symptoms among health care workers handling HLDs. The researcher observed work practices and interviewed 53 health care workers in 19 different locations from five hospitals in Canada about the frequency of HLD spills, use of PPE, and HLD-exposure symptoms. The researcher found that only 15% (n = 8) of the workers used face protection when handling HLDs. Almost 50% (n = 26) reported experiencing at least one chemical spill in the previous 12 months. The researcher concluded that monitoring and verifying compliance with safe work practices could significantly reduce worker exposure and health effects caused by exposure to HLDs.

12.3 **Participate in ongoing quality assurance and performance improvement activities related to manual chemical high-level disinfection by**
- **monitoring quality;**
- **developing strategies for compliance,**
- **establishing benchmarks to evaluate quality indicators,**
- **collecting data related to the levels of performance and quality indicators,**
- **evaluating practice based on the cumulative data collected,**
- **taking action to improve compliance, and**
- **assessing the effectiveness of the actions taken.**

[Recommendation]

Participating in ongoing quality assurance and performance improvement activities is a primary responsibility of health care personnel engaged in clinical practice.

12.4 **Report and document adverse events and occupational exposure incidents related to manual chemical high-level disinfection after each event according to the health care organization's policy and procedure and review these for potential opportunities for improvement.**[20,24,110] *[Recommendation]*

Reporting and reviewing adverse events and near misses can be useful for identifying actions that may prevent similar occurrences and revealing opportunities for improvement.

Glossary

Activation: The process by which a high-level disinfectant becomes chemically operative after combination with another chemical.

Chemical-resistant gloves: Gloves with varying levels of resistance to challenge chemicals based on the glove manufacturer's test data for breakthrough time, degree of degradation, and permeation rate.

Critical water: Water that is extensively treated to remove microorganisms and other materials.

Endotoxin: A toxic substance that is released when a bacterial cell disintegrates.

High-level disinfection: A process that deactivates all types of microorganisms with the exception of bacterial spores and prions.

Instrument air: A medical gas that falls under the general requirements for medical gases as defined by the *NFPA 99: Health Care Facilities Code,* is not respired, is compliant with the *ANSI/ISA S-7.0.01: Quality Standard for Instrument Air,* and is filtered to 0.01 μm, free of liquids and hydrocarbon vapors, and dry to a dew point of -40 F (-40 C).

Minimum effective concentration: The minimum concentration of a liquid chemical germicide that achieves the claimed microbicidal activity as determined by dose-response testing.

Minimum recommended concentration: The minimum concentration at which the manufacturer tested the product and validated its performance.

Pseudo-outbreak: An episode of false increased disease incidence due to enhanced surveillance (eg, microbiological culturing) or other factor (eg, laboratory contamination, false positive test).

Purging: The removal of visible moisture from a device after rinsing.

Reuse life: The period of time an activated high-level disinfectant solution can be used, provided the concentration of the active ingredient remains at or above the manufacturers' specified minimum recommended concentration.

Semicritical items: Items that contact mucous membranes or nonintact skin.

Shelf-life: The period of time during which a stored product remains effective, useful, or suitable for use.

Threshold limit value: The airborne concentration of a substance not to be exceeded during any part of the working exposure.

Utility water: Water obtained directly from a faucet that has not been purified, distilled, or otherwise treated. Synonym: tap water.

References

1. Rutala WA, Weber DJ; Healthcare Infection Control Practices Advisory Committee. *Guideline for Disinfection and Sterilization in Healthcare Facilities, 2008.* Washington, DC: Centers for Disease Control and Prevention; 2008. https://www.cdc.gov/infectioncontrol/pdf/guidelines/disinfection-guidelines.pdf. Updated February 2017. Accessed October 5, 2017. [IVA]

2. Spaulding EH, Lawrence CA, Block SS, Reddish GF. Chemical disinfection of medical and surgical materials. In: Lawrence CA, Block SS, Reddish GF, eds. *Disinfection, Sterilization, and Preservation.* Philadelphia, PA: Lea & Febiger; 1968:517-531. [VA]

3. Rutala WA, Weber DJ. Reprocessing semicritical items: current issues and new technologies. *Am J Infect Control.* 2016;44(5):e53-e62. [VA]

4. Rutala WA, Weber DJ. Cleaning, disinfection, and sterilization in healthcare facilities. In: *APIC Text of Infection Control and Epidemiology.* Arlington, VA: Association for Professionals in Infection Control and Epidemiology; 2016. [IVB]

5. Improperly sterilized or HLD equipment—a growing problem. *Quick Safety.* 2017(33):1-5. https://www.jointcommission.org/assets/1/23/qs_33a_2017.pdf. Accessed October 5, 2017. [VC]

6. *Guideline for Use of High-Level Disinfectants & Sterilants in the Gastroenterology Setting.* Chicago, IL: Society of Gastroenterology Nurses and Associates, Inc; 2017:13. [IVB]

7. 29 CFR 1910.1200: Hazard communication: toxic and hazardous substances. Occupational Safety and Health Administration. https://www.osha.gov/pls/oshaweb/owadisp.show_document?p_table=standards&p_id=10099. Accessed October 5, 2017.

8. Guideline for processing flexible endoscopes. In: *Guidelines for Perioperative Practice.* Denver, CO: AORN, Inc; 2017:717-800. [IVA]

9. Tosh PK, Disbot M, Duffy JM, et al. Outbreak of *Pseudomonas aeruginosa* surgical site infections after arthroscopic procedures: Texas, 2009. *Infect Control Hosp Epidemiol.* 2011;32(12):1179-1186. [IIIA]

10. Rutala WA, Weber DJ. Disinfection and sterilization in health care facilities: an overview and current issues. *Infect Dis Clin North Am.* 2016;30(3):609-637. [VA]

11. Rutala WA, Weber DJ. Gastrointestinal endoscopes: a need to shift from disinfection to sterilization? *JAMA.* 2014;312(14):1405-1406. [VA]

12. McDonnell G, Burke P. Disinfection: is it time to reconsider Spaulding? *J Hosp Infect.* 2011;78(3):163-170. [VA]

13. Lorena NS, Pitombo MB, Cortes PB, et al. *Mycobacterium massiliense* BRA100 strain recovered from postsurgical infections: resistance to high concentrations of glutaraldehyde and alternative solutions for high level disinfection. *Acta Cir Bras.* 2010;25(5):455-459. [IIIB]

14. Duarte RS, Lourenco MC, Fonseca Lde S, et al. Epidemic of postsurgical infections caused by *Mycobacterium massiliense.* *J Clin Microbiol.* 2009;47(7):2149-2155. [IIIB]

15. Tschudin-Sutter S, Frei R, Kampf G, et al. Emergence of glutaraldehyde-resistant *Pseudomonas aeruginosa.* *Infect Control Hosp Epidemiol.* 2011;32(12):1173-1178. [VA]

16. Meyers J, Ryndock E, Conway MJ, Meyers C, Robison R. Susceptibility of high-risk human papillomavirus type 16 to clinical disinfectants. *J Antimicrob Chemother.* 2014;69(6):1546-1550. [IIIB]

17. Ofstead CL, Wetzler HP, Snyder AK, Horton RA. Endoscope reprocessing methods: a prospective study on the impact of human factors and automation. *Gastroenterol Nurs.* 2010;33(4):304-311. [IIIA]

18. Ubhayawardana DL, Kottahachchi J, Weerasekera MM, Wanigasooriya IW, Fernando SS, De Silva M. Residual bioburden in reprocessed side-view endoscopes used for endoscopic retrograde cholangiopancreatography (ERCP). *Endosc Int Open.* 2013;1(1):12-16. [IIIB]

19. Best practices for the safe use of glutaraldehyde in health care. 2006. Occupational Safety and Health Administration. http://www.osha.gov/Publications/3258-08N-2006-English.html. Accessed October 5, 2017. [VA]

20. Cohen NL, Patton CM. Worker safety and glutaraldehyde in the gastrointestinal lab environment. *Gastroenterol Nurs.* 2006;29(2):100-104. [VB]

21. ECRI. Ethylene oxide, formaldehyde, and glutaraldehyde. *Operating Room Risk Management.* 2012;1A. [VB]

22. Pala G, Moscato G. Allergy to ortho-phthalaldehyde in the healthcare setting: advice for clinicians. *Expert Rev Clin Immunol.* 2013;9(3):227-234. [VA]

23. Nayebzadeh A. The effect of work practices on personal exposure to glutaraldehyde among health care workers. *Ind Health.* 2007;45(2):289-295. [IIIB]

24. Weber DJ, Consoli SA, Rutala WA. Occupational health risks associated with the use of germicides in health care. *Am J Infect Control.* 2016;44(5):e85-e89. [IIIB]

25. Alfa MJ. Intra-cavitary ultrasound probes: cleaning and high-level disinfection are necessary for both the probe head and handle to reduce the risk of infection transmission. *Infect Control Hosp Epidemiol.* 2015;36(5):585-586. [VA]

26. Guidelines for cleaning and preparing external- and internal-use ultrasound probes between patients, safe handling, and use of ultrasound coupling gel. The American Institute of Ultrasound in Medicine. http://www.aium.org/officialStatements/57. Approved May 2017. Accessed October 5, 2017. [IVC]

27. Westerway SC, Basseal JM, Brockway A, Hyett JA, Carter DA. Potential infection control risks associated with ultrasound equipment—a bacterial perspective. *Ultrasound Med Biol.* 2017;43(2):421-426. [IIIB]

28. Shokoohi H, Armstrong P, Tansek R. Emergency department ultrasound probe infection control: challenges and solutions. *Open Access Emerg Med.* 2015;7:1-9. [VB]

29. Leroy S, M'Zali F, Kann M, Weber DJ, Smith DD. Impact of vaginal-rectal ultrasound examinations with covered and low-level disinfected transducers on infectious transmissions in France. *Infect Control Hospital Epidemiol.* 2014;35(12):1497-1504. [IIIB]

30. Casalegno JS, Le Bail Carval K, Eibach D, et al. High risk HPV contamination of endocavity vaginal ultrasound probes: an underestimated route of nosocomial infection? *Plos One.* 2012;7(10):e48137. [IIIB]

31. M'Zali F, Bounizra C, Leroy S, Mekki Y, Quentin-Noury C, Kann M. Persistence of microbial contamination on transvaginal ultrasound probes despite low-level disinfection procedure. *Plos One.* 2014;9(4):e93368. [IIIB]

32. Ngu A, McNally G, Patel D, Gorgis V, Leroy S, Burdach J. Reducing transmission risk through high-level disinfection of transvaginal ultrasound transducer handles. *Infect Control Hosp Epidemiol.* 2015;36(5):581-584. [IIIB]

33. Combs CA, Fishman A. A proposal to reduce the risk of transmission of human papilloma virus via transvaginal ultrasound. *Am J Obstet Gynecol.* 2016;215(1):63-67. [VA]

34. Chu K, Obaid H, Babyn P, Blondeau J. Bacterial contamination of ultrasound probes at a tertiary referral university medical center. *AJR Am J Roentgenol.* 2014;203(5):928-932. [VB]

35. Ryndock E, Robison R, Meyers C. Susceptibility of HPV16 and 18 to high level disinfectants indicated for semi-critical ultrasound probes. *J Med Virol.* 2016;88(6):1076-1080. [IIIB]

36. *ANSI/AAMI ST58:2013 Chemical Sterilization and High-Level Disinfection in Health Care Facilities.* Arlington, VA: Association for the Advancement of Medical Instrumentation; 2013. [IVC]

37. Guideline for medical device and product evaluation. In: *Guidelines for Perioperative Practice.* Denver, CO: AORN, Inc; 2017:e135-e142. [IVB]

38. FDA-cleared sterilants and high level disinfectants with general claims for processing reusable medical and dental devices—March 2015. US Food and Drug Administration. http://www.fda.gov/MedicalDevices/DeviceRegulationandGuidance/ReprocessingofReusableMedicalDevices/ucm437347.htm. Accessed October 5, 2017.

39. Wallace CA. New developments in disinfection and sterilization. *Am J Infect Control.* 2016;44:e23-e27. [VB]

40. Hawley B, Casey ML, Cox-Ganser JM, Edwards N, Fedan KB, Cummings KJ. Notes from the field: Respiratory symptoms and skin irritation among hospital workers using a new disinfection product—Pennsylvania, 2015. *MMWR Morb Mortal Wkly Rep.* 2016;65(15):400-401. [VB]

41. Abdulla FR, Adams BB. Ortho-phthalaldehyde causing facial stains after cystoscopy. *Arch Dermatol.* 2007;143(5):670. [VC]

42. Anderson SE, Umbright C, Sellamuthu R, et al. Irritancy and allergic responses induced by topical application of ortho-phthalaldehyde. *Toxicol Sci.* 2010;115(2):435-443. [IIIA]

43. Suneja T, Belsito DV. Occupational dermatoses in health care workers evaluated for suspected allergic contact dermatitis. *Contact Derm.* 2008;58(5):285-290. [IIB]

44. Warshaw EM, Schram SE, Maibach HI, et al. Occupation-related contact dermatitis in North American health care workers referred for patch testing: cross-sectional data, 1998 to 2004. *Dermatitis.* 2008;19(5):261-274. [IIIB]

45. Fujita H, Ogawa M, Endo Y. A case of occupational bronchial asthma and contact dermatitis caused by ortho-phthalaldehyde exposure in a medical worker. *J Occup Health.* 2006;48(6):413-416. [VB]

46. Arif AA, Delclos GL. Association between cleaning-related chemicals and work-related asthma and asthma symptoms among healthcare professionals. *Occup Environ Med.* 2012;69(1):35-40. [IIIB]

47. Robitaille C, Boulet LP. Occupational asthma after exposure to ortho-phthalaldehyde (OPA). *Occup Environ Med.* 2015;72(5):381. [VB]

48. Walters GI, Moore VC, McGrath EE, Burge PS, Henneberger PK. Agents and trends in health care workers' occupational asthma. *Occup Med (Lond).* 2013;63(7):513-516. [IIIB]

49. Bakerly ND, Moore VC, Vellore AD, Jaakkola MS, Robertson AS, Burge PS. Fifteen-year trends in occupational asthma: data from the shield surveillance scheme. *Occup Med (Lond).* 2008;58(3):169-174. [IIIB]

50. Copeland S, Nugent K. Persistent and unusual respiratory findings after prolonged glutaraldehyde exposure. *Int J Occup Environ Med.* 2015;6(3):177-183. [VB]

51. Donnay C, Denis MA, Magis R, et al. Under-estimation of self-reported occupational exposure by questionnaire in hospital workers. *Occup Environ Med.* 2011;68(8):611-617. [IIIB]

52. Ryu M, Kobayashi T, Kawamukai E, Quan G, Furuta T. Cytotoxicity assessment of residual high-level disinfectants. *Biocontrol Sci.* 2013;18(4):217-220. [IIIB]

53. Suzukawa M, Yamaguchi M, Komiya A, Kimura M, Nito T, Yamamoto K. Ortho-phthalaldehyde-induced anaphylaxis after laryngoscopy. *J Allergy Clin Immunol.* 2006;117(6):1500-1501. [VB]

54. Rideout K, Teschke K, DimichWard H, Kennedy SM. Considering risks to healthcare workers from glutaraldehyde alternatives in high-level disinfection. *J Hosp Infect.* 2005;59(1):4-11. [IIIB]

55. Guideline for cleaning and care of surgical instruments. In: *Guidelines for Perioperative Practice.* Denver, CO: AORN, Inc; 2017:815-850. [IVA]

56. American Society for Healthcare Engineering, Facility Guidelines Institute. *Guidelines for Design and Construction of Hospitals and Outpatient Facilities.* Chicago, IL: American Society for Healthcare Engineering; 2014. [IVC]

57. Guidelines interpretations. Facility Guidelines Institute. https://www.fgiguidelines.org/guidelines/interpretations-2/. Accessed October 5, 2017. [VA]

58. Hota S, Hirji Z, Stockton K, et al. Outbreak of multidrug-resistant *Pseudomonas aeruginosa* colonization and infection secondary to imperfect intensive care unit room design. *Infect Control Hosp Epidemiol.* 2009;30(1):25-33. [VB]

59. Siegel JD, Rhinehart E, Jackson M, Chiarello L; the Healthcare Infection Control Practices Advisory Committee. 2007 Guideline for isolation precautions: preventing transmission of infectious agents in healthcare settings. Centers for Disease Control and Prevention. https://www.cdc.gov/infectioncontrol/guidelines/isolation/. Updated 2017. Accessed October 5, 2017. [IVA]

60. HSE National Decontamination of Reusable Invasive Medical Devices Advisory Group, ed. *Health Service Executive Standards and Recommended Practices for Endoscope Reprocessing Units.* Version 2.2. Tipperary, Ireland: Health Service Executive; 2012. [IVB]

61. Bringhurst J. Special problems associated with reprocessing instruments in outpatient care facilities. *Am J Infect Control.* 2016;44:e63-e67. [VA]

62. Roberts CG. The role of biofilms in reprocessing medical devices. *Am J Infect Control.* 2013;41(5 Suppl):S77-S80. [VA]

63. 29 CFR 1910.1030: Bloodborne pathogens. US Government Publishing Office. https://www.ecfr.gov/cgi-bin/text-idx?SID=a71fad4cc5d7ca4d71154a2c80a4f88f&mc=true&node=se29.6.1910_11030&rgn=div8. Accessed October 5, 2017.

64. Merritt K, Hitchins VM, Brown SA. Safety and cleaning of medical materials and devices. *J Biomed Mater Res.* 2000;53(2):131-136. [IIB]

65. Rutala WA, Weber DJ. Disinfection, sterilization, and antisepsis: an overview. *Am J Infect Control.* 2016;44:e1-e6. [VA]

66. Gray RA, Williams PL, Dubbins PA, Jenks PJ. Decontamination of transvaginal ultrasound probes: review of national practice and need for national guidelines. *Clin Radiol.* 2012;67(11):1069-1077. [IIIB]

67. Sanz GE, Theoret J, Liao MM, Erickson C, Kendall JL. Bacterial contamination and cleanliness of emergency department ultrasound probes. *CJEM.* 2011;13(6):384-389. [IIIB]

68. Alfa MJ. Current issues result in a paradigm shift in reprocessing medical and surgical instruments. *Am J Infect Control.* 2016;44:e41-e45. [VA]

69. Kampf G, Bloss R, Martiny H. Surface fixation of dried blood by glutaraldehyde and peracetic acid. *J Hosp Infect.* 2004;57(2):139-143. [IIIB]

70. Alfa MJ, Olson N, DeGagne P, Jackson M. A survey of reprocessing methods, residual viable bioburden, and soil levels in patient-ready endoscopic retrograde choliangiopancreatography duodenoscopes used in Canadian centers. *Infect Control Hosp Epidemiol.* 2002;23(4):198-206. [IIIA]

71. Alfa MJ. Monitoring and improving the effectiveness of cleaning medical and surgical devices. *Am J Infect Control.* 2013;41(5 Suppl):S56-S59. [VA]

72. Yasuhara H, Fukatsu K, Komatsu T, Obayashi T, Saito Y, Uetera Y. Prevention of medical accidents caused by defective surgical instruments. *Surgery.* 2012;151(2):153-161. [IIIA]

73. Parada SA, Grassbaugh JA, Devine JG, Arrington ED. Instrumentation-specific infection after anterior cruciate ligament reconstruction. *Sports Health.* 2009;1(6):481-485. [IIIB]

74. Federal insecticide, fungicide, and rodenticide act [as amended through P.L. 112–177, effective Sept. 28, 2012]. US Senate Committee on Agriculture, Nutrition, & Forestry. https://www.agriculture.senate.gov/imo/media/doc/FIFRA.pdf. Accessed October 5, 2017.

75. Summary of the federal insecticide, fungicide, and rodenticide act. US Environmental Protection Agency.https://www.epa.gov/laws-regulations/summary-federal-insecticide-fungicide-and-rodenticide-act. Accessed October 5, 2017.

76. *State Operations Manual Appendix A—Survey Protocol, Regulations and Interpretive Guidelines for Hospitals.* Rev 151; 2015 Centers for Medicare & Medicaid Services. https://www.cms.gov/Regulations-and-Guidance/Guidance/Manuals/downloads/som107ap_a_hospitals.pdf. Accessed October 5, 2017.

77. *State Operations Manual Appendix L—Guidance for Surveyors: Ambulatory Surgical Centers.* Rev. 137; 2015. Centers for Medicare & Medicaid Services. https://www.cms.gov/Regulations-and-Guidance/Guidance/Manuals/downloads/som107ap_l_ambulatory.pdf. Accessed October 5, 2017.

78. 42 CFR 482. Conditions of participation for hospitals. 2011. Government Publishing Office. https://www.gpo.gov/fdsys/granule/CFR-2011-title42-vol5/CFR-2011-title42-vol5-part482. Accessed October 5, 2017.

79. 42 CFR 416. Ambulatory surgical services. 2011. Government Publishing Office. https://www.gpo.gov/fdsys/granule/CFR-2011-title42-vol3/CFR-2011-title42-vol3-part416. Accessed October 5, 2017.

80. IC.02.02.01: The hospital reduces the risk of infections associated with medical equipment, devices, and supplies. In: *Hospital Accreditation Standards.* Oakbrook Terrace, IL: Joint Commission Resources; 2017.

81. SS.1: Organization. In: *NIAHO Interpretive Guidelines and Surveyor Guidance.* Version 11. Milford, OH: DNV-GL Healthcare; 2014:80-82.

82. IC.02.02.01: The organization reduces the risk of infections associated with medical equipment, devices, and supplies. In: *Standards for Ambulatory Care.* Oakbrook Terrace, IL: Joint Commission Resources; 2017.

83. Infection prevention and control and safety. In: *Accreditation Handbook for Ambulatory Health Care.* Skokie, IL: Accreditation Association for Ambulatory Health Care, Inc.; 2016:54-57.

84. Operating room policy, environment, and procedures. In: *Regular Standards and Checklist for Accreditation of Ambulatory Surgery Facilities.* Version 14.5. Gurnee, IL: American Association for Accreditation of Ambulatory Surgery Facilities, Inc; 2017:24-36.

85. High-level disinfection and sterilization: know your process. *Jt Comm Perspect.* 2014;34(2):9. [VB]

86. Howie R, Alfa MJ, Coombs K. Survival of enveloped and non-enveloped viruses on surfaces compared with other micro-organisms and impact of suboptimal disinfectant exposure. *J Hosp Infect.* 2008;69(4):368-376. [IIIB]

87. Maillard JY. Innate resistance to sporicides and potential failure to decontaminate. *J Hosp Infect.* 2011;77(3):204-209. [VB]

88. Rutala WA, Gergen MF, Weber DJ. Disinfection of a probe used in ultrasound-guided prostate biopsy. *Infect Control Hosp Epidemiol.* 2007;28(8):916-919. [IIIB]

89. Kac G, Podglajen I, Si-Mohamed A, Rodi A, Grataloup C, Meyer G. Evaluation of ultraviolet C for disinfection of endocavitary ultrasound transducers persistently contaminated despite probe covers. *Infect Control Hosp Epidemiol.* 2010;31(2):165-170. [IIIB]

90. Bloc S, Mercadal L, Garnier T, et al. Evaluation of a new disinfection method for ultrasound probes used for regional anesthesia: ultraviolet C light. *J Ultrasound Med.* 2011;30(6):785-788. [IIIC]

91. Vickery K, Gorgis VZ, Burdach J, Patel D. Evaluation of an automated high-level disinfection technology for ultrasound transducers. *J Infect Public Health.* 2014;7(2):153-160. [IIIB]

92. Rutala WA, Gergen MF, Sickbert-Bennett E. Effectiveness of a hydrogen peroxide mist (trophon) system in inactivating healthcare pathogens on surface and endocavitary probes. *Infect Control Hosp Epidemiol.* 2016;37(5):613-614. [IIIB]

93. Johnson S, Proctor M, Bluth E, et al. Evaluation of a hydrogen peroxide-based system for high-level disinfection of vaginal ultrasound probes. *J Ultrasound Med.* 2013;32(10):1799-1804. [IIIB]

94. Rutala WA, Gergen MF, Bringhurst J, Weber DJ. Effective high-level disinfection of cystoscopes: is perfusion of channels required? *Infect Control Hosp Epidemiol.* 2016;37(2):228-231. [IIB]

95. Unal M, Yucel I, Akar Y, Oner A, Altin M. Outbreak of toxic anterior segment syndrome associated with glutaraldehyde after cataract surgery. *J Cataract Refract Surg.* 2006;32(10):1696-1701. [VA]

96. Karpelowsky JS, Maske CP, Sinclair-Smith C, Rode H. Glutaraldehyde-induced bowel injury after laparoscopy. *J Pediatr Surg.* 2006;41(6):e23-e25. [VB]

97. Nazik H, Bodur S, Api M, Aytan H, Narin R. Glutaraldehyde-induced bowel injury during gynecologic laparoscopy. *J Minim Invasive Gynecol.* 2012;19(6):756-757. [VB]

98. *AAMI TIR 34: 2014. Water for the Reprocessing of Medical Devices.* Arlington, VA: Association for the Advancement of Medical Instrumentation; 2014. [IVC]

99. Gillespie JL, Arnold KE, Noble-Wang J, et al. Outbreak of *Pseudomonas aeruginosa* infections after transrectal ultrasound-guided prostate biopsy. *Urology.* 2007;69(5):912-914. [VB]

100. Wendelboe AM, Baumbach J, Blossom DB, Frank P, Srinivasan A, Sewell CM. Outbreak of cystoscopy related infections with *Pseudomonas aeruginosa*: New Mexico, 2007. *J Urol.* 2008;180(2):588-592. [IIIB]

101. Guideline for sterile technique. In: *Guidelines for Perioperative Practice.* Denver, CO: AORN, Inc; 2017:75-104. [IVA]

102. Stigt JA, Wolfhagen MJ, Smulders P, Lammers V. The identification of *Stenotrophomonas maltophilia* contamination in ultrasound endoscopes and reproduction of decontamination failure by deliberate soiling tests. *Respiration.* 2015;89(6):565-571. [VB]

103. Guideline for a safe environment of care, part 1. In: *Guidelines for Perioperative Practice.* Denver, CO: AORN, Inc; 2017:243-268. [IVA]

104. 29 CFR 1910.151: Medical services and first aid. Occupational Safety and Health Administration https://www.osha.gov/pls/oshaweb/owadisp.show_document?p_table=STANDARDS&p_id=9806. Accessed October 5, 2017.

105. *ANSI/ISEA Z358.1-2014 American National Standard for Emergency Eyewash and Shower Equipment.* Arlington, VA: International Safety Equipment Association; 2014. [IVC]

106. Occupational safety and health act of 1970 (PL 91-596). Occupational Safety and Health Administration. https://www.osha.gov/pls/oshaweb/owadisp.show_document?p_table=OSHACT&p_id=2743. Accessed October 5, 2017.

107. Overview of health care HVAC systems. In: *HVAC Design Manual for Hospitals and Clinics.* Atlanta, GA: American Society of Heating, Refrigerating and Air-Conditioning Engineers; 2013:1-18. [IVC]

108. *Industrial Ventilation: A Manual of Recommended Practice for Design.* Cincinnati, OH: American Conference of Governmental Industrial Hygienists; 2016. [IVC]

109. Guideline for a safe environment of care, part 2. In: *Guidelines for Perioperative Practice.* Denver, CO: AORN, Inc; 2017:269-294. [IVA]

110. National Institute for Occupational Safety and Health, ed. *Evaluation of Ortho-phthalaldehyde in Eight Healthcare Facilities.* HHE report no. 2006-0238-3239. Cincinnati, OH: US Department of Health and Human Services, Centers for Disease Control and Prevention, National Institute for Occupational Safety and Health; 2015. [IIIA]

111. TLV / BEI introduction. American Conference of Governmental Industrial Hygienists. http://www.acgih.org/tlv-bei-guidelines/tlv-bei-introduction. Accessed October 5, 2017.

112. OSHA occupational chemical database. Occupational Safety and Health Administration. https://www.osha.gov/chemicaldata/. Accessed October 5, 2017.

113. 29 CFR 1910.134: Personal protective equipment: respiratory protection. Occupational Safety and Health Administration. https://www.osha.gov/pls/oshaweb/owadisp.show_document?p_table=STANDARDS&p_id=12716. Accessed October 5, 2017.

114. 29 CFR 1910.133: Personal protective equipment: eye and face protection. US Government Publishing Office. http://www.ecfr.gov/cgi-bin/text-idx?SID=138cf8e943da8b05e30a2d25732e5a51&mc=true&node=se29.5.1910_1133&rgn=div8. Accessed October 5, 2017.

115. 29 CFR 1910.132: Personal protective equipment: general requirements. Occupational Safety and Health Administration. https://www.osha.gov/pls/oshaweb/owadisp.show_document?p_table=STANDARDS&p_id=9777. Accessed October 5, 2017.

116. 29 CFR 1910.138: Personal protective equipment: hand protection. Occupational Safety and Health Administration. https://www.osha.gov/pls/oshaweb/owadisp.show_document?p_table=STANDARDS&p_id=9788. Accessed October 5, 2017.

117. Guideline for prevention of transmissible infections. In: *Guidelines for Perioperative Practice.* Denver, CO: AORN, Inc; 2017:507-542. [IVA]

118. Guideline for surgical attire. In: *Guidelines for Perioperative Practice.* Denver, CO: AORN, Inc; 2017:105-128. [IVA]

119. Resource conservation and recovery act (RCRA) laws and regulations. US Environmental Protection Agency. https://www.epa.gov/rcra. Accessed October 5, 2017.

120. 42 USC 6901: Congressional findings. US Government Publishing Office. https://www.gpo.gov/fdsys/pkg/USCODE-2011-title42/html/USCODE-2011-title42-chap82.htm. Accessed October 5, 2017.

121. 42 USC 6926: Authorized state hazardous waste programs. US Government Publishing Office. https://www.gpo.gov/fdsys/granule/USCODE-2010-title42/USCODE-2010-title42-chap82-subchapIII-sec6926. Accessed October 5, 2017.

122. Introduction to hospital waste management. In: *Healthcare Risk Control.* Vol 3. Plymouth Meeting, PA: ECRI, Inc; 2011:1-13. [VB]

123. Management of hazardous chemicals and waste. In: *Healthcare Risk Control.* Vol 3. Plymouth Meeting, PA: ECRI, Inc; 2017:1-15. [VB]

124. Guideline for patient information management. In: *Guidelines for Perioperative Practice.* Denver, CO: AORN, Inc; 2017:591-616. [IVA]

125. RC.01.01.01: The hospital maintains complete and accurate medical records for each individual patient. In: *Hospital Accreditation Standards.* Oakbrook Terrace, IL: Joint Commission Resources; 2017.

126. MS.16: Medical record maintenance. In: *NIAHO Interpretive Guidelines and Surveyor Guidance.* Version 11. Milford, OH: DNV-GL Healthcare; 2014:37.

127. RC.01.01.01: The organization maintains complete and accurate clinical records. In: *Standards for Ambulatory Care.* Oakbrook Terrace, IL: Joint Commission Resources; 2017.

128. Clinical records and health information. In: *Accreditation Handbook for Ambulatory Health Care.* Skokie, IL: Accreditation Association for Ambulatory Health Care, Inc; 2016:51-53.

129. Medical records: operating room records. In: *Regular Standards and Checklist for Accreditation of Ambulatory Surgery Facilities.* Version 14.5. Gurnee, IL: American Association for Accreditation of Ambulatory Surgery Facilities; 2017:60-63.

130. Medical records: procedure room records. In: *Procedural Standards and Checklist for Accreditation of Ambulatory Surgery Facilities.* Version 3. Gurnee, IL: American Association for Accreditation of Ambulatory Surgery Facilities, Inc; 2011:64-66.

131. HR.01.05.03: Staff participate in ongoing education and training. In: *Comprehensive Accreditation Manual: CAMH for Hospitals.* Oakbrook Terrace, IL: Joint Commission Resources; 2017.

132. MS.10: Continuing education. In: *NIAHO Interpretive Guidelines and Surveyor Guidance.* Version 11. Milford, OH: DNV-GL Healthcare; 2014:30.

133. HR.01.05.03: Staff participate in ongoing education and training. In: *Comprehensive Accreditation Manual: CAMAC for Ambulatory Care.* Oakbrook Terrace, IL: Joint Commission Resources; 2017.

134. Governance. In: *Accreditation Handbook for Ambulatory Health Care.* Skokie, IL: Accreditation Association for Ambulatory Health Care, Inc; 2016:33-40.

135. Personnel: personnel records; individual personnel files. In: *Regular Standards and Checklist for Accreditation of Ambulatory Surgery Facilities.* Gurnee, IL: American Association for Accreditation of Ambulatory Surgery Facilities, Inc; 2017:74-75.

136. Henn SA, Boiano JM, Steege AL. Precautionary practices of healthcare workers who disinfect medical and dental devices using high-level disinfectants. *Infect Control Hosp Epidemiol.* 2015;36(2):180-185. [IIIB]

137. Taneja N, Gill SS, Biswal M, et al. Working awareness of healthcare workers regarding sterilisation, disinfection, and transmission of bloodborne infections and device-related infections at a tertiary care referral centre in north India. *J Hosp Infect.* 2010;75(3):244-245. [IIIC]

138. Bailey C, Kay R, Starling P, et al. A health system approach to improving high level disinfection practices. *Am J Infect Control.* 2015;43:S14. [VC]

139. Rettig SL, Hoegg CL, Teszner E, Smathers SA, Satchell L, Sammons J. Ensuring competency of high-level disinfection (HLD) practices in non-central processing department (CPD) locations. *Am J Infect Control.* 2015;43:S22. [VB]

140. LD.04.01.07: The hospital has policies and procedures that guide and support patient care, treatment and services. In: *Hospital Accreditation Standards.* Oakbrook Terrace, IL: Joint Commission Resources; 2017.

141. LD.04.01.07: The organization has policies and procedures that guide and support patient care, treatment, or services. In: *Standards for Ambulatory Care.* Oakbrook Terrace, IL: Joint Commission Resources; 2017.

142. Personnel: personnel records. In: *Procedural Standards and Checklist for Accreditation of Ambulatory Surgery Facilities.* Version 3. Gurnee, IL: American Association for Accreditation of Ambulatory Surgery Facilities, Inc; 2011:77-79.

143. Steege AL, Boiano JM, Sweeney MH. NIOSH health and safety practices survey of healthcare workers: training and awareness of employer safety procedures. *Am J Ind Med.* 2014;57(6):640-652. [IIIA]

144. PI.03.01.01: The hospital improves performance on an ongoing basis. In: *Hospital Accreditation Standards.* Oakbrook Terrace, IL: Joint Commission Resources; 2017.

145. QM.1: Quality management system. In: *NIAHO Interpretive Guidelines and Surveyor Guidance.* Version 11. Milford, OH: DNV-GL Healthcare; 2014:10-17.

146. PI.03.01.01: The organization improves performance. In: *Standards for Ambulatory Care.* Oakbrook Terrace, IL: Joint Commission Resources; 2017.

147. Quality management and improvement. In: *Accreditation Handbook for Ambulatory Health Care.* Skokie, IL: Accreditation Association for Ambulatory Health Care, Inc; 2016:46-50.

148. Quality assessment/quality improvement: quality improvement. In: *Regular Standards and Checklist for Accreditation of Ambulatory Surgery Facilities.* Version 14.5. Gurnee, IL: American Association for Accreditation of Ambulatory Surgery Facilities, Inc; 2017:64.

Acknowledgments

Lead Author

Sharon A. Van Wicklin, MSN, RN, CNOR, CRNFA(E), CPSN-R, PLNC, FAAN
Senior Perioperative Practice Specialist
AORN Nursing Department
Denver, Colorado

The author and AORN thank Gerald McDonnell, BSc, PhD, Senior Director, Johnson & Johnson Family of Companies, Raritan, New Jersey; Susan G. Klacik, BS, CRCST, ACE, CHL, FCS, President, Klacik Consulting LLC, Canfield, Ohio; Judith L. Goldberg, DBA, MSN, RN, CNOR, CSSM, CHL, Director, Perioperative and Procedural Services, Lawrence & Memorial Hospital, Waterford, Connecticut; Marie A. Bashaw, DNP, RN, NEA-BC, CNOR, Assistant Professor, Wright State University, Dayton, Ohio; Susan Ruwe, MSN, RN, CPHQ, CIC, Senior Infection Preventionist, Carle Foundation Hospital, Urbana, Illinois; Bernard C. Camins, MD, MSc, Associate Professor of Medicine, University of Alabama at Birmingham; Dawn Myers Yost, MSN, RN, CNOR, CSSM, Manager, Training and Development Surgical Services/Business Manager, West Virginia University Hospitals/West Virginia University Medicine, Morgantown; and Jane Flowers, MSN, RN, CNOR, NEA-BC, CRCST, Manager, Sterile Processing, University of Maryland Shore Regional Health, Easton, for their assistance in developing this guideline.

Publication History

Originally published August 1980, *AORN Journal,* as AORN "Recommended practices for sterilization and disinfection."

Format revision July 1982; revised February 1987.

Revised October 1992 as "Recommended practices for disinfection"; published as proposed recommended practices for September 1994 as "Recommended practices for chemical disinfection."

Revised 1998 as "Recommended practices for high-level disinfection"; published March 1999, *AORN Journal.*

Revised November 2004; published in *Standards, Recommended Practices, and Guidelines,* 2005 edition. Reprinted February 2005, *AORN Journal.*

Revised November 2008; published in *Perioperative Standards and Recommended Practices,* 2009 edition.

Minor edition revisions made in November 2009 for publication in *Perioperative Standards and Recommended Practices,* 2010 edition.

Reformatted September 2012 for publication in *Perioperative Standards and Recommended Practices,* 2013 edition.

Minor editing revisions made in November 2014 as "Guideline for high-level disinfection" in *Guidelines for Perioperative Practice,* 2015 edition.

Revised January 2018 for publication in *Guidelines for Perioperative Practice,* 2018 edition.

Evidence ratings revised and minor editorial changes made to conform to the current AORN Evidence Rating model, September 2019, for online publication in *Guidelines for Perioperative Practice.*

HYPOTHERMIA

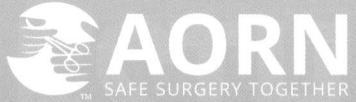

TABLE OF CONTENTS

P *indicates a recommendation or evidence relevant to pediatric care.*

MEDICAL ABBREVIATIONS & ACRONYMS

ASPAN – American Society of PeriAnesthesia Nurses
ERAS – Enhanced Recovery After Surgery
FDA – US Food and Drug Administration
IV – Intravenous
NICE – National Institute for Health and Clinical Excellence

OR – Operating room
PACU – Postanesthesia care unit
MHAUS – Malignant Hyperthermia Association of the United States
RCT – Randomized controlled trial

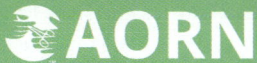
GUIDELINE FOR
PREVENTION OF HYPOTHERMIA

The Guideline for Prevention of Hypothermia was approved by the AORN Guidelines Advisory Board and became effective as of July 1, 2019. The recommendations in the guideline are intended to be achievable and represent what is believed to be an optimal level of practice. Policies and procedures will reflect variations in practice settings and/or clinical situations that determine the degree to which the guideline can be implemented. AORN recognizes the many diverse settings in which perioperative nurses practice; therefore, this guideline is adaptable to all areas where operative or other invasive procedures may be performed.

Purpose

All perioperative patients are at risk for developing unplanned **hypothermia**. This document provides guidance to the perioperative team for measuring the patient's body temperature, selecting methods for the prevention or treatment of unplanned hypothermia, and implementing the selected warming interventions.

In this document, hypothermia is defined as a core body temperature of < 36° C (< 96.8° F).[1] Although the definition of hypothermia varies among sources, it is frequently stated as body temperature lower than 35° C or 36° C (95° F or 96.8° F).[2,3] Hypothermia may be further delineated as

- mild (32° C to 35.9° C [89.6° F to 96.6° F]),
- moderate (28.1° C to 31.9° C [82.6° F to 89.4° F]), or
- severe (< 28° C [< 82.4° F]).[4]

The human body has two thermal compartments: the core and the peripheral.[5] The core body compartment includes primarily the trunk and head, which have a nearly constant temperature in a wide range of environments and thermoregulatory responses. The peripheral thermal compartment is composed of tissues that are mostly in the arms and legs, and the temperatures in these tissues are typically lower than core body temperature. The core temperature is normally tightly regulated, but the peripheral temperature may vary over a wider range. A change in the core or peripheral temperature normally leads to a behavioral or an autonomic response. A behavioral response to a temperature decrease may be moving into a warmer environment or putting on more clothing. The primary autonomic responses to a decrease in core body temperature are vasoconstriction and shivering. Anesthesia (eg, general, neuraxial, regional) prevents or alters these behavioral and autonomic responses, which results in a decrease in the patient's core temperature.[5-17]

General anesthesia blocks the autonomic response of vasoconstriction, which causes redistribution of body heat from the core to the periphery.[6,9] This redistribution is responsible for approximately 80% of the decrease in core body temperature during the first hour after initiation of general anesthesia. During this time period, the patient's core temperature can decrease by 0.5° C to 1.5° C (0.9° F to 2.7° F). General anesthesia also decreases metabolic heat production by about 15% to 30% and slightly increases cutaneous heat loss, which exaggerates temperature loss. After the first hour, the temperature continues to drop, but the rate at which it drops declines. The decrease in temperature during this time is generally caused by the heat loss exceeding metabolic heat production. After a period of time, the autonomic response will be reactivated, resulting in the temperature reaching a plateau. Neuraxial anesthesia (eg, spinal, epidural) also blocks the autonomic responses of shivering and vasoconstriction, but only in the anesthetized part of the body.[5]

To a lesser degree, hypothermia is caused by **radiant**, **evaporative**, **convective**, and **conductive heat loss**. Heat loss occurs because of low perioperative room temperature, the patient wearing little or no clothing, exposure of the patient's internal organs and tissue to the environment, air moving at a high velocity over the patient, administration of room-temperature IV and irrigation fluids, and the evaporation of skin preparation solutions.[5-17]

Adverse patient outcomes from unplanned hypothermia may include myocardial events, wound infections, poor wound healing, postoperative pain, increased blood loss and need for blood transfusion, reversible coagulopathy (ie, platelet dysfunction), impaired renal function, decreased drug metabolism, increased peripheral vascular resistance, postoperative protein catabolism, altered mental status, pressure ulcers, increased postanesthesia care unit (PACU) length of stay, prolonged hospitalization, and death.[1,3,4,8,9,13,14,16,18-72] However, some studies have not found an association between hypothermia and the patient outcomes of surgical site infection, blood loss, wound complications, death, increased length of hospitalization, or increased length of time in the PACU.[19,27,52,64,73-87] Further research is needed to determine the association between unplanned patient hypothermia and patient outcomes.

Although thermal comfort is an important patient outcome and is noted in several studies, it has not been found to be an accurate reflection of patient temperature.[88] Patients who have received regional anesthesia may be hypothermic but report their thermal comfort as "warm."[5]

Shivering, an autonomic thermoregulatory response to hypothermia, is also an important adverse patient outcome. Shivering may exacerbate surgical site pain, raise intracranial and intraocular pressure, and increase oxygen

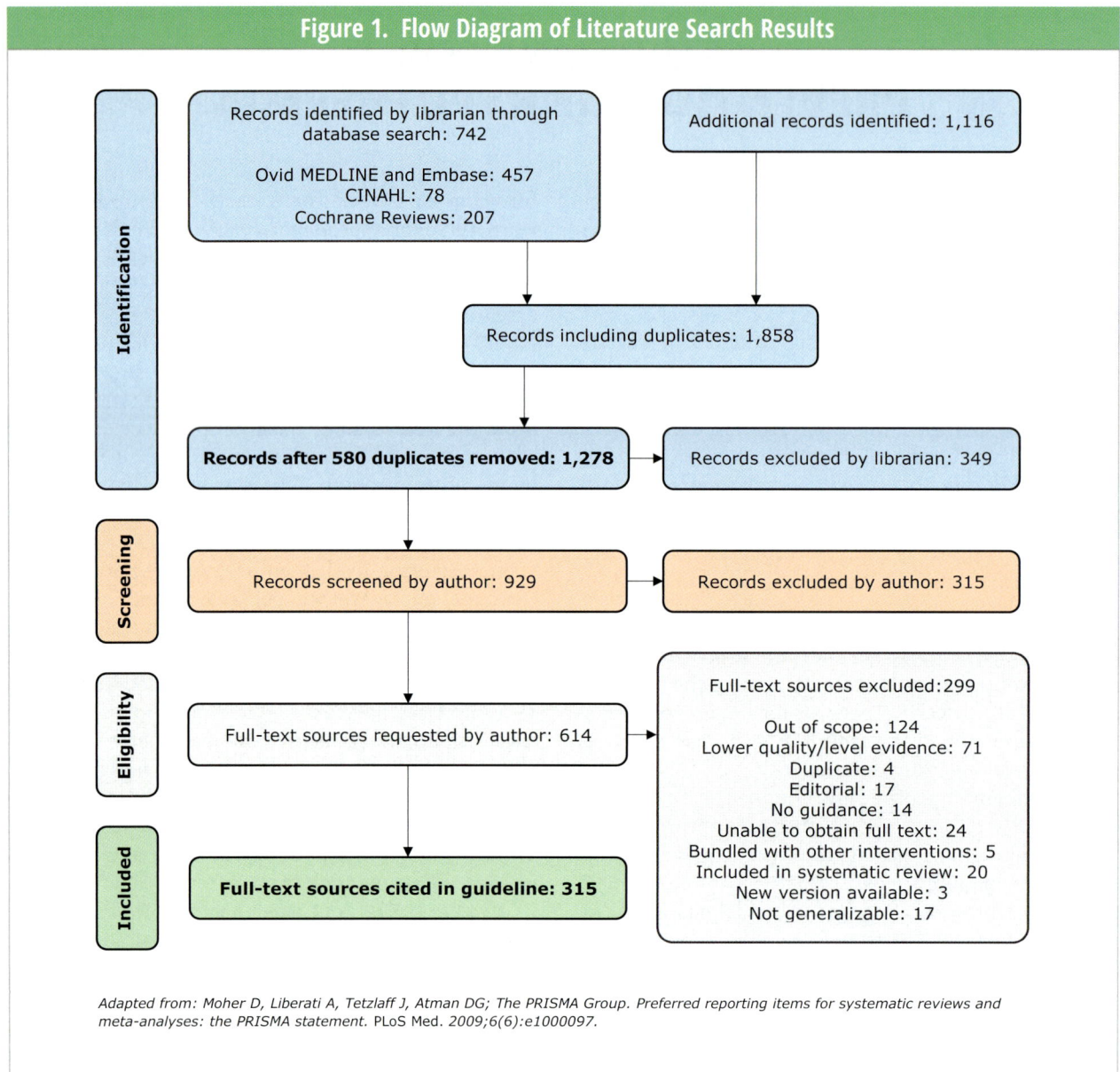

Figure 1. Flow Diagram of Literature Search Results

Adapted from: Moher D, Liberati A, Tetzlaff J, Atman DG; The PRISMA Group. Preferred reporting items for systematic reviews and meta-analyses: the PRISMA statement. PLoS Med. 2009;6(6):e1000097.

consumption.[89] Shivering can be minimized by **active warming methods** and by medications. The selection of medication for treatment of shivering is beyond the scope of this document because it requires an order from a prescriber.

These topics are also beyond the scope of this guideline:

- planned, intentional, or therapeutic hypothermia;
- rewarming after intentionally induced hypothermia;
- pharmacological agents used for prevention of hypothermia (eg, amino acids, fructose, carbohydrates);
- treatment for accidental or extreme hypothermia related to trauma or conditions outside of a health care facility;
- a cost-benefit analysis of treatment methods; and
- care and treatment of patients experiencing a malignant hyperthermia crisis. For guidance in handling malignant hyperthermia, contact the Malignant Hyperthermia Association of the United States (MHAUS) Hotline at (800) 644-9737 or access https://www.mhaus.org.

Evidence Review

A medical librarian with a perioperative background conducted a systematic search of the databases Ovid MEDLINE®, Ovid Embase®, EBSCO CINAHL®, and the Cochrane Database of Systematic Reviews. The search was limited to literature published in English from September 2013 through May 2018. At the time of the initial search, weekly alerts were created on the topics included in that search. Results from these alerts were provided to the lead author until September 2018. The lead author requested additional articles that either did not fit the original search criteria or were discovered during the evidence appraisal process. The lead author and the medical librarian also identified relevant guidelines from government agencies, professional organizations, and standards-setting bodies.

Search terms included *hypothermia, accidental/unplanned/inadvertent/unintentional/core/redistribution hypothermia, normothermia, shivering, trembling, shaking, shuddering, heat distribution, body temperature regulation, thermal management, thermoregulatory response threshold, thermoregulatory vasoconstriction/vasodilation/vasodilatation, rewarming, heating, thermogenesis, preoperative/intraoperative/comfort warming, warming technique, warming blanket, thermal pad, forced air/convective warming, negative pressure rewarming, circulating-water garment, cutaneous warming system, resistive heating, inspired gas humidification, intravenous infusion warming, warming irrigation, warmed solution, heat production, heat loss, adaptive/nonshivering/facultative thermogenesis, thermoregulation, monitoring (intraoperative), thermography, thermometers, temperature mapping, skin-surface temperature gradient, skin/esophageal/tympanic/temporal artery/oral/axillary/rectal thermometers, skin/esophageal/tympanic/temporal artery/oral/axillary/rectal temperatures, prewarming, temperature reporting, intraoperative care, operating room nursing, perioperative care, surgical procedures (operative), intraoperative/postoperative complications, operative surgical procedures,* and *operative procedures.*

Included were research and non-research literature in English, complete publications, and publications with dates within the time restriction when available. Historical studies were also included. Excluded were non-peer-reviewed publications and older evidence within the time restriction when more recent evidence was available. Editorials, news items, and other brief items were excluded. Low-quality evidence was excluded when higher-quality evidence was available, and literature outside the time restriction was excluded when literature within the time restriction was available (Figure 1).

Articles identified in the search were provided to the project team for evaluation. The team consisted of the lead author and one evidence appraiser. The lead author and the evidence appraiser reviewed and critically appraised each article using the AORN Research or Non-Research Evidence Appraisal Tools as appropriate. A second appraiser was consulted if there was a disagreement between the lead author and the primary evidence appraiser. The literature was independently evaluated and appraised according to the strength and quality of the evidence. Each article was then assigned an appraisal score. The appraisal score is noted in brackets after each reference as applicable.

Each recommendation rating is based on a synthesis of the collective evidence, a benefit-harm assessment, and consideration of resource use. The strength of the recommendation was determined using the AORN Evidence Rating Model and the quality and consistency of the evidence supporting a recommendation. The recommendation strength rating is noted in brackets after each recommendation.

Note: The evidence summary table is available at http://www.aorn.org/evidencetables/.

Editor's note: MEDLINE is a registered trademark of the US National Library of Medicine's Medical Literature Analysis and Retrieval System, Bethesda, MD. Embase is a registered trademark of Elsevier B.V., Amsterdam, The Netherlands. CINAHL, Cumulative Index to Nursing and Allied Health Literature, is a registered trademark of EBSCO Industries, Birmingham, AL.

1. Body Temperature Measurement

1.1 **Measure and monitor the patient's temperature during all phases of perioperative care.** [Recommendation] P

Clinical practice guidelines from professional organizations recommend temperature monitoring.[90-99]

The clinical practice guideline from the American Society of Anesthesiologists states that "every patient receiving anesthesia shall have temperature monitored when clinically significant changes in body temperature are intended, anticipated or suspected."[100(p3)]

Low-quality evidence also supports the importance of monitoring the patient's temperature during perioperative care.[13,14,25,27,30,33,35,36,101-103]

1.2 **Select the temperature measurement site and method in collaboration with the perioperative team based on the requirements of the procedure, anesthesia type, anesthesia delivery method, accessibility of the body site for measurement, and invasiveness of the method.** [Recommendation] P

The selection of a site and method for temperature measurement will depend on many patient- and procedure-specific factors. Low-quality evidence supports core body temperature as the most accurate way to assess the patient's thermal status but does not indicate one site and method that will be applicable in all clinical situations.[5,12,30] The sites that measure core body temperature include the pulmonary artery, cutaneous sites when measured with **zero-heat-flux** or **double-sensor thermometry**, the distal esophagus, the nasopharynx with the probe inserted 10 cm to 20 cm, and the tympanic membrane when measured with a probe using contact **thermistor** or **thermocouple** mechanisms. Table 1 and Table 2 show methods for measuring core and peripheral temperatures.[104-139]

Multiple clinical practice guidelines provide recommendations for the selection of a temperature measurement site and method.

The National Institute for Health and Care Excellence (NICE) guidelines[98] recommend using a site that is considered either a direct measurement or a direct estimate of core body temperature, including

Table 1. Core Temperature Measurement Sites and Methods

Sites and Methods	Notes
Pulmonary artery using a catheter	• Preferred site for measuring core temperature[103] • Very invasive[31,34] • Costly[34]

Cutaneous site using zero-heat-flux thermometry	• Noninvasive
	• May be used for core body temperature measurement[104-106]
	• Measurements correlate closely to temperature taken from
	  ○ rectal and bladder sites[107]
	  ○ the pulmonary artery site when body temperature is above 34° C (93.2° F)[108]
	  ○ the esophageal site when body temperature is above 32° C (89.6° F)[108]
	  ○ the esophageal or iliac arterial sites[109]
	  ○ nasopharyngeal and sublingual sites[110]

Cutaneous using double-sensor thermometry	• Noninvasive • May be used for measuring core body temperature[111] • Comparable to measurement at the distal esophageal and bladder sites[112]
Distal esophagus using a probe	• Minimally invasive and easy to use[94] • May be used for measuring core body temperature[34,102,113] • More reliable than the rectal site for measuring core body temperature[114] • May be affected by general anesthesia administered with humidified gases if the probe is not inserted correctly[31,94] • May be more accurate than measurement at the nasopharyngeal site[115]
Nasopharynx using a probe	• Correlates closely to core body temperature[34,102] • Reflects change in temperature more slowly than core sites[116] • May be less accurate than measurement at the distal esophagus[115]
Tympanic membrane using a probe with contact thermistor or thermocouple mechanisms	• May be used for measuring core temperature[102,113] • Measurements correlate more closely to arterial blood temperature than bladder or rectal sites do[117]

the pulmonary artery, distal esophagus, urinary bladder, cutaneous (ie, deep forehead using zero-heat-flux thermometry), sublingual, axillary, and rectal sites. The NICE guidelines also recommend against using indirect estimates of core body temperature, which is defined as a reading produced by a thermometer after a correction factor has been applied (eg, infrared tympanic, infrared temporal, infrared forehead, forehead strips). Furthermore, the NICE guidelines state that there may be inaccuracies in core body temperature estimation when using peripheral sites (eg, sublingual, axillary) for patients whose core body temperature is not in the normothermic range (36.5° C to 37.5° C [97.7° F to 99.5° F]).

The MHAUS guideline recommends using the following sites for continuous core body temperature monitoring: esophagus, nasopharynx, tympanic membrane (with the probe in contact with the membrane), bladder, and pulmonary artery.[91]

The American Society of PeriAnesthesia Nurses (ASPAN) guideline for promotion of perioperative normothermia state that temperatures taken at the near-core (ie, peripheral) sites are approximately equivalent to core body temperatures but may not be reliable when measuring extreme values (eg, < 35° C [< 95° F], > 39° C [102.2° F]).[140] These guidelines also state that the temporal artery temperature approximates core body temperature but may not be accurate for measuring extreme values.

The American College of Critical Care Medicine and the Infectious Diseases Society of America recommend choosing "the most accurate and reliable method to measure temperature based on the clinical circumstances of the patient."[97(p1332)]

A clinical practice guideline endorsed by the Canadian Association of General Surgeons recommends using esophageal or oral temperature monitoring in all surgical patients and avoiding use of infrared tympanic membrane thermometry if a more reliable method is available.[93] A European multinational guideline recommends using the core body temperature as the reference site.[92] The guideline states that oral thermometry is the most reliable noninvasive site, but other less-invasive sites also suited for perioperative use include nasopharyngeal, oropharyngeal, esophageal, vesical, or

Table 2. Peripheral Temperature Measurement Sites and Methods

Sites and Methods	Notes
Oral site using a thermometer or probe	• Noninvasive • May be used for measuring core body temperature in adult patients[118-120,126] • Measurements correlate with tympanic temperature in awake and anesthetized patients[121] • May be affected by intubation[126]
Bladder using a urinary catheter with a temperature sensor	• Invasive and poses risk for development of a catheter-associated urinary tract infection • Reflects change in temperature more slowly than core sites[118] • More reliable than using an electronic thermometer rectally to measure core body temperature[114] • May be affected by a low urine output[31,34,94,122] • May be affected by lower abdominal procedures[31,34] • Measurements are more closely correlated to pulmonary artery temperature than infrared tympanic temperature is[123]
Axilla using a thermometer	• Noninvasive • May be used for postoperative temperature measurement when the oral site is not accessible • Measurements correlate closely to bladder temperature[118] • Measurements may be lower than at nasopharynx and temporal artery sites[124] • Recommended for neonates[125] • Generally adequate[103] • Intubation may affect accuracy[126]
Rectum using a thermometer or probe	• Reflects change in temperature more slowly than core sites[34] • More accurate than inguinal and axillary sites for measuring core body temperature[114] • May be affected by the presence of stool[34] • May be inaccurate[103]

Tympanic membrane using an infrared sensor	• Not recommended for use in perioperative patients because of inaccuracy[102,120,123,126-128]
	• Results within seconds, noninvasive, easy to use
	• Measurements are less closely correlated to pulmonary artery temperature than bladder temperature is[123]
	• When measuring using an ear piece, is comparable to measurement at the esophageal[129] and nasopharyngeal[130] sites
	• In pediatric patients:
	  ○ Good for screening of fever[131]
	  ○ Superior to the axillary site for detection of mild hypothermia (< 36° C [< 96.8° F])[132]
	  ○ Measurements are more closely correlated to rectal temperature than temporal artery temperature is[133] P

Cutaneous site using a liquid crystal temperature strip	• Noninvasive[31] • May be affected by ambient temperature in the operating room and changes in cutaneous blood flow caused by the effects of anesthesia[31,134] • When the temperature drops, the variance between the cutaneous strip measurement and the pulmonary artery measurement increases[104] • Should not be used when temperatures outside of normothermia are expected[43,102]
Temporal artery using a thermometer	• Noninvasive core body temperature measurement that may be used for adults undergoing colorectal or gynecologic surgery[119,135] • Faster than using an electronic thermometer at oral or axillary sites[135] • Reflects pulmonary artery temperature more accurately than tympanic membrane measurement using an infrared sensor[126] • Can be affected by technique and cleanliness of the lens[136] • Measurements correlate closely to oral[137] and nasopharyngeal[124] temperature • Measurements correlate with bladder temperatures during normothermia but do not correlate when the patient has hypothermia or hyperthermia[138] • Superior to measurement at the axillary site for detection of mild hypothermia (< 36° C [< 96.8° F])[132] • Good for screening of fever in pediatric patients[131] • Lack of agreement with oral[128] and bladder temperatures[88,139] • Diaphoresis and airflow across the face may affect measurements[126]

direct tympanic membrane temperature measurement, and their use is determined by the surgical site.[92]

The Society of Pediatric Nurses recommends the using

- temporal artery thermometry for infants younger than 3 months without fever and for patients older than 3 months with or without fever, ill or well;
- rectal thermometry for infants younger than 3 months unless contraindicated by diagnosis;
- tympanic methods for children 6 months of age or older, with correct positioning of the ear; and
- oral methods for children 6 months of age or older when the patient can cooperate.[141]

1.3 **Use the same site and method of temperature measurement throughout the perioperative phases when clinically feasible.** *[Recommendation]* **P**

Clinical practice guidelines recommend using the same site and method for temperature measurement.[92,94,140]

Moderate-quality evidence indicates that temperature measurements can vary significantly when temperatures are measured at different sites or by different methods.[36,115,132,142-144]

In a randomized controlled trial (RCT), Erdling and Johansson[115] found that temperature measurements taken at the nasopharyngeal site were 0.2° C (0.36° F) higher than those taken at the esophageal site in 43 patients who underwent colorectal surgery. The temperature differences were statistically significant.

1.4 **Determine the frequency of patient temperature measurement based on the individual patient assessment and the health care organization's policies and procedures.** *[Conditional Recommendation]* **P**

Low-quality evidence for temperature monitoring frequency and monitoring based on procedure duration conflicts, with recommendations ranging from 15 to 60 minutes.[25,28,34,101,145-147]

The American Association of Nurse Anesthetists clinical practice guidelines state that "when clinically significant changes in body temperature are intended, anticipated, or suspected, monitor body temperature."[96(p3)]

Clinical practice guidelines from the American Society of Anesthesiologists state that "every patient receiving anesthesia shall have temperature monitored when clinically significant changes in body temperature are intended, anticipated or suspected."[100(p3)] Continually is defined as repeated regularly and frequently in rapid succession.

The NICE guidelines recommend intraoperative temperature measurement every 30 minutes.[98]

The Association of Surgical Technologists guidelines recommend that temperature be taken with the same frequency as other vital signs and at least every 30 minutes.[94]

A multinational European guideline recommends taking the temperature 1 to 2 hours before the start of anesthesia and either continuously or every 15 minutes during surgery.[92]

For temperature monitoring based on procedure duration, NICE[98] and MHAUS[91] recommend monitoring temperature during procedures that are 30 minutes or longer.

1.5 **Calibrate the selected temperature-monitoring device according to the manufacturer's written instructions for use.** *[Recommendation]* **P**

Calibration is recommended in a clinical practice guideline from the American College of Critical Care Medicine and the Infectious Diseases Society of America.[97]

1.6 **Document the site and method of temperature measurement and the value of the patient's temperature in the patient's record.** *[Recommendation]* **P**

Documentation serves as a method of communication among all care providers involved in planning, implementing, and evaluating patient care. Documenting patient care activities provides a description of the care administered and the status of patient outcomes on transfer of care.[96,148]

Documentation of the patient's temperature is recommended in clinical practice guidelines from the American Association of Nurse Anesthetists.[96,148]

1.7 **Communicate the patient's most recent temperature during transitions of care (eg, preoperative to intraoperative, intraoperative to postoperative).**[159] *[Recommendation]* **P**

1.8 **When the patient's temperature is outside the normothermic range, communicate the patient's temperature to the perioperative team.**[149] *[Recommendation]* **P**

When team members are aware that the patient's temperature is outside of the normothermic range, they can institute the hypothermia treatment measures specific to their role.

2. Prevention Methods

2.1 **Implement methods for preventing or treating hypothermia for all patients during all phases of perioperative care.** *[Recommendation]* **P**

All perioperative patients are at risk for developing hypothermia. Maintaining **normothermia** by preventing hypothermia is supported by clinical practice guidelines.[99,150-152]

2.2 Select the method for preventing hypothermia (ie, active warming, passive insulation, a combination of methods) preoperatively in collaboration with the perioperative team members (eg, perioperative registered nurse, anesthesia professional, surgeon, scrub person) based on the following criteria:

- patient-specific factors:
  - age (eg, premature and other low-birth-weight infants, older than 65 years),
  - sex (ie, female),
  - low body-surface area or weight,
  - congestive heart failure,
  - cardiac vessel disease,
  - previous cardiac surgery,
  - preexisting medical conditions (eg, hypothyroidism, hypoglycemia; malnourishment, burns, trauma, infantile neuronal ceroid lipofuscinosis, neurologic disorders),
  - hypotension, and
  - history of organ transplantation;
- type and duration of the surgical procedure[1,3,38,43,63,103,153-157];
- type and duration of the planned anesthesia[3,7,17,34-36,43,98,140,158,159];
- patient positioning;
- use of a pneumatic tourniquet[153,160];
- use of an intermittent pneumatic compression device[161];
- warming equipment constraints (eg, access to the surgical site, skin surface area contact, device size)[24]; and
- potential for adverse events associated with the use of warming equipment.

[Recommendation] **P**

Patient assessment is a standard of perioperative nursing practice.[162] Although all perioperative patients are at risk for developing hypothermia, some patients may be at increased risk due to the listed patient-specific factors.[1,3,4,6,7,15,35,36,38,43,46,53,88,153-157,159,163-167]

A clinical practice guideline from ASPAN[140] supports the selection of the patient warming method based on an assessment.

Although several patient- and procedure-specific factors have been associated with unplanned hypothermia, the evidence cannot be synthesized because it varies by surgical procedure and outcomes studied.[1,3,7,17,24,34-36,38,43,103,153-159,164,168]

In a prospective study, Hoda and Popken[157] found a correlation between lower core temperatures and longer surgical procedure duration, but no difference in patient temperatures between open or laparoscopic urologic procedures. The patients (N = 300) were warmed intraoperatively with a combination of an upper- and lower-body forced-air warmer and a single warming blanket. The researchers measured core body temperature pre-operatively, at induction of anesthesia, and at the beginning and end of the surgery.

Conversely, in a retrospective study, Mehta and Barclay[158] found that patients who underwent open colorectal surgery (n = 150) had a mean core body temperature that was significantly lower (0.2° C [0.36° F]) than those who underwent laparoscopic procedures (n = 105). A limitation of this study is that the patient warming methods for the two groups were not clearly described in the article.

2.3 A combination of active warming methods or active and passive insulation methods may be used. *[Conditional Recommendation]* **P**

Moderate-quality evidence supports the use of a combination of warming methods.[87,169-172] Three RCTs investigated various combinations of warming methods to prevent hypothermia.[87,171,172]

Pagnocca et al[171] compared use of a circulating-water mattress to a combination of a circulating-water mattress and a forced-air warming device in patients undergoing exploratory laparotomy under general anesthesia. The group that received the combined warming method (n = 19) had a higher temperature at the end of anesthesia and the end of surgery than the group that received the single warming method (n = 24).

Smith et al[87] compared warmed cotton blankets (n = 180) to a combination of intravenous (IV) fluid warming and convective warming (n = 156) in patients undergoing elective ambulatory gynecologic, orthopedic, urologic, and general surgery scheduled for longer than 30 minutes. The researchers found that the combination of IV fluid warming and convective warming was more effective in maintaining normothermia than the application of warmed cotton blankets. However, warming the patient did not decrease the time spent in the PACU or improve the patient satisfaction score, but it did increase costs.

Okeke[172] compared the use of room-temperature irrigation and IV fluids, the use of room-temperature irrigation fluids and warmed IV fluids, and the use of warmed irrigation and IV fluids in patients undergoing transurethral resection of the prostate. Patients who received warmed irrigation and room-temperature IV fluids (n = 40) experienced a significantly smaller temperature decrease than patients who received room-temperature IV and irrigation fluids (n = 40). Patients who received warmed IV and irrigation fluids (n = 40) had no significant change in the mean body temperature, and no patient in this group stated he or she felt cold or shivered.[171]

2.4 When active warming is indicated, prewarm the patient with the selected method. *[Recommendation]* **P**

Although high-quality evidence supports prewarming the patient,[52,64,158,173-193] some researchers did not find a difference in the incidence of hypothermia or intraoperative core body temperatures after preoperative warming of the patient.[75,194-199]

The authors of five systematic reviews concluded that there were benefits to prewarming patients.[176,179,181,183,193] The articles reviewed used various active warming methods.

In addition to the studies included in the systematic reviews, 9 RCTs support prewarming.[115,173,175,180, 185,186,188,190,191] The studies involved a total of 1,784 patients and compared no preoperative warming to prewarming using a variety of active warming methods. The researchers found that patients who were prewarmed experienced

- higher postoperative temperatures,[186]
- higher core body temperatures during the procedure,[115,173,185,188] and
- a lower rate of hypothermia.[175,180,190,191]

Four RCTs involving 267 patients found no benefits to prewarming.[194,197-199] The researchers found that patients who were prewarmed did not have higher intraoperative or postoperative core body temperatures or a difference in the incidence of hypothermia compared to those who were not prewarmed. Despite these findings, patients who were prewarmed with a forced-air warming device reported an increased sensation of warmth preoperatively and postoperatively.

Clinical practice guidelines recommend prewarming the patient as an intervention for preventing unplanned hypothermia.[92,93,98,140,200,201]

2.5 Determine the minimum amount of time for prewarming the patient before anesthesia induction. *[Conditional Recommendation]* **P**

Moderate-quality evidence supports prewarming the patient for a minimum of 10 minutes.[183,193]

A systematic review by Connelly et al[193] included 14 studies, 11 of which were RCTs. The studies included 1,240 patients who underwent various types of surgeries and compared no prewarming to various prewarming methods. The review authors found two studies that compared different time frames for prewarming; one study compared core temperatures of patients who received prewarming for zero, 20, 40, 60, or 80 minutes and the other study compared temperatures for patients who received prewarming for zero, 10, 20, or 30 minutes. The review authors found the average prewarming time to be 30 minutes, although a minimum of 10 minutes was sufficient to significantly reduce the rates of hypothermia.

Llewellyn[183] performed a systematic review of two RCTs. The studies involved 98 patients who underwent elective spinal or abdominal surgery and compared the effects of pre-warming with a forced-air warming device for a period of 60 minutes to no prewarming intervention. One study compared temperatures taken at 15-minute intervals and the other study used 30-minute intervals. The review author recommended prewarming and that further research be done to determine a prewarming time frame.

Other studies supporting prewarming used a set time frame instead of comparing various time frames. The minimum prewarming times were 15 minutes,[202,203] 20 minutes,[186,199] 30 minutes,[182,187,188] 45 minutes,[192] 60 minutes,[198,204] 86 minutes,[175] and 2 hours.[189]

2.6 When hypothermia is identified before surgery, initiate interventions to normalize the patient's core body temperature before the patient's transfer to the operating room (OR), if possible. *[Recommendation]* **P**

Normalizing the patient's core body temperature preoperatively may prevent worsening of the hypothermic condition because it may not be possible to warm the patient intraoperatively. However, the benefits or harms to the patient may vary depending on the clinical situation. Further research on this topic is needed.

Low-quality evidence supports normalizing the patient's core body temperature before the patient's transfer to the OR.[17,25,36,102,113]

In a nonexperimental study involving 147 patients, Kim and Yoon[17] identified a low preoperative body temperature as a risk factor for intraoperative hypothermia. The patients in this study underwent abdominal surgery under general anesthesia. The researchers found a significant relationship between a low preoperative core body temperature and the incidence of hypothermia at 1 hour after the administration of anesthesia.

Clinical practice guidelines from NICE[98] and ASPAN[140] recommend normalizing the patient's core body temperature before the patient's transfer to the OR.

3. Passive Insulation Methods

3.1 When indicated, use one or more of the following passive insulation methods during all phases of perioperative care:
- cotton blankets,
- surgical drapes,
- plastic sheeting,

- thermal clothing,
- a non-linting wrap, or
- blankets or garments made of reflective composite fabric (eg, space blankets).

[Recommendation] P

The use of passive insulation methods for prevention of hypothermia is recommended in clinical practice guidelines,[92,94,98,140] although further research is needed to compare the different passive methods. Passive methods provide insulation against heat loss, one of the mechanisms that causes hypothermia, but they are not an effective means of treating hypothermia.[29]

Warttig et al[205] performed a systematic review of 11 RCTs that involved 699 patients, to compare different methods of rewarming patients after surgery, including thermal insulation. The patients underwent various types of procedures. The risk of bias was high or unclear in most of the studies. The review authors found no significant difference in rewarming time when either thermal insulation or cotton blankets were used.

Alderson et al[206] performed a systematic review of 22 studies involving 1,256 patients older than 18 years who underwent routine or emergency surgery. The studies compared the use of reflective blankets or clothing against normal care, use of non-reflective blankets or clothing, and use of forced-air warming against use of reflective blankets or clothing. The review authors concluded that the risk of bias was unclear, but there was a high risk for performance bias and a low risk for attrition bias in the majority of the studies. The review authors determined that most of the evidence was of low quality with a high potential for skewed results related to personnel changing their behavior because of an awareness of the method being tested. They concluded there was no clear evidence that the use of a reflective blanket or clothing increases a person's temperature compared to usual care.

Additional evidence regarding the use of reflective blankets that was not included in either of these systematic reviews is of low to moderate quality and varies in results. The evidence consists of three RCTs and one quasi-experimental study involving a total of 660 patients having various types of surgery lasting 1 hour or less; unilateral total hip or knee arthroplasty; and various procedures using sedation, spinal, epidural, or general anesthesia.[207-210] The researchers compared the use of reflective blankets to cotton blankets[208-210] or application of a forced-air warming device.[207] They found that patients who received a reflective blanket

- had a significantly smaller drop in the temperature gradient between the temporal artery tem-

perature and the foot temperature and a significant increase in the foot temperature[209];
- had no significant differences in temperature compared to patients who received warmed cotton blankets[208,210]; and
- had no significant differences in sublingual temperatures compared to patients who received a forced-air warming device.[207]

In a quasi-experimental study involving 72 patients who underwent spinal surgery, Lee et al[211] investigated the use of warmed socks as a passive insulation method. The participants were assigned in equal numbers to either a group that received warmed socks or a group that did not. The researchers found that the temperature in the group that received warmed socks was significantly higher than in the group that did not receive warmed socks.

4. Active Warming Methods

4.1 When indicated, warm the patient with one or more of the following active warming methods during all phases of perioperative care:
- a forced-air warming device (eg, blanket, gown),
- a water-filled mattress,
- a circulating-water garment,
- an electric warming blanket,
- a carbon-fiber blanket,
- a resistive polymer blanket,
- a thermal exchange chamber,
- a negative pressure warming system,
- warmed anesthesia gases,
- warmed IV fluids,
- warmed irrigation fluids,
- radiant warming, and
- warmed insufflation gases.

[Recommendation] P

High-quality evidence supports the use of active warming for prevention of unplanned hypothermia,[43,52,64,67,69,72,157,169,212-216] although further research is needed to compare the different methods of active warming.

Some evidence specifically supports the use of active warming methods in the PACU.[1,33,36,205,217,218] Numerous studies indicate that active warming methods are more effective in preventing hypothermia than passive methods.[169,180,206,212,214,218-225]

In a systematic review with meta-analysis, Shaw et al[214] reviewed 25 RCTs to determine whether the type of warming intervention influenced the frequency or severity of inadvertent perioperative hypothermia in surgical patients receiving neuraxial anesthesia. The results showed that during neuraxial anesthesia, active forced-air warming was more effective than passive methods in preventing hypothermia. The review authors concluded that more research is needed to compare the different methods of active warming.

Sultan et al[215] performed a systematic review with meta-analysis of 13 RCTs involving 789 patients who underwent elective cesarean delivery. The review authors found warming decreased shivering and the incidence of hypothermia, increased the patient's temperature at the end of surgery, and increased thermal comfort. The review authors concluded that active warming by warming IV fluids, using forced-air warming, or using a combination of methods reduced patient temperature change and improved thermal comfort. The review authors suggested that active warming be performed during cesarean deliveries.

Guedes Lopes et al[169] systematically reviewed seven articles (ie, one meta-analysis, one case-control study, and five correlational and randomized clinical trials) to evaluate the effectiveness of active warming systems compared to passive systems in preventing hypothermia. The review authors concluded that active warming methods were more effective than passive methods in maintaining normothermia and that forced-air warming and circulating-water devices were the most effective of the active methods.

Benson et al[18] conducted an RCT that involved 30 patients who underwent total knee arthroplasty. The patients were randomly and equally assigned to either a control group that received a gown and cotton blanket or an experimental group that was warmed using a patient-controlled, forced-air warming gown. The researchers found pain scores were not significantly different between the two groups, but the patients in the experimental group had higher temperatures in the PACU, used fewer opioids postoperatively, and were more satisfied with their thermal comfort than those in the control group. The researchers recommended that all patients receive active warming, especially those with compromised thermoregulatory systems and those undergoing surgeries considered to be exceptionally painful.

Use of active warming is also recommended in a number clinical practice guidelines.[92,95,98,140,200,201]

4.2 Forced-air warming systems (eg, over- and under-body blankets, warm-air gowns) may be used. [Conditional Recommendation] P

Although high-quality evidence supports the use of forced-air warming systems for prevention and treatment of hypothermia,[18,44,87,176,179,195,205,206,219,224-242] there is important variation in the study results. Some evidence indicates that other active warming devices may be equally effective to[169,207,242-252] or more effective than[175,242,252-259] forced-air warming devices in maintaining normothermia.

In a systematic review with meta-analysis, Nieh and Su[242] reviewed 29 RCTs that involved 1,875 surgical patients. The studies compared forced-air warming to passive insulation, circulating-water mattresses, resistive heating blankets, and radiant warming systems. The review authors concluded that forced-air warming was more effective in reducing perioperative hypothermia than passive insulation and circulating-water mattresses, but equally as effective as circulating-water garments, resistive heating blankets, and radiant warming systems. The authors also found the thermal comfort scores were higher for forced-air warming compared to passive insulation, resistive heating blankets, and radiant warming systems, but lower than those for circulating-water mattresses.

Warttig et al[205] performed a systematic review of 11 RCTs published between 1990 and 2012 that involved 699 patients. They found that the mean time to achieve normothermia was less when forced-air warming was applied than when warm or room-temperature blankets or circulating hot water devices were used. The authors concluded there was a clinically significant reduction in the time to return to normothermia when an active warming device, particularly forced-air warming, was used.

However, in another systematic review of 14 RCTs published from January 2000 through April 2007, Galvao et al[252] found moderate evidence that forced-air warming devices were equal in effectiveness to carbon-fiber blankets and less effective than circulating-water garments for maintaining normothermia. The studies involved 1,191 patients 18 years of age or older who underwent non-emergency surgery. The review authors recommended future research regarding costs of purchasing and maintaining warming systems.

Fourteen RCTs published more recently than these systematic reviews support forced-air warming. The studies involved a total of 728 patients who underwent cesarean deliveries; cleft lip and palate procedures; and gynecologic, plastic, orthopedic, and general surgeries.[87,179,219,224,225,233-241] The studies compared forced-air warming to the application of blankets, reflective insulation, a circulating-water mattress, an electric heating pad, and a circulating-water pad wrapped around a single extremity with a vacuum applied. The researchers found that the use of a forced-air warming device resulted in a significant increase in thermal comfort scores and a decrease in the

- incidence of hypothermia (ie, a core temperature below 36° C [96.8° F]),[87,179,219,224,233-238,240]
- rate of shivering,[87,233,236,238]
- rate of complications,[233,238]

- length of time from dressing application to extubation,[239]
- time for restoring the initial temperature decrease after induction,[224,225,233,238] and
- rate of hypothermia but not until 90 minutes after induction.[238]

Other research not included in the systematic reviews supports various products as being more effective in maintaining normothermia or thermal comfort than forced-air warming devices. This evidence consists of 10 RCTs and one quasi-experimental study involving a total of 462 patients who underwent orthopedic, general, laparoscopic colorectal, and off-pump coronary artery bypass grafting surgery; burn treatment; and cesarean deliveries.[175,253-262] These studies compared multiple interventions to forced-air warming, including self-warming blankets, carbon-fiber blankets, warm water–circulating devices, and warmed IV fluids. The researchers found that

- patients who were warmed with a forced-air warming device
  - had no difference in incidence of hypothermia,[258]
  - had a higher occurrence of adverse outcomes (ie, more blood loss, lower core body temperatures, longer overall hospital stays) than patients warmed with a circulating-water device,[258]
  - returned to baseline temperatures of 37° C (98.6° F) more slowly than patients warmed with a warm water and pulsating negative-pressure device,[254]
  - had lower final core body temperatures than patients warmed with a circulating-water device or an electric heating blanket,[260] and
  - had a lower warming rate than patients warmed with a conductive/resistive warming blanket in addition to a warming mattress[261];
- patients warmed with a forced-air warming device combined with warmed IV fluids had a lower temperature increase compared to patients warmed with a combination of a circulating-water warming device and warmed IV fluids[258];
- patients warmed with a forced-air warming device applied preoperatively did not have a significant difference in the end-of-surgery temperatures[259];
- patients warmed with a forced-air warming device applied after skin antisepsis had significantly lower temperatures than patients warmed with a self-warming blanket for a median of 86 minutes before entering the OR[175];
- patients warmed with a lower-body forced-air warming blanket had significantly lower temperatures at the end of the procedure than patients warmed with circulating water leg wraps combined with a full-length circulating water mattress[257]; and
- patients warmed with an upper-body forced-air warming device had significantly lower rectal and esophageal temperatures at incision, 1 hour after incision, at skin closure, and immediately after surgery than patients warmed with a water garment warming system that permitted active warming of both the upper and lower extremities and the back.[262]

Evidence about the negative effects of forced-air warming systems is not consistent. This evidence consists of a systematic review[263] and simulation-based studies in a laboratory setting.[264-268]

Haeberle et al[263] conducted a systematic review that evaluated the infection risk of using forced-air warming devices in the orthopedic population. The authors reviewed eight studies consisting of three RCTs, one of which involved canines; two laboratory studies; two quasi-experimental studies; and one retrospective study. The review authors concluded that there is no evidence in the current orthopedic literature that establishes a link between forced-air warming devices and an increase in surgical site infections.

Studies not included in this systematic review indicate that there may be a risk for an increase in air particle counts or a disruption in the airflow with the use of a forced-air warming system.[264-268] Three of these studies also found contamination internally in the machines.[265-267] However, other studies did not find a correlation between forced-air warming and a disruption in the airflow, an increase in bacterial counts on the sterile field, or air particle counts.[269-272]

Several clinical practice guidelines recommend use of forced-air warming devices for procedures longer than 30 minutes or for patients at a high risk for inadvertent hypothermia.[92,93,98,140,200,201]

4.2.1 **Use forced-air warming devices with the manufacturer-designated blanket attached to the hose and according to the manufacturer's instructions for use.** *[Recommendation]* **P**

Following the manufacturer's instructions for use of forced-air warming devices reduces the risk of burning the patient. The temperature at the hose can range from 41.5° C to 47.7° C (106.7° F to 117.9° F), which may cause burns. The temperature of the air leaving the blanket is 2.5° C to 16.9° C (4.5° F to 30.4° F) lower than when it comes out of the hose.

Low-quality evidence also supports using a forced-air warming device attached to the manufacturer-designated blanket.[273-276]

4.2.2 When using a forced-air warming blanket with a head drape, arrange the drape in a manner that allows the air to flow freely from under the drape, and keep the blower activated while the drape is in place. *[Conditional Recommendation]* **P**

Loosely tucking the head drape reduces the risk of creating an oxygen-enriched atmosphere that would increase the potential for a fire. A quality improvement project conducted by Chapp and Lange[277] supports placing the drape in a manner that allows the air to flow freely from under the drape. The authors measured the amount of oxygen that accumulated under the head drape of a forced-air warming device. The source of the oxygen was a leak in the anesthesia tubing. They found that an oxygen-enriched atmosphere was created under a tucked, forced-air warming device head drape within 5 to 10 minutes. They also noted that the time was decreased when the oxygen flow was higher, the drape was tucked tightly, and the blower was turned off.

4.3 Warm water–circulating devices may be used. *[Conditional Recommendation]* **P**

Although there is some high-quality evidence supporting the use of warm water–circulating devices for prevention of hypothermia,[257,258,260,278] there is also some supporting low-quality evidence[169,243,253-255,279,280] and important variation in the study results. Two studies indicate that water-circulating devices may be as effective as forced-air warming devices in maintaining normothermia,[250,280] and three other studies indicate that other products may be more effective in maintaining normothermia than a warm water–circulating device.[237,242,281]

Galvao et al[252] performed a systematic review with meta-analysis consisting of 14 RCTs published between January 2000 and the end of April 2007. The review authors found that circulating-water garments were more effective in maintaining normothermia than carbon-fiber blankets or forced-air warming devices.

The studies supporting use of warm water–circulating devices involved 264 patients having surgery for burn treatment, off-pump coronary artery bypass grafting, electrophysiology surgery, and general surgery.[255,257,258,262,278] The studies compared warm water–circulating devices to forced-air warming devices, warmed IV fluids, and several combinations of active warming methods. The researchers found that

- patients who were warmed with a warm water–circulating device
  - had significantly higher core body temperatures, less blood loss, and shorter overall hospital stays than patients warmed with a forced-air warming device[258] and
  - returned to a temperature of 37° C (98.6° F) faster than patients warmed with a forced-air warming device[253];
- patients warmed with a warm water–circulating device combined with warm IV fluids had a mean temperature increase of 1.4° C (2.5° F), which was the highest temperature increase compared to other combinations of active warming methods, including a forced-air warming mattress plus warmed IV fluids, a forced-air warming blanket with a radiator ceiling, and a bed warmer[255];
- patients warmed with a warm water gel pad were significantly less likely to be hypothermic at the end of the procedure compared with patients placed on a non-activated gel pad[278];
- patients warmed with circulating-water leg wraps combined with a full-length circulating-water mattress set at 42° C (107.6° F) had significantly higher temperatures at the end of the procedure than patients warmed by a lower-body forced-air blanket[257]; and
- patients warmed with a water garment warming system that permitted active warming of both the upper and lower extremities and the back had significantly higher rectal and esophageal temperatures at incision, 1 hour after incision, at skin closure, and immediately after surgery than patients warmed with an upper-body forced-air warming device.[262]

Perez-Protto et al[280] conducted an RCT to determine whether a circulating-water garment alone was more effective than a circulating-water mattress used in combination with a forced-air warming device. The study included 36 patients who underwent abdominal surgery who were randomly assigned to either a group warmed with a circulating-water garment (n = 16) or a group warmed with a circulating-water mattress used in combination with a forced-air warming device (n = 20). The researchers found the core body temperatures increased significantly in both groups during the first 3 hours of surgery. They concluded that the circulating-water garment was comparably effective to the combination of the circulating-water mattress and forced-air warming device.

Ruetzler et al[250] conducted a quasi-experimental study involving patients who underwent open abdominal surgery who were warmed with either circulating warm water in a pad wrapped around a single extremity together with a vacuum applied to the limb (n = 37) or an upper-body forced-air warming device (n = 34). The difference in mean temperatures was never more than approximately 0.2° C (0.36° F). The researchers concluded that the systems transfer comparable amounts of heat and both appear suitable for use even during long surgeries or surgeries involving large surface areas.

Clinical practice guidelines from ASPAN[140] and the ERAS® (Enhanced Recovery After Surgery) Society[201] recommend use of warm water–circulating devices.

4.4 **Conductive/resistive warming** devices (eg, electric heating pads, carbon-fiber resistive-heating blankets, conductive warming mattresses, self-warming blankets) may be used. [*Conditional Recommendation*]

Although high-quality evidence supports the use of conductive/resistive devices for prevention of hypothermia,[176,220-222,231,282-285] there is important variation in the study results. Some of the evidence indicates that forced-air warming devices may be equally effective to conductive/resistive devices in maintaining normothermia,[242-244,247-249,251,252,286,287] and other evidence indicates that other products may be more effective in maintaining normothermia than conductive/resistive devices.[236,257]

Munday et al[176] conducted a systematic review of the literature involving a total of 719 participants in 12 studies. The review authors found that an under-body carbon-polymer mattress was effective in preventing hypothermia, and the effectiveness of this device was increased when it was applied before surgery.

Seven RCTs not included in this systematic review also support the use of conductive/resistive warming devices.[220-222,260,282,284,285] These studies involved a total of 749 patients having orthopedic; gynecologic; spinal; cesarean delivery; head and neck; ear, nose, and throat; or unspecified day surgery lasting less than 40 minutes. These studies compared conductive/resistive warming devices (ie, an active self-warming blanket, a conductive warming mattress, a resistive warming mattress, an electric carbon-polymer warming blanket) to cotton blankets, sheets, hospital duvets, warmed IV fluids, inactivated warming mattresses, and increased ambient room temperature. The researchers found that

- patients warmed with an active self-warming blanket had a significantly lower rate of hypothermia compared to those receiving passive thermal insulation[220];
- patients warmed with a combination of an activated self-warming blanket, warmed IV fluids, cotton blankets, and an OR temperature of 22° C to 23° C (71.6° F to 73.4° F) had significantly higher temperatures at 30 minutes after admission and at discharge from the OR compared to

a group warmed with the same combination but without the activated self-warming blanket[282];
- patients warmed with an activated resistive warming mattress had a lower rate of hypothermia (12.5%) compared to patients with no warming mattress (34.2%)[285];
- patients warmed with an activated conductive warming mattress had higher temperatures in the PACU compared to patients who had an inactivated mattress[221];
- patients warmed with a combination of a conductive warming mattress and a hospital duvet had a significantly lower rate of hypothermia compared to patients using only a hospital duvet[284]; and
- patients warmed with a combination of an electric carbon-polymer warming blanket, blankets, and sheets had a lower rate of hypothermia (24%) compared to patients using blankets and sheets only (39%).[222]

A clinical practice guideline from NICE[112] and a multinational European guideline[105] also recommend use of conductive/resistive warming devices.

Other studies support different products as being equally effective to conductive/resistive warming devices in maintaining normothermia.[244,247,248,251,286,287] These studies involved a total of 274 patients who underwent major open abdominal and orthopedic surgery and compared conductive/resistive warming devices (ie, a carbon-fiber resistive warming device, an under-body resistive heating device, a resistive polymer system, a conductive warming mattress) to forced-air warming devices. The researchers found that

- patients who were warmed with an under-body resistive heating device did not have significantly different core body temperatures compared to patients warmed with an upper-body forced-air warming blanket,[251]
- patients warmed with a carbon-fiber resistive warming device did not have lower average core body temperatures compared to patients warmed with a forced-air warming system,[248]
- patients warmed with a resistive warming device did not have a significantly different end of surgery temperature or intraoperative core temperature compared to patients warmed with a forced-air warming system,[244,247,287] and
- patients warmed with a conductive mattress did not have a significant difference in mean core temperature on admission to the recovery room compared to patients warmed with a forced-air warming device or warmed IV fluids.[286]

In an RCT, Hofer et al[260] found that conductive/resistive warming devices were more effective than forced-air warming devices, but less effective than circulating-water devices. The study involved 90 patients having elective multiple off-pump coronary artery bypass grafting procedures. The mean final body core temperature was 34.7° C (94.5° F) for patients warmed with the forced-air warming device, 35.6° C (96.1° F) for patients warmed with conductive/resistive warming devices, and 36.5° C (97.7° F) for patients warmed with the circulating-water device.

4.5 **Warmed anesthesia gases may be used to warm the patient as an adjunct to other active warming or passive insulation methods.** [Conditional Recommendation] **P**

Although high-quality evidence supports the use of warmed anesthesia gases,[43,288-292] the evidence may not be generalizable to all patients. The research supporting warming of anesthesia gases involved 362 patients who underwent orthopedic, general, and spine surgery and liver transplantation. The studies compared the use of warmed and humidified anesthesia gases using a heat-and-moisture exchanger (ie, passive warming) to gases warmed using a heated humidifier (ie, active warming) and to room-temperature gases. The researchers found that patients who received actively warmed anesthesia gases

- had a significantly lower rate and duration of hypothermia compared to patients who received passive warming methods;[292]
- still experienced hypothermia, but to a lesser degree of severity, and had higher core body temperatures compared to patients who did not receive the actively warmed gases;[186,289,291] and
- had significantly lower rates of hypothermia compared to patients who received room-temperature gases.[290]

Further research is needed to determine the potential harms of using warmed anesthesia gases, especially in pediatric patients.

4.6 **Warmed IV fluids may be used as an adjunct to other active warming methods.** [Conditional Recommendation] **P**

Although there is high-quality evidence supporting the use of warmed IV fluids,[165,172,176,285,286,293-297] the evidence does not clearly show that this is an effective intervention for prevention of unplanned hypothermia when used without other interventions. Two studies support the administration of warmed IV fluids as an adjunct to other warming methods.[51,255]

The use of warmed IV and irrigation fluids is supported in a systematic review of the literature performed by Campbell et al.[297] The review included 17 studies involving warming of IV fluids that were published between 1986 and 2014 and involved a total of 840 participants. The risk of bias was either high or unclear related to inappropriate or unclear randomization and blinding procedures. The outcome measured was mean core body temperature.

The researchers who conducted the reviewed studies found the temperature of the participants who received the warmed IV fluids was about 0.5° C (0.9° F) warmer than of those who received room-temperature IV fluids at 30, 60, 90, and 120 minutes and at the end of surgery. The review authors concluded that administration of warmed IV fluids appears to keep patients warmer intraoperatively when compared to use of room-temperature IV fluids. The remainder of the results were expressed as warming of fluids and not specifically to the warming of IV or irrigation fluids. The review authors were unable to determine whether the actual differences in temperature were clinically meaningful, whether there are other benefits or harms associated with the use of warmed fluids, and whether using fluid warming in addition to other warming methods increases the benefits because a ceiling effect may occur with the use of multiple methods of warming. The review authors also could not determine whether warming of fluids alone could reduce the number of complications.[298]

Munday et al[176] performed a systematic review of 12 studies with a total of 719 participants and found IV fluid warming to be effective in decreasing the rate of hypothermia. The review authors recommended warming IV fluid by any method for all cesarean deliveries and applying preoperative warming strategies when possible.

Seven RCTs published more recently than these systematic reviews also support the use of warmed IV fluids.[172,285,286,293-296] These studies involved 601 patients who underwent elective cesarean delivery under spinal anesthesia, orthopedic surgery, general surgery, and short ambulatory urologic procedures. The studies compared warmed IV fluids to room-temperature IV fluids and to combinations with forced-air warming devices and a conduction mattress. The researchers found that patients who received warmed IV fluids experienced

- a significantly shorter time to spontaneous breathing, eye opening, consciousness recovery, and extubation[293];
- a reduction in the incidence of postoperative shivering and postoperative cognitive dysfunction[293];
- a significantly higher temperature during or at the end of anesthesia[172,285,294,296];
- a lower rate of hypothermia (14%) compared with those who received room-temperature IV fluids (32%)[295]; and
- no maternal hypothermia and no significant differences in maternal or neonatal core body temperature on admission to the PACU.[286]

However, Choi et al[298] suggested that warmed IV fluids were not effective for prevention of unplanned hypothermia. This RCT involved 52 patients who underwent laparoscopic colorectal surgery. The participants were randomly assigned to either a control group that received room-temperature IV fluids or an experimental group that received warmed IV fluids. The researchers found a significantly smaller drop in core body temperature in the IV fluid warming group at 2 hours postinduction. However, they concluded that the temperature difference between the two groups at the end of the procedure was too small to recommend warming of IV fluids as an effective method for preventing hypothermia.

Clinical practice guidelines support warming of IV fluids.[92,93,98,140]

4.6.1 **Use US Food and Drug Administration (FDA)–cleared technology that is designed for warming IV fluids in accordance with the manufacturer's written instructions for use.** [*Recommendation*]

Using FDA-cleared technology that is designed for warming IV fluids reduces the risk of burning the patient.

A systematic review by Holtzclaw[43] and a multinational European guideline[92] recommend using technology designed for warming IV fluids.

The evidence comparing whether in-line warmers or fluid warming cabinets are more effective is inconclusive, and further research is needed. Andrzejowski et al[295] conducted an RCT and did not find significant differences in patient temperatures when using fluids warmed by in-line warmers, fluids warmed in fluid-warming cabinets, or room-temperature fluids. This study involved 76 surgical patients undergoing day surgery lasting less than 30 minutes who were to receive at least 1 L of IV fluids. The tympanic membrane temperature of those receiving room-temperature fluids was 0.4° C (0.72° F) lower than those receiving fluids warmed in the warming cabinet. Fourteen percent of those patients who received warmed fluid became hypothermic compared to 32% of those who received the room-temperature fluid. A limitation of this study is the very short time frame within which the fluids must be administered.

4.7 **Warmed irrigation solutions (33° C to 40° C [91.4° F to 104° F]) may be used.** [*Conditional Recommendation*] **P**

Although there is some high-quality evidence supporting the use of warmed irrigation solutions for prevention of hypothermia,[172,297,299-302] there is also some supporting low-quality evidence[303,304] and important variation in the study results. It is unclear whether the use of warmed irrigation solutions is an effective intervention for prevention of unplanned hypothermia when used without other interventions.

Campbell et al[297] conducted a systematic review and did not find significant differences in core body temperatures between patients who received warmed or room-temperature irrigation fluids. The review included five studies involving the use of warmed irrigation fluids that were published between 1986 and 2014 and involved a total of 310 participants. The risk of bias was either high or unclear related to inappropriate or unclear randomization and blinding procedures. Some of the studies described the use of warmed fluids but did not specify the fluid type as IV or irrigation fluid. The review authors were unable to determine whether the actual differences in temperature were clinically meaningful, whether there are other benefits or harms associated with the use of warmed IV fluids, and whether using fluid warming in addition to other warming methods increases the benefits.

Jin et al[302] performed a systematic review of 13 RCTs that compared the rate of hypothermia in patients receiving room-temperature irrigation solution to those receiving warmed solution. The studies included a total of 686 patients who underwent endoscopic surgery. The review authors found that the patients who received warmed irrigation solution had a lower rate of hypothermia compared with those who received room-temperature solution. The authors recommended warming irrigation solution to between 33° C and 40° C (91.4° F and 104° F).

Three RCTs,[172,300,301] two quasi-experimental studies,[299,303] and one nonexperimental study[304] published after these systematic reviews support the use of warmed irrigation fluids. These studies involved 246 patients who underwent orthopedic or urologic surgeries. The researchers compared warmed irrigation fluids to room-temperature irrigation fluids and combinations of warmed and room-temperature IV fluids. The researchers found that patients who received warmed irrigation fluids were less likely to experience hypothermia and a decrease in core body temperature than those who received room-temperature irrigation fluids.

However, Oh et al[305] did not find any benefit to using warmed irrigation solutions. In an RCT that involved 72 patients undergoing arthroscopic shoulder surgery, the researchers compared warmed irrigation fluid to room-temperature irrigation fluid. No other methods of active warming were used during the study. The researchers found no difference in the rate of hypothermia (temperature lower than 36° C [96.8° F]) between patients who received warmed irrigation fluids and those who received room-temperature fluids.

Warming of irrigation fluids to 38° C to 40° C (100.4° F to 104° F) is recommended in clinical practice guidelines.[92,98,140]

4.8 Radiant warming devices may be used. *[Conditional Recommendation]* P

In a quasi-experimental study, Yang et al[218] compared the time required for rewarming by applying warm cotton blankets to the time required for rewarming with the application of a radiant warming device for 130 hypothermic patients in the PACU. The researchers found that the time required for rewarming was shorter for the radiant warmer group than for the warm blanket group. The researchers concluded that the radiant warmer was more effective than warm cotton blankets for warming hypothermic patients.

Kadam et al[249] conducted an RCT that involved 29 patients undergoing laparoscopic cholecystectomy. The patients were warmed by a forced-air warmer (n = 15) or a radiant warming device applied to the face (n = 14). The researchers found no significant difference between the groups at 15 or 90 minutes, but four of the patients warmed with the radiant warming device experienced postoperative headaches. The researchers concluded the devices were equivalent in respect to the warming abilities.

Further research is needed to evaluate these study results and to evaluate the use of radiant warmers intraoperatively for the prevention of unplanned hypothermia.

4.9 Warm insufflation gases may be used as an adjunct to other active warming methods. *[Conditional Recommendation]* P

High-quality evidence regarding the warming of insufflation gases is inconclusive and may not be generalizable to all patients.[306-308]

In a systematic review of the literature, Birch et al[307] reviewed 22 RCTs that involved a total of 1,428 participants. The risk of bias was unclear in 10 studies, high in one, and low in 11. The review authors found no significant differences between the warmed and non-warmed groups in pain scores, morphine use 6 hours after surgery, time in the PACU, length of hospitalization, lens fogging, length of surgery, or frequency of major adverse events. Fourteen of the studies compared the intraoperative core body temperatures of patients insufflated with heated and humidified gas to those insufflated with room-temperature gas. These studies showed a higher temperature in the warmed groups, but when the analysis was limited to the eight studies with a low risk of bias, the difference became insignificant.

The review authors concluded there was a smaller decrease in core body temperature with the use of heated, humidified insufflation gas, but it did not result in an improvement in patient outcomes. The review authors stated that the results should be interpreted with caution because there were variations in study design related to varying insufflation gas temperatures, humidity ranges, gas volumes, and temperature probe locations.

In a systematic review published in 2008, Sajid et al[308] reviewed 10 RCTs involving 565 patients. The studies examined the effects of room-temperature carbon dioxide insufflation gas compared to warm humidified carbon dioxide insufflation gas on postoperative pain, risk of hypothermia, analgesic requirement, total hospital stay, and lens fogging. The studies showed the warmed gas group had significantly less postoperative pain, a lower incidence or no difference in the incidence of hypothermia, lower analgesia requirements, and no difference in length of hospital stay or lens fogging. The review authors concluded that warmed, humidified insufflation gases should be considered as the first choice for laparoscopic procedures.

However, in a nonexperimental study, Roth et al[306] used calorimetrics to determine the benefits of warming and humidifying insufflation gases and concluded they had very little effect on core body temperature. The researchers recommended that the decision to warm insufflation gases be based primarily on costs and consideration of other risks and benefits.

A clinical practice guideline from NICE[309] states that use of a warming device for insufflation gases during abdominal surgery shows promise, but there is insufficient evidence to recommend routine adoption of this technique for prevention of hypothermia.

4.10 Ambient room temperatures may be increased as an adjunct to other active warming methods. *[Conditional Recommendation]* P

Although there is some high-quality evidence regarding increasing ambient room temperature for prevention of hypothermia,[51,185,310-314] there is important variation in the study results. The greatest positive impact was seen in the pediatric population.

Cassey et al[185] conducted an RCT that involved children 6 weeks to 15 years of age scheduled for elective surgery lasting at least 20 minutes. The ambient temperature in the induction room was set at 21° C (69.8° F) for the control group (n = 30) and at 26° C (78.8° F) for the experimental group (n = 30). The patients' approximate length of stay in the induction room was 30 minutes and the duration of the anesthetic ranged from 20 to 50 minutes. The researchers found that the experimental group had a significantly higher core body temperature at 20 and 30 minutes postinduction.

Deren et al[312] conducted an RCT in which 66 patients who underwent elective knee or minimally invasive hip arthroplasty were randomly and equally assigned to an experimental or control group. The experimental room was prewarmed to a temperature of 24° C (75.2° F) for a period of 15 minutes before the patient arrived, and the temperature was decreased to 17° C (62.6° F) after induction, positioning, and application of an upper-body forced-air warming blanket. The control room was set at 17° C (62.6° F) for the entire procedure and an upper-body forced-air warming blanket was applied after positioning. The researchers found a marginally significant difference in the patients' temperatures between the prewarmed and control rooms when the forced-air warming blanket was activated and at the surgery start time but found no significant difference between the groups for the last recorded temperatures. The researchers concluded that prewarming the OR had minimal effect on preventing intraoperative hypothermia. A limitation of this study is that the researchers examined the effect of prewarming and not an increase in the ambient temperature for the entire procedure.

In a prospective study measuring the correlation between ambient OR temperature and the core body temperature in patients undergoing emergent surgery for trauma, Inaba et al[310] found that ambient OR temperature had no effect on core body temperature. The study involved 118 patients, of whom 29.7% had an admission temperature of > 35° C (> 95° F). All patients received warmed IV fluids, irrigation fluids, and anesthesia gases. A forced-air warming blanket was applied when possible. The ORs were set at a temperature between 20° C and 27° C (68° F and 80.6° F). Thirty-nine percent of the patients experienced a decrease in core body temperature, while 61% either maintained or experienced an increase in temperature.

A clinical practice guideline from ASPAN[140] and a multinational European guideline[92,140] also recommend increasing the OR ambient temperature.

4.11 **Document measures taken to maintain patient normothermia in the patient's medical record, including the warming method used, warming device identifier, and temperature settings when applicable.** [*Recommendation*] P

Documentation serves as a method of communication among all care providers involved in planning, implementing, and evaluating patient care. Documenting nursing activities provides a description of the perioperative nursing care administered and the status of patient outcomes on transfer of care.[148]

Glossary

Active warming method: A method that warms the patient by application of heat to the surface of the skin, blood, or internal structures and may be categorized as convective or conductive.

Electronic thermometer: A device used to measure the body temperature of a patient by means of a transducer coupled with an electronic signal amplification, conditioning, and display unit. The transducer may be in a detachable probe with or without a disposable cover.

Conductive heat loss: Body heat that is transferred from the body to another object by direct physical contact.

Conductive/resistive warming: A method of warming that uses electricity passing through a conductor to generate heat. Conductive systems transfer heat directly to the patient through contact with warm blankets or pads. Some systems use heated water circulating inside pads that wrap around the patient or conductive polymers or fabrics inside mattresses or blankets that do not contain heating elements, so the heat is dispersed evenly throughout the blanket with no hot or cold spots. Synonym: Resistive warming method.

Convective heat loss: Body heat lost when air moves across the skin.

Convective warming: A method of warming using a device that transfers heat to the body by warming the air surrounding the patient.

Double-sensor thermometry: A noninvasive method of measuring temperature using dual-sensor heat flux technology. Temperature is measured by a self-adhesive sensor placed on the patient's forehead.

Evaporative heat loss: Body heat lost through water evaporation from the skin and mucous membranes.

Hypothermia: Core body temperature below 36° C (96.8° F).

Liquid crystal temperature strip: A device applied to the forehead that changes color corresponding to the variation in the surface temperature of the skin. The liquid crystals, which are cholesteric esters, are sealed in plastic.

Normothermia: Normal core body temperature between 36° C and 38° C (96.8° F and 100.4° F).

Passive insulation method: A device used to prevent patient heat loss (eg, insulating garment, warm blanket).

Radiant heat loss: Body heat transferred to the environment when the environment is cooler than the body.

Reflective composite fabric: A fabric that reduces the amount of body heat lost through radiation and convection.

Thermocouple: A temperature sensor in which a pair of wires of dissimilar metals are joined, and the free ends of the wires are connected to an instrument that measures the difference in potential created at the junction of the two metals. A thermocouple produces a temperature-dependent voltage as a result of the thermoelectric effect, and this voltage can be interpreted to measure temperature.

Thermistor: A temperature sensor that uses a semi-conductor whose resistance varies sharply in a known manner with the temperature.

Zero-heat-flux thermometry: A noninvasive method for measuring core temperature in which a thermosensoric patch is applied to the lateral forehead.

References

1. Paulikas CA. Prevention of unplanned perioperative hypothermia. *AORN J.* 2008;88(3):358-365. [VC]

2. Beltramini AM, Salata RA, Ray AJ. Thermoregulation and risk of surgical site infection. *Infect Control Hosp Epidemiol.* 2011;32(6):603-610. [VB]

3. Journeaux M. Peri-operative hypothermia: implications for practice. *Nurs Stand.* 2013;27(45):33-38. [VA]

4. Mitchell JC, D'Angelo M. Implications of hypothermia in procedural areas. *J Radiol Nurs.* 2008;27(2):70-73. [VC]

5. Sessler DI. Perioperative thermoregulation and heat balance. *Lancet.* 2016;387(10038):2655-2664. [VA]

6. Lenhardt R. The effect of anesthesia on body temperature control. *Front Biosci (Schol Ed).* 2010;2:1145-1154. [VA]

7. Sessler DI. Perioperative heat balance. *Anesthesiology.* 2000;92(2):578-590. [VA]

8. Sessler DI. Thermoregulatory defense mechanisms. *Crit Care Med.* 2009;37(7 Suppl):S203-S210. [VA]

9. Sessler DI. Temperature monitoring and perioperative thermoregulation. *Anesthesiology.* 2008;109(2):318-338. [VA]

10. Matsukawa T, Sessler DI, Sessler AM, et al. Heat flow and distribution during induction of general anesthesia. *Anesthesiology.* 1995;82(3):662-673. [IIIA]

11. Kuht J, Farmery AD. Body temperature and its regulation. *Anaesth Intensive Care Med.* 2014;15(6):273-278. [VC]

12. Durel YP, Durel JB. A comprehensive review of thermoregulation and intraoperative hypothermia. *Curr Rev Nurse Anesth.* 2000;22(22):249. [VC]

13. Carrero EJ, Fàbregas N. Thermoregulation and neuroanesthesia. *Saudi J Anaesth.* 2012;6(1):5-7. [VC]

14. Burns SM, Wojnakowski M, Piotrowski K, Caraffa G. Unintentional hypothermia: implications for perianesthesia nurses. *J Perianesth Nurs.* 2009;24(3):167-173. [VB]

15. Kurz A. Physiology of thermoregulation. *Best Pract Res Clin Anaesthesiol.* 2008;22(4):627-644. [VA]

16. Lantry J, Dezman Z, Hirshon JM. Pathophysiology, management and complications of hypothermia. *Br J Hosp Med.* 2012;73(1):31-37. [VB]

17. Kim EJ, Yoon H. Preoperative factors affecting the intraoperative core body temperature in abdominal surgery under general anesthesia: an observational cohort. *Clin Nurse Spec.* 2014;28(5):268-276. [IIIB]

18. Benson EE, McMillan DE, Ong B. The effects of active warming on patient temperature and pain after total knee arthroplasty. *Am J Nurs.* 2012;112(5):26-33. [IC]

19. Lista F, Doherty CD, Backstein RM, Ahmad J. The impact of perioperative warming in an outpatient aesthetic surgery setting. *Aesthet Surg J.* 2012;32(5):613-620. [VB]

20. Vanamoorthy P, Pandia MP, Bithal PK, Valiaveedan SS. Refractory hypotension due to intraoperative hypothermia during spinal instrumentation. *Indian J Anaesth.* 2010;54(1):56-58. [VA]

21. Lau AW, Chen CC, Wu RS, Poon KS. Hypothermia as a cause of coagulopathy during hepatectomy. *Acta Anaesthesiol Taiwan.* 2010;48(2):103-106. [VA]

22. Niday LM. Intraoperative hypothermia and delayed awakening. *Int Student J Nurse Anesth.* 2011;10(1):34-39. [VB]

23. Kapetanopoulos A, Katsetos MC, Kluger J. Intraoperative hypothermia increased defibrillation energy requirements. *J Cardiovasc Med.* 2007;8(9):741-743. [VC]

24. John M, Ford J, Harper M. Peri-operative warming devices: performance and clinical application. *Anaesthesia.* 2014;69(6):623-638. [VC]

25. Torossian A. Thermal management during anaesthesia and thermoregulation standards for the prevention of inadvertent perioperative hypothermia. *Best Pract Res Clin Anaesthesiol.* 2008;22(4):659-668. [VB]

26. Reynolds L, Beckmann J, Kurz A. Perioperative complications of hypothermia. *Best Pract Res Clin Anaesthesiol.* 2008;22(4):645-657. [VA]

27. da Silva AB, Peniche Ade C. Perioperative hypothermia and incidence of surgical wound infection: a bibliographic study. *Einstein (Sao Paulo).* 2014;12(4):513-517. [VC]

28. Putzu M, Casati A, Berti M, Pagliarini G, Fanelli G. Clinical complications, monitoring and management of perioperative mild hypothermia: anesthesiological features. *Acta Biomed Ateneo Parmense.* 2007;78(3):163-169. [VB]

29. Kumar S, Wong PF, Melling AC, Leaper DJ. Effects of perioperative hypothermia and warming in surgical practice. *Int Wound J.* 2005;2(3):193-204. [VA]

30. Esnaola NF, Cole DJ. Perioperative normothermia during major surgery: is it important? *Adv Surg.* 2011;45:249-263. [VB]

31. Sohn VY, Steele SR. Temperature control and the role of supplemental oxygen. *Clin Colon Rectal Surg.* 2009;22(1):21-27. [VC]

32. Dickinson A, Qadan M, Polk HC Jr. Optimizing surgical care: a contemporary assessment of temperature, oxygen, and glucose. *Am Surg.* 2010;76(6):571-577. [VB]

33. Diaz M, Becker DE. Thermoregulation: physiological and clinical considerations during sedation and general anesthesia. *Anesth Prog.* 2010;57(1):25-32. [VC]

34. Kurz A. Thermal care in the perioperative period. *Best Pract Res Clin Anaesthesiol.* 2008;22(1):39-62. [VA]

35. Hernandez M, Cutter TW, Apfelbaum JL. Hypothermia and hyperthermia in the ambulatory surgical patient. *Clin Plast Surg.* 2013;40(3):429-438. [VB]

36. Hart SR, Bordes B, Hart J, Corsino D, Harmon D. Unintended perioperative hypothermia. *Ochsner J.* 2011;11(3):259-270. [VA]

37. Heier T, Caldwell JE. Impact of hypothermia on the response to neuromuscular blocking drugs. *Anesthesiology.* 2006;104(5):1070-1080. [VC]

38. Pearce B, Christensen R, Voepel-Lewis T. Perioperative hypothermia in the pediatric population: prevalence, risk factors and outcomes. *J Anesth Clin Res.* 2010;1:102. [IIIC]

39. Jeyadoss J, Thiruvenkatarajan V, Watts RW, Sullivan T, van Wijk RM. Intraoperative hypothermia is associated with an increased intensive care unit length-of-stay in patients undergoing elective open abdominal aortic aneurysm surgery: a retrospective cohort study. *Anaesth Intensive Care.* 2013;41(6):759-764. [IIIC]

40. Uzoigwe CE, Khan A, Smith RP, et al. Hypothermia and low body temperature are common and associated with high mortality in hip fracture patients. *Hip Int.* 2014;24(3):237-242. [IIIC]

41. Qadan M, Gardner SA, Vitale DS, Lominadze D, Joshua IG, Polk HC Jr. Hypothermia and surgery: immunologic mechanisms for current practice. *Ann Surg.* 2009;250(1):134-140. [IIIC]

42. Caldwell JE, Heier T, Wright PM, et al. Temperature-dependent pharmacokinetics and pharmacodynamics of vecuronium. *Anesthesiology.* 2000;92(1):84-93. [VC]

43. Holtzclaw BJ. Managing inadvertent and accidental hypothermia. *Online J Clin Innov.* 2008;10(2):1-58. [IIIA]

44. Mahoney CB, Odom J. Maintaining intraoperative normothermia: a meta-analysis of outcomes with costs. *AANA J.* 1999;67(2):155-163. [IIIB]

45. Fred C, Ford S, Wagner D, Vanbrackle L. Intraoperatively acquired pressure ulcers and perioperative normothermia: a look at relationships. *AORN J.* 2012;96(3):251-260. [IIIB]

46. Hannan EL, Samadashvili Z, Wechsler A, et al. The relationship between perioperative temperature and adverse outcomes after off-pump coronary artery bypass graft surgery. *J Thorac Cardiovasc Surg.* 2010;139(6):1568-1575. [IIIA]

47. Quiroga E, Tran NT, Hatsukami T, Starnes BW. Hypothermia is associated with increased mortality in patients undergoing repair of ruptured abdominal aortic aneurysm. *J Endovasc Ther.* 2010;17(3):434-438. [IIIB]

48. Morehouse D, Williams L, Lloyd C, et al. Perioperative hypothermia in NICU infants: its occurrence and impact on infant outcomes. *Adv Neonatal Care.* 2014;14(3):154-164. [IIIB]

49. Yamasaki H, Tanaka K, Funai Y, et al. The impact of intraoperative hypothermia on early postoperative adverse events after radical esophagectomy for cancer: a retrospective cohort study. *J Cardiothorac Vasc Anesth.* 2014;28(4):955-959. [IIIA]

50. Moslemi-Kebria M, El-Nashar SA, Aletti GD, Cliby WA. Intraoperative hypothermia during cytoreductive surgery for ovarian cancer and perioperative morbidity. *Obstet Gynecol.* 2012;119(3):590-596. [IIIA]

51. Coon D, Michaels J5, Gusenoff JA, Chong T, Purnell C, Rubin JP. Hypothermia and complications in postbariatric body contouring. *Plast Reconstr Surg.* 2012;130(2):443-448. [IIIA]

52. Poveda VB, Nascimento AS. The effect of intraoperative hypothermia upon blood transfusion needs and length of stay among gastrointestinal system cancer surgery. *Eur J Cancer Care (Engl).* 2017;26(6). [IIIB]

53. Billeter AT, Hohmann SF, Druen D, Cannon R, Polk HC Jr. Unintentional perioperative hypothermia is associated with severe complications and high mortality in elective operations. *Surgery.* 2014;156(5):1245-1252. [IIIA]

54. Sim R, Hall NJ, de Coppi P, Eaton S, Pierro A. Core temperature falls during laparotomy in infants with necrotizing enterocolitis. *Eur J Pediatr Surg.* 2012;22(1):45-49. [IIIB]

55. Konstantinidis A, Inaba K, Dubose J, et al. The impact of nontherapeutic hypothermia on outcomes after severe traumatic brain injury. *J Trauma.* 2011;71(6):1627-1631. [IIIB]

56. Seamon MJ, Wobb J, Gaughan JP, Kulp H, Kamel I, Dempsey DT. The effects of intraoperative hypothermia on surgical site infection: an analysis of 524 trauma laparotomies. *Ann Surg.* 2012;255(4):789-795. [IIIB]

57. Karalapillai D, Story DA, Calzavacca P, Licari E, Liu YL, Hart GK. Inadvertent hypothermia and mortality in postoperative intensive care patients: retrospective audit of 5050 patients. *Anaesthesia.* 2009;64(9):968-972. [IIIA]

58. Sumer BD, Myers LL, Leach J, Truelson JM. Correlation between intraoperative hypothermia and perioperative morbidity in patients with head and neck cancer. *Arch Otolaryngol Head Neck Surg.* 2009;135(7):682-686. [IIIB]

59. Sun Z, Honar H, Sessler DI, et al. Intraoperative core temperature patterns, transfusion requirement, and hospital duration in patients warmed with forced air. *Anesthesiology.* 2015;122(2):276-285. [IIIA]

60. Karalapillai D, Story D, Hart GK, et al. Postoperative hypothermia and patient outcomes after elective cardiac surgery. *Anaesthesia.* 2011;66(9):780-784. [IIIA]

61. Flaifel HA, Ayoub F. Esophageal temperature monitoring. *Middle East J Anesthesiol.* 2007;19(1):123-147. [IIIB]

62. Romlin B, Petruson K, Nilsson K. Moderate superficial hypothermia prolongs bleeding time in humans. *Acta Anaesthesiol Scand.* 2007;51(2):198-201. [IIIB]

63. Emmert A, Franke R, Brandes IF, et al. Comparison of conductive and convective warming in patients undergoing video-assisted thoracic surgery: a prospective randomized clinical trial. *Thorac Cardiovasc Surg.* 2017;65(5):362-366. [IIIB]

64. Yi J, Lei Y, Xu S, et al. Intraoperative hypothermia and its clinical outcomes in patients undergoing general anesthesia: national study in China. *Plos One.* 2017;12(6):e0177221. [IIIA]

65. Kiekkas P, Theodorakopoulou G, Stefanopoulos N, Tsotas D, Baltopoulos GI. Postoperative hypothermia and mortality in critically ill adults: review and meta-analysis. *Aust J Adv Nurs.* 2011;28(4):60-67. [IIIB]

66. Frisch NB, Pepper AM, Jildeh TR, Shaw J, Guthrie T, Silverton C. Intraoperative hypothermia during surgical fixation of hip fractures. *Orthopedics.* 2016;39(6):e1170-e1177. [IIIB]

67. Scott EM, Buckland R. A systematic review of intraoperative warming to prevent postoperative complications. *AORN J.* 2006;83(5):1090-1113. [IA]

68. Rajagopalan S, Mascha E, Na J, Sessler DI. The effects of mild perioperative hypothermia on blood loss and transfusion requirement. *Anesthesiology.* 2008;108(1):71-77. [IA]

69. Kurz A, Sessler DI, Lenhardt R. Perioperative normothermia to reduce the incidence of surgical-wound infection and shorten hospitalization. Study of Wound Infection and Temperature Group. *N Engl J Med.* 1996;334(19):1209-1215. [IA]

70. Winkler M, Akca O, Birkenberg B, et al. Aggressive warming reduces blood loss during hip arthroplasty. *Anesth Analg.* 2000;91(4):978-984. [IB]

71. Schmied H, Kurz A, Sessler DI, Kozek S, Reiter A. Mild hypothermia increases blood loss and transfusion requirements during total hip arthroplasty. *Lancet.* 1996;347(8997):289-292. [IB]

72. Frank SM, Fleisher LA, Breslow MJ, et al. Perioperative maintenance of normothermia reduces the incidence of morbid cardiac events. A randomized clinical trial. *JAMA.* 1997;277(14):1127-1134. [IB]

73. Baucom RB, Phillips SE, Ehrenfeld JM, et al. Defining intraoperative hypothermia in ventral hernia repair. *J Surg Res.* 2014;190(1):385-390. [IIIA]

74. Young H, Bliss R, Carey JC, Price CS. Beyond core measures: identifying modifiable risk factors for prevention of surgical site infection after elective total abdominal hysterectomy. *Surg Infect (Larchmt).* 2011;12(6):491-496. [IIIB]

75. Constantine RS, Kenkel M, Hein RE, et al. The impact of perioperative hypothermia on plastic surgery outcomes: a multivariate logistic regression of 1062 cases. *Aesthet Surg J.* 2015;35(1):81-88. [IIIB]

76. Karalapillai D, Story D, Hart GK, et al. Postoperative hypothermia and patient outcomes after major elective noncardiac surgery. *Anaesthesia.* 2013;68(6):605-611. [IIIB]

77. Fecho K, Lunney AT, Boysen PG, Rock P, Norfleet EA. Postoperative mortality after inpatient surgery: Incidence and risk factors. *Ther Clin Risk Manag.* 2008;4(4):681-688. [IIIA]

78. Lehtinen SJ, Onicescu G, Kuhn KM, Cole DJ, Esnaola NF. Normothermia to prevent surgical site infections after gastrointestinal surgery: Holy grail or false idol? *Ann Surg.* 2010;252(4):696-704. [IIIA]

79. Melton GB, Vogel JD, Swenson BR, Remzi FH, Rothenberger DA, Wick EC. Continuous intraoperative temperature measurement and surgical site infection risk: analysis of anesthesia information system data in 1008 colorectal procedures. *Ann Surg.* 2013;258(4):606-612; discussion 612-613. [IIIA]

80. Baucom RB, Phillips SE, Ehrenfeld JM, et al. Association of perioperative hypothermia during colectomy with surgical site infection. *JAMA Surg.* 2015;150(6):570-575. [IIIA]

81. Brown MJ, Curry TB, Hyder JA, et al. Intraoperative hypothermia and surgical site infections in patients with class I/clean wounds: a case-control study. *J Am Coll Surg.* 2017;224(2):160-171. [IIIA]

82. Geiger TM, Horst S, Muldoon R, et al. Perioperative core body temperatures effect on outcome after colorectal resections. *Am Surg.* 2012;78(5):607-612. [IIIB]

83. Tedesco NS, Korpi FP, Pazdernik VK, Cochran JM. Relationship between hypothermia and blood loss in adult patients undergoing open lumbar spine surgery. *J Am Osteopath Assoc.* 2014;114(11):828-838. [IIIA]

84. Long KC, Tanner EJ, Frey M, et al. Intraoperative hypothermia during primary surgical cytoreduction for advanced ovarian cancer: risk factors and associations with postoperative morbidity. *Gynecol Oncol.* 2013;131(3):525-530. [IIIA]

85. Linam WM, Margolis PA, Staat MA, et al. Risk factors associated with surgical site infection after pediatric posterior spinal fusion procedure. *Infect Control Hosp Epidemiol.* 2009;30(2):109-116. [IIIA]

86. Salazar F, Donate M, Boget T, et al. Intraoperative warming and post-operative cognitive dysfunction after total knee replacement. *Acta Anaesthesiol Scand.* 2011;55(2):216-222. [IA]

87. Smith CE, Sidhu RS, Lucas L, Mehta D, Pinchak AC. Should patients undergoing ambulatory surgery with general anesthesia be actively warmed? *Internet J Anesthesiol.* 2007;12(1). [IB]

88. Winslow EH, Cooper SK, Haws DM, et al. Unplanned perioperative hypothermia and agreement between oral, temporal artery, and bladder temperatures in adult major surgery patients. *J Perianesth Nurs.* 2012;27(3):165-180. [IIIA]

89. Rightmyer J, Singbartl K. Preventing perioperative hypothermia. *Nursing.* 2016;46(9):57-60. [VC]

90. Nygren J, Thacker J, Carli F, et al. Guidelines for perioperative care in elective rectal/pelvic surgery: Enhanced Recovery After Surgery (ERAS®) society recommendations. *Clin Nutr.* 2012;31(6):801-816. [IVA]

91. Temperature monitoring during surgical procedures. Malignant Hyperthermia Association of the United States. https://www.mhaus.org/mhau001/assets/File/Temperature%20Monitoring%20during%20Surgical%20Procedures.pdf. Developed 2012. Accessed March 23, 2019. [IVB]

92. Torossian A, Brauer A, Hocker J, Bein B, Wulf H, Horn EP. Preventing inadvertent perioperative hypothermia. *Dtsch Arztebl Int.* 2015;112(10):166-172. [IVA]

93. Forbes SS, Eskicioglu C, Nathens AB, et al. Best Practice in General Surgery Committee, University of Toronto. Evidence-based guidelines for prevention of perioperative hypothermia. *J Am Coll Surg.* 2009;209(4):492-503. [IVA]

94. *AST Standards of Practice for Maintenance of Normothermia in the Perioperative Patient.* Littleton, CO: Association of Surgical Technologists; 2015. [IVB]

95. Gustafsson UO, Scott MJ, Schwenk W, et al. Guidelines for perioperative care in elective colonic surgery: Enhanced Recovery After Surgery (ERAS®) Society recommendations. *Clin Nutr.* 2012;31(6):783-800. [IVA]

96. *Standards for Nurse Anesthesia Practice.* Park Ridge, IL: American Association of Nurse Anesthetists; 2019. [IVB]

97. O'Grady NP, Barie PS, Bartlett JG, et al. Guidelines for evaluation of new fever in critically ill adult patients: 2008 update from the American College of Critical Care Medicine and the Infectious Diseases Society of America. *Crit Care Med.* 2008;36(4):1330-1349. [IVB]

98. National Collaborating Centre for Nursing and Supportive Care. *The Management of Inadvertent Perioperative Hypothermia in Adults* (NICE Clinical Guidelines, No. 65). London, UK: Royal College of Nursing; 2008. https://www.ncbi.nlm.nih.gov/books/NBK53797/. Accessed April 3, 2019. [IVC]

99. Neft M, Quraishi JA, Greenier E. A closer look at the standards for nurse anesthesia practice. *AANA J.* 2013;81(2):92-96. [IVC]

100. Standards for basic anesthetic monitoring. American Society of Anesthesiologists. https://www.asahq.org/standards-and-guidelines/standards-for-basic-anesthetic-monitoring. Amended 2015. Accessed April 3, 2019. [IVC]

101. Sessler DI. Temperature monitoring: the consequences and prevention of mild perioperative hypothermia. *South Afr J Anaesth Analg.* 2014;20(1):25-31. [VB]

102. Singh A. Strategies for the management and avoidance of hypothermia in the perioperative environment. *J Perioper Pract.* 2014;24(4):75-78. [VB]

103. Aksu C, Kuş A, Gürkan Y, Solak M, Toker K. Survey on postoperative hypothermia incidence in operating theatres of Kocaeli University. *Turk Anesteziyoloji ve Reanimasyon Dernegi Dergisi.* 2014;42(2):66-70. [IIIB]

104. Eshraghi Y, Nasr V, Parra-Sanchez I, et al. An evaluation of a zero-heat-flux cutaneous thermometer in cardiac surgical patients. *Anesth Analg.* 2014;119(3):543-549. [IIIB]

105. *Bair Hugger for Measuring Core Temperature During Perioperative Care.* MedTech Innovation Briefing. London, England: National Institute for Health and Care Excellence; 2017. [VA]

106. Brandes IF, Perl T, Bauer M, Brauer A. Evaluation of a novel noninvasive continuous core temperature measurement system with a zero heat flux sensor using a manikin of the human body. *Biomed Tech (Berl).* 2015;60(1):1-9. [IIIC]

107. Schell-Chaple HM, Liu KD, Matthay MA, Puntillo KA. Rectal and bladder temperatures vs forehead core temperatures measured with SpotOn monitoring system. *Am J Crit Care.* 2018;27(1):43-50. [IIIB]

108. Mäkinen M, Pesonen A, Jousela I, et al. Novel zero-heat-flux deep body temperature measurement in lower extremity vascular and cardiac surgery. *J Cardiothorac Vasc Anesth.* 2016;30(4):973-978. [IIIC]

109. Dahyot-Fizelier C, Lamarche S, Kerforne T, et al. Accuracy of zero-heat-flux cutaneous temperature in intensive care adults. *Crit Care Med.* 2017;45(7):e715-e717. [IIIB]

110. Iden T, Horn EP, Bein BF, Böhm RF, Beese JF, Höcker J. Intraoperative temperature monitoring with zero heat flux technology (3M SpotOn sensor) in comparison with sublingual and nasopharyngeal temperature: an observational study. *Eur J Anaesthesiol.* 2015;32(6):387-391. [IIIB]

111. Kimberger O, Thell R, Schuh M, Koch J, Sessler DI, Kurz A. Accuracy and precision of a novel non-invasive core thermometer. *Br J Anaesth.* 2009;103(2):226-231. [IIB]

112. Kimberger O, Saager L, Egan C, et al. The accuracy of a disposable noninvasive core thermometer. *Can J Anaesth.* 2013;60(12):1190-1196. [IIB]

113. Hardcastle TC, Stander M, Kalafatis N, Hodgson RE, Gopalan D. External patient temperature control in emergency centres, trauma centres, intensive care units and operating theatres: a multi-society literature review. *S Afr Med J.* 2013;103(9):609-611. [VA]

114. Lefrant JY, Muller L, de La Coussaye JE, et al. Temperature measurement in intensive care patients: comparison of urinary bladder, oesophageal, rectal, axillary, and inguinal methods versus pulmonary artery core method. *Intensive Care Med.* 2003;29(3):414-418. [IIIB]

115. Erdling A, Johansson A. Core temperature—the intraoperative difference between esophageal versus nasopharyngeal temperatures and the impact of prewarming, age, and weight: a randomized clinical trial. *AANA J.* 2015;83(2):99-105. [IB]

116. Pawley MD, Martinsen P, Mitchell SJ, et al. Brachial arterial temperature as an indicator of core temperature: proof of concept and potential applications. *J Extra Corpor.* 2013;45(2):86-93. [IIIB]

117. Gobolos L, Philipp A, Ugocsai P, et al. Reliability of different body temperature measurement sites during aortic surgery. *Perfusion.* 2014;29(1):75-81. [IIIB]

118. Langham GE, Maheshwari A, Contrera K, You J, Mascha E, Sessler DI. Noninvasive temperature monitoring in postanesthesia care units. *Anesthesiology.* 2009;111(1):90-96. [IIB]

119. Calonder EM, Sendelbach S, Hodges JS, et al. Temperature measurement in patients undergoing colorectal surgery and gynecology surgery: a comparison of esophageal core, temporal artery, and oral methods. *J Perianesth Nurs.* 2010;25(2):71-78. [IIB]

120. Hooper VD, Andrews JO. Accuracy of noninvasive core temperature measurement in acutely ill adults: the state of the science. *Biol Res Nurs.* 2006;8(1):24-34. [IIIA]

121. Hocker J, Bein B, Bohm R, Steinfath M, Scholz J, Horn EP. Correlation, accuracy, precision and practicability of perioperative measurement of sublingual temperature in comparison with tympanic membrane temperature in awake and anaesthetised patients. *Eur J Anaesthesiol.* 2012;29(2):70-74. [IIB]

122. Sato H, Yamakage M, Okuyama K, et al. Urinary bladder and oesophageal temperatures correlate better in patients with high rather than low urinary flow rates during noncardiac surgery. *Eur J Anaesthesiol.* 2008;25(10):805-809. [IB]

123. Moran JL, Peter JV, Solomon PJ, et al. Tympanic temperature measurements: are they reliable in the critically ill? A clinical study of measures of agreement. *Crit Care Med.* 2007;35(1):155-164. [IIIA]

124. Sahin SH, Duran R, Sut N, Colak A, Acunas B, Aksu B. Comparison of temporal artery, nasopharyngeal, and axillary temperature measurement during anesthesia in children. *J Clin Anesth.* 2012;24(8):647-651. [IIB]

125. Smith J. Methods and devices of temperature measurement in the neonate: a narrative review and practice recommendations. *Newborn Infant Nurs Rev.* 2014;14(2):64-71. [VA]

126. Lawson L, Bridges EJ, Ballou I, et al. Accuracy and precision of noninvasive temperature measurement in adult intensive care patients. *Am J Crit Care.* 2007;16(5):485-496. [IIIB]

127. Farnell S, Maxwell L, Tan S, Rhodes A, Philips B. Temperature measurement: comparison of non-invasive methods used in adult critical care. *J Clin Nurs.* 2005;14(5):632-639. [IIIB]

128. Frommelt T, Ott C, Hays V. Accuracy of different devices to measure temperature. *MEDSURG Nursing.* 2008;17(3):171-174. [IIA]

129. Kiya T, Yamakage M, Hayase T, Satoh J, Namiki A. The usefulness of an earphone-type infrared tympanic thermometer for intraoperative core temperature monitoring. *Anesth Analg.* 2007;105(6):1688-1692. [IIIB]

130. Masamune T, Yamauchi M, Wada K, et al. The usefulness of an earphone-type infrared tympanic thermometer

during cardiac surgery with cardiopulmonary bypass: clinical report. *J Anesth.* 2011;25(4):576-579. [IIB]

131. Apa H, Gözmen S, Bayram N, et al. Clinical accuracy of tympanic thermometer and noncontact infrared skin thermometer in pediatric practice: an alternative for axillary digital thermometer. *Pediatr Emerg Care.* 2013;29(9):992-997. [IIIB]

132. Drake-Brockman TFE, Hegarty M, Chambers NA, Von Ungernsternberg BS. Monitoring temperature in children undergoing anaesthesia: a comparison of methods. *Anaesth Intensive Care.* 2014;42(3):315-320. [IIIA]

133. Minzola DJ, Keele R. Relationship of tympanic and temporal temperature modalities to core temperature in pediatric surgical patients. *AANA J.* 2018;86(1):19-26. [IIIB]

134. Eyelade OR, Orimadegun AE, Akinyemi OA, Tongo OO, Akinyinka OO. Esophageal, tympanic, rectal, and skin temperatures in children undergoing surgery with general anesthesia. *J Perianesth Nurs.* 2011;26(3):151-159. [IIIB]

135. Barringer LB, Evans CW, Ingram LL, Tisdale PP, Watson SP, Janken JK. Agreement between temporal artery, oral, and axillary temperature measurements in the perioperative period. *J Perianesth Nurs.* 2011;26(3):143-150. [IIIA]

136. Furlong D, Carroll DL, Finn C, Gay D, Gryglik C, Donahue V. Comparison of temporal to pulmonary artery temperature in febrile patients. *Dimens Crit Care Nurs.* 2015;34(1):47-52. [IIIB]

137. McConnell E, Senseney D, George SS, Whipple D. Reliability of temporal artery thermometers. *Medsurg Nurs.* 2013;22(6):387-392. [IIIA]

138. Kimberger O, Cohen D, Illievich U, Lenhardt R. Temporal artery versus bladder thermometry during perioperative and intensive care unit monitoring. *Anesth Analg.* 2007;105(4):1042-1047. [IIIB]

139. Stelfox HT, Straus SE, Ghali WA, Conly J, Laupland K, Lewin A. Temporal artery versus bladder thermometry during adult medical-surgical intensive care monitoring: an observational study. *BMC Anesthesiol.* 2010;10:13. [IIIA]

140. Hooper VD, Chard R, Clifford T, et al. ASPAN's evidence-based clinical practice guideline for the promotion of perioperative normothermia: second edition. *J Perianesth Nurs.* 2010;25(6):346-365. [IVA]

141. Asher C, Northington LK. *SPN Position Statement: Temperature Measurement.* Chicago, IL: Society of Pediatric Nurses; 2016. http://www.pedsnurses.org/p/cm/ld/fid=220&tid=28&sid=1574. Accessed April 3, 2019. [IVC]

142. Counts D, Acosta M, Holbrook H, et al. Evaluation of temporal artery and disposable digital oral thermometers in acutely ill patients. *Medsurg Nurs.* 2014;23(4):239-250. [IIIA]

143. Fetzer SJ, Lawrence A. Tympanic membrane versus temporal artery temperatures of adult perianesthesia patients. *J Perianesth Nurs.* 2008;23(4):230-236. [IIIB]

144. Washington GT, Matney JL. Comparison of temperature measurement devices in post anesthesia patients. *J Perianesth Nurs.* 2008;23(1):36-48. [IIIA]

145. Collins JB, Verheyden CN, Mahabir RC. Core measures: implications for plastic surgery. *Plast Reconstr Surg.* 2013;131(6):1266-1271. [VB]

146. Arshad M, Qureshi WA, Ali A, Haider SZ. Frequency of hypothermia during general anaesthesia. *Pak J Med Health Sci.* 2011;5(3):549-552. [IIIC]

147. Horosz B, Malec-Milewska M. Methods to prevent intraoperative hypothermia. *Anaesthesiol Intensive Ther.* 2014;46(2):96-100. [VA]

148. Guideline for health care information management. In: *Guidelines for Perioperative Practice.* Denver, CO: AORN, Inc; 2019:371-400. [IVB]

149. Guideline for team communication. In: *Guidelines for Perioperative Practice.* Denver, CO: AORN, Inc; 2019:1093-1120. [IVA]

150. Yokoe DS, Anderson DJ, Berenholtz SM, et al. A compendium of strategies to prevent healthcare-associated infections in acute care hospitals: 2014 updates. *Infect Control Hosp Epidemiol.* 2014;35(8):967-977. [IVB]

151. Fleisher LA, Fleischmann KE, Auerbach AD, et al. 2014 ACC/AHA guideline on perioperative cardiovascular evaluation and management of patients undergoing noncardiac surgery: a report of the American College of Cardiology/American Heart Association Task Force on Practice Guidelines. *Circulation.* 2014;130(24):2215-2245. [IVA]

152. Berrios-Torres SI, Umscheid CA, Bratzler DW, et al. Centers for Disease Control and Prevention guideline for the prevention of surgical site infection, 2017. *JAMA Surg.* 2017;152(8):784-791. [IVA]

153. Chon JY, Lee JY. The effects of surgery type and duration of tourniquet inflation on body temperature. *J Int Med Res.* 2012;40(1):358-365. [IIIA]

154. Khan SA, Aurangzeb M, Zarin M, Khurshid M. Temperature monitoring and perioperative heat loss. *J Postgrad Med Inst.* 2010;24(2):85-90. [IIIC]

155. Leijtens B, Koeter M, Kremers K, Koeter S. High incidence of postoperative hypothermia in total knee and total hip arthroplasty: a prospective observational study. *J Arthroplasty.* 2013;28(6):895-898. [IIIB]

156. Parodi D, Tobar C, Valderrama J, et al. Hip arthroscopy and hypothermia. *Arthroscopy.* 2012;28(7):924-928. [IIIB]

157. Hoda MR, Popken G. Maintaining perioperative normothermia during laparoscopic and open urologic surgery. *J Endourol.* 2008;22(5):931-938. [IIB]

158. Mehta OH, Barclay KL. Perioperative hypothermia in patients undergoing major colorectal surgery. *ANZ J Surg.* 2014;84(7-8):550-555. [IIIB]

159. de Brito Poveda V, Galvão C, Santos CB. Factors associated to the development of hypothermia in the intraoperative period. *Rev Lat Am Enfermagem.* 2009;17(2):228-233. [IIIB]

160. Guideline for care of patients undergoing pneumatic tourniquet-assisted procedures. In: *Guidelines for Perioperative Practice.* Denver, CO: AORN, Inc; 2019:607-636. [IVB]

161. Guideline for prevention of venous thromboembolism. In: *Guidelines for Perioperative Practice.* Denver, CO: AORN, Inc; 2019:1123-1152. [IVB]

162. Standards of perioperative nursing. In: *Guidelines for Perioperative Practice.* Denver, CO: AORN, Inc; 2015:693-708. https://www.aorn.org/guidelines/clinical-resources/aorn-standards. Accessed April 3, 2019. [IVB]

163. Huh J, Cho YB, Yang MK, Yoo YK, Kim DK. What influence does intermittent pneumatic compression of the lower limbs intraoperatively have on core hypothermia? *Surg Endosc.* 2013;27(6):2087-2093. [IA]

164. Han SB, Gwak MS, Choi SJ, et al. Risk factors for inadvertent hypothermia during adult living-donor liver transplantation. *Transplant Proc.* 2014;46(3):705-708. [IIIB]

165. Araz C, Pirat A, Unlukaplan A, et al. Incidence and risk factors of intraoperative adverse events during donor lobectomy for living-donor liver transplantation: a retrospective analysis. *Exp Clin Transplant.* 2012;10(2):125-131. [IIIA]

166. Talley HC, Talley CH. AANA Journal course update for nurse anesthetists—part 5: evaluation of older adults. *AANA J.* 2009;77(6):451-460. [VB]

167. Yang R, Wolfson M, Lewis MC. Unique aspects of the elderly surgical population: an anesthesiologist's perspective. *Geriatr Orthop Surg Rehabil.* 2011;2(2):56-64. [VA]

168. Maintaining perioperative normothermia. *J Perioper Pract.* 2017;27(1):4-9. [VB]

169. Guedes Lopes I, Sousa Magalhães AM, Abreu dS, Batista dA. Preventing perioperative hypothermia: an integrative literature review. *Revista de Enfermagem Referência.* 2015;8(1):147-155. [IIIC]

170. Eich C, Zink W, Schwarz SKW, Radke O, Bräuer A. A combination of convective and conductive warming ensures pre- and post-bypass normothermia in paediatric cardiac anaesthesia. *Appl Cardiopulm Pathophysiol.* 2009;13(1):3-10. [IIIC]

171. Pagnocca ML, Tai EJ, Dwan JL. Temperature control in conventional abdominal surgery: Comparison between conductive and the association of conductive and convective warming. *Rev Bras Anestesiol.* 2009;59(1):56-66. [IB]

172. Okeke LI. Effect of warm intravenous and irrigating fluids on body temperature during transurethral resection of the prostate gland. *BMC Urol.* 2007;7:15. [IB]

173. Cho YJ, Lee SY, Kim TK, Hong DM, Jeon Y, eds. Effect of prewarming during induction of anesthesia on microvascular reactivity in patients undergoing off-pump coronary artery bypass surgery: a randomized clinical trial. *Plos One.* 2016;11(7):e0159772. [IC]

174. Minchin I. Management of temperature & major abdominal surgery. *Dissector.* 2009;37(3):13-15. [IIC]

175. Koc BB, Schotanus MGM, Kollenburg JAPAC, Janssen MJA, Tijssen F, Jansen EJP. Effectiveness of early warming with self-warming blankets on postoperative hypothermia in total hip and knee arthroplasty. *Orthop Nurs.* 2017;36(5):356-360. [IC]

176. Munday J, Hines S, Wallace K, Chang AM, Gibbons K, Yates P. A systematic review of the effectiveness of warming interventions for women undergoing cesarean section. *Worldviews Evid Based Nurs.* 2014;11(6):383-393. [IB]

177. Gorges M, Ansermino JM, Whyte SD. A retrospective audit to examine the effectiveness of preoperative warming on hypothermia in spine deformity surgery patients. *Paediatr Anaesth.* 2013;23(11):1054-1061. [IIIB]

178. Gorges M, West NC, Cheung W, Zhou G, Miyanji F, Whyte SD. Preoperative warming and undesired surgical and anesthesia outcomes in pediatric spinal surgery—a retrospective cohort study. *Paediatr Anaesth.* 2016;26(9):866-875. [IIIB]

179. Moola S, Lockwood C. Effectiveness of strategies for the management and/or prevention of hypothermia within the adult perioperative environment. *Int J Evid Based Healthc.* 2011;9(4):337-345. [IA]

180. Perl T, Peichl LH, Reyntjens K, Deblaere I, Zaballos JM, Bräuer A. Efficacy of a novel prewarming system in the prevention of perioperative hypothermia. A prospective, randomized, multicenter study. *Minerva Anestesiol.* 2014;80(4):436-443. [IA]

181. de Brito Poveda V, Clark AM, Galvão CM. A systematic review on the effectiveness of prewarming to prevent perioperative hypothermia. *J Clin Nurs.* 2013;22(7-8):906-918. [IA]

182. Rosenkilde C, Vamosi M, Lauridsen J, Hasfeldt D. Efficacy of prewarming with a self-warming blanket for the prevention of unintended perioperative hypothermia in patients undergoing hip or knee arthroplasty. *J Perianesth Nurs.* 2017;32(5):419-428. [IIB]

183. Llewellyn L. Effect of pre-warming on reducing the incidence of inadvertent peri-operative hypothermia for patients undergoing general anaesthesia: a mini-review. *British Journal of Anaesthetic & Recovery Nursing.* 2013;14(1-2):3-10. [IA]

184. Roberson MC, Dieckmann LS, Rodriguez RE, Austin PN. A review of the evidence for active preoperative warming of adults undergoing general anesthesia. *AANA J.* 2013;81(5):351-356. [IIB]

185. Cassey JG, King RA, Armstrong P. Is there thermal benefit from preoperative warming in children? *Paediatr Anaesth.* 2010;20(1):63-71. [IB]

186. Jo YY, Chang YJ, Kim YB, Lee S, Kwak HJ, eds. Effect of preoperative forced-air warming on hypothermia in elderly patients undergoing transurethral resection of the prostate. *Urol J.* 2015;12(5):2366-2370. [IB]

187. Melling AC, Ali B, Scott EM, Leaper DJ. Effects of preoperative warming on the incidence of wound infection after clean surgery: a randomised controlled trial. *Lancet.* 2001;358(9285):876-880. [IA]

188. Shin KM, Ahn JH, Kim IS, et al. The efficacy of prewarming on reducing intraprocedural hypothermia in endovascular coiling of cerebral aneurysms. *BMC Anesthesiol.* 2015;15:8. [IA]

189. Wong PF, Kumar S, Bohra A, Whetter D, Leaper DJ. Randomized clinical trial of perioperative systemic warming in major elective abdominal surgery. *Br J Surg.* 2007;94(4):421-426. [IB]

190. Horn EP, Bein B, Broch O, et al. Warming before and after epidural block before general anaesthesia for major abdominal surgery prevents perioperative hypothermia: a randomised controlled trial. *Eur J Anaesthesiol.* 2016;33(5):334-340. [IB]

191. Wasfie TJ, Barber KR. Value of extended warming in patients undergoing elective surgery. *Int Surg.* 2015;100(1):105-108. [IB]

192. D'Angelo Vanni SM, Castiglia YM, Ganem EM, et al. Preoperative warming combined with intraoperative skin-surface warming does not avoid hypothermia caused by spinal anesthesia in patients with midazolam premedication. *Sao Paulo Med J.* 2007;125(3):144-149. [IB]

193. Connelly L, Cramer E, DeMott Q, et al. The optimal time and method for surgical prewarming: a comprehensive review of the literature. *J Perianesth Nurs.* 2017;32(3):199-209. [IIIA]

194. Nicholson M. A comparison of warming interventions on the temperatures of inpatients undergoing colorectal surgery. *AORN J.* 2013;97(3):310-322. [IC]

195. Rowley B, Kerr M, Van Poperin J, Everett C, Stommel M, Lehto RH. Perioperative warming in surgical patients: a comparison of interventions. *Clin Nurs Res.* 2015;24(4):432-441. [IIC]

196. Adriani MB, Moriber N. Preoperative forced-air warming combined with intraoperative warming versus intraoperative warming alone in the prevention of hypothermia during gynecologic surgery. *AANA J.* 2013;81(6):446-451. [IIA]

197. Shukry M, Matthews L, de Armendi AJ, et al. Does the covering of children during induction of anesthesia have an effect on body temperature at the end of surgery? *J Clin Anesth.* 2012;24(2):116-120. [IA]

198. Akhtar Z, Hesler BD, Fiffick AN, et al. A randomized trial of prewarming on patient satisfaction and thermal comfort in outpatient surgery. *J Clin Anesth.* 2016;33:376-385. [IA]

199. Munday J, Osborne S, Yates P, Sturgess D, Jones L, Gosden E. Preoperative warming versus no preoperative warming for maintenance of normothermia in women receiving intrathecal morphine for cesarean delivery: a single-blinded, randomized controlled trial. *Anesth Analg.* 2018;126(1):183-189. [IB]

200. Lassen K, Soop M, Nygren J, et al. Consensus review of optimal perioperative care in colorectal surgery: Enhanced Recovery After Surgery (ERAS) group recommendations. *Arch Surg.* 2009;144(10):961-969. [IVC]

201. Lassen K, Coolsen M, Slim K, et al. Guidelines for perioperative care for pancreaticoduodenectomy: Enhanced Recovery After Surgery (ERAS®) Society recommendations. *Clin Nutr.* 2012;31(6):817-830. [IVA]

202. Horn EP, Schroeder F, Gottschalk A, et al. Active warming during cesarean delivery. *Anesth Analg.* 2002;94(2):409-414. [IA]

203. Chung SH, Lee BS, Yang HJ, et al. Effect of preoperative warming during cesarean section under spinal anesthesia. *Korean J Anesthesiol.* 2012;62(5):454-460. [IB]

204. Andrzejowski J, Hoyle J, Eapen G, Turnbull D. Effect of prewarming on post-induction core temperature and the incidence of inadvertent perioperative hypothermia in patients undergoing general anaesthesia. *Br J Anaesth.* 2008;101(5):627-631. [IB]

205. Warttig S, Alderson P, Campbell G, Smith AF. Interventions for treating inadvertent postoperative hypothermia. *Cochrane Database of Syst Rev.* 2014;11:CD009892. [IA]

206. Alderson P, Campbell G, Smith AF, Warttig S, Nicholson A, Lewis SR. Thermal insulation for preventing inadvertent perioperative hypothermia. *Cochrane Database Syst Rev.* 2014:6:CD009908. [IA]

207. Tjoakarfa C, David V, Ko A, Hau R. Reflective blankets are as effective as forced air warmers in maintaining patient normothermia during hip and knee arthroplasty surgery. *J Arthroplasty.* 2017;32(2):624-627. [IC]

208. Koëter M, Leijtens B, Koëter S. Effect of thermal reflective blanket placement on hypothermia in primary unilateral total hip or knee arthroplasty. *J Perianesth Nurs.* 2013;28(6):347-352. [IC]

209. Koenen M, Passey M, Rolfe M. "Keeping them warm"—a randomized controlled trial of two passive perioperative warming methods. *J Perianesth Nurs.* 2017;32(3):188-198. [IB]

210. Kurnat-Thoma E, Roberts MM, Corcoran EB. Perioperative heat loss Prevention—a feasibility trial. *AORN J.* 2016;104(4):307-319. [IIB]

211. Lee HY, Kim G, Shin Y. Effects of perioperative warm socks-wearing in maintaining core body temperature of patients undergoing spinal surgery. *J Clin Nurs.* 2018;27(7):1399-1407. [IIC]

212. Cobb B, Cho Y, Hilton G, Ting V, Carvalho B. Active warming utilizing combined IV fluid and forced-air warming decreases hypothermia and improves maternal comfort during cesarean delivery: a randomized control trial. *Anesth Analg.* 2016;122(5):1490-1497. [IC]

213. Madrid E, Urrútia G, Roqué i Figuls M, et al. Active body surface warming systems for preventing complications caused by inadvertent perioperative hypothermia in adults. *Cochrane Database Syst Rev.* 2016;4: CD009016. [IA]

214. Shaw CA, Steelman VM, DeBerg J, Schweizer ML. Effectiveness of active and passive warming for the prevention of inadvertent hypothermia in patients receiving neuraxial anesthesia: a systematic review and meta-analysis of randomized controlled trials. *J Clin Anesth.* 2017;38:93-104. [IA]

215. Sultan P, Habib AS, Cho Y, Carvalho B. The effect of patient warming during caesarean delivery on maternal and neonatal outcomes: a meta-analysis. *Br J Anaesth.* 2015;115(4):500-510. [IA]

216. Allen GS. Intraoperative temperature control using the Thermogard system during off-pump coronary artery bypass grafting. *Ann Thorac Surg.* 2009;87(1):284-288. [IB]

217. Pikus E, Hooper VD. Postoperative rewarming: are there alternatives to warm hospital blankets. *J Perianesth Nurs.* 2010;25(1):11-23. [IIIB]

218. Yang HI, Lee HF, Chu TL, Su YY, Ho LH, Fan JY. The comparison of two recovery room warming methods for hypothermia patients who had undergone spinal surgery. *J Nurs Scholarsh.* 2012;44(1):2-10. [IIB]

219. Yoo HS, Park SW, Yi JW, Kwon MI, Rhee YG. The effect of forced-air warming during arthroscopic shoulder surgery with general anesthesia. *Arthroscopy.* 2009;25(5):510-514. [IB]

220. Torossian A, Van Gerven E, Geertsen K, Horn B, Van de Velde M, Raeder J. Active perioperative patient warming using a self-warming blanket (BARRIER EasyWarm) is superior to passive thermal insulation: a multinational, multicenter, randomized trial. *J Clin Anesth.* 2016;34:547-554. [IA]

221. Chakladar A, Dixon MJ, Crook D, Harper CM. The effects of a resistive warming mattress during caesarean section: a randomised, controlled trial. *Int J Obstet Anesth.* 2014;23(4):309-316. [IA]

222. Sharma M, Dixon M, Eljelani F, Crook D, Harper M. A randomised controlled trial to determine the influence of carbon-polymer warming blankets on the incidence of perioperative hypothermia during and after short, day-case operations. *J One Day Surg.* 2014;24(4):92-99. [IB]

223. Allen PB, Salyer SW, Dubick MA, Holcomb JB, Blackbourne LH. Preventing hypothermia: comparison of current devices

used by the US army in an in vitro warmed fluid model. *J Trauma.* 2010;69(Suppl 1):S154-61. [IIB]

224. Horn EP, Bein B, Steinfath M, Ramaker K, Buchloh B, Hocker J. The incidence and prevention of hypothermia in newborn bonding after cesarean delivery: a randomized controlled trial. *Anesth Analg.* 2014;118(5):997-1002. [IA]

225. Borms SF, Engelen SL, Himpe DG, Suy MR, Theunissen WJ. Bair Hugger forced-air warming maintains normothermia more effectively than Thermo-lite insulation. *J Clin Anesth.* 1994;6(4):303-307. [IB]

226. Sato H, Yamakage M, Okuyama K, et al. Forced-air warming effectively prevents midazolam-induced core hypothermia in volunteers. *Eur J Anaesthesiol.* 2009;26(7):566-571. [IIC]

227. Zeba S, Surbatovic M, Marjanovic M, et al. Efficacy of external warming in attenuation of hypothermia in surgical patients. *Vojnosanit pregl.* 2016;73(6):566-571. [IC]

228. Panossian C, Simoes CM, Milani WR, Baranauskas MB, Margarido CB. The intraoperative use of warming blankets in patients undergoing radical prostatectomy is related with a reduction in post-anesthetic recovery time. *Rev Bras Anestesiol.* 2008;58(3):220-226. [IIIC]

229. Witt L, Dennhardt N, Eich C, et al. Prevention of intraoperative hypothermia in neonates and infants: results of a prospective multicenter observational study with a new forced-air warming system with increased warm air flow. *Paediatr Anaesth.* 2013;23(6):469-474. [IIIB]

230. Shorrab AA, El-Sawy ME, Othman MM, Hammouda GE. Prevention of hypothermia in children under combined epidural and general anesthesia: a comparison between upper- and lower-body warming. *Paediatr Anaesth.* 2007;17(1):38-43. [IIB]

231. Steelman VM. Conductive skin warming and hypothermia: an observational study. *AANA J.* 2017;85(6):461-468. [IIIB]

232. de Bernardis RC, Siaulys MM, Vieira JE, Mathias LA, eds. Perioperative warming with a thermal gown prevents maternal temperature loss during elective cesarean section. A randomized clinical trial. *Braz J Anesthesiol.* 2016;66(5):451-455. [IB]

233. Nieh HS, Shu-Fen. Forced-air warming for rewarming and comfort following laparoscopy: a randomized controlled trail. *Clin Nurs Res.* 2018;27(5):540-559. [IA]

234. Pu Y, Cen G, Sun J, et al. Warming with an underbody warming system reduces intraoperative hypothermia in patients undergoing laparoscopic gastrointestinal surgery: a randomized controlled study. *Int J Nurs Stud.* 2014;51(2):181-189. [IA]

235. Kim YS, Jeon YS, Lee JA, et al. Intra-operative warming with a forced-air warmer in preventing hypothermia after tourniquet deflation in elderly patients. *J Int Med Res.* 2009;37(5):1457-1464. [IA]

236. Leung KK, Lai A, Wu A. A randomised controlled trial of the electric heating pad vs forced-air warming for preventing hypothermia during laparotomy. *Anaesthesia.* 2007;62(6):605-608. [IB]

237. Ihn CH, Joo JD, Chung HS, et al. Comparison of three warming devices for the prevention of core hypothermia and post-anaesthesia shivering. *J Int Med Res.* 2008;36(5):923-931. [IB]

238. Rajan S, Halemani KR, Puthenveettil N, Baalachandran R, Gotluru P, Paul J. Are active warming measures required

during paediatric cleft surgeries? *Indian J Anaesth.* 2013;57(4):377-380. [IB]

239. Su S, Nieh H. Efficacy of forced-air warming for preventing perioperative hypothermia and related complications in patients undergoing laparoscopic surgery: A randomized controlled trial. *Int J Nurs Pract.* [IA]

240. Fleisher LA, Metzger SE, Lam J, Harris A. Perioperative cost-finding analysis of the routine use of intraoperative forced-air warming during general anesthesia. *Anesthesiology.* 1998;88(5):1357-1364. [IB]

241. Moysés AM, dos Santos Trettene A, Navarro LH, Ayres JA. Hypothermia prevention during surgery: Comparison between thermal mattress and thermal blanket. *Rev Esc Enfermagem USP.* 2014;48(2):226-252. [IB]

242. Nieh HC, Su FS. Meta-analysis: effectiveness of forced-air warming for prevention of perioperative hypothermia in surgical patients. *J Adv Nurs.* 2016;72(10):2294-2314. [IA]

243. de Brito Poveda V, Martinez EZ, Galvão CM. Active cutaneous warming systems to prevent intraoperative hypothermia: a systematic review. *Rev Lat Am.* 2012;20(1):183-191. [IC]

244. Fanelli A, Danelli G, Ghisi D, Ortu A, Moschini E, Fanelli G. The efficacy of a resistive heating under-patient blanket versus a forced-air warming system: a randomized controlled trial. *Anesth Analg.* 2009;108(1):199-201. [IC]

245. Sandoval MF, Mongan PD, Dayton MR, Hogan CA. Safety and efficacy of resistive polymer versus forced air warming in total joint surgery. *Patient Saf Surg.* 2017;11:11. [VA]

246. Kimberger O, Held C, Stadelmann K, et al. Resistive polymer versus forced-air warming: comparable heat transfer and core rewarming rates in volunteers. *Anesth Analg.* 2008;107(5):1621-1626. [IB]

247. Tanaka N, Ohno Y, Hori M, Utada M, Ito K, Suzuki T. A randomised controlled trial of the resistive heating blanket versus the convective warming system for preventing hypothermia during major abdominal surgery. *J Perioper Pract.* 2013;23(4):82-86. [IB]

248. Egan C, Bernstein E, Reddy D, et al. A randomized comparison of intraoperative PerfecTemp and forced-air warming during open abdominal surgery. *Anesth Analg.* 2011;113(5):1076-1081. [IB]

249. Kadam VR, Moyes D, Moran JL. Relative efficiency of two warming devices during laparoscopic cholecystectomy. *Anaesth Intensive Care.* 2009;37(3):464-468. [IB]

250. Ruetzler K, Kovaci B, Guloglu E, et al. Forced-air and a novel patient-warming system (vitalHEAT vH2) comparably maintain normothermia during open abdominal surgery. *Anesth Analg.* 2011;112(3):608-614. [IIB]

251. Ng V, Lai A, Ho V. Comparison of forced-air warming and electric heating pad for maintenance of body temperature during total knee replacement. *Anaesthesia.* 2006;61(11):1100-1104. [IA]

252. Galvão CM, Marck PB, Sawada NO, Clark AM. A systematic review of the effectiveness of cutaneous warming systems to prevent hypothermia. *J Clin Nurs.* 2009;18(5):627-636. [IA]

253. Wadhwa A, Komatsu R, Orhan-Sungur M, et al. New circulating-water devices warm more quickly than forced-air in volunteers. *Anesth Analg.* 2007;105(6):1681-1687. [IC]

254. Rein EB, Filtvedt M, Walloe L, Raeder JC. Hypothermia during laparotomy can be prevented by locally applied warm water and pulsating negative pressure. *Br J Anaesth.* 2007;98(3):331-336. [IC]

255. Kjellman BM, Fredrikson M, Glad-Mattsson G, Sjöberg F, Huss FR. Comparing ambient, air-convection, and fluid-convection heating techniques in treating hypothermic burn patients, a clinical RCT. *Ann Surg Innov Res.* 2011;5(1):4. [IC]

256. Butwick AJ, Lipman SS, Carvalho B. Intraoperative forced air-warming during cesarean delivery under spinal anesthesia does not prevent maternal hypothermia. *Anesth Analg.* 2007;105(5):1413-1419. [IC]

257. Hasegawa K, Nakagawa F, Negishi C, Ozaki M. Core temperatures during major abdominal surgery in patients warmed with new circulating-water garment, forced-air warming, or carbon-fiber resistive-heating system. *J Anesth.* 2012;26(2):168-173. [IIA]

258. Calcaterra D, Ricci M, Lombardi P, Katariya K, Panos A, Salerno TA. Reduction of postoperative hypothermia with a new warming device: a prospective randomized study in off-pump coronary artery surgery. *J Cardiovasc Surg.* 2009;50(6):813-817. [IA]

259. De Witte JL, Demeyer C, Vandemaele E. Resistive-heating or forced-air warming for the prevention of redistribution hypothermia. *Anesth Analg.* 2010;110(3):829-833. [IA]

260. Hofer CK, Worn M, Tavakoli R, et al. Influence of body core temperature on blood loss and transfusion requirements during off-pump coronary artery bypass grafting: a comparison of 3 warming systems. *J Thorac Cardiovasc Surg.* 2005;129(4):838-843. [IC]

261. Sugai H, Koizumi T, Sumita S, Yamakage M. Relative clinical heat transfer effectiveness: forcedair warming vs. conductive fabric electric warming, A randomized controlled trial. *J Anesth Surg.* 2018;5(2):123-126. [IC]

262. Janicki PK, Higgins MS, Janssen J, Johnson RF, Beattie C. Comparison of two different temperature maintenance strategies during open abdominal surgery: upper body forced-air warming versus whole body water garment. *Anesthesiology.* 2001;95(4):868-874. [IB]

263. Haeberle HS, Navarro SM, Samuel LT, et al. No evidence of increased infection risk with forced-air warming devices: a systematic review. *Surg Technol Int.* 2017;31:295-301. [IIIC]

264. Dasari KB, Albrecht M, Harper M. Effect of forced-air warming on the performance of operating theatre laminar flow ventilation. *Anaesthesia.* 2012;67(3):244-249. [IIB]

265. Reed M, Kimberger O, McGovern PD, Albrecht MC. Forced-air warming design: evaluation of intake filtration, internal microbial buildup, and airborne-contamination emissions. *AANA J.* 2013;81(4):275-280. [IIIB]

266. Albrecht M, Gauthier RL, Belani K, Litchy M, Leaper D. Forced-air warming blowers: an evaluation of filtration adequacy and airborne contamination emissions in the operating room. *Am J Infect Control.* 2011;39(4):321-328. [IIIB]

267. Albrecht M, Gauthier R, Leaper D. Forced-air warming: a source of airborne contamination in the operating room? *Orthop Rev (Pavia).* 2009;1(2):e28. [IIIB]

268. He X, Karra S, Pakseresht P, Apte SV, Elghobashi S. Effect of heated-air blanket on the dispersion of squames in an operating room. *Int J Numer Method Biomed Eng.* 2018;34(5):e2960. [IIIB]

269. Zink RS, Iaizzo PA. Convective warming therapy does not increase the risk of wound contamination in the operating room. *Anesth Analg.* 1993;76(1):50-53. [IIC]

270. Huang JK, Shah EF, Vinodkumar N, Hegarty MA, Greatorex RA. The Bair Hugger patient warming system in prolonged vascular surgery: an infection risk? *Crit Care.* 2003;7(3):R13-R16. [IIIB]

271. Kellam MD, Dieckmann LS, Austin PN. Forced-air warming devices and the risk of surgical site infections. *AORN J.* 2013;98(4):354-366. [IIIB]

272. Sessler DI, Olmsted RN, Kuelpmann R. Forced-air warming does not worsen air quality in laminar flow operating rooms. *Anesth Analg.* 2011;113(6):1416-1421. [IIB]

273. Sikka RS, Prielipp RC. Forced air warming devices in orthopaedics: a focused review of the literature. *J Bone Joint Surg Am.* 2014;96(24):e200. [VB]

274. Chung K, Lee S, Oh SC, Choi J, Cho HS. Thermal burn injury associated with a forced-air warming device. *Korean J Anesthesiol.* 2012;62(4):391-392. [VC]

275. Wu X. The safe and efficient use of forced-air warming systems. *AORN J.* 2013;97(3):302-308. [VB]

276. Brauer A, Quintel M. Forced-air warming: technology, physical background and practical aspects. *Curr Opin Anaesthesiol.* 2009;22(6):769-774. [VA]

277. Chapp K, Lange L. Warming blanket head drapes and trapped anesthetic gases: understanding the fire risk. *AORN J.* 2011;93(6):749-760. [VB]

278. Wagner K, Smith CE, Quan KJ. Prevention of hypothermia during interventional cardiology procedures in adults. *Internet J Anesthesiol.* 2010;23(2). [IB]

279. Kiridume K, Hifumi T, Kawakita K, et al. Clinical experience with an active intravascular rewarming technique for near-severe hypothermia associated with traumatic injury. *J Intensive Care.* 2014;2(1):11. [VB]

280. Perez-Protto S, Sessler DI, Reynolds LF, et al. Circulating-water garment or the combination of a circulating-water mattress and forced-air cover to maintain core temperature during major upper-abdominal surgery. *Br J Anaesth.* 2010;105(4):466-470. [IC]

281. Trentman TL, Weinmeister KP, Hentz JG, Laney MB, Simula DV. Randomized non-inferiority trial of the vitalHEAT temperature management system vs the Bair Hugger warmer during total knee arthroplasty. *Can J Anaesth.* 2009;56(12):914-920. [IB]

282. Dostálová V, Schreiberova J, Bartoš M, et al. Thermal management in patients undergoing elective spinal surgery in prone position—a prospective randomized trial. *Cesk Slov Neurol N.* 2017;80/113(5):553-560. [IC]

283. Engelen S, Berghmans J, Borms S, Suy-Verburg M, Himpe D. Resistive heating during off-pump coronary bypass surgery. *Acta Anaesthesiol Belg.* 2007;58(1):27-31. [IIC]

284. Perl T, Rhenius A, Eich CB, Quintel M, Heise D, Bräuer A. Conductive warming and insulation reduces perioperative hypothermia. *Cent Eur J Med.* 2012;7(3):284-289. [IA]

285. Paris LG, Seitz M, McElroy KG, Regan M. A randomized controlled trial to improve outcomes utilizing various warming techniques during cesarean birth. *J Obstet Gynecol Neonatal Nurs.* 2014;43(6):719-728. [IA]

286. Chebbout R, Newton RS, Walters M, Wrench IJ, Woolnough M. Does the addition of active body warming to in-line intravenous fluid warming prevent maternal hypothermia during elective caesarean section? A randomised controlled trial. *Int J Obstet Anesth.* 2017;31:37-44. [IC]

287. Brandt S, Oguz R, Hüttner H, et al. Resistive-polymer versus forced-air warming: comparable efficacy in orthopedic patients. *Anesth Analg.* 2010;110(3):834-838. [IA]

288. Jo YY, Kim HS, Chang YJ, Yun SY, Kwak HJ. The effect of warmed inspired gases on body temperature during arthroscopic shoulder surgery under general anesthesia. *Korean J Anesthesiol.* 2013;65(1):14-18. [IA]

289. Anaegbu N, Olatosi O, Tobi K. Effectiveness of heat moisture exchangers (hmes) in preventing perioperative hypothermia among adult patients undergoing abdominal surgery under general endotracheal anaesthesia. *J West Afr Coll Surg.* 2013;3(3):16-32. [IB]

290. Lee Y, Kim H. The effects of heated humidified gases on body temperature and shivering in patients under general anesthesia. *Int J Biosci Biotechnol.* 2013;5(4):61-72. [IIB]

291. Lee HK, Jang YH, Choi KW, Lee JH. The effect of electrically heated humidifier on the body temperature and blood loss in spinal surgery under general anesthesia. *Korean J Anesthesiol.* 2011;61(2):112-116. [IB]

292. Han SB, Gwak MS, Choi SJ, et al. Effect of active airway warming on body core temperature during adult liver transplantation. *Transplant Proc.* 2013;45(1):251-254. [IB]

293. Ma H, Lai B, Dong S, et al, eds. Warming infusion improves perioperative outcomes of elderly patients who underwent bilateral hip replacement. *Medicine (Baltimore).* 2017;96(13):e6490. [IC]

294. Kim G, Kim MH, Lee SM, Choi SJ, Shin YH, Jeong HJ. Effect of pre-warmed intravenous fluids on perioperative hypothermia and shivering after ambulatory surgery under monitored anesthesia care. *J Anesth.* 2014;28(6):880-885. [IA]

295. Andrzejowski JC, Turnbull D, Nandakumar A, Gowthaman S, Eapen G. A randomised single blinded study of the administration of pre-warmed fluid vs active fluid warming on the incidence of peri-operative hypothermia in short surgical procedures. *Anaesthesia.* 2010;65(9):942-945. [IA]

296. Hong-xia X, Zhi-jian Y, Hong Z, Zhiqing L. Prevention of hypothermia by infusion of warm fluid during abdominal surgery. *J Perianesth Nurs.* 2010;25(6):366-370. [IB]

297. Campbell G, Alderson P, Smith AF, et al. Warming of intravenous and irrigation fluids for preventing inadvertent perioperative hypothermia. *Cochrane Database Syst Rev.* 2015;(4):CD009891. [IIA]

298. Choi JW, Kim DK, Lee SW, Park JB, Lee GH. Efficacy of intravenous fluid warming during goal-directed fluid therapy in patients undergoing laparoscopic colorectal surgery: a randomized controlled trial. *J Int Med Res.* 2016;44(3):605-612. [IA]

299. Parodi D, Valderrama J, Tobar C, et al. Effect of warmed irrigation solution on core body temperature during hip arthroscopy for femoroacetabular impingement. *Arthroscopy.* 2014;30(1):36-41. [IIA]

300. Pan X, Ye L, Liu Z, Wen H, Hu Y, Xu X. Effect of irrigation fluid temperature on core body temperature and inflammatory response during arthroscopic shoulder surgery. *Arch Orthop Trauma Surg.* 2015;135(8):1131-1139. [IB]

301. Tekgul ZT, Pektas S, Yildirim U, et al. A prospective randomized double-blind study on the effects of the temperature of irrigation solutions on thermoregulation and postoperative complications in percutaneous nephrolithotomy. *J Anesth.* 2015;29(2):165-169. [IA]

302. Jin Y, Tian J, Sun M, Yang K. A systematic review of randomised controlled trials of the effects of warmed irrigation fluid on core body temperature during endoscopic surgeries. *J Clin Nurs.* 2011;20(3-4):305-316. [IB]

303. Board TN, Srinivasan MS. The effect of irrigation fluid temperature on core body temperature in arthroscopic shoulder surgery. *Arch Orthop Trauma Surg.* 2008;128(5):531-533. [IIC]

304. Mirza S, Panesar S, AuYong KJ, French J, Jones D, Akmal S. The effects of irrigation fluid on core temperature in endoscopic urological surgery. *J Perioper Pract.* 2007;17(10):494-503. [IIIC]

305. Oh JH, Kim JY, Chung SW, et al. Warmed irrigation fluid does not decrease perioperative hypothermia during arthroscopic shoulder surgery. *Arthroscopy.* 2014;30(2):159-164. [IA]

306. Roth JV, Sea S. An assessment by calorimetric calculations of the potential thermal benefit of warming and humidification of insufflated carbon dioxide. *Surg Laparosc Endosc Percutan Tech.* 2014;24(3):e106-e109. [IIIB]

307. Birch DW, Dang JT, Switzer NJ, et al. Heated insufflation with or without humidification for laparoscopic abdominal surgery. *Cochrane Database Syst Rev.* 2016;10:CD007821. [IA]

308. Sajid MS, Mallick AS, Rimpel J, Bokari SA, Cheek E, Baig MK. Effect of heated and humidified carbon dioxide on patients after laparoscopic procedures: a meta-analysis. *Surg Laparosc Endosc Percutan Tech.* 2008;18(6):539-546. [IB]

309. *HumiGard for Preventing Inadvertent Perioperative Hypothermia (Medical Technologies Guidance [MTG31]).* London, UK: National Institute for Health and Care Excellence; 2017. [IVC]

310. Inaba K, Berg R, Barmparas G, et al. Prospective evaluation of ambient operating room temperature on the core temperature of injured patients undergoing emergent surgery. *J Trauma Acute Care Surg.* 2012;73(6):1478-1483. [IIIB]

311. Cheng KW, Wang CH, Chen CL, et al. Decreased fresh gas flow cannot compensate for an increased operating room temperature in maintaining body temperature during donor hepatectomy for living liver donor hepatectomy. *Transplant Proc.* 2010;42(3):703-704. [IIIB]

312. Deren ME, Machan JT, DiGiovanni CW, Ehrlich MG, Gillerman RG. Prewarming operating rooms for prevention of

intraoperative hypothermia during total knee and hip arthroplasties. *J Arthroplasty.* 2011;26(8):1380-1386. [IA]

313. Ozer AB, Tosun F, Demirel I, Unlu S, Bayar MK, Erhan OL. The effects of anesthetic technique and ambient temperature on thermoregulation in lower extremity surgery. *J Anesth.* 2013;27(4):528-534. [IIB]

314. Kent AL, Williams J. Increasing ambient operating theatre temperature and wrapping in polyethylene improves admission temperature in premature infants. *J Paediatr Child Health.* 2008;44(6):325-331. [IIB]

Guideline Development Group

Lead Author: Byron L. Burlingame[1], MS, BSN, RN, CNOR, Senior Perioperative Nursing Specialist, AORN Nursing
Methodologist: Amber Wood[2], MSN, RN, CNOR, CIC, FAPIC, Editor-in-Chief, Guidelines for Perioperative Practice, AORN, Denver, Colorado
Evidence Appraisers: Byron L. Burlingame[1]; Doreen Wagner[3], PhD, RN, CNOR, Professor, Kennesaw State University, Kennesaw, Georgia; and Amber Wood[2]
Subject Matter Expert: Doreen Wagner[3]

Guidelines Advisory Board Members:

- Donna A. Pritchard[4], MA, BSN, RN, NE-BC, CNOR, Director of Perioperative Services, Interfaith Medical Center, Brooklyn, New York
- Mary C. Fearon[5], MSN, RN, CNOR, Service Line Director Neuroscience, Overlake Medical Center, Sammamish, Washington
- Brenda G. Larkin[6], MS, ACNS-BC, CNS, CNOR, Clinical Nurse Specialist, Aurora Lakeland Medical Center, Lake Geneva, Wisconsin
- Elizabeth S. Pincus[7], MSN, MBA, RN, ACNS-BC, CNS-CP, CNOR, Clinical Nurse, St Francis Hospital, Roslyn, New York
- Darlene B. Murdock[8], BSN, BA, RN, CNOR, Clinical Staff Nurse IV, Memorial Herman Texas Medical Center, Houston, Texas

Guidelines Advisory Board Liaisons:

- Leslie Ann Jeter[9], MSNA, RN, CRNA, Staff CRNA, Ambulatory Anesthesia of Atlanta, Georgia
- Craig S. Atkins[10], DNP, CRNA, Chief Nurse Anesthetist, Belmar ASC, LLC, Denver, Colorado
- Lynn J. Reede[11], DNP, MBA, CRNA, FNAP, Senior Director, Professional Practice, American Association of Nurse Anesthetists, Des Plaines, Illinois
- Cassie Dietrich[12], MD, Anesthesiologist, Anesthesia Associate of Kansas City, Overland Park, Kansas
- Brian J. Cammarata[13], MD, Partner & Director of Risk Management, Old Pueblo Anesthesia, Tucson, Arizona

External Review: Expert review comments were received from individual members of the American Association of Nurse Anesthetists (AANA), American College of Surgeons (ACS) and the American Society of Anesthesiologists (ASA). Their responses were used to further refine and enhance this guideline; however, their responses do not imply endorsement. The draft was also open for a 30-day public comment period.

Financial Disclosure and Conflicts of Interest

This guideline was developed, edited, and approved by the AORN Guidelines Advisory Board without external funding being sought or obtained. The guideline was financially supported entirely by AORN and was developed without any involvement of industry. Potential conflicts of interest for all Guidelines Advisory Board members were reviewed before the annual meeting and each monthly conference call. None of the members of the Guideline Development Group reported a potential conflict of interest.[1-13]

Publication History

Originally published as Recommended Practices for the Prevention of Unplanned Perioperative Hypothermia in *Perioperative Standards and Recommended Practices, 2008* edition.

Minor editing revisions made to omit PNDS codes; reformatted September 2012 for publication in *Perioperative Standards and Recommended Practices*, 2013 edition.

Minor editing revision made in November 2014 for publication as Guideline for Prevention of Unplanned Perioperative Hypothermia in *Guidelines for Perioperative Practice*, 2015 edition.

Revised November 2015 for online publication as Guideline for Prevention of Unplanned Patient Hypothermia in *Guidelines for Perioperative Practice.*

Revised 2019 for online publication in Guidelines for *Perioperative Practice.*

Scheduled for review in 2024.

INFORMATION MANAGEMENT

TABLE OF CONTENTS

[P] *indicates a recommendation or evidence relevant to pediatric care.*

MEDICAL ABBREVIATIONS & ACRONYMS

ARRA – American Recovery and Reinvestment Act
CDI – Clinical documentation improvement
CMS – Centers for Medicare & Medicaid Services
EHR – Electronic health record
EMR – Electronic medical record
FTP – File transfer protocol
HIPAA – Health Insurance Portability and Accountability Act

HITECH – Health Information Technology for Economic and Clinical Health
ONC – Office of the National Coordinator for Health Information Technology
PNDS – Perioperative Nursing Data Set
RN – Registered nurse
SNOMED-CT – Systematized Nomenclature of Medicine—Clinical Terms

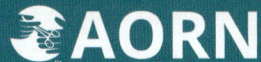

GUIDELINE FOR
PATIENT INFORMATION MANAGEMENT

The Guideline for Patient Information Management was approved by the AORN Guidelines Advisory Board and became effective July 1, 2016. It was presented as a proposed guideline for comments by members and others. The recommendations in the guideline are intended to be achievable and represent what is believed to be an optimal level of practice. Policies and procedures will reflect variations in practice settings and/or clinical situations that determine the degree to which the guideline can be implemented. AORN recognizes the many diverse settings in which perioperative nurses practice; therefore, this guideline is adaptable to all areas where operative or other invasive procedures may be performed.

Purpose

This document provides guidance to assist perioperative nurses in documenting and managing patient care information within the perioperative practice setting. Highly reliable data collection is not only necessary to chronicle the patient's response to nursing interventions, but also to demonstrate the health care organization's progress toward improving health care outcomes. Health care data collection and retention is rapidly transitioning from traditional paper formats to standardized electronic applications that incorporate criteria from statutes and regulations, accreditation requirements, and standards-setting bodies. Whether patient data are captured using paper or electronic formats, the nursing process should be completed for each surgical or procedural intervention performed.[1,2]

The nursing process is a formalized systematic approach to providing and documenting patient care that is embedded within perioperative patient care workflow (ie, clinical workflow). Comprehensive perioperative documentation accurately reflects the patient experience and is essential for the continuity of goal-directed nursing care and for effective comparison of realized versus anticipated patient outcomes.[3,4]

This document should be viewed as a conceptual outline that can be used to create a comprehensive documentation platform. It is not inclusive of all documentation elements, nor should it be seen as the only guideline that may be used when developing or revising a clinical documentation system.

The following topics are outside the scope of this document: **electronic health record** (EHR) adoption, accreditation requirements for health information technology criteria, EHR certification, EHR human factors science, establishing health information exchanges and interoperability requirements, submission of mandatory quality reporting criteria, hand-off communication requirements, perioperative team communications, requirements to complete data analytics, and patient access to personal health information.

Evidence Review

A medical librarian conducted a systematic search of the databases MEDLINE®, CINAHL®, and the Cochrane Database of Systematic Reviews. The librarian also conducted a nonsystematic search of the Scopus® database. Results were limited to literature published in English from January 2011 to June 2015. During the development of the guideline, the lead author requested additional articles that either did not fit the original search criteria or were discovered during the evidence appraisal process, and the lead author and the medical librarian identified relevant guidelines from government agencies and standards-setting bodies. At the time of the initial search, the librarian established weekly alerts on the search topics and until October 2015, presented relevant alert results to the lead author.

Search terms included the subject headings and keywords *medical informatics, nursing informatics, documentation, information management, medical records, electronic health records, computerized patient records, information storage and retrieval, forms and records control, computer-assisted decision making, operating room information systems, hospital information systems, health information exchange, clinical decision support systems, interoperability, systems integration, data mining,* and *informed consent.* The concepts of **standardized terminologies** were included with a broad subject-heading controlled vocabulary as well as individual headings and keywords for relevant standardized terminologies. Subject headings and keywords related to government regulations included *government regulation, meaningful use, Health Insurance Portability and Accountability Act, HIPAA, Health Information Technology for Economic and Clinical Health, American Recovery and Reinvestment Act, Affordable Care Act,* and *Medicare and Medicaid Electronic Health Care Record.* The keywords *big data,* **electronic signature**, *charting by exception, variance charting, electronic medical record, EHR, Health Level Seven International, HL7,* and *EMR* also were included in the search, as were terms related to the concepts of data collection, retention, storage, and governance.

Articles identified by the search were provided to the lead author and an evidence appraiser. Excluded were non-peer-reviewed publications and evidence from other disciplines when evidence from the perioperative setting was available **(Figure 1)**. The lead author and the evidence appraiser reviewed and critically appraised each article using the AORN Research or Non-Research Evidence

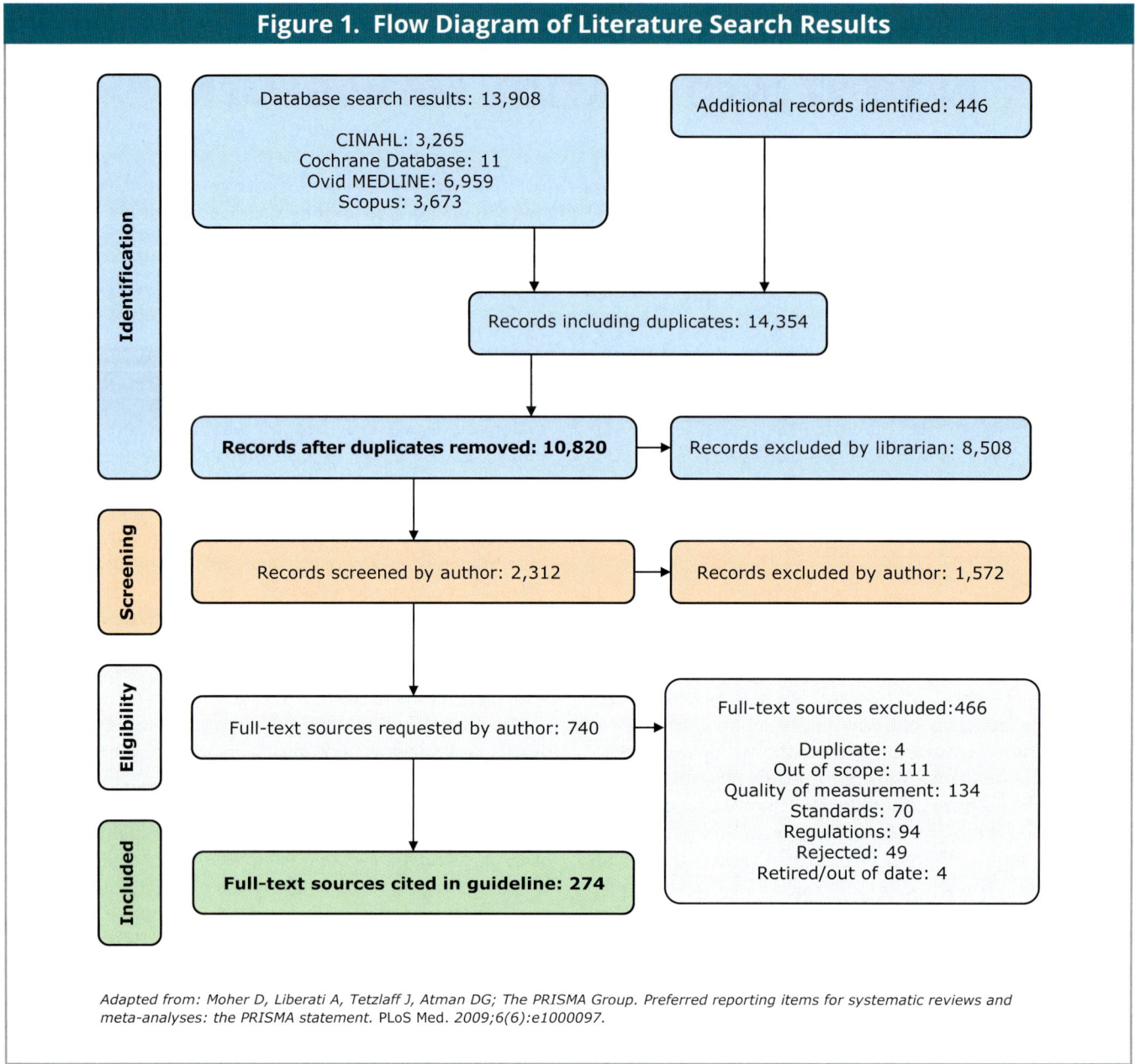

Figure 1. Flow Diagram of Literature Search Results

Database search results: 13,908

CINAHL: 3,265
Cochrane Database: 11
Ovid MEDLINE: 6,959
Scopus: 3,673

Additional records identified: 446

Records including duplicates: 14,354

Records after duplicates removed: 10,820

Records excluded by librarian: 8,508

Records screened by author: 2,312

Records excluded by author: 1,572

Full-text sources requested by author: 740

Full-text sources excluded: 466

Duplicate: 4
Out of scope: 111
Quality of measurement: 134
Standards: 70
Regulations: 94
Rejected: 49
Retired/out of date: 4

Full-text sources cited in guideline: 274

Identification
Screening
Eligibility
Included

Adapted from: Moher D, Liberati A, Tetzlaff J, Atman DG; The PRISMA Group. Preferred reporting items for systematic reviews and meta-analyses: the PRISMA statement. PLoS Med. 2009;6(6):e1000097.

Appraisal Tools as appropriate. The literature was independently evaluated and appraised according to the strength and quality of the evidence. Each article was then assigned an appraisal score. The appraisal score is noted in brackets after each reference, as applicable.

Each recommendation rating is based on a synthesis of the collective evidence, a benefit-harm assessment, and consideration of resource use. The strength of the recommendation was determined using the AORN Evidence Rating Model and the quality and consistency of the evidence supporting a recommendation. The recommendation strength rating is noted in brackets after each recommendation.

Note: The evidence summary table is available at http:// www.aorn.org/evidencetables/.

Editor's note: MEDLINE is a registered trademark of the US National Library of Medicine, Bethesda, MD. CINAHL, Cumulative Index to Nursing and Allied Health Literature, is a registered trademark of EBSCO Industries, Birmingham, AL. Scopus is a registered trademark of Elsevier B.V., Amsterdam, The Netherlands.

1. Patient Health Care Records

1.1 As part of the **legal health record**, the perioperative patient health care record should reflect the plan of care, including assessment, nursing diagnosis, outcome identification, planning, implementation of interventions, and evaluation of progress toward the expected outcome.[3-6] *[Recommendation]*

The nursing process provides the guiding framework for documenting perioperative nursing care. When the nursing process is used in perioperative practice settings, it demonstrates the critical-thinking skills practiced by the registered nurse (RN) in caring for the patient undergoing operative or other invasive procedures.[3-5,7,8] Documentation includes information about the patient's current and past health status, nursing diagnoses and interventions, expected outcomes, and evaluation of the patient's response to perioperative nursing care.[7,9-11]

1.2 **Record assessment findings (eg, physical, psychosocial, cultural, spiritual) in the patient health care record before the operative or other invasive procedure.** *[Recommendation]*

The patient assessment forms a baseline for identifying the patient's health status, developing nursing diagnoses, and establishing an individualized plan of care. Recurring assessments throughout the patient's perioperative experience contribute to continuity in the delivery of care.[5,11-13]

Intraoperative nursing interventions are embedded within the delivery of care but are not consistently reflected in clinical documentation.[8,14,15] In a systematic review of nursing documentation literature, Wang et al[16] found that inadequacies in the use of nursing process structure within clinical documentation resulted in one or more deficiencies in the application of the assessment process. In a subsequent qualitative content analysis of nursing communication and documentation patterns, Keenan et al[17] identified that inconsistent nursing documentation practices contributed to discrepancies in the transfer of information, causing vulnerabilities for serious and undetectable clinical errors.

1.3 **Record the nursing interventions performed, the time at which they were performed, the location of care, and the name and role of the person performing the care.**[4,6,12] *[Recommendation]*

Clinical judgments are based on actual or potential patient problems (eg, nursing diagnoses) that determine the nursing interventions to be implemented to achieve expected perioperative patient outcomes.[4,5,11] Documenting nursing interventions promotes continuity of patient care and improves the exchange of patient care information between health care team members. Researchers who conducted a qualitative study of eight medical-surgical settings across four hospitals identified discrepancies in interdisciplinary information exchange and what nurses documented about patient care. They

recommended capturing core patient information to increase consistency in care planning and accessibility of information for the patient care team.[17]

1.4 **Record expected and interim patient outcomes in the patient health care record.**[3,5,11] *[Recommendation]*

The goals for nursing interventions are to prevent potential patient injury or complications and treat actual patient problems (eg, nursing diagnoses). Identified nursing diagnoses contribute to interim and expected patient outcomes for the planned surgical or procedural intervention.[9] Expert consensus indicates that nurses who associate the patient diagnoses with planned interventions are more outcome focused than task oriented.[18]

1.5 **The patient health care record should reflect continuous reassessment and evaluation of perioperative nursing care and the patient's response to implemented nursing interventions.**[3,5,12,13,19] *[Recommendation]*

The nursing process directs perioperative nurses to evaluate the effectiveness of nursing interventions toward attaining desired patient outcomes. Reassessment throughout the patient's perioperative experience contributes to continuity in the delivery of care.[3,5,11]

The evaluation process provides information for continuity of care, performance improvement activities, perioperative nursing research, and management of risk. Professional nursing associations have determined that documentation provides a mechanism for comparing actual versus expected outcomes.[3,5,9]

1.5.1 **Patient data must be collected concurrently with each assessment, reassessment, or evaluation and recorded in the patient health care record.**[20,21] *[Regulatory Requirement]*

Continuous evaluation of the patient's condition establishes a baseline to determine fluctuations in the patient's status.[5,3,12] Appropriately captured patient data contribute to a centralized repository that members of the health care team can use to monitor the patient's status, coordinate prescribed treatments, and evaluate the effectiveness of care rendered.[19,22-25]

2. Documentation and Nursing Workflow

2.1 **Synchronize perioperative nursing documentation with the nursing workflow.**[26-29] *[Recommendation]*

Nursing workflow represents the cognitive process of nursing care activities and establishes the approach for patient care data collection. Documentation of nursing activities is dictated by health care organization policy and by regulatory and accrediting agency requirements and is necessary to inform other health care professionals involved in the patient's care. To accurately represent the patient's experience and promote quality delivery of care, data aggregation should be coordinated with clinical workflow.[4,14,26,30] Hayrinen et al[31] conducted a retrospective, descriptive study in which they examined 489 nursing care plans. They found that the incorporation of nursing process workflow into the framework of clinical documentation platforms improved documentation completeness and compliance with regulatory requirements.

2.2 **Facilitate data capture using a format designed to support clinical workflow activities while eliminating redundancy in data entry.**[2,27,29,32,33] *[Recommendation]*

High-quality evidence indicates that work inefficiencies, such as the format or the location where clinical data are captured within documentation systems, have a negative correlation on clinical reasoning and decision making.[30,34-38]

The burden of clinical documentation has been associated with decreased nursing attention to patient care activities, which has been shown to adversely affect patient safety. In a time-motion study spanning 274 health systems in 15 states, Hendrich et al[39] found that when nursing time was divided between patient care responsibilities and transferring patient information between different information systems, the frequency of transcription errors, fragmentation of care, and duplication of effort increased and resulted in an inefficient measurement of nursing care quality.

Several studies have shown that interruption during established clinical processes results in competition for cognitive resources and may contribute to an adverse event or patient harm by reducing situational awareness.[40-42] Redundancy in the design of documentation activities further reduces the nurse's ability to focus on the clinical environment and may create a risk for error.[33,43] The authors of a Cochrane Review on the effects of using nursing record systems on nursing practice and health care outcomes identified that when processes are simplified and data capture is standardized and organized, there is a reduction in the reliance on memory to complete tasks, thereby potentially eliminating harmful events.[15]

In a single-site observational study on nursing workflow, Cornell et al[43] examined the percentage of time nurses dedicated to patient care and documentation activities. They found that nursing time was focused primarily on patient care (eg, assessment, interventions) with documentation being completed in intervals and not concurrently with patient care. This, along with frequent switching between patient care and documentation, was correlated with nursing cognitive disruption, which resulted in slower performance and increased the potential for error.

In a subsequent follow-up observational and randomized investigation, Cornell et al[44] examined the effect of new electronic documentation implementation on nursing activities and workflow. Findings indicated that the repeated clustering of patient care and documentation activities, evenly distributed, affected nursing workflow by increasing the amount of time dedicated to electronic documentation without negatively affecting direct patient care time.

2.2.1 **Clinical documentation should reflect patient-focused care.**[45-48] *[Recommendation]* **P**

Clinical (eg, nursing) documentation systems often do not support health care personnel in accommodating the specific needs of the individual (eg, teaching needs, age-specific criteria, self-care requirements).[45,49,50] Health care currently relies on the technology-centered medical model of care, and patient-centric, evidence-based care is often not represented within documentation platforms. Researchers have identified discrepancies between care delivered and what is captured in patient care documentation; thus, efforts to improve and ensure the accuracy of patient care data capture are necessary.[51,52]

2.2.2 **Incorporate all necessary patient care data important to ongoing and transitional care into the patient's health care record.** *[Recommendation]*

Despite the efficiencies in the quality and quantity of patient care information captured by electronic documentation systems, the reliance on asynchronous information transfer to communicate continuing patient care needs means critical elements necessary to ensure a comprehensive treatment plan are often lacking. A recent systematic literature review that explored the role that electronic patient records have on shift hand over (ie, hand off) identified that omissions of detailed care information and communication errors occurred frequently during the hand-over period.[53] The authors concluded that the completion of documentation fields resulted in less missing data and the quality of information was more accurate and current, resulting in improved clinician synchronous communications and care continuity.

The quality of information available to clinicians affects the quality of care provided. Nurse scientists conducted an exploratory study on the characteristics of clinical health care decision making as influenced by data collection and information processing.[54] Findings from this small qualitative study of patient records at one hospital suggest that the type of data captured in the clinical documentation produced the necessary information for therapeutic interventions.

A comparative study of nursing verbal communications and related documentation for care transitions revealed that synchronous oral exchanges during hand overs incorporated more contextual information related to the current and future needs of the patient, while associated documentation reflected only the clinical observations of care interventions.[55]

2.2.3 Evaluate perioperative electronic documentation systems for their effect on clinical workflow and patient safety and their ability to accommodate the organization's objectives for the implementation site. Provide input and recommendations for improvement to the information technology team.[15,16,26,27,56]

Clinical information systems should address

- clinical workflow,[26,27,57-61]
- information needs of the patient care environment,[46,58,60]
- patient population characteristics,[45,47,49,60] and
- clinician and provider usability requirements.[40,42,50,58,59,62]

[Recommendation] **P**

High-quality evidence indicates that effective information systems collect, store, and organize patient information to allow real-time updates and support clinical decision making and are accessible to health care professionals when needed.[61,63,64] Research on the effect of health information technology implementation has shown that changes in contextual clinical work processes made to accommodate clinical information systems have both positive and negative influences on clinical workflow and patient safety.[37,42,50,58,65] Technology can more positively affect clinical workflow, data availability, patient outcomes, and health care provider satisfaction when clinicians are involved in the selection and implementation of the information system.[15,51,66]

3. Structured Vocabularies

3.1 Use the Perioperative Nursing Data Set (PNDS) and other structured vocabularies inclusive of the nursing process workflow with discrete representation of each phase of the perioperative patient care continuum (ie, preadmission, preoperative, intraoperative, postoperative).[31,67,68] *[Recommendation]*

The use of a structured vocabulary facilitates the capture of expressed observations, treatments, and patient responses within the clinical domain of care. A structured vocabulary describes patient care using controlled (ie, standardized) and unambiguous terms that are interpreted with consistent meaning by health care clinicians.[31,69,70] Patient information gathered from the collection of standardized data creates the knowledge perioperative RNs use to provide individualized patient care. The synthesis of knowledge for patient care interventions is in turn documented, resulting in the wisdom of perioperative nursing practice.[70,71]

Using structured nursing data elements (eg, the PNDS) that include nursing diagnoses, interventions, and outcomes in clinical documentation demonstrates perioperative nursing contributions to patient outcomes and represents professional nursing practice.[4,8,72,73]

3.2 Incorporate the PNDS into the documentation platform.[8,9,72] *[Recommendation]*

The PNDS is a controlled, structured, and coded nursing language that describes perioperative nursing influence on the effectiveness and safety of patient care delivery and the contributions of perioperative nursing to patient outcomes. Although a gap exists in the current literature regarding clinical application of the PNDS, the existing evidence demonstrates that clinical documentation systems that incorporate standardized language provide patient care data that can be aggregated and analyzed to determine clinical efficiencies, examine operational metrics, and create new evidence for sustainable improvements in health care quality.[9,11,26,68]

3.2.1 Incorporate nursing process workflow and unambiguous representation of the patient experience in each phase of perioperative nursing documentation.[74-76] *[Recommendation]*

The phases of perioperative patient care collectively represent the unique domain of perioperative nursing. Standardization of patient care information improves the quality of the data[77] and can be used to support the extraction and interpretation of data for

- clinical **decision support**,[78-80]
- improved quality metrics,[31,80,81]
- information exchange,[80,81]
- research,[81,82]
- policy making,[31,81] and
- nursing visibility.[4,8,9,31,67,69,74,83,84]

3.3 Implement a documentation system that includes a standardized perioperative electronic framework. *[Recommendation]*

Standardization in documentation platforms promotes uniformity in comprehensive patient care data capture among health care organizations and creates a foundation for sharing health care data.[85,86] The burgeoning cost of health care and the drive for improved quality have created urgency for implementation of **electronic medical records** (EMRs) and **interoperable** EHR systems.[87-89] Adoption of EHR systems is a component of the **American Recovery and Reinvestment Act** (ARRA) of 2009[22] to facilitate access to quality care and improve patient safety[79,86] through high-reliability processes using data analysis to evaluate performance and outcomes.[90] **Data quality** facilitated by the adoption of an EHR and established by compliance with laws, clinical practice standards, and national quality measures adds to the relevance of efficiency benchmarks. Experts agree that the adoption of EHR technology also will lead to quantifiable improvements in reducing the time required for patient care data capture by nurses.[77,81,88,91]

Inpatient and ambulatory EHR implementation has been stimulated by the ARRA incentives for EHR adoption and subsequent analysis and dissemination of performance metrics.[86] Achieving success with the national **Health Information Technology for Economic and Clinical Health** (HITECH)[86] agenda for comparative analysis among health care organizations can be accomplished by implementing an electronic documentation framework (eg, AORN Syntegrity®) embedded with standardized sets of documentation values applicable across multiple perioperative settings to increase the confidence in data quality and research validity.[77,81,92]

3.3.1 The health care documentation system must incorporate the standardized clinical terminologies identified by the US government to promote interoperability of health care data.[80,93,94] *[Regulatory Requirement]*

To accomplish the national health care strategy of promoting the availability of patient care data between and across health care organizations and providers, the Health Information Technology Standards Committee established by the Office of the National Coordinator for Health Information Technology (ONC) has identified clinical terminologies to standardize EHR data for interoperability **(Table 1)**.[80,95] Experts assert that the standardization of EHR data allows the electronic sharing of vital patient care information and thereby supports the continuity of uninterrupted ongoing care.[85]

The PNDS is incorporated into the ONC clinical vocabulary standards through the Systematized Nomenclature of Medicine–Clinical Terms (SNOMED-CT®).[9] The incorporation of the PNDS into the US government vocabulary standards enables measurement of the perioperative nursing contribution to the quality and outcomes of population health.

3.3.2 Structured data collected using a standardized perioperative electronic framework should allow for data aggregation and be extractable for use in research and analytics. *[Recommendation]*

The ability to mine standardized clinical data fuels the development of new knowledge to transform practice and improve patient outcomes.[96] Structured data made available for direct import into statistical applications expands the capacity to generate and analyze observational evidence that can be generalizable to all perioperative settings.[96,97] Standardized data are more easily integrated into larger data sets, facilitating the reuse of de-identified clinical data for predictive analytics that improve the detection of disease processes and facilitate earlier interventions and improvements in the quality and efficiency of health care delivery.[98,99]

4. Comprehensive Representation of Care

4.1 Structure perioperative nursing documentation to meet professional and regulatory compliance requirements for a comprehensive representation of patient care.[20,21,100-102] *[Recommendation]*

Patient care information collected and entered into the health care record is a tool for monitoring and evaluating the patient's health status and response to care, a resource for evaluating compliance with regulatory requirements, and a method for aligning provision of services with reimbursement.[4,103,104]

4.2 Perioperative nursing documentation must correspond to the elements of regulatory statutes,

Table 1. Office of the National Coordinator for Health Information Technology Clinical Vocabulary Standards for Interoperability

Vocabulary	Data Type
CVX Codes for Vaccines Administered	Vaccines (administered)
CPT Current Procedural Terminology	Medical, surgical, and diagnostic services rendered for claims
CDC PHIN/VADS Centers for Disease Control and Prevention Public Health Information Network/Vocabulary Access and Distribution System	Patient characteristic (administrative gender, date of birth)
HCPCS* Healthcare Common Procedure Coding System	Medical, surgical, and diagnostic services rendered for claims
ICD-9 CM* International Statistical Classification of Diseases and Related Health Problems—Clinical Modification (9th ed)	Diagnoses and assessments
ICD-9 PCS* International Statistical Classification of Diseases and Related Health Problems—Procedural Coding System (9th ed)	Diagnoses and assessments
ICD-10 CM International Statistical Classification of Diseases and Related Health Problems—Clinical Modification (10th ed)	Diagnoses and assessments
ICD-10 PCS International Statistical Classification of Diseases and Related Health Problems—Procedural Coding System (10th ed)	Diagnoses and assessments
ICF International Classification of Functioning, Disability, and Health	Functional status
ISO-639 International Organization for Standardization – Standard 639	Representation of languages and language groups
LOINC® Logical Observation Identifiers, Names, and Codes	Outcomes and assessments
RxNORM	Normalized clinical drug names
SNOMED-CT® Systematized Nomenclature of Medicine Clinical Terms	Diagnoses, interventions, and outcomes
UCUM The Unified Code for Units of Measure	Units of measure for results

LOINC is a registered trademark of Regenstrief Institute, Inc, Indianapolis, IN. SNOMED-CT is a registered trademark of the International Health Terminology Standards Development Organisation, Copenhagen, Denmark.

* ICD-9 is being discontinued from US mandatory quality reporting beginning calendar year 2017.

Adapted from A Blueprint for the CMS Measures Management System. Version 11.1 ed. Washington, DC: Centers for Medicare & Medicaid Services; August 2015. https://www.cms.gov/Medicare/Quality-Initiatives-Patient-Assessment-Instruments/MMS/Downloads/Blueprint111.pdf. Accessed April 20, 2016.

health care accreditation measures, national practice standards, and mandatory quality and reimbursement for quality performance criteria.[20,105]
[Regulatory Requirement]

Clinical documentation serves as the legal record of care delivery (ie, legal health record) and assists with cross-disciplinary patient care coordination.[21,103,106]

4.2.1 Include the following components in clinical documentation:
- assessments;
- clinical problems;
- communications with other health care professionals regarding the patient;
- communication with and education of the patient, the patient's family members, the patient's designated support person, and other third parties;
- medication records;
- order acknowledgement, implementation, and management;
- patient care interventions;
- patient clinical parameters;

- patient responses and outcomes, including changes in the patient's status; and
- plans of care that reflect the social and cultural framework of the patient.[4]

[Recommendation]

4.2.2 Perioperative nursing documentation frameworks should correspond to professional guidelines and standards. [Recommendation]

Organizations that provide guidelines and standards relevant to perioperative practice settings include the

- Association of periOperative Registered Nurses,
- American Association of Blood Banks,
- American Association of Nurse Anesthetists,
- American Health Information Management Association,
- Agency for Healthcare Research and Quality,
- American National Standards Institute,
- American Society of Anesthesiologists,
- Association for the Advancement of Medical Instrumentation,
- Association of PeriAnesthesia Nurses,
- Institute for Safe Medication Practices,
- Malignant Hyperthermia Association of the United States,
- National Fire Protection Agency,
- National Institute for Occupational Safety and Health,
- National Quality Forum,
- US Pharmacopeia, and
- United Network for Organ Sharing.

Examples of guidance from professional standards-setting agencies that may be considered for incorporation into perioperative documentation include

- national patient safety guidelines,
- organ and tissues tracking guidelines,
- perioperative recommendations for safe patient care,
- safe medication administration guidelines, and
- timing of clinical events.

As licensed health care professionals, perioperative RNs have a responsibility to maintain the established standards of perioperative nursing care. The standards of nursing practice require documentation to be based on the patient's condition or needs and the relationship to the proposed intervention and to be relevant to the period of patient care (eg, preadmission testing, preoperative, intraoperative, postoperative care).[4,5,107] National practice standards cross all disciplines of nursing care and are applicable to perioperative nursing practice.

4.2.3 Perioperative nursing documentation should correspond to established guidelines and practices for perioperative nursing care.[107] Elements of perioperative guidelines that should be incorporated into clinical documentation include

- aseptic technique maintenance[76,108-111];
- local anesthesia administration[23,101,112-122];
- medication administration practices (eg, use of abbreviations)[23,112,113,115,118,123-126];
- moderate sedation/analgesia administration[23,101-121,127-129];
- patient care considerations (eg, latex allergy, implanted electronic device, dentures)[20,76,100,113,118,130-137];
- patient positioning[76,101,114,118,132,138];
- patient information exchanged[3,100-102,118,120,121,136,139-143];
- safety precautions, including
  - electrical safety precautions,[118,136,142-147]
  - equipment use precautions (eg, laser, pneumatic tourniquet, magnetic resonance imaging),[133,147-151]
  - fire prevention,[76,100,118,124,130,141,144,146,150,152-154]
  - human tissue procurement, processing, and preservation precautions,[76,118,120-122,155-160]
  - infection prevention,[76,112,114,118,124,125,142,152,161-168]
  - tissue protection,[30,114,118,124,150,152,169-172]
  - radiation exposure prevention,[170]
  - retained surgical items prevention,[115,118,173,174]
  - correct site, side, person surgery processes,[76,88,100,116,120,121,124,135,136,138,145,175-181] and
  - skin preparation and antisepsis[23,76,101,114,115,117,118,124,128,142,153,164,168,182,183];
- specimen and tissue management[20,76,114,118,121,122,155,158,174,180];
- sterilization/disinfection practices[76,114,118,128,130,131,145,146,153,166,179,180,184-188]; and
- traffic control measures.[76,130,141,152,153,166]

[Recommendation]

The AORN guidelines for perioperative nursing practice are nationally recognized as the standard of care for all operative or invasive procedure patient care settings. Perioperative recommendations for practice are not mandatory nursing care criteria but have been incorporated into regulatory and other standards-setting agencies' guidelines and have been used to support judicial decisions.[189-195]

4.2.4 Perioperative nursing documentation must correspond to local, state, and federal regulatory requirements. [Regulatory Requirement]

State and federal regulations are a collection of general and permanent rules (ie, laws) established to protect the welfare of the public and fortify the guiding principles of the nation. Many statutes or laws are established at the national level and may be amplified at the state level. The amplified statute would become the mandatory authority for the state. An example of this would be document retention requirements that vary among states. Failure to comply with the final law-making authority could result in monetary penalties for the offending organization or monetary penalties or incarceration for the offending individual. Agencies with regulatory authority include the

- Centers for Disease Control and Prevention,
- Centers for Medicare & Medicaid Services (CMS),
- Department of Health and Human Services,
- Occupational Safety and Health Administration, and
- US Food and Drug Administration.

Criteria identified by regulatory agencies for patient care documentation include

- allergies,[21,76,100,102,106,182,196]
- cultural variables,[21,100,106,116,135,197]
- equipment used for patient care (eg, type, model number),[76,100-102,115,134,135,144,145,174,182,196,198]
- names of legal guardian(s) and patient support person(s),[76,102,116,135,196]
- nutritional considerations,[20,100,102,196]
- ordered tests and services provided,[76,100,134,199]
- patient and family education and engagement,[21,100,106,135,196,200]
- patient identifiers and demographics,[20,76,100,134,174]
- patient attributes and status (eg, immunizations, disabilities)[20-22,76,100,101,106,135,176,177,196,201]
- safety precautions,[21,76,106,144,163,199]
- surgical consent(s),[76,100,135,177] and
- surgical implants and explants, including unique identifiers.[21,76,100,106,134,157,198,201-204]

4.2.5 **Perioperative nursing documentation must correspond to health care accreditation organization requirements.** *[Regulatory Requirement]*

Compliance with state or national health care accreditation agency criteria is mandatory for organizations seeking CMS reimbursement or striving to meet established patient safety goals.[20,105] Accrediting bodies review documentation for compliance to the minimum standards for an element of performance. The following accreditation agencies currently have **deemed status**:

- the American Association for Accreditation of Ambulatory Surgery Facilities, Inc[143];

- the Accreditation Association for Ambulatory Health Care, Inc[142];
- State CMS[205];
- DNV-GL[206];
- the Healthcare Facilities Accreditation Program[207]; and
- The Joint Commission.[208,209]

Elements of performance identified by accreditation agencies may include evidence of[20,105]

- blood and tissue tracking;
- compliance with The Joint Commission's National Patient Safety Goals;
- elimination of nationally identified unacceptable abbreviations, acronyms, and symbols;
- hand-over communications;
- identification of implantable objects;
- identification of designated support person(s);
- infection control practices;
- medication reconciliation;
- patient care elements (eg, care plans, tests, services provided);
- pain management interventions;
- education of the patient, the patient's family members, and the patient's designated support person;
- patient demographics; and
- the presence of a current history and physical.

4.2.6 **Perioperative nursing documentation must incorporate mandatory reporting criteria for quality performance reimbursement.** *[Regulatory Requirement]*

To improve population health, the US government is coordinating evidence-based standards development to be incorporated into the national agenda on health care reform. These efforts are incentivized through inclusion within the CMS reimbursement programs and made public through national reporting forums (eg, Hospital Compare[210]). Agencies responsible for national standards development or reimbursement for quality performance criteria include, but are not limited to, the

- Centers for Disease Control and Prevention,
- National Quality Forum, and
- Agency for Healthcare Research and Quality.

Measurement criteria for quality performance reimbursement are included in the following regulations and reporting requirements:

- Ambulatory Surgical Center Payment System,[211]
- Deficit Reduction Act of 2005,[174]
- Hospital Inpatient Prospective Payment System,[211]
- Hospital Outpatient Prospective Payment System,[211]

- national quality reporting metrics,[211] including the
  - Hospital Inpatient Quality Reporting Program, inclusive of the Surgical Care Improvement Project measures,
  - Hospital Acquired Condition Reduction Program,
  - Hospital Value-based Purchasing Program,
  - Hospital Outpatient Quality Reporting Program, and
  - Ambulatory Surgical Center Quality Reporting Program.

4.3 Perioperative documentation must include all patient care orders given in the perioperative patient care setting.[20,100] *[Regulatory Requirement]*

The CMS requires that patient care orders be documented.

4.3.1 Enter patient care orders into the clinical documentation system close to the time when the order is communicated or the intervention is initiated. *[Recommendation]*

4.3.2 All orders, including verbal orders, standing orders, orders included on surgeon preference cards, and order sets must be dated, timed, and authenticated by the ordering health care practitioner with prescriptive authority.[100,208,209,212-215] *[Regulatory Requirement]*

4.3.3 To prevent patient harm from occurring as a result of outdated, incomplete, or erroneous entries, standing orders and preprinted order sets in the documentation framework should[216-219]

- not use unacceptable abbreviations,
- not use trailing zeros in medication dosages,
- use standardized names and terms to describe treatments and interventions (eg, brand names versus generic names for medications, device instructions), and
- be reviewed by the attending surgeon for accuracy of information for the intended procedure.

[Recommendation]

The use of preprinted standing orders that have been updated and do not have any of the problems in the bulleted list above has been shown to reduce medication errors and improve documentation compliance.[220]

4.3.4 Document verbal orders when they are communicated and verify the orders using a read-

back process that involves the ordering health care practitioner.[215-218,221] *[Recommendation]*

4.4 The patient care record must include a complete and accurate informed patient consent for each operative or invasive procedure to be performed.[100,116,177,213] The informed consent process must be documented for procedures and treatments that are identified in the health care facility's medical staff policies as requiring informed consent.[21,100,177] Unless designated as an emergency situation in the health care facility's informed consent policy, a "properly executed informed consent"[116] must include[20,21,106]

- the name of the health care facility providing the surgery or invasive procedure;
- the specific name of the intervention to be performed;
- indications for the proposed intervention;
- the name of the responsible health care provider performing the intervention;
- a statement identifying the risks and benefits associated with the proposed intervention and indication of discussion with the patient or patient's legal representative;
- the signature of the patient or the patient's legal representative;
- the date and time the patient or the patient's legal representative signed the informed consent document;
- the date and time and the signature of the person who witnessed the patient or the patient's legal representative signing the informed consent document; and
- the signature of the responsible health care provider who executed the informed consent discussion with the patient or the patient's legal representative.

[Regulatory Requirement]

The patient or the patient's legal representative is entitled to participate in the informed decision-making process for planning care and treatment, including the right to request or refuse treatment.[116,213]

4.4.1 Additional content that may be identified on the informed consent document and may be regulated by state statutes and administrative rules includes[20,21,106]

- identification of assisting physicians including, but not limited to, medical residents who will be contributing significantly to the proposed intervention and
- identification of assisting health care personnel who are not physicians but who are performing within their scope of practice (eg, RN first assistant, nurse

practitioner) and who will be contributing significantly to the proposed intervention. *[Regulatory Requirement]*

4.5 The names, roles, and credentials of individuals participating in the patient's perioperative care, as well as those not directly involved in the scheduled surgical or procedural intervention, must be recorded in the patient health care record.[21,106] *[Regulatory Requirement]*

Individuals participating in the patient's perioperative care experience may include
- surgical or procedural patient care team members,
- identified legal representatives,
- identified patient support person(s),
- recipients of patient care information on behalf of the patient,
- health care professionals contributing to the patient's care (eg, pathologist, x-ray technician, approved health care student),
- industry representatives,
- law enforcement officers (eg, prison guards), or
- approved observers.

A comprehensive patient-centric record of care reflects interactions between the patient's health care team and those individuals legally representing or providing physical, spiritual, or other support services to the patient.[21,106] Documentation of interactions provides the groundwork for transparency in care planning through effective representation of the patient's involvement in the plan of care and contributions made toward the treatment plan.

4.6 Clinical documentation platforms (ie, paper, electronic) should support the collection of **tailored health care information** using a format that accommodates and is **customized** to the clinical environment.[49] *[Recommendation]* **P**

Tailoring patient health information allows the collection of unique patient care data (eg, communicable diseases, responses to medications, psychosocial considerations) that may affect the planned operative or other invasive procedure. The collection of tailored health care information is standardized to the clinical setting (eg, surgical versus interventional radiology) but may vary by the requirements of the environment where perioperative care is delivered (eg, pediatric hospital, cancer treatment center, ambulatory surgery center).[49,50]

4.6.1 Select formats for the collection of tailored patient care information that were established based on nationally recognized standards of practice that outline the nurse's responsibilities to the patient.[4,104] *[Recommendation]*

4.6.2 The health care organization's risk management and legal representatives should format and review charting by exception processes.[222,223] *[Recommendation]*

The minimum criteria for charting by exception should include
- identifying objective physical assessment criteria for the patient population being served (eg, endoscopy patients, orthopedic patients);
- identifying and defining what constitutes normal findings;
- describing the process for documenting normal findings (eg, "within normal limits");
- describing the process for identifying, describing, and documenting objective abnormal or key findings;
- listing the practice standards, care guidelines, and clinical pathways used to guide patient care;
- listing a rationale, including decisions and interventions, for deviations from established guidance for patient care;
- setting the frequency of documentation entries; and
- adhering to state or national statutory requirements (eg, record **authentication**).[104,194,224]

Short[225] reported that charting by exception, also known as variance charting, was successfully implemented at one medical center. When charting by exception, the nurses' documentation time was significantly reduced when used with a comprehensively designed documentation system.

A well-designed documentation system corresponds to the health care organization's policy for charting by exception and allows for an indisputable description of the patient's condition. Charting by exception may lead to litigious situations when organizational policy has not been well formulated or updated for changes in statutory requirements or when the nurse has not followed the established guidance for charting by exception.[104,194,222]

4.7 Cognitive processes used in patient care should be supported by **clinical support technologies** (eg, AORN Syntegrity) that are embedded within electronic clinical documentation systems.[37,226,227] *[Recommendation]*

The processes within perioperative patient care are classified as cognitive performance or the intellectual processing of information to complete a finite task.[226] Multitasking, environmental stimulation, and availability of information contribute to the nurse's ability or inability to accommodate needed adjustments in patient care activities. The collective evidence indicates that use of poorly designed clinical information systems, those not conforming to national data standards, or those that do not incorporate clinical workflow and work process requirements may contribute to patient harm.[30,37,56,226-229] Alternately, clinical information systems that incorporate technology innovations (eg, order entry, decision support, clinical alerts) and support the cognitive processes of patient care have been found to enhance health care worker performance and result in improved patient safety and quality patient outcomes.[30,37,63,226-229]

5. Security and Confidentiality

5.1 Patient information must be secure, held confidential, and protected from unauthorized disclosure.[230] *[Regulatory Requirement]*

The Health Insurance Portability and Accountability Act (HIPAA) of 1996 guarantees the privacy of individuals receiving health services and the confidentiality of "individually identifiable health information."[230] Updated to correspond with the HITECH Act, HIPAA now includes security standards for protecting electronic health information (ie, Security Rule) and regulations that specify compliance, investigation, payments, and penalties (ie, Enforcement Rule) that were established in 1996.[230,231]

5.2 Access to patient health information must be limited to authorized individuals based on the health care role (eg, surgeon, RN, perfusionist), responsibility, and function (eg, postanesthesia care unit RN assisting in the endoscopy unit).[20,230-232] *[Regulatory Requirement]*

Controlling access to the patient's health information prevents privacy and security breaches for HIPAA-covered entities.[230-232] The health care organization has a legal responsibility to establish procedures to prevent unauthorized access to sensitive patient health information and to execute a plan for data breach notification practices should a breach occur.[230,231,233]

5.2.1 Implement the following risk-reduction strategies to proactively mitigate potential access violations[224,232]:
- establish perioperative information management policies that include remote access protocols, on-/off-site information storage practices, and employee exit strategies that are reviewed and updated

as the environment changes (eg, new regulations, transitions from paper to electronic documentation platforms);
- identify procedures for the use of organizational and personal mobile devices (eg, cell phones, tablet technologies, video imaging) within the perioperative care environment;
- establish awareness and sensitivity to data security and privacy by reinforcing the existing health care organization's information security policy for monitoring and auditing access to patient health information;
- restrict access to electronic health information to users with individualized, unique authorization credentials that are associated with time-sensitive passwords using alphanumeric-symbol combinations; and
- hold competency-based education programs on information access and sharing for all employees upon hire, when changes are made for documentation practices, and when problems are identified within the perioperative care environment.

[Recommendation]

5.2.2 Ambulatory surgery centers must have a person designated to oversee the protection of clinical records. This individual is responsible not only for the confidentiality, security, and physical safety of the clinical records, but also for maintaining a method of tracking who has access to the records and identifying designated locations of paper records throughout the facility in an effort to prevent unauthorized access.[20,230,231,234] *[Regulatory Requirement]*

5.2.3 Any significant medical advice given to a patient via text, email, or telephone must be permanently entered in the patient's clinical record and signed and dated.[20,234] *[Regulatory Requirement]*

5.3 Comply with the health care organization's information policies for sharing electronic patient information. The organization's information policies should include[224,235,236] processes for
- determining that electronic patient health information, either to or from outside organizations or shared with the patient, meets current requirements for information exchange and security (eg, **malware** protection);
- validating original source authenticity and the accuracy of transmitted information; and

- evaluating electronically transmitted content (eg, email, text, file transfer protocol [FTP]) for potential corruption. *[Recommendation]*

Electronic transmission of patient health information is held to the same privacy and security criteria as facility-based EHRs. Sensitive patient information in paper, electronic text, or image formatting can be exposed to unintended or unauthorized disclosure if effective sharing safeguards are not in place.[230,231,236] Authors of a systematic review of the literature on the security and privacy of EHRs found that compliance with the standards and federal regulations for sharing protected patient information has been accomplished by using interchange script language, using multi-agent hierarchical architecture, adding precision access control with on-demand revocation to access control processes, and employing systems that gather disparate patient data while preserving patient anonymity during communications.[232] Electronic transmission of patient health information by e-mail, mobile storage media, or other formats may introduce malicious software into the health care information system.

5.3.1 Establish policies and procedures for verifying electronic patient health information for authenticity and accuracy and for evaluating content for potential corruption.[224,231,236,237] *[Recommendation]*

5.3.2 The patient must have a signed consent for release of information in the health care record before graphic imaging takes place and before the release of patient-specific information, including remote access to and relocation of health information from the treating organization.[177,230,231,238,239] Nonconsented disclosure of sensitive patient health information requires execution of the data breach notification process by the health care organization.[230,231,237,240] *[Regulatory Requirement]*

5.3.3 To complete full disclosure and reporting, the organization's information technology and risk management personnel should collaborate to discover all patient care records that were involved in a non-consented disclosure.[240,241] *[Recommendation]*

5.4 Documentation entries made into the patient health care record must include an authentication process at the completion of the documentation process or according to the organization's established policies.[80,86,100,101,224,242,243] Health care records must accurately reflect the patient care experience, be completed promptly, and be associated with an author identification procedure to ensure the **integrity** of the content.[20,100,105] *[Regulatory Requirement]*

Authentication identifies the author of the documentation entry and indicates responsibility for the interventions performed and patient information collected. Authentication legally binds the owner of the signature with the responsibility for the accuracy of the content within the document.[224]

5.4.1 The authentication process may include, but is not limited to,[224,233,244]

- using an electronic or **digital signature** or a **code key** in the format designated by the health care organization as the legal representation of an individual's written signature for the EHR.
- completing a pen-to-paper signature, using initials with a **signature legend** on the same document, or a rubber signature stamp for paper-based documentation platforms (eg, faxed, scanned documents) and as permitted by the health care organization's policy.
  - Initials with a signature legend should be avoided on narrative documentation (eg, comments, patient quotes, consultation), assessment data collection, or when a signature is required by law (eg, patient informed consent).
  - **Digitized inked signatures** (ie, signature image) should only be used when deemed acceptable by the health care organization and allowed by state or federal reimbursement regulations.
- using a countersignature demonstrating accuracy of content entered into a patient health care record; once countersigned, the content is legally considered the cosigner's entry (eg, cosigned nursing student entry).

[Regulatory Requirement]

5.4.2 Authentication of verbal orders must occur within the time frame specified by state statutory guidelines. If state law does not specify a time frame, the federal mandate applies for verbal orders to be authenticated by the responsible physician within 48 hours of entering the order.[100] *[Regulatory Requirement]*

5.5 The patient care record must be retained in the original or a legally reproducible format for the

Table 2. US Federal Minimum Retention Guidelines	
Source	**Retention Period**
Ambulatory surgical services[1]	Not specified
Hospitals[2]	5 years from the date of discharge
Hospitals, critical access[3]	6 years from date of last entry or longer as mandated by state statutory guidelines or as necessary for legal proceedings
Department of Veterans Affairs operation log file (including type of surgery, date, patient's name, surgeon, assistant scrub person, anesthetist, agent, method, sponge count, preoperative and postoperative diagnoses, complications, and other information)[4]	Destroy after 20 years
Department of Veterans Affairs (date surgery was performed, members of the surgical and nursing teams, and other information pertaining to the surgery of a patient)[4]	Destroy after 3 years

References

1. *42 CFR §416.47. Condition of participation: medical records. Centers for Medicare & Medicaid Services. Department of Health and Human Services. https://www.gpo.gov/fdsys/granule/CFR-2007-title42-vol3/CFR-2007-title42-vol3-sec416-47. Accessed April 20, 2016.*
2. *42 CFR §482.24. Condition of participation: medical record services. Centers for Medicare & Medicaid Services. Department of Health and Human Services. https://www.gpo.gov/fdsys/granule/CFR-2011-title42-vol5/CFR-2011-title42-vol5-sec482-24/content-detail.html. Accessed April 20, 2016.*
3. *42 CFR §485.638. Conditions of participation: clinical records. Centers for Medicare & Medicaid Services. Department of Health and Human Services. https://www.gpo.gov/fdsys/granule/CFR-2011-title42-vol5/CFR-2011-title42-vol5-sec485-638. Accessed April 21, 2016.*
4. Department of Veterans Affairs Records Control Schedule 10-1. *Washington, DC: Veterans Health Administration; 2016. http://www1.va.gov/vhapublications/RCS10/rcs10-1.pdf. Accessed April 21, 2016.*

minimum allocation of time dictated by federal regulations and state statutes of limitations. Organizational policies may address other time frames for record retention based on the patient population served (eg, pediatric patients, oncology patients), facility demographics (eg, research, trauma, academic), media used to store patient data (eg, paper, microfilm, optical disc), or operational requirements (eg, regulatory compliance).[20,76,105,215,224,245,246] *[Regulatory Requirement]* **P**

The American Health Information Management Association recommends retaining operative indexes for a minimum of 10 years and the register of surgical procedures permanently.[215] The minimum retention guidelines for perioperative information according to US federal regulations are detailed in **Table 2**.

5.6 Electronic documentation platforms should have an alternate data entry and backup process.[247-250] Formalize a complete **downtime** process that addresses hardware, operating system, and network disruptions to preserve data accuracy and uninterrupted health care processes, including strategies to
- facilitate an uninterrupted patient care schedule (eg, paper forms, documentation backup media),
- identify changes to existing workflows (eg, how new orders are communicated, clinical resources),

- recover potential loss of patient care data, and
- incorporate patient care data that are captured using alternate documentation platforms (eg, paper forms) into the electronic information system.[41,247,251]

[Recommendation]

Backup processes will mitigate interruptions in patient care that could result from technology failures. Dependence on technology can significantly influence the effectiveness and efficiency of patient care delivery when systems are interrupted.[41,247,251]

5.6.1 Provide education on the policies, procedures, and alternate workflows associated with the downtime or technology performance issues.[41,247,251] *[Recommendation]*

6. Modifying Existing Records

6.1 Modifications to existing content in the patient health care record should comply with federal and state regulations, health care accreditation requirements, and national practice guidelines.[4,224] *[Recommendation]*

The patient care record is a legal representation of services provided by the health care organization. Perioperative nurses are obligated to accurately represent the patient's care within the health care record.[100,105,230]

6.2 Only make **amendments**, **corrections**, or **addendums** to the patient care record to present an accurate description of the care provided or to protect the patient's interest.[252,253] *[Recommendation]*

Using inappropriate methods to correct, clarify, or change existing entries in the patient health care record may expose the health care organization or clinicians to liability for falsification of patient care information.[4,19] After conducting a meta-study of the essentials of quality nursing documentation, Jefferies et al[104] recommended recording patient care activities as they occur and avoiding late entries, duplication of events, unnecessary information, or controversial information that could lead to modifications of the patient care record.

6.3 In the health care organization's information management policy, outline the processes for making legally acceptable modifications to the patient care record.[224,252] *[Recommendation]*

Corrections, amendments, and addendums are limited by the functionality of the documentation platform used.

6.3.1 Follow established organizational policies and procedures when making amendments or addendums to the patient care record. Perform corrections, amendments, and addendums in paper records by[6,12,224,254]

- placing a single line through the incorrect entry, being careful not to obliterate the inaccurate information;
- writing "error," "mistaken entry," or "omit" next to the incorrect text as determined by organizational policy;
- providing the rationale for the correction above the inaccurate entry if room is available or adding it to the margin of the document;
- signing and dating the entry; and
- entering the correct information in the next available space or adjacent to the acknowledged inaccurate information.

[Recommendation]

6.3.2 Corrections, amendments, and addendums in EHRs should[224,252]

- have a **versioning** or "track corrections" function (eg, an electronic strikethrough with a time stamp) to identify the alterations made to an entry that has been authenticated;
- automatically date-, time-, and author-stamp each entry;
- generate a symbol or other notation to identify when an alteration has been

made to existing content that creates a new version of the document;
- retain and link the original document version to the newly created version; and
- reflect corrections made to the EHR on the paper copy.

[Recommendation]

6.3.3 Corrections completed after a final signature or authentication process has occurred should be consistent with the functionality of the information system and established organizational policies and procedures. *[Recommendation]*

6.3.4 Corrections completed before the final signature or authentication process might not be classified as a "correction" according to organizational policy and the information system in place. *[Conditional Recommendation]*

6.3.5 Complete addendums within the original document using the source information system when available and include the addendums in the permanent patient care record or **data repository** system. *[Recommendation]*

6.3.6 Make deletions and retractions of content from a closed EHR system according to organizational policies and procedures and the functionality of the information system in place. *[Recommendation]*

7. Education

7.1 Provide initial and ongoing education and competency verification on understanding of the principles and performance of the processes for documenting patient care and of best practices for maintaining the security of patient care information.[4,255,256] *[Recommendation]*

Initial and periodic competency-based education programs to maintain proficiency in the application of knowledge and use of the documentation platform improve the effectiveness of documentation practices and reinforce strategies to avert unintentional disclosure of patient care information.[257] In a non-experimental study conducted in the United Kingdom, fewer than half of the responding clinicians (n = 141) reported having received any form of data protection training. The researchers suggested that this could increase the risk for mishandling patient data.[258] Bruylands et al[259] conducted a mixed-method study on the quality of nursing care with the use of electronic nursing documentation. They identified that skill in using documentation tools deteriorated without subsequent education and reinforcement of practices.

7.2 Incorporate the health care organization's policies for information management and the procedures for documentation processes and activities into orientation and ongoing education for personnel in the perioperative care environment.[5,107,260] *[Recommendation]*

Perioperative personnel who receive ongoing education and participate in periodic review of policies and procedures develop the knowledge, skills, and attitudes that affect patient outcomes.[107]

7.2.1 Provide education on the significance and use of structured vocabularies for clinical documentation. At a minimum, include the following[4,9,31,68,72]:
- the value structured terminology brings to clinical documentation;
- an overview of the PNDS;
- the contributions of the PNDS to perioperative nursing practice and patient outcomes; and
- how standardized documentation facilitates benchmarking, comparative analysis, predictive analytics, and efficiency reporting.

[Recommendation]

7.2.2 Include a review of the following in education and competency verification for perioperative RNs[261-263]:
- national and organizational documentation standards, guidelines, and requirements;
- procedures for completing amendments, addendums, and corrections;
- procedures for sharing patient information securely while maintaining patient privacy;
- procedures for initiating breach notification;
- compliance requirements for health care data capture; and
- legal implications for failure to comply with documentation standards.

[Recommendation]

7.2.3 Incorporate demonstration of the following minimum skills in education and competency verification for users of perioperative information systems, a component of the EHR[261,263,264]:
- accessing and closing the patient care record;
- the information system's functionality (eg, data entry, order acknowledgment);

- the authentication processes;
- downtime procedures including alternate workflows to accommodate patient care; and
- compliance requirements for health care data capture.

[Recommendation]

8. Policies and Procedures

8.1 Develop policies and procedures for perioperative information management, review them periodically, revise them as necessary, and make them readily available in the practice setting. As new evidence emerges, policies and procedures should evolve to accommodate best practices and technology developments.[260] *[Recommendation]*

Policies and procedures establish authority, responsibility, and accountability and serve as operational guidelines that are used to minimize patient risk factors, standardize practice, direct health care personnel, and establish guidelines for continuous performance improvement activities.

8.2 Have a multidisciplinary team develop and establish a perioperative services information management policy that complements and reinforces existing organization-wide policies (ie, risk management, quality improvement, health information privacy and security) and includes the unique considerations of the perioperative care environment.[260] *[Recommendation]*

A collaborative approach to policy development and the provision of access to policies for all health care personnel results in improved communication and compliance with established practices within the health care organization.

8.2.1 Include the following guidance in information management policies and documentation procedures for EHR systems[252,253,260,265]:
- forwarding addendums to each destination where patient information is retained,
- editing content before a final signature or authentication process occurs,
- using cut-copy-paste and "carry forward" functionality to populate the patient care record,
- completing corrections in an active or locked patient care record,
- rectifying a misidentification of patient health information (ie, wrong name association),
- amending clinical content in an active or locked patient care record,

- completing a delayed entry and updating the long-term record or data repository,
- deleting or retracting information from a locked patient care record while maintaining the **integrity** of the record, and
- defining components that are required for record completion.

[*Recommendation*]

8.3 Policies and procedures must include information on data privacy and security and identify risk-reduction strategies to proactively mitigate potential violations of patient health information access.[230,231] [*Regulatory Requirement*]

8.3.1 Implement the following risk-reduction strategies[224,235,253,262]:
- establish remote access protocols, onsite/off-site information storage practices, and employee exit strategies to protect patient health information;
- frequently review and update policies as the health care information environment changes (eg, new regulations, transitions from paper to electronic documentation platforms);
- identify procedures for using mobile devices (eg, cell phone, tablet technologies, video imaging) within the perioperative care environment;
- reinforce the existing health care organization's information security policy for monitoring and auditing access to patient health information within the perioperative care environment;
- restrict access to electronic health information by user type with individualized unique authorization credentials associated with time-sensitive passwords using alpha-numeric-symbol combinations; and
- hold annual competency-based education programs on information access and sharing for all employees in the perioperative care environment.

[*Recommendation*]

9. Quality

9.1 Develop and implement a quality management program that focuses on the integrity of the data within the patient health care record.[260]
[*Recommendation*]

Regularly monitoring and validating documentation processes is necessary for variance reporting, which supports process and performance measure-ment to quantify organizational effectiveness and nursing influence on patient outcomes.[4,107]

9.2 Participate in the organization-wide clinical documentation improvement (CDI) program. [*Recommendation*]

Participation in a CDI program facilitates data and documentation analysis while providing a structured framework to achieve consistency in quality processes that affect patient satisfaction, accreditation standing, and reimbursement status.[261] Representation of perioperative RNs in the CDI program will allow concerns specific to perioperative practice to be addressed and areas for improvement identified.

9.2.1 Review the perioperative CDI program for[16,224,255]
- use of acceptable abbreviations,
- timeliness and chronology of patient information,
- legibility,
- use of clear and specific language,
- blank spaces or data fields,
- content omissions (eg, missing informed consent),
- delayed entries (eg, next day entry),
- inconsistencies (eg, conflicting assessment findings, procedure start times),
- inappropriate information (eg, communications with attorneys),
- authentication of verbal orders,
- absence of signatures or counter-signature,
- approved documentation practices (eg, charting by exception/variance charting), and
- alterations to clinical content.

[*Recommendation*]

9.3 Incorporate validation procedures for the perioperative information system into the quality management program and comprehensive strategies for EHR system security and maintenance.[250,266] Data quality may be determined by periodic validation of the information system for the integrity of[224,250,252]
- collected patient care information,
- report generation,
- file storage and retrieval,
- data security, and
- control for document versioning.

[*Recommendation*]

Perioperative information systems are complex systems that contribute to improved care or may add to error-prone documentation processes.[250,267-269] Validation procedures help to maintain the integrity of patient health information.

9.3.1 Establish audits performed as a part of a quality-driven information management program. Retain audit trails and place on a retention schedule following the state statute of limitations and needs of the health care organization.[224,270] Audit trails may include[224,270,271]

- paper-based sign-out processes,
- logbook activities,
- EHR access and operations performed,
- EHR metadata,
- electronic tracking system, and
- data mining activities.

[Recommendation]

Auditing procedures help to establish user and organizational accountability for the legal integrity of the patient health care record.

9.3.2 Include perioperative information systems in the organizational information technology risk mitigation plan.[250,268,272] Collaborate with the organization's risk manager, information services department, and engineering department to coordinate efforts to plan for[250,268,272-274]

- perioperative information system upgrades and maintenance;
- system redundancies (eg, remote patient care record access, backup generators);
- unanticipated access to and theft of patient health care information; and
- organizational information technology network infrastructure maintenance, upgrades, and conversions to the perioperative information system.

[Recommendation]

Proactive multidisciplinary contingency planning for information system failures and disaster response procedures will help maintain continuity in patient care activities.

Editor's note: AORN Syntegrity is a registered trademark of AORN, Inc, Denver, CO. SNOMED-CT is a registered trademark of the International Health Terminology Standards Development Organisation, Copenhagen, Denmark.

Glossary

Addendum: New documentation used to add information to an original documentation entry of patient health information.

Amendment: Additional documentation completed to clarify a preexisting entry of patient health information.

American Recovery and Reinvestment Act (ARRA): An economic stimulus package enacted by the US Congress in 2009 with a defined purpose of stimulating jobs, investments, and consumer spending. The ARRA contains provisions for improving health care quality through the use of health information technology.

Authentication: A security measure to establish the validity of an electronic transmission, message, or original source (eg, author) or to verify the authorization of an individual to receive specific information. Authentication is used to confirm that an individual or system is who or what it claims to be.

Clinical information systems: Computer technology used in the patient care environment for collecting patient health care information.

Clinical support technologies: Assorted technologies used in the patient care environment to facilitate the clinician's ability to provide safe, comprehensive interventions for the delivery of quality health care.

Code key: A computer code used to authenticate entries in an electronic health record as permitted by state, federal, and reimbursement regulations.

Correction: A change made to the documented patient health information meant to clarify the entry after the document has been authenticated.

Customize: To specifically select or set preferences or options for health care information.

Data mining: The process of extracting and analyzing data for usable information from relationships, patterns, information clusters, and data trends. The new information may be used for predictive modeling in decision support processes for clinical, operational, and research utilization.

Data quality: Data remaining unchanged from their original meaning; data are complete, correct, comprehensive, and consistent for the intended use.

Data repository: A central location where health care data (eg, clinical, financial, operational) and files are stored and maintained for later retrieval and use.

Decision support: An interactive computer-based program that provides reminders, advice, or interpretation of patient data at a specific point in time.

Deemed status: The "deeming" authority granted to national accreditation organizations (eg, The Joint Commission, DNV-GL) by the Centers for Medicare & Medicaid Services (CMS) to determine, on CMS's behalf, whether a health care provider organization is in compliance with the regulations to provide and receive payment for Medicare services. Six areas are deemable: quality assurance, antidiscrimination, access to services, confidentiality and accuracy of enrollee records, information on advance directives, and provider participation rules.

Digital signature: A cryptographic signature (ie, digital key) used to authenticate the user, provide legal ownership, and ensure integrity of the unit of information.

Digitized inked signature: A handwritten signature using a pen pad to create an electronic representation of the actual signature.

Downtime: Periods of time when the clinical information system (ie, electronic health record) is unavailable because of scheduled maintenance or upgrades or technology failure, power outage, or another unscheduled event.

Electronic health record: An electronic record of health-related information for an individual that conforms to nationally recognized interoperability standards and that can be created, managed, and consulted by authorized clinicians and staff members across more than one health care organization.

Electronic medical record: An electronic record of health-related information for an individual that can be created, gathered, managed, and consulted by authorized clinicians and staff members within one health care organization.

Electronic signature: The technology-neutral electronic process used to sign (ie, attest) content for authorship and legal responsibility for a section of information. The electronic signature format is determined by the technology used to collect or create the signature.

Health Information Technology for Economic and Clinical Health: A component of the American Recovery and Reinvestment Act of 2009 that addresses the use of electronic health information technology to improve health care quality, coordination of care, and health information privacy and security.

Integrity: The accuracy, consistency, and reliability of information content, processes, and systems.

Interoperable: The ability for health information systems to exchange or share health information within and across organizational boundaries.

Legal health record: The medical record generated at or for a health care organization as its business record or released upon request, which represents an exact duplicate of the original record.

Malware: Software considered harmful to a computer system including but not limited to viruses, worms, Trojan horses, spyware, and unauthorized adware.

Metadata: The descriptive data that characterizes other data to create a clearer understanding of their meaning and to achieve greater reliability and quality of information (eg, name, address, and telephone number of a patient).

Signature legend: A document that identifies an author's full signature and title when initials are used to authenticate entries in the health care record.

Standardized terminology: Terminology developed according to specific characteristics so that each data element is expressed as a single, clear and unambiguous concept. Standardized terminology concepts maintain their meaning permanently.

Tailored health care information: The unique patient characteristics based on multiple factors influencing health status and health behaviors and collected to inform individualized nursing interventions.

Versioning: The process of assigning a unique version name or number to an electronic heath record and used to identify revisions occurring to previously documented content.

References

1. Chow M, Beene M, O'Brien A, et al. A nursing information model process for interoperability. *J Am Med Inform Assoc.* 2015;22(3):608-614. [VB]

2. Gugerty B, Maranda MJ, Beachley M, et al. *Challenges and Opportunities in Documentation of the Nursing Care of Patients.* Baltimore, MD: Maryland Nursing Workforce Commission, Documentation Work Group; 2007. [IIIB]

3. Standards of perioperative nursing. In: *Guidelines for Perioperative Practice.* Denver, CO: AORN, Inc, 2015:693-708. [IVA]

4. *ANA Principles for Documentation.* Silver Spring, MD: American Nurses Association; 2010. [IVA]

5. *Nursing: Scope and Standards of Practice.* Silver Spring, MD: American Nurses Association; 2010. [IVA]

6. Peterson AM. Medical record as a legal document part 2: meeting the standards. *J Legal Nurse Consult.* 2013;24(1):4-10. [VA]

7. *Nursing's Social Policy Statement: The Essence of the Profession.* Silver Spring, MD: American Nurses Association; 2010. [IVA]

8. Beyea SC. Describing professional nursing through a universal record in perioperative settings. *Int J Nurs Terminol Classif.* 2003;14(S4):23. [IIIB]

9. Petersen C, ed. *Perioperative Nursing Data Set.* 3rd ed. Denver, CO: AORN; 2011. [IVA]

10. Kuc JA, Iyer PW, Levin BL, Shea MA. Perioperative records. In: Iyer PW, Levin BL, Shea MA, eds. *Medical Legal Aspects of Medical Records.* Tucson, AZ: Lawyers & Judges Publishing Company; 2006:657-677. [IVA]

11. Junttila K, Hupli M, Salanterä S. The use of nursing diagnoses in perioperative documentation. *Int J Nurs Terminol Classif.* 2010;21(2):57-68. [IIIB]

12. Guido GW. *Legal & Ethical Issues in Nursing.* 5th ed. Boston, MA: Pearson; 2010. [VA]

13. Exhibit B: Perioperative explications for the ANA Code of Ethics for Nurses. In: *Guidelines for Perioperative Practice.* Denver, CO: AORN, Inc; 2015:711-732. [IVB]

14. Staggers N, Clark L, Blaz JW, Kapsandoy S. Why patient summaries in electronic health records do not provide the cognitive support necessary for nurses' handoffs on medical and surgical units: insights from interviews and observations. *Health Informatics J.* 2011;17(3):209-223. [IIIB]

15. Urquhart C, Currell R, Grant MJ, Hardiker NR. Nursing record systems: effects on nursing practice and healthcare outcomes. *Cochrane Database Syst Rev.* 2009: (1):CD002099. [IA]

16. Wang N, Hailey D, Yu P. Quality of nursing documentation and approaches to its evaluation: a mixed-method systematic review. *J Adv Nurs.* 2011;67(9):1858-1875. [IIA]

17. Keenan G, Yakel E, Dunn Lopez K, Tschannen D, Ford YB. Challenges to nurses' efforts of retrieving, documenting, and communicating patient care information. *J Am Med Inform Assoc.* 2013;20(2):245-251. [IIIA]

18. Micek WT, Berry L, Gilski D, Kallenbach A, Link D, Scharer K. Patient outcomes: the link between nursing diagnoses and interventions. *J Nurs Adm.* 1996;26(11):29-35. [VA]

19. Monarch K. Documentation, part 1: principles for self-protection. Preserve the medical record—and defend yourself. *Am J Nurs.* 2007;107(7):58-60. [VB]

20. 42 CFR §416.47. Condition of participation: medical records. Centers for Medicare & Medicaid Services. Department of Health and Human Services. https://www.gpo.gov/fdsys/granule/CFR-2007-title42-vol3/CFR-2007-title42-vol3-sec416-47. Accessed April 20, 2016. [IA]

21. 42 CFR §482. Conditions of participation for hospitals. Centers for Medicare & Medicaid Services. Department of Health and Human Services. https://www.gpo.gov/fdsys/granule/CFR-2011-title42-vol5/CFR-2011-title42-vol5-part482/content-detail.html. Accessed April 20, 2016. [IA]

22. 42 USC § 18001. Patient Protection and Affordable Care Act. January 7, 2011. https://www.gpo.gov/fdsys/granule/USCODE-2010-title42/USCODE-2010-title42-chap157-subchapI-sec18001. Accessed April 20, 2016. [IA]

23. Guideline for medication safety. In: *Guidelines for Perioperative Practice.* Denver, CO: AORN, Inc; 2016:289-332. [IVB]

24. Barney L, Jackson JJ, Ollapally VM, Savarise MT, Senkowski CK. Documentation of services provided in the postoperative global period. *Bull Am Coll Surg.* 2013;98(5):48-51. [IVB]

25. Ammenwerth E, Rauchegger F, Ehlers F, Hirsch B, Schaubmayr C. Effect of a nursing information system on the quality of information processing in nursing: an evaluation study using the HIS-monitor instrument. *Int J Med Inf.* 2011;80(1):25-38. [IIA]

26. Whittenburg L. Workflow viewpoints: analysis of nursing workflow documentation in the electronic health record. *J Healthc Inf Manag.* 2010;24(3):71-75. [VB]

27. Lee S, McElmurry B. Capturing nursing care workflow disruptions: comparison between nursing and physician workflows. *Comput Inform Nurs.* 2010;28(3):151-599. [IIIB]

28. *Better EHR: Usability, Workflow and Cognitive Support in Electronic Health Records.* Houston, TX: National Center for Cognitive Informatics & Decision Making; 2014. [IVA]

29. Colligan L, Potts HW, Finn CT, Sinkin RA. Cognitive workload changes for nurses transitioning from a legacy system with paper documentation to a commercial electronic health record. *Int J Med Inf.* 2015;84(7):469-476. [IIA]

30. Institute of Medicine; Page A, eds. *Keeping Patients Safe: Transforming the Work Environment of Nurses.* Washington, DC: National Academies Press; 2004. [IVA]

31. Hayrinen K, Lammintakanen J, Saranto K. Evaluation of electronic nursing documentation—nursing process model and standardized terminologies as keys to visible and transparent nursing. *Int J Med Inform.* 2010;79(8):554-564. [IIIB]

32. Keohane CA, Bane AD, Featherstone E, et al. Quantifying nursing workflow in medication administration. *J Nurs Adm.* 2008;38(1):19-26. [IIIB]

33. Capuano T, Bokovoy J, Halkins D, Hitchings K. Workflow analysis: eliminating non-value-added work. *J Nurs Adm.* 2004;34(5):246-256. [IIIA]

34. Roberson D, Connell M, Dillis S, et al. Cognitive complexity of the medical record is a risk factor for major adverse events. *Permanente J.* 2014;18(1):4-8. [IB]

35. Ahmed A, Chandra S, Herasevich V, Gajic O, Pickering BW. The effect of two different electronic health record user interfaces on intensive care provider task load, errors of cognition, and performance. *Crit Care Med.* 2011;39(7):1626-1634. [IB]

36. Potter P, Boxerman S, Dunagan C, et al. An analysis of nurses' cognitive work: a new perspective for understanding medical errors. *Adv Patient Saf.* 2005;1:39-51. [IIA]

37. Karsh BT, Holden RJ, Alper SJ, Or CK. A human factors engineering paradigm for patient safety: designing to support the performance of the healthcare professional. *Qual Saf Health Care.* 2006;15(Suppl 1):i59-i65. [VB]

38. Benner P, Sheets V, Uris P, Malloch K, Schwed K, Jamison D. Individual, practice, and system causes of errors in nursing: a taxonomy. *J Nurs Adm.* 2002;32(10):509-523. [IIIB]

39. Hendrich A, Chow M, Skierczynski BA, Lu Z. A 36-hospital time and motion study: how do medical-surgical nurses spend their time? *Permanente J.* 2008;12(3):25-34. [IIIA]

40. Ash JS, Berg M, Coiera E. Some unintended consequences of information technology in health care: the nature of patient care information system-related errors. *J Am Med Inform Assoc.* 2004;11(2):104-112. [IIIA]

41. Bloomrosen M, Starren J, Lorenzi NM, Ash JS, Patel VL, Shortliffe EH. Anticipating and addressing the unintended consequences of health IT and policy: a report from the AMIA 2009 Health Policy Meeting. *J Am Med Inform Assoc.* 2011;18(1):82-90. [IVB]

42. Harrison MI, Koppel R, Bar-Lev S. Unintended consequences of information technologies in health care—an interactive sociotechnical analysis. *J Am Med Inform Assoc.* 2007;14(5):542-549. [VA]

43. Cornell P, Herrin-Griffith D, Keim C, et al. Transforming nursing workflow, part 1: the chaotic nature of nurse activities. *J Nurs Adm.* 2010;40(9):366-373. [IIIB]

44. Cornell P, Riordan M, Herrin-Griffith D. Transforming nursing workflow, part 2: the impact of technology on nurse activities. *J Nurs Adm.* 2010;40(10):432-439. [IIB]

45. Irwin RS, Richardson ND. Patient-focused care: using the right tools. *Chest.* 2006;130(1 Suppl):73S-82S. [VA]

46. Allan J, Englebright J. Patient-centered documentation: an effective and efficient use of clinical information systems. *J Nurs Adm.* 2000;30(2):90-95. [VB]

47. Nailon RE. The assessment and documentation of language and communication needs in healthcare systems: current practices and future directions for coordinating safe, patient-centered care. *Nurs Outlook.* 2007;55(6):311-317. [VA]

48. Institute of Medicine. *Crossing the Quality Chasm: A New Health System for the 21st Century.* Washington, DC: National Academies Press; 2001. [IVA]

49. Spooner SA; Council on Clinical Information Technology American Academy of Pediatrics. Special requirements of electronic health record systems in pediatrics. *Pediatrics.* 2007;119(3):631-637. [IVB]

50. Park EJ, McDaniel A, Jung MS. Computerized tailoring of health information. *Comput Inform Nurs.* 2009;27(1):34-43. [VA]

51. Payne TH, tenBroek AE, Fletcher GS, Labuguen MC. Transition from paper to electronic inpatient physician notes. *J Am Med Inform Assoc.* 2010;17(1):108-111. [VC]

52. Korst LM, Eusebio-Angeja AC, Chamorro T, Aydin CE, Gregory KD. Nursing documentation time during implementation of an electronic medical record. *J Nurs Adm.* 2003;33(1):24-30. [IIIB]

53. Flemming D, Hübner U. How to improve change of shift handovers and collaborative grounding and what role does the electronic patient record system play? Results of a systematic literature review. *Int J Med Inf.* 2013;82(7):580-592. [IIIA]

54. Andreia Neves da Mota L, Soares Pereira FM, Ferreira de Sousa PA. Nursing information systems: exploration of information shared with physicians. *Refencia.* 2014;4(1):83-89. [IIIB]

55. Jefferies D, Johnson M, Nicholls D. Comparing written and oral approaches to clinical reporting in nursing. *Contemp Nurse.* 2012;42(1):129-138. [IIIA]

56. Ammenwerth E, Eichstadter R, Haux R, Pohl U, Rebel S, Ziegler S. A randomized evaluation of a computer-based nursing documentation system. *Methods Inf Med.* 2001;40(2):61-68. [IA]

57. Harrington L. Electronic health record workflow: why more work than flow? *AACN Adv Crit Care.* 2015;26(1):5-9. [VC]

58. Asaro PV, Boxerman SB. Effects of computerized provider order entry and nursing documentation on workflow. *Acad Emerg Med.* 2008;15(10):908-915. [IIB]

59. Ay F, Polat Ş. The belief and opinions of nurses on the electronic patient record system. *Int J Caring Sci.* 2014;7(1):258-268. [IIIB]

60. Mahler C, Ammenwerth E, Wagner A, et al. Effects of a computer-based nursing documentation system on the quality of nursing documentation. *J Med Syst.* 2007;31(4):274-282. [IIA]

61. Stead WW, Lin HS, eds. *Computational Technology for Effective Health Care: Immediate Steps and Strategic Directions.* Washington, DC: National Academies Press; 2009. [IVA]

62. Poissant L, Pereira J, Tamblyn R, Kawasumi Y. The impact of electronic health records on time efficiency of physicians and nurses: a systematic review. *J Am Med Inform Assoc.* 2005;12(5):505-516. [IIA]

63. Amarasingham R, Plantinga L, Diener-West M, Gaskin DJ, Powe NR. Clinical information technologies and inpatient outcomes: a multiple hospital study. *Arch Intern Med.* 2009;169(2):108-114. [IIB]

64. Shojania KG, Jennings A, Mayhew A, Ramsay CR, Eccles MP, Grimshaw J. The effects of on-screen, point of care computer reminders on processes and outcomes of care. *Cochrane Database Syst Rev.* 2009;(3):CD001096. [IA]

65. Harrington L, Kennerly D, Johnson C. Safety issues related to the electronic medical record (EMR): synthesis of the literature from the last decade, 2000-2009. *J Healthc Manag.* 2011;56(1):31-43. [IIIB]

66. *ANA Position Statement: Electronic Health Record.* December 11, 2009. http://nursingworld.org/MainMenuCategories/Policy-Advocacy/Positions-and-Resolutions/ANAPosition Statements/Position-Statements-Alphabetically/Electronic-Health-Record.html. Accessed April 20, 2016. [IVB]

67. Kim H, Dykes P, Mar P, Goldsmith D, Choi J, Goldberg H. Towards a standardized representation to support data reuse: representing the ICNP semantics using the HL7 RIM. *Stud Health Technol Inform.* 2009;146:308-313. [IIIB]

68. Lundberg C, Warren J, Brokel J, et al. Selecting a standardized terminology for the electronic health record that reveals the impact of nursing on patient care. *Online J Nurs Inform.* 2008;12(2). [IVA]

69. Zielstorff RD. Characteristics of a good nursing nomenclature from an informatics perspective. *Online J Nurs Inform.* 1998;3(2). [VC]

70. Tastan S, Linch GC, Keenan GM, et al. Evidence for the existing American Nurses Association-recognized standardized nursing terminologies: a systematic review. *Int J Nurs Stud.* 2014;51(8):1160-1170. [IIIA]

71. Graves JR, Corcoran S. The study of nursing informatics. *Image J Nurs Sch.* 1989;21(4):227-231. [IVB]

72. Beyea SC. Standardized language—making nursing practice count. *AORN J.* 1999;70(5):831-838. [IVB]

73. Carrington JM. The usefulness of nursing languages to communicate a clinical event. *Comput Inform Nurs.* 2012;30(2):82-88. [IIIA]

74. Saba VK, Taylor SL. Moving past theory: use of a standardized, coded nursing terminology to enhance nursing visibility. *Comput Inform Nurs.* 2007;25(6):324-331. [IVB]

75. Dykes PC, DaDamio RR, Goldsmith D, Kim HE, Ohashi K, Saba VK. Leveraging standards to support patient-centric interdisciplinary plans of care. *AMIA Annual Symp Proc.* 2011; 2011:356-363. [IIIB]

76. 42 CFR §482.51. Condition of participation: surgical services. Centers for Medicare & Medicaid Services. Department of Health and Human Services. https://www.gpo.gov/fdsys/granule/CFR-2010-title42-vol5/CFR-2010-title42-vol5-sec482-51. Accessed April 20, 2016. [IA]

77. Westra BL, Subramanian A, Hart CM, et al. Achieving "meaningful use" of electronic health records through the integration of the Nursing Management Minimum Data Set. *J Nurs Adm.* 2010;40(7-8):336-343. [IVB]

78. Mangalmurti SS, Murtagh L, Mello MM. Medical malpractice liability in the age of electronic health records. *N Engl J Med.* 2010;363(21):2060-2067. [IVA]

79. Centers for Medicare & Medicaid Services (CMS) HHS. Medicare and Medicaid programs; changes in provider and supplier enrollment, ordering and referring, and documentation requirements; and changes in provider agreements. Final rule. *Fed Regist.* 2012;77(82):25284-25318. [IA]

80. 42 CFR Part 495 Medicare and Medicaid programs; Electronic Health Record Incentive Program—modifications to meaningful use in 2015 through 2017. Proposed rule. *Fed Regist.* 2015;80(72):20346-20399. [IA]

81. Hayrinen K, Saranto K, Nykanen P. Definition, structure, content, use and impacts of electronic health records: a review of the research literature. *Int J Med Inform.* 2008;77(5):291-304. [IIIA]

82. Hyun S, Bakken S. Toward the creation of an ontology for nursing document sections: mapping section names to the

LOINC semantic model. *AMIA Annu Symp Proc.* 2006;2006:364-368. [IIIB]

83. National Quality Forum. Executive summary. In: *Health Information Technology Automation of Quality Measure: Quality Data Set and Data Flow.* Washington, DC: NQF;2009:iii-vi. [IA]

84. Goossen WT, Ozbolt JG, Coenen A, et al. Development of a provisional domain model for the nursing process for use within the Health Level 7 reference information model. *J Am Med Inform Assoc.* 2004;11(3):186-194. [IIIB]

85. Adler-Milstein J, Jha AK. Sharing clinical data electronically: a critical challenge for fixing the health care system. *JAMA.* 2012;307(16):1695-1696. [VA]

86. Centers for Medicare & Medicaid Services (CMS) HHS. Medicare and Medicaid programs; electronic health record incentive program—stage 2. Final rule. *Fed Regist.* 2012;77(171):53967-54162. [IA]

87. Jha AK, DesRoches CM, Campbell EG, et al. Use of electronic health records in US hospitals. *N Engl J Med.* 2009;360(16):1628-1638.

88. Brown DS, Donaldson N, Burnes Bolton L, Aydin CE. Nursing-sensitive benchmarks for hospitals to gauge high-reliability performance. *J Healthc Qual.* 2010;32(6):9-17. [IVB]

89. US Department of Health and Human Services. *Report to Congress: Medicare Ambulatory Surgical Center Value-Based Purchasing Implementation Plan.* Washington, DC: Centers for Medicare & Medicaid Services; 2011. https://www.cms.gov/Medicare/Medicare-Fee-for-Service-Payment/ASCPayment/Downloads/C_ASC_RTC-2011.pdf. Accessed April 20, 2016. [IA]

90. *Becoming a High Reliability Organization: Operational Advice for Hospital Leaders.* Rockville, MD: Agency for Healthcare Research and Quality; 2008. [IVB]

91. Thompson D, Johnston P, Spurr C. The impact of electronic medical records on nursing efficiency. *J Nurs Adm.* 2009;39(10):444-451. [VB]

92. Shekelle PG, Morton SC, Keeler EB. *Costs and Benefits of Health Information Technology.* Evidence Report/Technology Assessment No. 132. (Prepared by the Southern California Evidence-based Practice Center under Contract No. 290-02-0003.). Rockville, MD: Agency for Healthcare Research and Quality; 2006. [IVA]

93. Department of Veterans Affairs. Sharing information between the Department of Veterans Affairs and the Department of Defense. Interim final rule. *Fed Regist.* 2011;76(203):65133-65135.

94. Office of the National Coordinator for Health Information Technology (ONC) Department of Health and Human Services. 2014 Edition Release 2 Electronic Health Record (EHR) certification criteria and the ONC HIT Certification Program; regulatory flexibilities, improvements, and enhanced health information exchange. Final rule. *Fed Regist.* 2014;79(176):54429-54480. [IA]

95. A Blueprint for the CMS Measures Management System. Version 11.1 ed. Washington, DC: Centers for Medicaid Services; August 2015. https://www.cms.gov/Medicare/Quality-Initiatives-Patient-Assessment-Instruments/MMS/Downloads/Blueprint111.pdf. Accessed April 20, 2016. [IA]

96. Murdoch TB, Detsky AS. The inevitable application of big data to health care. *JAMA.* 2013;309(13):1351-1352. [VA]

97. Al-Rawajfah OM, Aloush S, Hewitt JB. Use of electronic health-related datasets in nursing and health-related research. *West J Nurs Res.* 2015;37(7):952-983. [IIIA]

98. *Transforming Health Care Through Big Data.* New York, NY: Institute for Health Technology Transformation; 2013. [VB]

99. Sun J, Hu J, Luo D, et al. Combining knowledge and data driven insights for identifying risk factors using electronic health records. *AMIA Annu Symp Proc.* 2012;2012:901-910. [IIA]

100. 42 CFR §482.24. Condition of participation: medical record services. Centers for Medicare & Medicaid Services. Department of Health and Human Services. https://www.gpo.gov/fdsys/granule/CFR-2011-title42-vol5/CFR-2011-title42-vol5-sec482-24/content-detail.html. Accessed April 20, 2016. [IA]

101. 42 CFR §482.23. Condition of participation: nursing services. Centers for Medicare & Medicaid Services. Department of Health and Human Services. https://www.gpo.gov/fdsys/granule/CFR-2011-title42-vol5/CFR-2011-title42-vol5-sec482-23/content-detail.html. Accessed April 20, 2016. [IA]

102. 42 CFR §416.46. Condition for Coverage—Nursing services. Centers for Medicare & Medicaid Services. Department of Health and Human Services. https://www.gpo.gov/fdsys/granule/CFR-2007-title42-vol3/CFR-2007-title42-vol3-sec416-46. Accessed April 20, 2016. [IA]

103. Scruth EA. Quality nursing documentation in the medical record. *Clin Nurse Spec.* 2014;28(6):312-314. [VC]

104. Jefferies D, Johnson M, Griffiths R. A meta-study of the essentials of quality nursing documentation. *Int J Nurs Pract.* 2010;16(2):112-124. [IIIA]

105. 42 CFR §485.638. Conditions of participation: clinical records. Centers for Medicare & Medicaid Services. Department of Health and Human Services. https://www.gpo.gov/fdsys/granule/CFR-2011-title42-vol5/CFR-2011-title42-vol5-sec485-638. Accessed April 21, 2016. [IA]

106. 42 CFR §416. Ambulatory surgical services. Centers for Medicare & Medicaid Services. Department of Health and Human Services. https://www.cms.gov/Regulations-and-Guidance/Legislation/CFCsAndCoPs/ASC.html. Accessed April 21, 2016. [IA]

107. Guidelines for Perioperative Practice. Denver, CO: AORN, Inc; 2016. [IVA]

108. 42 CFR §416.51. Conditions for coverage: infection control. Centers for Medicare & Medicaid Services. Department of Health and Human Services. https://www.gpo.gov/fdsys/granule/CFR-2012-title42-vol3/CFR-2012-title42-vol3-sec416-51. Accessed April 21, 2016. [IA]

109. NPSG.07.05.01: Implement evidence-based practices for preventing surgical site infections. In: *Comprehensive Accreditation Manual for Hospitals.* Oakbrook Terrace, IL: The Joint Commission; 2015. [IVA]

110. IC.01.05.01: The hospital has an infection prevention and control plan. In: *Comprehensive Accreditation Manual for Hospitals.* Oakbrook Terrace, IL: The Joint Commission; 2015. [IVA]

111. IC.02.01.01: The hospital implements its infection prevention and control plan. In: *Comprehensive Accreditation Manual for Hospitals.* Oakbrook Terrace, IL: The Joint Commission; 2015. [IVA]

112. Guideline for care of the patient receiving local anesthesia. In: *Guidelines for Perioperative Practice.* Denver, CO: AORN, Inc; 2016:577-588. [IVB]

113. Krenzischek DA, Wilson L; ASPAN. ASPAN pain and comfort clinical guideline. *J Perianesth Nurs.* 2003;18(4):232-236. [IVC]

114. ASPAN. *2015-2017 Perianesthesia Nursing Standards, Practice Recommendations and Interpretive Statements.* Cherry Hill, NJ: American Society of PeriAnesthesia Nurses; 2015. [IVB]

115. 42 CFR §416.48. Condition for coverage: pharmaceutical services. Centers for Medicare & Medicaid Services. Department of Health and Human Services. https://www.gpo.gov/fdsys/granule/CFR-2007-title42-vol3/CFR-2007-title42-vol3-sec416-48/content-detail.html. Accessed April 21, 2016. [IA]

116. Centers for Medicare & Medicaid Services. Department of Health and Human Services. Condition of participation: patient's rights. 42 CFR §482.13. http://www.ecfr.gov/cgi-bin/text-idx?rgn=div5;node=42:5.0.1.1.1;cc=ecfr. Accessed April 21, 2016. [IA]

117. Medication management. In: *Comprehensive Accreditation Manual for Hospitals.* Oakbrook Terrace, IL: The Joint Commission; 2015. [IVA]

118. Provision of care, treatment, and services. In: *Comprehensive Accreditation Manual for Hospitals.* Oakbrook Terrace, IL: The Joint Commission; 2015. [IVA]

119. Medical records: 600.040.010. In: *Medicare Standards and Checklist for Accreditation of Ambulatory Surgery Facilities.* 6.5 ed. Gurnee, IL: American Association for Accreditation of Ambulatory Surgery Facilities; 2014:89. [IVA]

120. Clinical records and health information. In: *Accreditation Handbook for Ambulatory Health Care.* Skokie, IL: Accreditation Association for Ambulatory Health Care Inc; 2015:49-51. [IVA]

121. Quality of care provided. In: *Accreditation Handbook for Ambulatory Health Care.* Skokie, IL: Accreditation Association for Ambulatory Health Care Inc; 2015:42-43. [IVA]

122. 29 CFR §1910.1030. Bloodborne pathogens. US Department of Labor, Occupational Safety and Health Standards. http://www.osha.gov/pls/oshaweb/owadisp.show_document?p_table=standards&p_id=10051. Accessed April 21, 2016. [IA]

123. *AORN Position Statement: Preventing Wrong-Patient, Wrong-Site, Wrong-Procedure Events.* AORN, Inc. https://www.aorn.org/guidelines/clinical-resources/position-statements. Accessed April 20, 2016. [IVB]

124. Guideline for preoperative patient skin antisepsis. In: *Guidelines for Perioperative Practice.* Denver, CO: AORN, Inc; 2016:41-64. [IVA]

125. Rights and responsibilities of the individual. In: *Comprehensive Accreditation Manual for Hospitals.* Oakbrook Terrace, IL: The Joint Commission; 2015. [IVA]

126. NPSG.03.06.01: Maintain and communicate accurate patient medication information. In: *Comprehensive Accreditation Manual for Hospitals.* Oakbrook Terrace, IL: The Joint Commission; 2015. [IVA]

127. Guideline for prevention of transmissible infections. In: *Guidelines for Perioperative Practice.* Denver, CO: AORN, Inc; 2016:471-506. [IVA]

128. Postanesthetic care unit (PACU). In: *Regular Standards and Checklist for Accreditation of Ambulatory Surgery Facilities.* 14.4 ed. Gurnee, IL: American Association for Accreditation of Ambulatory Surgery Facilities; 2016:43-45. [IVB]

129. Guideline for care of the patient receiving moderate sedation/analgesia. In: *Guidelines for Perioperative Practice.* Denver, CO: AORN, Inc; 2016:617-648. [IVB]

130. Guideline for a safe environment of care, part 1. In: *Guidelines for Perioperative Practice.* Denver, CO: AORN, Inc; 2016:237-262. [IVA]

131. Guideline for prevention of unplanned patient hypothermia. In: *Guidelines for Perioperative Practice.* Denver, CO: AORN, Inc; 2016:531-554. [IVB]

132. Guideline for prevention of deep vein thrombosis. In: *Guidelines for Perioperative Practice.* Denver, CO: AORN, Inc; 2016:521-530. [IVB]

133. Guideline for positioning the patient. In: *Guidelines for Perioperative Practice.* Denver, CO: AORN, Inc; 2016:649-668. [IVB]

134. 42 CFR §482.27. Condition of participation: laboratory services. Centers for Medicare & Medicaid Services. Department of Health and Human Services. https://www.gpo.gov/fdsys/granule/CFR-2011-title42-vol5/CFR-2011-title42-vol5-sec482-27/content-detail.html. Accessed April 21, 2016. [IA]

135. 42 CFR §416.52. Conditions for coverage: patient admission, assessment and discharge. Centers for Medicare & Medicaid Services. Department of Health and Human Services. https://www.gpo.gov/fdsys/granule/CFR-2011-title42-vol3/CFR-2011-title42-vol3-sec416-52. Accessed April 21, 2016. [IA]

136. Record of care, treatment, and services. In: *Comprehensive Accreditation Manual for Hospitals.* Oakbrook Terrace, IL: The Joint Commission; 2015. [IVA]

137. Guideline for complementary care interventions. In: *Guidelines for Perioperative Practice.* Denver, CO: AORN, Inc; 2016:507-520. [IVA]

138. Universal Protocol. In: *Comprehensive Accreditation Manual for Hospitals.* Oakbrook Terrace, IL: The Joint Commission; 2015. [IVA]

139. Quality and performance improvement standards for perioperative nursing. In: *Guidelines for Perioperative Practice.* Denver, CO: AORN, Inc; 2015:761-770. [IVB]

140. Guideline for transfer of patient care information. In: *Guidelines for Perioperative Practice.* Denver, CO: AORN, Inc; 2016:669-674. [IVB]

141. Surgical and related services. In: *Accreditation Handbook for Ambulatory Health Care.* Skokie, IL: Accreditation Association for Ambulatory Health Care Inc; 2015:64-71. [IVA]

142. Accreditation Association for Ambulatory Health Care. *Accreditation Handbook for Ambulatory Health Care.* Skokie, IL: The Association; 2015. [IVA]

143. *Regular Standards and Checklist for Accreditation of Ambulatory Surgery Facilities.* Version 14.4. Gurnee, IL: American Association for Accreditation of Ambulatory Surgery Facilities; 2016. [IVA]

144. 42 CFR §482.41. Condition of participation: physical environment. Centers for Medicare & Medicaid Services. Department of Health and Human Services. https://www.gpo.gov/fdsys/granule/CFR-2011-title42-vol5/CFR-2011-title42-vol5-sec482-41. Accessed April 21, 2016. [IA]

145. 42 CFR §416.44. Condition for coverage: environment. Centers for Medicare & Medicaid Services. Department of Health and Human Services. https://www.gpo.gov/fdsys/granule/CFR-2012-title42-vol3/CFR-2012-title42-vol3-sec416-44. Accessed April 21, 2016. [IA]

146. Environment of care. In: *Comprehensive Accreditation Manual for Hospitals*. Oakbrook Terrace, IL: The Joint Commission; 2015. [IVA]

147. Guideline for electrosurgery. In: *Guidelines for Perioperative Practice*. Denver, CO: AORN, Inc; 2016:119-136. [IVB]

148. Guideline for care of patients undergoing pneumatic tourniquet-assisted procedures. In: *Guidelines for Perioperative Practice*. Denver, CO: AORN, Inc; 2016:151-176. [IVA]

149. Guideline for minimally invasive surgery. In: *Guidelines for Perioperative Practice*. Denver, CO: AORN, Inc; 2016:589-616. [IVB]

150. Guideline for laser safety. In: *Guidelines for Perioperative Practice*. Denver, CO: AORN, Inc; 2016:137-150. [IVB]

151. Guideline for sharps safety. In: *Guidelines for Perioperative Practice*. Denver, CO: AORN, Inc; 2016:417-440. [IVA]

152. Guideline for a safe environment of care, part 2. In: *Guidelines for Perioperative Practice*. Denver, CO: AORN, Inc; 2016:263-288. [IVA]

153. Infection prevention and control. In: *Comprehensive Accreditation Manual for Hospitals*. Oakbrook Terrace, IL: The Joint Commission; 2015. [IVA]

154. *ANSI/AAMI ST79:2010, A1, A2, A3 & A4:2013: Comprehensive Guide to Steam Sterilization and Sterility Assurance in Health Care Facilities*. Arlington, VA: Association for the Advancement of Medical Instrumentation; 2013. [IVA]

155. Medical records: 600.010.060. In: *Medicare Standards and Checklist for Accreditation of Ambulatory Surgery Facilities*. 6.5 ed. Gurnee, IL: American Association for Accreditation of Ambulatory Surgery Facilities; 2014:79. [IVA]

156. Guideline for autologous tissue management. In: *Guidelines for Perioperative Practice*. Denver, CO: AORN, Inc; 2016:185-236. [IVA]

157. 24 CFR §482.45. Condition of participation: organ, tissue, and eye procurement. Centers for Medicare & Medicaid Services. Department of Health and Human Services. https://www.gpo.gov/fdsys/granule/CFR-2011-title42-vol5/CFR-2011-title42-vol5-sec482-45. Accessed April 21, 2016. [IA]

158. Guideline for specimen management. In: *Guidelines for Perioperative Practice*. Denver, CO: AORN, Inc; 2016. [IVA]

159. *Policy on Standardized Packaging of Human Organs and Tissue Typing Materials*. Richmond, VA: Organ Procurement and Transplantation Network; 2010. [IA]

160. Transplant safety. In: *Comprehensive Accreditation Manual for Hospitals*. Oakbrook Terrace, IL: The Joint Commission; 2015. [IVA]

161. Guideline for processing flexible endoscopes. In: *Guidelines for Perioperative Practice*. Denver, CO: AORN, Inc; 2016:675-758. [IVB]

162. Guideline for cleaning and care of surgical instruments. In: *Guidelines for Perioperative Practice*. Denver, CO: AORN, Inc; 2016:773-808. [IVA]

163. Quality Indicators. Agency for Healthcare Research and Quality. http://www.qualityindicators.ahrq.gov/. Accessed April 21, 2016. [IA]

164. Mangram AJ, Horan TC, Pearson ML, Silver LC, Jarvis WR. Guideline for prevention of surgical site infection, 1999. Hospital Infection Control Practices Advisory Committee. *Infect Control Hosp Epidemiol*. 1999;20(4):247-278. [IVA]

165. 42 CFR §482.43. Condition of participation: discharge planning. Centers for Medicare & Medicaid Services. Department of Health and Human Services. https://www.gpo.gov/fdsys/granule/CFR-2011-title42-vol5/CFR-2011-title42-vol5-sec482-43/content-detail.html. Accessed April 21, 2016. [IA]

166. National Patient Safety Goal 7: Reduce the risk of health care-associated infections. In: *Comprehensive Accreditation Manual for Hospitals*. Oakbrook Terrace, IL: The Joint Commission; 2015. [IVA]

167. SCIP-Inf-4: Cardiac surgery patients with controlled 6 a.m. postoperative blood glucose. In: *The Specifications Manual for National Hospital Inpatient Quality Measures*. Version 3.3. Washington, DC: Centers for Medicare & Medicaid Services and Joint Commission; 2011. http://www.wicheckpoint.org/Docs/STK_Q2-11_Manual_CMSTJC.pdf. Accessed April 21, 2016.

168. SCIP-Inf-6: Surgery patients with appropriate hair removal. In: *The Specifications Manual for National Hospital Inpatient Quality Measures*. Version 3.3. Washington, DC: Centers for Medicare & Medicaid Services and Joint Commission; 2011. http://www.wicheckpoint.org/Docs/STK_Q2-11_Manual_CMSTJC.pdf. Accessed April 21, 2016. [IA]

169. General safety in the facility. General. In: *Regular Standards and Checklist for Accreditation of Ambulatory Surgery Facilities*. 14.4 ed. Gurnee, IL: American Association for Accreditation of Ambulatory Surgery Facilities; 2016:45-50. [IVB]

170. Guideline for radiation safety. In: *Guidelines for Perioperative Practice*. Denver, CO: AORN, Inc; 2016:333-368. [IVB]

171. *ANSI Z136.4-2010: American National Standard Recommended Practice for Laser Safety Measurements for Hazard Evaluation*. Orlando, FL: Laser Institute of America; 2010. [IVA]

172. *ANSI Z136.7-2008: American National Standard for Testing and Labeling of Laser Protective Equipment*. Orlando, FL: Laser Institute of America; 2008. [IVA]

173. Guideline for prevention of retained surgical items. In: *Guidelines for Perioperative Practice*. Denver, CO: AORN, Inc; 2016:369-416. [IVA]

174. 109th US Congress. Deficit Reduction Act of 2005. Pub L 109-171. February 8, 2006. https://www.gpo.gov/fdsys/pkg/PLAW-109publ171/html/PLAW-109publ171.htm. Accessed April 21, 2016. [IA]

175. *AORN Position Statement: Creating a Practice Environment of Safety*. AORN, Inc. http://www.aorn.org/guidelines/clinical-resources/position-statements. Accessed April 20, 2016. [IVB]

176. 42 CFR §482.22. Condition of participation: medical staff. Centers for Medicare & Medicaid Services. Department of Health and Human Services. http://www.gpo.gov/fdsys/pkg/CFR-2010-title42-vol5/pdf/CFR-2010-title42-vol5-sec482-22.pdf. Accessed April 21, 2016. [IA]

177. 42 CFR §416.42. Condition for coverage: surgical services. Centers for Medicare & Medicaid Services. Department of Health and Human Services. https://www.gpo.gov/fdsys/granule/CFR-2007-title42-vol3/CFR-2007-title42-vol3-sec416-42/content-detail.html. Accessed April 21, 2016. [IA]

178. 42 CFR §416.49. Condition for coverage: laboratory and radiologic services. Centers for Medicare & Medicaid Services. Department of Health and Human Services. https://www.gpo.gov/fdsys/granule/CFR-2010-title42-vol3/CFR-2010-title42-vol3-sec416-49. Accessed April 21, 2016. [IA]

179. Anesthesia. Pre-anesthesia care. In: *Regular Standards and Checklist for Accreditation of Ambulatory Surgery Facilities.* 14.4 ed. Gurnee, IL: American Association for Accreditation of Ambulatory Surgery Facilities; 2016:79-81. [IVB]

180. General environment—additional Medicare standards. In: *Medicare Standards and Checklist for Accreditation of Ambulatory Surgery Facilities.* 6.5 ed. Gurnee, IL: American Association for Accreditation of Ambulatory Surgery Facilities; 2014:37. [IVA]

181. Operating suite: 200.010.005. In: *Medicare Standards and Checklist for Accreditation of Ambulatory Surgery Facilities.* 6.5 ed. Gurnee, IL: American Association for Accreditation of Ambulatory Surgery Facilities; 2014:9. [IVA]

182. 42 CFR §482.25. Condition of participation: pharmaceutical services. Centers for Medicare & Medicaid Services. Department of Health and Human Services. https://www.gpo.gov/fdsys/granule/CFR-2011-title42-vol5/CFR-2011-title42-vol5-sec482-25. Accessed April 21, 2016. [IA]

183. National Patient Safety Goal 2: Improve the effectiveness of communication among caregivers. In: *Comprehensive Accreditation Manual for Hospitals.* Oakbrook Terrace, IL: The Joint Commission; 2015. [IVA]

184. Operating room policy, environment and procedures. Sterilization. In: *Medicare Standards and Checklist for Accreditation of Ambulatory Surgery Facilities.* 6.5 ed. Gurnee, IL: American Association for Accreditation of Ambulatory Surgery Facilities; 2014:13-15. [IVA]

185. Quality control. In: *ANSI/AAMI ST79:2010, A1, A2, A3 & A4:2013: Comprehensive Guide to Steam Sterilization and Sterility Assurance in Health Care Facilities.* Arlington, VA: Association for the Advancement of Medical Instrumentation; 2013:97-138. [IVA]

186. Guideline for high-level disinfection. In: *Guidelines for Perioperative Practice.* Denver, CO: AORN, Inc; 2016:759-772. [IVA]

187. Clinical practice guideline 1: ASPAN's evidence-based clinical practice guideline for the promotion of perioperative normothermia. In: *Perianesthesia Nursing Standards and Practice Recommendations 2010-2012.* Cherry Hill, NJ: American Society of PeriAnesthesia Nurses; 2010:24-45. [IVA]

188. Operating room policy, environment and procedures. Procedures—sterilization. In: *Regular Standards and Checklist for Accreditation of Ambulatory Surgery Facilities.* 14.4 ed. Gurnee, IL: American Association for Accreditation of Ambulatory Surgery Facilities; 2016:27-28. [IVA]

189. Beyond the count: preventing the retention of foreign objects during interventional radiology procedures. *Pa Patient Saf Advis.* 2008;5(1):24-27. [IVB]

190. ECRI Institute. Sales representatives and other outsiders in the OR. *Operating Room Risk Management.* 2013;1. [IVB]

191. Use of blunt-tip suture needles to decrease percutaneous injuries to surgical personnel: safety and health information bulletin. National Institute for Occupational Safety and Health. http://www.cdc.gov/niosh/docs/2008-101/. Accessed April 20, 2016. [IA]

192. Rutala WA, Weber DJ; Healthcare Infection Control Practices Advisory Committee (HICPAC). *Guideline for Disinfection and Sterilization in Healthcare Facilities, 2008.* Atlanta, GA: Centers for Disease Control and Prevention; 2008.

193. Pommier v ABC Insurance Company, 715 So2d 1270, 1297-1342 (La.App.3dCir. 1998). [IA]

194. Lama v Borras, 1994 16 F3d 473 (United States Court of Appeals, First Circuit, February 25, 1994). http://law.justia.com/cases/federal/appellate-courts/F3/16/473/491880/. Accessed April 21, 2016. [IA]

195. Ledesma v Shashoua, 2007 WL 2214650 (Tex App, August 3, 2007). [IA]

196. 42 CFR §482.52. Condition of participation: anesthesia services. Centers for Medicare & Medicaid Services. Department of Health and Human Services. https://www.gpo.gov/fdsys/granule/CFR-2011-title42-vol5/CFR-2011-title42-vol5-sec482-52/content-detail.html. Accessed April 21, 2016. [IA]

197. 42 CFR §482.28. Condition of participation: food and dietetic services. Centers for Medicare & Medicaid Services. Department of Health and Human Services. https://www.gpo.gov/fdsys/granule/CFR-2011-title42-vol5/CFR-2011-title42-vol5-sec482-28. Accessed April 21, 2016. [IA]

198. 21 CFR §821. Medical device tracking requirements. US Food and Drug Administration. Department of Health and Human Services. https://www.gpo.gov/fdsys/granule/CFR-2011-title21-vol8/CFR-2011-title21-vol8-part821. Accessed April 21, 2016. [IA]

199. 42 CFR §482.26. Condition of participation: radiologic services. Centers for Medicare & Medicaid Services. Department of Health and Human Services. https://www.gpo.gov/fdsys/granule/CFR-2011-title42-vol5/CFR-2011-title42-vol5-sec482-26. Accessed April 21, 2016. [IA]

200. Andreae C, Ekstedt M, Snellman I. Patients' participation as it appears in the nursing documentation, when care is ruled by standardized care plans. *ISRN Nurs.* 2011;2011:707601. [IIIB]

201. Social Security Act, 42 USC 1396d §1905, Pub L No. 74-271. [IA]

202. Medical device tracking; guidance for industry and FDA staff. US Food and Drug Administration. http://www.fda.gov/MedicalDevices/DeviceRegulationandGuidance/GuidanceDocuments/ucm071756.htm. Accessed April 21, 2016. [IA]

203. Food and Drug Administration Modernization Act of 1997, S 830, 105th Cong, 1st Sess (1997), Pub L No 105-115. [IA]

204. UDI Compliance Initiative Summary. Scituate, MA: Strategic Marketplace Initiative; 2015. [VC]

205. Survey & Certification—certification & compliance. Centers for Medicare & Medicaid Services. https://www.cms.gov/Medicare/Provider-Enrollment-and-Certification/CertificationandComplianc/index.html. Accessed April 21, 2016. [IA]

206. *NIAHO Interpretive Guidelines and Surveyor Guidance.* 10.1 ed. Milford, OH: DNV Healthcare Inc; 2012. [IVA]

207. Overview. Healthcare Facilities Accreditation Program. http://www.hfap.org/about/overview.aspx. Accessed April 21, 2016. [IVA]

208. *Comprehensive Accreditation Manual for Ambulatory Care.* Oakbrook Terrace, IL: The Joint Commission; 2015. [IVA]

209. *Comprehensive Accreditation Manual for Hospitals.* Oakbrook Terrace, IL: The Joint Commission; 2015. [IVA]

210. Hospital compare. Medicare.gov. https://www.medicare.gov/hospitalcompare/search.html?. Accessed April 21, 2016. [IA]

211. Centers for Medicare & Medicaid Services (CMS) HHS. Medicare and Medicaid programs: hospital outpatient prospective payment and ambulatory surgical center payment systems and quality reporting programs; Hospital Value-Based Purchasing Program; organ procurement organizations; quality improvement organizations; Electronic Health Records (EHR) Incentive Program; provider reimbursement determinations and appeals. Final rule with comment period and final rules. *Fed Regist.* 2013;78(237):74825-75200. [IA]

212. Straube BM. *Letter to David T. Tayloe Jr.* [written communication]. Baltimore, MD: Department of Health & Human Services; 2010. [IA]

213. 42 CFR §416.50. Condition for coverage: patient rights. Centers for Medicare & Medicaid Services. US Department of Health and Human Services. https://www.gpo.gov/fdsys/granule/CFR-2011-title42-vol3/CFR-2011-title42-vol3-sec416-50. Accessed April 21, 2016. [IA]

214. RC.02.03.07: Qualified staff receive and record verbal orders. In: Comprehensive Accreditation Manual for Ambulatory Care. Oakbrook Terrace, IL: The Joint Commission; 2015. [IVA]

215. Bryant G, DeVault K, Ericson C, et al. Guidance for clinical documentation improvement programs. *J AHIMA.* 2010;81(5):45-50. [IVB]

216. Dawson A, Orsini MJ, Cooper MR, Wollenburg K. Medication safety—reliability of preference cards. *AORN J.* 2005; 82(3):399-407. [IIB]

217. MM.04.01.01: Medication orders are clear and accurate. In: *Comprehensive Accreditation Manual for Hospitals.* Oakbrook Terrace, IL: The Joint Commission; 2015. [IVA]

218. Cole LM. Med report. Documenting to reduce medication errors. *OR Nurse.* 2008;2(7):17-19. [IVC]

219. Brunetti L, Santell JP, Hicks RW, Stevenson JG. USP Medication Safety Forum. The impact of abbreviations on patient safety. *Jt Comm J Qual Patient Saf.* 2007;33(9):576-583. [IIIA]

220. Broussard M, Bass PF 3rd, Arnold CL, McLarty JW, Bocchini JA Jr. Preprinted order sets as a safety intervention in pediatric sedation. *J Pediatr.* 2009;154(6):865-868. [IIB]

221. MM.04.01.01: Medication orders are clear and accurate. In: *Comprehensive Accreditation Manual for Ambulatory Care.* Oakbrook Terrace, IL: The Joint Commission; 2015. [IVA]

222. Murphy EK. Charting by exception. *AORN J.* 2003;78(5):821-823. [VA]

223. Kerr N. "Creating a protective picture": a grounded theory of RN decision making when using a charting-by-exception documentation system. *Medsurg Nurs.* 2013;22(2):110-118. [IIIA]

224. AHIMA e-HIM Work Group on Maintaining the Legal EHR. Maintaining a legally sound health record: paper and electronic. *J AHIMA.* 2005;76(10):64A-64L. [IVB]

225. Short MS. Charting by exception on a clinical pathway. *Nurs Manage.* 1997;28(8):45-46. [IIIB]

226. Holden RJ. Cognitive performance-altering effects of electronic medical records: an application of the human factors paradigm for patient safety. *Cogn Technol Work.* 2011;13(1):11-29. [IIIB]

227. *Driving Quality and Performance Measurement—A Foundation for Clinical Decision Support: A Consensus Report.* Washington, DC: NQF; 2010.

228. Committee on Data Standards for Patient Safety Board on Health Care Services Institute of Medicine of the National Academies. *Key Capabilities of an Electronic Health Record System. Letter Report.* Washington, DC: National Academies Press; 2003. [IVA]

229. Institute of Medicine. *Digital Infrastructure for the Learning Health System: The Foundation for Continuous Improvement in Health and Health Care: Workshop Series Summary.* Washington, DC: The National Academies Press; 2011. [IVA]

230. Health Insurance Portability and Accountability Act of 1996, 42 USC §201 (1996), Pub L No. 104-191, 110 Stat 1936. [IA]

231. Modifications to the HIPAA Privacy, Security, Enforcement, and Breach Notification rules under the Health Information Technology for Economic and Clinical Health Act and the Genetic Information Nondiscrimination Act; other modifications to the HIPAA rules. *Fed Regist.* 2013;78(17):5565-5702. [IA]

232. Fernandez-Aleman JL, Senor IC, Lozoya PA, Toval A. Security and privacy in electronic health records: a systematic literature review. *J Biomed Inform.* 2013;46(3):541-562. [IB]

233. 21 CFR §11. Electronic records; electronic signatures. US Food and Drug Administration. Department of Health and Human Services. http://www.ecfr.gov/cgi-bin/text-idx?SID=801a6a66afbc46f404bcd011da79ab5e&mc=true&tpl=/ecfrbrowse/Title21/21cfrv1_02.tpl#0. Accessed April 21, 2016. [IA]

234. Accreditation Association for Ambulatory Health Care. Clinical records and health information. In: *Accreditation Handbook for Ambulatory Health Care.* Skokie, IL: The Association; 2015:49-51.

235. US Department of Health and Human Services. *Nationwide Privacy and Security Framework for Electronic Exchange of Individually Identifiable Health Information.* Washington, DC: Office of the National Coordinator for Health Information Technology; 2008. https://www.healthit.gov/sites/default/files/nationwide-ps-framework-5.pdf. Accessed April 21, 2016. [IA]

236. Connecting for Health Work Group on Consumer Access Policies for Networked Personal Health Information. *Security and Systems Requirements.* New York, NY: Markle Foundation; 2008. [IVA]

237. 16 CFR §318. Health breach notification rule. US Federal Trade Commission. https://www.ftc.gov/enforcement/rules/rulemaking-regulatory-reform-proceedings/health-breach-notification-rule. Accessed April 21, 2016. [IA]

238. RI.01.03.03: The hospital honors the patient's right to give or withhold informed consent to produce or use recordings, films, or other images of the patient for purposes other than his or her care. In: *Comprehensive Accreditation Manual for Hospitals.* Oakbrook Terrace, IL: The Joint Commission; 2015. [IVA]

239. RI.01.03.01: The hospital honors the patient's right to give or withhold informed consent. In: *Comprehensive Accreditation Manual for Hospitals.* Oakbrook Terrace, IL: The Joint Commission; 2015. [IVA]

240. The AMA Code of Medical Ethics' opinion on computerized medical records. *Virtual Mentor.* 2011;13(3):161-162. [IVB]

241. *Nursing Informatics: Scope and Standards of Practice.* 2nd ed. Silver Spring, MD: American Nurses Association; 2014. [IVA]

242. RC.01.02.01. Entries in the clinical record are authenticated. In: *Comprehensive Accreditation Manual for Ambulatory Care.* Oakbrook Terrace, IL: The Joint Commission; 2015. [IVA]

243. RC.01.04.01: The hospital audits its medical records. In: *Comprehensive Accreditation Manual for Hospitals.* Oakbrook Terrace, IL: The Joint Commission; 2015. [IVA]

244. Public Law 106-229: Electronic Signatures in Global and National Commerce Act. https://www.gpo.gov/fdsys/pkg/PLAW-106publ229/content-detail.html. Accessed April 21, 2016. [IA]

245. RC.01.05.01: The hospital retains its medical records. In: *Comprehensive Accreditation Manual for Hospitals.* Oakbrook Terrace, IL: The Joint Commission; 2015. [IVA]

246. RC.01.05.01: The organization retains its clinical records. In: *Comprehensive Accreditation Manual for Ambulatory Care.* Oakbrook Terrace, IL: The Joint Commission; 2015. [IVA]

247. Campbell EM, Sittig DF, Guappone KP, Dykstra RH, Ash JS. Overdependence on technology: an unintended adverse consequence of computerized provider order entry. *AMIA Annu Symp Proc.* 2007: 94-98. [IIIB]

248. Drass R, Free J. Planning for the unknown: maintaining your network infrastructure during a disaster. *Health Manag Technol.* 2014;35(2):18-20.

249. Rector M. Improving disaster recovery outcomes. Healthcare data must be protected to conform to HIPAA requirements, which active archive supports through the expanded role of tape. *Health Manag Technol.* 2012;33(3):16-17. [VB]

250. *SAFER Guide: High Priority Practices.* HealthIT.gov. http://www.healthit.gov/sites/safer/files/guides/safer_highpriority practices _sg001_form_0.pdf. Accessed April 20, 2016. [IA]

251. Agrawal A, Glasser AR. Barcode medication. Administration implementation in an acute care hospital and lessons learned. *J Healthc Inf Manag.* 2009;23(4):24-29. [VA]

252. *Amendments, Corrections, and Deletions in the Electronic Health Record Toolkit.* Chicago, IL: American Health Information Management Association; 2009. [IVB]

253. Weis JM, Levy PC. Copy, paste, and cloned notes in electronic health records; prevalence, benefits, risks, and best practice recommendations. *Chest.* 2014;145(3):632-638. [VA]

254. Peterson AM. Medical record as a legal document part 1: setting the standards. *J Legal Nurse Consult.* 2012;23(2):9-17. [VA]

255. Medical records. *Operating Room Risk Management.* 2008;1(Medical Records 3). [IVB]

256. Bredfeldt CE, Awad EB, Joseph K, Snyder MH. Training providers: beyond the basics of electronic health records. *BMC Health Serv Res.* 2013;13:503. [IIB]

257. Sittig DF, Singh H. Rights and responsibilities of users of electronic health records. *CMAJ.* 2012;184(13):1479-1483. [IVB]

258. Tahim A, Sabharwal S, Dhokia R, Bajekal R, Kyriacou S. Data protection training improves data handling. *Clinical Teacher.* 2012;9(6):403-407. [IIIB]

259. Bruylands M, Paans W, Hediger H, Muller-Staub M. Effects on the quality of the nursing care process through an educational program and the use of electronic nursing documentation. *Int J Nurs Knowl.* 2013;24(3):163-170. [IIA]

260. Clark JS, Delgado VA, Demorsky S, et al. Assessing and improving EHR data quality (updated). *J AHIMA.* 2013;84(3):48-53. [IVB]

261. Russo R; American Health Information Management Association. *Clinical Documentation Improvement.* Chicago, IL: AHIMA, American Health Information Management Association; 2010. [IVB]

262. Agaku IT, Adisa AO, Ayo-Yusuf OA, Connolly GN. Concern about security and privacy, and perceived control over collection and use of health information are related to withholding of health information from healthcare providers. *J Am Med Inform Assoc.* 2014;21(2):374-378. [IIIA]

263. Gajanayake R, Iannella R, Sahama T. Privacy oriented access control for electronic health records. *Electronic Journal of Health Informatics.* 2014;8(2):e15. [IIIB]

264. Berretoni A, Bochantin F, Brown T, et al. HIM functions in healthcare quality and patient safety. *J AHIMA.* 2011;82(8): 42-45. [IVB]

265. Hersh W. Copy and paste. AHRQ WebM&M [serial online]. https://psnet.ahrq.gov/webmm/case/157. Published July/August 2007. Accessed April 21, 2016. [VA]

266. Singh H, Ash JS, Sittig DF. Safety Assurance Factors for Electronic Health Record Resilience (SAFER): study protocol. *BMC Med Inform Decis Mak.* 2013;13:46. [VA]

267. Clancy CM. Nursing, system design, and health care quality. *AORN J.* 2009;90(4):581-583. [VA]

268. SAFER Guide: Organizational Responsibilities. HealthIT.gov. https://www.healthit.gov/safer/guide/sg002. Accessed April 21, 2016. [IA]

269. Magrabi F, Ong M-S, Runciman W, Coiera E. An analysis of computer-related patient safety incidents to inform the development of a classification. *J Am Med Inform Assoc.* 2010;17(6):663-670. [IIA]

270. Nunn S. Managing audit trails. *J AHIMA.* 2009;80(9):44-45. [VC]

271. Haugen MB, Herrin B, Slivochka S, Tolley LM, Warner D, Washington L. Rules for handling and maintaining metadata in the EHR. *J AHIMA.* 2013;84(5):50-54. [IVB]

272. *SAFER Guide: Contingency Planning.* HealthIT.gov. https://www.healthit.gov/safer/guide/sg003. Accessed April 21, 2016. [IA]

273. *SAFER Guide: System Interfaces.* HealthIT.gov. https://www.healthit.gov/safer/guide/sg005. Accessed April 21, 2016. [IA]

274. Zoraster RM, Burkle CM. Disaster documentation for the clinician. *Disaster Med Public Health Prep.* 2013;7(4):354-360. [VA]

Acknowledgments

Lead Author

Sharon Giarrizzo-Wilson, MS, RN-BC, CNOR
President and CEO
SymQuality Consulting, LLC
Denver, Colorado

Contributing Author

Ramona L. Conner, MSN, RN, CNOR
Editor-in-Chief, Guidelines for Perioperative Practice
AORN Nursing Department
Denver, Colorado

The authors and AORN thank Janice Neil, PhD, RN, CNE, Associate Professor, College of Nursing, East Carolina University, Greenville, North Carolina; Lisa Spruce, DNP, RN, CNS-CP, ACNS, ACNP, CNOR, FAAN, Director of Evidence-based Perioperative Practice, AORN Nursing Department, Denver, Colorado; Martha Stratton, MSN, MHSA, RN, CNOR, NEA-BC, Vice President of Perioperative Services, Doctors Hospital, Augusta, Georgia; Missi Merlino, MHA, RN-BC, CNOR, Staff Nurse II, Baylor Scott & White Health, Temple, Texas; and Nathalie Walker, MBA, BS, RN, CNOR, Member of the Louisiana Nursing Supply and Demand Commission, a subcommittee of the Health Works Commission of Louisiana, Metairie, Louisiana, for their assistance in developing this guideline.

Publication History

Originally published March 1982, *AORN Journal,* as "Recommended practices for documentation of perioperative nursing care."

Format revision July 1982.

Revised March 1987; revised September 1991; revised November 1995; published June 1996.

Revised; published January 2000, *AORN Journal.*

Reformatted July 2000.

Revised November 2011; published online as "Recommended practices for perioperative health care information management" in *Perioperative Standards and Recommended Practices.*

Reformatted September 2012 for publication in *Perioperative Standards and Recommended Practices,* 2013 edition.

Minor editing revisions made in November 2014 for publication as "Guideline for health care information management" in *Guidelines for Perioperative Practice,* 2015 edition.

Revised July 2016 for online publication in *Guidelines for Perioperative Practice.*

Evidence ratings revised and minor editorial changes made to conform to the current AORN Evidence Rating model, September 2019, for online publication in *Guidelines for Perioperative Practice.*

INSTRUMENT CLEANING

AORN
SAFE SURGERY TOGETHER

TABLE OF CONTENTS

MEDICAL ABBREVIATIONS & ACRONYMS

ASC – Ambulatory surgery center
ASHRAE – American Society of Heating, Refrigerating
  and Air-Conditioning Engineers
ATP – Adenosine triphosphate
CDBAC – Coco alkyl dimethylbenzyl ammonium chloride
CDC – Centers for Disease Control and Prevention
CHG – Chlorhexidine gluconate
CJD – Creutzfeldt-Jakob disease
CRE – Carbapenemase-resistant *Enterobacteriaceae*
DI – Deionized
EO – Ethylene oxide
FDA – US Food and Drug Administration
EPA – Environmental Protection Agency
HVAC – Heating, ventilation, and air conditioning
ICU – Intensive care unit
IFU – Instructions for use
IUSS – Immediate use steam sterilization
NaOH – Sodium hydroxide

OOSS – Ophthalmic Outpatient Surgery Society
OR – Operating room
OSHA – Occupational Safety and Health Administration
OV – Ophthalmic viscoelastic
OVD – Ophthalmic viscosurgical device
PPE – Personal protective equipment
RLU – Relative light units
RN – Registered nurse
RO – Reverse osmosis
SDS – Safety data sheet
SHEA – Society for Healthcare Epidemiology of America
SSI – Surgical site infection
TASS – Toxic anterior segment syndrome
TDS – Total dissolved solids
TSE – Transmissible spongiform encephalopathy
vCJD – Variant Creutzfeldt-Jakob disease
WHO – World Health Organization

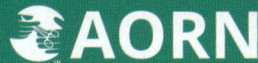

GUIDELINE FOR
CARE AND CLEANING OF SURGICAL INSTRUMENTS

The Guideline for Care and Cleaning of Surgical Instruments was approved by the AORN Guidelines Advisory Board and became effective as of October 12, 2020. The recommendations in the guideline are intended to be achievable and represent what is believed to be an optimal level of practice. Policies and procedures will reflect variations in practice settings and/or clinical situations that determine the degree to which the guideline can be implemented. AORN recognizes the many diverse settings in which perioperative nurses practice; therefore, this guideline is adaptable to all areas where operative or other invasive procedures may be performed.

Purpose

This document provides guidance for **cleaning** surgical instruments, including point-of-use treatment, transport, **decontamination**, inspection, and general care of reusable medical devices (eg, surgical instruments). Guidance is also provided for selection of cleaning chemicals (eg, detergent, enzymatic, disinfectant), selection of decontamination equipment, monitoring and control of water quality, and the use of personal protective equipment (PPE) that must be worn during cleaning and care of instruments. Special considerations are addressed for processing ophthalmic instruments, processing laryngoscope blades and handles, and minimizing the risk for transmitting prion diseases from contaminated reusable medical devices. The recommendations are general recommendations; specific guidance for care and cleaning of each instrument can be found in the instrument's US Food and Drug Administration (FDA)-cleared manufacturer-validated instructions for use (IFU).[1]

Failure to correctly clean and decontaminate surgical instruments and other medical devices used in invasive procedures can lead to subsequent failures in high-level disinfection and sterilization that put patients at risk for developing a surgical site infection (SSI).[2] Approximately 50% of SSIs are deemed to be preventable with the use of evidence-based strategies.[3] Effective decontamination[2,4] and subsequent sterilization are essential SSI prevention measures.[2,5] The number of SSIs that can be attributed to inadequate medical device processing is unknown because this is not often investigated as the cause.[6]

Sterilization, packaging for sterilization, high-level disinfection, processing of flexible endoscopes, and reprocessing of single-use devices are outside the scope of this document. Guidance for these topics is provided in the AORN Guideline for Sterilization,[7] Guideline for High-Level Disinfection,[8] Guideline for Sterilization Packaging Systems,[9] and Guideline for Processing Flexible Endoscopes.[10]

Evidence Review

A medical librarian with a perioperative background conducted a systematic search of the databases Ovid MEDLINE®, Ovid Embase®, EBSCO CINAHL®, and the Cochrane Database of Systematic Reviews. The search was limited to literature published in English from January 2014 through August 2019. At the time of the initial search, weekly alerts were created on the topics included in that search. Results from these alerts were provided to the lead author until November 2019. The lead author requested additional articles that either did not fit the original search criteria or were discovered during the evidence appraisal process. The lead author and the medical librarian also identified relevant guidelines from government agencies, professional organizations, and standards-setting bodies.

Search terms included *adenosine triphosphate, antineoplastic agents, arthroscopic shavers, asepsis, bacteria, bacterial adhesion, bacterial load, biofilms, biofoul, borescopes, cart washers, case cart, central services department, chemical safety, cleaning verification, corrosion, Creutzfeldt-Jakob syndrome, cross infection, cytotoxic, decontamination, detergents, disinfection, disinfection and sterilization, endotoxins, enzymatic detergents, equipment and supplies, equipment contamination, equipment reuse, evaluation studies as topic, guidelines as topic, impingement, infection control, instrument air, instrument cleaning, instrument coating, instrument dipping, instrument disinfectant, instrument drying, instrument marking, instrument tape, insulation test, ionized water, laryngoscopes, leaching, luciferases, luminescent measurements, magnification, maintenance, medical device reprocessing, microbial sensitivity tests, mitomycin, occupational hazards, occupational exposure, powered surgical equipment, printing (three-dimensional), prion diseases, protein test, rigid endoscopes, risk management, robotic instruments, satellite sterile processing, sterile water, sterile processing department, sterilization, surgical equipment and supplies, surgical instruments, surgical procedures (operative), surgical wound infection, TOSI test, toxic anterior segment syndrome, toxic endothelial cell destruction, ultrasonic, washer disinfector, washing system, water microbiology, water purification,* and *water supply.*

Included were research and non-research literature in English, complete publications, and publications with dates within the time restriction when available. Excluded were non-peer-reviewed publications and older evidence within the time restriction when more recent evidence was available. Editorials, news items, and other brief items were

Figure 1. Flow Diagram of Literature Search Results

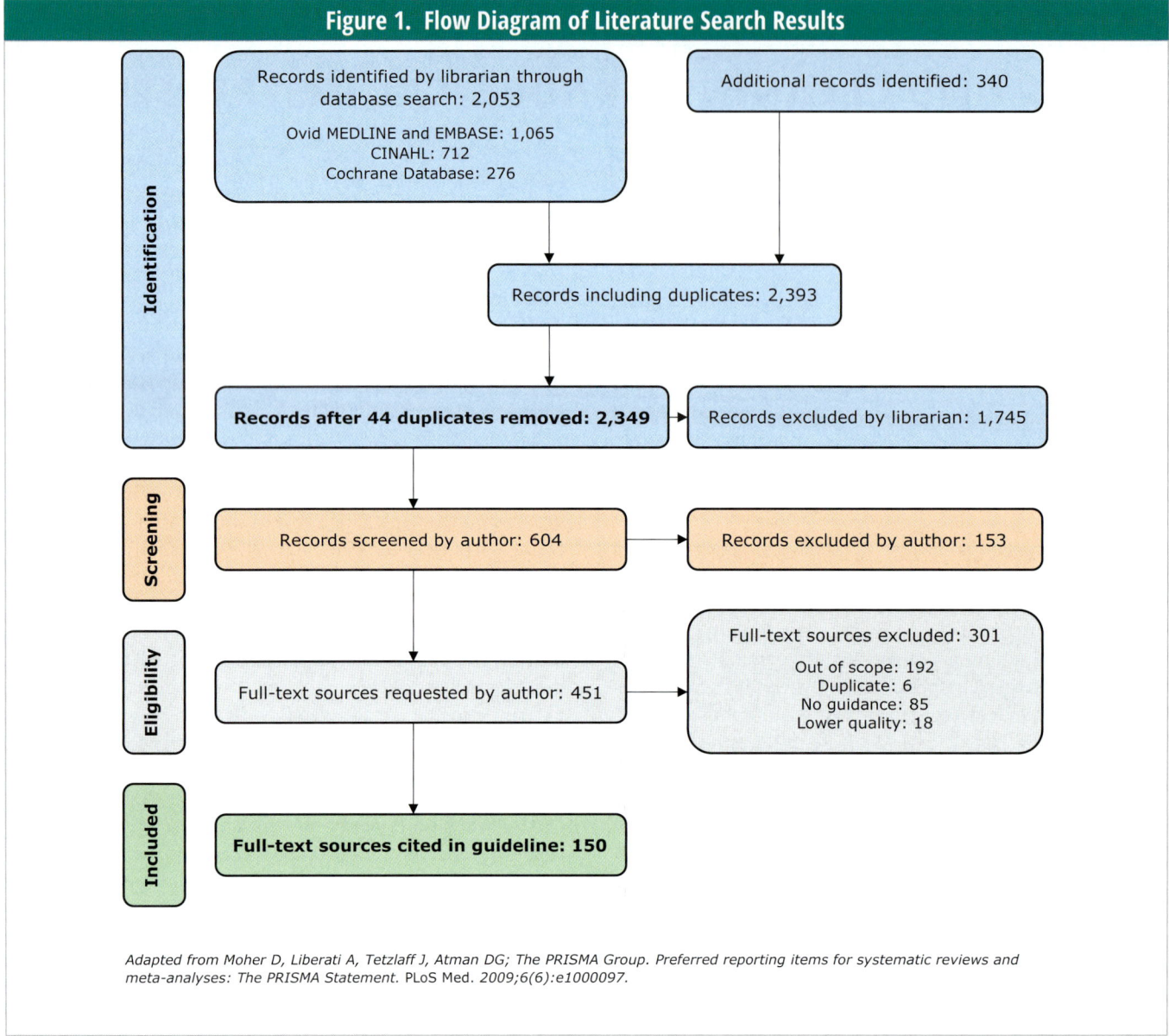

Identification

Records identified by librarian through database search: 2,053

Ovid MEDLINE and EMBASE: 1,065
CINAHL: 712
Cochrane Database: 276

Additional records identified: 340

Records including duplicates: 2,393

Records after 44 duplicates removed: 2,349

Records excluded by librarian: 1,745

Screening

Records screened by author: 604

Records excluded by author: 153

Eligibility

Full-text sources requested by author: 451

Full-text sources excluded: 301

Out of scope: 192
Duplicate: 6
No guidance: 85
Lower quality: 18

Included

Full-text sources cited in guideline: 150

Adapted from Moher D, Liberati A, Tetzlaff J, Atman DG; The PRISMA Group. Preferred reporting items for systematic reviews and meta-analyses: The PRISMA Statement. PLoS Med. 2009;6(6):e1000097.

excluded. Low-quality evidence was excluded when higher-quality evidence was available, and literature outside the time restriction was excluded when literature within the time restriction was available. Articles that discussed antimicrobial multifunctional surface coatings were considered and determined to be out of scope for this document and therefore were excluded **(Figure 1)**.

Articles identified in the search were provided to the project team for evaluation. The team consisted of the lead author and one evidence appraiser. The lead author and the evidence appraiser reviewed and critically appraised each article using the AORN Research or Non-Research Evidence Appraisal Tools as appropriate. The literature was independently evaluated and appraised according to the strength and quality of the evidence. Each article was then assigned an appraisal score. The appraisal score is noted in brackets after each reference as applicable.

Each recommendation rating is based on a synthesis of the collective evidence, a benefit-harm assessment, and consideration of resource use. The strength of the recommendation was determined using the AORN Evidence Rating Model and the quality and consistency of the evidence supporting a recommendation. The recommendation strength rating is noted in brackets after each recommendation.

Note: The evidence summary table is available at http://www.aorn.org/evidencetables/.

Editor's note: MEDLINE is a registered trademark of the US National Library of Medicine's Medical Literature Analysis and Retrieval System, Bethesda, MD. CINAHL, Cumulative Index to Nursing and Allied Health Literature, is a registered trademark of EBSCO Industries, Birmingham, AL.

1. Pre-Purchase Evaluation

1.1 Use only FDA-cleared surgical instruments that have written, manufacturer-validated IFU for care, cleaning, and decontamination. *[Recommendation]*

Surgical instruments and devices are classified according to their use[11] and are subject to FDA clearance under current premarket approval requirements[12] or premarket notification 510(k) requirements.[13] Manufacturers of FDA-cleared instruments and devices provide **validated**[1] IFU that cover cleaning and decontamination and how to process reusable devices between uses.[1,6,14,15] Instructions for use provide users with validated techniques for processing instruments, and these validated techniques are required for reliable decontamination.[2,14,16,17]

1.2 Before initial purchase and use, convene an interdisciplinary team to develop a standardized process for evaluating and selecting

- reusable medical devices (eg, surgical instruments and devices) and
- equipment and supplies that will be used for processing.[18]

[Recommendation]

Interdisciplinary teams solicit input from personnel with broad expertise to inform optimal decision making.[18] A standardized product evaluation and selection process that includes input from key personnel facilitates selection of functional and reliable products that are safe, cost-effective, and environmentally friendly; promote quality care; and prevent duplication or rapid obsolescence.[18]

1.2.1 Include the following members in the interdisciplinary team responsible for pre-purchase evaluation of surgical instruments, medical devices, equipment, and supplies used for reprocessing:

- sterile processing personnel,
- a perioperative registered nurse(s) (RN[s]),
- a surgeon(s),
- a surgical technologist(s),
- an infection preventionist(s),
- an anesthesia professional(s),
- biomedical engineering personnel,
- facility engineering personnel, and
- other stakeholders determined by the health care organization (eg, an industrial hygienist, materials management personnel, stakeholders outside the perioperative setting).

[Recommendation]

Representatives of different disciplines can contribute expertise that influences the organization's successful integration of new medical devices in clinical practice. The infrastructure in the facility and the capabilities of the biomedical engineering service may influence purchasing decisions.

1.3 Before purchase and use of reusable surgical instruments and other medical devices, determine whether the resources are available for performance of the processing methods provided in the manufacturer's validated IFU, including

- medical device processing personnel who can understand and use the IFU (ie, education and competency needs are met)[19];
- the time needed to complete all processing steps;
- a water supply of the specified quality;
- other utilities (eg, electricity, ventilation, steam supply, drains, **instrument air**);
- facility infrastructure (eg, space; sinks; lighting; heating, ventilation, and air conditioning [HVAC] controls)
- decontamination equipment;
- inspection equipment (eg, endoscopic camera, **borescope**, lighted magnification);
- space for device disassembly;
- accessories (eg, adaptors to connect the device and decontamination equipment);
- accessories for cleaning **lumens**, ports, and internal parts (eg, flushing and cleaning supplies);
- cleaning chemicals (ie, detergent, enzymatic, disinfectant) with the recommended characteristics and compatibility;
- procedures for processing steps (eg, pretreatment, cleaning, decontamination, inspection); and
- any required lubricants or treatments.[1,14-16]

[Recommendation]

The instrument manufacturers' IFU provide instructions for cleaning and processing that are required to achieve the validated results.[14] **See Section 15. Education** for more information about education and competency.

1.3.1 In the environment in which the surgical instrument will be used, evaluate the

- instrument's quality[20] (eg, material, structural durability),
- instrument's performance in surgical procedure(s),
- equipment needed for transport,
- transport methods to the decontamination area,
- cleaning and decontamination practices,

- inspection and functionality testing practices, and
- environmental conditions required for handling and storage.

[Recommendation]

Cleaning, decontamination, and handling instructions recommended by device manufacturers can vary widely. Some instruments may require special cleaning, packaging, sterilization, or maintenance procedures that cannot be provided by the facility without modifications to existing space, processes, and equipment.[5,14]

The manufacturer's IFU contain details the user needs to determine the needed environment, time, equipment, and supplies for proper processing of the medical device.

2. Sterile Processing Area

2.1 The sterile processing area should be designed for unidirectional functional workflow patterns as described in the AORN Guideline for Design and Maintenance of the Surgical Suite.[21]
[Recommendation]

The requirements for processing reusable surgical instruments do not vary by location. Equivalent procedures, supplies, and equipment are needed in all locations where sterile processing is performed.[22,23]

Refer to the AORN Guideline for Design and Maintenance of the Surgical Suite,[21] Guideline for Sterilization Packaging Systems,[9] and Guideline for Sterilization[7] for additional information.

2.2 Perform cleaning and decontamination in an area separate from locations where clean items are handled.[5,21-24] *[Recommendation]*

Physical separation of decontamination areas from areas where clean items are handled minimizes the risk of cross contamination. Cross contamination can result when soiled items are placed near clean items or are placed on surfaces upon which clean items are later placed. Droplets and **aerosols** created during cleaning of soiled instruments can contaminate nearby clean items or surfaces.[21,25]

2.3 Do not clean or decontaminate instruments in sinks where eyewash stations are located or hand hygiene (ie, hand washing, surgical hand antisepsis) is performed. *[Recommendation]*

Cleaning soiled instruments can contaminate the sink and faucet, which can contaminate the person using the sink for clean activities, such as hand washing, surgical hand antisepsis, or flushing his or her eyes.

2.4 The decontamination area must contain
- an eyewash station[5,26] and
- a dedicated hand hygiene sink.[27]

[Regulatory Requirement]

The Occupational Safety and Health Administration (OSHA) requires that an eyewash station be provided where chemicals that are hazardous to the eyes are located.[26] Hand hygiene facilities are required by OSHA for use after removal of PPE.[27] See the AORN Guideline for a Safe Environment of Care, Section 10. Chemicals, for more information.

2.5 The decontamination area should be equipped with
- multiple sinks that are
  - designated for soaking and cleaning, intermediate rinse, and final rinse;
  - large enough to accommodate instrument trays;
  - at an ergonomically correct height; and
  - marked at the water level needed for cleaning solution measurement;
- storage space for PPE and cleaning supplies;
- automated equipment (eg, washer-disinfector, **ultrasonic cleaner**) consistent with the types of instruments to be cleaned and decontaminated;
- adaptors and accessories to connect instruments with cleaning equipment and utilities; and
- utilities that support decontamination, drying, inspection, and documentation, including
- access to **critical water** for rinsing instruments (See Section 3. Water Quality);
  - a pressure-regulated, instrument air supply[5];
  - electrical capacity to power all equipment at the same time; and
  - data lines to support electronic equipment for documentation of processing steps.

[Recommendation]

Automated decontamination provides an effective level of cleaning that is more easily replicated than manual decontamination methods alone.[28-30] Utilities to support decontamination processes are needed in the decontamination area.[5] Instrument air forced through the lumen eliminates moisture that can serve as a medium for microbial growth.[5] Pressure regulation of the instrument air protects the reusable surgical instrument from damage caused by using too much pressure.[5] The instrument manufacturer's IFU provide the required pressure for drying with instrument air.

2.6 Stock the decontamination area with the accessories and supplies needed to clean and decontaminate instruments in accordance with the manufacturers' written IFU,[5] including
- brushes or other devices designed to remove organic material and debris from lumens, with

a diameter and length described in the manufacturer's IFU;

- chemicals for cleaning and disinfecting in accordance with the manufacturer's IFU for the instruments and devices to be processed and equipment used for processing (eg, detergents, enzymatic solutions, ethyl alcohol, isopropyl alcohol);
- clean, soft, nonlinting cloths;
- equipment and supplies for functionality testing;
- a source of critical water (eg, deionized [DI], **reverse osmosis** [RO], filtered);
- a thermometer; and
- a device to measure or an automated method to dispense cleaning solutions.

[Recommendation]

Using brushes or devices that are intended for cleaning medical devices, are of the correct size, and are used in accordance with the brush and device manufacturer's IFU can facilitate cleaning of lumens. The instrument manufacturer's IFU may recommend specific cleaning chemicals. Soft, nonlinting cleaning cloths may prevent scratches to the surface of instruments and prevent lint from adhering to the surface of instruments.

Critical water is used for final rinsing. Impurities in untreated water can leave residues on instruments that may lead to corrosion, pitting, or staining.[5,31,32] A thermometer is used to monitor that cleaning solution temperatures are within the correct range as described in the cleaning solution manufacturer's IFU. Devices to measure volume are used to mix detergents at the concentration specified by the detergent manufacturer's written IFU.

2.7 Maintain the decontamination area HVAC system within the HVAC design parameters that were applicable according to regulatory and professional guidelines at the time of design or most recent renovation of the HVAC system.[5,21] *[Recommendation]*

The HVAC system controls the air quality, temperature, humidity, and pressure of the room in comparison with the surrounding areas.[21] The HVAC system is designed in accordance with the American Society of Heating, Refrigerating and Air-Conditioning Engineers (ASHRAE) and local regulatory requirements to reduce the number of environmental contaminants and to provide a comfortable environment for occupants in the area.[21]

2.7.1 An interdisciplinary team that includes an infection preventionist(s), a perioperative RN(s), sterile processing personnel, a representative(s) from facility maintenance, an anesthesia professional(s), and other stakeholders representing the health care organization should develop and implement a systematic process for monitoring HVAC performance parameters in the decontamination area and a mechanism for resolving variances. *[Recommendation]*

The ASHRAE guidelines related to room temperature ranges for the decontamination area are the accepted professional guidelines for HVAC systems in the United States.[33] Negative pressure helps prevent contaminated air from entering into positive-pressure, clean areas. The evidence on the effect of relative humidity on bacterial, fungal, and viral growth is inconclusive. Further research is warranted to determine optimal relative humidity levels to control environmental contamination.

2.7.2 Room temperature may be intentionally adjusted to accommodate the individual comfort needs of the occupants.[22,23] *[Conditional Recommendation]*

Personnel working in the decontamination area and wearing PPE may become uncomfortably warm at room temperatures above 72° F (22° C). Lower room temperatures may contribute to the comfort and improve the task performance of personnel wearing PPE.[34]

2.7.3 Report an unintentional variance in the predetermined HVAC system parameters (ie, a variance other than an intentional temperature adjustment) according to the health care organization's policy and procedure.[24] *[Recommendation]*

Rapid communication between affected and responsible personnel may help facilitate resolution of the variance.

2.7.4 In the event of an HVAC parameter variance, perform a risk assessment and take measures to restore the functionality of the area after the variance has been corrected.[24] *[Recommendation]*

3. Water Quality

3.1 In collaboration with clinical engineering personnel, facility engineering personnel, and infection preventionists, establish a process and frequency for monitoring the quality of water (eg, **utility water**, critical water) used in decontamination processes as part of the organization's water management program.[35-37] *[Recommendation]*

Table 1. Water Quality Values

Hardness/Total Dissolved Solids	Utility Water	Critical Water
CaCO$_3$ content (mg/L)	< 150	< 1
Conductivity (µS/cm)	< 500	< 10
pH	6-9	5-7
Chloride (mg/L)	< 250	< 1
Iron (mg/L)	n/a	< 0.2
Copper (mg/L)	n/a	< 0.1
Manganese (mg/L)	n/a	< 0.1
Bacteria (CFU/mL)	n/a	< 10
Endotoxin (EU/mL)	n/a	< 10
Total organic carbon (mg/mL)	< 1	< 1
Color and turbidity	Colorless, clear, no visible residues	

Hospital water systems are susceptible to bacterial contamination.[35-40] Routine quality evaluation can detect water quality issues that can impede decontamination and sterilization processes.[32] Water quality that does not meet the requirements specified in the detergent or the cleaning equipment manufacturers' IFU can adversely affect the efficacy of cleaning chemistries[5,32,41] and can contain waterborne bacteria, including *Legionella*[36,37,40,42-46] and *Pseudomonas* species.[42,47]

In a nonexperimental study, Alfa et al[28] investigated the effectiveness of a commercially available test for determining the presence of organic soil on instruments that had been cleaned in automated washers. An objective of the researchers was to determine the level of protein, hemoglobin, carbohydrate, and **endotoxin** on surgical instruments before and after cleaning in an automated washer. The researchers evaluated five types of surgical instruments from plastic-surgery trays for residuals both before and after cleaning. Of a total of 25 instruments tested, 21 (84%) had substantially higher carbohydrate levels and 15 (60%) had higher endotoxin levels after cleaning than before cleaning. The researchers concluded that endotoxins remaining on surgical instruments after cleaning in automated washers may be related to water quality. The researchers recommended water quality monitoring.

The authors of an organizational experience report described water quality testing strategies employed in the hospital, including measurement of total dissolved solids (TDS), chlorine, and water microbiology.[48] Using these three water-quality measurements, the organization detected *Pseudomonas aeruginosa* in the hospital RO water supply and high TDS (60-70 ppm versus < 10 ppm expected) in the water used in the reusable surgical instrument decontamination area. Corrective measures were taken and no surgical complications (eg, SSI) were reported. The authors concluded that regular assessment of water quality is a relatively inexpensive and simple technology that can be valuable in hospital infection control programs.

3.2 **Water should be monitored and controlled to the values in Table 1.**[32,49] *[Recommendation]*

Poor water quality can
- reduce the effectiveness of some disinfectants and cleaning chemicals by interacting with them to form insoluble precipitates,
- create deposit buildup blockages in valves and filters,
- leave a white-grey residue on instruments after drying, and
- cause irreparable damage to instruments.[49]

Chloride is damaging to stainless steel and can cause pitting corrosion.[32]

3.2.1 **Monitor and control the quality of the water utility that is supplied to decontamination equipment (eg, washer-disinfectors).** *[Recommendation]*

An increase in pH, within the limits specified in **Table 1**, can improve the antimicrobial activity of some disinfectants (ie, glutaraldehyde, quaternary ammonium compounds) but decreases the antimicrobial activity of others (eg, phenols, hypochlorites, and iodine) by altering the disinfectant molecule or the cell surface.[2] The manufacturer's IFU provide guidance for water requirements for the specific equipment.

3.2.2 **Monitor and control the quality of critical water in holding tanks.** *[Recommendation]*

Critical water (eg, RO, DI) in holding tanks is vulnerable to contamination. When waterborne bacteria form **biofilms** inside critical water holding tanks, removing the biofilm becomes extremely difficult.[31] Preventive maintenance plays a key role in the quality control of critical water.[31]

The World Health Organization (WHO) recommends cleaning reservoirs used to hold critical water every 2 months.[49]

3.2.3 **Evaluate water quality after major maintenance and repairs of the water supply system (eg, changes to the water distribution system that require utility shut-off).** *[Recommendation]*

Water supply maintenance can influence water quality. Evaluation facilitates determination of water quality relative to the requirements for cleaning as specified in the detergent and cleaning equipment manufacturers' written IFU.[32]

4. Cleaning Products and Equipment

4.1 **Convene an interdisciplinary team (See Recommendation 1.2.1) to establish and implement a procedure for evaluating and selecting cleaning products (eg, pretreatment products, detergents, enzymatic cleaners, disinfectants) and decontamination equipment.** *[Recommendation]*

The chemical actions of cleaning products vary, and products are intended for different applications. Some cleaning products include enzymes and target specific types of bioburden[2,50,51] **(Table 2)**. Others are intended for general purpose cleaning.

Some cleaning products contain one or more enzymes to break up soil and facilitate its removal.[14,50] Enzymes are specific in terms of the soils they remove.[14] Some enzymatic detergents contain more than one enzyme and are intended to be multipurpose; others are intended for a specific type of soil.[14] Protease enzymes target blood and body salts.[14] Amylases target carbohydrates, starches, and sugars.[14] Lipases break down fats and oils.[14] The pH and the rinsability of cleaning products vary. Cleaning equipment manufacturers' IFU for cleaning solutions also vary.

4.1.1 **Use only FDA-cleared mechanical washer-disinfectors.** *[Recommendation]*

Medical washers and medical washer-disinfectors are class II medical devices regulated by the FDA.[52]

4.2 **Select compatible products by reviewing the validated manufacturers' IFU for the**

- **surgical instrument or other medical device to be cleaned and decontaminated,**
- **cleaning chemical (ie, detergent, enzymatic, disinfectant), and**
- **cleaning equipment.**
[Recommendation]

The intended use of cleaning solutions and cleaning equipment varies. Following the manufacturers' validated[1] IFU facilitates correct selection and use of cleaning solutions and equipment, thereby preventing potential damage to instruments.[14]

4.2.1 **Use neutral detergents that are low foaming and easy to remove during rinsing for manual or mechanical cleaning, unless contraindicated by the device or cleaning equipment manufacturer's IFU.** *[Recommendation]*

Detergents facilitate soil removal from the surface of instruments. Neutral pH or slightly alkaline detergents are compatible with most instruments and work well with enzymes that may be added to detergents to help break down and facilitate removal of organic materials.[2] Detergents that are low foaming facilitate visual observation of the cleaning process.[16]

4.2.2 **Select cleaning products that**
- **are compatible with and do not cause damage to the instruments and devices they will be used to clean,**[14,53]
- **are nonabrasive,**[14]
- **are low foaming,**[14]
- **are easy to remove during rinsing,**[14]
- **are biodegradable,**[14]
- **are environmentally preferable,**[54]
- **are nontoxic in the specific-use dilution,**[14]
- **are effective for removing soils under specified conditions,**[14]
- **have a long shelf life,**[14]

Table 2: Enzymes and Target Soils

Enzyme Type	Targeted Soil
Proteases[1]	Organic material
Amylases[1]	Carbohydrates, starches, and sugars
Lipases[1]	Fats and oils
Cellulases[2]	Cellulose

References
1. Rutala WA, Weber DJ; Healthcare Infection Control Practices Advisory Committee (HICPAC). *Guideline for Disinfection and Sterilization in Healthcare Facilities, 2008.* Atlanta, GA: Centers for Disease Control and Prevention; 2008. https://www.cdc.gov/infectioncontrol/guidelines/disinfection/. Accessed August 10, 2020.
2. Juturu V, Wu JC. Microbial cellulases: engineering, production and applications. *Renew Sust Energ Rev.* 2014;33:188-203.

- are cost-effective,[14] and
- can be tested for effective concentration.[14]
[Recommendation]

Cleaning products that are nonabrasive can help protect the surface of instruments from damage. Cleaning products that are low foaming are less likely to interfere with the action of mechanical cleaning equipment. Cleaning products that are easy to remove facilitate removal of detergent during rinsing.[14] Cleaning products that are nontoxic contribute to personnel safety. Use of cleaning products that are effective on clinically relevant soils may increase the efficacy of the cleaning and subsequent disinfection and, when indicated, sterilization processes. An Environmental Protection Agency (EPA) Safer Choice label indicates that the product has been scientifically evaluated and determined to contain ingredients that pose the least concern among chemicals in their class.[55]

4.3 Cleaning solution must be handled according to its corresponding safety data sheet (SDS) and the product manufacturer's IFU. The SDS must be readily accessible to employees within the workplace.[56] [Regulatory Requirement]

Highly acidic or alkaline cleaning agents are corrosive and can cause injury to skin or mucus membranes.[14] Exposure to enzymatic detergents can cause respiratory illness such as asthma.[2] Access to the cleaning product IFU and SDS helps personnel to use the product correctly and obtain information useful for implementing processes that prevent injury.[24]

4.4 Follow the cleaning product manufacturer's written IFU for
- water quality,
- solution concentration and dilution,
- water temperature,
- contact time,
- conditions of storage (eg, temperature, distance to equipment for automated dispensers), and
- shelf life and use life.[2,5]
[Recommendation]

Water quality, including temperature, hardness, and pH, can affect the effectiveness of cleaning products.[32] Using the product in the concentration recommended by the manufacturer's IFU facilitates correct cleaning chemistry.[5] The manufacturer has validated the correct temperature and contact time to achieve effective and reliable cleaning with the specific product. Using the product at a temperature other than that specified in the IFU can render the product ineffective.[14]

4.4.1 An automated titration unit may be used to dispense cleaning and disinfection solutions. [Conditional Recommendation]

The concentration of the solution can vary when it is mixed manually. Use of a titration unit can aid in accurate measurement of the chemical during preparation of the cleaning solution and help personnel to consistently obtain the recommended concentration of the cleaning product.

4.5 Do not use abrasive devices and products to clean instruments unless their use is specified in the device manufacturer's written IFU. [Recommendation]

Abrasive devices and products, such as metal scouring pads, scouring powders, and sodium hypochlorite can cause permanent damage to instrument surface integrity and can result in pitting that can harbor microorganisms and soil.[5]

4.6 Use brushes or other items that meet the specifications (eg, diameter, length, materials) in the instrument or medical device manufacturer's IFU to clean crevices and lumens. [Recommendation]

Soil can become lodged in crevices, box locks, lumens, and other areas of instruments. Use of a brush intended for these difficult-to-clean areas facilitates removal of soil.[5,57]

4.6.1 To clean lumens, use brushes that
- meet the requirement for cleaning as specified in the instrument or device manufacturer's written IFU,[5]
- are long enough to clean the entire length of the lumen and exit at the distal end,
- contact the inner surface of the lumen without collapsing,
- have a rounded or smooth tip and bristles soft enough to prevent damage to the internal lumen surface, and
- are either designed for single use and discarded after each use or are reusable and cleaned and decontaminated after each use.[5]
[Recommendation]

Brushes that are too short to exit the distal length of a lumen can push debris to a point in the lumen but fail to remove it. Brushes with bristles that are too small or too large in diameter can prevent thorough cleaning. Bristles that are abrasive can damage instruments.

Reusable brushes that are not cleaned and decontaminated can cause contaminants to be transferred from one device to another. Use of single-use disposable brushes eliminates the risk of using a contaminated brush.

5. Processing Before Use

5.1 Before use, process (ie, clean, decontaminate, inspect, perform functionality testing, package, high-level disinfect or sterilize) all new, repaired, refurbished, and loaned instruments and reusable surgical instruments according to the device manufacturer's IFU. *[Recommendation]*

Failure to clean, inspect, disinfect, or sterilize an item may lead to transmission of pathogenic microorganisms from a contaminated device and create a risk for patient injury, including SSI.[58] Cleaning and decontamination removes soil and renders devices safe to handle and prepares them for subsequent processing (eg, high-level disinfection, sterilization).[2,5] Incomplete or ineffective cleaning can inhibit effectiveness of subsequent disinfection and sterilization.[4,5,58-61] It is not possible to verify how all new, repaired, refurbished, and loaned instruments and devices have been handled, cleaned, inspected, or processed before receipt in the facility.

Surgical instruments are cleaned after manufacturing by the manufacturer, but these cleaning processes do not meet the same standards of cleaning and decontamination before first use of a new device in the health care facility. An example of how manufacturers' cleaning practices can fail can be found in a recent FDA Class 2 Device Recall.[62] The reason given for the recall was "potentially insufficient cleaning processes or potential inadequate process monitoring for cleaning parameters."[62]

5.2 Provide the manufacturer's IFU to personnel responsible for processing instruments and reusable medical devices in a format that they can read and understand.[5,19] *[Recommendation]*

Instructions for use identify the processes necessary to achieve effective decontamination and sterility.[5]

5.2.1 The manufacturer's IFU may be provided in either written or electronic format at the point of use for processing personnel. *[Recommendation]*

5.2.2 Establish a process for regular review of the instrument or medical device manufacturers' IFU to verify that processing practices comply with the most current manufacturers' IFU. *[Recommendation]*

Manufacturers may make modifications to their IFU when new technology becomes available, when regulatory requirements change, or when modifications are made to a device.

5.3 Verify that accessories specified by the reusable surgical instrument manufacturer for all processing steps are accessible before use, and use them in accordance with the manufacturer's IFU. *[Recommendation]*

Using accessories that are designed and manufactured to the device manufacturer's specifications facilitates performance of the required cleaning and processing procedures.[14]

5.4 Remove reusable surgical instruments from external shipping containers and web-edged or corrugated cardboard boxes before transfer into the sterile processing area. *[Recommendation]*

External shipping containers and web-edged cardboard boxes may become contaminated during transport and can carry contaminants into the facility.[5,7]

5.5 Inspect instruments for defects and correct function upon receipt, and verify
- lack of damage,
- completeness of sets,
- tip integrity and alignment,
- surface integrity (eg, free from visible cracks and pitting),
- security of screws,
- ability to be disassembled and reassembled (if applicable),
- ratchet function,
- cutting edges sharpness,
- box lock integrity,
- free motion of moveable parts, and
- insulation integrity (for instruments used for electrosurgery).

[Recommendation]

Inspecting instruments before processing may minimize the risk of damaged, nonfunctioning, or incorrectly functioning instruments being used in patient care.

5.6 An interdisciplinary team (See Recommendation 1.2.1) appointed by the health care organization should establish standard operating procedures for managing loaned reusable surgical instruments, to include
- a process for requesting, approval, and communication for **loaned items**;
- preprocedure requirements for the lender of the items, including
  - instrument or reusable medical device delivery (eg, timing, location, documentation, communication) and
  - manufacturers' IFU delivery;
- shared responsibilities of the lender and the health care organization, including

- education for personnel before processing and use;
- a method for obtaining processing accessories required by the manufacturer's IFU;
- inventory requirements and a process for taking inventory;
- processes for handling, decontaminating, inspecting, packaging, and sterilizing the items before use;
- instrument set weight limits;
- processes for point-of-use treatment;
- processes for postprocedure decontamination;
- procedures for returning the item(s) to the lender; and
- documentation of processes and transactions related to loaned instruments; and
- postprocedure responsibilities of the lender, including time requirements for vendor retrieval.

[Recommendation]

A successful loaned instrument management program begins with clear and detailed policies and procedures developed in collaboration with all stakeholders.[63]

5.6.1 Consider all loaned reusable surgical instruments to be contaminated and deliver them directly to the decontamination area for decontamination, inspection, and packaging before sterilization for patient use. *[Recommendation]*

It is not possible to know under what conditions instruments were processed at another facility or for the receiving facility to monitor or control events that may contaminate items during transport.[5] Conditions of transport vary, and an event could occur during transport that could compromise sterility or cause damage to the instruments before they are received at the facility. The receiving facility is responsible for providing the surgical patient with sterile products and is therefore responsible for monitoring the cleaning and sterilization process. Cleaning always precedes disinfection and sterilization.[2,64] Inspection verifies that the instruments have no visible defects or damage. Parameters of inhouse sterilization can be verified immediately after a cycle is complete. Even if the instruments have been sterilized in another health care facility, the user will have no record of the previous sterilization process in the event of a recall.

In a laboratory study, Costa et al[65] evaluated the condition of loaned orthopedic instrument sets containing implants. The researchers collected flexible medullary reamers, depth gauges, and screws used for intermedullary nailing that were in clinical use for less than 1 year. The instruments were assessed for residual adenosine triphosphate (ATP), protein, bacterial contamination, endotoxin, and biofilm upon delivery to the hospital and after cleaning and steam sterilization. Before cleaning, the researchers observed that blood and tests for ATP, protein, and bacteria revealed high levels of contamination. Visible soil was released during lumen brushing. Using scanning electron microscopy, the researchers observed biofilm and fragments that appeared to be bone on the screws within the set. The researchers concluded that complex-design loaned instrument sets require a multi-disciplinary management approach that enables complete decontamination.

5.6.2 Loaned reusable surgical instruments should be delivered to the health care facility to allow time for inventorying and processing in accordance with the organization's standard operating procedures and the manufacturer's IFU. *[Recommendation]*

Insufficient time to process instruments according to the manufacturer's written IFU, presents a patient safety risk.[5] Management of loaned instruments requires planning. Requesting the instruments well in advance of the surgical procedure allows adequate time for the vendor to deliver the instruments and for facility personnel to perform the required cleaning; decontamination; inspection; sterilization; and if needed, **product quality assurance testing** procedures.

5.6.3 Obtain and review the manufacturers' written IFU for cleaning before processing and preferably before receipt of loaned instruments. *[Recommendation]*

When instructions are received in advance, preparations can be made for cleaning and sterilization before the arrival of the instruments. Advance preparation can prevent potential delays in patient care and facilitate correct cleaning and sterilization procedures. Review of processing instructions before receipt of the instruments may improve the efficiency and effectiveness of processing.

5.6.4 Obtain the accessories needed to process loaned instruments according to the manufacturer's written IFU before processing. *[Recommendation]*

Accessories specified in the manufacturer's written IFU are those the manufacturer has determined are needed to perform required cleaning procedures.[14,16]

5.6.5 Inventory and record the type and quantity of loaned instruments and confirm receipt with the lender upon delivery. [Recommendation]

Inventory lists of instruments, a photographic inventory, or use of automated inventory systems help provide verification that the instrument set is complete upon receipt. Taking inventory is critical to verifying that all required instruments have been received and are available for use during the procedure. When an inventory is not performed, it is not possible to determine whether the instruments that were intended to be delivered were received and that all instruments are returned to the lender. If an instrument critical to the procedure is not available when needed, the surgeon may not be able to perform the procedure as planned and patient care may be compromised or delayed.

5.6.6 After use, process (ie, clean, decontaminate, and disinfect or sterilize) loaned instruments before returning them to the vendor or lending facility.[5,7] [Recommendation]

Instruments used in procedures may be contaminated with blood, body fluids, or other potentially infectious materials and may pose a safety risk to health care and other personnel if they are not handled or cleaned and decontaminated correctly.[5]

6. Point-of-Use Treatment

6.1 Begin preparation for instrument decontamination at the point of use.[5] [Recommendation]

Moistening and removing **gross soil** at the point of use can help prevent organic material and debris from drying on instruments.[2,4,5] Organic material and debris are more difficult to remove from surgical instruments when they are allowed to dry,[29] and residual soil can affect the efficacy of subsequent disinfection and sterilization processes.[2,5,29,66] Removal of organic material and debris at the point of use can improve the efficacy and effectiveness of cleaning and decontamination.[2,5,14,29,65]

Soil that is allowed to dry on surgical instrument surfaces promotes the formation of a dry biofilm, which is difficult to remove and is more resistant to inactivation by steam sterilization than a hydrated biofilm.[67] Penetration of antimicrobials and disinfectants into biofilms do not necessarily kill the embedded cells[68]; therefore, preventing biofilm formation is a priority.

A report of an outbreak investigation[69] of SSIs following craniotomy procedures details the importance of point-of-use treatment. Before the outbreak,

the surgical power tool used for tumor resection was disassembled and rinsed, and point-of-use treatment was performed in the operating room (OR) before the device was sent to the decontamination area. Surgical site infection rates ranged from 0.6% to 4.4% during the time this disassembly and point-of-use treatment occurred in the OR. An outbreak (SSI rate 8.75%) followed a change in reprocessing protocols that eliminated point-of-use treatment in the OR, with no other contributing practice changes found. The researchers concluded that infections were transmitted by inadequate cleaning processes.

Bezek et al[70] conducted a laboratory-based study to evaluate the effect of various factors (ie, glucose concentration, temperature, stainless steel roughness) on biofilm formation by four common pathogens (ie, *Escherichia coli, Staphylococcus aureus, Pseudomonas aeruginosa, Listeria monocytogenes*). The aim of the study was to identify variables that can be manipulated to decrease the incidence of bacterial adhesion and biofilm formation on stainless steel surfaces in both the food and medical industries. The researchers found that the untreated stainless steel surface was more susceptible to **biofouling** than polished, brushed, or electroplated surfaces. Each pathogen, except *P aeruginosa,* showed decreased biofouling with the addition of glucose to the growth medium. *P aeruginosa* was greatly influenced by glucose concentration, with significantly higher biofouling potential when 5% glucose was added to the growth medium. For all tested pathogens, low temperature (40° F [4° C]) reduced biofouling.

6.1.1 During the procedure, remove gross soil from instrument surfaces with a sterile radiopaque surgical sponge moistened with sterile water. Do not use saline to wipe instrument surfaces. [Recommendation]

Soil (eg, blood, body fluids) and the sodium chloride in saline are damaging to instrument surfaces because they can cause corrosion, rusting, and pitting.[5,32] These materials, especially when dry, can be difficult to remove[66] from surfaces during the cleaning and decontamination process, reducing the efficacy of the subsequent sterilization process.[5,14] Dried blood represents a significant challenge to cleaning surgical instruments.[29]

In a randomized controlled trial, Lindgren et al[71] compared bacterial growth in 100 basins containing solutions used for intraoperative removal of gross soil from instruments during total hip arthroplasty and total knee arthroplasty procedures. The control solution (n = 47) was sterile water and the experimental solution (n = 53) contained 0.05% chlorhexidine (CHG). Among the control group, 9% (n = 4) had bacterial growth including *Micrococcus luteus, Staphylococcus hominis,* and gram-variable coccobacilli, and one had "unidentifiable" gram-positive rods. The experimental solution had no bacterial growth.

The researchers also studied wound complications including wound drainage (one in the control group), superficial infection (two in the control group), and deep infection (one in the experimental group). This study had important limitations. First, the researchers stated they were unable to correlate the presence of bacteria with a subsequent wound complication because the study was not powered to make this correlation. Second, the researchers did not evaluate the effects of using the experimental 0.05% CHG solution on instrument surface integrity. They concluded that a solution of 0.05% CHG in sterile water appears to be effective in eliminating bacterial growth in solutions used for intraoperative instrument gross soil removal, but they were not able to correlate this contamination with postoperative wound complications including deep infection. [70]

6.1.2 Use sterile water to irrigate instruments with lumens at frequent intervals during the procedure. *[Recommendation]*

Irrigating instrument lumens throughout a procedure removes gross soil[66] and may reduce the risk of biofilm formation. Biofilm can form on many surfaces but is particularly problematic when it forms in lumens because it is difficult to see and remove. After a biofilm forms, mechanical action is required to remove it.

In a 2015 organizational experience report, Lucas et al[72] described bone cement retention in a variety of orthopedic reusable surgical instruments after soiling and cleaning. The analysis included use of red dye and microcomputed tomography to assess the amount and location of bone cement debris in these orthopedic devices. Significantly more bone cement was retained in the more complex reusable surgical instruments. The researchers concluded that device design characteristics including narrow lumens, hinges, inaccessible cracks and crevices, and complex configuration are difficult to clean. This study emphasizes the importance of removing soil from complex-design devices beginning at the point of use.

If not removed, soil, biofilm, and buildup biofilm can impede subsequent disinfection or sterilization processes.[2,5]

6.2 Sharp instruments must be separated from other instruments and confined in a puncture-resistant container before transport to the decontamination area.[27] *[Regulatory Requirement]*

Segregation of sharps from other instruments minimizes the risk of injury to personnel handling instruments during cleaning and decontamination and is an OSHA requirement.[27] See the AORN Guideline for Sharps Safety.[73]

6.2.1 Disposable sharps (eg, scalpel blades, suture needles) must be removed and discarded into a closeable, puncture-resistant container that is leak-proof on its sides and bottom and is labeled or color coded as biohazardous.[27,73] *[Regulatory Requirement]*

6.3 Protect delicate instruments (eg, fiberoptic cords, endoscopes, microsurgical instruments, robotic instruments) from damage during transport to a decontamination area by segregating them into different containers or by placing them on top of heavier instruments.[5] *[Recommendation]*

Instruments may shift during transport, causing heavy instruments to damage more delicate instruments.

6.4 Keep instruments moist until they are cleaned by using either saturation with an enzymatic pretreatment product or a towel moistened with water placed over the instruments. Do not use saline. *[Recommendation]*

Keeping instruments moist helps prevent soil (eg, blood, body fluids) from drying and adhering to the instruments. Dried soil can make instruments more difficult to clean and potentially lead to the formation of dry-surface biofilm.[29,67] Prolonged exposure of instruments to chloride in sodium chloride (saline) can cause pitting.[5,32] Treating instruments with an enzymatic pretreatment at the point of use can help prevent rusting and corrosion; prevent blood, organic materials, and debris from drying on the instruments; and inhibit dry-surface biofilm formation.[5,67]

6.4.1 Before transporting instruments, discard liquids used for point-of-use treatment in accordance with local, state, and federal regulations. *[Recommendation]*

6.4.2 When disposing of the solution before transport is not feasible, it must be transported in a leak-proof, puncture-resistant container to the disposal area.[40] *[Regulatory Requirement]*

Contaminated liquids may be spilled during transport, presenting a risk of contaminating the environment and exposing personnel to blood, body fluids, and other potentially infectious materials.[10,12,40]

7. Transport to the Decontamination Area

7.1 Transport contaminated instruments to the decontamination area as soon as possible after completion of the procedure. *[Recommendation]*

Removal of soil from instruments becomes more difficult after the instruments have dried.[2,5]

7.2 Contaminated instruments must be transported to the decontamination area in a closed container or enclosed transport cart that is
- leak proof,
- puncture resistant,
- large enough to contain all contents, and
- labeled with a fluorescent orange or orange-red label containing a biohazard legend.[27] *[Regulatory Requirement]*

Containing contaminated instruments decreases the potential for injury to personnel or their exposure to blood, body fluids, or other potentially infectious materials[27] and helps prevent damage to the instruments during transport.[5]

Transporting soiled instruments in a manner that prevents exposing personnel to bloodborne pathogens and other potentially infectious materials is an OSHA requirement.[27]

Labeling the transport containment device communicates to others that the contents are potentially infectious.[5,27]

7.2.1 A red bag or red container may be used to cover the leak-proof, puncture-resistant container instead of a label for biohazard identification.[27] *[Conditional Recommendation]*

7.2.2 If the exterior of the containment device becomes contaminated, it must either be cleaned and disinfected or placed inside another biohazard-labeled container.[27,44] *[Regulatory Requirement]*

Contact with contaminated surfaces can transmit potentially infectious microorganisms.[27] Refer to the AORN Guideline for Transmission-Based Precautions[74] for additional guidance.

7.3 Separate contaminated items from clean and sterile supplies before transporting contaminated items to the processing area. Clean and sterile supplies that are not separated from con-taminated items should be considered contaminated. *[Recommendation]*

Separation of contaminated items from clean and sterile supplies minimizes the risk of cross contamination.[5]

8. Personal Protective Equipment

8.1 Personnel working in the decontamination area and handling contaminated instruments must wear PPE consistent with their risk of exposure, including
- a fluid-resistant gown with sleeves,
- general purpose utility gloves with a cuff that extends beyond the cuff of the gown,
- a mask with fluid barrier protection,
- eye protection or a full-face shield, and
- shoe covers or boots designed for use as PPE.[27] *[Regulatory Requirement]*

Contaminated instruments are a potential source of transmissible pathogens. Personnel in the decontamination area are at risk for exposure to blood, body fluids, and other potentially infectious materials. Personal protective equipment helps to protect the individual from exposure to infectious materials.

Splashes, splatters, and skin contact can be reasonably anticipated by personnel handling contaminated instruments. Fluid-resistant gowns can prevent transfer of microorganisms from contaminated items to skin.[5] Utility gloves can protect the wearer from punctures, cuts, and nicks and exposure of the hands to blood, body fluids, and other potentially infectious materials.[5] Utility glove cuffs that extend beyond the cuff of the gown provide fluid protection during manual instrument cleaning. A mask and eye protection or a full face shield can protect the face and eyes from droplets, splatter, aerosols, and chemicals used for cleaning purposes.[5] Fluid-resistant shoe covers can protect shoes from contaminants and splashes, splatters, and spills.

8.1.1 Personal protective equipment should be immediately available to personnel entering an area in which there is a risk of exposure to transmissible pathogens. *[Recommendation]*

There is potential for exposure to transmissible pathogens in the decontamination area, and OSHA requires the employer to provide PPE.[27] Placing PPE in an area where it is readily available to decontamination area personnel can facilitate compliance with OSHA requirements for wearing PPE when there is danger of exposure to blood, body fluids, or other potentially infectious materials.[27]

8.2 Remove PPE in a manner that minimizes exposure to the outside, contaminated area of the PPE. *[Recommendation]*

Self-contamination is possible during PPE doffing. Following correct procedures can protect personnel from inadvertent exposure to pathogens when doffing PPE. See the AORN Guideline for Transmission-Based Precautions for additional guidance.[74]

8.3 Personnel must perform hand hygiene after doffing PPE.[27] *[Regulatory Requirement]*

Perforations can occur in gloves, and hands can become contaminated during removal of PPE; OSHA requires hand hygiene after removal of PPE.[27]

8.4 Reusable PPE must be cleaned and decontaminated and its integrity confirmed between uses. *[Regulatory Requirement]*

Reusable gloves, gowns, aprons, face shields, and eyewear can become contaminated and their integrity compromised during use.[27] Decontamination and confirmation of integrity helps to protect the wearer from exposure.

9. Cleaning and Decontamination

9.1 Clean and decontaminate instruments as soon as possible after use. *[Recommendation]*

Cleaning instruments as soon as possible after use can help prevent formation of biofilm and dried blood and body fluids.[2,4,5,59-61] When blood or other bioburden dries on instruments, it can become more difficult to remove.[2,4,5,29,59-61] The presence of bioburden, biofilm, and buildup biofilm interferes with the effectiveness of disinfection or sterilization.[2,4,5,59-61,75]

9.2 Clean and decontaminate all instruments that were open in the OR or procedure room.[5] *[Recommendation]*

Items that are open in the OR are at risk for contamination. See the AORN Guideline for Sterile Technique for more information.[76]

9.3 Clean and decontaminate surgical instruments and equipment according to the manufacturer's validated, written IFU.[1,5] *[Recommendation]*

Cleaning, which involves the removal of organic and inorganic soil, is the first step in decontamination and can be accomplished through manual or mechanical processes.[5,14,77,78] The instrument and equipment manufacturers have determined the manual or mechanical steps and processes necessary to effectively clean a device.[5,14,77] Decontamination may require use of a disinfectant.

9.4 Before processing, disassemble instruments and devices composed of more than one piece according to the manufacturer's written IFU. *[Recommendation]*

When surfaces cannot be contacted by cleaning solutions, thorough cleaning cannot be achieved; thus, these surfaces can retain organic material and debris. The retained debris can prevent contact of cleaning solutions and disinfecting or sterilizing agents with instrument surfaces, reduce the effectiveness of subsequent disinfection or sterilization processes,[2,5] and cause patient injury if the debris is not removed before sterilization.[69,79-85]

9.4.1 After disassembly, arrange the instrument or medical device components in a manner that will permit contact of cleaning solutions with all surfaces of the item. *[Recommendation]*

The manufacturer's IFU provides specific guidance on optimal cleaning procedures.

9.4.2 In preparation for manual cleaning, disassemble instruments and open ports, valves, stopcocks, ratchets, and joints.[5] *[Recommendation]*

Opening and disassembling instruments facilitates contact of the cleaning solution with all surfaces of the instruments.

9.4.3 Rinse instruments in cool water before manual cleaning.[5,14] *[Recommendation]*

Hot water can denature blood proteins, which makes them more difficult to remove.[5] Cool water can help prevent coagulation of blood on instruments and can help remove gross soil from lumens, joints, and crevices.[2,6,10] Rinsing with cool water can wash away water-soluble blood proteins and prevent denaturing.[5]

9.4.4 Unless contraindicated in the device manufacturer's IFU, submerge the device in a cleaning solution that is compatible with the device and is mixed according to the cleaning solution manufacturer's IFU.[5] *[Recommendation]*

Full submersion of the instrument in the cleaning solution reduces the risk of splashing potentially contaminated cleaning solution onto personnel and into the environment. The concentration and temperature of the cleaning solution specified in the detergent IFU have been validated by the detergent manufacturer as necessary for the detergent to be effective.[14]

9.4.5 Flush lumens with cleaning solution and brush them with a brush of the length, diameter, type, and material specified in the device manufacturer's IFU.[14] *[Recommendation]*

Brushing is necessary to facilitate detergent contact of the cleaning solution within lumens. Brushes that are too short cannot contact the entire lumen. Brushes with a diameter that is too small will not contact all surfaces within the lumen.[2,5] Brushes with a diameter that is too large will collapse within the lumen, which can result in ineffective cleaning.[2,5]

9.4.6   **Perform brushing under the surface of the water during manual cleaning.** *[Recommendation]*

Brushing under water reduces the risk of aerosolization of chemicals and contaminants during manual cleaning.[14]

9.5   **Perform manual cleaning as specified in the instrument manufacturer's written IFU for instruments that cannot tolerate mechanical cleaning.** *[Recommendation]*

Manual cleaning is often recommended for devices that cannot tolerate the action of mechanical cleaning or cannot be immersed (eg, power drills, delicate microsurgical instruments, flexible endoscopes, cameras). Seals on lensed instruments can be damaged when processed through ultrasonic equipment.[5] Mechanical cleaning of devices when the manufacturer's written IFU recommend against it can result in damage to instruments and can limit the associated warranty.

9.6   **Change the cleaning solution per the cleaning solution manufacturer's IFU or between each use if the manufacturer's IFU does not make a recommendation.** *[Recommendation]*

Bioburden is deposited in the cleaning solution during the cleaning process and can interfere with cleaning process effectiveness.[5] Frequent changes of the cleaning solution can help to minimize bioburden.

9.6.1   **Change the cleaning solution when the temperature of the solution does not meet the temperature specified in the manufacturer's IFU.** *[Recommendation]*

Adding water to the existing solution changes cleaning solution concentration and therefore is not permissible.

9.7   **Establish a process and frequency for cleaning sinks and sink drains in the decontamination area.** *[Recommendation]*

Sinks and basins can be reservoirs for pathogen transmission. Decontaminating sinks used for manual cleaning between uses is a mechanism for reducing risk of transmission. Refer to the AORN Guideline for Environmental Cleaning for more information.[86]

A case report describes *Pseudomonas aeruginosa* colonization and biofilm formation in sink drains that was associated with an outbreak in three wards in the hospital.[87] The organization scheduled plumbing replacement. Some of the plumbing could not be immediately replaced and these sink drains were treated with 250 mL of 24% acetic acid once weekly and incubated 30 minutes before flushing until they were replaced. Cultures were taken every fourth week immediately before the next treatment, and culture results were negative in all but one instance. The authors concluded that mature *Pseudomonas* biofilm may be completely eradicated with acetic acid at a concentration as low as 0.5% as a strategy for preventing *Pseudomonas* species transmission. As it relates to the decontamination environment, this study is important because it reveals information about potential for sink drain contamination with gram-negative bacteria. Gram-negative waterborne bacteria could remain on reusable surgical instruments that are hand washed and lead to medical devices harboring endotoxins after complete processing and sterilization or high-level disinfection.

In an epidemiological analysis to investigate infection and colonization control of patients and the environment for carbapenemase-resistant *Enterobacteriaceae* (CRE) in an intensive care unit (ICU) in Belgium, Smolders et al[88] found a positive and significant relationship between contaminated sinks and CRE in patients admitted to ICU rooms. While this study is not specific to the decontamination area for instrument processing, it is important in that the researchers determined that decontaminating sink drains with acetic acid (ie, 250 mL 25% acetic acid three times weekly) was an effective strategy.

9.8   **For instruments that require lubrication, use a type of lubricant that is compatible with the instrument and subsequent sterilization method.** *[Recommendation]*

Instruments require different types of lubricant depending on the design of the device or the sterilization method.[5,14,77] Oil- or silicone-based lubricants may coat the instrument and reduce the effectiveness of some sterilization methods including steam and ethylene oxide (EO), and they may provide nutrients for microbial growth.[1] Following the device manufacturer's instructions for lubrication can facilitate selection and use of the correct lubricant.

9.8.1   **For instruments that are not compatible with lubricant (eg, orthopedic implants) in a mechanical washer, use cycles that exclude the use of lubricants.** *[Recommendation]*

9.9 After manual cleaning, use mechanical methods (eg, ultrasonic cleaner, <u>washer-disinfector/ decontaminator</u>) for cleaning instruments and medical devices unless otherwise specified in the manufacturers' IFU.[14,16,28] *[Recommendation]*

Mechanical cleaning after manual cleaning is preferred over manual cleaning alone because mechanical cleaning is reproducible and provides consistent cleaning solution concentrations, temperature control, and washing and rinsing processes. Manual cleaning alone is subject to variation among personnel.[16,28,89] Mechanical cleaning reduces the risk to personnel of exposure to blood, body fluids, other potentially infectious materials, and other hazards.[14,16] Mechanical cleaning is more easily monitored for quality than manual cleaning.[14,16]

9.9.1 Use indicated accessories (eg, flushing ports and tubing for minimally invasive surgery instruments) according to the equipment and device manufacturers' IFU.[14,16] *[Recommendation]*

9.10 Ultrasonic cleaners may be used to remove soil from hard-to-access areas of instruments unless otherwise specified in the manufacturer's IFU.[5] *[Conditional Recommendation]*

Ultrasonic cleaners use **cavitation** as the mechanism of cleaning action and can provide an effective means of removing soil from hard-to-reach areas, such as lumens, joints, and crevices.[5,14,16,72] Ultrasonic cleaners vary by design, intended use, operation, and maintenance. Some ultrasonic cleaners are designed and intended for use on specific instruments and will have specific manufacturers' IFU for these specific instruments.[90,91]

9.10.1 Use cleaning solutions that are compatible with the ultrasonic cleaner. *[Recommendation]*

Cleaning solutions that are not compatible with the ultrasonic cleaner can interfere with the cavitation process and result in incomplete cleaning.

9.10.2 Use accessories that are compatible with the ultrasonic cleaner (eg, metal open weave basket). *[Recommendation]*

Porous material such as silicone mats can absorb the cavitation, thus negating the effect of the cavitation.[5]

9.10.3 When required in the ultrasonic cleaning device manufacturers' IFU, perform degassing of the cleaning solution before instrument processing. *[Recommendation]*

Degassing removes air bubbles that can interfere with the cavitation process.[5]

9.10.4 Remove gross soil and cleaning solutions used during manual cleaning from instruments before they are placed in the ultrasonic cleaner. *[Recommendation]*

Ultrasonic cleaners are not designed to remove gross soil. They are designed to remove small debris from joints, crevices, lumens, and hard-to-reach areas.[5]

9.10.5 Do not mix instruments composed of brass, copper, aluminum, or chrome with instruments made of stainless steel in an ultrasonic cleaner.[14] Instruments made of similar metals may be combined in the ultrasonic cleaner unless otherwise specified in the instrument manufacturer's written IFU.[5] *[Recommendation]*

Placing instruments made of dissimilar metals in the ultrasonic cleaner can cause the transfer of ions from one instrument to another, which is known as **electroplating**, and can result in etching and pitting of the instrument. Damage to the finish of the instrument can create surface imperfections that can harbor microorganisms and debris.[14,16]

9.10.6 Only instruments that are compatible with the ultrasonic cleaning process should be subjected to ultrasonic cleaning. *[Recommendation]*

Some instruments are not compatible with ultrasonic cleaning and will sustain damage if cleaned in an ultrasonic cleaner.[5,14,16] Lenses may loosen, internal components of air-powered drills may sustain damage if immersed, and chrome plating can loosen.[5]

9.10.7 Submerge and fill instrument lumens with cleaning solution. Alternatively, if the ultrasonic cleaner includes adaptors or connections for internal lumen flushing, attach these to lumens to be cleaned. *[Recommendation]*

The presence of air prevents the cleaning solution from contacting the inner lumen of instruments and affects the cavitation process.[5,14,16]

9.10.8 Rinse instruments thoroughly with critical water after ultrasonic cleaning. *[Recommendation]*

Rinsing removes the cleaning solution and any debris that can be deposited on the instruments as they are removed from the ultrasonic cleaning device.[5]

9.10.9 **Close the lid when the ultrasonic cleaner is in use.** *[Recommendation]*

A closed lid contains any aerosolized contaminants that may be produced during cavitation in an ultrasonic cleaner.[5] Many ultrasonic cleaners feature an auto-close lid.

9.10.10 **Change the cleaning solution after each use in the ultrasonic cleaner as directed in the ultrasonic cleaner manufacturer's IFU and cleaning solution manufacturer's IFU.**[5] *[Recommendation]*

Organic material and debris that is lifted from instruments during the ultrasonic processing is deposited in the solution and can become a growth medium for bacteria and other microorganisms. Cleaning effectiveness can be diminished when the cleaning solution is heavily soiled. Some manufacturers' IFU specify using a fresh cleaning solution each time an ultrasonic cycle is run.

9.10.11 **Empty, clean, disinfect, rinse, and dry ultrasonic cleaners at least each day the ultrasonic cleaner is used or, preferably, after each use according to the manufacturer's IFU.**[5] *[Recommendation]*

Fluid in the ultrasonic cleaner can harbor gram-negative bacteria. Growth of these bacteria can result in the production of endotoxins, which are heat resistant and are not deactivated or removed by steam sterilization.[65]

9.10.12 **Perform cavitation testing for ultrasonic cleaning devices each day it is used, according to the manufacturer's IFU.** *[Recommendation]*

Effective cavitation is essential for ultrasonic cleaning device function. Daily testing provides verification that the device is functioning at the time of the test.[5]

9.11 **If allowed in the manufacturer's written IFU, use mechanical washer-disinfectors/decontaminators according to the manufacturer's IFU for instruments and medical devices.** *[Recommendation]*

Using mechanical methods to clean and disinfect surgical instruments and medical devices is a more thorough and reliable method than manual cleaning alone for those items that can withstand mechanical cleaning and disinfection.[5] Mechanical washer-disinfectors combine mechanical action with chemical cleaning agents in a staged cleaning cycle designed to thoroughly clean and disinfect surgical instruments.[29] To function properly, these machines must be performing at targeted mechanical efficiency and deliver the correct chemical cleaning agents at the correct temperature and at the correct dosage for the correct duration.[29] The results of washer-disinfector performance testing are used for validation of washer-disinfector performance and in the FDA clearance process. Washer-disinfector equipment designs vary among manufacturers and models.[5] Following the manufacturer's written IFU facilitates correct equipment use.

9.11.1 **Position surgical instruments and their containment devices and accessories in the washer-disinfector in a manner that facilitates contact of the cleaning solution with all surfaces of the items by**[5]
- **disassembling items composed of more than one part according to the manufacturer's IFU and securing small parts,**
- **placing instruments in open mesh-bottom pans,**
- **opening ports and stopcocks,**
- **removing stylets from lumened instruments,**
- **placing instrument ratchets in the open position,**
- **arranging items to prevent water pooling, and**
- **separating sharp instruments from electrical cords and insulated instruments.**

[Recommendation]

Preparing and positioning items as described above facilitates contact of the cleaning solution with all surfaces of the instrument. Contact with the cleaning solution is essential for effective cleaning and decontamination.[5] Securing small parts helps to prevent loss. Placing items on their edge helps prevent water retention on horizontal surfaces. Sharp items can damage the softer material of cords and cables and can damage insulation coverings.

9.11.2 **Follow the instrument manufacturer's written IFU during use of automated cleaning equipment, including placement of the instrument within mechanical washers, cycle parameters, and any other specific cleaning requirements.** *[Recommendation]*

The variety of equipment available and the complexity of devices make it essential to consult and follow the manufacturer's IFU to achieve optimal cleaning effectiveness.[5]

9.11.3 **Before processing implants in automated cleaning equipment, consult the implant manufacturer's IFU for implant compatibility, including whether the lubricant cycle should be used.** *[Recommendation]*

Lubricant retained on implants that are sterilized by the organization (eg, as part of an orthopedic fixation set) may not be biocompatible and can cause inflammation when implanted into the patient.

9.11.4 **Consult with the mechanical washer manufacturer's written IFU to determine**
- **the level of decontamination that is achieved (eg, low level, intermediate) and**
- **how to monitor the cycle to determine that the parameters necessary to render the processed items safe to handle are met** (See Section 16. Quality).

[Recommendation]

9.12 **Use the type of water for cleaning that is consistent with the manufacturers' written IFU and the intended use of the equipment and cleaning product.**[5,14,32] *[Recommendation]*

Water quality is affected by the presence of dissolved minerals, solids, chlorides, and other impurities and by its acidity and alkalinity (ie, pH).[32] Minerals can cause deposits, scale, or water spots to form on instruments.[32,92] Excessive chlorides can cause pitting.[32] The pH level affects the performance of enzymatic and detergent agents.[32] Untreated water quality fluctuates over time, varies with geographic location and season, and can affect the outcome of cleaning actions[28,32] (See Section 3. Water Quality).

9.13 **Perform the final rinse with critical water.**[5] *[Recommendation]*

Untreated water can contain contaminants, including endotoxins, which can be deposited on instruments during the final rinse. Rinsing with critical water can prevent deposits of impurities or contaminants on instruments.[5,28,32] Critical water can prevent spotting, stains, deposits, and corrosion on the surfaces of instruments.[32]

Endotoxins are heat stable and are not eradicated by subsequent steam sterilization. Endotoxins on surgical instruments can cause severe tissue inflammation[32] (See Section 3. Water Quality).

10. Cleaning Verification and Inspection

10.1 **An interdisciplinary team** (See Recommendation 1.2.1) **should establish and implement a cleaning verification testing protocol.** *[Recommendation]*

Currently, there is no single standard of clean, nor is there a standard test for soil for surgical instruments.[16,93] Efficacy of cleaning has traditionally been evaluated through visual inspection.[5] Visual inspection is subjective, and pathogens and soils are not visible without microscopic examination. Even under ideal cleaning conditions, instruments may retain soil that is not visible. There are, however, a number of tests that can be used to assess cleaning efficiency.[64,94,95] Manufacturers may establish "benchmark cutoffs" for manual cleaning of instruments (eg, flexible endoscopes) that users can employ so that any instrument failing this quantitative cutoff after cleaning is re-cleaned before disinfection/sterilization.[96] Quantitative testing can be used in a quality monitoring program to observe for trends and to monitor performance of washer-disinfectors and manual processes.

Reusable surgical instruments with complex designs (eg, powered devices, robotic instruments, instruments with narrow lumens) can present challenges to decontamination processes, and cleaning verification may be useful to evaluate cleaning effectiveness in these devices.[64,93,97,98]

Saito et al[99] conducted a nonexperimental study designed to evaluate instruments used for robotic surgery (N = 41) for residual protein (using Micor BCA Protein Assay Kit; Thermo Fisher Scientific) in 2017. The evaluation included measurement of protein release following the procedure using an ultrasonic cleaner, to quantify protein after the procedure, and after in-house cleaning (ie, manual brushing followed 15-minute ultrasonication with enzymatic detergent) at one, two, and three repetitions.

Robotic instruments were contaminated with 72.3×10^3 µg protein/instrument after the procedure. Resulting protein release was 650 µg, 550 µg, and 530 µg per robotic instrument, respectively, after the three repetitions of in-house cleaning. The researchers concluded that even after meticulous cleaning in accordance with manufacturers' instructions, residual protein remained on robotic instruments, and that serial ultrasonication and repeated measures of residual protein to evaluate residual contamination may be warranted.[98]

In an organizational experience report, Kurley[100] describes a pilot program in which ATP was used to evaluate cleanliness of surgical instruments after decontamination and before sterilization. The author selected a handheld ATP testing device that designates "pass" (0-10 relative light units [RLU]), "caution" (11-30 RLU), and "fail" (> 30 RLU) levels and determined that "pass" levels would be required for progression to sterilization. Failures to pass ATP testing led the author to evaluate cleaning protocols by contacting the device manufacturer to clarify IFU, which the author described as "vague and difficult to interpret." The organization made many constructive changes to cleaning protocols as a result of ATP cleaning verification and concluded that the ATP testing program resulted in significant improvements to cleaning processes.

10.1.1 **Cleaning effectiveness may be evaluated by testing for one or more markers, including**
- protein,
- carbohydrate,
- hemoglobin,
- endotoxin,
- lipid,
- sodium ion,
- bioburden, and
- ATP.[5]

[Conditional Recommendation]

10.2 **Use lighted magnification to inspect surgical instruments and other reusable medical devices after decontamination.** *[Recommendation]*

An instrument that appears clean to the naked eye may harbor debris that cannot be seen without magnification.[5]

10.2.1 **Repeat the decontamination process if retained soil is seen or detected with cleaning verification tests.** *[Recommendation]*

10.3 **Inspect and evaluate items for**
- cleanliness;
- completeness (ie, no missing parts);
- correct alignment;
- surface integrity;
- sharpness of cutting edges;
- integrity of insulation on insulated devices;
- integrity of cords and cables;
- clarity of lenses;
- integrity of seals and gaskets;
- integrity of instrument labels (eg, instrument tape) and similar products, if present;
- correct functioning; and
- absence of
  - corrosion, pitting, burrs, nicks, and cracks;
  - wear and chipping of inserts and plated surfaces;
  - moisture; and
  - any other defects.

[Recommendation]

Use of instruments that are not thoroughly cleaned, are damaged, or do not function correctly poses a risk to patients.[2,4]

10.3.1 **Verify that powered equipment can be switched on and off and is functioning as intended. Attach powered equipment to the power source for testing as specified in the manufacturer's IFU.** *[Recommendation]*

Power that does not cease when a powered device is turned off can cause harm to personnel or patients.[14] Verifying that instruments requiring a power source are functioning as intended facilitates patient and personnel safety when this verification occurs during device processing.

10.3.2 **Before inspection, assemble instruments that require assembly. After inspection, disassemble instruments before packaging them for sterilization unless the instrument manufacturer's IFU indicates that the item can be sterilized when assembled.** *[Recommendation]*

Disassembling items before sterilization facilitates sterilant contact of all surfaces of the item being sterilized.[2,4] Assembly for inspection allows the user to confirm correct fit and that mechanisms (eg, locking, articulation) function as intended.[5]

10.3.3 **Inspect the internal channels of reusable arthroscopic shavers using an endoscopic camera or borescope.** *[Recommendation]*

It is not possible to visually inspect arthroscopic shaver channels without a device that can penetrate the channel. Retained organic material or debris in lumens can harbor pathogens and ultimately lead to patient injury.[96,101]

In a 2007 case-control study, Tosh et al[102] reported on an outbreak of *Pseudomonas aeruginosa* SSI in seven patients on whom the same arthroscopic shaver was used. During investigation, the researchers found debris in a lumen of the shaver although the shaver had undergone repeated decontamination and sterilization procedures. The researchers concluded that the retained surgical debris allowed the bacteria to survive the sterilization process, and the subsequent use of the shaver was likely related to the SSI outbreak.

10.3.4 **An endoscopic camera or borescope may be used to inspect other lumened devices.** *[Conditional Recommendation]*

While it is not known if lumened devices other than reusable arthroscopic shavers have been implicated in SSI outbreaks, an endoscopic camera or borescope can facilitate identification of retained soil. Clinical soil retained after cleaning can impede subsequent disinfection and sterilization.[5]

10.3.5 **Visually examine insulated devices and test them using equipment designed to detect insulation failure.** *[Recommendation]*

Electrode insulation damage caused during use or processing may create an alternate pathway for the electrical current to leave the active electrode and cause patient injury.[103] Some insulation failures are not visible. Damage to insulation may not be seen during visual inspection.[103]

Serious patient injury, such as thermal bowel injury, can occur when instruments with insulation defects are used. See the Guideline for Electrosurgical Safety[103] for more information.

10.4 **Test insulated equipment for current leakage before use and after decontamination.** *[Recommendation]*

Testing before use and after decontamination allows a defective device to be replaced before use or sterilization and provides an opportunity for corrective action in advance of the surgical procedure.[103]

10.5 **Identify defective reusable surgical instruments and remove them from service for repair or disposal.**[5] *[Recommendation]*

Identification of defective instruments and removal from service facilitates segregation of these instruments from instruments to be used when assembling sets. Removing defective instruments from service reduces the risk that defective instruments will be used.[5]

10.5.1 An interdisciplinary team (See Recommendation 1.2.1) should determine a standardized communication strategy and actions to perform when a reusable surgical instrument is removed from service.[103] *[Recommendation]*

10.5.2 Include the following in the standardized communication:
- the communication pathway between sterile processing and surgical personnel,
- physician notification (eg, a one-of-a-kind item is unavailable and no replacement is available)
- whether an instrument may be substituted for the instrument that is out of service,
- device disposition (eg, how the device is handled when sent for repair), and
- documentation according to facility policy and procedure.[103]

[Recommendation]

10.6 **Thoroughly dry instruments before they are assembled and packaged for sterilization.**[5] *[Recommendation]*

Moisture can interfere with sterilization processes.[5] Excess moisture on instrument surfaces can alter the content of steam and can pose a challenge for effective heating of the instrument during steam sterilization.[5] Hydrogen peroxide vapor and hydrogen peroxide gas plasma sterilization cycles may fail in the presence of excess moisture.[59] Ethylene oxide combines with water to form ethylene glycol (ie, antifreeze), which is toxic and is not removed during aeration.[61]

11. Intraocular Ophthalmic Instruments

11.1 **Take special precautions when processing intraocular ophthalmic instruments.**[104] *[Recommendation]*

Most instances of **toxic anterior segment syndrome** (TASS) appear to be related to instrument processing[31,104-108]; however, the incidence of TASS has decreased in the past few years.[106,109] This decrease may be attributed to technological advances and better mitigation measures.

11.2 **Immediately after use during the procedure, wipe ophthalmic instruments with sterile water and a sterile lint-free sponge or cloth and flush or immerse them in sterile water according to the manufacturer's written IFU.**[5] *[Recommendation]*

Keeping the ophthalmic **viscoelastic** (OV) and organic material moist helps facilitate removal.[5] Ophthalmic viscoelastic material can harden and dry within minutes, making subsequent removal difficult.[5] Keeping OV or other organic material moist can prevent drying and hardening of such material on ophthalmic devices.[104] Biofilm adheres to the surfaces of instruments and is very difficult to remove.[5]

11.3 **Clean intraocular instruments in a designated cleaning area, separately from general surgical instruments.**[5] *[Recommendation]*

Procedures for processing ophthalmic instruments differ from those for general surgical instruments.[104,110] Cleaning intraocular instruments separately from general surgical instruments can help prevent cross contamination with bioburden from heavily soiled nonophthalmic surgical instruments.[5]

11.4 **Use single-use disposable cannulae whenever possible.** *[Recommendation]*

Effective cleaning of very small lumens in these devices is difficult.

11.5 **At the close of the procedure, use sterile water to flush the phacoemulsification**
- **irrigation and aspiration ports,**
- **irrigation/aspiration hand pieces, and**

- **accessory reusable tips and tubing according to the manufacturer's IFU before disconnecting the hand piece from the unit.** [Recommendation]

When OV material dries on phacoemulsification hand pieces, it is difficult to remove.[104] Flushing immediately after the procedure can help prevent OV material from drying.[104]

11.6 **Select and use cleaning products for intraocular instruments in accordance with the instrument manufacturer's written IFU.**[5] [Recommendation]

Some experts recommend against using enzymatic detergents.[104,105]

In 2014, a survey developed by the American Society of Cataract and Refractive Surgery, the American Academy of Ophthalmology, and the Ophthalmic Outpatient Surgery Society (OOSS) was sent to OOSS-member ophthalmic single-specialty ambulatory surgery centers (ASCs) with questions about cleaning and sterilization practices for intraocular instruments.[104] Complete responses were received from 182 ASCs. A majority (55.5%) did not use enzyme for intraocular instrument decontamination. The average self-reported rate of endophthalmitis was 0.021% for non-enzyme-using facilities compared to 0.027% for enzyme-using facilities.

11.7 **After cleaning, rinse intraocular instruments with a copious amount of utility or critical water.** [Recommendation]

Tamashiro et al[108] conducted a laboratory study in 2013 to evaluate the cytotoxicity of reusable cannulas for ophthalmic surgery after the cannulas were filled with an ophthalmic viscosurgical device (OVD) and cleaned with an enzymatic detergent. The researchers used 30 reusable 25-gauge injection cannulas, 20 mm in length, whose lumens were filled with an OVD solution for 50 minutes (to simulate a worst-case clinical scenario). The cannulas were processed according to recommendations by presoaking, washing the lumen using a high-pressure water jet, backwashing with enzymatic detergent in an ultrasonic cleaner, preliminary rinsing with tap water, final rinsing with sterile **distilled water**, drying with compressed filtered air, packaging for sterilization, and sterilization using saturated steam under pressure (134° C [273° F] for 4 minutes).

The researchers found that a longer washing duration of the lumen was needed than was prescribed in the protocol (a 7- versus 5-second lumen wash with a high-pressure water jet) to remove the OVD solution. The cleaning protocol used in this study removed residues of OVD solution and enzymatic detergent as shown by the lack of cytotoxicity of all sample extracts on evaluation with US Pharma-copeia 32. The researchers concluded that this cleaning protocol (ie, a 7-second lumen wash with a high-pressure water jet) has the potential to minimize the occurrence of TASS associated with residues of OVD solutions and enzymatic detergents.[108]

In a laboratory-based study, Tsaousis et al[111] evaluated the alterations in the morphology and elemental composition of reusable phacoemulsification tips after cleaning and sterilization. The researchers studied two types of reusable phacoemulsification needles with one tip of each kind undergoing one, two, and three sterilization cycles using saturated steam under pressure after cleaning, followed by thorough rinsing with sterile water between cycles. Another set of tips underwent the same procedure but without rinsing. These intraocular instruments were then examined through scanning electron microscopy and energy-dispersive x-ray spectroscopy to assess morphologic changes and surface deposits. The researchers found smaller and fewer residues in tips after sterilization with the use of enzymes and thorough rinsing. They concluded that rinsing significantly reduced the size and number of residues after use of enzymatic detergents but detergent residues were detected even after thorough rinsing with sterile water.

11.7.1 **Perform a final rinse including lumens with critical or sterile water.**[104] [Recommendation]

Untreated water may contain endotoxins, which are heat stable and as such will remain biologically active after sterilization and which have been implicated in occurrences of TASS.[104] Residual enzymes and detergents not rinsed from instruments have been associated with TASS incidence.[105,107]

11.7.2 **Dry lumens with pressure-regulated instrument air.** [Recommendation]

Instrument air forced through the lumen eliminates moisture that can serve as a medium for microbial growth.[5] Pressure regulation of the instrument air protects the reusable surgical instrument from damage caused by using too much pressure.[5] The instrument manufacturer's IFU provides the required pressure for drying with instrument air.

11.8 **If an ultrasonic cleaner is used for intraocular ophthalmic instruments, empty, clean, disinfect, rinse, and dry the ultrasonic cleaner after use for non-intraocular ophthalmic instruments and at least daily or, preferably, after each use.**[5] **If not contraindicated by the ultrasonic cleaner manufacturer's written IFU, wipe the chamber with**

70% to 90% alcohol and dry it with a lint-free cloth.[104] *[Recommendation]*

Inadequately cleaned ultrasonic cleaners and endotoxins have been associated with TASS. Fluid in the ultrasonic cleaner can harbor gram-negative bacteria. Growth of these bacteria can result in the production of endotoxins. Alcohol promotes drying, inhibits microbial growth, and can prevent biofilm formation. Cleaning and disinfecting the ultrasonic cleaner before use for intraocular ophthalmic instruments reduces the risk of cross contamination.[104] Some intraocular instrument manufacturers' IFU may require dedicated ultrasonic cleaners that are not used for other types of instruments.

11.9 **After decontamination, inspect instruments that have been in contact with OV material under magnification,[104] preferably lighted magnification, for residual OV material.** *[Recommendation]*

Retained OV material has been associated with TASS.[104] Viscoelastic material is difficult to remove during cleaning, especially if it has been allowed to dry. Inspection under magnification can facilitate detection of residual materials. Although studies conducted on rabbits showed that OV material alone, even if denatured by steam sterilization, did not cause ocular inflammation, the presence of endotoxin in OV material can cause severe ocular reaction.[104]

11.10 **Maintain records of all processing procedures, decontamination equipment, and cleaning solutions used with ophthalmic instruments.** *[Recommendation]*

Records of cleaning methods and solutions can assist in surveillance efforts and be used to facilitate investigation of any suspected or confirmed cases of TASS.

12. Laryngoscope Blades and Handles

12.1 **Clean, decontaminate, dry, and store reusable laryngoscope blades and their handles in a manner that reduces the risk of exposing patients and personnel to potentially pathogenic microorganisms.** *[Recommendation]*

Laryngoscope blades and handles may be a source of contamination. In a 2014 prospective descriptive study, Choi et al[112] described microbial analysis of reusable laryngoscope blades and handles stored in emergency crash carts. Among the 291 samples, the researchers found bacterial contamination of blades (18.2%), handle tops (5.6%), and handles with rough surfaces (28.2%). The microbial contaminants included 18 types of bacteria and two unidentified molds. Some but not all of

the laryngoscope blades and handles were packaged in the cart. The researchers concluded that laryngoscope microbial transmission remains a risk factor for health care–associated infection and suggest that organizations develop stricter standards for high-level disinfection and consider using single-use, one-piece laryngoscopes with blades that are not folded.

In a comprehensive integrative review, Negri de Sousa et al[113] identified 77 articles that addressed the laryngoscope blade or handle as a potential source of contamination. Based on the quality of the research, the authors selected 20 articles for further review. In five of the studies, blood was found on the laryngoscope blade. None of the studies that investigated the handles found blood.

12.1.1 **Convene an interdisciplinary team (See Recommendation 1.2.1) to establish and implement standardized procedures for processing laryngoscope blades and handles.** *[Recommendation]*

12.2 **After each use, clean reusable laryngoscope blades and high-level disinfect or sterilize them according to the manufacturer's IFU.[2]** *[Recommendation]*

Cleaning and disinfection minimizes the risk of pathogen transmission.[2] Laryngoscope blades are considered semicritical items that require a minimum of high-level disinfection because they contact mucous membranes.[2]

12.3 **Clean and low-level disinfect reusable laryngoscope handles after each use. Reusable laryngoscope handles may be high-level disinfected or sterilized if specified in the manufacturer's IFU.** *[Recommendation]*

Laryngoscope handles are classified as noncritical items according to the Spaulding Classification.[2] Noncritical items are those that contact intact skin.[2] According to the Centers for Disease Control and Prevention (CDC), low-level disinfectants are used for noncritical items.[2] Although the laryngoscope handle by itself is a noncritical device, the laryngoscope consists of two parts that are handled concurrently. In a comprehensive, integrative review, Negri de Sousa et al[113] recommended that both parts of the laryngoscope be classified as semicritical. Laryngoscope handles have a knurled surface (ie, a series of small ridges cut into the metal) to facilitate grip; the rough surface can accumulate soil and harbor pathogens.[113] When the laryngoscope blade is folded closed, the tip of the blade contacts the handle. Studies have demonstrated the presence of microorganisms on laryngoscope handles.[112,113]

Howell et al[114] conducted a series of laboratory studies to evaluate effectiveness of germicidal wipes and residual effect after disinfection using two disinfectant wipes (ie, coco alkyl dimethyl-benzyl ammonium chloride [CDBAC], 2% chlorhexidine gluconate [CHG]) on laryngoscope handles. The CHG group showed low levels of bacterial growth compared to the CDBAC group. The researchers concluded that CHG germicidal wipes were superior to CDBAC wipes and that if laryngoscope handles were disinfected using wipes, sterilization at established intervals is also indicated.

Other researchers cited in the literature review evaluated costs and life cycle assessment in 2018, comparing per-use costs and environmental effects of laryngoscopes, including reusable low-level disinfected ($0.58/use), reusable high-level disinfected ($0.98/use), reusable sterilized ($2.39/use), and single use ($10.66/use).[115] The researchers found that reusable laryngoscope handles and blades had a lesser degree of environmental impact than single use, with high-level disinfection being the least toxic to the environment.[116]

Recommendations for processing vary within the published literature;[113] however, the Association of Anaesthetists of Great Britain and Ireland suggested that laryngoscope handles become contaminated with bacteria and blood during use and as such recommended that they be cleaned, disinfected, and sterilized after every use.[117]

In a literature review, Van Wicklin[116] discussed contamination of laryngoscope blades and handles, disinfection practices, and environmental concerns surrounding use of single-use laryngoscopes. The author included seven international studies published between January 2012 and May 2018 in the review and concluded that while more research is warranted, the literature supported current recommendations for practice.

12.4 **Package and store reusable laryngoscope blades and handles that have been high-level disinfected or sterilized in a manner that prevents contamination and identifies them as ready for use.** *[Recommendation]*

Packaging assists in preventing recontamination of items that have been high-level disinfected.[112] Packaging of laryngoscope blades to prevent recontamination is a CDC recommendation.[2]

In a retrospective chart review, Nielsen et al[118] compared outcomes for upper aerodigestive tract procedures before and after implementation of airway cart instrument packaging. The researchers compared 100 patient records before and after implementation and found there were four infections in each group, no deaths, and no significant differences in length of stay or complications. However, the set-up time was significantly different (46.6 seconds versus 95.5 seconds). The researchers concluded that packaging instruments did not result in better outcomes but may contribute to risk associated with a longer set-up time for airway emergencies.[118]

13. Prion Disease Transmission Precautions

13.1 **Take special precautions to minimize the risk of transmission of prion diseases from contaminated reusable surgical instruments.**[119] *[Recommendation]*

Prions are a unique class of infectious proteins that cause fatal neurological diseases known as **transmissible spongiform encephalopathies** (TSEs).[119] Examples of prion diseases are Gerstmann-Sträussler-Scheinker syndrome, fatal familial insomnia syndrome, and **Creutzfeldt-Jakob disease** (CJD).[119] **Variant Creutzfeldt-Jakob disease** (vCJD) is acquired from cattle with bovine spongiform encephalopathy or "mad cow disease."[119] Transmissible spongiform encephalopathies have been described in a number of animal species. To date, with the exception of cattle, there is no evidence of transmission of TSEs to humans from animals.[119] Iatrogenic transmission of CJD has been reported in more than 250 cases worldwide linked to contaminated human growth hormone, dura mater and corneal grafts, and neurosurgical instruments.[120] Six cases were linked to the use of contaminated equipment, neurosurgical instruments in four cases and stereotactic electroencephalogram depth electrodes in two cases.[120]

Prions are resistant to conventional physical and chemical sterilization.[119] Special precautions and protocols are required to inactivate prions[119,121] and these precautions are not limited to acute care settings; the presence of prions has been reported in the ambulatory surgery environment.[25]

13.2 **An interdisciplinary team (See Recommendation 1.2.1) should establish, document, and implement evidence-based policies and procedures to minimize the risk of prion disease transmission between patients. These processes should be based on**
- **the patient's prion disease status or risk of having a prion disease;**
- **the level of infectivity of the tissue involved, as defined by the *WHO Tables on Infectivity Distribution in Transmissible Spongiform Encephalopathies*[122]; and**
- **the intended use of the reusable surgical instrument.**
[Recommendation]

A defined protocol based on available evidence provides guidance to protect patients and health care workers from prion transmission.

The WHO has published clinical diagnostic criteria for CJD.[121] These criteria are used to identify patients at risk of having or developing CJD. Patients at high risk include those with

- progressive dementia consistent with CJD in whom a diagnosis has not been confirmed or ruled out,
- a familial history of a prion disease,
- a history of dura mater transplants, or
- a history of receiving cadaveric-derived pituitary hormone.[119]

Although all prion diseases are infectious, the risk of infection is not the same for all tissue. Based on successful experimental transmission, the risk of infection from tissue types is categorized as high, low, or no risk.[122] Tissue from the posterior eye retina or optic nerve, brain, pituitary gland, and spinal cord are categorized as high risk.[122] Liver, lung, spleen, kidney, and lymph nodes are categorized as low risk, as are body fluids, blood, and urine.[122]

13.3 **If the need for a surgical implant is anticipated, only deliver the implant essential for the specific patient to the sterile field. Discard all implants opened to the field during the procedure and do not process them for subsequent use.** [Recommendation]

Discarding potentially contaminated implants eliminates the risk of implanting a prion-contaminated implant into a patient. Implants, such as screws, are often supplied in racks that hold multiple implants. When sets containing multiple implants are open, there is a risk of cross contamination of implants that are not used. Removing implants that will not be needed for the patient before sterilizing the tray decreases the amount of implant inventory that will need to be discarded.

13.4 **Use instruments designed for single use on high-risk tissue of patients who are known or suspected to be infected with prion disease and discard them after use.**[120] **If single-use instruments are not available, limit reusable instruments to those that are easy to clean. Keep the number of instruments used to a minimum.** [Recommendation]

Prions are highly resistant to conventional disinfection and sterilization processes.[5,119] Discarding these devices eliminates the risk of transmission through these devices.

Use of single-use instruments eliminates the need to implement special processing protocols and eliminates the risk of instruments contaminated with prions being used on another patient.[123] Use of single-use instruments also eliminates the risk of exposure of personnel who process instruments.

The CDC recommends that all disposable instruments that come into contact with high-infectivity tissues and low-infectivity tissues of suspected or conformed TSE patients should be disposed of by incineration.[120]

According to the National Institute for Health and Care Excellence,[124] tonsillectomy procedures in Europe were considered high-risk for prion disease transmission through reusable instruments, and single-use instruments were required for all tonsillectomy procedures. An audit of tonsillectomy procedures indicated that single-use instruments were associated with a more than 100% increase in complication rates. Primary hemorrhage resulting in return to the OR doubled from a baseline rate of 0.6% with reusable instruments to 1.2% when single-use instruments were introduced. The rates returned to baseline levels after implementation of purchase decisions that considered quality of the single-use instruments. The investigators also conducted two separate and detailed audits of suppliers of single-use tonsillectomy instruments in the United Kingdom, which showed considerable variation in the quality and consistency of the single-use instruments available. Careful specification and quality control of instruments are identified in this audit as key requirements to ensure patient safety when using single-use instruments.

Successful cleaning is a critical step in processing instruments exposed to high-risk tissue. When instruments are difficult to clean thoroughly, the potential for incomplete cleaning is increased. The challenge to cleaning is reduced when easy-to-clean devices are used.

13.4.1 **If it is necessary to use reusable instruments on high-risk tissue of patients suspected of having prion disease, use instruments that are easy to clean and will tolerate exposure to an extended steam sterilization cycle.**[119] [Recommendation]

Depending on the cleaning management before sterilization (eg, cleaning process, cleaning product), extended steam sterilization cycles may not be necessary. However, at the time of this publication and based on current knowledge, an extended cycle steam sterilization is recommended as the option for sterilization that provides the greatest margin of safety.[119]

13.4.2 **For all patients undergoing brain biopsy, use only single-use brain biopsy sets.** [Recommendation]

Creutzfeldt-Jakob disease is often definitively diagnosed by brain biopsy, and whether the patient has a prion disease may not be known at the time of surgery.

Commercial single-use brain biopsy sets are available, or sets can be assembled using instruments at the end of their useful life and discarding them after use.

13.4.3 **When reusable neuroendoscopes are needed for patients with known or suspected prion disease, use rigid neuroendoscopes.**[124] *[Recommendation]*

Flexible neuroendoscopes contain narrow lumens that are difficult to clean. Neuroendoscopes may not be compatible with the cleaning procedures and extended steam sterilization cycles recommended for items contaminated with prions.

13.4.4 **Do not use power drills and saws for patients with known or suspected prion disease.** *[Recommendation]*

Power drills and saws create aerosols and may splatter potentially infectious material. Although there are no reported cases of occupational transmission of prion disease through exposure to aerosols, much about prions and their infectivity is unknown.[119]

Power drills are difficult to clean, and the cleaning and sterilization methods recommended to eliminate prion infectivity may damage them.

13.5 **Process reusable instruments that have contacted high-risk tissue from patients known or suspected to have a prion disease in accordance with the most current infection prevention guidelines.**[119] *[Recommendation]*

Reducing infectivity is crucial to providing instruments that are safe to use on patients. When a potentially contaminated device can be cleaned and prion tissue removed, the risk of prion disease transmission is minimized. There is currently no consensus on the best method of managing instruments that are likely to be contaminated with prions. Until recently, the most referenced guidelines for managing prevention of TSEs were the *WHO Infection Control Guidelines for Transmissible Spongiform Encephalopathies*.[121] These were published in 1999 and were based on studies that

- did not incorporate conventional cleaning procedures that reduce protein contamination,
- investigated inactivation using tissue **homogenates** dried onto carriers, and
- investigated inactivation using various strains and concentrations of prions and a variety of tissue.[5]

Although they are effective, the WHO guidelines for managing instruments contaminated with prions[121] are impractical and are corrosive to instruments. The more current Society for Healthcare Epidemiology of America (SHEA) "Guideline for disinfection and sterilization of prion-contaminated medical instruments,"[119] published in 2010, reflects research conducted after the WHO publication. This guideline identifies practices that can eliminate prion infectivity with a wide margin of safety.[119]

13.6 **Identify instruments that require special prion processing procedures in a manner that alerts personnel who handle and process instruments that the instruments are contaminated or potentially contaminated with prions.**[5] *[Recommendation]*

Awareness that instruments are contaminated or potentially contaminated with prions reduces the risk of these instruments being ineffectively processed and subsequently used on other patients.

13.6.1 **Use an instrument-tracking process or system that provides for tracking of surgical instruments used on high-risk tissue (eg, spinal and brain tissue).** *[Recommendation]*

Instrument tracking systems identify items used during the procedure and identify the patient for whom the items were used.

13.7 **Do not use instruments that cannot be cleaned or that require sterilization using low-temperature technologies, or discard them after use.**[63] *[Recommendation]*

For reusable surgical instruments that contact high-risk tissues in procedures for patients with known or suspected prion disease, steam sterilization for an extended cycle time is the only sterilization method recommended in national guidelines at this time.[63] Low-temperature sterilization technologies have not been incorporated into WHO[121] and CDC[120] guidance for inactivating prions.

Research into the effectiveness of gaseous hydrogen peroxide for inactivating prions is ongoing. Several studies have demonstrated that hydrogen peroxide vapor and some hydrogen peroxide gas plasma technologies in combination with specific cleaning agents are effective in inactivating prions, and researchers have suggested that sterilization with gaseous hydrogen peroxide protocols will be practical and widely used in the future.[119]

In a quasi-experimental study designed to test the effectiveness of a gaseous hydrogen peroxide sterilization process to inactivate prions, Fichet et al[125] contaminated stainless steel wires with prion-infected brain homogenates and then exposed them to gaseous hydrogen peroxide sterilization. Sterilization parameters included a vacuum process at 86° F (30° C) for three or six pulses. The researchers concluded that exposure under these conditions demonstrated that gaseous hydrogen peroxide was effective in inactivating prions.

In a quasi-experimental study to test effectiveness of decontamination methods to inactivate prions, Yan et al[126] contaminated stainless steel wires with prion-infected brain homogenate material and subjected them to a variety of decontamination and sterilization procedures including exposure to gaseous hydrogen peroxide, steam sterilization, sodium hydroxide, enzymatic detergent, enzymatic detergent plus gaseous hydrogen peroxide, peracetic acid, alkaline detergent, alkaline detergent plus ortho phthalaldehyde, alkaline detergent plus steam sterilization, and alkaline detergent plus gaseous hydrogen peroxide. The researchers injected the wires into the brains of living hamsters. Successful processing was defined as a total group survival time of 18 months after implantation. After 18 months, only those hamsters incubated with wires reprocessed with an alkaline detergent followed by sterilization with a four injection gaseous hydrogen peroxide cycle showed no clinical signs of prion disease.

In a quasi-experimental study to determine the effectiveness of hydrogen peroxide gas plasma for inactivating animal and human prions, Rogez-Kreuz et al[127] decontaminated prion-contaminated steel wires with combinations of enzymatic or alkaline detergents and gaseous hydrogen peroxide. The researchers found that gaseous hydrogen peroxide decreased the infectivity of the prions; however, its efficacy was dependent on the concentration of the hydrogen peroxide and the systems used to deliver it. Only one specific model of a hydrogen peroxide gas plasma sterilizer was 100% effective in inactivating prions.

13.8 **Keep instruments moist until they are cleaned and decontaminated.**[119] **Instruments may be kept moist by immersion in water, a wet cloth draped over the instruments, or pretreatment product application.**[119] *[Recommendation]*

When prions dry on instruments, they become highly resistant to removal.[119,128,129] Dried films of tissue are more resistant to prion inactivation by steam sterilization than tissue that is kept moist.[119,128,129]

Prions are **hydrophobic** and in the absence of moisture can strongly attach to surfaces, particularly stainless steel.[129] Keeping instruments moist until cleaning and decontamination can help reduce the tenacity of prions to adhere to surfaces.

13.9 **Decontaminate instruments in a mechanical washer as soon as possible after use.**[119] *[Recommendation]*

Mechanical washing is preferred because process consistency is more likely than with manual washing, and the mechanical process is more easily monitored. Automation of cleaning facilitates reproducibility of the cleaning process. Mechanical washers employ a validated cycle that is not possible with manual cleaning.

Stainless steel has a high affinity for prion **adsorption**. The longer prion-contaminated instruments are permitted to dry, the greater the adsorption and the more difficult the prion removal.[119,128,129]

13.9.1 **Follow the mechanical washer-disinfector manufacturer's IFU for decontaminating the mechanical washer-disinfector after processing instruments that may be contaminated with prions.** *[Recommendation]*

No studies were found that address cleaning and disinfecting the mechanical washer after processing instruments that may be contaminated with prions.

13.9.2 **Use cleaning chemicals that have evidence of inactivating prion infectivity and that are compatible with the instruments to be cleaned.**[119] *[Recommendation]*

It is important that product selection decisions take into consideration the combined effect of point-of-use treatment, cleaning, disinfection, and sterilization and effectiveness against other infectious diseases and not just the ability to inactivate prions. The EPA considers prions to be "pests."[130] As such, EPA registration for pesticides that are effective in inactivating prions are subject to testing requirements.[131] To date, there are no EPA-registered pesticides that are effective for inactivating prions.[132]

The WHO recommendation to soak instruments in 1 N sodium hydroxide (NaOH)[121] is effective at eliminating prion infectivity but, because of incompatibility with most instruments, is impractical. Several alkaline and enzymatic cleaning agents in combination with steam sterilization have been shown to be effective as well and are compatible with instruments.[119]

Cleaning formulas have a varying ability to remove and inactivate prions. However, research has shown that some cleaning agents such as phenolic formulations may increase the resistance of prions to subsequent steam sterilization.[133,134] Research to identify effective cleaning verification tools that measure effective deactivation of prions has been conducted,[135] but further study is needed.

In a laboratory-based study, Botsios et al[136] evaluated a protocol using cavitation with an ultrasonic cleaner with a combination of thio-urea, urea and 4M guanidine hydrochloride (GdnHCl) at 72° F (22° C). The researchers found that the protocol resulted in a 4-log reduction for both CJD and scrapie proteins.

In an investigative study of the effectiveness of innovative physical and chemical methods of prion inactivation, Fichet et al[134] subjected prion-contaminated stainless steel wires to a variety of cleaning chemistries and steriliza-tion technologies. The researchers found that one phenolic formulation increased the resis-tance of prions to inactivation.

In a quasi-experimental study, McDonnell et al[133] found that cleaning with certain chemical formulations, alkaline formulations in particular, in combination with steam sterilization was an effective prion-decontamination process. The researchers found that low-temperature gaseous hydrogen peroxide sterilization reduced infectiv-ity in both the presence and absence of cleaning.

In a randomized controlled trial to determine effectiveness of prion inactivation, Schmitt et al[137] subjected prion-contaminated stainless steel wires to either an automated decontamination procedure developed for prion decontamination, or a routine automated alkaline disinfection pro-cess used for sterile processing in Germany. The routine procedure included an alkaline wash and thermal disinfection. The specially designed prion decontamination process included an alkaline wash, thermal disinfection, and an oxidizing pro-cess using hydrogen peroxide combined with an alkaline detergent. After processing, the research-ers implanted the wires into the brains of eight hamsters. The researchers found that the spe-cially designed process was more effective than conventional alkaline cleaning, was as effective as exposure to a steam sterilization process at 273° F (134° C) for 2 hours, and left no detectable prion infectivity. The researchers also found that although the alkaline cleaning resulted in signifi-cant reduction of prion infectivity, it did not elim-inate prion infectivity in six of the eight animals in which the stainless steel wires were implanted.

13.10 **After decontamination, use one of the following three methods recommended by SHEA to steam sterilize instruments exposed to high-risk tissue:**
- **prevacuum sterilization at 273° F (134° C) for 18 minutes**[119]**;**

- **gravity displacement sterilization at 270° F (132° C) for 60 minutes**[119]**; or**
- **immersion in 1 N NaOH for 60 minutes, then removal, rinsing with water, and sterilization using one of the cycles noted above (1 N NaOH is a solution of 40 g NaOH in 1 L water).**[119]
[Recommendation]

These measures have demonstrated safety and efficacy.[119]

The SHEA guidelines state "it is unclear from the published literature which of these options is best for complete inactivation of prions because some studies have revealed excellent but not complete inactivation of the test prions with autoclaving only . . . and the same result for use of NaOH and autoclaving. . . ."[119(p111)]

A fourth option described in the SHEA guidelines is to immerse the contaminated instruments in 1 N NaOH for 60 minutes and heat them in a gravity displacement sterilizer at 250° F (121° C) for 30 min-utes, then clean and subject the instruments to rou-tine sterilization.[119] This option is effective for prion inactivation; however, it can damage many devices, especially anodized aluminum-containing devices (depending on the quality and finish of the materi-als used) and therefore is not recommended by many device manufacturers.[133]

13.10.1 **Do not use immediate use steam sterilization (IUSS) for instruments used for procedures on patients with known or suspected prion disease.**[5] *[Recommendation]*

Steam sterilization cycles for IUSS of surgical instruments are different from those recom-mended by SHEA for prion inactivation.[119] The steam sterilization cycles recommended by SHEA for instruments exposed to high-risk tis-sue are supported by prion investigational stud-ies and have been shown to inactivate prions.[119]

13.11 **Process semicritical and critical devices contami-nated with low-risk tissue from high-risk patients using processing procedures recom-mended in the device manufacturer's IFU.**[119] *[Recommendation]*

Instruments contaminated with low-risk tissue are unlikely to transmit infection after processing using conventional protocols because those instruments would not be used in the central nervous system.[119]

The SHEA guidelines make no recommendation regarding processing of devices exposed to low-risk tissue.[119] Studies to determine the risk associated with low-risk tissues are ongoing, and until evidence indi-cates that special processing protocols are required to prevent transmission of infection, SHEA makes no recommendation. Transmission of infection from low-risk tissue has only been demonstrated in animal studies of direct inoculation into the brain.[119]

13.12 **Instruments used for treatment of patients with suspected or diagnosed CJD and those whose diagnosis is unclear should be promptly identified, isolated, and processed by following the most current guidelines for prion inactivation.**[119,123,138] *[Recommendation]*

Inadequately cleaned and decontaminated instruments may pose a risk to subsequent patients who have contact with the instruments.[120,122,124,129,138-140] According to Belay et al,[138] multiple reports to the CDC of patient exposure to inadequately processed prion-contaminated surgical instruments in the United States occurred during a neurosurgical procedure for a patient whose CJD diagnosis was confirmed after the procedure.

Brown and Farrell[141] described instrument handling procedures as part of a multimodal approach to avoiding iatrogenic CJD from invasive instruments. In addition to patient diagnostic testing, the authors recommended using a regional set of dedicated instruments for all neurosurgical patients with proven or highly probable CJD and instruments that are quarantined after the procedure for any neurosurgical patient with dementia or cerebellar signs, which are the signature presentations of CJD. The authors suggest that a regional set of instruments could be shared by participating hospitals. If after surgery the patient was confirmed negative for CJD, the instruments could then be returned to general use. If the patient were postoperatively diagnosed with CJD, the instruments used would be returned to the dedicated set for CJD suspected patients.

The current SHEA Guidelines[119] describe six cases of CJD transmitted by neurosurgical instruments in Europe between 1952 through 1976, demonstrating prion survival of several years. Two of these cases occurred in 1967. These patients developed CJD 15 and 18 months after stereotactic electroencephalographic explorations using electrodes that had been implanted earlier in a patient with CJD and sterilized with 70% alcohol and formaldehyde vapor. Two years later, the electrodes were retrieved and implanted into the brain of a chimpanzee who then developed CJD.[119]

14. Records Maintenance

14.1 **Maintain records of instrument cleaning and disinfection processes.** *[Recommendation]*

Instrument cleaning and disinfection process records provide data for the identification of trends

and demonstration of compliance with regulatory requirements and accreditation agency standards.[25]

14.1.1 **The following information may be included in cleaning and decontamination records:**
- date,
- time,
- identification of instruments,
- method and verification of cleaning and results of cleaning audits,
- number or identifier of the mechanical instrument washer and results of washer efficacy testing,
- name of the person performing the cleaning and decontamination,
- lot numbers of cleaning agents,
- testing results for insulated instruments,
- applicable cleaning verification test used,
- disposition of defective equipment, and
- maintenance of cleaning equipment.

[Conditional Recommendation]

Record maintenance enables traceability in the event of a failure.[5] The use of automated instrument tracking systems can facilitate the capture of these data elements. Records of washer testing provide a source of evidence for review during investigation of clinical issues, including SSIs. Records of equipment maintenance provide evidence that equipment has been maintained.

14.1.2 **Maintain records for a time period specified by the health care organization and in compliance with local, state, and federal regulations.**[5,7] *[Recommendation]*

15. Education

15.1 **Provide education and verify competency of team members with responsibilities for cleaning and care of instruments used in surgery.** *[Recommendation]*

It is the responsibility of the health care organization to provide initial and ongoing education and to verify the competency of perioperative team members.[142] Initial and ongoing education of perioperative personnel about cleaning and care of instruments facilitates the development of knowledge, skills, and attitudes that affect safe patient care.[143]

15.1.1 **Provide education and verify competency for specific knowledge and skills related to cleaning and care of surgical instruments including the following:**
- location and understanding[19] of manufacturers' IFU for the

- o reusable surgical instrument or medical device,
- o decontamination equipment (eg, washer-disinfectors, ultrasonic cleaners),
- o cleaning chemicals and disinfectants,
- o inspection equipment, and
- o cleaning verification tools;
- organizational procedures for decontamination and cleaning verification;
- selection and safe use of cleaning chemicals and decontamination equipment;
- washer-disinfector cleaning efficacy testing procedures;
- PPE use during instrument processing;
- risks and hazards associated with instruments contaminated with biohazardous materials[27];
- risks and hazards associated with chemical exposure (ie, exposure plan)[56];
- location of and how to use emergency exposure equipment (eg, eye wash stations);
- location of and how to read SDS[56];
- risks associated with prion-contaminated instruments and procedures for their decontamination;
- measures to minimize risks of exposure to transmissible pathogens[27];
- TASS and strategies to prevent its occurrence;
- process failure response protocols;
- handling new reusable surgical instruments or medical devices and decontamination supplies; and
- handling loaned instruments and instrument sets.

[Recommendation]

Ongoing development of knowledge and skills and documentation of personnel participation is a regulatory requirement for both hospital and ambulatory settings.[142,144,145]

16. Quality

16.1 The health care organization's quality management program should evaluate the cleaning, decontamination, and care of instruments. [Recommendation]

Quality assurance and performance improvement programs can facilitate the identification of problem areas and assist personnel in evaluating and improving the quality of patient care and formulating plans for corrective actions.[146] These programs provide data that may be used to determine whether an individual organization is within benchmark goals and, if not, to identify areas that

may require corrective actions. A quality management program[146] provides a mechanism to evaluate effectiveness of processes, compliance with manufacturers' written IFU, sterile processing policies and procedures, and function of equipment.

Collecting data to monitor and improve patient care, treatment, and services is a regulatory requirement for both hospital and ambulatory settings.[144,145]

16.1.1 An interdisciplinary team (See Recommendation 1.2.1) should establish and maintain the quality management program in the health care organization. [Recommendation]

Instrument cleaning and care involves collaboration among these personnel. Interdisciplinary perspectives are especially important when establishing and implementing quality management programs for improving quality for work that is dependent on interdisciplinary team collaboration.

16.2 The quality management program should include quality objectives development and regular review of performance improvement of these areas. [Recommendation]

Identification of quality management and performance improvement objectives can focus efforts of the interdisciplinary team on the areas that are at greatest risk of process failure or the areas in greatest need for improvement. Clearly identifying these objectives facilitates the development of a performance improvement plan that can be integrated into the overall quality program for the health care organization.[146]

16.3 The quality management program must include evaluation of worker safety practices related to bloodborne pathogen safety and chemical safety annually. [Regulatory Requirement]

Organizations where employees perform duties that place them at risk for exposure to bloodborne pathogens are required to develop and maintain an exposure control plan.[27] All employers with hazardous chemicals in their workplaces are required to have labels and SDS for potentially exposed workers and to train workers to handle the chemicals safely.[56]

16.4 The quality management program should include monitoring of manual and mechanical cleaning. [Recommendation]

Cleaning is an essential component of instrument processing and can affect the efficacy of a subsequent sterilization processes. Ineffective cleaning can impede subsequent sterilization.[2,5,147,148]

16.4.1 **Test mechanical cleaners (eg, washer-disinfectors/decontaminators, ultrasonic cleaners) for correct function on installation, at least weekly (preferably daily) during routine use, after major repairs, and after significant changes in cleaning parameters (eg, changing cleaning solutions).**[5] *[Recommendation]*

Thorough cleaning is dependent on how the equipment is used, how instruments are placed in the machine, and whether the equipment is functioning correctly. Monitoring washer function provides information about whether the equipment is functioning correctly. Testing washer-disinfectors/decontaminators on a regular basis verifies that the equipment is functioning correctly or identifies an opportunity for corrective action.

16.4.2 **Evaluate manual cleaning using objective measures (eg, chemical reagent tests for detecting clinically relevant soils [eg, protein]) when new types of instruments requiring manual cleaning are processed and periodically at intervals determined by the health care facility.** *[Recommendation]*

Manual cleaning is a learned skill and is subject to human error.

16.4.3 **When verifying the effectiveness of manual cleaning, evaluate the instruments that are the most difficult to clean.** *[Recommendation]*

Evaluating the most difficult instruments to clean provides a robust measure of cleaning effectiveness.

16.5 **Preventive maintenance and repairs should be performed by qualified personnel as specified by the manufacturer's IFU for each piece of equipment used for cleaning, decontamination, and drying of surgical instruments and other medical devices.** *[Recommendation]*

Preventive maintenance requirements or recommendations are what the device manufacturer has determined are necessary to keep instruments and equipment in optimal working order.[5] Providing instruments and equipment in optimal working order is essential for patient and user safety.

16.5.1 **In consultation with the manufacturer's IFU, an interdisciplinary team (See Recommendation 1.2.1) should determine and implement the schedule for preventive maintenance of all equipment.** *[Recommendation]*

16.6 **Maintenance and service of instruments and other medical devices used in invasive proce-**dures should be performed by qualified personnel only. *[Recommendation]*

Instruments and other medical devices used in surgery are complex. Having qualified personnel service instruments and equipment increases the probability that repair and service will be performed correctly.

16.6.1 **Maintain records of instrument, equipment, and other medical device maintenance and service.** *[Recommendation]*

Records of maintenance can be used to determine compliance with the IFU and records of service can provide information useful in determining whether equipment needs to be replaced.

16.7 **Report adverse events related to surgical instruments according to the health care organization's policy and procedure and use this information for process improvement.** *[Recommendation]*

Surgical site infection has been reported as a result of inadequate cleaning of surgical instruments.[69,79,82,104,149,150] Reports of near misses can be used to identify actions that should be taken to prevent actual adverse events and can reveal opportunities for improvement.

16.7.1 **During investigation of SSIs, have infection preventionists, perioperative RNs, and designated sterile processing personnel review the cleaning process records.**

16.7.2 **Investigate near misses (ie, unplanned events that do not result in injury, such as organic or inorganic material discovered in a processed instrument tray) and take corrective action to prevent serious adverse events.**

Glossary

Adsorption: The adhesion of extremely thin layers of molecules to the solid surfaces they contact.

Aerosol: A suspension of fine solid or liquid particles in air.

Biofilm: An accumulated biomass of bacteria and extracellular material that is tightly adhered to a surface, making it difficult to remove.

Biofouling: The formation of bacterial biofilm combined with subsequent loading of dead cell debris and growth medium residues.

Borescope: A device used to inspect the inside of an instrument through a small opening or lumen of the instrument.

Cavitation: A process that uses high-frequency sound waves to form microscopic bubbles that become unstable and implode, creating tiny vacuums capable of removing debris from instrument surfaces and crevices.

Cleaning: A process that uses friction, detergent, and water to remove organic debris; the process by which any type of soil, including organic debris, is removed to the extent necessary for further processing or for the intended use. Cleaning removes rather than kills microorganisms.

Creutzfeldt-Jakob disease: A fatal degenerative neurological disease caused by a prion.

Critical water: Water that is treated to remove microorganisms, organic, and inorganic material from water (eg, treated with filtration, reverse osmosis, deionization, sterilization) and meets predetermined water quality parameters.

Decontamination: The use of physical or chemical means to remove, inactivate, or destroy bloodborne pathogens on a surface or item to render them no longer capable of transmitting infectious particles and render the surface or item safe for handling, use, or disposal.

Distilled water: Water that has been boiled, vaporized, cooled, and condensed to remove impurities.

Electroplating: A process whereby electrical current reduces dissolved metal cations that then form a coating on an electrode, causing a change in the surface properties of a device.

Endotoxin: A heat-stable toxin present in the bacterial cell wall, primarily in gram-negative organisms that are pyrogenic and increase capillary permeability.

Gross soil: Organic material (eg, blood, tissue, bone) and debris (eg, bone cement) that accumulates on surgical instruments during operative or other invasive procedures.

Homogenate: A tissue that is or has been made homogenous, as by grinding cells into a creamy consistency for laboratory studies. A homogenate usually lacks cell structure.

Hydrophobic: Absence of affinity to water.

Instrument air: A medical gas that falls under the general requirements for medical gases as defined by NFPA 99 (Health care facilities code), is not respired, is compliant with the ANSI/ISA 7.0.01 (Quality standard for instrument air), and is filtered to 0.01 microns, free of liquids and hydrocarbon vapors, and dry to a dew point of -40° C (-40° F).

Loaned items: Reusable surgical instruments and other medical devices used in health care facilities that are not owned by the facility.

Lumen: A channel or path through a tubular structure.

Product quality assurance testing: A quality assurance process used to verify that a device manufacturer's instructions for sterile processing can be achieved in the health care setting.

Reverse osmosis: A water-purifying process whereby water under pressure is passed through a semi-permeable membrane to eliminate impurities.

Toxic anterior segment syndrome: A complication of ophthalmic surgery involving a severe, noninfectious inflammation of the anterior segment of the eye, caused by various contaminants in solutions, medications, steam, and residue on surgical instruments and supplies.

Transmissible spongiform encephalopathies: Fatal prion diseases that affect the brain and nervous system. The development of tiny holes in the brain cause it to appear like a sponge, hence the term "spongiform."

Ultrasonic cleaner: A processing unit that transmits ultrasonic waves through the cleaning solution in a mechanical process known as cavitation. Ultrasonic cleaning is particularly effective in removing soil deposits from hard-to-reach areas.

Validated: A documented procedure performed by manufacturers for obtaining, recording, and interpreting the results required to establish that a process will consistently yield product that complies with predetermined specifications.

Variant Creutzfeldt-Jakob disease: A fatal degenerative neurological disease caused by a prion; the human form of bovine spongiform encephalopathy (ie, mad cow disease).

Viscoelastic: A gel injected into the anterior chamber during ophthalmic surgery to maintain the depth of the chamber, protect the corneal endothelium, and stabilize the vitreous.

Washer-disinfector/decontaminator: A processing unit that, by use of either single or multiple chambers, automatically cleans and decontaminates surgical instruments. It employs a cool water rinse, hot water wash, rinse, drying, and thermal disinfection. An ultrasonic cleaning feature and lubricant rinse may be added.

Utility water: Water from the utility tap that may require further treatment to achieve specifications; mainly used for flushing and washing.

References

1. *Reprocessing Medical Devices in Health Care Settings: Validation Methods and Labeling. Guidance for Industry and Food and Drug Administration Staff.* Rockville, MD: US Department of Health and Human Services, Food and Drug Administration, Center for Devices and Radiological Health, Center for Biologics Evaluation and Research; March 17, 2015. https://www.fda.gov/regulatory-information/search-fda-guidance-documents/reprocessing-medical-devices-health-care-settings-validation-methods-and-labeling. Accessed August 10, 2020.

2. Rutala WA, Weber DJ; Healthcare Infection Control Practices Advisory Committee (HICPAC). *Guideline for Disinfection and Sterilization in Healthcare Facilities, 2008.* Atlanta, GA: Centers for Disease Control and Prevention; 2008. https://www.cdc.gov/infectioncontrol/guidelines/disinfection/. Accessed August 10, 2020. [IVA]

3. Berrios-Torres SI, Umscheid CA, Bratzler DW, et al. Centers for Disease Control and Prevention guideline for the prevention of surgical site infection, 2017. *JAMA Surg.* 2017;152(8):784-791. [IVA]

4. Jinadatha C, Bridges A. Cleaning, disinfection, and sterilization. In: *APIC Text of Infection Control and Epidemiology.* Arlington, VA: Association for Professionals in Infection Control and

Epidemiology; 2018. http://text.apic.org/toc/basic-principles-of-infection-prevention-practice/cleaning-disinfection-and-sterilization. Accessed August 10, 2020. [IVA]

5. *ANSI/AAMI ST79: Comprehensive Guide to Steam Sterilization and Sterility Assurance in Health Care Facilities.* Arlington, VA: Association for the Advancement of Medical Instrumentation (AAMI); 2017. [IVC]

6. Reprocessing of reusable medical devices. US Food and Drug Administration. https://www.fda.gov/medical-devices/products-and-medical-procedures/reprocessing-reusable-medical-devices. Accessed August 10, 2020.

7. Guideline for sterilization. In: *Guidelines for Perioperative Practice.* Denver, CO: AORN, Inc; 2020:959-988. [IVA]

8. Guideline for high-level disinfection. In: *Guidelines for Perioperative Practice.* Denver, CO: AORN, Inc; 2020:299-326. [IVA]

9. Guideline for sterilization packaging systems. In: *Guidelines for Perioperative Practice.* Denver, CO: AORN, Inc; 2020:551-570. [IVA]

10. Guideline for processing flexible endoscopes. In: *Guidelines for Perioperative Practice.* Denver, CO: AORN, Inc; 2020:183-272. [IVA]

11. 21 CFR 860: Medical device classification procedures. https://www.ecfr.gov/cgi-bin/text-idx?SID=fee96239054dab44b0eab0045392d3b1&mc=true&tpl=/ecfrbrowse/Title21/21cfr860_main_02.tpl. Accessed August 10, 2020.

12. 21 CFR 814: Premarket approval of medical devices. https://www.ecfr.gov/cgi-bin/text-idx?SID=fee962390 54dab44b0eab0045392d3b1&mc=true&tpl=/ecfrbrowse/Title21/21cfr814_main_02.tpl. Accessed August 10, 2020.

13. 21 CFR 807.81-100. Subpart E—Premarket notification procedures. https://www.ecfr.gov/cgi-bin/text-idx?SID=c0bb7f852d0f89888f63a20b427f609a&mc=true&node=sp21.8.807.e&rgn=div6. Accessed August 10, 2020.

14. *AAMI TIR12: 2010 Designing, Testing, and Labeling Reusable Medical Devices for Reprocessing In Health Care Facilities: A Guide for Medical Device Manufacturers.* Arlington, VA: Association for the Advancement of Medical Instrumentation; 2010. [IVC]

15. *ANSI/AAMI/ISO 17664:2017: Processing of Health Care Products—Information to be Provided by the Medical Device Manufacturer for the Processing of Medical Devices.* Arlington, VA: Association for the Advancement of Medical Instrumentation; 2017. [IVC]

16. *AAMI TIR30:2011/(R)2016: A Compendium of Processes, Materials, Test Methods, and Acceptance Criteria for Cleaning Reusable Medical Devices.* Arlington, VA: Association for the Advancement of Medical Instrumentation; 2016. [IVC]

17. *ASTM E2314-03(2014): Standard Test Method for Determination of Effectiveness of Cleaning Processes for Reusable Medical Instruments Using a Microbiologic Method (Simulated Use Test).* West Conshohocken, PA: ASTM International; 2014. [IVC]

18. Guideline for medical device and product evaluation. In: *Guidelines for Perioperative Practice.* Denver, CO: AORN, Inc; 2020:705-714. [IVA]

19. *AAMI TIR55:2014/(R)2017: Human Factors Engineering for Processing Medical Devices.* Arlington, VA: Association for the Advancement of Medical Instrumentation; 2017. [IVC]

20. Moss R, Prescott DM, Spear JM. Instrument manufacturing: implications for perioperative teams. *AORN J.* 2020;112(1):15-29. [VB]

21. Guideline for design and maintenance of the surgical suite. In: *Guidelines for Perioperative Practice.* Denver, CO: AORN, Inc; 2020:51-82. [IVA]

22. Facility Guidelines Institute. *Guidelines for Design and Construction of Hospitals.* Chicago, IL: American Society for Healthcare Engineering; 2018. [IVA]

23. Facility Guidelines Institute. *Guidelines for Design and Construction of Outpatient Facilities.* Chicago, IL: American Society for Healthcare Engineering; 2018. [IVA]

24. Guideline for a safe environment of care. In: *Guidelines for Perioperative Practice.* Denver, CO: AORN, Inc; 2020:115-150. [IVA]

25. ASCs must work harder to prevent aerosol infectants: human version of mad cow disease is one risk. *Same Day Surg.* 2018;42(2):13-16. [VA]

26. 29 CFR 1910.151: Medical services and first aid. https://www.ecfr.gov/cgi-bin/text-idx?SID=388646509705aeefe60fb39193d0be16&mc=true&node=sp29.5.1910.k&rgn=div6. Accessed August 10, 2020.

27. 29 CFR 1910.1030: Bloodborne pathogens. https://www.ecfr.gov/cgi-bin/text-idx?SID=72702951fccf826f45871ad7fdb3593f&mc=true&node=se29.6.1910_11030&rgn=div8. Accessed August 10, 2020.

28. Alfa MJ, Olson N, Al-Fadhaly A. Cleaning efficacy of medical device washers in North American healthcare facilities. *J Hosp Infect.* 2010;74(2):168-177. [IIIA]

29. *ASTM D7225-13(2019)e1: Standard Guide for Blood Cleaning Efficiency of Detergents and Washer-Disinfectors.* West Conshohocken, PA: ASTM International; 2019. [IVC]

30. Rutala WA, Gergen MF, Weber DJ. Efficacy of a washer-disinfector in eliminating healthcare-associated pathogens from surgical instruments. *Infect Control Hosp Epidemiol.* 2014;35(7):883-885. [IIA]

31. Uetera Y, Kishii K, Yasuhara H, et al. A 5 year longitudinal study of water quality for final rinsing in the single chamber washer-disinfector with a reverse osmosis plant. *PDA J Pharm Sci Technol.* 2013;67(4):399-411. [IIIA]

32. *AAMI TIR34: 2014/(R)2017: Technical Information Report: Water for the Reprocessing of Medical Devices.* Arlington, VA: Association for the Advancement of Medical Instrumentation; 2017. [IVC]

33. American Society of Heating, Refrigerating and Air-Conditioning Engineers. Infection control. In: *HVAC Design Manual for Hospitals and Clinics.* Atlanta, GA: American Society of Heating, Refrigerating and Air-Conditioning Engineers, Inc (ASHRAE); 2013:19–34. [IVC]

34. Piil JF, Lundbye-Jensen J, Trangmar SJ, Nybo L. Performance in complex motor tasks deteriorates in hyperthermic humans. *Temperature (Austin).* 2017;4(4):420-428. [IIIB]

35. *ASHRAE 188-2018: Legionellosis: Risk Management for Building Water Systems.* Atlanta, GA: ASHRAE; 2018. [IVA]

36. *Requirement to Reduce Legionella Risk in Healthcare Facility Water Systems to Prevent Cases and Outbreaks of Legionnaires' Disease.* Washington, DC: Department of Health and Human

Services; 2017. https://www.cms.gov/Medicare/Provider-Enrollment-and-Certification/SurveyCertificationGenInfo/Policy-and-Memos-to-States-and-Regions-Items/Survey-And-Cert-Letter-17-30-. Accessed August 10, 2020.

37. Perkins KM, Reddy SC, Fagan R, Arduino MJ, Perz JF. Investigation of healthcare infection risks from water-related organisms: summary of CDC consultations, 2014–2017. *Infect Control Hosp Epidemiol.* 2019;40(6):621-626. [IVA]

38. Hsu MS, Wu MY, Huang YT, Liao CH. Efficacy of chlorine dioxide disinfection to non-fermentative gram-negative bacilli and non-tuberculous mycobacteria in a hospital water system. *J Hosp Infect.* 2016;93(1):22-28. [IVB]

39. Walker J, Moore G. Safe water in healthcare premises. *J Hosp Infect.* 2016;94(1):1. [VA]

40. *Developing a Water Management Program to Reduce Legionella Growth and Spread in Buildings: A Practical Guide to Implementing Industry Standards.* Version 1.1. Washington, DC: US Department of Health and Human Services, Centers for Disease Control and Prevention; 2017. [VA]

41. Marek A, Smith A, Peat M, et al. Endoscopy supply water and final rinse testing: five years of experience. *J Hosp Infect.* 2014;88(4):207-212. [VA]

42. Borella P, Bargellini A, Marchegiano P, Vecchi E, Marchesi I. Hospital-acquired *Legionella* infections: an update on the procedures for controlling environmental contamination. *Ann Ig.* 2016;28(2):98-108. [VA]

43. Casini B, Buzzigoli A, Cristina ML, et al. Long-term effects of hospital water network disinfection on *Legionella* and other waterborne bacteria in an Italian university hospital. *Infect Control Hosp Epidemiol.* 2014;35(3):293-299. [IIIA]

44. D'Alessandro D, Fabiani M, Cerquetani F, Orsi GB. Trend of *Legionella* colonization in hospital water supply. *Ann Ig.* 2015;27(2):460-466. [IIB]

45. Demirjian A, Lucas CE, Garrison LE, et al. The importance of clinical surveillance in detecting legionnaires' disease outbreaks: a large outbreak in a hospital with a *Legionella* disinfection system–Pennsylvania, 2011-2012. *Clin Infect Dis.* 2015;60(11):1596-1602. [IIIB]

46. Marinelli L, Cottarelli A, Solimini AG, Del Cimmuto A, De Giusti M. Evaluation of timing of re-appearance of VBNC *Legionella* for risk assessment in hospital water distribution systems. *Ann Ig.* 2017;29(5):431-439. [IIIB]

47. Moore G, Stevenson D, Thompson K, et al. Biofilm formation in an experimental water distribution system: the contamination of non-touch sensor taps and the implication for healthcare. *Biofouling.* 2015;31(9-10):677-687. [IIA]

48. Bhalchandra R, Chandy M, Ramanan VR, et al. Role of water quality assessments in hospital infection control: experience from a new oncology center in eastern India. *Indian J Pathol Microbiol.* 2014;57(3):435-438. [VA]

49. *Decontamination and Reprocessing of Medical Devices for Health-care Facilities.* Geneva, Switzerland: World Health Organization and the Pan American Health Organization; 2016. [IVB]

50. Stiefel P, Mauerhofer S, Schneider J, Maniura-Weber K, Rosenberg U, Ren Q. Enzymes enhance biofilm removal efficiency of cleaners. *Antimicrob Agents Chemother.* 2016;60(6):3647-3652. [IIIA]

51. Juturu V, Wu JC. Microbial cellulases: engineering, production and applications. *Renew Sust Energ Rev.* 2014;33:188-203. [VA]

52. *Medical Washers and Medical Washer-Disinfectors—Class II Special Controls Guidance for the Medical Device Industry and FDA Review Staff.* Rockville, MD: US Department of Health and Human Services, Food and Drug Administration, Center for Devices and Radiological Health; 2002. https://www.fda.gov/medical-devices/guidance-documents-medical-devices-and-radiation-emitting-products/medical-washers-and-medical-washer-disinfectors-class-ii-special-controls-guidance-document-medical. Accessed August 11, 2020.

53. Crawford M. How clean is clean? Chemistry can damage medical equipment in the quest to meet stringent guidelines. *Biomed Instrum Technol.* 2014;48(4):260-263. [VB]

54. *Final Guidance on Environmentally Preferable Purchasing. 1999.* US Environmental Protection Agency. https://www.epa.gov/sites/production/files/2015-09/documents/finalepp guidance.pdf. Accessed August 11, 2020.

55. *EPA's Safer Choice Standard.* US Environmental Protection Agency. https://www.epa.gov/sites/production/files/2013-12/documents/standard-for-safer-products.pdf. Revised February 2015. Accessed August 11, 2020.

56. 29 CFR 1910.1200: Toxic and hazardous substances. https://www.osha.gov/laws-regs/regulations/standardnumber/1910/1910.1200. Accessed August 10, 2020. [VB]

57. Basile RJ, Kovach S, Drosnock MA. Guidelines for selecting a cleaning brush. *Biomed Instrum Technol.* 2019;53(s2):49-54. [VB]

58. Rutala WA, Weber DJ. Disinfection and sterilization: an overview. *Am J Infect Control.* 2013;41(5 Suppl):S2-S5. [VA]

59. *ANSI/AAMI ST58:2013/(R)2018: Chemical Sterilization and High-Level Disinfection in Health Care Facilities.* Arlington, VA: Association for the Advancement of Medical Instrumentation; 2018. [IVC]

60. *ANSI/AAMI ST91:2015: Flexible and Semi-Rigid Endoscope Processing in Healthcare Facilities.* Arlington, VA: Association for the Advancement of Medical Instrumentation; 2015. [IVC]

61. *ANSI/AAMI ST41:2008/(R)2018: Ethylene Oxide Sterilization in Health Care Facilities: Safety and Effectiveness.* Arlington, VA: Association for the Advancement of Medical Instrumentation; 2018. [IVC]

62. Class 2 device recall BIOMET Orthopedics. US Food & Drug Administration. https://www.accessdata.fda.gov/scripts/cdrh/cfdocs/cfRes/res.cfm?ID=180539. February 26, 2020. Accessed August 11, 2020.

63. Seavey R. High-level disinfection, sterilization, and antisepsis: current issues in reprocessing medical and surgical instruments. *Am J Infect Control.* 2013;41(5 Suppl):S111-S117. [VA]

64. Veiga-Malta I. Preventing healthcare-associated infections by monitoring the cleanliness of medical devices and other critical points in a sterilization service. *Biomed Instrum Technol.* 2016;50(Suppl 3):45-52. [IIIC]

65. Costa DM, Lopes LKO, Vickery K, et al. Reprocessing safety issues associated with complex-design orthopaedic loaned

surgical instruments and implants. *Injury.* 2018;49(11):2005-2012. [IIB]

66. *AST Standards of Practice for the Decontamination of Surgical Instruments.* Littleton, CO: Association of Surgical Technologists; 2009. https://www.ast.org/uploadedFiles/Main_Site/Content/About_Us/Standard_Decontamination_%20Surgical_Instruments_.pdf. Accessed August 10, 2020. [IVC]

67. Almatroudi A, Tahir S, Hu H, et al. *Staphylococcus aureus* dry-surface biofilms are more resistant to heat treatment than traditional hydrated biofilms. *J Hosp Infect.* 2018;98(2):161-167. [IIA]

68. Araújo PA, Mergulhão F, Melo L, Simões M. The ability of an antimicrobial agent to penetrate a biofilm is not correlated with its killing or removal efficiency. *Biofouling.* 2014;30(6):675-683. [IIIB]

69. Sheitoyan-Pesant C, Alarie I, Iorio-Morin C, Mathieu D, Carignan A. An outbreak of surgical site infections following craniotomy procedures associated with a change in the ultrasonic surgical aspirator decontamination process. *Am J Infect Control.* 2017;45(4):433-435. [VB]

70. Bezek K, Nipič D, Torkar KG, et al. Biofouling of stainless steel surfaces by four common pathogens: the effects of glucose concentration, temperature and surface roughness. *Biofouling.* 2019;35(3):273-283. [IIA]

71. Lindgren KE, Pelt CE, Anderson MB, Peters CL, Spivak ES, Gililland JM. A chlorhexidine solution reduces aerobic organism growth in operative splash basins in a randomized controlled trial. *J Arthroplasty.* 2018;33(1):211-215. [IB]

72. Lucas AD, Nagaraja S, Gordon EA, Hitchins VM. Evaluating device design and cleanability of orthopedic device models contaminated with a clinically relevant bone test soil. *Biomed Instrum Technol.* 2015;49(5):354-362. [IIIC]

73. Guideline for sharps safety. In: *Guidelines for Perioperative Practice.* Denver, CO: AORN, Inc; 2020:859-882. [IVA]

74. Guideline for transmission-based precautions. In: *Guidelines for Perioperative Practice.* Denver, CO: AORN, Inc; 2020:1071-1098. [IVA]

75. Almatroudi A, Hu H, Deva A, et al. A new dry-surface biofilm model: an essential tool for efficacy testing of hospital surface decontamination procedures. *J Microbiol Methods.* 2015;117:171-176. [IIA]

76. Guideline for sterile technique. In: *Guidelines for Perioperative Practice.* Denver, CO: AORN, Inc; 2020:917-958. [IVA]

77. *ASTM F1744-96(2016): Standard Guide for Care and Handling of Stainless Steel Surgical Instruments.* West Conshohocken, PA: ASTM International; 2016. [IVB]

78. Spruce L. Back to basics: instrument cleaning. *AORN J.* 2017;105(3):292-299. [VA]

79. Baruque Villar G, de Mello Freitas FT, Pais Ramos J, et al. Risk factors for *Mycobacterium abscessus* subsp. *bolletii* infection after laparoscopic surgery during an outbreak in Brazil. *Infect Control Hosp Epidemiol.* 2015;36(1):81-86. [IIIC]

80. Weber DJ, Rutala WA. Assessing the risk of disease transmission to patients when there is a failure to follow recommended disinfection and sterilization guidelines. *Am J Infect Control.* 2013;41(5 Suppl):S67-S71. [VA]

81. Roth V, Espino-Grosso P, Henriksen C, Canales B. Cost and UTI rate following office cystoscopy before and after implementing new standardized handling and storage practices. *J Urol.* 2019;201(Suppl 4):e1137. [VA]

82. Bilavsky E, Pfeffer I, Tarabeia J, et al. Outbreak of multidrug-resistant Pseudomonas aeruginosa infection following urodynamic studies traced to contaminated transducer. *J Hosp Infect.* 2013;83(4):344-346. [VA]

83. Scorzolini L, Mengoni F, Mastroianni CM, et al. Pseudo-outbreak of *Mycobacterium gordonae* in a teaching hospital: importance of strictly following decontamination procedures and emerging issues concerning sterilization. *New Microbiol.* 2016;39(1):25-34. [VA]

84. Dupont C, Terru D, Aguilhon S, et al. Source-case investigation of *Mycobacterium wolinskyi* cardiac surgical site infection. *J Hosp Infect.* 2016;93(3):235-239. [VA]

85. Kumarage J, Khonyongwa K, Khan A, Desai N, Hoffman P, Taori SK. Transmission of multi-drug resistant Pseudomonas aeruginosa between two flexible ureteroscopes and an outbreak of urinary tract infection: the fragility of endoscope decontamination. *J Hosp Infect.* 2019;102(1):89-94. [VA]

86. Guideline for environmental cleaning. In: *Guidelines for Perioperative Practice.* Denver, CO: AORN, Inc; 2020:151-182. [IVA]

87. Stjärne Aspelund A, Sjöström K, Olsson Liljequist B, Mörgelin M, Melander E, Påhlman LI. Acetic acid as a decontamination method for sink drains in a nosocomial outbreak of metallo-β-lactamase-producing *Pseudomonas aeruginosa*. *J Hosp Infect.* 2016;94(1):13-20. [VA]

88. Smolders D, Hendriks B, Rogiers P, Mul M, Gordts B. Acetic acid as a decontamination method for ICU sink drains colonized by carbapenemase-producing *Enterobacteriaceae* and its effect on CPE infections. *J Hosp Infect.* 2019;102(1):82-88. [IIIA]

89. Alfa MJ, Olson N. Comparison of washer-disinfector cleaning indicators: impact of temperature and cleaning cycle parameters. *Am J Infect Control.* 2014;42(2):e23-e26. [IIA]

90. Czyrko C. Effective infection control procedures: ultrasonic cleaners. *Dent Nurs.* 2015;11(8):469-471. [VC]

91. Di Blasio A, Barenghi L. Pitfalls of cleaning controls in ultrasonic washers. *Am J Infect Control.* 2015;43(12):1374-1375. [VA]

92. Kean R, Johnson R, Doyle M. Code grey: stained surgical instruments and their impact on one Canadian health authority. *Healthc Q.* 2017;20(3):65-68. [VA]

93. Moi LL, Joo TL, Meh MG. Cleaning verification in medical device reprocessing: is this required? *Can J Infect Control.* 2015;30(4):237-238. [IIIB]

94. Huang Y, Chen Y, Chen M, et al. Comparing visual inspection, aerobic colony counts, and adenosine triphosphate bioluminescence assay for evaluating surface cleanliness at a medical center. *Am J Infect Control.* 2015;43(8):882-886. [IIIB]

95. Schmitt C, Pires Maciel AL, Boszczowski I, et al. Evaluation of adenosine triphosphate test for cleaning assessment of gastroscopes and the effect on workload in a busy endoscopy center. *Am J Infect Control.* 2018;46(10):1110-1114. [IIIA]

96. Alfa MJ. Monitoring and improving the effectiveness of cleaning medical and surgical devices. *Am J Infect Control.* 2013;41(5 Suppl):S56-S59. [VA]

97. Saito Y, Yasuhara H, Murakoshi S, Komatsu T, Fukatsu K, Uetera Y. Novel concept of cleanliness of instruments for robotic surgery. *J Hosp Infect.* 2016;93(4):360-361. [VA]

98. Gillespie E, Othman N, Irwin L. Using ultraviolet visible markers in sterilizing departments. *Am J Infect Control.* 2014;42(12):1343. [VB]

99. Saito Y, Yasuhara H, Murakoshi S, Komatsu T, Fukatsu K, Uetera Y. Challenging residual contamination of instruments for robotic surgery in Japan. *Infect Control Hosp Epidemiol.* 2017;38(2):143-146. [IIIB]

100. Kurley B. ATP testing: an anecdotal look at its use in an office-based plastic surgery setting. *Plast Surg Nurs.* 2014;34(4):167-170. [VA]

101. *Important Information for Infection Preventionists Regarding Media Attention on an Outbreak Involving Reusable Surgical Instruments.* Washington, DC: Association for Professionals in Infection Control and Epidemiology (APIC); 2012. [VA]

102. Tosh PK, Disbot M, Duffy JM et al. Outbreak of *Pseudomonas aeruginosa* surgical site infections after arthroscopic procedures: Texas, 2009. *Infect Control Hosp Epidemiol.* 2011;32(12):1179-1186. [IIIA]

103. Guideline for electrosurgical safety. In: *Guidelines for Perioperative Practice.* Denver, CO: AORN, Inc; 2020. [IVA]

104. Chang DF, Mamalis N; Ophthalmic Instrument Cleaning and Sterilization Task Force. Guidelines for the cleaning and sterilization of intraocular surgical instruments. *J Cataract Refract Surg.* 2018;44(6):765-773. [IVB]

105. Mamalis N. Toxic anterior segment syndrome: role of enzymatic detergents used in the cleaning of intraocular surgical instruments. *J Cataract Refract Surg.* 2016;42(9):1249-1250. [VA]

106. Shorstein NH, Lucido C, Carolan J, Liu L, Slean G, Herrinton LJ. Failure modes and effects analysis of bilateral same-day cataract surgery. *J Cataract Refractive Surg.* 2017;43(3):318-323. [VA]

107. Mamalis N, Edelhauser HF. Enzymatic detergents and toxic anterior segment syndrome. *Ophthalmology.* 2013;120(3):651-652. [VA]

108. Tamashiro NSM, Souza RQ, Gonçalves CR, et al. Cytotoxicity of cannulas for ophthalmic surgery after cleaning and sterilization: evaluation of the use of enzymatic detergent to remove residual ophthalmic viscosurgical device material. *J Cataract Refract Surg.* 2013;39(6):937-941. [IIIC]

109. Valdez-García JE, Climent A, Chávez-Mondragón E, Lozano-Ramírez JF. Anterior chamber bacterial contamination in cataract surgery. *BMC Ophthalmol.* 2014;14:57. doi:10.1186/1471-2415-14-57. [IIIA]

110. Junk AK, Chen PP, Lin SC, et al. Disinfection of tonometers: a report by the American Academy of Ophthalmology. *Ophthalmology.* 2017;124(12):1867-1875. [IIIB]

111. Tsaousis KT, Werner L, Reiter N, et al. Comparison of different types of phacoemulsification tips. II. Morphologic alterations induced by multiple steam sterilization cycles with and without use of enzyme detergents. *J Cataract Refract Surg.* 2016;42(9):1353-1360. [IIB]

112. Choi JH, Cho YS, Lee JW, Shin HB, Lee IK. Bacterial contamination and disinfection status of laryngoscopes stored in emergency crash carts. *J Prev Med Pub Health.* 2017;50(3):158-164. [IIIA]

113. Negri de Sousa AC, Levy CE, Freitas MIP. Laryngoscope blades and handles as sources of cross-infection: an integrative review. *J Hosp Infect.* 2013;83(4):269-275. [VA]

114. Howell V, Thoppil A, Young H, Sharma S, Blunt M, Young P. Chlorhexidine to maintain cleanliness of laryngoscope handles: an audit and laboratory study. *Eur J Anaesthesiol.* 2013;30(5):216-221. [IIIA]

115. Sherman J, Raibley LA 4th, Eckelman MJ. Life cycle assessment and costing methods for device procurement: comparing reusable and single-use disposable laryngoscopes. *Anesth Analg.* 2018;127(2):434-443. [IIIA]

116. Van Wicklin SA. Contamination and disinfection of rigid laryngoscopes: a literature review. *AORN J.* 2019;110(1):49-59. [VA]

117. *Guidelines: Infection Prevention and Control 2020.* London, UK: Association of Anaesthetists of Great Britain and Ireland; 2020. [IVA]

118. Nielsen SW, Stevens JR, Stevens GJ, Patel J, Eller RL. Mandated wrapping of airway cart instruments: limited access without the intended safety benefits. *Laryngoscope.* 2019;129(3):715-719. [IIIA]

119. Rutala WA, Weber DJ; Society for Healthcare Epidemiology of America. Guideline for disinfection and sterilization of prion-contaminated medical instruments. *Infect Control Hosp Epidemiol.* 2010;31(2):107-117. [IVA]

120. Infection control: iatrogenic transmission of CJD. Centers for Disease Control and Prevention. https://www.cdc.gov/prions/cjd/infection-control.html. Accessed August 11, 2020. [VA]

121. *WHO Infection Control Guidelines for Transmissible Spongiform Encephalopathies: Report of a WHO Consultation, Geneva, Switzerland, 23-26 March 1999.* World Health Organization. https://www.who.int/csr/resources/publications/bse/WHO_CDS_CSR_APH_2000_3/en/. Accessed August 11, 2020. [IVA]

122. *WHO Tables on Tissue Infectivity Distribution in Transmissible Spongiform Encephalopathies.* Geneva, Switzerland: WHO Press; 2010. https://www.who.int/bloodproducts/tablestissueinfectivity.pdf?ua=1s. Accessed August 11, 2020. [IVA]

123. Thomas JG, Chenoweth CE, Sullivan SE. Iatrogenic Creutzfeldt-Jakob disease via surgical instruments. *J Clin Neurosci.* 2013;20(9):1207-1212. [VA]

124. *Patient Safety and Reduction of Risk of Transmission of Creutzfeldt-Jakob Disease (CJD) via Interventional Procedures.* London, UK: National Institute for Health and Care Excellence; 2006. [IVA]

125. Fichet G, Antloga K, Comoy E, Deslys JP, McDonnell G. Prion inactivation using a new gaseous hydrogen peroxide sterilisation process. *J Hosp Infect.* 2007;67(3):278-286. [IIB]

126. Yan ZX, Stitz L, Heeg P, Pfaff E, Roth K. Infectivity of prion protein bound to stainless steel wires: a model for testing decontamination procedures for transmissible spongiform encephalopathies. *Infect Control Hosp Epidemiol.* 2004;25(4):280-283. [IIB]

127. Rogez-Kreuz C, Yousfi R, Soufflet C, et al. Inactivation of animal and human prions by hydrogen peroxide gas plasma sterilization. *Infect Control Hosp Epidemiol.* 2009;30(8):769-777. [IIB]

128. Secker TJ, Hervé R, Keevil CW. Adsorption of prion and tissue proteins to surgical stainless steel surfaces and the efficacy of decontamination following dry and wet storage conditions. *J Hosp Infect.* 2011;78(4):251-255. [IIIA]

129. Smith A, Winter S, Lappin D, et al. Reducing the risk of iatrogenic Creutzfeldt-Jakob disease by improving the cleaning of neurosurgical instruments. *J Hosp Infect.* 2018;100(3):e70-e76. [IIIA]

130. Record of decision by principal deputy AA/OPPTS regarding status of prions under FIFRA. US Environmental Protection Agency. https://www.epa.gov/sites/production/files/2015-09/documents/records_of_decision_on_prions.pdf. April 29, 2004. Accessed August 11, 2020.

131. *Product Performance Test Guidelines. OCSPP 810.2700: Products with Prion-Related Claims.* US National Service Center for Environmental Publications (NSCEP). Environmental Protection Agency. https://nepis.epa.gov/Exe/ZyPDF.cgi/P100IJB7.PDF?Dockey=P100IJB7.PDF. December 2012. Accessed August 11, 2020.

132. Search for registered pesticide products. US Environmental Protection Agency. https://www.epa.gov/safepestcontrol/search-registered-pesticide-products. Updated June 19, 2017. Accessed August 11, 2020.

133. McDonnell G, Dehen C, Perrin A, et al. Cleaning, disinfection and sterilization of surface prion contamination. *J Hosp Infect.* 2013;85(4):268-273. [IIIA]

134. Fichet G, Comoy E, Duval C, et al. Novel methods for disinfection of prion-contaminated Imedical devices. *Lancet.* 2004;364(9433):521-526. [IIB]

135. Belondrade M, Nicot S, Beringue V, Coste J, Lehmann S, Bougard D. Rapid and highly sensitive detection of variant Creutzfeldt-Jakob disease abnormal prion protein on steel surfaces by protein misfolding cyclic amplification: application to prion decontamination studies. *PLoS One.* 2016;11(1):e0146833. doi:10.1371/journal.pone.0146833. [IIIA]

136. Botsios S, Tittman S, Manuelidis L. Rapid chemical decontamination of infectious CJD and scrapie particles parallels treatments known to disrupt microbes and biofilms. *Virulence.* 2015;6(8):787-801. [IIA]

137. Schmitt A, Westner IM, Reznicek L, Michels W, Mitteregger G, Kretzschmar HA. Automated decontamination of surface-adherent prions. *J Hosp Infect.* 2010;76(1):74-79. [IA]

138. Belay ED, Blase J, Sehulster LM, Maddox RA, Schonberger LB. Management of neurosurgical instruments and patients exposed to Creutzfeldt-Jakob disease. *Infect Control Hosp Epidemiol.* 2013;34(12):1272-1280. [IIIA]

139. López FJG, Ruiz-Tovar M, Almazán-Isla J, Alcalde-Cabero E, Calero M, de Pedro-Cuesta J. Risk of transmission of sporadic Creutzfeldt-Jakob disease by surgical procedures: systematic reviews and quality of evidence. *Euro Surveill.* 2017;22(43). doi:10.2807/1560-7917.ES.2017.22.43.16-00806. [IIIA]

140. Smyth EG, Farrell M, Healy DG, et al. Managing the consequences of neurosurgical intervention in a patient with previously undiagnosed Creutzfeldt-Jakob disease. *Infect Control Hosp Epidemiol.* 2014;35(7):907-908. [VA]

141. Brown P, Farrell M. A practical approach to avoiding iatrogenic Creutzfeldt-Jakob disease (CJD) from invasive instruments. *Infect Control Hosp Epidemiol.* 2015;36(7):844-848. [VA]

142. Standards of perioperative nursing practice. AORN, Inc. https://www.aorn.org/guidelines/clinical-resources/aorn-standards. Revised 2009. Accessed August 10, 2020. [IVB]

143. Duro M. Improving device reprocessing through education and audits. *AORN J.* 2016;103(1):P13-P14. [VA]

144. *State Operations Manual Appendix A: Survey Protocol, Regulations and Interpretive Guidelines for Hospitals.* Rev. 200, 02-21-20. Centers for Medicare & Medicaid Services. https://www.cms.gov/Regulations-and-Guidance/Guidance/Manuals/downloads/som107ap_a_hospitals.pdf. Accessed August 11, 2020.

145. *State Operations Manual Appendix L: Guidance for Surveyors: Ambulatory Surgical Centers.* Rev. 200, 02-21-20. Centers for Medicare & Medicaid Services. https://www.cms.gov/Regulations-and-Guidance/Guidance/Manuals/downloads/som107ap_l_ambulatory.pdf. Accessed August 11, 2020.

146. *ANSI/AAMI ST90:2017: Processing of Health Care Products: Quality Management Systems for Processing in Health Care Facilities.* Arlington, VA: Association for the Advancement of Medical Instrumentation; 2017. [IVC]

147. Smith K, Araoye I, Gilbert S, et al. Is retained bone debris in cannulated orthopedic instruments sterile after autoclaving? *Am J Infect Control.* 2018;46(9):1009-1013. [IIB]

148. Davis J. Retained bioburden on surgical instruments after reprocessing: are we just scraping the surface? *Pennsylvania Patient Safety Advisory.* 2017;14(2):71-75. [VA]

149. Boyle MA, O'Donnell MJ, Russell RJ, Galvin N, Swan J, Coleman DC. Overcoming the problem of residual microbial contamination in dental suction units left by conventional disinfection using novel single component suction handpieces in combination with automated flood disinfection. *J Dent.* 2015;43(10):1268-1279. [IIIC]

150. Southworth PM. Infections and exposures: reported incidents associated with unsuccessful decontamination of reusable surgical instruments. *J Hosp Infect.* 2014;88(3):127-131. [VA]

Guideline Development Group and Acknowledgements

Lead Author: Erin Kyle[1], DNP, RN, CNOR, NEA-BC, Editor-in-Chief, Guidelines for Perioperative Practice, AORN, Denver, Colorado

Methodologist: Amber Wood[2], MSN, RN, CNOR, CIC, FAPIC, Senior Perioperative Practice Specialist, AORN, Denver, Colorado

Evidence Appraiser: Erin Kyle[1]; Marie Bashaw[3], DNP, RN, NEA-BC, Professor and Director of Nursing, Wittenberg University, Springfield, Ohio

Guidelines Advisory Board Members:

- Susan Lynch[4], PhD, RN, CSSM, CNOR, Associate Director, Surgical Services, Penn Medicine-Chester County Hospital, West Chester, Pennsylvania

- Donna A. Pritchard[5], MA, BSN, RN, NE-BC, CNOR, Director of Perioperative Services, Interfaith Medical Center, Brooklyn, New York
- Bernard C. Camins[6], MD, MSc, Medical Director, Infection Prevention, Mount Sinai Health System, New York, New York
- Jennifer Hanrahan[7], DO, Medical Director of Infection Prevention, Metrohealth Medical Center, Cleveland, Ohio
- Elizabeth (Lizz) Pincus[8], MSN, RN, CNS-CP, CNOR, Clinical Nurse, Regional Medical Center of San Jose, San Jose, California
- David Wyatt[9], PhD, MA, MPH, BSN, RN, NEA-BC, CNOR, Chief Nursing Officer, University Hospitals at the University of Texas Southwestern Medical Center, Dallas.

Guidelines Advisory Board Liaisons:
- Cassie Dietrich[10], MD, Anesthesiologist, Anesthesia Associates of Kansas City, Overland Park, Kansas
- Susan G. Klacik[11], BS, CRCST, FCS, Clinical Educator, International Association of Healthcare Central Service Materiel Management (IAHCSMM), Chicago, Illinois
- Susan Ruwe[12], MSN, RN, CPHQ, CIC, Senior Infection Preventionist, Carle Foundation Hospital, Argenta, Illinois

External Review: Expert review comments were received from individual members of the American Association of Nurse Anesthetists (AANA), American College of Surgeons (ACS), Association for Professionals in Infection Control and Epidemiology (APIC), American Society of Anesthesiologists (ASA), International Association of Healthcare Central Service Materiel Management (IAHCSMM), the Society for Healthcare Epidemiology of America (SHEA), and the Surgical Infection Society (SIS). Their responses were used to further refine and enhance this guideline; however, their responses do not imply endorsement. The draft was also open for a 30-day public comment period.

Financial Disclosure and Conflicts of Interest

This guideline was developed, edited, and approved by the AORN Guidelines Advisory Board without external funding being sought or obtained. The Guidelines Advisory Board was financially supported entirely by AORN and was developed without any involvement of industry.

Potential conflicts of interest for all Guidelines Advisory Board members were reviewed before the annual meeting and each monthly conference call. None of the members of the Guideline Development Group reported a potential conflict of interest.[1-9] If any conflicts of interest had emerged during the development of this guideline, the advisory board concluded that individuals with potential conflicts could remain on the advisory board if they reminded the advisory board of potential conflicts before any related discussion and recused themselves from a related discussion if requested.

Publication History

Originally published February 1988, *AORN Journal*. Revised March 1992.

Revised November 1996; published January 1997, *AORN Journal*.

Reformatted July 2000.

Revised November 2001; published March 2002, *AORN Journal*.

Revised 2007; published in *Perioperative Standards and Recommended Practices*, 2008 edition.

Minor editing revisions made to omit PNDS codes; reformatted September 2012 for publication in *Perioperative Standards and Recommended Practices*, 2013 edition.

Revised September 2014 for online publication in *Perioperative Standards and Recommended Practices*.

Minor editing revisions made in November 2014 for publication in *Guidelines for Perioperative Practice*, 2015 edition.

Evidence ratings revised in *Guidelines for Perioperative Practice*, 2018 edition, to conform to the current AORN Evidence Rating Model.

Evidence ratings revised and minor editorial changes made to conform to the current AORN Evidence Rating model, September 2019, for online publication in *Guidelines for Perioperative Practice*.

Revised October 2020 for online publication in *Guidelines for Perioperative Practice*.

Scheduled for review in 2024.

LASER SAFETY

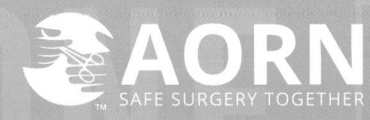

TABLE OF CONTENTS

MEDICAL ABBREVIATIONS & ACRONYMS

ANSI – American National Standards Institute
CO2 – Carbon dioxide
DLSO – Deputy laser safety officer
ET – Endotrachael
FDA – US Food and Drug Administration
IFU – Instructions for use
KTP – Potassium titanyl phosphate
LSO – Laser safety officer

LSSC – Laser safety site contact
MAUDE – Manufacturer and User Device Experience
Nd – Neodymium
O2 – Oxygen
OSHA – Occupational Safety and Health Administration
PPE – Personal protective equipment
PVC – Polyvinyl chloride
YAG – Yttrium aluminum garnet

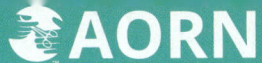

GUIDELINE FOR
LASER SAFETY

The Guideline for Laser Safety was approved by the AORN Guidelines Advisory Board and became effective as of July 29, 2020. The recommendations in the guideline are intended to be achievable and represent what is believed to be an optimal level of practice. Policies and procedures will reflect variations in practice settings and/or clinical situations that determine the degree to which the guideline can be implemented. AORN recognizes the many diverse settings in which perioperative nurses practice; therefore, this guideline is adaptable to all areas where operative or other invasive procedures may be performed.

Purpose

This document provides guidance to the perioperative team on the safe use of **lasers**, the roles and responsibilities of personnel, and the educational requirements for personnel involved with use of a **laser system** for medical procedures.

The laser system consists of the laser, a delivery system that directs the output of the laser, a power supply with control and calibration functions, the mechanical housing, and the medium.[1] The light produced by a laser is a portion of the electromagnetic spectrum and may be infrared, visible, or ultraviolet. The type of light produced depends on the type of diode[2] or the material or medium inside the laser (eg, solid, liquid, gas).[3,4] The solid medium may be yttrium aluminum garnet (YAG) with neodymium (Nd), or it may be **doped** with holmium. The liquid medium is usually a dye, and the gas may be carbon dioxide (CO_2) or excimer.[4] The medium that is present is frequently used as a descriptor of the laser system (eg, Nd:YAG, CO_2).

The word "laser" is an acronym for light amplification by stimulated emission of radiation. Lasers are classified as 1, 1C, 1M, 2, 2M, 3R, 3B, or 4, which is based on the accessible laser radiation.[5,6] The majority of the lasers used in health care facilities are class 3R, 3B, and 4[1]:

- Class 3R laser systems present a low risk for injury, although the eye may be injured if it is focused and stable and the beam enters the eye directly or via **specular reflection**.[1] The **diffuse reflection** is usually not a hazard. Class 3R lasers are not hazardous to the skin and do not normally present a fire hazard.[1]
- Class 3B laser systems may be hazardous when the beam enters the eye directly or via specular reflection, but they do not normally cause a diffuse reflection or act as an ignition source.[1] The diffuse reflection is usually not a hazard. Class 3B lasers are not hazardous to the skin and do not normally present a fire hazard.[1]

- Class 4 laser systems are hazardous to the skin and to the eye when the beam enters the eye directly. They may be hazardous when the beam enters the eye via a diffuse reflection. Class 4 lasers also can present a fire hazard and may produce laser-generated air contaminants and hazardous plasma radiation.[1]

Lasers are used in a wide variety of settings (eg, offices, clinics, ambulatory surgery centers, hospitals) and procedures, including gynecologic, orthopedic, dermatologic, ophthalmologic, urologic, neurosurgical, cardiovascular, otolaryngologic, and cosmetic procedures.[1,7-13]

When the laser is activated, the beam can be reflected, scattered, transmitted, or absorbed. Reflection can be either diffuse or specular. The scattered beam may be absorbed or it may be **backscattered**. Absorption results in thermal damage to the tissue. The amount of thermal damage depends on the laser wavelength, beam fluence, radiance, chromophore consistency, water content of the tissue, the length of time of the application, and the temperature to which the tissue is heated.[5,12] The effects of the laser on the target tissue may be either a **photothermal interaction**, a **photochemical interaction**, or a **photomechanical/ photoacoustic interaction**.[1,5,14]

The patient may experience various adverse effects or complications from laser treatment, depending on the area being treated. Adverse effects or complications include pain, edema, bleeding, purpura, infection, air embolism, hemorrhage, surgical emphysema, cellular damage around the area of laser impingement, skin pigmentation, scarring, reticulate erythema, ocular complications, and burns.[7,10,15-20] In a review of the Manufacturer and User Facility Device Experience (MAUDE) database, Zelickson et al[21] found 494 adverse events caused by the use of various lasers in dermatological settings between 2007 and 2011. The reported injuries to patients included blistering, burns, scarring, pigmentation damage, and infection.

The effects of the laser are considered beneficial if the laser beam reaches the intended target, but if it reaches a non-intended target, the effect can be an injury, and the beam is then considered hazardous. The hazards are generally categorized as beam hazards or non-beam hazards. Beam hazards can cause ocular and cutaneous injury. Non-beam hazards originate within the laser device itself or are created by the laser beam's interaction with materials in the surgical environment; these include laser plume hazards, fire hazards, and electrical hazards inherent in a high-voltage system.[22-24] The hazards to patients and personnel can be minimized by the use of personal protective equipment (PPE) and engineering, administrative, procedural, and special controls (eg, signage).[6,25]

Unintentional exposure to the laser beam may result in injuries to the eyes or the skin of the patient or health care personnel.[4,6,12,26] The type of injury will vary based on the classification of the laser.[4,26]

Another hazard associated with the use of a laser is fire.[27] Smith and Roy[28] surveyed 8,523 members of the American Academy of Otolaryngology—Head and Neck Surgery to obtain information regarding the characteristics and the frequency of OR fires in otolaryngology. Eighty-eight of the 349 surgeons who responded to the survey reported having witnessed at least one OR fire during their career. For the total of 106 fires reported, the ignition source was an electrosurgical unit (59%), a laser (32%), or a light cord (7%). In an analysis of 5,297 surgical malpractice claims from 1985 to 2009 in the American Society of Anesthesiologists Closed Claims Database, Mehta et al[29] found 103 claims related to surgical fires. Lasers were found to be the ignition source in nine of the claims. The remaining sources of ignition were electrosurgical devices (n = 93) and a defibrillator (n = 1).

A limitation of the evidence is that randomized controlled trials related to laser injury prevention may expose patients to harm and, as such, would not be ethical. A limited number of other types of studies have been conducted and contribute valuable knowledge to the field. However, interpretation of these studies is limited by the nature of this type of research, which can only show association among study variables and cannot determine causation. Because of a lack of research on interventions to prevent injury from the use of lasers, much of the available evidence is based on generally accepted practices and expert opinion.

The following topics are outside the scope of this document:

- general fire safety (See the AORN Guideline for a Safe Environment of Care[30]),
- surgical smoke safety (See the AORN Guideline for Surgical Smoke Safety[31]),
- credentialing and educational requirements for physicians and allied health practitioners,
- laser use in the dental setting,
- the selection of lasers,
- the selection of a method of ventilation, and
- power and energy settings.

Evidence Review

A medical librarian with a perioperative background conducted a systematic search of the databases Ovid MEDLINE®, Ovid Embase®, EBSCO CINAHL®, and the Cochrane Database of Systematic Reviews. The search was limited to literature published in English from January 2009 through March 2019. At the time of the initial search, weekly alerts were created on the topics included in that search. Results from these alerts were provided to the lead author until May 2019. The lead author requested additional articles that either did not fit the original search criteria or were dis-

covered during the evidence appraisal process. The lead author and the medical librarian also identified relevant guidelines from government agencies, professional organizations, and standards-setting bodies.

Search terms included *ablation techniques, access control, accident prevention, accidental activation, airway fires, airway laser, airway stents, anesthesia, awake patients, balloon dilation, bronchoscopy, burns, catheter ablation, CO₂ laser, cosmetic techniques, diode laser, distribution of safety glasses, documentation, double lumen tube, durable medical equipment, electric power supplies, electric wiring, electrical equipment and supplies, endobronchial surgery, endoscopy, endotracheal tube, equipment and supplies (hospital), equipment contamination, equipment failure, equipment failure analysis, equipment safety, eye burns, eye injuries, eye protective devices, filtering criteria, fire extinguisher, fire management, fire safety, fires, goggles, intraoperative complications, laryngeal disease, laryngeal neoplasms, laser ablation, laser audit, laser calibration, laser debulking, laser documentation, laser fiber, laser hazard analysis, laser hazards, laser knife, laser malfunction, laser operator, laser photoablation, laser power setting, laser safety, laser safety audit, laser safety committee, laser safety education, laser safety officer, laser safety program, laser scalpel, laser surgery, laser therapy, laser treatment area, laser vaporization, laser-related burns, lasers, misdirection, nonablative laser treatment, nominal hazard zone, nurses, occupational exposure, occupational hazards, occupational injuries, occupational safety, ocular adnexa, ocular laser injuries, operative microscope, patient safety, perioperative nursing, personal protective equipment, postoperative complications, power sources and settings, preoperative care, protective clothing, pulsed laser, pulsed tissue ablation, rigid bronchoscopy, risk management, safety glasses, safety lenses, sedated patients, shared airway procedures, shared airway safety, surgical equipment, surgical fires,* and *veins.*

Included were research and non-research literature in English, complete publications, and publications with dates within the time restriction when available. Historical studies also were included. Excluded were non-peer-reviewed publications and older evidence within the time restriction when more recent evidence was available. Editorials, news items, and other brief items were excluded. Low-quality evidence was excluded when higher-quality evidence was available, and literature outside the time restriction was excluded when literature within the time restriction was available (Figure 1).

Articles identified in the search were provided to the project team for evaluation. The team consisted of the lead author and one evidence appraiser. The lead author and the evidence appraiser reviewed and critically appraised each article using the AORN Research or Non-Research Evidence Appraisal Tools as appropriate. A second appraiser was consulted in the event of a disagreement between the lead author and the primary evidence appraiser. The literature was independently evaluated and appraised according to the strength and quality of the evidence. Each article was

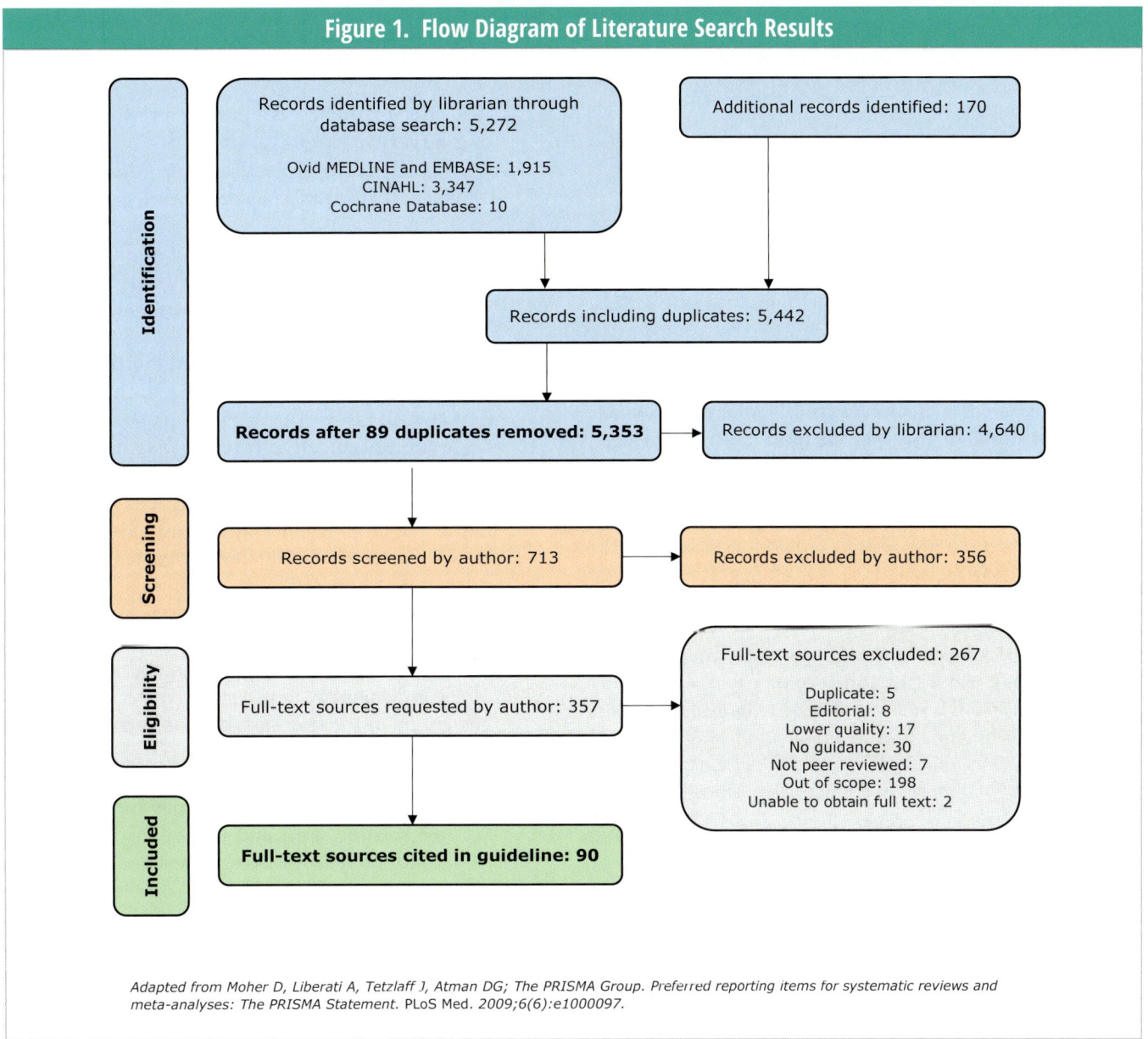

Figure 1. Flow Diagram of Literature Search Results

Records identified by librarian through database search: 5,272

Ovid MEDLINE and EMBASE: 1,915
CINAHL: 3,347
Cochrane Database: 10

Additional records identified: 170

Identification

Records including duplicates: 5,442

Records after 89 duplicates removed: 5,353

Records excluded by librarian: 4,640

Screening

Records screened by author: 713

Records excluded by author: 356

Eligibility

Full-text sources requested by author: 357

Full-text sources excluded: 267

Duplicate: 5
Editorial: 8
Lower quality: 17
No guidance: 30
Not peer reviewed: 7
Out of scope: 198
Unable to obtain full text: 2

Included

Full-text sources cited in guideline: 90

Adapted from Moher D, Liberati A, Tetzlaff J, Atman DG; The PRISMA Group. Preferred reporting items for systematic reviews and meta-analyses: The PRISMA Statement. PLoS Med. 2009;6(6):e1000097.

then assigned an appraisal score. The appraisal score is noted in brackets after each reference as applicable.

Each recommendation rating is based on a synthesis of the collective evidence, a benefit-harm assessment, and consideration of resource use. The strength of the recommendation was determined using the AORN Evidence Rating Model and the quality and consistency of the evidence supporting a recommendation. The recommendation strength rating is noted in brackets after each recommendation.

Note: *The evidence summary table is available at http:// www.aorn.org/evidencetables/.*

Editor's note: *MEDLINE is a registered trademark of the US National Library of Medicine's Medical Literature Analysis and Retrieval System, Bethesda, MD. Embase is a registered trademark of Elsevier B.V., Amsterdam, The Netherlands. CINAHL,*

Cumulative Index to Nursing and Allied Health Literature, is a registered trademark of EBSCO Industries, Birmingham, AL.

1. Precautions to Mitigate Hazards

1.1 **Laser warning signs must be placed in visible locations at all entrances to the room when lasers are in use.**[32] *[Regulatory Requirement]*

The Occupational Safety and Health Administration (OSHA) requires placement of warning signs.[32]

1.1.1 **Use warning signs that are specific to the type of laser being used and that meet the American National Standards Institute (ANSI) criteria as described in ANSI Z-136.1**[25] **and ANSI Z136.3.**[1] *[Recommendation]*

A clinical guideline recommends the use of laser-specific warning signs.[1] Warning signs alert everyone in the vicinity that a laser is in use.[9,12]

1.2 Close doors in the **nominal hazard zone**.[1] *[Recommendation]*

A clinical guideline recommends keeping doors closed in the nominal hazard zone.[1] Closing doors assists with defining the nominal hazard zone and preventing laser beams from migrating beyond the room.[12,13,33,34]

1.3 Cover windows in the nominal hazard zone with a barrier that blocks transmission of the beam as applicable to the type of laser being used (eg, color dependent).[1,35,36] *[Recommendation]*

Clinical guidelines recommend keeping windows, including door windows, covered as described.[1,35,36] Covering the windows assists with preventing the laser beams from migrating beyond the room.[4,9,12,18,22,33,34,37]

1.4 Place the laser in stand-by mode, turn off the laser, or use beam shutters or caps when laser transmission is not required.[1,35,36] *[Recommendation]*

Clinical guidelines recommend placing the laser in stand-by mode, turning off the laser, or using beam shutters or caps when laser transmission is not required.[1,35,36] These actions assist with preventing unintentional activation of the laser.[18,33,37-39]

1.5 Disable the laser when it is not in use by removing the laser key and placing the key in a designated secure location.[1,35,36] *[Recommendation]*

Clinical guidelines recommend disabling the laser when it is not in use.[1,35,36]

1.6 Restrict access to the laser activation security code or laser keys to authorized personnel.[1] *[Recommendation]*

A clinical guideline recommends restricting access as described.[1] Restricting access to the laser activation security code or laser keys assists with preventing unauthorized personnel from activating the laser.[9,33]

1.7 Perform calibration or aiming beam alignment testing before each procedure according to the manufacturer's instructions for use (IFU).[1,35,36,40,41] *[Recommendation]*

Fukuda et al[42] tested 60 laser devices for agreement between the setting and the power delivered. Eight of the devices had agreement between the setting and the power delivered, but 52 did not. The researchers recommended periodic calibration.

Clinical guidelines also recommend calibration and aiming testing.[1,35,36,40,41]

1.8 Use laser-resistant teeth protectors when performing surgery in the oral cavity.[22,43] *[Recommendation]*

Use of a tooth protector assists with protecting the teeth from damage by the laser.[22,43]

1.9 Limit traffic into the OR to the patient and those trained in laser safety.[1] *[Recommendation]*

A clinical guideline recommends limiting traffic.[1]

1.10 Complete a laser safety checklist approved by the health care organization before each procedure involving a laser.[36] *[Recommendation]*

A clinical guideline recommends using a laser safety checklist.[36] A laser safety checklist may assist personnel in following safe practices before, during, and after procedures involving a laser.[9,36]

Alidina et al[44] conducted a free-text comment survey in 11 hospitals in which a surgical safety checklist was implemented. There were 54 respondents before and 50 respondents after implementation. The researchers found the number of responses reporting complications decreased after the implementation of the checklist, but the decrease did not reach statistical significance.

1.10.1 The laser safety checklist may include equipment to be used and personnel and patient safety interventions (eg, presence of eyewear, signage placed, calibration completed).[36] *[Conditional Recommendation]*

1.11 Perform a laser time out before the start of the laser procedure. *[Recommendation]*

A clinical guideline recommends performing a laser time out.[36] Performing a time out may assist with improving team communication.[21,23]

1.11.1 The laser time out may
- be included in the preprocedural time out or be independent,
- include the components of the laser checklist or state that the laser checklist was completed, and
- include fire safety if not included as a portion of the preprocedural time out.

[Conditional Recommendation]

2. Eye Protection

2.1 Eye protection applicable to the specific wavelength and **optical density** of the laser in use must be worn in the nominal hazard zone.[45,46] *[Regulatory Requirement]*

Eye protection is required by OSHA.[45,46] Eye injury can occur in less than the **aversion response time** of 0.25 seconds.[37,47] The area of the eye that is at risk for injury depends on the wavelength of the laser.[18,22,48-50]

2.1.1 Eye protection for personnel may include goggles; face shields; and spectacles or prescription eyewear with special filter materials, reflective coating, or a combination of both.[1] *[Conditional Recommendation]*

A clinical guideline recommends using the applicable type of eye protection.[1]

2.1.2 Select eye protection based on the

- laser manufacturer's protective eyewear specifications,[4,33]
- wavelength of laser emission,[4,9,12,22,24,33,48,51,52]
- optical density of the eyewear recommended by the laser manufacturer's IFU,[9,12,22,24,33,48,51,53]
- type of procedure,[1]
- radiant exposure limits,[22,24]
- need for corrective lenses,
- restriction of peripheral vision,
- fit,[33] and
- comfort.[33,54]

[Recommendation]

Using these criteria to determine the type of eye protection assists with selecting the correct type of eyewear.[4,9,12,22,24,33,48,51,53] The **laser user** may not be able to wear protective eyewear for certain procedures, such as when using an indirect ophthalmoscope and laser delivered by a microscope.

2.1.3 Inspect protective eyewear before use for

- pitting, crazing, cracking, and discoloration[1,36,52];
- mechanical integrity of the frame[1,36];
- wear or damage to straps or other retaining devices[1,36];
- light leaks[1,36]; and
- coating damage.[1,36]

[Recommendation]

Clinical guidelines recommend inspection of eyewear.[1,36,52] Defects in eyewear may allow the laser beam to enter the eye.[33,51]

2.1.4 Protective eyewear must be removed from use if damaged or faded.[46] *[Regulatory Requirement]*

Removal of defective eyewear is required by OSHA.[46]

2.1.5 Place protective eyewear at the entrances to every room where a laser is in use.[1] *[Recommendation]*

A clinical guideline recommends placing protective eyewear at the entrance to every room where a laser is in use.[1] Having protective eyewear at the entrance makes it readily available for all who enter the room.[4,9,13,55]

2.1.6 A color-coded or other type of label may be placed on protective eyewear to match the corresponding laser. *[Conditional Recommendation]*

This practice is intended to make it easier to choose the correct protective eyewear.[9]

2.2 When wearing laser goggles, use precautions when administering medication (eg, by verifying the contents of the medication vial with another person).[56] *[Recommendation]*

Tinted laser goggles may alter the color of medication labels, which may increase the risk for a medication error.[56]

2.3 Use laser shutters or filters with the appropriate optical density on microscopes and microscope accessory oculars.[1] *[Recommendation]*

A clinical guideline supports the use of shutters and laser filters to protect the laser user from laser exposure.[1] Use of proper shutters or filters decreases the risk for eye injury.[9]

2.3.1 Verify proper function of the shutter or filter before use.[1] *[Recommendation]*

A clinical guideline recommends verifying proper functioning of the shutter or filter before use.[1]

2.4 Protect the patient's eyes and eyelids from injury using a method approved by the **laser safety officer** (LSO), including

- providing goggles or glasses designated for the type of laser being used to patients who remain awake during laser procedures[1,36];
- applying wet eye pads, laser-specific eye shields, opaque barrier blocks, or other devices approved by the LSO to patients who undergo general anesthesia[1,36,52];
- applying metal corneoscleral eye shields of appropriate size that are approved by the US Food and Drug Administration (FDA) for use during laser procedures to patients undergoing laser treatments on or around the eyelids[1]; or
- use water soluble eye lubricants and occlusive metal protective eyewear for any procedures performed on the face.[1]

[Recommendation]

Clinical guidelines recommend providing protective eyewear to protect the patients eyes from the laser beams.[1,36,52] Using the listed methods of eye protection may prevent or decrease the potential for injury to the patient's eyes.[4,9,12,13,18,22,33,57-61]

2.4.1 **Chose the method of protection based on the intended procedure, target tissue site, laser wavelength, patient position, and type of anesthesia.**[1,36,52] *[Recommendation]*

Clinical guidelines recommend selecting the method of protection based on all or some of the criteria listed.[1,36,52] Use of eye protection based on the listed criteria may prevent or decrease the potential for injury to the patient's eyes.[9,18,22,33]

2.5 **Clean, disinfect, and store protective eyewear according to the manufacturer's written IFU.**[1,36] *[Recommendation]*

Clinical guidelines recommend cleaning, disinfecting, and storing protective eyewear according to the manufacturer's IFU.[1,36]

3. Fire Prevention

3.1 **Use only accessories compatible with the laser system, and use them in accordance with the manufacturer's IFU.**[1,36] *[Recommendation]*

Clinical guidelines recommend using only compatible accessories in surgery.[1,36]

3.2 **Use technologies other than laser devices (eg, bipolar electrosurgery, coblation technology, non-energy-applying instruments) when feasible and indicated by the fire risk assessment.**[62] *[Recommendation]*

Use of technologies other than laser devices when indicated by the fire risk assessment may decrease the potential for a fire.[62]

3.3 **Use water-soluble lubricants (eg, eye lubricant) near the surgical site.**[63,64] *[Recommendation]*

Petroleum-based eye lubricants are flammable and therefore a fuel source.[34,62]

3.4 **Stop delivery of oxygen (O_2) or decrease the percentage to the lowest tolerable level before activating the laser near the patient's head, face, or neck.** *[Recommendation]*

Dhar et al[64] conducted a descriptive laboratory study to determine the difference in time to ignition of a moistened neurosurgical patty at 50%, 75%, and 100% O_2 using 5 W of power. The mean time to ignition of the wet neurosurgical patties

was 63.06 seconds at 50% O_2, 54.1 seconds at 75% O_2, and 33.85 seconds at 100% O_2. Similar results were found at 7.5 W and 10 W. The researchers recommended using the lowest possible percentage of O_2.

In a laboratory study, Stuermer et al[63] measured the amount of time to ignition for fat, muscle, and cartilage using a CO_2 laser at 2 W, 4 W, 6 W, and 8 W. The tests were carried out at O_2 concentrations of 21%, 30%, 40%, 50%, 70%, and 100%. The researchers found the ignition time decreased for all three fuels as the O_2 concentration increased. The average time to ignition was decreased by 14% without smoke exhaustion and 36% with smoke exhaustion for every 10% increase in O_2.

A clinical guideline recommends stopping the delivery of O_2 or decreasing the percentage to the lowest tolerable level before activating the laser near the patient's head, face, or neck.[65]

3.5 **Protect exposed tissues around the surgical site with moist materials (eg, towels, sponges), and remoisten them as needed.**[64] *[Recommendation]*

In a descriptive laboratory study, Hammons et al[66] used a CO_2 laser to determine the results of reflection off of various surfaces onto surgical field materials. They found there was no reflection off wet gauze. The researchers recommended using a tongue blade covered with a moistened sponge to prevent reflection of the laser beam.

Dhar et al[64] conducted a descriptive laboratory study to determine the difference in time to ignition of dry and moistened neurosurgical patties. At 5 W of laser power and 50% O_2, the dry patties ignited in an average of 2.3 seconds and the moist patties ignited in an average of 63.9 seconds. The researchers recommended that only moist patties be used near the laser target area.

Clinical guidelines also recommend protecting exposed tissue around the surgical site with saline-saturated materials.[35,36,65]

3.6 **Use moistened radiopaque sponges or towels for rectal packing or for covering the anus during perineal surgery.**[1] *[Recommendation]*

A clinical guideline recommends using moist rectal packs.[1] Methane gas is highly flammable and potentially explosive. Moist packing prevents the release of methane gas from the rectum.[9]

3.7 **Keep a basin of saline or water on the sterile field or within easy reach of the scrub person or the laser user if no scrub person is present.**[36] *[Recommendation]*

Having water or saline within reach provides a means for extinguishing a fire.[22,23,33,53] A clinical guideline recommends having a basin of saline or water accessible on the back table in case of a fire.[36]

3.8 Instruct patients to avoid using hair styling products (eg, hair spray, styling gel, mousse) on the day of surgery.[22,33] [Recommendation]

A clinical guideline recommends against using hair styling products.[36] Many hair styling products are petroleum based and flammable.[22,33]

4. Laser Shared Airway Procedures

4.1 Use an FDA-approved, laser-retardant endotracheal (ET) tube during laser procedures involving the airway.[67-69] [Recommendation]

Ahmed et al[69] conducted a laboratory study using a CO_2 laser to determine the amount of time it would take to penetrate the wall and cuff of a standard polyvinyl chloride (PVC) ET tube. The researchers found at 2 W of power, the time to penetration was less than 1 second at a 90-degree angle. The researchers recommended using a laser-resistant ET tube.

In a laboratory study, Coughlan and Verma[68] examined the time to penetrate or ignite three different laser-resistant ET tubes and a PVC ET tube using a potassium titanyl phosphate (KTP) laser in pulsed and continuous mode. The laser immediately penetrated the outer covering of the laser-resistant tube but did not penetrate the inner lining. A spark was produced when the beam interacted with the black marking on the PVC tube, but perforation did not occur. The researchers concluded that laser-resistant tubes are safe to use during procedures performed with the KTP laser.

Roy and Smith[67] compared the time to ignition of a reinforced, laser safe ET tube and a traditional ET tube when a CO_2 laser was aimed directly at the tube with 21% to 60% O_2 flowing through it. The researchers fired the laser until the time of ignition or a maximum of 2 minutes, whichever was longer. The traditional tube ignited in 1 second to 8 seconds. The time to ignition was shorter when a higher percentage of O_2 was flowing through the tube. The reinforced, laser safe ET tube did not ignite when the CO_2 laser was fired directly at the tube but did ignite when the laser was aimed at the non-reinforced tip of the tube. The researchers recommended using the reinforced, laser-safe ET tube during surgeries performed with a CO_2 laser and noted that fires ignite faster with higher concentrations of O_2.

Polyvinylchloride ET tubes are contraindicated any time there is a potential for contact with a laser.[1]

Clinical guidelines recommend using a laser-resistant ET tube.[1,36,65]

4.1.1 Use an ET tube that has been tested for the type of laser to be used, as found in the manufacturer's IFU.[1] [Recommendation]

A clinical guideline recommends using an ET tube that has been tested for the type of laser used.[1]

4.1.2 Inflate ET tube cuffs with sterile water or saline during procedures involving laser treatment of the patient's airway or aerodigestive tract.[6] [Recommendation]

Clinical guidelines recommend inflating the ET tube cuff as described.[1,36,65] The cuffs of the laser-resistant ET tube may not be laser retardant, and inflating the cuff with a liquid may help decrease the potential for the tube to ignite or may serve as an extinguisher.[8]

Li et al[70] reviewed the records of 704 patients undergoing surgery with a CO_2 laser and found 127 adverse events related to the use of the laser. The adverse events included the PVC ET tube bursting, sparks, dense smoke, and burning smells. The researchers also conducted an in vitro experiment to determine whether an ET tube cuff filled with water was more resistant to bursting than a cuff filled with air when exposed to a laser beam. The researchers pointed the laser beam at ET tube cuffs that were inflated with air or filled with water. They found the water-filled cuffs to be more resistant to bursting than the air-filled cuffs. The researchers recommended inflating the ET tube cuffs with water instead of air.

4.1.3 Methylene blue may be added to the sterile water or saline.[6] [Conditional Recommendation]

Adding methylene blue to the saline may help identify a tube-cuff rupture.[8]

4.1.4 Place moistened packs around the ET tube when possible and keep them continuously moist during procedures involving the patient's airway or aerodigestive tract.[64,68,69,71] [Recommendation]

In a laboratory setting, Ahmed et al[69] compared the time to penetration of wet and dry neurosurgical patties using a CO_2 laser. Using 2 W of power, the dry patties were penetrated in less than 1 second and the wet patties were penetrated in 180 seconds. The researchers recommended using a wet patty to cover the ET tube during laser surgery and keeping the patty moist.

In a laboratory study, Coughlan and Verma[68] examined the time to penetrate or ignite the blue radiopaque strip and the white sponge portion of dry and wet surgical patties with a KTP laser in continuous and pulsed modes. The blue strip on the dry patties was penetrated in an average of 3 seconds in a continuous mode and 4.8 seconds in a pulsed mode. When the laser, in the continuous mode, was aimed at the blue strip on a wet patty, a flame resulted but no penetration occurred; in the pulsed mode there was a spark with no penetration. When the laser in the continuous mode was aimed at the white sponge portion of the dry patty, penetration occurred in 15 seconds, but the moist patty was not penetrated. When the laser in the pulsed mode was aimed at the white sponge portion, no penetration occurred with either the dry or wet patty. The researchers recommended that the patties be kept moist.

Dhar et al[64] performed a laboratory study to test the time to ignition of wet and dry neurosurgical patties placed around an ET tube in a cadaveric porcine model. The ignition source was a CO_2 laser. The researchers found the average ignition time for the dry patties was 2.3 seconds, whereas the average ignition time for the wet patties was 63.9 seconds. The researchers concluded that moist neurosurgical patties may be used to help prevent airway fires, but they need to be kept moist and changed frequently.

Roy and Smith[71] conducted a laboratory study to examine the rate of perforation of ET tubes during laser use. The researchers found that tube perforation occurred even with moist pledgets in place. The researchers surmised that the pledgets may not have covered the area where the perforation occurred, or the laser may have penetrated the pledget. The researchers concluded that moistened pledgets may help protect the ET tube from the laser beam.

A clinical guideline recommends using moistened packs around the ET tube.[36]

5. Fiberoptic Procedures

5.1 **Cover the end of the laser fiber with a moist sponge or towel when the laser is not in use.**[1] *[Recommendation]*

A clinical guideline recommends covering the end of the laser fiber with a moist sponge when it is not in use.[1]

5.2 **Secure the working end of the laser fiber in a holster-type device before and between uses.** *[Recommendation]*

The benefits of holstering include keeping the fiber on the sterile field and possible prevention of fires on the drapes or patient burns related to accidental activation.[72]

5.3 **Take precautions to avoid breaking a laser fiber, including by not**
- **leaning against a fiber,**
- **clamping a fiber,**[38] **or**
- **stressing or bending a fiber beyond what is specified as acceptable in the manufacturer's IFU.**[23,73]
[Recommendation]

Taking these precautions may assist with decreasing the risk of breaking the fiber.[23,38] Breaking a fiber may result in a fire, damage to instruments, or injury to the patient or personnel.[54]

5.4 **During a procedure involving a laser fiber and a laser catheter sheath, the scrub person should**
- **inspect the laser catheter sheath and laser fiber for damage before and after the procedure**[13,40,59,74,75]**;**
- **confirm before the procedure that the catheter sheath meets the manufacturer's labeled length and the laser fiber is of sufficient length to extend beyond the catheter**[73-76]**;**
- **confirm that the catheter sheath and the laser fiber are intact and complete after each removal from the patient**[13,73-76]**; and**
- **remove the sheath and catheter from service, implement the organization's policy for retained surgical items, and make the surgical team aware of the missing fiber or fiber portion before the patient leaves the surgical suite if the catheter or sheath fails inspection.**[74-76]
[Recommendation]

A clinical guideline recommends performing all or some of the precautions listed to prevent retention of a laser fiber.[40] Breakage of the fiber and puncturing of the insertion catheter have been reported in case reports.[73,75,77,78]

6. Instrumentation

6.1 **Minimize the use of reflective surfaces during laser surgery.**[66] *[Recommendation]*

Clinical guidelines recommend minimizing the use of reflective surfaces during surgery.[1,35,36] The laser beam may reflect off surfaces onto non-target tissues, potentially causing skin or eye injury.[1,4,35]

In a laboratory descriptive study, Hammons et al[66] used a CO_2 laser to determine the results of reflection off of various surfaces onto surgical field materials. The researchers found that the reflection off sandblasted and polished surfaces created a hole in a glove and a flame on a surgical gown. The researchers concluded that there is a risk for damage to surgical field materials from reflected laser beams.

6.2 Use **anodized**-, dull-, non-reflective-, or matte-finished instruments near the laser site.[1,36] *[Recommendation]*

In a laboratory descriptive study, Hammons et al[66] used a CO_2 laser to determine the results of reflection off of various surfaces onto surgical field materials. The researchers found that the reflection off sandblasted and polished surfaces created a hole in a glove and a flame on a surgical gown. The researchers concluded that there is a risk of damage to surgical field materials from reflected laser beams.

Clinical guidelines also recommend use of anodized-, dull-, non-reflective-, or matte-finished instruments near the laser site.[1,36]

6.3 Cover reflective instruments that cannot be anodized with materials that will not reflect and will not ignite when exposed to the laser beam (eg, saline saturated radiopaque towels, radiopaque sponges).[1] *[Recommendation]*

A clinical guideline recommends covering reflective instruments.[1] Performing this action may decrease the risk of beam reflection.[13,33]

6.4 Inspect instruments that have been coated (ie, **ebonized**) for damage to the integrity of the coating before use, after use, and before packaging for sterilization.[36] *[Recommendation]*

A clinical guideline recommends inspecting coated instruments.[36]

6.4.1 Remove the instrument from service if damaged. *[Recommendation]*

Damage or scratches to the coating may allow the laser beam to reflect off the instrument, potentially causing skin or eye injury.

6.5 Use a shielding device (eg, backstop or guard) during CO_2 laser surgery inside of a body cavity.[1,36,41] *[Recommendation]*

Clinical guidelines recommend the use of shielding devices.[1,36,41] The CO_2 laser beam continues to move through the tissue after it cuts or coagulates. A backstop or guard may prevent the laser beam from affecting non-targeted tissue.[9,38]

7. Foot Pedal

7.1 Place the laser foot pedal in a position convenient to the user and in a position where it will not be confused with other foot pedals.[1,36] *[Recommendation]*

Clinical guidelines recommend placing the foot petal as described.[1,36] Accidental activation or misdirection of the laser beam may cause eye and skin injury to the patient and health care personnel. Attention to placement of the foot switch may reduce the potential for unintended activation of the laser beam.[9,33]

7.2 Encase the foot pedal in a fluid-resistant cover when there is potential for fluid spills. *[Recommendation]*

7.3 The person in control of the delivery device should be the only person to activate the laser foot pedal.[35,36] *[Recommendation]*

Clinical guidelines recommend that the person in control of the laser hand piece should be the only person to activate the foot pedal.[35,36] Having only the person in control of the delivery device activate the laser decreases the risk of unintentional activation.[33,38]

7.4 Place or manipulate the foot petal by handling the foot petal itself and not using the cord. *[Recommendation]*

8. Service and Maintenance

8.1 Lasers must be inspected, tested, and maintained.[79] *[Regulatory Requirement]*

The Centers for Medicare & Medicaid Services (CMS) requires that lasers be inspected, tested, and maintained.[79]

8.1.1 Follow the laser manufacturers' IFU regarding inspection, testing, and maintenance. *[Recommendation]*

8.2 Lasers must be placed on the critical equipment list in hospitals.[80] *[Regulatory Requirement]*

The CMS requires hospitals to place lasers on the critical equipment list.[80]

8.3 A designated and trained individual (eg, a biomedical engineering services representative, a manufacturer's service representative, a third-party service representative) must inspect lasers before initial use within the facility and perform periodic preventive maintenance and repair in accordance with the manufacturer's IFU.[79,80] *[Regulatory Requirement]*

The CMS requires having a trained individual perform laser maintenance.[79,80]

8.4 Documentation of the training received by the individual performing the inspections and maintenance must be retained by the facility.[79,80] *[Regulatory Requirement]*.

The CMS requires retention of the inspection and maintenance documentation.[79,80]

8.5 Document inspection, preventive maintenance, and repair in accordance with the health care organization's policy.[1,41] *[Recommendation]*

Documentation provides a retainable record of any inspection, preventive maintenance, and repair performed.[12] Clinical guidelines recommend documenting inspection, maintenance, and repairs as described in policy.[1,41]

8.6 Perform inspection, preventive maintenance, and repair in a temporary laser-controlled area. *[Recommendation]*

A clinical guideline recommends performing inspection, preventive maintenance, and repair in a temporary laser-controlled area.[1] Performing these duties in a temporary laser-controlled area helps prevent injury to bystanders or people passing by.

9. Laser Safety Program

9.1 Develop and implement a laser safety program that
- applies to all owned, leased, rented, or borrowed laser equipment;
- applies in any location where lasers are used; and
- includes the following components:
  - description of the interdisciplinary laser safety committee, which may be the same as a facility-wide safety committee;
  - usage criteria and authorized procedures for all health care personnel working in laser nominal hazard zones;
  - laser hazards and applicable controls (eg, beam and non-beam);
  - requirements for monitoring compliance with applicable administrative, engineering, and procedural control measures;
  - the type and frequency of medical examinations for personnel;
  - education requirements (eg, competency verification, certification, participating personnel qualifications);
  - description of quality processes, including audits; and
  - policies and procedures covering use of lasers.[1]

[Recommendation]

A clinical guideline recommends implementing a laser safety program.[1] A laser safety program establishes requirements for the safe operation of lasers in all locations and provides guidance to minimize laser hazards.[4,9,11,33]

10. Health Care Organization Responsibilities

10.1 The health care organization should
- define the qualifications for the LSO;
- appoint the LSO;
- provide to the LSO a letter of "authority to suspend, restrict, or terminate the operation of a laser system if he/she deems that the laser hazard controls are inadequate"[1(p7)];
- appoint a **deputy laser safety officer** (DLSO) and **laser safety site contact** (LSSC) if these positions are determined to be required;
- appoint a health care professional trained in laser safety (ie, a **laser safety specialist**) to supervise every **laser treatment–controlled area**;
- appoint a specific laser safety committee or assign the responsibilities of the laser safety committee to an associated committee;
- delegate the administration of the laser program to the laser safety committee and LSO or designated alternates;
- credential and maintain a list of the credentialed personnel involved with laser delivery;
- establish a plan for handling accidental exposure incidents;
- provide education and training to all personnel that is commensurate with the job description and applicable to the lasers used in the facility; and
- define the scope of responsibilities for those credentialed to perform laser procedures.[1,36,41]

[Recommendation]

Low-quality evidence[8,9,11,13,33] and clinical guidelines[1,36,41] support the responsibilities listed.

10.1.1 The health care organization must credential laser users.[79,80] *[Regulatory Requirement]*

The CMS requires credentialing.[79,80]

10.1.2 The health care organization must provide PPE as applicable to each type of laser in use.[45,55] *[Regulatory Requirement]*

Employers are required by OSHA to provide a safe work environment for employees.[45,55]

11. Laser Safety Committee

11.1 Form an interdisciplinary laser safety committee, which may be a portion of the facility-wide safety committee, that includes the following individuals or departmental representatives:
- administrators,
- the LSO,
- a biomedical engineer and/or clinical/biomedical engineer,
- a physician representative from each specialty group that uses lasers,
- anesthesia professionals,
- perioperative services administrators,
- a perioperative educator,
- medical staff education/credentialing personnel,
- quality department personnel,
- surgical technologists,
- the laser safety specialist, and
- a DLSO if deemed necessary.[1,36]

[Recommendation]

Low-quality evidence[9] and clinical guidelines[1,36] support forming an interdisciplinary team.

11.1.1 One person may represent more than one department or role based on the organizational staffing plan. *[Conditional Recommendation]*

11.2 Delegate the following responsibilities to the laser safety committee:
- conducting strategic planning for and acquisition of laser-related technology (eg, technology assessment, cost analysis, product evaluation, review of marketing information from laser vendors);
- establishing requirements for credentialing;
- verifying that any physician who operates a laser has completed the health care organization–required education on laser operation and safety precautions and coursework in basic laser physics, laser-tissue interaction, and clinical applications for the specific laser for which privileges are sought;
- establishing and maintaining a laser safety program;
- establishing requirements for hazard evaluation;
- developing and enforcing laser-related policy and procedures;
- overseeing laser-related education and competency verification;
- establishing staffing requirements;
- establishing a quality assurance and improvement program;

- appointing and delegating authority and responsibility for supervising laser safety to an LSO; and
- overseeing third-party laser services.[1,36]

[Recommendation]

Low-quality evidence[4,9] and clinical guidelines[1,36] support delegating all or some of these responsibilities to the laser safety committee.

12. Laser Safety Officer (LSO)

12.1 Establish the qualifications for the LSO, which may include
- education and experience in laser operations, clinical applications, and safety;
- completion of a formal medical laser safety course;
- completion of a formal medical laser safety officer course; or
- certification as a medical laser safety officer.

[Conditional Recommendation]

12.2 Delegate the following responsibilities to the LSO:
- enforcing, monitoring, and overseeing the laser safety program;
- verifying that protective equipment is available, used correctly, and maintained in working order;
- verifying that ANSI-compliant warning signs are posted in locations where lasers are in use;
- verifying that changes to the policies and procedures are completed, if necessary, after any modifications are made during service or system updates;
- verifying that the type of fire extinguisher needed for each specific laser, based on the manufacturer's IFU, is available and located as defined by the health care organization's policy and procedure;
- verifying that all operators including third-party operators are properly credentialed according to the health care organization's policy;
- verifying all third-party-provided equipment is compliant with facility policies and procedures and governmental regulations including documentation of inspection, preventive maintenance, and repair;
- maintaining education records;
- maintaining records on the laser's maintenance and service;
- performing a laser hazard evaluation before initial use in the facility;
- performing periodic safety audits;
- performing adverse event investigations;

- determining the laser treatment–controlled area and nominal hazard zone for each laser used;
- maintaining a laser inventory including classifications of laser;
- determining the laser classification of each system and reassessing if it is not provided by the manufacturer;
- restricting, suspending, or terminating the operation of any laser system when the hazard controls are not in compliance;
- obtaining and maintaining any regulatory requirements such as licenses;
- obtaining approved written, operating, maintenance, service, and calibration procedures from the manufacturer or distributor;
- communicating to the laser user any imminent danger from a laser hazard;
- overseeing the implementation of control measures listed in the laser manufacturer's IFU in the nominal hazard zone and the laser treatment–controlled area;
- administering policies and procedures for control of laser hazards, maintenance, service, and use of lasers;
- approving equipment installation according to the manufacturer's safety recommendations;
- ensuring that maintenance of equipment is performed by qualified personnel;
- coordinating laser safety education programs; and
- designating a DLSO or LSSC if indicated by the facility staffing pattern.

[Recommendation]

Low-quality evidence[9,11,33,34,51] and clinical guidelines[1,36,40,41] support assigning all or some of these responsibilities to the LSO.

12.2.1 The LSO may fulfill multiple roles (eg, **laser operator**) within the health care organization, depending on the scope of services provided.[1] *[Conditional Recommendation]*

A clinical guideline supports the option of having the LSO fulfill multiple roles.[1]

12.2.2 The LSO may delegate responsibilities to a qualified individual (eg, the DLSO) as applicable to the job description.[1] *[Conditional Recommendation]*

A clinical guideline supports the option of having the LSO delegate responsibilities.[1]

12.3 Educate, train, and verify the competency of the LSO on the following topics:
- laser terminology,

- laser-specific information (eg, wave lengths, pulse shapes, modes, power/energy, classification, controlled areas),
- radiometric units and measurement devices,
- steps and requirements for performing a laser hazard evaluation,
- fundamentals of lasers and optics,
- laser tissue interactions,
- beam and non-beam hazards and appropriate control measures,
- regulatory requirements and standards of practice,
- laser safety program administration,
- maximum permissible exposure values,
- laser/optical radiation bioeffects, and
- hazard classification.

[Recommendation]

Low-quality evidence[11,81,82] and a clinical guideline[25] support incorporating the listed components in the education for the LSO.

13. Deputy Laser Safety Officer (DLSO)

13.1 The DLSO may function as the laser safety officer in the absence of the LSO. The DLSO may also be the laser user, laser operator, or other trained individual.[1] *[Conditional Recommendation]*

Low-quality evidence[33] and a clinical guideline[1] support these responsibilities for the DLSO.

14. Laser Safety Site Contact (LSSC)

14.1 Delegate the following responsibilities to the LSSC:
- overseeing laser use for each site when lasers are used in multiple sites in a health care organization (eg, ambulatory surgery unit, eye clinic),
- troubleshooting equipment malfunctions,
- monitoring compliance with laser policies and procedures,
- reviewing laser-related documentation (eg, logs, laser manufacturers' IFU),
- acting as a resource to personnel,
- assessing needs for continuing education and training, and
- assisting with data gathering and quality monitoring for the facility (eg, education, credentialing, licensure).[1]

[Recommendation]

A clinical guideline recommends that the LSSC have these responsibilities.[1]

14.2 The LSSC may not be needed when the laser is used in only one location and the LSO is available.

The LSSC may also serve as the laser user or operator.[1] *[Conditional Recommendation]*

A clinical guideline recommends these criteria for the LSSC.[1]

14.3 Educate and train the LSSC as applicable to the type of lasers used in the facility and based on job responsibilities.[1] *[Recommendation]*

A clinical guideline recommends educating the LSSC.[1]

15. Laser Safety Specialist

15.1 Delegate the following responsibilities to the laser safety specialist:

- overseeing the safety of laser use in each room where a laser is used,
- supervising laser usage in a room,
- acting as a liaison between the clinical laser users and the LSO,
- troubleshooting equipment problems,
- monitoring compliance with the health care organization's laser policies and procedures,
- reviewing laser-related documentation (eg, logs, laser manufacturers' IFU),
- acting as a resource to staff members and laser users, and
- assessing needs for continuing education and training.

[Recommendation]

15.1.1 A laser safety specialist may not be needed where the laser is used in only one location and the LSO is available. *[Recommendation]*

16. Laser Operator

16.1 Assign a laser operator who has no competing responsibilities that would require leaving the laser unattended to every procedure in which a laser is used, including when the laser has a foot pedal with an activation button. *[Recommendation]*

A clinical guideline recommends that the laser operator have no conflicting duties.[1]

16.1.1 The laser operator may not be required when the laser console is controlled by the laser user. *[Conditional Recommendation]*

16.2 Delegate the following responsibilities to the laser operator:

- setting up and calibrating the laser according to the manufacturer's IFU before each use,

- confirming the power settings with the laser user before the laser is activated,
- operating the console under the direction of the laser user,
- placing the laser in stand-by mode when it is not in active use,
- removing the keys at the end of the procedure,
- assisting in the documentation of the laser parameters and safety controls as defined by facility policy and procedure,
- ensuring that appropriate PPE is being used during the procedure, and
- overseeing the safety hazards controls during operation.[1,35,40,41]

[Recommendation]

Low-quality evidence[4,9,83] and clinical guidelines[1,35,40,41] recommend all or some of the listed responsibilities.

16.3 Educate, train, and verify competency of the laser operator as applicable to the type of lasers used in the facility and based on job responsibilities, including

- laser operation principles;
- clinical applications;
- potential risks to the patient and health care personnel;
- safety procedures including the location and operation of the emergency stop button;
- care of the laser, safety equipment, and accessories; and
- hands-on use of the laser (eg, setup, testing, control panel use).[1]

[Recommendation]

A clinical guideline recommends education on this content.[1]

17. Laser User

17.1 The laser user must be credentialed by the health care organization as applicable to laser used.[79,80] *[Regulatory Requirement]*

The CMS requires credentialing of laser users.[79,80]

17.2 The laser user should only activate the laser system when in direct control of the laser hand piece.[1] *[Recommendation]*

Control of activation by the laser user assists with decreasing the risk of unintentional discharge of laser energy and minimizes the potential for patient or health care personnel injury.[9]

A clinical guideline recommends control of activation by the laser user.[1]

18. Audits

18.1 Complete a laser safety audit at least annually, or more frequently as determined by the LSO.[1] *[Recommendation]*

Low-quality evidence[9,33] and a clinical guideline[1] support conducting an audit.

18.1.1 Include the following in the laser audit:
- examining all laser-related equipment and safety devices (eg, eyewear, warning signs, inspection tracking indicators) for any damage,
- examining the laser for appropriate labeling,
- reviewing preventive maintenance and service records,
- confirming appropriate storage condition,
- verifying physical plant and use areas,
- verifying competency of the personnel in laser safety, and
- observing personnel performance of tasks related to laser use for compliance with the health care organization's written policies and procedures.[1]

[Recommendation]

A clinical guideline recommends including these steps in the audit process.[1] A laser safety audit helps verify that safety measures are in place and that safe practices are being followed.[9,33]

18.1.2 Report the results of the laser safety audit, including a proposed correction plan for any identified deficits, to the facility-designated committee or administration.[1] *[Recommendation]*

A clinical guideline recommends reporting the audit results.[1]

19. Unintentional Exposure/ Equipment Failure

19.1 When patient or personnel injuries or equipment failures occur,
- remove the device from service;
- retain all accessories and packaging if possible;
- report the adverse event details according to the health care organization's policy and procedures, including device identification and maintenance and service information; and
- follow organizational policy and procedures for seeking medical care for laser-related injuries.[1,36]

[Recommendation]

Retaining the device, accessories, and packaging assists with a complete incident investigation.[84]

Clinical guidelines recommend seeking the care of the physician after injury.[1,36]

19.2 The facility must establish a policy and procedure for labeling laser equipment that is out of service.[85] *[Regulatory Requirement]*

Developing a program and procedures for use of **lockout/tagout devices** is an OSHA requirement.[85]

19.3 The health care organization must report to the FDA and the manufacturer when a medical device is suspected to have contributed to a death or serious injury.[86] *[Regulatory Requirement]*

19.3.1 The health care organization must report to other regulatory bodies as defined by state or local regulations. *[Regulatory Requirement]*

20. Third-Party Laser Vendors

20.1 Apply all components of the laser safety program to all situations in which a laser is brought into the facility by a third-party laser vendor. *[Recommendation]*

20.2 The laser safety committee should oversee all aspects of third-party laser services and define the role of the representative from a third party. *[Recommendation]*

20.3 The LSO should
- verify that all third-party operators are properly credentialed according to the health care organization's policy;
- verify that all third-party-provided equipment is compliant with facility policies and procedures and governmental regulations, including documentation of inspection, preventive maintenance, and repair;
- maintain third-party operators' education records; and
- maintain records on the maintenance and service of third-party owned lasers.

[Recommendation]

A clinical guideline supports giving the LSO the listed responsibilities.[1]

20.4 Obtain and retain documentation of inspection, preventive maintenance, and repair for lasers brought into the facility by a third-party vendor. *[Recommendation]*

A clinical guideline supports obtaining and retaining the listed documentation.[1]

21. Education and Competency Assessment

21.1 Education, training, and competency verification must be completed for all individuals involved in laser use.[45] Education must be specific to the laser used and procedures performed; applicable to the job responsibilities; and performed periodically and when new laser equipment, accessories, or safety equipment is brought into the practice.[45] *[Regulatory Requirement]*

Education is required by OSHA.[45,46]

21.1.1 Participate in laser education at least every 5 years.[1] *[Recommendation]*

A clinical guideline recommends renewing education at least every 5 years.[1]

21.1.2 The education must include
- safety precautions for each type of laser used and
- PPE:
  o what is required;
  o when is it required;
  o how to don, doff, adjust, and wear it;
  o limitations;
  o proper care and maintenance;
  o useful life; and
  o disposal.[45,46]

[Regulatory Requirement]

Education on PPE and laser safety precautions is an OSHA requirement.[45,46]

21.1.3 The education should include
- the laser safety program and departmental policies,
- laser operation as applicable to the job responsibilities,
- hazards associated with lasers and measures to control the hazards,
- reporting of adverse events,
- instrumentation,
- emergency laser shut off,
- window coverings,
- warning signs and alarms,
- electrical safety, and
- fire prevention and management of fires.[35,41,87]

[Recommendation]

Low-quality evidence[4,9,11,12,27,33,88,89] and clinical guidelines[35,41,87] support education on laser use and precautions.

22. Documentation

22.1 Document in the patient's medical record in a manner consistent with the health care organization's policies and procedures, and include the
- wavelength used,
- safety measures implemented during laser use,
- total energy used if available and applicable,
- total activation time if available,
- on and off time for head and neck procedures,
- laser device identification (eg, serial or biomedical number), and
- patient protection used (eg, type of eyewear, eye shield).[8,9,11,33]

[Recommendation]

Documentation serves as a method of communication among all care providers involved in planning, implementing, and evaluating patient care. Documentation of nursing activities provides a description of the perioperative nursing care administered and the status of patient outcomes on transfer of care.[8,9,11,33,90]

Glossary

Anodized: A matte finish applied to metal surgical instruments to decrease reflectivity.

Aversion response time: The amount of time it takes for closure of the eyelid, eye movement, pupillary constriction, or movement of the head to avoid exposure to a bright light.

Backscatter: The reflection of the laser beam back in the direct from which it came.

Deputy laser safety officer: The person who assumes the role of the laser safety officer when the laser safety officer is not available.

Diffuse reflection: Reflection of the laser beam off a shiny object in multiple outgoing directions and at many angles, such as 30, 45, and 60 degrees.

Doped: The addition of small quantities of an element (an impurity) to a pure semiconductor to change its electrical conductivity characteristics.

Ebonized: A black finish applied to metal surgical instruments to decrease reflectivity.

Lasers: Devices that produce an intense, coherent, directional beam of light by stimulating electronic or molecular transitions to lower energy levels. An acronym for light amplification by stimulated emission of radiation.

Laser operator: The person who sets up the laser and operates the laser console to control the laser parameters under the supervision of the laser user.

Laser safety officer: The person responsible for effecting the knowledgeable evaluation of laser hazards and authorized and responsible for monitoring and overseeing the control of laser hazards.

Laser safety site contact: The designated person responsible for oversight of safe laser use in each area where a laser is used. Works under the supervision of the laser safety officer.

Laser safety specialist: The designated employee responsible for oversight of safe laser use in each room where a laser is used. Works under the supervision of the laser safety officer.

Laser system: The combination of the laser or lasers, a delivery system, a power supply, control console, mechanical housing, associated liquids and gases required for the operation of the laser, and optical components.

Laser treatment–controlled area: The room in which the laser is used. Laser-specific personal protective equipment is required in this area.

Laser user: The person credentialed by the facility to control the application of the laser for its intended purpose within the user's scope of practice, license, education, and experience.

Lockout/tagout devices: Devices that are applied to a piece of equipment that prevent it from being activated and alert everyone that the machine has malfunctioned.

Nominal hazard zone: The space in which the level of direct, reflected, or scattered radiation used during normal laser operation exceeds the applicable maximum permissible exposure. Exposure levels beyond the boundary of the nominal hazard zone are below the appropriate maximum permissible exposure level of the laser. Special eye and skin precautions must be enforced in the nominal hazard zone.

Optical density: The value that defines the ability of a filter to absorb a specific laser wavelength.

Photochemical interaction: Produced by absorption of the light into the chromophores, resulting in a biological cascade of events that relieves pain and reduces inflammation.

Photomechanical/photoacoustic interaction: Produced by a laser that uses shorter pulses of power and thermal expansion, creating acoustic waves that fracture the target tissue into smaller particles.

Photothermal interaction: Produced by a laser that uses prolonged energy exposure, leading to an increase in chromophore temperature and cellular vaporization.

Specular reflection: Reflection of the laser beam off a shiny object in a single outgoing direction at a single angle, such as 30 degrees.

References

1. American National Standards Institute; Laser Institute of America. *ANSI Z136.3-2018: American National Standard for Safe Use of Lasers in Health Care.* Orlando, FL: Laser Institute of America; 2018. [IVC]

2. Ripley PM. The physics of diode lasers. *Laser Med Sci.* 1996;11(2):71-78. [VC]

3. Müller A, Marschall S, Jensen OB, et al. Diode laser based light sources for biomedical applications. *Laser & Photonics Reviews.* 2013;7(5):605-627. [VC]

4. Mary S. Laser safety: practical measures and latest legislative requirements. *J Perioper Pract.* 2011;21(9):299-303. [VC]

5. Appendix B: Lasers used in medicine and surgery. In: American National Standards Institute; Laser Institute of America. *ANSI Z136.3-2018: American National Standard for Safe Use of Lasers in Health Care.* Orlando, FL: Laser Institute of America; 2018:54-60. [VC]

6. Section III: Chapter 6. Laser hazards. In: *OSHA Technical Manual.* Occupational Safety and Health Administration. https://www.osha.gov/dts/osta/otm/otm_iii/otm_iii_6.html. Accessed March 31, 2020. [VB]

7. Sankaranarayanan G, Resapu RR, Jones DB, Schwaitzberg S, De S. Common uses and cited complications of energy in surgery. *Surg Endosc.* 2013;27(9):3056-3072. [VA]

8. Appendix D: Use of lasers in specialties. In: American National Standards Institute; Laser Institute of America. *ANSI Z136.3-2018: American National Standard for Safe Use of Lasers in Health Care.* Orlando, FL: Laser Institute of America; 2018:72-103. [VC]

9. Laser use and safety. ECRI Institute. https://www.ecri.org/components/HRC/Pages/SurgAn17.aspx. Published September 26, 2017. Accessed March 31, 2020. [VB]

10. Vano-Galvan S, Jaen P. Complications of nonphysician-supervised laser hair removal: case report and literature review. *Can Fam Physician.* 2009;55(1):50-52. [VB]

11. Plauntz L. Guidelines for staff administering laser therapy in an office setting. *Plast Surg Nurs.* 2013;33(1):29-35. [VA]

12. De Felice E. Shedding light: laser physics and mechanism of action. *Phlebology.* 2010;25(1):11-28. [VB]

13. Technology background: surgical lasers. ECRI Institute. https://www.ecri.org/components/HDJournal/Pages/Tech-Background-Surgical-Lasers.aspx#. Published November 30, 2016. Accessed March 31, 2020. [VC]

14. Jacques SL. Laser-tissue interactions: photochemical, photothermal, and photomechanical. *Surg Clin North Am.* 1992;72(3):531-558. [VB]

15. Bahammam MA. Treatment of a gingival injury from a cosmetic laser burn: a case report. *Compend Contin Educ Dent.* 2018;39(4):238-243. [VB]

16. Zhang AY, Obagi S. Diagnosis and management of skin resurfacing-related complications. *Oral Maxillofac Surg Clin North Am.* 2009;21(1):1-12. [VB]

17. Yan Y, Olszewski AE, Hoffman MR, et al. Use of lasers in laryngeal surgery. *J Voice.* 2010;24(1):102-109. [VB]

18. Cao LY, Taylor JS, Vidimos A. Patient safety in dermatology: a review of the literature. *Dermatol Online J.* 2010;16(1):3. [VA]

19. Srinivas CR, Kumaresan M. Lasers for vascular lesions: standard guidelines of care. *Indian J Dermatol Venereol Leprol.* 2011;77(3):349-368. [IVC]

20. Tremaine AM, Avram MM. FDA MAUDE data on complications with lasers, light sources, and energy-based devices. *Lasers Surg Med.* 2015;47(2):133-140. [VA]

21. Zelickson Z, Schram S, Zelickson B. Complications in cosmetic laser surgery: a review of 494 Food and Drug Administration Manufacturer and User Facility Device Experience reports. *Dermatol Surg.* 2014;40(4):378-382. [VB]

22. Dudelzak J, Goldberg DJ. Laser safety. *Curr Probl Dermatol.* 2011;42:35-39. [VC]

23. Best C. Anesthesia for laser surgery of the airway in children. *Paediatr Anaesth.* 2009;19(Suppl 1):155-165. [VC]

24. Pierce JS, Lacey SE, Lippert JF, Lopez R, Franke JE, Colvard MD. An assessment of the occupational hazards related to medical lasers. *J Occup Environ Med.* 2011;53(11):1302-1309. [VA]

25. American National Standards Institute; Laser Institute of America. *ANSI Z136.1: American National Standard for Safe Use of Lasers.* Orlando, FL: Laser Institute of America; 2014. [IVC]

26. Barkana Y, Belkin M. Laser eye injuries. *Surv Ophthalmol.* 2000;44(6):459-478. [VB]

27. Wöllmer W, Schade G, Kessler G. Endotracheal tube fires still happen—a short overview. *Med Laser Appl.* 2010;25(2):118-125. [VA]

28. Smith LP, Roy S. Operating room fires in otolaryngology: risk factors and prevention. *Am J Otolaryngol.* 2011;32(2):109-114. [IIIB]

29. Mehta SP, Bhananker SM, Posner KL, Domino KB. Operating room fires: a closed claims analysis. *Anesthesiology.* 2013;118(5):1133-1139. [VB]

30. Guideline for a safe environment of care. In: *Guidelines for Perioperative Practice.* Denver, CO: AORN, Inc; 2020:115-150. [IVA]

31. Guideline for surgical smoke safety. In: *Guidelines for Perioperative Practice.* Denver, CO: AORN, Inc; 2020:1007-1038. [IVA]

32. 29 CFR 1926—Safety and health regulations for construction. Electronic Code of Federal Regulations. https://www.ecfr.gov/cgi-bin/retrieveECFR?gp=1&SID=63ef827aff4a5dca23aaaedc7e9e8aa1&ty=HTML&h=L&mc=true&n=pt29.8.1926&r=PART. Accessed March 31, 2020.

33. Smalley PJ. Laser safety: risks, hazards, and control measures. *Laser Ther.* 2011;20(2):95-106. [VB]

34. Thomas G, Isaacs R. Basic principles of lasers. *Anaesth Intensive Care Med.* 2011;12(12):574-577. [VC]

35. Dhepe N. Minimum standard guidelines of care on requirements for setting up a laser room. *Indian J Dermatol Venereol Leprol.* 2009;75(Suppl S2):101-110. [IVC]

36. *AST Standards of Practice for Laser Safety.* Littleton, CO: Association of Surgical Technologists; 2019. [IVC]

37. Adelman MR, Tsai LJ, Tangchitnob EP, Kahn BS. Laser technology and applications in gynaecology. *J Obstet Gynaecol.* 2013;33(3):225-231. [VC]

38. Dhar P, Malik A. Anesthesia for laser surgery in ENT and the various ventilatory techniques. *Trends in Anaesthesia and Critical Care.* 2011;1(2):60-66. [VB]

39. Seifert PC, Peterson E, Graham K. Crisis management of fire in the OR. *AORN J.* 2015;101(2):250-263. [VA]

40. Kaneko S. Safety guidelines for diagnostic and therapeutic laser applications in the neurosurgical field. *Laser Ther.* 2012;21(2):129-136. [IVC]

41. National Fire Protection Association Technical Committee on Laser Fire Protection. *NFPA 115: Standard for Laser Fire Protection.* Quincy, MA: NFPA; 2020. [IVC]

42. Fukuda TY, Jesus JF, Santos MG, Cazarini Junior C, Tanji MM, Plapler H. Calibration of low-level laser therapy equipment. *Rev Bras Fisioter.* 2010;14(4):303-308. [IIIB]

43. Grant DG, Tierney PA, Hinni ML. Custom thermoplastic mouth guard for endoscopic laser surgery. *Clin Otolaryngol.* 2009;34(5):499-500. [VC]

44. Alidina S, Hur HC, Berry WR, et al. Narrative feedback from OR personnel about the safety of their surgical practice before and after a surgical safety checklist intervention. *Int J Qual Health Care.* 2017;29(4):461-469. [IIIB]

45. 29 CFR 1910.133 - Eye and face protection. Occupational Safety and Health Administration. https://www.osha.gov/laws-regs/regulations/standardnumber/1910/1910.133. Accessed March 31, 2020.

46. 29 CFR 1910.132 - General requirements. Occupational Safety and Health Administration. https://www.osha.gov/laws-regs/regulations/standardnumber/1910/1910.132. Accessed March 31, 2020.

47. Kontadakis GA, Karagiannis D, Kandarakis AS. Macular injury with rapid onset of choroidal neovascularization from laser epilation. *JAMA Ophthalmol.* 2015;133(4):488-490. [VB]

48. Paulausky C. Laser safety: the eyes have it! *Occup Health Saf.* 2014;83(8):10-12. [VC]

49. Thach AB, Lopez PF, Snady-Mccoy LC, Golub BM, Frambach DA. Accidental Nd:YAG laser injuries to the macula. *Am J Ophthalmol.* 1995;119(6):767-773. [VB]

50. Lin LT, Liang CM, Chiang SY, Yang HM, Chang CJ. Traumatic macular hole secondary to a Q-switch alexandrite laser. *Retina.* 2005;25(5):662-665. [VB]

51. van As G. The diode laser—the importance of laser eye safety. *Dent Today.* 2011;30(6):128. [VC]

52. Guidelines for office-based laser procedures. American Society for Laser Medicine and Surgery, Inc. https://www.aslms.org/for-professionals/professional-resources/standards-of-practice/guidelines-for-office-based-laser-procedures. Published August 2, 2012. Accessed March 31, 2020. [IVC]

53. Minkis K, Whittington A, Alam M. Dermatologic surgery emergencies: complications caused by systemic reactions, high-energy systems, and trauma. *J Am Acad Dermatol.* 2016;75(2):265-284. [VB]

54. Althunayan AM, Elkoushy MA, Elhilali MM, Andonian S. Adverse events resulting from lasers used in urology. *J Endourol.* 2014;28(2):256-260. [VC]

55. PL 91-596: Occupational Safety and Health Act of 1970, as amended January 1, 2004. Occupational Safety and Health Administration. https://www.osha.gov/laws-regs/oshact/completeoshact. Accessed March 31, 2020.

56. Park JC, Herbert EN. Laser goggles alter the perceived colour of drug labels, increasing the risk for drug errors. *Can J Ophthalmol.* 2013;48(2):e27-e28. [VC]

57. Lin CC, Tseng PC, Chen CC, Woung LC, Liou SW. Iritis and pupillary distortion after periorbital cosmetic alexandrite laser. *Graefes Arch Clin Exp Ophthalmol.* 2011;249(5):783-785. [VB]

58. Halkiadakis I, Skouriotis S, Stefanaki C, et al. Iris atrophy and posterior synechiae as a complication of eyebrow laser epilation. *J Am Acad Dermatol.* 2007;57(2 Suppl):S4-S5. [VB]

59. Mueller NM, Mueller EJ. KTP photoselective laser vaporization of the prostate: indications, procedure, and nursing implications. *Urol Nurs.* 2004;24(5):373-379. [VC]

60. Hammes S, Augustin A, Raulin C, Ockenfels HM, Fischer E. Pupil damage after periorbital laser treatment of a port-wine stain. *Arch Dermatol.* 2007;143(3):392-394. [VB]

61. Huang A, Phillips A, Adar T, Hui A. Ocular injury in cosmetic laser treatments of the face. *J Clin Aesthet Dermatol.* 2018;11(2):15-18. [VA]

62. Dennis E. Decreasing airway fires. *OR Nurse 2012.* 2012;6(2):37-40. [VB]

63. Stuermer KJ, Ayachi S, Gostian AO, Beutner D, Hüttenbrink KB. Hazard of CO_2 laser-induced airway fire in laryngeal surgery: experimental data of contributing factors. *Eur Arch Otorhinolaryngol.* 2013;270(10):2701-2707. [IIIC]

64. Dhar V, Young K, Nouraei SA, et al. Impact of oxygen concentration and laser power on occurrence of intraluminal fires during shared-airway surgery: an investigation. *J Laryngol Otol.* 2008;122(12):1335-1338. [IIIB]

65. Apfelbaum JL, Caplan RA, Barker SJ, et al. Practice advisory for the prevention and management of operating room fires: an updated report by the American Society of Anesthesiologists Task Force on Operating Room Fires. *Anesthesiology.* 2013;118(2):271-290. [IVA]

66. Hammons MA, Ramey NA, Stinnett S, Woodward JA. Effects of reflected CO_2 laser energy on operative field materials: risks to patients and operating room personnel. *Ophthalmic Plast Reconstr Surg.* 2010;26(5):386-388. [IIIB]

67. Roy S, Smith LP. Prevention of airway fires: testing the safety of endotracheal tubes and surgical devices in a mechanical model. *Am J Otolaryngol.* 2015;36(1):63-66. [IIIB]

68. Coughlan CA, Verma SP. Evaluating the effects of a 532-nm fiber-based KTP laser on transoral laser surgery supplies. *Otolaryngol Head Neck Surg.* 2013;149(5):739-744. [IIIB]

69. Ahmed F, Kinshuck AJ, Harrison M, et al. Laser safety in head and neck cancer surgery. *Eur Arch Otorhinolaryngol.* 2010;267(11):1779-1784. [IIIC]

70. Li S, Chen L, Tan F. Laryngeal surgery using a CO_2 laser: is a polyvinylchloride endotracheal tube safe? *Am J Otolaryngol.* 2012;33(6):714-717. [IIIA]

71. Roy S, Smith LP. Surgical fires in laser laryngeal surgery: are we safe enough? *Otolaryngol Head Neck Surg.* 2015;152(1):67-72. [IIIB]

72. Recommendations to reduce surgical fires and related patient injury: FDA Safety Communication. US Food and Drug Administration. https://www.fda.gov/medical-devices/safety-communications/recommendations-reduce-surgical-fires-and-related-patient-injury-fda-safety-communication. Updated July 18, 2018. Accessed March 30, 2020. [VB]

73. van den Bos RR, Neumann M, Nijsten T. Laser fibre stabs the catheter: a serious complication of endovenous laser ablation. *Phlebology.* 2011;26(3):119-120. [VB]

74. Ren S, Liu P, Wang W, Yang Y. Retained foreign body after laser ablation. *Int Surg.* 2012;97(4):293-295. [VB]

75. Lekich C, Hannah P. Retained laser fibre: Insights and management. *Phlebology.* 2014;29(5):318-324. [VB]

76. Lun Y, Shen S, Wu X, Jiang H, Xin S, Zhang J. Laser fiber migration into the pelvic cavity: a rare complication of endovenous laser ablation. *Phlebology.* 2015;30(9):641-643. [VA]

77. Bozoglan O, Mese B, Inci MF, Eroglu E. A rare complication of endovenous laser ablation: intravascular laser catheter breakage. *BMJ Case Rep.* 2013;2013. [VC]

78. Sarioglu S, Polat A, Erentug V. Retained laser fiber during endovenous laser ablation. *Chirurgia.* 2014;27(3):177-178. [VB]

79. *State Operations Manual Appendix L: Guidance for Surveyors: Ambulatory Surgical Centers.* Rev. 200, 02-21-20. Centers for Medicare & Medicaid Services. https://www.cms.gov/media/423701. Accessed March 31, 2020.

80. *State Operations Manual Appendix A: Survey Protocol, Regulations and Interpretive Guidelines for Hospitals.* Rev. 200, 02-21-20. Centers for Medicare & Medicaid Services. https://www.cms.gov/media/423601. Accessed March 31, 2020.

81. Edwards B, Sams B. Overview of the Board of Laser Safety's professional certification programs for laser safety officers. *Med Laser Appl.* 2010;25(2):70-74. [VB]

82. Appendix G: Laser safety and training programs. In: American National Standards Institute; Laser Institute of America. *ANSI Z136.3-2018: American National Standard for Safe Use of Lasers in Health Care.* Orlando, FL: Laser Institute of America; 2018:108-113. [VC]

83. Ohshiro T, Ohshiro T, Sasaki K, et al. Correct calibration procedure for the Q-switched ruby laser and checking the treatment irradiation pattern. *Laser Ther.* 2013;22(3):171-180. [VB]

84. Appendix I: Medical examinations. In: American National Standards Institute; Laser Institute of America. *ANSI Z136.3-2018: American National Standard for Safe Use of Lasers in Health Care.* Orlando, FL: Laser Institute of America; 2018:117-118. [VC]

85. 29 CFR 1910.147 - The control of hazardous energy (lockout/tagout). https://www.osha.gov/laws-regs/regulations/standardnumber/1910/1910.147. Occupational Safety and Health Administration. Accessed March 31, 2020.

86. Medical Device Reporting (MDR): How to report medical device problems. US Food and Drug Administration. https://www.fda.gov/medical-devices/medical-device-safety/medical-device-reporting-mdr-how-report-medical-device-problems. Updated July 8, 2019. Accessed March 30, 2020.

87. The nurse's role in the use of laser, light, and energy emitting devices. *J Dermatol Nurses Assoc.* 2013;5(5):289-290. [IVC]

88. Wang HM, Lee KW, Tsai CJ, Lu IC, Kuo WR. Tracheostomy tube ignition during microlaryngeal surgery using diode laser: a case report. *Kaohsiung J Med Sci.* 2006;22(4):199-202. [VB]

89. AlNomair N, Nazarian R, Marmur E. Complications in lasers, lights, and radiofrequency devices. *Facial Plast Surg.* 2012;28(3):340-346. [VB]

90. Guideline for patient information management. In: *Guidelines for Perioperative Practice.* Denver, CO: AORN, Inc; 2020:357-386. [IVA]

Guideline Development Group

Lead Author: Byron L. Burlingame[1], MS, BSN, RN, CNOR, Senior Perioperative Practice Specialist, AORN, Denver, Colorado

Methodologist: Amber Wood[2], MSN, RN, CNOR, CIC, FAPIC, Editor-in-Chief, Guidelines for Perioperative Practice, AORN, Denver, Colorado

Evidence Appraisers: Byron L. Burlingame[1] and Marie A. Bashaw[3], DNP, RN, NEA-BC, Assistant Professor, Wright State University, Dayton, Ohio

Subject Matter Experts:

- Vangie V. Dennis[4], MSN, RN, CNOR, CMLSO, Executive Director Perioperative Services, WellStar Atlanta Medical Center & Atlanta Medical Center South, Georgia
- Patricia A. Owens[5], MHA, BSN, RN, CNOR, CMLSO, Laser Specialist and Management Consultant, AestheticMed Consulting International, LLC, Indio, California

Guidelines Advisory Board Members:

- Donna A. Pritchard[6], MA, BSN, RN, NE-BC, CNOR, Director of Perioperative Services, Interfaith Medical Center, Brooklyn, New York
- Brenda G. Larkin[7], MS, ACNS-BC, CNS, CNOR, Clinical Nurse Specialist, Aurora Lakeland Medical Center, Lake Geneva, Wisconsin[7]
- Elizabeth S. Pincus[8], MSN, MBA, RN, ACNS-BC, CNS-CP, CNOR, Clinical Nurse, St Francis Hospital, Roslyn, New York

External Review: Expert review comments were received from individual members of the American Association of Nurse Anesthetists (AANA), American College of Surgeons (ACS), Association for Professionals in Infection Control and Epidemiology (APIC), American Society of Anesthesiologists (ASA), International Association of Healthcare Central Service Materiel Management (IAHC-SMM), Society for Healthcare Epidemiology of America (SHEA), and the Surgical Infection Society (SIS). Their responses were used to further refine and enhance this guideline; however, their responses do not imply endorsement. The draft was also open for a 30-day public comment period.

Financial Disclosure and Conflicts of Interest

This guideline was developed, edited, and approved by the AORN Guidelines Advisory Board without external funding being sought or obtained. The Guidelines Advisory Board was entirely supported financially by the AORN and was developed without any involvement of industry.

Potential conflicts of interest for all advisory board members were reviewed before the annual meeting and each monthly conference call. Six members of the guideline development group reported no potential conflict of interest.[1-3,6-8] Two members[4,5] disclosed potential conflicts of interest. After review and discussion of these disclosures, the advisory board concluded that individuals with potential conflicts could remain on the advisory board if they reminded the advisory board of potential conflicts before any related discussion and recused themselves from a related discussion if requested.

Publication History

Originally published November 1989, *AORN Journal*, as Recommended Practices: Laser Safety in the Practice Setting. Revised November 1993.

Revised November 1997; published January 1998, *AORN Journal*, as Recommended Practices for Laser Safety in Practice Settings. Reformatted July 2000.

Revised November 2003; published in *Standards, Recommended Practices, and Guidelines*, 2004 edition. Reprinted April 2004, *AORN Journal*.

Revised October 2010 as Recommended Practices for Laser Safety in Perioperative Practice Settings for online publication in *Perioperative Standards and Recommended Practices*. Reformatted September 2012 for publication in *Perioperative Standards and Recommended Practices*, 2013 edition.

Minor editing revisions made in November 2014 for publication as Guideline for Laser Safety in *Guidelines for Perioperative Practice*, 2015 edition.

Revised and combined with the Guideline for Electrosurgery, as Guideline for Safe Use of Energy-Generating Devices, September 2016, for online publication in *Guidelines for Perioperative Practice*.

Evidence ratings revised and minor editorial changes made to conform to the current AORN Evidence Rating model, September 2019, for online publication in *Guidelines for Perioperative Practice*.

Revised July 2020 for publication in *Guidelines for Perioperative Practice* online.

Scheduled for review in 2024.

AORN GUIDELINES FOR
PERIOPERATIVE PRACTICE,
2022 EDITION

LOCAL ANESTHESIA

TABLE OF CONTENTS

[P] *indicates a recommendation or evidence relevant to pediatric care.*

MEDICAL ABBREVIATIONS & ACRONYMS

AANA – American Association of Nurse Anesthetists
ACLS - Advanced cardiac life support
ANA – American Nurses Association
ASA – American Society of Anesthesiologists
ASPAN – American Society of PeriAnesthesia Nurses
ASRA – American Society of Regional Anesthesia and Pain Medicine
CBC – Complete blood count

CNS – Central nervous system
CVS – Cardiovascular system
LAST – Local anesthetic systemic toxicity
OR – Operating room
RN – Registered nurse
SpO$_2$ – Blood oxygen level
WALANT – Wide awake local anesthesia no tourniquet

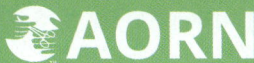

GUIDELINE FOR
CARE OF THE PATIENT RECEIVING
LOCAL-ONLY ANESTHESIA

The Guideline for Care of the Patient Receiving Local-Only Anesthesia was approved by the AORN Guidelines Advisory Board and became effective as of November 9, 2020. The recommendations in the guideline are intended to be achievable and represent what is believed to be an optimal level of practice. Policies and procedures will reflect variations in practice settings and/or clinical situations that determine the degree to which the guideline can be implemented. AORN recognizes the many diverse settings in which perioperative nurses practice; therefore, this guideline is adaptable to all areas where operative or other invasive procedures may be performed.

Purpose

This document provides guidance for the perioperative registered nurse (RN) caring for a patient receiving local-only anesthesia by injection, infiltration, **tumescent infiltration**, or topical application. This document includes guidance about patient assessment, patient monitoring, and documentation of patient care as well as guidance on recognition, assessment, and treatment of adverse reactions to local anesthesia, including **local anesthetic systemic toxicity** (LAST), local anesthetic allergies, and other adverse reactions (eg, **methemoglobinemia**). It is not the intent of this guideline to address situations that require the services of an anesthesia professional or to substitute the services of a perioperative RN in those situations that require the services of an anesthesia professional.

Local anesthetics have been in use for more than 100 years.[1] In 1884, the first surgery in which the surgeon used a local anesthetic, a cocaine solution, was performed for a patient with glaucoma.[2] Because cocaine had undesirable effects (eg, toxicity, addiction), new local anesthetics were sought to replace it.

A local anesthetic that appeared to be safer than cocaine, novocaine, was discovered in Germany in 1905. However, novocaine produced adverse effects (eg, allergic reaction) and had a short duration of action,[3] so the search continued. Lidocaine, which has a rapid onset of action and a lower toxicity incidence, was developed in the 1940s and was quickly followed by the development of mepivacaine, bupivacaine, prilocaine, etidocaine, and articaine.[2] The addition of epinephrine to local anesthetics produced the desirable effect of vasoconstriction, which extended the duration of anesthesia, reduced systemic absorption, and reduced toxicity.[4]

Epinephrine has historically been associated with causing tissue necrosis related to vasoconstriction of end arteries, particularly the digits.[5,6] The critical evaluation of the literature and investigation into the safe use of epinephrine in fingers and toes,[7] the current use of lidocaine with epinephrine by hand surgeons, and the introduction of the epinephrine vasoconstriction rescue agent, phentolamine, contributed to the increased use of the wide awake local anesthesia no tourniquet (WALANT) technique for hand surgeries.[8] The benefits of the WALANT technique include no tourniquet pain,[8,9] cost savings,[8,10-19] no preoperative testing,[8,12] no need for fasting,[8] less procedure and postanesthesia care time,[8,16,18,20-22] decreased use of supplies,[23,24] increased patient satisfaction,[12,17,25,26] and decreased anesthesia-related complications (eg, adverse effects of opiates, sedation for patients with comorbidities).[8,21] Potential risks of using the WALANT technique include vasoconstrictor-induced ischemia, bleeding, and reduced visibility at the surgical site.[27] The WALANT technique is successfully used for carpal tunnel release[13,26,28-30]; trigger finger release[9,13,29]; ganglion excision[21,29]; open reduction internal fixation radius fracture[31-34]; hardware removal[13,20]; tendon reconstruction[35]; open reduction internal fixation ankle fractures[36]; knee arthroscopy[22]; wrist arthroscopy[37]; and fracture fixation of the hand,[38] ulna,[39] and olecranon.[40]

The goal of the perioperative team is to provide safe care while minimizing pain and anxiety to the patient receiving local anesthesia. Local anesthesia is safe and effective, although, rarely, a patient may have a toxic systemic, allergic, or adverse reaction to the local anesthetic. Local anesthetic systemic toxicity may occur as serum levels of the local anesthetic increase. The symptoms of LAST may present as central nervous system (CNS) or cardiovascular system (CVS) complications or both.[41-47] Although the incidence of LAST is rare,[48-52] the consequences may be severe and potentially fatal.[41,43] Historically, allergic reactions to local anesthetics are also rare, occurring in less than 1% of all patients who receive a local anesthetic,[1,4,5,53,54] but allergic contact dermatitis from lidocaine is increasing, with a prevalence of 2.4%.[55] This increase is likely due to the increase in the number of over-the-counter medications containing lidocaine.[55]

The topics of moderate sedation analgesia; regional anesthesia; use of local anesthetics as an adjunct to general, regional, or moderate sedation; postoperative pain pumps; dental procedures; and the use of intravenous intralipid for drug toxicities resulting from non-local anesthetic medications are outside the scope of this document. Guidance for medication administration and documentation is provided in the Guideline for Medication Safety.[56]

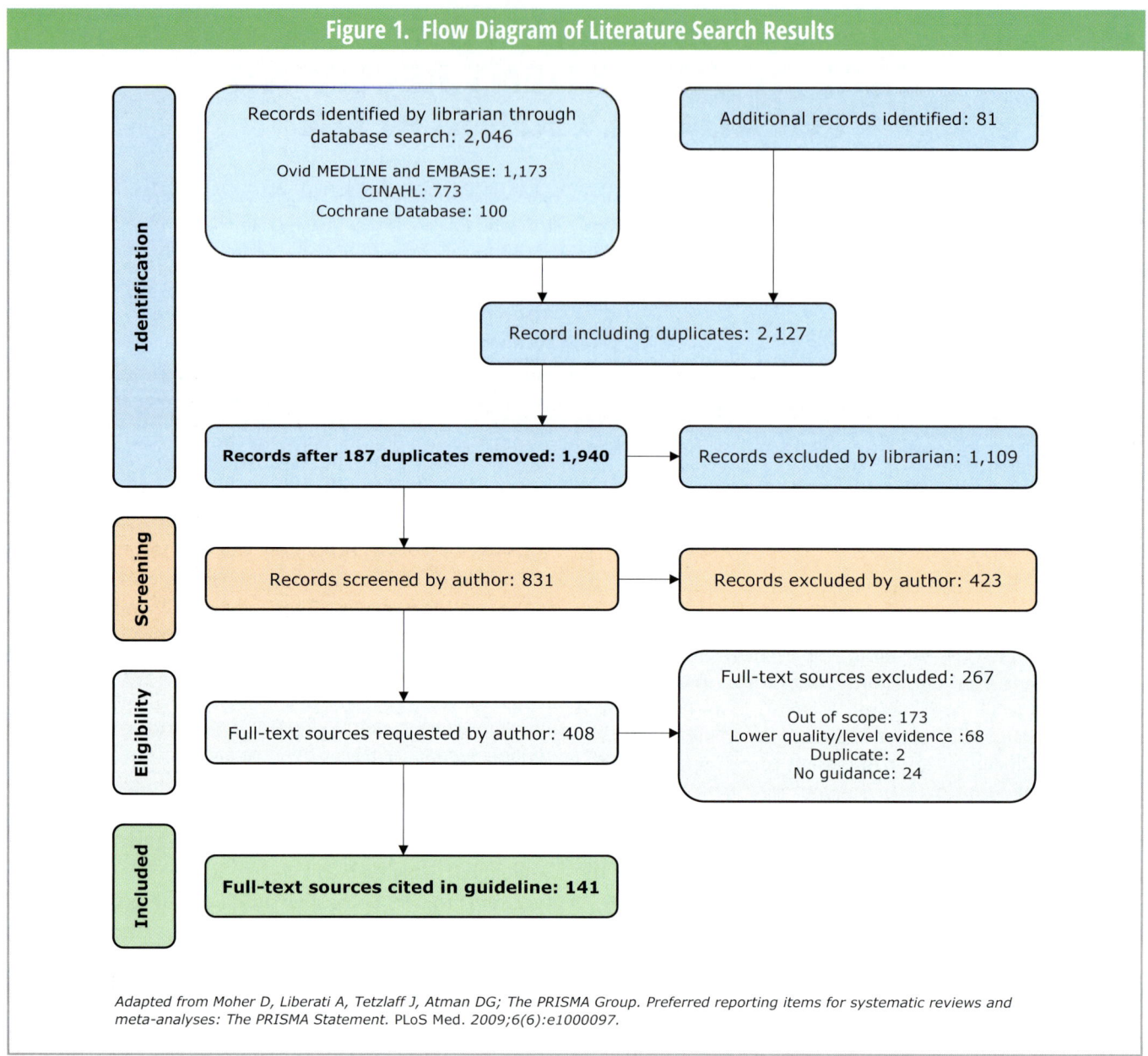

Figure 1. Flow Diagram of Literature Search Results

Records identified by librarian through database search: 2,046

Ovid MEDLINE and EMBASE: 1,173
CINAHL: 773
Cochrane Database: 100

Additional records identified: 81

Record including duplicates: 2,127

Records after 187 duplicates removed: 1,940

Records excluded by librarian: 1,109

Records screened by author: 831

Records excluded by author: 423

Full-text sources requested by author: 408

Full-text sources excluded: 267

Out of scope: 173
Lower quality/level evidence :68
Duplicate: 2
No guidance: 24

Full-text sources cited in guideline: 141

Identification

Screening

Eligibility

Included

Adapted from Moher D, Liberati A, Tetzlaff J, Atman DG; The PRISMA Group. Preferred reporting items for systematic reviews and meta-analyses: The PRISMA Statement. PLoS Med. 2009;6(6):e1000097.

Evidence Review

A medical librarian with a perioperative background conducted a systematic search of the databases Ovid MEDLINE®, Ovid Embase®, EBSCO CINAHL®, and the Cochrane Database of Systematic Reviews. The search was limited to literature published in English from January 2013 through August 2019. At the time of the initial search, weekly alerts were created on the topics included in that search. Results from these alerts were provided to the lead author until January 2020. Additional articles were requested by the lead author that were not identified in the original search (ie, did not fit the search criteria) or were discovered during the evidence appraisal process. The lead author and the medical librarian also identified relevant guidelines from government agencies, professional organizations, and standards-setting bodies.

Search terms included *ACLS, ACLS certified, advanced cardiac life support, allergic reaction, allergy, ambulatory surgical procedures, analgesia, anaphylactic reaction, anaphylaxis, anesthesia (local), anesthetics (local), blood pressure, blood pressure determination, bupivacaine, complications (intraoperative), complications (postoperative), drug hypersensitivity, elective surgical procedures, epinephrine, Exparel, heart rate, heart rate determination, hypersensitivity, infiltration anesthesia, intraoperative complications, LAST assessment, lidocaine, lidocaine with epinephrine, liposomal bupivacaine, liposomal lidocaine, local anesthesia, local anesthetic systemic toxicity, local only anesthesia, Marcaine, minor surgical procedures, monitoring (physiologic), nurse's role, nurse's scope of practice, patient monitoring, perioperative nursing, physical examination, physical reaction, physiologic monitoring, postoperative complications, pulse, risk assessment, SALANT, Sensorcaine, sodium bicarbonate, straight local* procedures no anesthesia provider, surgeon administered local or regional anesthesia, surgery (elective), surgery (operative), surgical nursing, surgical procedures (operative), topical anesthesia, vital signs, WALANT, wide awake local anesthesia, and Xylocaine.

Included were research and non-research literature in English, complete publications, and publications with dates within the time restriction when available. Excluded were non-peer-reviewed publications and those published prior to January 2013 when more recent evidence was available. Editorials, news items, and other brief items were excluded. Low-quality evidence was excluded when higher-quality evidence was available (Figure 1).

Articles identified in the search were provided to the project team for evaluation. The team consisted of the lead author and one evidence appraiser. The lead author and the evidence appraiser reviewed and critically appraised each article using the AORN Research or Non-Research Evidence Appraisal Tools as appropriate. The literature was independently evaluated and appraised according to the strength and quality of the evidence. Each article was then assigned an appraisal score. The appraisal score is noted in brackets after each reference as applicable.

Each recommendation rating is based on a synthesis of the collective evidence, a benefit-harm assessment, and consideration of resource use. The strength of the recommendation was determined using the AORN Evidence Rating Model and the quality and consistency of the evidence supporting a recommendation. The recommendation strength rating is noted in brackets after each recommendation.

Note: The evidence summary table is available at http://www.aorn.org/evidencetables/.

Editor's note: MEDLINE is a registered trademark of the US National Library of Medicine's Medical Literature Analysis and Retrieval System, Bethesda, MD. Embase is a registered trademark of Elsevier B.V., Amsterdam, The Netherlands. CINAHL, Cumulative Index to Nursing and Allied Health Literature, is a registered trademark of EBSCO Industries, Birmingham, AL. Exparel is a registered trademark of Pacira Pharmaceuticals, Inc, Parsippany-Troy Hills, NJ. Marcaine is a registered trademark of Hospira, Inc, Lake Forest, IL. Sensorcaine and Xylocaine are registered trademarks of Fresenius Kabi, Lake Zurich, IL.

1. Preoperative Care

1.1 **Perform and document a preoperative nursing assessment for the patient receiving local-only anesthesia.** *[Recommendation]*

The American Nurses Association (ANA) *Nursing: Scope and Standards of Practice*[57] and the AORN *Standards of Perioperative Nursing*[58] direct the RN to collect patient health data that are relevant to the patient's care. Performing a patient assessment

before an intervention is one standard of perioperative nursing practice.[58]

The benefits of performing a nursing assessment include the opportunity to identify allergies and comorbidities that might affect the absorption of the local anesthetic; to obtain baseline measures of vital signs, pain, and anxiety; and to evaluate the patient's level of consciousness. No research studies were found that specifically addressed preoperative nursing assessment of the patient receiving local-only anesthesia. Research is needed to define the essential elements of patient assessment that will promote safe and effective use of local-only anesthesia in surgical procedures.

1.2 **During the preoperative nursing assessment, review the patient's**
- **allergies and sensitivities (eg, medications, tape, latex)**[59-61];
- **age;**
- **height, weight, and body mass index**[59];
- **current medications and use of alternative/ complementary therapies**[56,59];
- **NPO status**[59];
- **medical history (eg, history and physical, progress notes)**[61,62];
- **laboratory test results**[59,60];
- **diagnostic test results**[59,60];
- **baseline cardiac status (eg, heart rate, blood pressure)**[59,60];
- **baseline respiratory status (eg, rate, rhythm, blood oxygen level [SpO$_2$])**[59,60];
- **baseline skin condition (eg, rash, breaks, ecchymosis)**[59,60];
- **baseline neurological status (eg, cognitive ability, mental status)**[59,60];
- **sensory impairments (eg, visual, auditory)**[59,60];
- **physical impairments (eg, difficulty walking, history of falls)**[59];
- **ability to tolerate the required operative position with draping for the duration of the procedure**[60];
- **anxiety level**[60,61];
- **pain level**[59,60];
- **previous surgery and anesthesia**[59];
- **perceptions of surgery**[60]**; and**
- **need for intravenous access.**

[Recommendation]

The American Society of PeriAnesthesia Nurses (ASPAN) *Perianesthesia Nursing Standards, Practice Recommendations and Interpretive Statements* recommends an assessment before a surgical procedure.[59] The preoperative assessment integrates the physical findings and helps identify any risk factors that may lead to complications.[63] Preoperative vital signs provide a baseline reference for comparison if there is an adverse reaction to the local anesthetic.

1.2.1 **Identify patients at increased risk for LAST before using local anesthetics. Patient factors that increase the risk for LAST include**
- **extremes of age (ie, younger than 16 years, older than 60 years**[44]**),**[45,64]
- **low muscle mass**[45] **(eg, neonates, infants, debilitated older adults),**[64]
- **frailty,**[65]
- **female sex,**[64]
- **cardiac disease (eg, conduction abnormalities, arrhythmias, ischemia, congestive heart failure, low ejection fraction**[64,65]**),**[45,64]
- **metabolic disease (eg, diabetes mellitus, mitochondrial disease),**[64,65]
- **liver disease,**[45,65]
- **CNS diseases,**[64]
- **low plasma binding (eg, liver disease, malnourishment, infancy, pregnancy),**[64]
- **acidosis,**[65] **and**
- **use of medications that inhibit sodium channels.**[65]

[Recommendation]

The assessment provides important information regarding underlying conditions (eg, cardiac, hepatic, renal) that may affect the patient's ability to metabolize the local anesthetic and place him or her at risk for developing LAST.

1.3 **A physical acuity assessment tool (eg, the American Society of Anesthesiologists [ASA] Physical Status Classification**[66] **[Table 1]) may be used to determine patient acuity.**[62] *[Conditional Recommendation]*

Use of a physical assessment tool with interrater reliability provides an objective and consistent means for assessing the patient's acuity.

1.3.1 **If there is a concern regarding the patient's acuity or anxiety level, consult with the surgeon or anesthesia provider to determine the plan of care.** *[Recommendation]*

Moderate-quality evidence supports consulting a surgeon or anesthesia provider about the patient's acuity or anxiety level.

Tantri et al[67] retrospectively reviewed 270 cataract surgeries performed under local anesthesia and monitored by RNs. During the presurgical evaluation, patients were classified as ASA I (n = 1), ASA II (n = 150), and ASA III (n = 119). Anesthesia consultation was requested in 24 cases (8.9%); no consultations were requested for the ASA I patient, five consultations were requested for ASA II patients,

Table 1. Physical Status Classification		
Status	**Definition of Patient Status**	**Example**
P1	A normal healthy patient	No physiologic, psychological, biochemical, or organic disturbance.
P2	A patient with mild systemic disease	Cardiovascular disease, asthma, chronic bronchitis, obesity, or diabetes mellitus.
P3	A patient with severe systemic disease	Cardiovascular or pulmonary disease that limits activity; severe diabetes with systemic complications; history of myocardial infarction, angina pectoris, or poorly controlled hypertension.
P4	A patient with severe systemic disease that is a constant threat to life	Severe cardiac, pulmonary, renal, hepatic, or endocrine dysfunction.
P5	A moribund patient who is not expected to survive without the operation	Surgery is done as a last recourse or resuscitative effort; major multi-system or cerebral trauma, ruptured aneurysm, or large pulmonary embolus.
P6	A declared brain-dead patient whose organs are being removed for donor purposes	

Reproduced with permission from the American Society of Anesthesiologists, Park Ridge, IL.

and 19 consultations were requested for ASA III patients. Most anesthesia consultations resulted in no intervention. Only one patient with an ASA III classification required anesthesia services of monitored anesthesia care due to complications of vitreous loss, bullous subconjunctival hemorrhage, and eye pain. In this study, cataract surgery performed with RN monitoring was associated with a low rate of anesthesia consultations. The ASA III patients were more likely than the ASA II patients to require anesthesia consultation and intervention.

Mitchell[68] surveyed 214 patients undergoing outpatient surgery with local or regional anesthesia and found that 77% of the patients experienced preoperative anxiety. Causes of the apprehension included how long the anesthetic would last and how long the numbness of the anesthetic would last. Intraoperative concerns included needing more than one injection, being awake during the procedure, and hearing what the physicians and nurses were saying during the procedure.

1.4 **Provide patient education regarding perioperative care during local-only anesthesia, including**

- the expected sequence of events[68,69] before, during, and immediately after the procedure;
- instructions on completing a pain-level assessment (eg, visual analog scale, pain score);
- how to request additional pain relief measures during and after the procedure;
- intraoperative symptoms (eg, tinnitus, metallic taste, lightheadedness, dizziness, anxiety) to report to the perioperative team, and
- postoperative symptoms to report to a designated health care provider.

[Recommendation] P

One of a nurse's primary responsibilities is providing patient education.[58] Three moderate-quality studies demonstrated the importance of preoperative education and communication to reduce patient anxiety about undergoing a surgical procedure with a local-only anesthetic.

El Hachem et al[70] used self-administered questionnaires to evaluate the distress of 388 children undergoing dermatologic surgery under local anesthesia. The children and their parents received oral and written therapeutic education measures that included structured information and a cartoon brochure illustrating the procedure. The authors concluded that specific measures for therapeutic pediatric patient education may be helpful in limiting discomfort, anxiety, and pain perception associated with procedures performed under local anesthesia. Further controlled studies are required to evaluate the benefits of specific therapeutic education measures.

Mitchell[69] surveyed 214 adult surgical patients regarding their surgical experience. The author concluded that providing information about the intraoperative care (eg, operating room [OR] environment, communication during the procedure, the length of the anesthetic) helps to reduce the anxiety of the surgical patient. Benefits include the potential for increased patient cooperation, compliance with postoperative instructions, and management of anxiety and pain. In another article describing the same study, Mitchell[68] reported that 54% of the patients stated it would be calming to have the nurses explain the events.

1.4.1 Use teaching strategies that are appropriate to the patient's and designated caregiver's learning needs and style,[59] language preference,[59] culture,[59] health literacy,[71] cognitive ability, and developmental level.[58] [Recommendation] P

1.4.2 Allow time for the patient's and designated caregiver's questions.[72] [Recommendation] P

1.4.3 Assess the patient's and designated caregiver's comprehension of new information.[60] [Recommendation] P

2. Intraoperative Care

2.1 Monitor and document the patient's physiological and psychological responses, identify nursing diagnoses based on patient assessment, and implement the plan of care. [Recommendation]

Patient assessment, diagnosis, and implementation are standards of perioperative nursing practice.[58] The ANA Nursing: Scope and Standards of Practice[57] and the AORN Standards of Perioperative Nursing[58] direct the RN to collect patient health data that are relevant to the patient's situation (eg, surgical or invasive procedure), analyze the assessment data, and implement nursing interventions.

2.1.1 Determine the plan of care based on the patient's condition and needs and the procedure to be performed, including
- the parameters to be monitored (eg, heart rate and rhythm, blood pressure, level of consciousness),
- monitoring frequency (eg, baseline, after local anesthetic administration, every 5 minutes, post procedure, before discharge[73]), and
- documentation.

[Recommendation]

Moderate-quality evidence and guidelines, including the ASA Standards for Basic Anesthetic Monitoring[74] and the American Association of Nurse Anesthetists (AANA) Standards for Nurse Anesthesia Practice,[75] support monitoring during general anesthesia, regional anesthesia, and monitored anesthesia care. Additionally, the ASA standards recommend monitoring the adequacy of ventilation by continual observation of qualitative clinical signs during regional anesthesia with no sedation and local anesthesia with no sedation.[74] A limitation of the evidence for local-only anesthesia is a lack of studies identifying the parameters to monitor or the optimal frequency for monitoring during local-only anesthesia procedures. Monitoring parameters and frequency are unresolved issues that warrant further research.

Kruger et al[76] conducted a retrospective review to investigate the relationship between prolonged noninvasive blood pressure measurement intervals and the incidence of hypotension during procedures performed with general anesthesia. Their analysis showed that noninvasive blood pressure measurement intervals longer than 6 minutes and

10 minutes were associated with approximately a fourfold greater incidence of hypotension.

The ASA standards require the continual (ie, "repeated, regularly and frequently in steady rapid succession"[74(p4)]) evaluation of the patient's oxygenation, ventilation, and circulation.[74]

In the case of *Messer v Martin,* the court upheld the standard of care to monitor the patient's vital signs during and after a procedure performed with the patient under local anesthesia. In this case, a patient underwent a surgical procedure with local anesthesia and then fainted in the elevator after leaving the clinic. The patient filed suit against the physician, the clinic, and the professional liability carrier for neglecting to monitor her postoperative vital signs and was granted a summary judgment. An RN acting as an expert witness stated in a deposition that the standard of care was to monitor the patient's vital signs (ie, blood pressure, pulse). The assigned nurse had failed to monitor the vital signs during or after the procedure.[73]

The benefits of patient monitoring during local-only anesthesia procedures include early detection and recognition of a deviation from the patient's baseline and opportunity to implement corrective actions.

2.1.2 **Baseline and intraoperative patient assessment, monitoring, and documentation may include**

- **pulse(s),**
- **blood pressure,**[65,74]
- **heart rhythm and rate,**[65,74]
- **respiratory rate,**[62]
- **SpO$_2$ by pulse oximetry,**[62,65,74]
- **pain level,**
- **anxiety level, and**
- **level of consciousness.**
[Conditional Recommendation]

The American Society of Regional Anesthesia and Pain Medicine (ASRA) *Checklist for Treatment of Local Anesthetic Systemic Toxicity*[65] recommends using the standard ASA monitors during procedures performed with local anesthesia. The AANA recommends monitoring, evaluating, and documenting the patient's physiologic conditions.[75] The ASA requires the continual evaluation of the patient's oxygenation, ventilation, and circulation.[74]

Patient anxiety may manifest as a needle phobia, a panic attack, or a vasovagal response.[4] A vasovagal response may occur any time before, during, or after the procedure and present as lightheadedness, nausea, diaphoresis, tinnitus, visual disturbance, confusion, pallor, bradycardia, and hypotension.[5]

There is a lack of evidence on monitoring physiological parameters and documentation during local-only anesthesia procedures.[74] The benefits of patient monitoring during local-only procedures include early recognition of a deviation from the patient's baseline and the opportunity to implement corrective actions.

2.2 **Calculate and identify the patient-specific local anesthetic maximum dose**[77,78] **by consulting with the licensed independent practitioner, the health care organization's medication formulary, a pharmacist, the product information sheet, and published reference material before administering the local anesthetic.**[56] *[Recommendation]*

Each local anesthetic has a recommended maximum safe dose (ie, mg/Kg). Patient factors (eg, cardiac, renal, hepatic dysfunction) may alter the total local anesthetic dose calculations.[79,80]

2.2.1 **During the preoperative briefing, verify the patient-specific maximum dose and discuss the patient's risk factors for developing LAST.**[64,77,78] *[Recommendation]*

Patient factors can reduce the threshold for developing LAST so that even a normally safe serum concentration of local anesthetic can lead to symptoms of instability. Local anesthetic systemic toxicity can result from the interaction of patient-specific factors, the peak plasma anesthetic concentration, and the properties of the local anesthetic being used.[79]

Tanawuttiwat et al[81] reported on the case of a patient undergoing implantation of an internal cardioverter defibrillator under local anesthesia. The surgical site at the left infraclavicular area was infiltrated with 20 mL 2% lidocaine followed by an additional 10 mL 2% lidocaine to relieve the patient's discomfort. A contrast venogram showed an obstruction in the axillary-subclavian system, causing the team to attempt the procedure on the right side. The new surgical site was infiltrated with 30 mL 2% lidocaine. While the surgeon was closing the new surgical site, the patient suffered a tonic-clonic seizure followed by pulseless electrical activity. The patient was successfully resuscitated. The patient's lidocaine level drawn during resuscitation was 8.7 mcg/mL. The normal value at this organization ranged from 1.5 mcg/mL to 5.0 mcg/mL. Factors contributing to this patient's lidocaine toxicity were advanced heart failure and age and mixed metabolic and respiratory acidosis. The authors recommended that risk factors for lidocaine toxicity be identified before surgery.[81]

2.2.2 Use the lowest effective dose of local anesthetic specific for each delivery method (eg, injection, topical) to achieve the desired effect.[64,65] [Recommendation]

The ASRA Practice Advisory on Local Anesthetic Systemic Toxicity[64] recommends using the lowest effective dose of local anesthetic as a means of preventing LAST.

2.3 Monitor the patient during and after completion of the local anesthetic administration according to the health care organization's policy.[65] [Recommendation] P

Signs of clinical toxicity may be delayed 30 minutes or longer depending on patient-specific characteristics (eg, pediatric, geriatric) and the type of local anesthetic administration (eg, topical, injection).[65]

3. Adverse Reactions

3.1 Implement strategies for assessing, monitoring, treating, and preventing LAST. [Recommendation]

The ASRA *Practice Advisory on Local Anesthetic Systemic Toxicity,*[64] the Association of Anesthetists of Great Britain and Ireland *AAGBI Safety Guideline: Management of Severe Local Anaesthetic Toxicity,*[82] and the Japanese Society of Anesthesiologists "Practical guide for the management of systemic toxicity caused by local anesthetics"[83] describe the signs and symptoms of LAST. The classic description is that LAST is typified by early signs of subjective symptoms of CNS excitement such as agitation, auditory changes, metallic taste, or an abrupt onset of psychiatric symptoms. The early symptoms are followed by seizures, CNS depression (ie, drowsiness, coma, respiratory arrest), and initial signs of cardiac toxicity (eg, hypertension, tachycardia, ventricular arrhythmias) followed by cardiac depression (eg, bradycardia, conduction block, asystole, decreased contractility, hypotension).[64]

3.1.1 Assess the patient for local anesthetic systemic toxicity, including[65]
- CNS signs and symptoms:
  - metallic taste,[64,65,83]
  - perioral numbness (eg, tongue, lips),[42,65,83]
  - auditory changes (eg, tinnitus),[48,64,65,83]
  - agitation,[48,64,65,83]
  - dizziness,[48,65,83]
  - diplopia,[65]
  - dysarthria (eg, slurred speech),[42,48,83]
  - shivering,[79]
  - tremors,[48,79]
  - delirium,[42,83]
  - syncope,[48,83]
  - seizures,[48,64,65,83]
  - respiratory arrest,[64] and
  - coma[64,65]; and
- CVS signs and symptoms:
  - bradycardia/hypotension or tachycardia/hypertension (initially),[64,65]
  - bradycardia/progessive hypotension (with increased toxicity),[64,65] and
  - ventricular arrhythmias (ventricular tachycardia, Torsades de Pointes, ventricular fibrillation, or asystole).[48,64]

[Recommendation]

The timing of LAST symptoms varies. Symptoms that occur in less than 60 seconds after injection suggest intravascular injection of local anesthetic with direct access to the brain. Symptoms that occur 1 to 5 minutes after injection suggest intermittent intravascular injection, lower extremity injection, or delayed tissue absorption.[64]

Approximately one-third of patients present with both CNS and CVS signs and symptoms (eg, hypertension or hypotension and electrocardiogram changes), 43% present with only CNS symptoms (eg, seizure, loss of consciousness, prodromes, agitation), and 24% present with only CVS symptoms (eg, bradycardia/hypotension, dysrhythmias, conduction delay, cardiac arrest).[64]

The CNS signs and symptoms of LAST can be divided into three phases: initial, excitation, and depression.[84] During the initial stages of LAST, the patient may exhibit prodromal symptoms, such as a metallic taste,[64,65,83] numbness of the tongue and lips,[65,83] auditory changes (eg, tinnitus),[64,65,83] dizziness,[65,83] and seizures.[64,65,83,84] During the excitation phase, patients may experience tonic-clonic convulsions. During the depression phase, patients may experience unconsciousness, CNS depression, and respiratory arrest.[84]

The CVS signs and symptoms of LAST also can be divided into three phases.[84] The initial phase includes hypertension and tachycardia during the CNS excitation phase.[84] The intermediate phase includes myocardial depression, decreased cardiac output, and mild to moderate hypotension.[84] The third, terminal phase, includes peripheral vasodilation, profound hypotension, sinus bradycardia, conduction defects, ventricular dysrhythmias, and cardiovascular collapse.[84]

The incidence of LAST is rare, but it remains a serious complication of local anesthetic use.[64] The reported incidence of LAST comes from registry studies, administrative databases, case reports, and case series.[41] Moderate-level studies have examined the incidence of LAST in orthopedic patients receiving peripheral nerve blocks.[49,50,52]

Mörwald et al[50] identified 238,473 patients from a large administrative database who had received a peripheral nerve block for total joint arthroplasty between 2006 and 2014. The cumulative rate of all studied outcomes (eg, cardiac arrest, seizures) in all procedures (ie, total hip replacement, total knee replacement, total shoulder replacement) during the study period was 1.8 per 1,000 peripheral nerve blocks. The authors concluded that improvements in the application of peripheral nerve blocks (eg, use of ultrasound guidance) have led to a decreased rate of LAST and the related complications; however, because LAST may cause significant harm to the patient, appropriate resources should be available wherever regional anesthesia is performed.

Rubin et al[52] studied 710,327 patients who underwent hip, knee, or shoulder arthroplasty with a peripheral nerve block between 1998 and 2013. The average adjusted incidence of LAST was 1.04 per 1,000 peripheral nerve blocks, with a decreasing trend during the 15-year study period. Peripheral nerve blocks used in conjunction with shoulder arthroplasty had the highest incidence of LAST compared to hip and knee arthroplasty. Local anesthetic systemic toxicity continues to be a rare, clinically relevant complication of peripheral nerve blocks.

Awareness, knowledge, and understanding of LAST has increased from clinical cases reports, laboratory investigations, studies, literature reviews, and education programs.[48] Based on case reports,[48,85,86] LAST can occur after the inadvertent intravascular injection of a local anesthetic,[87-91] topical administration of a local anesthetic[92,93,94] (eg, oropharyngeal spray[95,96]), and local anesthetic overdose.[77,97]

Byrne and Engelbrecht[84] reviewed the toxicity of local anesthetic agents and concluded that no dose of local anesthetic is safe if administered incorrectly (eg, intravascularly, intra-arterially). The authors found that toxicity is dependent on the absolute plasma level and the rate of the rise in the plasma level. Most incidences of toxicity are caused by intravascular injection of local anesthetic, but an intra-arterial injection is more dangerous than an intravascular injection. Bupivacaine, levobupivacaine, and ropivacaine are more toxic than lidocaine and prilocaine. In 17 of 20 case reports about LAST, the local anesthetic used was ropivacaine or bupivacaine.

Di Gregorio et al[98] retrospectively reviewed 93 reports of LAST published during a 30-year period from 1979 to 2009. The cases were analyzed for onset of toxicity and signs and symptoms. The onset of LAST generally occurred after a single injection of a local anesthetic. Onset occurred in less than 1 minute in more than 50% of the cases and in less than 5 minutes in 75% of the cases. The median time for onset of signs of toxicity was 52.5 seconds. In 25% of the cases, symptoms occurred 5 minutes or more after initial injection. In a single case, the symptoms of LAST occurred at 60 minutes. Central nervous system symptoms were the most common manifestation of LAST, occurring in 44% of the reports; CVS symptoms occurred in 11% of the reports, and a combination of CNS and CVS symptoms occurred in 45% of the reports.

Wolfe and Butterworth[99] reviewed the mechanisms and toxicity of LAST and concluded that short-acting and lower-potency local anesthetics (eg, lidocaine, mepivacaine) depressed cardiac contractility without causing cardiac arrhythmias. The authors further concluded that longer-acting and higher-potency local anesthetics (eg, bupivacaine, levobupivacaine, ropivacaine) produced conduction defects and cardiac arrhythmias with or without reduced contractile function. A lower-ratio dose of bupivacaine, levobupivacaine, and ropivacaine can produce cardiovascular toxicity versus CNS toxicity. Central nervous system toxicity from local anesthetics is generally easier to manage and provides better chances for recovery than treatment of cardiovascular toxicity. The outcomes of cardiovascular toxicity from local anesthetics may be serious injury or death.

3.1.2 **If LAST is suspected or if signs and symptoms of LAST occur,**
- **stop the administration of the local anesthetic;**[43,65,82,83]
- **call for help (eg, code team, anesthesia professional, 911, LAST rescue kit**[100]**);**[65,82,83]
- **maintain the airway;**[43,64,82,83]
- **ventilate with 100% oxygen;**[43,65,82,83]
- **assist with resuscitation (ie, basic or advanced cardiac life support [See Recommendation 6.2.2]);**[82,83]
- **be prepared to establish or assist with IV access;**[82,83,101] **and**
- **be prepared to assist with the administration of 20% lipid emulsion therapy (Table 2).**[65,82]

[Recommendation]

Prompt and effective airway management is important for preventing hypoxia, hypercapnia, and acidosis, which can potentiate LAST.[64] The ASRA Practice Advisory on Local Anesthetic

Table 2. Treatment for Local Anesthetic Systemic Toxicity (LAST)

- Infuse lipid emulsion therapy at first sign of LAST after airway management.[1,2]
  - 20% lipid emulsion bolus
- 100 mL over 2 to 3 minutes if the patient weighs more than 70 kg (154 lb) and
- 1.5 mL/kg over 2 to 3 minutes if the patient weighs less than 70 kg[1,2]
  - 20% lipid emulsion infusion
- 200 mL to 250 mL over 15 to 20 minutes if the patient weighs more than 70 kg and
- 0.25 mL/kg/minute if the patient weighs less than 70 kg[1,2]
  - Continue infusion for at least 10 minutes after attaining circulatory stability.[1]
- Reduce individual epinephrine doses to ≤ 1mcg/kg[1,2]
- Avoid vasopressin, calcium channel blockers, beta blockers, or local anesthetics[1,2]
- Control seizures, benzodiazepines preferred[1,2]
- Avoid large doses of propofol in patients showing signs of cardiovascular instability[2]

References

1. Neal JM, Barrington MJ, Fettiplace MR, et al. The third American Society of Regional Anesthesia and Pain Medicine practice advisory on local anesthetic systemic toxicity: executive summary 2017. Reg Anesth Pain Med. 2018;43(2):113-123.
2. Checklist for treatment of local anesthetic systemic toxicity (LAST). https://www.asra.com/content/documents/asra_last_checklist_2018.pdf. Accessed August 31, 2020.

Systemic Toxicity,[64] the Association of Anesthetists of Great Britain and Ireland AAGBI Safety Guideline: Management of Severe Local Anaesthetic Toxicity,[82] the Japanese Society of Anesthesiologists "Practical guide for the management of systemic toxicity caused by local anesthetics,"[83] and the American Heart Association guidelines for cardiac arrest in special situations[102] provide guidance for treating LAST.

The use of lipid emulsion therapy for the effective treatment of LAST started with animal testing in 1998 followed by reports of the first clinical uses in 2006.[103] Current recommendations have evolved from low levels of evidence (eg, laboratory studies,[104-106] case reports[77,87-89,91-93,97,107]) of lipid emulsion treatment for LAST. At the first signs of LAST, ASRA recommends managing the airway and then administering 20% lipid emulsion therapy.[64,65]

3.1.3 Store LAST rescue kits where they are immediately available to areas where local anesthetics are used (eg, regional block areas, ORs).[100] Include the following in the kit:

- lipid emulsion 20% (1 L total),[100]
- large syringes (eg, 50 mL) and needles for administration,
- IV administration supplies (eg, tubing, catheters), and
- the ASRA LAST Checklist.[65,100]

[Recommendation]

Low-quality evidence details the contents of a LAST rescue kit.[65,100] Berrío Valencia and Vargas Silva[100] described placing the LAST res-

cue kits in the area where regional blocks are performed and in the OR storage area (eg, OR medication room) for quick access.

3.1.4 Continue monitoring the patient for 4 to 6[43] hours after a cardiovascular event and at least 2 hours after a CNS event.[65] *[Recommendation]*

The ASRA Checklist for Treatment of Local Anesthetic Systemic Toxicity[65] recommends prolonged monitoring of 4 to 6 hours after a cardiovascular event and at least 2 hours after a CNS event. Cardiovascular depression caused by local anesthetics can persist or recur after treatment.[65] A case study also supports the intervention. After the successful resuscitation with cardiopulmonary resuscitation and lipid emulsion of a patient who received an accidental intravascular injection of bupivacaine, Marwick et al[108] reported cardiac toxicity 40 minutes after the cessation of lipid emulsion therapy. The authors attributed the cardiovascular instability to a recurrence of LAST after lipid rescue.

3.1.5 Implement LAST prevention strategies when administering local anesthetics, including

- using the lowest effective dose to achieve the desired effect,[64,65]
- injecting the local anesthetic incrementally,[64,65]
- aspirating the needle and syringe before each injection,[64,65]
- being aware of the additive effect of local anesthetics,[64]

- using ultrasound guidance when performing peripheral nerve blocks,[49,51] and
- discussing the dosing parameters of the local anesthetic in the preoperative briefing.[64,65]

[Recommendation]

The ASRA Practice Advisory on Local Anesthetic Systemic Toxicity[64] and the Checklist for Treatment of Local Anesthetic Systemic Toxicity (LAST)[65] recommend risk-reduction strategies to prevent LAST.

3.2 Implement strategies for assessing and treating an allergic reaction to the local anesthetic. [Recommendation]

Allergic reactions to local anesthetics are rare, occurring in less than 1% of all patients who receive a local anesthetic.[54,109,110] The primary symptoms of an immediate allergic reaction to a local anesthetic are cutaneous and occur within a few minutes of the injection, although symptoms may occur as late as 1 month after the injection.[111] An adverse reaction to a local anesthetic mimicking an allergy may be caused by anxiety, intravascular administration of the local anesthetic, intravascular absorption of epinephrine, local anesthetic overdose, toxic levels caused by a lack of metabolism, and intolerance.[4] Anxiety, fear of needles, and fear of injection-site pain can trigger a vasovagal response (eg, lightheadedness, diaphoresis, nausea, bradycardia, hypotension) that can present similarly to allergic reactions.[5]

Moderate-quality evidence varies regarding the frequency of an allergy to a local anesthetic. To et al[55] retrospectively reviewed the charts of 1,819 patients who underwent patch testing for suspected allergic contact dermatitis. The overall prevalence of allergic contact dermatitis was 2.4%. Benzocaine had the highest prevalence followed by lidocaine. The authors found that allergic contact dermatitis from lidocaine is increasing. Because lidocaine is the active ingredient in several over-the-counter pain or itch relief lotions, creams, sprays, and drops, the authors attributed the increase to the growing number of these products and the aging population that frequently uses these preparations.

Moderate-level studies found occurrences of local anesthetic allergy were rare.[109,112,113] Two retrospective reviews led by Kvisselgaard[114,115] in Denmark demonstrated that none of the patients referred to the regional allergy clinic for a suspected immediate-type allergy to local anesthetics reacted to local anesthetics on provocation. Limitations of these two studies is generalizability. Moderate-quality evidence supports allergy testing and evaluation (eg, intradermal skin testing, provocation) to make a final diagnosis of an allergy to a local anesthetic.[116-119]

3.2.1 Recognize and assess the signs and symptoms of an allergic reaction to a local anesthetic, including

- anxiety,[112]
- bronchospasm,[112]
- dizziness,[61,109,112]
- dyspnea,[112]
- erythema,[109,113]
- edema,[109,112,113]
- heart arrhythmias (ie, tachycardia,[5,61,112] bradycardia[5,112]),[109]
- hypertension,[61,109]
- hypotension,[5,109,112,113]
- nausea,[109,112]
- ocular reactions,[61]
- palpitations,[109,112,113]
- pruritus,[109,112,113]
- rash,[109,112]
- syncope,[61,109,112,113] and
- urticaria.[5,109,112,113]

[Recommendation]

Moderate-quality studies[109,112,113] and lower-level evidence (eg, a literature review[110], case reports[120-129]) describe the systemic and local signs and symptoms of an allergic reaction to a local anesthetic.

3.2.2 Notify the licensed independent practitioner if the patient exhibits any signs and symptoms of an allergic reaction. [Recommendation]

3.2.3 Provide treatment ordered by the licensed independent practitioner (eg, medications [eg, antihistamine, epinephrine]). [Recommendation]

3.2.4 Document the allergic symptom development in relation to the time the local anesthetic was administered and treatment.[4] [Recommendation]

3.3 Implement strategies for assessing and treating methemoglobinemia after the use of a local anesthetic. [Recommendation]

3.3.1 Recognize and assess the signs and symptoms of methemoglobinemia following an injection of a local anesthetic, including

- anxiety,[130]
- lightheadedness,[130]
- headache,[130]
- tachycardia,[130]
- fatigue,[130]
- confusion,[130]
- dizziness,[130]
- tachypnea,[130]
- low pulse oximetric readings,[131]

- cyanosis,[130,131]
- cardiac arrythmias,[130]
- acidosis,[130]
- coma,[130] and
- seizures.[130]

[Recommendation]

Methemoglobinemia is a rare and unusual complication in which the iron (Fe^{2+}) in hemoglobin is oxidized to the ferric (Fe^{3+}) state. Methemoglobinemia can be triggered by lidocaine and other local anesthetics.[130,131] In the ferric state, it is unable to bind oxygen, leading to tissue hypoxia and possibly death. Methemoglobinemia may be caused by a hereditary deficiency of intrinsic cytochrome b5-MetHb reductase or by the presence of congenital hemoglobin M. Hemoglobin M is a form of hemoglobin that is unable to bind to oxygen. Acquired methemoglobinemia is a result of exposure to common oxidants such as lidocaine and prilocaine.[130]

The symptoms of methemoglobinemia typically develop within 20 to 60 minutes after exposure to local anesthetics but may occur as much as 2 hours later.[132] Case reports link methemoglobinemia to the application of lidocaine-prilocaine cream[132,133] and the use of benzocaine spray during bronchoscopies[134] and transesophageal echocardiograms.[131]

Patients with comorbidities that impair oxygen transport (eg, anemia, heart disease, pulmonary disease [eg, chronic obstructive pulmonary disease, pneumonia]) are at a higher risk for methemoglobinemia.[130]

3.3.2 Closely monitor patients with liver cirrhosis and neonates for methemoglobinemia.[130] [Recommendation]

3.3.3 If a diagnosis of methemoglobinemia is suspected,
- discontinue the use of the local anesthetic (eg, lidocaine, prilocaine, benzocaine),[130-132]
- administer high-flow oxygen and titrate as needed,[130-132]
- be prepared to establish intravenous access,
- be prepared to administer methylene blue intravenously if ordered by the physician,[130-132]
- be prepared for laboratory testing (eg, arterial blood gas analysis,[131] complete blood count [CBC][132]),
- repeat methylene blue administration as needed and ordered,[130,131] and
- monitor the patient for signs of recurrence,[130]

- use multiple wavelength CO-oximetry,[132] and
- monitor the patient for signs of adverse reactions to the methylene blue administration (eg, chest pains, dyspnea, hypertension, diaphoresis, paradoxical increase of MetHb, hemolytic anemia) or overdose.[132]

[Recommendation]

Diagnosis is crucial for the best clinical outcomes. Diagnosis of methemoglobinemia is based on laboratory tests (eg, arterial blood gas analysis,[131] CBC[132]) and clinical presentation. Standard pulse oximetry is unable to differentiate between oxyhemoglobin and MetHb. MetHb absorbs light at both wavelengths used to differentiate oxyhemoglobin from deoxyhemoglobin.[130] Multiple wavelength CO-oximetry can detect accurate measurements of the true oxygen-carrying status.[132]

3.4 Implement strategies for assessing and treating (eg, phentolamine injection) WALANT technique complications (eg, vasoconstrictor-induced ischemia).[8,27] [Recommendation]

Using epinephrine as part of the WALANT technique provides temporary hemostasis and prolongs the effect of the local anesthetic.[4,27] A potential complication of using epinephrine is vasoconstrictor-induced ischemia.[4,27] The reversal for the vasoconstrictive effects of epinephrine is a subcutaneous injection of phentolamine (1 mg/mL).[8,27]

4. Postoperative Care

4.1 Postoperatively monitor and document the patient's
- pulse,[59]
- heart rhythm and rate,[59]
- blood pressure,[59]
- respiratory rate,[59]
- SpO$_2$ by pulse oximetry.[59]

[Conditional Recommendation]

The ASPAN *Perianesthesia Nursing Standards, Practice Recommendations and Interpretive Statements*[59] recommends initial and ongoing monitoring and documentation of vital signs.

4.2 Postoperatively assess and document the patient's level of pain,[59] anxiety, and the condition of dressings and visible incisions.[59] [Conditional Recommendation]

The ASPAN *Perianesthesia Nursing Standards, Practice Recommendations and Interpretive Statements*[59] recommends assessing and documenting pain, anxiety, and the condition of dressings and visible incisions.

4.3 If the patient received lipid emulsion therapy for LAST, continue monitoring the patient for signs of cardiovascular instability for 2 to 6 hours (See Recommendation 3.1.4).[65] [Recommendation]

4.4 Evaluate the patient for discharge readiness based on specific discharge criteria (eg, stable vital signs, adequate pain control) developed by an interdisciplinary team (eg, surgeons, perioperative RNs). [Recommendation]

4.4.1 In accordance with the health care organization's discharge criteria, a qualified provider defined by and authorized under the health care organization's guidelines and policies may be required to discharge the patient. [Conditional Recommendation]

4.4.2 Provide the patient with verbal and written discharge instructions.[135-137] [Recommendation]

5. Education

5.1 Provide initial and ongoing education and competency verification activities related to local anesthesia pharmacology (eg, recommended dose, onset, duration of action), calculation of total dose, contraindications, desired effects, adverse reactions (eg, LAST, allergic reaction, methemoglobinemia), electrocardiogram rhythm interpretation, and resuscitation. [Recommendation]

Low-quality evidence supports the importance of promoting knowledge and awareness of LAST among physicians.[138-140] Sagir an Guyal[138] surveyed 200 postgraduate residents of various specialties. Twenty-seven percent correctly identified the toxic dose of lidocaine, and 25% identified the toxic dose of lidocaine with epinephrine. Only 7% were aware of the toxic dose of bupivacaine. Seventy percent of the residents responded that local anesthetics could be toxic, and 81% of this group correctly identified the signs and symptoms of cardiotoxicity. Two percent knew about lipid emulsion as treatment for LAST. The authors concluded that there is a need to increase awareness about detection and treatment of LAST among all medical practitioners who regularly use local anesthetics.

No studies were found that have investigated the perioperative RN's knowledge of local anesthetics as a risk factor for the patient's development of LAST or an allergic reaction. Further research is needed to define the role of the perioperative RN in early detection and treatment of LAST and adverse medication reactions (eg, allergy).

The benefits of the perioperative RN knowing the local anesthetic medication's indications for use, contraindications, desired effects, and adverse effects include the potential for early detection and treatment of LAST and allergic reactions.[139]

6. Policies and Procedures

6.1 Convene an interdisciplinary team that includes pharmacist(s), surgeon(s), perioperative RN(s), anesthesia professional(s), and other stakeholders identified by the organization to develop and implement policies and procedures for care of the patient receiving local-only anesthesia. [Recommendation]

Policies and procedures assist in the development of patient safety, quality assessment, and performance improvement activities. Policies and procedures establish authority, responsibility, and accountability within the organization. Policies and procedures also serve as operational guidelines that are used to minimize patient risk for injury or complications, standardize practice, direct perioperative personnel, and establish continuous performance improvement programs.

The Centers for Medicare & Medicaid Services requires health care organizations that provide care to patients covered by Medicare and Medicaid to establish policies and procedures for patient care.[136,137]

6.2 Address the following in policies and procedures regarding the care of the patient receiving local-only anesthesia:

- patient selection criteria for local-only anesthesia;
- patient assessment criteria (See Recommendation 1.2);
- personnel qualifications, competencies, and certifications (eg, certified basic life support, certified advanced cardiovascular life support);
- staffing requirements[141];
- monitoring (ie, parameters, frequency);
- risk assessment and criteria for consultation with an anesthesia professional;
- recovery and discharge criteria;
- documentation requirements (eg, vital signs, anxiety level, medication response);
- medication supplies (eg, lipid emulsion, methylene blue, resuscitation medications);
- emergency equipment (eg, supplemental oxygen, suction apparatus, resuscitation);
- emergency procedures; and
- emergency transfer protocols.

[Recommendation]

6.2.1 **At a minimum, personnel should be competent in basic life support.**[82,83] *[Recommendation]*

Serious cardiac or respiratory complications can occur abruptly after the administration of local anesthetic medications. If the medication enters the bloodstream directly, seizures, circulatory and respiratory distress, cardiovascular collapse, or even death can result. The initial treatment of LAST is maintaining an airway and basic life support.[82,83]

6.2.2 **Convene an interdisciplinary team to determine advanced cardiac life support (ACLS) certification requirements in the practice setting based on regulatory standards**[136,137] **and the acuity of the patients.** *[Recommendation]*

Considerations for requiring ACLS may include competency to recognize common arrhythmias and immediate availability of additional support (eg, code team, anesthesia professional). Personnel available to assist in an emergency can vary depending in the facility type and staffing (eg, charge anesthesia provider, charge RN, code team) present in the facility. In a hospital-based OR, the code team and additional anesthesia providers may be readily available. In an ASC or office-based OR, the call for help may be to 911.

6.3 **Develop the health care organization's policy and procedure for staffing requirements during local-only anesthesia procedures by identifying the number of perioperative RNs needed to implement the plan of care (eg, RN circulator, additional RN to monitor) based on the patient's assessment, patient's acuity,**[141] **and the type of procedures performed.**[135] *[Recommendation]*

6.3.1 **At a minimum, one perioperative RN circulator should be dedicated to each patient undergoing an operative or other invasive procedure and should be present during that patient's entire intraoperative experience.**[141] *[Recommendation]*

AORN is committed to the provision of safe perioperative nursing care by ensuring that every patient undergoing an operative or other invasive procedure is cared for by minimum of one RN in the circulating role. The perioperative RN works collaboratively with other perioperative professionals (eg, surgeons, anesthesia professionals, surgical technologists) to meet patient needs, and is accountable for the patient's outcomes resulting from the nursing care provided during the operative or other invasive procedure. Using clinical knowledge, judgment, and clinical-reasoning skills based on scientific principles, the perioperative RN plans and implements nursing care to address the physical, psychological, and spiritual responses of the patient undergoing an operative or other invasive procedure.[141]

Glossary

CO-oximetry: A clinical test that quantifies carboxyhemoglobin and methemoglobin and calculates the content of oxygen bound to hemoglobin.

Local anesthetic systemic toxicity: An uncommon, potentially fatal, toxic reaction that occurs when the threshold blood levels of a local anesthetic are exceeded by an inadvertent, intravascular injection or slow systemic absorption of a large, extravascular volume of local anesthetic.

Methemoglobinemia: A rare and unusual complication in which the iron (Fe^{2+}) in hemoglobin is oxidized to the ferric (Fe^{3+}) state. Methemoglobinemia can be triggered by lidocaine and other local anesthetics.

Tumescent infiltration: A technique involving the infiltration of large amounts of fluid containing a dilute local anesthetic (eg, lidocaine) that results in swelling and firmness of the surgical area. Tumescent infiltration is used during liposuction, varicose vein, and dermatologic procedures.

References

1. Lirk P, Hollmann MW, Strichartz G. The science of local anesthesia: basic research, clinical application, and future directions. *Anesth Analg.* 2017;126(4):1381-1392. [VA]

2. Calatayud J, González A. History of the development and evolution of local anesthesia since the coca leaf. *Anesthesiology.* 2003;98(6):1503-1508. [VA]

3. Gordh T, Lindqvist K. Lidocaine: the origin of a modern local anesthetic. 1949. *Anesthesiology.* 2010;113(6):1433-1437. [VA]

4. Volcheck GW, Mertes PM. Local and general anesthetics immediate hypersensitivity reactions. *Immunol Allergy Clin North Am.* 2014;34(3):525-546. [VA]

5. Fathi R, Serota M, Brown M. Identifying and managing local anesthetic allergy in dermatologic surgery. *Dermatol Surg.* 2016;42(2):147-156. [VA]

6. Zhang JX, Gray J, Lalonde DH, Carr N. Digital necrosis after lidocaine and epinephrine injection in the flexor tendon sheath without phentolamine rescue. *J Hand Surg Am.* 2017;42(2):e119-e123. [VA]

7. Thomson CJ, Lalonde DH, Denkler KA, Feicht AJ. A critical look at the evidence for and against elective epinephrine use in the finger. *Plast Reconstr Surg.* 2007;119(1):260-266. [VA]

8. Lalonde DH. Conceptual origins, current practice, and views of wide awake hand surgery. *J Hand Surg Eur Vol.* 2017;42(9):886-895. [VA]

9. Mohd Rashid MZ, Sapuan J, Abdullah S. A randomized controlled trial of trigger finger release under digital anesthesia with (WALANT) and without adrenaline. *J Orthop Surg (Hong Kong).* 2019;27(1). doi: 10.1177/2309499019833002. [IB]

10. Rhee PC. The current and possible future role of wide-awake local anesthesia no tourniquet hand surgery in military health care delivery. *Hand Clin.* 2019;35(1):13-19. [VA]

11. Tang JB, Xing SG, Ayhan E, Hediger S, Huang S. Impact of wide-awake local anesthesia no tourniquet on departmental settings, cost, patient and surgeon satisfaction, and beyond. *Hand Clin.* 2019;35(1):29-34. [VA]

12. Van Demark RE Jr, Becker HA, Anderson MC, Smith VJS. Wide-awake anesthesia in the in-office procedure room: lessons learned. *Hand (N Y).* 2018;13(4):481-485. [VA]

13. Rhee PC, Fischer MM, Rhee LS, McMillan H, Johnson AE. Cost savings and patient experiences of a clinic-based, wide-awake hand surgery program at a military medical center: a critical analysis of the first 100 procedures. *J Hand Surg Am.* 2017;42(3):e139-e147. [IIIB]

14. Caggiano NM, Avery DM, Matullo KS. The effect of anesthesia type on nonsurgical operating room time. *J Hand Surg Am.* 2015;40(6):1202-1209. [IIIB]

15. Kazmers NH, Presson AP, Xu Y, Howenstein A, Tyser AR. Cost implications of varying the surgical technique, surgical setting, and anesthesia type for carpal tunnel release surgery. *J Hand Surg Am.* 2018;43(11):971-977. [IIIB]

16. Alter TH, Warrender WJ, Liss FE, Ilyas AM. A cost analysis of carpal tunnel release surgery performed wide awake versus under sedation. *Plast Reconstr Surg.* 2018;142(6):1532-1538. [IIIB]

17. Rabinowitz J, Kelly T, Peterson A, Angermeier E, Kokko K. In-office wide-awake hand surgery versus traditional surgery in the operating room: a comparison of clinical outcomes and healthcare costs at an academic institution. *Curr Orthop Pract.* 2019;30(5):429-434. [IIIB]

18. Codding JL, Bhat SB, Ilyas AM. An economic analysis of MAC versus WALANT: a trigger finger release surgery case study. *Hand (N Y).* 2017;12(4):348-351. [IIIB]

19. Kazmers NH, Stephens AR, Presson AP, Yu Z, Tyser AR. Cost implications of varying the surgical setting and anesthesia type for trigger finger release surgery. *Plast Reconstr Surg Glob Open.* 2019;7(5):e2231. [IIIB]

20. Poggetti A, Del Chiaro A, Nicastro M, Parchi P, Piolanti N, Scaglione M. A local anesthesia without tourniquet for distal fibula hardware removal after open reduction and internal fixation: the safe use of epinephrine in the foot. A randomized clinical study. *J Biol Regul Homeost Agents.* 2018;32(6 Suppl 1):57-63. [IB]

21. Saleem Z, Azhar MJ, Arain SH, Chohan ZA. Excision of dorsal wrist ganglia under local anesthesia with adrenaline without tourniquet, and with evacuation of the cyst during dissection for the ease and completeness of the excision. *Pak J Med Health Sci.* 2017;11(1):447-449. [IIIB]

22. Barroso Rosa S, James D, Matthews BD. Is knee arthroscopy under local anaesthetic a patient-friendly technique? A prospective controlled trial. *Eur J Orthop Surg Traumatol.* 2016;26(6):633-638. [IIB]

23. Lalonde DH. Latest advances in wide awake hand surgery. *Hand Clin.* 2019;35(1):1-6. [VA]

24. Van Demark RE Jr, Smith VJS, Fiegen A. Lean and green hand surgery. *J Hand Surg Am.* 2018;43(2):179-181. [VA]

25. Lalonde D. Minimally invasive anesthesia in wide awake hand surgery. *Hand Clin.* 2014;30(1):1-6. [VA]

26. Via GG, Esterle AR, Awan HM, Jain SA, Goyal KS. Comparison of local-only anesthesia versus sedation in patients undergoing staged bilateral carpal tunnel release: a randomized trial. *Hand (N Y).* 2019. doi: 10.1177/1558944719836237. [IB]

27. Ruxasagulwong S, Kraisarin J, Sananpanich K. Wide awake technique versus local anesthesia with tourniquet application for minor orthopedic hand surgery: a prospective clinical trial. *J Med Assoc Thai.* 2015;98(1):106-110. [IB]

28. Diaz-Abele J, Luc M, Dyachenko A, Aldekhayel S, Ciampi A, McCusker J. Lidocaine with epinephrine versus bupivacaine with epinephrine as local anesthetic agents in wide-awake hand surgery: a pilot outcome study of patient's pain perception. *J Hand Surg Glob Online.* 2020;2(1):1-6. [IB]

29. Gunasagaran J, Sean ES, Shivdas S, Amir S, Ahmad TS. Perceived comfort during minor hand surgeries with wide awake local anaesthesia no tourniquet (WALANT) versus local anaesthesia (LA)/tourniquet. *J Orthop Surg (Hong Kong).* 2017;25(3). doi: 10.1177/2309499017739499. [IB]

30. Kang SW, Park HM, Park JK, et al. Open cubital and carpal tunnel release using wide-awake technique: reduction of postoperative pain. *J Pain Res.* 2019;12:2725-2731. [IIIB]

31. Orbach H, Rozen N, Rubin G. Open reduction and internal fixation of intra-articular distal radius fractures under wide-awake local anesthesia with no tourniquet. *J Int Med Res.* 2018;46(10):4269-4276. [IIC]

32. Huang YC, Hsu CJ, Renn JH, et al. WALANT for distal radius fracture: open reduction with plating fixation via wide-awake local anesthesia with no tourniquet. *J Orthop Surg Res.* 2018;13(1):195. [IIIB]

33. Huang YC, Chen CY, Lin KC, Yang SW, Tarng YW, Chang WN. Comparison of wide-awake local anesthesia no tourniquet with general anesthesia with tourniquet for volar plating of distal radius fracture. *Orthopedics.* 2019;42(1):e93-e98. [IIIB]

34. Ahmad AA, Yi LM, Ahmad AR. Plating of distal radius fracture using the wide-awake anesthesia technique. *J Hand Surg Am.* 2018;43(11):1045.e1-1045.e5. [VB]

35. Nakanishi Y, Omokawa S, Kobata Y, et al. Ultrasound-guided selective sensory nerve block for wide-awake forearm tendon reconstruction. *Plast Reconstr Surg Glob Open.* 2015;3(5):e392. [IIC]

36. Li YS, Chen CY, Lin KC, Tarng YW, Hsu CJ, Chang WN. Open reduction and internal fixation of ankle fracture using wide-awake local anaesthesia no tourniquet technique. *Injury.* 2019;50(4):990-994. [IIIB]

37. Liu B, Ng CY, Arshad MS, Edwards DS, Hayton MJ. Wide-awake wrist and small joints arthroscopy of the hand. *Hand Clin.* 2019;35(1):85-92. [VA]

38. Hyatt BT, Rhee PC. Wide-awake surgical management of hand fractures: technical pearls and advanced rehabilitation. *Plast Reconstr Surg.* 2019;143(3):800-810. [VA]

39. Ahmad AA, Ikram MA. Plating of an isolated fracture of shaft of ulna under local anaesthesia and periosteal nerve block. *Trauma Case Rep.* 2017;12:40-44. [VB]

40. Ahmad AA, Sabari SS, Ruslan SR, Abdullah S, Ahmad AR. Wide-awake anesthesia for olecranon fracture fixation. *Hand (N Y).* 2019. doi: 10.1177/1558944719861706. [VB]

41. Wolfe RC, Spillars A. Local anesthetic systemic toxicity: reviewing updates from the American Society of Regional

Anesthesia and Pain Medicine Practice Advisory. *J Perianesth Nurs.* 2018;33(6):1000-1005. [VA]

42. Gitman M, Fettiplace MR, Weinberg GL, Neal JM, Barrington MJ. Local anesthetic systemic toxicity: a narrative literature review and clinical update on prevention, diagnosis, and management. *Plast Reconstr Surg.* 2019;133(3):783-795. [VA]

43. McEvoy MD, Thies KC, Einav S, et al. Cardiac arrest in the operating room: part 2—special situations in the perioperative period. *Anesth Analg.* 2018;126(3):889-903. [VA]

44. Waldinger R, Weinberg G, Gitman M. Local anesthetic toxicity in the geriatric population. *Drugs Aging.* 2020;37(1):1-9. [VA]

45. El-Boghdadly K, Pawa A, Chin KJ. Local anesthetic systemic toxicity: current perspectives. *Local Reg Anesth.* 2018;11:35-44. [VA]

46. El-Boghdadly K, Chin KJ. Local anesthetic systemic toxicity: continuing professional development. *Can J Anaesth.* 2016;63(3):330-349. [VA]

47. Jayanthi R, Nasser K, Monica K. Local anesthetics systemic toxicity. *J Assoc Physicians India.* 2016;64(3):92-93. [VC]

48. Vasques F, Behr AU, Weinberg G, Ori C, Di Gregorio G. A review of local anesthetic systemic toxicity cases since publication of the American Society of Regional Anesthesia recommendations: to whom it may concern. *Reg Anesth Pain Med.* 2015;40(6):698-705. [IIIB]

49. Barrington MJ, Kluger R. Ultrasound guidance reduces the risk of local anesthetic systemic toxicity following peripheral nerve blockade. *Reg Anesth Pain Med.* 2013;38(4):289-299. [IIIA]

50. Mörwald EE, Zubizarreta N, Cozowicz C, Poeran J, Memtsoudis SG. Incidence of local anesthetic systemic toxicity in orthopedic patients receiving peripheral nerve blocks. *Reg Anesth Pain Med.* 2017;42(4):442-445. [IIIB]

51. Liu SS, Ortolan S, Sandoval MV, et al. Cardiac arrest and seizures caused by local anesthetic systemic toxicity after peripheral nerve blocks: should we still fear the reaper? *Reg Anesth Pain Med.* 2016;41(1):5-21. [IIIA]

52. Rubin DS, Matsumoto MM, Weinberg G, Roth S. Local anesthetic systemic toxicity in total joint arthroplasty: incidence and risk factors in the United States from the National Inpatient Sample 1998-2013. *Reg Anesth Pain Med.* 2018;43(2):131-137. [IIIA]

53. Jenerowicz D, Polańska A, Glińska O, Czarnecka-Operacz M, Schwartz RA. Allergy to lidocaine injections: comparison of patient history with skin testing in five patients. *Postepy Dermatol Alergol.* 2014;31(3):134-138. [VA]

54. Malinovsky JM, Chiriac AM, Tacquard C, Mertes PM, Demoly P. Allergy to local anesthetics: reality or myth? *Presse Med.* 2016;45(9):753-757. [VA]

55. To D, Kossintseva I, de Gannes G. Lidocaine contact allergy is becoming more prevalent. *Dermatol Surg.* 2014;40(12):1367-1372. [IIIB]

56. Recommended practices for medication safety. In: *Perioperative Standards and Recommended Practices.* Denver, CO: AORN, Inc; 2020:333-482. [IVB]

57. *Nursing: Scope and Standards of Practice.* 3rd ed. Silver Spring, MD: American Nurses Association; 2015. [IVB]

58. *Standards of Perioperative Nursing.* AORN, Inc. https://www.aorn.org/guidelines/clinical-resources/aorn-standards. Accessed August 31, 2020. [IVB]

59. *Perianesthesia Nursing Standards, Practice Recommendations and Interpretive Statements.* Cherry Hill, NJ: American Society of PeriAnesthesia Nurses; 2019/2020. [IVB]

60. Petersen C, ed. *Perioperative Nursing Data Set.* 3rd ed. Denver, CO: AORN, Inc; 2011. [IVB]

61. Liu W, Yang X, Li C, Mo A. Adverse drug reactions to local anesthetics: a systematic review. *Oral Surg Oral Med Oral Pathol Oral Radiol.* 2013;115(3):319-327. [IIIB]

62. Treasure T, Bennett J. Office-based anesthesia. *Oral Maxillofac Surg Clin North Am.* 2007;19(1):45-57. [VB]

63. Kost M. Nursing considerations for procedural sedation and analgesia: this first in a two-part series reviews patient assessment, red flags, and pharmacologic agents. *Am Nurse Today.* 2019;14(5):6-11. [VA]

64. Neal JM, Barrington MJ, Fettiplace MR, et al. The third American Society of Regional Anesthesia and Pain Medicine practice advisory on local anesthetic systemic toxicity: executive summary 2017. *Reg Anesth Pain Med.* 2018;43(2):113-123. [IVA]

65. Checklist for treatment of local anesthetic systemic toxicity (LAST). American Society of Regional and Pain Medicine. https://www.asra.com/content/documents/asra_last_checklist_2018.pdf. Accessed August 31, 2020. [VA]

66. ASA physical status classification system. American Society of Anesthesiologists. https://www.asahq.org/standards-and-guidelines/asa-physical-status-classification-system. Accessed August 31, 2020. [VA]

67. Tantri A, Clark C, Huber P, et al. Anesthesia monitoring by registered nurses during cataract surgery: assessment of need for intraoperative anesthesia consultation. *J Cataract Refract Surg.* 2006;32(7):1115-1118. [IIIB]

68. Mitchell M. Patient anxiety and conscious surgery. *J Perioper Pract.* 2009;19(6):168-173. [IIIB]

69. Mitchell M. Conscious surgery: influence of the environment on patient anxiety. *J Adv Nurs.* 2008;64(3):261-271. [IIIB]

70. El Hachem M, Carnevale C, Diociaiuti A, et al. Local anesthesia in pediatric dermatologic surgery: evaluation of a patient-centered approach. *Pediatr Dermatol.* 2018;35(1):112-116. [IIIB]

71. *Informed Consent for Anesthesia Care: Policy and Practice Considerations.* Park Ridge, IL: American Association of Nurse Anesthetists; 2016. [IVB]

72. Davis-Evans C. Alleviating anxiety and preventing panic attacks in the surgical patient. *AORN J.* 2013;97(3):354-364. [VB]

73. Failure to monitor local anesthesia pt. before discharge. Case on point: Messer v. Martin, 2004 WL 1171736 N.W.2d -WI(2004). *Nurs Law Regan Rep.* 2004;45(1):2. [VB]

74. Standards for basic anesthetic monitoring. American Society of Anesthesiologists. https://www.asahq.org/~/media/sites/asahq/files/public/resources/standards-guidelines/standards-for-basic-anesthetic-monitoring.pdf. Last affirmed October 28, 2015. Accessed August 31, 2020. [IVB]

75. Standards for nurse anesthesia practice. American Association of Nurse Anesthetists. https://www.aana.com/docs/default-source/practice-aana-com-web-documents-(all)/standards-for-nurse-anesthesia-practice.pdf. 2019. Accessed August 31, 2020. [IVA]

76. Kruger GH, Shanks A, Kheterpal S, et al. Influence of non-invasive blood pressure measurement intervals on the occurrence of intra-operative hypotension. *J Clin Monit Comput.* 2018;32(4):699-705. [IIIA]

77. Buck D, Kreeger R, Spaeth J. Case discussion and root cause analysis: bupivacaine overdose in an infant leading to ventricular tachycardia. *Anesth Analg.* 2014;119(1):137-140. [VA]

78. Garcia-Rodriguez L, Spiegel JH. Are surgeons overdosing patients with lidocaine? *Am J Otolaryngol.* 2018;39(3):370-371. [VA]

79. Khatri KP, Rothschild L, Oswald S, Weinberg G. Current concepts in the management of systemic local anesthetic toxicity. *Adv Anesth.* 2010;28(1):147-159. [VA]

80. Petrar S, Montemurro T. Total local anesthetic administered is integral to the syndrome of local anesthetic systemic toxicity. *Anesthesiology.* 2014;121(5):1130-1131. [VA]

81. Tanawuttiwat T, Thisayakorn P, Viles-Gonzalez JF. LAST (local anesthetic systemic toxicity) but not least: systemic lidocaine toxicity during cardiac intervention. *J Invasive Cardiol.* 2014;26(1):E13-E15. [VB]

82. AAGBI safety guideline: management of severe local anaesthetic toxicity. 2010. Association of Anaesthetists of Great Britain and Ireland. https://anaesthetists.org/Home/Resources-publications/Guidelines/Management-of-severe-local-anaesthetic-toxicity. Accessed August 31, 2020. [IVB]

83. Safety Committee of Japanese Society of Anesthesiologists. Practical guide for the management of systemic toxicity caused by local anesthetics. *J Anesth.* 2019;33(1):1-8. [IVB]

84. Byrne K, Engelbrecht C. Toxicity of local anaesthetic agents. *Trends Anaesth Crit Care.* 2013;3(1):25-30. [VB]

85. Gitman M, Barrington MJ. Local anesthetic systemic toxicity: a review of recent case reports and registries. *Reg Anesth Pain Med.* 2018;43(2):124-130. [VA]

86. Özer AB, Erhan ÖL. Systemic toxicity to local anesthesia in an infant undergoing circumcision. *Agri.* 2014;26(1):43-46. [VA]

87. Aydin G. Unexpected local anesthesia toxicity during the ultrasonography-guided peripheral nerve block. *J Clin Anesth.* 2018;50:26. [VA]

88. Kien NT, Giang NT, Van Manh B, et al. Successful intralipid-emulsion treatment of local anesthetic systemic toxicity following ultrasound-guided brachial plexus block: case report. *Int Med Case Rep J.* 2019;12:193-197. [VA]

89. Eizaga Rebollar R, García Palacios MV, Morales Guerrero J, Torres Morera LM. Lipid rescue in children: the prompt decision. *J Clin Anesth.* 2016;32:248-252. [VA]

90. Najafi N, Veyckemans F, Du Maine C, et al. Systemic toxicity following the use of 1% ropivacaine for pediatric penile nerve block. *Regional Anesth Pain Med.* 2016;41(4):549-550. [VB]

91. Shenoy U, Paul J, Antony D. Lipid resuscitation in pediatric patients—need for caution? *Paediatr Anaesth.* 2014;24(3):332-334. [VA]

92. Nicholas E, Thornton MD. Lidocaine toxicity during attempted epistaxis cautery. *J Emerg Med.* 2016;51(3):303-304. [VB]

93. Musielak M, McCall J. Lipid rescue in a pediatric burn patient. *J Burn Care Res.* 2016;37(4):e380-e382. [VA]

94. Hoda S, O'Brien J, Gamble J. Intractable seizures in a toddler after application of an over-the-counter local anesthetic cream. *CMAJ.* 2016;188(14):1030-1032. [VA]

95. Mittal S, Mohan A, Madan K. Ventricular tachycardia and cardiovascular collapse following flexible bronchoscopy: lidocaine cardiotoxicity. *J Bronchology Interv Pulmonol.* 2018;25(2):e24-e26. [VA]

96. Bacon B, Silverton N, Katz M, et al. Local anesthetic systemic toxicity induced cardiac arrest after topicalization for transesophageal echocardiography and subsequent treatment with extracorporeal cardiopulmonary resuscitation. *J Cardiothorac Vasc Anesth.* 2019;33(1):162-165. [VA]

97. Whiteman DM, Kushins SI. Successful resuscitation with intralipid after Marcaine overdose. *Aesthet Surg J.* 2014;34(5):738-740. [VA]

98. Di Gregorio G, Neal JM, Rosenquist RW, Weinberg GL. Clinical presentation of local anesthetic systemic toxicity: a review of published cases, 1979 to 2009. *Reg Anesth Pain Med.* 2010;35(2):181-187. [VA]

99. Wolfe JW, Butterworth JF. Local anesthetic systemic toxicity: update on mechanisms and treatment. *Curr Opin Anaesthesiol.* 2011;24(5):561-566. [VB]

100. Berrío Valencia MI, Vargas Silva JF. Protocolo y necesidad de kit para toxicidad sistémica por anestésicos locales [Protocol and importance of using the kit for local anesthetic systemic toxicity]. *Rev Colomb Anestesiol.* 2013;41(4):274-279. [VA]

101. Gosselin S, Hoegberg LCG, Hoffman RS, et al. Evidence-based recommendations on the use of intravenous lipid emulsion therapy in poisoning. *Clin Toxicol (Phila).* 2016;54(10):899-923. [IIIB]

102. Lavonas EJ, Drennan IR, Gabrielli A, et al. Part 10: Special circumstances of resuscitation. 2015 American Heart Association guidelines update for cardiopulmonary resuscitation and emergency cardiovascular care. *Circulation.* 2015;132(18 Suppl 2):S501-S518. [IVA]

103. Fettiplace MR, Weinberg G. Past, present, and future of lipid resuscitation therapy. *JPEN J Parenter Enteral Nutr.* 2015;39(1 Suppl):72S-83S. [VA]

104. Fettiplace MR, Akpa BS, Ripper R, et al. Resuscitation with lipid emulsion: dose-dependent recovery from cardiac pharmacotoxicity requires a cardiotonic effect. *Anesthesiology.* 2014;120(4):915-925. [IIC]

105. Fettiplace MR, Ripper R, Lis K, Feinstein DL, Rubinstein I, Weinberg G. Intraosseous lipid emulsion: an effective alternative to IV delivery in emergency situations. *Crit Care Med.* 2014;42(2):e157-60. [IC]

106. Gonca E, Çatlı D. The effects of lidocaine with epinephrine on bupivacaine-induced cardiotoxicity. *Turk J Anaesthesiol Reanim.* 2018;46(6):447-452. [IIC]

107. Hayaran N, Sardana R, Nandinie H, Jain A. Unusual presentation of local anesthetic toxicity. *J Clin Anesth.* 2017;36:36-38. [VA]

108. Marwick PC, Levin AI, Coetzee AR. Recurrence of cardiotoxicity after lipid rescue from bupivacaine-induced cardiac arrest. *Anesth Analg.* 2009;108(4):1344-1346. [VA]

109. Batinac T, Sotošek Tokmadžić V, Peharda V, Brajac I. Adverse reactions and alleged allergy to local anesthetics: analysis of 331 patients. *J Dermatol.* 2013;40(7):522-527. [IIIA]

110. Bhole MV, Manson AL, Seneviratne SL, Misbah SA. IgE-mediated allergy to local anaesthetics: separating fact from perception: a UK perspective. *Br J Anaesth.* 2012;108(6):903-911. [VA]

111. Fuzier R, Lapeyre-Mestre M, Mertes PM, et al. Immediate- and delayed-type allergic reactions to amide local anesthetics: clinical features and skin testing. *Pharmacoepidemiol Drug Saf.* 2009;18(7):595-601. [IIIC]

112. Harboe T, Guttormsen AB, Aarebrot S, Dybendal T, Irgens A, Florvaag E. Suspected allergy to local anaesthetics: follow-up in 135 cases. *Acta Anaesthesiol Scand.* 2010;54(5):536-542. [IIIB]

113. Grzanka A, Misiołek H, Filipowska A, Miśkiewicz-Orczyk K, Jarząb J. Adverse effects of local anaesthetics—allergy, toxic reactions or hypersensitivity. *Anestezjol Intens Ter.* 2010;42(4):175-178. [IIIB]

114. Kvisselgaard AD, Krøigaard M, Mosbech HF, Garvey LH. No cases of perioperative allergy to local anaesthetics in the Danish Anaesthesia Allergy Centre. *Acta Anaesthesiol Scand.* 2017;61(2):149-155. [IIIA]

115. Kvisselgaard AD, Mosbech HF, Fransson S, Garvey LH. Risk of immediate-type allergy to local anesthetics is overestimated-results from 5 years of provocation testing in a Danish allergy clinic. *J Allergy Clin Immunol Pract.* 2018;6(4):1217-1223. [IIIA]

116. Brinca A, Cabral R, Gonçalo M. Contact allergy to local anaesthetics-value of patch testing with a caine mix in the baseline series. *Contact Dermatitis.* 2013;68(3):156-162. [IIIA]

117. Trautmann A, Stoevesandt J. Differential diagnosis of late-type reactions to injected local anaesthetics: inflammation at the injection site is the only indicator of allergic hypersensitivity. *Contact Dermatitis.* 2019;80(2):118-124. [IIIB]

118. Yllmaz I, Özdemir SK, Aydin Ö, Çelik GE. Local anesthetics allergy: who should be tested? *Eur Ann Allergy Clinical Immunol.* 2018;50(2):66-71. [IIIB]

119. Trautmann A, Goebeler M, Stoevesandt J. Twenty years' experience with anaphylaxis-like reactions to local anesthetics: genuine allergy is rare. *J Allergy Clin Immunol Pract.* 2018;6(6):2051-2058. [IIIB]

120. Kvisselgaard AD, Melchiors BB, Krøigaard M, Garvey LH. Lidocaine as a rare and hidden allergen in the perioperative setting: a case report. *A A Pract.* 2019;12(11):430-432. [VA]

121. Dickison P, Smith SD. Biting down on the truth: a case of a delayed hypersensitivity reaction to lidocaine. *Australas J Dermatol.* 2019;60(1):66-67. [VA]

122. Vega F, Argíz L, Bazire R, Las Heras P, Blanco C. Delayed urticaria due to bupivacaine: a new presentation of local anesthetic allergy. *Allergol Int.* 2016;65(4):498-500. [VA]

123. Russo PAJ, Banovic T, Wiese MD, Whyte AF, Smith WB. Systemic allergy to EDTA in local anesthetic and radiocontrast media. *J Allergy Clin Immunol Pract.* 2014;2(2):225-229. [VA]

124. McGarry DP, Kim YM, Casselman J, et al. Ocular desensitization in the face of local anesthetic hypersensitivity. *J Allergy Clin Immunol Pract.* 2017;5(3):819-820. [VA]

125. Presman B, Vindigni V, Tocco-Tussardi I. Immediate reaction to lidocaine with periorbital edema during upper blepharoplasty. *Int J Surg Case Rep.* 2016;20:24-26. [VB]

126. Kumar A. Diffuse epithelial keratopathy following a single instillation of topical lignocaine: the damaging drop. *Cutan ocul toxicol.* 2016;35(2):173-175. [VB]

127. Halabi-Tawil M, Kechichian E, Tomb R. An unusual complication of minor surgery: contact dermatitis caused by injected lidocaine. *Contact Dermatitis.* 2016;75(4):253-255. [VB]

128. Domínguez-Ortega J, Phillips-Angles E, González-Muñoz M, Heredia R, Fiandor A, Quirce S. Allergy to several local anesthetics from the amide group. *J Allergy Clin Immunol Pract.* 2016;4(4):771-772. [VB]

129. Al-Dosary K, Al-Qahtani A, Alangari A. Anaphylaxis to lidocaine with tolerance to articaine in a 12 year old girl. *Saudi Pharm J.* 2014;22(3):280-282. [VB]

130. Barash M, Reich KA, Rademaker D. Lidocaine-induced methemoglobinemia: a clinical reminder. *J Am Osteopath Assoc.* 2015;115(2):94-98. [VA]

131. Kane GC, Hoehn SM, Behrenbeck TR, Mulvagh SL. Benzocaine-induced methemoglobinemia based on the Mayo Clinic experience from 28 478 transesophageal echocardiograms: incidence, outcomes, and predisposing factors. *Arch Intern Med.* 2007;167(18):1977-1982. [IIIA]

132. Shamriz O, Cohen-Glickman I, Reif S, Shteyer E. Methemoglobinemia induced by lidocaine-prilocaine cream. *Isr Med Assoc J.* 2014;16(4):250-254. [VA]

133. Larson A, Stidham T, Banerji S, Kaufman J. Seizures and methemoglobinemia in an infant after excessive EMLA application. *Pediatr Emerg Care.* 2013;29(3):377-379. [VA]

134. Brown C, Bowling M. Methemoglobinemia in bronchoscopy: a case series and a review of the literature. *J Bronchology Interv Pulmonol.* 2013;20(3):241-246. [IIIC]

135. Committee on Ambulatory Surgical Care. Guidelines for ambulatory anesthesia and surgery. American Society of Anesthesiologists. https://www.asahq.org/standards-and-guidelines/guidelines-for-ambulatory-anesthesia-and-surgery. Reaffirmed October 17, 2018. Accessed August 31, 2020. [IVB]

136. *State Operations Manual Appendix A—Survey Protocol, Regulations and Interpretive Guidelines for Hospitals.* Rev. 200, 02-21-20. Centers for Medicare & Medicaid Services. https://www.cms.gov/Regulations-and-Guidance/Guidance/Manuals/downloads/som107ap_a_hospitals.pdf. Accessed August 31, 2020.

137. *State Operations Manual Appendix L—Guidance for Surveyors: Ambulatory Surgical Centers.* Rev. 200, 02-21-20. Centers for Medicare & Medicaid Services. https://www.cms.gov/Regulations-and-Guidance/Guidance/Manuals/downloads/som107ap_l_ambulatory.pdf. Accessed August 31, 2020.

138. Sagir A, Goyal R. An assessment of the awareness of local anesthetic systemic toxicity among multi-specialty postgraduate residents. *J Anesth.* 2015;29(2):299-302. [IIIB]

139. Barrington MJ, Weinberg GL, Neal JM. A call to all readers: educating all surgeons on preventing and treatment of local anaesthetic systemic toxicity. *ANZ J Surg.* 2016;86(9):636-637. [VA]

140. Urfalıoğlu A, Urfalıoğlu S, Öksüz G. The knowledge of eye physicians on local anesthetic toxicity and intravenous lipid treatment: questionnaire study. *Turk J Ophthalmol.* 2017;47(6):320-325. [IIIB]

141. AORN position statement on perioperative registered nurse circulator dedicated to every patient undergoing an operative or other invasive procedure. AORN, Inc. https://www.aorn.org/guidelines/clinical-resources/position-statements. Accessed August 31, 2020. [IVB]

Guideline Development Group and Acknowledgements

Lead Author: Mary J. Ogg[1], MSN, RN, CNOR, Senior Perioperative Practice Specialist, AORN, Denver, Colorado

Methodologist: Erin Kyle[2], DNP, RN, CNOR, NEA-BC, Editor-in-Chief, Guidelines for Perioperative Practice, AORN, Denver, Colorado

Evidence Appraiser: Marie Bashaw[3], DNP, RN, NEA-BC, Professor and Director of Nursing, Wittenberg University, Springfield, Ohio

Guidelines Advisory Board Members:

- Donna A. Pritchard[4], MA, BSN, RN, NE-BC, CNOR, Director of Perioperative Services, Interfaith Medical Center, Brooklyn, New York
- Kate McGee[5], BSN, RN, CNOR, Staff Nurse, Aurora West Allis Medical Center, East Troy, Wisconsin

Guidelines Advisory Board Liaisons:

- Craig S. Atkins[6], DNP, CRNA, Chief Nurse Anesthetist, Belmar Ambulatory Surgical Center, Lakewood, Colorado
- Cassie Dietrich[7], MD, Anesthesiologist, Anesthesia Associates of Kansas City, Overland Park, Kansas
- Juan Sanchez[8], MD, MPA, FACS, FACHE, Associate Professor of Surgery, Johns Hopkins University School of Medicine, Baltimore, Maryland
- Doug Schuerer[9], MD, FACS, FCCM, Professor of Surgery, Trauma Director, Washington University School of Medicine, St Louis, Missouri

External Review: Expert review comments were received from individual members of the American Association of Nurse Anesthetists (AANA), American College of Surgeons (ACS), Association for Professionals in Infection Control and Epidemiology (APIC), American Society of Anesthesiologists (ASA), International Association of Healthcare Central Service Materiel Management (IAHCSMM), the Society for Healthcare Epidemiology of America (SHEA), and the Surgical Infection Society (SIS). Their responses were used to further refine and enhance this guideline; however, their responses do not imply endorsement. The draft was also open for a 30-day public comment period.

Financial Disclosure and Conflicts of Interest

This guideline was developed, edited, and approved by the AORN Guidelines Advisory Board without external funding being sought or obtained. The Guidelines Advisory Board was financially supported entirely by AORN and was developed without any involvement of industry.

Potential conflicts of interest for all Guidelines Advisory Board members were reviewed before the annual meeting and each monthly conference call. None of the members of the Guideline Development Group reported a potential conflict of interest.[1-9]

Publication History

Originally published May 1984, *AORN Journal.*

Revised September 1989. Revised August 1993.

Revised November 1997; published February 1998.

Reformatted July 2000.

Revised November 2001; published April 2002, *AORN Journal.*

Revised 2006; published in *Standards, Recommended Practices, and Guidelines,* 2007 edition.

Minor editing revisions made to omit Perioperative Nursing Data Set codes; reformatted September 2012 for publication in *Perioperative Standards and Recommended Practices,* 2013 edition.

Revised October 2014; published in *Guidelines for Perioperative Practice,* 2015 edition.

Evidence ratings revised in *Guidelines for Perioperative Practice,* 2018 edition, to conform to the current AORN Evidence Rating Model.

Evidence ratings revised and minor editorial changes made to conform to the current AORN Evidence Rating model, September 2019, for online publication in *Guidelines for Perioperative Practice.*

Minor revisions to clarify symptoms of LAST made in June 2021 for online publication *in Guidelines for Perioperative Practice.*

Scheduled for review in 2025.

MEDICATION SAFETY

TABLE OF CONTENTS

Ⓐ *indicates additional information is available in the Ambulatory Supplement.*

Ⓟ *indicates a recommendation or evidence relevant to pediatric care.*

MEDICAL ABBREVIATIONS & ACRONYMS

ASC – Ambulatory surgery center
CMS – Centers for Medicare & Medicaid Services
HIPEC – Hyperthermic intraperitoneal chemotherapy
PPE – Personal protective equipment

PRN – As needed
RN - Registered nurse
SDS – Safety data sheet

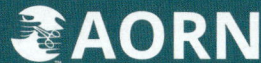
GUIDELINE FOR
MEDICATION SAFETY

The Guideline for Medication Safety was approved by the AORN Guidelines Advisory Board and became effective September 1, 2017. It was presented as a proposed guideline for comments by members and others. The recommendations in the guideline are intended to be achievable and represent what is believed to be an optimal level of practice. Policies and procedures will reflect variations in practice settings and/or clinical situations that determine the degree to which the guideline can be implemented. AORN recognizes the many diverse settings in which perioperative nurses practice; therefore, this guideline is adaptable to all areas where operative or other invasive procedures may be performed.

Purpose

This document provides guidance to perioperative team members for developing, implementing, and evaluating safety precautions that may assist with decreasing **medication errors** throughout the six phases of the medication use process. The medication use process includes procuring medication, prescribing medication, transcribing medication orders, dispensing medication, administering medication, and monitoring patient outcomes. The dispensing of medications from the pharmacy to the caregiver or patient is considered to be outside the role of the perioperative registered nurse (RN) and is not covered in this document.

Medication errors can occur at any point in the medication use process and may or may not be detected before administration of the medication. Errors detected before administration are commonly referred to as **near miss** errors.[1] Reports of medication errors show that errors can be influenced by many factors and may be connected to any person who is involved in the process. Results of medication errors can include substantial threats to patients, increased health care costs, and compromised patient confidence in the health care system.[2]

Although the phases of the medication use process are the same in all practice settings where medications are administered, there are unique considerations specific to the perioperative setting, including the following:

- The transcription and documentation phase may be omitted or modified.
- Medication is removed from the original manufacturer's packaging for aseptic delivery to the sterile field.
- An intermediary (eg, scrub person) in sterile attire receives and transfers dispensed medications to the proceduralist or assistant who is in sterile attire.

- Medications dispensed to the sterile field may be handled by multiple individuals before administration.
- Medications may be ordered and administered by multiple health care providers.
- Medications may be labeled one way on the sterile field and a different way off the sterile field.
- Sensory distractions are intrinsic to the environment.[3]

The following topics are outside the scope of this document:

- adverse drug reactions,
- drug-drug interactions,
- dosing recommendations,
- drug diversion prevention,
- medication-specific recommendations for prescribing,
- recommendations for manufacturers (eg, labeling),
- recommendations for specific components of a computerized order entry system,
- interventions that apply to the pharmacy,
- situations involving products contaminated at the manufacturer or compounder,
- regulations and recommendations based on laws that do not apply in the United States,
- antibiotic and anticoagulant stewardship programs,
- situations involving prescription of potentially inappropriate medications,
- dispensing errors,
- management of drug shortages,
- selection and administration of anesthetic agents and medication,
- medication-specific disposal methods,
- the effect of culture on reporting of medication errors,
- off-label use of medications, and
- recommendations for implementation of bar coding.

Evidence Review

A medical librarian conducted a systematic search of the databases Ovid MEDLINE®, EBSCO CINAHL®, Scopus®, and the Cochrane Database of Systematic Reviews. The search was limited to literature published in English from January 2011 through April 2016. The lead author requested additional articles that either did not fit the original search criteria or were discovered during the evidence appraisal process. The lead author and the medical librarian also identified relevant guidelines from government agencies, professional organizations, and standards-setting bodies.

Search terms included subject headings such as *operating rooms, drug storage, adverse drug event, medication systems, drug labeling, medication errors, medical waste disposal, compounding, and drug administration.* Additional keywords and phrases

Figure 1. Flow Diagram of Literature Search Results

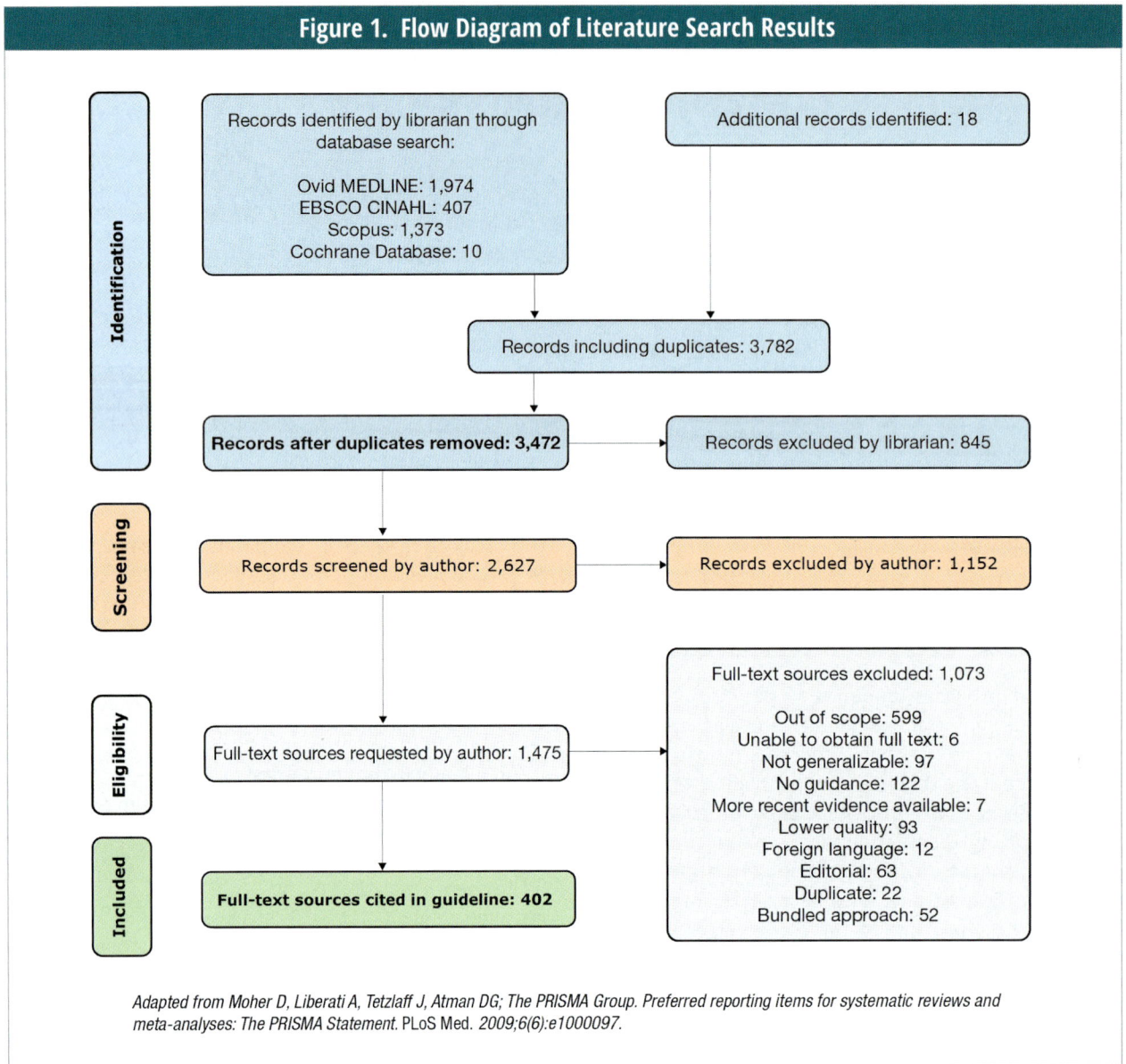

Identification

Records identified by librarian through database search:

Ovid MEDLINE: 1,974
EBSCO CINAHL: 407
Scopus: 1,373
Cochrane Database: 10

Additional records identified: 18

Records including duplicates: 3,782

Records after duplicates removed: 3,472

Records excluded by librarian: 845

Screening

Records screened by author: 2,627

Records excluded by author: 1,152

Eligibility

Full-text sources requested by author: 1,475

Full-text sources excluded: 1,073

Out of scope: 599
Unable to obtain full text: 6
Not generalizable: 97
No guidance: 122
More recent evidence available: 7
Lower quality: 93
Foreign language: 12
Editorial: 63
Duplicate: 22
Bundled approach: 52

Included

Full-text sources cited in guideline: 402

Adapted from Moher D, Liberati A, Tetzlaff J, Atman DG; The PRISMA Group. Preferred reporting items for systematic reviews and meta-analyses: The PRISMA Statement. PLoS Med. 2009;6(6):e1000097.

included *drug diversion, name differentiation, verbal order, drug storage, medication reconciliation,* and *medication cart.*

Included were research and non-research literature in English, complete publications, and publications with dates within the time restriction when available. Excluded were non-peer-reviewed publications and older evidence within the time restriction when more recent evidence was available. Editorials, news items, and other brief items were excluded. Low-quality evidence was excluded when higher-quality evidence was available, and literature outside the time restriction was excluded when literature within the time restriction was available. Also excluded were articles that presented a bundled approach, articles that described medication errors and corrective situations involving nursing students, and prevalence studies with no interventions for correction. Some international studies were excluded because the results are not generalizable to the United States **(Figure 1)**.

Articles identified in the search were provided to the project team for evaluation. The team consisted of the lead author and three evidence appraisers. The lead author divided the search results into topics and assigned members of the team to review and critically appraise each article using the AORN Research or Non-Research Evidence Appraisal Tools as appropriate. The literature was independently evaluated and appraised according to the strength and quality of the evidence. Each article was then assigned an appraisal score. The appraisal score is noted in brackets after each reference as applicable.

Each recommendation rating is based on a synthesis of the collective evidence, a benefit-harm assessment, and consideration of resource use. The strength of the recommendation was determined using the AORN Evidence Rating Model and the quality and consistency of the evidence supporting a recommendation. The recommendation strength rating is noted in brackets after each recommendation.

Note: The evidence summary table is available at http://www.aorn.org/evidencetables/.

Editor's note: MEDLINE is a registered trademark of the US National Library of Medicine's Medical Literature Analysis and Retrieval System, Bethesda, MD. CINAHL, Cumulative Index to Nursing and Allied Health Literature, is a registered trademark of EBSCO Industries, Birmingham, AL. Scopus is a registered trademark of Elsevier B.V., Amsterdam, The Netherlands.

1. Medication Management Plan

1.1 Establish a multidisciplinary team to be responsible for the oversight of the medication management plan. [Recommendation]

The multidisciplinary team may be commonly known as the pharmacy and therapeutics committee or medication safety committee. Including representatives from all disciplines involved in the process strengthens policies and procedures, contributes to interprofessional collaboration, and may enhance teamwork and compliance. Moderate quality evidence supports a multidisciplinary team approach to medication management and error prevention.[4-15]

1.2 Include the following representatives on the multidisciplinary team:
- perioperative RNs,
- **licensed independent practitioners**,
- anesthesia professionals,[16]
- pharmacists,[11,17]
- risk management/quality personnel,
- purchasing personnel,
- infection preventionists, and
- administrators.

[Recommendation]

Involving all health care professionals who participate in the medication use process assists with identifying medication error risk factors from a variety of perspectives.

1.2.1 One individual may represent more than one discipline, based on organizational staffing. [Conditional Recommendation]

Health care organizations may assign multiple roles and responsibilities to a single individual.

1.3 The multidisciplinary team should develop, oversee the implementation, and conduct an evaluation of the perioperative medication management plan. [Recommendation]

Developing a medication management plan that incorporates structures, processes, and professional responsibilities into each of the six phases of the medication use process allows for identification of latent and active failures and provides a guideline for performing the steps of the medication use process.

1.3.1 Include the following processes in the medication management plan:
- procuring, storing, and disposing of all medications[11,18] (See Recommendations 2 and 11);
- administering medication (See Recommendation 5);
- performing **medication reconciliation** (See Recommendation 6);
- managing **hazardous medications**, when applicable (See Recommendation 10)[19];
- transcribing medication orders (See Recommendation 13);
- monitoring quality assurance and improvement (See Recommendation 15);
- managing look-alike and sound-alike medications;
- managing medication shortages, discontinuations, or recalls[14,20,21];
- managing **high-alert medications**[22]; and
- creating, maintaining, and reviewing preference cards and standing order forms.

[Recommendation]

1.3.2 Align the perioperative medication plan with the facility or health care organization medication plan. [Recommendation]

1.3.3 Communicate the medication management plan to all members of the perioperative team. [Recommendation]

Increasing the perioperative team's awareness of the health care organization's medication management plan disseminates a broader picture of medication risk-reduction strategies and can help communicate the interdependence of the team's actions.[14]

1.3.4 Implement the medication management plan consistently in all areas where operative and other invasive procedures are performed. [Recommendation]

1.4 The multidisciplinary team should
- establish, monitor, and review the portion of the formulary unique to the perioperative services[11,23];
- establish, monitor, and review medications that are routinely stocked at par level in perioperative medication storage areas;
- establish the frequency of the review of the formulary and medication stock;

- establish the type of labels to be used, including preprinted labels for use on the sterile field[24];
- define the scope, role, orientation, and assessment of competency for supplemental personnel (eg, temporary personnel, contracted pharmacist) as related to the medication use process; and
- standardize medication-related perioperative documents.

[Recommendation]

The author of an organizational experience report found compliance with labeling of medications improved with the use of preprinted labels.[25]

1.5 **The multidisciplinary team should select technological devices (eg, bar-code systems, computerized prescriber order entry system, biometrics, pharmacy automation, radio-frequency identification systems, electronic medication storage and inventory systems, electronic medication administration records, electronic medication reconciliation tools) to be used during all phases of the medication use process based primarily on the safety aspects incorporated into each device.** *[Recommendation]*

High-quality evidence supports the use of technological devices to decrease medication errors[26-47] or the potential for errors.[48-51] In addition, the evidence establishes other benefits for the use of technological devices, including providing nurses with more patient contact time,[52] improving medication order turnaround time,[53-55] and decreasing prescribing time.[55-58]

The use of computerized ordering systems has also been shown to result in fewer illegible and incomplete prescriptions.[59-61] Meisenberg et al[62] conducted a quality study that found preprinted orders contained fewer errors than handwritten orders, and orders entered in a computerized prescriber order entry system contained even fewer errors. Eighty-five (91%) of the 93 physicians who responded to a survey believed that computerized order entry decreased the number of medication errors compared to handwritten prescriptions.[63] In addition, in other nonexperimental studies, use of automated dispensing cabinets has been shown to decrease the number of medication selection and preparation errors[64,65] and increase efficiency.[66]

Conversely, some of the literature documents situations in which medication errors continued to occur or new errors occurred following implementation of computerized medication information systems (eg, selection of the wrong medication from the list on the computer).[47,62,67-84] In addition, in an observational, cross-sectional comparative study, Hinojosa-Amaya et al[85] found that the number of errors decreased but the severity of the errors

increased when a computerized prescriber order entry system was instituted. The severity of errors was measured on a 9-point scale ranging from "capacity to cause error" to "contributes to or causes death."

In a review of the literature, Fischer[34] found that the number of errors decreased when computerized order entry was used, but the author could not determine whether there was an association between the errors and patient harm. Another review of the literature identified that some of the medication errors connected with computerized order entry include wrong-patient errors; duplicate orders; and selection of the wrong dose, wrong route, wrong timing, and wrong drug.[86] In a quasi-experimental study, Leung et al[87] found a 45% decrease in the number of preventable adverse drug events with the use of a computerized order entry system with advanced clinical decision support, but the number of potential adverse drug events increased significantly.

In a qualitative study, Hoonakker et al[88] found that computerized prescriber order entry systems disrupted the quality of physician–nurse communication for the short term (ie, 3 months), but the quality of communication returned to pre-implementation levels in the long term (ie, 12 months).

Tschannen et al[89] reviewed the effects of the implementation of a computerized order entry system on nursing workflow and found that the process to confirm orders was lengthened and there was a reduction in communication between medical and nursing personnel. The researchers theorized this could lead to an increase in medication errors.

1.6 **The multidisciplinary team should develop and review a list of do-not-use abbreviations and symbols that are inappropriate for inclusion in documentation.** *[Recommendation]*

Two studies found that even with a "do not use" list, problems persisted because prescribers continued to use other error-prone abbreviations that were not on the list.[90,91]

1.7 **The health care organization must provide resources to the perioperative team, such as up-to-date online reference materials and access to drug information centers.**[23] *[Regulatory Requirement]*

Regulatory and professional guidelines, a review of the literature, and a descriptive study of medication errors in an intensive care unit emphasize the importance of having various resources available to help prevent medication errors.[9,23,92,93]

1.8 **Involve pharmacists in all phases of medication management.** *[Recommendation]*

There is general agreement worldwide that benefits are realized when a pharmacist is involved in all phases of the medication use process. These benefits include a decrease in readmissions, decreased medication discrepancies upon discharge, identification of medication errors before administration, and decreased costs.[9,11,94-122] Two studies involving critical access facilities found fewer dispensing errors when the dispensing was done by a pharmacist compared to a telepharmacy service[65] and fewer medication errors when a pharmacist was present at least 40 hours per week.[123]

Conversely, McCoy et al[124] conducted a randomized clinical trial that sought to determine whether pharmacy surveillance of patients with acute kidney injury would detect and prevent medication errors that were not corrected by the electronic clinical support system. The researchers did not find a significant decrease in the number of errors and concluded that pharmacy surveillance did not show an incremental benefit over the clinical decision support systems already in place.

Evidence supports the involvement of a pharmacist in medication reconciliation.[102,125,126] Some of the evidence supports medication reconciliation being performed by a pharmacist instead of nurses,[127,128] a resident/intern,[129] or a pharmacy technician.[128] Aag et al[130] found that the medication reconciliation process was completed in less time by the pharmacist than by a nurse, but there was not a significant difference in the number of discrepancies found. Zemaitis et al[131] found a decrease in readmission rates when a pharmacist performed medication reconciliation.

1.8.1 **The health care organization may contract with a pharmacist to provide consultative services onsite or via telepharmacy.**[23,132,133] *[Conditional Recommendation]*

The Centers for Medicare & Medicaid Services (CMS) Conditions of Participation states that "Hospitals must provide pharmaceutical services that meet the needs of their patients."[23] The CMS Conditions for Coverage for ambulatory surgery centers (ASCs) states that a specific licensed health care professional is required to provide direction to the ASC's pharmaceutical service unless the ASC is performing activities that under state law may only be performed by a licensed pharmacist.[132] **(A)**

2. Procurement and Storage

2.1 **Take precautions to mitigate the risks associated with medication and medication-related supply procurement and storage.** *[Recommendation]*

The literature, including regulatory requirements, describes several strategies for safe procurement and storage of medication.[14,23,132,134-137]

2.2 **Procure medications**
- **as single-dose units if available,**
- **in a size as close as possible to the anticipated dose,**
- **in prefilled syringes if available, and**
- **in limited concentrations.**

[Recommendation]

Procurement of single-dose vials in the smallest available size produces less waste,[134-136] and prefilled syringes eliminate the potential for relabeling errors.[137]

2.3 **All medications and related supplies must be stored securely in areas with limited access, including refrigerated areas, anesthesia carts, and emergency carts.**[14,23,138] *[Regulatory Requirement]*

The CMS states,

The operating room suite is considered secure when the suite is staffed and staff are actively providing patient care. When the suite is not in use (e.g., weekends, holidays and after hours), it would not be considered secure. A hospital may choose to lock the entire suite, lock non-mobile carts containing drugs and biologicals, place mobile carts in a locked room, or otherwise lock drugs and biologicals in a secure area. If an individual operating room is not in use, the hospital is expected to lock non-mobile carts, and ensure mobile carts are in a locked room. . . . Due to their mobility, mobile nursing medication carts, anesthesia carts, epidural carts and other medication carts containing drugs or biologicals . . . must be locked in a secure area when not in use.[23]

2.4 **Store medications according to the specifications (eg, temperature) stated in the medication manufacturer's instructions for use.**[11,14,23] *[Recommendation]*

Medications may have sensitive formulations that require storage at specific temperature ranges to maintain stability or avoid inactivation. Failure to control the temperature of medication storage areas may result in decreased therapeutic levels caused by inactivation, a change in pH, a change in concentration, or spoilage. Temperature-sensitive medications have been shown to deteriorate when stored outside of the recommended temperature ranges.[139]

2.4.1 **Medications that require refrigeration must be stored in a segregated area of the refrigerator with restricted access.**[132] *[Regulatory Requirement]*

2.5 All Class II, III, IV, and V medications must be stored in a locked location.[23,132] *[Regulatory Requirement]* Ⓐ

2.6 Organize medications in the storage areas including emergency and specialty carts in a standardized manner using safety considerations, including
- separating medications by generic name and packaging;
- separating high-alert medications;
- providing separate bins or dividers for all medications in storage;
- labeling storage bins, using **tall man lettering** when possible, with both the medication's generic and brand names;
- positioning medication containers so that the labels are visible; and
- avoiding alphabetical storage.

[Recommendation]

Placing medications in storage areas using these safety considerations may assist in selection of the correct medication and decrease the potential for medication errors.[140,141]

2.6.1 Separate sound-alike and look-alike medications in storage locations.[10,137,142] *[Recommendation]*

Incidents of the wrong medication being selected because of look-alike containers and labels have been reported in the literature.[77,137,140,143-149]

3. Prescribing Phase

3.1 Take precautions to mitigate the risk for medication errors in the prescribing phase of the medication use process. *[Recommendation]*

Moderate-quality evidence establishes that medication errors occur during the prescribing phase. The reported errors are related to the use of incorrect abbreviations, illegible handwriting, and incomplete information.[6,70,79,82,150-152]

3.2 All medications must be prescribed by a licensed independent practitioner in accordance with state and federal regulatory requirements. *[Regulatory Requirement]*

Regulatory requirements direct prescriptive authority.[11,14,23,132,153-155]

3.3 In medication orders,
- do not use trailing zeros;
- use leading zeros, if the dose is less than 1 unit of the selected unit of measure; and
- use only approved abbreviations.[91,155-157]

[Recommendation]

Clinical guidelines provide recommendations for the required elements of medication orders.[9,17,154,158,159] In a nonexperimental study of medication administration, Gimenes et al[82] found that 91.3% of the prescriptions contained abbreviations. The researchers recommended using no abbreviations or acronyms.

3.3.1 When hand writing medication orders, write legibly and include a legible signature of the prescriber initiating the order. *[Recommendation]* Ⓐ

3.4 Pick lists, preference cards, and protocols that contain orders for medications may be considered preprinted orders if so defined in the facility or health care organization policy and procedure. When considered to be a preprinted order, place the item in the patient's medical record unless the order is recorded by another means. *[Conditional Recommendation]*

No evidence defining pick lists, preference cards, or protocols was found in the literature review for this guideline. Use of standing orders is a commonly accepted practice throughout the United States. The literature did not reveal any specific evidence related to medications included in standing orders; however, there are regulatory requirements for documentation of medication orders.[23,132]

3.4.1 Preprinted orders must be reviewed for accuracy by the prescribing licensed independent practitioner at least annually and after every change.[23,132,159,160] *[Regulatory Requirement]*

3.4.2 A written order to reflect items requiring a prescriber's order must be placed in the patient's medical record.[23] *[Regulatory Requirement]*

3.5 For verbal medication orders, which must only be used when required by clinical necessity,
- allow only authorized persons to receive and carry out the order, consistent with federal and state law and the health care organization policy and procedures;
- confirm the order by reading back the order to the prescriber digit by digit and spelling out the medication name if necessary;
- immediately record the order in the patient's record;
- have the prescriber review, validate, and sign the order as close as possible to the time of the medication administration;
- have the person documenting the order sign it legibly; and

- verify the order contains all components of a written order. *[Regulatory Requirement]*

The CMS regulations and professional practice guidelines identify the necessary elements for safe use of verbal orders.[14,23,132,161,162] Verbal orders can be misinterpreted for a number of reasons, including but not limited to, regional dialects, background noise, muffled voices behind surgical masks, and orders involving sound-alike or commonly confused medication names. Verbal orders have been the source of medication errors.[161]

4. Preparation

4.1 Take precautions to mitigate the risk of medication errors occurring when the medication is obtained and prepared. *[Recommendation]*

Grou Volpe et al[8] conducted a descriptive study of medication errors that involved 484 medication administrations; 293 of the administrations (61%) contained errors that occurred during the preparation phase. Preparation errors were defined as any discrepancy that occurred during the preparation and formulation of the medication. The preparation errors included incorrect dilution, mixing of two incompatible medications, and inadequate packaging. The researchers did not define "inadequate packaging."

4.2 Retrieve medications from storage bins, automated dispensing storage systems, or a satellite pharmacy for only one patient at a time. *[Recommendation]*

Retrieving medications for more than one patient at a time may increase the risk for error. Medication administration errors have occurred because a perioperative nurse retrieved the wrong product from an automated dispensing system.[163] If a restocking error has occurred, it is more likely to be detected if the nurse is focused on each medication required for the individual patient at the time the medication is being retrieved.

4.2.1 Verify all medications obtained from storage against the original medication order. *[Recommendation]*

The original medication order, including preprinted order forms, prescriptions, or preference cards, establishes what medication the prescriber intended the patient to receive. Automated dispensing storage systems have been reported to have up to a 5% misfill rate.[164] As medications are obtained, an additional visual confirmation of the order and product will help establish accuracy in administering the correct medication.

4.3 Use compounded medications prepared by a compounding pharmacy that meets the standards specified in USP 797 when available.[165] *[Recommendation]*

Moderate-quality evidence supports medication **compounding** in a pharmacy and under sterile conditions to decrease the potential for contamination.[17,165-167]

4.4 When medications compounded by a compounding pharmacy that meets the standards specified in USP 797 are not available, medications may be compounded in the perioperative suite for immediate use.[165] *[Conditional Recommendation]*

4.4.1 Perioperative personnel performing compounding in the perioperative suite must
- have completed competency verification;
- combine no more than three medications together;
- perform hand hygiene before compounding;
- disinfect nonsterile surfaces including the medication container;
- use aseptic technique;
- use dispensing equipment or a sterile syringe for removal of medication from the container;
- verify the correct medication, amount, and concentration;
- visually inspect the compounded medication for absence of particulate material; and
- apply a label unless the medication is being immediately administered or verify the label applied by the scrub person if medication is transferred to the sterile field.[23,165]

[Regulatory Requirement]

4.4.2 Administration of medications compounded in the perioperative suite must begin within 1 hour of compounding.[23,165] *[Regulatory Requirement]*

Medications compounded in the perioperative suite are considered to be at high risk for contamination because they have been compounded in a location where room air quality is less than ISO Class 5.[165]

4.4.3 Medications compounded in the perioperative suite must be under continuous observation if not administered immediately. *[Regulatory Requirement]*

Continuous observation reduces the potential for contamination or confusion with other compounded preparations.[23,165]

4.5 Label compounded preparations prepared off the sterile field with
- patient identification information,
- the names and amounts of all ingredients,
- the name or initials of the person who prepared the compound,
- the date of preparation, and
- the beyond-use date and time (See Recommendation 7 for labeling requirements on the sterile field).[9,23,137,168]

[*Recommendation*]

4.5.1 When a medication is compounded off the sterile field and will be either administered immediately or delivered immediately to the sterile field, labeling is not required. [*Recommendation*]

4.5.2 When a medication is prepared in multiple concentrations, use labels that are different colors.[166] [*Recommendation*]

4.5.3 Include the full medication name on the medication label; do not abbreviate the name.[169] [*Recommendation*]

4.5.4 Use tall man lettering on labels placed on containers (eg, syringes, sterile medication cups, IV bags) if medications have look-alike or sound-alike names (See Recommendation 7.6.1). [*Recommendation*]

The evidence supports the use of tall man lettering to increase name differentiation between look-alike medication names.[9,10,16,17,24,140,142,170-175]

5. Administration

5.1 Take precautions to mitigate the risk for errors during medication administration. [*Recommendation*]

Moderate-quality evidence describes the causes of medication errors that occur during the administration phase.[8,70,168,176] Causes include dosage miscalculation,[6,177] name mix-ups,[77,143,178-182] omissions errors,[6,8,150,151] wrong time,[6,8,150] and syringe swap.[183]

5.2 Administer all medications according to the manufacturer's instructions for use. [*Recommendation*] Ⓐ

Manufacturer's instructions for use provide specific instructions for dosage and administration.

5.3 Before administering medication, verify the
- right patient using at least two patient identifiers,
- right medication,
- right dose,
- right route,
- right time,
- right strength or concentration,
- right medication administration rate, and
- infusion pump settings, if applicable.[3,23,141]

[*Recommendation*]

5.3.1 Verify the compatibility of medications administered through a single IV line before concurrent administration. [*Recommendation*]

In a descriptive study, Kanji et al[184] reviewed 434 simultaneously administered medication infusions and found that 68% contained medications that were considered to be incompatible but were administered simultaneously through the same IV tubing. The researchers did not report on the outcomes of the patients in the study.

5.3.2 A dosage calculation tool may be used to calculate maximum dose limits, especially for high-alert medications. [*Conditional Recommendation*]

5.4 Verify that the patient is not allergic to the medication. [*Recommendation*]

Adverse events have been reported because allergies were not verified.[185]

5.5 Verify that the medication dose is correctly adjusted to the patient's weight. [*Recommendation*] Ⓟ

Adverse events have been reported because the dosage was not appropriate for the weight of the patient.[9,186]

5.6 Develop and use a double-checking system (eg, independent double check) performed by two licensed individuals for predetermined high-alert and high-risk medications (eg, insulin, heparin). [*Recommendation*]

Low-quality evidence supports double checking of high-alert and high-risk medications to decrease medication administration errors.[9,17,137,141,155,168,187-190] However, after conducting a systematic literature review, Alsulami et al[191] concluded that there was insufficient evidence to support or refute the practice of double checking. The review consisted of 16 studies including three qualitative studies and one randomized controlled trial. The researchers recommended that more studies be completed to determine the efficacy of double checking high-alert and high-risk medications.

5.7 Confirm preoperatively that the patient has taken or discontinued medications and herbal supplements on the day of surgery or the designated number of days before surgery as ordered by the licensed independent practitioner. *[Recommendation]*

5.7.1 Notify the physician and anesthesia professional if the patient has not taken or has not discontinued medications as ordered. *[Recommendation]*

5.8 Do not interrupt or distract personnel who are preparing and administering medications. *[Recommendation]*

Moderate-quality evidence supports preventing interruptions and distractions during medication administration because interruptions have been shown to be a cause of medication errors.[7,176,192-201]

5.8.1 Use a distraction- and interruption-free zone when available.[202] *[Recommendation]*

5.8.2 Use a do-not-interrupt signal method (eg, a "do not disturb" sign, vest, verbal cue) during medication administration. *[Recommendation]*

The use of do-not-interrupt signals to indicate when the person administering or preparing medications should not be disturbed has been shown to contribute to decreasing medication errors.[10,192,193,200-204]

5.8.3 A standard phrase, such as "I cannot be interrupted now," established by the health care organization's policy and procedure may be used to help prevent interruptions during medication administration.[201,202] *[Conditional Recommendation]*

5.9 Use single-dose/single-use vials and single-use dispensing devices on only one patient. *[Recommendation]*

Low-quality evidence contains reports of infections being transmitted by the reuse of single-patient vials and single-use dispensing devices (eg, insulin pens) on more than one patient.[134,205-208] The contamination of single-use medication vials has also been demonstrated in laboratory studies.[209] In a nonexperimental study, Baniasadi et al[210] examined opened single and **multidose vials** that were within their use date and found both types of vials were contaminated after the initial medication withdrawal.

5.9.1 Use a sterile needle and a sterile syringe each time a medication is withdrawn from a single-dose/single-use vial. *[Recommendation]*

A Joint Commission *Sentinel Event Alert* and a case study contain reports of bacterial and viral (eg, hepatitis B and C) infections being spread by the reuse of needles and syringes.[134,211]

5.10 Use multidose vials for only one patient when medication is prepared at the point of use. *[Recommendation]*

Low-quality evidence contains reports of infections being spread by use of a multidose vial for more than one patient.[134,212-214]

5.10.1 Use a sterile needle and a sterile syringe each time a medication is withdrawn from a multidose vial. *[Recommendation]*

The literature contains reports of infections being spread by the use of a multidose vial for more than one patient and recommends use of a sterile needle and a sterile syringe each time a vial is entered.[134,211,215,216]

5.10.2 Label multidose vials at the time of first use with a beyond-use date of 28 days or as specified by the manufacturer.[165] *[Recommendation]*

When a product has been opened or a vial cap has been punctured or removed, the manufacturer's expiration date is no longer valid unless it is within the 28-day limit.[134]

5.10.3 When a multidose vial is supplied with individual applicator tips, change the applicator tip between uses for different patients. *[Recommendation]*

One nonexperimental study showed no contamination of the solution when a fresh tip was used.[217]

5.11 Store multidose vials outside the immediate patient treatment area when possible.[134] *[Recommendation]*

5.12 Use alcohol to disinfect the rubber septum on all vials and allow vials to dry before each entry. *[Recommendation]*

Moderate-quality evidence supports disinfecting the rubber septum to remove any contaminant present on the stopper.[134,218]

5.13 Use a syringe and needle only once to administer a medication to a single patient, then discard the syringe and needle. *[Recommendation]*

5.13.1 When administering incremental doses to a single patient from the same syringe is an integral part of the procedure, the same syringe and needle may be reused, with strict adherence to aseptic technique. *[Conditional Recommendation]*

5.13.2 Do not leave the syringe unattended and discard it immediately at the end of the procedure. *[Recommendation]*

509

5.14 Carefully read the labels on all containers before removing the contents for preparation or administration. [*Recommendation*]

The literature contains reports of medication errors resulting from syringe swaps and clearly labeled syringes not being read carefully by the person administering the medication.[137,168,219] Wearing colored lenses, such as laser goggles, may distort the wearer's ability to determine the color of the label.[220]

5.15 Discard all medication containers (eg, vials, ampules) for which the sterility has been compromised.[134] [*Recommendation*]

5.16 Discard unused, opened irrigation or IV solutions at the end of the procedure. [*Recommendation*]

Irrigation and IV containers and supplies are considered to be for single-patient use. Using surplus volume from any irrigation or IV solution containers or supplies for more than one patient increases the risk of cross contamination.

5.17 Discard medications that are removed from the original package and found in a secondary container without a label. [*Recommendation*]

Medications that are removed from the original package and not labeled cannot be verified before administration, which may increase the risk for administering the wrong medication.

5.18 Puncture (eg, spike) intravenous solution containers within 1 hour of the initiation of administration. [*Recommendation*]

The Association for Professionals in Infection Control and Epidemiology supports beginning administration within 1 hour of the medication being spiked.[221]

Haas et al[222] tested lactated Ringer's solution for bacterial contamination at various times (ie, at the time of spiking; 1, 2, 4, and 8 hours after spiking) and found no bacterial growth at any of the time points. The mean number of bags sampled was 16 (range, 15 to 17) at each time point. A limitation of this study is that the test was not conducted on any other solutions used in the clinical setting.

5.19 Take precautions to mitigate the risk for errors associated with tubing by
- tracing all tubing to the point of origin and point of insertion,
- labeling all tubing and injection ports with the point of exit (eg, epidural, arterial, venous),
- avoiding the use of y-port extension tubing,
- aligning tubing to avoid tangling and to facilitate easy identification,

- avoiding use of standard Luer-lock syringes for medications intended for oral or enteric administration,
- allowing only individuals who have been deemed competent to manage connections and lines, and
- using only non-Luer-lock connectors on spinal, epidural, and combined spinal/epidural devices.[168]

[*Recommendation*]

The literature contains reports of medication errors related to tubing misconnections and tubing mixups that support the use of the precautions listed.[17,146,189,223-230]

5.20 Retain all used medication vials and delivery devices in the OR or invasive procedure room until the completion of the procedure.[188] [*Recommendation*]

6. Transitions of Care

6.1 Take precautions to mitigate the risk for errors during the transitions of care between phases of perioperative care. [*Recommendation*]

High-quality evidence from national and international sources supports the use of **medication reconciliation** as a method for detecting potential medication errors, reducing hospital admissions,[155,231,232] and creating financial savings.[128,231-233] The errors consist of omissions,[234] medications prescribed without indication,[235] incorrect routes, and incorrect dosages.[231,236-259] Conversely, a systematic review of the literature and a quasi-experimental study did not find a benefit to medication reconciliation.[260,261] Medication errors have been reported to occur during all phases of perioperative care.[262,263] This recommendation specifies the role of the perioperative nurse in the reconciliation process and includes the information that should be shared at the time of a transition of care.

6.2 Obtain a baseline medication history at admission.[262] [*Recommendation*]

6.2.1 Include the following in the medication history:
- the patient's allergies and symptoms of reaction and
- all products taken regularly or as needed and administered via all routes, including prescribed and nonprescribed medications and herbal and dietary supplements.

[*Recommendation*]

An analysis of medication errors supports including these components in a medication history.[253] This list of medications is the first step in the medication reconciliation process and provides information necessary for reconciling the patient's medications at the time of discharge.[262] Many patients take herbal remedies that may interact with prescribed medications and affect postprocedure patient outcomes.[264]

6.2.2 Include the name, dose, frequency, route, purpose, and date and time of the last dose taken for each item listed in the medication history. *[Recommendation]*

6.2.3 Obtain the medication history by interview with the patient or caregivers and, if information is missing, consult additional sources (eg, the primary physician's office, pharmacy, primary caregivers including home health nurses). *[Recommendation]*

High-quality evidence supports obtaining the list of medications by interview instead of by using only the existing medical record because discrepancies have been found between medical records and patient-stated lists.[265] Moderate-quality evidence also supports use of other sources because inaccuracies have been discovered in medication histories obtained strictly from patients.[266]

6.3 The medication history and medications administered during each phase of care should be communicated to the receiving caregiver by a person designated by the health care organization. *[Recommendation]*

Sharing of information regarding the medication history and medications administered may decrease medication errors.

6.3.1 Include the following in the information provided to the receiving caregiver using the means described in the facility or health care organization policy and procedure:
- Preoperative to intraoperative phase:
  - medication allergies and reaction,
  - preoperative medication history including the last dose taken,
  - medications administered during the preoperative phase including the dose and time, and
  - effects of medications administered during the preoperative phase.
- Intraoperative change of personnel:
  - medication allergies and reactions,
  - preoperative medication history including the last dose taken,

  - medications administered during the preoperative phase including the dose and time,
  - effects of medications administered during the preoperative phase,
  - medications administered during intraoperative phase including the dose and time,
  - IV and irrigation fluids administered intraoperatively,
  - anesthesia type and route,
  - current or pending laboratory or other test results that relate to medications, and
  - medications present on the sterile field.
- Intraoperative to postoperative phase I or phase II:
  - medication allergies and reaction,
  - preoperative medication history including the last dose taken,
  - medications received during the preoperative phase including the dose and time,
  - effects of medications received during the preoperative phase,
  - medications administered during the intraoperative phase including the dose and time,
  - patient responses to medications administered during the intraoperative phase,
  - IV and irrigation fluids administered,
  - anesthesia type and route,
  - current or pending laboratory or other test results that relate to medications,
  - infusion pump settings if applicable, and
  - surgeon's orders for medications if present.
- Postoperative phase I to postoperative phase II or to an inpatient caregiver:
  - medication allergies,
  - preoperative medication history including the last dose taken,
  - medications received during the preoperative phase including the dose and time,
  - effects of medications received during the preoperative phase,
  - medications administered during the intraoperative phase including the dose and time,
  - effects of medications received during the intraoperative phase,
  - IV and irrigation fluids administered,
  - anesthesia type and route,
  - current or pending laboratory or other test results that relate to medications,
  - infusion pump settings if applicable,
  - surgeon's orders for medications if present,

- medications administered during the postoperative phase including the dose and time,
- the patient's responses to medications administered during the postoperative phase, and
- IV fluids administered.

[Recommendation]

6.4 Complete the medication reconciliation process before the patient is discharged. *[Recommendation]*

Moderate-quality evidence supports performing medication reconciliation during all phases of care to decrease medication errors and unintentional discrepancies.[4,14,216,245,253,262,267-275] The evidence specific to the perioperative setting is limited; however, the evidence derived from other settings is relevant to perioperative care. Some of the literature revealed that medication errors do occur after medication reconciliation[276]; however, the reported errors did not affect patient outcomes.[277]

6.4.1 Compare the medication history to the post-discharge medication instructions and verify that medications ordered are indicated and dosages are appropriate. *[Recommendation]*

6.4.2 Consult with or alert the prescriber if discrepancies between the admission history and the discharge medication list are found. *[Recommendation]*

6.4.3 Document the results of the consultation. *[Recommendation]*

6.5 The medication reconciliation process should
- be standardized for all patients,
- include the use of a standardized medication reconciliation form that may be electronic with a scripted list of questions or prompts,[234] and
- engage patients and their caregivers.[31,278-281]

[Recommendation]

7. Transfer to the Sterile Field

7.1 Take precautions to mitigate the risk for errors during transfer of medications to the sterile field and handling of medications on the sterile field. *[Recommendation]*

The literature contains reports of errors including incorrect medications being drawn up from unlabeled bowls and incorrect medications being administered from unlabeled syringes on the sterile field.[16,24,282]

7.2 Before transferring medication to the sterile field, check the expiration date and visually inspect the medication for any indication that the medication was compromised during the storage process (eg, particulates, discoloration). If there is any question of compromise, do not transfer the item to the sterile field and discard it according to facility or health care organization policy and procedure. *[Recommendation]*

7.3 The RN circulator transferring the medication to the sterile field and the person receiving the medication should concurrently verify the medication name, strength, dosage, and expiration date by reading the label aloud.[16,24,140,283] *[Recommendation]*

7.4 Use aseptic technique during transfer of medications to the sterile field.[284] *[Recommendation]*

7.4.1 Do not remove rubber stoppers from vials unless they are designed to be removed. *[Recommendation]*

7.4.2 Use a commercially available sterile transfer device (eg, sterile vial spike, filter straw, plastic catheter) to deliver medications to the sterile field. *[Recommendation]*

Medication vials are not designed to pour the contents aseptically into a secondary container on the sterile field. Transfer devices are designed to minimize splashing, spilling, and the need to reach over the sterile field, which may cause contamination of the sterile field.

7.5 Transfer only one medication at a time to the sterile field and apply a label immediately, before another medication or solution is transferred.[16,24,283] *[Recommendation]*

7.6 Label containers and syringes on the sterile field that contain medications, solutions, chemicals, and reagents immediately after they are received[141]
- with the medication name, strength, dilution and diluent if used, date, and time accepted on to the sterile field[141];
- with no abbreviations or only approved abbreviations and dose expressions[175]; and
- without unnecessary information.[175]

[Recommendation]

7.6.1 Use tall man lettering on labels placed on containers (eg, syringes, sterile medication cups, IV bags) and shelving and bins containing products with look-alike names. *[Recommendation]*

Moderate-quality evidence supports the use of tall man lettering to increase name differentiation between look-alike medication names.[9,10,16,17,24,140,142,170-175] Or and Wang[285] found that tall man lettering increased differentiation accuracy, but other typographic styles were also effective.

7.7 **The RN circulator transferring the medication to the sterile field and the person receiving the medication should concurrently verify the label on the medication container on the sterile field.** *[Recommendation]*

7.8 **Verify the label of the medications, solutions, chemicals, and reagents at the time of relief of the RN circulator or the scrub person.**[24,283] *[Recommendation]*

Hand overs involving multiple personnel increase the risk for miscommunication. Enhancing communication among perioperative team members may help reduce medication errors.

7.9 **Discard unlabeled solutions on the sterile field.**[24] *[Recommendation]*

7.10 **Deliver medications, solutions, chemicals, and reagents to the sterile field as close as possible to the time they will be administered.**[24,283] *[Recommendation]*

7.11 **If there is no designated scrub person, the licensed person delivering the medication to the sterile field should confirm the medication visually and verbally with the licensed independent practitioner performing the procedure.** *[Recommendation]*

7.12 **Give verbal confirmation when a medication is passed to the licensed independent practitioner for subsequent administration, even when only one medication is on the sterile field.** *[Recommendation]*

A standardized method of communication may help reduce the risk for error involving medications on the sterile field.

8. Patient Monitoring

8.1 **Perioperative team members who are responsible for medication administration must monitor the patient for therapeutic effect or adverse reactions to medications.**[23] *[Regulatory Requirement]*

Adverse patient outcomes as a result of inadequate monitoring after medication administration are reported in the literature.[6,70,178,286] Assessing the patient's response to medication provides information related to dose effectiveness and the identifi-

cation of symptoms of a potential medication-related adverse effect (eg, anaphylaxis, toxicity), which facilitates a timely and effective response. Monitoring the patient for effects of medications is consistent with professional standards associated with the medication use process.[287]

8.2 **Perioperative team members who are responsible for medication administration should monitor and document the patient's physiological and psychological responses. The physiological and psychological responses monitored (eg, heart rate and rhythm, blood pressure, level of consciousness) should be based on the patient's condition and needs and the procedure performed. The frequency should be as described in the facility policy and procedure.**[17,23,288,289] *[Recommendation]*

8.2.1 **Document patient responses as close as possible to the time the medication was administered and the response was observed.** *[Recommendation]*

8.3 **Include the patient's medication regimen in the postprocedure assessment (eg, postdischarge telephone call) completed by the perioperative RN or pharmacist.** *[Recommendation]*

Including the patient's medication regimen in the postprocedure assessment provides an opportunity to confirm the patient's status, response to medications, actual adverse conditions (eg, nausea, vomiting, ineffective pain control, inability to perform activities of daily living), and knowledge and compliance with the medication regimen.

9. Education

9.1 **Education regarding the preoperative and postoperative medication regimen must be provided to the patient, caregivers, and other individuals involved in the patient's care.**[23,132] *[Regulatory Requirement]*

Moderate-quality evidence supports patient education and shows patients may not understand their medication regimen.[242] Education is connected with decreasing adverse drug events related to medications improperly self-administered by the patient after discharge[182] and helps decrease readmissions.[117,127]

9.1.1 **In the preprocedure education, include which medications are to be held and which medications are to be taken.**[290] *[Recommendation]*

9.1.2 In the postprocedure education, include
- a list of medications to be taken;
- when to discontinue medications;
- when to resume medications that were being taken;
- a list of discontinued medications;
- the method of measurement and self-administration of medications, including injection techniques if injectable medications are prescribed;
- medication safety precautions (eg, medications should be taken only as prescribed, medications should not be shared, medications should be secured);
- when to obtain medication-related laboratory tests;
- potential adverse effects and when to seek medical attention;
- the method of storage and handling;
- the method of disposal for unused medications;
- use of patient-controlled administration devices;
- the importance of keeping a list of current allergies and current medications; and
- sources for additional information and ongoing education.[134,155,242,273,291-298]

[Recommendation]

In addition, high-quality evidence suggests that patient education at discharge improves patient satisfaction and medication adherence.[299] Valente and Murray[300] found that after 500 patients returning for care in a physician's office received educational materials on the significance of allergies, 340 of the patients submitted amended forms listing allergies not previously included on their medical records. They concluded that the education resulted in an improvement in the accuracy of the allergies listed on the medical records. Patient education is also supported in the ASHP guidelines on preventing medication errors with chemotherapy and biotherapy.[9]

9.2 Patient medication instructions should be
- provided verbally and in written format[301];
- tailored to the needs of the patient,[301] including
  ○ age-specific requirements (eg, large print),
  ○ special population needs (eg, non-English speaking, hearing impaired),
  ○ readability or level of comprehension (eg, 5th grade, 8th grade, college), and
  ○ health literacy level;
- provided to the patient, support persons, and any additional care providers[155]; and
- documented on the patient record.[154]

[Recommendation]

9.2.1 Standardize and print written medication instruction sheets.[290] *[Recommendation]*

10. Hazardous Medications

10.1 Take precautions to mitigate the risks related to handling hazardous medications. *[Recommendation]*

The literature contains reports of harmful effects resulting from handling hazardous medications and supports the use of safety measures.[302-308] Absorption of hazardous medications occurs via the dermal route, inhalation, ingestion, accidental injection, and exposure to excreta from patients receiving chemotherapy.[309] In a nonexperimental study, Gulten et al[310] demonstrated that use of personal protective equipment (PPE) and engineering precautions have preventive effects on genotoxicity caused by handling of antineoplastic drugs.

10.2 The health care organization must create a hazardous medication management plan.[311] *[Regulatory Requirement]* Ⓐ

10.2.1 Include the following in the hazardous medication management plan:
- a list of hazardous medications administered in the facility[19,312];
- safe work practices, including facility and engineering controls to be used when handling hazardous medications;
- role-specific educational requirements;
- when PPE is to be used and by whom; and
- processes for handling and disposing of waste.[14,309,313,314]

[Recommendation]

10.2.2 Review and update the plan annually and when new hazardous medications are introduced.[309] *[Recommendation]*

10.3 The health care organization should provide
- policies and procedures based on the most current evidence related to handling of hazardous medications,
- primary engineering controls (eg, ventilation hood),
- supplemental engineering controls (eg, closed-system transfer devices),
- PPE as applicable to the hazardous medication,
- discipline-specific education as applicable to the hazardous medication,
- instructions for patients and caregivers,
- provisions for hazardous waste disposal, and
- spill kits.[309,312,315,316]

[Recommendation]

Table 1. Resources for Handling Hazardous Medications	
Organization	**Website**
National Institute for Occupational Safety and Health	https://www.cdc.gov/niosh/topics/antineoplastic/ https://www.cdc.gov/niosh/hhe/hheprogram.html
Occupational Safety and Health Administration	https://www.osha.gov/SLTC/hazardousdrugs/index.html
US Pharmacopeial Convention	http://www.usp.org/frequently-asked-questions/hazardous-drugs-handling-healthcare-settings

10.4 The health care organization should provide allowances for personnel of childbearing age (eg, assignments that do not include handling of hazardous medications).[309,312] *[Recommendation]*

Lawson et al[317] conducted a descriptive study that included 7,482 pregnant nurses, of whom 775 experienced a spontaneous abortion at less than 20 weeks of pregnancy. Of these 775 nurses, 48 (6.1%) had handled antineoplastic medications. Of the 6,707 nurses who gave birth to live infants, 254 (3.8%) had handled antineoplastic medications. After adjusting for age, parity, shift work, and hours worked, the researchers concluded that nurses who were exposed to antineoplastic medications during pregnancy had a two-fold increased risk of spontaneous abortion.

10.5 Store hazardous medications in compliance with USP 800 and applicable regulatory requirements.[313] *[Recommendation]*

10.6 Handle hazardous medications according to manufacturer's instructions for use, regulatory requirements, and advisories from professional organizations (Table 1). *[Recommendation]*

10.6.1 Personal protective equipment must be worn during handling of hazardous medications.[311] *[Regulatory Requirement]*

Moderate-quality evidence supports the wearing of PPE.[309,310,312,313,318-320] In a nonexperimental study, Villarini et al[321] found less DNA damage occurred in health care workers involved in preparation, transportation, administration, and disposal of anticancer agents when PPE was worn.

10.6.2 Select personal protective equipment based on the risk of exposure and the activities to be performed including receipt, storage, transport, compounding, administration, deactivation, spill control, and waste disposal of hazardous medications.[309] *[Recommendation]*

10.6.3 Wear two pairs of powder-free chemotherapy gloves (or other gloves as described in the manufacturer's instructions for use) that are inspected before use to verify the absence of physical defects for handling all hazardous medications. *[Recommendation]*

Powder-free gloves help to reduce the potential for work area contamination caused by the dispersal of contaminated powder from the gloves.[312,313,319] Hazardous medications may permeate a single layer of gloves, allowing skin to be exposed to the medication.[309,312,322]

10.6.4 Change gloves every 30 minutes unless otherwise stated in the glove manufacturer's instructions for use. *[Recommendation]*

Professional guidelines specify changing gloves every 30 minutes when handling chemotherapeutic agents.[309,313,320]

10.6.5 Wear a single-use chemotherapy gown during handling of hazardous medications. Use a sterile gown for personnel in the sterile field and nonsterile gown for personnel not in the sterile field.[323] *[Recommendation]*

Professional guidelines recommend wearing a gown that
- is for single use,
- is lint free,
- is impermeable to hazardous medications,
- is long sleeved,
- fastens in the back,
- has elastic or knit cuffs, and
- does not have seams or closures that are permeable to the medication being handled.[309,312,313]

10.6.6 Goggles or goggles with full face shields must be worn when handling hazardous medications.[309] *[Regulatory Requirement]*

Eye glasses or safety glasses with side shields do not provide adequate eye protection. Face shields in combination with goggles provide protection to the face and eyes. Face shields alone do not provide full eye and face protection.[312,313,319]

10.6.7 **An N95 respirator or more-protective respirator that meets the Occupational Safety Health Administration requirements for respiratory protection must be worn when there is a risk that airborne powder or aerosol will be generated.**[312,313,319,324] *[Regulatory Requirement]*

An N95 mask provides protection from aerosolized hazardous medication but provides little or no protection from vapors or gases.[313]

10.6.8 **Dispose of personal protective equipment worn while handling hazardous medications in a hazardous disposal container.**[309] *[Recommendation]*

10.6.9 **Wash hands with soap and water as soon as possible after doffing PPE.**[322] *[Recommendation]*

10.7 **Use a hazardous medication container that is sealed, leak proof, resistant to breakage, and labeled with the applicable hazard warnings and the same components as any other medication container.**[309,312,313,320] *[Recommendation]*

10.8 **A safety data sheet (SDS) must be present and readily accessible for each hazardous medication present in the facility.**[19,309,311,313] *[Regulatory Requirement]*

10.9 **Contain hazardous medication spills and clean contaminated surfaces according to the instructions provided in the SDS.**[313] *[Recommendation]*

10.9.1 **Make spill kits accessible in all areas where the potential for a spill exists.**[313,322] *[Recommendation]*

10.9.2 **Personal protective equipment appropriate for the type of medication must be worn during the spill cleanup process.**[311,313] *[Regulatory Requirement]*

10.9.3 **Document the details of the spill, including the name of the medication, time of exposure, and names of those exposed according to facility policy and procedure.**[313] *[Recommendation]*

10.9.4 **Seek immediate medical attention if exposed to hazardous medications.**[313] *[Recommendation]*

10.10 **Use single-use instruments, if available, for administration of hazardous medications.** *[Recommendation]*

The use and disposal of single-use instruments eliminates the need to institute special protocols for deactivation and decontamination and may reduce the risk of exposing personnel to hazardous medications. The process of deactivating the medication and removing the medication from the instrument may be harmful to the instrument.

10.11 **For instruments and surfaces contaminated with hazardous medications, deactivate, clean, and decontaminate with agents indicated for the type of contaminant and the surface to be cleaned or decontaminated per the manufacturer's cleaning instructions.**[309] *[Recommendation]*

Moderate-quality evidence shows chemotherapeutic medications are found on many surfaces where hazardous medications are prepared, stored, and administered and supports removal from the surfaces.[310,313,325,326]

10.11.1 **Select and use agents for deactivation, cleaning, and decontamination based on the surface and medication manufacturers' instructions for use and the SDS.** *[Recommendation]*

The efficacy of cleaning agents varies with the surface to be cleaned and the hazardous medication present on the surface.[327-329]

10.11.2 **Do not apply agents with a spray device.** *[Recommendation]*

A spray application may aerosolize the hazardous medication residue.[313]

10.11.3 **Personal protective equipment must be worn during the deactivation, cleaning, and decontamination process.**[311,313] *[Regulatory Requirement]*

10.12 **Take precautions in preparation for and during administration of chemotherapeutic medication for hyperthermic intraperitoneal chemotherapy (HIPEC) procedures, including**
- **conducting education on the process and potential areas of contamination preprocedure,**
- **wearing two pairs of sterile chemotherapy gloves,**
- **wearing sterile chemotherapy-protective gowns,**
- **minimizing splashing during internal organ manipulation,**
- **cleaning up any spilled solution and properly disposing of materials used for cleanup,**
- **careful cleaning of the HIPEC device following the manufacturer's instructions for use,**
- **wearing an N95 respirator or more-protective respirator, and**
- **using infusion bags instead of syringes to inject medication.**

[Recommendation]

A National Institute for Occupational Safety and Health health hazard evaluation and a descriptive study involving six German hospitals and 19 HIPEC procedures support the recommendations listed above for cisplatin used in intraperitoneal surgical procedures.[330,331] The evidence is limited, and further research is needed, especially related to respiratory protection.

10.13 Wear personal protective equipment during handling of excreta from patients who have received hazardous medications within the past 48 hours.[309] *[Recommendation]*

10.14 Hazardous medications and associated devices (eg, tubing, syringes, needles, IV bags, drapes contaminated by hazardous medications) must be disposed of according to federal, state, and local regulations.[322,332] *[Regulatory Requirement]*

10.14.1 Use collection containers that are dedicated for chemotherapy waste.[320] *[Recommendation]*

10.15 The health care organization must provide role-specific education related to hazardous medications.[311] *[Regulatory Requirement]*

Moderate-quality evidence supports the education of personnel who could be exposed to hazardous medications.[9,155,309,312,313,315,318-320,333-338] In a nonexperimental study, Hon et al[339] found there was a lack of knowledge about hazardous medications among all health care personnel, and the lack of knowledge was greater in those who were not responsible for preparing or administering medication. In another nonexperimental study, Hon et al[308] found higher amounts of a chemotherapeutic medication in the urine of personnel who handled hazardous medications but did not receive education regarding the safety measures for handling those medications compared with personnel who did receive the education.

10.15.1 Include the following information in education on hazardous medication safety practices:
- hazardous medications present and the associated risks,
- the hazardous medication plan,
- the use of PPE and engineering controls,
- hazardous medication exposure response,
- spill management,
- precautions for administration,
- handling of contaminated patient excreta, and
- handling of contaminated waste.

[Recommendation]

10.16 The health care organization must establish and implement policies and procedures for handling hazardous medications.[309,313] *[Regulatory Requirement]*

10.16.1 In the policies and procedures, define the precautions to be taken during
- receiving;
- storage;
- transport;
- preparation;
- administration;
- spill cleanup;
- waste handling, including deactivation, cleaning, and decontamination including agents to be used, and dilutions if required;
- handling of patient excreta;
- disposal of hazardous medications; and
- use of PPE.[11,309,315,318]

[Recommendation]

10.17 Establish a medical surveillance program and follow-up program for all personnel potentially exposed to hazardous medication. *[Recommendation]*

Moderate-quality evidence recommends that a medical surveillance program be instituted. A relationship has been established between being exposed to hazardous medications and abnormalities in the blood of those exposed.[304,305,308,309,313,319,336,340,341]

11. Medication Disposal

11.1 Medications must be disposed of according to local, state, and federal regulations and the medication manufacturer's instructions for use.[332,342-344] *[Regulatory Requirement]*

Certain medications may be classified as controlled substances or medical hazardous waste, and there may be specific federal, state, or local requirements for disposal.

11.2 Review the SDS and collaborate with a pharmacist to determine the correct method for disposing of medications. *[Recommendation]*

The SDS provides specific information regarding methods of safe handling and disposal.

11.2.1 Medications may be discarded by returning them to the manufacturer; using a third party disposal system; incinerating them, sending them to the landfill, or if permitted, flushing them into the sanitary sewer. *[Conditional Recommendation]*

Disposal of medications into the sanitary sewer can lead to the presence of medications (eg, controlled substances, chemotherapeutic agents) in hospital waste water. Some of these substances are thought to be ecotoxic, but the definitive effect is unknown.[18,294,345,346] Chiarello et al[345] performed a descriptive study at a Brazilian hospital in which the contents of the hospital sewage was tested for the presence of medications. The researchers found that current methods of sewage treatment only eliminated some medications, and those medications were eliminated with varying success.

11.3 Collaborate with pharmacy personnel to determine the proper methods for returning unused and unopened medications in medication storage areas to the pharmacy. *[Recommendation]*

Returning medications to the pharmacy increases the accuracy for accounting for unused medications. Returning unopened medications to the pharmacy may increase the chances for exchanging the medications to avoid outdates and consequent waste.

12. Education

12.1 Provide education and verify competency regarding precautions to be taken to mitigate the risk for medication errors. *[Recommendation]*

Initial and periodic education on safe medication practices provides direction for personnel in providing safe patient care. Additional periodic educational programs provide opportunities to reinforce previous learning and introduce new information on adjunct technology, its use, and potential risks. Competency verification serves as an indicator that personnel have an understanding of safe medication practices. Moderate-quality evidence identifies education as a means for decreasing medication errors.[8,9,347-353]

12.2 Include the following in role-specific[9] education and competency verification activities:
- the medication use process, including reconciliation;
- pharmacology, including medication intent for use and contraindications;
- medication allergies and treatment;
- medication disposal;
- handling and administering high-alert medications;
- using technology for medication error prevention,[13,30,354,355] and administration[23];
- methods to decrease interruptions;
- methods for handling and preventing near-miss incidents[356];
- calculations[192];
- injection techniques[134];

- tubing types and correct methods for connection;
- use of abbreviations[90];
- review of policies and procedures;
- double-checking processes;
- methods of and significance of reporting adverse drug events;
- medications associated with emergency care;
- use of medication-related education tools for patients and their support persons;
- regulations relevant to safe medication practices;
- identifying distinct pairs for look-alike and sound-alike medications;
- storage requirements for look-alike and sound-alike medications;
- applicable storage requirements (eg, temperature control) for medications;
- rotating stock;
- securing medication inventory (ie, both scheduled and nonscheduled products);
- receiving and processing verbal, written, or electronic orders;
- maintaining preference cards and standing order forms;
- retrieving or returning medications from medication storage areas, including outdated medications;
- patient age-related requirements when obtaining, preparing, and administering medications;
- using visual and verbal validation when placing a medication on the sterile field;
- labeling medications when outside of their original container (eg, on the sterile field);
- safe dosage limits and dosage calculations;
- use of medication containers, adjunct equipment, and supplies;
- documentation requirements; and
- monitoring patients' responses to medications.

[Recommendation]

Moderate-quality evidence establishes that medication errors are reduced when education is provided.[5,7,9,12,18,69,82,91,134,135,140,154,189,192,193,202,223,225,300,350-352,357-370]

12.3 The health care organization should provide medication reference materials to personnel.[353,371] *[Recommendation]*

12.3.1 Reference materials should
- be readily accessible;
- be current;
- be applicable to the population served; and
- provide information on drug dosing, appropriateness of use, contraindications, adverse effects, drug-drug interactions, drug formula interactions, nursing considerations, and monitoring parameters.[371]

[Recommendation]

13. Documentation

13.1 Take precautions to mitigate the risk for errors associated with medication documentation, including during the transcription phase. *[Recommendation]*

Documentation throughout the medication use process is a professional medicolegal standard and provides data for identifying trends and demonstrating compliance with regulatory requirements and accreditation standards. Documentation also facilitates continuity of patient care through clear communication and supports collaboration among health care team members.

The literature contains reports of errors occurring during documentation and transcription. The errors reported include weight-dependent medications ordered without the patient's weight being recorded.[70,150,152,176,372]

13.2 Document medications administered in a manner that
- is legible and easily accessible,
- is free of unapproved abbreviations and acronyms, and
- is timely.

[Recommendation]

Documentation that occurs in real time has been reported to lower the number of medication errors.[372] Immediate documentation of untoward effects is a medicolegal standard and contributes to planning, intervening, and supporting continuity of care. Documentation also serves as a means for systems review to improve processes related to medication use. In a nonexperimental study, Hartel et al[59] found documentation errors in 3.5% of 1,934 prescriptions. The handwriting readability was rated as being moderate in 42%, poor in 52%, and unreadable in 4% of the prescriptions. The researchers concluded the transcription errors were the result of the poor level of readability.

13.2.1 Use a consistent format for documenting medication administration, including the
- medication name,
- total amount of medication administered when multiple injections of the same medication (eg, lidocaine) are administered during a procedure,
- route of administration,
- administration rate,
- date and time administration began,
- concentration of the medication and solutions administered,
- duration of administration or time that treatment was completed, and

- identity of the person administering the medication.

[Recommendation]

Requirements for documentation of medication administration are detailed in regulatory requirements[17,23] and professional practice guidelines.[9,16,154]

13.2.2 Use a consistent format for documentation related to medication administration when applicable, including
- patient responses, including any adverse effects observed or reported by the patient during or after administration;
- communications with patients, health care providers, and caregivers, including the dates and times the events occurred, names of persons involved, and steps taken to resolve questions and problems; and
- discharge instructions.

[Recommendation]

13.2.3 Use a consistent format for documenting medication history, including the
- patient's current medications including dosage, frequency, and last dose received;
- patient's allergies[23,132,140] and
- patient's weight in both pounds and kilograms.

[Recommendation]

13.2.4 Have a second person who possesses the competency for managing medications verify medication orders for accuracy after transcription and before administration to the patient. *[Recommendation]*

Errors have been reported to occur during the transcription phase including transcription into an incorrect patient record, transcription into an incorrect location in the electronic medical record, and transcription of the dosage incorrectly.[164,373]

13.3 Take precautions to prevent transmission and receipt of incorrect or partial orders when electronically transmitting or copying, including
- placing only one sheet on the copier screen at a time,
- numbering pages, and
- requesting order confirmation.

[Recommendation]

A case report describes an error that occurred when an order containing three pages was placed on a fax machine to be transmitted to the pharmacy. The error occurred because only two of the pages were transmitted, and the medications on the page that was not transmitted were not given to the patient.[374]

14. Policies and Procedures

14.1 Develop policies and procedures that address all phases of the medication use process in all phases of perioperative care. Revise policies and procedures as necessary and make them readily available in the practice setting in which they are used. *[Recommendation]*

Policies and procedures assist in the development of patient safety, quality assessment, and performance improvement activities. Policies and procedures also serve as operational guidelines to minimize patients' risk for injury or complications, standardize practice, and direct personnel. Policies and procedures establish authority, responsibility, and accountability within the practice setting.

14.2 Policies and procedures must address
- roles and responsibilities of each discipline (eg, RN, certified RN anesthetist, physician assistant) regarding who may administer medications, the types of medication, routes of administration, and techniques for administration and
- education and training for all personnel who administer medications.[9,23]
[Regulatory Requirement]

14.3 Address the following in policy and procedures related to medication:
- culturally sensitive medication practices for the communities served, including
  o age-specific populations,
  o special populations (eg, women's practices, ophthalmology, oncology), and
  o ethnically diverse populations;
- handling of hazardous medications[19] (See Recommendation 10);
- use of a patient-controlled analgesia device[355];
- prevention of tubing misconnections[225];
- managing medication shortages[14]; and
- the acceptable types of orders, including
  o verbal orders,[23]
  o **as needed (PRN) orders**,
  o **standing orders**,
  o **automatic stop orders**,
  o **titrating orders**,
  o **taper orders**,
  o **range orders**, and
  o **signed and held orders**;
- medication order content;
- medication disposal;

- labeling;
- storage requirements;
- documentation of all medications administered and postadministration monitoring performed;
- handling of containers from which medication has been removed;
- parameters for monitoring after administration; and
- the medication reconciliation process.
[Recommendation]

14.3.1 The policy and procedure for verbal orders should
- describe when verbal orders may be used,
- provide a means to determine the validity/authenticity of the prescriber,
- list the required contents of a complete verbal order,
- list who may give and receive verbal orders, and
- define criteria for read-back techniques.[162]
[Recommendation]

15. Quality

15.1 Establish a quality plan that includes evaluation of all phases of the medication use process. *[Recommendation]*

Quality assurance and performance improvement programs can facilitate the identification of problem areas and assist personnel in evaluating and improving the quality of patient care and formulating plans for corrective action. These programs provide data that may be used to determine whether an individual organization is within benchmark goals, and if not, to identify areas that may require corrective action. A quality management program provides a mechanism to evaluate effectiveness of processes and compliance with medication safety policies and procedures. Low-quality evidence supports the use of a quality plan to analyze all data collected on medication errors (eg, causes, frequency, severity), and assist with determining corrective interventions.[14,375,376]

15.2 Use a mechanism to determine and analyze medication errors, near misses, and adverse drug events, which may include
- **trigger tools**,[377-380]
- self-reporting tools (eg, electronic, paper),[9,176,381]
- direct observation with immediate feedback,[382]
- chart review, and
- a combination of mechanisms.[7,383-385]
[Recommendation]

In a nonexperimental retrospective study, Elliot et al[386] compared the use of an electronic reporting tool to a paper method. The researchers found the use of the electronic system resulted in an increase in the number of reported occurrences, and occurrences were reported earlier. The researchers also found that users thought the system was easier to use, was more accessible, and was more consistent than the paper system.

In a systematic literature review, Meyer-Massetti et al[387] identified strengths and weaknesses for all of the mechanisms listed above. The reviewers concluded the trigger tools were the most effective method and required less labor, while the incident report review was the most effective at identifying the severity of the medication events.

15.3 **Include the following components in the quality plan:**
- **clearly defined quality metrics that address preventable adverse events, medication errors, and technology;**
- **metrics that can lead to specific interventions (eg, if a stocking error is the metric, the intervention is to change the method of stocking);**
- **metrics that are applicable to the facility;**
- **a method for analyzing medication errors (eg, failure mode, effects, and criticality analysis; healthcare failure mode effect analysis; plan, do, check, act; define, measure, analyze, improve, control; audit and feedback process);**
- **a method to assess technology workarounds and solutions for workarounds if technology is used, and**
- **a method to identify medication errors that occur during medical emergencies.**[9,203,354,388-397]
[Recommendation]

The literature contains reports of workarounds that have been created that could interfere with the purpose of the technology[72,369,398,399] or have negative effects on patient safety.

Niazkhani et al[400] conducted a qualitative study in The Netherlands and found that when the labels for the medication administration record did not arrive in a timely manner, the medication information was handwritten in, and this resulted in the medication being administered to patients twice. A descriptive study by Gokhman et al[361] recommends that emergency situations be included in the quality monitoring program.

15.4 **Medication administration errors must be reported immediately to the attending physician and, if appropriate, to the health care organization's quality program.**[23,132] *[Regulatory Requirement]*

15.5 **Share quality data, reports, and action plans with all involved personnel (eg, pharmacy, physicians, nursing, purchasing, governing board).** *[Recommendation]*

Sharing the information with all involved personnel can result in interventions occurring at all phases of the medication use process to correct the identified problem areas.[193,401,402]

Glossary

As needed (PRN) orders: Orders acted on based on the occurrence of a specific indication or symptom.

Automatic stop orders: Orders that include a date or time to discontinue a medication.

Compounding: The process of combining two or more different medications. Compounding does not include mixing, reconstituting, or similar acts that are performed in accordance with the directions contained in approved labeling provided by the product's manufacturer or other manufacturer directions consistent with that labeling.

Hazardous medication: Any medication that is identified to meet one of the following criteria: carcinogenicity, teratogenicity, or developmental toxicity; reproductive toxicity in humans; organ toxicity at low doses in humans or animals; and genotoxicity or a new medication that mimics existing hazardous medications in structure or toxicity.

High-alert medication: A medication that has a heightened risk of causing significant patient harm when used in error.

Licensed independent practitioner: Any individual permitted by law and the organization to provide care and services without direction or supervision, within the scope of the individual's license and consistent with individually granted clinical privileges.

Medication error: A preventable event that occurs during any phase of the medication use process including procuring, prescribing, transcribing, dispensing, administering, or monitoring. The event may or may not lead to patient harm or inappropriate medication use.

Medication reconciliation: The process of comparing the patient's current medications at the time of admission or at the time of arrival at the present point of care to the list of medications ordered at the time of transfer of care or discharge. This reconciliation process begins at the point of admission to the perioperative care area and ends at the point of discharge from the perioperative care area.

Multidose vial: Defined by the Safe Injection Practices Coalition as a bottle of injectable medication that contains more than one dose of medication and has a label to indicate approval by the US Food and Drug Administration for use on more than one person.

Near miss: A variation in a normal process that, if continued, could result in negative patient outcome.

Range orders: Medication orders in which the dose or dosing interval varies over a prescribed range, depending on the situation or patient's status.

Signed and held orders: New prewritten (held) medication orders and specific instructions from a licensed independent practitioner to administer medication(s) to a patient in clearly defined circumstances that become active upon the release of the orders on a specific date(s) and time(s).

Standing order: A prewritten medication order and specific instructions from the licensed independent practitioner to administer a medication to a person in clearly defined circumstances.

Tall man lettering: The capitalization of the dissimilar portion of the name of a medication that distinguishes it from a similar drug name (Examples: vinblastine – vinBLAStine; vincristine – vinCRIStine).

Taper order: A medication order in which the dose is decreased by a particular amount with each dosing interval.

Titrating order: A medication order in which the dose is either progressively increased or decreased in response to the patient's status.

Trigger tool: A software tool that reviews a patient's record looking for clues, events, or sentinel words (eg, the ordering of certain drugs, orders for antidotes, certain abnormal laboratory values, abrupt stop orders) to identify potential adverse events. When the program identifies the established clue, event, or sentinel word on a patient's chart, a notice is sent to the designated person to initiate a more detailed chart audit. The messages received may be called alerts or notifications.

References

1. Boeker EB, de Boer M, Kiewiet JJS, Lie-A-Huen L, Dijkgraaf MGW, Boermeester MA. Occurrence and preventability of adverse drug events in surgical patients: a systematic review of literature. *BMC Health Serv Res.* 2013;13:364. [IIIA]

2. ASHP guidelines on preventing medication errors in hospitals. *Am J Hosp Pharm.* 1993;50(2):305-314. [IVC]

3. Hicks RW, Wanzer L, Goeckner B. Perioperative pharmacology: a framework for perioperative medication safety. *AORN J.* 2011;93(1):136-142. [VB]

4. Seidling HM, Stutzle M, Hoppe-Tichy T, et al. Best practice strategies to safeguard drug prescribing and drug administration: an anthology of expert views and opinions. *Int J Clin Pharm.* 2016;38(2):362-373. [IIIB]

5. Adhikari R, Tocher J, Smith P, Corcoran J, MacArthur J. A multi-disciplinary approach to medication safety and the implication for nursing education and practice. *Nurse Educ Today.* 2014;34(2):185-190. [IIIB]

6. Cousins DH, Gerrett D, Warner B. A review of medication incidents reported to the national reporting and learning system in England and Wales over 6 years (2005-2010). *Br J Clin Pharmacol.* 2012;74(4):597-604. [IIIB]

7. Härkänen M, Turunen H, Vehviläinen-Julkunen K. Differences between methods of detecting medication errors: a secondary analysis of medication administration errors using incident reports, the global trigger tool method, and observations. *J Patient Saf.* March 24, 2016. Epub ahead of print. [IIIA]

8. Grou Volpe CR, Moura Pinho DL, Morato Stival M, De Oliveira Karnikowski MG. Medication errors in a public hospital in Brazil. *Br J Nurs.* 2014;23(11):552-559. [IIIC]

9. Goldspiel B, Hoffman JM, Griffith NL, et al. ASHP guidelines on preventing medication errors with chemotherapy and biotherapy. *Am J Health Syst Pharm.* 2015;72(8):e6-e35. [IVC]

10. Anderson P, Townsend T. Preventing high alert medication errors in hospital patients. *Am Nurse Today.* 2015;10(5):18-23. [VC]

11. ASHP guidelines: minimum standard for pharmacies in hospitals. *Am J Health Syst Pharm.* 2013;70(18):1619-1630. [IVC]

12. Sanchez SH, Sethi SS, Santos SL, Boockvar K. Implementing medication reconciliation from the planner's perspective: a qualitative study. *BMC Health Serv Res.* 2014;14:290. [IIIB]

13. Mandrack M, Cohen MR, Featherling J, et al. Nursing best practices using automated dispensing cabinets: nurses' key role in improving medication safety. *Medsurg Nurs.* 2012;21(3):134-144. [VB]

14. Buxton JA, Babbitt R, Clegg CA, et al. ASHP guidelines: minimum standard for ambulatory care pharmacy practice. *Am J Health Syst Pharm.* 2015;72(14):1221-1236. [IVB]

15. Zhao RY, He XW, Shan YM, Zhu LL, Zhou Q. A stewardship intervention program for safe medication management and use of antidiabetic drugs. *Clin Interv Aging.* 2015;10:1201-1212. [VA]

16. Merry AF, Shipp DH, Lowinger JS. The contribution of labelling to safe medication administration in anaesthetic practice. *Best Pract Res Clin Anaesthesiol.* 2011;25(2):145-159. [VB]

17. May SK, Park S. Risk factors and strategies for prevention of medication errors in patients with subarachnoid hemorrhage. *Hosp Pharm.* 2013;48(Suppl 5):S10-S20. [VB]

18. Mankes RF, Silver CD. Quantitative study of controlled substance bedside wasting, disposal and evaluation of potential ecologic effects. *Sci Total Environ.* 2013;444:298-310. [IIIB]

19. ASHP guidelines on handling hazardous drugs. *Am J Health Syst Pharm.* 2006;63(12):1172-1193. [IVC]

20. De Oliveira GSJ, Theilken LS, McCarthy RJ. Shortage of perioperative drugs: implications for anesthesia practice and patient safety. *Anesth Analg.* 2011;113(6):1429-1435. [VB]

21. Golembiewski J. Drug shortages in the perioperative setting: causes, impact, and strategies. *J Perianesth Nurs.* 2012;27(4):286-292. [VB]

22. Engels MJ, Ciarkowski SL. Nursing, pharmacy, and prescriber knowledge and perceptions of high-alert medications in a large, academic medical hospital. *Hosp Pharm.* 2015;50(4):287-295. [IIIA]

23. Centers for Medicare & Medicaid Services (CMS), DHHS. Medicare and Medicaid programs; hospital conditions of participation: requirements for history and physical examinations; authentication of verbal orders; securing medications; and postanesthesia evaluations. Final rule. *Fed Regist.* 2006;71(227):68671-68695.

24. Cohen MR, Smetzer JL. No unlabeled containers anywhere, ever! Where did this come from? *Hosp Pharm.* 2015; 50(3):185-188. [VC]

25. Erbe B. Safe medication administration in the operating room. *Tar Heel Nurse.* 2011;73(1):10-13. [VB]

26. Bonkowski J, Carnes C, Melucci J, et al. Effect of barcode-assisted medication administration on emergency department medication errors. *Acad Emerg Med.* 2013;20(8):801-806. [IIB]

27. Bonkowski J, Weber RJ, Melucci J, Pesavento T, Henry M, Moffatt-Bruce S. Improving medication administration safety in solid organ transplant patients through barcode-assisted medication administration. *Am J Med Qual.* 2014;29(3):236-241. [IIB]

28. Sethuraman U, Kannikeswaran N, Murray KP, Zidan MA, Chamberlain JM. Prescription errors before and after introduction of electronic medication alert system in a pediatric emergency department. *Acad Emerg Med.* 2015;22(6):714-719. [IIIB]

29. Ching JM, Williams BL, Idemoto LM, Blackmore CC. Using lean "automation with a human touch" to improve medication safety: a step closer to the "perfect dose." *Jt Comm J Qual Patient Saf.* 2014;40(8):341-350. [IIB]

30. Armada ER, Villamanan E, Lopez-de-Sa E, et al. Computerized physician order entry in the cardiac intensive care unit: effects on prescription errors and workflow conditions. *J Crit Care.* 2014;29(2):188-193. [IIIB]

31. Allison GM, Weigel B, Holcroft C. Does electronic medication reconciliation at hospital discharge decrease prescription medication errors? *Int J Health Care Qual Assur.* 2015;28(6):564-573. [IIIB]

32. Charles K, Cannon M, Hall R, Coustasse A. Can utilizing a computerized provider order entry (CPOE) system prevent hospital medical errors and adverse drug events? *Perspect Health Inf Manag.* 2014;11:1b. [IIB]

33. Connor AJ, Hutton P, Severn P, Masri I. Electronic prescribing and prescription design in ophthalmic practice. *Eur J Ophthalmol.* 2011;21(5):644-648. [IIIB]

34. Fischer JR. The impact of health care technology on medication safety. *S D Med.* 2014;67(7):279-280. [VC]

35. Green RA, Hripcsak G, Salmasian H, et al. Intercepting wrong-patient orders in a computerized provider order entry system. *Ann Emerg Med.* 2015;65(6):679-686. [IIB]

36. Henneman PL, Marquard JL, Fisher DL, et al. Barcode verification: reducing but not eliminating medication errors. *J Nurs Adm.* 2012;42(12):562-566. [IIIB]

37. Hernandez F, Majoul E, Montes-Palacios C, et al. An observational study of the impact of a computerized physician order entry system on the rate of medication errors in an orthopaedic surgery unit. *Plos One.* 2015;10(7):e0134101. [IIB]

38. Hassink JJM, Jansen MMPM, Helmons PJ. Effects of bar code-assisted medication administration (BCMA) on frequency, type and severity of medication administration errors: a review of the literature. *Eur J Hosp Pharm Sci Pract.* 2012;19(5):489-494. [VB]

39. Khammarnia M, Kassani A, Eslahi M. The efficacy of patients' wristband bar-code on prevention of medical errors: a meta-analysis study. *Appl Clin Inform.* 2015;6(4):716-727. [IIA]

40. Leung AA, Schiff G, Keohane C, et al. Impact of vendor computerized physician order entry on patients with renal impairment in community hospitals. *J Hosp Med.* 2013;8(10): 545-552. [IIB]

41. Manias E, Kinney S, Cranswick N, Williams A, Borrott N. Interventions to reduce medication errors in pediatric intensive care. *Ann Pharmacother.* 2014;48(10):1313-1331. [IIIA]

42. Nuckols TK, Smith-Spangler C, Morton SC, et al. The effectiveness of computerized order entry at reducing preventable adverse drug events and medication errors in hospital settings: a systematic review and meta-analysis. *Syst Rev.* 2014;3:56. [IIIA]

43. Roberts DL, Noble B, Wright MJ, Nelson EA, Shaft JD, Rakela J. Impact of computerized provider order entry on hospital medication errors. *J Clin Outcomes Manag.* 2013;20(3):109-115. [IIA]

44. Sanchez Cuervo M, Rojo Sanchis A, Pueyo Lopez C, Gomez De Salazar Lopez De Silanes E, Gramage Caro T, Bermejo Vicedo T. The impact of a computerized physician order entry system on medical errors with anti-neoplastic drugs 5 years after its implementation. *J Clin Pharm Ther.* 2015;40(5):550-554. [IIA]

45. Shawahna R, Rahman N, Ahmad M, Debray M, Yliperttula M, Decleves X. Electronic prescribing reduces prescribing error in public hospitals. *J Clin Nurs.* 2011;20(21-22):3233-3245. [IIB]

46. Truitt E, Thompson R, Blazey-Martin D, NiSai D, Salem D. Effect of the implementation of barcode technology and an electronic medication administration record on adverse drug events. *Hosp Pharm.* 2016;51(6):474-483. [IIB]

47. Westbrook JI, Li L, Georgiou A, Paoloni R, Cullen J. Impact of an electronic medication management system on hospital doctors' and nurses' work: a controlled pre-post, time and motion study. *J Am Med Inform Assoc.* 2013;20(6):1150-1158. [IIIB]

48. Jozefczyk KG, Kennedy WK, Lin MJ, et al. Computerized prescriber order entry and opportunities for medication errors: comparison to tradition paper-based order entry. *J Pharm Pract.* 2013;26(4):434-437. [IIB]

49. Buus A, Nyvang L, Heiden S, Pape-Haugaard L. Quality assurance and effectiveness of the medication process through tablet computers? *Stud Health Technol Inform.* 2012; 180:348-352. [IIIB]

50. McComas J, Riingen M, Chae Kim S. Impact of an electronic medication administration record on medication administration efficiency and errors. *Comput Inform Nurs.* 2014; 32(12):589-595. [IIIB]

51. Seibert HH, Maddox RR, Flynn EA, Williams CK. Effect of barcode technology with electronic medication administration record on medication accuracy rates. *Am J Health Syst Pharm.* 2014;71(3):209-218. [IIA]

52. Dwibedi N, Sansgiry SS, Frost CP, et al. Bedside barcode technology: impact on medication administration tasks in an intensive care unit. *Hosp Pharm.* 2012;47(5):360-366. [IIIB]

53. Abbass I, Mhatre S, Sansgiry SS, Tipton J, Frost C. Impact and determinants of commercial computerized prescriber order entry on the medication administration process. *Hosp Pharm.* 2011;46(5):341-348. [IIIA]

54. Stroud D. Preventing medication administration errors: lockable, computerized medication administration carts help hospitals avoid errors and reduce costs. *Health Manag Technol.* 2013;34(11):18-19. [VC]

55. Aziz MT, Ur-Rehman T, Qureshi S, Bukhari NI. Reduction in chemotherapy order errors with computerised physician order entry and clinical decision support systems. *HIM J.* 2015;44(3):13-22. [IIIB]

56. Maat B, Rademaker CMA, Oostveen MI, Krediet TG, Egberts TCG, Bollen CW. The effect of a computerized prescribing and calculating system on hypo- and hyperglycemias and on prescribing time efficiency in neonatal intensive care patients. *JPEN J Parenter Enteral Nutr.* 2013;37(1):85-91. [IIB]

57. Hollister DJ, Messenger A. Implementation of computerized physician order entry at a community hospital. *Conn Med.* 2011;75(4):227-233. [VB]

58. Morley C, McLeod E, McKenzie D, et al. Reducing dose omission of prescribed medications in the hospital setting: a narrative review. *Drugs Ther Perspect.* 2016;32(5):203-208. [VB]

59. Hartel MJ, Staub LP, Roder C, Eggli S. High incidence of medication documentation errors in a Swiss university hospital due to the handwritten prescription process. *BMC Health Serv Res.* 2011;11:199. [IIIB]

60. Albarrak AI, Al Rashidi EA, Fatani RK, Al Ageel SI, Mohammed R. Assessment of legibility and completeness of handwritten and electronic prescriptions. *Saudi Pharm J.* 2014;22(6):522-527. [IB]

61. Abramson EL, Barron Y, Quaresimo J, Kaushal R. Electronic prescribing within an electronic health record reduces ambulatory prescribing errors. *Jt Comm J Qual Patient Saf.* 2011;37(10):470-478. [IIB]

62. Meisenberg BR, Wright RR, Brady-Copertino CJ. Reduction in chemotherapy order errors with computerized physician order entry. *J Oncol Pract.* 2014;10(1):e5-e9. [VA]

63. Al-Rowibah FA, Younis MZ, Parkash J. The impact of computerized physician order entry on medication errors and adverse drug events. *J Health Care Finance.* 2013;40(1):93-102. [IIIB]

64. Fanning L, Jones N, Manias E. Impact of automated dispensing cabinets on medication selection and preparation error rates in an emergency department: a prospective and direct observational before-and-after study. *J Eval Clin Pract.* 2016;22(2):156-163. [IIIB]

65. Cochran GL, Barrett RS, Horn SD. Comparison of medication safety systems in critical access hospitals: combined analysis of two studies. *Am J Health Syst Pharm.* 2016;73(15):1167-1173. [IIIA]

66. Tsao NW, Lo C, Babich M, Shah K, Bansback NJ. Decentralized automated dispensing devices: systematic review of clinical and economic impacts in hospitals. *Can J Hosp Pharm.* 2014;67(2):138-148. [IIIB]

67. Turchin A, Shubina M, Goldberg S. Unexpected effects of unintended consequences: EMR prescription discrepancies and hemorrhage in patients on warfarin. *AMIA Annu Symp Proc.* 2011;2011:1412-1417. [IIIB]

68. Sparnon E. Spotlight on electronic health record errors: errors related to the use of default values. *Penn Patient Saf Advis.* 2013;10(3):92-95. [IIIB]

69. Rodriguez-Gonzalez CG, Herranz-Alonso A, Martin-Barbero ML, et al. Prevalence of medication administration errors in two medical units with automated prescription and dispensing. *J Am Med Inform Assoc.* 2012;19(1):72-78. [IIIB]

70. Stultz JS, Nahata MC. Preventability of voluntarily reported or trigger tool-identified medication errors in a pediatric institution by information technology: a retrospective cohort study. *Drug Saf.* 2015;38(7):661-670. [IIIB]

71. Wetterneck TB, Walker JM, Blosky MA, et al. Factors contributing to an increase in duplicate medication order errors after CPOE implementation. *J Am Med Inform Assoc.* 2011;18(6):774-782. [IIIB]

72. Van Der Sijs H, Rootjes I, Aarts J. The shift in workarounds upon implementation of computerized physician order entry. *Stud Health Technol Inform.* 2011;169:290-294. [IIIB]

73. Joy A, Davis J, Cardona J. Effect of computerized provider order entry on rate of medication errors in a community hospital setting. *Hosp Pharm.* 2012;47(9):693-699. [VA]

74. Nelson CE, Selbst SM. Electronic prescription writing errors in the pediatric emergency department. *Pediatr Emerg Care.* 2015;31(5):368-372. [IIIA]

75. Schwartzberg D, Ivanovic S, Patel S, Burjonrappa SC. We thought we would be perfect: medication errors before and after the initiation of computerized physician order entry. *J Surg Res.* 2015;198(1):108-114. [IIB]

76. Naunton M, Gardiner HR, Kyle G. Look-alike, sound-alike medication errors: a novel case concerning a Slow-Na, Slow-K prescribing error. *Int Med Case Rep J.* 2015;8:51-53. [VC]

77. Cohen MR, Smetzer JL. ISMP medication error report analysis—tretinoin confused with isotretinoin; death from intravenous nimodipine; incorrect medication names selected during order entry; reduce Ambien dose in order sets; confusion between levothyroxine and liothyronine. *Hosp Pharm.* 2013;48(6):455-457. [VC]

78. Maat B, Au YS, Bollen CW, van Vught AJ, Egberts TCG, Rademaker CMA. Clinical pharmacy interventions in paediatric electronic prescriptions. *Arch Dis Child.* 2013;98(3):222-227. [IIIA]

79. Tully MP. Prescribing errors in hospital practice. *Br J Clin Pharmacol.* 2012;74(4):668-675. [VB]

80. Villamanan E, Larrubia Y, Ruano M, et al. Potential medication errors associated with computer prescriber order entry. *Int J Clin Pharm.* 2013;35(4):577-583. [IIIB]

81. Warrick C, Naik H, Avis S, Fletcher P, Franklin BD, Inwald D. A clinical information system reduces medication errors in paediatric intensive care. *Intensive Care Med.* 2011;37(4):691-694. [IIB]

82. Gimenes FRE, Marques TC, Teixeira TCA, Mota MLS, Silva AE, Cassiani SH. Medication wrong-route administrations in relation to medical prescriptions. *Rev Lat Am Enfermagem.* 2011;19(1):11-17. [IIIB]

83. Redwood S, Rajakumar A, Hodson J, Coleman JJ. Does the implementation of an electronic prescribing system create unintended medication errors? A study of the sociotechnical context through the analysis of reported medication incidents. *BMC Med Inform Decis Mak.* 2011;11:29. [IIIB]

84. Westbrook JI, Reckmann M, Li L, et al. Effects of two commercial electronic prescribing systems on prescribing error rates in hospital in-patients: a before and after study. *Plos Med.* 2012;9(1):e1001164. [IIA]

85. Hinojosa-Amaya JM, Rodríguez-Garcia FG, Yeverino-Castro SG, Sánchez-Cárdenas M, Villarreal-Alarcón MÁ, Galarza-Delgado DÁ. Medication errors: electronic vs. paper-based prescribing. Experience at a tertiary care university hospital. *J Eval Clin Pract.* 2016;22(5):751-754. [IIA]

86. Electronic prescribing: the risk of errors and adverse effects. *Prescrire Int.* 2016;25(167):24-27. [VB]

87. Leung AA, Keohane C, Amato M, et al. Impact of vendor computerized physician order entry in community hospitals. *J Gen Intern Med.* 2012;27(7):801-807. [IIB]

88. Hoonakker PLT, Carayon P, Walker JM, Brown RL, Cartmill RS. The effects of computerized provider order entry implementation on communication in intensive care units. *Int J Med Inform.* 2013;82(5):e107-e117. [IIIB]

89. Tschannen D, Talsma A, Reinemeyer N, Belt C, Schoville R. Nursing medication administration and workflow using computerized physician order entry. *Comput Inform Nurs.* 2011;29(7):401-410. [IIIB]

90. Samaranayake NR, Cheung DST, Lam MPS, et al. The effectiveness of a "do not use" list and perceptions of healthcare professionals on error-prone abbreviations. *Int J Clin Pharm.* 2014;36(5):1000-1006. [VB]

91. Samaranayake NR, Dabare PRL, Wanigatunge CA, Cheung BMY. The pattern of abbreviation use in prescriptions: a way forward in eliminating error-prone abbreviations and standardisation of prescriptions. *Curr Drug Saf.* 2014;9(1):34-42. [IIIB]

92. Flannery AH, Parli SE. Medication errors in cardiopulmonary arrest and code-related situations. *Am J Crit Care.* 2016;25(1):12-20. [VB]

93. Thomas AN, Taylor RJ. An analysis of patient safety incidents associated with medications reported from critical care units in the north west of England between 2009 and 2012. *Anaesthesia.* 2014;69(7):735-745. [IIIB]

94. Alex S, Adenew AB, Arundel C, Maron DD, Kerns JC. Medication errors despite using electronic health records: the value of a clinical pharmacist service in reducing discharge-related medication errors. *Qual Manag Health Care.* 2016;25(1):32-37. [VA]

95. Abbasinazari M, Hajhossein Talasaz A, Eshraghi A, Sahraei Z. Detection and management of medication errors in internal wards of a teaching hospital by clinical pharmacists. *Acta Med Iran.* 2013;51(7):482-486. [IIIA]

96. Cesarz JL, Steffenhagen AL, Svenson J, Hamedani AG. Emergency department discharge prescription interventions by emergency medicine pharmacists. *Ann Emerg Med.* 2013;61(2):209-214. [IIIB]

97. Ernst AA, Weiss SJ, Sullivan A4, et al. On-site pharmacists in the ED improve medical errors. *Am J Emerg Med.* 2012;30(5):717-725. [IIIB]

98. Ho L, Akada K, Messner H, Kuruvilla J, Wright J, Seki JT. Pharmacist's role in improving medication safety for patients in an allogeneic hematopoietic cell transplant ambulatory clinic. *Can J Hosp Pharm.* 2013;66(2):110-117. [VA]

99. Jiang S, Zheng X, Li X, Lu X. Effectiveness of pharmaceutical care in an intensive care unit from china. A pre- and post-intervention study. *Saudi Med J.* 2012;33(7):756-762. [IIIB]

100. Jiang SP, Zhu ZY, Wu XL, Lu XY, Zhang XG, Wu BH. Effectiveness of pharmacist dosing adjustment for critically ill patients receiving continuous renal replacement therapy: a comparative study. *Ther Clin Risk Manag.* 2014;10:405-412. [IIIB]

101. Mergenhagen KA, Blum SS, Kugler A, et al. Pharmacist-versus physician-initiated admission medication reconciliation: impact on adverse drug events. *Am J Geriatr Pharmacother.* 2012;10(4):242-250. [IIB]

102. ASHP statement on the pharmacist's role in medication reconciliation. *Am J Health Syst Pharm.* 2013;70(5):453-456. [IVC]

103. Phatak A, Prusi R, Ward B, et al. Impact of pharmacist involvement in the transitional care of high-risk patients through medication reconciliation, medication education, and postdischarge call-backs (IPITCH Study). *J Hosp Med.* 2016;11(1):39-44. [IB]

104. Lenssen R, Heidenreich A, Schulz JB, et al. Analysis of drug-related problems in three departments of a German university hospital. *Int J Clin Pharm.* 2016;38(1):119-126. [IIIB]

105. Ibanez-Garcia S, Rodriguez-Gonzalez CG, Martin-Barbero ML, Sanjurjo-Saez M, Herranz-Alonso A; iPharma. Adding value through pharmacy validation: a safety and cost perspective. *J Eval Clin Pract.* 2016;22(2):253-260. [IIIB]

106. Fernandez-Llamazares CM, Calleja-Hernandez M, Manrique-Rodriguez S, Perez-Sanz C, Duran-Garcia E, Sanjurjo-Saez M. Prescribing errors intercepted by clinical pharmacists in paediatrics and obstetrics in a tertiary hospital in Spain. *Eur J Clin Pharmacol.* 2012;68(9):1339-1345. [IIIA]

107. Zaal RJ, Jansen MMPM, Duisenberg-van Essenberg M, Tijssen CC, Roukema JA, van den Bemt PMLA. Identification of drug-related problems by a clinical pharmacist in addition to computerized alerts. *Int J Clin Pharm.* 2013;35(5):753-762. [IIIB]

108. Kuo GM, Touchette DR, Marinac JS. Drug errors and related interventions reported by United States clinical pharmacists: the American College of Clinical Pharmacy practice-based research network medication error detection, amelioration and prevention study. *Pharmacotherapy.* 2013;33(3):253-265. [IIIB]

109. Caroff DA, Bittermann T, Leonard CE, Gibson GA, Myers JS. A medical resident-pharmacist collaboration improves the rate of medication reconciliation verification at discharge. *Jt Comm J Qual Patient Saf.* 2015;41(10):457-461. [IIA]

110. Graabaek T, Kjeldsen LJ. Medication reviews by clinical pharmacists at hospitals lead to improved patient outcomes: a systematic review. *Basic Clin Pharmacol Toxicol.* 2013;112(6):359-373. [IIIB]

111. Han J, Ah Y, Suh SY, et al. Clinical and economic impact of pharmacists' intervention in a large volume chemotherapy preparation unit. *Int J Clin Pharm.* 2016;38(5):1124-1132. [IIIB]

112. Khalili H, Farsaei S, Rezaee H, Dashti-Khavidaki S. Role of clinical pharmacists' interventions in detection and prevention of medication errors in a medical ward. *Int J Clin Pharm.* 2011;33(2):281-284. [IIIB]

113. Hohmann C, Neumann-Haefelin T, Klotz JM, Freidank A, Radziwill R. Drug-related problems in patients with ischemic stroke in hospital. *Int J Clin Pharm.* 2012;34(6):828-831. [IIIB]

114. Galvin M, Jago-Byrne M, Fitzsimons M, Grimes T. Clinical pharmacist's contribution to medication reconciliation on admission to hospital in Ireland. *Int J Clin Pharm.* 2013;35(1):14-21. [IIIB]

115. Pal A, Babbott S, Wilkinson ST. Can the targeted use of a discharge pharmacist significantly decrease 30-day readmissions? *Hosp Pharm.* 2013;48(5):380-388. [IIB]

116. Reis WCT, Scopel CT, Correr CJ, Andrzejevski VMS. Analysis of clinical pharmacist interventions in a tertiary teaching hospital in Brazil. *Einstein.* 2013;11(2):190-196. [IIIB]

117. Warden BA, Freels JP, Furuno JP, Mackay J. Pharmacy-managed program for providing education and discharge instructions for patients with heart failure. *Am J Health Syst Pharm.* 2014;71(2):134-139. [IIB]

118. Stasiak P, Afilalo M, Castelino T, et al. Detection and correction of prescription errors by an emergency department pharmacy service. *Can J Emerg Med.* 2014;16(3):193-206. [IIIA]

119. Balling L, Erstad BL, Weibel K. Impact of a transition-of-care pharmacist during hospital discharge. *J Am Pharm Assoc.* 2015;55(4):443-448. [IIIC]

120. Tripathi S, Crabtree HM, Fryer KR, Graner KK, Arteaga GM. Impact of clinical pharmacist on the pediatric intensive care practice: an 11-year tertiary center experience. *J Pediatr Pharmacol Ther.* 2015;20(4):290-298. [IIIB]

121. Sebaaly J, Parsons LB, Pilch NAW, Bullington W, Hayes GL, Easterling H. Clinical and financial impact of pharmacist involvement in discharge medication reconciliation at an academic medical center: a prospective pilot study. *Hosp Pharm.* 2015;50(6):505-513. [IIIB]

122. Hamblin S, Rumbaugh K, Miller R. Prevention of adverse drug events and cost savings associated with PharmD interventions in an academic level I trauma center: an evidence-based approach. *J Trauma Acute Care Surg.* 2012;73(6):1484-1490. [IIIB]

123. Cochran GL, Haynatzki G. Comparison of medication safety effectiveness among nine critical access hospitals. *Am J Health Syst Pharm.* 2013;70(24):2218-2224. [IIIC]

124. McCoy AB, Cox ZL, Neal EB, et al. Real-time pharmacy surveillance and clinical decision support to reduce adverse drug events in acute kidney injury: a randomized, controlled trial. *Appl Clin Inform.* 2012;3(2):221-238. [IA]

125. van den Bemt PMLA, van der Schrieck-de Loos EM, van der Linden C, Theeuwes AMLJ, Pol AG; Dutch CBO WHO High 5s Study Group. Effect of medication reconciliation on unintentional medication discrepancies in acute hospital admissions of elderly adults: a multicenter study. *J Am Geriatr Soc.* 2013;61(8):1262-1268. [IIA]

126. Bishop MA, Cohen BA, Billings LK, Thomas EV. Reducing errors through discharge medication reconciliation by pharmacy services. *Am J Health Syst Pharm.* 2015;72(17 Suppl 2):S120-S126. [IIIB]

127. Gardella JE, Cardwell TB, Nnadi M. Improving medication safety with accurate preadmission medication lists and postdischarge education. *Jt Comm J Qual Patient Saf.* 2012;38(10):452-458. [VA]

128. Kramer JS, Stewart MR, Fogg SM, et al. A quantitative evaluation of medication histories and reconciliation by discipline. *Hosp Pharm.* 2014;49(9):826-838. [IIIB]

129. Beckett RD, Crank CW, Wehmeyer A. Effectiveness and feasibility of pharmacist-led admission medication reconciliation for geriatric patients. *J Pharm Pract.* 2012;25(2):136-141. [IB]

130. Aag T, Garcia BH, Viktil KK. Should nurses or clinical pharmacists perform medication reconciliation? A randomized controlled trial. *Eur J Clin Pharmacol.* 2014;70(11):1325-1332. [IA]

131. Zemaitis CT, Morris G, Cabie M, Abdelghany O, Lee L. Reducing readmission at an academic medical center: results of a pharmacy-facilitated discharge counseling and medication reconciliation program. *Hosp Pharm.* 2016;51(6):468-473. [IIIB]

132. Centers for Medicare & Medicaid Services. *State Operations Manual Appendix L—Guidance for Surveyors: Ambulatory Surgical Centers.* Rev. 137; 2015. https://www.cms.gov/Regulations-and-Guidance/Guidance/Manuals/downloads/som107ap_l_ambulatory.pdf. Accessed July 12, 2017.

133. Cole SL, Grubbs JH, Din C, Nesbitt TS. Rural inpatient telepharmacy consultation demonstration for after-hours medication review. *Telemed J E Health.* 2012;18(7):530-537. [IIB]

134. The Joint Commission. Preventing infection from the misuse of vials. *Sentinel Event Alert.* June 16, 2014;52. https://www.jointcommission.org/sea_issue_52/. Accessed July 12, 2017. [VB]

135. Horvath G, MacGregor RL. Is your facility properly managing pharmaceutical waste? *OR Nurse.* 2013;7(5):8-12. [VB]

136. Buck D, Subramanyam R, Varughese A. A quality improvement project to reduce the intraoperative use of single-dose fentanyl vials across multiple patients in a pediatric institution. *Paediatr Anaesth.* 2016;26(1):92-101. [VA]

137. Yadav G, Gupta SK, Bharti AK, Khuba S, Jain G, Singh DK. Case report: syringe swap and similar looking drug containers: a matter of serious concern. *Anaesth Pain Intensive Care.* 2013;17(2):205-207. [VC]

138. Fry RA, Wilton N, Boyes G. Unusual volatile agent switch: implications for checking unsealed volatile agent containers. *Anaesth Intensive Care.* 2015;43(3):419-420. [VC]

139. De Winter S, Vanbrabant P, Vi NTT, et al. Impact of temperature exposure on stability of drugs in a real-world out-of-hospital setting. *Ann Emerg Med.* 2013;62(4):380-387. [IIIB]

140. Grissinger M. Ambulatory surgery facilities: a comprehensive review of medication error reports in Pennsylvania. *Penn Patient Saf Advis.* 2011;8(3):85-93. [IIIB]

141. Tobias JD, Yadav G, Gupta SK, Jain G. Medication errors: a matter of serious concern. *Anaesth Pain Intensive Care.* 2013;17(2):111-114. [VB]

142. Anto B, Barlow D, Oborne CA, Whittlesea C. Incorrect drug selection at the point of dispensing: a study of potential predisposing factors. *Int J Pharm Pract.* 2011;19(1):51-60. [IIIB]

143. Medication safety. *J Pharm Pract Res.* 2011;41(2):139-143. [VC]

144. Medication safety. *J Pharm Pract Res.* 2011;41(1):52-56. [VC]

145. Cote V, Prager JD. Iatrogenic phenol injury: a case report and review of medication safety and labeling practices

with flexible laryngoscopy. *Int J Pediatr Otorhinolaryngol.* 2014; 78(10):1769-1773. [VC]

146. Cohen MR, Smetzer JL. ISMP medication error report analysis—FDA advise-ERR: FDA approves hydromorphone labeling revisions to reduce medication errors; differentiating penicillin from penicillamine; infusion reconnected to the wrong patient; spell out acetaminophen on. *Hosp Pharm.* 2012;47(1):10-13. [VC]

147. Cohen MR, Smetzer JL. ISMP medication error report analysis—drug stability and compatibility; proper use of single-dose vials; what drugs are present on nursing units?; Arixtra—not a hemostat; Pradaxa-Plavix mix-up. *Hosp Pharm.* 2012;47(8):578-582. [VC]

148. Butala BP, Shah VR, Bhosale GP, Shah RB. Medication error: subarachnoid injection of tranexamic acid. *Indian J Anaesth.* 2012;56(2):168-170. [VC]

149. Koczmara C, Hyland S. Drug name alert: potential for confusion between Pradaxa and Plavix. *Dynamics.* 2011;22(3): 25-26. [VB]

150. Vazin A, Zamani Z, Hatam N. Frequency of medication errors in an emergency department of a large teaching hospital in southern Iran. *Drug Healthc Patient Saf.* 2014;6:179-184. [IIIB]

151. Zeraatchi A, Talebian M, Nejati A, Dashti-Khavidaki S. Frequency and types of the medication errors in an academic emergency department in Iran: the emergent need for clinical pharmacy services in emergency departments. *J Res Pharm Pract.* 2013;2(3):118-122. [IIIB]

152. Manias E, Kinney S, Cranswick N, Williams A. Medication errors in hospitalised children. *J Paediatr Child Health.* 2014;50(1):71-77. [IIIB]

153. 21 USC 13: Drug Abuse Prevention and Control. Subchapter I: Control and enforcement (sections 801-904). US Government Publishing Office. https://www.gpo.gov/fdsys/granule/USCODE-2011-title21/USCODE-2011-title21-chap13/content-detail.html. Accessed July 12, 2017.

154. Guideline for patient information management. In: *Guidelines for Perioperative Practice.* Denver, CO: AORN, Inc; 2017:591-616. [IVA]

155. Neuss MN, Polovich M, McNiff K, et al. 2013 updated American society of clinical oncology/oncology nursing society chemotherapy administration safety standards including standards for the safe administration and management of oral chemotherapy. *J Oncol Pract.* 2013;9(2 Suppl):5s-13s. [IVB]

156. Shawahna R, Rahman N, Ahmad M, Debray M, Yliperttula M, Decleves X. Impact of prescriber's handwriting style and nurse's duty duration on the prevalence of transcription errors in public hospitals. *J Clin Nurs.* 2013;22(3-4):550-558. [IIIB]

157. Cohen MR, Smetzer JL. Dangerous close call with wintergreen oil; are 10 mL syringes needed when giving drugs via venous access devices?; use of "NoAC" abbreviation; unsafe frequency notation; 2014-15 targeted medication safety best practices for hospitals. *Hosp Pharm.* 2014;49(4):325-328. [VC]

158. Paul IM, Neville K, Galinkin JL, et al. Metric units and the preferred dosing of orally administered liquid medications. *Pediatrics.* 2015;135(4):784-787. [IVC]

159. ISMP guidelines for standard order sets. Institute for Safe Medication Practices. http://www.ismp.org/Tools/guidelines/StandardOrderSets.asp. Accessed July 12, 2017. [IVC]

160. Sakushima K, Umeki R, Endoh A, Ito YM, Nasuhara Y. Time trend of injection drug errors before and after implementation of bar-code verification system. *Technol Health Care.* 2015;23(3):267-274. [IIIB]

161. Al-Shaiji TF. Achieving detumescence of ischemic priapism with intra-cavernosal injection of fentanyl: an unexpected outcome of miscommunication error. *Curr Drug Saf.* 2011;6(3):194-196. [VC]

162. Recommendations to reduce medication errors associated with verbal medication orders and prescriptions. National Coordinating Council for Medication Error Reporting and Prevention. http://www.nccmerp.org/recommendations-reduce-medication-errors-associated-verbal-medication-orders-and-prescriptions. Adopted February 20, 2001. Revised May 1, 2015. Accessed July 12, 2017. [IVC]

163. Hicks RW, Becker SC, Windle PE, Krenzischek DA. Medication errors in the PACU. *J Perianesth Nurs.* 2007;22(6):413-419. [IIIC]

164. Hicks RW, Becker SC, Cousins DD. *MEDMARX Data Report: A Chartbook of Medication Error Findings from the Perioperative Settings from 1998-2005.* Rockville, MD: US Pharmacopeia; 2007. [IIIC]

165. Pharmaceutical compounding—sterile preparations (797). In: *USP Compounding Compendium.* Rockville, MD: US Pharmacopeial Convention; 2016:40-85. [IVB]

166. Matousek P, Kominek P, Garcic A. Errors associated with the concentration of epinephrine in endonasal surgery. *Eur Arch Otorhinolaryngol.* 2011;268(7):1009-1011. [VC]

167. Dehmel C, Braune SA, Kreymann G, et al. Do centrally pre-prepared solutions achieve more reliable drug concentrations than solutions prepared on the ward? *Intensive Care Med.* 2011;37(8):1311-1316. [IIIB]

168. Patel S, Loveridge R. Obstetric neuraxial drug administration errors: a quantitative and qualitative analytical review. *Anesth Analg.* 2015;121(6):1570-1577. [IIIB]

169. Cohen MR, Smetzer JL. ISMP medication error report analysis—important change with heparin labels; Benadryl dispensed instead of vitamins for home parenteral nutrition; potassium and sodium acetate injection mix-ups; don't truncate, stem, or shorten drug names. *Hosp Pharm.* 2013;48(4):267-269. [VC]

170. Cohen M, Smetzer J. ISMP medication error report analysis—preventing mix-ups between various formulations of amphotericin B; Arixtra is not a hemostat; measurement mix-up; drug names too close for comfort; new vaccine errors reporting program. *Hosp Pharm.* 2013;48(2):95-98. [VC]

171. Emmerton L, Rizk MFS, Bedford G, Lalor D. Systematic derivation of an Australian standard for tall man lettering to distinguish similar drug names. *J Eval Clin Pract.* 2015;21(1):85-90. [IIIB]

172. Darker IT, Gerret D, Filik R, Purdy KJ, Gale AG. The influence of "tall man" lettering on errors of visual perception in the recognition of written drug names. *Ergonomics.* 2011;54(1):21-33. [IIIB]

173. DeHenau C, Becker MW, Bello NM, Liu S, Bix L. Tallman lettering as a strategy for differentiation in look-alike, sound-alike drug names: the role of familiarity in differentiating drug doppelgangers. *Appl Ergon*. 2016;52:77-84. [IIIB]

174. Or CKL, Chan AHS. Effects of text enhancements on the differentiation performance of orthographically similar drug names. *Work*. 2014;48(4):521-528. [IIIB]

175. Trudeau M, Green E, Cosby R, et al. Key components of intravenous chemotherapy labeling: a systematic review and practice guideline. *J Oncol Pharm Pract*. 2011;17(4):409-424. [IVB]

176. Harkanen M, Turunen H, Saano S, Vehvilainen-Julkunen K. Detecting medication errors: analysis based on a hospital's incident reports. *Int J Nurs Pract*. 2015;21(2):141-146. [IIIB]

177. Barak M, Greenberg Z, Danino J. Delayed awakening following inadvertent high-dose remifentanil infusion in a 13 year old patient. *J Clin Anesth*. 2011;23(4):322-324. [VC]

178. Cohen MR, Smetzer JL. ISMP medication error report analysis—tragedy in the postanesthesia care unit; mix-ups between risperidone and ropinirole. *Hosp Pharm*. 2013;48(7):538-541. [VC]

179. Medication safety. *J Pharm Pract Res*. 2014;44(1):38-43. [VC]

180. Cohen MR, Smetzer JL. ISMP medication error report analysis—leucovorin-levoleucovorin mix-up; two error-reduction principles, one change; syringe pull-back method of verifying IV admixtures is unreliable; fleet enema saline is not just saline; ISMP processes health IT. *Hosp Pharm*. 2013;48(10):803-806. [VC]

181. Cohen MR, Smetzer JL. U-500 insulin safety concerns mount; improved labeling needed for camphor product; cardizem-cardene mix-up; initiative to eliminate tubing misconnections. *Hosp Pharm*. 2014;49(2):117-120. [VC]

182. Cohen MR, Smetzer JL. ISMP medication error report analysis. *Hosp Pharm*. 2015;50(5):347-350. [VC]

183. Shridhar Iyer U, Fah KK, Chong CK, Macachor J, Chia N. Survey of medication errors among anaesthetists in Singapore. *Anaesth Intensive Care*. 2011;39(6):1151-1152. [IIIC]

184. Kanji S, Lam J, Goddard RD, et al. Inappropriate medication administration practices in Canadian adult ICUs: a multicenter, cross-sectional observational study. *Ann Pharmacother*. 2013;47(5):637-643. [IIIA]

185. Zhou L, Dhopeshwarkar N, Blumenthal KG, et al. Drug allergies documented in electronic health records of a large healthcare system. *Allergy*. 2016;71(9):1305-1313. [IIIB]

186. Echeta G, Moffett BS, Checchia P, et al. Prescribing errors in adult congenital heart disease patients admitted to a pediatric cardiovascular intensive care unit. *Congenit Heart Dis*. 2014;9(2):126-130. [IIIB]

187. Modic MB, Albert NM, Sun Z, et al. Does an insulin double-checking procedure improve patient safety? *J Nurs Adm*. 2016;46(3):154-160. [IB]

188. Girard NJ. Vial mistakes involving heparin. *AORN J*. 2011;94(6):644, -554. [VB]

189. Gilbar PJ, Seger AC. Fatalities resulting from accidental intrathecal administration of bortezomib: strategies for prevention. *J Clin Oncol*. 2012;30(27):3427-3428. [VC]

190. Kellett P, Gottwald M. Double-checking high-risk medications in acute settings: a safer process. *Nurs Manag (Harrow)*. 2015;21(9):16-22. [VC]

191. Alsulami Z, Conroy S, Choonara I. Double checking the administration of medicines: what is the evidence? A systematic review. *Arch Dis Child*. 2012;97(9):833-837. [IIIB]

192. Ofosu R, Jarrett P. Reducing nurse medicine administration errors. *Nurs Times*. 2015;111(20):12-14. [VB]

193. Murphy M, While A. Medication administration practices among children's nurses: a survey. *Br J Nurs*. 2012;21(15):928-933. [IIIB]

194. McLeod M, Barber N, Franklin BD. Facilitators and barriers to safe medication administration to hospital inpatients: a mixed methods study of nurses' medication administration processes and systems (the MAPS study). *Plos One*. 2015;10(6):e0128958. [IIIB]

195. Raban MZ, Westbrook JI. Are interventions to reduce interruptions and errors during medication administration effective?: a systematic review. *BMJ Qual Saf*. 2014;23(5):414-421. [IIA]

196. Williams T, King MW, Thompson JA, Champagne MT. Implementing evidence-based medication safety interventions on a progressive care unit. *Am J Nurs*. 2014;114(11):53-62. [VB]

197. Choo J, Johnston L, Manias E. Nurses' medication administration practices at two Singaporean acute care hospitals. *Nurs Health Sci*. 2013;15(1):101-108. [IIIB]

198. Bower R, Jackson C, Manning JC. Interruptions and medication administration in critical care. *Nurs Crit Care*. 2015;20(4):183-195. [IIIB]

199. Verweij L, Smeulers M, Maaskant JM, Vermeulen H. Quiet please! Drug round tabards: are they effective and accepted? A mixed method study. *J Nurs Scholarsh*. 2014;46(5):340-348. [IIIB]

200. Fore AM, Sculli GL, Albee D, Neily J. Improving patient safety using the sterile cockpit principle during medication administration: a collaborative, unit-based project. *J Nurs Manag*. 2013;21(1):106-111. [VB]

201. Bravo K, Cochran G, Barrett R. Nursing strategies to increase medication safety in inpatient settings. *J Nurs Care Qual*. 2016;31(4):335-341. [IIIB]

202. Pape TM. The effect of a five-part intervention to decrease omitted medications. *Nurs Forum*. 2013;48(3):211-222. [VB]

203. Capasso V, Johnson M. Improving the medicine administration process by reducing interruptions. *J Healthc Manag*. 2012;57(6):384-390. [VC]

204. Craig J, Clanton F, Demeter M. Reducing interruptions during medication administration: the white vest study. *J Res Nurs*. 2014;19(3):248-261. [IIB]

205. Fabbri G, Panico M, Dallolio L, et al. Outbreak of ampicillin/piperacillin-resistant *Klebsiella pneumoniae* in a neonatal intensive care unit (NICU): investigation and control measures. *Int J Environ Res Public Health*. 2013;10(3):808-815. [VC]

206. Branch-Elliman W, Weiss D, Balter S, Bornschlegel K, Phillips M. Hepatitis C transmission due to contamination of multidose medication vials: summary of an outbreak and a call to action. *Am J Infect Control*. 2013;41(1):92-94. [VC]

207. De Smet B, Veng C, Kruy L, et al. Outbreak of *Burkholderia cepacia* bloodstream infections traced to the use of Ringer lactate solution as multiple-dose vial for catheter flushing, Phnom Penh, Cambodia. *Clin Microbiol Infect*. 2013;19(9):832-837. [VC]

208. Cohen M, Smetzer J. ISMP medication error report analysis—error prevention strategies for strong iodine solution; do not use an insulin pen for multiple patients. *Hosp Pharm*. 2012;47(4):260-263. [VC]

209. Jog M, Sachidananda R, Saeed K. Risk of contamination of lidocaine hydrochloride and phenylephrine hydrochloride topical solution: in vivo and in vitro analyses. *J Laryngol Otol*. 2013;127(8):799-801. [IIIB]

210. Baniasadi S, Dorudinia A, Mobarhan M, Karimi Gamishan M, Fahimi F. Microbial contamination of single- and multiple-dose vials after opening in a pulmonary teaching hospital. *Braz J Infect Dis*. 2013;17(1):69-73. [IIIB]

211. Moore ZS, Schaefer MK, Hoffmann KK, et al. Transmission of hepatitis C virus during myocardial perfusion imaging in an outpatient clinic. *Am J Cardiol*. 2011;108(1):126-132. [VA]

212. Drezner K, Antwi M, Del Rosso P, Dorsinville M, Kellner P, Ackelsberg J. A cluster of methicillin-susceptible *Staphylococcus aureus* infections at a rheumatology practice, New York City, 2011. *Infect Control Hosp Epidemiol*. 2014;35(2):187-189. [VC]

213. King CA, Ogg M. Safe injection practices for administration of propofol. *AORN J*. 2012;95(3):365-372. [VB]

214. Kundra S, Singh RM, Grewal A, Gupta V, Chaudhary AK. Necrotizing fasciitis after spinal anesthesia. *Acta Anaesthesiol Scand*. 2013;57(2):257-261. [VB]

215. Ersoz G, Uguz M, Aslan G, Horasan ES, Kaya A. Outbreak of meningitis due to *Serratia marcescens* after spinal anaesthesia. *J Hosp Infect*. 2014;87(2):122-125. [VC]

216. Coyle JR, Goerge E, Kacynski K, et al. Hepatitis C virus infections associated with unsafe injection practices at a pain management clinic, Michigan, 2014-2015. *Pain Med*. 2017;18(2):322-329. [VC]

217. Rashid M, Karagama YG. Study of microbial spread when using multiple-use nasal anaesthetic spray. *Rhinology*. 2011;49(3):281-285. [IIIB]

218. Hilliard JG, Cambronne ED, Kirsch JR, Aziz MF. Barrier protection capacity of flip-top pharmaceutical vials. *J Clin Anesth*. 2013;25(3):177-180. [IIIB]

219. Laha B, Hazra A. Medication error report: intrathecal administration of labetalol during obstetric anesthesia. *Indian J Pharmacol*. 2015;47(4):456-458. [VC]

220. Park JC, Herbert EN. Laser goggles alter the perceived colour of drug labels, increasing the risk for drug errors. *Can J Ophthalmol*. 2013;48(2):e27-e28. [VC]

221. Dolan SA, Arias KM, Felizardo G, et al. APIC position paper: safe injection, infusion, and medication vial practices in health care. *Am J Infect Control*. 2016;44(7):750-757. [IVB]

222. Haas RE, Beitz E, Reed A, et al. No bacterial growth found in spiked intravenous fluids over an 8-hour period. *Am J Infect Control*. 2017;45(4):448-450. [IIIB]

223. Preventing catheter/tubing misconnections: much needed help is on the way! *Alta RN*. 2011;67(2):24-25. [VC]

224. Paparella SF, Wollitz A. Mix-ups and misconnections: avoiding intravenous line errors. *J Emerg Nurs*. 2014;40(4):382-384. [VC]

225. Simmons D, Phillips MS, Grissinger M, Becker SC; USP Safe Medication Use Expert Committee. Error-avoidance recommendations for tubing misconnections when using Luer-tip connectors: a statement by the USP safe medication use expert committee. *Jt Comm J Qual Patient Saf*. 2008;34(5):293-296, 245. [VB]

226. Döring M, Brenner B, Handgretinger R, Hofbeck M, Kerst G. Inadvertent intravenous administration of maternal breast milk in a six-week-old infant: a case report and review of the literature. *BMC Res Notes*. 2014;7:17. [VC]

227. Cohen MR, Smetzer JL. ISMP medication error report analysis. *Hosp Pharm*. 2011;46(2):82-86. [VC]

228. Cohen MR, Smetzer JL. ISMP medication error report analysis—avoiding inadvertent intravenous injection of oral liquids; medication within intravenous tubing may be overlooked; searching by drug name gives information on wrong drug. *Hosp Pharm*. 2012;47(11):825-828. [VC]

229. Shenoi AN, Fortenberry JD, Kamat P. Accidental intra-arterial injection of propofol. *Pediatr Emerg Care*. 2014;30(2):136. [VC]

230. Ross MJ, Wise A. Accidental epidural administration of Syntocinon. *Int J Obstet Anesth*. 2012;21(2):203-204. [VC]

231. Kilcup M, Schultz D, Carlson J, Wilson B. Postdischarge pharmacist medication reconciliation: impact on readmission rates and financial savings. *J Am Pharm Assoc*. 2013;53(1):78-84. [IIB]

232. Ghatnekar O, Bondesson A, Persson U, Eriksson T. Health economic evaluation of the Lund Integrated Medicines Management model (LIMM) in elderly patients admitted to hospital. *BMJ Open*. 2013;3(1). [IIB]

233. Feldman LS, Costa LL, Feroli ERJ, et al. Nurse-pharmacist collaboration on medication reconciliation prevents potential harm. *J Hosp Med*. 2012;7(5):396-401. [IIIB]

234. Gimenez Manzorro A, Zoni AC, Rodriguez Rieiro C, et al. Developing a programme for medication reconciliation at the time of admission into hospital. *Int J Clin Pharm*. 2011;33(4):603-609. [IIB]

235. Selcuk A, Sancar M, Okuyan B, Demirtunc R, Izzettin FV. The potential role of clinical pharmacists in elderly patients during hospital admission. *Pharmazie*. 2015;70(8):559-562. [IIIB]

236. Dodds LJ. Optimising pharmacy input to medicines reconciliation at admission to hospital: lessons from a collaborative service evaluation of pharmacy-led medicines reconciliation services in 30 acute hospitals in England. *Eur J Hosp Pharm Sci Pract*. 2014;21(2):95-101. [IIIA]

237. Lee Y, Kuo L, Chiang Y, et al. Pharmacist-conducted medication reconciliation at hospital admission using information technology in Taiwan. *Int J Med Inf*. 2013;82(6):522-527. [IIIA]

238. Marotti SB, Kerridge RK, Grimer MD. A randomised controlled trial of pharmacist medication histories and supplementary prescribing on medication errors in postoperative medications. *Anaesth Intensive Care*. 2011;39(6):1064-1070. [IB]

239. Mekonnen AB, McLachlan AJ, Brien JE. Effectiveness of pharmacist-led medication reconciliation programmes on

clinical outcomes at hospital transitions: a systematic review and meta-analysis. *BMJ Open.* 2016;6(2):e010003. [IIB]

240. Becerra-Camargo J, Martinez-Martinez F, Garcia-Jimenez E. The effect on potential adverse drug events of a pharmacist-acquired medication history in an emergency department: a multicentre, double-blind, randomised, controlled, parallel-group study. *BMC Health Serv Res.* 2015;15:337. [IB]

241. Gattari TB, Krieger LN, Hu HM, Mychaliska KP. Medication discrepancies at pediatric hospital discharge. *Hosp Pediatr.* 2015;5(8):439-445. [IIIB]

242. Ziaeian B, Araujo KLB, Van Ness PH, Horwitz LI. Medication reconciliation accuracy and patient understanding of intended medication changes on hospital discharge. *J Gen Intern Med.* 2012;27(11):1513-1520. [IIIB]

243. Wolf O, Aberg H, Tornberg U, Jonsson KB. Do orthogeriatric inpatients have a correct medication list? A pharmacist-led assessment of 254 patients in a Swedish university hospital. *Geriatr Orthop Surg Rehabil.* 2016;7(1):18-22. [IIIB]

244. Yi SB, Shan JCP, Hong GL. Medication reconciliation service in Tan Tock Seng Hospital. *Int J Health Care Qual Assur.* 2013;26(1):31-36. [IIIC]

245. González-García L, Salmerón-García A, García-Lirola M, Moya-Roldán S, Belda-Rustarazo S, Cabeza-Barrera J. Medication reconciliation at admission to surgical departments. *J Eval Clin Pract.* 2016;22(1):20-25. [IIIB]

246. Hohn N, Langer S, Kalder J, Jacobs MJ, Marx G, Eisert A. Optimizing the pharmacotherapy of vascular surgery patients by medication reconciliation. *J Cardiovasc Surg.* 2014;55(2 Suppl 1):175-181. [IIIB]

247. Knez L, Suskovic S, Rezonja R, Laaksonen R, Mrhar A. The need for medication reconciliation: a cross-sectional observational study in adult patients. *Respir Med.* 2011;105(Suppl 1):S60-S66. [IIIB]

248. Mendes AE, Lombardi NF, Andrzejevski VS, Frandoloso G, Correr CJ, Carvalho M. Medication reconciliation at patient admission: a randomized controlled trial. *Pharm Pract.* 2016;14(1):656. [IB]

249. Holland DM. Interdisciplinary collaboration in the provision of a pharmacist-led discharge medication reconciliation service at an Irish teaching hospital. *Int J Clin Pharm.* 2015;37(2):310-319. [IIIB]

250. Belda-Rustarazo S, Cantero-Hinojosa J, Salmeron-Garcia A, Gonzalez-Garcia L, Cabeza-Barrera J, Galvez J. Medication reconciliation at admission and discharge: an analysis of prevalence and associated risk factors. *Int J Clin Pract.* 2015;69(11):1268-1274. [IIIB]

251. Bemt PMLA, Schrieck-de Loos EM, Linden C, Theeuwes AMLJ, Pol AG. Effect of medication reconciliation on unintentional medication discrepancies in acute hospital admissions of elderly adults: a multicenter study. *J Am Geriatr Soc.* 2013;61(8):1262-1268. [IIA]

252. Benson JM, Snow G. Impact of medication reconciliation on medication error rates in community hospital cardiac care units. *Hosp Pharm.* 2012;47(12):927-932. [IIA]

253. Gao T, Gaunt MJ. Breakdowns in the medication reconciliation process. *Penn Patient Saf Advis.* 2013;10(4):125-136. [IIIA]

254. Rubio CB, Garrido PN, Segura BM, Ferrit M, Calderón AC, Catalá PRM. Medication reconciliation at admission in old patients. *Aten Farm.* 2014;16(1):13-22. [IIIB]

255. Gaspar Carreño M, Gavião Prado C, Costa Nogueira J, et al. Medication reconciliation on admission. *Aten Farm.* 2014; 16(4):273-281. [IIIB]

256. Hellstrom LM, Bondesson A, Hoglund P, Eriksson T. Errors in medication history at hospital admission: prevalence and predicting factors. *BMC Clin Pharmacol.* 2012;12:9. [IIIA]

257. Young L, Barnason S, Hays K, Do V. Nurse practitioner-led medication reconciliation in critical access hospitals. *J Nurse Pract.* 2015;11(5):511-518. [IIB]

258. Bell CM, Brener SS, Gunraj N, et al. Association of ICU or hospital admission with unintentional discontinuation of medications for chronic diseases. *JAMA.* 2011;306(8):840-847. [IIIB]

259. Magalhães GF, Santos GN, Rosa MB, Noblat Lde A. Medication reconciliation in patients hospitalized in a cardiology unit. *Plos One.* 2014;9(12):e115491. [IIIB]

260. Hellstrom LM, Hoglund P, Bondesson A, Petersson G, Eriksson T. Clinical implementation of systematic medication reconciliation and review as part of the Lund Integrated Medicines Management model—impact on all-cause emergency department revisits. *J Clin Pharm Ther.* 2012;37(6):686-692. [IIA]

261. Lehnbom EC, Stewart MJ, Manias E, Westbrook JI. Impact of medication reconciliation and review on clinical outcomes. *Ann Pharmacother.* 2014;48(10):1298-1312. [IIIB]

262. Cortelyou-Ward K, Swain A, Yeung T. Mitigating error vulnerability at the transition of care through the use of health IT applications. *J Med Syst.* 2012;36(6):3825-3831. [VB]

263. Treiber LA, Jones JH. Medication errors, routines, and differences between perioperative and non-perioperative nurses. *AORN J.* 2012;96(3):285-294. [IIIB]

264. Gallo E, Pugi A, Lucenteforte E, et al. Pharmacovigilance of herb-drug interactions among preoperative patients. *Altern Ther Health Med.* 2014;20(2):13-17. [IIIA]

265. Lee A, Varma A, Boro M, Korman N. Value of pharmacist medication interviews on optimizing the electronic medication reconciliation process. *Hosp Pharm.* 2014;49(6):530-538. [IIB]

266. Meyer C, Stern M, Woolley W, Jeanmonod R, Jeanmonod D. How reliable are patient-completed medication reconciliation forms compared with pharmacy lists? *Am J Emerg Med.* 2012;30(7):1048-1054. [IIIB]

267. Lu Y, Clifford P, Bjorneby A, et al. Quality improvement through implementation of discharge order reconciliation. *Am J Health Syst Pharm.* 2013;70(9):815-820. [VB]

268. Richards M, Ashiru-Oredope D, Chee N. What errors can be identified by pharmacy-led medicines reconciliation? A prospective study. *Acute Med.* 2011;10(1):18-21. [IIIB]

269. Karapinar-Carkit F, Borgsteede SD, Zoer J, Egberts TCG, van den Bemt PMLA, van Tulder M. Effect of medication reconciliation on medication costs after hospital discharge in relation to hospital pharmacy labor costs. *Ann Pharmacother.* 2012;46(3):329-338. [IIIB]

270. Philbrick AM, Harris IM, Schommer JC, Fallert CJ. Medication discrepancies associated with subsequent

pharmacist-performed medication reconciliations in an ambulatory clinic. *J Am Pharm Assoc.* 2015;55(1):77-80. [IIIB]

271. Leguelinel-Blache G, Arnaud F, Bouvet S, et al. Impact of admission medication reconciliation performed by clinical pharmacists on medication safety. *Eur J Intern Med.* 2014;25(9):808-814. [IIIB]

272. Mekonnen AB, McLachlan AJ, Brien JE. Pharmacy-led medication reconciliation programmes at hospital transitions: a systematic review and meta-analysis. *J Clin Pharm Ther.* 2016;41(2):128-144. [IIA]

273. Deitelzweig S. Care transitions in anticoagulation management for patients with atrial fibrillation: an emphasis on safety. *Ochsner J.* 2013;13(3):419-427. [VB]

274. Zoni AC, Duran Garcia ME, Jimenez Munoz AB, Salomon Perez R, Martin P, Herranz Alonso A. The impact of medication reconciliation program at admission in an internal medicine department. *Eur J Intern Med.* 2012;23(8):696-700. [IIC]

275. Andreoli L, Alexandra J, Tesmoingt C, et al. Medication reconciliation: a prospective study in an internal medicine unit. *Drugs Aging.* 2014;31(5):387-393. [IIIB]

276. Cornu P, Steurbaut S, Leysen T, et al. Effect of medication reconciliation at hospital admission on medication discrepancies during hospitalization and at discharge for geriatric patients. *Ann Pharmacother.* 2012;46(4):484-494. [IIIB]

277. Shiu JR, Fradette M, Padwal RS, et al. Medication discrepancies associated with a medication reconciliation program and clinical outcomes after hospital discharge. *Pharmacotherapy.* 2016;36(4):415-421. [IIIB]

278. Lee KP, Hartridge C, Corbett K, Vittinghoff E, Auerbach AD. "Whose job is it, really?" Physicians', nurses', and pharmacists' perspectives on completing inpatient medication reconciliation. *J Hosp Med.* 2015;10(3):184-186. [IIIB]

279. De Winter S, Vanbrabant P, Spriet I, et al. A simple tool to improve medication reconciliation at the emergency department. *Eur J Intern Med.* 2011;22(4):382-385. [IIA]

280. Cullinan S, O'Mahony D, Byrne S. Application of the structured history taking of medication use tool to optimise prescribing for older patients and reduce adverse events. *Int J Clin Pharm.* 2016;38(2):374-379. [IIIB]

281. Henneman EA, Tessier EG, Nathanson BH, Plotkin K. An evaluation of a collaborative, safety focused, nurse-pharmacist intervention for improving the accuracy of the medication history. *J Patient Saf.* 2014;10(2):88-94. [IIA]

282. Narendra PL, Biradar PA, Rao AN. Vanishing bowl of local anesthetics: a lesson for sterile labeling. *Anesth Essays Res.* 2014;8(3):407-409. [VC]

283. Medication safety. *J Pharm Pract Res.* 2015;45(1):86-92. [VC]

284. Guideline for sterile technique. In: *Guidelines for Perioperative Practice.* Denver, CO: AORN, Inc; 2017:75-104. [IVA]

285. Or CKL, Wang H. A comparison of the effects of different typographical methods on the recognizability of printed drug names. *Drug Saf.* 2014;37(5):351-359. [IIIB]

286. Sakuma M, Ida H, Nakamura T, et al. Adverse drug events and medication errors in Japanese paediatric inpatients: a retrospective cohort study. *BMJ Qual Saf.* 2014;23(10):830-837. [IIIA]

287. Standards for perioperative nursing. In: *Guidelines for Perioperative Practice.* Denver, CO: AORN, Inc; 2015:693-708. [IVC]

288. Cohen MR, Smetzer JL. ISMP medication error report analysis—fatal patient-controlled anesthesia adverse events; name confusion with new cancer drugs; medication safety officer group to become a part of ISMP. *Hosp Pharm.* 2013;48(9):715-724. [VC]

289. Guideline for care of the patient receiving local anesthesia. In: *Guidelines for Perioperative Practice.* Denver, CO: AORN, Inc; 2017:617-628. [IVA]

290. Pfeifer K, Slawski B, Manley A, Nelson V, Haines M. Improving preoperative medication compliance with standardized instructions. *Minerva Anestesiol.* 2016;82(1):44-49. [VA]

291. Chien HY, Ko JJ, Chen YC, et al. Study of medication waste in Taiwan. J Exp Clin Med. 2013;5(2):69-72. [IIIB]

292. Warle-van Herwaarden MF, Kramers C, Sturken-boom MC, van den Bemt PMLA, De Smet PAGM; Dutch HARM-Wrestling Task Force. Targeting outpatient drug safety: recommendations of the Dutch HARM-Wrestling Task Force. *Drug Saf.* 2012;35(3):245-259. [IVB]

293. Manworren RCB, Gilson AM. CE: Nurses' role in preventing prescription opioid diversion. *Am J Nurs.* 2015;115(8):34-40. [VB]

294. Strauch KA. Invisible pollution: the impact of pharmaceuticals in the water supply. *AAOHN J.* 2011;59(12):525-533. [VB]

295. Trovato JA, Tuttle LA. Oral chemotherapy handling and storage practices among veterans affairs oncology patients and caregivers. *J Oncol Pharm Pract.* 2014;20(2):88-92. [VA]

296. Perks S, Robertson S, Haywood A, Glass B. Clozapine repackaged into dose administration aids: a common practice in Australian hospitals. *Int J Pharm Pract.* 2012;20(1):4-8. [IIIB]

297. Beckett VL, Tyson LD, Carroll D, Gooding NM, Kelsall AW. Accurately administering oral medication to children isn't child's play. *Arch Dis Child.* 2012;97(9):838-841. [IIIB]

298. Armor BL, Wight AJ, Carter SM. Evaluation of adverse drug events and medication discrepancies in transitions of care between hospital discharge and primary care follow-up. *J Pharm Pract.* 2016;29(2):132-137. [IIIB]

299. Sarangarm P, London MS, Snowden SS, et al. Impact of pharmacist discharge medication therapy counseling and disease state education: pharmacist assisting at routine medical discharge (project PhARMD). *Am J Med Qual.* 2013;28(4):292-300. [IIB]

300. Valente S, Murray LP. Creative strategies to improve patient safety: allergies and adverse drug reactions. *J Nurses Staff Dev.* 2011;27(1):E1-E5. [VB]

301. Borgsteede SD, Karapinar-Carkit F, Hoffmann E, Zoer J, van den Bemt PMLA. Information needs about medication according to patients discharged from a general hospital. *Patient Educ Couns.* 2011;83(1):22-28. [IIIB]

302. Bouraoui S, Brahem A, Tabka F, Mrizek N, Saad A, Elghezal H. Assessment of chromosomal aberrations, micronuclei and proliferation rate index in peripheral lymphocytes from Tunisian nurses handling cytotoxic drugs. *Environ Toxicol Pharmacol.* 2011;31(1):250-257. [IIIB]

303. Connor TH, Lawson CC, Polovich M, McDiarmid MA. Reproductive health risks associated with occupational

exposures to antineoplastic drugs in health care settings: a review of the evidence. *J Occup Environ Med.* 2014;56(9):901-910. [IIIB]

304. El-Ebiary AA, Abuelfadl AA, Sarhan NI. Evaluation of genotoxicity induced by exposure to antineoplastic drugs in lymphocytes of oncology nurses and pharmacists. *J Appl Toxicol.* 2013;33(3):196-201. [IIIB]

305. Gomez-Olivan LM, Miranda-Mendoza GD, Cabrera-Galeana PA, et al. Oxidative stress induced in nurses by exposure to preparation and handling of antineoplastic drugs in Mexican hospitals: a multicentric study. *Oxid Med Cell Longev.* 2014;2014:858604. [IIIB]

306. Hon C, Abusitta D. Causes of health care workers' exposure to antineoplastic drugs: an exploratory study. *Can J Hosp Pharm.* 2016;69(3):216-223. [IIIB]

307. Musak L, Smerhovsky Z, Halasova E, et al. Chromosomal damage among medical staff occupationally exposed to volatile anesthetics, antineoplastic drugs, and formaldehyde. *Scand J Work Environ Health.* 2013;39(6):618-630. [IIIB]

308. Hon C, Teschke K, Shen H, Demers PA, Venners S. Antineoplastic drug contamination in the urine of Canadian healthcare workers. *Int Arch Occup Environ Health.* 2015;88(7):933-941. [IIIB]

309. Controlling occupational exposure to hazardous drugs. Occupational Safety and Health Administration. https://www.osha.gov/SLTC/hazardousdrugs/controlling_occex_hazardousdrugs.html. Accessed July 13, 2017.

310. Gulten T, Evke E, Ercan I, Evrensel T, Kurt E, Manavoglu O. Lack of genotoxicity in medical oncology nurses handling antineoplastic drugs: effect of work environment and protective equipment. *Work.* 2011;39(4):485-489. [IIIB]

311. Occupational Safety and Health Administration. 29 CFR §1910.1200. Hazard communication. US Government Publishing Office. http://www.ecfr.gov/cgi-bin/text-idx?SID=3a88b79bbd5ccb9689a55025239c3ff8&mc=true&node=se29.6.1910_11200&rgn=div8. Accessed July 13, 2017.

312. Easty AC, Coakley N, Cheng R, et al. Safe handling of cytotoxics: guideline recommendations. *Curr Oncol.* 2015;22(1):e27-e37. [IVB]

313. Hazardous drugs—handling in healthcare settings (800). In: *USP Compounding Compendium.* Rockville, MD: US Pharmacopeial Convention; 2016:86-103. [IVC]

314. Bussieres J, Tanguay C, Touzin K, Langlois E, Lefebvre M. Environmental contamination with hazardous drugs in Quebec hospitals. *Can J Hosp Pharm.* 2012;65(6):428-435. [IIIA]

315. Ensuring healthcare worker safety when handling hazardous drugs. *Oncol Nurs Forum.* 2015;42(3):217-218. [IVB]

316. Boiano JM, Steege AL, Sweeney MH. Adherence to precautionary guidelines for compounding antineoplastic drugs: a survey of nurses and pharmacy practitioners. *J Occup Environ Hyg.* 2015;12(9):588-602. [IIIB]

317. Lawson CC, Rocheleau CM, Whelan EA, et al. Occupational exposures among nurses and risk of spontaneous abortion. *Am J Obstet Gynecol.* 2012;206(4):327.e1-327.e8. [IIIA]

318. Leduc-Souville B, Bertrand E, Schlatter J. Risk management of excreta in a cancer unit. *Clin J Oncol Nurs.* 2013;17(3):248-252. [IIIB]

319. Meade E. Avoiding accidental exposure to intravenous cytotoxic drugs. *Br J Nurs.* 2014;23(16):S34. [VA]

320. Vyas N, Yiannakis D, Turner A, Sewell GJ. Occupational exposure to anti-cancer drugs: a review of effects of new technology. *J Oncol Pharm Pract.* 2014;20(4):278-287. [VB]

321. Villarini M, Dominici L, Piccinini R, et al. Assessment of primary, oxidative and excision repaired DNA damage in hospital personnel handling antineoplastic drugs. *Mutagenesis.* 2011;26(3):359-369. [IIIB]

322. Menonna-Quinn D. Safe handling of chemotherapeutic agents in the treatment of nonmalignant diseases. *J Infus Nurs.* 2013;36(3):198-204. [VB]

323. *PB70: Liquid Barrier Performance and Classification of Protective Apparel and Drapes Intended for use in Health Care Facilities.* Arlington, VA: Association for the Advancement of Medical Instrumentation; 2012. [IVC]

324. Occupational Safety and Health Administration. 29 CFR §1910.134. Respiratory protection. https://www.osha.gov/pls/oshaweb/owadisp.show_document?p_table=standards&p_id=12716. Accessed July 13, 2017.

325. Hon C, Teschke K, Chua P, Venners S, Nakashima L. Occupational exposure to antineoplastic drugs: identification of job categories potentially exposed throughout the hospital medication system. *Saf Health Work.* 2011;2(3):273-281. [IIIB]

326. Hon C, Teschke K, Chu W, Demers P, Venners S. Antineoplastic drug contamination of surfaces throughout the hospital medication system in Canadian hospitals. *J Occup Environ Hyg.* 2013;10(7):374-383. [IIIB]

327. Queruau Lamerie T, Nussbaumer S, Decaudin B, et al. Evaluation of decontamination efficacy of cleaning solutions on stainless steel and glass surfaces contaminated by 10 antineoplastic agents. *Ann Occup Hyg.* 2013;57(4):456-469. [IIIB]

328. Walton AML, Mason S, Busshart M, et al. Safe handling: implementing hazardous drug precautions. *Clin J Oncol Nurs.* 2012;16(3):251-254. [VB]

329. Bohlandt A, Groeneveld S, Fischer E, Schierl R. Cleaning efficiencies of three cleaning agents on four different surfaces after contamination by gemcitabine and 5-fluorouracile. *J Occup Environ Hyg.* 2015;12(6):384-392. [IIIB]

330. Schierl R, Novotna J, Piso P, Bohlandt A, Nowak D. Low surface contamination by cis/oxaliplatin during hyperthermic intraperitoneal chemotherapy (HIPEC). *Eur J Surg Oncol.* 2012;38(1):88-94. [IIIB]

331. Couch J, Burr G, Niemeier MT. Evaluation of exposures to healthcare personnel from cisplatin during a mock interperitoneal operation for cancer treatment. *J Assoc Occup Health Prof Healthc.* 2011;31(2):17-19. [VA]

332. Solid Waste Disposal Act [as amended through Pub L No 107-377, December 31, 2002].

333. Souza Oliveira AD, Câmara Alves AE, Silva JA, Silva Oliveira LF, Medeiros SM. Occupational risks of the nursing team's exposure to chemotherapeutic agents: integrative literature review. *Rev Enferm UFPE.* 2013;7(3):794-802. [IIIB]

334. Hennessy KA, Dynan J. Improving compliance with personal protective equipment use through the model for improvement and staff champions. *Clin J Oncol Nurs.* 2014;18(5):497-500. [VB]

335. Boiano JM, Steege AL, Sweeney MH. Adherence to safe handling guidelines by health care workers who administer antineoplastic drugs. *J Occup Environ Hyg.* 2014;11(11):728-740. [IIIB]

336. Jeong KW, Lee B, Kwon MS, Jang J. Safety management status among nurses handling anticancer drugs: nurse awareness and performance following safety regulations. *Asian Pac J Cancer Prev.* 2015;16(8):3203-3211. [IIIB]

337. Polovich M, Gieseker KE. Occupational hazardous drug exposure among non-oncology nurses. *Medsurg Nurs.* 2011; 20(2):79-85. [VA]

338. Hon C, Teschke K, Demers PA, Venners S. Antineoplastic drug contamination on the hands of employees working throughout the hospital medication system. *Ann Occup Hyg.* 2014;58(6):761-770. [IIIB]

339. Hon C, Teschke K, Shen H. Health care workers' knowledge, perceptions, and behaviors regarding anti-neoplastic drugs: survey from British Columbia, Canada. *J Occup Environ Hyg.* 2015;12(10):669-677. [IIIA]

340. Ladeira C, Viegas S, Padua M, et al. Assessment of genotoxic effects in nurses handling cytostatic drugs. *J Toxicol Environ Health A.* 2014;77(14-16):879-887. [IIIB]

341. Santovito A, Cervella P, Delpero M. Chromosomal damage in peripheral blood lymphocytes from nurses occupationally exposed to chemicals. *Hum Exp Toxicol.* 2014;33(9):897-903. [IIIB]

342. Drug Enforcement Administration (DEA), Department of Justice. Disposal of controlled substances. Final rule. *Fed Regist.* 2014;79(174):53519-53570.

343. Unused Pharmaceuticals in the Health Care Industry: Interim Report. Washington, DC: Environmental Protection Agency; 2008. https://nepis.epa.gov/Exe/ZyPDF.cgi/P100165B.PDF?Dockey=P100165B.PDF. Accessed July 13, 2017. [VB]

344. Federal Water Pollution Control Act [as amended through Pub L No 107-303, November 27, 2002].

345. Chiarello M, Minetto L, Giustina SVD, Beal LL, Moura S. Popular pharmaceutical residues in hospital wastewater: quantification and qualification of degradation products by mass spectroscopy after treatment with membrane bioreactor. *Environ Sci Pollut Res Int.* 2016;23(16):16079-16089. [IIIB]

346. Frédéric O, Yves P. Pharmaceuticals in hospital wastewater: their ecotoxicity and contribution to the environmental hazard of the effluent. *Chemosphere.* 2014;115(1):31-39. [IIIC]

347. Nguyen H, Pham H, Vo D, et al. The effect of a clinical pharmacist-led training programme on intravenous medication errors: a controlled before and after study. *BMJ Qual Saf.* 2014;23(4):319-324. [IIB]

348. Laukaityte E, Bruyere M, Bull A, Benhamou D. Accidental injection of patent blue dye during gynaecological surgery: lack of knowledge constitutes a system error. *Anaesth Crit Care Pain Med.* 2015;34(1):57-60. [VC]

349. Westbrook JI, Rob MI, Woods A, Parry D. Errors in the administration of intravenous medications in hospital and the role of correct procedures and nurse experience. *BMJ Qual Saf.* 2011;20(12):1027-1034. [IIIB]

350. Karavasiliadou S, Athanasakis E. An inside look into the factors contributing to medication errors in the clinical nursing practice. *Health Sci J.* 2014;8(1):32-44. [VB]

351. Zyoud AH, Abdullah NAC. The effect of individual factors on the medication error. *Glob J Health Sci.* 2016;8(12):57756. [IIIB]

352. Thornton P. Medication safety. *J Pharm Pract Res.* 2015;45(4):450-458. [VC]

353. Niemann D, Bertsche A, Meyrath D, et al. A prospective three-step intervention study to prevent medication errors in drug handling in paediatric care. *J Clin Nurs.* 2015;24(1-2):101-114. [IIIB]

354. Samaranayake NR, Cheung STD, Chui WCM, Cheung BMY. Technology-related medication errors in a tertiary hospital: a 5-year analysis of reported medication incidents. *Int J Med Inform.* 2012;81(12):828-833. [IIIB]

355. Hicks RW, Hernandez J, Wanzer LJ. Perioperative pharmacology: patient-controlled analgesia. *AORN J.* 2012;95(2):255-262. [VB]

356. Speroni KG, Fisher J, Dennis M, Daniel M. What causes near-misses and how are they mitigated? *Nursing.* 2013; 43(4):19-24. [IIIB]

357. Abbotoy JL, Sessanna L. Hands-on BCMA education for direct care nurses. *Nurs Manage.* 2012;43(11):15-18. [VC]

358. Cleary-Holdforth J, Leufer T. The strategic role of education in the prevention of medication errors in nursing: part 2. *Nurse Educ Pract.* 2013;13(3):217-220. [VB]

359. Leufer T, Cleary-Holdforth J. Let's do no harm: medication errors in nursing: part 1. *Nurse Educ Pract.* 2013;13(3):213-216. [VB]

360. Lu M, Yu S, Chen I, Wang KK, Wu H, Tang F. Nurses' knowledge of high-alert medications: a randomized controlled trial. *Nurse Educ Today.* 2013;33(1):24-30. [IB]

361. Gokhman R, Seybert AL, Phrampus P, Darby J, Kane-Gill SL. Medication errors during medical emergencies in a large, tertiary care, academic medical center. *Resuscitation.* 2012;83(4):482-487. [IIIA]

362. Lap FT, Tak KY, So Yuen AS. How to change nurses' behavior leading to medication administration errors using a survey approach in United Christian Hospital. *J Nurse Educ Pract.* 2014;4(12):17-26. [IIIB]

363. Sears K, Goodman WM. Risk factors for increased severity of paediatric medication administration errors. *Healthc Policy.* 2012;8(1):e109-e126. [IIIB]

364. Abbasinazari M, Zareh-Toranposhti S, Hassani A, Sistanizad M, Azizian H, Panahi Y. The effect of information provision on reduction of errors in intravenous drug preparation and administration by nurses in ICU and surgical wards. *Acta Med Iran.* 2012;50(11):771-777. [IIB]

365. Haw C, Stubbs J, Dickens G. Medicines management: an interview study of nurses at a secure psychiatric hospital. *J Adv Nurs.* 2015;71(2):281-294. [IIIB]

366. Haseeb A, Winit-Watjana W, Bakhsh AR, et al. Effectiveness of a pharmacist-led educational intervention to reduce the use of high-risk abbreviations in an acute care setting in Saudi Arabia: a quasi-experimental study. *BMJ Open.* 2016;6(6):e011401. [IIB]

367. Chedoe I, Molendijk H, Hospes W, Van den Heuvel ER, Taxis K. The effect of a multifaceted educational intervention on medication preparation and administration errors in neonatal intensive care. *Arch Dis Child Fetal Neonatal Ed.* 2012;97(6):F449-F455. [IIB]

368. Lohmann K, Ferber J, Haefeli MF, et al. Knowledge and training needs of nurses and physicians on unsuitable drugs for patients with dysphagia or feeding tubes. *J Clin Nurs.* 2015;24(19-20):3016-3019. [IIIC]

369. Keane K. Reducing medication errors by educating nurses on bar code technology. *Medsurg Nurs.* 2014;23(5 Suppl 1):10-11. [VC]

370. Alsulami Z, Choonara I, Conroy S. Nurses' knowledge about the double-checking process for medicines administration. *Nurs Child Young People.* 2014;26(9):21-26. [IIIB]

371. Dabliz R, Levine S. Medication safety in neonates. *Am J Perinatol.* 2012;29(1):49-56. [VC]

372. Implementing real-time point of care documentation: a QI project to address medication administration errors. *Online J Nurs Inform.* 2014;18(3):1-1. [VB]

373. Bucsi R. Documentation errors related to electronic health records. *Insight.* 2012;37(3):19. [VB]

374. Order scanning systems (and fax machines) may pull multiple pages through the scanner at the same time, leading to drug omissions. *Alta RN.* 2011;67(1):24-25. [VC]

375. Perez-Garcia MdC, Soria-Aledo V, Collantes F. Implementation and evaluation of the medication management in nursing units of a university hospital by means of a quality improvement cycle. *Appl Nurs Res.* 2016;29:148-156. [VB]

376. Nwasor EO, Sule ST, Mshelia DB. Audit of medication errors by anesthetists in north western Nigeria. *Niger J Clin Pract.* 2014;17(2):226-231. [IIIC]

377. Burch KJ. Using a trigger tool to assess adverse drug events in a children's rehabilitation hospital. *J Pediatr Pharm Ther.* 2011;16(3):204-209. [IIIC]

378. Carnevali L, Krug B, Amant F, et al. Performance of the adverse drug event trigger tool and the global trigger tool for identifying adverse drug events: experience in a Belgian hospital. *Ann Pharmacother.* 2013;47(11):1414-1419. [IIIB]

379. Nobre C, McKay C. Surveillance of adverse drug events in a large tertiary-care hospital. *Conn Med.* 2012;76(2):91-94. [VB]

380. Harkanen M, Kervinen M, Ahonen J, Voutilainen A, Turunen H, Vehvilainen-Julkunen K. Patient-specific risk factors of adverse drug events in adult inpatients—evidence detected using the global trigger tool method. *J Clin Nurs.* 2015;24(3-4):582-591. [IIIC]

381. Kung K, Carrel T, Wittwer B, Engberg S, Zimmermann N, Schwendimann R. Medication errors in a Swiss cardiovascular surgery department: a cross-sectional study based on a novel medication error report method. *Nurs Res Pract.* 2013;2013:671820. [IIIB]

382. Donaldson N, Aydin C, Fridman M, Foley M. Improving medication administration safety: using naive observation to assess practice and guide improvements in process and outcomes. *J Healthc Qual.* 2014;36(6):58-68. [IIIB]

383. Taghon T, Elsey N, Miler V, McClead R, Tobias J. A medication-based trigger tool to identify adverse events in pediatric anesthesiology. *Jt Comm J Qual Patient Saf.* 2014;40(7):326-334. [VB]

384. Erstad BL, Patanwala AE, Theodorou AA. Comparison of methods for the detection of medication safety events in the critically ill. *Curr Drug Saf.* 2012;7(3):238-246. [IIIB]

385. Davies K, Mitchell C, Coombes I. The role of observation and feedback in enhancing performance with medication administration. *J Law Med.* 2015;23(2):316-321. [VB]

386. Elliott P, Martin D, Neville D. Electronic clinical safety reporting system: a benefits evaluation. *JMIR Med Inform.* 2014;2(1):e12. [IIB]

387. Meyer-Massetti C, Cheng CM, Schwappach DLB, et al. Systematic review of medication safety assessment methods. *Am J Health Syst Pharm.* 2011;68(3):227-240. [IIIB]

388. Cronrath P, Lynch TW, Gilson LJ, et al. PCA oversedation: application of healthcare failure mode effect (HFMEA) analysis. *Nurs Econ.* 2011;29(2):79-87. [IIB]

389. Velez-Diaz-Pallares M, Delgado-Silveira E, Carretero-Accame ME, Bermejo-Vicedo T. Using healthcare failure mode and effect analysis to reduce medication errors in the process of drug prescription, validation and dispensing in hospitalised patients. *BMJ Qual Saf.* 2013;22(1):42-52. [IIB]

390. Curatolo N, Gutermann L, Devaquet N, Roy S, Rieutord A. Reducing medication errors at admission: 3 cycles to implement, improve and sustain medication reconciliation. *Int J Clin Pharm.* 2014;37(1):113-120. [IIIB]

391. Ashley L, Dexter R, Marshall F, McKenzie B, Ryan M, Armitage G. Improving the safety of chemotherapy administration: an oncology nurse-led failure mode and effects analysis. *Oncol Nurs Forum.* 2011;38(6):E436-E444. [VB]

392. Cheng C, Chou C, Wang P, Lin H, Kao C, Su C. Applying HFMEA to prevent chemotherapy errors. *J Med Syst.* 2012;36(3):1543-1551. [VB]

393. Nguyen C, Cote J, Lebel D, et al. The AMELIE project: Failure mode, effects and criticality analysis: a model to evaluate the nurse medication administration process on the floor. *J Eval Clin Pract.* 2013;19(1):192-199. [VB]

394. Beckett RD, Yazdi M, Hanson LJ, Thompson RW. Improving medication safety through the use of metrics. *J Pharm Pract.* 2014;27(1):61-64. [IIIA]

395. de Boer M, Ramrattan MA, Boeker EB, Kuks PFM, Boermeester MA, Lie-A-Huen L. Quality of pharmaceutical care in surgical patients. *Plos One.* 2014;9(7):e101573. [IIIB]

396. Smeulers M, Verweij L, Maaskant JM, et al. Quality indicators for safe medication preparation and administration: a systematic review. *Plos One.* 2015;10(4):e0122695. [IIIB]

397. Rodriguez-Gonzalez CG, Martin-Barbero ML, Herranz-Alonso A, et al. Use of failure mode, effect and criticality analysis to improve safety in the medication administration process. *J Eval Clin Pract.* 2015;21(4):549-559. [VB]

398. Miller DF, Fortier CR, Garrison KL. Bar code medication administration technology: characterization of high-alert

medication triggers and clinician workarounds. *Ann Pharmacother.* 2011;45(2):162-168. [IIIA]

399. Rack LL, Dudjak LA, Wolf GA. Study of nurse workarounds in a hospital using bar code medication administration system. *J Nurs Care Qual.* 2012;27(3):232-239. [IIIB]

400. Niazkhani Z, Pirnejad H, van der Sijs H, Aarts J. Evaluating the medication process in the context of CPOE use: the significance of working around the system. *Int J Med Inf.* 2011;80(7):490-506. [IIIB]

401. Coleman JJ, Hodson J, Brooks HL, Rosser D. Missed medication doses in hospitalised patients: a descriptive account of quality improvement measures and time series analysis. *Int J Qual Health Care.* 2013;25(5):564-572. [VA]

402. Munn Z, Scarborough A, Pearce S, et al. The implementation of best practice in medication administration across a health network: a multisite evidence-based audit and feedback project. JBI *Database System Rev Implement Rep.* 2015;13(8):338-352. [IIB]

Acknowledgments

Lead Author

Byron L. Burlingame, MS, RN, BSN, CNOR
Senior Perioperative Practice Specialist
AORN Nursing Department
Denver, Colorado

Contributing Author

Ramona L. Conner, MSN, RN, CNOR, FAAN
Editor-in-Chief, Guidelines for Perioperative Practice
AORN Nursing Department
Denver, Colorado

The authors and AORN thank Janice Neil, PhD, RN, CNE, Associate Professor, College of Nursing, East Carolina University, Greenville, North Carolina; Mary Lamonte, MPH, MSN, RN, CNOR, Staff Nurse, Stamford Surgical Center, Stamford, Connecticut; Rodney W. Hicks, PhD, RN, FNP-BC, FAANP, Professor, Western University of Health Sciences, Pomona, California; Diana L. Wadlund, MSN, ACNP-C, CRNFA, Nurse Practitioner, Paoli Hospital, Paoli, Pennsylvania; Leslie Jeter, MSNA, RN, CRNA, Staff CRNA, Ambulatory Anesthesia of Atlanta, Georgia; Bernard C. Camins, MD, MSc, Associate Professor of Medicine Division of Infectious Diseases, University of Alabama at Birmingham Healthcare Epidemiologist, UAB Health System Medical Director, UAB Hospital Employee Health and UA HSF Employee Health, Birmingham; Jocelyn M. Chalquist, BSN, RN, CNOR, Surgical Services Educator, Aurora Medical Center-Kenosha, Kenosha, Wisconsin; Judith L. Goldberg, DBA, MSN, RN, CNOR, CSSM, CHL, Director, Patient Care Services, Perioperative and Procedural Services, Lawrence + Memorial Hospital, New London, Connecticut; Lisa Spruce, DNP, RN, CNS-CP, ACNS, ACNP, CNOR, FAAN, Director of Evidence-based Perioperative Practice, AORN Nursing Department, Denver, Colorado; Colleen Peralta, MSN, RN, Professor, College of Nursing, Long Beach City College, Long Beach, California; Vicki Barnett, MSN, RN, CNOR, Executive Director, Department of Surgical Services, Northside Hospital, Atlanta, Georgia; Evangeline (Vangie) Dennis, BSN, RN, CNOR, CMLSO, Director of Patient Care Practice, Emory Healthcare and Ambulatory Surgery Centers, Atlanta, Georgia; Brenda G. Larkin, MS, RN, CNOR, ACNS-BC, Clinical Nurse Specialist for Perioperative Services, Aurora Lakeland Medical Center and Aurora Memorial Hospital Burlington, Elkhorn, Wisconsin; and James (Jay) Bowers, BSN, RN, CNOR, TNCC, Clinical Educator, West Virginia Healthcare, Morgantown, for their assistance in developing this guideline.

Publication History

Originally published online December 2011 in *Perioperative Standards and Recommended Practices.*

Reformatted September 2012 for publication in *Perioperative Standards and Recommended Practices,* 2013 edition.

Minor editing revisions made in November 2014 for publication as "Guideline for medication safety" in *Guidelines for Perioperative Practice,* 2015 edition.

Revised September 2017 for online publication in *Guidelines for Perioperative Practice.*

Evidence ratings revised and minor editorial changes made to conform with the current AORN Evidence Rating model, September 2019, for online publication in *Guidelines for Perioperative Practice.*

AMBULATORY SUPPLEMENT: MEDICATION SAFETY

1. Medication Management Plan

1.8.1 **The health care organization may contract with a pharmacist to provide consultative services onsite or via telepharmacy.**[A1-A3]

The Centers for Medicare & Medicaid Services (CMS) Conditions of Participation states that "Hospitals must provide pharmaceutical services that meet the needs of their patients."[A1] The CMS Conditions for Coverage for ambulatory surgery centers (ASCs) states that a specific licensed health care professional is required to provide direction to the ASC's pharmaceutical service unless the ASC is performing activities that under state law may only be performed by a licensed pharmacist.[A2]

Ⓐ If an on-site pharmacist is not available, pharmaceutical services provided by the organization should be directed and overseen by a licensed pharmacist, or when appropriate, by a physician or dentist who is qualified to assume responsibility for the pharmaceutical services rendered.[A1,A4]

Ⓐ When required by law and regulation or the policy of the organization, if a medication has been recalled there must be a process by which patients are notified that the medication was recalled for safety reasons by the manufacturer or the US Food and Drug Administration.[A5]

2. Procurement and Storage

2.5 **All Class II, III, IV, and V medications must be stored in a locked location.**[A1,A2]

Ⓐ In accordance with the Comprehensive Drug Abuse Prevention and Control Act of 1970, if Class II, III, IV, and V drugs are used, records of receipt and disposition of the drugs must be maintained. Accountability procedures must be in place to ensure control of the distribution, use, and disposition of all scheduled drugs.

Ⓐ Records to trace the movement of scheduled drugs throughout the ASC must be current and maintained, and any discrepancies in count must be reconciled promptly. Scheduled drugs must be tracked from the point of entry into the ASC to the point of departure, either through administration, destruction, or return to the manufacturer.

Ⓐ The ASC must have a system in place to readily identify loss or diversion of all controlled substances, and the system should minimize the time between the actual loss or diversion and the time of detection.[A1]

Ⓐ The ASC must maintain a current medication formulary that includes the strength and dosage for dispensing and administering the medications. The medication formulary must be readily available to those involved in medication management. There must be a process to select and procure medications that are not on the formulary.[A5] Medications on the formulary that are dispensed or administered should be reviewed annually based on emerging safety and efficacy information.

3. Prescribing Phase

3.3.1 **When hand writing medication orders, write legibly and include a legible signature of the prescriber initiating the order.**

Ⓐ Prescription pads should be controlled and secured from unauthorized patient access, and should not be pre-signed and/or postdated.[A4]

5. Administration

5.2 **Administer all medications according to the manufacturer's instructions for use.**

Ⓐ Records must be maintained to ensure the control and safe dispensing of sample drugs in compliance with federal and state law.[A4]

10. Hazardous Medications

10.2 **The health care organization must create a hazardous medication management plan.**[A6]

Ⓐ The ASC must identify, in writing, its hazardous medications and its process for managing hazardous medications. This is also applicable to sample medications.[A2]

References

A1. Centers for Medicare & Medicaid Services (CMS), DHHS. Medicare and Medicaid programs; hospital conditions of participation: requirements for history and physical examinations; authentication of verbal orders; securing medications; and postanesthesia evaluations. Final rule. *Fed Regist.* 2006;71(227):68671–68695.

A2. *State Operations Manual Appendix L—Guidance for Surveyors: Ambulatory Surgical Centers.* Rev. 137; 2015. Centers for Medicare & Medicaid Services. https://www.cms.gov/Regulations-and-Guidance/Guidance/Manuals/downloads/som107ap_l_ambulatory.pdf. Accessed July 12, 2017.

A3. Cole SL, Grubbs JH, Din C, Nesbitt TS. Rural inpatient telepharmacy consultation demonstration for after-hours medication review. *Telemed J E Health.* 2012;18(7):530–537. [IIB]

A4. ASHP guidelines: minimum standard for pharmacies in hospitals. *Am J Health Syst Pharm.* 2013;70(18):1619–1630. [IVC]

A5. MM.05.01.17. In: *Standards for Ambulatory Care.* Oak Brook Terrace, IL: The Joint Commission; 2017.

A6. Occupational Safety and Health Administration. 29 CFR §1910.1200. Hazard communication. US Government Publishing Office. http://www.ecfr.gov/cgi-bin/text-idx?SID=3a88b79bbd5ccb9689a55025239c3ff8&mc=true&node=se29.6.1910_11200&rgn=div8. Accessed July 13, 2017.

Acknowledgments

Contributing Author
Jan Davidson, MSN, RN, CNOR, CASC
Director, Ambulatory Surgery Division
AORN, Inc
Denver, Colorado

Publication History

Originally published in *Perioperative Standards and Recommended Practices,* 2014 edition.

Revised September 2017 for publication in *Guidelines for Perioperative Practice,* 2018 edition.

Minor editorial changes made to conform with revised guideline format, September 2019, for online publication in *Guidelines for Perioperative Practice.*

AORN GUIDELINES FOR
PERIOPERATIVE PRACTICE,
2022 EDITION

MINIMALLY INVASIVE SURGERY

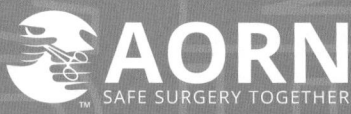

TABLE OF CONTENTS

P *indicates a recommendation or evidence relevant to pediatric care.*

MEDICAL ABBREVIATIONS & ACRONYMS

3D – Three dimensional
AAGL – American Association of Gynecologic Laparoscopists
ACR – American College of Radiology
ASGE – American Society of Gastrointestinal Endoscopy
CO_2 – Carbon dioxide
CT – Computed tomography
FGI – Facility Guidelines Institute
HFMEA – Health Failure Mode and Effects Analysis
IAFE – Intraabdominal fluid extravasation
IR – Interventional radiology

MIS – Minimally invasive surgery
MRI – Magnetic resonance imaging
N_2O – Nitrous oxide
OR – Operating room
RAPTOR – Resuscitation with angiography percutaneous treatments and operative resuscitations
RN – Registered nurse
TAVR – Transthoracic aortic valve replacement
TUR – Transurethral resection
TURP – Transurethral resection of the prostate
VA – Department of Veterans Affairs

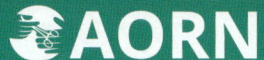
GUIDELINE FOR
MINIMALLY INVASIVE SURGERY

The Guideline for Minimally Invasive Surgery was approved by the AORN Guidelines Advisory Board and became effective December 15, 2016. It was presented as a proposed guideline for comments by members and others. The recommendations in the guideline are intended to be achievable and represent what is believed to be an optimal level of practice. Policies and procedures will reflect variations in practice settings and/or clinical situations that determine the degree to which the guideline can be implemented. AORN recognizes the many diverse settings in which perioperative nurses practice; therefore, this guideline is adaptable to all areas where operative or other invasive procedures may be performed.

Purpose

This document provides guidance for creating a safe environment of care for patients undergoing minimally invasive surgical procedures. The guideline addresses distension media used during endoscopic procedures, **hybrid operating rooms** (ORs), magnetic resonance imaging (MRI) hybrid ORs, navigation-guided procedures, and robotic-assisted surgery. The document provides guidance to

- perioperative personnel to reduce risks to patients and perioperative team members during **minimally invasive surgery** (MIS) and **computer-assisted technology** procedures;
- perioperative registered nurses (RNs) to assist in managing distension media (eg, gas, fluid) and irrigation fluid; and
- health care organizations for incorporating advancements in technology with consideration for workplace safety and ergonomics.

Minimally invasive surgery is a technique used in most surgical specialties. This guideline was initially developed to provide guidance during the emergence of endoscopic procedures in the 1990s but has been expanded to include other emerging technologies. Computer science development has led to advances in computer software and hardware for medical devices that allow the surgeon to perform surgery through smaller incisions or no incisions by using digital images and data. Use of these new technologies requires multidisciplinary teams and departments to merge knowledge and skill mix in new environments to enhance patient outcomes. *Digital OR* is a new term used to describe the complex environment of endoscopic suites, hybrid ORs, and computer-assisted surgeries. The technological enhancements allow for improved efficiencies and management of surgical areas.

The following topics are outside the scope of this document:
- flexible endoscopic gastrointestinal procedures,
- care and cleaning of instruments and related equipment (See the AORN Guideline for Processing Flexible Endoscopes[1] and the AORN Guideline for Cleaning and Care of Surgical Instruments[2]),
- design of the physical environment (See the AORN Guideline for a Safe Environment of Care, Part 2[3]),
- surgical smoke safety (See the AORN Guideline for Surgical Smoke Safety[4]),
- fluid warming (See the AORN Guideline Prevention of Unplanned Patient Hypothermia[5] and the AORN Guideline for a Safe Environment of Care, Part 1[6]),
- patient positioning (See the AORN Guideline for Patient Positioning[7]),
- energy-generating devices (See the AORN Guideline for Safe Use of Energy-Generating Devices[8]), and
- surgical technique (eg, trocar entry techniques).

Evidence Review

In January 2016, a medical librarian conducted systematic searches of the databases MEDLINE®, CINAHL®, and Scopus® and the Cochrane Database of Systematic Reviews, limiting the results to articles published in English after 2009. During the development of this guideline, the lead author requested supplementary searches for topics not included in the original search as well as articles and other sources that were discovered during the evidence appraisal process. The lead author and the medical librarian also identified relevant guidelines from government agencies and standards-setting bodies.

Search terms included the subject headings and keywords *minimally invasive surgical procedures, robotic surgical procedures, angioscopy, morcellation, interventional magnetic resonance imaging, interventional radiography, interventional ultrasonography, angioplasty, endoscopy, cholangiography,* and *hybrid operating room,* as well as headings and keywords identifying specific procedures. Patient monitoring and procedural complications were addressed by headings and keywords that included *nursing assessment, intraoperative and postoperative complications, intraoperative and physiologic monitoring, fluid monitoring, insufflation, extravasation, pneumoperitoneum, intraabdominal pressure, TUR syndrome,* and *compartment syndrome.* Occupational risks related to minimally invasive surgery were included in the search with terms such as *human engineering, occupational injuries, ergonomics, musculoskeletal injuries,* and *occupational accidents.*

Excluded were non-peer-reviewed publications and lower-level or lower-quality evidence when higher-level or higher-quality evidence was available. Surgical techniques (eg, open

Figure 1. Flow Diagram of Literature Search Results

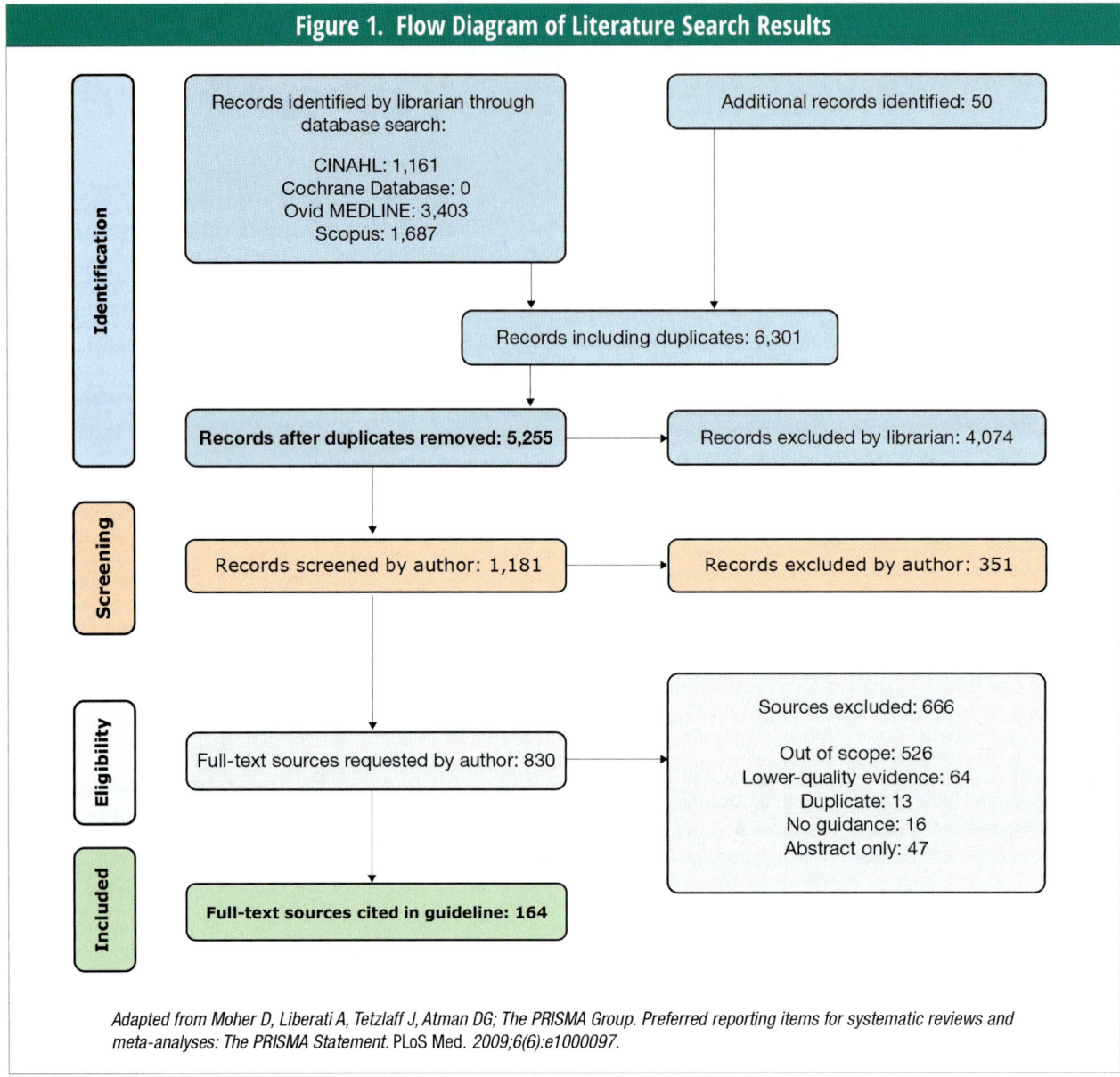

Adapted from Moher D, Liberati A, Tetzlaff J, Atman DG; The PRISMA Group. Preferred reporting items for systematic reviews and meta-analyses: The PRISMA Statement. PLoS Med. 2009;6(6):e1000097.

versus closed technique, trocar insertion, natural orifice technique, single-incision laparoscopic surgery) and anesthesia techniques (eg, goal-directed fluid therapy), endoclip migration, future product development and applications, equipment prototypes, enhanced recovery after surgery, dental navigation-guided surgery, and gastrointestinal endoscopy procedures also were excluded (Figure 1).

Articles identified in the search were provided to the project team for evaluation. The team consisted of the lead author and four evidence appraisers. The lead author divided the search results into topics and assigned members of the team to review and critically appraise each article using the AORN Research or Non-Research Evidence Appraisal Tools as appropriate. The literature was independently evaluated and appraised according to the strength and quality of the evidence. Each article was then assigned an appraisal score. The appraisal score is noted in brackets after each reference as applicable.

Each recommendation rating is based on a synthesis of the collective evidence, a benefit-harm assessment, and consideration of resource use. The strength of the recommendation was determined using the AORN Evidence Rating Model and the quality and consistency of the evidence supporting a recommendation. The recommendation strength rating is noted in brackets after each recommendation.

Note: The evidence summary table is available at http://www.aorn.org/evidencetables/.

Editor's note: MEDLINE is a registered trademark of the US National Library of Medicine's Medical Literature Analysis and Retrieval System, Bethesda, MD. CINAHL, Cumulative Index to Nursing and Allied Health Literature, is a registered trademark of EBSCO Industries, Birmingham, AL. Scopus is a registered trademark of Elsevier B.V., Amsterdam, The Netherlands.

1. Safe Environment

1.1 **Establish a multidisciplinary team to create an efficient, safe environment for minimally invasive procedures.** *[Recommendation]*

Experts agree on the need for a multidisciplinary team to plan the design and workflow of the minimally invasive OR environment.[3,9-12]

Strong et al[13] described creating a committee composed of representatives from hospital administration and physician and nursing leadership to review ethical considerations for implementing new technologies and new techniques in surgery. In an effort to improve quality, this committee reviewed new devices and procedures, approved the introduction of new devices into the health care system, provided uniform credentialing standards, and reviewed early patient outcomes.

1.2 **The multidisciplinary team, including perioperative RNs, physicians, surgical technologists, infection preventionists, biomedical engineers, and other members of the health care team, should plan the room configuration.** *[Recommendation]*

In describing their experience with developing an endoscopic surgical suite at the International Neuroscience Institute in Hanover, Germany, Samii and Gerganov[9] stated that "a dedicated endoscopic OR should provide work flow optimization, ergonomics, and highest safety standards for the patient."

In a literature review regarding endourology ORs, Sabnis et al[10] provided a description of an optimal endoscopy suite. The review authors recommended a surgical suite 60 m² to 70 m² in size to provide adequate space for multiple ceiling booms, **fluoroscopy** equipment, an ultrasonography machine, a laser machine, irrigation pumps, and an integrated technologies system to record and archive data from cameras and imaging equipment. The authors described advances in data relay systems that create a seamless two-way communication between the ORs and electronic medical records, a radiological picture archiving and communication system, and classrooms or auditoriums anywhere in the world. The authors recommended installing ceiling-mounted equipment booms to improve efficiency, reduce clutter, and interconnect equipment. They also recommended reducing tripping hazards by providing electrical outlets close to the location of the equipment stored on the shelves and providing video display monitors in all four quadrants of the room for nurses, assistants, surgical technologists, and anesthesiologists to keep the team focused on the surgical procedure.

1.2.1 Include the following in the room configuration plan:

- access to the patient and surgical field;
- placement of equipment booms, video monitors, and overhead lights to reduce distractions[11] and ergonomic hazards specific to MIS (ie, slips, trips, falls in low lighting, collisions);
- an adequate quantity of dedicated electrical circuits and appropriate placement and connection of power cords and cables;
- systems to evacuate and filter surgical smoke during the MIS procedure and at the end of the procedure when the **pneumoperitoneum** is released;
- methods to control and minimize traffic; and
- collaboration with vendors to achieve medical device intraoperability.

[Recommendation]

Equipment booms provide shelving, electrical outlets, and medical gas ports to improve ergonomics and safety related to the multiple cords and tubing required to perform minimally invasive procedures. Installation of overhead ceiling-mounted arms to support the video monitors improves the ability of the surgical team to view the endoscopic images. Integration systems used for routing and switching images to and from the OR environment also provide archiving capabilities that can be used for patient teaching, remote viewing, and creating educational materials for the health care team members. The focus of the multidisciplinary team is to use these technologies to enhance the quality and safety of surgery.[9,10]

Problems with equipment may be a source of distraction for the surgical team. In a facility observation of endourological procedures, Persoon et al[11] measured the level of observed interference with the main task of the surgical team. The authors also interviewed eight urologists and seven residents on the effects of distracting factors. During the 78 procedures that were observed, a median of 20 distracting events occurred per procedure. The researchers calculated that there was one distraction every 1.8 minutes during the procedure. Equipment problems (ie, availability and failure) were the most frequently observed distraction and were identified by the physicians as a source of distraction. The problem of equipment failure in **endoscopic surgery** demonstrates the need for education, policies, and programs to introduce new technologies to the perioperative team.

Moderate-quality evidence identified the need to improve ergonomics in laparoscopic procedures.[14-16]

Choi[14] performed a literature review of the ergonomic challenges of laparoscopic surgery. Surgical personnel encounter physical stress in the head, neck, and shoulders caused by static postures and awkward body positions. Items that create ergonomic challenges include the OR bed position, the position of monitor(s), hand held instruments, the position of foot pedal(s), cognitive challenges (eg, lack of direct viewing of the surgical field and interpretation of the camera angle to images on the video monitor), and the position of equipment cart(s). The author provided a table summarizing the literature on ergonomic considerations for the laparoscopic OR. This review highlighted the need to understand the effects of advanced technology in the OR.

Stavroulis et al[15] conducted a cross sectional survey of 27 theatre personnel at a tertiary referral hospital in the United Kingdom about their experiences with working in integrated and nonintegrated operating theatres. The respondents rated survey items from 1 (poor) to 10 (excellent) regarding everyday tasks, interaction with the medical team, perception of teamwork, stress, and overall satisfaction. The theatre team members had high satisfaction scores related to working in the integrated theatre and believed that this environment resulted in greater efficiency, better teamwork, and reduced stress levels. The limitations of this study were a small sample size and that the questionnaire was not a validated tool.

1.3 **Consult a representative of the health care organization's information technology department to identify information system requirements before new technologies are purchased.** *[Recommendation]*

The American Society of Gastrointestinal Endoscopy (ASGE) Technology Committee reviewed existing, new, and emerging endoscopic technologies.[17] The review featured information about image quality, storage and retrieval systems, ease of use, and safety considerations. The authors recommended that hospitals assess device compatibility with existing systems, type of image capture (eg, standard definition versus high definition), integration with electronic medical record systems, and centralized storage and archiving systems when purchasing an image management system.

Medical devices usually have proprietary interfaces, and it can be a challenge to manage a system that contains components from multiple manufacturers. Rockstroh et al[18] developed a concept for a data storage system to address the inability to easily retrieve data collected from multiple sources in the intraoperative environment. The researchers developed a surgical data recorder prototype to be used in neurosurgical procedures for removal of brain tumors. Data were transmitted and collected from the microscope, navigation equipment, intraoperative ultrasound, and electrophysiological workstation for measurement of evoked potentials. The surgical data recorder was able to store the generated data correctly, completely, and quickly even when more data than expected were sent to the system. The data could be stored in one location for easier retrieval and analysis. Working with the information technology representative for the health care facility early in the product selection process can provide insight into the compatibility of the equipment within the existing system.

1.3.1 **The image capture system must comply with Health Insurance Portability and Accountability Act requirements.**[19-21] *[Regulatory Requirement]*

1.3.2 **Identify remote telecommunications technology requirements that meet the health care organization strategic plan.** *[Recommendation]*

Low-quality evidence describes the benefits of telecommunication and telementoring in training, mentoring, and teaching.[17,22-25]

Anderson et al[22] described the use of integrated endourology suites for remote monitoring and supervision of urology residents. The researchers surveyed 100 patients on their satisfaction after surgery in which a junior urology resident performed the procedure and the attending surgeon observed the procedure in a control room equipped with live visual, audio, and **telestration** communication. The patient satisfaction mean scores were 9.5 out of 10 (ie, highly satisfied) regarding their comfort with having the procedure performed under remote monitoring and supervision. The researchers reported that most patients scored their satisfaction as greater than 7 for comfort with hearing the conversation between the supervising surgeon and resident over the speakers, having a urology resident perform the procedure, having a video camera in the room, and having other residents and medical students watch the procedure and with the privacy provided during the procedure. The researchers proposed using an integrated endourology suite and remote monitoring and supervision as an option to meet training criteria for residents and to promote efficiency, regulatory compliance, safety, and productivity.

Telecommunication has emerged as an alternative to physical presence as a mentoring tool. Santomauro et al[23] studied the use of teleconferencing for proctoring and mentoring surgeons. The authors proposed a pathway for adoption of a telementoring system for surgeon learning. They described the benefits of this technology in providing support and increasing surgeon confidence. They reported that extensive evidence demonstrated that surgeon volume affected outcomes (ie, a surgeon who performs a high volume of a procedure will have fewer complications). Allowing the high-volume surgeon access to an integrated OR via video and two-way communication provides support to and promotes confidence in a surgeon who may perform fewer procedures (eg, robotic-assisted prostatectomy). Current limitations in telecommunication systems include lag time of signals, insufficient virtual private network bandwidth, inaccuracy of telestration marks on tissue, and medicolegal issues. Improvement in these areas could widen the adoption of a telementoring system.

1.4 **Create a room layout with equipment positions for MIS systems based on procedure type(s), physical configuration, and recommendations by the equipment manufacturers.** [*Recommendation*]

The increase in equipment needed to provide minimally invasive procedures presents challenges to the perioperative team. Moderate-quality evidence reflects a need to standardize room setups to improve efficiency, decrease distractions, and improve the safety of patient care.[9-11,14-17,26-34]

The use of ceiling-mounted booms and video monitors is one solution. Nocco and del Torchio[27] conducted a survey of 17 surgeons and nine nurses at one facility in Italy before and after the installation of an integrated OR. The participants agreed that the features of the integrated OR improved quality, reduced risk, and reduced surgical time.

Al-Hakim[29] observed MIS surgeries (N = 17) in one facility and recorded all events that disrupted the operative time. The researchers divided the disruptive events into general categories: prerequisite requirements, work design, communication, and other. Work design events included problems with the OR bed and patient positioning, arrangement of instrumentation and materials, poor lighting, visual quality of monitors, and clothing (eg, lead aprons). The analysis showed that disruptions in the work design, such as an incorrect patient position or equipment failure, prolonged operative time and were recorded most frequently as disruptions to the procedure. The operative time was affected 15% of the time from personnel failure to follow work design protocols.

Klein et al[35] conducted a two-part randomized controlled trial to examine coping strategies associated with the performance of laparoscopic skills. Strain coping was defined as straining to use cognitive resources under stressful conditions. The researchers enlisted 48 undergraduate students as participants to help ensure an adequate sample size and variability (n = 24 men, n = 24 women). The students were tasked with performing a laparoscopic maneuver using a simulator. The researchers studied the coping skills of one group of students during a 45-minute peg-transfer task under a low-strain condition with a top camera view of 90 degrees. The second group worked under a high-strain condition with the camera view was rotated to 135 degrees. The 135-degree view created distortion and increased the difficulty of completing the peg maneuver in the specified time frame. Participants experienced strain coping in the group that worked with the extreme camera angle.

In the second part of the study, the researchers assessed the effects of monitoring displayed vital signs on the ability to complete the peg maneuver in the specified time frame. Three 33.02-cm monitors were located 59 cm behind the trainer box, 104.14 cm above the ground, and approximately 124 cm from the participant's eyes. The students were randomly assigned into groups of four men and four women to one of three different display conditions: control, split screen, and separated monitor screens. The control group performed the wood peg maneuver as in Part I, whereas the other groups were introduced to vital sign information.[35]

In the split-screen group, all information was displayed on the middle monitor with the simulator wooden box displayed on the top left, the oxygen value on the bottom left, and the heart rate value on top right quadrant of the screen. The third group saw the information in the same sequence but with each image displayed on a separate screen. Visual scanning by participants in the split screen view required minimal head movement whereas the participants in the separated monitor group were required to move their heads 65 degrees to see the vital signs on the different monitors. Monitoring critical signals resulted in slowed peg transfer compared with no monitoring.[35]

The researchers recommended that displays showing fluctuating information be positioned close together to minimize the effects of visual scanning. The participants using the split screen display did not differ statistically in performance from the participants using separated displays but the results showed a correlation in increased straining and frustration for the group using separated monitors. Using-split screen technology may reduce the number of monitors required. The researchers concluded that the laparoscopic environment induces strain coping and that visual scanning can impair detection of a critical signal (eg, vital sign data).[35]

Further research is needed on the positioning of equipment to enhance the performance of perioperative personnel during minimally invasive procedures.

1.5 **Prepare endoscopic equipment (eg, camera, light source, insufflation device) and instrumentation according to the manufacturer's instructions for use and physician preference.** [Recommendation]

1.5.1 Inspect MIS equipment and instrumentation before use, remove defective items from service, and send the item for repair or replacement according to the health care organization's policy and procedures. Inspect items for
- cleanliness;
- function and alignment of instrumentation;
- corrosion, pitting, burrs, nicks, and cracks;
- sharpness of cutting edges;
- wear and chipping of instruments and plated surfaces;
- missing parts;
- integrity of insulation on insulated devices;
- integrity of cables;
- clarity of lenses;
- integrity of seals and gaskets; and
- other defects.[2,36,37]

[Recommendation]

1.6 **Be prepared to convert a laparoscopic procedure to an open procedure.** [Recommendation]

A systematic review of the literature and a case series article[38,39] reported complications of vessel or organ injury caused by obtaining access during laparoscopic procedures. Evidence is limited about best practices in preparing for these emergencies. In a literature review of bowel injury in gynecological procedures, Llarena et al[38] reported that the overall incidence of bowel injury is one in 769 but the rate increases with surgical complexity. Levy et al[39] reported the incidence of iatrogenic injuries in laparoscopic surgeries to be low and described six case studies of bladder injury in laparoscopic procedures performed under urgent conditions (ie, three cases of appendicitis, two diagnostic laparoscopies for abdominal pain, and one ectopic pregnancy). Research is needed to determine best practices for preparing for emergent conversion to an open procedure.

2. Gas Insufflation Media

2.1 **Identify potential patient injuries and complications associated with gas insufflation media used during MIS procedures, and establish practices that reduce the risk for injuries and complications.** [Recommendation]

Gas distension media is used during MIS procedures for creating a pneumoperitoneum or space to visualize the surgical field with the endoscope. Carbon dioxide (CO_2) is the most commonly used gas, but other gases can be used, such as air, nitrogen, nitrous oxide (N_2O), argon, and helium.[40,41] The gas distension media is chosen based on the properties of the gas media, the procedure, and the patient's history.

Carbon dioxide is colorless, odorless, inexpensive, nonflammable, and easily dissolved in the bloodstream.[40,42,43] It is most frequently used to create a pneumoperitoneum, but is also used in other procedures, such as endovein harvest procedures,[40,44] esophageal endoscopic submucosal dissections,[45] robotic-assisted endoscopic thyroidectomy,[46] and diagnostic hysteroscopy in physician offices.[47] Carbon dioxide has been reported to have metabolic, hemodynamic, and cardiovascular adverse effects, especially among older adults and patients with preexisting medical conditions. Low-quality evidence indicates that the use of CO_2 for insufflation is safe but can result in hypercarbia, acidosis, peritoneal irritation, gas emboli, and cardiac arrhythmias. However, these complications occur at a rate of less than 1%.[40,42,43,48]

Nitrous oxide has many of the same benefits as CO_2, but its use has historically been considered a safety concern because of fear of combustion. Rammohan et al[49] conducted a randomized controlled trial of 77 patients undergoing laparoscopic surgery during an 8-week period and randomly assigned them to one of two groups. For group I (n = 38), the gas distension medium was N_2O, and for group II (n = 39), the gas distension medium was CO_2. The researchers found that there were significant differences between the two groups in heart rate changes and mean arterial pressure changes during the pneumoperitoneum. The N_2O group did not experience the same initial rise in these vital signs that the CO_2 group did. The patients in the N_2O insufflation group had lower pain scores than the patients in the CO_2 insufflation group.

A Cochrane review conducted by Cheng et al[41] compared CO_2 pneumoperitoneum with N_2O pneumoperitoneum in a review of three randomized controlled trials with a total of 100 participants and found no significant differences between the groups in any surgical outcomes. None of the trials reported any serious adverse events in the N_2O group; however, none of the studies had the statistical power to establish the safety of N_2O in pneumoperitoneum. In this same Cochrane review, the authors compared CO_2 and helium for creating a pneumoperitoneum. There were no significant differences in outcomes related to cardiopulmonary complication or morbidity. The safety of helium is still a large concern due to reports of serious adverse events related to subcutaneous emphysema in the scrotum, face, and cervical areas.

Air, helium, and N_2O are less soluble in blood than CO_2 and, therefore, it takes longer for a gas embolism to absorb in the bloodstream, which makes use of these gases less optimal for managing serious adverse effects.

2.2 **Take precautions to mitigate the risk for injury associated with gas insufflation during MIS.** *[Recommendation]*

2.2.1 **Set the insufflation flow rate according to the surgeon's specification and the manufacturer's instructions for use.**[50] *[Recommendation]*

The manufacturer's instructions for use provide specification for flow rate and trocar, filter, and tubing diameter for achieving best insufflation results. The gas flow rate is dependent on the smallest diameter in the insufflation system. Doubling the radius in the lumen of the system will increase gas flow rates. Decreasing the radius will increase resistance. Placing a 10-mm laparoscope in a 10-mm sheath that is also delivering the insufflation gas will decrease the diameter and increase the resistance to insufflation gas flow, which may result in inadequate insufflation. In situations where high gas flow is required, a system with low resistance and a large diameter will improve the gas flow rate.[50]

2.2.2 **Review and follow the manufacturers' instructions for use of insufflation equipment and make the instructions readily available to users.**[50] *[Recommendation]*

2.2.3 **Elevate the insufflator above the level of the surgical cavity if possible.** *[Recommendation]*

Elevating the insufflator and tubing decreases the risk of body fluids backing up into the insufflator device.[50]

2.2.4 **Flush the insufflator and insufflation tubing with the selected gas before the tubing is connected to the cannula (eg, Veress needle).** *[Recommendation]*

Flushing the tubing removes room air from the tubing. Filling the insufflation tubing with the selected insufflation gas reduces the risk for an air embolism.[50,51]

2.2.5 **Verify that a hydrophobic filter is in place between the insufflator and the insufflation tubing, and that the filter is compatible with the insufflator.** *[Recommendation]*

A filter helps prevent contaminants from flowing through the insufflator into the surgical cavity, prevents backflow of abdominal fluids and particulates that could contaminate the insufflator, and prevents cross contamination. When the filter is compatible with the insufflator, it does not interfere with the flow rate.[50]

2.2.6 **During a hysteroscopy, use insufflators designed and intended for hysteroscopy.** *[Recommendation]*

The American College of Obstetricians and Gynecologists recommends that insufflators designed for use in laparoscopic procedures not be used for hysteroscopy procedures. The small uterine cavity requires an insufflator that insufflates at high pressures with low volume. Laparoscopic insufflators insufflate at low pressures with large volumes and are therefore not recommended for hysteroscopy procedures.[47]

2.2.7 **Turn on endoscopic gas insufflator alarms and make them sufficiently audible to be heard above competing noise.**[3] *[Recommendation]*

2.3 **When a gas cylinder is used, check the cylinder to verify that it contains the selected gas and that it is not empty before the procedure begins. Have a second full cylinder readily available for immediate replacement of an empty cylinder.** *[Recommendation]*

2.4 **Maintain insufflation pressure at the lowest level necessary to achieve pneumoperitoneum within the specification of the surgeon.** *[Recommendation]*

Moderate-quality evidence[52-60] supports maintaining a pneumoperitoneum pressure of less than 15 mmHg. In a randomized controlled trial, Eryilmaz et al[53] tested the liver function of patients during laparoscopic cholecystectomy procedures. The patients were randomly assigned to either a group with a pneumoperitoneum at 10 mmHg (n = 20) or a group with a pneumoperitoneum at 14 mmHg (n = 23). The researchers found that the group with pneumoperitoneum at 14 mmHg had decreased blood flow to the liver and increased postoperative first hour serum aspartate aminotransferase. The researchers concluded that using a 10 mmHg pneumoperitoneum in laparoscopic cholecystectomy procedures is safe.

2.4.1 **Monitor gas insufflation pressures for maintenance of pressure at the desired level.** *[Recommendation]*

2.5 **Be prepared to detect and implement interventions to manage a gas embolism.** *[Recommendation]*

The occurrence of gas embolism in laparoscopic surgery is rare and is rapidly reversed due to the high gaseous solubility of CO_2.[40,57] The increased intraabdominal pressure and open blood vessels in abdominal laparoscopic surgery increase the chances for gas entrapment into an injured vein, artery, or solid organ. A gas embolus becomes a life-threatening event when large volumes of gas are introduced into the system and migrate to the right ventricle or pulmonary artery.[40] Incidents of gas embolism have been reported in procedures using CO_2 insufflation, such as abdominal laparoscopic procedures,[55] endoscopic vein harvesting,[40] and endoscopic thyroidectomy.[61]

Park et al[40] performed a review of the literature and described the incidence, pathophysiology, clinical signs, diagnosis, prevention, and treatment of CO_2 embolism during all types of laparoscopic surgery. The authors reported varied rates of embolism occurrence in laparoscopic surgeries using CO_2 insufflation.

2.5.1 **In the event of a gas embolism, the RN circulator should assist with immediate treatment.** *[Recommendation]*

Treatment to prevent the embolus from blocking circulation to vital organs may include

- discontinuation of the insufflation gas[40];
- discontinuation of the anesthetic agents and ventilation of the patient with 100% oxygen in an attempt to wash out the insufflation gas from the lungs and improve ventilation perfusion mismatch and hypoxemia;
- hyperventilation to assist in the removal of a CO_2 embolus[62];
- changing the patient's position (eg, from supine to Trendelenburg or left lateral position) to favor permanence of air in the appendage of the right atrium, therefore allowing blood flow under the air bubble[62];
- infusion of large amounts of IV fluids in an attempt to push the blocked airlock into the lungs where it can be absorbed (volume expansion will increase the central venous pressure and may reduce further gas entry)[40,62];

- administration of inotropes, vasopressors, and vasodilators specific to pulmonary circulation[40,62]; and
- cardiopulmonary resuscitation.[40]

3. Irrigation and Distension Media

3.1 **Identify potential injuries and complications associated with fluid used for irrigation or as distension media during MIS and computer-assisted procedures.** *[Recommendation]*

Fluid media is used in MIS procedures for distension to improve visualization of the cavity or irrigation in a joint. The fluid may be instilled under gravity or pressure or with an infusion pump. Complications from fluid **extravasation** or **intravasation** are rare but can be life threatening. Fluid extravasation can lead to edema in the surrounding tissue, abdominal distension, or intraabdominal compartment syndrome.[63] Fluid intravasation occurs when the irrigation fluid is absorbed into the patient's bloodstream, leading to physiological changes such as hyponatremia, hypervolemia, and cardiovascular and pulmonary complications. This is also referred to as **transurethral resection (TUR) syndrome** because it was first reported during transurethral resection of the prostate (TURP) procedures.[47,64]

Fluid distension-related complications occur in less than 1% of procedures but the risks increase with the length of the procedure and the degree of dissection of the surrounding tissues. For example, a diagnostic hysterectomy has a lower risk of fluid absorption than a resectoscopic myomectomy.[65]

Moderate-quality evidence[47,63-75] indicates that complications in the use of fluid media used to distend the cavity or improve visualization can result in intravasation or extravasation of the fluid. The use of improper or excessive amounts of fluid for irrigation or distension media can lead to hypervolemia and hyponatremia.

Several authors have reported cases of airway compromise caused by extravasation of irrigation fluid during shoulder arthroscopy procedures.[66,68,69] Cases have also been reported of complications in hysteroscopy procedures from irrigation fluid, including fluid overload,[74] hypotonic hyponatremia, heart failure, and cerebral and pulmonary edema.[65,67,70-72]

Kocher et al[63] conducted a survey of hip arthroscopists in the Multicenter Arthroscopy of the Hip Outcomes Research Network to evaluate the incidence of intraabdominal fluid extravasation (IAFE) in patients undergoing hip arthroscopies. Fifteen arthroscopists (88%) responded to the survey. The respondents provided a retrospective review of patient medical records to answer the survey questions related to the number of hip arthroscopies performed and symptomatic IAFE cases they encountered. A total of 25,648 procedures performed between 1984 and 2010 were reported, and 40 patients (0.16%) were reported to have an IAFE complication occur during the procedure.

Prevention of IAFE includes close observation for abdominal distension, a decrease in core body temperature, and hemodynamic instability. Higher arthroscopic fluid pump pressure and iliopsoas tenotomy had a significant correlation as risk factors in the patients who experienced IAFE. The mean pump pressures for reported cases of symptomatic IAFE were 45 mmHg to 90 mmHg. The 15 survey respondents stated they generally used a pump pressures of 30 mmHg to 80 mmHg. Iliopsoas tenotomy was reported to be performed only 25% of the time during hip arthroscopy. In the 40 IAFE cases, 25 patients had an iliopsoas tenotomy performed. The authors recommended early detection of intraabdominal fluid with computed tomography (CT) or ultrasound to prevent adverse outcomes and provided an algorithm for treatment after intraabdominal or retroperitoneal fluid extravasation has been established after hip arthroscopy.[63]

3.2 **Select the irrigation or distension fluid in consultation with the surgeon based on procedure type, patient assessment, and instruments to be used (eg, energy-generating devices).** [*Recommendation*]

Moderate-quality evidence[36,37,47,64,65,75-78] indicates that fluid distension media should be selected based on the medium least likely to cause complications in the event of excess fluid absorption and on compatibility with energy-generating devices. **Table 1** provides information about fluids used for irrigation or distension media in MIS procedures.

Nonelectrolyte and low viscosity media, such as 1.5% glycine, 3% sorbitol, or 5% mannitol, are most often selected when monopolar instrumentation is required for gynecological and urologic endoscopic procedures. These hypotonic solutions without electrolytes can cause TUR syndrome, although healthy adults typically can accommodate the fluid and electrolyte imbalance created by excess absorption of these solutions. Age and comorbidities, such as cardiovascular and renal dysfunction, may increase a patient's risk for developing hyponatremia and fluid overload.[47,65]

The American Association of Gynecologic Laparoscopists (AAGL) notes that new evidence has led to careful consideration of use of these fluids in premenopausal women. Hyponatremia occurs after surgeries using these solutions with equal frequency in men and women, but premenopausal women who develop hyponatremia and encephalopathy are 25 times more likely to die or have permanent brain damage than men or postmenopausal women.[47]

Normal saline 0.9% is most frequently selected as the distension fluid and can be used in procedures during which bipolar instrumentation will be used. This is an isotonic solution containing electrolytes and can be safer when large amounts of fluid are absorbed. The AAGL recommends using normal saline for hysteroscopy procedures in which bipolar resection is used, to reduce the risk of hyponatremia and hypo-osmolality.[47]

High-viscosity fluid media, such as 32% dextran 70, does not mix or blend with blood, so it is better for visibility in the presence of bleeding during endoscopic procedures. However, dextran can draw six times its own volume into the bloodstream, resulting in vascular overload and subsequent heart failure and pulmonary edema. Munro and Christianson[65] reported limiting the infusion amount of this fluid to between 300 mL and 500 mL. The high sugar content of dextran requires immediate rinsing of the instrumentation to decrease the damage that can occur from the use of this fluid media.[47,65]

Yousef et al[64] compared glycine 1.5%, glucose 5%, and normal saline 0.9% as irrigating solutions during TURP procedures in 360 patients enrolled in a randomized prospective controlled trial. Patients were randomly assigned to one of three groups of 120 patients. The medical and nursing personnel involved in the postoperative care of the patient were blinded to the type of irrigation used during the procedure. Seventeen patients in the glycine group developed TUR syndrome, which occurs when there is excessive absorption of irrigating fluid. The researchers defined TUR syndrome as a sodium level of 125 mmol/L or less after a TURP and two or more symptoms including nausea, vomiting, bradycardia, hypotension, chest pain, mental confusion, anxiety, paresthesia, and visual disturbance.

Traditionally, glycine 1.5% has been used for TURP because it is a nonelectrolyte fluid and is safe to use with monopolar energy-generating devices. Because of the advancement of bipolar resection devices, normal saline can now be used during TURP procedures. The researchers concluded that bipolar resection with saline and monopolar resection with glucose 5% resulted in fewer complications than monopolar resection with glycine 1.5%.[64]

3.2.1 **During the preoperative nursing risk assessment related to fluid management, assess the patient's**
- **skin color and turgor,**
- **weight and age,**
- **allergies and sensitivities to medications,**

549

Table 1. Fluids Used for Irrigation or Distension Media

Solution	Electrolyte Solution	Uses	Potential Contraindications	Adverse Reactions
0.9% Sodium chloride[1]	Yes	General irrigation, hysteroscopy, use with laser and bipolar electrosurgery, urologic procedures[2,3]	Monopolar electrosurgery	Hypervolemia, pulmonary edema, abdominal cramping, nausea and vomiting, diarrhea
Ringer's lactate[4]	Yes	General irrigation	Monopolar electrosurgery	Fluid shift from intracellular to extracellular compartment, hypervolemia
Dextran[5]	No	Hysteroscopy; volume generally limited to 300 mL and not to exceed 500 mL[5]	Hypersensitivity to dextran or any component of the formulation, hemostatic defects (eg, thrombocytopenia, hypofibrinogenemia), cardiac decompensation, renal disease with severe oliguria or anuria, hepatic impairment[2]	Plasma expander leading to fluid or solute overload; disseminated intravascular coagulation; overdose, marked by pulmonary edema, increased bleeding time, and decreased platelet function[2]
Glycine 1.5%[6]	No	Urologic irrigation, hysteroscopy, and resectoscopy with monopolar electrosurgery[3]	Severe cardiopulmonary or renal dysfunction, decreased liver function; additives may be incompatible, consult with a pharmacist	Aggravated pre-existing hyponatremia caused by shifts from intracellular to extracellular compartment; fluid and electrolyte disturbances (eg, edema, marked diuresis, pulmonary congestion); impaired liver function leading to accumulation of ammonia in the blood; allergic reactions, which are rare[2]
Mannitol 5%[7]	No	Urologic irrigation, hysteroscopy and resectoscopy with monopolar electrosurgery[2,8]	Severe cardiopulmonary or renal dysfunction	Aggravated pre-existing hyponatremia caused by shifts from intracellular to extracellular compartment, fluid and electrolyte disturbances (eg, edema, marked diuresis, pulmonary congestion), hypernatremia caused by loss of water and excess of electrolytes from continuous administration
Sorbitol 3%[9]	No	Urological irrigation	Severe cardiopulmonary or renal dysfunction, fructose intolerance	Aggravated pre-existing hyponatremia caused by shifts from intracellular to extracellular compartment, hypernatremia caused by loss of water and excess of electrolytes from continuous administration, hyperglycemia in patients with diabetes mellitus, allergic reactions (eg, urticaria)[8]

	Table 1 Continued. Fluids Used for Irrigation or Distension Media			
Solution	**Electrolyte Solution**	**Uses**	**Potential Contraindications**	**Adverse Reactions**
Sorbitol 3% / Mannitol 0.5%[10]	No	Urologic irrigation	Severe cardiopulmonary or renal dysfunction, fructose intolerance	Aggravated pre-existing hyponatremia caused by shifts from intracellular to extracellular compartment, hypernatremia caused by loss of water and excess of electrolytes from continuous administration, hyperglycemia in patients with diabetes mellitus, hyperlactatemia in patients who are metabolically compromised caused by metabolism of sorbitol[8,10]
Sterile water[11]	No	General irrigation, washing, rinsing, and dilution purposes; transurethral resection of the prostate[11]	Continuous irrigation, as a distension medium; additives may be incompatible, consult with a pharmacist	Hemolysis when absorbed into the bloodstream

Editor's note: This table presents irrigation solutions that are in common use; however, it is not all inclusive. Use of other irrigation solutions may be indicated in certain patient populations and for certain conditions.

References

1. Sodium chloride for irrigation [package insert]. Bethlehem, PA: B. Braun Medical, Inc; 2014.
2. AAGL Advancing Minimally Invasive Gynecology Worldwide; Munro MG, Storz K, Abbott JA, et al. AAGL Practice Report: Practice Guidelines for the Management of Hysteroscopic Distending Media: (replaces Hysteroscopic Fluid Monitoring Guidelines. J Am Assoc Gynecol Laparosc. 2000;7:167-168.). J Minim Invasive Gynecol. 2013;20(2):137-148.
3. Darwish AM, Hassan ZZ, Attia AM, Abdelraheem SS, Ahmed YM. Biological effects of distension media in bipolar versus monopolar resectoscopic myomectomy: a randomized trial. J Obstet Gynaecol Res. 2010;36(4):810-817.
4. Lactated Ringers for irrigation [package insert]. Lake Forrest, IL: Hospira; 2014.
5. Dextran [package insert]. Lake Forrest, IL: Hospira; 2014.
6. 1.5% glycine irrigation [package insert]. Irvine, CA: B. Braun Medical, Inc; 2014.
7. 5% mannitol irrigation [package insert]. Irvine, CA: B. Braun Medical, Inc; 2014.
8. Park JT, Lim HK, Kim S, Um DJ. A comparison of the influence of 2.7% sorbitol-0.54% mannitol and 5% glucose irrigating fluids on plasma serum physiology during hysteroscopic procedures. Korean J Anesthesiol. 2011;61(5):394-398.
9. Sorbitol - sorbitol irrigant. Irvine, CA: B. Braun Medical, Inc; 2010.
10. Sorbitol - mannitol irrigation [package insert]. Lake Forrest, IL: Hospira; 2009.
11. Sterile water for irrigation [package insert]. Lake Forest, IL: Hospira; 2004.

- conditions or diseases that may predispose or exacerbate the seriousness of hyponatremia or hypervolemia, and
- medications that may predispose or exacerbate the seriousness of hyponatremia or hypervolemia.[47,79]

[Recommendation]

The use of improper or excessive amounts of fluid for irrigation or distension media can lead to hypervolemia and hyponatremia. Patients who have congestive heart failure, liver cirrhosis, or renal diseases are more susceptible to hypervolemia and hyponatremia. The main causes of hyponatremia in hypoosmolar patients are inappropriate antidiuretic hormone secretion, renal disorders, endocrine deficiencies, and certain medications.[47,79]

3.3 Monitor the amount of fluid dispensed and collected during the procedure in collaboration with the anesthesia professional. *[Recommendation]*

Moderate-quality evidence suggests that intravasation[47,64,65,67,70-72,80,81] or extravasation[63,66,68,69,82-85] of irrigation and distension fluid used during MIS procedures can occur rapidly with only subtle warning signs. Monitoring the amount of fluid infused and collected during the procedure helps determine whether the patient is at risk for complications.

Kumar and Kumar[81] studied the differences between intravasation rates and fluid deficit rates. Intravasation of fluid occurs from the pressure of the irrigation fluid entering the systemic circulation through the cut ends of the traumatized blood vessels. It is influenced by cavity pressure and hemostatic mechanisms, which can change frequently during a procedure and vary from patient to patient. Fluid deficit is the amount of irrigation fluid in milliliters already absorbed by the patient.

The researchers studied 41 hysteroscopic procedures used a controller-operated pump to measure the intravasation rate. When there was a sudden rise in the intravasation rate, the pressure was lowered in the uterine cavity. In some cases, the fluid deficit was within normal limits, but the intravasation rate increased. The researchers suggested that patient safety is increased if intravasation rate monitoring is performed along with conventional fluid deficit monitoring.[81]

The evidence review found only one study that examined all endoscopic procedures (ie, endoscopic prostate surgery, hysteroscopy, bladder, knee and shoulder arthroscopy). Silva et al[79] conducted a cohort study on endoscopic procedures performed at one facility in Brazil. The researchers reviewed 142 patient records and completed a three-part questionnaire collecting data about the preoperative, intraoperative, and postoperative phases of patient care. They reported a 21.8% complication rate. In their analysis of the factors associated with complications, they found age, sodium level at the end of the procedure, and total fluid administered to be statistically correlated with complications in cardiovascular, respiratory, neurological, gastrointestinal, and kidney function. This study is limited by the size and the observational nature of the data collection.

Kocher et al[63] reported that 15 arthroscopists who were members of the Multicenter Arthroscopy of the Hip Outcomes Research Network completed a survey to retrospectively collect data on hip arthroscopies they had performed. Forty cases of IAFE were reported out of the overall 25,648 hip arthroscopies reviewed by the senior author. Preventative measures suggested by the arthroscopists surveyed included lowering the pump settings, maintaining core temperature, monitoring pH and cardiac function, and periodically monitoring intraoperative abdominal distension.

3.3.1 **The RN circulator should report fluid deficit to the anesthesia professional and surgeon at regular intervals throughout the procedure.** [*Recommendation*]

The AAGL practice guideline for the management of hysteroscopic distending media recommends that an automated fluid management system and media management protocol be in place to assist with assessment of risk factors leading to complications from fluid overload. Moderate-quality evidence supports the team monitoring the fluid deficit and establish-

ing criteria for treatment and termination of a procedure.[47,63,70]

3.3.2 **Monitor the patient for physiologic changes, including core temperature, laboratory test results (eg electrolytes, coagulation studies), and potential fluid retention in the abdomen, face, and neck.** [*Recommendation*]

Multiple cases have been reported of complications from fluid intravasation and extravasation in MIS procedures using fluid for irrigation and distension media.[66,68,69,82,84-87] The authors collectively reported early detection through monitoring electrolyte levels, physiologic responses, and core temperature in prevention of these complications. Transurethral resection syndrome is well documented in the literature as a complication from excessive absorption of nonelectrolyte fluid during TURP. Transurethral resection syndrome is used as a common term to describe fluid overload[47] and is identified when the patient experiences more than two of these symptoms: hyponatremia (serum sodium of 125 mmol/L or less), nausea, vomiting, bradycardia, hypotension, chest pain, mental confusion, anxiety, paraesthesia, or visual disturbance.[86] This syndrome is rare but can be life threatening.[47,64,86]

Patients undergoing hip and shoulder arthroscopy procedures are at risk for fluid extravasation and complications of compression to surrounding tissue. Verma and Sekiya[85] reported a case of fluid extravasation in hip arthroscopy in a healthy 21-year-old patient who presented with shortness of breath 24 hours after surgery. An abdominal CT revealed fluid in the patient's abdomen. In their literature review, the authors of this report found three other case studies with similar complications. They suggested five early warning signs: inability to distend the joint, increase in fluid required to distend the joint, frequent cut-off of the pump, abdominal and thigh distension, and acute hypothermia.

Stafford et al[84] reviewed the cases of 36 patients undergoing hip arthroscopy performed by one physician in one facility. The volume of irrigation fluid infused, operating time, fluid pressures, and volumes of fluid recovered were measured in all 36 procedures. They found the mean loss of fluid into the peri-articular tissues was 1,132 mL. There was a correlation between the volume of extravasated fluid and both the length of surgery and the volume of infused fluid used. The authors concluded that reduced operative times (< 90 minutes) and fluid pressure at low rates (< 50 mmHg) reduced the risk of fluid extravasation.

Reported cases of fluid leaking into surrounding tissue during shoulder arthroscopy are common, and this generally does not cause harm to the patient. Airway compromise from edema and tracheal compression have been reported.[66,68]

Wegmuller et al[70] described a case of a patient experiencing life-threatening laryngeal edema during a hysteroscopy. When the patient became symptomatic, it was discovered that 76 L of fluid was used, which exceeded the normal amount of 4 L to 7 L. An exact fluid balance was not available during the procedure. The authors calculated a fluid overload of 11 L. Their recommendation from this experience was to ensure there is good communication on clinical observations between the patient (when regional anesthesia is used), anesthesia professional, nurse, and surgeon. An agreement should be determined for measurement of fluid balance and termination of the procedure if fluid absorption reaches 1,000 mL. Based on their literature search and experience, they also recommended keeping resection time to less than 60 minutes to reduce the risk for fluid overload.

Jo et al[67] published a case report of a 34-year-old woman who had elective hysteroscopy and suffered extreme hyponatremia caused by an electrolyte-free sorbitol/mannitol solution used as distension irrigation fluid. During the procedure, 2 L sorbitol/mannitol solution were infused. The author reported difficulty in measuring the fluid absorption rate due to the large amount of fluid leakage through the uterine cervix. The patient's temperature dropped, her pulse oximetry declined to 85%, and her end-tidal CO_2 decreased to 22 mmHg. The surgeon stopped the procedure, and the patient was managed for fluid overload and transferred to the intensive care unit. The patient suffered mild brain swelling without pontine myelinolysis and pulmonary edema. She was discharged on postoperative day four and remained asymptomatic at the 6-month follow-up appointment. The authors concluded that intraoperative fluid balance should be maintained, and early detection and prompt management of suspected fluid absorption are important.

3.3.3 **Monitor the patient for adverse reactions when medications are added to fluids used for irrigation or distension media.[88]** [*Recommendation*]

3.4 **Contain fluids used for irrigation or as distension media.** [*Recommendation*]

The AAGL recommends that the surgical team account for all fluid used as distension media.[47] The team should accurately monitor all input and output, including fluid returned from the hysteroscope, spilled from the vagina, and lost to the floor.

Moderate-quality evidence[47,63,89] suggests that a measurement system should be used for accurate monitoring of input and output of fluids in MIS procedures.

3.4.1 **Use drapes that capture as much fluid return as possible.** [*Recommendation*]

Drapes designed for collection facilitate the accurate measurement of fluid. Fluid absorption is determined by subtracting the amount of fluid recovered from the amount of fluid instilled. The volumetric calculation does not take into consideration extraneous fluid losses (eg, fluid loss on the floor, on the drape), which cannot be accurately quantified; nor does it consider additives, such as blood.[47,63,89]

3.4.2 **Collect as much irrigation or distension fluid as possible in a closed-container system.** [*Recommendation*]

Estimating the fluid deficit can be very difficult for the surgical team. Boyd and Stanley[89] studied the accuracy of fluid measurement by the surgical team. Four RN circulators were asked to estimate the initial volume of fluid in the irrigating fluid bag, the remaining volume of irrigating fluid in the bag, fluid volume in kick buckets, fluid lost on the floor, and fluid in the suction canister for gynecological procedures in a simulated OR. The researchers found that fluid collected in rigid suction canisters was most consistently measured accurately. Partially emptied bags, fluid on the floor, and fluid in kick buckets were measured inaccurately.

The researchers also measured the fluid in eleven 3-L bags of 1.5% glycine and found all were overfilled by 2.8% (mean of 84 mL, range 62 mL to 125 mL), which the authors stated was consistent with other research demonstrating that 3-L bags of commonly used media may be overfilled by 2.8% to 6%. The authors concluded that surgical team members' estimates of the level of fluid left in a bag can vary, which also compounds the problem of fluid measurement inaccuracy. Fluids can also be lost in the drapes and on the floor, making it difficult to estimate output.[89]

3.4.3 Prevent fluids used for irrigation or as distension media from coming into contact with electrical equipment. *[Recommendation]*

Containing fluid used during a procedure prevents contact with electrical outlets, switches, and the internal components of electrical equipment, including electrosurgical electrodes. Preventing fluid contact with electrical equipment minimizes the risk of burns, fires, and damage to the equipment.[8,36]

3.5 Use automated fluid management systems in a manner that minimizes the potential for injury. *[Recommendation]*

Automated fluid management systems calculate the amount of fluid dispensed to the patient and compare this with the amount returned to the system. The deficit is measured, and an alarm alerts the user to potential fluid overload. This timely notification of a deficit provides an opportunity to take corrective action before physiologic compromise of the patient.[47,79,81,89]

3.5.1 Use fluid for the distension media that is compatible with the fluid management system and the endoscope manufacturer's instructions for use.[36] *[Recommendation]*

3.5.2 Use accessories (eg, tubing, collection canisters) that are compatible with the fluid management system.[36] *[Recommendation]*

3.5.3 Fluid management equipment safety features should include
- clearly labeled control settings,
- a quick setting reference chart attached to the equipment,
- audible alarms,
- a display with measurement of fluid instilled and returned to the regulator (ie, fluid deficit), and[81]
- a display of measurement of cavity pressure.[47]

[Recommendation]

3.5.4 Verify the fluid pump settings for fluid distension with the surgeon before administration and continually monitor the settings throughout the procedure.[47] *[Recommendation]*

Moderate-quality evidence[47,63,65,79,81] supports monitoring pump pressures, inflow volumes, and outflow volumes of fluids used during MIS procedures.

3.5.5 Initiate corrective action in response to audible alarms from the fluid management system and notify the surgeon and anesthesia professional if corrective actions do not result in a reduction of the fluid volume deficit to a safe level. *[Recommendation]*

3.6 Report, investigate, and take corrective action when an adverse event or near miss related to fluid management equipment occurs. *[Recommendation]*

Reporting adverse events and near misses through an adverse event reporting and investigation system provides a mechanism to determine trends and potential risk factors and evaluate the effectiveness of corrective actions.[90]

4. Energy-Generating Devices

4.1 Take precautions to mitigate the risk for injury associated with the use of energy-generating devices during MIS. *[Recommendation]*

The use of bipolar versus monopolar electrosurgery is a physician preference guided by the procedure, tissue type, and choice of distension media.[91-102] Risk for thermal injury from **active electrodes** has been reported in the literature.[93,95,103] Carbon dioxide is the most commonly used gas distension media because it is nonflammable and presents the least risk for complications from air embolism.[40]

Culp et al[94] studied the clinical implications of CO_2 and air as insufflation media by measuring the spark gap in a biological model. The researchers did not find a difference in the electrocautery function between CO_2 and air. They recommended the use CO_2 over the use of air as an insufflation gas in electrosurgery due to the favorable properties of CO_2 gas as insufflation media.

Fluid distension media can be either conductive or nonconductive. The use of a monopolar active electrode in conductive fluid, such as sodium chloride, has been shown to cause heat transfer and damage to surrounding tissue.[93,95,97] Glycine 1.5%, mannitol 5%, and sorbitol 3% are nonconductive fluids that are most frequently used in urologic and hysteroscopic procedures; however, these fluids have a high risk of producing TUR syndrome.[78]

4.2 Take safety precautions for reducing the risk for injury when using energy-generating devices during MIS, including
- selection of the lowest power setting that achieves the desired result,
- activation of the active electrode only when it is in close proximity to the tissue, and
- activation of the energy-generating device foot pedal only by the person in control of the

energy-delivering hand piece (eg, electrosurgical unit active electrode, laser hand piece, ultrasonic wand).[8,37] *[Recommendation]*

4.3 Select electrosurgical unit-activated instrumentation (ie, active electrodes) and accessories to include technology that minimizes or eliminates the risk for insulation failure and **capacitive-coupling** injuries.[8,37,76] *[Recommendation]*

4.3.1 Use conductive trocar systems.[8] *[Recommendation]*

4.3.2 Examine active electrodes for impaired insulation before and after use and, if reusable, during decontamination and package assembly.[2,37] *[Recommendation]*

4.4 Verify the properties of the selected distension media to minimize risks related to electrosurgery. *[Recommendation]*

Collateral tissue injury secondary to increased fluid temperatures can occur if the distension media is conductive.[8,95]

4.4.1 Use nonflammable insufflation gas.[94] *[Recommendation]*

4.4.2 Use nonelectrolyte distension fluids when monopolar electrosurgery is used.[47,65,73] *[Recommendation]*

5. Computer-Assisted Surgical Procedures

5.1 Identify potential risks for injury and complications associated with computer-assisted surgical procedures and implement safe practices. *[Recommendation]* **P**

Computer-assisted robotic surgery began with research conducted by the National Aeronautics and Space Administration in the 1980s to investigate providing surgical care in remote locations through surgeon-directed controls on Earth.[104] The evolution of robotic technology has been similar to the advancement of endoscopic surgery. Both began in urology and gynecology with a steep learning curve and longer surgical times compared with routine procedures. These technologies later began to be used in general, cardiothoracic,[105] colorectal, pediatric,[106] and head and neck procedures.[104,107] The robotic system provides three-dimensional (3D), high-definition views of the surgical field. Wristed laparoscopic instruments allow the surgeon 7 degrees of freedom of movement.

The system eliminates hand tremors and provides motion scaling and improved ergonomics for the surgeon.[23,104,108-111]

Computer-assisted navigation procedures provide a means for the surgical team to navigate with digital 3D images through minimally invasive techniques.[112-117] Navigation can be done with CT-based systems, fluoroscopy-based systems, or imageless systems. Computed tomography-based navigation is performed by scanning an area of the body and using the data to construct a 3D image. Scans can be performed preoperatively or intraoperatively in a hybrid room with a CT scanner or in an OR with a portable CT scanner.

Fluoroscopy-based navigation uses markers based on anatomic landmarks on the patient. The portable fluoroscopy unit can take arbitrary images during the procedure that are sent to the navigation unit by a computer program that relates the images to the surgical field in space and identifies the position of the surgical instruments.

An imageless system is a computer platform with a tracking system (usually an optical camera) and infrared markers on anatomical landmarks; a probe acquires surface points to create triangulation for navigation.[116,118,119] The radiologic 3D images provide the surgical team with the ability to visualize the internal structures for planning the operative approach and navigating with surgical instrumentation. This technology is similar to global positioning systems for orientation and direction. The use of navigation in MIS procedures may improve accuracy and reduce radiation exposure. Navigational minimally invasive approaches are used in neurosurgical, orthopedic, otorhinolaryngology, liver resection, thoracic, and maxillofacial surgical procedures. The registration and planning can be time consuming but promotes accuracy and decreases the invasiveness of surgery.[116] Research is needed on the complications and risks associated with using advanced technologies for all surgical specialties.

5.2 Safely position the patient in a manner that will facilitate the use of the computer-assisted equipment. *[Recommendation]*

Positioning the patient for computer-assisted procedures requires using the extreme Trendelenburg or reverse Trendelenburg position. The gravitational effect of these positions allows the patient's organs to move away from the surgical field. The Trendelenburg position increases venous return and increases the risk for cardiac or respiratory congestion. The reverse Trendelenburg position reduces venous return and cardiac output, increases peripheral and pulmonary resistance, and has the potential to result in misalignment of the patient's extremities.[36,105,108,120-123] (See the AORN Guideline for Positioning the Patient[7] for additional guidance).

5.3 **The perioperative RN circulator should delegate, supervise, and evaluate the activities for setting up the computer-assisted equipment.** *[Recommendation]*

Computer-assisted robotic equipment consists of a

- patient cart,
- surgeon console, and
- vision cart.

The computer-assisted robotic system is complex, necessitating coordination by the team members to reduce the risk of error and potential injury. The robotic patient cart consists of robotic arms to which instruments are attached, and these instruments are inserted into the body cavity through trocars. The instruments mimic the surgeon's hand movement, with wristed servant tools connected to the robotic arms. An endoscope that provides 3D images to the surgeon console and vision cart is also connected to the robotic arms. "Docking" the patient cart refers to moving the system over the sterile field and attaching the instruments to the robotic arms. This maneuver requires two perioperative personnel, a nonsterile person to move the cart and a sterile person to guide the equipment and prevent a collision with surrounding equipment.[121,124,125]

Computer-assisted surgical navigation equipment includes[116]

- infrared cameras,
- advanced digital images of the patient for use with the navigation software, and
- interactive display monitors.

5.3.1 **Follow the manufacturers' instructions for use for all equipment used in computer-assisted robotic minimally invasive procedures.** *[Recommendation]*

5.3.2 **The RN circulator should assist the surgeon with the registration process, which consists of**[112,116,117]

- **ensuring the preoperative radiologic studies are available,**
- **positioning the patient,**
- **positioning the navigation system so that the surgical field is in view of the tracking system (eg, infrared camera),**
- **attaching the patient antenna,**
- **collect data points from anatomical landmarks or fiducial markers,**
- **registering additional instruments if needed, and**
- **verifying the accuracy of the registration.**

[Recommendation]

Patient registration is the most important step in ensuring the accuracy of the navigation system. Kaduk et al[116] reported on a facility experience with the use of surgical navigation in maxillofacial surgery. The authors recommend using checklists to help ensure all steps are followed to improve the accuracy of the navigation system. They developed five checklists: preoperative, preoperative planning, OR, intraoperative imaging, and postoperative. These checklists define what is needed in each phase of the process and help ensure the correct images are available on the day of surgery.

5.3.3 **Notify the surgeon if the patient is moved after registration in computer-assisted navigation or after the robotic arms have been docked, and coordinate corrective action.**[105,121] *[Recommendation]*

6. Hybrid ORs

6.1 **Determine the requirements for the design and operation of the hybrid OR for surgical or invasive procedures.** *[Recommendation]*

Advancements in technology have led to changes and enhancements in OR design and equipment. One development has been the creation of the hybrid OR. The Facilities Guidelines Institute (FGI) defines a hybrid OR as "a room that meets the definition of an operating room and is also equipped to enable diagnostic imaging before, during and after surgical procedures."[126] The room design combines surgical environmental requirements and imaging equipment to accommodate patient care in one location for diagnostic and surgical procedures. The FGI notes that the use of portable imaging technology in an OR does not make the room a hybrid OR.

Low-quality evidence[76,127-135] supports the use of hybrid OR designs as defined by the FGI guidelines. Imaging equipment is selected based on the types of procedures that will be done in the hybrid OR. Permanently fixed imaging equipment may be single-plane, bi-plane multi-axial rotational angiography systems, CT equipment, or MRI equipment.[133] Fixed radiologic equipment requires that the hybrid OR have lead-lined shielding. Generally, there are four to six flat-screen monitors for projecting digital images to all four quadrants in the room. A large 40-inch to 56-inch flat-panel monitor is also used to show the digital data acquired from the imaging system and monitoring other vital signs.[132,135]

The hybrid OR may be located outside the traditional surgical suite. An OR is designated as a **restricted area** that can only be accessed through a **semi-restricted area**.[126] Hybrid ORs have been developed in cardiac catheterization suites, interventional suites, and surgical suites; regardless of location, the design requirements are the same. Meeting the requirements for installing fixed imaging equipment within a surgical environment can be challenging in an existing room or in conversion of an existing area because it requires additional space, equipment, and ceiling supports. A multidisciplinary team that collaborates with imaging personnel and perioperative personnel is key to creating a successful workflow design and a safe patient care environment.

The hybrid OR concept may optimize efficiency by decreasing transport of the patient and minimizing the number of patient hand overs.[133] Combining the efforts of cardiologists, interventional radiologists, and cardiac surgeons has benefitted patients who were not candidates for open heart surgery but were candidates for a less-invasive, lower-risk intervention, such as a transcatheter aortic valve replacement procedure.[131,133] Trauma patients can be sent straight to the hybrid OR, where angiography can be done to assess the extent of the injury and initiate treatment more quickly.[128,136] The hybrid OR is used by practitioners in all specialties (eg, cardiovascular, peripheral vascular, neurovascular, interventional radiology, cardiac catheterization, electrophysiology, orthopedic, trauma). Traditional models provide care separately for each procedure, and patients are transported from the interventional radiology suite or catheterization laboratory to the OR. The construction of the hybrid OR may be new construction or conversion of an existing interventional room or OR. The hybrid OR can be located in the surgical department, cardiac catheterization laboratory, or interventional radiology department. Combining these work areas can be challenging for health care providers, but creates a more efficient treatment option for the patient.[76,127,129-132,134]

6.2 Establish a multidisciplinary team including perioperative and radiology RNs, interventional radiologists, surgeons, first assistants, surgical technologists, anesthesia professionals, infection preventionists, and other involved personnel to develop the design of new construction or renovation of existing space to create a hybrid OR. *[Recommendation]*

Organizational experience reports have identified challenges of high cost, complex planning among multiple specialties, space requirements, schedule coordination, location, personnel training, team development, and credentialing criteria in designing a hybrid OR.[127,129,131-133,135,137,138]

Hybrid OR construction and design can be complicated by locating the room outside the surgical suite. **Table 2** shows the various procedures reported in the literature to be performed in a hybrid OR. Aston[127] described organizational experiences from various hospitals in which a hybrid OR had recently been installed. One facility described the need to reduce silos developed in traditional care where patients are scheduled for procedures in separate departments. The need to eliminate traditional silos of care by merging personnel and technologies into one location can create an unsettled culture.[129,133] Elimination of multiple hand overs, transportation delays, and possibly multiple anesthetic events benefits the patient.

In an expert opinion article, Schaadt and Landau[135] addressed planning, design, and use of the hybrid OR and suggested that the design should meet the strategic vision and budget and maximize operational efficiencies to promote the same standard of care for all patients.

6.2.1 The multidisciplinary team should
- **develop the design of new construction or renovation of existing space in compliance with federal, state, and local building regulatory requirements;**
- **identify and define the roles and responsibilities of team members; and**
- **establish safe processes and practices for working in the hybrid OR.**

[Recommendation]

Organizational experiences describe various approaches to creating a hybrid OR and personnel from multiple disciplines working together.[127-129,131-133,135,139-141] Collectively, the authors describe the hybrid OR project to be the first time interventional or cardiac catheterization laboratory personnel have worked with OR personnel. Each team member provides valuable knowledge of his or her normal workflow and, by describing their experience of aseptic technique, traffic flow, wire management, contrast injector placement, movement of the imaging system, and bed controls, the team members create a new workflow within the hybrid OR environment. The members of this team develop the collaborative culture required for the new environment.

Kirkpatrick et al[128] described creating a mock-up space before construction, where the team could visualize and walk through the normal routine of a surgical procedure. Creating cardboard screens and bringing in movable surgical equipment allowed the team to determine the best placement for ceiling-mounted

Table 2. Examples of Procedures Performed in a Hybrid OR

Cardiovascular	Cardiothoracic	Neurovascular	Other
Abdominal aortic aneurysm repair[1]	Transcatheter valve replacement (TAVR)[1-3]	Coil embolization or microsurgical clipping of cerebral aneurysms[1,5]	Hemorrhage control in trauma patients[10-12]
Aortic stent grafting[1]	Percutaneous removal of cardiac device leads[1]	Intracranial stenting of cerebral arteries[1,5]	High-risk obstetric procedures[13]
Carotid stent grafting[1]	Minimally invasive endoscopic bypass surgery[3]	Cerebral balloon angioplasty[1,6]	Orthopedic trauma[13,14]
Endovascular aortic repair (EVAR)[2,3]	Minimally invasive direct coronary artery bypass grafting[1,3]	Microneurosurgical resection of brain tumors[1,7]	
Thoracic endovascular aortic repair (TEVAR)[2,3]	Robotically enhanced minimally invasive direct coronary artery bypass[3]	Combined carotid surgical cutdown followed by endovascular coiling for bypass of tortuous anatomy[1,8]	
	Pediatric aortic and pulmonary stenosis[1,3]	Combined arteriovenous malformation embolization followed by microneurosurgical resection.[1,5,9]	
	Hypoplastic left heart syndrome treatment[1]	Cerebral vascular tumors[6]	
	Off-pump coronary artery bypass[1]	Spinal vascular tumors[6]	
	Atrial fibrillation/flutter abalation[3]		
	Hybrid maze procedure[3,4]		

References

1. Odle TG. Managing transition to a hybrid operating room. Radiol Technol. 2011;83(2):165-181.
2. Kaneko T, Davidson MJ. Use of the hybrid operating room in cardiovascular medicine. Circulation. 2014;130(11):910-917.
3. Kpodonu J. Hybrid cardiovascular suite: the operating room of the future. J Card Surg. 2010;25(6):704-709.
4. Los-Meyer A. Navigating the mini-maze procedure. Nurse Pract. 2010;35(5):7-10.
5. Murayama Y, Arakawa H, Ishibashi T, et al. Combined surgical and endovascular treatment of complex cerebrovascular diseases in the hybrid operating room. J Neurointerv Surg. 2013;5(5):489-493.
6. Gemmete JJ, Chaudhary N, Pandey AS, et al. Initial experience with a combined multidetector CT and biplane digital subtraction angiography suite with a single interactive table for the diagnosis and treatment of neurovascular disease. J Neurointerv Surg. 2013;5(1):73-80.
7. Childs S, Bruch P. Successful management of risk in the hybrid OR. AORN J. 2015;101(2):223-234.
8. Miguel K, Hirsch JA, Sheridan RM. Team training: a safer future for neurointerventional practice. J NeuroInterv Surg. 2011;3(3):285-287.
9. Kotowski M, Sarrafzadeh A, Schatlo B, et al. Intraoperative angiography reloaded: a new hybrid operating theater for combined endovascular and surgical treatment of cerebral arteriovenous malformations: a pilot study on 25 patients. Acta Neurochir (Wien). 2013;155(11):2071-2078.
10. D'Amours SK, Rastogi P, Ball CG. Utility of simultaneous interventional radiology and operative surgery in a dedicated suite for seriously injured patients. Curr Opin Crit Care. 2013;19(6):587-593.
11. Kirkpatrick AW, Vis C, Dube M, et al. The evolution of a purpose designed hybrid trauma operating room from the trauma service perspective: the RAPTOR (resuscitation with angiography percutaneous treatments and operative resuscitations). Injury. 2014;45(9):1413-1421.
12. Tan H, Zhang LY, Guo QS, et al. "One-stop hybrid procedure" in the treatment of vascular injury of lower extremity. Indian J Surg. 2015;77(1):75-78.
13. Clark A, Farber MK, Sviggum H, Camann W. Cesarean delivery in the hybrid operating suite: a promising new location for high-risk obstetric procedures. Anesth Analg. 2013;117(5):1187-1189.
14. Richter PH, Yarboro S, Kraus M, Gebhard F. One year orthopaedic trauma experience using an advanced interdisciplinary hybrid operating room. Injury. 2015;46(Suppl 4):S129-S134.

imaging equipment, monitors, shields, and equipment booms. A mock-up bed with the dimensions and fixed table mounts helped determine how the team would position the patient during procedures. The mocked up space also provided a means to test the length of the boom arms and collision factors for reaching optimal locations. The fixed floor mount of imaging equipment is a factor in designing the bed location relative to placement of anesthesia equipment.[127,135]

6.2.2 Select the imaging system and adjunct technologies that meet the identified requirements associated with the scope of services. [Recommendation] P

Input from physicians and health care personnel is important when making the decision about the type of imaging system to install in a hybrid OR. The imaging system is the most expensive component of building a hybrid OR.[135] New technologies in the digital manipulation of the images acquired by the system should be considered. Adjunct technologies in the hybrid OR may be 3D imaging reconstruction, echocardiography, intravascular ultrasound, digital subtraction angiography, video integration systems with picture archiving, and audiovisual recording systems.

Angiography is the most common imaging modality used in a hybrid OR. Single-plane, bi-plane, and multi-axial robotic angiography are options for the imaging system. The system may be ceiling mounted or floor mounted. Cardiac and peripheral vascular hybrid procedures require only a single-plane image. Bi-plane systems have two C-arms, one mounted on the floor and one on tracks in the ceiling. A bi-plane system is capable of acquiring images from two reference point at the same time. This system is most often used for smaller vessel angiography in pediatrics and neuroangiography. Using the two C-arms reduces the amount of radiation exposure and contrast media use. The multi-axial robotic angiography system is a single-plane, floor-mounted system with eight rotational axes that can provide more images at different angles without using the biplane technology.[135]

Computed tomography and MRI are other imaging systems that may be installed in a hybrid OR. Odle[133] described the use of CT scanners in an intermittent mode to decrease radiation exposure during CT-guided interventional procedures. Magnetic resonance imaging hybrid ORs may house the scanner between two rooms, allowing it to be brought into the room via a track system. The scanner can be used in conjunction with angiography to assist in planning the surgery or to determine during the procedure whether further resection is needed.

Childs and Bruch[142] described the benefits of an MRI hybrid OR as allowing practitioners to perform preoperative scans in the diagnostic room or in the MRI/OR suite for planning neurosurgical navigation, performing real-time monitoring of laser thermocoagulation of tumors, performing vessel wall imaging studies requiring embolization and operative intervention, and avoiding repeated same-day intubation of pediatric patients.

6.3 Establish standardized room setups. *[Recommendation]*
Standardized room setups may assist in preventing collisions with the imaging system and other equipment (eg, monitors, lead shielding, equipment booms).

Standardized room setups for each procedure will assist personnel in positioning monitors, overhead lights, lead shields, and booms in the appropriate loca-

tion for each procedure. Standardized room setup eliminates delays caused by team members having differing opinions about equipment placement. The positioning of the patient or side of the approach will also determine the location of bed controls, monitors, and equipment. The location of the imaging controls on the table side or on a remote trolley is determined by physician preference.[127,129,135,143,144]

6.3.1 Establish the no-fly zone according to the imaging system manufacturer recommendation, patient position, room configuration, and region of the body being imaged.[135] *[Recommendation]*
Schaadt and Landau[135] described the need for personnel knowledge of the imaging system and required clearances as important in the anticipation and prevention of potential serious collisions that can occur when people or equipment cross over into areas designated as no-fly zones while the imaging equipment is in operation. Some imaging systems have collision-detection devices and will stop moving if a possible collision is detected.

6.3.2 Assign responsibility for moving or securing equipment before initiation of the imaging system. *[Recommendation]*
In combination procedures with open surgical incisions and interventions requiring imaging, equipment booms and OR lights may have been moved into the no-fly zone. When imaging acquisition is required, all equipment should be moved out of the no-fly zone.[135]

6.3.3 Position the imaging bed control in an accessible location.[135] *[Recommendation]*

6.4 An RN circulator should be assigned to every patient undergoing an operative or other invasive procedure in a hybrid OR. *[Recommendation]*
Staffing for the perioperative setting is dynamic in nature and depends on clinical judgment, critical thinking, and the administrative skills of the perioperative RN administrator. Patients undergoing operative and other invasive procedures require perioperative nursing care provided by a perioperative RN, regardless of the setting.

AORN maintains that every surgical patient deserves a perioperative RN for the duration of any operative or other invasive procedure and actively promotes laws and regulation to ensure the supervisory presence of the professional RN in the perioperative setting. A minimum of one perioperative RN circulator dedicated to each patient undergoing an operative or other invasive procedure facilitates the provision of safe, quality patient care in the perioperative setting.[145]

6.4.1 Assign additional personnel depending on the type of procedure and the skill mix required. [*Recommendation*]

Low-quality evidence evidence[133,139,144,146-150] reflects the complexity of the patient care provided for the combined interventional and surgical procedures. The skill mix required is dependent on the procedure and requires unique coordination of ensuring the right personnel are in the room at the correct time due to the phasing of most procedures. More research is needed in this area.

The perioperative team in a hybrid room may include a
- perioperative circulating RN,
- radiology circulating RN,
- surgical scrub person (ie, RN or surgical technologist),
- radiology technologist,
- surgeon,
- surgical first assistant,
- anesthesia professional,
- radiology technician,
- interventional cardiologist, and
- perfusionist.

Katzen et al[147] described the facility experience at Baptist Cardiac and Vascular Institute after 16 years of having a hybrid OR located in the interventional lab area. A multidisciplinary team was convened to evaluate the program. Review of operating expenses revealed that labor cost was high because of the historic staffing pattern of two OR staff members and two interventional radiology staff members for every endovascular aortic repair procedure. The multidisciplinary team proposed a cross-training program for existing interventional radiology (IR) nurses and technologists to perform the function of the OR staff members.

To understand the scope of practice for each specialty, a team of OR and IR directors, managers, and educators met to perform a cross-walk of roles and responsibilities. The facility created a 15-week training program based on AORN guidelines and trained the IR nurses to achieve competence in traffic patterns, environmental cleaning, aseptic technique, and surgical attire. More studies are needed to review the cross training of roles to provide highly collaborative work team where personnel can work within their scopes of practice and maximize operational efficiencies.[147]

The Department of Veteran Affairs (VA) evaluated the complexities of developing a transtho-

racic aortic valve replacement (TAVR) program in their system. Since the approval of the TAVR procedure by the US Food and Drug Administration in 2002, more than 20,000 TAVR procedures have been performed, and there is minimal guidance on where the procedure is performed and who is directing the care of the TAVR program.[144] The VA, as a system, decided to develop a standardized approach to review applications for implementation of a structural heart program at any one of their facilities. A centralized team and the use of the Health Failure Mode and Effects Analysis (HFMEA) provided a systematic approach to help ensure room readiness and personnel competency for this complex program. The HFMEA provides a mechanism for identifying high-risk situations and hazard analysis. The personnel in the hybrid room provided unique understanding of roles and the ability to accurately perform their jobs during critical events. They performed drills to identify areas of crossover between roles and the skill level of each role.[144]

D'Amours et al[146] addressed the challenge of working in hybrid rooms on evening, nights, and weekends in a literature review. They described a Canadian study that demonstrated that 78% of major traumas occur in the evening, at nights, and on weekends. The resources required for staffing and coordinating the call schedules can be labor intensive. Clear understanding of clinical leadership and each team member's role is key to the coordination of care for a trauma patient in the hybrid room.

6.5 Determine what emergency supplies and equipment should be available before the procedure begins (eg, crash cart, supplies for converting to an open procedure, fire extinguisher, gas shutoff valves) based on the location of the hybrid OR and procedure. [*Recommendation*]

Evidence about the emergencies associated with combination procedures in a hybrid OR is limited. Research is needed about coordinating the care of patients in the complex hybrid OR environment. The hybrid OR can create efficiencies by decreasing the number of patient transfers and hand overs, but the multiple disciplines involved in the procedure can also create delays in treatment if the team is not well orchestrated.[128]

Kirkpatrick et al[128] and D'Amours et al[146] reported on the use of the hybrid OR for trauma procedures. The authors suggest that using the RAPTOR (resuscitation with angiography percutaneous treatments and operative resuscitations) concept in a hybrid OR provides a safer and more efficient environment for care of trauma patients. Kirkpatrick et al[128] described the design, build, and operation of the RAPTOR hybrid OR. In their facility, this suite was designed to serve the needs in caring for exsanguinating patients. The authors stated that the future is development of resuscitative ORs where patients can be transported to one location for evaluation and treatment without wasting critical time coordinating transport and patient care hand overs. The patient can have the diagnostic angiography to determine the extent of damage and bleeding. A minimally invasive repair may be adequate, but if more extensive surgery is required, the team can quickly move to an open procedure in the hybrid OR.[146]

6.6 **Radiation safety policies and procedures should be established, implemented, and reviewed periodically (See the AORN Guideline for Radiation Safety[151]).** *[Recommendation]*

6.7 **Identify structure, process, and clinical outcomes performance measures for procedures performed in the hybrid OR.** *[Recommendation]*

Patel et al[139] compared the error rate during the open phase versus the endovascular phase in the repair of aortic aneurysms in a hybrid OR. Two independent observers recorded errors that were defined as having potential to cause harm (ie, danger) or potential to disrupt the procedure (ie, delay). After observing nine procedures and recording the error rate, the researchers determined that more errors occurred during the endovascular phase of the procedure than during the open phase of the procedure (7.6/hour versus 3.75/hour, respectively).

A focus group was convened that devised a structured mental rehearsal to be performed at the beginning of each procedure. The error rate was then observed with the same tool during six procedures in which the mental rehearsal strategy was used. The error rate was significantly lower after the intervention (2.5/hour after the intervention versus 7.6/hour before the mental rehearsal). Danger and delay errors also decreased after the intervention, with 1.2 danger errors/total errors and 1.3 delay errors/total errors after the intervention compared to 1.75 danger errors/total errors and 2.0 delay errors/total errors before the intervention. The mental rehearsal requires all team members (eg, surgeon, anesthesia professional, radiologist, radiographer, nurses) to be present at the start of the radiological phase of combined procedures. The lead endovascular specialist summarizes the main steps of the radiologic phase and equipment needs for each stage. The nurse verbally confirms that equipment is available and present, and if not, it is retrieved from the supply cart. The lead endovascular specialist confirms that all team members understand and agree to proceed.[139]

A limitation of this study was that it included only a small population (N = 15 procedures) in one facility. Randomization is difficult to achieve because of the ethical dilemma of not providing the same intervention to all patients. A partial solution suggested by the researchers is to include multiple centers and randomly assign individual centers to either have the intervention or not. Further research in error prevention and patient safety will improve the coordination of care in this complex environment.[139]

Using change management strategies in the development of the team working in a hybrid room can be beneficial to the success of the program. The multidisciplinary team can assist in the development of and adherence to standards to help ensure that everyone is aware of the new structure for clinical, infection control, and radiation protocols.[133,152,153]

7. Intraoperative MRI

7.1 **Identify risks for injury and complications associated with intraoperative MRI procedures and establish safe practices regardless of magnet format or field strength.** *[Recommendation]*

Low-quality evidence describes the MRI hybrid OR as creating specific challenges for the perioperative team and requiring the following considerations:

- MRI-compatible equipment to provide safety to personnel and the patient,
- safety training before any team member (eg, clinical personnel, custodial workers, engineers, building maintenance personnel) is assigned to work in the environment,
- a safety checklist and time-out procedures to help ensure proper preparation of the environment, and
- screening tools for MRI personnel and patients to help prevent adverse events.[142,154-160]

The magnetic field can cause metal implants in the body to heat up or induce current, causing patient burns, twisting of implant wires, or even malfunction of the implant.[155]

7.2 **Prominently display zones and signs denoting the presence of an MRI scanner by posting outside the MRI suite and on the door leading to the scanner room.** *[Recommendation]*

The MRI area is usually divided into four zones. Zone I is uncontrolled and can be accessed by the public or if in the surgical suite, can be accessed by all personnel. Zone II is the interface between zones I and III. Zone III is a strictly controlled area containing the control room or vestibule for screened patients and personnel. Zone IV is the scanner room and is restricted to all screened personnel and patients because of the strong magnetic force in this zone.[142,154,155,157]

7.3 Appoint an MRI director to be responsible for ensuring

- policy development and review,
- consistent practice for MRI safety in all locations,
- review of reported adverse events, and
- continuous quality improvement.[155]
[Recommendation]

The American College of Radiology (ACR) published guidance on MRI safe practices developed by a multidisciplinary team of experts in 2013.[155] The MRI director provides consistency in safety practices in all areas where an MRI scanner is present.[155]

7.4 Assign an MRI technician for every procedure requiring MRI imaging to function as the MRI safety officer during the procedure. *[Recommendation]*

The ACR described personnel working in an MRI scanner environment as Level 1 and 2. Level 1 MRI personnel have minimal safety training and work within zones I to III. Level 2 MRI personnel (eg, MRI technicians) have more extensive training and supervise all non-MRI personnel in zones III and IV.[155]

7.5 All patients and personnel wishing to enter Zone III should first pass an MRI safety screening process.[155] *[Recommendation]*

7.5.1 Screen personnel with cardiac devices, stents, filters, grafts, cochlear implants, pumps, nerve stimulators, or metal foreign bodies (ie, bullets, pellets, shrapnel) for MRI safety. Document a screening checklist for personnel working in zones III and IV.[155] *[Recommendation]*

7.5.2 Screen patients with cardiac devices, stents, filters, grafts, cochlear implants, pumps, nerve stimulators, or metal foreign bodies (ie, bullets, pellets, shrapnel) for MRI safety. Document a screening checklist for every patient scheduled for surgery in the MRI hybrid OR.[155] *[Recommendation]*

7.5.3 The MRI director should establish a process for further investigation and approval for scanning a patient screened with any implants, foreign bodies, or other devices that are identified as MRI incompatible.[155] *[Recommendation]*

7.6 Use magnetic resonance imaging-safe (eg, non-ferromagnetic) equipment in all procedures, including

- cardiac and respiratory monitoring devices,

- oxygen tanks and fire extinguishers,
- room equipment (eg, chairs, gurneys, IV poles),
- instruments, and
- positioning equipment.[154,155,157]
[Recommendation]

Items such as oxygen tanks, IV poles, and anesthesia machines can become lethal projectiles, causing harm to personnel and patients or damage to the scanner.[154,155]

7.6.1 Use a safety checklist that confirms that MRI-incompatible equipment has been moved outside the 5 gauss line before the scanner is moved into the hybrid OR. *[Recommendation]*

Childs and Bruch[142] described the design of two hybrid ORs with a shared MRI system, where the magnet is housed between them in the diagnostic room (ie, a garage). The MRI system is brought into the hybrid OR via a track system. The room was designed with markings on the floor to designate the 5 gauss line to alert personnel to where the magnetic force is strongest when the magnet is in the room. All MRI-incompatible equipment is located outside this circle. The authors described the challenges for the team in performing an intraoperative scan and maintaining the integrity of the sterile field for neurosurgical procedures. The authors provided samples of safety checklists used for patient screening, room check before opening the garage door, and a compatibility check of all items before draping.

7.7 In the event of an emergency, initiate basic cardiopulmonary resuscitation and move the patient out of zone IV to prevent an MRI-incompatible device from entering the room.[157] *[Recommendation]*

Low-quality evidence[142,154,155,157] describes the risk of resuscitating any person in zone IV. The consensus of experts is to initiate basic cardiopulmonary resuscitation and then move the patient to a designated location to run the code. Moving the MRI scanner into the holding bay will also eliminate the risk and allow other personnel to enter the room.[142]

7.7.1 All persons who respond to an emergency situation should be trained in MRI safety, including police and fire responders.[154,155] *[Recommendation]*

7.7.2 Establish and implement a procedure for using the quench button that includes defining situations for use. *[Recommendation]*

A quench button is located in the control room and will turn off the magnet. Quenching the MRI machine can cause damage because the superconduction coils are no longer being cooled by the system. Use of the quench button should be limited and situations for its use should be defined in the procedure.[142,155,157]

7.7.3 **Drills may be used to help the team define and rehearse emergency response protocols.** [Conditional Recommendation]

8. Education

8.1 **Provide education and competency verification activities in the perioperative nursing care of patients who undergo MIS and computer-assisted procedures.** [Recommendation]

Minimally invasive surgery and computer-assisted systems are complex, can pose a safety risk, and require a steep learning curve for the surgeon and the perioperative team. Low-quality evidence supports education and competency verification of the perioperative personnel participating in MIS and computer-assisted surgical procedures and credentialing of physician and surgical assistants.[90,106,111,121,161]

8.2 **Provide initial and ongoing education and competency verification activities related to MIS procedures, including**

- **selection criteria, contraindications, and risks related to distension media;**
- **knowledge of the use and location of instrumentation and specialized equipment;**
- **preparation for and response to emergency events (eg, air embolism, conversion to an open procedure); and**
- **reporting of adverse events.**

[Recommendation]

Initial and ongoing education of perioperative personnel facilitates the development of knowledge, skills, and attitudes that affect safe patient care. Competency validation measures individual performance and provides a mechanism for documentation. Error may be minimized with education, training, and competency demonstration.

8.3 **Provide education and competency verification activities for perioperative team members participating in computer-assisted robotic procedures.** [Recommendation]

Low-quality evidence supports that a comprehensive training program and dedicated perioperative personnel are required for safe robotic programs.[106,109,111,118,161-163] Training programs include manufacturer-sponsored or private programs and include opportunities to practice on cadaveric tissue as well as in simulation trainers.

Seder et al[164] developed a triphasic model for a training program with cardiothoracic residents in robotic surgery. They studied the use of a basic algorithm that started with individual preclinical learning (ie, a module and simulation lab for practicing instrument manipulation and suturing), followed by mentored preclinical exercises (ie, cadaveric experiences and a simulation lab), and ending in progressive clinical responsibilities (ie, table-side assisting and second-console assisting with guidance from a trained surgeon). The researchers measured surgical outcomes and reported a 20% complication rate with no 90-day mortality. They discussed the need to look at different outcomes that could more appropriately assess individual competency, such as by measuring the time required for proper port placement, docking, instrument insertion, taking down the inferior pulmonary ligament, or isolating the pulmonary veins. Measuring these specific competencies can help the surgeon assess the area of difficulty and decrease the surgeon's and surgical team's frustration during the steep learning period for computer-assisted procedures.

Larson et al[111] described five ethical considerations concerning safety in robotic-assisted surgery credentialing guidelines: knowledge of laparoscopic physiology, access and management of minimally invasive complications, case selection for robotic skill mix, conversion to an open procedure as an acceptable solution by the facility with a plan for conversion to an open procedure, and having industry representatives advise only on equipment functioning and not make clinical decisions.

Expert opinion and facility experience reports describe the challenges of training, credentialing, and maintenance of competencies for a robotics program.[90,106,111,121,161] In a Pennsylvania Patient Safety Advisory reviewing the complications reported to the Pennsylvania Patient Safety Authority team training, education, and credentialing were identified as key strategies for implementing a robotic surgery program. Of 722 safety concerns reported in relation to robotic-assisted surgery, 545 (75.5%) were categorized as incidents that may or may not have reached the patient but did not result in harm, and 131 (24.0%) were attributed to equipment, supplies, or devices. Serious events were defined as resulting in patient injury (n = 177) including death (n = 10). Hospitals also provided information about contributing factors from their review of the incident. In two of the reported serious events, inexperienced staff members or issues of staff proficiency were identified as a contributing factor. Education and training of personnel were recommended for prevention of serious events.[90]

8.3.1 Include the following in education and competency verification for computer-assisted procedures:
- care, handling, and proper use of the robot and accompanying consoles and video equipment;
- troubleshooting equipment problems (eg, emergency shut off, equipment failure); and
- docking and undocking the robot. [P]
[Recommendation]

Corrigan[106] described the development of a pediatric robotic program in which a multidisciplinary team of nurses, surgeons, and anesthesiologists were provided with online education modules and simulation training. After several years of using the program, the team developed standardized protocols and a competency checklist for the perioperative personnel at their facility.

Ramsey[161] also described using standardized training and protocols to enhance efficiency and safety in a robotic program. At her facility, the perioperative team was able to demonstrate a reduced turnover time by standardizing preference cards, standardizing positioning, and creating a dedicated team for the robotic program. The author reported that turnover time for gynecologic robotic surgery was reduced to 23.2 minutes from an average of 24.8 minutes, Implementation of this process improvement allowed this facility to schedule an additional robotic procedure per day, and as many as six procedures could be completed by a single surgeon per day.

Zender and Thell[121] described the importance of educating personnel in maintaining safety in the care of patients undergoing robotic surgery. They emphasized the importance of the proficiency of the perioperative nurses in setup, connection, and positioning of the robotic patient cart. Steenwyk and Lyerly[105] recommended that the thoracic robotic team at their facility be able to perform the emergency undocking procedure in less than 60 seconds so they could quickly perform advanced cardiac life support if required.

8.3.2 Complete education and competency training and verification in assisting in the registration of the patient to the computer-assisted navigation system. [Recommendation]

8.4 Provide education and competency verification activities for radiation safety[151] and operating the imaging table, controls, and accessories in the hybrid OR. [Recommendation]

Fixed imaging system table tops are mounted on a fixed base. The **isocenter** and collision detectors are determined from the fixed base. The table tops can be changed to meet the needs of the procedure. They have different weight tolerances and two additional positioning capabilities: transverse and longitudinal. Schaadt and Landau[135] describe "driving the bed" as terminology used in the imaging departments to describe the movement of the table top during the procedure with the bed controls. Determining who drives the bed is dependent on physician preference, the equipment being used, and how the equipment and bed are configured.

There are advances in table top designs that now provide for flexible positioning with breaks in the table top, rails for bed attachments, and varying pad thicknesses.[135]

8.5 Provide education to personnel (eg, RN circulators, scrub personnel, housekeeping personnel, surgeons, anesthesia providers, MRI technologists) about working in and managing a hybrid OR with MRI imaging equipment, including
- MRI safety procedures,
- emergency procedures, and
- screening protocols.[142,154,155]
[Recommendation]

9. Policies and Procedures

9.1 Develop policies and procedures for MIS and computer-assisted procedures, review them periodically, revise them as necessary, and make them readily available in the practice setting in which they are used. [Recommendation]

Policies and procedures assist in the development of patient safety, quality assessment, and improvement activities. Policies and procedures also serve as operational guidelines used to minimize patients' risk for injury or complications, standardize practice, direct personnel, and establish continuous performance improvement programs. Policies and procedures establish authority, responsibility, and accountability within the practice setting.

9.2 Include the following in policies regarding MIS and computer-assisted equipment:
- required qualifications and credentials for operating specific equipment or devices (eg, radiologic equipment, MRI equipment) and
- procedure scheduling related to equipment availability.
[Recommendation]

Compromised patient safety, delay in care, or cancelation of the procedure may result when required equipment or qualified personnel are not available.

9.2.1 **Develop and implement policies and procedures for managing loaned MIS and computer-assisted equipment or instruments.**[2] *[Recommendation]*

Glossary

Active electrode: An electrosurgical unit accessory that directs current flow to the surgical site (eg, pencil, various pencil tips).

Capacitive coupling: The transfer of electrical current from the active electrode through intact insulation to adjacent conductive items (eg, tissue, trocars).

Computer-assisted technologies: Robotic, interventional radiology, voice-recognition, or other computer technologies used to enhance minimally invasive surgery.

Endoscopic surgery: Surgical procedures performed using endoscopic instrumentation inserted through a natural orifice or through one or more small incisions.

Extravasation: To pass by infiltration or effusion from a proper vessel or channel (eg, a blood vessel) into surrounding tissue.

Fluoroscopy: Observation of the internal features of an object by means of the fluorescence produced on a screen by x-rays transmitted through the object.

Hybrid operating room: An operating room designed with numerous imaging technologies (eg, 3-D angiography, computed tomography, magnetic resonance imaging, positron-emission tomography, intravascular ultrasound) to support surgical procedures that require multiple care providers with varied expertise to provide patient care in one location.

Insufflation: The act of blowing gas into a body cavity for the purpose of visual examination.

Intravasation: The entrance of foreign material or solution into a blood vessel.

Isocenter: The point in space through which the central ray of radiation beams pass.

Minimally invasive surgery: Surgical procedures performed through one or more small incisions using endoscopic instruments, radiographic and magnetic resonance imaging, computer-assisted devices, robotics, and other technologies.

No-fly zone: A zone defined by the imaging manufacturer that refers to workflow and the restriction of positioning dynamic equipment into this space during the operation of the imaging equipment.

Pneumoperitoneum: The presence of air or gas within the peritoneal cavity of the abdomen, often induced for diagnostic purposes.

Restricted area: Includes the OR and procedure room, the clean core, and scrub sink areas. People in this area are required to wear full surgical attire and cover all head and facial hair, including sideburns, beards, and necklines.

Semi-restricted area: Includes the peripheral support areas of the surgical suite and has storage areas for sterile and clean supplies, work areas for storage and processing of instruments, and corridors leading to the restricted areas of the surgical suite.

Telestration: A freehand sketch over a video image.

Transurethral resection syndrome: A mild to moderately severe absorption of nonelectrolyte solution following transurethral resection.

References

1. Guideline for processing flexible endoscopes. In: *Guidelines for Perioperative Practice.* Denver, CO: AORN, Inc; 2016:675-758. [IVA]

2. Guideline for cleaning and care of surgical instruments. In: *Guidelines for Perioperative Practice.* Denver, CO: AORN, Inc; 2016:773-808. [IVB]

3. Guideline for a safe environment of care, part 2. In: *Guidelines for Perioperative Practice.* Denver, CO: AORN, Inc; 2016:263-288. [IVB]

4. Guideline for surgical smoke safety. In: *Guidelines for Perioperative Practice.* Denver, CO: AORN, Inc; 2016:e77-e106. [IVA]

5. Guideline for prevention of unplanned patient hypothermia. In: *Guidelines for Perioperative Practice.* Denver, CO: AORN, Inc; 2016:531-554. [IVA]

6. Guideline for a safe environment of care, part 1. In: *Guidelines for Perioperative Practice.* Denver, CO: AORN, Inc; 2016:237-262. [IVB]

7. Guideline for positioning the patient. In: *Guidelines for Perioperative Practice.* Denver, CO: AORN, Inc; 2016:649-668. [IVB]

8. Guideline for safe use of energy-generating devices. In: *Guidelines for Perioperative Practice.* Denver, CO: AORN, Inc; 2016:e49-e76. [IVA]

9. Samii A, Gerganov VM. The dedicated endoscopic operating room. *World Neurosurg.* 2013;79(2 Suppl):S15.e19-e22. [VB]

10. Sabnis R, Ganesamoni R, Mishra S, Sinha L, Desai MR. Concept and design engineering: endourology operating room. *Curr Opin Urol.* 2013;23(2):152-157. [VB]

11. Persoon MC, Broos HJ, Witjes JA, Hendrikx AJ, Scherpbier AJ. The effect of distractions in the operating room during endourological procedures. *Surg Endosc.* 2011;25(2):437-443. [VA]

12. Koninckx PR, Stepanian A, Adamyan L, Ussia A, Donnez J, Wattiez A. The digital operating room and the surgeon. *Gynecol Surg.* 2013;10(1):57-62. [VB]

13. Strong VE, Forde KA, MacFadyen BV, et al. Ethical considerations regarding the implementation of new technologies and techniques in surgery. *Surg Endosc.* 2014;28(8):2272-2276. [VB]

14. Choi SD. A review of the ergonomic issues in the laparoscopic operating room. *J Healthc Eng.* 2012;3(4):587-603. [IIB]

15. Stavroulis A, Cutner A, Liao L-M. Staff perceptions of the effects of an integrated laparoscopic theatre environment on teamwork. *Gynecol Surg.* 2013;10(3):177-180. [IIIB]

16. Tjiam IM, Goossens RH, Schout BM, et al. Ergonomics in endourology and laparoscopy: an overview of musculoskeletal problems in urology. *J Endourol.* 2014;28(5):605-611. [IIIA]

17. Murad FM, Banerjee S, Barth BA, et al. Image management systems. *Gastrointest Endosc.* 2014;79(1):15-22. [VA]

18. Rockstroh M, Franke S, Neumuth T. Requirements for the structured recording of surgical device data in the digital operating room. *Int J Comput Assist Radiol Surg.* 2014;9(1):49-57. [IIIC]

19. 45 CFR 162 Subpart F—Standard Unique Employer Identifier. 2016. US Government Publishing Office. http://www.ecfr.gov/cgi-bin/text-idx?SID=cae9c2c6e308e3d431bcaaf2c5a1207a&mc=true&node=sp45.1.162.f&rgn=div6. Accessed October 26, 2016.

20. 45 CFR 162 Subpart D—Standard Unique Health Identifier for Health Care Providers. 2016. US Government Publishing Office. http://www.ecfr.gov/cgi-bin/text-idx?SID=60c2bd4a007fc0d54110ea2f89d6dab9&mc=true&node=pt45.1.162&rgn=div5#sp45.1.162.d. Accessed October 26, 2016.

21. 45 CFR 160 Subpart C—Compliance and Investigations. 2016. US Government Publishing Office. http://www.ecfr.gov/cgi-bin/text-idx?SID=60c2bd4a007fc0d54110ea2f89d6dab9&mc=true&node=pt45.1.160&rgn=div5#sp45.1.160.c. Accessed October 26, 2016.

22. Anderson SM, Kapp BB, Angell JM, et al. Remote monitoring and supervision of urology residents utilizing integrated endourology suites—a prospective study of patients' opinions. *J Endourol.* 2013;27(1):96-100. [IIIC]

23. Santomauro M, Reina GA, Stroup SP, L'Esperance JO. Telementoring in robotic surgery. *Curr Opin Urol.* 2013;23(2):141-145. [VB]

24. Haidegger T, Sándor J, Benyó Z. Surgery in space: the future of robotic telesurgery. *Surg Endosc.* 2011;25(3):681-690. [VB]

25. Nalugo M, Craner DR, Schwachter M, Ponsky TA. What is "telemedicine" and what does it mean for a pediatric surgeon? *Eur J Pediatr Surg.* 2014;24(4):295-302. [VB]

26. Buzink SN, van Lier L, de Hingh IHJT, Jakimowicz JJ. Risk-sensitive events during laparoscopic cholecystectomy: the influence of the integrated operating room and a preoperative checklist tool. *Surg Endosc.* 2010;24(8):1990-1995. [IIB]

27. Nocco U, del Torchio S. The integrated OR: efficiency and effectiveness evaluation after two years use, a pilot study. *Int J Comput Assist Radiol Surg.* 2011;6(2):175-186. [VA]

28. Schmitz PM, Gollnick I, Modemann S, Rothe A, Niegsch R, Strauss G. An improved instrument table for use in functional endoscopic sinus surgery. *Med Sci Monit Basic Res.* 2015;21:131-134. [IIC]

29. Al-Hakim L. The impact of preventable disruption on the operative time for minimally invasive surgery. *Surg Endosc.* 2011;25(10):3385-3392. [IIIC]

30. Held RT, Hui TT. A guide to stereoscopic 3D displays in medicine. *Acad Radiol.* 2011;18(8):1035-1048. [VB]

31. Kong SH, Oh BM, Yoon H, et al. Comparison of two- and three-dimensional camera systems in laparoscopic performance: a novel 3D system with one camera. *Surg Endosc.* 2010;24(5):1132-1143. [IIIA]

32. Kranzfelder M, Schneider A, Gillen S, Feussner H. New technologies for information retrieval to achieve situational awareness and higher patient safety in the surgical operating room: the MRI institutional approach and review of the literature. *Surg Endosc.* 2011;25(3):696-705. [VB]

33. Pluyter JR, Buzink SN, Rutkowski AF, Jakimowicz JJ. Do absorption and realistic distraction influence performance of component task surgical procedure? *Surg Endosc.* 2010;24(4):902-907. [IIA]

34. Shukla PJ, Maharaj R, Fingerhut A. Ergonomics and technical aspects of minimal access surgery in acute surgery. *Eur J Trauma Emerg Surg.* 2010;36(1):3-9. [VB]

35. Klein MI, DeLucia PR, Olmstead R. The impact of visual scanning in the laparoscopic environment after engaging in strain coping. *Hum Factors.* 2013;55(3):509-519. [IIA]

36. Morton PJ. Implementing AORN recommended practices for MIS: Part II. *AORN J.* 2012;96(4):378-392. [VA]

37. Ulmer BC. Best practices for minimally invasive procedures. *AORN J.* 2010;91(5):558-572. [VB]

38. Llarena NC, Shah AB, Milad MP. Bowel injury in gynecologic laparoscopy: a systematic review. *Obstet Gynecol.* 2015;125(6):1407-1417. [IIA]

39. Levy BF, De Guara J, Willson PD, Soon Y, Kent A, Rockall TA. Bladder injuries in emergency/expedited laparoscopic surgery in the absence of previous surgery: a case series. *Ann R Coll Surg Engl.* 2012;94(3):e118-e120. [VC]

40. Park EY, Kwon JY, Kim KJ. Carbon dioxide embolism during laparoscopic surgery. *Yonsei Med J.* 2012;53(3):459-466. [VB]

41. Cheng Y, Lu J, Xiong X, et al. Gases for establishing pneumoperitoneum during laparoscopic abdominal surgery. *Cochrane Database Syst Rev.* 2013(1):CD009569. [IA]

42. Binda MM. Humidification during laparoscopic surgery: overview of the clinical benefits of using humidified gas during laparoscopic surgery. *Arch Gynecol Obstet.* 2015;292(5):955-971. [VA]

43. Lee KC, Kim JY, Kwak HJ, Lee HD, Kwon IW. The effect of heating insufflation gas on acid-base alterations and core temperature during laparoscopic major abdominal surgery. *Korean J Anesthesiol.* 2011;61(4):275-280. [IA]

44. Najam O, Krishnamoorthy B, Kadir I, et al. Scrotal distension after endoscopic harvesting of the saphenous vein in patients with inguinal hernia. *Ann Thorac Surg.* 2011;92(2):733-735. [VC]

45. Maeda Y, Hirasawa D, Fujita N, et al. A pilot study to assess mediastinal emphysema after esophageal endoscopic submucosal dissection with carbon dioxide insufflation. *Endoscopy.* 2012;44(6):565-571. [IA]

46. Kim JA, Kim JS, Chang MS, Yoo YK, Kim DK. Influence of carbon dioxide insufflation of the neck on intraocular pressure during robot-assisted endoscopic thyroidectomy: a comparison with open thyroidectomy. *Surg Endosc.* 2013;27(5):1587-1593. [IIIB]

47. AAGL Advancing Minimally Invasive Gynecology Worldwide; Munro MG, Storz K, Abbott JA, et al. AAGL Practice Report:

Practice Guidelines for the Management of Hysteroscopic Distending Media: (replaces Hysteroscopic Fluid Monitoring Guidelines. J Am Assoc Gynecol Laparosc. 2000;7:167-168.). *J Minim Invasive Gynecol.* 2013;20(2):137-148. [IVB]

48. Hayden P, Cowman S. Anaesthesia for laparoscopic surgery. *Contin Educ Anaesth Crit Care Pain.* 2011;11(5):177-180. [VC]

49. Rammohan A, Manimaran AB, Manohar RR, Naidu RM. Nitrous oxide for pneumoperitoneum: no laughing matter this! A prospective single blind case controlled study. *Int J Surg.* 2011;9(2):173-176. [IA]

50. Jacobs VR, Morrison JE Jr, Kiechle M. Twenty-five simple ways to increase insufflation performance and patient safety in laparoscopy. *J Am Assoc Gynecol Laparosc.* 2004;11(3):410-423. [VA]

51. Olsen M, Avery N, Khurana S, Laing R. Pneumoperitoneum for neonatal laparoscopy: how safe is it? *Paediatr Anaesth.* 2013;23(5):457-459. [VC]

52. Aran T, Unsal MA, Guven S, Kart C, Cetin EC, Alver A. Carbon dioxide pneumoperitoneum induces systemic oxidative stress: a clinical study. *Eur J Obstet Gynecol Reprod Biol.* 2012;161(1):80-83. [IIIB]

53. Eryilmaz HB, Memis D, Sezer A, Inal MT. The effects of different insufflation pressures on liver functions assessed with LiMON on patients undergoing laparoscopic cholecystectomy. *The Scientific World Journal.* 2012;2012:172575. [IA]

54. Kim HY, Kim TY, Lee KC, et al. Pneumothorax during laparoscopic totally extraperitoneal inguinal hernia repair—a case report. *Korean J Anesthesiol.* 2010;58(5):490-494. [VC]

55. Otsuka Y, Katagiri T, Ishii J, et al. Gas embolism in laparoscopic hepatectomy: what is the optimal pneumoperitoneal pressure for laparoscopic major hepatectomy? *J Hepatobiliary Pancreat Sci.* 2013;20(2):137-140. [VB]

56. Liu F, Zhu S, Ji Q, Li W, Liu J. The impact of intra-abdominal pressure on the stroke volume variation and plethysmographic variability index in patients undergoing laparoscopic cholecystectomy. *Biosci Trends.* 2015;9(2):129-133. [IIIB]

57. Lasersohn L. Anaesthetic considerations for paediatric laparoscopy. *S Afr J Surg.* 2011;49(1):22-26. [VB]

58. Mura P, Cossu AP, Musu M, et al. Pituitary apoplexy after laparoscopic surgery: a case report. *Eur Rev Med Pharmacol Sci.* 2014;18(22):3524-3527. [VC]

59. Hackethal A, Brennan D, Rao A, et al. Consideration for safe and effective gynaecological laparoscopy in the obese patient. *Arch Gynecol Obstet.* 2015;292(1):135-141. [VB]

60. Meftahuzzaman SM, Islam MM, Chowdhury KK, et al. Haemodynamic and end tidal CO_2 changes during laparoscopic cholecystectomy under general anaesthesia. *Mymensingh Med J.* 2013;22(3):473-477. [IIIB]

61. Kim SH, Park KS, Shin HY, Yi JH, Kim DK. Paradoxical carbon dioxide embolism during endoscopic thyroidectomy confirmed by transesophageal echocardiography. *J Anesth.* 2010;24(5):774-777. [VC]

62. Pandey V, Varghese E, Rao M, et al. Nonfatal air embolism during shoulder arthroscopy. *Am J Orthop (Belle Mead NJ).* 2013;42(6):272-274. [VC]

63. Kocher MS, Frank JS, Nasreddine AY, et al. Intra-abdominal fluid extravasation during hip arthroscopy: a survey of the MAHORN group. *Arthroscopy.* 2012;28(11):1654-1660. [IIIB]

64. Yousef AA, Suliman GA, Elashry OM, Elsharaby MD, Elgamasy AEK. A randomized comparison between three types of irrigating fluids during transurethral resection in benign prostatic hyperplasia. *BMC Anesthesiol.* 2010;10:7. [IB]

65. Munro MG, Christianson LA. Complications of hysteroscopic and uterine resectoscopic surgery. *Clin Obstet Gynecol.* 2015;58(4):765-797. [VB]

66. Edwards DS, Davis I, Jones NA, Simon DW. Rapid tracheal deviation and airway compromise due to fluid extravasation during shoulder arthroscopy. *J Shoulder Elbow Surg.* 2014;23(7):e163-e165. [VC]

67. Jo YY, Jeon HJ, Choi E, Choi YS. Extreme hyponatremia with moderate metabolic acidosis during hysteroscopic myomectomy—a case report. *Korean J Anesthesiol.* 2011;60(6):440-443. [VC]

68. Khan F, Padmanabha S, Shantaram M, Aravind M. Airway compromise due to irrigation fluid extravasation following shoulder arthroscopy. *J Anaesthesiol Clin Pharmacol.* 2013;29(4):578-579. [VC]

69. Manjuladevi M, Gupta S, Upadhyaya KV, Kutappa AM. Postoperative airway compromise in shoulder arthroscopy: a case series. *Indian J Anaesth.* 2013;57(1):52-55. [VC]

70. Wegmuller B, Hug K, Meier Buenzli C, Yuen B, Maggiorini M, Rudiger A. Life-threatening laryngeal edema and hyponatremia during hysteroscopy. *Crit Care Res Pract.* 2011;2011:140381. [VC]

71. Woo YC, Kang H, Cha SM, et al. Severe intraoperative hyponatremia associated with the absorption of irrigation fluid during hysteroscopic myomectomy: a case report. *J Clin Anesth.* 2011;23(8):649-652. [VC]

72. Yang BJ, Feng LM. Symptomatic hyponatremia and hyperglycemia complicating hysteroscopic resection of intrauterine adhesion: a case report. *Chin Med J.* 2012;125(8):1508-1510. [VC]

73. Stocker L, Umranikar A, Moors A, Umranikar S. An overview of hysteroscopy and hysteroscopic surgery. *Obstet Gynaecol Reprod Med.* 2013;23(5):146-153. [VB]

74. Van Kruchten PM, Vermelis JMFW, Herold I, Van Zundert AAJ. Hypotonic and isotonic fluid overload as a complication of hysteroscopic procedures: two case reports. *Minerva Anestesiol.* 2010;76(5):373-377. [VC]

75. Rademaker BMP, van Kesteren PJM, de Haan P, Rademaker D, France C. How safe is the intravasation limit in hysteroscopic surgery? *J Minim Invasive Gynecol.* 2011;18(3):355-361. [IIIB]

76. Morton PJ. Implementing AORN recommended practices for minimally invasive surgery: part I. *AORN J.* 2012;96(3):295-314. [VA]

77. Darwish AM, Hassan ZZ, Attia AM, Abdelraheem SS, Ahmed YM. Biological effects of distension media in bipolar versus monopolar resectoscopic myomectomy: a randomized trial. *J Obstet Gynaecol Res.* 2010;36(4):810-817. [IB]

78. Park JT, Lim HK, Kim SG, Um DJ. A comparison of the influence of 2.7% sorbitol-0.54% mannitol and 5% glucose irrigating fluids on plasma serum physiology during hysteroscopic procedures. *Korean J Anesthesiol.* 2011;61(5):394-398. [IIC]

79. Silva JM Jr, Barros MA, Chahda MAL, Santos IM, Marubayashi LY, Malbouisson LM. Risk factors for perioperative complications in endoscopic surgery with irrigation. *Braz J Anesthesiol.* 2013;63(4):327-333. [IIIA]

80. Bergeron ME, Ouellet P, Bujold E, et al. The impact of anesthesia on glycine absorption in operative hysteroscopy: a randomized controlled trial. *Anesth Analg.* 2011;113(4):723-728. [IA]

81. Kumar A, Kumar A. New hysteroscopy pump to monitor real-time rate of fluid intravasation. *J Minim Invasive Gynecol.* 2012;19(3):369-375. [VA]

82. Ladner B, Nester K, Cascio B. Abdominal fluid extravasation during hip arthroscopy. *Arthroscopy.* 2010;26(1):131-135. [VC]

83. Cavaignac E, Pailhe R, Reina N, Chiron P, Laffosse JM. Massive proximal extravasation as a complication during arthroscopic anterior cruciate ligament reconstruction. *Knee Surg Rel Res.* 2013;25(2):84-87. [VC]

84. Stafford GH, Malviya A, Villar RN. Fluid extravasation during hip arthroscopy. *Hip Int.* 2011;21(6):740-743. [VA]

85. Verma M, Sekiya JK. Intrathoracic fluid extravasation after hip arthroscopy. *Arthroscopy.* 2010;26(9 Suppl):S90-S94. [VC]

86. Hermanns T, Fankhauser CD, Hefermehl LJ, et al. Prospective evaluation of irrigation fluid absorption during pure transurethral bipolar plasma vaporisation of the prostate using expired-breath ethanol measurements. *BJU Int.* 2013;112(5):647-654. [IIIB]

87. Lee KC, Kim HY, Lee MJ, Koo JW, Lim JA, Kim SH. Abdominal compartment syndrome occurring due to uterine perforation during a hysteroscopy procedure. *J Anesth.* 2010;24(2):280-283. [VC]

88. Guideline for medication safety. In: *Guidelines for Perioperative Practice.* Denver, CO: AORN, Inc; 2016:289-332. [IVA]

89. Boyd HR, Stanley C. Sources of error when tracking irrigation fluids during hysteroscopic procedures. *J Am Assoc Gynecol Laparosc.* 2000;7(4):472-476. [VA]

90. Dubeck D. Robotic-assisted surgery: focus on training and credentialing. *Penn Patient Saf Advis.* 2014;11(3):93-101. [VA]

91. Aubé C, Schmidt D, Brieger J, et al. Influence of NaCl concentrations on coagulation, temperature, and electrical conductivity using a perfusion radiofrequency ablation system: an ex vivo experimental study. *Cardiovasc Intervent Radiol.* 2007;30(1):92-97. [IIA]

92. Brace CL, Laeseke PF, Prasad V, Lee FT. Electrical isolation during radiofrequency ablation: 5% dextrose in water provides better protection than saline. *Conf Proc IEEE Eng Med Biol Soc.* 2006;1:5021-5024. [IIB]

93. Closon F, Tulandi T. Future research and developments in hysteroscopy. *Best Pract Res Clin Obstet Gynaecol.* 2015;29(7):994-1000. [VA]

94. Culp WC Jr, Kimbrough BA, Luna S, Maguddayao AJ, Eidson JL, Paolino DV. Use of the electrosurgical unit in a carbon dioxide atmosphere. *J Med Eng Technol.* 2016;40(2):29-34. [IIB]

95. Curtin B, Friebe I. Dermal burn during hip arthroscopy. *Orthopedics.* 2014;37(8):e746-e749. [VA]

96. Deffieux X, Gauthier T, Menager N, Legendre G, Agostini A, Pierre F. Hysteroscopy: guidelines for clinical practice from the French College of Gynaecologists and Obstetricians. *Eur J Obstet Gynecol Reprod Biol.* 2014;178:114-122. [IVA]

97. Faul P, Schlenker B, Gratzke C, Stief CG, Reich O, Gustaw Hahn R. Clinical and technical aspects of bipolar transurethral prostate resection. *Scand J Urol Nephrol.* 2008;42(4):318-323. [VB]

98. Groenman FA, Peters LW, Rademaker BMP, Bakkum EA. Embolism of air and gas in hysteroscopic procedures: pathophysiology and implication for daily practice. *J Minim Invasive Gynecol.* 2008;15(2):241-247. [VA]

99. Huang S, Gateley D, Moss ALH. Accidental burn injury during knee arthroscopy. *Arthroscopy.* 2007;23(12):1363.e1-1363.e3. [VB]

100. Laeseke PF, Sampson LA, Brace CL, Winter TC III, Fine JP, Lee FT Jr. Unintended thermal injuries from radiofrequency ablation: protection with 5% dextrose in water. *Am J Roentgenol.* 2006;186(5 Suppl):S249-S254. [IIA]

101. Ubee SS, Philip J, Nair M. Bipolar technology for transurethral prostatectomy. *Expert Rev Med Devices.* 2011;8(2):149-154. [VA]

102. Vilos GA, Newton DW, Odell RC, Abu-Rafea B, Vilos AG. Characterization and mitigation of stray radiofrequency currents during monopolar resectoscopic electrosurgery. *J Minim Invasive Gynecol.* 2006;13(2):134-140. [VA]

103. Craciunas L, Sajid MS, Howell R. Carbon dioxide versus normal saline as distension medium for diagnostic hysteroscopy: a systematic review and meta-analysis of randomized controlled trials. *Fertil Steril.* 2013;100(6):1709-1714. [IA]

104. Mandapathil M, Teymoortash A, Güldner C, Wiegand S, Mutters R, Werner JA. Establishing a transoral robotic surgery program in an academic hospital in Germany. *Acta Otolaryngol.* 2014;134(7):661-665. [VC]

105. Steenwyk B, Lyerly R 3rd. Advancements in robotic-assisted thoracic surgery. *Anesthesiol Clin.* 2012;30(4):699-708. [VB]

106. Corrigan K. Pediatric robotic surgery program requires multidisciplinary team collaboration. *AORN J.* 2014;99(3):7-8. [VB]

107. Pandey R, Garg R, Chandralekha, et al. Robot-assisted thoracoscopic thymectomy: perianaesthetic concerns. *Eur J Anaesthesiol.* 2010;27(5):473-477. [VA]

108. Best J, Day L, Ingram L, Musgrave B, Rushing H, Schooley B. Comparison of robotic vs standard surgical procedure on postoperative nursing care of women undergoing total abdominal hysterectomy. *Medsurg Nurs.* 2014;23(6):414-421. [IIIA]

109. Nayeemuddin M, Daley SC, Ellsworth P. Modifiable factors to decrease the cost of robotic-assisted procedures. *AORN J.* 2013;98(4):343-352. [VB]

110. Yuh B. The bedside assistant in robotic surgery—keys to success. *Urol Nurs.* 2013;33(1):29-32. [VB]

111. Larson JA, Johnson MH, Bhayani SB. Application of surgical safety standards to robotic surgery: five principles of ethics for nonmaleficence. *J Am Coll Surg.* 2014;218(2):290-293. [VB]

112. Christie S. Electromagnetic navigational bronchoscopy and robotic-assisted thoracic surgery. *AORN J.* 2014;99(6):750-763. [VB]

113. Kawachi H, Kawachi Y, Ikeda C, Takagi R, Katakura A, Shibahara T. Oral and maxillofacial surgery with computer-assisted navigation system. *Bull Tokyo Dent Coll.* 2010;51(1):35-39. [VC]

114. Metz P, Adam J, Gerken M, Jalali B. Compact, transmissive two-dimensional spatial disperser design with application in

simultaneous endoscopic imaging and laser microsurgery. *Appl Opt.* 2014;53(3):376-382. [VA]

115. Muns A, Meixensberger J, Arnold S, et al. Integration of a 3D ultrasound probe into neuronavigation. *Acta Neurochir.* 2011;153(7):1529-1533. [VA]

116. Kaduk WMH, Podmelle F, Louis PJ. Surgical navigation in reconstruction. *Oral Maxillofac Surg Clin North Am.* 2013;25(2):313-333. [VB]

117. Young PS, Findlay H, Patton JTS, Mahendra A. (iii) Computer assisted navigation in musculoskeletal oncology. *Orthop Trauma.* 2014;28(5):294-302. [VB]

118. Mavrogenis AF, Savvidou OD, Mimidis G, et al. Computer-assisted navigation in orthopedic surgery. *Orthopedics.* 2013;36(8):631-642. [VA]

119. Kenngott HG, Wagner M, Gondan M, et al. Real-time image guidance in laparoscopic liver surgery: first clinical experience with a guidance system based on intraoperative CT imaging. *Surg Endosc.* 2014;28(3):933-940. [VA]

120. Zullo MD, McCarroll ML, Mendise TM, et al. Safety culture in the gynecology robotics operating room. *J Minim Invasive Gynecol.* 2014;21(5):893-900. [IIA]

121. Zender J, Thell C. Developing a successful robotic surgery program in a rural hospital. *AORN J.* 2010;92(1):72-86. [VB]

122. Gkegkes ID, Karydis A, Tyritzis SI, Iavazzo C. Ocular complications in robotic surgery. *Int J Med Robot.* 2015;11(3):269-274. [VA]

123. Hung CF, Yang CK, Cheng CL, Ou YC. Bowel complication during robotic-assisted laparoscopic radical prostatectomy. *Anticancer Res.* 2011;31(10):3497-3501. [VA]

124. Sarmanian JD. Robot-assisted thoracic surgery (RATS): perioperative nursing professional development program. *AORN J.* 2015;102(3):241-253. [VB]

125. Quinn D, Moohan J. Optimal laparoscopic ergonomics in gynaecology. *Obstet Gynaecol.* 2015;17(2):77-82. [VB]

126. Facility Guidelines Institute; American Society for Healthcare Engineering. *Guidelines for Design and Construction of Hospitals and Outpatient Facilities.* Chicago, IL: American Society for Healthcare Engineering; 2014. [IVA]

127. Aston G. The hybrid OR. *Hosp Health Netw.* 2014;88(3):34-37. [VC]

128. Kirkpatrick AW, Vis C, Dube M, et al. The evolution of a purpose designed hybrid trauma operating room from the trauma service perspective: the RAPTOR (resuscitation with angiography percutaneous treatments and operative resuscitations). *Injury.* 2014;45(9):1413-1421. [VB]

129. Baillie J. Dual hybrid suite "a first" for the UK. *Health Estate.* 2014;68(7):53-58. [VC]

130. Kleiman N. Room considerations with TAVR. *Methodist Debakey Cardiovasc J.* 2012;8(2):19-21. [VC]

131. Knudson L. Hybrid ORs set the stage for cutting-edge care. *AORN J.* 2012;96(2):C1, C8-C9. [VC]

132. Kpodonu J. Hybrid cardiovascular suite: the operating room of the future. *J Card Surg.* 2010;25(6):704-709. [VB]

133. Odle TG. Managing transition to a hybrid operating room. *Radiol Technol.* 2011;83(2):165-181. [VB]

134. Tsagakis K, Konorza T, Dohle DS, et al. Hybrid operating room concept for combined diagnostics, intervention and surgery in acute type A dissection. *Eur J Cardiothorac Surg.* 2013;43(2):397-404. [VB]

135. Schaadt J, Landau B. Hybrid OR 101: a primer for the OR nurse. *AORN J.* 2013;97(1):81-100. [VB]

136. Richter PH, Yarboro S, Kraus M, Gebhard F. One year orthopaedic trauma experience using an advanced interdisciplinary hybrid operating room. *Injury.* 2015;46(Suppl 4):S129-S134. [VB]

137. Klein LW, Miller DL, Balter S, et al. Occupational health hazards in the interventional laboratory: time for a safer environment. *J Radiol Nurs.* 2010;29(3):75-82. [VA]

138. Lauck S, Achtem L, Boone RH, et al. Implementation of processes of care to support transcatheter aortic valve replacement programs. *Eur J Cardiovasc Nurs.* 2013;12(1):33-38. [VB]

139. Patel SR, Gohel MS, Hamady M, et al. Reducing errors in combined open/endovascular arterial procedures: influence of a structured mental rehearsal before the endovascular phase. *J Endovasc Ther.* 2012;19(3):383-389. [IIA]

140. Shunk KA, Zimmet J, Cason B, Speiser B, Tseng EE. Development of a Veterans Affairs hybrid operating room for transcatheter aortic valve replacement in the cardiac catheterization laboratory. *JAMA Surg.* 2015;150(3):216-222. [VC]

141. Urbanowicz JA. The hybrid suite—sweet. *J Radiol Nurs.* 2011;30(2):62-66. [VB]

142. Childs S, Bruch P. Successful management of risk in the hybrid OR. *AORN J.* 2015;101(2):223-234. [VB]

143. Varu VN, Greenberg JI, Lee JT. Improved efficiency and safety for EVAR with utilization of a hybrid room. *Eur J Vasc Endovasc Surg.* 2013;46(6):675-679. [VA]

144. Speiser B, Dutra-Brice C. Transcatheter aortic valve replacement. *Dimens Crit Care Nurs.* 2014;33(5):262-274. [VB]

145. *AORN Position Statement on One Perioperative Registered Nurse Circulator Dedicated to Every Patient Undergoing an Operative or Other Invasive Procedure.* AORN, Inc. http://www.aorn.org/guidelines/clinical-resources/position-statements. Accessed October 26, 2016.

146. D'Amours SK, Rastogi P, Ball CG. Utility of simultaneous interventional radiology and operative surgery in a dedicated suite for seriously injured patients. *Curr Opin Crit Care.* 2013;19(6):587-593. [VB]

147. Katzen BT, Kiah J, Smith D, Denny D, Stoia M. Hybrid interventional radiology. *Perioper Nurs Clin.* 2010;5(2):215-227. [VB]

148. Karkos CD, Menexes GC, Patelis N, Kalogirou TE, Giagtzidis IT, Harkin DW. A systematic review and meta-analysis of abdominal compartment syndrome after endovascular repair of ruptured abdominal aortic aneurysms. *J Vasc Surg.* 2014;59(3):829-842. [IIA]

149. Contrera P, Cushing M. Transcatheter aortic valve replacement. *AANA J.* 2013;81(5):399-408. [VB]

150. Smeltzer HG, Scott JR, Frey SA, et al. Collaboration between interventional neurosurgery and vascular surgery in the hybrid operating room. *J Radiol Nurs.* 2014;33(3):127-131. [VC]

151. Guideline for radiation safety. In: *Guidelines for Perioperative Practice.* Denver, CO: AORN, Inc; 2016:333-368. [IVA]

152. Mason SL, Kuruvilla S, Riga CV, et al. Design and validation of an error capture tool for quality evaluation in the vascular and endovascular surgical theatre. *Eur J Vasc Endovasc Surg.* 2013;45(3): 248-254. [IIIA]

153. Robbins DA. Current modalities for abdominal aortic aneurysm repair: implications for nurses. *J Vasc Nurs.* 2010;28(4):136-146. [IIB]

154. Practice advisory on anesthetic care for magnetic resonance imaging: an updated report by the American Society of Anesthesiologists task force on anesthetic care for magnetic resonance imaging. *Anesthesiology.* 2015;122(3):495-520. [VA]

155. ACR guidance document on MR safe practices: 2013. *J Magn Reson Imaging.* 2013;37(3):501-530. [VA]

156. Zhao Y, Chen X, Wang F, et al. Integration of diffusion tensor-based arcuate fasciculus fibre navigation and intraoperative MRI into glioma surgery. *J Clin Neurosci.* 2012;19(2):255-261. [VA]

157. Ocazionez D, Dicks DL, Favinger JL, et al. Magnetic resonance imaging safety in cardiothoracic imaging. *J Thorac Imaging.* 2014;29(5):262-269. [VB]

158. Henrichs B, Walsh RP. Intraoperative MRI for neurosurgical and general surgical interventions. *Curr Opin Anaesthesiol.* 2014;27(4):448-452. [VB]

159. Hemingway M, Kilfoyle M. Safety planning for intraoperative magnetic resonance imaging. *AORN J.* 2013;98(5):508-524. [VB]

160. Oluigbo CO, Rezai AR. Magnetic resonance imaging safety of deep brain stimulator devices. *Handb Clin Neurol.* 2013; 116:73-76. [VB]

161. Ramsey R. Robotic gynecologic surgery: trends and nurse involvement at a regional hospital. *OR Nurse.* 2012;6(2):41-44. [VC]

162. Korb W, Geisler N, Straus G. Solving challenges in inter- and trans-disciplinary working teams: lessons from the surgical technology field. *Artif Intell Med.* 2015;63(3):209-219. [VA]

163. Taylor D. The implementation of a da Vinci Surgical System at The Royal Wolverhampton NHS Trust. *J Perioper Pract.* 2014;24(3):4-12. [VC]

164. Seder CW, Cassivi SD, Wigle DA. Navigating the pathway to robotic competency in general thoracic surgery. *Innovations (Phila).* 2013;8(3):184-189. [VC]

Acknowledgments

Lead Author
Mary C. Fearon, MSN, RN, CNOR
AORN Department of Nursing
Perioperative Practice Specialist
Denver, Colorado

Contributing Author
Ramona Conner, MSN, RN, CNOR, FAAN
Editor-in-Chief, Guidelines for Perioperative Practice
AORN Department of Nursing
Denver, Colorado

The authors and AORN thank Barbara L. Nalley, MSN, CRNP, CNOR, Manager, Jackson Surgical Assistants, Crofton, Maryland; David R. Urbach, MD, Clinical Epidemiology MSc, University Health Network, Toronto, Canada; James (Jay) Bowers, BSN, RN, CNOR, TNCC, Clinical Educator, West Virginia University Healthcare, Morgantown; Janice A. Neil, PhD, CNE, RN, Associate Professor, East Carolina College of Nursing, Greenville, North Carolina; Lisa Spruce, DNP, RN, CNS-CP, CNOR, ACNS, ACNP, FAAN, Director, Evidence-based Perioperative Practice, Department of Nursing, AORN, Denver, Colorado; and Sharon A. Van Wicklin, MSN, RN, CNOR, CRNFA(E), CPSN-R, PLNC, Senior Perioperative Practice Specialist, Department of Nursing, AORN, Denver, Colorado, for their assistance in developing this guideline.

Publication History

Originally published as proposed recommended practices February 1994, *AORN Journal.*

Revised November 1998; published February 1999, *AORN Journal.* Reformatted July 2000.

Revised November 2004; published as Recommended Practices for Endoscopic Minimally Invasive Surgery in *Standards, Recommended Practices, and Guidelines,* 2005 edition. March 2005, *AORN Journal.*

Revised October 2009 for online publication in *Perioperative Standards and Recommended Practices.*

Editorial revision July 2012. Recommendation IV.j revised and approved by the Recommended Practices Advisory Board. Reformatted September 2012 for publication in *Perioperative Standards and Recommended Practices,* 2013 edition.

Minor editing revisions made in November 2014 for publication in *Guidelines for Perioperative Practice,* 2015 edition, as Guideline for Minimally Invasive Surgery.

Revised December 2016 for online publication in *Guidelines for Perioperative Practice.*

Evidence ratings revised and minor editorial changes made to conform to the current AORN Evidence Rating model, September 2019, for online publication in *Guidelines for Perioperative Practice.*

MODERATE SEDATION/ ANALGESIA

TABLE OF CONTENTS

P indicates a recommendation or evidence relevant to pediatric care.

MEDICAL ABBREVIATIONS & ACRONYMS

AANA – American Association of Nurse Anesthetists
ACLS – Advanced cardiac life support
ANA – American Nurses Association
ARD – Acute respiratory distress
ASA – American Society of Anesthesiologists
BIPAP – Bilevel positive airway pressure
BIS – Bispectral index
BMI – Body mass index
CAD – Coronary artery disease
CO_2 – Carbon dioxide
COPD – Chronic obstructive pulmonary disease
CPAP – Continuous positive airway pressure
CRNA - Certified registered nurse anesthetist
CVA – Cerebrovascular accident
DIC – Disseminated intravascular coagulation
DM – Diabetes mellitus
ECMO – Extracorporeal membrane oxygenation
EGD – Esophagogastroduodenoscopy
ERCP – Endoscopic retrograde cholangiopancreatography

ESRD – End-stage renal disease
FDA – US Food and Drug Administration
HTN – Hypertension
ICAPS – International Committee for the Advancement of Procedural Sedation
MI – Miocardial infarction
NORA – Non-OR anesthesia
OSA – Obstructive sleep apnea
PACU – Postanesthesia care unit
PALS – Pediatric advanced life support
PCA – Postconceptual age
P-SAP – Perioperative sleep apnea prediction
RCT – Randomized controlled trial
RN – Registered nurse
SAMBA – Society for Ambulatory Anesthesia
SpO_2 – Oxygen saturation as detected by pulse oximeter
STBUR – Snoring, Trouble Breathing, Un-Refreshed
TIA – Transient ischemic attack

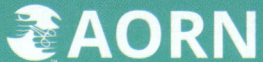
GUIDELINE FOR
CARE OF THE PATIENT RECEIVING MODERATE SEDATION/ANALGESIA

The Guideline for Care of the Patient Receiving Moderate Sedation/Analgesia was approved by the AORN Guidelines Advisory Board and became effective as of July 15, 2021. The recommendations in the guideline are intended to be achievable and represent what is believed to be an optimal level of practice. Policies and procedures will reflect variations in practice settings and/or clinical situations that determine the degree to which the guideline can be implemented. AORN recognizes the many diverse settings in which perioperative nurses practice; therefore, this guideline is adaptable to all areas where operative or other invasive procedures may be performed.

Purpose

This document provides guidance for care of the patient receiving **moderate sedation/analgesia** administered by a registered nurse (RN) in the perioperative practice setting. Guidance is provided for determining the scope of nursing practice related to administration of moderate sedation/analgesia, patient selection criteria, pre-sedation patient assessment (eg, airway, difficult mask ventilation, obstructive sleep apnea), intraoperative **continual** patient monitoring, staffing, medication administration, and postoperative discharge criteria.

The aim of moderate sedation/analgesia is to achieve a drug-induced, mild depression of consciousness with the use of sedatives or a combination of sedatives and analgesic medications, most often administered intravenously, and titrated to achieve a desired effect. The primary goal of moderate sedation/analgesia i15s to reduce the patient's anxiety and discomfort so that they can tolerate diagnostic, therapeutic, and invasive procedures. The patient can experience some degree of amnesia.[1,2]

Moderate sedation produces a condition in which the patient exhibits a mildly depressed level of consciousness and an altered perception of pain. The four distinct characteristics of moderate sedation/analgesia are the following:

- The patient is able to respond purposefully to verbal commands or light tactile stimulation.
- The patient maintains protective reflexes and is able to communicate verbally.
- The patient maintains adequate, spontaneous ventilation.
- There are minimal variations in the patient's vital signs.[1,2]

Depth of sedation occurs across a continuum from minimal sedation to moderate sedation/analgesia, to **deep sedation/analgesia**, and finally general anesthesia. Patients' responses to the medications for moderate sedation/analgesia are unpredictable. The patient may slip into a deeper level of sedation than intended; therefore, practitioners who administer moderate sedation/analgesia need to be able to rescue a patient who enters deep sedation/analgesia.[1,2]

The following topics are outside the scope of this document: local anesthesia, local monitored anesthesia care, general anesthesia, regional anesthesia (eg, spinal, epidural), total intravenous anesthesia, minimal sedation, deep sedation, endotracheal intubation, laryngoscopy, awake intubation, fospropofol, etomidate, chloral hydrate, nitrous oxide, RN-administered continuous infusion of sedatives, propofol administration in the emergency room and intensive care unit, sedation for intubated and mechanically ventilated patients, palliative care, premedication for general anesthesia, pain management following discharge from the postanesthesia care unit (PACU), surgical or procedural techniques, target-controlled infusion, and computer-assisted personalized sedation. It is not the intent of this guideline to address situations that require the services of an anesthesia professional or to substitute the services of a perioperative RN in those situations that require the services of an anesthesia professional.

The term *moderate sedation/analgesia* is used throughout this document in the recommendations and activities. Other terms may be used in the rationales if the cited literature refers to moderate sedation/analgesia by another term, such as *moderate sedation, conscious sedation, nurse-administered procedural sedation, nurse-administered propofol sedation,* or *procedural sedation and analgesia.*

Evidence Review

A medical librarian with a perioperative background conducted a systematic search of the databases Ovid MEDLINE, Ovid Embase, EBSCO CINAHL, and the Cochrane Database of Systematic Reviews. The search was limited to literature published in English from January 2015 through May 2020. At the time of the initial search, weekly alerts were created on the topics included in that search. Results from these alerts were provided to the lead author until September 2020. The lead author requested additional articles that either did not fit the original search criteria or were discovered during the evidence appraisal process. The lead author and the medical librarian also identified relevant guidelines from government agencies, professional organizations, and standards-setting bodies.

Search terms included *airway management, airway obstruction, Aldrete recovery score, antianxiety/anti-anxiety*

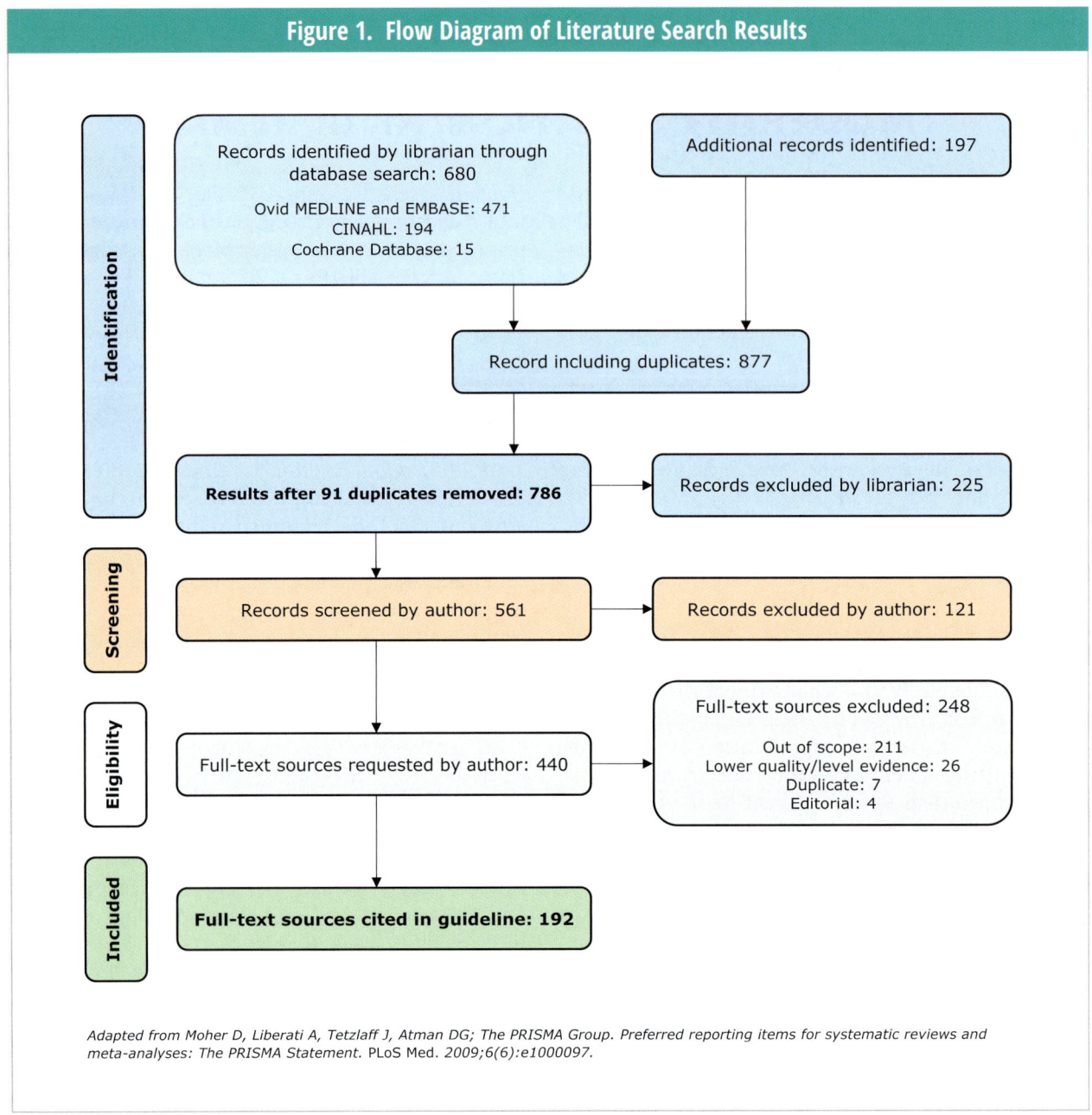

Figure 1. Flow Diagram of Literature Search Results

Records identified by librarian through database search: 680

Ovid MEDLINE and EMBASE: 471
CINAHL: 194
Cochrane Database: 15

Additional records identified: 197

Identification

Record including duplicates: 877

Results after 91 duplicates removed: 786

Records excluded by librarian: 225

Screening

Records screened by author: 561

Records excluded by author: 121

Eligibility

Full-text sources requested by author: 440

Full-text sources excluded: 248

Out of scope: 211
Lower quality/level evidence: 26
Duplicate: 7
Editorial: 4

Included

Full-text sources cited in guideline: 192

Adapted from Moher D, Liberati A, Tetzlaff J, Atman DG; The PRISMA Group. Preferred reporting items for systematic reviews and meta-analyses: The PRISMA Statement. PLoS Med. 2009;6(6):e1000097.

agents, ASA Continuum of Sedation Scale, ASA Physical Status Classification System, assess*, Berlin questionnaire, bispectral index, capnography, computer assisted personalized sedation, conscious sedation, consciousness monitors, depth of sedation, dexmedetomidine, difficult airway, difficult mask ventilation, discharge readiness criteria, fasting guidelines, fentanyl, flumazenil, ketamine, Mallampati classification, Mallampati score, Mallampati test, midazolam, moderate analgesia, moderate sedation, Modified Observer's Assessment of Alertness/Sedation Scale, naloxone, nitrous oxide, NPO, nurse-administered sedation, obstructive sleep apnea, obstructive sleep apnea assess*, post-anesthetic discharge scoring system, preoperative fasting, preprocedural fasting, propofol, Ramsay Sedation Scale, sleep apnea (obstructive), Sedasys, sedation plan, STOP-Bang, tracheobronchomalacia, and thyromental distance test.

Included were research and non-research literature in English, complete publications, and publications with dates within the time restriction when available. Historical studies were also included. Excluded were non-peer-reviewed publications and older evidence within the time restriction when more recent evidence was available. Editorials, news items, and other brief items were excluded. Low-quality evidence was excluded when higher-quality evidence was available, and literature outside the time restriction was excluded when literature within the time restriction was available (Figure 1).

Articles identified in the search were provided to the project team for evaluation. The team consisted of the lead author and one evidence appraiser. The lead author and the evidence appraiser reviewed and critically appraised each article using the AORN Research or Non-Research Evidence Appraisal Tools as appropriate. A second appraiser was consulted in the event of a disagreement between the lead author and the primary evidence appraiser. The literature was independently evaluated and appraised according to the strength and quality of the evidence. Each article was then assigned an appraisal score. The appraisal score is noted in brackets after each reference as applicable.

Each recommendation rating is based on a synthesis of the collective evidence, a benefit-harm assessment, and consideration of resource use. The strength of the recommendation was determined using the AORN Evidence Rating Model and the quality and consistency of the evidence supporting a recommendation. The recommendation strength rating is noted in brackets after each recommendation.

Note: The evidence summary table is available at http://www.aorn.org/evidencetables/.

1. Scope of Nursing Practice

1.1 **The perioperative RN administering moderate sedation/analgesia must practice within the scope of nursing practice as defined by the applicable state board of nursing and should comply with state advisory opinions, declaratory rules, and other regulations that direct the practice of the registered nurse.** *[Regulatory Requirement]*

The RN's scope of practice is determined by the state's nurse practice act and the state board of nursing. All states and territories have enacted a nurse practice act passed by the state's legislature. Each state's nurse practice act establishes a board of nursing. The board of nursing develops specific rules, regulations, and other guidance such as declaratory rulings and advisory opinions that clarify the law. The state board of nursing grants a license to practice nursing to a competent individual with the skills necessary to perform within a specified scope of practice.[3-6] The state's nurse practice act and its rules protect individuals receiving nursing care from licensed practitioners

1.2 **Consult with the state board of nursing for declaratory rulings and other guidelines that relate to the RN's role and responsibility when administering moderate sedation/analgesia.** *[Recommendation]*

The professional obligation of the perioperative RN to safeguard patients is grounded in the ethical obligation to the patient, the profession, and society, and guided by the American Nurses Association (ANA) *Nursing: Scope and Standards of Practice,*[3] AORN's *Standards of Perioperative Nursing,*[4]

AORN's *Perioperative Explications for the ANA Code of Ethics for Nurses,*[7] and state nurse practice acts.

1.2.1 **Review the medication manufacturer's instructions for use to determine whether administering the medication is within the scope of nursing practice.** *[Recommendation]*

Use of propofol is limited to persons trained in the administration of general anesthesia and not involved in the conduct of the surgical/diagnostic procedure.[8]

1.2.2 **Verify that administering the medications for moderate sedation/analgesia is within the scope of nursing practice as defined by the state board of nursing, state advisory opinions, declaratory rules, and other regulations that direct the practice of the RN.** *[Recommendation]*

Each state board of nursing regulates which medications (eg, propofol) are within the scope of practice for non-anesthesia providers to administer.

High-quality evidence supports that it is safe and efficacious for RNs to administer sedation/analgesia medications (eg, fentanyl,[9-19] meperidine,[20-22] dexmedetomidine[21,23]) alone or in combination with midazolam during gastrointestinal endoscopy,[11,12,14-17,20-22] bronchoscopy,[13,19,23] abortion,[9,18] and radiology procedures.[10]

In a 2004 joint statement, the American Association of Nurse Anesthetists (AANA) and the American Society of Anesthesiologists (ASA) urged caution during use of propofol:

> *Because sedation is a continuum, it is not always possible to predict how an individual patient will respond. Due to the potential for rapid, profound changes in sedative/analgesia depth and the lack of antagonistic medications, agents such as propofol require special attention.*
>
> *Whenever propofol is used for sedation/anesthesia, it should be administered only by persons trained in the administration of general anesthesia, who are not simultaneously involved in these surgical or diagnostic procedures. This restriction is concordant with specific language in the propofol insert, and failure to follow these recommendations could put patients at increased risk of significant injury or death.*
>
> *Similar concerns apply when other intravenous induction agents are used for sedation, such as thiopental, methohexital or etomidate.*[24]

The AORN Board of Directors endorsed this statement in 2005.

The ASA amended its Statement on Safe Use of Propofol in 2019. If an anesthesiologist is not caring for the patient,

non-anesthesia personnel who administer propofol should be qualified to rescue patients whose level of sedation becomes deeper than initially intended and who enter, if briefly, a state of general anesthesia.[25]

The statement additionally delineates the roles and responsibilities of the physician responsible for moderate sedation/analgesia and the practitioner administering propofol and provides specific guidance for education, training, airway management, cardiovascular management, monitoring, and staffing requirements.

Propofol is a sedative that is intended for general anesthesia.[1] The US Food and Drug Administration (FDA)–cleared propofol medication label warns against administration of propofol by persons who are not trained in the administration of general anesthesia and are involved in the conduct of the surgical/diagnostic procedure.[8] Despite this warning, high-quality studies have been conducted to evaluate the safety of nurse-administered propofol sedation in the endoscopy[11,26-36] and bronchoscopy settings.[37-39] A limitation of the evidence is that these studies were published only in gastroenterology and pulmonology journals, respectively.

In a subgroup analysis of a systematic review, Wadhwa et al[26] found there was no difference in adverse events when sedation was administered or supervised by a gastroenterologist compared to when sedation was administered by other practitioners (ie, anesthesiologists, critical care physicians). However, a limitation in the interpretation of this evidence is that it was derived secondarily from the study methodologies and may not have been an intended outcome of the studies.

In a systematic review with meta-analysis, Singh et al[40] found only one randomized controlled trial (RCT) that compared propofol administration by anesthesiologists to administration by non-anesthesia practitioners and found no difference in procedure time or patient satisfaction. They concluded that there is insufficient high-quality evidence comparing propofol administration by anesthesiologists to administration by other practitioners (ie, endoscopists).

A multisociety position statement from the American Association for the Study of Liver Diseases, American College of Gastroenterology, American Gastroenterological Association, and American Society for Gastrointestinal Endoscopy supports that it is safe for nurses to administer propofol sedation.[41]

The benefits of RN-administered propofol for moderate sedation/analgesia may not outweigh the potential harms. The benefits may include cost-effective care, improved efficiency, and increased access to care. The harms may include the sequalae of oversedation (eg, life-threatening respiratory or circulatory compromise) if the patient enters a deeper level of sedation than intended due to the narrow therapeutic window of propofol. The RN may not have the skills to rescue a patient who enters deep sedation/analgesia or general anesthesia.

1.3 An anesthesia professional (ie, anesthesiologist, certified registered nurse anesthetist [CRNA]) or other qualified licensed independent practitioner (eg, surgeon, endoscopist, dentist, podiatrist) should directly supervise the perioperative RN who is administering moderate sedation/analgesia.[42-44] *[Recommendation]*

Several clinical practice guidelines recommend that a qualified practitioner directly supervise the perioperative RN caring for the patient receiving moderate sedation/analgesia.[42-47]

1.3.1 The supervising practitioner should be physically present and immediately available in the procedure suite for diagnosis, treatment, and management of complications while the patient is sedated.[43,44] *[Recommendation]*

Clinical practice guidelines support the continued presence of the supervising practitioner.[43,44] The non-anesthesiologist sedation practitioner is responsible for all aspects of the sedated patient's care before, during, and after the surgical procedure.[43]

1.3.2 When the supervising practitioner is not an anesthesia professional, the practitioner should be qualified by education, training, credentialing, and licensure to administer moderate sedation/analgesia.[2,42,44] *[Recommendation]*

1.4 Provide the same standard of care (eg, patient monitoring, equipment) for patients who are receiving moderate sedation/analgesia in non-operating room anesthesia locations (eg, interventional cardiology, endoscopy, dental, radiology, office-based surgery) as for patients receiving moderate sedation/analgesia in the OR.[48-56] *[Recommendation]*

Clinical practice guidelines[49,57,58] and moderate-quality evidence[48,50-56] support providing the same standard of care when moderate sedation/analgesia is administered to patients outside of a traditional OR setting. There are significant patient safety concerns for sedation in non-OR anesthesia (NORA) locations because procedure types and complexity in these settings continue to expand rapidly, with increasing patient acuity that requires more invasive monitoring and deeper sedation.[50]

In a nonexperimental study of patient procedures registered in the National Anesthesia Clinical Outcomes Registry Database (N = 12,252,846), Chang et al[48] found that patients who had procedures performed in NORA locations had lower morbidity and mortality rates than those who had OR procedures, but there were increased complication rates in cardiology and radiology locations. The researchers recommended that providers ensure proper monitoring of patients and hold NORA locations to the same standard of care as is used in the OR.

Woodward et al[50] reviewed 10,357 claims in the Anesthesia Closed Claims Project database and found that although sedation in NORA settings seems to be safe overall, poor patient outcomes were more often related to suboptimal care and nonadherence to basic safe practices established by the ASA. The researchers recommended always being prepared for emergencies because complications are exceedingly difficult to manage in NORA environments.

2. Pre-sedation Patient Assessment

2.1 Perform a pre-sedation patient assessment and document the assessment before administering moderate sedation/analgesia. *[Recommendation]*

Assessing the patient before administering sedation/analgesia is recommended by the ASA[1] and AANA.[2] A pre-sedation assessment may reduce the patient's risk of experiencing an adverse event by determining whether the patient is a candidate for RN-administered moderate sedation or if the patient is at risk for adverse outcomes and requires additional interventions to minimize identified risks. The assessment also provides baseline measures of vital signs, pain, anxiety, and level of consciousness for comparison during and after the procedure.[2]

2.2 In the pre-sedation patient assessment, include a review of the patient's
- allergies and sensitivities (eg, medications, food, environment, adhesives, latex)[1,2,45,47,59-66];
- age[54,64,67-72];
- height, weight, and body mass index (BMI)[54,64-66,71,73];

- current medical and surgical history and physical examination (eg, history and physical)[1,2,45,46,60,64-66,71];
- current medications (eg, prescribed, over-the-counter, alternative/complementary therapies, supplements), dosage, last dose, and frequency[1,2,45,47,59-61,63-66,72,74];
- history of and current drug use (eg, street drugs, non-prescribed prescription drugs)[1,2,45,47,60,64,66,72,74];
- history and current cannabis use[1,2,45,47,60,64,66,75-79];
- history and current tobacco and alcohol use[1,45,60,61,64,66,70,80,81];
- laboratory test results (eg, serum electrolytes, coagulation studies)[1,2,46,64,66];
- diagnostic test results (eg, 12-lead electrocardiogram, echocardiogram, pulmonary function test)[2,46,64,66];
- baseline cardiac status (eg, heart rate, blood pressure)[1,2,46,47,64-66];
- baseline respiratory status (eg, rate, rhythm, blood oxygen level [SpO_2])[1,2,46,47,64-66];
- baseline neurological status (eg, level of consciousness)[46,60,64-66];
- airway (eg, obstructive sleep apnea, difficult mask ventilation)[1,2,47,59,64-66,71,72,82-85];
- physical limitations or sensory impairment (eg, visual, auditory, vocal)[64,66];
- level of anxiety[86];
- level of pain[66];
- pregnancy test results when applicable[45,66];
- NPO status[1,2,46,60,61,64-66,87];
- previous adverse experiences with anesthesia or moderate sedation, including
  - delayed emergence from anesthesia or sedation,
  - postprocedure nausea and/or vomiting,
  - reported adverse effects from anesthetic or sedative medications,
  - malignant hyperthermia, and
- airway or breathing problems[1,2,47,64,66];
- informed consent (ie, explaining the risks, benefits, and alternatives to sedation)[1,2,46,47,64]; and
- arrangement for a responsible adult caregiver to escort the patient home[46,66] or two adults (ie, driver and observer) for an infant or toddler riding home in a car safety seat.[47,88]

[Recommendation] **P**

Professional organizations recommend assessing the patient for the listed elements before administering sedation/analgesia.[1,2,45,47,59-61,64-66]

Low-quality evidence supports assessing the patient for marijuana (ie, cannabis) use before administering sedation.[75-79] Flisberg et al[75] conducted an RCT of 60 male patients undergoing day-case general anesthesia with laryngeal mask placement and found that cannabis use (ie, regular use at least once per week for at least the past 6 months) increased the dose of propofol required for anesthesia induction with insertion of a laryngeal mask. In a retrospective nonexperimental study of 250 patients who underwent endoscopic procedures, Twardowski et al[76] found that people who regularly used cannabis (ie, smoking or ingesting edible marijuana products on a daily or weekly basis) required a significantly higher amount of sedation for endoscopic procedures than nonusers (ie, no use of cannabis, sporadic use, topical use of cannabidiol oils or ointments). The researchers recommended assessing patients for cannabis use preoperatively to facilitate planning patient care and medication needs and to anticipate possible risks of increased sedative doses.

In an organizational experience report, Woo and Andrews[79] reported that long-term cannabis users had an increased requirement for sedation and experienced paradoxical agitation with adjunct anticholinergic medications. Karam et al[78] reported a case of a 35-year-old male patient with a physical status classification of ASA II, who was a chronic cannabis user (ie, smoking 3 to 4 times per week) and tobacco user (ie, smoking 5 to 6 cigarettes per day for the past 20 years) and had an increased narcotic dosage requirement during an emergency fasciotomy following right leg fracture. Huson et al[77] conducted a literature review and found that marijuana use may present anesthetic concerns, including an increased risk of cardiac arrhythmias, myocardial infarction, stroke, pulmonary obstruction, thromboembolism, or bleeding concerns.

Moderate-quality evidence supports assessing the patient for chronic **opioid** use before administering sedation.[72,74] Urman et al[72] conducted a nonexperimental study of 525,151 patients in a retrospective legal claims database of inpatient interventional radiology procedures with moderate sedation and found that risk factors for respiratory compromise included long-term opioid therapy use, active substance abuse, age older than 65 years, and sleep apnea. The researchers recommended assessing the patient for these factors preoperatively to guide monitoring to prevent respiratory compromise during the procedure, improve patient outcomes, and reduce costs. In a nonexperimental study of 239 patients who underwent colonoscopy, Patel et al[74] found that chronic daily opioid users required more sedation with fentanyl and midazolam than patients with a history of alcohol abuse and patients with no history of substance abuse.

| 2.2.1 | Assess older adult patients for |
| • **frailty**,[69,89]
| • **functional status**,[89-91] and
| • **cognitive impairment** (eg, delirium).[68,90-92]
[Recommendation]

Frailty is more reliable than chronological age as a predictor of surgical patient morbidity and mortality in older adults.[69,93] Older adults with a higher frailty score are at greater risk for surgical complications, longer hospital stays, discharge to a nursing home or an assisted living facility, hospital readmissions, and death.[89] Identifying frailty in the older adult may improve the patient's postoperative prognosis by facilitating shared decision making and identifying any **prehabilitation** opportunities.[69]

Preoperative functional impairment is a significant risk factor for poor surgical outcomes, especially in older adults, and is a predictor of mortality after major surgery.[91] The benefits of identifying impaired functional status in the older adult patient include identifying perioperative care needs, determining the ideal discharge location, and facilitating discharge planning.[90,91]

Preoperative cognitive impairment is associated with failure to arrive at scheduled procedures, increased use of emergency and rehabilitative services, prolonged hospitalization and complications, and elevated incidence of delirium.[90] The benefits of identifying cognitive impairment in the older adult patient include identifying the need for prehabilitation, facilitating discharge planning, and increasing perioperative monitoring.[68,90]

| 2.2.2 | An interdisciplinary team that includes the director of anesthesia services should determine additional assessment criteria for pediatric patients, such as
- history of premature birth,
- congenital anomalies,
- presence of autism spectrum disorder,
- behavioral issues,
- traumatic childhood experiences, and
- developmental or physical delays.[94]
[Recommendation] **P**

| 2.3 | A physical status classification tool (eg, the ASA Physical Status Classification [Table 1])[95] **may be used to determine patient acuity** [Conditional Recommendation]

A benefit of using a physical status classification tool is that it can provide an objective measurement of the patient's acuity. The ASA Physical Status Classification system is a widely used tool.[95] Patients classified as ASA I, ASA II, and medically stable ASA III are normally considered to be candidates for RN-administered moderate sedation/analgesia.[46,60,96]

Table 1. ASA Physical Status Classification System

Classification	Definition	Adult Examples	Pediatric Examples [P]
ASA I	A normal healthy patient	Healthy, non-smoking, no or minimal alcohol use	Healthy (no acute or chronic disease), normal BMI percentile for age
ASA II	A patient with mild systemic disease	Mild diseases only without substantive functional limitations. Examples include (but not limited to): current smoker, social alcohol drinker, pregnancy, obesity (30 < BMI < 40), well-controlled DM/HTN, mild lung disease	Asymptomatic congenital cardiac disease, well controlled dysrhythmias, asthma without exacerbation, well controlled epilepsy, non-insulin dependent diabetes mellitus, abnormal BMI percentile for age, mild/moderate OSA, oncologic state in remission, autism with mild limitations
ASA III	A patient with severe systemic disease	Substantive functional limitations; One or more moderate to severe diseases. Examples include (but not limited to): poorly controlled DM or HTN, COPD, morbid obesity (BMI ≥ 40), active hepatitis, alcohol dependence or abuse, implanted pacemaker, moderate reduction of ejection fraction, ESRD undergoing regularly scheduled dialysis, history (> 3 months) of MI, CVA, TIA, or CAD/stents	Uncorrected stable congenital cardiac abnormality, asthma with exacerbation, poorly controlled epilepsy, insulin dependent diabetes mellitus, morbid obesity, malnutrition, severe OSA, oncologic state, renal failure, muscular dystrophy, cystic fibrosis, history of organ transplantation, brain/spinal cord malformation, symptomatic hydrocephalus, premature infant PCA < 60 weeks, autism with severe limitations, metabolic disease, difficult airway, long term parenteral nutrition. Full term infants < 6 weeks of age
ASA IV	A patient with severe systemic disease that is a constant threat to life	Recent (< 3 months) MI, CVA, TIA, or CAD/stents, ongoing cardiac ischemia or severe valve dysfunction, severe reduction of ejection fraction, sepsis, DIC, ARD or ESRD not undergoing regularly scheduled dialysis	Symptomatic congenital cardiac abnormality, congestive heart failure, active sequelae of prematurity, acute hypoxic-ischemic encephalopathy, shock, sepsis, disseminated intravascular coagulation, automatic implantable cardioverter-defibrillator, ventilator dependence, endocrinopathy, severe trauma, severe respiratory distress, advanced oncologic state
ASA V	A moribund patient who is not expected to survive without the operation	Ruptured abdominal/thoracic aneurysm, massive trauma, intracranial bleed with mass effect, ischemic bowel in the face of significant cardiac pathology or multiple organ/system dysfunction	Massive trauma, intracranial hemorrhage with mass effect, patient requiring ECMO, respiratory failure or arrest, malignant hypertension, decompensated congestive heart failure, hepatic encephalopathy, ischemic bowel or multiple organ/system dysfunction
ASA VI	A declared brain-dead patient whose organs are being removed for donor purposes		

Reproduced with permission from the American Society of Anesthesiologists, Schaumburg, IL.

2.4 Assess the patient for characteristics that may indicate risk for difficulty with mask ventilation, including

- age > 55 years[85];
- obesity[1,71,85];
- a history of snoring, stridor, or sleep apnea[1,71,85];
- missing teeth, protruding incisors, loose teeth, dental appliances (eg, dentures, partials, veneers)[1,64,82,85];
- presence of a beard[71,85];
- a short neck[1,71,82,85];
- limited neck extension[1,71,82,85,97];
- cervical spine disease or trauma[1,85];
- presence of a neck mass[1,85];
- decreased hyoid-mental distance (eg, < 3 finger breadths in an adult)[1,71,82,85];
- dysmorphic facial features (eg, Pierre-Robin syndrome)[1,82,85];

- a small mouth opening (eg, < 3 cm in an adult)[1,85];
- a high, arched palate[1,82,85];
- macroglossia[1];
- a nonvisible uvula[1,82,85];
- a Mallampati classification of III or IV[71,85] (Figure 2);
- jaw abnormalities (eg, micrognathia, retrognathia)[1,85];
- a history of problems with anesthesia or sedation[1,64];
- advanced rheumatoid arthritis[1];
- chromosomal abnormality (eg, trisomy 21)[1,82]; and
- tonsillar hypertrophy.[1,82]

[Recommendation]

Clinical practice guidelines[1,64,82] and low-quality evidence[71,85,97] support using predictive factors to anticipate a difficult or impossible mask ventilation. The respiratory depressive effects of moderate sedation/analgesia medications may compromise respiration, and the ability to ventilate a patient with a mask is vital if there is an unanticipated compromised airway.[1] The potential harms to the patient associated with a difficult airway include death, brain injury, cardiopulmonary arrest, an unnecessary surgical airway, airway trauma, and damage to the teeth.[82]

Lee et al[98] conducted a systematic review and meta-analysis of 42 prospective observational studies of patients undergoing general anesthesia who had a preoperative Mallampati test assessment. They compared the results with the subsequent assessment rate of a difficult airway. The authors concluded that the Mallampati assessment was accurate in predicting difficult laryngoscopy and intubation but was not accurate in predicting difficult mask ventilation.

2.5 Assess the patient for risk of obstructive sleep apnea.[83,84,99-102] [Recommendation]

Clinical practice guidelines[83,84,101,102] and moderate-quality evidence[99,100] support the assessment and screening of patients for obstructive sleep apnea. Identifying patients with obstructive sleep apnea before surgery may provide opportunities for heightened awareness and implementation of interventions that reduce the patient's risk of experiencing adverse events.[84]

Obstructive sleep apnea is a sleep-related breathing disorder characterized by periodic, partial, or complete obstruction of the upper airway during sleep.[83,84,101] The repeated arousals from sleep to restore airway patency may cause

- daytime sleepiness,
- neurocognitive dysfunction (eg, attention/vigilance, delayed long-term visual and verbal memory),

- cerebrovascular disease,
- cardiovascular disorders (eg, hypertension, ischemic heart disease, arrhythmia, pulmonary hypertension, congestive heart failure),
- metabolic dysfunction, and
- depression.[83,84,101]

Moderate sedation/analgesia medications that affect the central nervous system may interfere with the normal respiratory compensatory mechanisms of hypoxemia and hypercarbia, and depressant medications may increase the risk of pharyngeal collapse in patients with obstructive sleep apnea.[102,103]

Complications associated with obstructive sleep apnea during perioperative care include oxygen desaturation, pulmonary complications, cardiac complications (eg, atrial fibrillation), and death.[84]

2.5.1 Use a screening tool that has been validated in surgical patients to assess the patient for obstructive sleep apnea,[84] such as the

- STOP-Bang tool,[100,101,104-107]
- Berlin questionnaire,[104,108]
- perioperative sleep apnea prediction (P-SAP) score,[109] and
- ASA checklist for the identification and assessment of obstructive sleep apnea.[83,104,108]

[Recommendation]

Obstructive sleep apnea screening tools are used to classify patients based on clinical symptoms and risk factors to determine high-risk patients who may need a referral to a higher level of care (eg, an anesthesia professional) or additional diagnostic testing (ie, polysomnography).[104] Representative questions in the screening tools ask about BMI, hypertension, loud snoring, apnea during sleep, tiredness during the day, and neck size. Although multiple researchers have investigated obstructive sleep apnea screening tools, many tools are not validated in surgical patient populations.[84]

Joshi et al[101] conducted a systematic review to develop the Society for Ambulatory Anesthesia (SAMBA) consensus statement on preoperative selection of adult patients with obstructive sleep apnea scheduled for ambulatory surgery. The SAMBA recommends use of the STOP-Bang questionnaire for obstructive sleep apnea screening because it is easy to administer and has a high sensitivity.

Abrishami et al[104] conducted a systematic review to identify and evaluate the available screening questionnaires for obstructive sleep apnea. The review included an analysis of nine prospective studies and one retrospective study with a total of 1,484 patients in the 10 studies. The authors found that the Wisconsin

Figure 2. Mallampati Classification

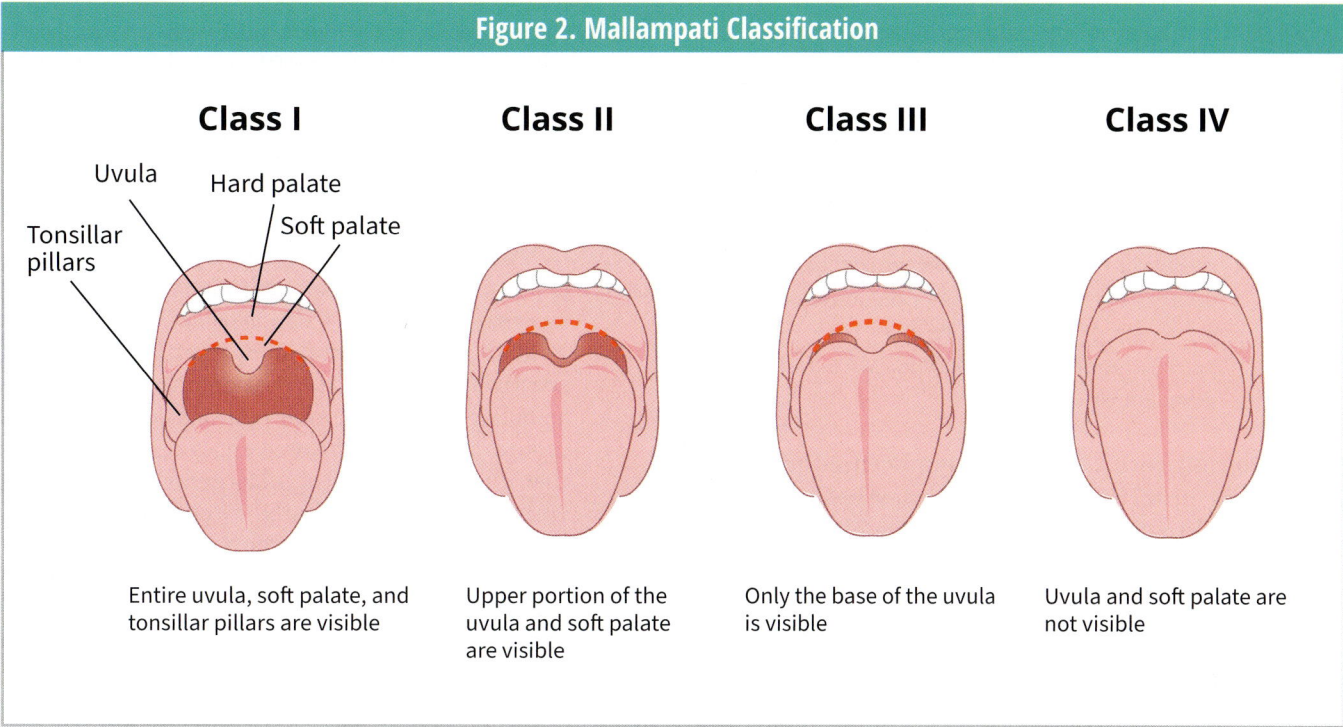

Class I	Class II	Class III	Class IV
Entire uvula, soft palate, and tonsillar pillars are visible	Upper portion of the uvula and soft palate are visible	Only the base of the uvula is visible	Uvula and soft palate are not visible

(Class I labels: Tonsillar pillars, Uvula, Hard palate, Soft palate)

and the Berlin questionnaires had the highest sensitivity and specificity for predicting the existence of obstructive sleep apnea. The STOP and the STOP-Bang questionnaires had the highest methodological validity, reasonable accuracy, and easy-to-use features. Based on these findings, the authors recommend the use of the STOP and STOP-Bang questionnaires to screen surgical patients for obstructive sleep apnea.

2.5.2 **Use a screening tool that has been validated in pediatric surgical patients (eg, Snoring, Trouble Breathing, Un-Refreshed [STBUR][110]) to assess the pediatric patient for obstructive sleep apnea.** *[Recommendation]* **P**

2.5.3 **Consult with the supervising licensed independent practitioner and an anesthesia professional if the patient presents with a history of obstructive sleep apnea or is identified during screening as at high risk for obstructive sleep apnea.** *[Recommendation]*

Patients who have severe obstructive sleep apnea may not be candidates for RN-administered moderate sedation/analgesia because they are at increased risk for difficult mask ventilation, and anesthetic and analgesic medications can interact with or affect consciousness, sleep, upper airway anatomy and physiology, arousal responses, muscle activation, and ventilatory drive.[1,83,102]

2.5.4 **Take additional precautions for patients who have obstructive sleep apnea, including**
- **being prepared for non-invasive positive pressure ventilation**[66,84,101,111] **(eg, continuous positive airway pressure [CPAP], bilevel positive airway pressure [BiPAP]); and**
- **careful titration of opioids**[1,99,102] **or non-opioid analgesia techniques.**[101]

[Recommendation]

Moderate sedation/analgesia medications may cause relaxation of the oropharyngeal structures, resulting in partial or total airway obstruction that may require positive pressure ventilation with CPAP or BiPAP.[1,83,84] In a quality improvement project, Willard et al[111] developed and implemented use of a nasal ventilation mask for patients with obstructive sleep apnea or obesity undergoing moderate or deep sedation for esophagogastroduodenoscopy (EGD) and colonoscopy procedures. The researchers found that the nasal ventilation mask offered supportive ventilation and had the ability to provide positive pressure assistive breaths.

Opioids, such as fentanyl, have depressant effects on the respiratory system, and patients who have obstructive sleep apnea may be at increased risk for respiratory complications from use of these medications.[102] Furthermore, opioid potency and pain perception may be augmented in patients who have obstructive sleep apnea because of chronic intermittent hypoxia and habitual sleep disruption.[102] Cozowicz et al[99] conducted a systematic review of 40 studies and found that patients with obstructive sleep apnea could be at increased risk for developing opioid-induced respiratory depression without overdosing. The initial 24 hours after opioid administration appeared to be the most critical for the development of life-threatening respiratory depression. The researchers recommended taking a cautious approach to opioid use, including patient monitoring, in patients with obstructive sleep apnea.

2.6 **Consult with the supervising licensed independent practitioner and an anesthesia professional to develop a perioperative plan of care if a patient presents with any of the following:**

- **previous difficulties with anesthesia or sedation, including difficult airway[1,60];**
- **obstructive sleep apnea or other airway-related issues (eg, obesity hypoventilation syndrome)[1,59,96];**
- **known history of respiratory instability[47] (eg, chronic obstructive pulmonary disease) or hemodynamic instability;**
- **history of coagulation abnormality[96];**
- **moderate to severe neurologic disease (eg, stroke, cerebrovascular accident, transient ischemic attack) or cardiac disease (eg, coronary artery disease, congestive heart failure, poorly controlled hypertension, implanted pacemaker, recent myocardial infarction);**
- **moderate to severe endocrine disease (eg, poorly controlled diabetes mellitus);**
- **history of renal disease (eg, acute renal failure, end stage renal disease) or liver disease (eg, active hepatitis, cirrhosis, liver failure) that may affect metabolism of medications administered for moderate sedation/analgesia;**
- **one or more significant comorbidities;**
- **pregnancy;**
- **inability to communicate (eg, aphasia);**
- **inability to tolerate the procedure[96];**
- **multiple drug allergies;**
- **use of medications with potential for drug interaction with sedative analgesics;**
- **polypharmacy[46,89,91,92];**
- **current substance abuse (eg, street drugs, alcohol, non-prescribed prescription drugs)[60];**
- **ASA physical status classification of ASA III[2,45,47,60]; or**
- **ASA physical status classification of ASA IV or above.[2,45,60,96]**

[Recommendation]

2.7 **Determine the patient's preference[112] and suitability for moderate sedation/analgesia based on the selection criteria developed by the collaboration of an interdisciplinary team (eg, perioperative RNs, anesthesia professionals, surgeons, endoscopists, quality and risk managers).** *[Recommendation]*

Moderate-quality evidence supports the importance of patient selection to facilitate optimal patient outcomes and prevent sedation failure.[30,51,96,113]

In a nonexperimental study, Chittle et al[112] retrospectively evaluated 198 patients who underwent ambulatory vascular interventional radiology procedures who were educated about sedation options then given the choice of undergoing the procedure with local anesthetic only, minimal sedation, or moderate sedation. The patients had variable preferences for sedation and venous access device placement, which the researchers identified as an opportunity for shared decision making to empower patients to select the option most aligned with their goals.

2.8 **Collaborate with the patient[112] and the supervising licensed independent practitioner to develop and implement the sedation plan.[2,64,114]** *[Recommendation]*

2.8.1 **Determine the need for IV access depending on the level of sedation intended; the route of medication administration (eg, intravenous, intranasal, oral); and organizational policy, procedure, and protocol.[1,2]** *[Recommendation]*

Intravenous administration of both a sedative to reduce anxiety and an analgesic to manage pain increases the probability of satisfactory moderate sedation/analgesia. Intravenous access provides a route for administration of rescue medications if needed.[1,2]

2.8.2 **No recommendation can be made for patient-controlled sedation.** *[No Recommendation]*

Although low-quality evidence supports the safe use of patient-controlled sedation,[10,115,116] further research is needed to evaluate the benefits and harms of patient-controlled sedation and establish patient selection criteria.

In a systematic review with meta-analysis of 13 RCTs that compared patient-controlled sedation with clinician-controlled sedation with propofol (N = 1,103 patients), Kreienbül et al[115] found that patient-controlled sedation in low- to medium-risk middle-aged nonobese patients had no impact on the risk of oxygen desaturation and significantly less use of rescue interventions for sedation-related adverse events. However, the researchers reported that the quality of the evidence was very low and that further high-quality research is needed to assess the risks and benefits of patient-controlled sedation. The researchers also noted that patient-controlled sedation may not be suitable for every patient, and that the patient must be able and willing to use a pump device and take responsibility for their own sedation.

Clements et al[10] conducted a RCT in Australia to compare radiologist-controlled sedation (n = 20), which was administered by a sedation nurse, and patient-controlled sedation (n = 20) with fentanyl and midazolam. The researchers found that there were no adverse events, and that patient-controlled sedation was not inferior to radiologist-controlled sedation for sedative dose and degree of sedation, with low cost and minimal additional training required for implementation.

In a literature review, Pambianco and Niklewski[116] found that use of patient-controlled sedation in endoscopy procedures produced differing results in patient satisfaction. They supported medication and patient selection as key elements to successful use of patient-controlled sedation.

2.8.3 A communication tool may be used to facilitate communication between the patient and the RN who is administering moderate sedation/analgesia. The tool may include

- a description of the procedure;
- the benefits and risks of the procedure;
- the adverse effects that may occur during or after the procedure;
- the choices that the patient can make for the sedation plan;
- a place for the patient to write down
  - benefits that are important to them,
  - their concerns about risks, and
  - questions or concerns about the options;
- a method for evaluating understanding; and
- a list of resources the patient can access for more information.[117]

[Conditional Recommendation]

In a literature review, Southerland et al[117] found that patients who will undergo anesthesia may benefit from using a tool (ie, patient decision aid) to support patient-centered care delivery and shared decision making. The benefits to the patient may include feeling better informed; having more knowledge; and having less anxiety, depression, and decisional conflict.

3. Continual Patient Monitoring

3.1 Before administering medication for moderate sedation/analgesia, obtain and document the patient's baseline physiological and psychological responses, including

- pulse,
- blood pressure,
- respiratory rate,
- SpO₂ by pulse oximetry,
- end-tidal carbon dioxide (CO_2) by capnography,
- pain level,
- anxiety level, and
- level of consciousness.[1,2,46,47,64-66,118,119]

[Recommendation]

Baseline preoperative vital signs provide a reference for comparison if the patient experiences any changes (eg, cardiac depression, respiratory depression) in response to the administration of medications for moderate sedation/analgesia.[1,2]

3.2 Continually monitor and observe the patient throughout the procedure.[1,2] *[Recommendation]*

Continual monitoring and observation of the patient's physiological and psychological status can lead to early detection of potential complications.[1,2]

3.3 The RN administering moderate sedation/analgesia should be in constant attendance with unrestricted immediate access to the patient and have no competing responsibilities that would compromise continual monitoring and assessment of the patient.[1,2,66] *[Recommendation]*

The care of the patient receiving moderate sedation/analgesia requires constant vigilance and monitoring to allow for an immediate response to any adverse reaction, complication, or need to titrate sedatives or analgesics.[1,2]

3.3.1 Two perioperative RNs should be assigned to care for the patient receiving moderate sedation/analgesia. One RN should administer the sedation medication and continually monitor the patient and the other RN should perform the circulating role. *[Recommendation]*

AORN maintains that every surgical patient needs the care of a perioperative RN for the duration of any operative or other invasive procedure and actively promotes laws and regulations to ensure the supervisory presence of the professional RN in the perioperative setting. A minimum of one perioperative RN circulator dedicated to each patient undergoing an operative or other invasive procedure facilitates the provision of safe, quality patient care in the perioperative setting.[120]

3.3.2 **The perioperative RN administering moderate sedation/analgesia may perform short, interruptible tasks (eg, opening additional suture, tying a gown) to assist the perioperative team, as long as these tasks do not compromise the continual monitoring of the patient and the RN remains within the operating or procedure room.[1,2,44,45,47,121]** *[Conditional Recommendation]*

Clinical practice guidelines support that the practitioner administering moderate sedation/analgesia can perform brief, interruptible tasks that do not compromise the continual monitoring of the patient.[1,2,44,45,47,121]

3.3.3 **The perioperative RN administering propofol for moderate sedation/analgesia should be completely dedicated to the task of monitoring the patient and should not perform any other tasks to assist the perioperative team.[25]** *[Recommendation]*

Propofol has a narrow therapeutic window, and there is potential for respiratory and cardiopulmonary complications, such as hypotension, bradycardia, apnea, and airway obstruction, that require early recognition and intervention by a practitioner who is completely dedicated to monitoring the patient.[25]

3.4 **Monitor and document the patient's physiological and psychological responses, identify nursing diagnoses based on assessment of the data, and implement the plan of care.[1,2]** *[Recommendation]*

The perioperative RN can detect the early signs of potential cardiorespiratory complications by continually monitoring and observing the patient's physiological and psychological status. Early recog-

nition and management of cardiac or respiratory depression may prevent hypoxic brain damage, cardiac arrest, or death.

3.4.1 **Include the following in intraoperative patient monitoring and documentation:**
- **cardiac rate and rhythm,**
- **blood pressure,**
- **respiratory rate,**
- **SpO$_2$ by pulse oximetry,**
- **end-tidal CO$_2$ by capnography,**
- **depth of sedation assessment** (Table 2)**,**
- **pain level,**
- **anxiety level, and**
- **level of consciousness.[1,2,46,47,64-66,118,119]**
[Recommendation]

Clinical practice guidelines support monitoring and documenting the patient's vital signs (eg, heart rate, blood pressure, SpO$_2$) when the patient is receiving moderate sedation/analgesia.[1,2,46,47,64-66,118,119] The early signs of cardiac and respiratory depression can be recognized by monitoring and documenting cardiac rate and rhythm, blood pressure, respiratory rate, oxygen saturation, end-tidal CO$_2$, depth of sedation, pain level, anxiety level, and level of consciousness.

High-quality evidence supports monitoring end-tidal CO$_2$ when the patient is receiving moderate sedation/analgesia.[122,123] Klare et al[122] conducted an RCT in Germany of 238 patients who underwent endoscopic retrograde cholangiopancreatography (ERCP) with midazolam and propofol sedation and either standard monitoring (n = 117) or capnographic monitoring (n = 121). The researchers found that apnea was more frequently detected with capnographic monitoring.

In a prospective cohort study, Barnett et al[123] compared sedation safety and patient

Table 2. Continuum of Depth of Sedation

	Minimal sedation anxiolysis	Moderate sedation/ analgesia ("conscious sedation")	Deep sedation/ analgesia	General anesthesia
Responsiveness	Normal response to verbal stimulation	Purposeful response to verbal or tactile stimulation	Purposeful response after repeated or painful stimulation	Unarousable even with painful stimulus
Airway	Unaffected	No intervention required	Intervention may be required	Intervention often required
Spontaneous ventilation	Unaffected	Adequate	May be inadequate	Frequently inadequate
Cardiovascular function	Unaffected	Usually maintained	Usually maintained	May be impaired

Reproduced with permission from the American Society of Anesthesiologists, Schaumburg, IL.

satisfaction in 966 patients before and after end-tidal CO_2 monitoring was implemented for outpatient colonoscopy with midazolam and fentanyl used for moderate sedation/analgesia. The researchers found that the addition of end-tidal CO_2 did not significantly improve patient safety or patient satisfaction, but it did increase cost. The researchers recommended reserving end-tidal CO_2 monitoring for patients at higher risk for adverse events since colonoscopy with moderate sedation is a low-risk procedure.

3.4.2 **Include the following in the postoperative assessment, monitoring, and documentation:**
- **cardiac rate and rhythm,**
- **blood pressure,**
- **respiratory rate,**
- **SpO₂,**
- **pain level,**
- **sedation level,**
- **level of consciousness,**
- **intravenous line (eg, patency, site, type of fluid),**
- **condition of the dressing and wound, and**
- **type and patency of drainage tubes.**[66]

[Recommendation]

3.4.3 **Assess the patient's level of consciousness by evaluating the patient's ability to respond purposefully to verbal commands either alone or with light tactile stimulation.**[1] *[Recommendation]*

Assessing the patient's level of consciousness by the patient's verbal responses at regular intervals during the procedure allows for quick determination of whether the patient is also breathing well. In addition, verbally reassuring the patient can divert the patient's attention and assist in reducing anxiety.

3.4.4 **Assess and document depth of sedation using an objective scale**[66] **that has been validated for use in surgical patients, such as the**
- **ASA Continuum of Sedation Scale,**[27,61,124]
- **Modified Observer's Assessment of Alertness/Sedation Scale,**[12,14,27-29,125,126]
- **Pasero Opioid-Induced Sedation Scale,**[127]
- **Ramsay Sedation Scale,**[27,30,31,128,129]
- **Modified Ramsay Sedation Scale,**[61,125]
- **Modified Richmond Agitation and Sedation**[125] **or**
- **Sedation Agitation Scale.**[130]

[Recommendation]

Several professional organizations[61,66,124,131] and moderate-quality evidence[127,130] have established the benefits of assessing and documenting the depth of sedation with an objective scale. It is important to use a scale that has been validated for use in surgical patients because many sedation scales were developed for use in critically ill patients who are sedated for different indications and for longer periods of time than surgical patients.

Nisbet and Mooney-Cotter[127] conducted a descriptive, survey-based study to determine validity and reliability of several sedation scales. They concluded that because sedation occurs on a continuum that is unknowable and unpredictable, it must be measured as accurately as possible. Changes in a patient's condition can be communicated with a valid, reliable, and easy-to-use sedation scale (eg, the Pasero Opioid-Induced Sedation Scale). Use of an objective scale facilitates timely recognition of advancing sedation and appropriate nursing actions of dose reduction, escalation of care, team communication, and management of treatment options.

In a retrospective study, Zhong et al[130] applied use of the Sedation Agitation Scale for assessment of sedation in pediatric patients who underwent bronchoscopy. The researchers found that it was a useful tool to guide individualized administration of midazolam to achieve ideal sedative effect and reduce adverse reactions.

Although several researchers used sedation scales as an objective measurement of sedation in their studies, investigation of the sedation scale was not an intended outcome of the study.[12,14,27-31,125,126,128,129]

3.4.5 **Bispectral index (BIS) monitoring may be used as adjunct technology to measure the patient's level of sedation when propofol is used.** *[Conditional Recommendation]*

When BIS monitoring is used, the National Institute for Health and Care Excellence supports using BIS monitors in combination with standard clinical monitoring to indicate the patient's response to anesthetic medications during surgery **(Table 3)**.[132]

Although BIS monitoring is more commonly used for general anesthesia, high-quality evidence supports using BIS monitoring when titrating propofol during endoscopy.[126] Park et al[126] conducted a systematic review and meta-analysis of 11 RCTs that included 1,039 patients who underwent gastrointestinal endoscopy

Table 3. Bispectral (BIS) Index Values[1-3]

Value*	Description
0	Coma, absence of cerebral electrical activity
0-40	Deep hypnotic state
40-60	General anesthesia
60-90	Varying levels of conscious sedation (ie, minimal to deep sedation)
90-100	Awake

The BIS is a direct measure of the effects of anesthetics and sedatives on the brain. The BIS is an integrated measure of cerebral electrical activity, derived from the electroencephalogram. Values for BIS range on a scale of zero to 100, with the numbers correlated to level of sedation.

Reference

1. *Depth of anaesthesia monitors – bispectral index (BIS), E-Entropy and Narcotrend-Compact M. National Institute for Health and Care Excellence (NICE). https://www.nice.org.uk/guidance/dg6/documents/depth-of-anaesthesia-monitors-eentropy-bis-and-narcotrend-diagnostics-consultation-document. Published November 21, 2012. Accessed June 17, 2021.*

under propofol sedation with and without BIS monitoring. The researchers found that total propofol consumption was significantly lower with BIS monitoring and recommended use of BIS monitoring as a safe and effective method for avoiding unnecessary administration of propofol during endoscopic procedures.

However, other evidence is inconclusive about whether BIS monitoring provides additional benefit when monitoring the patient who is receiving moderate sedation/analgesia.

Conway and Sutherland[133] conducted a systematic review and meta-analysis of 16 RCTs that included 2,138 patients who underwent procedural sedation and analgesia with propofol for endoscopy procedures and had depth of anesthesia monitoring with electroencephalogram devices, including BIS. The researchers found that use of the monitoring devices for adults reduced the amount of propofol administered but did not reduce adverse events cause by oversedation or reduce recovery duration.

Heo et al[29] conducted an RCT of 280 patients in South Korea who underwent moderate sedation with propofol administered by a nurse during colonoscopy. The patients were monitored with either BIS or a Modified Observer's Assessment of Alertness and Sedation scale. The researchers found that BIS monitoring was not effective for titrating the propofol dose when compared to use of the sedation scale.

In contrast, Jokelainen et al[125] conducted a prospective validation study in Finland of 200 patients who underwent sedation with propo-

fol for ERCP, to evaluate different methods of assessing depth of sedation, including BIS monitoring and multiple sedation scales (ie, Modified Observer's Assessment of Alertness and Sedation, Modified Ramsay Sedation, Modified Richmond Agitation/Sedation). The researchers found that a limitation of using the sedation scales was that they required the patient to respond to verbal or tactile stimuli, which impaired the ERCP procedure. Therefore, the researchers suggested that BIS monitoring may be preferrable in the clinical setting because the information is collected directly from the electroencephalogram rather than requiring the patient to respond.

In a nonexperimental study, Gelfand et al[134] retrospectively reviewed 55,210 intraoperative patient records and found that BIS monitoring was more likely to be used for complex procedures. These procedures included those for older adult patients, patients with a higher ASA physical status classification, and patients with extremes of BMI; procedures that used total intravenous anesthesia, a long-acting paralytic agent, or an endotracheal tube; emergency surgery; longer procedures; and procedures in certain surgical services.

Although there is a larger body of evidence on BIS monitoring during general anesthesia, further research is needed to evaluate the benefits and harms of BIS monitoring during RN-administered moderate sedation/analgesia, including the outcomes of anesthetic medication use, anesthesia awareness, postoperative complications (eg, delirium), ability to distinguish between moderate and deep sedation/analgesia, patient satisfaction, recovery time, and costs.

3.5 **Verify that monitoring equipment (eg, pulse oximetry, electrocardiogram, capnography, blood pressure measurement devices)[1,2,44,135]; oxygen source, tubing, cannulas and masks[1,2,44,49]; and suction source, tubing, and tips[1,2,44,49] are working properly, and are immediately available in the room where the procedure is being performed.** *[Recommendation]*

3.5.1 **Verify that clinical alarms of automatic monitoring devices are audible and set to alert the perioperative RN to critical changes in the patient's status.[1,45,62,66]** *[Recommendation]*

A clinical alarm (eg, cardiac monitor, capnography, pulse oximetry) is patient specific and used for the purpose of alerting team members to critical changes in the patient's condition. Patients have experienced injuries and near misses because alarms were turned off or inaudible.[62,136]

3.6 Verify that emergency resuscitation equipment and supplies are immediately available in every location in which moderate sedation/analgesia is administered.[1,2,44,45,47,57,66] *[Recommendation]*

Even though careful titration of sedation medications and analgesics to obtain the desired effect can make the use of short-acting agents very safe, respiratory depression, hypotension, or impaired cardiovascular function are common sequelae of sedation and analgesia.[1]

3.6.1 Emergency equipment and supplies should include
- resuscitation medications,[1,2,44,47,58,60,66]
- opioid and benzodiazepine antagonists,[1,66]
- age- and size-appropriate airway and ventilatory equipment (eg, laryngoscopes, endotracheal tubes, laryngeal mask airway, oral and nasal airways, mechanical positive bag-valve mask device),[1,2,44,47,58,66]
- defibrillators and defibrillation pads (eg, adult, pediatric),[1,2,44,47,58,66] and
- IV fluids and access equipment.[47,66]

[Recommendation] **P**

4. Medication Administration

4.1 The perioperative RN who is administering moderate sedation/analgesia should know the intended purpose, recommended dose, recommended dilution, onset, duration, effects, potential adverse reactions, drug compatibility, and contraindications for each medication used during moderate sedation/analgesia.[2,63,66] *[Recommendation]*

4.2 Before administering medications, verify the medication order, including the correct dosing parameters, and identify the patient-specific maximum dose by consulting either the health care organization's medication formulary, a pharmacist, a physician, or the product information sheet or other published reference material.[63] *[Recommendation]*

4.2.1 Adjust doses of sedatives and analgesics when caring for an older adult, as directed by the supervising practitioner.[67,137] *[Recommendation]*

Older adults who receive sedatives and analgesics, especially opioids and benzodiazepines, are at higher risk for overdose, severe sedation-related adverse events (eg, respiratory depression,[89] death), falls, fractures caused by falls, cognitive impairment, induced or worsened delirium, and worsened dementia.[67] Additionally, meperidine may have a higher risk of causing neurotoxicity, including delirium, than other opioids in older adults.[67] Because of these risks, the American Society for Gastrointestinal Endoscopy recommends administering fewer sedatives and analgesics at a slower rate with lower initial and cumulative doses.[137]

Moderate-quality evidence supports lowering medication dosages for older adults[138] and that older adults are more likely to experience a deeper level of sedation.[70]

In a review of sedation practices reported in the Clinical Outcomes Research Initiative endoscopic database (N = 1,385,436 patients who underwent colonoscopy), Childers et al[138] found that progressively less sedation was used in older patients.

Yeo et al[70] conducted a prospective study of 97 patients who underwent plastic surgical procedures under conscious sedation with midazolam and ketamine that was dosed according to the same perioperative sedation protocol. The researchers found that older age was significantly associated with a deeper level of sedation.

4.3 Administer intravenous medications one at a time, in incremental doses, and titrate to the desired effect (ie, moderate sedation that enables the patient to maintain protective reflexes, a patent airway, and spontaneous ventilation).[1,2] *[Recommendation]*

The incremental administration of agents decreases the risk for overdose and respiratory or circulatory depression because the person administering the agents can better observe the patient's response to the medications given.[1,2]

However, in a retrospective analysis of 1,665 patients who underwent colonoscopy, Finn et al[15] compared nurse-directed titration of sedation (n = 966) to physician-directed administration of bolus sedative (n = 699) and found that patients receiving the bolus had a significantly shorter sedation time, had a slightly longer colonoscopy time (25 minutes versus 24 minutes), received a lower weight-adjusted dose of fentanyl and midazolam, and had less risk for developing hypotension. There was no difference in patient satisfaction between the groups.

Further research is needed to compare bolus dosing with titration of sedation in patients receiving moderate sedation/analgesia.

4.4 When administering medications by a nonintravenous route (eg, oral, rectal, intramuscular, intranasal, transmucosal), allow sufficient time for drug absorption and onset before considering additional medication.[1,2] *[Recommendation]* **P**

The absorption rate of nonintravenous medications may be unpredictable because of delayed drug absorption and elimination.[1]

For pediatric patients, high-quality evidence establishes the benefit and safety of using nonintravenous medications, including intranasal[139-146] or oral[140,141,147-151] midazolam, intranasal dexmedetomidine,[152-157] intranasal fentanyl,[158,159] and intranasal ketamine.[142,149]

For adult patients, use of nonintravenous medications was studied in cataract surgery and dental procedures.

Chen et al[160] conducted an RCT of 156 patients older than 65 years who underwent cataract surgery with either oral diazepam (n = 73) or IV midazolam (n = 83). The researchers found that patients who received oral diazepam had less frequent undesired movement during surgery, although there was not a significant difference in cooperation, pain, or anxiety.

Rignell et al[161] retrospectively reviewed the records of 61 patients undergoing dental procedures who were sedated with oral midazolam and ranged in age from 62 to 93 years. The researchers found that sedation with oral midazolam was safe and effective in dental treatment of persons with major neurocognitive disorders (eg, memory problems, loss of intellectual abilities) who had a history of difficulty tolerating treatment.

Ryu et al[162] conducted an RCT of 240 patients ages 16 to 55 years who were sedated for third molar extraction with either local anesthesia only (n = 80), intranasal dexmedetomidine (n = 80), or IV dexmedetomidine (n = 80). The researchers found that although sedation was slightly deeper with the IV route, both IV and intranasal routes of dexmedetomidine administration were effective and safe for sedation in outpatient surgical procedures.

4.5 Under the direction of the supervising practitioner, the perioperative RN who is administering moderate sedation/analgesia should determine the necessity, method, and flow rate of oxygen administration based on the patient's optimal level of oxygen saturation as measured with pulse oximetry. *[Recommendation]*

High-quality evidence and clinical practice guidelines establish the benefit of using supplemental oxygen during moderate sedation/analgesia procedures.[1,2,45,163] Supplemental oxygen may decrease the patient's risk of oxygen desaturation during moderate sedation/analgesia.

Rozario et al[163] conducted a prospective, randomized, non-blinded study to evaluate the use of supplemental oxygen before and during EGD and colonoscopy procedures with moderate sedation and the occurrence of clinically significant desaturation events. Patients in the experimental group (n = 194) received low-flow oxygen at 2 L/minute before the administration of moderate sedation. The patients in the control group (n = 195) did not routinely receive oxygen unless an episode of desaturation (ie, oxygen saturation ≤ 95%) occurred. In the control group, 138 (70.8%) of the patients experienced a desaturation event compared with 24 (12.4%) in the experimental group. The experimental group was 98% less likely than the control group to experience any episode of desaturation. The researchers concluded that their results supported the routine use of supplemental oxygen at 2 L/minute to prevent desaturation during endoscopy procedures with moderate sedation.

4.6 Document the moderate sedation/analgesia medications administered, including the

- medication,
- strength,
- amount administered,
- route,
- time of each dose,
- patient response, and
- adverse reactions.[63,64]

[Recommendation]

4.7 Verify that opioid antagonists (eg, naloxone) and benzodiazepine antagonists (eg, flumazenil) are readily available before opioids and benzodiazepines are administered.[1,66] *[Recommendation]*

Moderate-quality evidence supports having naloxone and flumazenil available when opioids and benzodiazepines are administered for sedation.[164-166]

In a retrospective chart review, Hung et al[164] identified 45 cases of reversal agents (ie, naloxone, flumazenil) being used during a 6-year period that included 42,119 EGD procedures and 88,016 colonoscopies performed at a large teaching hospital, for a prevalence of 0.03% use of reversal agents. The researchers found that events triggering reversal use were oxygen desaturation, respiration changes, hypotension, and bradycardia. The patients who had a higher amount of reversal use were older, were female, had a higher ASA physical status classification, and had a higher Mallampati score.

4.7.1 Do not use sedation regimens that are intended to include routine administration of antagonists for reversal of sedatives or analgesics.[1] [Recommendation]

5. Discharge Readiness Criteria

5.1 Medical supervision of patient recovery and discharge after moderate sedation/analgesia should be the responsibility of the anesthesia professional or other qualified licensed independent practitioner.[1] [Recommendation]

The patient's risk for developing complications may extend into the postoperative period and may require the intervention of the medical practitioner.

5.1.1 A qualified provider defined by and authorized under the health care organization's guidelines and policies should be available in the facility to discharge the patient in accordance with the health care organization's discharge criteria.[2] [Recommendation]

5.2 Evaluate the patient for discharge readiness based on specific discharge criteria (eg, stable vital signs, adequate pain control) developed by an interdisciplinary team (eg, surgeons, perioperative RNs, anesthesia professionals).[1,2,47,66] [Recommendation]

The patient's recovery time will depend on the type and amount of sedation/analgesia administered, the procedure performed, and the health care organization's discharge criteria policy. Establishing discharge criteria minimizes the risk of an adverse outcome (eg, cardiorespiratory depression) after the patient has been discharged.[1,47]

5.2.1 Include the following in discharge readiness criteria:
- return to the preoperative baseline level of consciousness (eg, alert and oriented),[1,47,59,66,114,167]
- stable vital signs,[1,47,59,66,114,167]
- sufficient time interval (eg, 2 hours) since the last administration of an antagonist (eg, naloxone, flumazenil),[1,66]
- use of an objective patient assessment discharge scoring system (eg, Aldrete Recovery Score, Post-Anesthetic Discharge Scoring System),[1,66]
- absence of protracted nausea,[47,167]
- intact protective reflexes,[1,47,88]
- adequate pain control,[59,114,167]
- return of motor/sensory control,[47,167]

- at least 30 minutes after last sedative or analgesic medication by the intravenous route,[66] and
- arrangement for safe transport from the facility.[1,168]

[Recommendation]

5.2.2 Develop discharge criteria for each level of postanesthesia care (eg, phase I, phase II) when applicable.[66] [Recommendation]

5.3 Discharge may be delayed when the patient
- has obstructive sleep apnea,[66,83,99,101,103]
- receives medications by a nonintravenous route,[1]
- receives an antagonist,[1,66]
- experiences postoperative nausea and vomiting,[66]
- has a high frailty score,[69,89]
- has impaired functional status,[89-91] or
- has cognitive impairment (eg, delirium).[68,90-92]

[Conditional Recommendation]

Professional organizations[66,83,101] and moderate-quality evidence[99,103] support increased postoperative monitoring and longer stay in the PACU for patients with obstructive sleep apnea. The ASA[83] was unable to make a recommendation for the appropriate length of time to discharge, citing insufficient evidence, although they note that patients with obstructive sleep apnea may require a longer stay than patients who do not have obstructive sleep apnea because of the propensity to develop airway obstruction or central respiratory depression.

5.3.1 Pediatric patient discharge may be prolonged when
- the child receives a medication with a long half-life or
- only one responsible adult is accompanying a child recovering from moderate sedation/analgesia.[47]

[Conditional Recommendation] P

A guideline published by the American Academy of Pediatrics and the American Academy of Pediatric Dentistry recommends a longer period of observation before discharge of a child who has received a medication with a long half-life and before discharge of a child into the care of only one adult who is driving and thus has limited ability to observe the child.[47]

5.4 The perioperative RN must give the patient and their caregiver verbal and written discharge instructions.[1,2,47,88,169,170] [Regulatory Requirement]

Moderate sedation/analgesia medications may affect cognitive function, reducing the patient's ability to recall events during the perioperative period.[171-173] Veselis et al[171] conducted an RCT to study the effects of moderate sedation medications on conscious memory processes. The researchers randomly assigned healthy volunteers (N = 55) to five experimental groups that received sequential doses of a placebo (n = 11), thiopental (n = 11), propofol (n = 10), midazolam (n = 12), or dexmedetomidine (n = 11). Continual recognition task, delayed recognition task, and electroencephalogram testing occurred at specified intervals throughout the test period of 424 minutes. The medications increased reaction times and impaired memory on the continual recognition task equally, except for midazolam which had a greater effect. Via different mechanisms, both propofol and midazolam impair familiarity and recollection processes in recognition from long-term memory. The authors concluded that propofol and midazolam impaired recognition of event-related potentials from long-term memory but not working memory.

5.4.1 A copy of the written discharge instructions must be given to the patient and a copy should be placed in the patient's medical record.[169,170] *[Regulatory Requirement]*

5.4.2 The patient or a responsible adult should be able to verbalize an understanding of the discharge instructions. *[Recommendation]*

5.4.3 Include the following in discharge instructions given to the adults responsible for the care of an infant or toddler riding home in a car safety seat after receiving moderate sedation/analgesia:
- careful observation of the child's head position to avoid airway obstruction and
- care of two responsible adults (ie, driver and observer).[47,88]

[Recommendation] **P**

Clinical practice guidelines establish the importance of special instructions for observing the child's airway and of having two or more adults accompanying the child in the motor vehicle upon discharge.[47,88] The American Academy of Pediatrics and the American Academy of Pediatric Dentistry recommend special discharge instructions regarding prevention of airway obstruction after moderate sedation/analgesia for infants and toddlers riding home in a car safety seat.[47] The position of the child's head may cause airway obstruction when the head flexes forward on the body, leading to narrowing of the upper airway.

Infants who have received medications with a long half-life are at risk for airway obstruction when riding in a car safety seat.

6. Education

6.1 The perioperative RN must receive education and competency verification that addresses specialized knowledge and skills related to administering moderate sedation/analgesia.[169,170] *[Regulatory Requirement]*

Ongoing development of knowledge and skills and documentation of personnel participation is a regulatory and accreditation requirement for both hospitals and ambulatory settings.[169,170]

6.1.1 Include the following competencies related to administration of moderate sedation/analgesia:
- patient selection and assessment criteria (eg, obstructive sleep apnea, difficult mask ventilation)[2,131,174-177];
- use of the health care organization's selected assessment tools (eg, ASA Physical Status Classification, Mallampati classification, sedation scales, obstructive sleep apnea screening tools, frailty index, cognitive impairment screening tools);
- patient education and informed consent[2,131,176];
- selection, function, interpretation of measurements, and proficiency in the use of physiological monitoring equipment[2,30,131,174-176];
- pharmacology of the medications (eg, opioids, benzodiazepines, antagonists for opioids and benzodiazepines)[2,30,66,131,174,176,177];
- knowledge of airway anatomy and physiology[66,174];
- compromised airway management (eg, head-tilt, jaw-thrust, placement of oral and nasal airways, bag-mask ventilation)[1,30,38,41,66,131,175,176];
- basic dysrhythmia recognition and management[174];
- advanced cardiac life support (ACLS)[2,35,41,131,175] and pediatric advanced life support (PALS)[2,47,59,66,94] according to the patients served;
- recognition and management of complications associated with sedation/analgesia (eg, hypoxia, apnea, ability to rescue a patient whose level of sedation progresses to deep sedation)[1,2,66,131,174-176];
- selection and proficiency in the use of oxygen delivery devices[66,174];

- use of non-invasive positive pressure ventilation devices (eg, CPAP, BiPAP, nasal ventilation mask);
- postprocedure recovery monitoring and assessment for discharge criteria (eg, Aldrete Recovery Score, Post-Anesthetic Discharge Scoring System)[2,30,66,131,174,176]; and
- review of moderate sedation/analgesia policies and procedures.
  [Recommendation] [P]

6.1.2 Education and competency verification methods may include
- didactic content (eg, lectures, computer-based training modules),[30,35,38,131,174,176]
- simulation,[176]
- validation of skills (eg, assessment tool, return demonstration, observation),[30,38,174,176] and
- examination (eg, written, online).[131,176,178]
  [Conditional Recommendation]

6.2 **Competencies should reflect current regulations, nurse practice acts, standards, and guidelines related to the administration of moderate sedation/analgesia.** *[Recommendation]*

Regulations, nurse practice acts, standards, and guidelines affecting the administration of moderate sedation/analgesia are evolving and may change over time.

7. Policies and Procedures

7.1 **Develop moderate sedation/analgesia policies and procedures based on the state's medical and nurse practice acts, regulatory requirements, practice guidelines, professional organizations' statements, and accreditation requirements.** *[Recommendation]*

Numerous clinical practice guidelines support the benefit of following established criteria to develop safe practices for moderate sedation/analgesia policy and procedures.[1,2,45-47,59,66,121] These criteria are in the state's medical and nurse practice acts, regulatory requirements, practice guidelines, professional organizations' statements, and accreditation requirements. Policies and procedures assist in the development of patient safety, quality assessment, and performance improvement activities. Policies and procedures establish authority, responsibility, and accountability within the organization. Policies and procedures also serve as operational guidelines used to minimize patient risk for injury or complications, standardize practice, direct perioperative personnel, and establish continual performance improvement programs.

7.2 **The team developing the policies and procedures should include the director of anesthesia services[170] and representatives from all disciplines (eg, anesthesia, nursing, surgery, risk management, quality, pharmacy) with a role in the processes of moderate sedation/analgesia.** *[Recommendation]*

Involvement of an interdisciplinary team invites input from individuals in various disciplines and with unique perspectives. Inclusion of individuals who have a shared role in the care of patients receiving moderate sedation/analgesia in the development of policy and procedures facilitates the delivery of patient-centered, safe moderate sedation/analgesia.

7.3 **Include the following in policies and procedures for moderate sedation/analgesia:**
- patient selection and criteria for consultation (eg, ASA Physical Status Classification), including eligibility of pediatric patients (eg, age limit)[1,2,66];
- pre-sedation assessment requirements, including ordered laboratory and diagnostic tests based on information obtained from the patient health history and assessment, medical records, physical examination, and the type and invasiveness of the planned procedure[64];
- fasting guidelines[1,2,46,60,61,64-66,87];
- IV access requirements[1,2,66];
- continual patient monitoring parameters and frequency[1,2,66];
- permitted moderate sedation/analgesia medications and dosage guidelines, including
  - acceptable types of medication orders (eg, titrating orders[9])[63] and
  - patient controlled sedation[10,115,116];
- use of home equipment (eg, CPAP)[66,84,100];
- discharge criteria for each level of postanesthesia care (eg, phase I, phase II)[1,2,47,66];
- documentation (eg, parameters, frequency)[1,2,47,64,66];
- emergency equipment, medications, and procedures[1,2,44,45,47,57,66];
- staffing requirements[1,2,66];
- licensed independent practitioners' qualifications, education, and competency requirements for administering or supervising moderate sedation/analgesia[1,2,66];
- RN qualification, education, and competency requirements for administering moderate sedation/analgesia[1,2,66]; and
- criteria for transferring the patient to a higher level of care when the patient's acuity or level

of care required is outside the perioperative RN's capabilities or scope of practice.[1,2,66] *[Recommendation]* **P**

7.3.1 If the facility provides moderate sedation/analgesia for pediatric patients, develop pediatric-specific policies and procedures in collaboration with the interdisciplinary team and the director of anesthesia services. *[Recommendation]* **P**

7.3.2 Preoperative fasting requirements in the policy and procedure should include duration, type, and volume of permitted intake.[179] *[Recommendation]* **P**

Following fasting requirements that restrict food and fluid intake reduces the volume and pH of gastric contents.[179] Fasting reduces the risk of regurgitation, pulmonary aspiration, and pulmonary damage.[87,179]

The ASA practice guidelines for preoperative fasting recommend verifying compliance with the fasting requirements during the assessment.[87] The guideline defines preoperative fasting as a "prescribed period of time before a procedure when patients are not allowed the oral intake of liquids or solids."[87(p376)] The prescribed fasting periods allow healthy patients to have clear liquids up to 2 hours, breast milk up to 4 hours, infant formula up to 6 hours, a light meal or nonhuman milk up to 6 hours, and fatty foods 8 hours or more before an elective procedure.[87]

The International Committee for the Advancement of Procedural Sedation (ICAPS) found that fasting as currently practiced often substantially exceeds recommended time thresholds, which has known adverse consequences to the patient such as irritability, dehydration, and hypoglycemia.[180] The committee recommended an algorithm for fasting that allows each patient's aspiration risk to be stratified in the pre-sedation assessment using evidence-based factors related to patient characteristics, comorbidities, the nature of the procedure, and the nature of the anticipated sedation technique.

In a Cochrane review, Brady et al[179] systematically reviewed 38 RCTs that compared different preoperative fasting regimens for adult surgical patients and their effects on patient well-being (eg, thirst, hunger, aspiration, regurgitation, pain, nausea, vomiting, anxiety) and postoperative complications. The authors concluded there was no evidence to suggest that decreasing the amount of time that fluids

were allowed before surgery increased the risk of aspiration, regurgitation, or morbidity compared with the traditional fasting policy of nothing by mouth after midnight. Drinking water before surgery resulted in significantly lower gastric volumes. The authors concluded that the health care organization's fasting policy should be based on an appraisal of the evidence and a patient risk assessment (eg, history of gastrointestinal disease, autonomic neuropathy, pregnancy, older age).

In a similar Cochrane review for pediatric patients, Brady et al[181] systematically reviewed 25 RCTs that compared different preoperative fasting regimens for pediatric surgical patients at their effects on patient well-being and postoperative complications. The authors concluded that there was no evidence to suggest that children at normal risk of aspiration who are denied oral fluids for up to 6 hours before surgery have any benefit in gastric volume or pH compared to children who are allowed unlimited fluids up to 2 hours before surgery.

In a systematic review, Shaukat et al[182] included 40 studies that were conducted to investigate fasting and aspiration risk for elective colonoscopy procedures. The authors found that the incidence of aspiration requiring hospitalization during colonoscopy with moderate or deep sedation was very low, and that no study found that shorter fasting times were associated with an increased aspiration risk.

The benefits of preoperative fasting outweigh the harms. The benefits include a reduction in the incidence of aspiration, lung damage, death, nausea, and vomiting. The harms of preoperative fasting include the patient experiencing thirst, dehydration, hunger, hypoglycemia, irritability, pain (eg, sore throat, headache), nausea, vomiting, dizziness, anxiety, and stress.[87,179,180]

8. Quality

8.1 Participate in quality assurance and performance improvement activities that are consistent with the health care organization's plan to improve understanding of and compliance with the principles and skills of moderate sedation/analgesia administration.[66,114] *[Recommendation]*

Participating in ongoing quality assurance and performance improvement activities is a standard of perioperative nursing and a primary responsibility of the perioperative RN who is engaged in practice in the perioperative setting.[4]

8.2 The health care organization must report, track, and investigate adverse events related to moderate sedation/analgesia through the quality review process (eg, root cause analysis).[169,170] *[Regulatory Requirement]*

8.3 Quality assurance and performance improvement activities for moderate sedation/analgesia administration must include monitoring for compliance with the processes and outcomes of moderate sedation/analgesia administration. *[Regulatory Requirement]*

Collecting data to monitor and improve patient care, treatment, and services is a regulatory and accreditation requirement for both hospitals and ambulatory settings.[169,170]

Quality assurance and performance improvement programs assist in evaluating and improving the quality of patient care and formulating plans for corrective action. These programs provide data that may be used to determine whether an individual organization is within benchmark goals and, if not, to identify areas that may require corrective action.

8.3.1 Process measures related to moderate sedation/analgesia may include
- informed consent for the sedation and procedure completed;
- NPO status confirmed;
- history and physical completed;
- frailty, functional status, and cognitive impairment assessment completed for older adults;
- airway assessment completed[114];
- obstructive sleep apnea assessment completed, when indicated;
- adherence to required physiological monitoring (eg, frequency)[114];
- response to alarms[114];
- use of supplemental oxygen[114];
- use of a nonapproved sedation agent (eg, use of an anesthetic agent by a non-anesthesia provider);
- availability and proximity of emergency equipment[114];
- activation of emergency response teams[114];
- unplanned intervention by an anesthesia professional; and
- performance of an emergency procedure without an anesthesia professional or other qualified licensed independent practitioner present. *[Conditional Recommendation]*

8.3.2 Outcome measures related to moderate sedation/analgesia may include
- death[50,183-186];
- cardiac or respiratory arrest[16,54,183,185-187];
- aspiration[50,54,56,183,185,187];
- hypoxia leading to organ injury (eg, brain injury)[50,184,186,187];
- seizures[187];
- arrhythmia requiring cardioversion[185,187];
- prolonged amnesia, delirium, or postprocedure cognitive decline[114,187];
- posttraumatic stress disorder or emotional trauma[186,187];
- adverse reaction or allergy to a medication[183,185,188,189];
- use of an antagonist (ie, reversal agent)[114,183];
- level of sedation deeper than planned (ie, deep sedation, general anesthesia);
- unplanned transfer to a higher level of care[54,183];
- patient dissatisfaction[187]; and
- provider dissatisfaction.[187]

[Conditional Recommendation]

Moderate-quality evidence establishes the risks related to moderate sedation/analgesia, as well as the management and minimization of an associated adverse event.[16,50,54,185,186,190,191]

Many adverse events are caused by oversedation. In a retrospective review, Jones et al[190] found that the most common adverse events in 83 moderate sedation procedures were oversedation/apnea, hypoxemia, and aspiration. Karamnov et al[54] retrospectively reviewed 52 cases of patients who experienced moderate sedation safety incidents and found that the most common adverse events and unplanned interventions were related to oversedation. Stone et al[191] also found that oversedation was a contributing factor to most adverse events in 58 closed malpractice claims involving anesthesiologists in the endoscopy suite.

The International Sedation Task Force of the World Society of Intravenous Anesthesia[183] developed a tool to standardize sedation adverse event reporting and tracking. The authors listed common sedation adverse events and defined an adverse event as

Unexpected and undesirable response(es) to medication(s) and medical intervention used to facilitate procedural sedation and analgesia that threaten or cause patient injury or discomfort.[183]

The tool has a five-step process requiring the identification of a sedation event and description of the adverse event, the intervention performed, the outcome, and the severity of the event.[183]

As part of an organizational experience report, Lemay et al[192] developed an audit tool to evaluate safety, effectiveness, and communication during the use of procedural sedation for interventional radiology procedures. The authors recommended using the tool as a way to practically measure outcomes of procedural sedation.

Glossary

Benzodiazepine: A pharmacologic agent that has sedative, anxiolytic, amnesic, muscle relaxant, and anticonvulsant properties.

Cognitive impairment: Delirium or a neurodegenerative condition (eg, dementia, Alzheimer's disease, Parkinson's disease) that increases the risk for delirium. Common in older adults but differs from the cognitive changes of normal aging. Cognitive impairment is often assessed by a screening tool, such as the clock drawing test, Mini-Cog, mini-mental status exam, or short-orientation memory concentration test.

Continual: Repeated regularly and frequently in steady rapid succession.

Deep sedation/analgesia: A medication-induced depression of consciousness that allows patients to respond purposefully only after repeated or painful stimulation. The patient cannot be aroused easily, the ability to independently maintain a patent airway may be impaired, and spontaneous ventilation may be inadequate. Cardiovascular function usually is usually maintained.

Frailty: An age-related, multi-dimensional state of decreased physiologic reserve that results in diminished resilience, loss of adaptive capacity, and increased vulnerability to stressors. Frailty is most often measured by either the frailty index, frailty phenotype, or a screening tool that is based on these assessments (eg, Risk Analysis Index, Edmonton Frail Scale, modified frailty index, Clinical Frail Scale, FRAIL scale, single variable assessments).

Functional status: The assessment of an individual's ability to perform activities of daily living (eg, walking, bathing, eating, dressing) and instrumental activities of daily living (eg, transportation, cooking, housekeeping).

Licensed independent practitioner: A practitioner (eg, surgeon, endoscopist, dentist, podiatrist) who is permitted by law and the organization to provide supervision and oversight of the RN administering moderate sedation/analgesia, within the scope of the individual's license, and consistent with individually granted clinical privileges.

Moderate sedation/analgesia: A medication-induced depression of consciousness that allows patients to respond purposefully to verbal commands, either alone or accompanied by light tactile stimulation. No interventions are required to maintain a patent airway, and spontaneous ventilation is adequate. Cardiovascular function is usually maintained.

Older adult: A person aged 65 years or older. Further subdivided into

- **Young old:** ages 65 to 74 years;
- **Middle old:** ages 75 to 84 years;
- **Old old:** age 85 years and older.

Opioid: A pharmacologic agent that produces varying degrees of analgesia and sedation and relieves pain. Fentanyl, morphine, and hydromorphone are opioid analgesic medications that may be used for moderate sedation/analgesia.

Polypharmacy: The concurrent use of multiple medications by a patient to treat a single condition or multiple coexisting conditions, which may result in adverse drug interactions. Commonly defined as the use of five or more medications, but can vary from two to 11 or more concurrent medications.

Prehabilitation: The process of improving the functional capability of a patient before a surgical procedure so the patient can withstand any postoperative inactivity and associated decline.

Procedure suite: An area or areas of the building that contains the preoperative, intraoperative, and postoperative patient care areas and provisions for support areas.

References

1. Practice Guidelines for Moderate Procedural Sedation and Analgesia 2018: a report by the American Society of Anesthesiologists Task Force on Moderate Procedural Sedation and Analgesia, the American Association of Oral and Maxillofacial Surgeons, American College of Radiology, American Dental Association, American Society of Dentist Anesthesiologists, and Society of Interventional Radiology. *Anesthesiology.* 2018;128(3):437-479. [IVA]

2. *Non-Anesthesia Provider Procedural Sedation and Analgesia. Policy Considerations.* American Association of Nurse Anesthetists. https://www.aana.com/docs/default-source/practice-aana-com-web-documents-(all)/professional-practice-manual/non-anesthesia-provider-procedural-sedation-and-analgesia.pdf?sfvrsn=670049b1_4. Published 2016. Accessed June 17, 2021. [VA]

3. *Nursing: Scope and Standards of Practice.* 3rd ed. Silver Spring, MD: American Nurses Association; 2015. [IVB]

4. *Standards of Perioperative Nursing.* AORN, Inc. https://aorn.org/guidelines/clinical-resources/aorn-standards. Accessed June 17, 2021. [IVB]

5. About nursing licensure. National Council of State Boards of Nursing. https://www.ncsbn.org/licensure.htm. Accessed June 17, 2021. [VA]

6. *Nurse Practice Act Toolkit.* National Council of State Boards of Nursing. https://www.ncsbn.org/npa-toolkit.htm. Accessed June 17, 2021. [VA]

7. *AORN's Perioperative Explications for the* ANA Code of Ethics for Nurses with Interpretive Statements. AORN, Inc. https://aorn.org/guidelines/clinical-resources/code-of-ethics. Published 2017. Accessed June 17, 2021. [IVB]

8. DIPRIVAN (propofol) injectable emulsion, USP. US Food and Drug Administration. https://www.accessdata.fda.gov/drugsatfda_docs/label/2017/019627s066lbl.pdf. Revised April 2017. Accessed June 17, 2021.

9. Braaten KP, Urman RD, Maurer R, Fortin J, Goldberg AB. A randomized comparison of intravenous sedation using a dosing algorithm compared to standard care during first-trimester surgical abortion. *Contraception.* 2018;97(6):490-496. [IA]

10. Clements W, Sneddon D, Kavnoudias H, et al. Randomized and controlled study comparing patient controlled and radiologist controlled intra-procedural conscious sedation, using midazolam and fentanyl, for patients undergoing insertion of a central venous line. *J Med Imaging Radiat Oncol.* 2018;62(6):781-788. [IB]

11. Han SJ, Lee TH, Park SH, et al. Efficacy of midazolam- versus propofol-based sedations by non-anesthesiologists during therapeutic endoscopic retrograde cholangiopancreatography in patients aged over 80 years. *Dig Endosc.* 2017;29(3):369-376. [IB]

12. Han SJ, Lee TH, Yang JK, et al. Etomidate sedation for advanced endoscopic procedures. *Dig Dis Sci.* 2019;64(1):144-151. [IB]

13. Pastis NJ, Yarmus LB, Schippers F, et al. Safety and efficacy of remimazolam compared with placebo and midazolam for moderate sedation during bronchoscopy. *Chest.* 2019;155(1):137-146. [IA]

14. Sachar H, Pichetshote N, Nandigam K, Vaidya K, Laine L. Continued midazolam versus diphenhydramine in difficult-to-sedate patients: a randomized double-blind trial. *Gastrointest Endosc.* 2018;87(5):1297-1303. [IB]

15. Finn RT 3rd, Boyd A, Lin L, Gellad ZF. Bolus administration of fentanyl and midazolam for colonoscopy increases endoscopy unit efficiency and safety compared with titrated sedation. *Clin Gastroenterol Hepatol.* 2017;15(9):1419-1426. [IIIA]

16. Goudra B, Nuzat A, Singh PM, Gouda GB, Carlin A, Manjunath AK. Cardiac arrests in patients undergoing gastrointestinal endoscopy: a retrospective analysis of 73,029 procedures. *Saudi J Gastroenterol.* 2015;21(6):400-411. [IIIA]

17. Goudra B, Singh PM, Gouda G, Borle A, Carlin A, Yadwad A. Propofol and non-propofol based sedation for outpatient colonoscopy-prospective comparison of depth of sedation using an EEG based SEDLine monitor. *J Clin Monit Comput.* 2016;30(5):551-557. [IIB]

18. McLemore MR, Aztlan EA. Retrospective evaluation of the procedural sedation practices of expert nurses during abortion care. *J Obstet Gynecol Neonatal Nurs.* 2017;46(5):755-763. [IIIB]

19. Szczeklik W, Andrychiewicz A, Górka K, Konarska K, Soja J, Sladek K. Flexible bronchoscopy under conscious sedation with midazolam and fentanyl can be safely performed by nonanesthesiologists. *Pol Arch Med Wewn.* 2015;125(11):869-871. [IIIB]

20. Tu RH, Grewall P, Leung JW, et al. Diphenhydramine as an adjunct to sedation for colonoscopy: a double-blind randomized, placebo-controlled study. *Gastrointest Endosc.* 2006;63(1):87-94. [IB]

21. Kinugasa H, Higashi R, Miyahara K, et al. Dexmedetomidine for conscious sedation with colorectal endoscopic submucosal dissection: a prospective double-blind randomized controlled study. *Clin Transl Gastroenterol.* 2018;9(7):167. [IB]

22. Jin EH, Hong KS, Lee Y, et al. How to improve patient satisfaction during midazolam sedation for gastrointestinal endoscopy? *World J Gastroenterol.* 2017;23(6):1098-1105. [IIIB]

23. Riachy M, Khayat G, Ibrahim I, et al. A randomized double-blind controlled trial comparing three sedation regimens during flexible bronchoscopy: dexmedetomidine, alfentanil and lidocaine. *Clin Respir J.* 2018;12(4):1407-1415. [IB]

24. *AANA-ASA Joint Position Statement Regarding Propofol Administration.* American Association of Nurse Anesthetists. https://www.aana.com/docs/default-source/practice-aana-com-web-documents-(all)/professional-practice-manual/aana-asa-propofol-joint-ps.pdf?sfvrsn=f80049b1_4. Published April 14, 2004. Accessed June 17, 2021. [IVB]

25. *Statement on Safe Use of Propofol.* American Society of Anesthesiologists. https://www.asahq.org/standards-and-guidelines/statement-on-safe-use-of-propofol. Amended October 23, 2019. Accessed June 17, 2021. [IVB]

26. Wadhwa V, Issa D, Garg S, Lopez R, Sanaka MR, Vargo JJ. Similar risk of cardiopulmonary adverse events between propofol and traditional anesthesia for gastrointestinal endoscopy: a systematic review and meta-analysis. *Clin Gastroenterol Hepatol.* 2017;15(2):194-206. [IA]

27. Yoon SW, Choi GJ, Lee OH, et al. Comparison of propofol monotherapy and propofol combination therapy for sedation during gastrointestinal endoscopy: a systematic review and meta-analysis. *Dig Endosc.* 2018;30(5):580-591. [IB]

28. Kim EH, Park JC, Shin SK, Lee YC, Lee SK. Effect of the midazolam added with propofol-based sedation in esophago-gastroduodenoscopy: a randomized trial. *J Gastroenterol Hepatol.* 2018;33(4):894-899. [IB]

29. Heo J, Jung MK, Lee HS, et al. Effects of bispectral index monitoring as an adjunct to nurse-administered propofol combined sedation during colonoscopy: a randomized clinical trial. *Korean J Intern Med.* 2016;31(2):260-266. [IB]

30. López Muñoz C, Sánchez Yagüe A, Canca Sánchez JC, Reinaldo-Lapuerta JA, Moya Suárez AB. Quality of sedation with propofol administered by non-anesthetists in a digestive endoscopy unit: the results of a one year experience. *Rev Esp Enferm Dig.* 2018;110(4):231-236. [IIB]

31. Nonaka M, Gotoda T, Kusano C, Fukuzawa M, Itoi T, Moriyasu F. Safety of gastroenterologist-guided sedation with propofol for upper gastrointestinal therapeutic endoscopy in elderly patients compared with younger patients. *Gut Liver.* 2015;9(1):38-42. [IIIB]

32. Okeke FC, Shaw S, Hunt KK, Korsten MA, Rosman AS. Safety of propofol used as a rescue agent during colonoscopy. *J Clin Gastroenterol.* 2016;50(8):e77-e80. [IIIB]

33. Vargo JJ, Niklewski PJ, Williams JL, Martin JF, Faigel DO. Patient safety during sedation by anesthesia professionals during routine upper endoscopy and colonoscopy: an analysis of 1.38 million procedures. *Gastrointest Endosc.* 2017;85(1):101-108. [IIIA]

34. Ruiz-Curiel RE, Ydaly BH, Baptista A, Bronstein M. Sedation with propofol in digestive endoscopy administered by gastroenterologists. Experience in a Venezuelan hospital. *Rev Esp Enferm Dig.* 2018;110(4):246-249. [IIIB]

35. Lapidus A, Gralnek IM, Suissa A, Yassin K, Khamaysi I. Safety and efficacy of endoscopist-directed balanced propofol sedation during endoscopic retrograde cholangiopancreatography. *Ann Gastroenterol.* 2019;32(3):303-311. [IIIB]

36. Garewal D, Powell S, Milan SJ, Nordmeyer J, Waikar P. Sedative techniques for endoscopic retrograde cholangiopancreatography. *Cochrane Database Syst Rev.* 2012(6):CD007274. [IIA]

37. Chrissian AA, Bedi H. Bronchoscopist-directed continuous propofol infusion for targeting moderate sedation during endobronchial ultrasound bronchoscopy: a practical and effective protocol. *J Bronchology Interv Pulmonol.* 2015;22(3):226-236. [IIB]

38. Schulze M, Grande B, Kolbe M, et al. SafAIRway: an airway training for pulmonologists performing a flexible bronchoscopy with nonanesthesiologist administered propofol sedation: a prospective evaluation. *Medicine (Baltimore).* 2016;95(23):e3849. [IIB]

39. Khemasuwan D, Teerapuncharoen K, Griffin DC. Diagnostic yield and safety of bronchoscopist-directed moderate sedation with a bolus dose administration of propofol during endobronchial ultrasound bronchoscopy. *J Bronchology Interv Pulmonol.* 2018;25(3):181-188. [IIIB]

40. Singh H, Poluha W, Cheung M, Choptain N, Baron KI, Taback SP. Propofol for sedation during colonoscopy. *Cochrane Database Syst Rev.* 2008;(4):CD006268. [IA]

41. Vargo JJ, Cohen LB, Rex DK, Kwo PY; American Association for the Study of Liver Diseases; American College of Gasteroenterology; American Gastroenterological Association; American Society for Gastrointestinal Endoscopy. Position statement: nonanesthesiologist administration of propofol for GI endoscopy. *Gastroenterology.* 2009;137(6):2161-2167. [IVA]

42. *Statement on Granting Privileges for Administration of Moderate Sedation to Practitioners Who Are Not Anesthesia Professionals.* American Society of Anesthesiologists. https://www.asahq.org/standards-and-guidelines/statement-of-granting-privileges-for-administration-of-moderate-sedation-to-practitioners. Reaffirmed October 26, 2016. Accessed June 17, 2021. [IVB]

43. *Statement on the Anesthesia Care Team.* American Society of Anesthesiologists. https://www.asahq.org/-/media/sites/asahq/files/public/resources/standards-guidelines/statement-on-the-anesthesia-care-team.pdf?la=en&hash=9674E540AB92E575C1FD8AB9B48159F7656B9AEB. Last Amended October 23, 2019. Accessed June 17, 2021. [IVB]

44. Heneghan S, Myers J, Fanelli R, Richardson W, et al. Guidelines for Office Endoscopic Services. Society of American Gastrointestinal Endoscopic Surgeons (SAGES). https://www.sages.org/publications/guidelines/guidelines-for-office-endoscopic-services/. Approved November 2008. Accessed June 17, 2021. [IVB]

45. ASGE Standards of Practice Committee; Early DS, Lightdale JR, Vargo JJ 2nd, et al. Guidelines for sedation and anesthesia in GI endoscopy. *Gastrointest Endosc.* 2018;87(2):327-337. [IVA]

46. ACR-SIR Practice Parameter for Sedation/Analgesia. American College of Radiology/Society of Interventional Radiology. https://www.acr.org/-/media/acr/files/practice-parameters/sed-analgesia.pdf. Revised 2020. Accessed June 17, 2021. [IVB]

47. Coté CJ, Wilson S; American Academy of Pediatrics; American Academy of Pediatric Dentistry. Guidelines for monitoring and management of pediatric patients during and after sedation for diagnostic and therapeutic procedures. *Pediatrics.* 2019;143(6):e20191000. [IVB]

48. Chang B, Kaye AD, Diaz JH, Westlake B, Dutton RP, Urman RD. Interventional procedures outside of the operating room: results from the National Anesthesia Clinical Outcomes Registry. *J Patient Saf.* 2018;14(1):9-16. [IIIA]

49. *Guidelines for Office-Based Anesthesia.* American Society of Anesthesiologists; https://www.asahq.org/standards-and-guidelines/guidelines-for-office-based-anesthesia. Last amended October 23, 2019. Accessed June 17, 2021. [IVB]

50. Woodward ZG, Urman RD, Domino KB. Safety of non-operating room anesthesia: a closed claims update. *Anesthesiol Clin.* 2017;35(4):569-581. [IIIA]

51. Bhavani S. Non-operating room anesthesia in the endoscopy unit. *Gastrointest Endosc Clin N Am.* 2016;26(3):471-483. [VA]

52. Bouhenguel JT, Preiss DA, Urman RD. Implementation and use of anesthesia information management systems for non-operating room locations. *Anesthesiol Clin.* 2017;35(4):583-590. [VA]

53. Brovman EY, Preiss D, Urman RD, Gross WL. The challenges of implementing electronic health records for anesthesia use outside the operating room. *Curr Opin Anaesthesiol.* 2016;29(4):531-535. [VA]

54. Karamnov S, Sarkisian N, Grammer R, Gross WL, Urman RD. Analysis of adverse events associated with adult moderate procedural sedation outside the operating room. *J Patient Saf.* 2017;13(3):111-121. [IIIB]

55. Wong T, Georgiadis PL, Urman RD, Tsai MH. Non-operating room anesthesia: patient selection and special considerations. *Local Reg Anesth.* 2020;13:1-9. [VA]

56. Yeh T, Beutler SS, Urman RD. What we can learn from nonoperating room anesthesia registries: analysis of clinical outcomes and closed claims data. *Curr Opin Anaesthesiol.* 2020;33(4):527-532. [VA]

57. *Office Based Anesthesia: Position Statement.* American Association of Nurse Anesthetists. https://www.aana.com/docs/default-source/practice-aana-com-web-documents-(all)/professional-practice-manual/office-based-anesthesia.pdf?sfvrsn=503136ab_4. Accessed June 17, 2021. [IVB]

58. *Statement on Nonoperating Room Anesthetizing Locations.* American Society of Anesthesiologists. https://www.asahq.org/standards-and-guidelines/statement-on-nonoperating-room

-anesthetizing-locations. Reaffirmed October 17, 2018. Accessed June 17, 2021. [IVB]

59. *Sedation in Children and Young People: Sedation for Diagnostic and Therapeutic Procedures in Children and Young People.* National Institute for Health and Care Excellence. https://www.nice.org.uk/guidance/cg112/evidence/full-guideline-136287325. Updated February 2019. Accessed June 17, 2021. [IVA]

60. Cohen LB, Delegge MH, Aisenberg J, et al. AGA institute review of endoscopic sedation. *Gastroenterology.* 2007;133(2):675-701. [IVB]

61. Dumonceau JM, Riphaus A, Schreiber F, et al. Non-anesthesiologist administration of propofol for gastrointestinal endoscopy: European Society of Gastrointestinal Endoscopy, European Society of Gastroenterology and Endoscopy Nurses and Associates Guideline—updated June 2015. *Endoscopy.* 2015;47(12):1175-1189. [IVA]

62. Guideline for a safe environment of care. In: *Guidelines for Perioperative Practice.* Denver, CO: AORN, Inc; 2021:109-144. [IVA]

63. Guideline for medication safety. In: *Guidelines for Perioperative Practice.* Denver, CO: AORN, Inc; 2021:463-502. [IVA]

64. *Documenting Anesthesia Care: Practice and Policy Considerations.* American Association of Nurse Anesthetists. https://www.aana.com/docs/default-source/practice-aana-com-web-documents-(all)/professional-practice-manual/documenting-anesthesia-care.pdf?sfvrsn=ac0049b1_6. Published 2016. Accessed June 17, 2021. [IVB]

65. *Clinical Practice Guideline: Moderate Sedation and Analgesia.* Association of Radiologic & Imaging Nursing. https://www.arinursing.org/ARIN/assets/File/public/practice-guidelines/h_Moderate_Sedation_and_Analgesia.pdf. Revised 2009. Accessed June 17, 2021. [IVB]

66. *2019-2020 Perianesthesia Nursing Standards, Practice Recommendations and Interpretive Statements.* Cherry Hill, NJ: American Society of PeriAnesthesia Nurses; 2018. [IVB]

67. American Geriatrics Society 2019 updated AGS Beers Criteria® for potentially inappropriate medication use in older adults. *J Am Geriatr* Soc. 2019;67(4):674-694. [IVA]

68. Wiggins M, Arias F, Urman RD, et al. Common neurodegenerative disorders in the perioperative setting: recommendations for screening from the Society for Perioperative Assessment and Quality Improvement (SPAQI). *Perioper Care Oper Room Manag.* 2020;20:100092. [IVB]

69. Alvarez-Nebreda ML, Bentov N, Urman RD, et al. Recommendations for preoperative management of frailty from the Society for Perioperative Assessment and Quality Improvement (SPAQI). *J Clin Anesth.* 2018;47:33-42. [IVB]

70. Yeo H, Kim W, Park H, Kim H. Variables influencing the depth of conscious sedation in plastic surgery: a prospective study. *Arch Plast Surg.* 2017;44(1):5-11. [IIIB]

71. Tetzlaff JE, Maurer WG. Preprocedural assessment for sedation in gastrointestinal endoscopy. *Gastrointest Endosc Clin N Am.* 2016;26(3):433-441. [VA]

72. Urman RD, Moucharite M, Flynn C, Nuryyeva E, Ray CE Jr. Impact of respiratory compromise in inpatient interventional radiology procedures with moderate sedation in the *United States. Radiology.* 2019;292(3):702-710. [IIIA]

73. Horwitz G, Roncari D, Braaten KP, Maurer R, Fortin J, Goldberg AB. Moderate intravenous sedation for first trimester surgical abortion: a comparison of adverse outcomes between obese and normal-weight women. *Contraception.* 2018;97(1):48-53. [IIIA]

74. Patel R, Clayton S, Quintero E, Gill J. Chronic opioid users are more difficult to sedate than alcoholics and controls. *South Med J.* 2015;108(12):744-747. [IIIB]

75. Flisberg P, Paech MJ, Shah T, Ledowski T, Kurowski I, Parsons R. Induction dose of propofol in patients using cannabis. *Eur J Anaesthesiol.* 2009;26(3):192-195. [IB]

76. Twardowski MA, Link MM, Twardowski NM. Effects of cannabis use on sedation requirements for endoscopic procedures. *J Am Osteopath Assoc.* 2019;119(5):307-311. [IIIC]

77. Huson HB, Granados TM, Rasko Y. Surgical considerations of marijuana use in elective procedures. *Heliyon.* 2018;4(9):e00779. [VB]

78. Karam K, Abbasi S, Khan FA. Anaesthetic consideration in a cannabis addict. *J Coll Physicians Surg Pak.* 2015;25 Suppl 1:S2-S3. [VB]

79. Woo M, Andrews CN. Implications of cannabis use on sedation for endoscopic procedures. *Gastrointest Endosc.* 2019;90(4):656-658. [VC]

80. Wong J, An D, Urman RD, et al. Society for Perioperative Assessment and Quality Improvement (SPAQI) consensus statement on perioperative smoking cessation. *Anesth Analg.* 2020;131(3):955-968. [IVB]

81. Jeong S, Lee HG, Kim WM, et al. Increase of paradoxical excitement response during propofol-induced sedation in hazardous and harmful alcohol drinkers. *Br J Anaesth.* 2011;107(6):930-933. [IIIB]

82. Apfelbaum JL, Hagberg CA, Caplan RA, et al. Practice guidelines for management of the difficult airway: an updated report by the American Society of Anesthesiologists Task Force on Management of the Difficult Airway. *Anesthesiology.* 2013;118(2):251-270. [IVA]

83. American Society of Anesthesiologists Task Force on Perioperative Management of Patients with Obstructive Sleep Apnea. Practice guidelines for the perioperative management of patients with obstructive sleep apnea: an updated report by the American Society of Anesthesiologists Task Force on Perioperative Management of Patients with Obstructive Sleep Apnea. *Anesthesiology.* 2014;120(2):268-286. [IVA]

84. Chung F, Memtsoudis SG, Ramachandran SK, et al. Society of Anesthesia and Sleep Medicine Guidelines on Preoperative Screening and Assessment of Adult Patients with Obstructive Sleep Apnea. *Anesth Analg.* 2016;123(2):452-473. [IVA]

85. Zhou C, Chung F, Wong DT. Clinical assessment for the identification of the potentially difficult airway. *Periop Care Oper Room Manag.* 2017;9:16-19. [VA]

86. Kara D, Bayrak NA, Volkan B, Uçar C, Cevizci MN, Yildiz S. Anxiety and salivary cortisol levels in children undergoing esophago-gastro-duodenoscopy under sedation. *J Pediatr Gastroenterol Nutr.* 2019;68(1):3-6. [IIIB]

87. Practice guidelines for preoperative fasting and the use of pharmacologic agents to reduce the risk of pulmonary

aspiration: application to healthy patients undergoing elective procedures: an updated report by the American Society of Anesthesiologists Task Force on Preoperative Fasting and the Use of Pharmacologic Agents to Reduce the Risk of Pulmonary Aspiration. *Anesthesiology.* 2017;126(3):376-393. [IVA]

88. ASGE Standards of Practice Committee; Lightdale JR, Acosta R, Shergill AK, et al. Modifications in endoscopic practice for pediatric patients. *Gastrointest Endosc.* 2014;79(5):699-710. [IVA]

89. *AORN Position Statement on Care of the Older Adult in Perioperative Settings.* AORN, Inc. https://aorn.org/guidelines/clinical-resources/position-statements. Published 2015. Accessed June 17, 2021. [IVB]

90. Arias F, Wiggins M, Urman RD, et al. Rapid in-person cognitive screening in the preoperative setting: test considerations and recommendations from the Society for Perioperative Assessment and Quality Improvement (SPAQI). *J Clin Anesth.* 2020;62:109724. [IVB]

91. *Optimal Resources for Geriatric Surgery: 2019 Standards.* Chicago, IL: American College of Surgeons; 2019. [IVB]

92. *A Position Statement on the Older Adult.* American Society of PeriAnesthesia Nurses. https://www.aspan.org/Portals/6/docs/ClinicalPractice/PositionStatement/Current/PS_5.pdf?ver=2021-01-12-150828-397. Revised October 2019. Accessed June 17, 2021. [IVB]

93. Acosta A, Garzon MP, Urman RD. Screening and diagnosing frailty in the cardiac and noncardiac surgical patient to improve safety and outcomes. *Int Anesthesiol Clin.* 2019;57(3):111-122. [VA]

94. *A Position Statement on the Pediatric Patient.* American Society of PeriAnesthesia Nurses. https://www.aspan.org/Portals/6/docs/ClinicalPractice/PositionStatement/Current/PS_6.pdf?ver=2021-01-12-150828-537. Revised October 2019. Accessed June 17, 2021. [IVB]

95. ASA Physical Status Classification System. American Society of Anesthesiologists. https://www.asahq.org/standards-and-guidelines/asa-physical-status-classification-system. Amended December 13, 2020. Accessed June 17, 2021. [VA]

96. Seligson E, Beutler SS, Urman RD. Office-based anesthesia: an update on safety and outcomes (2017-2019). *Curr Opin Anaesthesiol.* 2019;32(6):756-761. [VA]

97. Prakash S, Mullick P. Airway management in patients with burn contractures of the neck. *Burns.* 2015;41(8):1627-1635. [VA]

98. Lee A, Fan LT, Gin T, Karmakar MK, Ngan Kee WD. A systematic review (meta-analysis) of the accuracy of the Mallampati tests to predict the difficult airway. *Anesth Analg.* 2006;102(6):1867-1878. [IIIA]

99. Cozowicz C, Chung F, Doufas AG, Nagappa M, Memtsoudis SG. Opioids for acute pain management in patients with obstructive sleep apnea: a systematic review. *Anesth Analg.* 2018;127(4):988-1001. [IIIA]

100. Szeto B, Vertosick EA, Ruiz K, et al. Outcomes and safety among patients with obstructive sleep apnea undergoing cancer surgery procedures in a freestanding ambulatory surgical facility. *Anesth Analg.* 2019;129(2):360-368. [IIIB]

101. Joshi GP, Ankichetty SP, Gan TJ, Chung F. Society for Ambulatory Anesthesia consensus statement on preoperative selection of adult patients with obstructive sleep apnea scheduled for ambulatory surgery. *Anesth Analg.* 2012;115(5):1060-1068. [IVA]

102. Memtsoudis SG, Cozowicz C, Nagappa M, et al. Society of Anesthesia and Sleep Medicine guideline on intraoperative management of adult patients with obstructive sleep apnea. *Anesth Analg.* 2018;127(4):967-987. [IVA]

103. Moos DD, Prasch M, Cantral DE, Huls B, Cuddeford JD. Are patients with obstructive sleep apnea syndrome appropriate candidates for the ambulatory surgical center? *AANA J.* 2005;73(3):197-205. [VA]

104. Abrishami A, Khajehdehi A, Chung F. A systematic review of screening questionnaires for obstructive sleep apnea. *Can J Anaesth.* 2010;57(5):423-438. [IIIA]

105. Cho J, Choi SM, Park YS, Lee CH, Lee SM, Lee J. Snoring during bronchoscopy with moderate sedation is a predictor of obstructive sleep apnea. *Tuberc Respir Dis (Seoul).* 2019;82(4):335-340. [IIIB]

106. May AM, Kazakov J, Strohl KP. Predictors of intraprocedural respiratory bronchoscopy complications. *J Bronchology Interv Pulmonol.* 2020;27(2):135-141. [IIIB]

107. Raveendran R, Wong J, Chung F. Morbid obesity, sleep apnea, obesity hypoventilation syndrome: are we sleepwalking into disaster? *Perioper Care Oper Room Manag.* 2017;9:24-32. [VA]

108. Chung F, Yegneswaran B, Liao P, et al. Validation of the Berlin questionnaire and American Society of Anesthesiologists checklist as screening tools for obstructive sleep apnea in surgical patients. *Anesthesiology.* 2008;108(5):822-830. [IIA]

109. Ramachandran SK, Kheterpal S, Consens F, et al. Derivation and validation of a simple perioperative sleep apnea prediction score. *Anesth Analg.* 2010;110(4):1007-1015. [IIIA]

110. Terry KL, Disabato J, Krajicek M. Snoring, Trouble Breathing, Un-Refreshed (STBUR) screening questionnaire to reduce perioperative respiratory adverse events in pediatric surgical patients: a quality improvement project. *AANA J.* 2015;83(4):256-262. [VA]

111. Willard CE, Rich AN, Broome ME, Silva SG, Muckler VC. Nasal ventilation mask for prevention of upper airway obstruction in patients with obesity or obstructive sleep apnea. *AANA J.* 2019;87(5):395-403. [VA]

112. Chittle MD, Oklu R, Pino RM, et al. Sedation shared decision-making in ambulatory venous access device placement: effects on patient choice, satisfaction and recovery time. *Vasc Med.* 2016;21(4):355-360. [IIIB]

113. McCain JD, Stancampiano FF, Bouras EP, et al. Creation of a score to predict risk of high conscious sedation requirements in patients undergoing endoscopy. *Gastrointest Endosc.* 2020;91(3):595-605. [IIIB]

114. Actionable Patient Safety Solutions (APSS): Moderate sedation. Patient Safety Movement. https://patientsafetymovement.org/clinical/surgical-and-procedural-safety/moderate-sedation/. Accessed June 17, 2021. [VA]

115. Kreienbühl L, Elia N, Pfeil-Beun E, Walder B, Tramèr MR. Patient-controlled versus clinician-controlled sedation with propofol: systematic review and meta-analysis with trial sequential analyses. *Anesth Analg.* 2018;127(4):873-880. [IA]

116. Pambianco D, Niklewski P. Computer-assisted and patient-controlled sedation platforms. *Gastrointest Endosc Clin N Am.* 2016;26(3):563-576. [VC]

117. Southerland WA, Beight LJ, Shapiro FE, Urman RD. Decision aids in anesthesia: do they help? *Curr Opin Anaesthesiol.* 2020;33(2):185-191. [VA]

118. *Standards for Basic Anesthesia Monitoring.* American Society of Anesthesiologists. https://www.asahq.org/standards-and-guidelines/standards-for-basic-anesthetic-monitoring. Last affirmed December 13, 2020. Accessed June 17, 2021. [IVB]

119. *Clinical Practice Guideline: Capnography.* Association or Radiologic and Imaging Nursing. https://www.arinursing.org/ARIN/assets/File/public/practice-guidelines/Capnography_CPG_FInal_031918.pdf. Accessed June 17, 2021. [IVB]

120. *AORN Position Statement on Perioperative Registered Nurse Circulator Dedicated to Every Patient Undergoing an Operative or Other Invasive Procedure.* AORN, Inc. https://aorn.org/guidelines/clinical-resources/position-statements. Revised March 2019. Accessed June 17, 2021. [IVB]

121. *Statement on the Use of Sedation and Analgesia in the Gastrointestinal Endoscopy Setting.* Society of Gastroenterology Nurses and Associates, Inc. https://www.sgna.org/Portals/0/Practice/Sedation/Sedation_FINAL.pdf?ver=2017-10-09-110940-983. Revised 2017. Accessed June 17, 2021. [IVB]

122. Klare P, Reiter J, Meining A, et al. Capnographic monitoring of midazolam and propofol sedation during ERCP: a randomized controlled study (EndoBreath Study). *Endoscopy.* 2016;48(1):42-50. [IA]

123. Barnett S, Hung A, Tsao R, et al. Capnographic monitoring of moderate sedation during low-risk screening colonoscopy does not improve safety or patient satisfaction: a prospective cohort study. *Am J Gastroenterol.* 2016;111(3):388-394. [IIA]

124. Committee on Quality Management and Departmental Administration. *Continuum of Depth of Sedation: Definition of General Anesthesia and Levels of Sedation/Analgesia.* American Society of Anesthesiologists. https://www.asahq.org/standards-and-guidelines/continuum-of-depth-of-sedation-definition-of-general-anesthesia-and-levels-of-sedation-analgesia. Last amended October 23, 2019. Accessed June 17, 2021. [VA]

125. Jokelainen J, Mustonen H, Kylänpää L, Udd M, Lindström O, Pöyhiä R. Assessment of sedation level for endoscopic retrograde cholangiopancreatography—a prospective validation study. *Scand J Gastroenterol.* 2018;53(3):370-375. [IIB]

126. Park SW, Lee H, Ahn H. Bispectral index versus standard monitoring in sedation for endoscopic procedures: a systematic review and meta-analysis. *Dig Dis Sci.* 2016;61(3):814-824. [IA]

127. Nisbet AT, Mooney-Cotter F. Comparison of selected sedation scales for reporting opioid-induced sedation assessment. *Pain Manag Nurs.* 2009;10(3):154-164. [IIIB]

128. Öztas S, Aka Aktürk Ü, Alpay LA, et al. A comparison of propofol-midazolam and midazolam alone for sedation in endobronchial ultrasound-guided transbronchial needle aspiration: a retrospective cohort study. *Clin Respir J.* 2017;11(6):935-941. [IIIB]

129. Ter Bruggen FFJA, Eralp I, Jansen CK, Stronks DL, Huygen FJPM. Efficacy of dexmedetomidine as a sole sedative agent in small diagnostic and therapeutic procedures: a systematic review. *Pain Pract.* 2017;17(6):829-840. [IA]

130. Zhong L, Shen K, Zhai S, et al. Application of sedation-agitation scale in conscious sedation before bronchoscopy in children. *Medicine (Baltimore).* 2019;98(1):e14035. [IIB]

131. American Association for Study of Liver Diseases; American College of Gastroenterology; American Gastroenterological Association Institute; et al. Multisociety sedation curriculum for gastrointestinal endoscopy. *Gastrointest Endosc.* 2012;76(1):e1-e25. [IVB]

132. Depth of anaesthesia monitors – bispectral index (BIS), E-Entropy and Narcotrend-Compact M. National Institute for Health and Care Excellence (NICE). https://www.nice.org.uk/guidance/dg6/documents/depth-of-anaesthesia-monitors-eentropy-bis-and-narcotrend-diagnostics-consultation-document. Published November 21, 2012. Accessed June 17, 2021. [IVB]

133. Conway A, Sutherland J. Depth of anaesthesia monitoring during procedural sedation and analgesia: a systematic review and meta-analysis. *Int J Nurs Stud.* 2016;63:201-212. [IA]

134. Gelfand ME, Gabriel RA, Gimlich R, Beutler SS, Urman RD. Practice patterns in the intraoperative use of bispectral index monitoring. *J Clin Monit Comput.* 2017;31(2):281-289. [IIIA]

135. ASGE Technology Committee; Gottlieb KT, Banerjee S, Barth BA, et al. Monitoring equipment for endoscopy. *Gastrointest Endosc.* 2013;77(2):175-180. [VA]

136. Impact of clinical alarms on patient safety: a report from the American College of Clinical Engineering Healthcare Technology Foundation. *J Clin Eng.* 2007;32(1):22-33. [VB]

137. ASGE Standards of Practice Committee; Chandrasekhara V, Early DS, Acosta RD, et al. Modifications in endoscopic practice for the elderly. *Gastrointest Endosc.* 2013;78(1):1-7. [IVA]

138. Childers RE, Williams JL, Sonnenberg A. Practice patterns of sedation for colonoscopy. *Gastrointest Endosc.* 2015;82(3):503-511. [IIIA]

139. Nemeth M, Jacobsen N, Bantel C, Fieler M, Sümpelmann R, Eich C. Intranasal analgesia and sedation in pediatric emergency care—a prospective observational study on the implementation of an institutional protocol in a tertiary children's hospital. *Pediatr Emerg Care.* 2019;35(2):89-95. [IIIB]

140. Conway A, Rolley J, Sutherland JR. Midazolam for sedation before procedures. *Cochrane Database Syst Rev.* 2016;(5):CD009491. [IA]

141. Gentz R, Casamassimo P, Amini H, Claman D, Smiley M. Safety and efficacy of 3 pediatric midazolam moderate sedation regimens. *Anesth Prog.* 2017;64(2):66-72. [IIB]

142. Alp H, Elmaci AM, Alp EK, Say B. Comparison of intranasal midazolam, intranasal ketamine, and oral chloral hydrate for conscious sedation during paediatric echocardiography: results of a prospective randomised study. *Cardiol Young.* 2019;29(9):1189-1195. [IB]

143. Stephen MC, Mathew J, Varghese AM, Kurien M, Mathew GA. A randomized controlled trial comparing intranasal midazolam and chloral hydrate for procedural sedation in children. *Otolaryngol Head Neck Surg.* 2015;153(6):1042-1050. [IB]

144. Tsze DS, Ieni M, Fenster DB, et al. Optimal volume of administration of intranasal midazolam in children: a randomized clinical trial. *Ann Emerg Med.* 2017;69(5):600-609. [IB]

145. Malia L, Laurich VM, Sturm JJ. Adverse events and satisfaction with use of intranasal midazolam for emergency department procedures in children. *Am J Emerg Med.* 2019;37(1):85-88. [VA]

146. Mellion SA, Bourne D, Brou L, et al. Evaluating clinical effectiveness and pharmacokinetic profile of atomized intranasal midazolam in children undergoing laceration repair. *J Emerg Med.* 2017;53(3):397-404. [IIB]

147. Ashley PF, Chaudhary M, Lourenço-Matharu L. Sedation of children undergoing dental treatment. *Cochrane Database Syst Rev.* 2018;(12):CD003877. [IA]

148. Khodadad A, Aflatoonian M, Jalilian R, et al. Comparison of oral midazolam with intravenous midazolam for sedation children during upper gastrointestinal endoscopy. *Acta Med Iran.* 2016;54(9):576-582. [IB]

149. Sado-Filho J, Viana KA, Corrêa-Faria P, Costa LR, Costa PS. Randomized clinical trial on the efficacy of intranasal or oral ketamine-midazolam combinations compared to oral midazolam for outpatient pediatric sedation. *PLoS One.* 2019;14(3):e0213074. [IB]

150. Chopra R, Marwaha M. Assessment of buccal aerosolized midazolam for pediatric conscious sedation. *J Investig Clin Dent.* 2015;6(1):40-44. [IIB]

151. Blumer S, Peretz B, Zisman G, Ratson T. Effect of sedation with midazolam and time to discharge among pediatric dental patients. *J Clin Pediatr Dent.* 2017;41(5):384-387. [IIIB]

152. Cao Q, Lin Y, Xie Z, et al. Comparison of sedation by intranasal dexmedetomidine and oral chloral hydrate for pediatric ophthalmic examination. *Paediatr Anaesth.* 2017;27(6):629-636. [IB]

153. Li BL, Zhang N, Huang JX, et al. A comparison of intranasal dexmedetomidine for sedation in children administered either by atomiser or by drops. *Anaesthesia.* 2016;71(5):522-528. [IB]

154. Xie Z, Shen W, Lin J, Xiao L, Liao M, Gan X. Sedation effects of intranasal dexmedetomidine delivered as sprays versus drops on pediatric response to venous cannulation. *Am J Emerg Med.* 2017;35(8):1126-1130. [IB]

155. Yuen VM, Li BL, Cheuk DK, et al. A randomised controlled trial of oral chloral hydrate vs. intranasal dexmedetomidine before computerised tomography in children. *Anaesthesia.* 2017;72(10):1191-1195. [IC]

156. Uusalo P, Guillaume S, Siren S, et al. Pharmacokinetics and sedative effects of intranasal dexmedetomidine in ambulatory pediatric patients. *Anesth Analg.* 2020;130(4):949-957. [IIB]

157. Mekitarian Filho E, Robinson F, de Carvalho WB, Gilio AE, Mason KP. Intranasal dexmedetomidine for sedation for pediatric computed tomography imaging. *J Pediatr.* 2015;166(5):1313-1315. [IIIC]

158. Fenster DB, Dayan PS, Babineau J, Aponte-Patel L, Tsze DS. Randomized trial of intranasal fentanyl versus intravenous morphine for abscess incision and drainage. *Pediatr Emerg Care.* 2018;34(9):607-612. [IB]

159. Adelgais KM, Brent A, Wathen J, et al. Intranasal fentanyl and quality of pediatric acute care. *J Emerg Med.* 2017;53(5):607-615. [IIB]

160. Chen M, Hill GM, Patrianakos TD, Ku ES, Chen ML. Oral diazepam versus intravenous midazolam for conscious sedation during cataract surgery performed using topical anesthesia. *J Cataract Refract Surg.* 2015;41(2):415-421. [IB]

161. Rignell L, Mikati M, Wertsén M, Hägglin C. Sedation with orally administered midazolam in elderly dental patients with major neurocognitive disorder. *Gerodontology.* 2017;34(3):299-305. [IIIB]

162. Ryu DS, Lee DW, Choi SC, Oh IH. Sedation protocol using dexmedetomidine for third molar extraction. *J Oral Maxillofac Surg.* 2016;74(5):926.e1-926.e7. [IB]

163. Rozario L, Sloper D, Sheridan MJ. Supplemental oxygen during moderate sedation and the occurrence of clinically significant desaturation during endoscopic procedures. *Gastroenterol Nurs.* 2008;31(4):281-285. [IB]

164. Hung A, Marshall J, Barnett S, Falchuk ZM, Sawhney M, Leffler DA. Risk factors and outcomes of reversal agent use in moderate sedation during endoscopy and colonoscopy. *J Clin Gastroenterol.* 2016;50(3):e25-e29. [IIIB]

165. Yonel Z, Asuni A, Taneja P. Defining over-sedation: literature review and national survey of dental hospitals within the United Kingdom. *SAAD Dig.* 2016;32:28-33. [VB]

166. Folland L, Brown E, Boyle C. A review of the use of flumazenil for the reversal of midazolam conscious sedation in dentistry. *SAAD Dig.* 2017;33:13-17. [VB]

167. *Standards for Perioperative Nursing in Australia.* Vol 1-2. 16th ed. Adelaide, SA: Australian College of Operating Room Nurses; 2020. [IVB]

168. *Discharge After Sedation or Anesthesia on the Day of the Procedure: Patient Transportation With or Without a Responsible Adult. Position Statement and Policy Considerations.* American Association of Nurse Anesthetists. https://www.aana.com/docs/default-source/practice-aana-com-web-documents-(all)/professional-practice-manual/discharge-after-sedation-or-anesthesia-on-the-day-of-the-procedure.pdf?sfvrsn=ed4a5bb1_2. Published 2018. Accessed June 17, 2021. [IVB]

169. 42 CFR 416: Ambulatory surgical services. Electronic Code of Federal Regulations. https://www.ecfr.gov/cgi-bin/text-idx?node=pt42.3.416&rgn=div5. Accessed June 17, 2021.

170. 42 CFR 482: Conditions of participation for hospitals. Electronic Code of Federal Regulations. https://www.ecfr.gov/cgi-bin/retrieveECFR?gp=1&SID=2bc06578c2ca4ab54fadf46e1fc4dfda&ty=HTML&h=L&mc=true&n=pt42.5.482&r=PART. Accessed June 17, 2021.

171. Veselis RA, Pryor KO, Reinsel RA, Li Y, Mehta M, Johnson R Jr. Propofol and midazolam inhibit conscious memory processes very soon after encoding: an event-related potential study of familiarity and recollection in volunteers. *Anesthesiology.* 2009;110(2):295-312. [IA]

172. Watkins TJ, Bonds RL, Hodges K, Goettle BB, Dobson DA, Maye JP. Evaluation of postprocedure cognitive function using 3 distinct standard sedation regimens for endoscopic procedures. *AANA J.* 2014;82(2):133-139. [IB]

173. Padmanabhan U, Leslie K, Eer AS, Maruff P, Silbert BS. Early cognitive impairment after sedation for colonoscopy: the effect of adding midazolam and/or fentanyl to propofol. *Anesth Analg.* 2009;109(5):1448-1455. [IC]

174. Dumonceau JM, Riphaus A, Beilenhoff U, et al. European curriculum for sedation training in gastrointestinal endoscopy: position statement of the European Society of Gastrointestinal Endoscopy (ESGE) and European Society of Gastroenterology and Endoscopy Nurses and Associates (ESGENA). *Endoscopy.* 2013;45(6):496-504. [IVB]

175. Tran TT, Beutler SS, Urman RD. Moderate and deep sedation training and pharmacology for nonanesthesiologists: recommendations for effective practice. *Curr Opin Anaesthesiol.* 2019;32(4):457-463. [VA]

176. Da B, Buxbaum J. Training and competency in sedation practice in gastrointestinal endoscopy. *Gastrointest Endosc Clin N Am.* 2016;26(3):443-462. [VB]

177. Kost M. Nursing considerations for procedural sedation and analgesia: part 1. *Am Nurse Today.* 2019;14(5):6-11. [VA]

178. Jensen JT, Savran MM, Møller AM, Vilmann P, Hornslet P, Konge L. Development and validation of a theoretical test in non-anaesthesiologist-administered propofol sedation for gastrointestinal endoscopy. *Scand J Gastroenterol.* 2016;51(7):872-879. [IIIB]

179. Brady M, Kinn S, Stuart P. Preoperative fasting for adults to prevent perioperative complications. *Cochrane Database Syst Rev.* 2003;(4):CD004423. [IA]

180. Green SM, Leroy PL, Roback MG, et al. An international multidisciplinary consensus statement on fasting before procedural sedation in adults and children. *Anaesthesia.* 2020;75(3):374-385. [IVA]

181. Brady M, Kinn S, Ness V, O'Rourke K, Randhawa N, Stuart P. Preoperative fasting for preventing perioperative complications in children. *Cochrane Database Syst Rev.* 2009;(4):CD005285. [IA]

182. Shaukat A, Malhotra A, Greer N, MacDonald R, Wels J, Wilt TJ. Systematic review: outcomes by duration of NPO status prior to colonoscopy. *Gastroenterol Res Pract.* 2017;2017:3914942. [IIIA]

183. Mason KP, Green SM, Piacevoli Q; International Sedation Task Force. Adverse event reporting tool to standardize the reporting and tracking of adverse events during procedural sedation: a consensus document from the World SIVA International Sedation Task Force. *Br J Anaesth.* 2012;108(1):13-20. [IVB]

184. Lee DH, Woo JH, Hong SE. Judicial precedent-based clinical practice guidelines of propofol in sedative esthetic surgery. *Aesthetic Plast Surg.* 2018;42(3):891-898. [VB]

185. Jani SR, Shapiro FE, Gabriel RA, et al. A comparison between office and other ambulatory practices: analysis from the National Anesthesia Clinical Outcomes Registry. *J Healthc Risk Manag.* 2016;35(4):38-47. [IIIB]

186. Ranum D, Beverly A, Shapiro FE, Urman RD. Leading causes of anesthesia-related liability claims in ambulatory surgery centers. *J Patient Saf.* 2017. doi: 10.1097/PTS.0000000000000431. [IIIB]

187. Ward DS, Williams MR, Berkenbosch JW, et al. Evaluating patient-centered outcomes in clinical trials of procedural sedation, part 2 safety: Sedation Consortium on Endpoints and Procedures for Treatment, Education, and Research Recommendations. *Anesth Analg.* 2018;127(5):1146-1154. [IVB]

188. Nguyen TT, Baker B, Ferguson JD. Allergic reaction to ketamine as monotherapy for procedural sedation. *J Emerg Med.* 2017;52(4):562-564. [VB]

189. Stone AB, Jones MR, Rao N, Urman RD. A dashboard for monitoring opioid-related adverse drug events following surgery using a national administrative database. *Am J Med Qual.* 2019;34(1):45-52. [VA]

190. Jones MR, Karamnov S, Urman RD. Characteristics of reported adverse events during moderate procedural sedation: an update. *Jt Comm J Qual Patient Saf.* 2018;44(11):651-662. [IIIB]

191. Stone AB, Brovman EY, Greenberg P, Urman RD. A medicolegal analysis of malpractice claims involving anesthesiologists in the gastrointestinal endoscopy suite (2007-2016). *J Clin Anesth.* 2018;48:15-20. [IIIB]

192. Lemay A, Shyn PB, Foley R, Beutler SS, Silverman SG, Urman RD. A procedural sedation quality improvement audit form tool for interventional radiology. *J Med Pract Manage.* 2015;30(6 Spec No):44-47. [VA]

Guideline Development Group

Lead Author: Amber Wood[1], MSN, RN, CNOR, CIC, FAPIC, Senior Perioperative Practice Specialist, AORN, Denver, Colorado

Methodologist: Erin Kyle[2], DNP, RN, CNOR, NEA-BC, Editor-in-Chief, *Guidelines for Perioperative Practice*, AORN, Denver, Colorado

Evidence Appraisers: Amber Wood[1]; Janice Neil[3], PhD, CNE, RN, Associate Professor, East Carolina College of Nursing, Greenville, North Carolina; and Erin Kyle[2]

Guidelines Advisory Board Members:

- Mary Fearon[4], MSN, RN, CNOR, Service Line Director Neuroscience, Overlake Medical Center, Sammamish, Washington
- Brenda G. Larkin[5], MS, ACNS-BC, CNS, CNOR, Clinical Nurse Specialist, Aurora Lakeland Medical Center, Lake Geneva, Wisconsin

Guidelines Advisory Board Liaisons:

- Craig S. Atkins[6], DNP, CRNA, Chief Nurse Anesthetist, Belmar Ambulatory Surgical Center, Lakewood, Colorado
- Cassie Dietrich[7], MD, Anesthesiologist, Anesthesia Associates of Kansas City, Overland Park, Kansas

External Review: Expert review comments were received from individual members of the American Association of Nurse Anesthetists (AANA), American College of Surgeons (ACS), Association for Professionals in Infection Control and Epidemiology (APIC), American Society of Anesthesiologists (ASA), International Association of Healthcare Central Service Materiel Management (IAHCSMM), the Society for Healthcare Epidemiology of America (SHEA), and the Surgical Infection Society (SIS). Their responses were used to further refine and enhance this guideline; however, their responses do not imply endorsement. The draft was also open for a 30-day public comment period.

Financial Disclosure and Conflicts of Interest

This guideline was developed, edited, and approved by the AORN Guidelines Advisory Board without external funding being sought or obtained. The Guidelines Advisory Board was financially supported entirely by AORN and was developed without any involvement of industry.

Potential conflicts of interest for all Guidelines Advisory Board members were reviewed before the annual meeting and each monthly conference call. None of the members of the Guideline Development Group reported a potential conflict of interest.[1-7]

Publication History

Originally published April 1993, *AORN Journal*, as "Recommended practices for monitoring the patient receiving intravenous conscious sedation."

Revised; published in January 1997, *AORN Journal*, as "Recommended practices for managing the patient receiving conscious sedation/analgesia." Reformatted July 2000.

Revised November 2001; published March 2002, *AORN Journal*, as "Recommended practices for managing the patient receiving moderate sedation/analgesia."

Revised 2007; published in *Perioperative Standards and Recommended Practices*, 2008 edition.

Minor editing revisions made to omit PNDS codes; reformatted September 2012 for publication in *Perioperative Standards and Recommended Practices*, 2013 edition.

Minor editing revisions made in November 2014 for publication as "Guideline for managing the patient receiving moderate sedation/analgesia" in *Guidelines for Perioperative Practice*, 2015 edition.

Revised December 2015 for online publication in *Guidelines for Perioperative Practice*.

Evidence ratings revised and minor editorial changes made to conform to the current AORN Evidence Rating model, September 2019, for online publication in *Guidelines for Perioperative Practice*.

Revised July 2021 for online publication in *Guidelines for Perioperative Practice*.

Scheduled for review in 2026.

PACKAGING SYSTEMS

TABLE OF CONTENTS

MEDICAL ABBREVIATIONS & ACRONYMS

BI – Biological indicator
CI – Chemical indicator
EO – Ethylene oxide
FDA – US Food and Drug Administration

IFU – Instructions for use
PI – Performance improvement
QA – Quality assurance

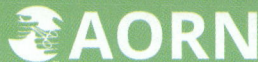
GUIDELINE FOR
STERILIZATION PACKAGING SYSTEMS

The Guideline for Sterilization Packaging Systems was approved by the AORN Guidelines Advisory Board and became effective as of October 1, 2019. The recommendations in the guideline are intended to be achievable and represent what is believed to be an optimal level of practice. Policies and procedures will reflect variations in practice settings and/or clinical situations that determine the degree to which the guideline can be implemented. AORN recognizes the many diverse settings in which perioperative nurses practice; therefore, this guideline is adaptable to all areas where operative or other invasive procedures may be performed.

Purpose

This document provides guidance to perioperative personnel for evaluating, selecting, and using sterilization **packaging systems** and for packaging the items to be sterilized and subsequently used in operative and other invasive procedures. Packaging systems are designed to permit sterilization of the contents within the package, protect the integrity of the sterilized contents, prevent contamination of the contents until the package is opened for use, and permit the aseptic delivery of the contents to the sterile field. Packaging systems include woven fabrics, single-use **nonwoven materials**, **paper-plastic pouches**, polyethylene material-plastic pouches, plastic-plastic pouches, and rigid **containment devices** (eg, sterilization containers, **instrument cases**, **cassettes**, **organizing trays**) composed of a variety of materials.

This guideline does not include recommendations for high-level disinfection, liquid chemical sterilization, processing flexible endoscopes, cleaning contaminated instruments, inspecting instruments, loading a sterilizer, sterilization, or aseptic presentation at the point of use. Refer to the AORN Guideline for Cleaning and Care of Surgical Instruments,[1] Guideline for High-Level Disinfection,[2] Guideline for Processing Flexible Endoscopes,[3] Guideline for Sterilization,[4] Guideline for Sterile Technique,[5] and the packaging system manufacturer's instructions for use (IFU) for more information.

Evidence Review

A medical librarian with a perioperative background conducted a systematic search of the databases Ovid MEDLINE®, Ovid Embase®, EBSCO CINAHL®, and the Cochrane Database of Systematic Reviews. The search was limited to literature published in English from January 2013 through October 2018. At the time of the initial search, weekly alerts were created on the topics included in that search. Results from these alerts were provided to the lead author until December 2018. The lead author requested additional articles that either did not fit the original search criteria or were discovered during the evidence appraisal process. The lead author and the medical librarian also identified relevant guidelines from government agencies, professional organizations, and standards-setting bodies.

Search terms included *barrier integrity, barrier properties, basket, biological indicators, central service department, central sterile processing, central supply (hospital), chemical indicators, clinical competence, colony count (microbial), condensation, cross infection, dental instruments, device packaging, disposable equipment, equipment and supplies, equipment contamination, equipment failure, equipment reuse, event-dependent, event-related, fabrics, flash sterilization, heat sealer, hospital central supply, hospital purchasing, humidity, immediate use steam sterilization, immediate use sterilization, indicators and reagents, infection control, instrument case, instrument cassette, instrument set, instrument tray, Kraft, loaner instruments, materials testing, medical packaging, microbial colony count, monitoring, Mylar, olefin, one tray, organizing tray, outdating, package integrity, packaging device, packaging material, packaging system, paper count sheets, peel pack, peel pouch, plastics, polypropene, polypropylene, pouch, product labeling, product packaging, purchasing department, quality control, reusable pack, rigid container, safety management, sequential wrapping, single use, steam, sterile instruments, sterile package, sterile packaging, sterile processing, sterile storage, sterile supplies, sterility maintenance cover, sterilization, sterilization and disinfection, sterilization container, sterilization wrap, surgical equipment, surgical equipment and supplies, surgical instruments, textiles, time-dependent, time-related,* and *Tyvek.*

Included were research and non-research literature in English, complete publications, and publications with dates within the time restriction when available. Excluded were non-peer-reviewed publications and older evidence within the time restriction when more recent evidence was available. Editorials, news items, and other brief items were excluded. Low-quality evidence was excluded when higher-quality evidence was available, and literature outside the time restriction was excluded when literature within the time restriction was available **(Figure 1)**.

Articles identified in the search were provided to the project team for evaluation. The team consisted of the lead author and one evidence appraiser. The lead author and the evidence appraiser reviewed and critically appraised each article using the AORN Research or Non-Research Evidence Appraisal Tools as appropriate. A second appraiser

Figure 1. Flow Diagram of Literature Search Results

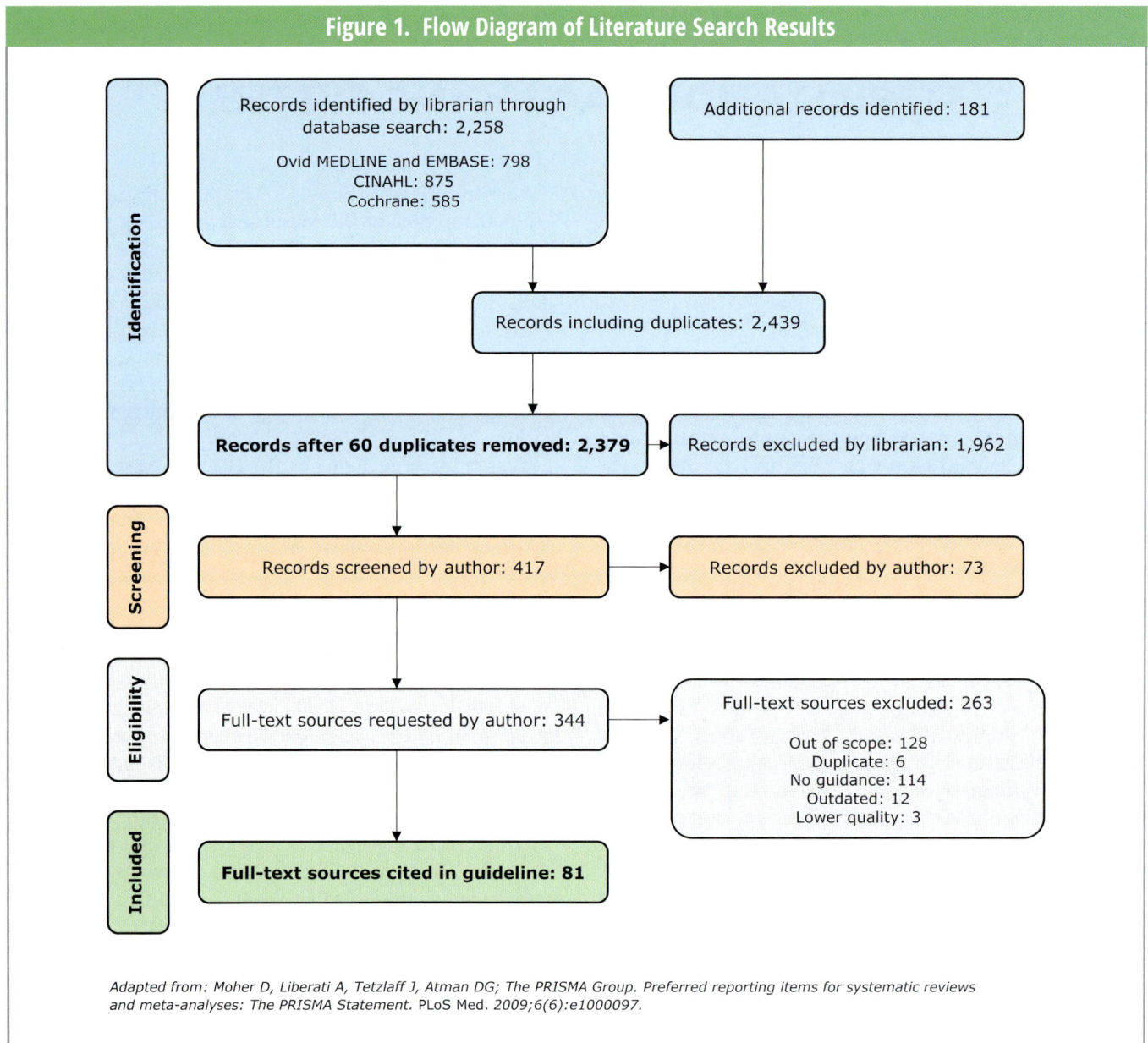

Adapted from: Moher D, Liberati A, Tetzlaff J, Atman DG; The PRISMA Group. Preferred reporting items for systematic reviews and meta-analyses: The PRISMA Statement. PLoS Med. 2009;6(6):e1000097.

was consulted if there was a disagreement between the lead author and the primary evidence appraiser. The literature was independently evaluated and appraised according to the strength and quality of the evidence. Each article was then assigned an appraisal score. The appraisal score is noted in brackets after each reference as applicable.

Each recommendation rating is based on a synthesis of the collective evidence, a benefit-harm assessment, and consideration of resource use. The strength of the recommendation was determined using the AORN Evidence Rating Model and the quality and consistency of the evidence supporting a recommendation. The recommendation strength rating is noted in brackets after each recommendation.

Note: The evidence summary table is available at http:// www.aorn.org/evidencetables/.

Editor's note: MEDLINE is a registered trademark of the US National Library of Medicine's Medical Literature Analysis and Retrieval System, Bethesda, MD. Embase is a registered trademark of Elsevier B.V., Amsterdam, The Netherlands. CINAHL, Cumulative Index to Nursing and Allied Health Literature, is a registered trademark of EBSCO Industries, Birmingham, AL. Mylar is a registered trademark of DuPont Tejin Films, Chester, VA. Tyvek is a registered trademark of DuPont, Wilmington, DE.

1. Pre-purchase Evaluation

1.1 Evaluate **sterilization packaging** before initial purchase and use. Packaging for sterilization of reusable medical devices and surgical instrumentation should

- have US Food and Drug Administration (FDA) clearance for performance claims and intended use[6-11];
- include clear and complete manufacturer's IFU[10-12];
- allow air removal to permit sterilant penetration of the package contents[10,12];
- provide a barrier to microorganisms during sterilization processing, handling, distribution, transport, and storage[10,13];
- resist tearing or puncture[10,12,13];
- have a sealing method that results in a complete seal that is tamper-evident and provides seal integrity[10,14,15];
- maintain protection for the sterile contents during storage and transport to the point of use[10,14-18];
- allow for aseptic presentation at the point of use[10,11,13-16,19];
- be free of toxic components and nonfast dyes[10,14,15];
- be nonlinting[10,12,14,15];
- be compatible with the intended methods of sterilization, sterilization parameters, and the devices to be sterilized[10,12-15]; and
- be easy to use.[17,20,21]

[Recommendation]

Before purchase, verifying that sterilization packaging is compatible with the sterilization method, equipment, and organizational handling and storage practices increases the likelihood that sterilization packaging will be effective in achieving and maintaining sterility during use in the organization.[10,12-15,18-20,22-29] For further guidance on pre-purchase evaluation, see the AORN Guideline for Medical Device and Product Evaluation.[30]

1.1.1 Review the manufacturers' IFU to verify that the packaging system and packaging material are intended for use with both the method(s) of sterilization and the specific equipment that will be used for sterilization in the organization.[10] *[Recommendation]*

The manufacturers' IFU provide detailed information that identifies correct use with the intended sterilization method(s) and equipment.[10,11]

1.1.2 Review the sterilization packaging manufacturer's **validation** information before purchase. *[Recommendation]*

The manufacturer validation testing information may include the extent of sterilant penetration, aeration times, maximum package content weight, level of resistance to tears and punctures, barrier performance, seal integrity

and strength, tensile properties, burst strength, use with extended steam sterilization cycles, sterility maintenance, and **shelf life**.[12,14,15,31-34]

1.1.3 Evaluate sterilization package performance in the environment in which it will be used, including these elements:
- product quality assurance testing results[10] (See Recommendation 10.2);
- barrier effectiveness[10-12,14,15];
- compatibility with the intended sterilization method(s) and cycles used within the facility[10];
- requirements for cleaning according to the IFU (eg, laundry for textiles, equipment for cleaning rigid containers)[11];
- biocompatibility[10,14,15];
- availability of an external **chemical indicator** (CI)[10-12,14,15];
- durability[10-12,14,15];
- **expected life of the device**, including all components[10-12,14,15];
- requirements for tracking use[10];
- method for tracking use[10];
- method for labeling[10];
- ability of the seal to maintain **package integrity**[10-12,14,15];
- requirements for disassembly, laundering, or cleaning[10];
- maintenance requirements[10];
- storage requirements[10];
- ease of use[12,20,23];
- weight[10];
- available sizes;
- ease of transport[12,20,23];
- ease of aseptic presentation[12,20,23];
- environmental impact[13,25,26,35-37]; and
- cost-effectiveness, including initial cost, cost to use, and cost to maintain.[13,38]

[Recommendation]

A sterilization packaging pre-purchase evaluation allows the organization to evaluate packaging performance in the work environment where it will be used.[10,30]

1.2 Select **environmentally preferable** sterilization packaging over other options when they are equivalent in performance.[13,22,25,26,35-37] *[Recommendation]*

Health care professionals have an ethical and professional responsibility to advocate for patients' health.[36] Because human health is dependent on the environment, by extension, it is important that nurses work to actively protect the environment by promoting and participating in initiatives that mitigate negative environmental impact.[36] Estimates of the amount of waste generated by health care facilities vary, with some estimates as high as 4 billion pounds annually. Much of that waste is generated in the operating room and consists of packaging and disposable supplies.[37] The manufacturing process requires use of raw materials and energy consumption and can result in varying levels of carbon and greenhouse gas emissions. Manufacturers of sterilization packaging can provide information regarding their sustainability practices. Some experts suggest that use of environmentally responsible packaging results in cost savings.[37]

1.2.1 Evaluate sterilization packaging for environmentally preferable criteria throughout the lifecycle of the product, including
- sustainable manufacturing,[22,25]
- reusability,[22,25,35-37]
- maintenance,[13,22,25,36]
- disposal (waste versus recycling),[13,22,25,26,35-37] and
- resource consumption to use the product.[22,25,35,36]
[Recommendation]

2. Compatibility with the Sterilization Method

2.1 Use sterilization packaging that is compatible with the specific sterilization method(s) and cycle(s) for which they will be used. [Recommendation]

The interaction among packaging systems, medical devices, and sterilizer technologies is complex. Not all packaging systems are suitable for all methods of sterilization.[1,4,8,10,14-16,19,24,34,39-43] The manufacturer's IFU provide detailed information for sterilization method and cycle type compatibility.[10,14,15,39,40]

2.1.1 For steam sterilization, use compatible packaging systems that are cleared by the FDA for steam sterilization and the sterilization cycle selected.[10,11] [Recommendation]

Packaging for steam sterilization may be cycle-specific, with some being validated for either gravity or dynamic air removal cycles. Packaging systems that are cleared by the FDA for use in steam sterilizers have been subjected to and passed extensive laboratory validation testing for use in steam sterilization cycles.[10,11]

2.1.2 For low-temperature hydrogen peroxide sterilization cycles (eg, vapor, gas plasma combination, ozone combination), use compatible sterilization packaging that is cleared by the FDA for these sterilization methods and intended cycle types.[11,39] [Recommendation]

Low-temperature **vaporized hydrogen peroxide sterilization** methods are affected by absorbent packaging materials (eg, cellulose-based packaging material, textile wrappers, paper-plastic pouches, porous wrap). Absorption of the sterilant (ie, hydrogen peroxide) by paper-plastic pouches or porous wrap has been shown to adversely affect the sterilization process.[11,39]

Ozone penetration can alter chemical and physical characteristics of some single-use packages, affecting durability.[43] Packaging materials that are most resistant to degradation are nonwoven pouches and reusable **rigid sterilization container systems**.[11,17,39]

2.1.3 For ethylene oxide (EO) sterilization, use compatible sterilization packaging that is cleared by the FDA for EO sterilization.[11,40] [Recommendation]

Woven, nonwoven, and peel-pouch packages and some rigid sterilization container systems can be permeated by 100% EO and allow aeration of the contents. However, some packaging materials can retain EO residuals, making the packaging difficult to aerate. Woven materials may absorb a large amount of relative humidity that is needed for EO sterilization and may not be suitable for EO sterilization cycles.[11,40]

Sufficient humidity helps maintain adequate hydration of microorganisms, thereby increasing their susceptibility to destruction by EO.[11,40]

3. Preparation for Packaging

3.1 Perform packaging for sterilization in an area intended, designed, and equipped for sterilization packaging. [Recommendation]

Competent personnel and equivalent environments, procedures, supplies, equipment, and quality assurance measures are needed in all locations where packaging is performed.[4] The requirements for packaging reusable medical devices for sterilization do not vary by location.[44-49]

3.2 Perform packaging for sterilization in a clean work area or room with restricted access (eg, the semi-restricted area of the perioperative suite), with physical separation from high-traffic hallways or other potential sources of contamination, such as sinks or waste containers. [Recommendation]

The presence of environmental contaminants[46] and extraneous objects in sterilized packages can be minimized when packaging occurs in a controlled environment.[10] See the AORN Guideline for Design and Maintenance of the Surgical Suite[48] for more information about semi-restricted area requirements.

3.3 **Store sterilization packaging materials in the environmental conditions specified in the manufacturer's IFU.**[10] *[Recommendation]*

The instructions included in the IFU have been validated by the manufacturer as part of the FDA clearance process. Some manufacturers of packaging materials may specify environmental storage condition requirements for their products.[10,14,15] Temperature and humidity equilibrium may be necessary to permit adequate sterilant penetration and to avoid **superheating**.[10] Storing wrap material in areas of low humidity may lead to superheating and sterilization failure.[10]

3.4 **Establish and follow standardized procedures for sterilization packaging.** *[Recommendation]*

Standardizing the process for packaging can reduce the risk for error related to human factors.[20,50,51] Sterile processing areas are unpredictable environments, with variations and interruptions that can disrupt work processes and lead to errors.[52] Establishing standardized procedures for sterilization packaging that are rooted in manufacturers' guidance for medical devices and sterilization packaging materials can streamline and clarify work-streams for personnel and teams. Errors in instrument trays (eg, missing instruments, absent CIs, extraneous items) can have significant effects at the point of use.[53] When work processes are standardized, personnel can more easily find their place when they return to work after an interruption or if other team members resume the work in their absence.

3.4.1 **Organizing accessories (See Recommendation 3.5) may be used to facilitate standardized organization of items within the tray or set.** *[Conditional Recommendation]*

Use of organizing accessories can assist personnel in applying standardized organization of items within trays and sets.[54,55]

3.5 **Determine compatibility of organizing accessories with sterile packaging systems before use.**[10,11] **Use only compatible organizing accessories.** *[Recommendation]*

Medical device manufacturers provide information about organizing-accessory compatibility in their IFU.[10,11]

3.5.1 **Use only organizing accessories (eg, trays, cassettes, silicone mats, towels, tray corners) that are permitted by the sterile pack-** aging system manufacturer's written IFU.[10,11] *[Recommendation]*

Adding materials to the container in a manner that is not in accordance with the manufacturer's IFU may inhibit sterilization and the performance of the container.[10,11]

3.5.2 **When permitted by the packaging and sterilizer manufacturers' IFU, use towels that are lint free, laundered (See Recommendation 5.1.1), and thoroughly rinsed.** *[Recommendation]*

Lint left on sterile instruments can become airborne particles that carry microorganisms. These particles can be transferred to the surgical wound and may cause a foreign-body reaction.[10] Rinsing the towels during the laundering process reduces the risk of transferring chemical residues to instruments.[10,39]

3.6 **Tip protectors may be used during processing of sharp items.** *[Conditional Recommendation]*

Tip protectors provide sharp items with a measure of protection from damage[10] and can protect personnel from sharps injuries.

3.6.1 **When used, tip protectors should be validated for the sterilization method.**[10] *[Recommendation]*

3.6.2 **When used, tip protectors should be colored or tinted (ie, not clear).** *[Recommendation]*

Tip protectors that are clear and colorless may be difficult for personnel to see on the sterile field, which poses a risk for a potential retained surgical item.[56]

3.7 **Verify that instruments and medical devices have been cleaned, inspected, dried, and assembled according to the instrument or medical device manufacturer's IFU prior to packaging.** *[Recommendation]*

Instruments and medical devices that have not been subjected to proper cleaning, inspection, and assembly as described in the IFU are not ready for packaging and subsequent sterilization.[10]

3.8 **Perform hand hygiene before handling instruments and medical devices for sterilization packaging.** *[Recommendation]*

Contaminants, oils, and soils transferred to instruments from the hands of personnel can compromise sterilization. Costa et al[57] conducted a laboratory-based study to determine the effect of hand hygiene and glove use on maintenance of surgical instrument cleanliness after decontamination and during inspection, assembly, and packaging of reusable surgical instruments. After manual and automated cleaning, 45 Halsted-mosquito forceps were assessed for adenosine triphosphate, protein, and microbial contamination after being handled with gloved or bare hands. Five groups were compared: nitrile gloved hands, bare hands immediately after hand hygiene, bare hands 1 hour after hand hygiene, bare hands 2 hours after hand hygiene, and bare hands 4 hours after hand hygiene.

The researchers found that bare hands that had not been washed immediately prior to handling instruments had significant increases in microbial load and protein contamination at each time interval. Gram-negative bacteria were among the organisms detected on the instruments, which presents a risk of endotoxin contamination. The researchers recommended that personnel who perform inspection, assembly, and packaging of reusable surgical instruments perform hand hygiene within the hour or wear clean gloves to perform these tasks.[57]

3.9   **Position items to be sterilized within packages in a way that facilitates sterilant contact with all surfaces and aseptic presentation of the package contents at the point of use.**[10] *[Recommendation]*

Sterilant contact is necessary for sterilization to be achieved, and incorrect packaging may prevent sterilization from occurring. Inappropriate handling can lead to loss of package integrity. Incorrect packaging can make aseptic delivery of the contents to the sterile field difficult or impossible.[58]

> **3.9.1**   **Place items to be sterilized into the container in a disassembled state unless the device manufacturer's IFU specifies that disassembly is not required.**[10] *[Recommendation]*
>
> Sterilization of assembled instruments can prevent exposure of some areas of the device to the sterilant.[10]

> **3.9.2**   **Place items to be sterilized in an open or unlatched position within the sterilization package.** *[Recommendation]*
>
> The open or unlatched position facilitates sterilant contact of all surfaces of the item.[10]

> **3.9.3**   **Racks, stringers, and V-shaped pouches designed and intended for sterilization may be used to maintain instruments in their open position.**[10,59] *[Conditional Recommendation]*

> **3.9.4**   **Position items that have concave or convex surfaces or lumens within sterilization packages in a manner that prevents water retention.**[10,16] *[Recommendation]*
>
> Preventing water retention can help avoid the occurrence of wet packs and sterilization

failure. Medical devices with lumens (eg, phacoemulsification hand pieces), especially those that are long, narrow, or closed on one end, pose a challenge to sterilization (See the AORN Guideline for Sterilization).[4] Although the device manufacturer's IFU provide instructions for orientation of the device within the sterilization container or the sterilizer, it is important to conduct verification testing of these complex devices to ensure there is no water retention following sterilization.

3.10   **Do not exceed 25 lb as total weight of the sterile packaging system and contents.**[10,11,60] *[Recommendation]*

Instrument sets weighing more than 25 lb are known to be difficult to dry without lengthy drying times and present an increased risk for ergonomic injury to health care personnel.[10,11,60]

3.11   **For loaner instrumentation and medical devices, use sterilization packaging that is described in the instrument or medical device manufacturer's written IFU.** *[Recommendation]*

Medical device manufacturers are responsible for ensuring that their devices are compatible with the recommended packaging methods and for providing written instructions for processing the device.[11]

> **3.11.1**   **If the loaner medical device manufacturer's IFU for sterilization packaging is not available in the organization, obtain it from the loaning vendor.** *[Recommendation]*
>
> Vendors that loan devices are responsible for providing manufacturers' IFU to users.

3.12   **Determine whether count sheets may be placed in instrument trays at the health care organization.** *[Conditional Recommendation]*

Instrument count sheets are used by perioperative teams for inventory control and for instrument counting during surgical procedures. There are no known reports of adverse events related to the use of sterilized count sheets contained within sterilized packages. However, there is limited research regarding the safety of subjecting toners, inks, and various papers to any sterilization method. Chemicals used in the manufacture of paper, toners, and inks pose a theoretical risk of reaction in some sensitized individuals.

A literature search related to cytotoxicity of count sheets yielded only one study. This laboratory-based study sought to evaluate cytotoxicity of ink transferred to instruments during steam sterilization.[61] The researchers created simulated count sheets using one copier, two printers, and 30% recycled copy paper. The copier and a laser printer used toner and the second printer used ink. The paper was printed with a solid 7.5 x 10-inch black block and was placed in direct contact with stainless steel instruments to maximize the potential for transfer during steam sterilization. All instrument sets were steam sterilized for 20 minutes at 121° C (249.8° F) under a prevacuum setting with a 10-minute dry time. Only the laser printer had visible transfer of the toner to the instruments. Cytotoxicity was measured using neutral red cytotoxicity assay for the printed paper before and after sterilization and for the instruments that had been exposed to the printed paper during steam sterilization. The researchers concluded that the label and toner ink transferred during sterilization was not cytotoxic but that further study is needed to incorporate a larger sample, various sterilization methods, and instruments of a variety of compositions.[61]

4. Chemical Indicator Placement

4.1 Select CIs specific to the sterilization method and cycle. *[Recommendation]*

External and internal CIs do not verify sterility of the contents. Internal CIs are used to verify that one or more of the conditions necessary for sterilization have been achieved for each package that has been exposed to a sterilization cycle.[10,16,19,39,40,62,63]

4.2 Place a CI on both the outside and inside of the package to be processed. Placing a CI on the outside of the package may not be necessary if the internal CI can be placed in the most challenging location within the package (See Recommendation 4.4) and remain readable through the package material after sterilization.[10,16,62] *[Recommendation]*

The purpose of external CIs is to visually identify that a package has been exposed to the sterilization process. External CIs are intended to differentiate processed from unprocessed packages.[10,16,62]

Internal CIs are used to verify that the sterilant has reached the contents of the package and that sterilization-method-specific critical variables of the sterilization process have been met.[10,16,62]

4.3 Place a **type 1 CI** (ie, process indicator) on the outside of the package.[10,16,62] *[Recommendation]*

Placing a type 1 CI on the outside of the package allows the user to identify whether it has been subjected to the sterilization process.[10,62] Examples of process indicators are indicator tape and indicator labels.

4.4 Place one or more of the following inside the package according to sterilization method selected and the manufacturer's IFU:
- **type 3 CI** (ie, single-parameter indicator),
- **type 4 CI** (ie, multiparameter indicator),
- **type 5 CI** (ie, integrating indicator), or
- **type 6 CI** (ie, emulating indicator).

[Recommendation]

4.4.1 Place the CI in an area within the package that presents the greatest challenge for air removal and sterilant contact. Consult the IFU from the CI manufacturer, the device manufacturer, and the containment device manufacturer for additional information.[4,10,62] *[Recommendation]*

The number and placement of internal CIs may be affected by the contents of the package, the configuration of the items within the set, and the packaging or containment device.[4,10,62] The package manufacturer's IFU provide information about the location that presents the greatest challenge for sterilization.[11]

4.4.2 When more than one internal CI is required for multilayered trays, place these according to the tray manufacturer's IFU and product quality assurance testing results (See Recommendation 10.2). *[Recommendation]*

The package manufacturer's IFU provide information about the location that presents the greatest challenge for sterilization in an empty container.[11] Containers are sometimes purchased empty and the organization builds the set according to the organization's needs. Sets that are customized pose sterilization challenges within the set based on the set configuration. Performing quality assurance product testing for these custom sets can assist in determining the location that is most challenging for sterilant contact and optimal CI placement.

4.5 Follow the CI manufacturer's IFU for storage and use.[10,62] *[Recommendation]*

The manufacturer's IFU provide instructions that have been validated for the product.[62] Some CIs are sensitive to light, and the manufacturer provides instructions to protect them from light.

5. Sterilization Wrap

5.1 Use reusable woven sterilization wrap according to the manufacturer's IFU in sterilization processes for which reusable woven materials are validated. *[Recommendation]*

Reusable woven sterilization wraps are not validated for all sterilization methods and cycles. Repeated laundering and sterilization cycles diminish barrier qualities of textile wraps.[10,41] The manufacturer's IFU provide details for correct use and maintenance of reusable woven sterilization wrap.

5.1.1 **Launder reusable woven sterilization wrap after each use in**

- **a health care–accredited laundry facility,**
- **the health care organization according to state regulatory requirements, or**
- **the health care organization according to Centers for Disease Control and Prevention recommendations for laundering[63] in the absence of state requirements.**
  [Recommendation]

Resterilization without relaundering may lead to superheating and could create a deterrent to sterilization. Overdrying, heat pressing (eg, ironing), and storage in areas of low humidity may lead to superheating and sterilization failure. In addition, when **woven textiles** are not rehydrated after sterilization or if repeated sterilization is attempted, the textiles may absorb the available moisture present in the steam, thereby possibly creating a dry or superheated steam effect.[10]

5.1.2 **De-lint textiles after washing and before packaging them.** *[Recommendation]*

Lint can become airborne particles that carry microorganisms. These particles can be transferred to the surgical wound and could cause a foreign-body reaction.[10]

5.1.3 **Inspect and monitor reusable woven sterilization wrap by**

- **visually inspecting it on a lighted table for defects (eg, holes, tears, worn spots)[10] and**
- **following the manufacturer's IFU for the number of times the reusable woven materials can be processed.[41]**
  [Recommendation]

The barrier qualities of woven materials are diminished by repeated laundering and sterilization cycles. Processes to evaluate material quality after each use are needed to determine suitability for continued use.

5.1.4 **When repairing reusable woven sterilization wrap, do not sew textiles with defects. Vulcanized patches may be used but should be kept to a minimum.** *[Recommendation]*

Sewing creates holes in the textile through which microbes can enter. Vulcanized patches do not permit penetration of most sterilants. Keeping the quantity and concentration of patches to a minimum may decrease the risk of compromised penetration of the sterilant.

5.2 **Use single-use nonwoven sterilization wrap according to the manufacturer's IFU in sterilization processes and cycles for which it is validated.** *[Recommendation]*

Single-use nonwoven sterilization wraps are not validated for all sterilization methods and cycles.[10,39,40] The manufacturer's IFU provide details for correct use and maintenance of single-use woven sterilization wrap.

5.2.1 **Inspect all single-use sterilization wrap for defects and cleanliness before use.[10] Do not use packaging materials with defects.[16]** *[Recommendation]*

Defective packaging materials can permit migration of pathogens into the package. In an observational study to determine susceptibility of packaging materials to bacterial transmission, Waked et al[64] used nails ranging in size from 1.1 mm to 10.0 mm that were contaminated with three colonies of skin flora to make holes in 90 samples of a polypropylene wrap. The researchers found that bacterial transmission occurred in all holes, regardless of size.

5.3 **When indicated, use tray corners for wrapped trays according to the manufacturers' IFU for the tray corners and the sterile barrier system.** *[Recommendation]*

Tray corners are designed and used to protect corners of wrapped trays from punctures and holes. The manufacturer's IFU provide information about how to use them and for which sterilization methods they are validated.

5.4 **Select the wrapping material size that completely covers the item(s) being packaged. Wrap the item(s) securely to prevent gapping, billowing, or formation of air pockets.[16]** *[Recommendation]*

Gapping, billowing, or air pockets may prevent sterilant contact with the surface of the device or allow penetration of contaminants into the package.[16]

5.5 **When indicated, use absorbent materials and tray liners for wrapped trays according to the manufacturers' IFU for the absorbent material/tray liner and the sterile barrier system.** *[Recommendation]*

Adding accessories to a sterile barrier system can inhibit air removal and sterilant penetration if these accessories are not used properly.[10] By following the manufacturers' IFU for the accessory and the sterile barrier system, the user can verify that the accessory is used properly.

5.6 Use wrapping materials labeled for single-use for only one sterilization cycle. *[Recommendation]*

Products labeled as single-use or disposable are intended for one use and are not intended to be reprocessed.[16]

5.7 Wrapping may be performed by either sequential wrapping with two single wraps or single wrapping with one double-bonded wrap. *[Conditional Recommendation]*

Sequential wrapping using two nonwoven, disposable, barrier-type wrappers provides a tortuous pathway to impede microbial migration and permits ease of presentation to the sterile field without compromising sterility.[10]

A fused or double-bonded, disposable, nonwoven single wrapper used according to the manufacturer's IFU provides a bacterial barrier comparable to a sequential double wrap.[12,65]

6. Peel Pouches

6.1 Use peel pouches (ie, paper-plastic, polyethylene material, polyester film) according to the manufacturer's IFU for sterilization methods and cycles that have been validated by the manufacturer.[10,14,15,24,39] *[Recommendation]*

Manufacturers' IFU provide steps that the manufacturers have determined should be followed to achieve and maintain sterility of the package contents.

6.2 Use peel pouches only for small, lightweight, low-profile items.[10] *[Recommendation]*

Heavy, sharp, large, or sharply angulated items (eg, drills, weighted vaginal speculums, large hand-held retractors) may compromise the package and seal integrity. The sterilization pouch manufacturer's IFU may provide details about sterilization pouch capacity limits.

6.3 Do not use peel pouches contained within wrapped sets or rigid containers unless this is allowed by the pouch manufacturer's IFU.[10] *[Recommendation]*

Peel pouch manufacturer's IFU provide information about orientation of the package within the sterilizer. A peel pouch with a plastic side may be difficult to position according to the manufacturer's IFU if it is contained within a wrapped set or rigid container. The impervious plastic side of a peel pouch in contact with devices within sets may prevent sterilant from contacting these devices.[10]

6.4 Do not use double pouching (ie, placing the item in one pouch and then placing this pouch inside another) unless the pouch manufacturer's IFU allows this practice.[10] *[Recommendation]*

Sterilization validation studies performed by the manufacturer provide confirmation that the pouch will perform as intended when two pouches are used in a single package.[10]

6.4.1 Unless otherwise specified in the manufacturer's IFU, when double pouching, place the sealed inner pouch
- **within the outer pouch without folding it and**
- **facing in the same direction as the outer pouch (ie, plastic or polyester film faces plastic or polyester film, and paper or polyethylene material faces paper or polyethylene material).**[10]
[Recommendation]

Folding the sealed inner pouch may entrap air and inhibit sterilant contact and can lead to polyethylene material seal failure at the fold.[10]

The plastic side of the pouch is impervious to sterilant penetration.[10] The paper side of the pouch permits sterilant penetration.[10] Facing the inner pouch in the same direction as the outer pouch results in contact through which the sterilant can penetrate.[10] If the paper side of the inner pouch is in contact with the plastic side of the outer pouch, penetration of the sterilant through the paper side of the inner pouch may be inhibited.[10]

7. Rigid Containers

7.1 Use rigid sterilization containers according to the manufacturer's written IFU for sterilization methods and cycles.[10,11] *[Recommendation]*

Rigid sterilization containers are medical devices and must be cleared by the FDA for use. The manufacturer's written IFU contain specific information about use and care of the rigid sterilization container. These instructions must be correctly followed because they represent the conditions that were tested in the medical device–clearance process in validation studies. Rigid sterilization container design and materials may affect compatibility with the sterilization process (eg, penetration of the sterilant, release of the sterilant and moisture). Directions related to the method of sterilization may vary by manufacturer. Manufacturers of rigid sterilization containers with FDA clearance have validated that their containers will permit sterilization using specific sterilization methods and cycle exposure times.

Rigid container manufacturers' IFU provide detailed information that identifies correct use with the intended sterilization method(s) and equipment, including

- safety precautions to be taken with routine use;
- recommended sterilization methods, cycle types, and cycle parameters;
- recommended types and placement of instruments and other medical devices;
- recommended load distribution and maximum weight for the package and contents;
- accessories intended for use that are specific to the sterilization method and cycle;
- accessories found to be incompatible during validation testing;
- stacking instructions and limitations;
- the most challenging location within the package for placement of internal CIs and internal biological indicators (BIs);
- instructions for cleaning, including recommended cleaning agents and cleaning methods;
- types of medical devices that the manufacturer included in validation studies of the sterile barrier system;
- authorized service companies if the reusable container requires repair; and
- instructions for inspection and routine maintenance, including
  - a schedule for implementing inspection and routine maintenance;
  - a caution that these procedures should be performed by trained personnel;
  - detailed directions concerning the maintenance of critical components; and
  - a recommended inspection protocol that allows the user to identify the end of the containment device's useful life.[10]

7.2 Clean rigid sterilization containers before each use according to the manufacturer's written IFU.[10] *[Recommendation]*

Cleaning instructions found in the manufacturer's IFU provide details about cleaning agents and methods that have been validated by the manufacturer for the rigid sterilization container.[10] Using cleaning agents or methods that are not described in the manufacturer's IFU can result in damage to the rigid container's components and can damage the seal or filter retention plates.

7.3 Inspect all parts of rigid sterilization containers before each use and on a scheduled basis, including that

- the mating surfaces and edges of the container and lid are free of dents and chips;
- the lid and container fit together properly and securely;
- the filter retention mechanisms and fasteners are secure and not distorted or burred;
- the latching mechanisms are functioning to maintain the seal;
- the handles are in working order;
- the integrity of the filter media is not compromised;
- the gaskets are pliable, securely fastened, and without breaks or cuts; and
- the valves are in working order.

[Recommendation]

Inspection of rigid sterilization containers is necessary to detect flaws and wear that may interfere with the sterilization process or sterility maintenance.

7.3.1 Do not use sterilization containers that do not pass the inspection. Remove damaged items from service for repair or replacement. *[Recommendation]*

Improperly maintained valves, worn gaskets, dents, or other damage may compromise both the integrity of the container and the ability of the container to seal. Ineffective seals can impede achievement and compromise maintenance of sterility.[10]

7.3.2 Establish and implement a schedule for routine rigid sterilization container inspection, maintenance, and repair. *[Recommendation]*

In addition to inspection prior to each use, scheduled routine inspection and maintenance of rigid sterilization containers can be a valuable tool for detecting defects and wear of rigid containers that may compromise sterility maintenance.

7.3.3 Inspect single-use and reusable filters before use, and use them only if they are intact. *[Recommendation]*

Filters that are not intact or are damaged can result in microbial ingress and failure to maintain sterility within a sterilized package.

7.4 Maintain and repair rigid containers according to the manufacturer's written IFU.[10,11] *[Recommendation]*

Seals, a latching mechanism, or filter retention plates that are not functioning properly can result in microbial ingress and failure to maintain sterility within a sterilized package. Because it is difficult to identify malfunctioning seals using visual inspection alone, it is important to adhere to stringent maintenance and repair protocols as described in the manufacturer's IFU.

7.5 **Evaluate the rigid sterilization container for sterilization and, if indicated, drying efficacy according to the manufacturer's written IFU.**[10] *[Recommendation]*

Rigid sterilization container systems vary widely in design, mechanics, and construction. Such variables affect the performance of the containers and their compatibility with sterilization methods.

Health care personnel are responsible for ensuring that rigid sterilization container systems are suitable for proposed sterilization uses and are compatible with sterilizers in the health care organization.

7.6 **Consult the container's manufacturer's IFU to determine limitations related to density of materials, weight, and distribution of contents before placing instruments or devices within rigid sterilization containers.**[10] *[Recommendation]*

Following the manufacturer's requirements for density of materials and weight and distribution of contents will facilitate sterilization and optimize the performance of the container.

8. Labeling

8.1 **Label packages to be sterilized with required information (See the AORN Guideline for Sterilization[4]). Package labels should**

- be visible and legible;
- be nontoxic and indelible;
- be written only on the nonporous portions of the package (eg, the plastic side of pouches, indicator tape or affixed labels on wrapped items);
- identify the sterilizer, cycle, and load number;
- identify the sterilization date;
- include a description of the contents;
- identify personnel who prepared and wrapped the package; and
- remain securely affixed to the package through handling, storage, and transport to the point of use.[4,10] *[Recommendation]*

Accurate labeling provides identification of the package contents as well as information that enables tracking of the sterilizer, sterilization cycle, personnel involved in the sterilization process, and the patient for whom the items were

used.[4] Package label information allows items to be identified or retrieved in the event of a sterilization processing error or equipment malfunction. For additional information, see the AORN Guideline for Sterilization.[4]

8.1.1 **When a marker is used to enter label information, use nontoxic, nonbleeding, and indelible ink. Write only on the indicator tape, affixed label, or plastic side of peel pouches.**[3] *[Recommendation]*

Use of a nontoxic ink will prevent toxins from being deposited on the package contents. The force of writing with a ballpoint pen or a pencil may cause perforation of the pouch.[3] Writing or placing a label on the paper side of the pouch may compromise the barrier properties by causing damage to the package.[3]

9. Education

9.1 **Provide education and competency verification activities that address specific knowledge and skills related to the selection and use of packaging systems.** *[Recommendation]*

Competency verification measures individual performance. Ongoing development of knowledge and skills and documentation of personnel participation are regulatory and accreditation requirements for both hospital and ambulatory settings.[66-70] Periodic education programs provide the opportunity to reinforce principles of packaging and packaging systems evaluation and may be used to introduce new equipment and relevant practices.[52,71-73]

9.1.1 **Include the following in education regarding sterilization packaging:**

- understanding and adhering to manufacturers' IFU,
- correct use of packaging systems,
- risks and potential hazards associated with packaging,
- environmental impact,
- measures to minimize risk,
- product quality assurance testing,
- corrective actions to employ in the event of a failure of the packaging system, and
- new information about changes in packaging technology and its compatibility with sterilization equipment and processes.

[Recommendation]

10. Quality

10.1 Conduct quality assurance (QA) and performance improvement (PI) activities consistent with the health care organization's plan for compliance with the principles and processes of selection and use of packaging systems. [*Recommendation*]

Quality assurance and PI programs assist in evaluating and improving the quality of packaging of items to be sterilized for operative and other invasive procedures.[74] Quality assurance programs provide information that can be used to determine whether packaging practices are in compliance with recognized standards and to identify areas that may require corrective action.

10.1.1 Establish QA and PI programs to monitor the workplace environment and practices associated with selection and use of packaging systems.[4,10,74] [*Recommendation*]

Monitoring the packaging processes allows comparison to a predetermined level of quality (ie, a benchmark). Opportunities to improve practice can be identified by this analysis.[75]

10.1.2 Monitor activities related to selection and use of packaging systems, including the following:
- using packaging systems according to their IFU;
- verifying the compatibility of packaging systems with sterilization processes;
- storing packaging materials;
- assembling, handling, and packaging wrapped, pouched, and containerized items;
- labeling packages for sterilization;
- storing sterilized items and evaluating event-related sterility (See the AORN Guideline for Sterilization[4]); and
- conducting product QA testing (See Recommendation 10.2).

[*Recommendation*]

Accreditation agencies seek verification that there is a process in place for sterilizing materials and that these materials are packaged, labeled, and stored in a manner that ensures sterility.[76]

10.1.3 Include the following elements in the QA and PI program:
- periodic review and evaluation activities to verify compliance or to identify the need for improvement,
- identification of corrective actions directed toward improvement priorities, and

- additional actions to take when improvement is not achieved or sustained.

[*Recommendation*]

Reviewing and evaluating QA and PI activities helps identify failure points that contribute to errors in the use of packaging systems and helps define actions for improvement and increasing competency.[75,77-79] Taking corrective actions may improve patient safety by enhancing understanding of the principles of and compliance with the processes for selection and use of packaging systems.

10.2 Perform product QA testing for new packaging, packaging accessories, and major changes in packaging type, changes in tray configuration or content density, and on a schedule defined in the manufacturers' IFU.[10,30] [*Recommendation*]

Product testing verifies the ability to achieve a sterile, dry package and contents in the health care facility.[10]

Product QA testing is used to verify that adherence to the device manufacturer's instructions for sterilization is achievable in the health care setting. Major changes to packaging type can affect sterilization performance in the practice setting.[10] Periodic QA monitoring is one way to measure performance of packaging systems and sterilizer function. Changes in packaging systems can result in unexpected process challenges in sterilization systems. For example, changing from using wrapping materials to using rigid sterilization containers may result in wet packs or other problems. Therefore, it is essential that product testing is done to evaluate sterilization packaging changes prior to use in patient care.

In a small laboratory-based study, Prince et al[80] evaluated sterilization parameters for dynamic air removal steam sterilization of 14 implant/instrument trays in rigid containers compared to the same 14 trays in "hospital wrap," which was not defined. Trays were selected based on density, complexity of the medical devices, number of levels within the tray, configuration of contents, and overall weight. Study trays ranged in weight from 8.9 lb to 30.6 lb. The researchers ran each tray in both maximum loads (ie, a full sterilizer chamber) and minimum loads (ie, the study tray alone in the sterilizer chamber) for comparison. They measured and recorded sterilization physical parameters for each run of each tray.

The researchers concluded that at least one tray (three-level system, density 0.018 lb/inch^3, total weight 23.5 lb) in a minimum load run resulted in measurement of low sterilization temperature within the tray (127.1° C [260.8° F]), which was lower than the expected parameters of 132° C +/- 2° C (269.6° F +/- 3.6° F). There was a positive BI in the middle of the three-tiered tray under a knob handle when sterilized with both minimum and maximum loads in a rigid sterilization container. When exposed to the same sterilization cycles but contained in a "hospital wrap," the same tray met sterilization temperature and had a negative BI. The researchers also concluded that placement of a rigid container in a minimally loaded sterilizer resulted in more difficulty to sterilize than in a maximally loaded chamber.[80] The results of this study are important because they reinforce the recommendation to perform product QA testing that is representative of how the products will be used in practice.

10.2.1 During product QA testing,
- place a BI and CI inside the set, tray, or pack being tested in the areas that present the greatest challenge to sterilant contact according to the manufacturer's IFU and
- run them in a full load.

[Recommendation]

10.2.2 Include the following in sterilization packaging product QA testing:
- evaluation of pass or fail results[10];
- evaluation of residual moisture on or in the package; and
- documentation of product testing activities, including
  - the date of the test,
  - a description of the package and contents,
  - the location of BIs and CIs within the test package, and
  - test results.[10]

[Recommendation]

10.2.3 Conduct QA testing of sterilization packaging and related equipment (eg, heat sealers) before initial use and on the schedule defined in the manufacturers' written IFU and according to organizational policy.[10]
[Recommendation]

Packaging systems and related equipment vary in design, mechanics, and construction. These variables affect the performance and compatibility of packaging systems with sterilization methods.[4,10]

10.2.4 Consult the packaging system manufacturer to determine the areas within the package that present the greatest challenge for sterilant contact.[10] *[Recommendation]*

10.2.5 During periodic product QA testing of packaging systems, evaluate sterilization efficacy and, if indicated, drying effectiveness for each sterilizer and cycle used.[4] *[Recommendation]*

Health care organizations are responsible for obtaining and maintaining manufacturers' documentation of methodology and performance testing for packaging systems.[4] Health care personnel are responsible for ensuring that packaging systems are suitable for proposed sterilization uses and compatible with existing sterilizers.[4]

10.2.6 Participate in ongoing QA and PI activities by
- identifying important elements for quality monitoring (eg, weight of containment devices not exceeding 25 lb),
- developing strategies for compliance,
- determining the frequency for periodic product QA testing,
- establishing benchmarks to evaluate quality indicators,
- collecting data related to levels of performance and quality indicators,
- evaluating practice based on the cumulative data collected,
- acting to improve compliance, and
- assessing the effectiveness of the actions taken.

[Recommendation]

Participating in ongoing QA and PI activities is a standard of perioperative nursing and a primary responsibility of the registered nurse who is engaged in practice in the perioperative setting.[81]

Glossary

Chemical indicators: Devices used to monitor exposure to one or more sterilization parameters.
- **Type 1**: A process indicator that demonstrates that the package has been exposed to the sterilization process to distinguish between processed and unprocessed packages.
- **Type 2**: A process indicator that is used for a specific purpose, such as the dynamic air removal test (Bowie-Dick test).
- **Type 3**: A single-parameter indicator that reacts to one of the critical parameters of sterilization.
- **Type 4**: A multiparameter indicator that reacts to one, two, or more of the critical parameters of sterilization.
- **Type 5** (integrating indicator): An indicator that reacts to all critical parameters of sterilization.
- **Type 6** (emulating indicator): An indicator that reacts to all critical parameters of a specified sterilization cycle.

Containment device: A reusable rigid sterilization container, instrument case, cassette, or organizing tray intended for the purpose of containing reusable devices for sterilization.

Environmentally preferable: Products or services that have a reduced negative effect on human health and the environment when compared to competing products or services that serve the same purpose.

Expected life of the device: The time that a device is expected to remain functional after it is placed into use. Although some implanted devices have specified "end of life" dates, other devices are not labeled as to their respective "end of life" but are expected to remain operational through activities such as maintenance, repairs, or upgrades, for an estimated period of time.

Instrument case/cassette: A sterilization container with a lid and a base, that permits air removal and sterilant penetration and removal. The devices require wrapping in packaging material if sterility of the contents is to be maintained.

Nonwoven material: Fabric made by bonding fibers together as opposed to weaving threads.

Organizing tray: A reusable metal or plastic tray that permits organization and protection of the contents. Some organizing trays have diagrams for the representative instruments etched onto the surface of the tray to facilitate their identification and placement within the tray.

Package integrity: Unimpaired physical condition of a final package.

Packaging system: The combination of the sterile barrier system and the protective packaging.

Paper-plastic pouch: A type of packaging made of a polyester film and paper that is suitable for packaging items to be sterilized in steam, or a type of packaging made of a polyester film and a polyethylene material that is suitable for packaging items to be sterilized in ethylene oxide, low-temperature hydrogen gas plasma, or hydrogen peroxide vapor. Synonym: peel pouch.

Peel pouch: A type of packaging made of a polyester film and paper that is suitable for packaging items to be sterilized in steam, or a type of packaging made of a polyester film and a polyethylene material that is suitable for packaging items to be sterilized in ethylene oxide, low-temperature hydrogen gas plasma, or hydrogen peroxide vapor. Synonym: paper-plastic pouch.

Rigid sterilization container system: Specifically designed heat-resistant, metal, plastic, or anodized aluminum receptacles used to package items, usually surgical instruments, for sterilization. The lids and/or bottom surfaces contain steam- or gas-permeable, high-efficiency microbial filters.

Sequential wrapping: A double-wrapping procedure that creates a package within a package.

Shelf life: When this term is used in conjunction with a sterile device, shelf life is considered to be the length of time a device is safe to use.

Sterile barrier system: The minimum package that prevents ingress of microorganisms and allows aseptic presentation of the product at the point of use.

Sterilization packaging: The organizers, accessories, and containment devices that, when combined, result in an organized tray or set that is contained within a sterile barrier system.

Sterilization validation studies: Tests performed by a device manufacturer that demonstrate that a sterilization process will consistently yield sterile product under defined parameters.

Superheating: A condition that occurs in steam sterilization when the temperature of the steam is higher than the temperature of the saturated steam, thereby creating a dry or superheated steam effect and adversely affecting the steam sterilization process.

Validation: A documented procedure for obtaining, recording, and interpreting the results required to establish that a process will consistently yield product that complies with predetermined specifications.

Vaporized hydrogen peroxide sterilization: A sterilization process in which vaporized hydrogen peroxide acts as a sterilant.

Woven textile: A reusable fabric constructed from yarns made of natural and/or synthetic fibers or filaments that are woven or knitted together to form a web in a repeated interlocking pattern.

References

1. Guideline for cleaning and care of surgical instruments. In: *Guidelines for Perioperative Practice.* Denver, CO: AORN, Inc; 2019:401-440. [IVA]

2. Guideline for manual chemical high-level disinfection. In: *Guidelines for Perioperative Practice.* Denver, CO: AORN, Inc; 2019:315-342. [IVA]

3. Guideline for processing flexible endoscopes. In: *Guidelines for Perioperative Practice.* Denver, CO: AORN, Inc; 2019:199-288. [IVA]

4. Guideline for sterilization. In: *Guidelines for Perioperative Practice.* Denver, CO: AORN Inc; 2019:973-1002. [IVA]

5. Guideline for sterile technique. In: *Guidelines for Perioperative Practice.* Denver, CO: AORN Inc; 2019:931-972. [IVA]

6. Overview of device regulation. US Food and Drug Administration. https://www.fda.gov/medicaldevices/deviceregulationandguidance/overview/default.htm. Accessed July 10, 2019.

7. The 510(k) Program: Evaluating Substantial Equivalence in Premarket Notifications [510k]. Guidance for Industry and Food and Drug Administration Staff. US Food and Drug Administration. https://www.fda.gov/medical-devices/guidance-documents-medical-devices-and-radiation-emitting-products/510k-program-evaluating-substantial-equivalence-premarket-notifications-510k-guidance-industry-and. Published July 28, 2014. Accessed July 10, 2019.

8. Reprocessing Medical Devices in Health Care Settings: Validation Methods and Labeling. Guidance for Industry and Food and Drug Administration Staff. US Food and Drug Administration. https://www.fda.gov/regulatory-information/search-fda-guidance-documents/reprocessing-medical-devices-health-care-settings-validation-methods-and-labeling. Published March 17, 2015. Accessed July 10, 2019.

9. Premarket approval (PMA). US Food and Drug Administration. https://www.fda.gov/MedicalDevices/DeviceRegulationandGuidance/HowtoMarketYourDevice/PremarketSubmissions/PremarketApprovalPMA/default.htm. Updated May 16, 2019. Accessed July 10, 2019.

10. ANSI/AAMI ST79: Comprehensive Guide to Steam Sterilization and Sterility Assurance in Health Care Facilities. Arlington, VA: Association for the Advancement of Medical Instrumentation; 2017. [IVC]

11. ANSI/AAMI ST77:2013/(R)2018: Containment Devices for Reusable Medical Device Sterilization. Arlington, VA: Association for the Advancement of Medical Instrumentation; 2018. [IVC]

12. Rutala WA, Weber DJ. Choosing a sterilization wrap for surgical packs. Infection Control Today. https://www.infectioncontroltoday.com/environmental-hygiene/choosing-sterilization-wrap-surgicalpacks. Published May 1, 2000. Accessed July 10, 2019. [VC]

13. Position Paper: Sterile Barrier Systems–Single Use or Reusables. Augsburg, Germany: Sterile Barrier Association; 2017. [IVC]

14. ANSI/AAMI/ISO 11607-1:2006/(R)2015: Packaging for Terminally Sterilized Medical Devices—Part 1: Requirements for Materials, Sterile Barrier Systems, and Packaging Systems. Arlington, VA: Association for the Advancement of Medical Instrumentation; 2015. [IVC]

15. ANSI/AAMI/ISO 11607-2:2006/(R)2015: Packaging for Terminally Sterilized Medical Devices – Part 2: Validation Requirements for Forming, Sealing, and Assembly Processes. Arlington, VA: Association for the Advancement of Medical Instrumentation; 2015. [IVC]

16. Rutala WA, Weber DJ; Healthcare Infection Control Practices Advisory Committee (HICAC). Guideline for Disinfection and Sterilization in Healthcare Facilities, 2008. Centers for Disease Control and Prevention. https://www.cdc.gov/infectioncontrol/pdf/guidelines/disinfection-guidelines-H.pdf. Updated May 2019. Accessed July 10, 2019. [IVA]

17. Mobley KS, Jackson JB 3rd. A prospective analysis of clinical detection of defective wrapping by operating room staff. Am J Infect Control. 2018;46(7):837-839. [IIIB]

18. Shaffer HL, Harnish DA, McDonald M, Vernon RA, Heimbuch BK. Sterility maintenance study: dynamic evaluation of sterilized rigid containers and wrapped instrument trays to prevent bacterial ingress. Am J Infect Control. 2015;43(12):1336-1341. [IIB]

19. AST Standards of Practice for Packaging Material and Preparing Items for Sterilization. Littleton, CO: Association of Surgical Technologists; 2009. [IVC]

20. Doyle PA, Gurses AP, Pronovost PJ. Mastering medical devices for safe use. Am J Med Qual. 2017;32(1):100-102. [VA]

21. Applying Human Factors and Usability Engineering to Medical Devices. Guidance for Industry and Food and Drug Administration Staff. US Food and Drug Administration. https://www.fda.gov/regulatory-information/search-fda-guidance-documents/applying-human-factors-and-usability-engineering-medical-devices. Published February 2016. Accessed July 10, 2019.

22. Final Guidance on Environmentally Preferable Purchasing. US Environmental Protection Agency. https://www.epa.gov/sites/production/files/2015-09/documents/finaleppguidance.pdf. Published August 1999. Accessed July 10, 2019. [IVA]

23. Spruce L. Back to basics: packaging systems. AORN J. 2018;107(5):602-610. [VA]

24. Seavey R. High-level disinfection, sterilization, and antisepsis: current issues in reprocessing medical and surgical instruments. Am J Infect Control. 2013;41(5 Suppl):S111-S117. [VA]

25. Brusco J, Ogg M. Health care waste management and environmentally preferable purchasing. AORN J. 2010;92(Suppl 6):S62-S69. [VB]

26. Conrardy J, Hillanbrand M, Myers S, Nussbaum GF. Reducing medical waste. AORN J. 2010;91(6):711-721. [VA]

27. Fayard C, Lambert C, Guimier-Pingault C, Levast M, Germi R. Assessment of residual moisture and maintenance of sterility in surgical instrument sets after sterilization. Infect Control Hosp Epidemiol. 2015;36(8):990-992. [IIB]

28. Puangsa-Ard Y, Thaweboon S, Jantaratnotai N, Pachimsawat P. Effects of resterilization and storage time on sterility of paper/plastic pouches. Eur J Dent. 2018;12(3):417-421. [IIB]

29. Diab-Elschahawi M, Blacky A, Bachhofner N, Koller W. Challenging the Sterrad 100NX sterilizer with different carrier materials and wrappings under experimental "clean" and "dirty"conditions. Am J Infect Control. 2010;38(10):806-810. [IIIB]

30. Guideline for medical device and product evaluation. In: Guidelines for Perioperative Practice. Denver, CO: AORN, Inc; 2019:715-724. [IVA]

31. Herman P, Larsen C. Measuring porous microbial barriers, part 1. Medical Device and Diagnostic Industry. https://www.mddionline.com/measuring-porous-microbial-barriers-part-1. Published May 1, 2008. Accessed July 10, 2019. [IVA]

32. Herman P, Larsen C. Measuring porous microbial barriers, part 2. Medical Device and Diagnostic Industry. https://www.mddionline.com/measuring-porous-microbial-barriers-part-2. Published June 1, 2008. Accessed July 10, 2019. [IVA]

33. AAMI TIR12: 2010 Designing, Testing, and Labeling Reusable Medical Devices for Reprocessing in Health Care Facilities: A Guide for Medical Device Manufacturers. Arlington, VA: Association for the Advancement of Medical Instrumentation; 2010. [IVC]

34. Wagner T, Scholla MH. Sterile barrier systems: managing changes and revalidations. Journal of Validation Technology. 2013;19(3):1-8. [VA]

35. Laustsen G. Reduce—recycle—reuse: guidelines for promoting perioperative waste management. AORN J. 2007;85(4):717-728. [VA]

36. AORN position statement on environmental responsibility. AORN, Inc. https://www.aorn.org/guidelines/clinical-resources/position-statements. Revised 2014. Accessed July 10, 2019. [IVB]

37. Lee RJ, Mears SC. Greening of orthopedic surgery. *Orthopedics.* 2012;35(6):e940-e944. [VB]

38. Krohn M, Fengler J, Mickley T, Flessa S. Analysis of processes and costs of alternative packaging options of sterile goods in hospitals—a case study in two German hospitals. *Health Econ Rev.* 2019;9(1):1. [IIIB]

39. *ANSI/AAMI ST58:2013: Chemical Sterilization and High-Level Disinfection in Health Care Facilities.* Arlington, VA: Association for the Advancement of Medical Instrumentation; 2013. [IVC]

40. *ANSI/AAMI ST41:2008/(R)2018: Ethylene Oxide Sterilization in Health Care Facilities: Safety and Effectiveness.* Arlington, VA: Association for the Advancement of Medical Instrumentation; 2018. [IVC]

41. *ANSI/AAMI ST65:2008/(R)2018: Processing of Reusable Surgical Textiles for Use in Health Care Facilities.* Arlington, VA: Association for the Advancement of Medical Instrumentation; 2018. [IVC]

42. Larrick K; AAMI. Examining the new AAMI standard . . . containment devices for reusable medical device sterilization. *Biomed Instrum Technol.* 2007;41(2):155-156. [VA]

43. Luqueta GR, Santos ED 2nd, Pessoa RS, Maciel HS. Evaluation of disposable medical device packaging materials under ozone sterilization. *Res Biomed Eng.* 2017;33(1):58-68. [IIIB]

44. Room design. In: *HVAC Design Manual for Hospitals and Clinics.* 2nd ed. Atlanta, GA: American Society of Heating, Refrigerating and Air-Conditioning Engineers (ASHRAE); 2013:151-202. [IVC]

45. *Guidelines for Design and Construction of Hospitals.* St Louis, MO: Facility Guidelines Institute; 2018. [IVC]

46. Veiga-Malta I. Preventing healthcare-associated infections by monitoring the cleanliness of medical devices and other critical points in a sterilization service. *Biomed Instrum Technol.* 2016;50(Suppl 3):45-52. [IIB]

47. Standards FAQ details. Temperature and humidity—monitoring requirements for sterile supply storage areas. The Joint Commission. https://www.jointcommission.org/standards_information/jcfaqdetails.aspx?StandardsFAQId=1686. Accessed July 10, 2019.

48. Guideline for design and maintenance of the surgical suite. In: *Guidelines for Perioperative Practice.* Denver, CO: AORN, Inc; 2019:73-104. [IVA]

49. *Guidelines for Design and Construction of Outpatient Facilities.* St Louis, MO: Facility Guidelines Institute; 2018. [IVC]

50. Take these steps to avoid issues with instruments. *Same Day Surg.* 2016;40(11):124-126. [VA]

51. Blackmore CC, Bishop R, Luker S, Williams BL. Applying lean methods to improve quality and safety in surgical sterile instrument processing. *Jt Comm J Qual Patient Saf.* 2013;39(3):99-105. [VA]

52. Sonstelie A, Dorval D, Pfeifer S. Bringing order to sterile processing through standardized processes. *Biomed Instrum Technol.* 2016;Spring(Suppl):29-31. [VA]

53. Stockert EW, Langerman A. Assessing the magnitude and costs of intraoperative inefficiencies attributable to surgical instrument trays. *J Am Coll Surg.* 2014;219(4):646-655. [VA]

54. Cuny E, Collins FM. Instrument processing, work flow and sterility assurance. *RDH.* 2013;33(6):69-77. [VB]

55. Kohn WJ, Collins AS, Cleveland JL, Harte JA, Eklund KJ, Malvitz DM; Centers for Disease Control and Prevention (CDC). Guidelines for infection control in dental health-care settings—2003. *MMWR Recomm Rep.* 2003;52(RR-17):1-61. [IVA]

56. Guideline for prevention of retained surgical items. In: *Guidelines for Perioperative Practice.* Denver, CO: AORN, Inc; 2019:765-814. [IVA]

57. Costa DM, Lopes LKO, Tipple AFV, et al. Effect of hand hygiene and glove use on cleanliness of reusable surgical instruments. *J Hosp Infect.* 2017;97(4):348-352. [IIA]

58. Trier T, Bello N, Bush TR, Bix L. The role of packaging size on contamination rates during simulated presentation to a sterile field. *Plos One.* 2014;9(7):e100414. [IIIB]

59. Papaioannou A. A review of sterilization, packaging and storage considerations for orthodontic pliers. *Int J Orthod Milwaukee.* 2013;24(3):19-21. [VC]

60. Guideline for safe patient handling and movement. In: *Guidelines for Perioperative Practice.* Denver, CO: AORN, Inc; 2019:817-868. [IVA]

61. Lucas AD, Chobin N, Conner R, et al. Steam sterilization and internal count sheets: assessing the potential for cytotoxicity. *AORN J.* 2009;89(3):521-531. [IIA]

62. *ANSI/AAMI/ISO 11140-1:2014: Sterilization of Health Care Products—Chemical Indicators—Part 1: General Requirements.* Arlington, VA: Association for the Advancement of Medical Instrumentation; 2014. [IVC]

63. *Guide to Infection Prevention for Outpatient Settings: Minimum Expectations for Safe Care.* Version 2.2. Atlanta, GA: Centers for Disease Control and Prevention; 2015. [IVA]

64. Waked WR, Simpson AK, Miller CP, Magit DP, Grauer JN. Sterilization wrap inspections do not adequately evaluate instrument sterility. *Clin Orthop Relat Res.* 2007;462:207-211. [IIB]

65. Webster J, Radke E, George N, Faoagali J, Harris M. Barrier properties and cost implications of a single versus a double wrap for storing sterile instrument packs. *Am J Infect Control.* 2005;33(6):348-352. [IIC]

66. Program: Ambulatory. HR.01.05.03: Staff participate in ongoing education and training. In: *The Joint Commission Comprehensive Accreditation and Certification Manual.* E-dition. Oakbrook Terrace, IL: The Joint Commission; 2018.

67. *State Operations Manual Appendix L—Guidance for Surveyors: Ambulatory Surgical Centers.* Rev 137; 2015. Centers for Medicare & Medicaid Services. https://www.cms.gov/Regulations-and-Guidance/Guidance/Manuals/Downloads/som107ap_l_ambulatory.pdf. Accessed July 10, 2019.

68. *State Operations Manual Appendix A—Survey Protocol, Regulations and Interpretive Guidelines for Hospitals.* Rev 183; 2017. Centers for Medicare & Medicaid Services. https://www.cms.gov/Regulations-and-Guidance/Guidance/Manuals/downloads/som107ap_a_hospitals.pdf. Accessed July 10, 2019.

69. Clinical records and health information. In: *Accreditation Handbook for Ambulatory Health Care.* Skokie, IL: Accreditation Association for Ambulatory Health Care, Inc; 2018:61-66.

70. Personnel: knowledge, skill & CME training. In: *Regular Standards and Checklist for Accreditation of Ambulatory Surgery Facilities.* Version 14.5. Gurnee, IL: American Association for Accreditation of Ambulatory Surgery Facilities; 2018:76-77.

71. Gould DJ, Hale R, Waters E, Allen D. Promoting health workers' ownership of infection prevention and control: using normalization process theory as an interpretive framework. *J Hosp Infect.* 2016;94(4):373-380. [IIIC]

72. Are staff pressured on sterilization? Intervene, or risk device compromise. *Same Day Surg.* 2012;36(5):49-51. [VA]

73. Benner P. *From Novice to Expert: Excellence and Power in Clinical Nursing Practice.* Upper Saddle River, NJ: Prentice Hall Health; 2001. [VA]

74. *ANSI/AAMI ST91:2015: Flexible and Semi-Rigid Endoscope Processing in Health Care Facilities.* Arlington, VA: Association for the Advancement of Medical Instrumentation; 2015. [IVC]

75. Swenson D. Why benchmarking is important to sterile processing. *Biomed Instrum Technol.* 2016;50(2):117-120. [VA]

76. Surgical services (SS). In: *NIAHO: National Integrated Accreditation for Healthcare Organizations: Interpretive Guidelines and Surveyor Guidance.* Version 11. Milford, OH: DNV GL Healthcare USA, Inc; 2014:80-91.

77. Seavey RE. Sterile processing accreditation surveys: risk reduction and process improvement. *AORN J.* 2015;102(4):358-368. [VA]

78. Knudson L. Identifying and eliminating sources of wet packs. *AORN J.* 2014;99(4):C1, C9-10. [VA]

79. IAHCSMM position paper on the management of loaner instrumentation. International Association of Healthcare Central Service Materiel Management. https://www.iahcsmm.org/images/Resources/Loaner_Instrument/Position-Paper.pdf. Accessed July 10, 2019. [IVA]

80. Prince D, Mastej J, Hoverman I, Chatterjee R, Easton D, Behzad D. Challenges to validation of a complex nonsterile medical device tray. *Biomed Instrum Technol.* 2014;48(4):306-311. [IIB]

81. Standards of perioperative nursing. In: *Guidelines for Perioperative Practice.* Denver, CO: AORN, Inc; 2015:693-708. [IVB]

Guideline Development Group

Lead Author: Erin Kyle[1], DNP, RN, CNOR, NEA-BC, Perioperative Practice Specialist, AORN, Denver, Colorado

Methodologist: Amber Wood[2], MSN, RN, CNOR, CIC, FAPIC, Editor-in-Chief, Guidelines for Perioperative Practice, AORN, Denver, Colorado

Evidence Appraisers: Erin Kyle[1]; Marie Bashaw[3], DNP, RN, NEA-BC, Assistant Professor, Director Nursing Administration and Health Care Master's Program, Wright State University College of Nursing and Health; and Amber Wood[2]

Guidelines Advisory Board Members:
- Heather A. Hohenberger[4], MSN, RN, CIC, CNOR, CPHQ, Administrative Director Surgical Services, IU Health Arnett Hospital, Lebanon, Indiana
- Jennifer Butterfield[5], MBA, RN, CNOR, CASC, Administrator, Lakes Surgery Center, West Bloomfield, Michigan
- Gerald McDonnell[6], PhD, BSc, Senior Director, Sterility Assurance, DePuy Synthes, Johnson & Johnson Family of Companies, Raritan, New Jersey
- Judith L. Goldberg[7], DBA, MSN, RN, CNOR, CSSM, CHL, CRCST, Director Nursing Excellence & Professional Development, Yale New Haven Health, Lawrence + Memorial Hospital, New London, Connecticut
- Elizabeth (Lizz) Pincus[8], MSN, RN, CNS-CP, CNOR, Clinical Nurse, Regional Medical Center of San Jose, San Jose, California
- Susan Lynch[9], PhD, RN, CSSM, CNOR, Associate Director Surgical Services, Chester County Hospital, Glen Mills, Pennsylvania
- Kristy Simmons[10], MSN, RN, CNOR, Clinical Nurse III, Woman's Hospital, Baton Rouge, Louisiana

Guidelines Advisory Board Liaisons:
- Susan Ruwe[11], MSN, RN, CPHQ, CIC, Senior Infection Preventionist, Carle Foundation Hospital, Argenta, Illinois
- Susan G. Klacik[12], BS, CRCST, FCS, Clinical Educator, International Association of Healthcare Central Service Materiel Management (IAHCSMM), Chicago, Illinois
- Julie K. Moyle[13], MSN, RN, Member Engagement Manager, Centura – Avista Adventist Hospital, Golden, Colorado

External Review: Expert review comments were received from individual members of the American Association of Nurse Anesthetists (AANA), American College of Surgeons (ACS), Association for Professionals in Infection Control and Epidemiology (APIC), American Society of Anesthesiologists (ASA), International Association of Healthcare Central Service Materiel Management (IAHCSMM), Practice Greenhealth, and the Society for Healthcare Epidemiology of America (SHEA). Their responses were used to further refine and enhance this guideline; however, their responses do not imply endorsement. The draft was also open for a 30-day public comment period.

Financial Disclosure and Conflicts of Interest

This guideline was developed, edited, and approved by the AORN Guidelines Advisory Board without external funding being sought or obtained. The Guidelines Advisory Board was financially supported entirely by AORN and was developed without any involvement of industry.

Potential conflicts of interest for all Guidelines Advisory Board members were reviewed before the annual meeting and each monthly conference call. Eleven members of the Guideline Development Group reported no potential conflict of interest.[1-3,5,7-12] Two members[4,6] disclosed potential conflicts of interest. After review and discussion of these disclosures, the advisory board concluded that individuals with potential conflicts could remain on the advisory board if they reminded the advisory board of potential conflicts before any related discussion and recused themselves from a related discussion if requested.

Publication History

Originally published February 1983, *AORN Journal.*

Revised November 1988, February 1992.

Revised November 1995; published May 1996, *AORN Journal.*

Revised and reformatted; published December 2000, *AORN Journal.*

Revised 2006; published in *Standards, Recommended Practices, and Guidelines,* 2007 edition.

Minor editing revisions made to omit PNDS codes; reformatted September 2012 for publication in *Perioperative Standards and Recommended Practices,* 2013 edition.

Revised September 2013 for online publication in *Perioperative Standards and Recommended Practices.*

Minor editing revisions made in November 2014 for publication in *Guidelines for Perioperative Practice,* 2015 edition.

Evidence ratings revised in *Guidelines for Perioperative Practice,* 2018 edition, to conform to the current AORN Evidence Rating Model.

Revised 2019 for online publication in *Guidelines for Perioperative Practice.*

Scheduled for review in 2024.

PATIENT SKIN ANTISEPSIS

AORN
SAFE SURGERY TOGETHER

TABLE OF CONTENTS

P   *indicates a recommendation or evidence relevant to pediatric care.*

MEDICAL ABBREVIATIONS & ACRONYMS

AAAAI – American Academy of Allergy, Asthma, and Immunology
ACS – American College of Surgeons
ANDA – Abbreviated New Drug Approval
ASA – American Society of Anesthesiologists
BCC – *Burkholderia cepacia* complex
BPO – Benzoyl peroxide
CDC – Centers for Disease Control and Prevention
CFU – Colony-forming units
CHG – Chlorhexidine gluconate
CIED – Cardiac implantable electronic device
CMS – Centers for Medicare & Medicaid Services
CoNS – Coagulase-negative staphylococci
ECG - Electrocardiogram
EPA – Environmental Protection Agency
ESU – Electrosurgical unit
FDA – US Food and Drug Administration
GRASE – Generally recognized as safe and effective
ICU – Intensive care unit
IFU – Instructions for use
IDSA – Infectious Diseases Society of America

MDRO – Multidrug-resistant organism
MIC – Minimum inhibitory concentration
MIC90 – 90% of the minimum inhibitory concentration
MRSA – Methicillin-resistant *Staphylococcus aureus*
MSSA – Methicillin-sensitive *Staphylococcus aureus*
MupR – Mupiricin resistant
NAON – National Association of Orthopaedic Nurses
NDA – New Drug Approval
NFPA – National Fire Protection Association
NICE – National Institute for Health and Care Excellence
OTC – Over the counter
PCMX – Chloroxylenol
PCR – Polymerase chain reaction
RCT – Randomized controlled trial
RN – Registered nurse
SDS – Safety data sheet
SHEA – Society for Healthcare Epidemiology of America
SIS – Surgical Infection Society
SSI – Surgical site infection
TSH – Thyroid stimulating hormone
WHO – World Health Organization

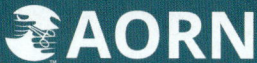
GUIDELINE FOR
PREOPERATIVE PATIENT SKIN ANTISEPSIS

The Guideline for Preoperative Patient Skin Antisepsis was approved by the AORN Guidelines Advisory Board and became effective as of May 13, 2021. The recommendations in the guideline are intended to be achievable and represent what is believed to be an optimal level of practice. Policies and procedures will reflect variations in practice settings and/or clinical situations that determine the degree to which the guideline can be implemented. AORN recognizes the many diverse settings in which perioperative nurses practice; therefore, this guideline is adaptable to all areas where operative or other invasive procedures may be performed.

Purpose

This guideline provides perioperative registered nurses (RNs) and other perioperative team members with evidence-based practice guidance for preoperative patient skin antisepsis to promote patient safety and reduce the risk of surgical site infection (SSI). Topics include **decolonization** for *Staphylococcus aureus*; **preoperative bathing**; hair removal; selection of surgical site antiseptics; application of surgical site **antiseptics**; safe handling, storage, and disposal of antiseptics; and skin antisepsis as part of SSI prevention **bundles**.

The goal of preoperative patient skin antisepsis is to reduce the patient's risk of developing an SSI by removing soil and transient microorganisms at the surgical site.[1] Reducing the amount of bacteria on the skin near the surgical incision lowers the risk of contaminating the surgical incision site.[1] As part of preparing the skin for antisepsis, preoperative decolonization, preoperative bathing, and hair management at the surgical site contribute to a reduction of microorganisms on the skin.[2-5] Effective skin antiseptics rapidly and persistently remove transient microorganisms and reduce resident microorganisms to subpathogenic levels with minimal skin and tissue irritation.[1]

Perioperative RNs play an essential role in developing protocols for preoperative decolonization and preoperative bathing; selecting and applying preoperative patient skin antiseptics; facilitating hair removal when necessary; and implementing SSI prevention bundles.

The following topics are outside the scope of this document: patient skin antisepsis after incision; antiseptic irrigation (See the AORN Guideline for Sterile Technique[6]); preoperative patient skin antisepsis with no incision; patient skin antisepsis for postoperative incision site care, including suture removal; patient bathing not intended for surgical preparation; decolonization for *Staphylococcus aureus* not intended for surgical preparation; mechanical

and oral antimicrobial bowel preparation; adhesive incise drapes (See the AORN Guideline for Sterile Technique[6]); and preoperative prophylactic antibiotic selection.

Evidence Review

A medical librarian with a perioperative background conducted a systematic search of the databases Ovid MEDLINE, Ovid Embase, EBSCO CINAHL, and the Cochrane Database of Systematic Reviews. The search was limited to literature published in English from January 2014 through January 2020. At the time of the initial search, weekly alerts were created on the topics included in that search. Results from these alerts were provided to the lead author until June 2020. The lead author requested additional articles that either did not fit the original search criteria or were discovered during the evidence appraisal process. The lead author and the medical librarian also identified relevant guidelines from government agencies, professional organizations, and standards-setting bodies.

Search terms included *administration (cutaneous), administration (topical), alcohol, anti-infective agents (local), antiseptic cloth, antiseptic shower, antiseptic solution, antisepsis, artificial nails, baby shampoo, bathing, benzalkonium chloride, Betadine, Betasept, body jewelry, body piercing, burns (chemical), care bundle, castile, cesarean section, chemical burns, ChloraPrep, chlorhexidine*, chlorhexidine alcohol, chlorhexidine wipe, chloroxylenol, clipp*, ClipVac, cost-benefit analysis, cross infection, depilat*, delivery of health care (integrated), dermatitis, disinfectant, Duraprep, ExCel AP, fingernails, fires, flammab*, Hyamine, hair removal, health care delivery (integrated), Hibiclens, impaired wound healing, infection prevention, iodine compounds, iodophors, jewelry, local anti-infective agents, male genitalia, mucous membrane, nail polish, nails, nasal cavity, nasal decolonization, nonshaved, Nozin, open wound, parachloroxylenol, patient care bundles, PCMX, penis, perioperative nursing, pHisoHex, post-natal infection, povidone-iodine, practice guidelines, practice guidelines as topic, preoperative antisepsis, preoperative bathing, preoperative care, preoperative shower, preoperative wash, program evaluation, prosthetic joint infection, PVP-I prep, quality improvement, razor, scrotum, shaving, shellfish, skin antisep*, skin paint, skin prep, skin scrub, skin sensitivity, sterile prep solution, sterile preparation, surgery (operative), surgical fires, surgical patients, surgical procedures, surgical procedures (operative), surgical site infection, surgical skin preparation, surgical wound infection, tape, Techni-Care, total joint replacement, treatment outcome, triclosan, vacuum hair, vagina, vaginal cleansing, vaginal irritation, vaginal vault, vaginitis, wound infection, ZuraGard, and 2-propanol.*

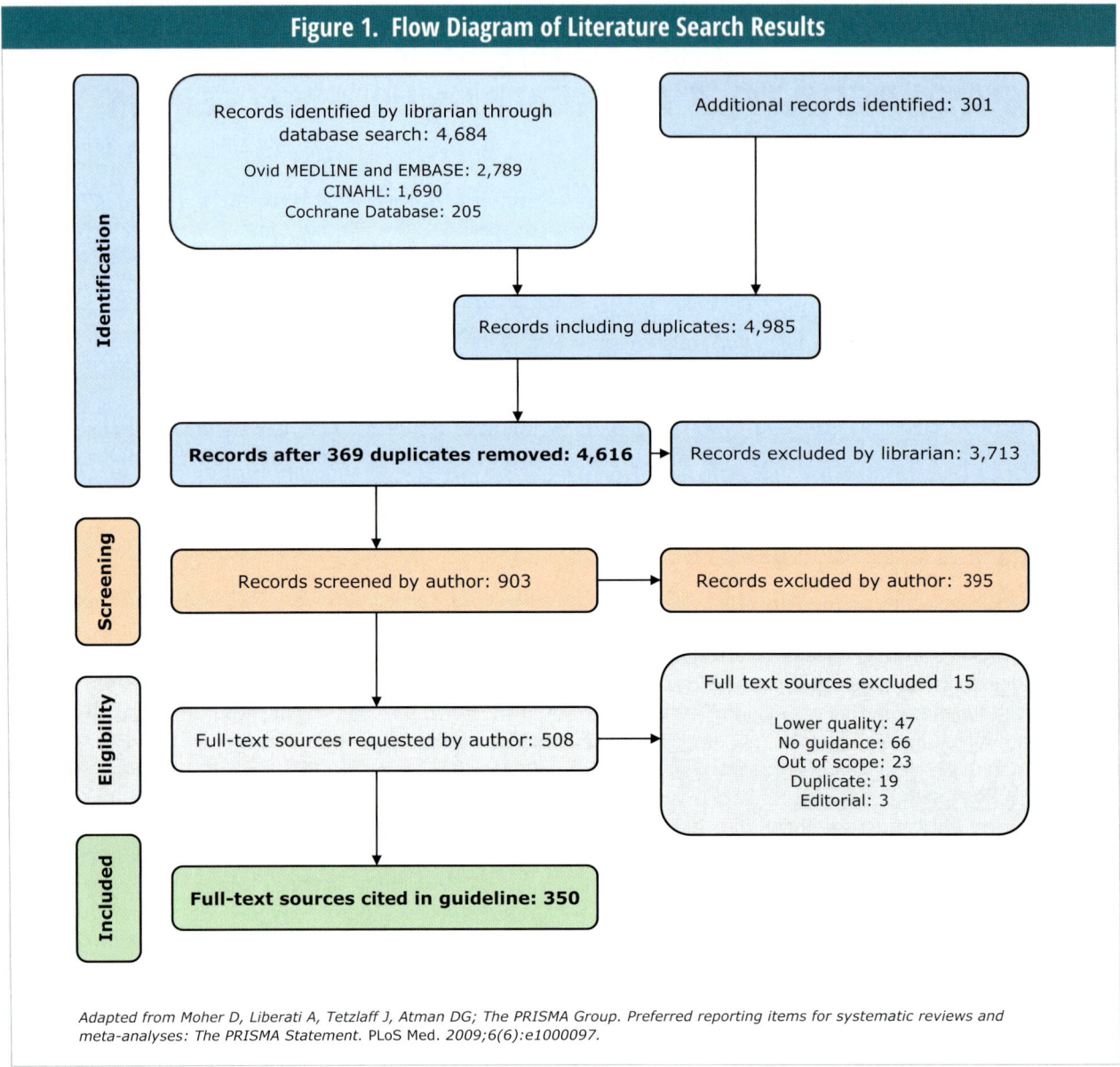

Figure 1. Flow Diagram of Literature Search Results

Adapted from Moher D, Liberati A, Tetzlaff J, Atman DG; The PRISMA Group. Preferred reporting items for systematic reviews and meta-analyses: The PRISMA Statement. PLoS Med. 2009;6(6):e1000097.

Included were research and non-research literature in English, complete publications, and publications with dates within the time restriction when available. Excluded were non-peer-reviewed publications and older evidence within the time restriction when more recent evidence was available. Editorials, news items, and other brief items were excluded. Low-quality evidence was excluded when higher-quality evidence was available, and literature outside the time restriction was excluded when literature within the time restriction was available (Figure 1).

Articles identified in the search were provided to the project team for evaluation. The team consisted of the lead author and one evidence appraiser. The lead author and the evidence appraiser reviewed and critically appraised each article using the AORN Research or Non-Research Evidence Appraisal Tools as appropriate. A second appraiser was consulted in the event of a disagreement between the lead author and the primary evidence appraiser. The literature was independently evaluated and appraised according to the strength and quality of the evidence. Each article was then assigned an appraisal score. The appraisal score is noted in brackets after each reference as applicable.

Each recommendation rating is based on a synthesis of the collective evidence, a benefit-harm assessment, and consideration of resource use. The strength of the recommendation was determined using the AORN Evidence Rating Model and the quality and consistency of the evidence supporting a recommendation. The recommendation strength rating is noted in brackets after each recommendation.

Note: The evidence summary table is available at http:// www.aorn.org/evidencetables/.

1. Decolonization

1.1 **Convene an interdisciplinary team (ie, one or more infection preventionists, epidemiologists, pharmacists, perioperative RNs, surgeons, microbiology laboratory personnel, and other stakeholders identified by the health care organization) to determine the need to implement a preoperative *Staphylococcus aureus* (methicillin-resistant *S aureus* [MRSA] and methicillin-sensitive *S aureus* [MSSA]) decolonization program within the organization.**[3,4,7-11] *[Recommendation]*

The objective of decolonization is to decrease the bacterial load, specifically of *S aureus*, on the patient's body and in the nares. This is a part of a multimodal approach for preventing SSIs.[12] *S aureus* colonizes the skin and intranasal cavities of approximately 30% of the population.[13] Patients colonized with *S aureus* have a two- to nine-fold increased risk for developing an SSI compared to patients not colonized with *S aureus*.[13-15] Eighty percent of *S aureus* SSIs can be attributed to the patient's own bacteria.[3,16] Given the burden *S aureus* infections impose on both the patient and health care system, decolonization can be an effective method for decreasing SSI risk for high-risk procedures and patients.[3]

In patients undergoing cardiothoracic, vascular, orthopedic, and general surgeries, high-quality evidence supports decolonization as protective against SSIs caused by MRSA and MSSA, whether the site of decolonization is the nares alone or a combination of nasal and skin decolonization.[16-18] Limitations of these studies were inconsistencies in monitoring compliance with the decolonization regimen, criteria used for identifying SSIs, and length of time for surveillance. Some studies used the Centers for Disease Control and Prevention (CDC) definitions identified by infection preventionists and epidemiologists, others used SSI definitions other than the CDC definitions, some relied on surgeon identification, and still others used the patient's assessment of the incision site.

Ma et al[17] conducted a systematic review and meta-analysis to evaluate the effectiveness of various preoperative decolonization treatments (eg, nasal, nasal and skin) for preventing SSIs in patients undergoing elective cardiac and orthopedic surgeries. The authors reviewed six randomized controlled trials (RCTs) (N = 4,213 patients) and 19 observational studies (N = 128,362 patients) published between 2002 and 2016. In the RCTs, the authors found a 41% improvement in *S aureus* SSI prevention with preoperative anti-staphylococcal decolonization compared to a placebo. The observational studies, which had greater variation in protocols, showed a significant decrease in SSIs caused by all organisms (51%) as well as those caused by *S aureus* (47%) when preoperative anti-staphylococcal decolonization was performed.

Schweizer et al[16] conducted a systematic review with meta-analysis that included five RCTs and 12 observational studies published between 1996 and 2010 to evaluate the effectiveness of decolonization on SSI reduction among patients undergoing cardiac and total joint replacement surgeries. Based on the study findings, the researchers concluded that SSIs caused by gram-positive bacteria, including *S aureus*, could be prevented by decolonizing patients who are nasal carriers of *S aureus*.

In a systematic review of 18 experimental and nonexperimental studies published between 2004 and 2015 that compared skin and nasal decolonization to no decolonization in both surgical and intensive care populations, George et al[19] found that decolonization resulted in reduction of *S aureus* SSIs, reduction of health care–associated MRSA infections, and eradication of *S aureus* nasal carriage.

In a randomized multi-center trial of patients undergoing cardiothoracic, vascular, orthopedic, and general surgical procedures who were screened and tested positive for *S aureus* nasal carriage, those who received a decolonization protocol had significantly lower incidence of health care–associated *S aureus* infection, specifically deep surgical site infections, compared to patients who received a placebo.[18] In a follow-up study, Bode et al[20] found that the 1-year mortality rate was three times lower among decolonized patients undergoing clean orthopedic, cardiac, vascular, and abdominal surgical procedures compared to the placebo group. The researchers concluded that decolonization not only reduced the incidence of *S aureus* SSIs but was beneficial beyond discharge and should be considered for patients undergoing clean surgical and other invasive procedures.

Conversely, in a systematic review and meta-analysis of two RCTs (N = 291) that evaluated the effect of nasal decolonization in *S aureus* carriers undergoing cardiac surgical procedures, the authors concluded that there was insufficient evidence to determine the benefit of decolonization in preventing SSIs and that larger RCTs with better-reported outcomes were needed.[21] Similarly, Ramos et al[22] evaluated the infection rates of colonized and noncolonized patients undergoing total hip, total knee, and spinal fusion procedures (N = 13,828) in a comparative study during a 5-year period. In the first half of the study, colonized patients received an antibiotic protocol (ie, mupirocin), and in the second half of study, patients received an antiseptic protocol (ie, povidone-iodine). Despite high

Table 1. Factors for Selecting Decolonization Strategies

Factor	Characteristics
Local Epidemiology	• The organization's baseline *Staphylococcus aureus* surgical site infection rate[4,7,10,11] • Community *S aureus* (ie, methicillin-resistant *S aureus* [MRSA] and methicillin-sensitive *S aureus* [MSSA]) colonization rates[8,10,11] • Regional antibiotic susceptibility profile[17]

Procedure-Specific Risk Factors	• High-risk procedures (eg, that have severe consequences if infection occurs)[4,7,38]
	  ○ Cardiothoracic[3,7,9,23-26,38,40]
	  ○ Hip fracture repair[3,7,9]
	  ○ Neurosurgery[38]
	  ○ Orthopedic[38]
	  ○ Spinal fusion[27,41]
	  ○ Total joint replacement[3,7,12,14,26,28-30,38,41]
	  ○ Traumatic lower extremity fracture repair[39]
	  ○ Vascular[10,31]
	  ○ Procedures identified as high risk by the health care organization[4,7]

Patient Risk Factors	• Age (usually refers to adults older than 65 years)[10,11,32]
	• Antibiotic exposure (eg, within the past 12 months,[10] particularly to fluoroquinolones[8])
	• Residing in a congregant setting (eg, skilled nursing, group housing, prison)[8]
	• Past *S aureus* infection[3]
	• *S aureus* colonization[3,4,10,22,33,34,40]
	• Indwelling medical device (eg, urinary catheter, endotracheal tubes)[8]
	• Hemodialysis or peritoneal dialysis[10]
	• History of cerebrovascular accident[10,35]
	• Hospitalization within the past 12 months[10,32]
	• Admission to a high-risk unit that exceeds 15 days (eg, an intensive care unit with a high multidrug-resistant organism infection rate)[8]
	• Prolonged hospital stay[8]
	• Obesity (eg, body mass index > 30)[10,24,35-37,40]
	• Presence of an underlying disease,[8] such as
	  ○ Asthma[36]
	  ○ End-stage liver disease[10]
	  ○ Diabetes[24]

Note: As more research occurs, additional risk factors for S aureus *carriage may be identified.*

adherence to the decolonization protocol by colonized patients, the rate of SSIs for colonized patients was 4.35% compared to 2.39% for noncolonized patients. According to the researchers, one possible explanation for these results is that *S aureus* colonization may be a marker for comorbidities that increase patient infection risk (eg, rheumatoid arthritis, obesity). The researchers concluded that decolonization may not be fully effective in preventing SSIs because the risk for infection after decolonization may not be lowered to the noncolonized patient level and more measures for SSI prevention may be necessary. Study limitations included a retrospective design and a large academic setting, which may have higher infection rates than smaller community hospitals.

1.1.1 Use a risk-based approach that includes local epidemiology, procedure-specific risk factors, and patient risk factors when determining *S aureus* decolonization strategies. [Recommendation]

Moderate-quality evidence[3,8-12,14,17,22-41] supports using a risk-based approach to determine decolonization protocols (Table 1).

1.1.2 Evaluate available resources and plan for expansion of services (eg, laboratory capacity, decolonization agent) that the decolonization strategy requires. [Recommendation]

Development of a preoperative *S aureus* decolonization program will require substantial institutional support and financial commitment.[3,8] Necessary components of a decolonization program include specialized lab equipment, microbiology laboratory personnel to process tests, the ability to disseminate results and provide the indicated treatment, and a mechanism for assuring compliance. Surgical patients may also incur the cost of lab testing and decolonization protocols; however, this cost should be weighed against the financial burden and human factors associated with an SSI.

Table 2. Characteristics of Targeted and Universal Perioperative Decolonization Strategies in One Organization

Characteristic	Universal Decolonization	Targeted Screening and Decolonization
Implementation of Strategy	Easy prescription of medication	Logistics can be challenging for screening, reporting of results, and prescription of medication
Sensitivity of Strategy	100% (*Staphylococcus aureus* carriers will not be missed)	Some patients may not be screened, the test procedure may not have 100% sensitivity, and nonnasal *S aureus* carriers may be missed
Volume of Mupirocin Use	Approximately 5 times that in the targeted strategy	For detected *S aureus* carriers only
Volume of Screening	No screening for the universal approach	All patients
Cost Components	Allocation of medication and mupirocin	Screening, reporting, allocation of medication, and mupirocin

Adapted with permission from Hetem DJ, Bootsma MC, Bonten MJ. Prevention of surgical site infections: decontamination with mupirocin based on preoperative screening for Staphylococcus aureus *carriers or universal decontamination.* Clin Infect Dis. *2016;62(5):631-636.*

1.2 **If indicated by the interdisciplinary team, establish a preoperative *S aureus* decolonization program.** *[Recommendation]*

The literature reveals a variety of strategies implemented with different degrees of intensity and surgical populations, leading to diverse outcomes. Local epidemiology, patient risk factors, health care resources, and operative or invasive procedure risk factors are key considerations for development of an optimal decolonization program.

1.2.1 **Select a horizontal, vertical, or blended implementation strategy for *S aureus* decolonization.**[12,42] *[Recommendation]*

Horizontal and vertical strategies are evidence-based approaches to preventing health care–associated infections.[12,42] A horizontal (ie, **universal decolonization**) approach focuses on reducing clinically relevant pathogens by using universal interventions, such as nasal decolonization, chlorhexidine gluconate (CHG) bathing, hand hygiene, and personal protective equipment for every member of a general population.[12,42] Vertical (ie, **targeted decolonization**) approaches are intended to reduce a specific pathogen (eg, *S aureus*) using targeted interventions, such as **active surveillance** (eg, screening for MRSA), nasal and skin decolonization, and contact precautions for a select population.[12,42] Blended approaches implement both horizontal and vertical strategies **(Table 2)**.[12]

Horizontal Approach: Universal Decolonization

A benefit of universal decolonization is the ability to eradicate a wide range of pathogens in a population, lessening the potential for cross transmission.[12] The time and resources for implementation are reduced when compared to targeted screening and decolonization, as it is not necessary to conduct testing or wait for results (eg, perform surveillance) before implementing the decolonization protocol. The risk of adopting the universal approach is the potential for development of resistance to the decolonizing agents (eg, mupirocin, CHG) and the cost of agents for administration to the whole surgical population.[11,12]

High-quality studies on universal decolonization for patients undergoing cardiac[23,24,40]; spine[27]; total joint[43,44]; combined orthopedic, plastic, and general abdominal[45]; and combined cardiac, total joint, and general orthopedic surgeries[16] found a significant decrease in

- *S aureus* SSIs,[16,27,40,43]
- all-cause SSIs,[43,45]
- superficial SSIs,[23]
- harvest site and sternal organ/space SSIs,[24]
- *S aureus* transmission,[45] and
- return to surgery and readmission to the hospital.[43]

However, no difference or decrease was found

- in causative SSI organisms,[24]
- deep incisional or organ/space SSIs,[23] and
- overall SSI rates.[24,44]

The studies did not evaluate resistance of *S aureus* to decolonizing agents. Additionally, patients may not have been subject to decolonization if undergoing an emergent procedure or may have failed to comply with the protocol. All studies had a before-and-after design with some using historical control groups, which can minimize confounding variable control, possibly contributing to false outcomes.

Three predictive model studies, two of cardiac procedures[46,47] and one of total joint arthroplasty procedures,[48] found that when compared to targeted or no decolonization, universal decolonization resulted in greater efficiency and lower cost as a result of the number of SSIs that would be prevented.

In a single-center survey of physicians and nurses (N = 55) regarding perceptions of and barriers to universal decolonization in total joint arthroplasty procedures, Masroor et al[49] found that most providers believed universal decolonization was cost-effective (67%) and more effective than selected decolonization (51%). However, 18% thought universal decolonization was neither beneficial nor necessary.

Vertical Approach: Targeted Decolonization

A benefit of targeted decolonization is that only those patients who test positive during screening receive treatment, thereby saving on cost for antiseptics and medications used in decolonization and, if antimicrobials are used, decreasing the chance of antimicrobial resistance.[12] In addition, by identifying the organism during screening, the optimal prophylactic antimicrobial can be selected.[50] Potential harms of a targeted nasal screening approach are that patients who are colonized with S aureus at other body sites may be missed, patients who are not S aureus carriers may not receive the benefits of decolonization for other colonizing bacteria and common skin commensal organisms, and additional cost and time is associated with screening.[12]

High-quality studies on the use of targeted decolonization for patients undergoing cardiothoracic,[25,31,51] cesarean delivery,[52] general,[53,54] neurologic,[55] orthopedic,[29,30,32,34,56,57] and both cardiac and orthopedic procedures[26] and ambulatory orthopedic, urologic, neurologic, cardiovascular, and general surgery procedures[58] found a significant decrease in

- incidence of revision procedures (eg, revision total joint arthroplasty for prosthetic joint infection),[30,57]
- deep incisional SSIs,[26,30]
- organ/space SSIs,[47]
- all-cause SSIs,[25,29,55]
- MRSA SSIs,[32]
- S aureus SSIs,[28,31]
- S aureus deep incisional and organ/space SSIs,[28] and
- S aureus colonization.[14,25,30,34,58]

However, eight studies found no difference or decrease in treated or untreated S aureus carriers in

- overall SSI rates,[28,34,52,53,56]
- S aureus SSIs,[3]
- MRSA SSIs,[54] and
- empyema incidence in pulmonary resections.[51]

A limitation of these studies is that all except three studies[52,56,58] had a before-and-after design with several using historical control groups, which may minimize control of confounding variables, leading to false outcomes. Additionally, some patients undergoing emergent surgeries may not have been screened and treated.

Tsang et al[30] conducted a survey of 85 patients undergoing total joint replacement procedures after completion of a targeted decolonization protocol, to gather feedback on acceptability of the protocol. Ninety-six percent of the patients strongly agreed that the protocol was painless and 79% strongly agreed that the treatment was acceptable.

In a literature review, Edmiston et al[10] found that targeted screening decolonization was effective for selective procedures that include cardiovascular, vascular with prosthetic graft, and orthopedic total joint procedures. However, the review authors concluded that the benefit in other device-related procedures is unknown.

The Society for Healthcare Epidemiology of America (SHEA) and the Infectious Diseases Society of America (IDSA),[7] the American Society of Health-System Pharmacists,[9] the World Health Organization (WHO),[3] the American College of Surgeons (ACS) and Surgical Infection Society (SIS),[11] and the National Association of Orthopaedic Nurses (NAON)[59] recommend a targeted decolonization protocol for preventing SSIs.

Blended Approach: Universal and Targeted Decolonization

Based on the surgical population, antibiotic resistance patterns, and community MRSA rates, facilities may decide to employ a universal strategy for high-risk procedures but a targeted approach for other surgical procedures. Blending of strategies for the same surgical procedure could include a targeted approach for nasal decolonization and universal CHG bathing.

In a literature review, Septimus and Schweizer[12] concluded that although the optimal implementation strategy for patients undergoing both elective and emergent surgical procedures are undetermined, a combination of targeted and universal decolonization approaches may be practical in the surgical patient population.

1.3 **Based on the selected implementation strategy, determine the screening method for S aureus.**[10,18,60] [Recommendation]

Screening methods for S aureus vary in time to receive results, performance (eg, specificity and sensitivity), and cost.[10] Nasal carriage of MRSA and MSSA can be detected with either a nasal culture or nasal polymerase chain reaction (PCR) method. Direct culture methods have a sensitivity of 80%, whereas molecular methods, such as PCR, have a sensitivity of 93%. The advantage of PCR over culturing is that PCR results are available within a few hours, whereas culturing can take from 1 to 2 days.[10] Therefore, PCR facilitates early identification of colonization, providing an opportunity for early eradication and interruption of a spread from the patient's nares to other body areas or to other hospitalized patients.[18,60] The disadvantage of PCR testing is that, according to Edmiston et al,[10] the cost of a PCR test can be more than three to 10 times the cost of traditional culture methods.

In a multi-center RCT, Bode et al[18] used nasal PCR screening to rapidly identify and decolonize *S aureus* carriers admitted to surgical and internal medicine floors, which resulted in a significant reduction in the rate of health care–associated *S aureus* infections. The researchers concluded that rapid nasal screening along with decolonization is an effective method for reducing health care–associated *S aureus* infections.

One disadvantage of performing nasal screening only, regardless of whether a traditional culture or PCR is used, is that patients can be colonized at sites other than the nares, and MRSA or MSSA may not be detected by a nasal culture or nasal PCR method. In a nonexperimental study, Bebko et al[60] compared both PCR tests and cultures taken at the preoperative visit and on the day of surgery from the groin and the nares of 140 patients undergoing orthopedic procedures with hardware implantation. The researchers found that PCR testing correctly identified all culture-positive samples, regardless of the collection site or resistance status of the organisms. Additionally, higher detection rates were noted when results from nose and groin sites were combined. The researchers suggested that the use of PCR could be beneficial when preadmission assessment by direct culture methods is impractical, such as when procedures are classified as urgent or emergent.

1.3.1 Determine a decolonization protocol specific to the implementation strategy, acknowledging that a physician order may be necessary.[12,15,21,22,24,27,41,44,61,62] *[Recommendation]*

Decolonization protocols generally include topical and intranasal antiseptics or antibiotics.[38] However, the literature search for this guideline did not find a standardized decolonization protocol. Nasal decolonization is most often performed by applying antibiotics (eg,

mupirocin) or antiseptics (eg, povidone-iodine, octenidine, alcohol-based) to the nares. The goal of nasal decolonization is to reduce the risk of SSI by preventing nasal cavity organisms from being transferred to the skin and surgical incision. The potential effectiveness of this method is believed to be dependent on both the antibiotic or antiseptic used and the application dose.[21] The patient's understanding of application instructions and compliance with those instructions also contribute to the effectiveness of nasal decolonization.[3]

Mupirocin is a topical antibacterial ointment that is effective against staphylococci, streptococci, and gram-negative organisms.[12] An alternative to nasal decolonization with mupirocin is the use of an antiseptic such as povidone-iodine (5%-10%),[15,22,39,41,44,45,61] octenidine,[24] or an alcohol-based antiseptic[27,62] (eg, 70% ethyl alcohol).

See Recommendation 1.5.2 and Recommendation 7.4 for more information on antibiotic and antiseptic tolerance and resistance.

The literature search found studies of four different nasal decolonization agents. Mupirocin nasal ointment was used under different regimens in 22 studies,[14,18,23,25,26,28-32,34,40,43,47,51-58] povidone-iodine in seven studies,[15,22,39,41,44,45,61] an alcohol-based antiseptic in two studies,[27,62] and octenidine in one study.[24]

Skin decolonization is often performed in conjunction with nasal decolonization to further reduce transfer of organisms to the surgical incision. Chlorhexidine gluconate was used for skin decolonization in the form of soap[14,18,23,25-27,29-32,34,39,40,43,47,51,53-56,58,62] or wipes[22,28,39,41,44,57,61] in all but four studies.[15,24,40,52] Three studies included hair shampoo, two with CHG[30,53] and one with octenidine.[24] Mouthwash with CHG was used in one study.[30]

The researchers in all studies except seven[18,27,31,45,47,58,62] reported using surgical antibiotic prophylaxis with different agents and frequency. Table 3 and Table 4 provide more information about these studies, the nasal decolonization agent, application protocol, skin antiseptic and application protocol (if used), antibiotic prophylaxis (if used), and study outcomes.

Clinical practice guidelines[3,4,7,9,11,38,59] from various health agencies and professional societies identify nasal antistaphylococcal agents (eg, mupirocin) as a decolonizing agent, but do not define optimal timing, dose, or duration (Table 5).

Table 3. Antibiotic Decolonization Protocols

Author, Year	Study Design	Procedure Type	Nasal Agent	Application Protocol	Skin Agent	Application Protocol	Antibiotic Prophylaxis	Outcomes
Agarwala et al,[32] 2016	Nonexperimental	Orthopedic implants*	Mupirocin 2%	Nares, axilla, and groin tid x 3 days	CHG 4%	Bath/shower on the night before operative procedures	Yes	No methicillin-resistant *Staphylococcus aureus* (MRSA) surgical site infections (SSIs)
Baratz et al,[34] 2015	Quasi-experimental	Total hip and knee replacement, including revision	Intervention Mupirocin 2% Comparator No treatment	Nares bid x 5 days	Intervention CHG 4% Comparator No CHG	Bath/shower daily x 5 days	Yes	Reduction in MRSA nasal carriage for the intervention group
Bode et al,[18] 2010	Randomized controlled trial (RCT)	Patients admitted to inpatient surgical and internal medicine services for at least 4 days	Intervention Mupirocin 2% Comparator Placebo	Nares bid x 5 days Nares bid x 5 days	Intervention CHG 4% Comparator Placebo	Bath/shower daily x 5 days Bath/shower daily x 5 days	Not indicated	Decrease in deep incisional SSIs Decrease in *S aureus* health care–associated infections Reduction in mean length of stay by ~ 2 days
del Diego Salas et al,[47] 2016	Quasi-experimental	Cardiac procedures**	Intervention Universal mupirocin 2% Comparator Targeted mupirocin 2%	Nares bid x 14 days Nares bid x 14 days	Intervention CHG 4% Comparator No CHG	Bath/shower night before procedure	Not indicated	Decrease in SSIs Cost savings related to fewer SSIs in intervention group
Grimmer et al,[51] 2014	Quasi-experimental	Pulmonary resection	Intervention Mupirocin 2% Comparator No treatment	Nares bid x 5 days	Intervention CHG 4% Comparator No CHG	Chest scrub on night before procedure	Yes	No reduction in empyema rate
Kline et al,[58] 2018	RCT	Ambulatory	Intervention Mupirocin 2% Comparator No treatment	Nares bid x 5 days	Intervention CHG 4% Comparator No CHG	Intervention Bath/shower daily x 5 days*** Comparator Bath/shower daily x 2 days	No	Reduction of *S aureus* nasal colonization at 4 body sites
Kohler et al,[23] 2015	Quasi-experimental	Cardiac procedures	Intervention Mupirocin 2% Comparator No treatment	Nares bid x 5 days	Intervention CHG 4% Comparator No CHG	Bath/shower daily x 5 days	Yes	Decrease in superficial SSIs
Langen-berg et al,[31] 2016	Quasi-experimental	Vascular procedures	Intervention Mupirocin 2% Comparator No treatment	Nares bid x 5 days	Intervention CHG 4% Comparator No CHG	Bath/shower daily x 5 days	Not indicated	Decrease in *S aureus* SSIs

Table 3 Continued. Antibiotic Decolonization Protocols

Author, Year	Study Design	Procedure Type	Nasal Agent	Application Protocol	Skin Agent	Application Protocol	Antibiotic Prophylaxis	Outcomes
Lefebvre et al,[56] 2017	Quasi-experimental	Deep brain stimulation	Intervention Mupirocin 2% Comparator No treatment	Nares tid x 5 days	Intervention CHG 4% Comparator Povidone-iodine 4%	Bath/shower daily x 5 days Bath/shower on evening before and day of procedure	Yes	Decrease in SSIs
Lemaignen et al,[40] 2018	Quasi-experimental	Cardiac procedures	Intervention Mupirocin 2% Comparator No treatment	Nares bid on the day of the procedure and 2 days after surgery	Intervention Polyvidone iodine Comparator No Polyvidone iodine	Bath/shower on night before procedure	Yes	Decrease in *S aureus* mediastinitis
Moroski et al,[14] 2015	Nonexperimental	Total hip and knee replacement procedures, including revision	Mupirocin 2%	Nares bid x 5 days	CHG 4%	Bath/shower daily x 3 days and before procedure	Yes	Reduction of MRSA and methicillin-susceptible *S aureus* nasal colonization
Romero-Palacios et al,[28] 2019	Quasi-experimental	Total hip and knee replacement, including revision	Intervention Mupirocin 2% Comparator No treatment	Nares bid x 5 days	Intervention CHG 2% Comparator No CHG	CHG wipes daily x 5 days	Yes	Decrease in deep incisional and organ/space *S aureus* prosthetic joint infections
Saraswat et al,[25] 2017	Quasi-experimental	Cardiac procedures	Intervention Mupirocin 2% Comparator No treatment	Nares bid x 5 days	Intervention CHG 4% Comparator No CHG	Bath/shower daily x 5 days	Yes	Decrease in coronary artery bypass graft SSIs Reduction of MRSA nasal colonization and transmission
Sasi et al,[53] 2015	Quasi-experimental	General procedures	Intervention Mupirocin 2% Comparator No treatment	Colonized site (nares, axilla, or groin) tid x 5 days	Intervention CHG 4% Comparator No CHG	Two baths/showers daily x 5 days, with shampoo with the second daily bath/shower	Yes, excluding clean procedures	No decrease in SSIs
Schweizer et al,[26] 2015	Quasi-experimental	Cardiac procedures, total hip replacements, total knee replacements	Intervention Mupirocin 2% Comparator No treatment	Nares bid x 5 days	Intervention CHG 4% Comparator No CHG	Bath/shower daily x 5 days	Yes	Decrease in deep incisional and organ/space SSIs
Shrem et al,[52] 2016	RCT	Cesarean delivery, elective and urgent	Intervention Mupirocin 2% Comparator No treatment	Nares bid x 5 days	None	None	Yes	No difference in SSI reduction between treated or untreated carriers Reduction in MRSA nasal colonization

Table 3 Continued. Antibiotic Decolonization Protocols

Author, Year	Study Design	Procedure Type	Nasal Agent	Application Protocol	Skin Agent	Application Protocol	Antibiotic Prophylaxis	Outcomes
Sousa et al,[56] 2016	RCT	Total hip replacements, total knee replacements	Intervention Mupirocin 2% Comparator No treatment	Nares bid x 5 days	Intervention CHG 4% Comparator No CHG	Bath/shower daily x 5 days	Yes	No difference in SSI reduction between treated or untreated carriers
Sporer et al,[29] 2016	Quasi-experimental	Total hip replacements, total knee replacements	Intervention Mupirocin 2% Comparator No treatment	Nares bid x 5 days	Intervention CHG 4% Comparator No CHG	Bath/shower daily x 5 days	Yes	Decrease in all-cause and *S aureus* SSIs
Stambough et al,[43] 2017	Quasi-experimental	Total hip replacements, total knee replacements	Intervention Universal mupirocin 2% Comparator Targeted mupirocin 2%	Nares bid x 5 days Nares bid x 5 days	Intervention CHG 4% Comparator CHG 4%	Bath/shower daily x 5 days Bath/shower daily x 5 days	Yes	Decrease in all-cause and *S aureus* SSIs Cost savings from limitation of future reoperations
Takahasi et al,[54] 2014	Quasi-experimental	Gastroenterological	Intervention Mupirocin 2% Comparator No treatment	Nares bid x 5 days	Intervention CHG 4% Comparator No CHG	Bath/shower daily x 5 days	Yes	Decrease in MRSA SSIs
Tsang et al,[30] 2018	Quasi-experimental	Total joint replacements	Intervention Mupirocin 2% Comparator No treatment	Nares tid x 5 days	Intervention CHG 4% Comparator No CHG	Bath/shower daily x 5 days including hair shampoo***	Yes	Decrease in deep incisional SSIs Decrease in revision surgeries Reduction in MRSA nasal and groin colonization

No procedure until negative for S aureus
**Hair removal performed on night before procedure*
***Included CHG mouthwash for intervention group*

1.3.2 **An *S aureus* decolonization protocol may be established for patients undergoing urgent procedures.**[26] *[Conditional Recommendation]*

Because of time sensitivity, patients undergoing urgent procedures often do not receive screening or begin a decolonization protocol.

In a quasi-experimental study, Schweizer et al[26] implemented a targeted decolonization bundle for patients undergoing cardiac and total joint procedures (N = 42,525) at 20 hospitals. All patients were screened, including those undergoing urgent procedures, but urgent procedure patients immediately began decolonization, and continued treatment until test results were known. If results were negative, decolonization was discontinued. However, the bundle resulted in a significant decrease in complex SSIs (ie, deep incisional, organ/space) for scheduled surgeries, but not for urgent procedures.

In a literature review, Septimus and Schweizer[12] concluded that facilities should study *S aureus* colonization rates in the community and in the specific surgical patient population to determine whether decolonization would be beneficial for urgent procedures in which a patient presents with unknown colonization status. The authors explained that, for surgical procedures, patients would receive a dose before the operative procedure and complete remaining doses after the procedure and that close collaboration between the infection preventionist, health care epidemiologist, and perioperative team would be necessary.

If a health care facility is using a targeted decolonization protocol, preoperative real-time PCR testing for high-risk patients undergoing urgent surgical procedures may be a consideration. Infection preventionists, microbiology laboratory personnel, and perioperative leaders may evaluate the feasibility of using this method.[12,18,25] As more rapid testing products become available; cost may decrease, making this option more accessible.

1.4 Implement the preoperative *S aureus* decolonization program as defined by the interdisciplinary team.[3] [Recommendation]

Identification and clear communication of implementation strategies is essential for a successful decolonization program. Acquisition of required resources, defined responsibilities, end-user buy-in, and administrative support are all vital components for success.[3]

1.4.1 Establish timing for initiation and completion of the decolonization protocol.[11] [Recommendation]

There is lack of evidence on optimal timing for nasal decolonization.[4] Many studies had at least one application of decolonizing agent completed in the immediate preoperative period. However, the number of applications and days on the protocol varied.

The application of nasal antibiotic decolonizing agents varied from two times a day for 5 days,[14,18,23,25,26,28,29,31,34,43,51,52,54,56,58] to two times a day for 14 days,[47] to three times a day for 3 days,[32] or three times a day for 5 days.[30,53,55] In four studies, the application continued after surgery. Lemaignen et al[40] applied the agent two times on the day of the procedure, as well as 2 days after the procedure. Kohler et al,[23] Saraswat et al,[25] and Sporer et al[29] continued the application two times a day after surgery if 10 doses were not completed before surgery.

The application of nasal antiseptic decolonizing agents on the day of the procedure varied from one,[39,61] to two,[15,41,44,45] to three times.[24,62] In one study, the agent was applied on the day of the procedure and application continued for 5 to 7 days after surgery.[27]

The ACS and SIS[11] recommend that decolonization protocols be completed as close as possible to the date of the procedure. The National Institute for Health and Care Excellence[4] (NICE) does not make a recommendation on timing because of a lack of evidence. The SHEA[7] recommends that screening and decolonization occur in the preoperative setting, and the WHO[3] and CDC[38] recommend perioperative application of decolonizing agents.

Saraswat et al[25] found a correlation between duration of preoperative decolonization and decreased frequency of postoperative *S aureus* colonization in patients undergoing cardiac operative procedures. Of 4,038 patients screened preoperatively by nasal PCR, 120 patients were found to be colonized with MRSA or MSSA. Fifty patients completed the 5-day skin and nasal decolonization preoperatively and 70 patients finished the decolonization regimen in the intensive care unit (ICU) after surgery. On postoperative ICU admission, all patients received nasal cultures for MRSA, and the incidence of MRSA for the previously colonized group was 20% (n = 24). The researchers concluded that for each additional day of preoperative decolonization, with a limit of 5 days, there was an associated 27% reduction in the risk of *S aureus* colonization for patients admitted postoperatively to the ICU.

Kohler et al[23] found that despite 14% of study participants beginning decolonization after operative procedures, there was no difference in SSI rate between those patients beginning the intervention before the operative procedure and those beginning treatment after the procedure.

Tsang et al[30] conducted a quasi-experimental study of patients undergoing elective orthopedic procedures who tested positive for *S aureus* and subsequently were decolonized. The researchers retested these patients 48 to 96 hours after treatment, at the time of the procedure, and at discharge. They concluded that the decolonization had lasting effects, for at least 10 days.

In contrast, Takahashi et al[54] found that targeted screening and decolonization for MRSA carriers undergoing gastroenterological operative procedures prevented MRSA SSIs. However, postoperative nasal colonization was a significant factor contributing to MRSA infection, and the benefit of decolonization in prevention varied according to the incidence of MRSA acquisition on the ward.

In a literature review of decolonization methods, Septimus and Schweizer[12] found that although long-term decolonization is challenging because some patients become recolonized within weeks of decolonization, surgical patients may benefit from relatively short-term decolonization or until the surgical incision has healed.

Table 4. Antiseptic Decolonization Protocols

Author, Year	Study Design	Procedure Type	Nasal Agent	Application Protocol	Skin Agent	Application Protocol	Additional Protocol	Antibiotic Prophylaxis	Outcome
Alcohol-Based Nasal Sanitizer									
Mullen et al,[27] 2017	Quasi-experimental	Spinal procedures	*Intervention* Alcohol-based nasal sanitizer *Comparator* Mupirocin 2%	Nares day of procedure and 5-7 days after surgery Nares bid x 5 days	*Intervention* CHG 4% *Comparator* CHG 4%	Frequency not indicated Frequency not indicated	Universal decolonization Surgical personnel voluntarily applied alcohol-based agent daily	Not indicated	Decrease in *Staphylococcus aureus* surgical site infections (SSIs)
Steed et al,[62] 2014	Randomized controlled trial (RCT)	Health care personnel	*Intervention* Alcohol-based nasal sanitizer *Comparator* Placebo	Nares tid, 1 day Nares tid, 1 day	None	None	None	No	Reduction in *S aureus* and total bacteria nasal carriage
Octenidine (OCT)									
Reiser et al,[24] 2017	Quasi-experimental	Coronary artery bypass graft	*Intervention* OCT nasal ointment *Comparator* No treatment	Nasal tid on day before procedure	*Intervention* OCT liquid soap *Comparator* No treatment	Bath/shower on night before and day of procedure, including hair shampoo	Universal decolonization	Yes	Decrease in harvest site and organ/space sternal SSIs
Povidone-Iodine (PI)									
Bebko et al,[61] 2015	Quasi-experimental	Orthopedic with implants	*Intervention* Nasal PI 5% *Comparator* No treatment	Nares day of procedure	*Intervention* CHG 2% *Comparator* No treatment	CHG wipes on night before and morning of procedure	Universal decolonization CHG 0.12% mouthwash on night before and morning of procedure	Yes	Decrease in 30-day SSIs Reduction in methicillin-resistant S aureus nasal carriage
Loftus et al,[45] 2020	RCT	Plastic, orthopedic, general abdominal	*Intervention* Universal nasal PI 5% *Comparator* Targeted mupirocin 2%	Nares within 1 hour of incision and after induction of anesthesia Nares bid x 5 days	*Intervention* CHG 2% *Comparator* CHG 2%	CHG wipes night before and morning of procedure CHG wipes daily x 5 days	Enhanced improvements in hand hygiene, vascular care, environmental cleaning	Not indicated	Decrease in *S aureus* transmission and SSIs
Phillips et al,[41] 2014	RCT	Spine fusion and joint replacements, including revision	*Intervention* Nasal PI 5% *Comparator* Mupirocin 2%	Nares day of procedure x 2 Nares bid x 5 days	*Intervention* CHG 2% *Comparator* CHG 2%	CHG wipes on night before and morning of procedure CHG wipes on night before and morning of procedure	Universal decolonization	Yes	Decrease in *S aureus* deep incisional SSIs
Rezapoor et al,[15] 2017	RCT	Orthopedic with implants, including revisions	*Intervention* Nasal PI 5% *Comparator* PI 10% *Comparator* Saline	Nares day of procedure x 2 Nares day of procedure x 2 Nares day of procedure x 2	None	None	Universal decolonization	Yes	Greatest reduction of nasal *S aureus* at 4 hours was with nasal PI 5%

Table 4 Continued. Antiseptic Decolonization Protocols

Author, Year	Study Design	Procedure Type	Nasal Agent	Application Protocol	Skin Agent	Application Protocol	Additional Protocol	Antibiotic Prophylaxis	Outcome
Torres et al,[44] 2016	Quasi-experimental	Total hip replacements and total knee replacements, including revision	*Intervention* Universal nasal PI 5% *Comparison* Targeted mupirocin 2%	Nares day of the procedure x 2 Nares bid x 5 days	*Intervention* CHG 4% CHG 2% *Comparison* CHG 4% CHG 2%	Bath/shower daily x 5 day and operative leg wipe day of procedure Bath/shower daily x 5 days and operative leg wipe day of procedure	None	Yes	No difference in SSIs Cost savings with PI
Urias et al,[39] 2018	Non-experimental	Trauma lower extremity fracture repair	*Intervention* Nasal PI 5%	Nares within 1 hour of incision	CHG 4% CHG 2%	If possible, bath/shower on night before surgery, but always on morning of surgery	Universal decolonization	Yes	Significant decrease in SSIs

1.4.2 Convene an interdisciplinary team that includes materials management personnel, senior administrators, finance managers, infection preventionists, and perioperative RNs to define a plan for procuring the decolonization agent.[3] *[Recommendation]*

Patient acquisition of decolonization agents may be difficult as this depends on the scheduling of the preoperative visit, time needed to obtain the lab result, cost of agents, and transportation availability. Successful decolonization strategies are budget conscious, reliable, easy, and provide continuous access methods that facilitate patient and personnel compliance with the protocol.[3]

In a quality improvement project, patients undergoing total joint arthroplasty procedures who tested positive for *S aureus* were notified by the preoperative clinic nurse 24 hours after the preoperative visit and asked to return to the clinic to receive a decolonization package at no charge.[28] In another quality improvement project with patients undergoing cardiac operative procedures who tested positive in the outpatient setting, an advanced practitioner (eg, physician assistant, nurse practitioner) ordered the medication and called the patients to provide them with instructions on how to purchase and use decolonizing agents. In the inpatient setting, personnel from the cardiac perioperative team ordered the agents preoperatively.[25]

In a 20-hospital quasi-experimental study to implement a decolonization bundle, 27.1% of the 328 patients who did not adhere to the protocol reported that problems obtaining the prescription or agent itself was the main barrier.[26]

In a single-center survey on barriers to universal decolonization implementation, both nurses and physicians identified difficulty in distributing a universal decolonization kit as a main barrier.[49] After implementation of universal decolonization, Phillips et al[41] conducted a follow-up patient survey, and 8% of patients reported it was difficult to purchase ointment because of the cost.

Rapid testing technology, such as the nasal PCR method, provides quick results and may allow for patients to be sent home with decolonizing agents. However, PCR testing is often more expensive than standard culture testing.[12]

1.4.3 Provide patients who will participate in the decolonization program with education about the benefits of decolonization and the patient's role in the decolonization protocol.[3,24,28,34,41,56,61,63,64] *[Recommendation]*

Education and engagement of patients is essential to the success of a decolonization protocol. Clear communication, instructions, and explanations are vital to ensuring adherence and advocacy. Participation and collaboration in the protocol provides a sense of ownership.[3]

In a nonexperimental study to evaluate patients' experience and satisfaction with nasal decolonization, patients undergoing total joint arthroplasty and spine fusion procedures (N = 1,679) were randomly assigned to either a single application of 5% povidone-iodine within 2 hours before the procedure or preoperative 2% mupirocin twice daily for 5 days, and were then interviewed upon treatment completion. More than two-thirds of the patients considered preoperative nasal decolonization with either povidone-iodine or mupirocin to be somewhat or very helpful in reducing SSIs. Being recruited as an active participant in SSI prevention was reported to be a

Table 5. Health Agency and Professional Society Decolonization Protocol Recommendations		
Entity	**Nasal Protocol**	**Skin Protocol**
American College of Surgeons and Surgical Infection Society, 2016[11]	Nasal mupirocin 2%	No recommendation
American Society of Health-System Pharmacists, 2013[9]	Nasal mupirocin 2%	No recommendation
Centers for Disease Control and Prevention, 2019[38]	Intranasal anti-staphylococcal antibiotic/antiseptic (eg, mupirocin or iodophor)	Chlorhexidine gluconate (CHG)
National Association of Orthopaedic Nurses, 2013[59]	Nasal mupirocin 2% bid until time of procedure	No recommendation
National Institute for Health and Care Excellence, 2019[4]	Nasal mupirocin 2%	CHG
Society for Healthcare Epidemiology of America/Infectious Diseases Society of America, 2014[7]	Anti-staphylococcal agent	No recommendation
World Health Organization, 2016[3]	Nasal mupirocin 2% with or without skin decolonization	If used, CHG

positive experience by 87.2% of patients who received mupirocin and 86.3% of patients who received povidone-iodine. The researchers concluded that including patients undergoing elective and urgent procedures in preoperative decolonization decisions and engagement as a team member in SSI prevention is beneficial.[63]

Several education modalities were used in studies where a decrease in SSIs and *S aureus* colonization were outcomes.[24,28,34,41,56,61] Sousa et al[56] convened patients who were *S aureus* positive 1 week before the procedure to provide education about the rationale for decolonization and application of decolonization protocol. Bebko et al[61] had patients watch an educational video on decolonization before receiving decolonizing agents. Reiser et al,[24] Baratz et al,[34] and Phillips et al[41] verbally instructed patients on how and when to apply the decolonizing agent. Phillips et al[41] also provided access to a 24-hour telephone number in case study participants had questions. Another modality was outlining instructions in an informational brochure that was given to each patient in an effort to maximize effectiveness of protocol and enhance compliance.[24,28,34,41]

1.4.4 **Provide health care personnel who will participate in the decolonization program with education on the benefits and details of the decolonization program used in the organization.[49,65]** *[Recommendation]*

In a single-center survey of physicians and nurses regarding perceptions and barriers to universal decolonization in total joint procedures, one identified barrier was the lack of education for both personnel and patients on the rationale and expected outcomes of universal

decolonization.[32] Tschelaut et al[65] conducted a survey of Austrian surgeons from multiple disciplines to determine the frequency of preoperative decolonization and assess current knowledge of decolonization. Of the 158 surgeons who completed the survey, 103 stated that decolonization did occur in the perioperative setting in their organizations, but the methods, antimicrobials, and personnel performing decolonization varied. They also reported that those educated on the benefit were most likely to institute the practice. The authors concluded more studies are needed that include education focused on decolonization.

1.5 **Monitor the decolonization regimen as part of an overall SSI surveillance and quality improvement program.[3]** *[Recommendation]*

Measurement of success and regular observation of processes can identify inconsistencies and areas for improvement.

1.5.1 **Assess patients' adherence to the decolonization regimen.[3,4,7-9,11,15,23,26-28,30,31,41,53,54,58,61]** *[Recommendation]*

The ACS and SIS state that, if followed, decolonization protocols are highly effective, and without adherence, there is no benefit.[11] Failure to adhere to protocol not only decreases the success rate for decolonization but also can increase the chance for resistance when antibiotic decolonization agents are used.

Schweizer et al[26] found a significant decrease in complex (eg, deep incisional, organ/space) *S aureus* rates for patients who were fully adherent to nasal mupirocin and CHG bathing protocols and no significant decrease for patients who were partially or nonadherent to the protocols. In patients with postoperative nasal MRSA acquisition, Takahashi et al[54] found that the preoperative compliance for mupirocin was 75% and for CHG bathing was 58.3%, resulting in a 44.4% eradication rate.

Monitoring patient adherence to the decolonization protocol as well as patient tolerance of decolonizing agents can be an implementation challenge, and many of the studies reviewed for this guideline did not include these measures. However, five high-quality studies with favorable outcomes did monitor patient adherence to decolonization.[26,28,30,41,58] The methods used included a daily diary to record the number and timing of applications,[30,58] an anonymous post-study survey,[28,41] and a compliance rating scale (ie, fully, partially, or not adherent).[26] Tsang et al[30] cautioned that when considering these implementation strategies, study participants are likely highly motivated and may be more adherent than those not participating in a study.

In other studies, because of a shorter length of treatment protocol[15,27,61] or patients hospitalized preoperatively,[23,31,53,54] compliance was measured by health care personnel directly observing or applying the decolonization protocol.

The WHO[3] recommends that when implementing a decolonization program, information on decolonization applications should be recorded in surveillance forms and health records, along with any adverse reactions.

1.5.2 **If using an antimicrobial (eg, mupirocin), include surveillance for antibiotic resistance as part of the antimicrobial stewardship program.**[3,4,8,9,11,26,42,66-68] *[Conditional Recommendation]*

A risk for inclusion of antimicrobial agents (eg, mupirocin) in decolonization regimens is the development of *S aureus* strains that are resistant to the antibiotic, thereby decreasing the efficacy of decolonization.[68] Implementing surveillance may allow for any increase in resistance to be identified.[4]

There are two known mupirocin resistant (MupR) phenotypes: low-level, defined as a **minimum inhibitory concentration** (MIC) between 8 mg/L and 64 mg/L, and high-level, defined as a MIC ≥ 512 mg/L.[67] In a study conducted at a large university hospital in Spain, Muñoz-Gallego et al[66] collected 64 blood and 358 nasal isolates during a 2-year period from patients hospitalized with invasive MRSA infections to determine the prevalence of mupirocin resistance. From the blood isolates, the researchers identified resistance in 15.6% of specimens, with low-level resistance in 4.7%

and high-level resistance in 10.9%. In the nasal isolates, the researchers found resistance in 15.1%, with low-level resistance in 3.1% and high-level resistance in 12%.

Deeny et al[67] estimated the relative transmissibility of MupR MRSA strains in the ICU and general patient population in Great Britain during a 5-year period and found that resistant strains were less transmissible than sensitive strains. However, the prevalence of mupirocin resistance increased 50% to 75% during universal decolonization and increased 10% during targeted decolonization, leading the authors to urge caution when adopting a widespread or universal approach to decolonization with mupirocin.

Hetem et al[42] conducted a study using universal decolonization with mupirocin and CHG bathing for patients undergoing orthopedic, cardiothoracic, and neurosurgical procedures in a teaching hospital in the Netherlands. Nasal cultures were collected before decolonization and 4 days after operative procedures in 935 patients to quantify the occurrence of mupirocin resistance in *S aureus* and coagulase-negative staphylococci (CoNS). Widespread mupirocin resistance was found in CoNS but no resistance was found in *S aureus*. As 97% of the co-colonizing bacteria acquired the mupirocin-resistant gene (mupA), the researchers recommended monitoring mupirocin-resistance development in *S aureus* when using mupirocin decolonization protocols.

In a study using targeted decolonization with mupirocin and CHG bathing for patients undergoing cardiac, hip, and knee procedures at 20 hospitals in the United States, Schweizer et al[26] found that only one of 36 isolates (2.8%) obtained from complex *S aureus* SSIs in this population showed high-level resistance to mupirocin.

To evaluate the risk of developing mupirocin resistance in targeted and universal decolonization strategies, Hetem et al[68] used published data on high-level mupirocin resistance in *S aureus* and CoNS, along with mathematical modeling and concluded that both strategies had an equally low risk for acquisition of MupR *S aureus*. However, the authors noted that as the prevalence of MupR *S aureus* increases, both strategies will become less successful.

When using mupirocin for decolonization, clinical practice guidelines from professional organizations recommend surveillance to detect emergence of resistance to the decolonizing agent.[3,4,8,9,11]

2. Preoperative Bathing

2.1 **Patients should perform preoperative bathing with either soap or an antiseptic before surgery or other invasive procedures.** [Recommendation] **P**

High-quality evidence supports that preoperative bathing may reduce the microbial flora on the patient's skin before a surgical or other invasive procedure.[69-75] Limitations of the evidence are that research has not confirmed the effect of preoperative bathing on SSI development. Additional research is needed to define optimal preoperative bathing procedures, including whether antiseptics are more effective than soaps (eg, plain, antimicrobial), whether bathing the whole body is more effective than bathing only the surgical site, the optimal timing of bathing before the procedure, and the optimal number of baths or showers before a procedure.[76]

The benefits of preoperative patient bathing outweigh the potential harms. Benefits include reduction of transient and resident microorganisms on the skin that may lower the patient's risk of developing an SSI.[2] The harms of preoperative patient bathing with an antiseptic may include skin irritation, allergic reaction, or unnecessary treatment with antiseptics.[2]

Soap versus Antiseptic

In a Cochrane systematic review of seven RCTs conducted between 1987 and 2014, Webster and Osborne[2] concluded that there was no clear benefit of preoperative bathing or showering with CHG over other skin antiseptic products in reducing the incidence of SSIs. Limitations to this review are that all but one of these studies were conducted before 1990, and since then, a number of SSI guidelines, bundles, and prevention strategies have been developed. Additionally, researchers in two other studies noted that there were no standardized interventions or outcome measurements found among the studies.[77,78]

The authors of a systematic review of eight RCTs published between 1983 and 2009 that compared the effects of 4% CHG to plain soap or 4% CHG to a placebo on the SSI rates of 10,655 patients undergoing Class I (clean) surgical procedures found SSI rates to be 7.1% for CHG, 9.1% for placebo, and 5.1% for plain soap. The authors concluded that the use of 4% CHG preoperatively cannot be recommended to reduce SSIs in clean surgical procedures.[79] Some limitations to this review were that all studies but one were conducted before 1992, and variation was found between studies in the number of baths, the amount of solution used, SSI definition, and the

period of follow-up. Additionally, clean surgical procedures have a lower incidence of SSIs, so a larger number of patients would be needed to see the true effect.

Evidence from two other systematic reviews is inconclusive. The authors of a systematic review with meta-analysis of eight RCTs and eight quasi-RCTs found that when compared to soap, placebo, or no bathing, routine preoperative whole-body bathing with CHG was not effective in preventing SSIs. The authors noted that details of CHG application were omitted from most of the studies and that even though additional research is needed, the low risk and low cost of preoperative bathing may be worth the marginal benefits of reducing SSI risk.[80] The authors of a systematic review of 20 studies including RCTs, quasi-experimental studies, and nonexperimental studies, found that antiseptic showers may reduce skin colonization and may prevent SSI, but data were inconclusive about which antiseptic was most effective.[71]

Similarly, evidence from RCTs is inconclusive. In an RCT of 100 patients scheduled for hepatectomy, Hsieh et al[81] assigned patients to receive either a 3-minute preoperative wash of the surgical site with 4% CHG soap or normal saline immediately preceding surgical skin preparation. Incision site cultures were taken before the wash, after surgical skin preparation, and after closure. No difference was found in microorganism eradication between solutions after skin preparation or after surgery, leading the authors to conclude there was no clear benefit for preoperative use of CHG. In an RCT of healthy volunteers (N = 60) in the United Kingdom, Tanner et al[70] found that CHG preoperative body washes were more effective than soap for reducing microbial growth immediately and at 6 hours after application, and that CHG had superior antibacterial activity in the groin area. Veiga et al[69] examined preoperative showers with 10% povidone-iodine 2 hours before surgery (n = 57) compared with no showering instruction (n = 57). This study found that the povidone-iodine showers effectively reduced *Staphylococcus* colonization of the skin for clean plastic surgical procedures of the thorax and abdomen.

In a quasi-experimental study of patients undergoing total hip and total knee arthroplasty procedures at two different hospitals, Colling et al[72] found a significant decrease in *S aureus* and MRSA SSIs in a group that bathed with 4% CHG soap the night before and morning of surgery compared to a group that did not complete preoperative bathing. The study groups were at two different locations, but univariate and multivariate analyses determined that the only variable associated with a decrease in SSIs was preoperative bathing with CHG.

Table 6. Health Agency and Professional Society Preoperative Bathing Recommendations

Entity	Bathing Agent	Frequency
American College of Obstetricians and Gynecologists, 2018[93]	Soap (plain or antimicrobial) or an antiseptic agent	At least night before surgery
American College of Surgeons and Surgical Infection Society, 2016[11]	Chlorhexidine gluconate, if not part of decolonization protocol	No recommendation
Centers for Disease Control and Prevention, 2017[76]	Either soap or an antiseptic agent	At least night before surgery
National Association of Orthopaedic Nurses, 2013[59]	Chlorhexidine gluconate	Evening before & morning of surgery
National Institute for Health and Care Excellence, 2019[4]	Soap	Dazzy before or day of surgery
Society for Healthcare Epidemiology of America/Infectious Diseases Society of America, 2014[7]	No recommendation, more research is needed	No recommendation
World Health Organization, 2016[3]	Plain or antimicrobial soap	Before surgery

Antiseptic Cloths

There is a growing body of evidence supporting the use of 2% CHG-impregnated cloth products; however, the results of studies involving the use of 2% CHG cloths for preoperative bathing conflict. The benefits of using 2% CHG-impregnated cloths are the ease of use for the applicant, a standardized amount of antiseptic in each cloth, and no rinsing requirement. Harms include the cost for multiple packets needed, which is dependent on body surface area, and the environmental effects of disposal.

Three systematic reviews support the practice of preoperative bathing with 2% CHG cloths.[73,82,83] Cai et al[73] conducted a systematic review with meta-analysis of one RCT and five retrospective studies published between 2010 and 2016 that compared preoperative use of 2% CHG-impregnated cloths to no preoperative bathing in patients undergoing total hip and total knee arthroplasty procedures. The researchers found a significant reduction in SSI rate, revision surgery rate, and length of stay after a procedure with preoperative use of the CHG-impregnated cloth. Karki and Cheng[82] evaluated four quasi-experimental studies that used two preoperative applications of CHG cloths in patients undergoing total joint arthroplasty, other orthopedic surgical procedures, and cesarean deliveries and found an association between use of the cloths and a reduction in SSIs. In a systematic review of 51 studies published between 1950 and 2017 to evaluate risk factors and measures for preventing infection in shoulder surgical procedures, Eck et al[83] found the strongest evidence (eg, Level I) for preventing SSI among patients undergoing surgical procedures of the shoulder was the use of 2% CHG cloths for preoperative bathing prior to the procedure.

Three RCTs[74,84,85] and five quasi-experimental studies[75,86-89] support the use of 2% CHG cloths for preoperative bathing. The limitations of two of the RCTs were that the studies were conducted in healthy volunteers and may not be generalizable to select patient populations.[84,85] Additionally, five of the studies were conducted in patients undergoing orthopedic procedures and may be limited in generalizability.[74,75,87-89]

In contrast to the supportive studies, researchers in two quasi-experimental studies[90,91] found no reduction in SSI with use of 2% CHG cloths before total joint arthroplasty[82] or pediatric urological and scrotal surgical procedures.[83]

In a quasi-experimental study to simulate the effect of preoperative bathing in patients undergoing posterior cervical spine procedures, Makhni et al[92] had 16 healthy volunteers wipe the right side of the neck with a 2% CHG-impregnated cloth after an evening shower and repeat cloth use in the morning. No cloths were applied to the left side of the neck. Bacterial swabs were used to obtain cultures from each side of the neck before and after the intervention. A decrease in bacterial counts was found on both sides of the neck; however, a significant difference was found on the CHG side.

A number of health agency and professional guidelines[3,4,7,11,59,76,93] make recommendations for preoperative bathing (Table 6).

2.1.1 **Wash or bathe patients who cannot perform preoperative bathing themselves.**[3,76] *[Recommendation].*

Physical limitations (ie, standing, range of motion) can interfere with the ability to apply soap or antiseptic to body surfaces. Whole-body coverage can be facilitated by the patient sitting or receiving assistance from a family member or caregiver and using a washcloth or cloth containing soap or antiseptic.

2.2 Patients should complete preoperative bathing at least once on the night before or the day of the operative or other invasive procedures.[3,4,59,72-76,83,93-95] [Recommendation]

Preoperative patient bathing before operative or other invasive procedures may reduce microbial skin contamination. Additional research is needed to determine the interval between bathing and the procedure and the optimal number of baths or showers.

In two RCTs, Edmiston et al[94,95] found that two or three applications of 4% CHG resulted in a significantly greater concentration of CHG at five anatomic sites compared to just one application. Five other studies found a significant decrease in SSI rate when participants performed two applications of 4% CHG soap[72] or 2% CHG-impregnated cloths[73-75,83] the night before and the day of the surgical procedure.

The number of preoperative baths or showers was the subject of a systematic review of 10 RCTs. Jakobsson et al[77] concluded that there was insufficient evidence to recommend a number of baths or showers to prevent SSIs. The authors reverted to a previous recommendation of three to five showers until more evidence becomes available.

The number and timing of applications recommended by health agencies and professional societies varies.[3,4,7,11,59,76,93]

2.3 Convene an interdisciplinary team that includes perioperative RNs, physicians, and infection preventionists to develop a mechanism for evaluating and selecting products for preoperative patient bathing.[96] [Recommendation]

Involvement of an interdisciplinary team facilitates input from all departments in which the product will be used and from personnel with clinical expertise.[96]

2.4 Develop a standardized protocol[97] for preoperative bathing that includes
- dose (ie, volume or amount of the product),[94,98]
- frequency (ie, number of applications),[78,94,95] and
- duration (ie, exposure time of skin to the antiseptic).[78,95]

[Recommendation]

A standardized regimen can achieve maximal antiseptic skin concentrations.[95,97] Operationalizing the process with clear instructions can provide a thorough and focused application process. To maximize the effects of an antiseptic, such as CHG, repeating application and pausing before rinsing enables the CHG to bind to the skin and prolongs its antimicrobial activity.[94]

To determine what dose, frequency, and timing would provide maximal CHG skin concentration, Edmiston et al conducted three RCTs with healthy volunteers, two using 4% CHG soap[94,95] and one using 2% CHG-impregnated cloths.[78] Varying protocols were used in each study, and within 3 hours of final application, skin swabs were taken from five anatomic sites: the right and left antecubital fossa, right and left popliteal fossa, and abdomen. Swabs were immediately placed into sealed test tubes and a colorimetric assay[99] was used to compare the swab solution color to freshly prepared CHG solution. The unit of measure for determining optimal skin concentration was 5 µ/mL, which is 90% of the minimum inhibitory concentration (MIC90) required to inhibit or kill skin staphylococci.[94]

In the first RCT, Edmiston et al[94] evaluated the effect of sending an electronic reminder to participants and a two- or three-shower regimen. A 118 mL bottle of 4% CHG soap was provided for each shower, and participants were asked to return bottles at the end of the study. Significantly higher skin concentrations were found in the groups that received electronic reminders, which had a mean CHG skin concentration of 30 µg/mL However, no significant difference was found in CHG skin concentration between the two- and three-shower groups. There was a wide variation in CHG soap use among participant groups, with an average of less than 50 mL used during each shower. The wide variance in the amount of product used led the researchers to conclude that a standardized regimen that includes the amount of product to use could maximize the effect of the protocol.

In the second RCT,[95] participants were asked to use a full bottle (118 mL) of 4% CHG soap for each of the two- or three-shower regimens and to complete either a no pause, a 1-minute pause, or a 2-minute pause before rinsing the soap. This protocol led to a mean CHG skin concentration of 970 µg/mL, which is well above the MIC90. The mean skin concentration was significantly higher with a 1- and 2-minute pause compared to no pause, but no significant difference was found between the 1- or 2-minute pause or the two- or three-shower groups.

In a third RCT to evaluate CHG surface concentration using 2% CHG-impregnated cloths, Edmiston et al[78] placed 100 volunteers into five groups of 20 study participants each with applications varying from one to five times. Six cloths were to be used for each shower, with each cloth used twice (front then back) with a 1-minute pause before switching cloth sides. Electronic reminders were sent to some volunteers; others did not receive reminders. After just two applications, the researchers found a mean composite CHG skin concentrations of 1,300 µg/mL. All application groups that received electronic reminders had increased mean CHG skin concentrations.

In a retrospective cohort study, Persichino et al[98] replaced 15 mL CHG soap packages with 118 mL of CHG for preoperative bathing for breast surgical procedures. The larger volumes of CHG resulted in a significant reduction in mastectomy SSI rates. In a regression analysis, body mass index, use of tissue expanders, and smaller volumes of CHG were identified as independent risk factors for infection in patients undergoing mastectomies.

2.4.1 **Electronic patient reminders for preoperative bathing protocols may be used.**[94] *[Conditional Recommendation]*

Edmiston et al[94] conducted an RCT to evaluate the effect of sending an electronic reminder to participants prior to scheduled preoperative bathing. The first group (N = 40) received an email, voicemail, or text message before each designated preoperative bathing time and the second group (N = 40) received no reminders. The researchers found significantly higher concentrations of CHG on the skin of participants who received electronic reminders compared to those participants who did not receive reminders.

2.5 **Provide clear verbal and written instructions for preoperative bathing to the patient and patient care provider.**[59,94,97,99,100] *[Recommendation]*

Achieving and maintaining optimal application protocols may be challenging; therefore, ongoing education, monitoring, and feedback is essential.[97]

In a qualitative study to capture the preoperative bathing experiences of 14 patients who underwent total hip arthroplasty procedures, Qvistgaard et al[100] discovered that patients often found it difficult to reach all required body areas for bathing or to simultaneously read bathing directions and complete bathing steps because of physical limitations. Additionally, if there was a long time between receiving verbal instructions and performing the bath, the information was often forgotten. Some patients were unsure or confused about the provided bathing instructions and found the assistance of a family member, caregiver, or health care personnel to be valuable.

The importance of education, clear instructions, and feedback were illustrated in two reports of organizational experiences to improve surgical outcomes through implementation of preoperative bathing.[94,99] After implementation of a hospital-wide preoperative bathing protocol to be completed the night before and morning of surgery, Edmiston et al[94] randomly selected 100 patients scheduled for orthopedic and general surgery procedures to determine whether they had successfully completed the protocol. The researchers found that close to 30% of the patients did not complete the protocol as instructed. Reasons for not completing the protocol were that the protocol benefit was not clearly communicated, the patient felt one bath was sufficient, or the patient forgot to bathe.

To improve preoperative bathing applications, Supple et al[99] completed a point prevalence survey to assess the patients' CHG skin concentration level at five anatomic sites (ie, neck, chest, abdomen, arm, leg) after use of 2% CHG cloths, as well as to obtain feedback on the education that was provided. The initial survey found low skin concentration and that education was inadequate or lacking. This feedback was shared with nursing personnel, who in turn provided standardized instruction sheets and rationale for bathing, which led to significantly improved CHG skin concentrations.

Guidelines from NAON[59] support the nursing practice of providing the patient with instructions for preoperative bathing protocols and advise providing written instructions.

2.5.1 **Instruct the patient to follow the manufacturer's instructions for safe use when applying the skin antiseptic product.** *[Recommendation]*

2.5.2 **After the preoperative bath or shower, instruct the patient not to apply**
- **alcohol-based hair or skin products,**
- **deodorant (when the axilla will be in the sterile field),**
- **lotions,**
- **emollients, or**
- **cosmetics.**

[Recommendation]

Surface agents can interfere with the effect of the antiseptic.[95]

The collective evidence does not support or refute this recommendation. Alcohol-based products in the hair or on the skin at the surgical site may pose a fire hazard when an ignition source is used near the site if the product is not dry. Lotions, emollients, cosmetics, and deodorants used at the surgical site may reduce the effectiveness of preoperative patient skin antiseptics or reduce the ability of patient monitors, adhesive surgical drapes, and adhesive dressings to adhere to the patient's skin.

2.5.3 **For patients undergoing procedures of the hand or foot, instruct the patient that the nails on the operative extremity should be clean and natural, without artificial nail surfaces (eg, extensions, overlays, acrylic, silk wraps, enhancements).**[101-103] *[Recommendation]*

Artificial nails or nail polish at the surgical site may harbor microorganisms, which could contaminate the surgical site or reduce the effectiveness of preoperative patient skin antisepsis.

The evidence review for this guideline found no cases of patient incision-site contamination related to the wearing of artificial nails or nail polish on the operative hand or foot. This is an unresolved issue that warrants additional research. However, in an RCT to evaluate nail varnish after completion of a surgical skin preparation, Kulkarni et al[104] randomly assigned adult patients undergoing dialysis (N = 43) to apply clear nail varnish to their dominant or nondominant hand 7 days before immersion of both hands in 10% povidone-iodine for 2 minutes. No significant difference was found in microbial count from fingers of varnished or unvarnished nails, leading the researchers to extrapolate that nail varnish would not be associated with increased risk for SSI.

The authors of a Cochrane review evaluated the effect of health care personnel's wearing of nail polish on surgical hand antisepsis and found insufficient evidence to determine whether the fresh or chipped nail polish of health care personnel increased the risk of the patient developing an SSI.[101] In a quasi-experimental study, McNeil et al[102] showed that the variety and amount of potentially pathogenic bacteria cultured from the fingertips of health care personnel wearing artificial nails was greater than for those with natural nails, both before and after surgical hand antisepsis. Although these studies showed nail contamination in health care personnel, these data may be extrapolated to the patient.

Removal of artificial nails or extenders that are near the surgical site may reduce contaminants on and under the nail. Refer to the AORN Guideline for Hand Hygiene[103] for additional guidance.

2.5.4 **Instruct patients undergoing procedures of the head or neck to shampoo their hair before surgery.**[105] *[Recommendation]*

The results from one RCT showed that shampooing with either 4% CHG or 7.5% povidone-iodine was effective in reducing resident flora on the scalp. No studies have compared shampoos with other types of antiseptics. The optimal preoperative shampoo product is an unresolved issue that warrants additional research.

Leclair et al[105] conducted an RCT of preoperative shampooing with a skin antiseptic by comparing scalp cultures, wound cultures, and SSI rates for 151 patients in four groups:

- preoperative shampoo and preoperative skin antisepsis with 4% CHG (n = 38),
- no preoperative shampoo and preoperative skin antisepsis with 4% CHG (n = 35),
- preoperative shampoo and preoperative skin antisepsis with 7.5% povidone-iodine (n = 37), and
- no preoperative shampoo and preoperative skin antisepsis with 7.5% povidone-iodine (n = 41).

Patients randomly assigned to a shampoo group were instructed to perform two preoperative shampoos with the assigned product at least 1 hour apart during the 2- to 24-hour period before surgery. All study patients had their hair clipped, scalp wetted with the assigned antiseptic, hair shaved with a razor, scalp scrubbed with the assigned antiseptic for a minimum of 5 minutes and blotted dry with a sterile towel, and an adherent plastic drape applied over the incision site. The researchers found that preoperative shampooing suppressed the emergence of resident flora on the scalp during neurosurgery and that CHG appeared to be superior to iodophors because of its residual antimicrobial activity.

Prescribing 4% CHG shampoo is a medical decision because it constitutes off-label use. This practice contradicts the 4% CHG manufacturer's instructions for use (IFU), which state that the product should not be used on the head. The benefits of using a 4% CHG shampoo may not outweigh the potential harms of CHG causing injury by contact with the eyes, ears, or mouth.

2.5.5 **For patients undergoing shoulder procedures, topical benzoyl peroxide (BPO) gel (eg, 5% with or without clindamycin) may be used as a skin decolonization agent in the days before surgery.**[106-109] *[Conditional Recommendation]*

Cutibacterium acnes, formerly called *Propionibacterium acnes*, resides in the sebaceous glands and hair bulbs of the dermis and is the main cause of SSIs in shoulder surgical procedures.[108,110,111] Benzol peroxide, a topical therapy for acnes vulgaris, has been used for many decades because of its ability to reduce C acnes.[108]

High-quality studies found that 5% BPO gel[107,108] or 5% BPO with 1.2% clindamycin gel[109] applied to a patient's shoulder 48 hours before shoulder surgery reduced *C acnes* colonization.

The number and location of BPO applications varied between studies. Sabetta et al[108] had participants apply gel five times to the shoulder and axilla. Kolakowski et al[107] had participants apply gel three times to the shoulder and axilla. Two studies followed the patients postoperatively. One study followed patients for 6 months,[107] and one followed patients for 2 months[108]; neither study found wound healing complication, infection, or unexplained pain during the follow-up time period.

Scheer et al[106] conducted a laboratory-based study to compare BPO with CHG showers for their ability to reduce *C acnes* at the site of application. Forty volunteers were randomized to two groups, 5% BPO or 4% CHG applied to the left shoulder. The treatment period was 3 days for both groups. In the BPO group, the 5% BPO gel was applied to a 5-cm strip of skin twice on the first day, twice the second day, and once prior to culturing on the third day. The CHG group had three showers over 2 days (two showers 2 hours apart on the first day and one shower on the day of culturing). On the trial day, the researchers performed surgical site preparation of the shoulder for 2 minutes with a 0.5% chlorhexidine solution in 70% ethanol prior to culturing. They found that BPO significantly reduced the presence of *C acnes* (ie, one of 20 in the BPO group versus seven of 20 in the CHG group). The researchers concluded that topical preparation with 5% BPO gel before shoulder surgery may be effective in reducing *C acnes* on the skin.

Hancock et al[112] found no decrease in presence of *C acnes* on the shoulder when BPO was applied immediately before surgical site skin preparation. This led the authors to conclude that multiple applications may be necessary to penetrate glands before surgical skin preparation, to see an effect.

Dizay et al[109] states that although all patients may benefit from BPO applied preoperatively, those at higher risk for infection with *C acnes* include patients with an existing shoulder prosthesis, patients undergoing shoulder revision surgery, and patients with a greater density of hair follicles and sebum.

Limitations of the evidence are that these studies were conducted using different procedure types (eg, joint arthroscopy, open shoulder procedures, total shoulder revision arthroplasty), patient populations, and methods of skin culture. A potential benefit of preoperative BPO application is reduction in *C acnes* burden at the surgical site. Potential harms include the cost and possible skin reactions to BPO.

3. Surgical Site Hair

3.1 **Leave hair at the surgical site in place unless hair removal is indicated.**[3-5,7,11,59,76,93,113-118] *[Recommendation]*

Moderate-quality evidence supports that hair at the surgical site should be left in place. The limitations of the evidence include that some studies had an inadequate sample size (ie, were underpowered) to determine the effect of hair removal on the development of SSI, the studies did not use a standardized definition of SSI, and the majority of the studies included in the systematic reviews were approximately 20 years old.

The benefits of leaving hair in place at the surgical site include preventing potential skin trauma from hair removal, potentially reducing the risk for SSI, and greater patient satisfaction.[113,118] The harms of leaving the hair in place at the surgical site include risk of fire when flammable skin antiseptics are used.[119]

Removing hair at the surgical site has long been believed to be associated with an increased rate of SSI. In a landmark nonexperimental study of 23,649 surgical wounds of all classifications (ie, clean, clean-contaminated, contaminated, and dirty), Cruse and Foord[114] found a 2.3% infection rate for surgical sites shaved with a razor, 1.7% for sites that were clipped, and 0.9% when no hair removal was performed. The researchers concluded that shaving should be kept to a minimum but did not suggest that hair should be left in place. Since this landmark study, a number of additional studies[5,113,115-118,120] have demonstrated that hair removal does not result in lower rates of SSI or bacterial burden.

In a systematic review of 19 RCTs published between 1971 and 2013 that evaluated the effect of hair removal on SSI reduction in different surgical specialties, Lefebvre et al[5] concluded that shaving resulted in significantly more SSIs than no hair removal, clipping, or chemical depilation. The researchers concluded that available data indicate hair removal should not be routine preoperative practice.

In systematic review of 21 studies, including RCTs, quasi-experimental studies, and nonexperimental studies, Broekman et al[115] did not find any evidence that shaving decreased the incidence of SSIs in neurosurgery procedures (ie, craniotomies, cerebral spinal fluid diversion, burr hole procedures, spinal procedures), with a possibility that, conversely, shaving increased infections in neurosurgical patients. The authors recommended additional research in this area.[115] The author of another systematic review evaluated 18 studies and found that scalp shaving in cranial surgeries did not result in fewer infections, leading the author to conclude that cranial surgeries should be performed without shaving.[116]

Marecek et al[117] conducted an RCT with 85 male volunteers to determine the effect of clipping axillary hair on *C acnes* bacterial load at the shoulder surgical site before and after surgical skin preparation. The researchers found a significantly higher *C acnes* burden in the clipped hair group compared to unclipped hair group before surgical site preparation and no difference in *C acnes* reduction between clipped and unclipped hair groups after surgical site preparation.

However, in a prospective RCT involving 1,543 patients undergoing general surgical procedures at a large teaching hospital to compare surgical site clipping (n = 768) to no clipping (n = 775), the researchers found that SSI rates were similar in both groups.[120] Of note, povidone-iodine was the only skin antiseptic used in the study, and participants included only patients undergoing general surgical procedures. The researchers concluded that generalization to procedures other than general surgical procedures cannot be assumed.

In a systematic review of 11 RCTs and three controlled clinical trials published between 1990 and 2016 that included 7,278 patients undergoing a variety of surgical procedures, Shi et al[118] found no significant difference in SSI rates between shaving, clipping, no hair removal, or use of depilatory cream. The authors concluded that shaving hair preoperatively most likely has no benefit for reducing SSIs, but more studies are needed to complete a robust meta-analysis.

Tanner et al[113] examined conflicting evidence in a Cochrane systematic review of 14 studies published between 1980 and 2011, including RCTs and quasi-RCTs, of a variety of procedure types. The authors concluded that the evidence sample sizes were too small and the studies were methodologically flawed, which prevented them from drawing strong conclusions that routine hair removal at the surgical site reduces the incidence of SSI.

Several health agencies and professional societies support the practice of leaving hair at the surgical site, unless the hair will interfere with the procedure (Table 7).[3,4,7,11,59,76,93]

3.1.1   **Instruct the patient to leave hair in place at the surgical site before operative or other invasive procedures.**[121] *[Recommendation]*

One nonexperimental study investigated patient compliance with not removing hair at the surgical site for planned cesarean deliveries. Ng et al[121] used an educational intervention campaign targeted toward prenatal patients to discourage pre-hospital hair removal after 36 weeks gestation. The researchers concluded that the patient education improved patient compliance with nonremoval of hair at the surgical site from 41% to 27% in a 3-year period. Although the researchers noted that other evidence-based practices for reduction of SSI rates, including switching to an alcohol-based skin antiseptic, were implemented during the time of this investigation, they also saw a reduction in SSIs for cesarean procedures and considered this educational campaign to be an important part of their multimodal approach to reducing SSI rates. Additional research is needed to determine whether hair removal by the patient has an effect on risk for SSI.[121]

3.2   **Hair at the surgical site may be removed when indicated based on individualized patient assessment. Hair removal may be indicated when the presence of hair**
- **interferes with vision in the surgical field,**
- **interferes with wound closure,**
- **causes the drape or dressing to not adhere, and**
- **creates a fire risk with use of alcohol-based skin antiseptics.**[113,119,122,123]

[Conditional Recommendation]

An individualized patient assessment is necessary to evaluate the proposed surgical incision, the presence of hair, and the amount of hair near the surgical site. Hair wet with alcohol-based skin antiseptics is flammable and can take up to an hour to dry thoroughly.[122,123]

3.2.1   **When hair removal is indicated, the amount of hair removed should be kept to a minimum. *[Recommendation]***

Two high-quality studies found that if hair removal is necessary, the amount of hair removal can be minimized.[124,125] In an RCT to evaluate different types of clipping with SSI rates in patients undergoing cranial procedures, Kose et al[124] clipped hair using a 2-cm-wide strip along the incision line (n = 50) or a 5-cm-wide strip along the incision line. (n = 50) The researchers found there was no difference in SSI rate between the groups; however, patients who received the wider clipped area reported a diminished self-image.

The authors of a Cochrane review of three RCTs published between 1992 and 2005 that included 1,039 women giving birth vaginally, compared perineal shaving to only clipping long pubic or perineal hair before skin preparation. The review authors found no difference in postpartum febrile incidences, wound infections, or

Table 7. Health Agency and Professional Society Hair Removal Recommendations	
Entity	**Recommendation**
American College of Obstetricians and Gynecologists, 2018[93]	Avoid, unless interferes with surgery; use clippers if necessary, immediately before surgical procedure
American College of Surgeons and Surgical Infection Society, 2016[11]	Avoid, unless interferes with surgery; use clippers if necessary
Centers for Disease Control and Prevention, 2017[76]	Avoid, unless interferes with surgery; use clippers if necessary, immediately before surgical procedure
National Association of Orthopaedic Nurses, 2013[59]	Use clippers if necessary, immediately before surgical procedure
National Institute for Health and Care Excellence, 2019[4]	Do not routinely remove; use clippers with a single-use head if necessary, on day of surgery
Society for Healthcare Epidemiology of America/Infectious Diseases Society of America, 2014[7]	Avoid, unless interferes with surgery; use clippers or depilatory agent if necessary, performed outside the OR
World Health Organization, 2016[3]	Avoid, use clippers if necessary

maternal satisfaction between the groups. The authors concluded that more evidence is needed before a recommendation can be made for routine perineal hair removal on admission for women in labor.[125]

3.2.2 **If indicated, remove hair at the surgical site by clipping or depilatory methods in a manner that minimizes injury to the skin.**[3-5,7,11,59,76,93,113,118,126,127] *[Recommendation]*

When hair removal is necessary, hair removal by clippers may be associated with lower risk of SSI than hair removal by razors.[113] Lefebvre et al[5] found that when compared to shaving, clipping and chemical depilation were associated with a lower risk of SSIs. The researchers also compared clipping directly with chemical depilation and found no difference in SSI rates between the methods but concluded that more RCTs are needed to confirm method equivalence. In systematic review, Shi et al[118] concluded that clipping is more effective in reducing SSIs than shaving or using depilatory cream.

Studies involving hair removal in the male genital area are limited and may conflict with recommendations to clip hair rather than shave hair with a razor, although additional research is needed. In an RCT of 217 procedures involving male genitalia, Grober et al[126] compared hair removal on the scrotum with clippers (n = 107) and razors (n = 108), with outcomes of quality of hair removal, skin trauma, and SSI events. The researchers concluded that hair removal by a razor on the scrotum prevented skin trauma and achieved better quality hair removal than clippers, with no apparent increase in infection rate. The study did not describe whether wet or dry methods were used for either clipping or shaving

and was limited by not being statistically powered to determine the effect on SSI. In a position statement by the Sexual Medicine Society of North America,[127] the authors state that because of the delicate, irregular, and elastic skin of male genitalia, surgeons should have a choice of using a razor or clipper for hair removal.

There is consensus among professional associations to recommend hair removal with clipping rather than shaving with a razor.[3,4,7,11,59,76,93]

3.2.3 **When hair removal is indicated, remove hair as close to the start of surgery as feasible in a location outside the OR or procedure room.**[4,5,7,59,76,113] *[Recommendation]*

A benefit of removing hair close to the time of surgery is that if a break in skin integrity occurs, the time is lessened for bacterial invasion before skin antisepsis occurs. The potential harms include additional time needed for preoperative preparation and that the patient's dignity may be compromised if privacy is not possible.

In a systematic review with meta-analysis, Lefebvre et al[5] found that regardless of the removal method employed, the risk of SSI was higher when hair removal occurred the day before surgery compared to the day of surgery. Conversely, a Cochrane systematic review by Tanner et al[113] found no significant difference in SSI rates between shaving or clipping the day before surgery or the day of surgery. However, the authors stated that the study populations were too small, and more research is needed to support this conclusion.

Regarding the timing of hair removal, both the SHEA and CDC recommend that, if indicated, hair should be removed immediately before the surgical procedure.[7,76] The NAON guidelines[59] recommend removing hair as close to the incision time as possible and the NICE[4] guidelines do not specify a timeframe but instead recommend that removal occurs on the day of surgery.

When hair is removed it can be dispersed and carried by air currents onto sterile supplies. The SHEA and IDSA recommend that, if hair clipping is necessary, it should be performed outside the procedural area.[7]

3.2.4 **When removing hair outside the OR or procedure room is not possible, remove the patient's hair in a manner that prevents dispersal of hair into the air of the OR or procedure room (eg, wet clipping, use of a vacuum device).[128,129]** *[Recommendation]*

Wetting the skin surface before clipping diminishes the amount of hair that is dispersed into the environment.

Edmiston et al[128] conducted an RCT in a simulated OR to evaluate the amount of loose hair particles and microbiological contamination at the surgical site with use of a clipper compared to a clipper with a vacuum device for hair removal. Eighteen male volunteers consented to the bilateral clipping of chest and groin hair using both methods. Before and during clipping, petri dishes were placed under the participant's chest and groin, and an airborne particle counter was hung on an IV pole placed near the clipping site. The researchers found a significantly lower amount of residual hair and microbiological contamination with use of the clipper and vacuum device. Additionally, the time to clip and clean up residual hair was significantly less with use of the clipper with vacuum device.

If using an adhesive method to remove excess hair, it is important to assess the method's adhesiveness and the condition of the patient skin (eg, loss of turgor, thinness, open wounds), as there is potential for skin injury.[128] Rolls of adhesive used for collecting hair on more than one patient can be a source of cross contamination. In a nonexperimental study, Harris et al[129] cultured 21 batches of three partially used tape rolls from three different hospitals and found multidrug-resistant organisms (MDROs), including MRSA, MSSA, and vancomycin-resistant enterococci on 11 of the batches. Visible contamination was also seen on the sides of tape rolls, leading the authors to conclude that single, sealed packets of adhesive should be used for individual patients and discarded after use.

3.2.5 **Use single-use clipper heads and dispose of them after each patient use.** *[Recommendation]*

Guidelines from NICE recommend using single-use clipper heads to reduce the risk of cross contamination of bloodborne pathogens between patients.[4] Three case reports epidemiologically linked the use of the same shaving razor on multiple patients to outbreaks of *Serratia marcescens*[130,131] and carbapenemase-producing *Klebsiella pneumoniae*[132] postoperative infections in patients undergoing neurological surgical procedures. In all three facilities, when the use of disposable razors[130,132] or disposable clippers[131] was implemented, no additional infections were reported.

3.2.6 **Disinfect the reusable clipper handle after each use, in accordance with the manufacturer's IFU.[4]** *[Recommendation]*

3.2.7 **When using depilatories for hair removal, follow the manufacturer's IFU, including testing skin for skin allergy and irritation reactions in an area away from the surgical site at least 24 hours before the surgical procedure.[5,113]** *[Recommendation]*

In two systematic reviews, the authors discussed that depilatories may cause skin irritation and allergic reactions and recommended patch testing at least 24 hours before the cream is applied.[5,113]

3.2.8 **Document in the patient's health care record the person performing hair removal, the hair removal method, time of removal, and area of hair removal.** *[Recommendation]*

4. Selection of the Surgical Site Antiseptic

4.1 **Convene an interdisciplinary team that includes one or more perioperative RNs, physicians, and infection preventionists to evaluate and select antiseptic products for surgical site preparation.[96]** *[Recommendation]*

Decisions about which preoperative skin antiseptic to use in the practice setting are complex. A variety of products may be necessary to meet the needs of various patient populations. Input from an interdisciplinary team with diverse experience and knowledge of skin antiseptics is helpful during review of the current research, clinical guidelines, and information provided by the manufacturers of surgical antiseptic agents.

Involvement of an interdisciplinary team also facilitates input from all departments in which the product will be used and from personnel with clinical expertise.[96]

In a 2015 Cochrane systematic review to evaluate skin antiseptics in clean surgical procedures, Dumville et al[1] found limited descriptions of interventions and inadequate sample sizes (ie, underpowered studies), making it difficult to interpret and have confidence in the study results. Therefore, until more robust studies can be conducted, the authors recommended that cost and potential adverse effects be considered when choosing among antiseptics.

4.1.1 **Identify the surgical site antisepsis plan (ie, select the antiseptic agent) prior to taking the patient to the operating room.** *[Recommendation]*

Patients may have allergies or other contraindications that prevent use of common skin antiseptics. When patient assessment is completed, developing an individualized plan of care contributes to patient safety.[64]

4.2 **Select an alcohol-based skin antiseptic for surgical site preparation unless contraindicated.**[1,3,76,83,133-135] *[Recommendation]*

Alcohol is bactericidal and effective for surgical skin preparation but does not have persistent activity when used alone.[7] Combining an alcohol-based solution with another antiseptic, such as CHG or povidone-iodine, provides a rapid, persistent, and cumulative effect.[7,11]

Two quasi-experimental studies that compared the use of isopropyl alcohol to CHG-alcohol in elective laparotomy[136] (N = 500) and sternotomies[137] (N = 2,985) found that CHG-alcohol was more effective in reducing SSIs and mediastinitis than isopropyl alcohol alone.

The benefit of using an alcohol-based antiseptic outweighs the harms. Alcohol-based antiseptics are broad spectrum and act immediately to lower the microbial count on skin. A potential harm is fire risk if the solution pools, vapors are trapped (eg, beneath drapes), the solution is not allowed to dry completely before activation of an electrosurgical device, or it is applied where it cannot dry easily (eg, to hair).[7]

Researchers have compared various skin antiseptic products, including aqueous povidone-iodine, aqueous CHG, CHG-alcohol, and iodine-based alcohol. However, the antiseptic formulation (aqueous or alcoholic), concentration, and application methods vary between studies. High-quality evidence was consistent in finding alcohol-based antiseptic solutions to be overall more effective than aqueous solutions in reducing the risk of SSIs and decreasing skin flora.

In a systematic review with meta-analysis of 17 RCTs, the authors of the *WHO Global Guidelines for the Prevention of Surgical Site Infection* found better clinical outcomes and antimicrobial effectiveness with alcohol-based antiseptics compared to aqueous solutions.[3] In a Cochrane systematic review with meta-analysis of 13 RCTs (N = 2,623) to evaluate the effect of a variety of skin antisepsis products used before clean surgeries, Dumville et al[1] found alcohol-containing products to have the highest probability of being effective in reducing SSI rates. However, the authors concluded that more quality research is needed to definitively identify one antiseptic as better than another for clean surgical procedure SSI prevention. In a systematic review to determine risk factors associated with SSIs in shoulder procedures, Eck et al[83] concluded that the only high-level evidence for SSI prevention was the use of alcohol-containing solutions to prep the skin at the time of surgery.

In a systematic review with meta-analysis of 13 RCTs and six observational studies published between 2000 and 2014, Privitera et al[138] evaluated aqueous and alcohol-containing solutions in all types of surgical procedures. The researchers found moderate-quality evidence to support the use of CHG for prevention of SSIs and high-quality evidence to support use of CHG for reduction of skin colonization compared to povidone-iodine. However, the authors acknowledged that more rigorous RCTs would provide stronger evidence to confirm the best antiseptic for surgical skin preparation.

Noorani et al[133] conducted a systematic review with meta-analysis of six studies (N = 5,031), in which all but two evaluated alcohol-based solutions, to determine the rate of postoperative SSIs in clean-contaminated procedures with various surgical skin preparation products. A significant difference in SSI rate was found with CHG (5.7%) compared to povidone-iodine (7.9%). Conversely, in a prospective cohort analysis of 47 hospitals, Hakkarainen et al[139] compared antiseptics with and without alcohol in clean-contaminated surgical procedures (N = 7,669) and found that one antiseptic was not more effective than another in reducing SSIs and a greater risk reduction did not occur with isopropyl alcohol-containing solutions.

A limitation of the literature review was a lack of studies comparing one alcohol-based antiseptic directly to another. Instead, most studies compared an alcohol-based antiseptic to an aqueous solution. However, in a systematic review and meta-analysis, Maiwald and Chan[140] concluded that the role of alcohol has been overlooked in the literature and that studies showing a perceived efficacy of CHG actually demonstrate the effectiveness of CHG-alcohol.

CHG in Alcohol-Based Solution versus Povidone-Iodine in Aqueous Solution

Three high-quality studies support the use of CHG-alcohol over aqueous povidone-iodine. The review authors of the CDC guideline for prevention of SSI conducted a separate systematic review with meta-analysis of five RCTs (N = 1,976) and concluded that CHG-alcohol was associated with a reduced risk of SSI compared to aqueous iodophor.[76] In a systematic review with meta-analysis of six RCTs (N = 2,080) published between 2008 and 2014 to compare the use of CHG-alcohol or aqueous povidone-iodine in clean, clean-contaminated, and contaminated surgical procedures, the researchers found significantly fewer SSIs and fewer positive skin cultures with CHG-alcohol.[135] Ayoub et al[134] conducted a similar systematic review with meta-analysis of six RCTs (N = 2,484) published between 2005 and 2013 and found CHG-alcohol to be more effective than aqueous povidone-iodine in reducing SSIs in clean and clean-contaminated surgical procedures. However, they determined that additional studies were needed to evaluate which solution is most effective in contaminated surgical procedures.

Alcohol-Based or Aqueous CHG

Conflicting results were found in two studies that compared alcoholic and aqueous CHG. In an RCT with 916 patients, researchers compared surgical skin preparation with CHG-alcohol (n = 454) to aqueous CHG (n = 462) and found no significant difference in SSI prevention or adverse events between the two groups.[141] A limitation of this study was that all procedures were performed in general practice offices as opposed to surgical suites. In a case-control study at a single facility to evaluate SSI risk factors in patients undergoing breast, colon, herniorrhaphy, open reduction internal fixation, total joint, spinal fusion, and prostate surgical procedures during a 9-month period, the researchers found that CHG with alcohol was associated with fewer SSIs than CHG used alone.[142]

Alcohol-Based or Aqueous Povidone-Iodine

Two independent systematic reviews with meta-analysis found low-quality evidence indicating that there was no significant difference between iodine-based alcohol solutions and povidone-iodine aqueous solutions.[3] Similarly, researchers in a historical-controlled interventional trial of 1,326 patient undergoing cardiac implantable electronic device (CIED) surgical procedures used aqueous povidone-iodine for one group and iodine-based alcohol solution for the other group. The authors found no difference in CIED infection rates with the use of either solution.[143]

Seven health agencies and professional organizations[3,4,7,11,59,76,93] recommend the use of alcohol-based antiseptics for surgical skin preparation (Table 8).

4.2.1 | **Select an alcohol-based antiseptic based on the patient assessment, and the surgical anatomic site.** [*Recommendation*]

Antiseptic skin preparation may be contraindicated for some patients.[76] Selecting a preoperative skin antiseptic based on an individual patient assessment may reduce the risk for patient complications. The authors of one literature review discussed various preoperative skin antiseptics and concluded that perioperative RNs should evaluate and select the optimal antiseptic for each patient.[144] Optimal skin antiseptics are effective in decreasing the microbial load on the skin, are safe to apply, prevent injury to the patient, have immediate and persistent action, and decrease the risk for SSI. The authors of another literature review concluded that the patient assessment was critical to selection of the most effective preoperative skin antiseptic.[145]

High-quality studies have compared alcohol combined with CHG to iodine-based antiseptics in a number of different surgical site preparation areas, but the study conclusions vary widely. Three high-quality studies favored CHG in combination with alcohol over iodine-based antiseptics for reducing SSIs in colorectal[146] and cardiac[147] surgical procedures and in reducing bacteria in foot and ankle surgeries.[148] Three high-quality studies supported use of iodine-based antiseptics in combination with alcohol over CHG for reducing SSIs in total joint[149] and general surgical procedures[150] and reducing organ/space SSIs in cardiac surgical procedures.[151]

However, five high-quality studies found similar overall SSI rates with either iodine-based or CHG-alcohol solutions in cardiac,[151] breast, colon, and vascular surgical procedures,[152] and cesarean deliveries.[153] Similar wound complications were found with either combination in foot,[154] total hip, and total knee surgical procedures.[149] Similar skin flora reduction was found for spinal surgical procedures.[155]

The recommendations from professional societies indicate evidence is lacking regarding the optimal antiseptic to combine with alcohol. The WHO states that although low-quality, the evidence shows a significant SSI reduction with use of an alcohol-based solution containing CHG.[3] The NICE guideline for surgical site infections states that an alcohol-based solution of CHG should be the first choice of antiseptic preparation.[4] Both the SHEA and CDC recommend the use of an alcohol-containing antiseptic but state that the most effective agent for combination is not clear.[7,76]

Table 8: Health Agency and Professional Society Skin Preparation Recommendations

Entity	Skin Preparation with Antiseptic
American College of Obstetricians and Gynecologists, 2018[93]	Alcohol-containing agents, unless contraindicated* Vaginally with 4% CHG or povidone-iodine before hysterectomy or vaginal surgery
American College of Surgeons and Surgical Infection Society, 2016[11]	Alcohol-containing agents, unless contraindicated* If no alcohol, chlorhexidine gluconate (CHG)
Centers for Disease Control and Prevention, 2017[76]	Alcohol-containing agents, unless contraindicated*
National Association of Orthopaedic Nurses, 2013[59]	Povidone-iodine, iodine-based alcohol, or CHG
National Institute for Health and Care Excellence, 2019[4]	Alcohol-based solution of CHG, unless contraindicated* or at a site next to a mucous membrane If next to a mucous membrane, use an aqueous solution of CHG
Society for Healthcare Epidemiology of America/ Infectious Diseases Society of America, 2014[7]	Alcohol-containing agents, unless contraindicated* The most effective antiseptic to combine with alcohol is unclear
World Health Organization, 2016[3]	Alcohol-based antiseptic solutions based on CHG

Contraindications for alcohol-based skin antiseptics include surfaces involving mucosa, cornea, ear, or large amounts of hair; use for preterm infants; and sensitivity or allergy to the drug or any ingredients.

4.3 **Select the antiseptic product based on the anatomical location of the surgical procedure.**[156,157]

[Recommendation]

Skin microbiota is dependent on the body site location (ie, moist, dry, sebaceous), with each site harboring a specific array of bacteria.[156] Consequently, each body part may have different responses to the same skin antiseptic.[157] Several high-quality studies evaluated the efficacy of antiseptic products based on procedure type; however, the evidence involving the various procedure-specific preoperative skin antisepsis selection yielded conflicting results, and this topic warrants additional research.

Abdominal Procedures

Several high-quality studies evaluated surgical site skin preparation of the abdomen in gynecological, general, and obstetric surgical procedures.

Two systematic reviews with meta-analysis evaluated abdominal surgical site preparation in patients undergoing cesarean delivery. In a review of four RCTs (N = 3,059) published between 2015 and 2017, that compared CHG-alcohol to povidone-iodine solutions with and without alcohol, Tolcher et al[158] found a significant reduction in SSI rates with CHG-alcohol. In a Cochrane review of 11 RCTs (N = 6,237) published between 1988 and 2017 that compared CHG-based to iodine-based antiseptics, Hadiati et al[159] found a slight reduction in SSI rates with CHG compared to povidone-iodine and little or no difference in the incidence of endometriosis or adverse skin reactions between antiseptic types.

In an RCT involving 661 patients undergoing gynecologic laparoscopic procedures using aqueous povidone-iodine (n = 221), iodine-based alcohol (n = 220), or CHG-alcohol (n = 220) for abdominal skin preparation, the researchers found no difference in SSI reduction between groups.[160]

In a prospective observational study, researchers found comparable SSI rates, skin irritation, and readmissions with either CHG-alcohol (n = 712) or aqueous povidone-iodine (n = 712) used for cesarean delivery surgical skin antisepsis.[161] Conversely, in a retrospective cohort study to evaluate abdominal surgical site preparation in patients undergoing abdominal hysterectomies with CHG-alcohol (n = 3,005) or aqueous povidone-iodine (n = 1,254), Uppal et al[162] found CHG-alcohol was associated with overall lower probability (44%) for SSI development.

In an RCT that involved 534 patients undergoing upper gastrointestinal or hepatobiliary-pancreatic surgical procedures with either aqueous CHG (n = 267) or aqueous povidone-iodine (n = 267) for abdominal surgical site preparation, Park et al[163] found no difference in the overall rate of SSIs between groups. Srinivas et al[164] conducted an RCT with 342 patients undergoing upper abdominal surgery and found SSI incidence was lower with CHG-alcohol (n = 158) than aqueous povidone-iodine (n = 184).

Researchers who conducted an RCT with 788 patients undergoing colorectal surgical procedures found a lower overall SSI rate with CHG-alcohol (n = 392) compared to iodine povacrylex-alcohol (n = 396) (15.9% to 18.7%).[146] Conversely, researchers in a multi-center retrospective study that compared CHG-alcohol (n = 425) to iodine povacrylex-alcohol (n = 115), and alcohol-based (n = 610) to non-alcohol-based antiseptics (n = 177) for abdominal preparation of patients undergoing colorectal procedures found no significant difference in SSI incidence or readmissions between groups.[165]

In a single-center quasi-experimental study, researchers compared three surgical skin antiseptics in three groups: aqueous povidone-iodine and isopropyl alcohol (n = 987), CHG-alcohol (n = 994), and iodine povacrylex-alcohol (n = 1,228). Study participants included patients undergoing general surgical procedures. Patients who received surgical site preparation with iodine povacrylex-alcohol had the lowest SSI rate (3.9 per 100 procedures) compared with patients who received aqueous povidone-iodine and alcohol (6.4 per 100 procedures) and CHG-alcohol (7.1 per 100 procedures).[150]

Because surgical site preparation of the abdomen includes the umbilicus, two studies evaluated the effect of skin antiseptic on umbilical microflora. In a quasi-experimental study of 93 patients undergoing elective abdominal surgery, aqueous povidone-iodine was applied to the abdomen for surgical site preparation. When the umbilical region was cultured, 25% of the patients still had umbilical microflora.[166] However, of seven patients who developed an SSI, only one had an SSI with the same causative agent as umbilical microflora.[166] In a nonexperimental study, patients undergoing laparoscopic cholecystectomy procedures (N = 162) who were cleansed with a CHG cloth and had a povidone-iodine-soaked cotton ball applied to the umbilicus preoperatively in addition to surgical skin preparation with aqueous povidone-iodine followed by CHG-alcohol had a significant reduction in port-site infections compared to patients who underwent standard surgical site preparation.[167]

Cardiothoracic Procedures

Eight moderate-quality studies evaluated surgical site preparation in cardiothoracic surgical procedures: three quasi-experimental studies of open heart surgical procedures,[147,151,168] two quasi-experimental and one nonexperimental study of CIED procedures,[143,169,170] and one RCT and one nonexperimental study of lower extremity preparation in vascular procedures.[171,172]

In a quasi-experimental study that compared aqueous povidone-iodine (n = 35) to CHG-alcohol (n = 35) in open heart procedures, the researchers found that preparation with aqueous povidone-iodine resulted in greater incidence of SSIs and skin organisms.[168] In a quasi-experimental study, Raja et al[151] found similar SSI rates with CHG-alcohol (n = 738) and iodine-based alcohol (n = 738). However, iodine-based alcohol was marginally more effective against organ/space SSIs.[151] Hannan et al[147] conducted a similar quasi-experimental study to evalu-

ate the effect of iodine-based alcohol (n = 364) and CHG-alcohol (n = 480), but provided standardized education on surgical site preparation for the CHG-alcohol group, which had a significantly lower SSI rate.

Da Costa et al[143] conducted a prospective observational study to compare aqueous povidone-iodine (n = 648) to iodine-based alcohol (n = 678) in patients undergoing CIED procedures. The researchers found CIED infection rates were equivalent with either antiseptic. In a quasi-experimental study, Qintar et al[169] compared CHG-alcohol (n = 1,450) to aqueous povidone-iodine (n = 1,390) in CIED procedures and found no significant difference in infection rate between the groups, leading the researchers to conclude that skin antiseptic did not play a role in SSI reduction. However, in a multi-center retrospective cohort study of 2,098 CIED procedures to determine factors associated with low risk of SSI, Asundi et al[170] found surgical site preparation with CHG to be an effective prevention measure compared to other antiseptics.

In an RCT of patients undergoing saphenous vein harvest who received surgical skin preparation with 0.5% CHG-alcohol (n = 41) or 2% CHG-alcohol (n = 44), the researchers found a lower incidence of superficial SSIs and detectable microorganisms on skin prepared with 2% CHG-alcohol.[171] In a retrospective analysis of 3,033 patients undergoing open lower extremity bypass to determine predicators of SSIs, iodine-based surgical skin preparation agents were identified as a contributing factor, leading the authors to recommend use of non-iodine skin preparation agents for reducing the risk of SSI in lower extremity bypass procedures.[172]

Hand Procedures

Researchers who conducted an RCT involving 240 patients undergoing clean soft tissue hand surgeries compared skin preparation with aqueous povidone-iodine (n = 80), iodine povacrylex-alcohol (n = 81), and CHG-alcohol (n = 79) and concluded that povidone-iodine alone and iodine povacrylex-alcohol were superior to CHG-alcohol in reducing bacterial counts on the hand.[173]

Foot and Ankle Procedures

In an RCT involving 49 patients undergoing clean foot surgical procedures, researchers compared skin preparation with CHG-alcohol (n = 26) to iodine-based alcohol (n = 23) and found no significant difference in postoperative infection rates or number of positive foot cultures between the groups.[154] However, Becerro de Bengoa Vallejo et al[174] conducted an RCT with 28 volunteers to compare four different skin preparation methods using aqueous CHG, aqueous povidone-iodine, and 70%

isopropyl alcohol. All participants underwent each of the following preparation methods:

- povidone-iodine scrub and paint,
- prewash with isopropyl alcohol followed by povidone-iodine scrub and paint,
- CHG scrub followed by isopropyl alcohol paint, and
- immersion in CHG, prewash with isopropyl alcohol, followed by povidone-iodine scrub and paint.[174]

Before and after skin preparation, cotton-tipped applicators were used to obtain aerobic cultures from the hallux nailfold and the web space between the first and second toes. The researchers found the greatest reduction in bacterial load on the foot occurred when alcohol was used with aqueous povidone-iodine.[174]

Authors of a systematic review with meta-analysis of eight RCTs and quasi-RCTs of 560 patients undergoing foot and ankle surgeries concluded that alcohol antiseptic solutions performed more effectively than aqueous iodine for reducing bacterial load of the foot, and CHG-alcohol was more effective than iodine-based alcohol for reducing foot flora.[148]

Lower Limb Trauma Procedures

Ritter et al[175] conducted an RCT involving 279 patients in Germany undergoing lower limb trauma procedures to compare CHG-alcohol (2% CHG and 70% isopropyl alcohol) (n = 112) to iodine-based alcohol (1% povidone-iodine and 50% 2-propanol) (n = 167) on the incidence of SSI and wound healing disorders. The SSI rate among participants in the povidone-iodine-alcohol group was 5.4% compared to an SSI rate of 1.8% in the CHG-alcohol group. Study participants in the povidone-iodine-alcohol group also experienced more wound healing disorders (7.2%) than those in the CHG-alcohol group (2.7%).

Hip and Knee Procedures

In a single-center RCT involving 780 patients undergoing hip or knee arthroplasties, researchers compared the use of CHG-alcohol skin antiseptics with povidone-iodine-alcohol skin antiseptics for effects on overall SSI rates. The researchers found that the povidone-iodine-alcohol group had a lower rate of overall SSIs (1.0%) compared to the CHG-alcohol group (3.1%); however, no difference was found in wound healing disorders between the two groups.[149]

Shoulder Procedures

Saltzman et al[110] conducted an RCT of 150 patients undergoing surgical procedures of the shoulder by comparing reduction of bacteria at the surgical site after surgical site preparation with three skin antiseptics: CHG-alcohol, iodine povacrylex-alcohol, and aqueous povidone-iodine. The researchers concluded that CHG-alcohol was the most effective for reducing overall bacteria in the shoulder area and povidone-iodine was the least effective for removing coagulase-negative *Staphylococcus* from the shoulder.

Heckman et al[176] conducted a quasi-experimental study with 12 volunteers to evaluate the effect of shoulder surgical skin preparation on eliminating *C acnes* presence in the dermal skin layer using three different protocols: aqueous CHG paint, aqueous CHG with mechanical scrub, and high-concentration CHG with mechanical scrub. The participants' shoulders were divided into three equal sections and each area was prepped using a different protocol. Punch biopsies of dermis were taken after skin preparation, and *C acnes* presence was found with all three protocols, with no significant differences between them. Lee et al[111] found similar results in a quasi-experimental study. The researchers obtained dermal biopsies from 10 male volunteers after surgical site preparation with CHG-alcohol and found *C acnes* presence in seven of the volunteers, yielding a 70% persistence rate.

However, Blonna et al[177] conducted a quasi-experimental study to compare a double surgical skin prep with aqueous CHG followed by iodine-based alcohol to a single surgical skin prep with iodine-based alcohol in 40 patients undergoing surgery for a displaced proximal humeral fracture. Each technique was applied to one-half of the patient's shoulder. The researchers found that both techniques significantly reduced *S aureus* and *C acnes* skin colonization.

Spine Procedures

In an RCT of 100 lumbar spine procedures, Savage et al[155] compared preoperative skin antisepsis with CHG-alcohol (n = 50) and iodine-based alcohol (n = 50). The researchers found that the antiseptics were equally effective in removing bacterial pathogens at the surgical site. They acknowledged that the skin flora of the lumbar spine differs from other locations of the body and that uniform application of an antiseptic may be easier than for other parts of the body (eg, foot, shoulder), which may allow antiseptics to be more effective on the spine.

In a prospective comparative study, Yoshii et al[178] found that CHG-alcohol (n = 98) and aqueous povidone-iodine (n = 92) were equally effective in eliminating the bacterial load at the surgical site in posterior spine surgeries. However, CHG-alcohol was found to have a longer lasting effect on bacterial reduction postoperatively. In a multi-center prospective study with more than 6,959 spinal surgery patients, Ghobrial et al[179] found that neither CHG-alcohol nor aqueous povidone-iodine produced a significant reduction in SSI rates. Of note, isopropyl alcohol was applied before each surgical skin preparation.

Chlorhexidine gluconate is contraindicated for use on meninges or neural tissue[180]; however, none of the studies reviewed evaluated neurotoxicity as an outcome measure. In a retrospective study of 11,095 patients who received 12,465 spinal anesthetics during a 4-year period to evaluate any new or progressive neurological effects with use of CHG-alcohol as surgical site preparation, Sviggum et al[181] found the rate to be less than 0.04%. The researchers concluded there was no added neurological risk with CHG-alcohol before spinal anesthesia. There are no published reports of neurotoxicity in humans. Ghobrial et al[179] purported that the risk of using CHG in spinal surgery may be limited to open spinal wounds, for which there are currently no human participant studies.

Gynecological Procedures

In an RCT, Eason et al[182] compared preoperative vaginal antisepsis with a povidone-iodine gel (n = 780) to no gel (n = 790) in abdominal hysterectomy procedures. The researchers found that the povidone-iodine gel group had a lower risk of developing abscesses, but there was no significant difference in infection rates.

Although it is considered off-label use,[180] researchers have evaluated CHG for vaginal surgical site preparation in gynecological procedures, which has yielded mixed outcomes. In a small single-center RCT of 123 hysteroscopy procedures, Rastogi et al[183] compared preoperative vaginal antisepsis with povidone-iodine (n = 63) to 4% CHG with 4% isopropyl alcohol (n = 60) and found that skin preparation with CHG-alcohol resulted in significantly more adverse vaginal and urinary symptoms in both the immediate and 24- to 48-hour postoperative period.

In an RCT of 50 patients undergoing vaginal hysterectomy procedures, Culligan et al[184] compared 4% CHG (n = 23) to povidone-iodine (n = 27) for preoperative vaginal antisepsis. The researchers found a significant decrease in vaginal flora bacterial colony counts 30 minutes after surgical skin preparation with CHG compared to povidone-iodine (22% to 63%) but no difference in incidence of SSIs or adverse symptoms.

In a quasi-experimental study of patients undergoing gynecological procedures (eg, abdominal hysterectomy, laparoscopic bilateral salpingo-oophorectomy) that included vaginal antisepsis with aqueous povidone-iodine (n = 64) or 2% CHG with a sterile water rinse after wound closure (n = 53), researchers compared overall SSI rates and patient-reported vaginal irritation. The researchers found no difference in SSI rates between the two groups. Study participants in the povidone-iodine group (3 of 64) reported more vaginal irritation than those in the CHG group (0 of 53) immediately after surgery. The researchers concluded that more RCTs are needed to determine the ideal antiseptic for SSI reduction for vaginal antisepsis in gynecological procedures.[185]

In a practice bulletin from the American College of Obstetricians and Gynecologists, the committee recommends vaginal antisepsis using povidone-iodine before hysterectomy or vaginal procedures, with off-label use of 4% CHG with low alcohol content (eg, 4%) as a safe and effective alternative when povidone-iodine is contraindicated or CHG is preferred by the surgeon.[93]

Two moderate-quality studies evaluated alternatives to vaginal povidone-iodine—sterile saline[186] and baby shampoo.[187] Both studies suggested that these alternatives were as effective as povidone-iodine for removing soil and transient microorganisms when used for vaginal surgical site preparation.

Obstetrical Procedures

High-quality evidence supports performing preoperative antisepsis of the vagina for cesarean deliveries. The authors of a Cochrane systematic review of 11 RCTS published between 1997 and 2017 with 3,403 patients found decreased rates of endometritis with povidone-iodine or CHG compared to saline or no vaginal cleansing. The researchers found the decrease was most prominent in patients with ruptured membranes.[188]

In a systematic review of 16 RCTs published between 1997 and 2016 with 4,837 patients, the researchers concluded that vaginal cleansing with 10% povidone-iodine reduced the risk of endometritis in women in labor or with ruptured membranes, but more research is needed for women who are not in labor.[189]

Two RCTs evaluated the effect of vaginal antisepsis in planned cesarean deliveries. Aref[190] randomly assigned 226 patients undergoing cesarean delivery to either vaginal antisepsis with povidone-iodine (n = 113) or no antisepsis (n = 113) and found a significant reduction in endometritis (2.8% to 11.8%) with povidone-iodine vaginal antisepsis. However, Lakhi et al[191] randomly assigned 1,114 patients undergoing nonemergent cesarean deliveries to either 4% CHG (n = 524) or 10% povidone-iodine (n = 590) antisepsis and found the rate of SSIs were significantly lower with CHG compared to povidone-iodine (0.6 to 2.0%). The rates of endometritis and vaginal mucosa irritation were similar between groups.

Conversely, in a quasi-experimental study to compare the rate of superficial or deep incisional SSIs in facilities with policies and procedures for vaginal antisepsis in women undergoing cesarean deliveries during labor (n = 523) to those facilities with no policy or procedure (n = 1,490), the researchers found that having a vaginal antisepsis policy did not result in lower rates of SSI.[192]

Eye Procedures

Three moderate-quality studies support preoperative eye antisepsis with 5% povidone-iodine ophthalmic solution irrigation to reduce rates of conjunctival bacterial load and risk of endophthalmitis from intraocular procedures.[193-195] A retrospective comparative study of 10,614 patients undergoing cataract surgical procedures compared three different surgical site preparations: 10% povidone-iodine to periocular skin and 5% povidone-iodine to conjunctiva (n = 8,650), 10% povidone-iodine to periocular skin only (n = 1,094), and 5% povidone-iodine to periocular skin and conjunctiva (n = 870).[194] The researchers concluded that preoperative skin disinfection with 10% povidone-iodine and conjunctival disinfection with 5% povidone-iodine significantly reduced the relative risk of postoperative endophthalmitis.[194] In a prospective study of 221 patients undergoing anterior segment intraocular procedures, Quiroga et al[193] found that conjunctival irrigation with 5% povidone-iodine solution effectively reduced conjunctival flora. In a nonexperimental study of 113 patients undergoing cataract surgical procedures, Baillif et al[195] found that antisepsis with 5% povidone-iodine to the ocular surface along with sterile technique resulted in low anterior chamber contamination.

The American Academy of Ophthalmology preferred practice guidelines recommend the use of topical povidone-iodine 5% drops instilled into the conjunctival sac preoperatively in adult patients undergoing cataract surgical procedures.[196]

Two high-quality studies found the use of 10% povidone-iodine effective in reducing conjunctival bacterial load with no adverse reactions.[197,198] Researchers who conducted an RCT of 271 cataract surgeries concluded that 10% povidone-iodine was more effective than 1% or 5% povidone-iodine solutions for reducing bacterial load of the eye.[197] In a prospective cohort study of 604 patients using 10% povidone-iodine with 3-minute exposure, Nguyen et al[198] found there were no adverse reactions or complications up to 1 month after surgery. However, researchers in Germany discussed safety concerns regarding high concentrations of povidone-iodine and recommended use of 1.25% povidone-iodine for ocular antisepsis, citing concern for exacerbating untreated hyperthyroidism and that additional research is needed to evaluate the effect of ophthalmic povidone-iodine on thyroid function.[199]

In an RCT to evaluate the reduction of bacterial load on eyelids in oculofacial procedures, Garcia et al[200] compared 10% povidone-iodine (n = 15), 70% isopropyl alcohol (n = 14), and baby shampoo (n = 20) and concluded that the reduction of bacterial counts was comparable among all three groups.

4.4 Select products for surgical site preparation that meet US Food and Drug Administration (FDA) requirements for over-the-counter (OTC) antiseptic products intended for use by health care professionals in a hospital or other health care situation outside the hospital.[201] *[Regulatory Requirement]*

The FDA Code of Federal Regulations Title 21 Part 310 mandates that the active ingredients in health care antiseptics be generally recognized as safe and effective (GRASE) by requiring testing that is consistent, up-to-date, and reflects current scientific knowledge and increasing use patterns. Antiseptic products that meet these testing requirements are identified as having **monograph** status. Antiseptic products that have not completed the testing requirements are considered new drugs and require FDA approval through new drug applications (NDA) or abbreviated new drug applications (ANDA). However, deferred rulemaking was granted for six active ingredients to allow for development and submission of new safety and effectiveness data for these ingredients:

- alcohol (ethanol),
- isopropyl alcohol,
- povidone-iodine,
- benzalkonium chloride,
- benzethonium chloride, and
- chloroxylenol (PCMX).[201]

The monograph or **nonmonograph** status of these active ingredients will be determined after completion and analysis of submitted studies.

4.4.1 Health care personnel should continue to adhere to facility infection control guidance for products containing the deferred six active ingredients. *[Recommendation]*

The FDA recommends no changes to health care personnel use of currently available products containing these active ingredients.[201]

4.4.2 Purchase selected skin antiseptic products packaged in single-use containers.[202] *[Recommendation]*

In November 2013, the FDA issued a Drug Safety Communication requesting that manufacturers package antiseptics indicated for preoperative skin preparation in single-use containers to reduce the risk of infection from improper antiseptic use and contamination of products during use.[202,203]

4.4.3 No recommendation can be made for selection of surgical skin preparation products labeled as sterile.[202,203] [No Recommendation]

The FDA Drug Communication issued in November 2013 encouraged manufacturers of OTC topical antiseptics for preoperative skin preparation to label their products as sterile or nonsterile. The Drug Communication clarifies that the term nonsterile on the product label does not indicate that the product contains harmful bacteria but designates that the product did not undergo a manufacturing process to eliminate all potential microorganisms. The FDA communication does not require manufacturers to produce sterile products or consumers to use only sterile products. Instead, the FDA continues to monitor and evaluate risks related to microbial contamination and recommends that health care professionals not dilute the products or use them beyond their expiration dates.[202,203]

In one RCT, researchers compared povidone-iodine skin antisepsis using both clean and sterile kits and found no difference in microbial counts on patients' skin.[204] This study has not been replicated, and no similar studies were found in the evidence review. This is an unresolved issue that warrants additional research.

When considering the purchase of sterile antiseptic products, it is important to confirm that no change in efficacy of the antiseptic occurred because of sterilization and to evaluate product cost.

4.4.4 Unless contraindicated (eg, antisepsis of split-thickness skin graft donor sites), select products for surgical site preparation that are tinted (ie, not clear).[205] [Recommendation]

Use of colored antiseptics is supported by a quasi-experimental study of skin preparation in upper-limb procedures.[205] This study showed that use of clear antiseptics resulted in more missed spots, mostly in finger areas, than did colored antiseptics.[205] Flammable clear antiseptics may also pose a fire or chemical burn hazard if unseen solution is allowed to drip or pool on or near the patient, although no studies were found that evaluated the effect of visibility on reducing fire or chemical hazards.

4.4.5 Select the tinted skin antiseptic that is most visible on the individual patient's skin.[206] [Recommendation]

McDaniel et al[206] conducted a quasi-experimental study to identify adequacy of skin preparation coverage using two tinted CHG-alcohol preparations on forearms of individuals with four different pigmentations: fair, medium-fair, medium-dark, and dark. The researchers found that orange tint was significantly easier to identify on fair and medium-fair skin tones, and teal tint was most visible on medium-dark and dark skin pigmentation.

4.5 Assess the patient for allergies and sensitivities to preoperative skin antiseptics before selecting the antiseptic.[4,207-219] [Recommendation] **P**

In an in vitro study, Quatresooz et al[207] found that the skin reacts differently to the action of chemicals in various anatomic sites of the body. The researchers found that, in the laboratory setting, povidone-iodine 100 mg/mL produced less irritation in the stratum corneum than two other antiseptics (ie, povidone-iodine 70 mg/mL, chlorhexidine digluconate 50 mg/mL), but in in vivo studies, the severity of skin irritation depends on individual susceptibility and the site of exposure.

In a case report, Sanders and Hawken[208] described three cases of chemical skin reactions to CHG that provide an example of how anatomic location may cause the skin to react differently to chemicals. In this report, three patients undergoing shoulder arthroscopy procedures developed partial thickness chemical burns on the shoulder from a CHG-alcohol preoperative skin antiseptic. The authors determined that the occurrences of chemical skin injury were related to alteration of the skin at the shoulder from traction and to local swelling from the procedure.

A 2004 position statement from the American Academy of Allergy Asthma and Immunology (AAAAI) asserted that fish or shellfish allergies do not indicate allergy to iodine. According to the position statement, contact dermatitis related to topically applied iodine antiseptics does not indicate an iodine allergy; rather, this is a reaction to chemicals in the product. Anaphylaxis caused by topical iodine antiseptic solutions is exceedingly rare and not proven to be related to iodine.[209] Limited evidence was found describing the relationship between seafood and iodine allergies. One nonexperimental survey study[211] and one literature review[210] support the assertion in the AAAAI position statement that seafood allergy is not related to iodine allergy.

Three case reports describe patients who developed anaphylactic reactions to povidone-iodine solution. Two reports are of broken skin in a pediatric patient[220] and a 56-year-old man,[214] and one is a report of vaginal application of povidone-iodine to a hypersensitized patient.[213]

In a 46-year period, the FDA received 43 reports of anaphylaxis with the use of CHG products applied to the skin.[219] As more than half of the cases reported were after 2010, the FDA issued a Drug Safety Communication in 2017 about the increased number of cases and requested that manufacturers add a warning addressing the risk to the Drug Facts label and that health care providers question patients about any history of allergy to antiseptic agents.[219]

In a literature review, Odedra and Farooque[215] concluded that caution should be taken when using CHG as an antiseptic in patients with a history of contact dermatitis and that clinicians should consider CHG allergy as a cause of perioperative anaphylaxis. Cases reports of anaphylaxis from CHG have been reported in the literature.[216-218]

4.5.1 **Use caution when selecting iodine and iodophor-based preoperative patient skin antiseptics for patients susceptible to iodism (eg, patients with burns, patients with thyroid disorders, pregnant women, lactating mothers).**[159,188,199,221-229] *[Recommendation]* **P**

Some patients are susceptible to iodism from preoperative skin antisepsis with iodine and iodophor-based antiseptics.[221]

Burns

Three reports demonstrate that repeated application of povidone-iodine to the skin of burn patients may cause iodine absorption,[222] induced hyperthyroidism,[223] and metabolic acidosis.[224] A review explained that the amount of iodine absorption from polyvinylpyrrolidone-iodine in patients with burns depends on the concentration applied, frequency of application, type and total surface area of the burn, and the patient's renal function.[225]

Thyroid Disorders

The author of a literature review concluded that most patients can tolerate excess quantities of iodine without negative effects, although iodine-induced hyperthyroidism may occur in patients with underlying hyperthyroidism or goiter.[225] In an RCT, Tomoda et al[226] compared preoperative patient skin antisepsis with povidone-iodine (n = 47) to CHG (n = 21) in patients with thyroid carcinoma who were on an iodine-restricted diet and undergoing total thyroidectomy. The researchers demonstrated that iodism resulted from a single application of povidone-iodine for skin antisepsis. In this study, postoperative iodine levels in the patients' urine were nearly seven times the preoperative levels. The researchers theorized that cutaneously absorbed iodine could potentially interfere with iodine therapy or cause thyroid dysfunction in susceptible patients.

Researchers in Germany cautioned that ophthalmic application of povidone-iodine may cause thyroid disturbances, specifically exacerbation of untreated hyperthyroidism.[199] The researchers recommended additional studies to evaluate the effect on the thyroid of ophthalmic povidone-iodine.

Patients Who Are Pregnant

The authors of a literature review recommended using iodine-based antiseptics with caution in women who are pregnant because iodine crosses the placental barrier.[225] In a Cochrane systematic review, Hadiati et al[159] discussed an abstract of one French RCT[227] (N = 22) in which the researchers compared CHG 0.5% with 70% alcohol to use of an antiseptic-impregnated adhesive incise drape. The researchers found a higher concentration of iodine in the cord blood of newborns in the group that received the antiseptic-impregnated adhesive incise drape but no significant difference in iodine of 48-hour urine or thyroid stimulating hormone blood levels on the fifth day. The authors of the systematic review did not make a recommendation based on this abstract.[159]

In a Cochrane systematic review that recommended the use of vaginal povidone-iodine antisepsis immediately before cesarean deliveries, Haas et al[188] did not discuss any risk of iodism in either the mother or the newborn.

In a nonexperimental study of women who were not pregnant (N = 12), Vorherr et al[228] demonstrated iodism after a 2-minute vaginal antisepsis with povidone-iodine, related to the high absorptivity of vaginal tissue. The researchers purported that since the vaginal tissue of women who are pregnant is hyperemic (ie, has an increased amount of blood in the tissues), povidone-iodine will be absorbed more efficiently than in women who are not pregnant. The researchers advised against treating vaginitis in pregnant women with repeated applications of povidone-iodine because of the risk for development of iodine-induced goiter and hypothyroidism in the fetus and newborn.

Patients Who Are Breastfeeding

The manufacturer's IFU of one iodine-based alcohol skin antiseptic recommend caution when using the product for women who are lactating because of potential **transient hypothyroidism** in the nursing newborn.[123] A case report by Kurtoğlu et al[229] describes an infant who developed hypothyroidism after receiving breast milk from its mother, who had been applying povidone-iodine to an episiotomy incision for 10 to 12 days postpartum

4.6 Convene an interdisciplinary team to determine which surgical skin antiseptics will be used for neonates. *[Recommendation]* **P**

Neonates, especially extremely premature neonates (ie, born prior to 32 weeks of gestation with very low birth weight [< 1,500 g] or extremely low birth weight [< 1,000 g]), are at an increased risk for skin irritation and chemical burns of the skin from both CHG and alcohol-based skin antiseptics[3,4,230-234] and may be at increased risk for transient hypothyroidism[225,229,231,235] or iodine-induced hyperthyroidism[236,237] when iodine-based antiseptics are used.

4.6.1 Use caution when selecting CHG and alcohol-based preoperative patient skin antiseptics for neonates. *[Recommendation]* **P**

Both WHO and NICE guidelines for the prevention of SSI emphasize the risk of chemical injury with the aqueous and alcoholic CHG antiseptics when used for surgical site preparation in neonates.[3,4]

The authors of three literature reviews[230-232] cited multiple case reports and studies that found an association between CHG and alcohol-based skin antisepsis and chemical burns in premature infants. The authors all concluded that use of single-use small-quantity applicators followed by removal of excess solution with normal saline and not covering the skin area with occlusive dressing after application can limit the chemical exposure to the neonate.[230-232] However, they agreed that additional studies are needed to determine the optimal antiseptic concentration and formulation, as well as possible adverse effects from different solutions. In a literature review, Sathiyamurthy et al[231] concluded that the use of CHG in neonates may be a better option than povidone-iodine because povidone-iodine use for neonates is associated with systemic absorption and hypothyroidism. They also noted that an alcohol-based preparation must be used with extreme caution in premature infants.

Authors of a case report of two extremely premature neonates with severe chemical burns as a result of 70% isopropyl alcohol applications for skin antisepsis found that pressure and decreased perfusion also played a role in the skin injury. The authors advised exercising extreme caution with use of alcohol for skin antisepsis in extremely premature infants.[233]

In another case report, Harpin and Rutter[234] described cutaneous alcohol absorption and hemorrhagic skin necrosis in a 27-week gestation twin premature infant from skin antisepsis with methylated spirits (95% ethanol and 5% wood naphtha, which is 60% methanol). In this case, the extremely premature neonate died. Although the role of alcohol intoxication in the neonate's death was unknown because blood alcohol levels were not drawn until 18 hours after the alcohol application, the authors suspected that the maximum alcohol level from cutaneous alcohol absorption was in the potentially fatal range.

4.6.2 Use caution when selecting povidone-iodine-based preoperative patient skin antiseptics for neonates. *[Recommendation]* **P**

In a prospective study, Smerdely et al[235] examined very low birth weight infants in neonatal ICUs at two hospitals: one in which iodine-containing antiseptics were used (n = 36) and one in which CHG-containing antiseptics were used (n = 27) for all invasive procedures. Urinary iodine excretion and thyrotropin (ie, thyroid stimulating hormone [TSH]) were significantly higher in the iodine-exposed group. Twenty-five percent of the infants in the iodine group developed transient neonatal hypothyroidism, with no development in the CHG infant group. The authors hypothesized that the selective development of hypothyroidism is related to gestational age, as the more premature an infant the greater the iodine absorption. As a result of this study, the use of iodine-containing antiseptics in the neonatal ICU was suspended.

However, in another prospective study, Yilmaz et al[238] evaluated the effect of exposure to a single dose of povidone-iodine or CHG antiseptics on thyroid functions (eg, TSH, thyroxine) and urinary iodine excretion in premature newborns (n = 30), full-term newborns (n = 40), and infants (n = 50). All participants received povidone-iodine–containing antiseptic on odd days and CHG-containing antiseptic on even days. Immediately after povidone-iodine application, the skin was wiped with alcohol to prevent long-term contact. The researchers found no significant difference in thyroid function between any of the three groups. However, urinary iodine excretion in premature and full-term groups was significantly elevated. The authors concluded that premature newborns, full-term newborns, and infants receiving a single dose of povidone-iodine for skin disinfection are not at risk for thyroid disorders.

One case of transient hypothyroidism was reported in an infant receiving cord care with iodine three times each day.[229] Two case reports of iodine-induced hyperthyroidism were reported, one in an infant born with giant omphalocele being treated with topical povidone-iodine dressings to promote escharification[236] and one in an infant after mediastinal lavage with povidone-iodine.[237]

4.7 **Before selecting a preoperative patient skin antiseptic product, assess the surgical site for**
- **skin integrity;**
- **presence of hair[239-241]; and**
- **proximity to mucosa, eyes, or ears.[3,4,242,243]**

[Recommendation]

Certain antiseptic products may be contraindicated on skin that is not intact; where large amounts of hair are present; and on mucosa, eyes, or ears. Assessment of the patient's skin, verification of the surgical site, and a review of product IFU are necessary components of safe patient care.

The presence of hair may contraindicate the use of flammable antiseptics according to manufacturers' IFU. A flammable antiseptic for preoperative skin antisepsis is contraindicated when the procedure involves an ignition source (eg, electrosurgical unit [ESU], laser) and the solution does not dry completely in hair. According to the Centers for Medicare & Medicaid Services (CMS), alcohol-based skin antiseptics that wick into the patient's hair result in prolonged drying times.[240,241] No evidence was found that describes the specific length or amount of hair that constitutes a fire risk during use of alcohol-based skin antiseptics.

In a case report, a patient described as having copious body hair was burned on the neck and shoulders while undergoing a tracheostomy.[239] After the patient's neck was prepared with an alcohol-based skin antiseptic, the surgical team allowed the solution to dry for 3 minutes before draping. Activation of the ESU ignited the fire, which was fueled by the skin antiseptic and the patient's body hair and oxidized in an oxygen-enriched environment. The authors of the case report recommended that the alcohol-based skin antiseptic product not be used for a hirsute patient because the hair can impede drying of the solution.[239]

In their SSI guidance documents, both the WHO and NICE state that alcohol should not be used on the mucosa or eyes.[3,4]

In a case report, Bever et al[242] described two neurosurgical cases, a cervical laminectomy and a craniotomy, where significant corneal damage occurred with use of 4% CHG despite occlusive dressings being placed over the patients' eyes before application of the skin antiseptic. Because of the potential for severe corneal toxicity, the authors recommended evaluating the use of CHG against the risk for SSI, and if CHG must be used, exercising great care to avoid contact with eyes.[242]

Singh and Blakley[243] conducted a systematic review to assess evidence on the safety of surgical antiseptic preparations in the ear. In 13 high-quality studies conducted in animal populations, six evaluated iodine-based solutions, five evaluated CHG and ethanol, and two evaluated hydrogen peroxide. Ototoxicity was measured through hearing, vestibular function, or histologic examination. The authors found iodine-based solution produced the least amount of ototoxicity, whereas CHG and a high concentration of alcohol-based solutions produced the greatest amount of ototoxicity. However, conclusive evidence regarding human toxicity from any solution was weak, leading the authors to conclude that iodine-based, nonalcoholic, nondetergent solutions appeared to have the least ototoxicity but should be used with caution.

4.8 **When FDA-approved (ie, monograph, NDA, ANDA) antiseptic products are contraindicated, collaboratively evaluate the risks and benefits of using nonmonograph antiseptics or alternative solutions (eg, soaps, saline) (See Recommendation 4.4).**

[Recommendation]

No evidence was found regarding the efficacy of alternative antiseptic products. When a patient has an allergy or a condition such as a large open wound, all available products approved by the FDA for antisepsis might be contraindicated. In this situation, the perioperative team is challenged to select a safe, effective alternative for the individual patient by weighing the potential benefits and harms.[96]

4.9 **Convene an interdisciplinary team to select skin markers for surgical site marking based on the**
- **effect on sterility of skin antisepsis (ie, no bacterial growth; does not transmit infection)[244-247];**
- **visibility on different skin types[248];**
- **visibility after surgical site preparation[248-251];**
- **non-transferability[248];**
- **non-sensitization[245,247,248]; and**
- **cost.[245]**

[Recommendation]

Marking the surgical site with a nonsterile permanent marker is a safe practice for identifying the surgical site. Researchers in two quasi-experimental studies, each of 20 healthy volunteers, evaluated the effect of site marking on the sterility of skin antisepsis.[244,245] The researchers concluded that skin marking with a nonsterile permanent marker did not affect the sterility of skin antisepsis with povidone-iodine, as evidenced by no culture growth at the treated areas.[244,245]

Researchers in a nonexperimental study investigated the potential for the surgical site marker to serve as a reservoir for transmissible infections. In this study, Wilson and Tate[246] compared two types of markers, water-based and alcohol-based, and determined that transmission of MRSA is feasible with water-based skin markers. They recommended against using water-based skin markers for multiple patients because of the theoretical risk of transmitting MRSA.

Bathla et al[248] conducted a quasi-experimental study to evaluate the visibility of 10 different skin markers after application of two surgical skin antiseptics (povidone-iodine and/or CHG) in five volunteers, each of whom represented one skin type on the Fitzpatrick skin type classification scale (ie, one volunteer in each classification between I and V). The researchers found that the volunteer with Fitzpatrick skin type V (ie, the darkest skin color) had less visible skin marking after application of the skin antiseptics. The researchers concluded that individuals with type V skin are more likely to have poor marking visibility with commercially available pens. They recommended that for optimal clarity when using skin marking pens, the ink color should be entirely different from both the color of the patient's skin and the color of skin antiseptic used. They also suggested that single-use marking pens be considered when there is a known infection risk, such as surgical procedure with implants.

Two experimental studies examined the erasure of the surgical site marking during preoperative patient skin antisepsis. Both studies involved permanent, alcohol-based markers and had a sample size of 20. The researchers found that a CHG-alcohol antiseptic product erased more site markings than did an iodine-based alcohol antiseptic product.[249,250]

For additional guidance on surgical site marking, see the AORN Guideline for Team Communication.[251]

5. Application of the Surgical Site Antiseptic

5.1 **Complete surgical site preparation with an antiseptic before beginning the surgical procedure.**[3,4,11,212] *[Recommendation]*

The purpose of surgical site preparation is to reduce the microbial load on the patient's skin and inhibit rapid rebound growth of microorganisms from the skin where the incision will be made. For optimal effectiveness of the antiseptic, it is necessary to adhere to the time allotment for application before the surgical procedure, as outlined in manufacturer's instructions.[212]

5.2 **Apply the preoperative patient skin antiseptic according to the manufacturer's IFU.**[251,252] *[Recommendation]*

Antiseptic manufacturers' IFU convey important safety and efficacy instructions to the user. Failure to adhere to manufacturers' IFU may result in patient harm or ineffectiveness of the preoperative patient skin antisepsis.

In an RCT to evaluate reduction in bacterial colony-forming units (CFU) with one application (n = 30) or two applications (n = 30) of aqueous CHG, Bajaj et al[252] found that the two applications recommended by the manufacturer's IFU substantially reduced CFU 10 minutes after surgical site preparation of the foot compared to one application. In another RCT involving 101 patients undergoing urological implant procedures, Malalasekera et al[253] found that a surgical site scrub with povidone-iodine led to a fourfold reduction in CFU at the groin compared to povidone-iodine paint alone. However, no difference was found in CFU reduction between a 5- or 10-minute scrub, leading the authors to conclude that a 5-minute scrub, as recommended by the manufacturer, may be satisfactory for urologic prosthetic procedures.

5.3 **Perform a standardized surgical site preparation protocol to include**
- **site preparation before application of the skin antiseptic,**
- **application of the skin antiseptic using sterile technique, and**
- **safety measures to prevent patient injury related to skin antiseptic use.**

[Recommendation]

Standardizing processes eliminates variability, resulting in less waste, fewer errors, and improved quality outcomes. In a quasi-experimental study, Lundberg et al[254] evaluated the compliance of 30 experienced health care professionals with surgical site preparation of the foot using the manufacturer's IFU for CHG-alcohol and povidone-iodine. Additionally, skin cultures of patients' first innerweb space and medial malleolus were obtained before and 30 minutes after skin preparation. Compliance with critical steps according to the manufacturer's IFU was 33.3% with use of povidone-iodine and 90% with use of CHG-alcohol, with no difference found in bacterial load regardless of compliance or health care professionals' years of experience. The authors recommended standardizing selection of antiseptics along with providing simple education to enhance protocol compliance.

The evidence review found a lack of procedure-specific clinical research evaluating the effectiveness of various surgical site preparation techniques.

5.3.1 Before application of a surgical skin antiseptic, complete the following:
- confirm the surgical site[251];
- assess the condition of the patient's skin[64];
- remove the patient's jewelry (eg, rings, piercings) within the area of surgical site preparation[101,103,255,256];
- verify that the skin is free of
  - soil or debris,[7,76,257-259]
  - emollients,
  - cosmetics,[95] and
  - alcohol-based products[260];
- if soiled, cleanse the areas in the surgical site that are of greater contamination than the surrounding area (ie, umbilicus, foreskin, under nails, intestinal or urinary stoma); and
- isolate highly contaminated areas (eg, anus, colostomy) near the surgical site with a sterile barrier drape.

[Recommendation]

The benefits of removing soil at the surgical site outweigh the harms. Organic and inorganic material in the umbilicus (eg, detritus) may reduce the effectiveness of the skin antiseptic and contaminate the surgical site for abdominal procedures. Areas under nails (ie, subungual areas) also may harbor organic and inorganic material, including microorganisms, that could limit the effectiveness of antisepsis for procedures involving the hand or foot. Similarly, surgical sites that include the penis may harbor microorganisms that accumulate in the area under the foreskin (ie, prepuce), if present, including organic material (ie, smegma). Intestinal or urinary stomas are also highly likely to contain organic material, such as mucin, that could render some antiseptics ineffective.

Jewelry present within the area of surgical site preparation may harbor microorganisms and trap these organisms on adjacent skin, which may contaminate the surgical site or reduce the effectiveness of preoperative patient skin antisepsis. Jewelry, including piercings, places patients undergoing operative and other invasive procedures at risk for electrical burns, trauma, and airway obstruction.[256] For additional guidance, see the AORN Guideline for Electrosurgical Safety.[261]

5.3.2 Apply surgical skin antiseptic using sterile technique, to include
- having a nonscrubbed perioperative team member apply the antiseptic[6];
- performing hand hygiene immediately before application of the antiseptic[103];
- wearing sterile gloves[6] (nonsterile gloves may be worn if the antiseptic applicator is long enough to prevent contact of the gloved hand with the skin antiseptic and the patient's skin);
- using sterile supplies[6,204];
- applying the antiseptic to an area large enough to accommodate
  - inadvertent shifting of the surgical drapes,
  - extension of the incision (eg, during conversion of a minimally invasive procedure to an open procedure),
  - potential additional incisions, and
  - all potential drain sites;
- starting at the incision site and moving toward the periphery of the surgical site;
- discarding the applicator after contact with a peripheral or contaminated area and using another sterile applicator for additional applications;
- prepping the area with a lower bacterial count first when the incision site is more highly contaminated than the surrounding skin (eg, anus, perineum, stoma, open wound, catheter, drain, axilla), then prepping the area of higher contamination (as opposed to working from the incision toward the periphery); and
- completing two separate surgical site preparations[6,259] and prepping the more contaminated site first[259,262] when performing procedures with different surgical wound classifications (eg, abdominal-perineal, abdominal-vaginal).

[Recommendation]

5.3.3 Arms may be covered during performance of preoperative patient skin antisepsis.[263-265]
[Conditional Recommendation]

In a quasi-experimental study, Markel et al[264] found the presence of particulates and shedding was decreased when arms were covered during surgical site antisepsis. Conversely, in a quasi-experimental study, Stapleton et al[264] found that wearing perioperative disposable jackets was not associated with SSI reduction for clean wounds and presented an additional financial burden. See the AORN Guideline for Surgical Attire for more information.[263]

5.3.4 When using aqueous povidone-iodine, either scrub (ie, 7.5% povidone-iodine) and paint (ie, 10% povidone-iodine) or paint alone may be used.[257,266,267] *[Conditional Recommendation]*

Evidence related to the comparison of scrub versus paint application techniques for preoperative patient skin antisepsis conflicts.

In an RCT of 150 patients undergoing clean surgical procedures, Vagholkar and Julka[266] compared three surgical site preparation techniques: a 3-minute scrub with paint, a 5-minute scrub with paint, and paint only. No significant difference in SSI rates was found between techniques, leading the researchers to conclude that no one method was superior. However, in a retrospective cohort study that compared scrubbing and painting (n = 1,004) with painting alone (n = 1,139) in patients undergoing cesarean deliveries, Weed et al[267] found that scrubbing and painting resulted in fewer SSIs and a shorter postoperative stay than painting alone. In another RCT involving 101 patients undergoing urological implant procedures, Malalasekera et al[253] found surgical site scrub with povidone-iodine led to a fourfold reduction in CFU at the groin compared to povidone-iodine paint alone.

In a systematic review with meta-analysis of five RCTs and two quasi-experimental studies (N = 1,352), Lefebvre et al[257] found no significant differences in SSI or positive skin culture rates between scrubbing before painting or painting alone. However, the authors concluded larger studies evaluating reduction of SSIs using both methods are needed.

5.3.5 Implement patient safety measures when performing surgical site preparation, to include

- following the manufacturer's instructions for maximum and minimum surface area per applicator when using a pre-filled antiseptic applicator[138,268];
- using radiopaque sponges when applicators are not available[269];
- applying the antiseptic with care (eg, gentle friction) on fragile tissue, burns, open wounds, or malignant areas[145];
- verifying antiseptic is applied to all surfaces between fingers or toes for surgical site preparation that includes the hand or foot[148,270-275];
- taking care to prevent patient aspiration of the skin antiseptic (eg, throat pack application) for surgical site preparation that includes the mouth[276-278];

- preventing prolonged contact with skin antiseptics by
  ○ protecting sheets, padding, and positioning equipment from the dripping or pooling of skin antiseptics beneath and around the patient[145,279-282];
  ○ protecting electrodes (eg, electrocardiogram [ECG], ESU dispersive electrode) and tourniquets from contact with skin antiseptics[279,281,283-285];
  ○ placing a fluid-resistant pad under the patient's buttocks during perineal preoperative patient skin antisepsis for patients in the lithotomy position[286-288]; and
  ○ removing the pad after the antiseptic is dry and before applying the sterile drape[145,279,281];
- removing any material near the patient that is in contact with the skin antiseptic, including electrodes (eg, ECG, ESU) and tourniquet materials (ie, cuff, padding), and replacing them as necessary[259]; and
- allowing the antiseptic to dry completely (ie, for the full time recommended in the manufacturer's IFU) before applying drapes.[119,212,289,290]

5.3.6 Implement personnel safety measures when lifting and holding the patient's extremity by

- using two hands to hold the extremity,
- obtaining assistance from another team member,
- using an assistive device, or
- using a combination of these methods.[291] *[Recommendation]*

Using these measures can minimize muscle fatigue for personnel who are performing surgical skin antisepsis. Minimizing muscle fatigue can be protective for both the health care worker (ie, can prevent an injury or strain) and the patient (ie, the person performing the prep is less likely to drop the extremity while applying the skin antiseptic). For additional guidance, see the AORN Guideline for Safe Patient Handling and Movement.[291]

5.4 When using flammable skin antiseptics, minimize the risk of fire by

- performing a fire risk assessment and communicating the use of flammable skin antiseptics before beginning the procedure,[119,292-294]
- minimizing oxygen delivery,[119]
- not heating flammable skin antiseptics,[259,295]

- using reusable or disposable sterile towels to absorb drips and excess solution during application,[293,296,297]
- wicking excess solution with a sterile towel or cotton tip applicator,[260,282,293,296,297]
- removing materials that are saturated with the skin antiseptic before the patient is draped,[259,260,282]
- moving flammable skin antiseptic–soaked materials away from the patient care vicinity,[240,241,260] and
- allowing time for the flammable skin antiseptic to dry completely and for fumes to dissipate before surgical drapes are applied or a potential ignition source is used.[260,280,292,293,296,297] [Recommendation]

Active communication regarding the use of flammable skin antiseptics alerts all perioperative team members to the inherent risks and facilitates taking collaborative precautions.[119]

Flammable skin antiseptics are a fuel source and pose a fire hazard. Preventing pooling of flammable skin antiseptics and allowing the antiseptic to dry completely to minimize the fire hazard is supported by CMS[240,241] and several clinical practice guidelines, including guidance from the National Fire Protection Association (NFPA),[260] the American Society of Anesthesiologists (ASA),[292] and the ECRI Institute.[296,297] Heating flammable antiseptics may pose a serious risk of fire. When the temperature of flammable chemicals increases, they become more unstable and may ignite easily.[259] Removal of any solution-soaked material from the immediate patient care vicinity decreases the chance of fire.

The practice of allowing fumes to dissipate before applying surgical drapes is supported by guidelines from the ASA,[292] the ECRI Institute,[296,297] and the NFPA.[293] The volatile fumes are flammable and may ignite without a connection between the ignition source and the actual skin antiseptic.[296,297]

Refer to the AORN Guideline for a Safe Environment of Care for additional guidance related to fire safety.[119]

5.4.1 **The risk of fire may be minimized by confining the hair with a water-soluble gel and non-metallic ties or with braids for longer hair.** [Conditional Recommendation]

No studies have evaluated the use of alternative hair management techniques or products to reduce the risk of fire. The AORN Guideline for a Safe Environment of Care recommends coating facial hair with water-soluble gel for surgical procedures that involve the head and neck to minimize the risk of combustion.[119]

5.4.2 **When an alcohol-based skin antiseptic is used for a procedure involving an ignition source and hair is present in surgical site preparation area, follow the antiseptic manufacturer's IFU.**[240,241] [Recommendation]

According to the CMS, alcohol-based antiseptics that wick into a patient's hair result in prolonged drying time.[240,241] The manufacturers' IFU for several alcohol-based antiseptics indicate that antiseptic applied to hair may take up to an hour to dry.[122,123]

5.5 **Do not apply microbial sealant after surgical skin preparation.** [Recommendation]

The benefits of using microbial sealants do not outweigh the potential harms. Researchers in two studies found no reduction in SSI rates after applying antimicrobial sealant immediately after skin preparation.[3,76] Potential harms associated with microbial sealant may include cost, sealants flaking off into the surgical wound, and hypersensitivity or allergic reaction to the sealant.[298,299]

5.6 **No recommendation can be made for sequential application of skin antiseptic before the incision is made.** [No Recommendation]

Limited and conflicting evidence exists regarding subsequent application of antiseptic before the incision is made. Additionally, the investigations did not use a consistent surgical antiseptic concentration, formulation, or application technique, making it difficult to evaluate the benefits and harms of repeated application and amplifying the necessity for additional research.

In a systematic review of 10 RCTs and quasi-experimental studies that evaluated sequential application of antiseptics, Mermel[300] concluded that sequential application of CHG and povidone-iodine antiseptics may reduce SSI risk more effectively than when either is applied alone. However, the review author noted that not all antiseptic concentrations were equal, some contained alcohol, and some were applied for a longer time or painted instead of scrubbed.

Two high-quality studies evaluated sequential application of antiseptics in total joint[301] and CIED[143] surgical procedures. In an RCT, Morrison et al[301] found a significant reduction in total joint SSIs when iodine-based alcohol was applied after surgical preparation with povidone-iodine scrub, povidone-iodine paint, and isopropyl alcohol. However, in a quasi-experimental study, Da Costa et al[143] found that CIED infection rates remained unaltered when either alcoholic or aqueous povidone-iodine was applied three times before surgical incision.

The authors of the NICE SSI guidelines identified sequential application of antiseptics as a key area for additional research, especially in regard to clinical and cost effectiveness.[4]

5.7 **At the end of the surgical procedure, remove the skin antiseptic from the patient's skin before application of an occlusive dressing or tape, unless otherwise indicated by the skin antiseptic manufacturer's IFU.**[145,218,302] *[Recommendation]*

The removal of skin antiseptics from the skin at the end of the surgical procedure is supported by one literature review,[145] one case report of a chemical burn from povidone-iodine,[302] and one case report of allergic reaction from CHG-alcohol[218] remaining on skin postoperatively. Residual skin antiseptics may cause skin irritation and contact dermatitis in sensitive individuals. Removing the solution as soon as possible after completion of the procedure minimizes the risk for on ongoing irritation.

5.8 **Assess the patient's skin for injury after the procedure.**[64] **A thorough evaluation of the patient's skin may be postponed until the patient is transferred to the postoperative area, depending on the patient's condition.** *[Recommendation]*

Evaluating the patient's progress toward attaining outcomes after an intervention is a standard of perioperative nursing practice.[64] Reassessing the patient's skin after the procedure is an important method of evaluating the patient for injury

5.9 **Document surgical site preparation in the patient's record, including the**
- **removal and disposition of any jewelry;**
- **assessment of the skin at the surgical site (eg, presence of rashes, skin eruptions, abrasions, redness, irritation, burns);**
- **antiseptic used;**
- **person performing surgical site preparation;**
- **area prepped; and**
- **postoperative skin assessment, including any skin irritation, hypersensitivity, or allergic response to preparation solutions.**

[Recommendation]

5.10 **Provide education and complete competency verification activities related to the principles and processes of skin antisepsis.** *[Recommendation]*

Incorporate topics for education and competency verification related to the principles and processes of skin antisepsis, including potential harms of antiseptics.[3]

5.10.1 **Provide education when new antiseptics or processes are introduced.** *[Requirement]*

6. Handling and Storage of Antiseptics

6.1 **Review and follow the skin antiseptic manufacturers' IFU and safety data sheets (SDS) for handling, storing, and disposing of skin antiseptics.**[303] *[Recommendation]*

Following the antiseptic manufacturer's IFU and the SDS is the safest method for handling, storing, and disposing of skin antiseptics. The evidence review identified a lack of research in the clinical setting for safe handling, storage, and disposal of skin antiseptics.

6.1.1 **Safety data sheets for all skin antiseptics used must be readily available in the practice area.**[303] *[Regulatory Requirement]*

The SDS provides information about the flammability of the antiseptic and the maximum safe storage temperature. The Occupational Safety and Health Administration requires that SDS be available for all chemicals used in the practice setting.[303] These documents outline the hazards related to the chemicals and actions to take in the event of a chemical exposure (eg, a splash to the eyes).

6.2 **Skin antiseptics must be stored in the original, single-use container.**[202,304-307] *[Regulatory Requirement]*

In November 2013, the FDA issued a drug safety communication requesting label changes and single-use packaging of OTC topical antiseptic products to decrease risk of infection.[202] Topical antiseptics are not required by the FDA to be manufactured as sterile, although most are manufactured with a sterile process. Nonsterile antiseptics may be contaminated with bacteria during or after manufacturing. As a result of reported outbreaks involving contaminated antiseptic products, the FDA requested that manufacturers package antiseptics for preoperative skin preparation in single-use containers, to be used only one time for one patient.[202]

Several case reports have linked antiseptics to patient infections, from both intrinsic[304,305,307] and extrinsic[306,307] contamination. In a laboratory study, Kim et al[308] evaluated the survival and susceptibility of *Burkholderia cepacia* complex (BCC), an opportunistic pathogenic bacteria occasionally recovered from antiseptics. The researchers found that BCC in water remained viable with low susceptibility to both CHG and benzalkonium chloride for 14 days. They recommended that improved detection methods and control measures for BCC contamination be considered during antiseptic manufacturing.

6.2.1 Single-use containers for skin antiseptics must be discarded after use and not be refilled.[202] *[Regulatory Requirement]*

6.3 Skin antiseptics must not be diluted.[202] *[Regulatory Requirement]*

In a drug safety communication, the FDA states that health care professionals should not dilute antiseptic products after opening them, to reduce the possibility that these products will become contaminated.[202]

6.4 Only warm nonflammable skin antiseptics if this is allowed in the manufacturer's IFU. Flammable skin antiseptics should not be warmed.[309,310] *[Recommendation]*

The benefits of warming nonflammable skin antiseptic may outweigh the potential harms. The benefits of heating nonflammable antiseptics may include improved patient satisfaction and body temperature maintenance. Wistrand et al[310] conducted an RCT involving 220 patients undergoing pacemaker and CIED implantation under local anesthesia to evaluate the effect of using a skin antiseptic warmed (36° C [97° F]) according to the manufacturer's IFU compared to room-temperature (20° C [68° F]) skin antiseptic on skin temperature and patient experience. The researchers found that preheated solution contributed to a more pleasant patient experience and significantly higher mean skin temperature.

The harms of heating antiseptics may include thermal or chemical burns, although no case reports of injury were found in the evidence review. Heating may alter the chemical composition and effectiveness of the skin antiseptic. In a 1985 expert opinion paper, Gottardi[309] described that the heating of povidone-iodine alters the equilibrium of the iodine content.

Review of the antiseptic manufacturer's instructions for the temperature limitation of antiseptic efficacy is essential to reducing infection risk and providing safe patient care.[202]

6.4.1 Do not warm skin antiseptics in a microwave oven or steam sterilizer. *[Recommendation]*

The evidence review found no literature to support or refute this recommendation. The temperature of the skin antiseptic is uncontrolled when heated in a microwave or steam sterilizer, and temperature extremes may result in a patient injury.

6.5 Storage of flammable skin antiseptics must comply with local, state, and federal regulations.[119,240,241,260,293,295] *[Regulatory Requirement]*

The CMS states in §482.41(c)(2) that "facilities, supplies, and equipment must be maintained to ensure an acceptable level of safety and quality," including storage in compliance with fire codes.[240,241] The NFPA has recommendations for storage of flammable solutions.[260,293,295] The AORN Guideline for a Safe Environment Care also recommends following local and state fire regulations for storage of flammable liquids, such as alcohol-based skin antiseptic solutions.[119]

6.6 Disposal of unused flammable skin antiseptics must be performed in a manner that decreases the risk of fire and is in accordance with local, state, and federal regulations.[119,240,241,311] *[Regulatory Requirement]*

Disposal of residual flammable antiseptics is regulated by the Environmental Protection Agency (EPA).[311] The CMS regulations state that trash must be stored and disposed of in accordance with federal, state, and local laws and regulations, including those from the EPA.[240,241]

There is a risk that fires can occur when flammable antiseptics are discarded in nonhazardous trash, and incineration or autoclaving of biohazardous waste can rapidly ignite flammable antiseptics. See the AORN Guideline for Safe Environment of Care for more guidance on disposal of flammable antiseptics.[119]

7. Quality

7.1 Bundled interventions that include preoperative skin antisepsis may be part of a quality improvement program to reduce SSIs.[93,312] *[Conditional Recommendation]* **P**

When evidence-based infection prevention interventions are implemented together, the most benefit is seen. The benefit of implementing bundled measures is the streamlining of efforts as one collaborative action instead of individual efforts. The collaborative nature of bundled measures makes it easier to educate health care personnel on implementation.

The use of bundled interventions provides a framework to facilitate implementation of a complex list of evidence-based practices in an organized manner.[93] The authors of a systematic review that compared patient outcomes before and after bundle implementation found that negative patient outcomes were less frequent after bundle implementation when compared to no care bundles or implementation of one evidence-based practice.[312]

Bundling preoperative, intraoperative, and postoperative care has been shown to decrease SSI rates. The authors of a systematic review with meta-analysis of 14 quasi-experimental studies from 2011 to 2017 on evidence-based bundles for cesarean delivery found that when three or more interventions were part of the bundle, there was an associated reduction in the overall SSI rate.[313]

High-quality evidence supports that the use of prevention bundles that included elements of preoperative patient skin antisepsis significantly reduced SSI rates in cardiothoracic,[314-316] pediatric cardiothoracic,[317] cataract,[318,319] colorectal,[320-324] cesarean delivery,[325,326] gynecological oncology,[327,328] orthopedic implant,[329,330] urologic,[331] and vascular[332] surgical procedures. When these bundles were applied to six different procedure groups[333] or cardiothoracic and orthopedic hardware surgical procedures,[17,26] significant reduction in SSI rates also occurred. Notably, some studies only measured reduction for one specific type of SSI, as opposed to overall SSI reduction.[318,320,321,331]

Reports of several organizational quality improvement programs noted a reduction of SSI rates with preoperative skin antisepsis as part of bundle implementation. Reduction of SSIs were found in pediatric cardiothoracic,[334] colorectal,[335,336] cesarean delivery,[337,338] pediatric neurology,[339] and orthopedic implant[340-342] surgical procedures. When bundle elements were applied to 10 different procedure groups,[343] general and orthopedic surgical procedures,[344] and pediatric cardiothoracic and neurology surgical procedures,[345] reduction in SSI rates also occurred.

7.1.1 The health care organization should use professional society guidelines to select preoperative patient skin antisepsis elements specific to their surgical population for inclusion in a bundle. *[Recommendation]*

Preoperative patient skin antisepsis elements may not yet be defined for all surgical procedures or patients.[346] Professional society guidelines provide evidence-based recommendations for SSI reduction.

Moderate-quality evidence supports including preoperative patient skin antisepsis elements as part of implemented bundles. Preoperative bundle elements included

- bathing or showering with soap or an antiseptic agent,[313-318,320-322,325,327-330,332,334-339,342,344]
- screening for *S aureus*,[17,26,316,330,334,339,342]
- decolonization of nares if the patient was *S aureus* positive,[17,26,339,342]
- decolonization of skin if the patient was *S aureus* positive,[17,26,339]
- decolonization of nares and skin for all patients,[316,329,334]

- hair management,[313,316,317,322,323,327,332,333,336-338,341,343-345]
- use of a skin antiseptic with CHG-alcohol,[316,317,320,321,326,327,329,331,332,334,336,338,340-345]
- use of a skin antiseptic with iodine-based alcohol,[314,329,331,341,343] and
- use of a skin antiseptic without alcohol.[318,319,324,325,328,329,337,338]

7.1.2 Determine outcome measures for selected bundled interventions. *[Recommendation]*

Identifying outcome measures provides an attainable goal, facilitates progress to be measured, and supports team engagement.

The outcome measure most frequently identified in the literature was SSI incidence reduction. Other outcomes measured with bundle implementation included

- patient satisfaction scores,[337]
- risk for wound complications,[326]
- readmissions,[328]
- incidence of postoperative sepsis,[321]
- facility SSI rate compared to rates in six similar studies,[329] and
- sustainment of SSI reduction.[322,330,340,343]

The multifactorial nature of SSI prevention makes it difficult to know which bundle element has the most significance. However, when elements are implemented together, the most benefit is seen, so it is likely the cumulative effect of all bundle components that produces the best outcome.[312]

7.2 Monitor adherence to and outcomes of bundled interventions.[11,93] *[Recommendation]*

An inverse association has been demonstrated between SSI rates and the number of bundle measures that are followed.[11,93] Compliance, relevant stakeholder buy-in, and incorporation of organizational culture are important elements for successful bundle implementation.[11,346]

High-quality studies that measured and obtained high patient and provider compliance found favorable results. Studies in which compliance with measures ranged between 75% and 90% showed significant reduction in SSI rates.[26,320,322,325,332] In a quasi-experimental study, Koek et al[333] implemented a bundle for six procedure groups and found significantly lower SSI risk for those surgeries in which there was complete bundle adherence. Mok et al[330] obtained 100% compliance with bundle measures and saw a reduction in SSI rates for patients undergoing hip procedures; patients were admitted the night before the procedure and elements were implemented by personnel.

Tanner et al[347] did not find a reduction in colorectal SSI rates after bundle implementation, even though some elements of the bundle were already part of the standard of care. The researchers found that compliance with these elements was low even before they were introduced as part of the bundle. The authors purported that increasing team member education and engagement may have led to different results and that studies evaluating the effectiveness of care bundles should include compliance with interventions both before and after bundle implementation.

In a nonexperimental study, Davis et al[348] evaluated implementation of a general surgery bundle at multiple hospitals and found that lower SSI rates were statistically correlated to compliance with bundle elements.

The SHEA recommends measuring compliance with process measures routinely and sharing the results with surgical team members, perioperative personnel, and the organization's leaders.[7]

7.3   **Evaluate and revise bundles when new interventions and evidence become available.**[8,93] *[Recommendation]*

No studies have shown the ideal actions to implement for prevention of SSIs in every surgical procedure, but there is a growing body of evidence in this area. Additionally, single interventions supported by evidence may not have been validated in combination with a group of interventions.[93] In the *Management of Multidrug-Resistant Organisms (MDROs) in Healthcare Settings,* Siegal et al[8] state that successful eradication and control of MDROs is dependent on periodic assessment and the addition of new and more stringent interventions.

7.4   **When CHG and mupirocin are part of the SSI bundle, surveillance for emergence of tolerance or resistance may be performed.**[4,97] *[Conditional Recommendation]*

Concern has been raised that the increased use of CHG may diminish its effects as a skin antiseptic and potentially cause cross resistance with antimicrobial agents.[97] However, the authors of three literature reviews concluded that there is little evidence to suggest increased CHG MIC concentrations have resulted in clinical resistance.[97,349,350] The authors concluded that ongoing surveillance is warranted and that efforts to prevent unnecessary and improper use of CHG should be implemented.[97,349,350] The NICE guidelines recommend that additional research be conducted to determine the association of CHG bathing with increased antimicrobial resistance.[4]

One risk for the inclusion of mupirocin in decolonization regimens is the development of *S aureus* strains that are resistant to mupirocin, thereby decreasing the efficacy of decolonization.[68] Imple-

menting surveillance may allow for any increase in resistance to be identified **(See Recommendation 1.5.2).**[4]

Glossary

Active surveillance: The practice of attempting to identify patients colonized with methicillin-susceptible *Staphylococcus aureus* and/or methicillin-resistant *S aureus.* Synonym: screening.

Antiseptic: A product with antimicrobial activity that is applied to the skin to reduce the number of microbial flora.

Bundle: Evidence-informed practices implemented simultaneously (ie, more than one intervention at a time) that are aimed at improving care outcomes when performed collectively.

Decolonization: The practice of treating patients who have known *Staphylococcus aureus* colonization with antimicrobial and/or antiseptic agents to eliminate *S aureus* colonization (See targeted decolonization, universal colonization).

Fitzpatrick skin type classification: A numerical categorization system for determining skin color, which ranges from very fair (skin type I) to very dark (skin type VI). Classification is based on an individual's hair and eye color, color of nonexposed skin, presence of freckles, sun exposure response, and tanning practices.

Iodism: Poisoning by iodine, a condition marked by severe rhinitis, frontal headache, emaciation, weakness, and skin eruptions. Caused by the administration of iodine or one of the iodides.

Monograph: A determination by the US Food and Drug Administration that an active ingredient is generally recognized as safe or effective (GRASE) for over-the-counter use because of evidence of effectiveness, safety, or both.

Microbial sealant: A film-forming protective barrier product designed to prevent bacteria migration (eg, cyanoacrylate liquid).

Microbiota: A community of microorganisms (ie, bacteria, yeast, viruses) that colonize the skin, nasal passages, throat, vagina, and gastrointestinal tract.

Minimum inhibitory concentration: The lowest concentration of an antimicrobial substance required to inhibit the growth of a microorganism.

Nonmonograph: A determination by the US Food and Drug Administration that an active ingredient is not generally recognized as safe or effective (GRASE) for over-the-counter use because of lack of evidence of effectiveness, safety, or both.

Patient care vicinity: A space in a location intended for the examination and treatment of patients that extends 1.8 m (6 ft) beyond the normal location of the bed, chair, table, treadmill, or other device that supports the patient during examination and treatment and extends vertically to 2.3 m (7 ft 6 inches) above the floor.

Preoperative bathing: A standardized regimen to reduce skin surface pathogens that is performed by showering or bathing/washing with an antiseptic or soap prior to surgical or other invasive procedures.

Sequential application: Repeating the entire surgical skin preparation with the same or a different antiseptic before the incision is made.

Surgical site preparation: Preoperative treatment of the patient's skin in the OR or procedure room that includes not only the immediate site of the intended surgical incision but also a broader area of the patient's skin.

Targeted decolonization: A vertical approach in which a specific organism, such as *S aureus,* is targeted for screening and laboratory testing before decolonization.

Transient hypothyroidism: Low serum thyroxine (T4) and high thyroid stimulating hormone (TSH) caused by a change in metabolism of the thyroid gland after iodine absorption.

Universal decolonization: A horizontal approach that entails nasal or body decolonization of high-risk patients regardless of their colonization status.

References

1. Dumville JC, McFarlane E, Edwards P, Lipp A, Holmes A, Liu Z. Preoperative skin antiseptics for preventing surgical wound infections after clean surgery. *Cochrane Database Syst Rev.* 2015;4:CD003949. [IA]

2. Webster J, Osborne S. Preoperative bathing or showering with skin antiseptics to prevent surgical site infection. *Cochrane Database Syst Rev.* 2015;2:CD004985. [IA]

3. *Global Guidelines on the Prevention of Surgical Site Infection.* Geneva, Switzerland: World Health Organization; 2016. [IVB]

4. *Surgical Site Infections: Prevention and Treatment.* London, UK: National Institute for Health and Care Excellence (NICE); 2019. [IVA]

5. Lefebvre A, Saliou P, Lucet JC, et al. Preoperative hair removal and surgical site infections: network meta-analysis of randomized controlled trials. *J Hosp Infect.* 2015;91(2):100-108. [IA]

6. Guideline for sterile technique. In: *Guidelines for Perioperative Practice.* Denver, CO: AORN, Inc; 2021:943-984. [IVA]

7. Compendium of strategies to prevent healthcare-associated infections in acute care hospitals: 2014 update. The Society for Healthcare Epidemiology of America. https://www.shea-online.org/index.php/practice-resources/41-current-guidelines/417-compendium-of-strategies-to-prevent-healthcare-associated-infections-in-acute-care-hospitals-2014-update. Accessed February 15, 2021. [IVA]

8. Siegel JD, Rhinehart E, Jackson M, Chiarello L, eds. *Management of Multidrug-Resistant Organisms in Health Care Settings, 2006.* Centers for Disease Control and Prevention. https://www.cdc.gov/infectioncontrol/pdf/guidelines/mdro-guidelines.pdf. Updated February 15, 2017. Accessed February 15, 2021. [IVA]

9. Bratzler DW, Dellinger EP, Olsen KM, et al. Clinical practice guidelines for antimicrobial prophylaxis in surgery. *Am J Health Syst Pharm.* 2013;70(3):195-283. [IVA]

10. Edmiston CE Jr, Ledeboer NA, Buchan BW, Spencer M, Seabrook GR, Leaper D. Is staphylococcal screening and suppression an effective interventional strategy for reduction of surgical site infection? *Surg Infect (Larchmt).* 2016;17(2):158-166. [VA]

11. Ban KA, Minei JP, Laronga C, et al. Executive summary of the American College of Surgeons/Surgical Infection Society Surgical Site Infection Guidelines—2016 update. *Surg Infect.* 2017;18(4):379-382. [IVB]

12. Septimus EJ, Schweizer ML. Decolonization in prevention of health care–associated infections. *Clin Microbiol Rev.* 2016;29(2):201-222. [VA]

13. Anderson MJ, David ML, Scholz M, et al. Efficacy of skin and nasal povidone-iodine preparation against mupirocin-resistant methicillin-resistant *Staphylococcus aureus* and *S. aureus* within the anterior nares. *Antimicrob Agents Chemother.* 2015;59(5):2765-2773. [IIB]

14. Moroski NM, Woolwine S, Schwarzkopf R. Is preoperative staphylococcal decolonization efficient in total joint arthroplasty. *J Arthroplasty.* 2015;30(3):444-446. [IIIB]

15. Rezapoor M, Nicholson T, Tabatabaee RM, Chen AF, Maltenfort MG, Parvizi J. Povidone-iodine-based solutions for decolonization of nasal *Staphylococcus aureus*: a randomized, prospective, placebo-controlled study. *J Arthroplasty.* 2017;32(9):2815-2819. [IB]

16. Schweizer M, Perencevich E, McDanel J, et al. Effectiveness of a bundled intervention of decolonization and prophylaxis to decrease gram positive surgical site infections after cardiac or orthopedic surgery: systematic review and meta-analysis. *BMJ.* 2013;346:f2743. [IIA]

17. Ma N, Cameron A, Tivey D, Grae N, Roberts S, Morris A. Systematic review of a patient care bundle in reducing staphylococcal infections in cardiac and orthopaedic surgery. *ANZ J Surg.* 2017;87(4):239-246. [IIA]

18. Bode LG, Kluytmans JA, Wertheim HF, et al. Preventing surgical-site infections in nasal carriers of *Staphylococcus aureus*. *N Engl J Med.* 2010;362(1):9-17. [IA]

19. George S, Leasure AR, Horstmanshof D. Effectiveness of decolonization with chlorhexidine and mupirocin in reducing surgical site infections: a systematic review. *Dimens Crit Care Nurs.* 2016;35(4):204-222. [IIA]

20. Bode LG, van Rijen MM, Wertheim HF, et al. Long-term mortality after rapid screening and decolonization of *Staphylococcus aureus* carriers: observational follow-up study of a randomized, placebo-controlled trial. *Ann Surg.* 2016;263(3):511-515. [IIIA]

21. Liu Z, Norman G, Iheozor-Ejiofor Z, Wong JK, Crosbie EJ, Wilson P. Nasal decontamination for the prevention of surgical site infection in *Staphylococcus aureus* carriers. *Cochrane Database Syst Rev.* 2017;5:CD012462. [IA]

22. Ramos N, Stachel A, Phillips M, Vigdorchik J, Slover J, Bosco JA. Prior *Staphylococcus aureus* nasal colonization: a risk factor for surgical site infections following decolonization. *J Am Acad Orthop Surg.* 2016;24(12):880-885. [IIIA]

23. Kohler P, Sommerstein R, Schönrath F, et al. Effect of perioperative mupirocin and antiseptic body wash on infection rate and causative pathogens in patients undergoing cardiac surgery. *Am J Infect Control.* 2015;43(7):e33-e38. [IIA]

24. Reiser M, Scherag A, Forstner C, et al. Effect of pre-operative octenidine nasal ointment and showering on surgical site infections in patients undergoing cardiac surgery. *J Hosp Infect.* 2017;95(2):137-143. [IIA]

25. Saraswat MK, Magruder JT, Crawford TC, et al. Preoperative *Staphylococcus aureus* screening and targeted decolonization in cardiac surgery. *Ann Thorac Surg.* 2017;104(4):1349-1356. [IIA]

26. Schweizer ML, Chiang HY, Septimus E, et al. Association of a bundled intervention with surgical site infections among patients undergoing cardiac, hip, or knee surgery. *JAMA.* 2015;313(21):2162-2171. [IIA]

27. Mullen A, Wieland HJ, Wieser ES, Spannhake EW, Marinos RS. Perioperative participation of orthopedic patients and surgical staff in a nasal decolonization intervention to reduce Staphylococcus spp surgical site infections. *Am J Infect Control.* 2017;45(5):554-556. [IIB]

28. Romero-Palacios A, Petruccelli D, Main C, Winemaker M, de Beer J, Mertz D. Screening for and decolonization of *Staphylococcus aureus* carriers before total joint replacement is associated with lower *S aureus* prosthetic joint infection rates. *Am J Infect Control.* 2020;48(5):534-537. [IIB]

29. Sporer SM, Rogers T, Abella L. Methicillin-resistant and methicillin-sensitive *Staphylococcus aureus* screening and decolonization to reduce surgical site infection in elective total joint arthroplasty. *J Arthroplasty.* 2016;31(9 Suppl):144-147. [IIA]

30. Tsang STJ, McHugh MP, Guerendiain D, et al. Evaluation of *Staphylococcus aureus* eradication therapy in orthopaedic surgery. *J Med Microbiol.* 2018;67(6):893-901. [IIA]

31. Langenberg JC, Thomas AR, Donker JM, van Rijen MM, Kluytmans JA, van der Laan L. Evaluation of *Staphylococcus aureus* eradication therapy in vascular surgery. *PLoS One.* 2016;11(8):e0161058. [IIB]

32. Agarwala S, Lad D, Agashe V, Sobti A. Prevalence of MRSA colonization in an adult urban Indian population undergoing orthopaedic surgery. *J Clin Orthop Trauma.* 2016;7(1):12-16. [IIIA]

33. Thakkar V, Ghobrial GM, Maulucci CM, et al. Nasal MRSA colonization: impact on surgical site infection following spine surgery. *Clin Neurol Neurosurg.* 2014;125:94-97. [IIIB]

34. Baratz MD, Hallmark R, Odum SM, Springer BD. Twenty percent of patients may remain colonized with methicillin-resistant *Staphylococcus aureus* despite a decolonization protocol in patients undergoing elective total joint arthroplasty. *Clin Orthop Relat Res.* 2015;473(7):2283-2290. [IIA]

35. Herwaldt LA, Cullen JJ, French P, et al. Preoperative risk factors for nasal carriage of *Staphylococcus aureus. Infect Control Hosp Epidemiol.* 2004;25(6):481-484. [IIIA]

36. Campbell KA, Cunningham C, Hasan S, Hutzler L, Bosco JA 3rd. Risk factors for developing *Staphylococcus aureus* nasal colonization in spine and arthroplasty surgery. *Bull Hosp Jt Dis* (2013). 2015;73(4):276-281. [IIIA]

37. Botelho-Nevers E, Berthelot P, Verhoeven PO, et al. Are the risk factors associated with *Staphylococcus aureus* nasal carriage in patients the same than in healthy volunteers? Data from a cohort of patients scheduled for orthopedic material implantation. *Am J Infect Control.* 2014;42(10):1121-1123.

38. Strategies to prevent hospital-onset *Staphylococcus aureus* bloodstream infections in acute care facilities. Centers for Disease Control and Prevention. https://www.cdc.gov/hai/prevent/staph-prevention-strategies.html#. Reviewed December 16, 2019. Accessed February 15, 2021. [IVB]

39. Urias DS, Varghese M, Simunich T, Morrissey S, Dumire R. Preoperative decolonization to reduce infections in urgent lower extremity repairs. *Eur J Trauma Emerg Surg.* 2018;44(5):787-793. [IIIB]

40. Lemaignen A, Armand-Lefevre L, Birgand G, et al. Thirteen-year experience with universal *Staphylococcus aureus* nasal decolonization prior to cardiac surgery: a quasi-experimental study. *J Hosp Infect.* 2018;100(3):322-328. [IIA]

41. Phillips M, Rosenberg A, Shopsin B, et al. Preventing surgical site infections: a randomized, open-label trial of nasal mupirocin ointment and nasal povidone-iodine solution. *Infect Control Hosp Epidemiol.* 2014;35(7):826-832. [IA]

42. Hetem DJ, Vogely HC, Severs TT, Troelstra A, Kusters JG, Bonten MJ. Acquisition of high-level mupirocin resistance in CoNS following nasal decolonization with mupirocin. *J Antimicrob Chemother.* 2014;70(4):1182-1184. [IIA]

43. Stambough JB, Nam D, Warren DK, et al. Decreased hospital costs and surgical site infection incidence with a universal decolonization protocol in primary total joint arthroplasty. *J Arthroplasty.* 2017;32(3):728-734. [IIA]

44. Torres EG, Lindmair-Snell JM, Langan JW, Burnikel BG. Is preoperative nasal povidone-iodine as efficient and cost-effective as standard methicillin-resistant *Staphylococcus aureus* screening protocol in total joint arthroplasty? *J Arthroplasty.* 2016;31(1):215-218. [IIIA]

45. Loftus RW, Dexter F, Goodheart MJ, et al. The effect of improving basic preventive measures in the perioperative arena on *Staphylococcus aureus* transmission and surgical site infections: a randomized clinical trial. *JAMA Netw Open.* 2020;3(3):e201934 [IA]

46. Hong JC, Saraswat MK, Ellison TA, et al. *Staphylococcus aureus* prevention strategies in cardiac surgery: a cost-effectiveness analysis. *Ann Thorac Surg.* 2018;105(1):47-53. [IIA]

47. del Diego Salas J, Orly de Labry Lima A, Espín Balbino J, Bermúdez Tamayo C, Fernández-Crehuet Navajas J. An economic evaluation of two interventions for the prevention of post-surgical infections in cardiac surgery. *Rev Calid Asist.* 2016;31(1):27-33. [IIA]

48. Williams DM, Miller AO, Henry MW, Westrich GH, Ghomrawi HMK. Cost-effectiveness of *Staphylococcus aureus* decolonization strategies in high-risk total joint arthroplasty patients. *J Arthroplasty.* 2017;32(9S):S91-S96. [IIIB]

49. Masroor N, Golladay GJ, Williams J, et al. Healthcare worker perceptions of and barriers to universal staphylococcal decolonization in elective orthopaedic joint surgeries. *Infect Control Hosp Epidemiol.* 2016;37(3):355-356. [IIIB]

50. Kavanagh KT, Calderon LE, Saman DM, Abusalem SK. The use of surveillance and preventative measures for methicillin-resistant *Staphylococcus aureus* infections in surgical patients. *Antimicrob Resist Infect Control.* 2014;3(1):18. [VA]

51. Grimmer LE, Stafford TS, Milman S, Ng T. Efficacy of preoperative nasal *Staphylococcus aureus* screening and chlorhexidine chest scrub in decreasing the incidence of post-resection empyema. *Surg Infect (Larchmt).* 2014;15(2):118-122. [IIB]

52. Shrem G, Egozi T, Naeh A, Hallak M, Walfisch A. Pre-cesarean *Staphylococcus aureus* nasal screening and decolonization: a prospective randomized controlled trial. *J Matern Fetal Neonatal Med.* 2016;29(23):3906-3911. [IA]

53. Sasi SP, Sistla SC, Sistla S, et al. Decolonisation of MRSA and its effect on surgical site infections—a study in a tertiary care institute. *Int J Clin Pract.* 2015;69(3):366-374. [IIA]

54. Takahashi Y, Takesue Y, Uchino M, et al. Value of pre- and postoperative meticillin-resistant *Staphylococcus aureus* screening in patients undergoing gastroenterological surgery. *J Hosp Infect.* 2014;87(2):92-97. [IIIB]

55. Lefebvre J, Buffet-Bataillon S, Henaux PL, Riffaud L, Morandi X, Haegelen C. *Staphylococcus aureus* screening and decolonization reduces the risk of surgical site infections in patients undergoing deep brain stimulation surgery. *J Hosp Infect.* 2017;95(2):144-147. [IIA]

56. Sousa RJ, Barreira PM, Leite PT, Santos AC, Ramos MH, Oliveira AF. Preoperative *Staphylococcus aureus* screening/decolonization protocol before total joint arthroplasty—results of a small prospective randomized trial. *J Arthroplasty.* 2016;31(1):234-239. [IB]

57. Malcolm TL, Robinson LD, Klika AK, Ramanathan D, Higuera CA, Murray TG. Predictors of *Staphylococcus aureus* colonization and results after decolonization. *Interdiscip Perspect Infect Dis.* 2016;2016:4367156. [IIIA]

58. Kline SE, Neaton JD, Lynfield R, et al. Randomized controlled trial of a self-administered five-day antiseptic bundle versus usual disinfectant soap showers for preoperative eradication of *Staphylococcus aureus* colonization. *Infect Control Hosp Epidemiol.* 2018;39(9):1049-1057. [IA]

59. Smith MA, Dahlen NR. Clinical practice guideline surgical site infection prevention. *Orthop Nurs.* 2013;32(5):242-248. [IVB]

60. Bebko SP, Byers P, Green DM, Awad SS. Identification of methicillin-susceptible or methicillin-resistant *Staphylococcus aureus* carrier status preoperatively using polymerase chain reaction in patients undergoing elective surgery with hardware implantation. *Infect Control Hosp Epidemiol.* 2015;36(6):738-741. [IIIB]

61. Bebko SP, Green DM, Awad SS. Effect of a preoperative decontamination protocol on surgical site infections in patients undergoing elective orthopedic surgery with hardware implantation. *JAMA Surg.* 2015;150(5):390-395. [IIA]

62. Steed LL, Costello J, Lohia S, Jones T, Spannhake EW, Nguyen S. Reduction of nasal *Staphylococcus aureus* carriage in health care professionals by treatment with a non-antibiotic, alcohol-based nasal antiseptic. *Am J Infect Control.* 2014;42(8):841-846. [IB]

63. Maslow J, Hutzler L, Cuff G, Rosenberg A, Phillips M, Bosco J. Patient experience with mupirocin or povidone-iodine nasal decolonization. *Orthopedics.* 2014;37(6):e576-e581. [IIIA]

64. Standards of perioperative nursing. AORN, Inc. https://www.aorn.org/guidelines/clinical-resources/aorn-standards. Accessed February 15, 2015. [IVB]

65. Tschelaut L, Assadian O, Strauss R, et al. A survey on current knowledge, practice and beliefs related to preoperative antimicrobial decolonization regimens for prevention of surgical site infections among Austrian surgeons. *J Hosp Infect.* 2018;100(4):386-392. [IIA]

66. Muñoz-Gallego I, Infiesta L, Viedma E, Perez-Montarelo D, Chaves F. Chlorhexidine and mupirocin susceptibilities in methicillin-resistant *Staphylococcus aureus* isolates from bacteraemia and nasal colonisation. *J Glob Antimicrob Resist.* 2016;4:65-69. [IIIA]

67. Deeny SR, Worby CJ, Tosas Auguet O, et al. Impact of mupirocin resistance on the transmission and control of healthcare-associated MRSA. *J Antimicrob Chemother.* 2015;70(12):3366-3378. [IIIA]

68. Hetem DJ, Bootsma MC, Bonten MJ. Prevention of surgical site infections: Decontamination with mupirocin based on preoperative screening for *Staphylococcus aureus* carriers or universal decontamination? *Clin Infect Dis.* 2016;62(5):631-636. [IIIB]

69. Veiga DF, Damasceno CAV, Veiga Filho JV, et al. Influence of povidone-iodine preoperative showers on skin colonization in elective plastic surgery procedures. *Plast Reconstr Surg.* 2008;121(1):115-118. [IA]

70. Tanner J, Gould D, Jenkins P, Hilliam R, Mistry N, Walsh S. A fresh look at preoperative body washing. *J Infect Prev.* 2012;13(1):11-15. [IB]

71. Kamel C, McGahan L, Polisena J, Mierzwinski-Urban M, Embil JM. Preoperative skin antiseptic preparations for preventing surgical site infections: a systematic review. *Infect Control Hosp Epidemiol.* 2012;33(6):608-617. [IIA]

72. Colling K, Statz C, Glover J, Banton K, Beilman G. Preoperative antiseptic shower and bath policy decreases the rate of *S. aureus* and methicillin-resistant *S. aureus* surgical site infections in patients undergoing joint arthroplasty. *Surg Infect (Larchmt).* 2015;16(2):124-132. [IIA]

73. Cai Y, Xu K, Hou W, Yang Z, Xu P. Preoperative chlorhexidine reduces the incidence of surgical site infections in total knee and hip arthroplasty: a systematic review and meta-analysis. *Int J Surg.* 2017;39:221-228. [IIA]

74. Kapadia BH, Elmallah RK, Mont MA. A randomized, clinical trial of preadmission chlorhexidine skin preparation for lower extremity total joint arthroplasty. *J Arthroplasty.* 2016;31(12):2856-2861. [IB]

75. Kapadia BH, Jauregui JJ, Murray DP, Mont MA. Does preadmission cutaneous chlorhexidine preparation reduce surgical site infections after total hip arthroplasty? *Clin Orthop Relat Res.* 2016;474(7):1583-1588. [IIA]

76. Berríos-Torres SI, Umscheid CA, Bratzler DW, et al. Centers for Disease Control and Prevention Guideline for the Prevention of Surgical Site Infection, 2017. *JAMA Surg.* 2017;152(8):784-791. [IVA]

77. Jakobsson J, Perlkvist A, Wann-Hansson C. Searching for evidence regarding using preoperative disinfection showers to prevent surgical site infections: a systematic review. *Worldviews Evid Based Nurs.* 2011;8(3):143-152. [IIA]

78. Edmiston CE, Krepel CJ, Spencer MP, et al. Preadmission application of 2% chlorhexidine gluconate (CHG): enhancing patient compliance while maximizing skin surface concentrations. *Infect Control Hosp Epidemiol.* 2016;37(3):254-259. [IB]

79. de Castro Franco LM, Cota GF, Pinto TS, Ercole FF. Preoperative bathing of the surgical site with chlorhexidine for infection prevention: systematic review with meta-analysis. *Am J Infect Control.* 2017;45(4):343-349. [IA]

80. Chlebicki MP, Safdar N, O'Horo JC, Maki DG. Preoperative chlorhexidine shower or bath for prevention of surgical site infection: a meta-analysis. *Am J Infect Control.* 2013;41(2):167-173. [IIA]

81. Hsieh CS, Cheng HC, Lin JS, Kuo SJ, Chen YL. Effect of 4% chlorhexidine gluconate predisinfection skin scrub prior to hepatectomy: a double-blinded, randomized control study. *Int Surg.* 2014;99(6):787-794. [IB]

82. Karki S, Cheng AC. Impact of non-rinse skin cleansing with chlorhexidine gluconate on prevention of healthcare-associated infections and colonization with multi-resistant organisms: a systematic review. *J Hosp Infect.* 2012;82(2):71-84. [IIIA]

83. Eck CF, Neumann JA, Limpisvasti O, Adams CR. Lack of level I evidence on how to prevent infection after elective shoulder surgery. *Knee Surg Sports Traumatol Arthrosc.* 2018;26(8):2465-2480. [IIIA]

84. Edmiston CE Jr, Seabrook GR, Johnson CP, Paulson DS, Beausoleil CM. Comparative of a new and innovative 2% chlorhexidine gluconate-impregnated cloth with 4% chlorhexidine gluconate as topical antiseptic for preparation of the skin prior to surgery. *Am J Infect Control.* 2007;35(2):89-96. [IB]

85. Edmiston CE Jr, Krepel CJ, Seabrook GR, Lewis BD, Brown KR, Towne JB. Preoperative shower revisited: can high topical antiseptic levels be achieved on the skin surface before surgical admission? *J Am Coll Surg.* 2008;207(2):233-239. [IB]

86. Graling PR, Vasaly FW. Effectiveness of 2% CHG cloth bathing for reducing surgical site infections. *AORN J.* 2013;97(5):547-551. [IIB]

87. Johnson AJ, Kapadia BH, Daley JA, Molina CB, Mont MA. Chlorhexidine reduces infections in knee arthroplasty. *J Knee Surg.* 2013;26(3):213-218. [IIB]

88. Zywiel MG, Daley JA, Delanois RE, Naziri Q, Johnson AJ, Mont MA. Advance pre-operative chlorhexidine reduces the incidence of surgical site infections in knee arthroplasty. *Int Orthop.* 2011;35(7):1001-1006. [IIB]

89. Johnson AJ, Daley JA, Zywiel MG, Delanois RE, Mont MA. Preoperative chlorhexidine preparation and the incidence of surgical site infections after hip arthroplasty. *J Arthroplasty.* 2010;25(6 Suppl):98-102. [IIB]

90. Farber NJ, Chen AF, Bartsch SM, Feigel JL, Klatt BA. No infection reduction using chlorhexidine wipes in total joint arthroplasty. *Clin Orthop Relat Res.* 2013;471(10):3120-3125. [IIA]

91. Berrondo C, Ahn JJ, Shnorhavorian M. Pre-operative skin antisepsis with chlorhexidine gluconate baths and wipes does not prevent postoperative surgical site infection in out-patient pediatric urologic inguinal and scrotal surgery. *J Pediatr Urol.* 2019;15(6):652.e1-652.e7. [IIA]

92. Makhni MC, Jegede K, Lombardi J, et al. No clear benefit of chlorhexidine use at home before surgical preparation. *J Am Acad Orthop Surg.* 2018;26(2):e39-e47. [IIC]

93. ACOG Practice Bulletin No. 195: Prevention of infection after gynecologic procedures. *Obstet Gynecol.* 2018;131(6): e172-e189. [IVB]

94. Edmiston CE Jr, Krepel CJ, Edmiston SE, et al. Empowering the surgical patient: a randomized, prospective analysis of an innovative strategy for improving patient compliance with preadmission showering protocol. *J Am Coll Surg.* 2014;219(2):256-264. [IB]

95. Edmiston CE Jr, Lee CJ, Krepel CJ, et al. Evidence for a standardized preadmission showering regimen to achieve maximal antiseptic skin surface concentrations of chlorhexidine gluconate, 4%, in surgical patients. *JAMA Surg.* 2015;150(11):1027-1033. [IB]

96. Guideline for medical device and product evaluation. In: *Guidelines for Perioperative Practice.* Denver, CO: AORN, Inc; 2021:719-728. [IVB]

97. Boyce JM. Best products for skin antisepsis. *Am J Infect Control.* 2019;47S:A17-A22. [VA]

98. Persichino J, Lee H, Sutjita M, Talavera K, San-Agustin G, Gnass S. Reducing the rate of surgical site infections after breast surgery with the use of larger volumes of 4% chlorhexidine gluconate solution as preoperative antiseptic showering. *Infect Control Hosp Epidemiol.* 2017;38(3):373-375. [IIB]

99. Supple L, Kumaraswami M, Kundrapu S, et al. Chlorhexidine only works if applied correctly: use of a simple colorimetric assay to provide monitoring and feedback on effectiveness of chlorhexidine application. *Infect Control Hosp Epidemiol.* 2015;36(9):1095-1097. [VB]

100. Qvistgaard M, Almerud Österberg S, Heikkilä K, Thorén A, Lovebo J. Patients' experiences with at-home preoperative skin disinfection before elective hip replacement surgery. *J Periop Pract.* 2017;27(7-8):162-166. [IIIB]

101. Arrowsmith VA, Taylor R. Removal of nail polish and finger rings to prevent surgical infection. *Cochrane Database Syst Rev.* 2014;8:CD003325. [IA]

102. McNeil SA, Foster CL, Hedderwick SA, Kauffman CA. Effect of hand cleansing with antimicrobial soap or alcohol-based gel on microbial colonization of artificial fingernails worn by health care workers. *Clin Infect Dis.* 2001;32(3):367-372. [IIA]

103. Guideline for hand hygiene. In: *Guidelines for Perioperative Practice.* Denver, CO: AORN, Inc; 2021:267-292. [IVB]

104. Kulkarni V, Murray A, Mittal R, Spence D, O'Kane G, Incoll I. Microbial counts in hands with and without nail varnish after surgical skin preparation: a randomized control trial. *J Hand Surg Eur Vol.* 2018;43(8):832-835. [IB]

105. Leclair JM, Winston KR, Sullivan BF, O'Connell JM, Harrington SM, Goldmann DA. Effect of preoperative shampoos on resident scalp flora. *Todays OR Nurse.* 1988;10(3):15-21. [IB]

106. Scheer VM, Bergman Jungeström M, Lerm M, Serrander L, Kalén A. Topical benzoyl peroxide application on the shoulder reduces *Propionibacterium acnes*: a randomized study. *J Shoulder Elbow Surg.* 2018;27(6):957-961. [IB]

107. Kolakowski L, Lai JK, Duvall GT, et al. Neer Award 2018: Benzoyl peroxide effectively decreases preoperative *Cutibacterium acnes* shoulder burden: a prospective randomized controlled trial. *J Shoulder Elbow Surg.* 2018;27(9):1539-1544. [IB]

108. Sabetta JR, Rana VP, Vadasdi KB, et al. Efficacy of topical benzoyl peroxide on the reduction of *Propionibacterium acnes* during shoulder surgery. *J Shoulder Elbow Surg.* 2015;24(7):995-1004. [IIB]

109. Dizay HH, Lau DG, Nottage WM. Benzoyl peroxide and clindamycin topical skin preparation decreases *Propionibacterium acnes* colonization in shoulder arthroscopy. *J Shoulder Elbow Surg.* 2017;26(7):1190-1195. [IIB]

110. Saltzman MD, Nuber GW, Gryzlo SM, Marecek GS, Koh JL. Efficacy of surgical preparation solutions in shoulder surgery. *J Bone Joint Surg Am.* 2009;91(8):1949-1953. [IA]

111. Lee MJ, Pottinger PS, Butler-Wu S, Bumgarner RE, Russ SM, Matsen FA 3rd. *Propionibacterium* persists in the skin despite standard surgical preparation. *J Bone Joint Surg Am.* 2014;96(17):1447-1450. [IIC]

112. Hancock DS, Rupasinghe SL, Elkinson I, Bloomfield MG, Larsen PD. Benzoyl peroxide + chlorhexidine versus chlorhexidine alone skin preparation to reduce *Propionibacterium acnes*: a randomized controlled trial. *ANZ J Surg.* 2018;88(11):1182-1186. [IB]

113. Tanner J, Norrie P, Melen K. Preoperative hair removal to reduce surgical site infection. *Cochrane Database Syst Rev.* 2011;11:CD004122. [IA]

114. Cruse PJ, Foord R. A five-year prospective study of 23,649 surgical wounds. *Arch Surg.* 1973;107(2):206-210.

115. Broekman ML, van Beijnum J, Peul WC, Regli L. Neurosurgery and shaving: what's the evidence? *J Neurosurg.* 2011;115(4):670-678. [IIIA]

116. Sebastian S. Does preoperative scalp shaving result in fewer postoperative wound infections when compared with no scalp shaving? A systematic review. *J Neurosci Nurs.* 2012;44(3):149-156. [IIIA]

117. Marecek GS, Weatherford BM, Fuller EB, Saltzman MD. The effect of axillary hair on surgical antisepsis around the shoulder. *J Shoulder Elbow Surg.* 2015;24(5):804-808. [IB]

118. Shi D, Yao Y, Yu W. Comparison of preoperative hair removal methods for the reduction of surgical site infections: a meta-analysis. *J Clin Nurs.* 2017;26(19-20):2907-2914. [IIA]

119. Guideline for a safe environment of care. In: *Guidelines for Perioperative Practice*. Denver, CO: AORN, Inc; 2021:109-144. [IVB]

120. Kowalski TJ, Kothari SN, Mathiason MA, Borgert AJ. Impact of hair removal on surgical site infection rates: a prospective randomized noninferiority trial. *J Am Coll Surg.* 2016;223(5):704-711. [IA]

121. Ng W, Alexander D, Kerr B, Ho MF, Amato M, Katz K. A hairy tale: successful patient education strategies to reduce prehospital hair removal by patients undergoing elective caesarean section. *J Hosp Infect.* 2013;83(1):64-67. [IIIB]

122. ChloraPrep One-step – chlorhexidine gluconate and isopropyl alcohol solution. NDC Code: 54365-400-12. US National Library of Medicine. DailyMed. https://dailymed.nlm.nih.gov/dailymed/drugInfo.cfm?setid=77a8858e-2b3e-4b13-83ed-c989b7cc554c. Accessed February 18, 2021.

123. 3M DuraPrep Surgical – iodine povacrylex and isopropyl alcohol solution. NDC Code: 17518-011-07. US National Library of Medicine. DailyMed. https://dailymed.nlm.nih.gov/dailymed/drugInfo.cfm?setid=22a10a54-6a04-48b3-9ec4-b26526183daf. Accessed February 18, 2021.

124. Kose G, Tastan S, Kutlay M, Bedir O. The effects of different types of hair shaving on the body image and surgical site infection in elective cranial surgery. *J Clin Nurs.* 2016;25(13-14):1876-1885. [IA]

125. Basevi V, Lavender T. Routine perineal shaving on admission in labour. *Cochrane Database Syst Rev.* 2014;11:CD001236. [IA]

126. Grober ED, Domes T, Fanipour M, Copp JE. Preoperative hair removal on the male genitalia: clippers vs. razors. *J Sex Med.* 2013;10(2):589-594. [IB]

127. Razors and Preoperative Preparation of the Male Genitalia. Sexual Medicine Society of North America, Inc. https://www.smsna.org/images/Razors.pdf. Revised January 2020. Accessed February 15, 2021. [IVB]

128. Edmiston CE Jr, Griggs RK, Tanner J, Spencer M, Seabrook GR, Leaper D. Perioperative hair removal in the 21st century: utilizing an innovative vacuum-assisted technology to safely expedite hair removal before surgery. *Am J Infect Control.* 2016;44(12):1639-1644. [IB]

129. Harris PN, Ashhurst-Smith C, Berenger SJ, Shoobert A, Ferguson JK. Adhesive tape in the health care setting: another high-risk fomite? *Med J Aust.* 2012;196(1):34. [IIIB]

130. Leng P, Huang WL, He T, Wang YZ, Zhang HN. Outbreak of Serratia marcescens postoperative infection traced to barbers and razors. *J Hosp Infect.* 2015;89(1):46-50. [VA]

131. Kim EJ, Park WB, Yoon JK, et al. Outbreak investigation of Serratia marcescens neurosurgical site infections associated with a contaminated shaving razors. *Antimicrob Resist Infect Control.* 2020;9(1):64. [VA]

132. Dai Y, Zhang C, Ma X, et al. Outbreak of carbapenemase-producing *Klebsiella pneumoniae* neurosurgical site infections associated with a contaminated shaving razor used for preoperative scalp shaving. *Am J Infect Control.* 2014;42(7):805-806. [VB]

133. Noorani A, Rabey N, Walsh SR, Davies RJ. Systematic review and meta-analysis of preoperative antisepsis with chlorhexidine versus povidone-iodine in clean-contaminated surgery. *Br J Surg.* 2010;97(11):1614-1620. [IIB]

134. Ayoub F, Quirke M, Conroy RM, Hill ADK. Chlorhexidine-alcohol versus povidone-iodine for pre-operative skin preparation: a systematic review and meta-analysis. *Int J Surg* Open. 2016. doi:10.1016/j.ijso.2016.02.002. [IA]

135. Anggrahita T, Wardhana A, Sudjatmiko G. Chlorhexidine-alcohol versus povidone-iodine as preoperative skin preparation to prevent surgical site infection: a meta-analysis. *Med J Indones.* 2017;26(1):54-61. [IA]

136. Harnoss JC, Assadian O, Kramer A, et al. Comparison of chlorhexidine-isopropanol with isopropanol skin antisepsis

for prevention of surgical-site infection after abdominal surgery. *Br J Surg.* 2018;105(7):893-899. [IIB]

137. Madej T, Plötze K, Birkner C, Jatzwauk L, Klaus M, Waldow T. Reducing mediastinitis after sternotomy with combined chlorhexidine-isopropyl alcohol skin disinfection: analysis of 3,000 patients. *Surg Infect.* 2016;17(5):552-556. [IIA]

138. Privitera GP, Costa AL, Brusaferro S, et al. Skin antisepsis with chlorhexidine versus iodine for the prevention of surgical site infection: a systematic review and meta-analysis. *Am J Infect Control.* 2017;45(2):180-189. [IIB]

139. Hakkarainen TW, Dellinger EP, Evans HL, et al. Comparative effectiveness of skin antiseptic agents in reducing surgical site infections: a report from the Washington State Surgical Care and Outcomes Assessment Program. *J Am Coll Surg.* 2014;218(3):336-344. [IIA]

140. Maiwald M, Chan ES. The forgotten role of alcohol: aa systematic review and meta-analysis of the clinical efficacy and perceived role of chlorhexidine in skin antisepsis. *PLoS One.* 2012;7(9):e42277. [IIA]

141. Charles D, Heal CF, Delpachitra M, et al. Alcoholic versus aqueous chlorhexidine for skin antisepsis: the AVALANCHE trial. *CMAJ.* 2017;189(31):E1008-E1016. [IA]

142. Young HL, Reese S, Knepper B, Miller A, Mauffrey C, Price CS. The effect of preoperative skin preparation products on surgical site infection. *Infect Control Hosp Epidemiol.* 2014;35(12):1535-1538. [IIIB]

143. Da Costa A, Tulane C, Dauphinot V, et al. Preoperative skin antiseptics for prevention of cardiac implantable electronic device infections: a historical-controlled interventional trial comparing aqueous against alcoholic povidone-iodine solutions. *Europace.* 2015;17(7):1092-1098. [IIA]

144. Digison MB. A review of anti-septic agents for pre-operative skin preparation. *Plast Surg Nurs.* 2007;27(4):185-189. [VB]

145. Murkin CE. Pre-operative antiseptic skin preparation. *Br J Nurs.* 2009;18(11):665-669. [VA]

146. Broach RB, Paulson EC, Scott C, Mahmoud NN. Randomized controlled trial of two alcohol-based preparations for surgical site antisepsis in colorectal surgery. *Ann Surg.* 2017;266(6):946-951. [IA]

147. Hannan MM, O'Sullivan KE, Higgins AM, et al. The combined impact of surgical team education and chlorhexidine 2% alcohol on the reduction of surgical site infection following cardiac surgery. *Surg Infect.* 2015;16(6):799-805. [IIB]

148. Yammine K, Harvey A. Efficacy of preparation solutions and cleansing techniques on contamination of the skin in foot and ankle surgery: a systematic review and meta-analysis. *Bone Joint J.* 2013;95-B(4):498-503. [IB]

149. Peel TN, Dowsey MM, Buising KL, Cheng AC, Choong PFM. Chlorhexidine-alcohol versus iodine-alcohol for surgical site skin preparation in an elective arthroplasty (ACAISA) study: a cluster randomized controlled trial. *Clin Microbiol Infect.* 2019;25(10):1239-1245. [IA]

150. Swenson BR, Hedrick TL, Metzger R, Bonatti H, Pruett TL, Sawyer RG. Effects of preoperative skin preparation on postoperative wound infection rates: a prospective study

of 3 skin preparation protocols. *Infect Control Hosp Epidemiol.* 2009;30(10):964-971. [IIB]

151. Raja SG, Rochon M, Mullins C, et al. Impact of choice of skin preparation solution in cardiac surgery on rate of surgical site infection: a propensity score matched analysis. *J Infect Prev.* 2018;19(1):16-21. [IIA]

152. Charehbili A, Swijnenburg RJ, van de Velde C, van den Bremer J, van Gijn W. A retrospective analysis of surgical site infections after chlorhexidine-alcohol versus iodine-alcohol for pre-operative antisepsis. *Surg Infect (Larchmt).* 2014;15(3): 310-313. [IIIA]

153. Ngai IM, Van Arsdale A, Govindappagari S, et al. Skin preparation for prevention of surgical site infection after cesarean delivery: a randomized controlled trial. *Obstet Gynecol.* 2015;126(6):1251-1257. [IA]

154. Shadid MB, Speth MJGM, Voorn GP, Wolterbeek N. Chlorhexidine 0.5%/70% alcohol and iodine 1%/70% alcohol both reduce bacterial load in clean foot surgery: a randomized, controlled trial. *J Foot Ankle Surg.* 2019;58(2):278-281. [IB]

155. Savage JW, Weatherford BM, Sugrue PA, et al. Efficacy of surgical preparation solutions in lumbar spine surgery. *J Bone Joint Surg Am.* 2012;94(6):490-494. [IA]

156. Carvajal J, Carvajal M, Hernández G. Back to basics: could the preoperative skin antiseptic agent help prevent biofilm-related capsular contracture? *Aesth Surg J.* 2019;39(8):848-859. [IIB]

157. Letzelter J, Hill JB, Hacquebord J. An overview of skin antiseptics used in orthopaedic surgery procedures. *J Am Acad Orthop Surg.* 2019;27(16):599-606. [VA]

158. Tolcher MC, Whitham MD, El-Nashar SA, Clark SL. Chlorhexidine–alcohol compared with povidone–iodine preoperative skin antisepsis for cesarean delivery: a systematic review and meta-analysis. *Am J Perinatol.* 2019;36(2):118-123. [IA]

159. Hadiati DR, Hakimi M, Nurdiati DS, Ota E. Skin preparation for preventing infection following caesarean section. *Cochrane Database Syst Rev.* 2014;9:CD007462 [IA]

160. Dior UP, Kathurusinghe S, Cheng C, et al. Effect of surgical skin antisepsis on surgical site infections in patients undergoing gynecological laparoscopic surgery: a double-blind randomized clinical trial. *JAMA Surg.* 2020;155(9):807-815. [IA]

161. Elshamy E, Ali YZA, Khalafallah M, Soliman A. Chlorhexidine-alcohol versus povidone-iodine for skin preparation before elective cesarean section: a prospective observational study. *J Matern Fetal Neonatal Med.* 2020;33(2):272-276. [IIA]

162. Uppal S, Bazzi A, Reynolds RK, et al. Chlorhexidine-alcohol compared with povidone-iodine for preoperative topical antisepsis for abdominal hysterectomy. *Obstet Gynecol.* 2017;130(2):319-327. [IIA]

163. Park HM, Han SS, Lee EC, et al. Randomized clinical trial of preoperative skin antisepsis with chlorhexidine gluconate or povidone-iodine. *Br J Surg.* 2017;104(2):e145-e150. [IA]

164. Srinivas A, Kaman L, Raj P, et al. Comparison of the efficacy of chlorhexidine gluconate versus povidone iodine as preoperative skin preparation for the prevention of surgical

site infections in clean-contaminated upper abdominal surgeries. *Surg Today.* 2015;45(11):1378-1384. [IA]

165. Kaoutzanis C, Kavanagh CM, Leichtle SW, et al. Chlorhexidine with isopropyl alcohol versus iodine povacrylex with isopropyl alcohol and alcohol- versus nonalcohol-based skin preparations: the incidence of and readmissions for surgical site infections after colorectal operations. *Dis Colon Rectum.* 2015;58(6):588-596. [IIIA]

166. Kleeff J, Erkan M, Jäger C, Menacher M, Gebhardt F, Hartel M. Umbilical microflora, antiseptic skin preparation, and surgical site infection in abdominal surgery. *Surg Infect (Larchmt).* 2015;16(4):450-454. [IIB]

167. Spaziani E, Di Filippo A, Orelli S, et al. Pre-operative skin antisepsis with chlorhexidine gluconate and povidone-iodine to prevent port-site infection in laparoscopic cholecystectomy: a prospective study. *Surg Infect (Larchmt).* 2018;19(3):334-338. [IIIB]

168. Said NS. Comparison between uses of chlorhexidine gluconate versus povidone iodine for skin preparation to prevent infection after cardiothoracic surgery. *IOSR J Nurs Health Sci.* 2017;6(2):72-80. [IIA]

169. Qintar M, Zardkoohi O, Hammadah M, et al. The impact of changing antiseptic skin preparation agent used for cardiac implantable electronic device (CIED) procedures on the risk of infection. *Pacing Clin Electrophysiol.* 2015;38(2):240-246. [IIB]

170. Asundi A, Stanislawski M, Mehta P, et al. Real-world effectiveness of infection prevention interventions for reducing procedure-related cardiac device infections: insights from the Veterans Affairs clinical assessment reporting and tracking program. *Infect Control Hosp Epidemiol.* 2019;40(8):855-862. [IIIA]

171. Casey A, Itrakjy A, Birkett C, et al. A comparison of the efficacy of 70% v/v isopropyl alcohol with either 0.5% w/v or 2% w/v chlorhexidine gluconate for skin preparation before harvest of the long saphenous vein used in coronary artery bypass grafting. *Am J Infect Control.* 2015;43(8):816-820. [IB]

172. Davis FM, Sutzko DC, Grey SF, et al. Predictors of surgical site infection after open lower extremity revascularization. *J Vasc Surg.* 2017;65(6):1769-1778. [IIIA]

173. Xu PZ, Fowler JR, Goitz RJ. Prospective randomized trial comparing the efficacy of surgical preparation solutions in hand surgery. *Hand* (N Y). 2017;12(3):258-264. [IB]

174. Becerro de Bengoa Vallejo R, Losa Iglesias ME, Alou Cervera L, Sevillano Fernández D, Prieto Prieto J. Preoperative skin and nail preparation of the foot: comparison of the efficacy of 4 different methods in reducing bacterial load. *J Am Acad Dermatol.* 2009;61(6):986-992. [IB]

175. Ritter B, Herlyn PKE, Mittlmeier T, Herlyn A. Preoperative skin antisepsis using chlorhexidine may reduce surgical wound infections in lower limb trauma surgery when compared to povidone-iodine: a prospective randomized trial. *Am J Infect Control.* 2020;48(2):167-172. [IB]

176. Heckmann N, Sivasundaram L, Heidari KS, et al. *Propionibacterium acnes* persists despite various skin preparation techniques. *Arthroscopy.* 2018;34(6):1786-1789. [IIB]

177. Blonna D, Allizond V, Bellato E, et al. Single versus double skin preparation for infection prevention in proximal

humeral fracture surgery. *Biomed Res Int.* 2018;2018:8509527. [IIB]

178. Yoshii T, Hirai T, Yamada T, et al. A prospective comparative study in skin antiseptic solutions for posterior spine surgeries: chlorhexidine-gluconate ethanol versus povidone-iodine. *Clin Spine Surg.* 2018;31(7):E353-E356. [IIB]

179. Ghobrial GM, Wang MY, Green BA, et al. Preoperative skin antisepsis with chlorhexidine gluconate versus povidone-iodine: a prospective analysis of 6959 consecutive spinal surgery patients. *J Neurosurg Spine.* 2018;28(2):209-214. [IIA]

180. Cardinal Health – chlorhexidine gluconate 4% liquid. NDC Code: 63517-061. US National Library of Medicine. DailyMed. https://dailymed.nlm.nih.gov/dailymed/drugInfo.cfm?setid=1b9c46b7-6515-1b9a-e054-00144ff88e88. Accessed February 18, 2021.

181. Sviggum HP, Jacob AK, Arendt KW, Mauermann ML, Horlocker TT, Hebl JR. Neurologic complications after chlorhexidine antisepsis for spinal anesthesia. *Reg Anesth Pain Med.* 2012;37(2):139-144. [IIIB]

182. Eason E, Wells G, Garber G, et al. Antisepsis for abdominal hysterectomy: a randomised controlled trial of povidone-iodine gel. *BJOG.* 2004;111(7):695-699. [IA]

183. Rastogi S, Glaser L, Friedman J, Carter IV, Milad MP. Tolerance of chlorhexidine gluconate vaginal cleansing solution: a randomized controlled trial. *J Gynecol Surg.* 2020;36(1):13-19. [IB]

184. Culligan PJ, Kubik K, Murphy M, Blackwell L, Snyder J. A randomized trial that compared povidone iodine and chlorhexidine as antiseptics for vaginal hysterectomy. *Am J Obstet Gynecol.* 2005;192(2):422-425. [IA]

185. Al-Niaimi A, Rice LW, Shitanshu U, et al. Safety and tolerability of chlorhexidine gluconate (2%) as a vaginal operative preparation in patients undergoing gynecologic surgery. *Am J Infect Control.* 2016;44(9):996-998. [IIB]

186. Amstey MS, Jones AP. Preparation of the vagina for surgery. A comparison of povidone-iodine and saline solution. *JAMA.* 1981;245(8):839-841. [IIIB]

187. Lewis LA, Lathi RB, Crochet P, Nezhat C. Preoperative vaginal preparation with baby shampoo compared with povidone-iodine before gynecologic procedures. *J Minim Invasive Gynecol.* 2007;14(6):736-739. [IIA]

188. Haas DM, Morgan S, Contreras K. Vaginal preparation with antiseptic solution before cesarean section for preventing postoperative infections. *Cochrane Database Syst Rev.* 2014;9:CD007892. [IA]

189. Caissutti C, Saccone G, Zullo F, et al. Vaginal cleansing before cesarean delivery: a systematic review and meta-analysis. *Obstet Gynecol.* 2017;130(3):527-538. [IA]

190. Aref NK. Vaginal cleansing prior to caesarian section: to do or not to do? A randomized trial. *J Gynecol Obstet Hum Reprod.* 2019;48(1):65-68. [IB]

191. Lakhi NA, Tricorico G, Osipova Y, Moretti ML. Vaginal cleansing with chlorhexidine gluconate or povidone-iodine prior to cesarean delivery: a randomized comparator-controlled trial. *Am J Obstet Gynecol MFM.* 2019;1(1):2-9. [IA]

192. La Rosa M, Jauk V, Saade G, et al. Institutional protocols for vaginal preparation with antiseptic solution and surgical

site infection rate in women undergoing cesarean delivery during labor. *Obstet Gynecol.* 2018;132(2):371-376. [IIA]

193. Quiroga LP, Lansingh V, Laspina F, et al. A prospective study demonstrating the effect of 5% povidone-iodine application for anterior segment intraocular surgery in Paraguay. *Arq Bras Oftalmol.* 2010;73(2):125-128. [IIA]

194. Wu PC, Li M, Chang SJ, et al. Risk of endophthalmitis after cataract surgery using different protocols for povidone-iodine preoperative disinfection. *J Ocul Pharmacol Ther.* 2006;22(1):54-61. [IIA]

195. Baillif S, Roure-Sobas C, Le-Duff F, Kodjikian L. Aqueous humor contamination during phacoemulsification in a university teaching hospital. *J Fr Opthalmol.* 2012;35(3):153-156. [IIIB]

196. Olson RJ, Braga-Mele R, Chen SH, et al. Cataract in the adult eye preferred practice pattern. *Ophthalmology.* 2017;124(2):P1-P119. [IVA]

197. Li B, Nentwich MM, Hoffmann LE, et al. Comparison of the efficacy of povidone-iodine 1.0%, 5.0%, and 10.0% irrigation combined with topical levofloxacin 0.3% as preoperative prophylaxis in cataract surgery. *J Cataract Refract Surg.* 2013;39(7):994-1001. [IA]

198. Nguyen CL, Oh LJ, Wong E, Francis IC. Povidone-iodine 3-minute exposure time is viable in preparation for cataract surgery. *Eur J Ophthalmol.* 2017;27(5):573-576. [VA]

199. Razavi B, Zollinger R, Kramer A, et al. Systemic iodine absorption associated with the use of preoperative ophthalmic antiseptics containing iodine. *Cutan Ocul Toxicol.* 2013;32(4):279-282. [IIB]

200. Garcia GA, Nguyen CV, Yonkers MA, Tao JP. Baby shampoo versus povidone-iodine or isopropyl alcohol in reducing eyelid skin bacterial load. Ophthalmic *Plast Reconstr Surg.* 2018;34(1):43-48. [IB]

201. Safety and effectiveness of health care antiseptics; topical antimicrobial drug products for over-the-counter human use. Final rule. *Fed Regist.* 2017;82(242):60474-60503.

202. FDA drug safety communication: FDA requests label changes and single-use packaging for some over-the-counter topical antiseptic products to decrease risk of infection. US Food and Drug Administration. https://www.fda.gov/drugs/drug-safety-and-availability/fda-drug-safety-communication-fda-requests-label-changes-and-single-use-packaging-some-over-counter. Accessed February 15, 2021.

203. Questions and answers: FDA requests label changes and single-use packaging for some over-the-counter topical antiseptic products to decrease risk of infection. US Food and Drug Administration. https://www.fda.gov/drugs/drug-safety-and-availability/questions-and-answers-fda-requests-label-changes-and-single-use-packaging-some-over-counter-topical. Accessed February 15, 2021.

204. Pearce BA, Miller LH, Martin MA, Roush DL. Efficacy of clean v sterile surgical prep kits. *AORN J.* 1997;66(3):464-470. [IB]

205. Sullivan PJ, Healy CE, Hirpara KM, Hussey AJ, Potter SM, Kelly JL. An assessment of skin preparation in upper limb surgery. *J Hand Surg Eur Vol.* 2008;33(4):513-514. [IIB]

206. McDaniel CM, Churchill RW, Argintar E. Visibility of tinted chlorhexidine gluconate skin preparation on varied skin pigmentations. *Orthopedics.* 2017;40(1):e44-e48. [IIC]

207. Quatresooz P, Xhauflaire-Uhoda E, Piérard-Franchimont C, Piérard GE. Regional variability in stratum corneum reactivity to antiseptic formulations. *Contact Dermatitis.* 2007;56(5):271-273. [IIIB]

208. Sanders TH, Hawken SM. Chlorhexidine burns after shoulder arthroscopy. *Am J Orthop (Belle Mead NJ).* 2012;41(4):172-174. [VB]

209. Sicherer SH. Risk of severe allergic reactions from the use of potassium iodide for radiation emergencies. *J Allergy Clin Immunol.* 2004;114(6):1395-1397. [IVB]

210. Schabelman E, Witting M. The relationship of radiocontrast, iodine, and seafood allergies: a medical myth exposed. *J Emerg Med.* 2010;39(5):701-707. [VA]

211. Huang SW. Seafood and iodine: an analysis of a medical myth. *Allergy Asthma Proc.* 2005;26(6):468-469. [IIIC]

212. Yasuda T, Hasegawa T, Yamato Y, et al. Optimal timing of preoperative skin preparation with povidone-iodine for spine surgery: a prospective, randomized controlled study. *Asian Spine J.* 2015;9(3):423-426. [IB]

213. Adachi A, Fukunaga A, Hayashi K, Kunisada M, Horikawa T. Anaphylaxis to polyvinylpyrrolidone after vaginal application of povidone-iodine. *Contact Dermatitis.* 2003;48(3):133-136. [VA]

214. Castelain F, Girardin P, Moumane L, Aubin F, Pelletier F. Anaphylactic reaction to povidone in a skin antiseptic. *Contact Dermatitis.* 2016;74(1):55-56. [VB]

215. Odedra KM, Farooque S. Chlorhexidine: an unrecognised cause of anaphylaxis. *Postgrad Med J.* 2014;90(1070):709-714. [VB]

216. Toomey M. Preoperative chlorhexidine anaphylaxis in a patient scheduled for coronary artery bypass graft: a case report. *AANA J.* 2013;81(3):209-214. [VA]

217. Khan RA, Kazi T, O'Donohoe B. Near fatal intra-operative anaphylaxis to chlorhexidine—is it time to change practice? *BMJ Case Rep.* 2011;bcr0920092300. [VA]

218. Dick AG, Dhinsa B, Walker RP, Singh S. Delayed allergic reaction to ChloraPrepTM in foot and ankle surgery. *J Foot Ankle Surg.* 2019;58(1):192-194. [VA]

219. FDA drug safety podcast: FDA warns about rare but serious allergic reactions with the skin antiseptic chlorhexidine gluconate. US Food and Drug Administration. https://www.fda.gov/drugs/fda-drug-safety-podcasts/fda-drug-safety-podcast-fda-warns-about-rare-serious-allergic-reactions-skin-antiseptic?source=govdelivery&utm_medium=email&utm_source=govdelivery. Accessed February 15, 2021.

220. Yoshida K, Sakurai Y, Kawahara S, et al. Anaphylaxis to polyvinylpyrrolidone in povidone-iodine for impetigo contagiosum in a boy with atopic dermatitis. *Int Arch Allergy Immunol.* 2008;146(2):169-173. [VB]

221. Leung AM, Braverman LE. Consequences of excess iodine. *Nat Rev Endocrinol.* 2014;10(3):136-142. [VA]

222. Lavelle KJ, Doedens DJ, Kleit SA, Forney RB. Iodine absorption in burn patients treated topically with povidone-iodine. *Clin Pharmacol Ther.* 1975;17(3):355-362. [VB]

223. Robertson P, Fraser J, Sheild J, Weir P. Thyrotoxicosis related to iodine toxicity in a paediatric burn patient. *Intensive Care Med.* 2002;28(9):1369. [VB]

224. Pietsch J, Meakins JL. Complications of povidone-iodine absorption in topically treated burn patients. *Lancet.* 1976;1(7954):280-282. [VA]

225. Zamora JL. Chemical and microbiologic characteristics and toxicity of povidone-iodine solutions. *Am J Surg.* 1986;151(3):400-406. [VA]

226. Tomoda C, Kitano H, Uruno T, et al. Transcutaneous iodine absorption in adult patients with thyroid cancer disinfected with povidone-iodine at operation. *Thyroid.* 2005;15(6):600-603. [IB]

227. Pello JY, Pons G, Leger FA, et al. Ioban 2 for cesarean section operative field: study of innocuity for the newborn. *Therapie.* 1990;45:85 [IIB]

228. Vorherr H, Vorherr UF, Mehta P, Ulrich JA, Messer RH. Vaginal absorption of povidone-iodine. *JAMA.* 1980;244(23):2628-2629. [IIIC]

229. Kurtoğlu S, Akın L, Akın MA, Çoban D. Iodine overload and severe hypothyroidism in two neonates. *J Clin Res Pediatr Endocrinol.* 2009;1(6):275-277. [VA]

230. Vanzi V, Pitaro R. Skin injuries and chlorhexidine gluconate-based antisepsis in early premature infants: a case report and review of the literature. *J Perinat Neonatal Nurs.* 2018;32(4):341-350. [VA]

231. Sathiyamurthy S, Banerjee J, Godambe SV. Antiseptic use in the neonatal intensive care unit—a dilemma in clinical practice: an evidence based review. *World J Clin Pediatr.* 2016;5(2):159-171. [VA]

232. Paternoster M, Niola M, Graziano V. Avoiding chlorhexidine burns in preterm infants. *J Obstet Gynecol Neonatal Nurs.* 2017;46(2):267-271. [VB]

233. Schick JB, Milstein JM. Burn hazard of isopropyl alcohol in the neonate. *Pediatrics.* 1981;68(4):587-588. [VB]

234. Harpin V, Rutter N. Percutaneous alcohol absorption and skin necrosis in a preterm infant. *Arch Dis Child.* 1982;57(6):477-479. [VA]

235. Smerdely P, Lim A, Boyages SC, et al. Topical iodine-containing antiseptics and neonatal hypothyroidism in very-low-birthweight infants. *Lancet.* 1989;2(8664):661-664. [IIIB]

236. Malhotra S, Kumta S, Bhutada A, Jacobson-Dickman E, Motaghedi R. Topical iodine-induced thyrotoxicosis in a newborn with a giant omphalocele. *AJP Rep.* 2016;6(2):e243-e245. [VA]

237. Bryant WP, Zimmerman D. Iodine-induced hyperthyroidism in a newborn. *Pediatrics.* 1995;95(3):434-436. [VB]

238. Yilmaz D, Teziç HT, Zorlu P, Firat S, Bilaloğlu E, Kutlu AO. Single dose povidone-iodine on thyroid functions and urinary iodine excretion. *Indian J Pediatr.* 2003;70(8):675-677. [IIIB]

239. Weber SM, Hargunani CA, Wax MK. DuraPrep and the risk of fire during tracheostomy. *Head Neck.* 2006;28(7):649-652. [VA]

240. *State Operations Manual Appendix A: Survey Protocol, Regulations and Interpretive Guidelines for Hospitals.* Rev. 200, 02-21-20. Centers for Medicare & Medicaid Services. https://www.cms.gov/Regulations-and-Guidance/Guidance/Manuals/downloads/som107ap_a_hospitals.pdf. Accessed February 16, 2021.

241. *State Operations Manual Appendix L: Guidance for Surveyors: Ambulatory Surgical Centers.* Rev. 200, 02-21-20. Centers for Medicare & Medicaid Services. https://www.cms.gov/Regulations-and-Guidance/Guidance/Manuals/downloads/som107ap_l_ambulatory.pdf. Accessed February 16, 2021.

242. Bever GJ, Brodie FL, Hwang DG. Corneal injury from presurgical chlorhexidine skin preparation. *World Neurosurg.* 2016;96:610.e1-610.e4. [VA]

243. Singh S, Blakley B. Systematic review of ototoxic presurgical antiseptic preparations—what is the evidence? *J Otolaryngol Head Neck Surg.* 2018;47(1):18. [IIB]

244. Cronen G, Ringus V, Sigle G, Ryu J. Sterility of surgical site marking. *J Bone Joint Surg Am.* 2005;87(10):2193-2195. [IIB]

245. Rooney J, Khoo OKS, Higgs AR, Small TJ, Bell S. Surgical site marking does not affect sterility. *ANZ J Surg.* 2008;78(8):688-689. [IIB]

246. Wilson J, Tate D. Can pre-operative skin marking transfer methicillin-resistant *Staphylococcus aureus* between patients? A laboratory experiment. *J Bone Joint Surg* Br. 2006;88(4):541-542. [IIIA]

247. Wollina U. Preoperative site marking in dermatosurgery. *J Cutan Aesthet Surg.* 2019;12(3):191-192. [VA]

248. Bathla S, Nevins EJ, Moori PL, Vimalachandran D. Which pen? A comparative study of surgical site markers. *J Perioper Pract.* 2018;28(1-2):21-26. [IIB]

249. Mears SC, Dinah AF, Knight TA, Frassica FJ, Belkoff SM. Visibility of surgical site marking after preoperative skin preparation. *Eplasty.* 2008;8:e35. [IIB]

250. Thakkar SC, Mears SC. Visibility of surgical site marking: a prospective randomized trial of two skin preparation solutions. *J Bone Joint Surg Am.* 2012;94(2):97-102. [IB]

251. Guideline for team communication. In: *Guidelines for Perioperative Practice.* Denver, CO: AORN; 2021:1065-1096. [IVB]

252. Bajaj TI, Loh C, Borgstrom D. Diluting chlorhexidine gluconate: one scrub or two? *Surg Infect (Larchmt).* 2014;15(5):544-547. [IB]

253. Malalasekera A, Louie-Johnsun M, Wang A, van Diepen DC, Gottlieb T, Chan L. Is a 10-minute surgical scrub necessary in urologic prosthetic surgery? A randomized study of the effect of a 5- vs 10-minute surgical scrub on bacterial colony counts in the genital skin. *Neurourol Urodyn.* 2019;38(3):990-995. [IB]

254. Lundberg PW, Smith AA, Heaney JB, et al. Pre-operative antisepsis protocol compliance and the effect on bacterial load reduction. *Surg Infect (Larchmt).* 2016;17(1):32-37. [IIB]

255. Trick WE, Vernon MO, Hayes RA, et al. Impact of ring wearing on hand contamination and comparison of hand hygiene agents in a hospital. *Clin Infect Dis.* 2003;36(11):1383-1390. [IIA]

256. Smith FD. Caring for surgical patients with piercings. *AORN J.* 2016;103(6):583-596. [VB]

257. Lefebvre A, Saliou P, Mimoz O, et al. Is surgical site scrubbing before painting of value? Review and meta-analysis of clinical studies. *J Hosp Infect.* 2015;89(1):28-37. [IIA]

258. Bonnevialle N, Geiss L, Cavalié L, Ibnoulkhatib A, Verdeil X, Bonnevialle P. Skin preparation before hip replacement in

emergency setting versus elective scheduled arthroplasty: bacteriological comparative analysis. *Orthop Traumatol Surg Res.* 2013;99(6):659-665. [IIA]

259. *AST Standards of Practice for Skin Prep of the Surgical Patient.* Association of Surgical Technologists. http://www.ast.org/uploadedfiles/main_site/content/about_us/standard_skin_prep.pdf. Accessed February 15, 2021. [IVC]

260. *NFPA 101: Life Safety Code.* Quincy, MA: National Fire Protection Association; 2021. [IVB]

261. Guideline for electrosurgical safety. In: *Guidelines for Perioperative Practice.* Denver, CO: AORN, Inc; 2021:83-108. [IVA]

262. Wood A. Clinical issues–January 2015. *AORN J.* 2015;101(1):149-157. [VA]

263. Guideline for surgical attire. In: *Guidelines for Perioperative Practice.* Denver, CO: AORN, Inc; 2021:1015-1032. [IVA]

264. Markel TA, Gormley T, Greeley D, Ostojic J, Wagner J. Wearing long sleeves while prepping a patient in the operating room decreases airborne contaminants. *Am J Infect Control.* 2018;46(4):369-374. [IIB]

265. Stapleton EJ, Frane N, Lentz JM, et al. Association of disposable perioperative jackets with surgical site infections in a large multicenter health care organization. *JAMA Surg.* 2019;155(1):15-20. [IIA]

266. Vagholkar K, Julka K. Preoperative skin preparation: which is the best method? *Internet J Surg.* 2012;28(4):1-8. [IA]

267. Weed S, Bastek JA, Sammel MD, Beshara M, Hoffman S, Srinivas SK. Comparing postcesarean infectious complication rates using two different skin preparations. *Obstet Gynecol.* 2011;117(5):1123-1129. [IIA]

268. Smid MC, Dotters-Katz SK, Silver RM, Kuller JA. Body mass index 50 kg/m2 and beyond: perioperative care of pregnant women with superobesity undergoing cesarean delivery. *Obstet Gynecol Surv.* 2017;72(8):500-510. [VA]

269. Guideline for prevention of retained surgical items. In: *Guidelines for Perioperative Practice.* Denver, CO: AORN, Inc; 2021:769-820. [IVA]

270. Naderi N, Maw K, Thomas M, Boyce DE, Shokrollahi K. A quick and effective method of limb preparation with health, safety and efficiency benefits. *Ann R Coll Surg Engl.* 2012;94(2):83-86. [IIB]

271. Chang A, Hughes A, du Moulin W, Mukerjee C, Molnar R. Randomised comparison of two skin preparation methods in foot and ankle surgery. *Foot Ankle Surg.* 2016;22(3):170-175. [IIB]

272. Dingemans SA, Spijkerman IJB, Birnie MFN, Goslings JC, Schepers T. Preoperative disinfection of foot and ankle: microbiological evaluation of two disinfection methods. *Arch Orthop Trauma Surg.* 2018;138(10):1389-1394. [IIC]

273. Best BA, Best TJ. Skin preparation in the hand surgery clinic: a survey of Canadian plastic surgeons and a pilot study of a new technique. *Can J Infect Control.* 2018;33(2):102-105. [IIB]

274. Seigerman DA, Rivlin M, Bianchini J, Liss FE, Beredjiklian PK. A comparison of two sterile solution application methods during surgical preparation of the hand. *J Hand Surg Am.* 2016;41(6):698-702. [IIB]

275. Syed UAM, Seidl AJ, Hoffman RA, Bianchini J, Beredjiklian PK, Abboud JA. Preoperative sterilization preparation of the

276. Chepla KJ, Gosain AK. Interstitial pneumonitis after betadine aspiration. *J Craniofac Surg.* 2012;23(6):1787-1789. [VA]

277. Choi WY, Park CW, Son KM, Cheon JS. Aspiration pneumonitis due to povidone-iodine aspiration during a facial bone fracture reduction operation. *J Craniofac Surg.* 2014;25(2):e172-e174. [VA]

278. Hitosugi T, Tsukamoto M, Yokoyama T. Pneumonia due to aspiration of povidone iodine after preoperative disinfection of the oral cavity. *Oral Maxillofac Surg.* 2019;23(4):507-511. [VA]

279. Stankiewicz M, Wyland M. A review of suspected intraoperative antiseptic burns: a quality improvement review. *J Periop Nurs.* 2017;30(4):25-29. [VB]

280. Sistema Espanol de Notificacion En Seguridad En Anestesia Y Reanimacion (SENSAR). Surgical burn secondary to the use of alcoholic chlorhexidine. *Rev Esp Anestesiol Reanim.* 2018;65(3):e1-e3. [VA]

281. Borrego L, Hernández N, Hernández Z, Peñate Y. Povidone-iodine induced post-surgical irritant contact dermatitis localized outside of the surgical incision area. Report of 27 cases and a literature review. *Int J Dermatol.* 2016;55(5):540-545. [VA]

282. Jones EL, Overbey DM, Chapman BC, et al. Operating room fires and surgical skin preparation. *J Am Coll Surg.* 2017;225(1):160-165. [IIB]

283. Chiang YC, Lin TS, Yeh MC. Povidone-iodine-related burn under the tourniquet of a child—a case report and literature review. *J Plast Reconstr Aesthet Surg.* 2011;64(3):412-415. [VA]

284. Palmanovich E, Brin YS, Laver L, Nyska M, Kish B. Third-degree chemical burns from chlorhexidine local antisepsis. *Isr Med Assoc J.* 2013;15(6):323-324. [VA]

285. Yang JH, Lim H, Yoon JR, Jeong HI. Tourniquet associated chemical burn. *Indian J Orthop.* 2012;46(3):356-359. [VA]

286. Hodgkinson DJ, Irons GB, Williams TJ. Chemical burns and skin preparation solutions. *Surg Gynecol Obstet.* 1978;147(4):534-536. [IIIB]

287. Lowe DO, Knowles SR, Weber EA, Railton CJ, Shear NH. Povidone-iodine-induced burn: case report and review of the literature. *Pharmacotherapy.* 2006;26(11):1641-1645. [VA]

288. Murthy MB, Krishnamurthy B. Severe irritant contact dermatitis induced by povidone iodine solution. *Indian J Pharmacol.* 2009;41(4):199-200. [VB]

289. Stinner DJ, Krueger CA, Masini BD, Wenke JC. Time-dependent effect of chlorhexidine surgical prep. *J Hosp Infect.* 2011;79(4):313-316. [IIIB]

290. Ryan SP, Adams SB, Allen N, Lazarides A, Wellman SS, Gage MJ. Intraoperative fire risk: evaluating the 3-minute wait after chlorhexidine-alcohol antiseptic scrub. *J Orthop Trauma.* 2021;35(1):e31-e33. [IIB]

291. Guideline for safe patient handling and movement. In: *Guidelines for Perioperative Practice.* Denver, CO: AORN; 2021:821-872. [IVB]

292. Apfelbaum JL, Caplan RA, Barker SJ, et al. Practice advisory for the prevention and management of operating room

fires: an updated report by the American Society of Anesthesiologists Task Force on Operating Room Fires. *Anesthesiology.* 2013;118(2):271-290. [IVA]

293. 16.13.3 germicides and antiseptics. In: *NFPA #99: Health Care Facilities Code Handbook.* Quincy, MA: National Fire Protection Association; 2018:99-145. [IVB]

294. Hempel S, Maggard-Gibbons M, Nguyen DK, et al. Wrong-site surgery, retained surgical items, and surgical fires: a systematic review of surgical never events. *JAMA Surg.* 2015;150(8):796-805. [IIIA]

295. *NFPA 30: Flammable and Combustible Liquids Code.* Quincy, MA: National Fire Protection Association; 2021. [IVB]

296. Surgical fire safety initiatives—part 1 of *ECRI Institute's Clinical Guide to Surgical Fire Prevention.* ECRI Institute. https://www.ecri.org/components/HDJournal/Pages/Fire-Safety-Initiatives-Clinical-Guide-to-Surgical-Fire-Prevention.aspx. Published October 1, 2009. Updated February 8, 2017. Accessed February 16, 2021. [IVC]

297. The team approach to surgical fire prevention—part 2 of *ECRI Institute's Clinical Guide to Surgical Fire Prevention.* ECRI Institute. https://www.ecri.org/components/HDJournal/Pages/Team-Approach-to-Fire-Prevention.aspx. Published October 1, 2009. Updated February 8, 2017. Accessed February 16, 2021. [IVC]

298. Wood A, Conner RL, Bruley ME, Lavanchy C, Horvath GM. Clinical issues–August 2014. *AORN J.* 2014;100(2):213-223. [VA]

299. Lipp A, Phillips C, Harris P, Dowie I. Cyanoacrylate microbial sealants for skin preparation prior to surgery. *Cochrane Database Syst Rev.* 2010;10:CD008062. [IA]

300. Mermel LA. Sequential use of povidone-iodine and chlorhexidine for cutaneous antisepsis: a systematic review. *Infect Control Hosp Epidemiol.* 2020;41(1):98-101. [IIA]

301. Morrison TN, Chen AF, Taneja M, Küçükdurmaz F, Rothman RH, Parvizi J. Single vs repeat surgical skin preparations for reducing surgical site infection after total joint arthroplasty: a prospective, randomized, double-blinded study. *J Arthroplasty.* 2016;31(6):1289-1294. [IA]

302. Rees A, Sherrod Q, Young L. Chemical burn from povidone-iodine: case and review. *J Drugs Dermatol.* 2011;10(4):414-417. [VB]

303. 29 CFR 1910.1200. Hazard Communication. Toxic and Hazardous Substances. Occupational Safety and Health Administration. https://www.osha.gov/laws-regs/regulations/standardnumber/1910/1910.1200. Accessed February 15, 2021.

304. Song JE, Kwak YG, Um TH, et al. Outbreak of Burkholderia cepacia pseudobacteraemia caused by intrinsically contaminated commercial 0.5% chlorhexidine solution in neonatal intensive care units. *J Hosp Infect.* 2018;98(3):295-299. [VA]

305. Ko S, An H, Bang JH, Park SW. An outbreak of *Burkholderia cepacia* complex pseudobacteremia associated with intrinsically contaminated commercial 0.5% chlorhexidine solution. *Am J Infect Control.* 2015;43(3):266-268. [VB]

306. O'Rourke E, Runyan D, O'Leary J, Stern J. Contaminated iodophor in the operating room. *Am J Infect Control.* 2003; 31(4):255-256. [VA]

307. Weber DJ, Rutala WA, Sickbert-Bennett EE. Outbreaks associated with contaminated antiseptics and disinfectants. *Antimicrob Agents Chemother.* 2007;51(12):4217-4224. [VA]

308. Kim JM, Ahn Y, LiPuma JJ, Hussong D, Cerniglia CE. Survival and susceptibility of Burkholderia cepacia complex in chlorhexidine gluconate and benzalkonium chloride. *J Ind Microbiol Biotechnol.* 2015;42(6):905-913. [IIB]

309. Gottardi W. The influence of the chemical behaviour of iodine on the germicidal action of disinfectant solutions containing iodine. *J Hosp Infect.* 1985;6 Suppl A:1-11. [VA]

310. Wistrand C, Söderquist B, Nilsson U. Positive impact on heat loss and patient experience of preheated skin disinfection: a randomised controlled trial. *J Clin Nurs.* 2016;25(21-22):3144-3151. [IB]

311. Summary of the Resource Conservation and Recovery Act. US Environmental Protection Agency. https://www.epa.gov/laws-regulations/summary-resource-conservation-and-recovery-act. Accessed February 15, 2021.

312. Lavallée JF, Gray TA, Dumville J, Russell W, Cullum N. The effects of care bundles on patient outcomes: a systematic review and meta-analysis. *Implement Sci.* 2017;12(1):142. [IIA]

313. Carter EB, Temming LA, Fowler S, et al. Evidence-based bundles and cesarean delivery surgical site infections: a systematic review and meta-analysis. *Obstet Gynecol.* 2017;130(4):735-746. [IIIA]

314. Chen HC, Chen MC, Chen YL, Tsai TH, Pan KL, Lin YS. Bundled preparation of skin antisepsis decreases the risk of cardiac implantable electronic device-related infection. *Europace.* 2016;18(6):858-867. [IIA]

315. Chien CY, Lin CH, Hsu RB. Care bundle to prevent methicillin-resistant *Staphylococcus aureus* sternal wound infection after off-pump coronary artery bypass. *Am J Infect Control.* 2014;42(5):562-564. [IIB]

316. Frenette C, Sperlea D, Tesolin J, Patterson C, Thirion DJG. Influence of a 5-year serial infection control and antibiotic stewardship intervention on cardiac surgical site infections. *Am J Infect Control.* 2016;44(9):977-982. [IIA]

317. Izquierdo-Blasco J, Campins-Martí M, Soler-Palacín P, et al. Impact of the implementation of an interdisciplinary infection control program to prevent surgical wound infection in pediatric heart surgery. *Eur J Pediatr.* 2015;174(7):957-963. [IIB]

318. Yang C, Chen A, Wang Y, Fang X, Ye R, Lin J. Prevention and control of perioperative incision infection in patients undergoing day cataract surgery. *Eye Sci.* 2014;29(3):182-185. [IIA]

319. Kwok RP, Yip WW, Jhanji V, Chan VC, Young AL. The incidence of postoperative endophthalmitis before and after a revised preoperative surgical site preparation protocol. *Asia Pac J Ophthalmol (Phila).* 2016;5(2):110-114. [IIA]

320. Gorgun E, Rencuzogullari A, Ozben V, et al. An effective bundled approach reduces surgical site infections in a high-outlier colorectal unit. *Dis Colon Rectum.* 2018;61(1):89-98. [IIA]

321. Keenan JE, Speicher PJ, Thacker JKM, Walter M, Kuchibhatla M, Mantyh CR. The preventive surgical site infection bundle in colorectal surgery: an effective approach to surgical

site infection reduction and health care cost savings. *JAMA Surg.* 2014;149(10):1045-1052. [IIB]

322. Weiser MR, Gonen M, Usiak S, et al. Effectiveness of a multidisciplinary patient care bundle for reducing surgical-site infections. *Br J Surg.* 2018;105(12):1680-1687. [IIA]

323. Albert H, Bataller W, Masroor N, et al. Infection prevention and enhanced recovery after surgery: a partnership for implementation of an evidence-based bundle to reduce colorectal surgical site infections. *Am J Infect Control.* 2019;47(6):718-719. [IIB]

324. Schiavone MB, Moukarzel L, Leong K, et al. Surgical site infection reduction bundle in patients with gynecologic cancer undergoing colon surgery. *Gynecol Oncol.* 2017;147(1):115-119. [IIB]

325. Davidson C, Enns J, Dempster C, Lundeen S, Eppes C. Impact of a surgical site infection bundle on cesarean delivery infection rates. *Am J Infect Control.* 2020;48(5):555-559. [IIA]

326. Temming LA, Raghuraman N, Carter EB, et al. Impact of evidence-based interventions on wound complications after cesarean delivery. *Am J Obstet Gynecol.* 2017;217(4):449.e1-449.e9. [IIIA]

327. Johnson MP, Kim SJ, Langstraat CL, et al. Using bundled interventions to reduce surgical site infection after major gynecologic cancer surgery. *Obstet Gynecol.* 2016;127(6):1135-1144. [IIB]

328. Lippitt MH, Fairbairn MG, Matsuno R, et al. Outcomes associated with a five-point surgical site infection prevention bundle in women undergoing surgery for ovarian cancer. *Obstet Gynecol.* 2017;130(4):756-764. [IIB]

329. Harold RE, Butler BA, Lamplot J, Luu HH, Lawton CD, Manning D. Multifaceted aseptic protocol decreases surgical site infections following hip arthroplasty. *Hip Int.* 2018;28(2):182-188. [IIA]

330. Mok WQ, Ullal MJ, Su S, et al. An integrative care bundle to prevent surgical site infections among surgical hip patients: a retrospective cohort study. *Am J Infect Control.* 2019;47(5):540-544. [IIA]

331. Vij SC, Kartha G, Krishnamurthi V, Ponziano M, Goldman HB. Simple operating room bundle reduces superficial surgical site infections after major urologic surgery. *Urology.* 2018;112:66-68. [IIB]

332. Fernández-Prada M, Martínez-Ortega C, Revuelta-Mariño L, Menéndez-Herrero Á, Navarro-Gracia JF. Evaluation of the bundle "zero surgical site infection" to prevent surgical site infection in vascular surgery. *Ann Vasc Surg.* 2017;41:160-168. [IIB]

333. Koek MBG, Hopmans TEM, Soetens LC, et al. Adhering to a national surgical care bundle reduces the risk of surgical site infections. *PLoS One.* 2017;12(9):e0184200. [IIA]

334. Hodge AB, Thornton BA, Gajarski R, et al. Quality improvement project in congenital cardiothoracic surgery patients: reducing surgical site infections. *Pediatr Qual Saf.* 2019;4(4):e188. [VA]

335. Deery SE, Cavallaro PM, McWalters ST, et al. Colorectal surgical site infection prevention kits prior to elective colectomy improve outcomes. *Ann Surg.* 2020;271(6):1110-1115. [VA]

336. DeHaas D, Aufderheide S, Gano J, Weigandt J, Ries J, Faust B. Colorectal surgical site infection reduction strategies. *Am J Surg.* 2016;212(1):175-177. [VA]

337. Holland C, Foster P, Ulrich D, Adkins K. A practice improvement project to reduce cesarean surgical site infection rates. *Nurs Womens Health.* 2016;20(6):544-551. [VA]

338. Money L, Eyer M, Duncan K. Creating a surgical site infection prevention bundle for patients undergoing cesarean delivery. *AORN J.* 2018;108(4):372-383. [VA]

339. Schaffzin JK, Simon K, Connelly BL, Mangano FT. Standardizing preoperative preparation to reduce surgical site infections among pediatric neurosurgical patients. *J Neurosurg Pediatr.* 2017;19(4):399-406. [VA]

340. Gallagher BJ, McMahon SE, Henderson K, Zachariah S, Wilson DS, Gallagher B. Reducing deep joint infection in hip hemiarthroplasty—a quality improvement project. *J Clin Outcomes Manag.* 2018;25(3):117-120. [VA]

341. Morris AJ, Roberts SA, Grae N, Hamblin R, Shuker C, Merry AF. The New Zealand Surgical Site Infection Improvement (SSII) Programme: a national quality improvement programme reducing orthopaedic surgical site infections. *N Z Med J.* 2018;131(1479):45-56. [VA]

342. Fornwalt L, Ennis D, Stibich M. Influence of a total joint infection control bundle on surgical site infection rates. *Am J Infect Control.* 2016;44(2):239-241. [VB]

343. Morris AJ, Jackways TM, Morgan A, Robertson R, McIntyre M. Reduction in surgical site infections in the Southern Cross Hospitals Network, 2004-2015: successful outcome of a long-term surveillance and quality improvement project. *N Z Med J.* 2018;131(1481):27-39. [VA]

344. Rozario D. Can surgical site infections be reduced with the adoption of a bundle of simultaneous initiatives? The use of NSQIP incidence data to follow multiple quality improvement interventions. *Can J Surg.* 2018;61(1):68-70. [VB]

345. Toltzis P, O'Riordan M, Cunningham DJ, et al. A statewide collaborative to reduce pediatric surgical site infections. *Pediatrics.* 2014;134(4):e1174-e1180. [VA]

346. Gómez-Romero FJ, Fernández-Prada M, Navarro-Gracia JF. Prevention of surgical site infection: analysis and narrative review of clinical practice guidelines. *Cir Esp.* 2017;95(9):490-502. [VA]

347. Tanner J, Kiernan M, Hilliam R, et al. Effectiveness of a care bundle to reduce surgical site infections in patients having open colorectal surgery. *Ann R Coll Surg Engl.* 2016;98(4):270-274. [IIB]

348. Davis CH, Kao LS, Fleming JB, Aloia TA; Texas Alliance for Surgical Quality Collaborative. Multi-institution analysis of infection control practices identifies the subset associated with best surgical site infection performance: a Texas Alliance for Surgical Quality Collaborative project. *J Am Coll Surg.* 2017;225(4):455-464. [IIIB]

349. Kampf G. Acquired resistance to chlorhexidine—is it time to establish an "antiseptic stewardship" initiative? *J Hosp Infect.* 2016;94(3):213-227. [VB]

350. George J, Klika AK, Higuera CA. Use of chlorhexidine preparations in total joint arthroplasty. *J Bone Jt Infect.* 2017;2(1):15-22. [VA]

Guideline Development Group

Lead Author: Karen deKay[1], MSN, RN, CNOR, CIC, Perioperative Practice Specialist, AORN, Denver, Colorado
Methodologist: Erin Kyle[2], DNP, RN, CNOR, NEA-BC, Editor-in-Chief, *Guidelines for Perioperative Practice*, AORN, Denver, Colorado
Evidence Appraisers: Janice Neal[3], PhD, RN, CNE, Associate Professor, East Carolina College of Nursing, Greenville, North Carolina; and Lisa Spruce[4], DNP, RN, ACNP, CNOR, CNS-CP, ACNS, FAAN, Director of Evidence-Based Perioperative Practice, AORN, Denver, Colorado

Guidelines Advisory Board Members:

- Linda Boley[5], MSN, BSN, RN, CNOR, Clinical Educator Surgical Services, Norton Women's and Children's Hospital, Louisville, Kentucky
- Crystal A. Bricker[6], MSN, RN, CNOR, Clinical Practice Partner, Perioperative Services, Advocate Health Care, Bloomington, Illinois
- Bernard Camins[7], MD, MSc, Health System Infection Prevention Medical Director, Mount Sinai Medical Center, New York, New York
- Mary Fearon[8], MSN, RN, CNOR, Service Line Director Neuroscience, Overlake Medical Center, Sammamish, Washington
- Elizabeth (Lizz) Pincus[9], MSN, RN, CNS-CP, CNOR, Clinical Nurse, Regional Medical Center of San Jose, California

Guidelines Advisory Board Liaisons:

- Shandra R. Day[10], MD, Assistant Professor, Infectious Disease, Ohio State University Wexner Medical Center, Columbus
- Jared M. Huston[11], MD, Director, Trauma Research, Northwell Health, Manhasset, New York

External Review: Expert review comments were received from individual members of the American Association of Nurse Anesthetists (AANA), American College of Surgeons (ACS), Association for Professionals in Infection Control and Epidemiology (APIC), American Society of Anesthesiologists (ASA), International Association of Healthcare Central Service Materiel Management (IAHCSMM), the Society for Healthcare Epidemiology of America (SHEA), and the Surgical Infection Society (SIS). Their responses were used to further refine and enhance this guideline; however, their responses do not imply endorsement. The draft was also open for a 44-day public comment period.

Financial Disclosure and Conflicts of Interest

This guideline was developed, edited, and approved by the AORN Guidelines Advisory Board without external funding being sought or obtained. The Guidelines Advisory Board was financially supported entirely by AORN and was developed without any involvement of industry.

Potential conflicts of interest for all Guidelines Advisory Board members were reviewed before the annual meeting and each monthly conference call. None of the members of the Guideline Development Group reported a potential conflict of interest.[1-11] If a conflict of interest had been disclosed, the Guidelines Advisory Board member would have recused themself from discussions about the topic for which the conflict existed.

Publication History

Originally published May 1976, *AORN Journal*, as "Standards for preoperative skin preparation of patients." Format revision March 1978, July 1982.

Revised February 1983, November 1988, November 1992, June 1996. Published November 1996, *AORN Journal;* reformatted July 2000.

Revised November 2001; published January 2002, *AORN Journal.*

Revised 2007; published as "Recommended practices for preoperative patient skin antisepsis" in *Perioperative Standards and Recommended Practices,* 2008 edition.

Minor editing revisions made to omit PNDS codes; reformatted September 2012 for publication in *Perioperative Standards and Recommended Practices,* 2013 edition.

Revised July 2014 for online publication in *Perioperative Standards and Recommended Practices.*

Minor editing revisions made in November 2014 for publication in *Guidelines for Perioperative Practice,* 2015 edition.

Evidence ratings revised in *Guidelines for Perioperative Practice,* 2018 edition, to conform to the current AORN Evidence Rating Model.

Evidence ratings revised and minor editorial changes made to conform to the current AORN Evidence Rating model, September 2019, for online publication in *Guidelines for Perioperative Practice.*

Revised May 2021 for online publication in *Guidelines for Perioperative Practice.*

Scheduled for review in 2026.

PNEUMATIC TOURNIQUETS

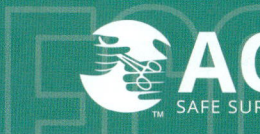

681

TABLE OF CONTENTS

🅟 *indicates a recommendation or evidence relevant to pediatric care.*

MEDICAL ABBREVIATIONS & ACRONYMS

AOP – Arterial occlusion pressure
BMI – Body mass index
DVT – Deep vein thrombosis
FDA – US Food and Drug Administration
IFU – Instructions for use
IVRA – Intravenous regional anesthesia
KTP – Tissue padding coefficient
LOP – Limb occlusion pressure

PVD – Peripheral vascular disease
QOF – Quality of field
RCT – Randomized controlled trial
SBP – Systolic blood pressure
SSI – Surgical site infection
TKA – Total knee arthroplasty
VTE – Venous thromboembolism

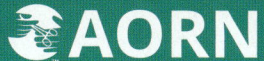
GUIDELINE FOR
PNEUMATIC TOURNIQUET SAFETY

The Guideline for Pneumatic Tourniquet Safety was approved by the AORN Guidelines Advisory Board and became effective as of May 11, 2020. The recommendations in the guideline are intended to be achievable and represent what is believed to be an optimal level of practice. Policies and procedures will reflect variations in practice settings and/or clinical situations that determine the degree to which the guideline can be implemented. AORN recognizes the many diverse settings in which perioperative nurses practice; therefore, this guideline is adaptable to all areas where operative or other invasive procedures may be performed.

Purpose

This document provides guidance to perioperative team members for the safe use of **pneumatic tourniquets** during operative or other invasive procedures. The guideline provides information about applying and removing tourniquet cuffs; monitoring a patient before, during, and after tourniquet inflation; and maintaining tourniquet equipment.

Pneumatic tourniquets are used to obtain a near bloodless field during extremity surgeries or to confine a bolus of **intravenous regional anesthesia** (IVRA) in an extremity. Pneumatic tourniquets provide arterial occlusion through an automated pressure regulator and are attached by tubing to a bladder in a cuff that fits the extremity circumferentially. Surgeons and anesthesia professionals continue to use pneumatic tourniquets,[1-5] although there is conflicting evidence as to whether complications such as increased estimated blood loss and increased blood transfusion rates outweigh the benefits of their use. Researchers define estimated blood loss in multiple ways and use varying terminology for blood loss during pneumatic tourniquet–assisted procedures, including measured, intraoperative, postoperative, calculated, and total blood loss. Many researchers have found that tourniquet use decreases intraoperative and measured blood loss, but there can be a paradoxical increase in postoperative blood loss, which may result in a total blood loss that is comparable to blood loss when no tourniquet is used.[6-8]

Some researchers have concluded that extremity surgery without a tourniquet can be safe and efficient for patients with certain conditions.[6-10] Although serious patient injuries related to the use of pneumatic tourniquets are uncommon, some patient conditions may increase the risk for complications associated with pneumatic tourniquet use. These conditions include diabetic neuropathy,[11] previous revascularization,[12] sickle cell anemia,[11,13] severe infection,[13] and a history of or current venous thromboembolism (VTE).[11,13] Complications that have been associated with pneumatic tourniquet use include uncomfortable skin redness,[14] chemical burns,[14-17] **compartment syndrome**,[18] femoral nerve palsy,[19] acute pulmonary edema,[20] cardiac arrest,[21] and fatal pulmonary edema.[22]

Tourniquets used for phlebotomy or traumatic bleeding (eg, field tourniquets) are outside the scope of this document. Other topics beyond the scope of this guideline include

- the use of medications to
  - prevent tourniquet complications (eg, heparin, steroids),
  - reduce ischemia damage (eg, dexamethasone, antioxidants),
  - alleviate pain during inflation (eg, oxygen, magnesium), and
  - facilitate hemostasis (eg, epinephrine, tranexamic acid);
- **preconditioning techniques**;
- **reperfusion techniques**;
- techniques for **staggered tourniquet deflation**; and
- prevention and management of local anesthetic systemic toxicity (See the AORN Guideline for Care of the Patient Receiving Local Anesthesia[23]).

Evidence Review

A medical librarian with a perioperative background conducted a systematic search of the databases Ovid MEDLINE®, Ovid Embase®, EBSCO CINAHL®, and the Cochrane Database of Systematic Reviews. The search was limited to literature published in English from January 2012 through February 2019. At the time of the initial search, weekly alerts were created on the topics included in that search. Results from these alerts were provided to the lead author until September 2019. The lead author requested additional articles that either did not fit the original search criteria or were discovered during the evidence appraisal process. The lead author and the medical librarian also identified relevant guidelines from government agencies, professional organizations, and standards-setting bodies.

Search terms included *acido*, acute capillary rupture syndrome, adductor canal block, adjustment pressure, ankle block, arm injur*, arterial occlusion pressure determination, arterial occlusion pressure estimation, arterial tourniquet, arthroplasty, avascular necrosis, Bier block, blood pressure, bloodless field, bloodless surgery, brachial plexus neuropath*, calcifications, carbon dioxide, cardiac output, chemoprophylaxis, compartment*

Figure 1. Flow Diagram of Literature Search Results

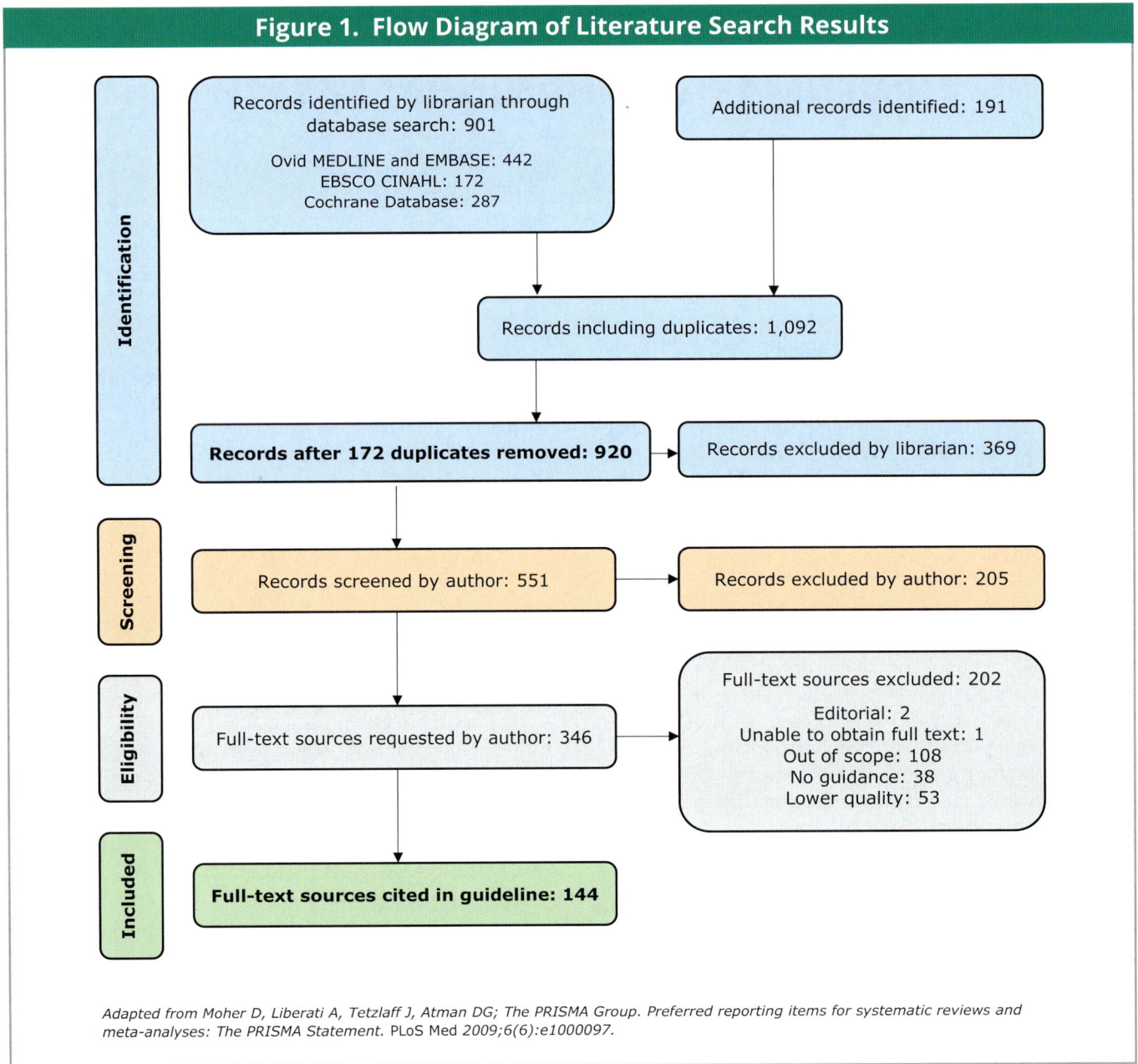

Records identified by librarian through database search: 901

Ovid MEDLINE and EMBASE: 442
EBSCO CINAHL: 172
Cochrane Database: 287

Additional records identified: 191

Identification

Records including duplicates: 1,092

Records after 172 duplicates removed: 920

Records excluded by librarian: 369

Screening

Records screened by author: 551

Records excluded by author: 205

Eligibility

Full-text sources requested by author: 346

Full-text sources excluded: 202

Editorial: 2
Unable to obtain full text: 1
Out of scope: 108
No guidance: 38
Lower quality: 53

Included

Full-text sources cited in guideline: 144

Adapted from Moher D, Liberati A, Tetzlaff J, Atman DG; The PRISMA Group. Preferred reporting items for systematic reviews and meta-analyses: The PRISMA Statement. PLoS Med 2009;6(6):e1000097.

syndromes, competencies, compression injur*, conduction an*thesia, conscious sedation, cuff injur*, cuff pain, damaged muscle tissue, digital block, disease transmission (infectious), distal tourniquet, DVT, elastic band, elastic bandages, elastic tourniquet cuff, elective surgical procedures, Esmarch bandage, exsanguinat*, extremities, extremity girth, fat embolism syndrome, foot injur*, functional outcomes, gauze bandage, hand injur*, hemodynamic effects, hemostasis (surgical), hidden blood loss, hyperemia, hypox*, iatrogenic fracture, inflation pressure, interface pressure, inter-tourniquet distances, intracranial pressure, intravenous regional an*sthesia, ischemi*, latex allergy, leg injur*, limb circumference, limb elevation, limb occlusion pressure determination, limb occlusion pressure estimation, limb surgery, local inflammation, lower extremity, maintain pressure, metabolic changes, metabolic effects, metabolic events, metabolic phenomena, microbial colonization of tourniquet, microvascular function, minimizing cuff pressure, muscle atrophy, musculoskeletal injur*, nerve injur*, nerve palsy, neuromuscular injur*, Northwick Park, nursing assessment, nursing care, nylon cuff, occlusion of vasculature, occlusion protocols, orthopedics, osteogenesis imperfecta, oxidative stress, oxygen consumption, pain measurement, paired tourniquet, paradoxical blood loss, paresthesia, patient comfort, patient experience, patient pain perception, patient positioning, patient preference, patient reported outcomes, patient satisfaction, performance metrics, perioperative assessment, perioperative care, peripheral block, peripheral nervous system diseases, phalange surgery, pneumatic tourniquet, postocclusive reactive hyperemia, postoperative anemia, postoperative complications, postoperative knee swelling, postoperative recovery, proximal tourniquet, pulmonary embolism, pulse, pulse oximetry monitoring, radial neuropath*, regulate pressure, reinflation, reperfusion injur*, respiration, rhabdomyolysis, Rhys Davies, routine practice, Rumpel-Leede phenomenon, sickle cell, silicon ring, simulated use of tourniquets, simulated training, skin integrity, skin lesions, soft tissue injur*, squeeze method, surgery (elective), surgery (operative), surgical hemostasis, surgical procedures (operative), systemic inflammation, systemic inflammatory response, thromboembolic events, tissue oxygen saturation, tourniquet, tourniquet width, tourniquet failure, tourniquet hypertension, tourniquet inflation, tourniquet injur*, tourniquet pain, tourniquet release timing, tourniquet time, tourniquet tolerance, tourniquet width, tourniquets, tumescent local an*thesia infiltration, two tourniquet sequential block, ulnar neuropath*, upper extremity, vascular injur*, venous congestion, venous occlusion technique, venous reflux, vital signs, and wide tourniquet cuff.

Included were research and non-research literature in English, complete publications, and publications with dates within the time restriction when available. Historical studies were also included. Excluded were non-peer-reviewed publications and older evidence within the time restriction when more recent evidence was available. Editorials, news items, and other brief items were excluded. Low-quality evidence was excluded when higher-quality evidence was available, and literature outside the time restriction was excluded when literature within the time restriction was available. Studies that evaluated **exsanguination** without the use of a pneumatic tourniquet were excluded (Figure 1).

Articles identified in the search were provided to the project team for evaluation. The team consisted of the lead author and one evidence appraiser. The lead author and the evidence appraiser reviewed and critically appraised each article using the AORN Research or Non-Research Evidence Appraisal Tools as appropriate. A second appraiser was consulted in the event of a disagreement between the lead author and the primary evidence appraiser. The literature was independently evaluated and appraised according to the strength and quality of the evidence. Each article was then assigned an appraisal score. The appraisal score is noted in brackets after each reference as applicable.

Each recommendation rating is based on a synthesis of the collective evidence, a benefit-harm assessment, and consideration of resource use. The strength of the recommendation was determined using the AORN Evidence Rating Model and the quality and consistency of the evidence supporting a recommendation. The recommendation strength rating is noted in brackets after each recommendation.

Note: *The evidence summary table is available at http://www.aorn.org/evidencetables/.*

Editor's note: *MEDLINE is a registered trademark of the US National Library of Medicine's Medical Literature Analysis and Retrieval System, Bethesda, MD. Embase is a registered trademark of Elsevier B.V., Amsterdam, The Netherlands. CINAHL, Cumulative Index to Nursing and Allied Health Literature, is a registered trademark of EBSCO Industries, Birmingham, AL.*

1. Preoperative Assessment

1.1 **During the preoperative briefing, determine whether the surgeon or anesthesia professional plans to use a pneumatic tourniquet.**[24] *[Recommendation]*

Discussing the plan of care for pneumatic tourniquet use during the briefing increases the team's ability to provide safe patient care.[24] Refer to the AORN Guideline for Team Communication[24] for additional guidance related to the briefing process.

Although high-quality evidence suggests that pneumatic tourniquet–assisted procedures can be performed safely,[6,7,9,10,25] there are important variations in the study results.[6,7,9,10,26-30] Evidence conflicts as to whether procedures performed with pneumatic tourniquets offer better, similar, or worse results than procedures performed without a tourniquet.[6,7,9,10,25,26,28,29,31-33] Further research is needed to assess the benefits and harms of tourniquet use.

Five systematic reviews[6,7,10,25,26] that included studies from 1991 to 2012 and seven more-recent randomized controlled trials (RCTs)[9,27-29,31,32,34] compared procedures in which tourniquets were or were not used. Researchers found that the benefits of pneumatic tourniquet use included

- better immediate implant efficacy,[9]
- decreased transfusion risk,[7]
- significantly less intraoperative blood loss,[6,7,10,25] and
- shorter operative time.[6,7,25]

The potential harms of pneumatic tourniquet use included

- decreased short-term **functional recovery** of the extremity,[7,25]
- increased analgesic use,[32]
- increased complication rates (eg, oozing, erythema, cellulitis, minor dehiscence, superficial infection, vessels injury, infection, wound dehiscence, hematoma requiring reoperation, manipulation under anesthesia,[8] skin vesicles, ecchymosis, nerve palsy, meralgia, ankylosis, foot drop, delayed incisional healing[7]),[7,25]
- increased incidence of deep vein thrombosis (DVT),[7,25]
- increased length of hospital stay,[26]
- increased postoperative blood loss,[10,31]
- increased postoperative numbness,[31]
- increased procedural revision,[27,32] and
- increased short-term pain.[9,26,27,32]

Although researchers found differences when comparing tourniquet use to no tourniquet use, there was conflicting evidence for the following outcomes:

- calculated blood loss,[9,25,31]
- complication rates,[6,26]
- DVT incidence,[26]

- length of stay,[7]
- long-term implant efficacy,[28,29]
- operative time,[10,26]
- pain[31,34] and long-term pain,[27,32]
- postoperative blood loss,[6,7]
- transfusion risk,[6,25] and
- swelling.[27,31]

Researchers did not find any differences between groups for the outcomes of field visibility,[31,32] metabolic processes,[34] or total blood loss.[6,7]

1.2 **Assess the patient's**
- **circulation in the extremity (eg, pulses, temperature, capillary refill),**
- **skin condition under and distal to the planned cuff site, and**
- **sensory and motor responses of the operative extremity compared to the contralateral extremity.**

[Recommendation]

Preoperative assessment provides a baseline to evaluate for skin or nerve injury and reperfusion of the extremity after tourniquet use.

1.3 **Assess the patient preoperatively for factors that may increase his or her risk of developing complications from pneumatic tourniquet use.**
[Recommendation]

The preoperative assessment provides information necessary to determine the individual patient's risk for pneumatic tourniquet complications and to identify preventive measures.

1.3.1 **Use pneumatic tourniquets with caution for an older adult patient.**[35-39] *[Recommendation]*

Low-quality evidence conflicts as to whether age older than 60 years increases the patient's risk for poor muscle recovery or other complications related to tourniquet use.[35-39] Researchers have correlated tourniquet-assisted procedures and increased patient age with
- delayed functional recovery,[37]
- increased atrophy,[38]
- increased risk for pulmonary embolism,[39]
- likelihood of neurological complications (ie, increased 0.7 times for every 10-year increase in age if inflation time is longer than 120 minutes,)[36] or
- no complications when the tourniquet fits well.[35]

1.3.2 **Use pneumatic tourniquets with caution for a patient with low preoperative hemoglobin.**[31-33,40,41] *[Recommendation]*

High-quality evidence indicates that tourniquet use in a patient with low preoperative

hemoglobin increases the patient's risk of requiring a postoperative blood transfusion related to symptomatic total blood loss.[31-33]

The findings of three RCTs[31-33] conflict as to whether using a tourniquet decreases the risk for transfusion related to blood loss. The researchers had varying conclusions, including that
- not using a tourniquet increased intraoperative blood loss[32];
- there was no difference in total blood loss, as measured by intraoperative hemoglobin change[31]; and
- tourniquet use significantly increased the risk for transfusion.[33]

Lower-quality studies also support using preoperative hemoglobin to predict risk for transfusion related to blood loss.[40,41] In a retrospective review of 366 primary total joint arthroplasties, Benjamin and Colgan[41] found that preoperative hemoglobin was a significant predictor for transfusion and women were six times more likely to require a transfusion. Boutsiadis et al[40] reviewed 150 consecutive uncemented total knee arthroplasties (TKAs) and found that for a 1 g/dL decrease in preoperative hemoglobin, the risk for transfusion quadrupled.

1.3.3 **Use pneumatic tourniquets with caution for a patient with an increased risk for VTE.**[42-45]
[Recommendation]

High-quality evidence conflicts as to whether tourniquet use alone increases the risk for VTE.[27,42] In an RCT that included 103 patients, Mori et al[42] found distal DVT incidence was higher for patients who had tourniquet-assisted procedures (n = 51) than for control group patients who had procedures with no tourniquet use (n = 52). Conversely, Liu et al[27] studied 52 patients and found no difference in DVT rates between legs in bilateral TKA procedures when a tourniquet was used on only one leg.

Lower-quality evidence also conflicts.[43-47] Researchers found
- a high incidence of DVT associated with tourniquet use during TKA procedures,[43,44]
- no difference in DVT incidence related specifically to tourniquet use during arthroscopic procedures,[46,47] and
- significantly lower DVT and proximal DVT incidence in an early-release tourniquet group compared to a late-release group.[45]

Refer to the AORN Guideline for Prevention of Venous Thromboembolism[48] for additional guidance related to patient-specific risk factors for VTE.

1.3.4 **Use pneumatic tourniquets with caution for a patient with a high body mass index (BMI).**[37,39,49-52] *[Recommendation]*

Moderate-quality evidence conflicts as to whether a patient's BMI increases his or her risk for injury with tourniquet use.[37,39,49-52] Further research on this topic is needed.

Researchers who conducted quasi-experimental[49] and nonexperimental[35,37,39,50,51,53] studies of tourniquet use in higher BMI patient populations found

- decreased functional recovery,[37,49]
- increased tourniquet inflation pressure,[50-52]
- increased risk for pulmonary embolism,[39] and
- increased swelling and pain.[49]

The researchers found no difference with tourniquet use for the following patient outcomes:

- DVT incidence,[49]
- infection,[49]
- implant efficacy,[49]
- length of hospital stay,[50] and
- overall complications.[35]

1.4 Assess the patient for potential contraindications to pneumatic tourniquet use and notify the prescriber (ie, the surgeon or anesthesia professional) of any identified contraindications.[24] *[Recommendation]*

Communication among perioperative team members facilitates care and decreases the risk for patient injury.[24]

1.4.1 Assess the patient for potential systemic contraindications to tourniquet use, including

- **arteriovenous grafts or fistulas,**[54]
- **diabetic neuropathy,**[11]
- **peripheral vascular disease (PVD),**[1,2,54-57]
- **previous revascularization,**[12]
- **sickle cell anemia,**[11,13]
- **severe infection,**[13] and
- **VTE or a history of VTE.**[11,13]

[Recommendation]

Patients with these systemic conditions may be excluded from participating in high-quality research studies because the risk for injury outweighs the potential benefits of tourniquet use.[54,55] In two RCTs, patients with PVD[54,55] or a previous arterial bypass graft[54] were excluded from the study population because these conditions were considered contraindications to tourniquet use. In contrast, some lower-quality evidence suggests that tourniquets may be used, with caution, for these patients.[11,58-60]

In a nonexperimental study, Walls et al[58] found no difference in postoperative vascular blood flow after observing tourniquet use in 40

patients diagnosed with PVD. Radiographic evidence of arterial calcification was seen on six patients' x-rays, although all participants were diagnosed preoperatively and sustained less than 50% vascular stenosis postoperatively. Woelfle-Roos et al[59] screened 765 patients for a diagnosis of vascular calcifications and found that for the 50 patients diagnosed, there was no difference for tourniquet failure rate or intraoperative blood loss compared to for patients without vascular calcifications. Koehler et al[60] also conducted a nonexperimental study and found no increased risk for incision-site complications or VTE after tourniquet use for 88 patients with an arterial calcification diagnosis compared to 285 patients who did not have arterial calcification.

In a literature review, Kumar et al[11] stated that tourniquet use in diabetic neuropathic patients requires extra caution to prevent complications. In another literature review, McMillan and Johnstone[13] stated that tourniquets could be used with caution with certain conditions (ie, PVD, arteriovenous fistula, previous vascular surgery, sickle cell disease, infection, reamed intramedullary nailing, previous thromboembolic event).

1.4.2 Assess the surgical site for potential contraindications to tourniquet use, including

- **malignancy,**
- **open fracture,**
- **severe crushing injuries,**[11]
- **severe scar tissue at the cuff location, or**
- **thigh circumference larger than 100 cm.**[55]

[Recommendation]

The pneumatic tourniquet manufacturer's instructions for use (IFU) may specify that these conditions are contraindications for tourniquet use. Mittal et al[55] conducted an RCT and excluded patients with a thigh circumference larger than 100 cm as a contraindication to tourniquet use. In a literature review, Kumar et al[11] recommended extra attention and care when using a pneumatic tourniquet on an extremity with a severe crush injury.

2. Tourniquet Application

2.1 **Verify the surgical site, including laterality, before tourniquet application.**[24] *[Recommendation]*

Verifying the tourniquet site can prevent placing the tourniquet on the wrong limb, which could result in a cascade of events leading to wrong-site surgery.

Refer to the AORN Guideline on Team Communication[24] for additional guidance related to wrong-site surgery prevention.

2.2 **Select the tourniquet cuff size to maintain pressure, fit, and field visibility according to the manufacturer's IFU.**[15,51] *[Recommendation]*

The findings of an observational study suggest that selecting the correct size and shape of the tourniquet cuff promotes consistent pressure, optimal overlap, and secure closure to reduce potential skin lesion complications.[51] Roth et al[51] observed pressure variations under the length of the tourniquet cuff in a sample of 25 patients and found unequal, higher pressures under the overlay of tourniquet cuffs on the patients' skin. The researchers recommended that the tourniquet overlap be as narrow as possible and noted that smaller leg circumferences require shorter cuffs for a snug fit. An important limitation of this study is that all tourniquet cuffs were inflated to 350 mmHg.

Additional low-quality evidence supports matching the tourniquet cuff shape (eg, **cylindrical tourniquet cuff**, **contoured tourniquet cuff**) to the extremity. Yang et al[15] reported on a case in which mismatching the shape of the tourniquet to the limb created friction that resulted in skin injury.

2.3 **Apply the tourniquet at the optimal location of the extremity based on the procedure.**[4,19,61] *[Recommendation]*

Low-quality evidence supports applying the tourniquet at the optimal location of the extremity to prevent patient injury while maintaining optimal field visibility.[4,19,61]

In 1995, Derner and Buckholz[61] retrospectively compared outcomes for 3,027 podiatry procedures and found that when ankle tourniquets were applied proximal to the malleolus, there were fewer complications than when thigh tourniquets were used. In 2013, Mingo-Robinet et al[19] concluded that using the most proximal and the greatest circumference of the extremity might decrease neuropathies related to case reports of tourniquet-use injuries.

2.4 **Use a contoured tourniquet cuff for extremities in which there is a tapering of the extremity between the upper and lower edge of the cuff.**[15,16,62] *[Recommendation]*

High-quality evidence supports use of contoured cuffs to confirm suitable fit around the extremity.[62]

In an RCT conducted in 2004, Younger et al[62] used an automated limb occlusion measurement tool and found that a wide, contoured cuff was associated with lower pressures compared to standard cuff pressures in 40 patients.

Lower-quality evidence also supports matching the cuff shape to the individual limb.[15,16] The authors of two case reports concluded that using the suitable tourniquet shape could have prevented maceration friction,[16] blistering, and scarring that required additional procedures to treat.[15]

2.5 **For patients with latex sensitivity or allergy, use pneumatic tourniquets, accessories, and supplies for exsanguination that are labeled as "not made with natural rubber latex."**[63,64] *[Recommendation]*

Low-quality evidence recommends having latex-free tourniquet and exsanguination supplies for use as needed.[63,64]

One literature review[63] and a clinical practice guideline[64] recommend reviewing the patient's allergies before surgery and removing latex tourniquet supplies to prevent potential harm to the patient when necessary.

Refer to the AORN Guideline for Safe Environment of Care[65] for additional guidance related to establishing a natural rubber latex-safe environment.

2.6 **Use a sterile tourniquet if the tourniquet will be positioned close to the surgical site.**[66] *[Recommendation]*

Low-quality evidence supports using single-use tourniquets when there is a short distance between the edge of the tourniquet and the surgical site, to decrease potential contamination and infection from reusable tourniquets.[66]

In 2011, Thompson et al[66] conducted a nonexperimental study to observe the rate of bacterial contamination on reusable tourniquet cuffs and found that 23 of 34 tourniquets were contaminated. A limitation of this study was the researchers' inability to examine direct associations with surgical site infection (SSI). The researchers recommended using sterile, single-use, disposable tourniquets to mitigate the potential for SSI from contaminated tourniquet cuffs.

2.7 **If a cuff position change is necessary, remove and reapply the cuff.**[15,16,19] *[Recommendation]*

Low-quality evidence supports completely removing the tourniquet cuff if reapplication is required.[15,16,19] The authors of three case reports found that reducing movement of the tourniquet cuff against the skin reduced friction and **shearing** that can result in skin damage.[15,16,19]

2.8 **Apply a low-linting, soft padding (eg, limb protection sleeve, two layers of stockinette) around the limb under the tourniquet cuff according to the cuff manufacturer's IFU.**[67,68] *[Recommendation]*

Moderate-quality evidence supports using padding under the tourniquet cuff,[67,68] although there is conflicting evidence regarding the type of material or whether this practice decreases the risk for harm. Several researchers have described the padding they used under the tourniquet, including wool,[27] cast padding,[69] single layers of padding,[27,70,71] double layers of padding,[72] or multiple layers in addition to stockinet.[73] Further research is needed.

Din and Geddes[67] published an RCT in 2004 that included 150 patients and found significantly lower skin complications with either cast padding or a skin drape compared to no skin protection under the tourniquet cuff.

In a 2006 RCT that included 92 patients, Olivecrona et al[68] found use of padding with a two-layer elastic stockinette resulted in a significantly lower number of blisters than use of cast padding or no padding.

More-recent evidence is of lower quality and has conflicting results. In a prospective, nonrandomized study of 174 patients that was published in 2018, Castillo Martin et al[74] found that application of a hyperoxygenated fatty-acid cream significantly reduced skin complications when placed on the skin and then covered with a plastic wrap under padding and the tourniquet cuff. Further research is needed regarding adjunct therapies that might be considered medication and require an order and additional medication safety practices.

Conversely, in a nonexperimental study published in 2014, Bosman and Robinson[75] reviewed 97 lower-extremity procedures in which padding was not used and found no significant increase in skin complications without padding when a contoured tourniquet cuff was inflated before application of the preoperative skin antiseptic.

In 2014, in two qualitative survey reports that included responses from a combined total of 251 surgeons, 94.8% of the respondents reported using cotton cast padding under tourniquet cuffs.[2,4]

2.8.1 **Verify that the padding is wrinkle-free and the tourniquet cuff does not pinch the skin.[76]** *[Recommendation]* **P**

Tredwell et al[76] conducted a nonexperimental study with two pediatric participants to compare the effect of different types of padding (ie, a sleeve, two types of cast padding, no padding) on the number and size of skin wrinkles that may lead to skin damage. The patient's limb that was protected with a sleeve had fewer and smaller wrinkles, and the researchers recommended applying a sleeve or two layers of stockinette stretched under the tourniquet cuff.

2.9 Use a physical barrier (eg, impervious adhesive drapes) to prevent fluid accumulation under the cuff and contamination of the tourniquet cuff.[2,14,15,17,66] *[Recommendation]* **P**

Low-quality evidence shows that fluid accumulation (eg, skin antiseptic, irrigation fluid) under the tourniquet cuff can produce chemical burns that result in unnecessary patient suffering and require additional treatment.[2,14,15,17]

Shah et al[2] conducted a survey of 40 surgeons and found that none used a fluid barrier during tourniquet-assisted procedures. The researchers found that 95.4% of the surgeons did not decontaminate the tourniquet after use, and 41.1% reported complications, including skin blisters. Yang et al[15] concluded in a case report that skin necrosis or blistering injuries were related to the antiseptic solution soaking the padding under the tourniquet cuff. The authors of two other case studies also concluded that skin injuries were related to fluid accumulation under tourniquet cuffs.[14,17]

Chiang et al[17] discussed a case in which a chemical burn was related to pressure and fluid maceration on a pediatric patient. The researchers concluded that the increased potential risk for skin injury in vulnerable pediatric populations requires more-stringent adherence to tourniquet protocols.

In an observational study, Thompson et al[66] found that all the reusable tourniquets they studied (N = 70) were contaminated. The researchers recommended using single-use sterile tourniquets to reduce the risk of infection.

2.10 **Position the cuff tubing on or near the lateral aspect of the extremity, facing away from the sterile field.** *[Recommendation]*

Although there is no evidence regarding complications from tourniquet cuff–induced pressure injuries, lateral placement of the cuff tubing alleviates the pressure of the patient's body on the tourniquet tubing, which could cause maceration and skin breakdown. Even when a sterile tourniquet is used, facing the tubing away from the sterile field increases the sterile field space and decreases the potential for tubing to occlude or contaminate the sterile field.

2.11 **Use tourniquet tubing and connectors that are incompatible with other tubing (eg, IV tubing) or are labeled to clearly identify that they are part of the tourniquet system.[77]** *[Recommendation]*

Clearly identifying different tubing in the perioperative setting may reduce confusion and prevent inaccurate connections.[77]

2.12 **Keep tourniquet tubing and electrical cords off the floor or covered and away from high-traffic areas to provide unobstructed pathways.[65]** *[Recommendation]*

Refer to the AORN Guideline for a Safe Environment of Care[65] for additional guidance related to safe use of electrical equipment.

3. Tourniquet Inflation

3.1 **When prophylactic antibiotics are ordered, time administration with the goal of achieving optimal tissue concentration.**[78-82] *[Recommendation]*

Moderate-quality evidence supports finding the optimal tissue concentration for prophylactic antibiotics based on the type of antibiotic and the procedure.[78-82]

In two studies published in 1994 and 1995 (N = 109), researchers found that administration of antibiotics 20 minutes before tourniquet inflation produced higher tissue concentrations than administration 4 hours before inflation.[81,82] However, three more-recent studies (N = 1,046) found no difference in SSI incidence when antibiotics were administered within 30 minutes before tourniquet inflation or administered 10 minutes before tourniquet deflation.[78-80]

In an RCT published in 2011, Akinyoola et al[78] found that administering cefuroxime prophylactically 1 minute after exsanguination and inflation resulted in significantly fewer deep infections, faster healing time, and higher surgeon satisfaction than administering antibiotics 5 minutes before exsanguination and inflation.

Soriano et al[79] conducted an RCT in 2008 to investigate the effects of giving 1.5 g cefuroxime either 10 to 30 minutes before tourniquet inflation (n = 442) or 10 minutes before deflation (n = 466) to 908 patients undergoing TKA. Both groups received a second dose of cefuroxime 6 hours after incision. The researchers found no difference in infection rates between the groups, but there was an increased risk of infection for patients with an American Society of Anesthesiologists physical status classification of III or IV and for patients who had a low hematocrit on postoperative day four.

In a nonexperimental study published in 2015, Prats et al[80] administered the antibiotic cefonicid to 32 TKA patients before they entered the operating room. The researchers took samples of synovial fluid to compare the concentration of cefonicid when the tourniquet was inflated to between 350 mmHg and 400 mmHg to the concentration after the prosthesis was implanted and the tourniquet was deflated. The researchers found that only one of the 32 patients began the procedure without reaching the minimum inhibitory concentration for antibiotic efficacy. For all the other patients, the antibiotic concentration levels fell but remained over the minimum inhibitory concentration level when the implantation was completed.

One literature review[83] and a clinical practice guideline[84] suggested that optimal tissue concentration of antibiotics can be achieved with administration of IV antibiotics either within 30 minutes before incision[83,84] or 10 minutes before tourniquet deflation.[84]

Although antibiotic timing was not the primary outcome, the researchers in 16 RCTs described the administration and timing of antibiotics in their study methodologies.[29,32,55,70,72,73,85-94] Further research on this topic is needed.

3.2 **Notify the OR team before the extremity is exsanguinated.** *[Recommendation]*

Adverse reactions are likely to occur close to the time of initial tourniquet inflation. Notifying the team before extremity exsanguination may facilitate the team members' response to any adverse reactions that could occur during this critical phase.

3.3 **Exsanguinate the extremity before inflation of the tourniquet.**[4,95] *[Recommendation]*

Exsanguinating the extremity before tourniquet cuff inflation facilitates a relatively bloodless field during extremity procedures.[95] Yalçinkaya et al[4] found that more than 95% of orthopedic surgeons and residents surveyed exsanguinated the extremity before inflating the tourniquet cuff.

3.3.1 **The extremity may be exsanguinated by elevation.**[95] *[Conditional Recommendation]*

Low-quality evidence indicates that the benefits of exsanguinating by elevation alone may outweigh the harms of elevating the extremity before inflating the tourniquet.[3,95]

Angadi et al[95] conducted a nonexperimental study in 2010 and found that in 50 patients, elevation required less time than exsanguination with an elastic wrap and there was no significant difference in tourniquet time or complications at 6 weeks after surgery.

Although exsanguination was not the primary outcome of the studies, some RCT researchers have reported using elevation alone for exsanguination in their study methodology section.[32,34,85,96-98] Further research is needed regarding the efficacy and safety of exsanguination methods.

3.3.2 **Elastic wrap (eg, an Esmarch bandage) may be used for exsanguination unless contraindicated (eg, by extended immobilization, infection, fracture, malignancy).**[22,99,100] *[Conditional Recommendation]*

Low-quality evidence indicates that the risk for harm may not outweigh the benefit of using an elastic wrap for exsanguination.[22,99,100] The potential harms include increased pain[100] and adverse events.[22,99]

Yalçinkaya et al[4] surveyed 211 orthopedic residents and surgeons in Turkey and reported that 173 surgeons used an elastic wrap or Esmarch bandage rather than elevation alone. Cunningham et al[3] surveyed orthopedic surgeons in Ireland about exsanguination techniques and found that these surgeons preferred using the Rhys-Davies exsanguinator over the use of elastic wraps or elevation alone. Among the respondents (N = 112), 6% of the surgeons used elastic wraps for upper extremity procedures and 10% of the surgeons used them for lower extremity procedures.[3]

Tanpowpong et al[100] conducted a quasi-experimental study to compare 23 healthy volunteers' responses to elevation and bandaging exsanguination and found that elevation significantly increased pain tolerance compared to elastic band exsanguination.

Desai et al[22] reported on a case in which the mechanical stress of elastic wrap exsanguination resulted in a pulmonary embolism in a patient who had surgery on the seventh day after sustaining a tibial plateau fracture. The authors recommended estimating the risk for existing DVT (eg, immobilization, planned use of a tourniquet) associated with elastic wraps and tourniquets to determine the use of either. Barron and McGrory[99] reported on a case in which not using mechanical exsanguination prevented a calcific myonecrosis mass rupture and allowed tourniquet use without adverse effects.

Many RCT researchers note the use of elastic wraps in their study methodologies but do not address outcomes specific to the use of elastic wraps.[9,27,54,71,73,89,94,101-104] Further research is needed to evaluate the benefits and harms associated with using elastic wraps for exsanguination.

3.3.3 Do not use a **hand-over-hand exsanguination technique**.[98] [Recommendation]

The potential harms of hand-over-hand exsanguination outweigh the potential benefits.

Zhang et al[98] conducted an RCT that included 236 patients and found that compared to exsanguination by elevating the extremity, a hand-over-hand squeeze exsanguination was associated with more skin tension blisters and increased postoperative pain.

3.4 Keep tourniquet inflation pressure to a minimum based on the individual patient's needs

instead of using a **standardized pressure**.[72,105,106] [Recommendation]

High-quality evidence supports that lower tourniquet pressure is associated with fewer postoperative complications.[72,105,106] The evidence supports using the lowest tourniquet pressure effective to achieve hemostasis, create a clear field of vision, and prevent excessive intraoperative blood loss based on individual patient factors.

In a systematic review, Ding et al[106] reviewed nine RCTs published between 2003 and 2017 that involved 1,200 surgical patients. The studies compared standard tourniquet pressures to individualized pressures and found no differences in operative time; however, lower pressures resulted in significantly better hemostatic effects as determined by field visibility and fewer complications.

In three RCTs[72,104,105] that were not included in this systematic review and included 440 patients, the researchers found that physician-specified pressures (eg, fixed pressure values, systolic blood pressure [SBP])[105] or pressures determined by SBP with a **safety margin**[72] using patient-specific methods were significantly associated with decreased intraoperative hyperemia,[104] fewer complications,[72,105] and increased postoperative functionality[72] compared to standardized inflation pressures.[104]

The researchers also found that using patient-specific methods for determining pressure resulted in no difference in tourniquet inflation time,[105] field visibility,[62,105] or pain.[72,104]

Lower-quality evidence also supports that lower inflation pressures decrease patients' pain[107] and protein degradation[35] in the tissue under the tourniquet cuff.

3.5 Measure the **limb occlusion pressure** (LOP) to determine initial tourniquet pressure.[72,104,105] [Recommendation]

High-quality evidence supports that using the LOP to determine tourniquet pressure could decrease complications related to higher pressures without jeopardizing the quality of field (QOF).[72,104,105]

Three RCTs that included 420 patients found that compared to other methods, using LOP resulted in lower pressures[72,104,105] but no difference in QOF[104,105] or intraoperative pain.[72,105] Tourniquet pressure based on the LOP was associated with

- a 2.9 times greater chance of an optimal QOF,[104]
- decreased short-term pain,[104]
- fewer skin blisters,[72,105] and
- fewer adverse events.[105]

Lower-quality evidence also supports that measuring the LOP results in lower pressure requirements than using a standardized pressure by limb or the patient's SBP with a safety margin.[62,72,104,105,108-113] These studies also found that the QOF visibility was acceptable with lower pressures, although further research is needed to determine potential adverse events related to lower pressures.

3.5.1 **Limb occlusion pressure may be measured manually using a Doppler ultrasound,[105] by using a US Food and Drug Administration (FDA)-cleared automatic system[108,114] in accordance with the manufacturer's IFU, or by using the arterial occlusion pressure (AOP) estimation formula.[53,103,109,115] [Conditional Recommendation]**

Techniques for measuring LOP have evolved, and the Doppler technique has been called the gold standard.[108,114] However, there are FDA-cleared automatic systems designed to remove the risk for human error associated with the Doppler technique.

Researchers using distal pulse oximetry sensory equipment[114] or pressure sensors within the tourniquet cuff[105] found no difference in measured LOP than when using the Doppler technique[108,114] and found lower pressures than standardized pressure[104] or surgeon-specified pressures.[72,116] Researchers who conducted studies of the AOP estimation formula concluded that lower pressure settings were required compared to those determined using the Doppler technique[103] or observed lower pressures[53,109]; however, one RCT was discontinued when researchers observed unsafe blood loss when the AOP estimation formula was used.[117]

Moderate-quality evidence supports measuring the LOP manually using Doppler ultrasound,[105] by using automatic distal pulse oximetry sensory,[114] by using pressure sensors within the tourniquet cuff,[108] or by using the AOP estimation formula.[53,103,109,115] Evidence regarding the AOP estimation formula efficacy conflicts,[103,117] and further research is needed.

Mu et al[105] conducted an RCT to compare surgeon-specified pressure to the patient-specific LOP by Doppler ultrasound and found significantly lower pressures and fewer adverse reactions (eg, blisters, swelling, pain, numbness) when pressures were patient specific.

In an RCT, McEwen et al[114] compared using the Doppler method to determine LOP to an automatic technique using a distal pulse sensor and found no difference. Several other researchers who conducted studies from 1993 to 2018 comparing the same automatic LOP technique used by McEwen et al[114] to the Doppler method found that using the automatic LOP

technique resulted in lower required tourniquet pressures.[62,72,104,116,118,119]

Masri et al[108] conducted an RCT to compare measuring the LOP by an automatic, continuous dual-purpose patient sensor and pneumatic effector with the Doppler technique. They found no significant difference between the two techniques.

Evidence conflicts on using the AOP estimation formula exclusively to guide pressure parameters.[53,103,109,115] Some evidence shows that using the AOP estimation formula resulted in lower pressures[53,109] compared to LOP determined by Doppler ultrasound[103] or standardized pressure.[115] However, the evidence conflicts regarding the QOF with use of the AOP estimation formula.[103,117]

Tuncalı et al[103] conducted an RCT that included 93 patients and found that compared to using the Doppler technique, the AOP formula took less time to estimate the LOP, resulted in 9% lower pressures, and resulted in no difference in tourniquet effectiveness. Conversely, Perez et al[117] stopped their RCT early after finding that pressures based on the estimated AOP with a safety margin produced an unacceptable QOF and surgeons were unable to complete the procedures safely.

In nonexperimental studies that included 471 participants, researchers observed that the calculated AOP estimation formula in addition to a safety margin was associated with low pressures and no complications.[53,109]

3.5.2 **Take the baseline SBP or LOP measurement when the patient's blood pressure is stabilized to the level expected during surgery; this may be done before or after induction of anesthesia.[119] [Recommendation]**

In 1993, Pedowitz et al[119] published an RCT that included 60 patients and recommended finding the LOP preoperatively, before the decrease in blood pressure that occurs during induction of anesthesia. However, the researchers acknowledged that the procedure to determine the LOP can cause pain and that finding the LOP after anesthesia and stabilization of blood pressure may mitigate unnecessary pain.

3.5.3 **Add a safety margin to the LOP based on the manufacturer's IFU when available.[62,72,113,119] [Recommendation]**

Although no studies compared safety margin parameters, moderate-quality evidence includes various methods for determining safety margin parameters to facilitate a bloodless operative field and account for any intraoperative variations in the patient's condition. Researchers used either a standardized pressure of 50 mmHg[113,119] or determined safety margins based on the LOP:

- 40-50 mmHg for LOP < 130 mmHg,
- 60-75 mmHg for LOP 131-190 mmHg and
- 80-100 mmHg for LOP > 190 mmHg.[62,72]

3.5.4 **Inflation pressure may be increased for limbs with larger circumferences.**[53] *[Conditional Recommendation]*

Low-quality studies have shown that limb circumference is only one of the many variables to consider when determining inflation pressure.[118] Conversely, Tuncalı et al[53] conducted a nonexperimental study to investigate the correlation of SBP and AOP in 193 patients and found that higher pressures were required for larger extremity circumferences that correlate with a higher SBPs, which led to higher AOP values.

3.6 **Inflate the tourniquet cuff in coordination with the surgeon and the anesthesia professional after verifying the pressure and position of the extremity.**[20] *[Recommendation]*

Santhosh et al[20] reported a case of a 20-year-old patient undergoing the removal of hemangioma who developed a pulmonary edema after exsanguination and 1 minute of tourniquet inflation to 250 mmHg. The patient's condition improved with tourniquet deflation, which confirmed that circulatory overload was caused by the fluid shift related to exsanguination. The authors concluded that the entire team needs to be attentive during exsanguination and inflation of the tourniquet to respond quickly to systemic effects of tourniquet use.

3.7 **When using multiple tourniquet cuffs on the same extremity, confirm whether**

- **a dual-bladder tourniquet cuff and extra connective tubing will be used,**
- **a higher pressure is planned to compensate for the narrow size of each cuff bladder, and**
- **the planned location on the extremity is wide enough to accommodate the additional width of the dual-bladder tourniquet cuff.**[102,120]

[Recommendation]

Moderate-quality evidence shows that higher pressures are necessary with narrow cuffs,[102] which are associated with an increased risk for patient injury.[120]

Haghighi et al[102] conducted an RCT with 80 patients and found that although Bier blocks are frequently completed with two narrow tourniquet cuffs inflated separately, using one wide cuff resulted in signifi-

cantly longer time to onset of pain and median time to reach maximum pain, with similar fentanyl consumption. However, patients who had two narrow cuffs consumed significantly fewer opioid medications. The double tourniquet group had significantly higher pressures, which were determined using the manual LOP technique. The researchers concluded that procedures shorter than 40 minutes in which a single, wide tourniquet is used can result in satisfactory pain relief with lower potential injury related to medication toxicity and higher pressures.

In 1998, Kokki et al[120] conducted an RCT of 28 patients in which the tourniquet manufacturer's IFU were followed to increase the pressure in a narrow cuff compared to a wide cuff. The researchers found that tourniquet use increased muscular injury regardless of which cuff was used.

3.7.1 **Clearly identify the cuff location, respective tubing, and equipment.** *[Recommendation]*

When there is more than one tourniquet or tourniquet bladder to be inflated, clearly identifying the cuffs, tubing, and equipment for the tourniquet location may reduce the risk of erroneously inflating or deflating the incorrect cuff.

3.7.3 **Clearly communicate the inflation sequence when using a dual-bladder cuff or when using two single-bladder cuffs together for IVRA.**[24] *[Recommendation]*

4. Monitoring During Inflation

4.1 **Keep pneumatic tourniquet inflation time to a minimum.**[8,121-125] *[Recommendation]* P

Although high-quality evidence supports reducing the length of time the tourniquet is inflated to prevent the potential harms associated with longer inflation times,[8,121-125] there are important variations in study results[8,70,71,91,97,121,124,126-128] and further research is needed.

Five systematic reviews that included studies published between 1997 and 2016,[8,121-124] and an additional six RCTs[69-71,96,97,126] and four quasi-experimental studies[91,125,127,128] reviewed the effects of early and late tourniquet release in 6,315 surgical patients. The benefits of **early release** included decreased time to functional recovery[123] and fewer complications.[8,121-125] Potential harms included increased

- calculated blood loss,[8,121,122,124]
- intraoperative blood loss,[123]
- postoperative blood loss,[121,122,124]
- total blood loss,[121-124] and
- blood transfusion rate.[8,121,124,128]

The researchers found no difference between early and **late release** for the following outcomes:

- postoperative analgesic consumption,[91]
- DVT incidence,[70,97,121,122]
- reduction in hemoglobin or hematocrit,[8,121,122,124] and
- implant efficacy.[96,125]

Although researchers found differences when comparing early and late tourniquet release, there was conflicting evidence for the following outcomes:

- blood loss,[8,71,97,121,124,126,127]
- complication rate,[71,97,124]
- functional recovery,[70,97,127]
- length of hospital stay,[70,91,127,128]
- postoperative pain,[97,126,127] and
- transfusion rate.[8,71,91,124,126]

Even with relatively short tourniquet inflation times (ie, 26 ± 8 minutes), researchers have found elevated markers of systemic inflammatory response when measured 15 minutes after tourniquet deflation.[129] In 1986, one group of researchers recommended that inflation times for pediatric patients should be less than 75 minutes.[130]

4.2 Monitor the patient for complications related to tourniquet inflation or duration.[14] *[Recommendation]*

Low-quality evidence suggests that visual monitoring of the tourniquet cuff may facilitate tourniquet problem identification before a patient injury occurs.[14]

Ellanti and Hurson[14] concluded in a case report that skin blisters and necrosis occurred when the tourniquet shifted distally. The authors suggested that regular inspection of the tourniquet site during the procedure could prevent patient injury when the fluid barrier has shifted.

4.2.1 Monitor the patient for normothermia during tourniquet inflation.[131-134] *[Recommendation]* **P**

Low-quality evidence[131-134] shows that tourniquet use can disrupt core body temperature.

Estebe et al[133] conducted an RCT in 1996 of 26 patients and found that patients' core temperatures increased during pneumatic tourniquet–assisted procedures correlating with the length of time the tourniquet was inflated, whereas patients undergoing procedures without a tourniquet did not have an increase in core temperature.

Chon and Lee[134] conducted a nonexperimental study in 2012 and found that prolonged tourniquet inflation time in 30 open procedures and 30 arthroscopic procedures was associated with a lower esophageal temperature 5 minutes after inflation. A limitation of this study is that the average preoperative core temperature in the arthroscopic group was significantly lower than in the open procedures

group. The researchers recommended more studies to find associations between temperature, procedure type, and duration of tourniquet inflation.

In 1986, Bloch[132] retrospectively examined significant increases in the body temperatures of pediatric patients undergoing unilateral limb procedures (n = 32), bilateral limb procedures (n = 24), and superficial procedures without a tourniquet (n = 14). Body temperatures increased 0.71° C and 1.33° C (1.3° F and 2.4° F) for unilateral and bilateral tourniquet–assisted procedures respectively.

In a 1992 quasi-experimental study, Bloch et al[131] found a significant increase in body temperature during tourniquet inflation in 47 pediatrics patients. There was no significant decrease in temperature after 15 minutes of deflation. These researchers recommended against aggressively warming pediatric patients during tourniquet-assisted procedures because the transient rise in temperature could be mistaken for malignant hyperthermia.

4.2.2 Monitor pediatric patients for respiratory acidosis.[130] *[Recommendation]* **P**

Low-quality evidence shows that respiratory acidosis may be an increased risk in pediatric populations when tourniquet inflation is longer than 75 minutes.[130]

In a 1986 nonexperimental study, Lynn et al[130] observed that in 15 pediatric patients, lactic acid was elevated for 10 minutes after tourniquet deflation. The researchers recommended assessing respiratory acidosis by blood gas tension in pediatric patients undergoing tourniquet-assisted procedures, especially if tourniquet inflation is longer than 75 minutes.

4.2.3 For regional and local anesthesia procedures, monitor the patient's tolerance (eg, pain) during inflation.[3,100] *[Recommendation]*

Low-quality evidence[3,100] shows that patients experience increased pain during tourniquet inflation.

In a nonexperimental study, Tanpowpong et al[100] found that neither elevation nor an elastic bandage was able to negate tourniquet-related pain in 23 healthy volunteers. All the volunteers reported that the maximal pain occurred under the tourniquet cuff after inflation.

Cunningham et al[3] surveyed 60 orthopedic surgeons in Ireland. Respondents reported that 54% of their patients undergoing upper extremity procedures tolerated tourniquet inflation poorly under local or regional anesthesia. Conversely,

71% of the respondents reported that lower extremity procedures were rarely or never tolerated poorly.

4.3 **Keep activation indicators and pressure displays visible to the entire OR team and keep audible alarms sufficiently loud to be heard above other sounds in the OR.**[65] *[Recommendation]*

Refer to the AORN Guideline for a Safe Environment of Care[65] for additional guidance related to clinical and alert alarms.

4.4 **Inform the surgeon of the tourniquet inflation time at regular, established intervals.**[135] *[Recommendation]*

A clinical practice guideline recommends informing the surgeon of the tourniquet time every 15 minutes after the 1-hour mark of inflation.[135]

5. Tourniquet Deflation

5.1 **Coordinate the timing of tourniquet deflation based on the surgical procedure and the anesthesia plan of care.**[24] *[Recommendation]*

Confirming, before tourniquet deflation, that any surgical interventions to occur during use of the tourniquet have been completed facilitates teamwork for safe patient care. Additional interventions may occur after the tourniquet is deflated.

5.2 **When tourniquets are used on two extremities, confirm the sequence and timing of the deflation of each of the tourniquets.**[136] *[Recommendation]*

Zarrouki et al[136] reviewed a case report of cardiac arrest after prescribed staggered inflation and deflation of bilateral tourniquets. The researchers recommended following duration and pressure limits for pneumatic tourniquets to allow safe bilateral procedures.

5.2.1 **Clearly communicate the deflation sequence when using multiple or dual-bladder tourniquet cuffs for IVRA.**[24] *[Recommendation]*

5.3 **Remove the cuff and padding from the extremity after deflation of the tourniquet.** *[Recommendation]*

5.4 Postoperatively assess the patient's
- circulation in the extremity (eg, pulses, temperature, capillary refill),
- skin condition under and distal to the cuff site, and
- sensory and motor response of the operative extremity compared to the contralateral extremity.[18]

[Recommendation]

Comparing the preoperative assessment to postoperative changes allows for evaluation of skin or nerve injury and reperfusion of the extremity after tourniquet use. Kindle et al[18] reported on a case in which excessive tourniquet pressure and time caused compartment syndrome after an anterior cruciate ligament repair that led to additional neurologic symptoms.

5.5 **Monitor the patient's vital signs after tourniquet deflation.**[21,136-138] *[Recommendation]*

Low-quality evidence shows that patients' vital signs are affected during deflation and warrant monitoring.[21,136-138] After tourniquet deflation, products of anaerobic metabolism (eg, lactate) enter the systemic circulation and may cause acidosis.

Huh et al[137] conducted a nonexperimental study involving 86 TKA patients and observed blood pressure changes and related **baroreflex autoregulation** during tourniquet deflation. Of 86 patients undergoing a TKA, 15 developed severe hypotension, and 10 of these patients required pharmaceutical intervention to correct hypotension during tourniquet deflation.

Panerai et al[138] conducted a nonexperimental study that included nine healthy volunteers and found a significant decrease in blood pressure and cerebral blood flow velocity after tourniquet deflation. The researchers concluded that systemic changes were only weakly associated with tourniquet use.

The authors of two case reports described cardiac arrest immediately after tourniquet deflation and concluded that the arrests were related to tourniquet deflation.[21,136]

5.6 **Monitor the patient for normothermia after tourniquet deflation.**[139] *[Recommendation]*

Tsunoda et al[139] compared a matched-cohort of 10 patients who underwent tourniquet-assisted procedures to 10 patients who underwent procedures without tourniquets. The tourniquet-assisted procedures group had significantly higher postoperative peak body temperatures, and both groups took 24 hours to return to preoperative body temperature.

5.7 **Assess the patient for tourniquet-associated pain after tourniquet deflation.**[9,27,32,33,140] *[Recommendation]*

High-quality evidence suggests that tourniquet use increases postoperative short-term pain and analgesic use.[9,27,32,33]

Researchers conducting RCTs found that compared to longer tourniquet inflation time, patients who underwent procedures without tourniquet assistance or with shorter duration of tourniquet inflation time
- had significantly more short-term pain,[9,27,32,33]
- used significantly fewer analgesics,[32] and
- did not have a difference in long-term pain.[32,33]

Kruse et al[140] observed that use of a tourniquet in 603 patients was associated with an increased use of postoperative opioids with a higher peak in severity of pain and a longer postanesthesia care unit stay. They concluded that antioxidants could attenuate the pain response.

5.8 **Report preoperative assessment, tourniquet intervention, and postoperative evaluation during the hand over to the recovery team.**[24] *[Recommendation]*

Hand-over communication facilitates the continuity of care and may prevent confusion and injury during the postoperative recovery phase. Refer to the AORN Guideline for Team Communication[24] for additional guidance related to hand-over procedures.

6. Equipment Safety

6.1 **Verify that the tourniquet and accessories are complete, clean or sterile, and functioning according to the manufacturer's IFU:**
- **confirm that the battery is fully charged, if applicable;**
- **inspect the cuff, tubing, connectors, and closure systems for damage or flaws;**
- **test the tourniquet for integrity and function; and**
- **use a pneumatic tourniquet regulator that is compatible with all associated components and secure the connections.**

[Recommendation]

6.1.1 **Clean and disinfect reusable cuffs and bladders after each use with a facility-approved disinfectant in accordance with the manufacturer's IFU, including dry time.**[141] *[Recommendation]*

In a nonexperimental study, Sahu et al[141] found that all 16 tourniquets examined had bacterial colonies, and the inside and proximal edges of tourniquets were the areas most contaminated with *Staphylococcus* species (77.9%), of which 74.6% were coagulase-negative staphylococci. Two different solutions were 90% effective in reducing tourniquet contamination. The researchers recommended using an alcohol-based solution to disinfect tourniquets.

6.2 **Maintain records of tourniquet maintenance, including**
- **biomedical equipment identification number or serial number,**
- **date of inspection, and**
- **preventive maintenance.**

[Recommendation]

Accreditation agencies require that medical devices be maintained.[142]

6.3 **When there is evidence of complications or adverse events related to the use of a pneumatic tourniquet,**
- **notify the OR team,**
- **obtain functioning equipment and supplies,**
- **replace faulty equipment and supplies under the direction of the operator, and**
- **document the actions taken.**

[Recommendation]

6.4 **The health care organization must report to the FDA and the manufacturer when a pneumatic tourniquet is suspected of having contributed to a death or serious injury.**[143] *[Regulatory Requirement]*

6.4.1 **The health care organization must report to other regulatory bodies as defined by state or local regulations.**[143] *[Regulatory Requirement]*

6.4.2 **When a patient injury occurs as a result of pneumatic tourniquet use, the user must**
- **remove the tourniquet supplies and equipment from service;**
- **retain all supplies if possible; and**
- **report the adverse event details,**[142] **including device identification and maintenance and service information, according to the health care organization's policy and procedures.**[143]

[Regulatory Requirement]

It is a Centers for Medicare & Medicaid Services requirement[142] to retain the pneumatic tourniquet equipment, regulator, cuff, and tubing accessories to facilitate an investigation and prevent future injuries.

7. Documentation

7.1 **Document the following:**
- **initial assessment of the operative extremity:**
  - **skin condition,**
  - **peripheral vasculature, and**
  - **neuromuscular and sensory responses;**
- **tourniquet cuff size and location;**
- **the person who applied the tourniquet;**
- **skin protection measures taken;**
- **cuff pressure settings;**
- **times of inflation and deflation;**
- **total time inflated;**
- **reperfusion time, if applicable;**
- **postoperative assessment of the operative extremity:**
  - **skin condition,**
  - **peripheral vasculature, and**
  - **neuromuscular and sensory responses;**

- systemic reactions to ischemia and reperfusion;
- communication of concerns (ie, to whom, what, and when); and
- system identification information.[144]

[Recommendation]

Documenting the cuff pressure settings provides a comprehensive representation of patient care. See the AORN Guideline for Patient Information Management for more information on documentation.[144]

8. Education

8.1 Provide education on the use of pneumatic tourniquets and the physiologic effects of pneumatic tourniquet use, including

- following all manufacturers' IFU for tourniquet equipment and accessories,
- identifying contraindications to pneumatic tourniquet use,
- identifying risks to patients and precautions to minimize these risks,
- selecting the appropriate tourniquet cuff based on patient assessment and plan of care,
- applying tourniquet and accessories safely,
- measuring initial tourniquet pressure settings and safety margins, and
- identifying corrective actions in the event of a patient injury.

[Recommendation]

8.2 Verify the competency of personnel responsible for the safety of patients undergoing pneumatic tourniquet–assisted procedures.

Glossary

Arterial occlusion pressure estimation formula: A tourniquet-pressure estimation formula that equals the systolic blood pressure + 10 divided by the tissue padding coefficient (KTP): [(SBP+10)/KTP].

Baroreflex autoregulation: A physiological response to control fluctuations in blood pressure.

Compartment syndrome: A pathologic condition caused by the progressive development of arterial compression and consequent reduction of blood supply. Clinical manifestations include swelling, restriction of movement, vascular compromise, and severe pain or lack of sensation.

Contoured tourniquet cuff: A pneumatic tourniquet cuff with a distal edge shorter than the proximal edge, creating a funnel-like shape when applied to a tapered extremity.

Cylindrical tourniquet cuff: A pneumatic tourniquet cuff with equal distal and proximal edges to fit non-tapered extremities.

Early release: Deflating the tourniquet any time before dressings are applied.

Exsanguination: The process of forcible expulsion of blood from an extremity before inflation of the pneumatic tourniquet.

Functional recovery: The process of rehabilitating the operative extremity to preoperative functional abilities.

Hand-over-hand exsanguination technique: The exsanguination technique of manually squeezing the patient's extremity by changing hands over each other, moving from the distal extremity toward the pneumatic tourniquet.

Intravenous regional anesthesia: The administration of intravenous anesthetic agents that is sometimes facilitated by a pneumatic tourniquet to localize medications distally to provide patients decreased sensory and motor function and to allow surgeons to perform extremity procedures under moderate sedation when general anesthesia is contraindicated or not desired.

Late release: Deflating the tourniquet after dressings are applied.

Limb occlusion pressure: The minimum pressure required to stop the flow of arterial blood into the limb distal to the pneumatic tourniquet cuff. Synonym: arterial occlusion pressure.

Pneumatic tourniquet: A tourniquet in which pressure is created with air inside a bladder cuff.

Preconditioning techniques: Techniques used to reduce oxidative stress and increase skeletal muscle ischemia tolerance related to tourniquet inflation by initiating anesthetic regimens or short intervals of temporary ischemia.

Reperfusion techniques: Techniques used to allow reperfusion of the extremity by deflating the pneumatic tourniquet for a period of time before reinflating the tourniquet to continue the operative procedure.

Reperfusion time: Time the tourniquet is deflated and reinflated during the procedure.

Safety margin: Additional pressure added to a pneumatic tourniquet inflation pressure to account for physiologic variations during the procedure to ensure the quality of field.

Shearing: A sliding movement of skin and subcutaneous tissue that leaves the underlying muscle stationary.

Staggered tourniquet deflation: A method of releasing and re-inflating a pneumatic tourniquet a few times before completely deflating the cuff at the end of a procedure with a goal of mitigating a physiological response to a sudden loss of blood volume.

Standardized pressure: Using a standard pneumatic tourniquet inflation pressure that is not based on patient-specific factors.

References

1. Boya H, Tuncalı B, Özcan Ö, Araç Ş, Tuncay C. Practice of tourniquet use in Turkey: a pilot study. *Acta Orthop Traumatol Turc.* 2016;50(2):162-170. [IIIB]

2. Shah FA, Mahmood K, Din SU, Mehsod WM, Qureshi AR, Babar IU. A survey of tourniquet use in limbs surgery among the orthopaedic surgeons of Peshawar. *Pak J Med Health Sci.* 2014;8(3):523-526. [IIIC]

3. Cunningham L, McCarthy T, O'Byrne J. A survey of upper and lower limb tourniquet use among Irish orthopaedic surgeons. *Ir J Med Sci.* 2013;182(3):325-330. [IIIB]

4. Yalçinkaya M, Sökücü S, Erdoğan S, Kabukçuoğlu YS. Tourniquet use in orthopedic surgery: a descriptive survey study among Turkish orthopedic surgeons and residents in Istanbul. *Acta Orthop Traumatol Turc.* 2014;48(5):483-490. [IIIB]

5. Daruwalla ZJ, Rowan F, Finnegan M, Fennell J, Neligan M. Exsanguinators and tourniquets: do we need to change our practice? *Surgeon.* 2012;10(3):137-142. [IIIC]

6. Yi S, Tan J, Chen C, Chen H, Huang W. The use of pneumatic tourniquet in total knee arthroplasty: a meta-analysis. *Arch Orthop Trauma Surg.* 2014;134(10):1469-1476. [IA]

7. Jiang F, Zhong H, Hong YC, Zhao GF. Use of a tourniquet in total knee arthroplasty: a systematic review and meta-analysis of randomized controlled trials. *J Orthop Sci.* 2015;20(1):110-123. [IA]

8. Zhang W, Liu A, Hu D, Tan Y, Al-Aidaros M, Pan Z. Effects of the timing of tourniquet release in cemented total knee arthroplasty: a systematic review and meta-analysis of randomized controlled trials. *J Orthop Surg Res.* 2014;9:125. [IA]

9. Pfitzner T, von Roth P, Voerkelius N, Mayr H, Perka C, Hube R. Influence of the tourniquet on tibial cement mantle thickness in primary total knee arthroplasty. *Knee Surg Sports Traumatol Arthrosc.* 2016;24(1):96-101. [IA]

10. Li X, Yin L, Chen ZY, et al. The effect of tourniquet use in total knee arthroplasty: grading the evidence through an updated meta-analysis of randomized, controlled trials. *Eur J Orthop Surg Traumatol.* 2014;24(6):973-986. [IA]

11. Kumar K, Railton C, Tawfic Q. Tourniquet application during anesthesia: "what we need to know?" *J Anaesthesiol Clin Pharmacol.* 2016;32(4):424-430. [VA]

12. Ducic I, Chang S, Dellon AL. Use of the tourniquet in reconstructive surgery in patients with previous ipsilateral lower extremity revascularization: is it safe? A survey. *J Reconstr Microsurg.* 2006;22(3):183-189. [IIIC]

13. McMillan TE, Johnstone AJ. Tourniquet uses and precautions. *Surgery.* 2017;35(4):201-203. [VB]

14. Ellanti P, Hurson C. Tourniquet-associated povidone-iodine-induced chemical burns. *BMJ Case Rep.* 2015;2015. [VC]

15. Yang JH, Lim H, Yoon JR, Jeong HI. Tourniquet associated chemical burn. *Indian J Orthop.* 2012;46(3):356-359. [VB]

16. Supradeeptha C, Shandilya SM, Naresh A, Satyaprasad J. Aqueous based povidone-iodine related chemical burn under the tourniquet (a case report) and literature review. *J Orthop.* 2013;10(3):152-154. [VB]

17. Chiang YC, Lin TS, Yeh MC. Povidone-iodine-related burn under the tourniquet of a child—a case report and literature review. *J Plast Reconstr Aesthet Surg.* 2011;64(3):412-415. [VC]

18. Kindle BJ, Murthy N, Stolp K. Compartment syndrome with mononeuropathies following anterior cruciate ligament reconstruction. *Am J Phys Med Rehabil.* 2015;94(5):e37-e41. [VC]

19. Mingo-Robinet J, Castañeda-Cabrero C, Alvarez V, Léon Alonso-Cortés JM, Monge-Casares E. Tourniquet-related iatrogenic femoral nerve palsy after knee surgery: case report and review of the literature. *Case Rep Orthop.* 2013;2013:368290. [VC]

20. Santhosh MC, Pai RB, Rao RP. Acute pulmonary edema following inflation of arterial tourniquet. *Rev Esp Anestesiol Reanim.* 2014;61(8):451-453. [VA]

21. Houng WR, Lee CL, Chiou HM, Wei YS. Cardiac arrest after tourniquet deflation in tibial plateau fracture surgery in a healthy man. *Formosan Journal of Musculoskeletal Disorders.* 2012;3(1):34-38. [VB]

22. Desai S, Prashantha PG, Torgal SV, Rao R. Fatal pulmonary embolism subsequent to the use of Esmarch bandage and tourniquet: a case report and review of literature. *Saudi J Anaesth.* 2013;7(3):331-335. [VB]

23. Guideline for care of the patient receiving local anesthesia. In: *Guidelines for Perioperative Practice.* Denver, CO: AORN, Inc; 2020:447-442. [IVA]

24. Guideline for team communication. In: *Guidelines for Perioperative Practice.* Denver, CO: AORN, Inc; 2020:1039-1070. [IVA]

25. Zhang W, Li N, Chen S, Tan Y, Al-Aidaros M, Chen L. The effects of a tourniquet used in total knee arthroplasty: a meta-analysis. *J Orthop Surg Res.* 2014;9(1):13. [IA]

26. Præstegaard M, Beisvåg E, Erichsen JL, Brix M, Viberg B. Tourniquet use in lower limb fracture surgery: a systematic review and meta-analysis. *Eur J Orthop Surg Traumatol.* 2019;29(1):175-181. [IB]

27. Liu PL, Li DQ, Zhang YK, et al. Effects of unilateral tourniquet used in patients undergoing simultaneous bilateral total knee arthroplasty. *Orthop Surg.* 2017;9(2):180-185. [IB]

28. Stetzelberger V, Obertacke U, Jawhar A. Tourniquet application during TKA did not affect the accuracy of implant positioning: a randomized clinical trial. *Knee Surg Sports Traumatol Arthrosc.* 2018;26(6):1728-1736. [IA]

29. Molt M, Harsten A, Toksvig-Larsen S. The effect of tourniquet use on fixation quality in cemented total knee arthroplasty a prospective randomized clinical controlled RSA trial. *Knee.* 2014;21(2):396-401. [IA]

30. Ejaz A, Laursen AC, Kappel A, Jakobsen T, Nielsen PT, Rasmussen S. Tourniquet induced ischemia and changes in metabolism during TKA: a randomized study using microdialysis. *BMC Musculoskelet Disord.* 2015;16:326. [IB]

31. Nakayama H, Yoshiya S. The effect of tourniquet use on operative performance and early postoperative results of anatomic double-bundle anterior cruciate ligament reconstruction. *J Orthop Sci.* 2013;18(4):586-591. [IB]

32. Ejaz A, Laursen AC, Kappel A, et al. Faster recovery without the use of a tourniquet in total knee arthroplasty. *Acta Orthop.* 2014;85(4):422-426. [IA]

33. Liu D, Graham D, Gillies K, Gillies RM. Effects of tourniquet use on quadriceps function and pain in total knee arthroplasty. *Knee Surg Relat Res.* 2014;26(4):207-213. [IB]

34. Tsarouhas A, Hantes ME, Tsougias G, Dailiana Z, Malizos KN. Tourniquet use does not affect rehabilitation, return to activities, and muscle damage after arthroscopic

meniscectomy: a prospective randomized clinical study. *Arthroscopy.* 2012;28(12):1812-1818. [IA]

35. Drolet BC, Okhah Z, Phillips BZ, et al. Evidence for safe tourniquet use in 500 consecutive upper extremity procedures. *Hand (N Y).* 2014;9(4):494-498. [IIIB]

36. Horlocker TT, Hebl JR, Gali B, et al. Anesthetic, patient, and surgical risk factors for neurologic complications after prolonged total tourniquet time during total knee arthroplasty. *Anesth Analg.* 2006;102(3):950-955. [IIIA]

37. Hoogeboom TJ, van Meeteren NL, Schank K, Kim RH, Miner T, Stevens-Lapsley JE. Risk factors for delayed inpatient functional recovery after total knee arthroplasty. *Biomed Res Int.* 2015;2015:167643. [IIIB]

38. Bailey AN, Hocker AD, Vermillion BR, et al. MAFbx, MuRF1, and the stress-activated protein kinases are upregulated in muscle cells during total knee arthroplasty. *Am J Physiol Regul Integr Comp Physiol.* 2012;303(4):R376-R386. [IIIC]

39. Lu K, Xu M, Li W, Wang K, Wang D. A study on dynamic monitoring, components, and risk factors of embolism during total knee arthroplasty. *Medicine (Baltimore).* 2017;96(51):e9303. [IIIB]

40. Boutsiadis A, Reynolds RJ, Saffarini M, Panisset JC. Factors that influence blood loss and need for transfusion following total knee arthroplasty. *Ann Transl Med.* 2017;5(21):418. [IIIB]

41. Benjamin JB, Colgan KM. Are routine blood salvage/preservation measures justified in all patients undergoing primary TKA and THA? *J Arthroplasty.* 2015;30(6):955-958. [IIIB]

42. Mori N, Kimura S, Onodera T, Iwasaki N, Nakagawa I, Masuda T. Use of a pneumatic tourniquet in total knee arthroplasty increases the risk of distal deep vein thrombosis: a prospective, randomized study. *Knee.* 2016;23(5):887-889. [IA]

43. Lai CK, Lee QJ, Wong YC, Wai YL. Incidence of deep vein thrombosis and its natural history following unilateral primary total knee replacement in local Chinese patients—a prospective study. *Journal of Orthopaedics, Trauma and Rehabilitation.* 2016;21:35-38. [IIIB]

44. Watanabe H, Kikkawa I, Madoiwa S, Sekiya H, Hayasaka S, Sakata Y. Changes in blood coagulation–fibrinolysis markers by pneumatic tourniquet during total knee joint arthroplasty with venous thromboembolism. *J Arthroplasty.* 2014;29(3):569-573. [IIIB]

45. Zan P, Mol MO, Yao JJ, et al. Release of the tourniquet immediately after the implantation of the components reduces the incidence of deep vein thrombosis after primary total knee arthroplasty. *Bone Joint Res.* 2017;6(9):535-541. [IIB]

46. Sun Y, Chen D, Xu Z, et al. Incidence of symptomatic and asymptomatic venous thromboembolism after elective knee arthroscopic surgery: a retrospective study with routinely applied venography. *Arthroscopy.* 2014;30(7):818-822. [IIIB]

47. Ye S, Dongyang C, Zhihong X, et al. The incidence of deep venous thrombosis after arthroscopically assisted anterior cruciate ligament reconstruction. *Arthroscopy.* 2013;29(4):742-747. [IIIB]

48. Guideline for prevention of venous thromboembolism. In: *Guidelines for Perioperative Practice.* Denver, CO: AORN, Inc; 2020:1101-1130. [IVA]

49. Li Z, Liu D, Long G, et al. Association of tourniquet utilization with blood loss, rehabilitation, and complications in Chinese obese patients undergoing total knee arthroplasty: a retrospective study. *Medicine (Baltimore).* 2017;96(49):e9030. [IIC]

50. Lozano LM, Tío M, Rios J, et al. Severe and morbid obesity (BMI ≥ 35 kg/m(2)) does not increase surgical time and length of hospital stay in total knee arthroplasty surgery. *Knee Surg Sports Traumatol Arthrosc.* 2015;23(6):1713-1719. [IIIB]

51. Roth KE, Mandryka B, Maier GS, et al. In-vivo analysis of epicutaneous pressure distribution beneath a femoral tourniquet—an observational study. *BMC Musculoskelet Disord.* 2015;16:1. [IIIB]

52. Tuncalı B, Boya H, Kayhan Z, Araç Ş. Obese patients require higher, but not high pneumatic tourniquet inflation pressures using a novel technique during total knee arthroplasty. *Eklem Hastalik Cerrahisi.* 2018;29(1):40-45. [IIIB]

53. Tuncalı B, Boya H, Kayhan Z, Araç Ş, Çamurdan MA. Clinical utilization of arterial occlusion pressure estimation method in lower limb surgery: effectiveness of tourniquet pressures. *Acta Orthop Traumatol Turc.* 2016;50(2):171-177. [IIIB]

54. Memtsoudis SG, Stundner O, Yoo D, et al. Does limb preconditioning reduce pain after total knee arthroplasty? A randomized, double-blind study. *Clin Orthop Relat Res.* 2014;472(5):1467-1474. [IA]

55. Mittal R, Ko V, Adie S, et al. Tourniquet application only during cement fixation in total knee arthroplasty: a double-blind, randomized controlled trial. *ANZ J Surg.* 2012;82(6):428-433. [IA]

56. Saied A, Ayatollahi Mousavi A, Arabnejad F, Ahmadzadeh Heshmati A. Tourniquet in surgery of the limbs: a review of history, types and complications. *Iran Red Crescent Med J.* 2015;17(2):e9588. [VA]

57. Parvizi J, Diaz-Ledezma C. Total knee replacement with the use of a tourniquet: more pros than cons. *Bone Joint J.* 2013;95-B(11 Suppl A):133-134. [VB]

58. Walls RJ, O'Malley J, O'Flanagan SJ, Kenny PJ, Leahy AL, Keogh P. Total knee replacement under tourniquet control: a prospective study of the peripheral arterial vasculature using colour-assisted duplex ultrasonography. *Surgeon.* 2015;13(6):303-307. [IIIB]

59. Woelfle-Roos JV, Dautel L, Mayer B, Bieger R, Woelfle KD, Reichel H. Vascular calcifications on the preoperative radiograph: harbinger of tourniquet failure in patients undergoing total knee arthroplasty? *Skeletal Radiol.* 2017;46(9):1219-1224. [IIA]

60. Koehler SM, Fields A, Noori N, Weiser M, Moucha CS, Bronson MJ. Safety of tourniquet use in total knee arthroplasty in patients with radiographic evidence of vascular calcifications. *Am J Orthop (Belle Mead NJ).* 2015;44(9):E308-E316. [IIIB]

61. Derner R, Buckholz J. Surgical hemostasis by pneumatic ankle tourniquet during 3027 podiatric operations. *J Foot Ankle Surg.* 1995;34(3):236-246. [IIIA]

62. Younger AS, McEwen JA, Inkpen K. Wide contoured thigh cuffs and automated limb occlusion measurement

allow lower tourniquet pressures. *Clin Orthop Relat Res.* 2004;(428):286-293. [IB]

63. Jensen J, Hicks RW, Labovitz J. Understanding and optimizing tourniquet use during extremity surgery. *AORN J.* 2019;109(2):171-182. [IVA]

64. Latex Allergy Management Guidelines. American Association of Nurse Anesthetists. https://www.aana.com/docs/default-source/practice-aana-com-web-documents-(all)/latex-allergy-management.pdf?sfvrsn=9c0049b1_8. September 2018. Accessed March 5, 2020. [IVB]

65. Guideline for a safe environment of care. In: *Guidelines for Perioperative Practice.* Denver, CO: AORN, Inc; 2020:115-150. [IVA]

66. Thompson SM, Middleton M, Farook M, Cameron-Smith A, Bone S, Hassan A. The effect of sterile versus non-sterile tourniquets on microbiological colonisation in lower limb surgery. *Ann R Coll Surg Engl.* 2011;93(8):589-590. [IIIC]

67. Din R, Geddes T. Skin protection beneath the tourniquet. A prospective randomized trial. *ANZ J Surg.* 2004;74(9):721-722. [IC]

68. Olivecrona C, Tidermark J, Hamberg P, Ponzer S, Cederfjäll C. Skin protection underneath the pneumatic tourniquet during total knee arthroplasty: a randomized controlled trial of 92 patients. *Acta Orthop.* 2006;77(3):519-523. [IB]

69. Kvederas G, Porvaneckas N, Andrijauskas A, et al. A randomized double-blind clinical trial of tourniquet application strategies for total knee arthroplasty. *Knee Surg Sports Traumatol Arthrosc.* 2013;21(12):2790-2799. [IB]

70. Zhang Y, Li D, Liu P, Wang X, Li M. Effects of different methods of using pneumatic tourniquet in patients undergoing total knee arthroplasty: a randomized control trial. *Irish J Med Sci.* 2017;186(4):953-959. [IA]

71. Yakumpor T, Panichkul P, Kanitnate S, Tammachote N. Blood loss in TKA with tourniquet release before and after wound closure. *J Med Assoc Thai.* 2018;101(10):1443-1449. [IA]

72. Olivecrona C, Ponzer S, Hamberg P, Blomfeldt R. Lower tourniquet cuff pressure reduces postoperative wound complications after total knee arthroplasty: a randomized controlled study of 164 patients. *J Bone Joint Surg Am.* 2012;94(24):2216-2221. [IA]

73. Na YG, Bamne AB, Won HH, Kim TK. After early release of tourniquet in total knee arthroplasty, should it be reinflated or kept deflated? A randomized trial. *Knee Surg Sports Traumatol Arthrosc.* 2017;25(9):2769-2777. [IA]

74. Martín BC, Martín JIC, Oliver JL, Gómez JD. The effect of hyperoxygenated fatty acids in preventing skin lesions caused by surgical pneumatic tourniquets. *Adv Skin Wound Care.* 2018;31(5):214-217. [IIB]

75. Bosman HA, Robinson AH. Pneumatic tourniquet use in foot and ankle surgery—is padding necessary? *Foot (Edinb).* 2014;24(2):72-74. [IIIB]

76. Tredwell SJ, Wilmink M, Inkpen K, McEwen JA. Pediatric tourniquets: analysis of cuff and limb interface, current practice, and guidelines for use. *J Pediatr Orthop.* 2001;21(5):671-676. [IIIC]

77. The Joint Commission. Managing risk during transition to new ISO tubing connector standards. *Sentinel Event Alert.* 2014(53):1-6.

78. Akinyoola AL, Adegbehingbe OO, Odunsi A. Timing of antibiotic prophylaxis in tourniquet surgery. *J Foot Ankle Surg.* 2011;50(4):374-376. [IB]

79. Soriano A, Bori G, García-Ramiro S, et al. Timing of antibiotic prophylaxis for primary total knee arthroplasty performed during ischemia. *Clin Infect Dis.* 2008;46(7):1009-1014. [IB]

80. Prats L, Valls J, Ros J, Jover A, Pérez-Villar F, Fernández-Martinez JJ. Influence of the ischaemic tourniquet in antibiotic prophylaxis in total knee replacement. *Rev Esp Cir Ortop Traumatol.* 2015;59(4):275-280. [IIIB]

81. Dounis E, Tsourvakas S, Kalivas L, Giamaçellou H. Effect of time interval on tissue concentrations of cephalosporins after tourniquet inflation. Highest levels achieved by administration 20 minutes before inflation. *Acta Orthop Scand.* 1995;66(2):158-160. [IIB]

82. Papaioannou N, Kalivas L, Kalavritinos J, Tsourvakas S. Tissue concentrations of third-generation cephalosporins (ceftazidime and ceftriaxone) in lower extremity tissues using a tourniquet. *Arch Orthop Trauma Surg.* 1994;113(3):167-169. [IIIB]

83. Bicanic G, Crnogaca K, Barbaric K, Delimar D. Cefazolin should be administered maximum 30 min before incision in total knee arthroplasty when tourniquet is used. *Med Hypotheses.* 2014;82(6):766-768. [VB]

84. Bratzler DW, Dellinger EP, Olsen KM, et al. Clinical practice guidelines for antimicrobial prophylaxis in surgery. *Am J Health Syst Pharm.* 2013;70(3):195-283. [VA]

85. Harsten A, Bandholm T, Kehlet H, Toksvig-Larsen S. Tourniquet versus no tourniquet on knee-extension strength early after fast-track total knee arthroplasty; a randomized controlled trial. *Knee.* 2015;22(2):126-130. [IA]

86. Reda W, ElGuindy AM, Zahry G, Faggal MS, Karim MA. Anterior cruciate ligament reconstruction; is a tourniquet necessary? A randomized controlled trial. *Knee Surg Sports Traumatol Arthrosc.* 2016;24(9):2948-2952. [IA]

87. Wu Y, Lu X, Ma Y, et al. Efficacy and safety of limb position on blood loss and range of motion after total knee arthroplasty without tourniquet: a randomized clinical trial. *Int J Surg.* 2018;60:182-187. [IA]

88. Chen S, Li J, Peng H, Zhou J, Fang H, Zheng H. The influence of a half-course tourniquet strategy on peri-operative blood loss and early functional recovery in primary total knee arthroplasty. *Int Orthop.* 2014;38(2):355-359. [IA]

89. Chiu FY, Hung SH, Chuang TY, Chiang SC. The impact of exsanguination by Esmarch bandage on venous hemodynamic changes in total knee arthroplasty—a prospective randomized study of 38 knees. *Knee.* 2012;19(3):213-217. [IB]

90. Fan Y, Jin J, Sun Z, et al. The limited use of a tourniquet during total knee arthroplasty: a randomized controlled trial. *Knee.* 2014;21(6):1263-1268. [IA]

91. Chang CW, Lan SM, Tai TW, Lai KA, Yang CY. An effective method to reduce ischemia time during total knee arthroplasty. *J Formos Med Assoc.* 2012;111(1):19-23. [IIB]

92. Ledin H, Aspenberg P, Good L. Tourniquet use in total knee replacement does not improve fixation, but appears to

reduce final range of motion. *Acta Orthopaedica.* 2012;83(5):499-503. [IA]

93. Dennis DA, Kittelson AJ, Yang CC, Miner TM, Kim RH, Stevens-Lapsley J. Does tourniquet use in TKA affect recovery of lower extremity strength and function? A randomized trial. *Clin Orthop Relat Res.* 2016;474(1):69-77. [IB]

94. Tarwala R, Dorr LD, Gilbert PK, Wan Z, Long WT. Tourniquet use during cementation only during total knee arthroplasty: a randomized trial. *Clin Orthop Relat Res.* 2014;472(1):169-174. [IA]

95. Angadi DS, Blanco J, Garde A, West SC. Lower limb elevation: useful and effective technique of exsanguination prior to knee arthroscopy. *Knee Surg Sports Traumatol Arthrosc.* 2010;18(11):1559-1561. [IIIC]

96. Vertullo CJ, Nagarajan M. Is cement penetration in TKR reduced by not using a tourniquet during cementation? A single blinded, randomized trial. *J Orthop Surg (Hong Kong).* 2017;25(1):2309499016684323. [IA]

97. Vaishya R, Agarwal AK, Vijay V, Tiwari MK. Short term outcomes of long duration versus short duration tourniquet in primary total knee arthroplasty: a randomized controlled trial. *J Clin Orthop Trauma.* 2018;9(1):46-50. [IA]

98. Zhang M, Liu G, Zhao Z, Wu P, Liu W. Comparison of lower limb lifting and squeeze exsanguination before tourniquet inflation during total knee arthroplasty. *BMC Musculoskelet Disord.* 2019;20(1):35. [IB]

99. Barron SL, McGrory BJ. Total knee arthroplasty in a patient with ipsilateral calcific myonecrosis. *Arthroplast Today.* 2018;4(4):421-425. [VA]

100. Tanpowpong T, Kitidumrongsook P, Patradul A. The deleterious effects of exsanguination with a tight bandage on tourniquet tolerance in the upper arm. *J Hand Surg Eur Vol.* 2012;37(9):839-841. [IIC]

101. Huang GS, Wang CC, Hu MH, et al. Bilateral passive leg raising attenuates and delays tourniquet deflation-induced hypotension and tachycardia under spinal anaesthesia: a randomised controlled trial. *Eur J Anaesthesiol.* 2014;31(1):15-22. [IA]

102. Haghighi M, Mardani-Kivi M, Mirbolook A, et al. A comparison between single and double tourniquet technique in distal upper limb orthopedic surgeries with intravenous regional anesthesia. *Arch Bone Jt Surg.* 2018;6(1):63-70. [IA]

103. Tuncalı B, Boya H, Kayhan Z, Araç Ş. Tourniquet pressure settings based on limb occlusion pressure determination or arterial occlusion pressure estimation in total knee arthroplasty? A prospective, randomized, double blind trial. *Acta Orthop Traumatol Turc.* 2018;52(4):256-260. [IB]

104. Sáenz-Jalón M, Ballesteros-Sanz MA, Sarabia-Cobo CM, et al. Assessment of the pneumatic ischemia technique using the limb occlusion pressure during upper limb surgery. *J Perianesth Nurs.* 2018;33(5):699-707. [IB]

105. Mu J, Liu D, Ji D, et al. Determination of pneumatic tourniquet pressure of lower limb by ultrasonic Doppler. *Ann Plast Surg.* 2018;80(3):290-292. [IA]

106. Ding L, Ding CY, Wang YL, et al. Application effect of pneumatic tourniquet with individualized pressure setting in orthopedic surgery of extremities: a meta-analysis. *J Adv Nurs.* 2019;75(12):3424-3433. [IB]

107. Lim E, Shukla L, Barker A, Trotter DJ. Randomized blinded control trial into tourniquet tolerance in awake volunteers. *ANZ J Surg.* 2015;85(9):636-638. [IB]

108. Masri BA, Day B, Younger AS, Jeyasurya J. Technique for measuring limb occlusion pressure that facilitates personalized tourniquet systems: a randomized trial. *J Med Biol Eng.* 2016;36(5):644-650. [IB]

109. Liu HY, Guo JY, Zhang ZB, Li KY, Wang WD. Development of adaptive pneumatic tourniquet systems based on minimal inflation pressure for upper limb surgeries. *Biomed Eng Online.* 2013;12:92. [IIIB]

110. Sato J, Ishii Y, Noguchi H, Takeda M. Safety and efficacy of a new tourniquet system. *BMC Surg.* 2012;12:17. [IIIB]

111. Anderson JG, Bohay DR, Maskill JD, et al. Complications after popliteal block for foot and ankle surgery. *Foot Ankle Int.* 2015;36(10):1138-1143. [IIIB]

112. Sarfani S, Cantwell S, Shin AY, Kakar S. Challenging the dogma of tourniquet pressure requirements for upper extremity surgery. *J Wrist Surg.* 2016;5(2):120-123. [IIC]

113. Lieberman JR, Staheli LT, Dales MC. Tourniquet pressures on pediatric patients: a clinical study. *Orthopedics.* 1997;20(12):1143-1147. [IIIB]

114. McEwen JA, Kelly DL, Jardanowski T, Inkpen K. Tourniquet safety in lower leg applications. *Orthop Nurs.* 2002;21(5):55-62. [IC]

115. Unver B, Karatosun V, Tuncalı B. Effects of tourniquet pressure on rehabilitation outcomes in patients undergoing total knee arthroplasty. *Orthop Nurs.* 2013;32(4):217-222. [IIB]

116. Olivecrona C, Blomfeldt R, Ponzer S, Stanford BR, Nilsson BY. Tourniquet cuff pressure and nerve injury in knee arthroplasty in a bloodless field: a neurophysiological study. *Acta Orthop.* 2013;84(2):159-164. [IIB]

117. Perez BA, Smith BA, Gugala Z, Lindsey R. The reduced cuff inflation protocol does not improve the tissue oxygen recovery after tourniquet ischemia. *J Anesth Clin Res.* 2014;5:474. [IB]

118. Graham B, Breault MJ, McEwen JA, McGraw RW. Occlusion of arterial flow in the extremities at subsystolic pressures through the use of wide tourniquet cuffs. *Clin Orthop Relat Res.* 1993;(286):257-261. [IIC]

119. Pedowitz RA, Gershuni DH, Botte MJ, Kuiper S, Rydevik BL, Hargens AR. The use of lower tourniquet inflation pressures in extremity surgery facilitated by curved and wide tourniquets and an integrated cuff inflation system. *Clin Orthop Relat Res.* 1993;(287):237-244. [IB]

120. Kokki H, Väätäinen U, Penttilä I. Metabolic effects of a low-pressure tourniquet system compared with a high-pressure tourniquet system in arthroscopic anterior crucial ligament reconstruction. *Acta Anaesthesiol Scand.* 1998;42(4):418-424. [IC]

121. Tie K, Hu D, Qi Y, Wang H, Chen L. Effects of tourniquet release on total knee arthroplasty. *Orthopedics.* 2016;39(4):e642-e650. [IB]

122. Zan PF, Yang Y, Fu D, Yu X, Li GD. Releasing of tourniquet before wound closure or not in total knee arthroplasty:

a meta-analysis of randomized controlled trials. *J Arthroplasty.* 2015;30(1):31-37. [IA]

123. Wang C, Zhou C, Qu H, Yan S, Pan Z. Comparison of tourniquet application only during cementation and long-duration tourniquet application in total knee arthroplasty: a meta-analysis. *J Orthop Surg Res.* 2018;13(1):216. [IB]

124. Huang Z, Ma J, Zhu Y, et al. Timing of tourniquet release in total knee arthroplasty. *Orthopedics.* 2015;38(7):445-451. [IA]

125. Rathod P, Deshmukh A, Robinson J, Greiz M, Ranawat A, Rodriguez J. Does tourniquet time in primary total knee arthroplasty influence clinical recovery? *J Knee Surg.* 2015;28(4):335-342. [IIC]

126. Wang K, Ni S, Li Z, et al. The effects of tourniquet use in total knee arthroplasty: a randomized, controlled trial. *Knee Surg Sports Traumatol Arthrosc.* 2017;25(9):2849-2857. [IA]

127. Huang ZY, Pei FX, Ma J, et al. Comparison of three different tourniquet application strategies for minimally invasive total knee arthroplasty: a prospective non-randomized clinical trial. *Arch Orthop Trauma Surg.* 2014;134(4):561-570. [IIB]

128. Abbas K, Raza H, Umer M, Hafeez K. Effect of early release of tourniquet in total knee arthroplasty. *J Coll Physicians Surg Pak.* 2013;23(8):562-565. [IIC]

129. Wakai A, Wang JH, Winter DC, Street JT, O'Sullivan RG, Redmond HP. Tourniquet-induced systemic inflammatory response in extremity surgery. *J Trauma.* 2001;51(5):922-926. [IB]

130. Lynn AM, Fischer T, Brandford HG, Pendergrass TW. Systemic responses to tourniquet release in children. *Anesth Analg.* 1986;65(8):865-872. [IIIC]

131. Bloch EC, Ginsberg B, Binner RA Jr, Sessler DI. Limb tourniquets and central temperature in anesthetized children. *Anesth Analg.* 1992;74(4):486-489. [IIB]

132. Bloch EC. Hyperthermia resulting from tourniquet application in children. *Ann R Coll Surg Engl.* 1986;68(4):193-194. [IIIC]

133. Estebe JP, Le Naoures A, Malledant Y, Ecoffey C. Use of a pneumatic tourniquet induces changes in central temperature. *Br J Anaesth.* 1996;77(6):786-788. [IC]

134. Chon JY, Lee JY. The effects of surgery type and duration of tourniquet inflation on body temperature. *J Int Med Res.* 2012;40(1):358-365. [IIIB]

135. *Standards, Guidelines, and Position Statements for Perioperative Registered Nursing Practice.* 12th ed. Bath, ON: Operating Room Nurses Association of Canada; 2015. [IVB]

136. Zarrouki Y, Abouelhassan T, Samkaoui MA. Cardiac arrest after tourniquet deflation in upper limb. *Trauma Case Rep.* 2017;7:1-2. [VC]

137. Huh IY, Kim DY, Lee JH, Shin SJ, Cho YW, Park SE. Relation between preoperative autonomic function and blood pressure change after tourniquet deflation during total knee replacement arthroplasty. *Korean J Anesthesiol.* 2012;62(2):154-160. [IIIB]

138. Panerai RB, Saeed NP, Robinson TG. Cerebrovascular effects of the thigh cuff maneuver. *Am J Physiol Heart Circ Physiol.* 2015;308(7):H688-H696. [IIIB]

139. Tsunoda K, Sonohata M, Kugisaki H, et al. The effect of air tourniquet on interleukin-6 levels in total knee arthroplasty. *Open Orthop J.* 2017;11:20-28. [IIC]

140. Kruse H, Christensen KP, Møller AM, Gögenur I. Tourniquet use during ankle surgery leads to increased postoperative opioid use. *J Clin Anesth.* 2015;27(5):380-384. [IIIA]

141. Sahu SK, Tudu B, Mall PK. Microbial colonisation of orthopaedic tourniquets: a potential risk for surgical site infection. *Indian J Med Microbiol.* 2015;33 Suppl:115-118. [IIB]

142. *State Operations Manual Appendix A: Survey Protocol, Regulations and Interpretive Guidelines for Hospitals.* Rev 183. 2018. Centers for Medicare & Medicaid Services. https://www.cms.gov/Regulations-and-Guidance/Guidance/Manuals/downloads/som107ap_a_hospitals.pdf. Accessed March 5, 2020.

143. Medical device reporting (MDR): How to report medical device problems. US Food and Drug Administration. https://www.fda.gov/medical-devices/medical-device-safety/medical-device-reporting-mdr-how-report-medical-device-problems. Accessed March 5, 2020.

144. Guideline for patient information management. In: *Guidelines for Perioperative Practice.* Denver, CO: AORN, Inc; 2020:357-386. [IVA]

Guideline Development Group

Lead Author: Mary Alice Anderson[1], MSN, RN, CNOR, Perioperative Practice Specialist, AORN, Denver, Colorado

Methodologist: Amber Wood[2], MSN, RN, CNOR, CIC, FAPIC, Editor-in-Chief, Guidelines for Perioperative Practice, AORN, Denver, Colorado

Evidence Appraisers: Mary Alice Anderson[1]; Marie Bashaw[3], DNP, RN, NEA-BC, Assistant Professor, Director Nursing Administration and Health Care Master's Program, Wright State University College of Nursing and Health, Dayton, Ohio; and Amber Wood[2]

Guidelines Advisory Board Members:
- Susan Lynch[4], PhD, RN, CSSM, CNOR, Associate Director, Surgical Services, Chester County Hospital, West Chester, Pennsylvania
- Darlene B. Murdock[5], BSN, BA, RN, CNOR, Clinical Staff Nurse IV, Memorial Herman Texas Medical Center, Houston
- Elizabeth (Lizz) Pincus[6], MSN, RN, CNS-CP, CNOR, Clinical Nurse, Regional Medical Center of San Jose, California
- Kristy Simmons[7], MSN, RN, CNOR, Clinical Nurse III, Woman's Hospital, Baton Rouge, Louisiana

Guidelines Advisory Board Liaisons:
- Craig S. Atkins[8], DNP, CRNA, Chief Nurse Anesthetist, Belmar Ambulatory Surgical Center, Lakewood, Colorado
- Doug Schuerer[9], MD, FACS, FCCM, Professor of Surgery, Trauma Director, Washington University School of Medicine, St Louis, Missouri

External Review: Expert review comments were received from individual members of the American Association of Nurse Anesthetists (AANA), American College of Surgeons (ACS), Association for Professionals in Infection Control and Epidemiology (APIC), American Society of Anesthesiologists (ASA), International Association of Healthcare Central Service Materiel Management (IAHCSMM), the Society for Healthcare Epidemiology of America (SHEA), and the Surgical Infection Society (SIS). Their responses were used to further refine and enhance this guideline; however, their responses do not imply endorsement. The draft was also open for a 30-day public comment period.

Financial Disclosure and Conflicts of Interest

This guideline was developed, edited, and approved by the AORN Guidelines Advisory Board without external funding being sought or obtained. The Guidelines Advisory Board was financially supported entirely by AORN and was developed without any involvement of industry.

Potential conflicts of interest for all Guidelines Advisory Board members were reviewed before the annual meeting and each monthly conference call. None of the members of the Guideline Development Group reported a potential conflict of interest.[1-9] Any conflicts of interest, had they arisen, would have been mitigated with recusal of the person having the conflict in the applicable topic.

Publication History

Originally published April 1984, *AORN Journal.* Revised November 1990.

Published as proposed recommended practices March 1994. Revised November 1998; published December 1998. Reformatted July 2000.

Revised November 2001; published February 2002, *AORN Journal.*

Revised 2006; published in *Standards, Recommended Practices, and Guidelines,* 2007 edition.

Minor editing revisions made to omit PNDS codes; reformatted September 2012 for publication in *Perioperative Standards and Recommended Practices,* 2013 edition.

Revised April 2013 for online publication in *Perioperative Standards and Recommended Practices.*

Evidence ratings revised 2013 to conform to the AORN Evidence Rating Model.

Minor editing revisions made in November 2014 for publication in *Guidelines for Perioperative Practice,* 2015 edition.

Evidence ratings revised in *Guidelines for Perioperative Practice,* 2018 edition, to conform to the current AORN Evidence Rating Model.

Evidence ratings revised and minor editorial changes made to conform to the current AORN Evidence Rating model, May 2019, for publication in *Guidelines for Perioperative Practice* online.

Revised May 2020 for online publication in *Guidelines for Perioperative Practice.*

Scheduled for review in 2025.

POSITIONING THE PATIENT

TABLE OF CONTENTS

[P] *indicates a recommendation or evidence relevant to pediatric care.*

MEDICAL ABBREVIATIONS & ACRONYMS

AANA – American Association of Nurse Anesthetists
ASA – American Society of Anesthesiologists
AWHONN – Association of Women's Health, Obstetric and Neonatal Nurses
BMI – Body mass index
CK – Creatinine kinase
CPAP – Continuous positive airway pressure
CPR – Cardiopulmonary resuscitation
DVT – Deep vein thrombosis
EPUAP – European Pressure Ulcer Advisory Panel
ETCO$_2$ – End-tidal carbon dioxide
FDA – US Food and Drug Administration

IFU – Instructions for use
IV – Intravenous
MAUDE – Manufacturer and User Facility Device Experience
NPUAP – National Pressure Ulcer Advisory Panel
OR – Operating room
PAO$_2$ – Pressure of oxygen in arterial blood
PPPIA – Pan Pacific Pressure Injury Alliance
RCT – Randomized controlled trial
RN – Registered nurse
SSEP – Somatosensory evoked potential
TCeMEP – Transcranial electrical motor evoked potential
VAE – Venous air embolism

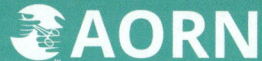

GUIDELINE FOR
POSITIONING THE PATIENT

The Guideline for Positioning the Patient was approved by the AORN Guidelines Advisory Board and became effective May 1, 2017. It was presented as a proposed guideline for comments by members and others. The recommendations in the guideline are intended to be achievable and represent what is believed to be an optimal level of practice. Policies and procedures will reflect variations in practice settings and/or clinical situations that determine the degree to which the guideline can be implemented. AORN recognizes the many diverse settings in which perioperative nurses practice; therefore, this guideline is adaptable to all areas where operative or other invasive procedures may be performed.

Purpose

This document provides guidance to perioperative team members for positioning patients undergoing operative and other invasive procedures in the perioperative practice setting. Guidance is provided for

- demonstrating respect and privacy during patient positioning;
- conducting preoperative and postoperative nursing assessments specific to patient positioning;
- identifying, selecting, maintaining, and using positioning equipment and devices;
- selecting and using pressure-redistributing support surfaces and prophylactic dressings to prevent pressure injury;
- using neurophysiological monitoring to identify and prevent potential positioning injuries;
- implementing safe practices for positioning patients in the supine, Trendelenburg, reverse Trendelenburg, lithotomy, sitting and semi-sitting, lateral, and prone positions and modifications of these positions;
- implementing safe practices for positioning patients who are pregnant or obese;
- documenting patient positioning and positioning-related activities;
- planning education and verifying competency of personnel responsible for patient positioning;
- developing policies and procedures related to patient positioning; and
- implementing quality improvement programs related to patient positioning.

A discussion of positions or devices used for anesthesia administration, positions for cardiopulmonary resuscitation (CPR), and positions that are preferred or modified for specific procedures are outside the scope of this document. Recommendations for patient moving and handling, trans-

port, transfer, and fall prevention are also outside of the scope of this document. Guidance for preventing deep vein thrombosis (DVT) is outside of the scope of this document; however, because some mechanical methods of DVT prophylaxis are inherently associated with patient positioning, guidance is provided relative to the use of mechanical DVT prophylaxis in combination with specific positions. Guidance related to positioning for robotic procedures is included with the relevant recommendation. There are a vast variety of surgical positions and of positioning equipment and devices, and it would not be possible to address them all in this document; therefore, the information in this guideline is limited to the most commonly used positions and positioning equipment and devices.

Positioning patients is one of the most important tasks performed by perioperative personnel[1,2] and is the responsibility of all members of the surgical team.[3-5] The goals of patient positioning include

- providing exposure of the surgical site[6];
- maintaining the patient's comfort and privacy;
- providing access to intravenous (IV) lines and monitoring equipment;
- allowing for optimal ventilation by maintaining a patent airway and avoiding constriction or pressure on the chest or abdomen;
- maintaining circulation and protecting muscles, nerves, bony prominences, joints, skin, and vital organs from injury;
- observing and protecting fingers, toes, and genitals; and
- stabilizing the patient to prevent unintended shifting or movement.

Positioning the patient is a team effort that includes the perioperative registered nurse (RN), the anesthesia professional, the surgeon, and other perioperative personnel (eg, first assistants, assistive personnel).[1,5,7-9] As patient advocates, perioperative team members are responsible for maintaining the patient's autonomy, dignity, and privacy and for representing the patient's interests throughout the procedure.[10] Some elements of patient positioning are core to anesthesia practice; therefore, the ability of the perioperative team to support the activities of the anesthesia professional is essential. All perioperative team members involved in positioning activities are responsible for

- understanding the physiologic changes that occur during operative and other invasive procedures[9,11-14];
- evaluating the patient's risk for injury based on an assessment of identified needs and the planned operative or invasive procedure[9,13];
- anticipating the surgeon's requirements for surgical access;
- gathering positioning equipment and devices;

- using positioning equipment and devices correctly;
- monitoring the patient during the procedure[1];
- applying principles of body mechanics and ergonomics during patient positioning;
- respecting the patient's individual positioning limitations; and
- implementing interventions to provide for the patient's comfort and safety and to protect the patient's circulatory, respiratory, musculoskeletal, neurological, and integumentary structures.[2,3,5,13,15]

Incorrectly positioning a surgical patient can result in serious injury to both personnel and the patient.[1,4] Performing patient positioning requires the application of lifting, pushing, or pulling forces and therefore presents a high risk for musculoskeletal injury to the lower back and shoulders of the team members performing these tasks.[16] Because of the effects of sedation, regional anesthesia, or general anesthesia, patients lack normal perception and protective reflexes and are thus at increased risk for positioning injury.[4,17]

Most positioning injuries are caused by mechanisms involving compression or stretching.[13] Stretching leads to nerve compression and ischemic changes from reduced blood flow.[13] Some surgical positions increase the risk for a stretching injury (eg, lateral neck rotation).[13] Compression reduces blood flow and disrupts cellular integrity, resulting in tissue edema, ischemia, and necrosis.[13] Positioning injuries can affect the skin and soft tissues, joints, ligaments and bones, eyes, nerves, and blood and lymph vessels.[4] A positioning injury can be temporary or permanent, and the effects of the injury can range from minor inconvenience to long-term functional restriction, secondary morbidity, or even death.[4,14]

Many positioning injuries are associated with prolonged procedures. The definition of a prolonged procedure is subjective, and the literature does not conclusively define a time parameter for prolonged surgery. The American Society of Anesthesiologists (ASA) Task Force on Perioperative Visual Loss[18] considers procedures to be prolonged when they exceed an average of 6.5 hours duration (range 2 hours to 12 hours).

Failing to provide appropriate positioning interventions for individuals undergoing operative or other invasive procedures may be deemed negligence or a failure to meet the duty of care owed to the patient.[19] When there is a positioning injury, the doctrine of *res ipsa loquitur* (ie, the thing speaks for itself) may be applicable.[11] Under this doctrine, there is an assumption that the event that caused the injury was under the control of the defendant (eg, surgeon, anesthesia professional, perioperative RN) and would not have occurred if proper care had been provided to the plaintiff (ie, patient).[11] The potential for a patient injury and for litigation underscores the importance of implementing positioning interventions to prevent nerve and tissue damage and thoroughly and accurately documenting the care provided.[11,12]

Evidence Review

A medical librarian conducted a systematic literature search of the databases Ovid MEDLINE®, EBSCO CINAHL®, Scopus®, and the Cochrane Database of Systematic Reviews. The search was limited to literature published in English from 2008 through February 2016. At the time of the initial search, weekly alerts were created for the topics included in that search. Results from these alerts were provided to the lead author until September 2016. The lead author requested a supplementary search on eye protection and requested additional articles that either did not fit the original search criteria or were discovered during the evidence appraisal process. The lead author and the medical librarian also identified relevant guidelines from government agencies, professional organizations, and standards-setting bodies.

Search terms included *positioning, positioning injury, compression injury, shear, friction, pressure, interface pressure, pressure ulcers, pressure reducing, pressure relieving, positioning surfaces, support surfaces, positioning equipment, positioning devices, safety straps, OR table, OR bed, OR mattress, alternating pressure mattresses, procedure table, padding, foam, gel, viscoelastic, supine, Fowler/Semi-Fowler/beach chair, lithotomy, lateral, prone, Trendelenburg/reverse Trendelenburg, jack-knife/Kraske,* and *robotic.* Other subject headings and keywords were included to address specific positioning devices, alternative terms for positions, patient-monitoring indicators, and risk assessment.

Excluded were non-peer-reviewed publications and low-quality evidence when higher-quality evidence was available. In total, 1,013 research and nonresearch sources of evidence were identified for possible inclusion, and of these, 529 are cited in the guideline (Figure 1).

Included articles were independently evaluated and critically appraised according to the strength and quality of the evidence. Articles identified in the search were provided to the project team for evaluation. The team consisted of the lead author and one evidence appraiser. The articles were reviewed and critically appraised using the AORN Research or Non-Research Evidence Appraisal Tools as appropriate. Each article was then assigned an appraisal score. The appraisal score is noted in brackets after each reference as applicable.

Each recommendation rating is based on a synthesis of the collective evidence, a benefit-harm assessment, and consideration of resource use. The strength of the recommendation was determined using the AORN Evidence Rating Model and the quality and consistency of the evidence supporting a recommendation. The recommendation strength rating is noted in brackets after each recommendation.

Note: The evidence summary table is available at http://www.aorn.org/evidencetables/.

Editor's note: Ovid MEDLINE is a registered trademark of the US National Library of Medicine's Medical Literature Analysis and Retrieval System, Bethesda, MD. CINAHL, Cumulative Index to Nursing and Allied Health Literature, is a registered trademark of

Figure 1. Flow Diagram of Literature Search Results

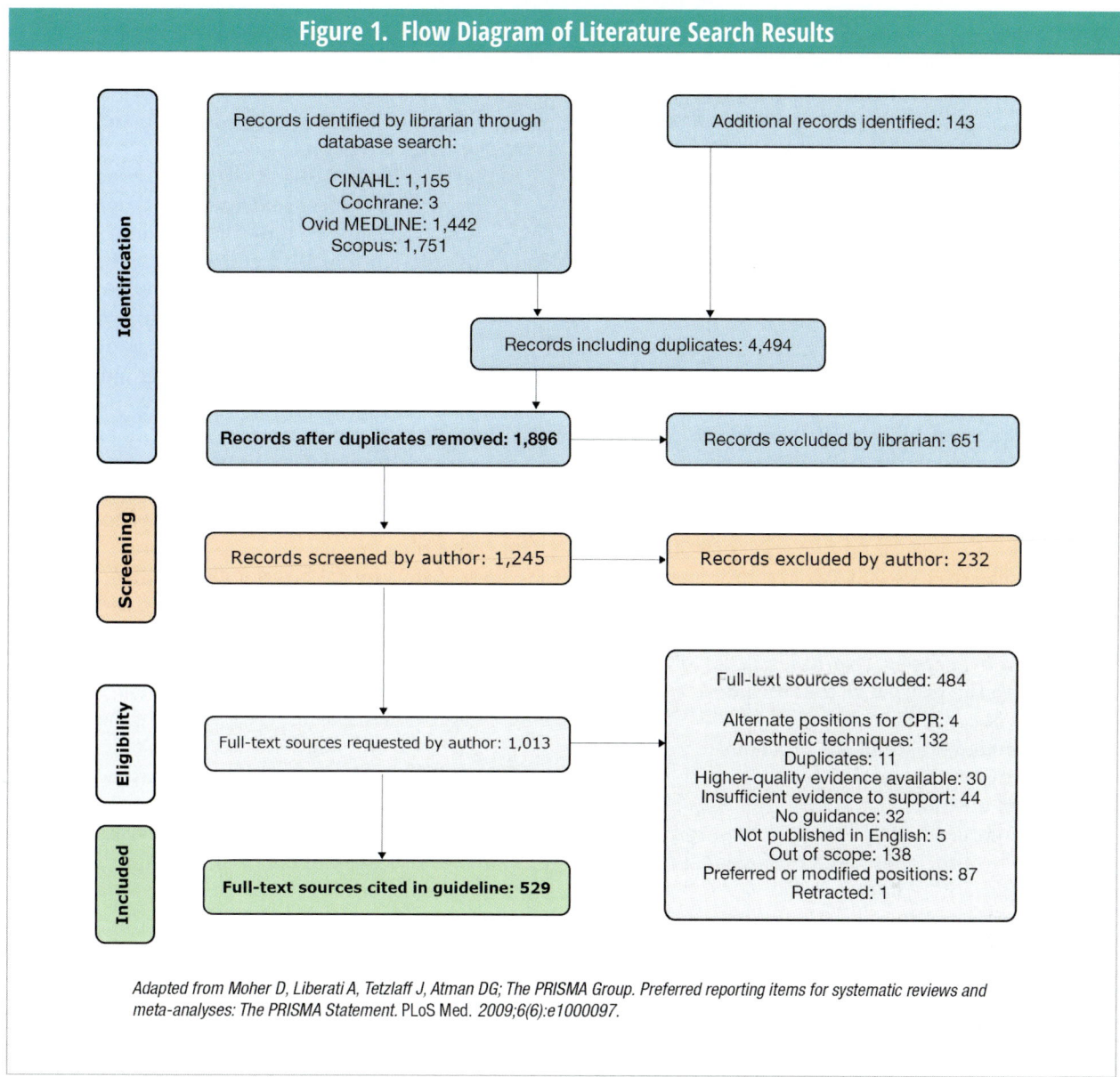

Adapted from Moher D, Liberati A, Tetzlaff J, Atman DG; The PRISMA Group. Preferred reporting items for systematic reviews and meta-analyses: The PRISMA Statement. PLoS Med. *2009;6(6):e1000097.*

EBSCO Industries, Birmingham, AL. Scopus is a registered trademark of Elsevier B.V., Amsterdam, The Netherlands.

1. Patient Privacy

1.1   **Provide care that respects the dignity and privacy of each patient**[10] **during patient positioning.** *[Recommendation]*

Perioperative team members are responsible for ensuring equitable, compassionate, and optimal care for all perioperative patients without bias or intolerance.[6,10] Some patients (eg, patients who are obese, patients with disabilities) present additional challenges during patient positioning, and a greater level of advocacy may be required to create an environment of respect and sensitivity.[6]

1.2   **Implement measures to provide privacy during patient positioning.** *[Recommendation]*

Maintaining the patient's privacy is essential to preserving the trust developed in the caregiver-patient relationship.[10] Perioperative team members have an obligation to protect patients from undue exposure or unwarranted invasions of privacy.[6,10]

1.2.1   **Provide privacy during patient positioning by**
- **keeping windows covered and doors closed in patient care areas,**
- **restricting access to perioperative patient care areas to authorized personnel only,**
- **limiting traffic in procedure rooms, and**
- **exposing only the areas of the patient's body necessary to provide care or access.**

[Recommendation]

Maintaining the patient's privacy is reflected by implementing processes to protect the patient's auditory and physical privacy.[10] Keeping the patient covered, unless specific exposure of an area of the body is required, will help to keep the patient warm as well as to maintain the patient's dignity during a vulnerable time.[20]

2. Assessment for Injury Risk

2.1 **Conduct a preoperative patient assessment to identify patients at risk for positioning injury, develop a plan of care, and implement interventions to prevent injury.** [*Recommendation*]

Patient assessment is a critical responsibility performed by the perioperative RN to help prevent injury related to patient positioning.[9,21-24] Identifying patients at risk for positioning injury and developing a plan of care is necessary for implementing preventive interventions.[19,23,25-27]

2.2 **Perform a preoperative assessment of factors related to the procedure that includes**
- **type of procedure**[21,28-30];
- **estimated length of the procedure**[21,25,28-34];
- **ability of the patient to tolerate the anticipated position**[35];
- **amount of surgical exposure required**[5];
- **ability of the anesthesia professional to access the patient**[21,28]; and
- **desired procedural position, potential change of position, and positioning devices required.**[5,26,29,30,32,34]

[*Recommendation*]

The type and estimated duration of the surgical procedure are significant factors in estimating the patient's risk for tissue damage.[12,15,30,32,36,37] Lumbley et al[29] found that the types of procedures with the most pressure injuries were abdominal, noncardiac thoracic, and orthopedic. Shaw et al[26] found that orthopedic procedures were a significant predictor of pressure injury. In a systematic review of 23 studies that examined sensory changes or nerve injury after abdominoplasty procedures, Ducic et al[14] found that most patient injuries occurred during surgeries that included more than one procedure type. The researchers noted that combining procedures increased operative time and the risk for positioning injury.[14]

Moderate-quality evidence varies as to the specific length of time after which a positioning injury would be expected to occur.[29,33,34,36,38,39] The risk for pressure injury is multifactorial and increases with the length of surgery.[32] In an analysis of 44 claims from the American Association of Nurse Anesthetists (AANA) Foundation Closed Malpractice Claims Database, Fritzlen et al[38] found that 57% (n = 25) of the injuries reported occurred during procedures that lasted longer than 2 hours. O'Connell[36] proposed that procedures lasting longer than 4 hours presented an increased risk for tissue damage in even the healthiest patients. Mills et al[39] conducted a review of records of adult urological robotic procedures and found the median time for procedures during which positioning injuries occurred was 5.5 hours.

The ASA Task Force on Prevention of Perioperative Peripheral Neuropathies[35] suggested that ascertaining whether the patient can tolerate the anticipated surgical position may be helpful to reduce the risk for nerve injury.

Providing sufficient surgical exposure may reduce surgical complications by improving visibility of the surgical site, easing access to the operative area and anatomic structures, and reducing operative time.[2,4,5]

Safe surgical positioning requires that the anesthesia professional assess the patient's range of motion, assess nerve and vascular impairment, participate in the positioning of the patient, have sufficient access to the patient to provide adequate depth of anesthesia, assess the position of the patient intraoperatively, maintain hemodynamic stability and oxygenation, and protect the patient through the use of noninvasive and invasive monitors.[4,5,15,40,41]

Some surgical positions and positioning devices increase the patient's risk for injury.[34] A key causative factor for pressure injury is external pressure on bony prominences for prolonged periods.[42] Pressure points vary based on the surgical position and placement of positioning devices. Straps or adhesive tape used to secure a patient in the desired position during a surgical procedure can be a source of pressure that results in injury.[43]

2.3 **Participate in the health care organization's pressure injury prevention program by conducting a preoperative assessment of the patient's risk for pressure injury.**[44] [*Recommendation*]

Prevention of pressure injury is an important aspect of perioperative patient care.[45] Surgical positioning presents a risk for skin breakdown and pressure injury.[22,34,46] Risk assessment provides a method for identifying individuals who are susceptible to pressure injuries and for implementing interventions to prevent pressure injury.[19,25,47,48] Use of the same processes and tools for pressure injury risk assessment throughout the health care organization promotes consistency in reporting and enhances communication among caregivers working in different areas or on different shifts.[49] The Centers for Medicare & Medicaid Services no longer pays for health services provided for care related to Stage 3 and Stage 4 pressure injuries that develop during a hospital admission.[50] This regulation provides strong impetus for perioperative RNs to be cognizant of risk factors that can contribute to pressure injury.[27]

2.3.1

Use a structured risk assessment tool for preoperative assessment of the patient's risk for pressure injury. [Recommendation]

High-quality evidence supports the use of a risk assessment tool.[3,19,51] Risk assessment tools provide

- practical frameworks for assessment,
- operational definitions of risk factors that have clinical relevance and can be reliably measured,
- clinical reminders of risks, and
- an auditable standard.[3,19,51]

Risk assessment tools do not necessarily include assessment of all key factors that may increase the patient's risk for pressure injury, and they are limited in their ability to determine the importance of one risk factor compared with another or to determine the cumulative effects of multiple risk factors.[19] The use of a risk assessment tool does not replace the need for a comprehensive patient assessment conducted by a qualified perioperative RN using sound clinical judgment.[19]

There is a lack of agreement as to which risk assessment tool is most effective for predicting the risk for pressure injury in perioperative patients.[19] Pressure injury risk assessment tools identified in the literature include the Braden Scale,[52] Munro Scale,[53,54] and Scott Triggers tool[55] **(Table 1)**.

The Braden Scale is widely used for pressure injury risk assessment, but it does not address risk factors specific to surgical patients.[56,57] In a meta-analysis of three pooled studies, He et al[57] found that the Braden Scale had a low predictive validity for assessing pressure injury risk in surgical patients. The Braden Scale has been used as a preoperative tool to assess older adult frailty,[23] which may be a predictor of postoperative complications because the older adult's frailty level is an indicator of vulnerability to stressors resulting from diminished physiologic reserves associated with the aging process.[23] The Munro Scale and the Scott Triggers tool were developed to help perioperative RNs identify surgical patients at risk for pressure injury.[53-55]

2.3.2

In the pressure injury risk assessment, include evaluation and documentation of the patient's

- **age,**[17,21,25,27,30,31,51,56]
- **nutritional status,**[19,21,23,25,30,37,44,51,58]
- **laboratory test values,**[17,19,21,25,37,59]
- **comorbidities affecting tissue perfusion (eg, diabetes, peripheral vascular disease),**[4,19,21,23,25,27,30,31,37,51,56,60,61]
- **skin condition (eg, color, turgor, integrity, temperature, moisture, pre-existing pressure injury),**[6,19,21,27,30,31,37,43,44,51,56,61-64]
- **ASA physical status classification,**[64,65]
- **body mass index (BMI),**[12,17,21,25,27,30-32,64] **and**
- **peripheral pulses (ie, rate, rhythm, symmetry, amplitude).**[37]

[Recommendation]

The risk for skin and pressure injury is high in both older and very young patients.[2] Patients 65 years and older are particularly vulnerable to positioning injury.[1,31,37,43] Older adults may also have conditions such as osteoporosis, osteoarthritis, or coronary artery disease that can increase their risk for positioning injury.[1,22,31]

Both inadequate nutritional intake and poor nutritional status can increase the risk for pressure injury.[19,38] Patients who are malnourished are at increased risk for pressure injury because they do not have the stored reserves that help the body promote effective healing and protect itself from injury.[19,43,49,66-68] Inadequate nutrition increases the risk for tissue damage, delayed wound healing, sepsis, and wound infection.[23] Undernourished and malnourished states may be more prevalent in the older adult population.[23] Despite the appearance of having a nutritional reserve, patients who are obese may be at risk for nutritional deficits.[58,69] Patients who have undergone previous weight loss surgery are also vulnerable to nutritional deficits that may increase their risk for pressure injury.[69]

Evidence related to the relevance of laboratory test values as indicators of malnutrition and pressure injury is limited.[19] Data have not clearly demonstrated specific laboratory markers of nutritional status that best predict pressure injury in perioperative patients.[42] Patients with low hematocrit (ie, < 38%) and hemoglobin levels (ie, < 14.1 g/dL) are at greater risk for positioning injury than patients with normal hematocrit (ie, men 40% to 54%; women 36% to 48%) and hemoglobin levels (ie, men 13.5 g/dL to 17.5 g/dL; women 12.0 g/dL to 15.5 g/dL).[2,15,19,42,49] Serum albumin and prealbumin levels are not considered reliable indicators of nutritional status[19]; however, low albumin levels (ie, 40 g/L ± 7.1 g/L) may interfere with healing, placing the patient at increased risk for pressure injury.[42] Reduced albumin levels may also be indicators of an inflammatory response that increases metabolism and secondarily increases the risk for malnutrition.[19]

Tool	Braden Scale	Munro Scale	Scott Triggers Tool
Table 1. Pressure Injury Risk Assessment Tools: Adult			
Indicators	• Sensory perception • Moisture • Activity • Mobility • Nutrition • Friction and shear[1]	**Preoperative** • Mobility • Nutritional status • Body mass index • Weight loss within the past 30 to 180 days • Age • Comorbidities[3] **Intraoperative** • American Society of Anesthesiologists physical status classification • Type of anesthesia • Temperature • Hypotension • Moisture • Surface/motion • Position[3] **Postoperative** • Length of perioperative duration • Blood loss[3]	• Age older than 62 years • Serum albumin level < 3.5 g/L or body mass index < 19 kg/m² or > 40 kg/m² • American Society of Anesthesiologists physical status classification of III or higher • Estimated surgery time longer than 180 minutes[5]
Scoring	Each indicator is assessed and scored from 1 to 4 for a total score of 6 to 23.[1] Lower scores are indicative of a greater risk for pressure injury.[1]	Preoperative, intraoperative, and postoperative indicators are scored as low, medium, and high risk for each phase of care.[4] The level of risk may change throughout the perioperative period.[4] The cumulative score reflects the patient's risk for pressure injury.[4]	Each indicator is considered a trigger. Patients with 2 or more triggers are considered to be at high risk for pressure injury.[5]
Patient Population	Validated tool for assessing the patient's risk for pressure injury.[1] Does not assess risk factors specific to surgical patients.[2]	Developed specifically for the perioperative patient.[3,4]	Developed specifically for the perioperative patient.[5]

References

1. *Bergstrom N, Braden BJ, Laguzza A, Holman V. The Braden Scale for Predicting Pressure Sore Risk.* Nurs Res. 1987;36(4):205-210.
2. *He W, Liu P, Chen HL. The Braden Scale cannot be used alone for assessing pressure ulcer risk in surgical patients: a meta-analysis.* Ostomy Wound Manage. 2012;58(2):34-40.
3. *Munro Pressure Ulcer Risk Assessment Scale for Perioperative Patients—Adults. AORN, Inc. https://www.aorn.org/-/media/aorn/guidelines/tool-kits/pressure-ulcer/munro-pressure-ulcer-risk-assessment-scale.xlsx?la=en. Accessed March 10, 2017.*
4. *Cardinal Health/AORN Pressure Ulcer Prevention Project. Instructions for the Munro Pressure Ulcer Risk Assessment Scale for Perioperative Patients for Adults. AORN, Inc. https://www.aorn.org/-/media/aorn/guidelines/tool-kits/pressure-ulcer/instructions-for-munro-risk-assessment-scale.pdf?la=en. Accessed March 10, 2017.*
5. *Scott SM. Progress and challenges in perioperative pressure ulcer prevention. J Wound Ostomy Continence Nurs. 2015;42(5):480-485.*

Comorbidities that affect tissue perfusion and oxygenation may increase the potential for pressure injury.[15,19,35,38,42,49,67,70] General anesthetics administered to surgical patients result in some degree of vasodilation that subsequently leads to hypotension and reduced tissue perfusion.[15,27,33,34,36,49,64,71,72] Hypoperfusion of tissue under pressure in an immobile patient can be a significant factor related to the development of pressure injury in a perioperative patient.[29] Patients with diabetes, respiratory disease, and vascular disease are at increased risk for injury as a result of reduced tissue perfusion and oxygenation.[42]

Patients with preexisting peripheral vascular disease have baseline limb ischemia and may not tolerate positions (eg, lithotomy position) that lead to additional reductions in perfusion.[73] In a retrospective review of 222 patients who developed pressure injuries after undergoing surgery lasting at least 2 hours, Lumbley et al[29] found that patient comorbidities affecting tissue perfusion in combination with malnutrition and cachexia resulted in a predisposition toward intraoperative pressure injuries. In an analysis of 44 cases from the AANA Foundation Closed Malpractice Claims Database, Fritzlen et al[38] found that 55% (n = 24) of the patients who were injured had preexisting pathological conditions that placed them at increased risk for injury. When abnormal body habitus (ie, BMI ≤ 21 kg/m^2 or BMI > 28 kg/m^2) was included as a preexisting condition, the percentage of patients who were injured increased to 70% (n = 31).

A skin risk assessment evaluates the condition of the patient's skin and factors that may put the patient at risk for pressure injury (eg, decreased turgor, cool temperature).[43] Preoperative visual assessment of the patient's skin, bony prominences, and body surfaces that will be subjected to pressure, friction, or shear force during the procedure may help direct interventions to prevent pressure injuries. A preoperative skin assessment establishes a baseline for comparison with a postoperative skin assessment.[31] Alterations in skin color, moisture, temperature, texture, mobility, and turgor may lead to the development of a pressure injury or the progression of an existing pressure injury.[19,22] Breaks in skin integrity increase a patient's risk for infection or pressure injury and can lead to psychological distress and challenges in pain management.[47]

The skin of older adults (ie, ≥ 65 years) is fragile and prone to shear injuries.[37] The skin of older adults is less elastic; the dermis is thin and has less collagen, muscle, and adipose tissue than the skin of younger adults.[22,31,36,41-43,56] These changes leave the older adult's skin more susceptible to pressure, bruising, skin tears, infection, impaired thermoregulation, and slow healing.[23,36,41,42,56,66] Skin assessments may be more difficult in patients who are obese because of the patient's size, lack of landmarks, and chronic conditions.[6,74]

The presence of excess moisture on the skin disrupts the skin's natural protective barrier and weakens the elasticity of the skin.[61] Moisture increases the potential for skin damage caused by skin maceration that intensifies the negative effects of pressure, shear, and friction.[19,31,56,61,75]

All surgical patients are at risk for pressure injury, but the presence of certain factors puts some patients at higher risk.[8,22,25,30,31,49,51,56,76] Mills et al[39] conducted a review of records of 334 adult urological robotic surgeries to identify risk factors associated with positioning injuries. The researchers found that ASA physical status classification was significantly associated with pressure injury. In a nonexperimental study to eval-

uate the number of injuries caused by surgical positioning and to identify risk factors predictive of pressure injury, Menezes et al[65] prospectively evaluated 172 patients undergoing elective surgery in the supine, lateral, and lithotomy positions for development of a pressure injury. The results of the study showed a significant association between pressure injury and patients with an ASA classification of II or III (n = 19; 90.5%) compared to patients with an ASA classification of I (n = 2; 9.5%).

In a case series with retrospective chart analysis and review of intraoperative neurophysiological monitoring data from 398 patients, Silverstein et al[77] found that BMI was a significant predictor of generalized upper extremity neural compromise. Patients who are obese may be at increased risk for positioning injury because they may not tolerate traditional surgical positions as well as patients of normal weight.[1,24,32,49] In the prospective study conducted by Menezes et al,[65] the results also showed a significant association between pressure injury and patients with a BMI ≥ 30 kg/m^2 (n = 15; 71.4%) compared to patients with a BMI < 30 kg/m^2 (n = 6; 28.6%). Patients who are thin or underweight and have decreased body mass are more susceptible to skin and pressure injury than patients of normal weight because they have less adipose tissue to protect nerves and bony prominences.[2,12,32,42,68]

Preoperative assessment of the rate, rhythm, symmetry, and amplitude of peripheral pulses provides a baseline for comparison after patient positioning and placement of positioning devices.

2.3.3 Use a structured pediatric risk assessment tool for preoperative assessment of the risk for pressure injury in pediatric patients.[44] [Recommendation] P

Using a risk assessment tool that is appropriate to the population may increase the accuracy of risk prediction.[19,44,47,78] Because of differences in anatomic structure, the sites most susceptible to pressure injury in the pediatric population differ from those in the adult population.[19,43,78] For example, the occipital region is at increased risk for skin breakdown in infants and toddlers in the supine position because they have a disproportionately large head size.[19,48]

Neonates are vulnerable to skin and pressure injuries because of an immature and underdeveloped epidermis and dermis.[15,19,78] The skin of children may be more resilient to normal and shear pressures than the skin of older adults because it is supported with sufficient collagen and elastin.[45] Neonates and children are at higher risk for nutritional deficiencies because of smaller appetites and dietary intake in combination with an increased nutritional requirement necessary to meet normal growth needs.[19]

Pediatric and neonatal pressure injury risk assessment tools identified in the literature include the Braden Q Scale,[45,47,48,79] the Braden Q + P Scale,[47] the Glamorgan Scale,[47,79,80] and the Neonatal Skin Risk Assessment Scale[81] (Table 2).

2.4 **Perform a preoperative assessment of patient-specific factors that may increase the patient's risk for positioning injury. Assess the patient for the presence of**
- **critical devices (eg, catheters, drains)[21,28];**
- **jewelry or body piercings[28];**
- **braided hair, hair accessories, or hair extensions;**
- **superficial implants (eg, dermal, iris) or implanted critical devices (eg, pacemaker, implantable chemotherapy port)[4,21,31]; and**
- **prosthetics (eg, prosthetic limb) or corrective devices (eg, orthopedic immobilizer).[28]**

[Recommendation] **P**

Critical devices are those for which there is a risk of significant clinical impact to the patient if the device is dislodged or does not perform as expected.[82] Examples of critical devices include vascular access devices, endotracheal tubes, nasogastric feeding tubes, and indwelling urinary catheters.[82] Pressure injuries can occur as a result of pressure on the skin from critical devices.[19] Critical devices may have tubes or other attachments that can become entrapped in skin folds, resulting in skin damage, especially in patients who are obese.[19] Critical devices may have been placed in locations that limit the ability for pressure to be redistributed.[83] Notably, children are particularly vulnerable to pressure injury from iatrogenic sources such as tubing, cardiac leads, probes, identification bands, and security tags.[15,43]

The presence of jewelry or body piercings may lead to surgical site infection, electrical burns, airway obstruction, or pressure injury.[63,84,85]

Braided hair or hair that has been secured in an accessory (eg, barrette, bobby pin, ponytail holder) may create an area of sufficient pressure to compress and injure the skin and soft tissue between the skull and the surface on which the patient's head is resting.[63,86] Hair accessories may have plastic or metal components, and hair extensions may be attached to the scalp with metal clips, tapes, or adhesives that could lead to pressure injuries.[86]

The presence of a superficial implant or implanted critical device can increase the patient's risk for injury from pressure on the implant or device.[87] Dermal implants are decorative shapes implanted under the skin to create a silhouette of the molded shape on the surface of the skin.[85,88,89] The implant can be made of silicone, Teflon®, or metal.[85,88,89] Subdermal implants have components that are completely embedded under intact skin and cannot be removed.[85,88,89] Transdermal and microdermal implants have anchors that lie under the skin with metal pieces that penetrate through the skin[85] to which jewelry can be attached.[88,89] In some cases, the attached jewelry can be removed.[88,89] Patients with dermal implants may be at increased risk for skin breakdown or pressure injury resulting from pressure at the implant site.[88,89] The damage from pressure at the implant site may not be immediately visible because the pressure injury may initially manifest in the deeper tissue.[89]

Patients with iris implants or eye jewelry who are positioned in the prone position may be at increased risk for ocular injury. Consultation with an ophthalmologist regarding methods for reducing direct pressure on the eye or preventing corneal abrasion may be necessary to prevent a position-related injury.[88]

Prosthetics or corrective devices may create pressure on the skin and soft tissue if left in place during the procedure.

2.4.1 **Remove the patient's jewelry, body piercings, hair accessories, or other items that may pose a risk for positioning injury before the patient is transferred to or positioned on the operating room (OR) bed.[21,28]** *[Recommendation]*

Some jewelry or piercings may interfere with the surgical site or become entangled in bedding or caught on equipment while the patient is being moved and can cause injuries as a result of accidental removal. Patients positioned on jewelry, body piercings, hair accessories, hair extensions, or braids may be subject to pressure injuries.[84-86,90]

2.4.2 **Do not position the patient directly on critical or superficial implanted devices.[19] When positioning the patient on a critical or implanted device cannot be prevented,**
- **reposition the patient and critical devices that are able to be repositioned during the procedure[15,19,63] and**
- **base repositioning interventions and repositioning intervals on the individual patient and the device(s).[19]**

[Recommendation]

Table 2. Pressure Injury Risk Assessment Tools: Pediatric and Neonatal P

Tool	Braden Q Scale	Braden Q + P Scale	Glamorgan Scale	Neonatal Skin Risk Assessment Scale
Indicators	• Mobility • Activity • Sensory perception • Moisture • Friction and shear • Nutritional status • Tissue perfusion[1]	• Height and weight • American Society of Anesthesiologists physical status classification • Surgical position • Length of procedure • Devices • Underlying condition • Sensory perception • Moisture • Mobility • Nutrition • Friction and shear • Tissue perfusion (ie, capillary refill > 2 seconds or oxygen saturation < 95%)[2]	• Mobility • Hard surfaces • Peripheral perfusion • Nutritional status • Anemia (ie, hemoglobin levels < 9.0 g/dL) • Pyrexia (ie, temperature > 100.4° F [38° C] more than 4 hours) • Low serum albumin levels (ie, < 3.5 g/L) • Weight (< 10th percentile) • Incontinence (inappropriate for age)[3]	• General skin condition • Mental state • Mobility • Activity • Nutritional status • Moisture[4]
Scoring	Each indicator is assessed and scored from 1 to 4 for a total score of 7 to 28.[1] Lower scores are indicative of a greater risk for pressure injury.[1]	Each indicator is assessed using a weighted yes/no scoring system.[2] Higher scores are indicative of a greater risk for pressure injury.[2]	Each indicator is assigned a weighted score.[3] Higher scores are indicative of a greater risk for pressure injury.[3]	Each indicator is assessed and scored from 1 to 4 for a total score of 6 to 24.[4] Lower scores are indicative of a greater risk for pressure injury.[4]
Patient Population	Validated tool for assessing the pediatric patient's risk for pressure injury.[1]	Developed specifically for the perioperative pediatric patient.[2]	Validated tool for assessing the pediatric patient's risk for pressure injury.[3]	Validated tool for assessing the neonatal patient's risk for pressure injury.[4]

References

1. *Quigley SM, Curley MA. Skin integrity in the pediatric population: preventing and managing pressure ulcers.* J Soc Pediatr Nurs. *1996;1(1):7-18.*
2. *Galvin PA, Curley MA. The Braden Q+P: a pediatric perioperative pressure ulcer risk assessment and intervention tool.* AORN J. *2012;96(3):261-270.*
3. *Willock J, Anthony D, Richardson J. Inter-rater reliability of the Glamorgan Paediatric Pressure Ulcer Risk Assessment Scale.* Paediatr Nurs. *2008;20(7):4-19.*
4. *Huffines B, Logsdon MC. The Neonatal Skin Risk Assessment Scale for predicting skin breakdown in neonates.* Issues Compr Pediatr Nurs. *1997;20(2):103-114.*

Pressure injuries can occur as a result of prolonged pressure on the skin from critical or implanted devices.[19,91] Repositioning the patient and critical device redistributes pressure from pressure points and from the device.[15,19,42,91] Simple position changes (eg, changing degree of lateral rotation, elevating the head of the bed) may be sufficient to redistribute pressure and prevent injury.[19]

2.4.3 **Support and secure critical devices in a manner that decreases pressure and tension and does not damage skin.**[19,83] *[Recommendation]*

Securing critical devices is paramount to patient safety.[82] Supporting critical devices may help to decrease pressure and prevent pressure injury.[19] Effectively supporting critical devices

may require the use of adhesive tape or medical adhesives. Although the tape or adhesive may successfully secure the device, the application process can cause tension to the surrounding tissue, increasing shear and causing pressure from the device onto the adjacent skin.[83] The use of adhesive tape or medical adhesives for securing and supporting critical devices can be especially damaging in very young and older patients who have fragile skin.[15]

2.4.4 **Prophylactic dressings may be used to prevent pressure injury from critical devices.**[19] *[Conditional Recommendation]* P

The evidence review did not reveal any studies specific to the use of prophylactic dressings for prevention of pressure injury from critical devices in perioperative patients; however, there is moderate-quality evidence to support the use of dressings as a prophylactic intervention to prevent pressure injury related to compression from critical devices (ie, tracheostomy tubes and ties, ventilation and nasal continuous positive airway pressure [CPAP] masks, nasotracheal tubes).[92-95] In a study to determine the efficacy of prophylactic dressings for preventing pressure injury in patients undergoing noninvasive ventilation applied through a face mask, Weng[92] concluded that the use of prophylactic dressings increased patient comfort and reduced the incidence of pressure injury.

Kuo et al[93] conducted a retrospective review of the records of 134 pediatric tracheostomy patients and concluded that the use of a silver-impregnated polyurethane foam dressing placed under the tracheostomy tube and ties reduced the occurrence of postoperative pressure injury from the tracheostomy tube and ties.

In a quasi-experimental study, Huang et al[94] found that the application of a dressing and cushioning material significantly reduced the size and severity of nasal ala pressure injuries attributable to nasotracheal intubation during oral and maxillofacial surgery.

Günlemez et al[95] investigated the efficacy of silicone gel sheeting applied to the nares of preterm infants ventilated with nasal CPAP. They concluded that the use of the silicone gel sheeting reduced the incidence and severity of nasal injury (ie, bleeding, crusting, excoriation, columella necrosis) associated with nasal CPAP.

2.5 Communicate with surgical team members regarding the patient's risk for positioning injury. [Recommendation]

Communication of the preoperative assessment findings to surgical team members is necessary for providing safe patient care.[88]

2.5.1 Collaborate with perioperative team members to determine interventions to be implemented to mitigate the patient's risk for injury.[28,29,62] [Recommendation]

Applying appropriate interventions (eg, changing the surgical approach or position, providing extra padding to redistribute pressure, collaborating with personnel from other departments [eg, radiology, ophthalmology] to determine contraindications or revisions to the plan of care) may help prevent patient injury.[88]

Ulm et al[96] retrospectively reviewed the records of 831 patients who underwent robotic gynecological surgery to determine the inci-

dence of position-related injury. The researchers found that only seven patients (0.8%) experienced a position-related injury. They concluded that the reason for the infrequent occurrence of position-related injury was the use of a collaborative team approach for preventing patient injury.

2.5.2 During the preoperative briefing, discuss interventions that will be implemented to prevent positioning injury[28] and review the effectiveness of these interventions during the postoperative debriefing. [Recommendation]

Collaborative preprocedure assessment and planning and postprocedure review may improve efficiency and communication among team members and may help to reduce or eliminate potential injuries associated with patient positioning.[3,6,97,98]

3. Providing Positioning Devices

3.1 Identify and provide the positioning equipment and devices required for the operative or invasive procedure.[21,23,24] [Recommendation]

Perioperative team members determine the equipment and devices to be used based on the planned procedure, surgeon's preferences, and risk factors identified during the preoperative patient assessment. Safe patient care requires that the patient's position

- provide optimal exposure for the surgical team[2,4,41];
- allow for the placement of positioning equipment and devices[21,41];
- incorporate modifications necessary to accommodate the patient's physical needs[21,41]; and
- provide sufficient access for the anesthesia professional to administer the necessary depth of anesthesia, maintain hemodynamic stability and oxygenation, and preserve and protect invasive infusion sites and monitoring devices.[4,5,15,40]

3.2 Before the patient's arrival in the procedure room, identify and resolve potential conflicts in the availability of positioning equipment. [Recommendation]

Procedures may be delayed and the patient's safety may be compromised when the equipment necessary to correctly and safely position the patient is not available.[6]

3.2.1 Confirm the availability of required positioning equipment when the procedure is scheduled. [Recommendation]

Verifying the availability of positioning equipment at the time of scheduling may help prevent delays in patient care.

3.3 **Confirm that the OR is set up correctly for the planned procedure before the patient arrives in the procedure room.**[24] *[Recommendation]*

Patient safety may be compromised when the room arrangement is not specific to the planned procedure and its laterality.[99]

3.4 **Verify the correct patient position and positioning equipment during the time out.**[100] *[Recommendation]*

The World Health Organization[100] recommends including a discussion of issues and concerns related to positioning equipment as part of the time out. Using effective methods to improve communication and involve all members of the perioperative team may help to reduce errors and improve patient safety.[99,101,102]

4. Maintenance of Devices

4.1 **Select, clean, inspect, and maintain positioning equipment, devices, and support surfaces and ensure they are repaired or replaced when damaged, defective, or obsolete.**[9,28] *[Recommendation]*

Clean and functional equipment and devices contribute to patient and personnel safety. Failures in surface integrity can contribute to bacterial growth and patient skin breakdown. Equipment, devices, and support surfaces may have a finite life span.[19] Use of damaged, defective, or obsolete equipment and devices poses a risk for injury to patients and personnel.

4.2 **Develop and implement processes and procedures for evaluating, selecting, and purchasing positioning equipment and devices.**[103] *[Recommendation]*

Patient and health care worker safety, quality, and cost containment are primary concerns of perioperative personnel as they participate in evaluating and selecting equipment and devices for use in the perioperative setting.[103] The technology used to design and create positioning equipment, devices, and support surfaces continues to evolve; therefore, it is important for perioperative team members to be informed by current evidence regarding the use of these products.

4.2.1 **Actively participate in the process of identifying and selecting positioning equipment and devices.**[6] *[Recommendation]*

Personnel who perform positioning activities are a reliable source of feedback regarding desired features, functionality, and safety design of positioning equipment and devices.

4.2.2 **Maintain an inventory of positioning equipment, devices, and support surfaces sufficient to meet the anticipated demand.**[4] *[Recommendation]*

Positioning needs vary with each patient. Without the necessary equipment, optimal positioning may not be possible. Working without the necessary equipment, substituting equipment of a lesser quality, or using equipment designed for other purposes increases the risk for injuries to patients and personnel. Having an adequate inventory of devices and equipment improves efficiency, lessens the potential for patient care to be delayed, and decreases the possibility of conflict that may arise when the needed equipment is not available.

In a nonexperimental study to examine problems associated with surgical patient positioning, Sørensen et al[8] sent an electronic questionnaire to 833 perioperative RNs employed at four public university hospitals in Denmark. There were 481 responses (57.7%) to the survey. The results showed there was an overall lack of OR beds, positioning equipment, and devices available for patient arm and leg support. The lack of available equipment unduly complicated the positioning process. At times, it was necessary for personnel to spend time and effort searching for equipment, particularly equipment and devices required for the prone and lateral positions. The inadequate supply of equipment and devices also required personnel to either compete for or share the equipment. The researchers concluded that the lack of sufficient quantities of positioning equipment and devices presented a risk to patient and personnel safety.

4.3 **Establish a multidisciplinary team to determine the type of support surfaces that will be used for perioperative patients. Multidisciplinary team members may include wound, ostomy, and continence care RNs; perioperative RNs; infection preventionists; supply chain managers; and other involved personnel.** *[Conditional Recommendation]*

Moderate-quality evidence regarding the most effective pressure-redistributing support surface is inconclusive, and further research is warranted to determine the effectiveness of support surfaces in the perioperative setting.[30,31,51,104-109]

In an effort to provide clinical guidance for selecting a support surface based on individual patient needs, the Wound, Ostomy and Continence Nurses

Society has developed an evidence- and consensus-based algorithm for support surface selection that uses the Braden Scale mobility and moisture subscale scores to drive selection of support surfaces.[109] The algorithm can be adapted to include specific products used by the health care organization.[109]

King and Bridges[105] conducted a quasi-experimental study to determine peak skin interface pressures when using three support surfaces—an OR bed mattress, a polyurethane convoluted foam overlay on an OR bed mattress, and a viscoelastic dry polymer gel overlay on an OR bed mattress—with participants in the supine and lateral positions. The researchers found that in the supine position, participants' sacral pressures were significantly higher on the OR bed mattress with the foam overlay than on the OR bed mattress alone or with the gel overlay. Heel pressures were significantly lower on the OR bed mattress with the foam overlay than on the OR bed mattress alone or with the gel overlay. In the lateral position, participants' trochanter pressures were significantly higher on the OR bed mattress with the foam overlay than on the OR bed mattress with the gel overlay. Most of the participants reported that the foam overlay was the most comfortable surface and the gel overlay was the least comfortable surface. The researchers concluded that adding a foam or gel overlay to an OR bed mattress did not reduce skin interface pressures.

Hoshowsky and Schramm[104] conducted a randomized controlled trial (RCT) to examine the effects of two OR bed mattresses—a vinyl-covered 2-inch (5.1-cm) foam mattress and a nylon fabric-covered 2-inch (5.1-cm) foam-and-gel mattress—and one viscoelastic dry polymer gel overlay on intraoperative pressure injury formation. The researchers found that both the foam-and-gel mattress and the viscoelastic gel overlay were significantly more effective than the foam mattress in preventing skin changes and pressure injury, but the viscoelastic gel overlay was the most effective surface for preventing pressure injury.

Scott[55] evaluated the efficacy of a 4-inch (10.2 cm) multi-layer pressure-redistributing surface compared with a 2-inch (5.1-cm) foam OR bed mattress. The author found that patients were eight times more likely to develop a pressure injury when positioned on the foam surface compared with the multi-layer pressure-redistributing surface.

Deane et al[110] conducted a quasi-experimental study to determine whether changes in skin interface pressures could be related to the OR bed surface material. The researchers measured the interface pressure between the participants' skin and an OR bed mattress, an OR bed mattress covered with a convoluted foam overlay, and an OR bed mattress covered with a viscoelastic gel overlay. They found the interface pressures for the OR bed mattress with the convoluted foam overlay were not statistically lower than for the OR bed mattress alone. The interface pressures for the OR bed mattress with the viscoelastic gel overlay were significantly higher than for the OR bed mattress with the convoluted foam overlay.

Wu et al[107] conducted a quasi-experimental study to evaluate the efficacy of high-density foam pads compared with viscoelastic polymer pads in the prevention of pressure injury. The researchers found that the average and peak pressures measured at the points padded with the viscoelastic polymer were significantly lower than at the points padded with high-density foam; however, there was not a significant difference in the number of pressure injuries.

Reddy[106] conducted a systematic review of 64 RCTs, systematic reviews, and observational studies to determine the effects of surfaces used to prevent pressure injuries. Based on evidence of a moderate quality, the researcher concluded that viscoelastic foam mattresses reduced the incidence of pressure injuries in people at risk compared with foam mattresses; however, the most effective mattress was undetermined. The researcher also concluded that using pressure-redistributing overlays on OR beds was more effective than no overlay for preventing pressure injuries, but this conclusion was supported by only very low-quality evidence.

In a Cochrane systematic review of support surfaces for pressure injury prevention, McInnes et al[108] analyzed 59 RCTs and quasi-randomized trials, published or unpublished, that assessed the effects of any support surface for prevention of pressure injury in any patient group or setting. The researchers found that foam alternatives (eg, viscoelastic foam) reduced the incidence of pressure injury in patients at risk for pressure injury. The researchers also found that pressure-redistributing overlays on the OR bed reduced the incidence of postoperative pressure injury.

In a nonexperimental study conducted in a university medical center in Canada, Pham et al[76] calculated the cost of using the existing OR bed mattress and supplemental padding compared with the cost of using a viscoelastic dry polymer gel overlay on top of the OR bed mattress. The researchers found that the use of the viscoelastic gel overlay during procedures lasting 90 minutes or longer decreased the incidence of postoperative pressure injury by 0.51% and resulted in an overall cost savings of $46 per patient ($38.23 in 2017 US dollars).

4.4 **Verify cleanliness, surface integrity, and correct function of positioning equipment, devices, and support surfaces before use.**[5,21,28,41] *[Recommendation]*

Positioning equipment and devices are exposed to direct patient contact and frequent hand contact and have the potential for surface contamination with microorganisms and body substances.[111,112] Application of rigorous environmental cleaning practices will assist in providing a clean environment for perioperative patients and minimize the risk for exposure of health care personnel and patients to potentially infectious microorganisms.[113]

Loss of surface integrity can create a reservoir for the collection of dirt and debris that may be difficult or impossible to remove during cleaning and can lead to bacterial growth. Surfaces that are irregular, wrinkled, or damaged can contribute to skin breakdown. Some support surfaces (eg, convoluted foam) can lose resilience, hold moisture, prevent air circulation, and harbor microorganisms if not replaced when soiled.[43] Inspection and evaluation provide an opportunity to identify and remove from service soiled or defective items that might put patients at risk for infection or injury.

4.4.1 **Remove soiled, damaged, or defective surfaces, devices, and equipment from service and have them cleaned, repaired, or replaced.** *[Recommendation]*

Removal from service, followed by cleaning, repair, and replacement of soiled, damaged, or defective equipment and devices helps prevent further damage from use and reduces the risk for patient infection or injury to patients or personnel.

4.5 **Have preventive maintenance and repair performed at established intervals on all equipment and devices used for patient positioning.**[28] *[Recommendation]*

Regular preventive maintenance promotes optimal functioning of equipment and devices and decreases the risk for injury to patients and personnel.

4.5.1 **Align the schedule for preventive maintenance and repair with the manufacturer's instructions for use (IFU).** *[Recommendation]*

The manufacturer is the most reliable source for determining preventive maintenance schedules. Between January 2009 and January 2016, the US Food and Drug Administration (FDA)[114] received more than 1,000 medical device reports associated with slippage or movement of neurosurgical head holders that resulted in more than 700 injuries. The FDA determined that slippage of the neurosurgical head holders was multifactorial and not specific to any manufacturer or brand of device; however, one cause of the slippage was found to be a lack of preventive maintenance. The FDA suggested the risk for injury

could be mitigated by following the manufacturer's instructions for cleaning, maintaining, and replacing the neurosurgical head holder based on the manufacturer's suggested life expectancy of the device (ie, number of uses or length of time the device has been in use). The FDA also recommended inspecting the neurosurgical head holder system before and after each use, removing any parts of the system that appear to be damaged, and returning defective items to the manufacturer for repair or replacement.

4.5.2 **Have qualified individuals perform preventive maintenance and repairs.** *[Recommendation]*

Preventive maintenance requires special skills and knowledge that includes systematic inspection, testing, measurement, adjustment, parts replacement, and detection and correction of device or equipment malfunction either before it occurs or before it develops into a major failure. Having qualified personnel perform preventive maintenance and repair increases the probability that repair and service will be performed correctly.

5. Correct Use of Devices

5.1 **Use OR beds, positioning equipment and devices, and support surfaces correctly.**[28] *[Recommendation]*

Patients and health care workers are at risk for injury if OR beds, positioning equipment and devices, and support surfaces are not used correctly.

5.2 **Use OR beds and attachments in accordance with the manufacturer's IFU.**[5,24] *[Recommendation]*

Patient injuries resulting from failure to follow the positioning equipment manufacturer's IFU have been reported.[115,116] Dauber and Roth[115] reported the case of an obese patient undergoing spinal fusion surgery in the prone position on a spinal table. When a slight axial rotational adjustment was made to the patient's position, the table rapidly tilted vertically, causing the patient to fall to the floor. The patient's vital signs remained stable, and neither the endotracheal tube nor the indwelling IV catheter became dislodged; however, the patient immediately developed a large subgaleal hematoma. During a root cause analysis of the event, it was determined that the incident was caused by a failure to correctly activate the table-locking mechanism.

Ahmad et al[116] reported two incidents of muscle necrosis and anterior thigh compartment syndrome caused by incorrect placement of Jackson table attachments. Both patients were injured as a result of a failure to follow the manufacturer's IFU.

The Jackson table has adjustable pads designed to support the iliac crest and thighs. The iliac crest pads are designed by the manufacturer to be higher than the thigh pads. When the thigh and iliac crest pads are reversed (either in error or deliberately to achieve a greater degree of lumbar lordosis, as was the reason in these cases), the higher iliac crest pad creates a greater degree of focal pressure on the thighs that can lead to patient injury.

5.2.1 **Pad and place the perineal post on the fracture table in accordance with the manufacturer's IFU.**[117] *[Recommendation]*

Incorrect placement of the perineal post of the fracture table can lead to perineal pressure injury, pudendal neuropathy, or erectile dysfunction.[36,117-119] Accurate post placement and sufficient padding around the perineal post can help to prevent these injuries.[36,117-120]

5.3 **Use positioning equipment and devices and support surfaces in accordance with the manufacturer's IFU.** *[Recommendation]*

In an expert opinion article, Chitlik[9] described an incident that illustrates the importance of following the manufacturer's IFU when using vacuum-packed positioning devices. Rather than disconnecting the suction and closing the valve on the device per the manufacturer's IFU, personnel were leaving the suction attached to the device during the procedure. This resulted in the device deflating during the procedure, losing its capacity to keep the patient in the desired position. When the device deflated, there was a tendency for the patient to slide toward the head of the bed, which necessitated repositioning interventions.

5.3.1 **Use positioning equipment and devices that are designed and intended for use in positioning surgical patients.**[63] *[Recommendation]*

Using equipment and devices intended for use in positioning surgical patients decreases the risk for injury to patients and personnel.

5.3.2 **Verify compatibility between positioning devices and support surfaces before use.** *[Recommendation]*

Manufacturers may permit or preclude the use of certain devices or surfaces with their products. Using products or surfaces that are not compatible with each other increases the risk for injury to patients or personnel.

5.3.3 **Use neurosurgical head holder systems and their accessories in accordance with the manufacturer's IFU.**[114] *[Recommendation]* **P**

Between January 2009 and January 2016, the FDA received more than 1,000 medical device reports associated with slippage or movement of neurosurgical head holders that resulted in more than 700 injuries.[114] These reports described injuries that included skull fractures, hematomas, and facial bruises and lacerations, as well as surgical procedures that were delayed, prolonged, or terminated. The FDA determined that slippage of the neurosurgical head holders was multifactorial and not specific to any manufacturer or brand of device; however, the FDA recommended that health care providers

- follow the manufacturer's IFU,
- use the manufacturer-recommended accessories with the neurosurgical head holder system, and
- report adverse events associated with the neurosurgical head holder system to the manufacturer and to the FDA through MedWatch: The FDA Safety Information and Adverse Event Reporting Program.[114,121]

The risk for adverse events associated with neurosurgical head holder systems may be greater in the pediatric population because of the varying thickness of the developing cranium.[122] In a survey of 164 neurosurgeons who treated pediatric patients, 158 (96%) of whom reported using cranial fixation pins in their practice, 89 (54%) of the neurosurgeons reported having experienced complications directly related to the use of cranial fixation pins, including cranial fracture, epidural or subdural hematoma, scalp laceration, or cerebrospinal fluid leak.[123]

Poli et al[122] reported the case of a 7-year-old boy who underwent a left suboccipital craniectomy in the prone position. The patient's head was fixed in a Mayfield neurosurgical head holder system. At the end of the procedure, a computerized axial tomography scan revealed a left hemispheric epidural hematoma with a small depressed skull fracture at the site of one of the pins. The patient underwent immediate surgical evacuation of the hematoma and was discharged 13 days later.

5.4 **Use OR beds and positioning equipment and devices that have the weight and size capacity and the articulation abilities necessary for safe movement and care of the patient.** *[Recommendation]*

Accommodating the unique needs of individual patients is necessary to prevent injury to patients and personnel.[6,74] Operating room bed and positioning device requirements may vary based on the patient's height and weight.

In a qualitative analysis of 863 perioperative incident reports from six institutions in the Midwest, Chappy[124] identified specific events that affected perioperative patient safety during a 3-year period. Sixteen incidents involved patient positioning (2%), and of these, 10 reports (63%) involved patients who were too heavy for the OR bed or bed attachment specifications. In all 10 of these procedures, the OR bed or attachment was used in spite of the weight restrictions because alternative OR beds or equipment were not available. Notably, in all procedures, there was a note in the perioperative record that the surgeon was informed of the weight restriction before the start of the procedure.

5.4.1 Designate facility personnel to ensure that positioning equipment and devices with a weight limit are clearly labeled. *[Recommendation]*

6. Avoiding Positioning Hazards

6.1 Identify potential hazards associated with positioning activities and establish safe practices. *[Recommendation]*

Positioning patients and using positioning equipment and devices during perioperative care can result in injury to both patients and personnel.[6,16,125] Identifying potential hazards and establishing safe practices may reduce the risk for patient and personnel injury.

6.2 Ensure an adequate number of personnel, devices, and equipment are available during patient positioning activities to promote patient and personnel safety.[4-6,41,58,125] *[Recommendation]*

Having a sufficient number of personnel to position the patient helps maintain the patient's physiologic body alignment and provide support for the patient's extremities[28] and also reduces the physical demands placed on the personnel performing the task.[16,41,58,125,126] In a qualitative study to capture the perceptions of perioperative team members related to patient and personnel safety during prone positioning, Asiedu et al[127] analyzed open-ended questionnaires and conducted interviews with members of the spine positioning team from a large midwestern teaching and research hospital. The participants reported that limited numbers of available personnel was one of the major challenges faced during prone positioning. The availability of personnel was affected by daily staffing patterns. When the number of personnel was limited (as sometimes occurred during lunch or dinner breaks or during emergency procedures performed outside of normal operating hours), perioperative team members were required to move patients without the number of personnel needed to move the patient safely.

The participants also reported that the difficulty of positioning very large patients could be a source of anxiety and stress to the positioning team and that the receiver role (ie, the person catching the patient during the flip from the supine position on the transport gurney to the prone position on the OR bed) was more challenging than the sender role (ie, the person flipping the patient away from himself or herself). The difficulty of the receiver role was increased with larger patients because it took longer, required more energy, and increased the risk for injury.[127]

6.3 At least one surgical team member should attend the patient on the OR bed at all times.[28] *[Recommendation]* **P**

A lack of clear communication about who is responsible for watching the patient after the safety straps are removed or before the patient is transferred to the OR bed has been reported as a contributing factor for patient falls in the perioperative setting.[128]

In an incident reported by Redman and McNatt,[129] an 8-month-old infant had been extubated and was lying quietly on the OR bed after an inguinal hernia repair. The anesthesia professional was standing at the head of the bed with her right hand on the child's head. Her body was turned to the left side as she manipulated the anesthesia machine with her left hand. The RN circulator had turned to observe the anesthesia professional when the child suddenly moved from a supine position and fell head-first off the left side of the bed. The RN circulator reacted quickly and was able to cushion the child's fall with her left hand. The child's body came to rest on the top of the RN's shoes. The child was immediately returned to the OR bed alert and awake with no evidence of injury.

Noting that gurneys and patient beds have side rails but OR beds do not, the authors developed a set of portable, cushioned side rails that could be attached to the OR bed to prevent pediatric patient falls. The authors proposed that using the side rails increased the margin of safety, but cautioned that the use of the side rails was not a substitute for constant attendance, vigilant observation, and other safety measures (eg, safety straps) commonly used to prevent patient falls.[129]

6.4 Coordinate positioning of the patient with team members by
- verifying that all team members are ready for positioning to occur or
- implementing a countdown to begin positioning.

[Recommendation]

Failure to coordinate positioning activities can result in sliding or pulling the patient and shear forces or friction on the patient's skin. Shearing occurs when the patient's skin remains stationary and the underlying tissues shift or move, as might occur when the patient is pulled or dragged without support to the skeletal system.[43,75] Shearing leads to blood vessel constriction that can increase the risk for ischemia and tissue necrosis.[75,130] Friction occurs when skin surfaces rub against a rough stationary surface,[43] leading to increased shedding of layers of epidermis and an increased susceptibility to pressure injury.[75,130]

Asiedu et al[127] analyzed open-ended questionnaires and conducted interviews with members of the spine positioning team from a large midwestern teaching and research hospital. The participants suggested implementing an audible and visual "pause" before any patient movement to ensure that equipment is set up correctly (eg, wheels locked) and that all positioning personnel are ready for the transfer or positioning to occur, as a method to prevent patient and personnel injury.

6.4.1 When the patient has critical devices (eg, catheters, drainage tubes),
- **communicate about the presence of the critical device,**
- **take measures to secure them during positioning, and**
- **confirm correct placement and patency after positioning.**
[Recommendation]

Positioning activities can dislodge critical devices.[131]

7. Pressure-Reducing Surfaces

7.1 **Position patients on surfaces that reduce the potential for pressure injury.** *[Recommendation]*

All perioperative patients are at risk for pressure injury because they are immobile during the procedure; placed on a relatively hard surface; unable to feel pain caused by pressure, friction, and shear forces; and unable to change position to relieve the pressure.[19] Before coming to the OR, a patient may have been transported to the emergency department by ambulance and may have waited for many hours on a hard surface.[31] A patient may have undergone a diagnostic procedure that required remaining in one position for a prolonged period. Some surgical procedures require that the patient be positioned on a hard surface (eg, vacuum-packed positioning device) to maintain the patient's position.[34] Patients are also at risk because of the use of vasoactive medications and the effects of anesthesia on hemodynamic status and tissue perfusion.[31]

7.2 **Position patients on surfaces that are smooth and wrinkle-free.**[4,22,61,118] *[Recommendation]*

Wrinkles in the surface beneath the patient can increase the risk for skin breakdown or pressure injury.[4,22,63]

7.3 **Do not position patients on multiple layers of sheets, blankets, or other materials.**[4,19,61-63,71,132] *[Recommendation]* **P**

Bed linen and other layers of material (eg, disposable incontinence pads) may be needed for patient comfort and to manage moisture or drainage[19]; however, placing blankets or other materials between the support surface and the patient reduces the pressure-redistributing effect of the support surface.[4,34,62,63,71,133]

In an organizational improvement project to establish the most effective method for preparing the surface of the OR bed to decrease pressure, Campbell[132] evaluated the sacral pressure readings of 20 patients undergoing peripheral vascular surgery. The author found that each layer of cloth or material placed between the patient and the OR bed mattress decreased the pressure-redistributing performance of the OR bed mattress and significantly increased sacral pressure readings. Increasing the number of layers of materials under the patient from three layers to nine layers increased pressure readings from an average of 41.2 mmHg to 73.8 mmHg. The author recommended decreasing the number of sheets and blankets beneath the patient.

7.4 **Do not position patients on warming blankets, if possible.**[25,132,134] *[Recommendation]* **P**

Warming blankets placed under surgical patients increase tissue metabolism and multiply the body's demand for oxygen, nutrients, and by-product removal. When patients are anesthetized, hypotensive, and immobile, they may not be able to meet this increased demand and are thus more susceptible to tissue damage.[25,132]

Grous et al[134] conducted a nonexperimental descriptive study to identify factors contributing to pressure injury in 33 patients undergoing operative procedures lasting longer than 10 hours. The researchers observed patient positioning and the placement of all positioning and warming devices. The patients were assessed for pressure injury within 48 hours after surgery. The researchers found that of the 15 patients (46%) who developed pressure injures, 12 (80%) had been placed on warming blankets during the procedure. The researchers recommended that warming blankets not be placed under patients undergoing surgical procedures.

Notably, in some patient populations (eg, neonates) there are limited options for placement of warming blankets, and positioning the patient on a warming blanket may be an effective method for preventing hypothermia. In these cases, it is necessary to evaluate the benefit of reducing the potential for pressure injury compared with the risk for hypothermia.

7.5 | **Position patients on surfaces that redistribute pressure.** *[Recommendation]*

Positioning perioperative patients on surfaces that redistribute pressure may reduce the risk for pressure injury.[15,31,51,118] Pressure redistribution is the ability of a supportive material to distribute the load over a broader surface or contact area.[75,109] Pressure redistribution is accomplished by envelopment and immersion.[75] Envelopment is the ability of the support surface to conform and shape itself to the patient's body.[19,75,109] An enveloping support surface increases contact area and reduces pressure.[19,75] Immersion is the depth that a patient's body descends into the support surface.[19,75,109] The greater the level of immersion, the greater the amount of body surface area that is contacted.[19,75] The greater the surface area, the lower the overall pressure.[19,75] Notably, the patient's body can be immersed too deeply into the surface, leading to a "bottoming out" effect.[75] Bottoming out occurs when the support surface becomes fully compressed under the weight of the patient's body, resulting in the patient lying directly on a hard surface.[75] To prevent bottoming out, it is important that support surfaces provide at least 1 inch (2.5 cm) of supportive material between the bed and the patient's body.[104,135]

Using surfaces that reduce tissue interface pressures may be effective in redistributing pressure and lowering the patient's risk for a pressure injury.[75,105] Interface pressures greater than 32 mmHg may occlude capillary blood flow and lead to diminished tissue perfusion and ischemic injury that later manifests as a pressure injury.[36,104,136] However, devices used to measure interface pressure may underestimate pressures at the point where deep tissue injury occurs.[137] In addition, because of variability in individual patients, interface pressure alone may not be sufficient to evaluate the effectiveness of a particular surface in redistributing pressure and preventing pressure injury.[43,75] The duration of pressure may be more of a contributing factor than the intensity of the pressure.[19,105] Pressure injuries may be caused by high pressures applied for short periods or low pressures applied for long periods.[138]

Support surfaces that are designed to redistribute pressure may be constructed of various materials or combinations of materials that include foam, gel, air, or fluid.[19,31,104] Support surfaces may also be designed with structures such as bladders or modules arranged in layers or zones.[19] Support surfaces may be static (ie, lacking in movement) or dynamic.[31,43,104] Dynamic support surfaces are powered to provide movement that alters the immersion and envelopment characteristics of the surface, controls the temperature and humidity between the support surface and the patient, and redistributes pressure.[19] Controlling the temperature and humidity slows metabolic activity, decreases circulatory demand, inhibits sweating, and reduces skin hydration to decrease the risk for pressure injury.[75]

Static surfaces such as viscoelastic polymer (ie, gel) overlays are designed to reduce shearing and to support the patient's weight without becoming fully compressed under the weight of the patient's body.[30,31,61] Gel overlays are radiolucent, latex-free, and reusable.[30]

Foam overlays come in various depths and densities.[30] Foam density (ie, kg/m³) affects the lifespan of the foam padding and its ability to support the weight that is placed on it during a specified period of time.[139] Indentation load deflection indicates how much weight is required to compress the foam padding to 25% of its original size.[139] No evidence exists regarding the optimal foam density and indentation load deflection for preventing pressure injury in perioperative patients. Using a 3-inch (7.6-cm) low-density foam may not be as effective as using a 2-inch (5.1-cm) high-density foam. Some foam products may be ineffective when used with a patient who is obese because of compression resulting from the patient's weight.[74] Most foam products have a weight limit of approximately 253.5 lb (115 kg); however, some viscoelastic foam mattresses can support up to 694.5 lb (315 kg).[62]

Static air overlays have multiple chambers that allow air exchange between compartments when the patient lies on the surface. Dynamic air overlays or powered devices include air overlays and mattress replacements that can be customized to fit the articulation of various OR bed sections. Alternating air overlays are designed to alternate inflation and deflation of chambers so that pressure points are constantly changing.[30,31]

Simulated fluid immersion technology maintains the patient in a simulated fluid environment designed to redistribute pressure and eliminate pressure points by displacing the patient's weight throughout a simulated fluid medium.[140,141] The system allows the immersion properties of the mattress to be adjusted to the individual patient.[141]

Worsley et al[141] found the simulated fluid immersion mattress provided a high level of pressure redistribution with low peak pressures over the body in supine, sitting, and lateral positions. Kirkland-Walsh et al[142] measured full-body interface pressures in four different support surfaces and found the simulated fluid immersion surface produced the lowest average sacral pressure (22.1 mmHg). Further research is needed to determine whether simulated surfaces reduce the risk for pressure injury in perioperative patients.[140-142]

There are a vast variety of pressure-redistributing surfaces available for use with perioperative patients. It is essential that perioperative patients be positioned on surfaces that redistribute pressure; however, selection of appropriate support surfaces for the perioperative practice setting is a complex process that warrants evaluation and review by a multidisciplinary team (See Recommendation 4.3).

7.5.1   **Do not use towels, sheets, and blankets as positioning devices.**[61-63] *[Recommendation]*

Using rolled or folded towels, sheets, or blankets as positioning devices increases pressure, contributes to friction injuries, and decreases the pressure-redistributing properties of the support surface.[6,25,61-63]

7.5.2   **Pillows may be used for patient positioning.** *[Conditional Recommendation]*

Notably, pillows provide only a minimal amount of pressure redistribution.[62,63]

7.5.3   **A vacuum-packed positioning device may be used.**[143] *[Conditional Recommendation]*

Using a vacuum-packed positioning device provides stability and helps maintain the patient in the desired position.[143] Vacuum-packed positioning devices are designed to reduce pressure injury by providing a surface on which the patient's weight is evenly distributed and supported.[144] However, after decompression, these devices can increase pressure on nerves and over bony prominences.[34,145] When a vacuum-packed positioning device is used to support a patient in the lateral position, the patient's circulatory system may be compromised not only by the tight restraint provided by the device, but also by the overall effects of gravity on the patient's body and the horizontal body posture.[34]

Stephenson et al[145] described the case of a 14-year-old boy who underwent thoracoscopic resection of a right-sided mediastinal mass in the left lateral position on a vacuum-packed positioning device. The procedure lasted 3 hours. During his follow up visit 6 days after surgery, the patient complained of a 2-day history of shooting and burning left-leg pain and an area of numbness on the lateral aspect of the thigh. He was limping because of the pain, but had no motor deficit. The patient was diagnosed with a lateral femoral cutaneous neuropathy. Six weeks after surgery the patient's pain and numbness had decreased but was still present.

7.5.4   **Place positioning devices (eg, shoulder supports) beneath the patient and not beneath the OR bed mattress or the overlay on top of the OR bed mattress.** *[Recommendation]*

Placing positioning devices beneath the OR bed mattress or overlay decreases the pressure-redistributing properties of the mattress or overlay.[31,63]

7.5.5   **Continue repositioning activities intended to prevent pressure injury in patients who are placed on pressure-redistributing surfaces.**[19,109] *[Recommendation]*

Repositioning is helpful for providing pressure relief and comfort even when a pressure-redistributing surface is used.[19] The damaging effects of pressure are related to both magnitude and duration.[109] Repositioning activities reduce the duration of pressure.[109]

7.6   **Position patients identified as being at high risk for pressure injury on high-specification reactive foam surfaces, if possible.** *[Recommendation]*

The National Pressure Ulcer Advisory Panel (NPUAP), European Pressure Ulcer Advisory Panel (EPUAP), and Pan Pacific Pressure Injury Alliance (PPPIA)[19] recommend the use of high-specification reactive foam surfaces for perioperative patients at high risk for pressure injury. High-specification surfaces are pressure-redistributing pads or mattresses composed of high-density or viscoelastic foam that conforms to the body contours.[146] These surfaces may include multiple layers of foams of various grades and types.[19,62] Properties of a high-specification foam mattress include

- a density of 35 kg/m^3,
- an indentation force deflection of 35 to 130,
- hardness (ie, the ability to push back and carry weight) of 130 Newtons,
- a support factor of 1.75 to 2.4,
- a depth of 5.9 inches (150 mm), and
- a mattress cover with a moisture vapor transmission rate of 33 g/m^2/24 hours.[19]

A reactive support surface is designed to reduce the risk for pressure injury by changing its load distribution in response to an applied load (ie, the patient's weight).[19] Reactive support surfaces provide deep immersion and a high degree of envelopment to reduce high pressure concentrations over bony prominences.[19] Using high-specification reactive foam surfaces may be an effective strategy to reduce the incidence of pressure injury in perioperative patients.[62,63]

In a Cochrane systematic review of support surfaces for pressure injury prevention, McInnes et al[108] analyzed 59 RCTs and quasi-randomized trials, published and unpublished, that assessed the effects of any support surface for prevention of pressure injury in any patient group or setting. The researchers concluded that the use of high-specification foam mattresses was indicated for patients at high risk for pressure injury.

7.6.1 **Place patients on high-specification reactive or alternating pressure support surfaces before and after surgery,[19] if possible.** [Recommendation]

The NPUAP, EPUAP, and PPPIA[19] recommend the use of high-specification reactive alternating pressure support surfaces for perioperative patients before and after surgery. Positioning a patient on a high-specification surface reduces the risk for pressure injury when the patient is immobile or sedated.

7.7 **Use additional pressure-redistributing padding to support the patient and redistribute pressure from bony prominences and other pressure points.**[6,19,23,28,51,58,147] [Recommendation]

Placing padding between the patient and hard surfaces and using additional padding on bony prominences and other pressure points increases patient comfort, helps redistribute pressure, and decreases the potential for nerve or pressure injury.[5,23,36,41,62,68,118,147] Patients who are obese may require additional padding because the excess weight of the patient puts additional pressure on areas that contact the OR bed or positioning devices used.[24] Older adults may have musculoskeletal diseases or deformities (eg, arthritis, kyphotic spines) that necessitate additional padding.[23,60]

Notably, the use of excessive padding that creates misalignment or additional pressure or is applied too tightly does not redistribute pressure and can cause pressure injury.[35,143]

7.8 **Prophylactic dressings may be applied to bony prominences (eg, heels, sacrum) or other areas subjected to pressure, friction, and shear.** [Conditional Recommendation]

There is moderate-quality evidence to support the use of prophylactic dressings for prevention of pressure injury[148-154]; however, further research is warranted regarding the use of prophylactic dressings in perioperative patients.

The use of prophylactic dressings may reduce the effects of pressure, shear, and friction on healthy skin at increased risk for pressure injury.[150] In a nonexperimental study to identify the modes of action by which prophylactic dressings prevented pressure injury, Call et al[151] tested nine commercially available dressings and found that the use of prophylactic dressings reduced the forces of shear, pressure, and friction placed on patients at risk for pressure injury. The researchers found that the dressings were able to effectively redirect these forces to wider areas and minimize the mechanical loads placed on skeletal structures. The use of prophylactic dressings significantly reduced the amount of shear delivered to the skin by several mechanisms, including

- displacing the shear force outside of the dressing area;
- using silicone adhesives to absorb shear;
- providing bulk to absorb shear;
- having multiple layers of foam to create a displacement plane for absorbing shear; and
- stretching, molding, and conforming to the skin surface to absorb pressure.

The researchers noted that adhesion was an important element of the effectiveness of the dressing because insufficient adhesion allowed the dressing to easily release from the skin, whereas excessive adhesion led to cell stripping or disruption of granulation when used over a healing wound. The researchers concluded that prophylactic dressings were useful to enhance but not replace pressure injury prevention programs.

In an RCT to investigate the effectiveness of multi-layered soft silicone border foam dressings in preventing pressure injury, Santamaria et al[148] randomly allocated 440 critically ill patients to either a control group (n = 221) that received the usual care for pressure injury prevention or an experimental group (n = 219) that received the usual care plus a silicone border foam dressing applied to the sacrum and a silicone border foam dressing applied to each of their heels. The researchers found there were significantly fewer patients with pressure injuries in the experimental group (n = 5; 3.1%) compared with the control group (n = 20; 13.1%). The researchers concluded that the multilayered soft silicone border foam dressings were effective in preventing pressure injuries in critically ill patients.

Moore and Webster[150] conducted a Cochrane systematic review of four RCTs to evaluate the efficacy of dressings in preventing pressure injury in people of any age without pre-existing pressure injury but considered to be at risk for pressure injury in any health care setting. The researchers concluded that although prophylactic dressings reduced the incidence of pressure injury, the results were compromised by the low quality of the trials included.

7.8.1 Establish a multidisciplinary team to determine the type of prophylactic dressings that will be used in the perioperative setting as part of the health care organization's pressure injury prevention program. Multidisciplinary team members may include wound specialists; wound, ostomy, and continence care RNs; infection preventionists; perioperative RNs; supply chain managers; and other involved personnel. *[Conditional Recommendation]*

There are numerous types of prophylactic dressings, including

- semipermeable film dressings (ie, a thin polyurethane membrane coated with a layer of acrylic adhesive),
- hydrocolloid dressings (ie, a dressing containing a dispersion of gelatin, pectin, and carboxymethylcellulose together with other polymers and adhesives that form a flexible wafer), and
- foam dressings (ie, open cell, hydrophobic, polyurethane foam sheet).[150]

The use of a prophylactic dressing alters the temperature and humidity of the skin surface.[155] The amount of moisture trapped next to the skin, the amount of moisture that escapes from the dressing, and the amount of heat that is trapped by the dressing can affect the suitability of the dressing for use in preventing pressure injury.[155]

Each dressing is unique and its effectiveness in preventing pressure injury is based on the materials from which it is constructed, the number of layers in the dressing, the presence of perforations or micropores in the films used, the concentration of thermally dense polymers, the amount of air entrapment in the foam, and the amount of moisture accumulated under the dressing.[155]

7.8.2 Size prophylactic dressings used for prevention of pressure injury according to the manufacturer's IFU. *[Recommendation]*

Correct sizing of the prophylactic dressing helps ensure effective redistribution of pressure, shear, and friction forces from areas of risk.[151]

7.8.3 Do not use multiple layers of prophylactic dressings.[83] *[Recommendation]*

Using multiple layers of prophylactic dressings can increase the amount of pressure, shear, and friction applied to the skin.[83,151]

7.8.4 Replace prophylactic dressings if damaged, displaced, loosened, or moist.[19] *[Recommendation]*

The effectiveness of the dressing may be compromised if damaged, displaced, loosened, or moist.

7.8.5 Continue safe positioning practices intended to prevent pressure injury in patients receiving prophylactic dressings.[19,153] *[Recommendation]*

The use of prophylactic dressings does not negate the need for positioning interventions to prevent pressure injury.[19,151]

8. Safe Positioning Practices

8.1 Implement safe positioning practices. *[Recommendation]*

Patients undergoing surgical procedures are at increased risk for injury caused by compression or stretching of tissues during positioning.[2,3,7] The patient who is sedated or has received a regional or general anesthetic may not be able to communicate or sense numbness, tingling, tissue temperature changes, or limitation of mobility; therefore, a proactive approach by the perioperative team is necessary to prevent positioning injury.[41]

8.2 Maintain the patient's head and neck in a neutral position without extreme lateral rotation.[28,118] *[Recommendation]*

Extreme lateral rotation of the patient's head and neck can result in a brachial plexus stretching injury.[5,7,11,41,68,118,143,156-161] Extreme lateral rotation of the neck can also compress and twist muscles and vessels.[160,162] Direct compression on the neck muscles can lead to compartment syndrome.[162] Reperfusion of the muscles after repositioning of the head to its neutral physiologic position can lead to facial and neck swelling, angioedema, upper airway edema, and muscular edema that further increases compartment pressures and worsens muscle ischemia.[162] Extreme neck rotation can also precipitate paraplegia in patients with preexisting spinal cord pathology.[163]

There have been reports of postoperative infection of the salivary glands (ie, sialadenitis), also known as "anesthesia mumps" associated with extreme lateral rotation and extension of the head.[164-168] Compression of the patient's tongue from the airway maintenance device in combination with lateral rotation and flexion of the head can occlude the Stensen duct, which drains the parotid gland, or the Wharton duct, which drains the submandibular gland, leading to salivary stasis and secondary bacterial infection.[164-168] Compression or kinking of the arterial or venous vasculature can obstruct venous return to the head and neck or decrease blood supply to the salivary glands, resulting in an ischemic sialadenitis.[160,165]

In some cases, the degree of lateral neck rotation required for visualization may be reduced by tilting the table away from the surgeon. Morrison et al[169] suggested that tilting the operating bed 15 degrees improved visibility and reduced pain and the risk for brachial plexus injury associated with lateral rotation of the neck for prolonged periods during rhytidectomy procedures.

8.3 | **Reposition the patient's head or take other actions (eg, removing the head strap) to reduce scalp pressure during the procedure, if possible.** [Recommendation]

Alopecia, resulting from ischemic changes in the scalp may occur after exposure to prolonged pressure during surgical procedures.[170,171] Repositioning the patient's head may help prevent pressure alopecia and occipital neuropathy; however, changing the patient's head position during the procedure may be difficult and could potentially dislodge or change the position of the airway maintenance device.

Multiple cases of alopecia have been reported that occurred following surgical procedures lasting longer than 4 hours.[170-177] In all cases, the authors suggested that the alopecia could have been prevented by repositioning of the patient's head during the procedure.

8.3.1 | **The patient's scalp may be massaged during the procedure.** [Conditional Recommendation]

Low-quality evidence suggests that massaging the patient's scalp during the procedure may be an effective method of preventing alopecia that occurs after prolonged surgery.[175-177] There are some benefits associated with massage (eg, encourages hyperemia, increases tissue suppleness, reduces edema); however, massage may also damage underlying tissue.[178] Further research is warranted.

8.4 | **Protect the patient's eyes when the patient is under general anesthesia.** [Recommendation]

Corneal abrasions or other ocular injuries can occur in anesthetized patients as a result of direct trauma to the unprotected eye or a failure of the eye to fully close.[179-181] General anesthesia reduces tear production and can lead to corneal drying.[179-181] Corneal abrasion can result from increased intraocular pressure and edema, as might occur when the patient is in the Trendelenburg position.[179-182]

In a literature review to determine the etiology of perioperative corneal abrasions and compare ocular protection strategies, Grixti et al[181] examined

eight RCTs and one historical controlled study. The authors found that passive closure of the eyelids did not provide sufficient protection of the eyes. They noted that an unprotected, closed eye requires constant vigilance by the anesthesia professional to prevent reopening, thus posing a distraction from other duties. Passive closure may also be impractical during certain types of surgical procedures because of the placement of surgical drapes or the position of the patient.

Moderate-quality evidence shows that none of the available methods of corneal protection for patients undergoing general anesthesia are completely effective, and all may be associated with adverse effects.[181,183] Kocatürk et al[183] assessed the efficacy of hypoallergenic adhesive tape, antibiotic ointment, artificial liquid tear gel, and ocular lubricant for perioperative protection of patients' eyes in 184 patients undergoing spinal surgery in the prone position. The researchers found that all of the methods were suitable for protecting against corneal injuries, but all methods resulted in temporary symptoms during the postoperative period (ie, adhesive lids, foreign body sensation, burning, stinging, photophobia, blurred vision, dryness, conjunctival congestion, chemosis).

8.4.1 | **The patient's eyelids may be taped closed.** [Conditional Recommendation]

Grixti et al[181] found that taping the eyelids with adhesive or cellophane provided ocular protection. They recommended horizontal taping rather than vertical taping because the patient's eyelids may open under vertical taping, whereas horizontal taping achieves complete closure of the eyes by apposition of the upper and lower eyelids. The authors also recommended taping the patient's eyelids immediately after induction (as soon as the eyelid reflex disappears) and before tracheal intubation to reduce the risk for mechanical trauma to the cornea (unless rapid-sequence induction is being performed).

Taping the eyelids provides protection but impedes the anesthesia professional's ability to perform direct observation of the eyes and assess pupillary reactions. There are also potential hazards associated with eyelid taping. If the tape is placed incorrectly, mechanical trauma or exposure keratopathy can occur. Ocular surface contact with the adhesive substance or the edge of the tape can denude the exposed cornea. Periodic monitoring of the tape is necessary to verify that it has not become displaced. Other undesirable reactions to eyelid taping may include allergy to the tape material, breakdown of eyelid skin, or trauma to the eyelashes. The authors suggested that the tape be removed from upper to lower eyelid before the patient's emergence from anesthesia to help prevent corneal abrasion and ocular injury that might occur if the patient opens his or her eyes prematurely under the tape.

8.4.2 **Transparent dressings may be used for eyelid closure.** [*Conditional Recommendation*]

The application of bio-occlusive transparent dressings provides complete and uniform lid closure and reduces tear film evaporation, thus creating a moist environment and preventing corneal desiccation.[181] The conformity of the transparent dressing also allows sealing at the periphery, reducing the risk of displacement.[181]

8.4.3 **The patient's eyes may be lubricated.** [*Conditional Recommendation*]

Ocular lubricants may not be necessary for the majority of patients because the decreased tear production associated with general anesthesia is not detrimental to the ocular surface, provided the eyelids are taped closed.[181] A patient with pre-existing dry eye syndrome or other ocular surface disorders may require ocular lubrication.[181] The use of ocular lubrication may also be necessary for a patient with facial burns or other facial injuries that preclude taping of the eyelids.[181] When deemed necessary, preservative-free, water-based formulations are indicated, as these have a low complication rate.[181] Repeated applications of lubricant at regular intervals during the procedure may compensate for diminished tear production, but may also present an increased risk for corneal abrasion.[181]

8.4.4 **Goggles may be used for ocular protection, except when the patient is in the prone position and a face positioner is used.**[184] [*Conditional Recommendation*]

Goggles provide mechanical protection against ocular surface trauma, but they are ineffective in preventing corneal desiccation.[181] When the patient is in the prone position and goggles are used in combination with a face positioner, the goggles can become displaced and cause pressure on the globe.[181,184]

8.5 **The anesthesia professional should check the patient's airway maintenance device after patient positioning and should implement corrective actions as indicated.** [*Recommendation*] **P**

Changes in patient position during positioning could lead to changes in airway maintenance device position or intracuff pressure. An increase in intra-

cuff pressure may cause damage to the tracheal mucosa.[185] A decrease in intracuff pressure may cause an air leak, resulting in inadequate ventilation and increased risk for aspiration.[185]

In a nonexperimental study to determine whether changes in head and neck position could lead to changes in endotracheal tube intracuff pressure, Olsen et al[185] measured intracuff pressures in 84 patients ages 0.9 years to 17 years undergoing adenotonsillectomy procedures. The researchers found the intracuff pressure increased in 46 patients (54.8%), decreased in 28 patients (33.3%), and remained constant in 10 patients (11.9%). The researchers concluded that regular monitoring of the endotracheal tube intracuff pressure and rechecking of intracuff pressure after positioning activities is indicated.

8.6 **Do not allow the patient's neck to be hyperextended for prolonged periods.** [*Recommendation*]

Hyperextension of the neck can stretch the brachial plexus,[186] lead to cardiovascular complications associated with compression or mechanical manipulation of the carotid sinus,[187] or injure the spinal cord.[188]

8.7 **Verify the patient's body is in physiologic alignment when the patient is positioned.** [*Recommendation*]

Maintaining the patient's physiologic body alignment and supporting extremities and joints reduces the potential for injury.[28,189]

8.8 **Prevent the patient's body from contacting metal portions of the OR bed and other hard surfaces.**[37] [*Recommendation*]

Ulnar or radial nerve injury can occur if the patient's arm is allowed to rest against the metal surface of the OR bed.[41,68,156]

8.9 **Prevent the patient's extremities from unintentionally dropping or hanging below level of the OR bed.** [*Recommendation*]

Allowing the patient's arm to fall or hang off the OR bed can cause radial (if supinated) or median (if pronated) nerve injury.[11,12,143] Allowing the patient's leg to fall or hang off the OR bed can injure the lateral femoral cutaneous nerve.[157]

In a qualitative analysis of 863 perioperative incident reports from six institutions in the Midwest, Chappy[124] identified specific events that affected perioperative patient safety during a 3-year period. Sixteen of the reported incidents involved patient positioning (2%). Three of these incidents (19%) involved patients' legs not being effectively secured to the OR bed and falling off the bed during the procedure. Notably, this was only discovered at the end of the procedure when the surgical drapes were removed.

8.10 **Monitor the location of patient's hands, fingers, feet, toes, and genitals during positioning activities, including changes in the configuration of the OR bed.** *[Recommendation]*

Monitoring the location of the patient's hands, fingers, feet, toes, and genitals ensures they are in a position that is clear of OR bed breaks, sources of compression, or other potential hazards.[36,37]

8.11 **Apply safety restraints and monitoring devices (eg, blood pressure cuffs, pulse oximetry sensors) in a manner that safely secures the patient and allows the accessory device to function effectively without nerve, tissue, or circulatory compression.**[6,58] *[Recommendation]*

Applying safety restraints reduces the patient's risk of falling off the OR bed. Any device, secured too tightly can result in patient injury.[190] Securing restraints or monitoring accessories too tightly or placing them over superficial nerves or bony prominences can occlude blood vessels or cause nerve or pressure injury.[38,41,143,191-195] Blood pressure cuffs applied too tightly can cause ulnar or radial nerve trauma.[28,143,156] The radial nerve is vulnerable to injury when the arms are secured too tightly to the arm boards.[28,156] The skin of older adults is fragile and may be prone to injury from tape, tight restraints, and monitoring accessories.[37]

8.11.1 **Verify placement, tightness, and security of safety restraints after positioning or repositioning activities, including changes in OR bed configuration, and take corrective actions as indicated.** *[Recommendation]*

Verifying placement, tightness, and security of safety restraints reduces the risk for patient injury from restraints that may have come undone or shifted during patient positioning.[196]

8.11.2 **Assess the patient's relevant pulses after securing safety straps, and implement corrective actions as indicated.** *[Recommendation]*

Checking the relevant pulses after securing safety straps verifies adequate perfusion and allows the perioperative RN to assess color, capillary refill time, and pulses and compare them to baseline levels.[191]

8.12 **Position patients with spinal cord lesions in a manner that prevents direct pressure on the lesion.**[197] *[Recommendation]* **P**

Preventing direct pressure on spinal cord lesions prevents injury to neural elements within the lesion and violation of the cerebrospinal fluid space.[197] Drummond et al[197] reported the case of a 32-year-old man with a history of spina bifida who underwent revision of an artificial urinary sphincter. The patient had a meningomyelocele that had been repaired when he was an infant. He had been diagnosed with a pseudomeningocele within the previous 3 years. The patient was positioned in the lithotomy position with additional padding placed under his left hip to minimize pressure on the pseudomeningocele. The procedure lasted 1.25 hours. When he arrived in the post-anesthesia care unit, the patient was confused, and during the next 5 hours he was oriented only to person and spoke in monosyllables.

Magnetic resonance imaging performed 2.5 months after the surgery revealed cerebral atrophy. The patient had persistent cognitive impairment, short-term memory impairment, and word-finding difficulty. The pseudomeningocele was predominantly to the left of the midline; therefore, the lithotomy position and the positioning devices used to reduce pressure on the pseudomeningocele had actually applied rather than relieved pressure. The pressure on the pseudomeningocele resulted in inadequate cerebral perfusion and a permanent injury to the patient. The authors concluded that preventing direct pressure on meningoceles or meningomyeloceles is essential for preventing patient injury.

8.13 **Neurophysiological monitoring may be used intraoperatively to identify potential positioning injuries.** *[Conditional Recommendation]*

Neurophysiological monitoring (eg, somatosensory evoked potential [SSEP], transcranial electrical motor evoked potential [TCeMEP]) is used during surgical procedures to detect changes in the electrophysiological conduction of peripheral nerves and central nervous system pathways that may signal nervous system damage.[77,198-203] The field has evolved from monitoring the function of the spinal cord to monitoring for neural compromise that can occur outside an operative field during a surgical procedure (eg, a positioning injury).[77] Peripheral nerves in the upper extremities or the brachial plexus can become entrapped, compressed, stretched, or ischemic from pressure (eg, arms on arm boards), stretching (eg, taping of shoulders in cervical spine surgeries), dislocation or subluxation of the shoulder, or compression (eg, arm tucking, use of blood pressure cuffs).[200] With the advent of electrophysiology in the OR, neural function can be monitored, and compromise can be detected before a potential injury becomes irreversible.[77,198,200,202,203] Implementing repositioning interventions to reverse neurological conduction changes identified by SSEP monitoring may prevent peripheral nerve injury.[161,198,200-203]

In a prospective cohort observational study to evaluate the use of SSEP monitoring to detect position-related brachial plexus injury during cranial surgery, Jellish et al[204] conducted a focused preoperative and postoperative neurological examination of the brachial plexus on 65 patients undergoing cranial surgery. The patients were positioned in the supine position with the head turned to the contralateral side and secured with a neurosurgical head holder system. The researchers found that six patients (9.2%) developed significantly decreased SSEP amplitude changes after positioning. All of the SSEP changes occurred within the first hour after positioning. The patients' arms were repositioned when the SSEP changes were noted, preventing a positioning injury. The researchers concluded that upper extremity nerve stress can be detected in real time using SSEP monitoring and that neurophysiological monitoring can be an effective method of protecting patients from position-related nerve injury.

In a nonexperimental study of 485 consecutive patients who underwent microvascular decompression surgery, Ying et al[205] evaluated the effectiveness of SSEP monitoring for detecting peripheral nerve and brachial plexus injuries caused by incorrect positioning. The researchers found that 14 patients (2.89%) experienced a significant change of SSEP (n = 6 ulnar nerve, n = 8 median nerve). All of the changes occurred within 10 minutes after positioning. The researchers concluded that continuous intraoperative SSEP monitoring was a useful and valid technique to minimize intraoperative neurological injuries.

Using TCeMEP monitoring in addition to SSEP monitoring may help to validate the SSEP findings and provide additional coverage for emerging motor nerve injury that is not detectable using SSEP monitoring alone.[199,206,207]

Schwartz et al[206] conducted a retrospective review of 3,806 patients who underwent anterior cervical spine surgery with neurophysiological monitoring consisting of SSEP, TCeMEP, and electromyography. The researchers found that 69 patients (1.8%) showed intraoperative evidence of potential neurological injury, prompting repositioning interventions that included releasing shoulder countertraction; repositioning the patient's arms; loosening the sheet used to tuck the patient's arms; reducing shoulder abduction; adding padding to support the shoulders, forearms, or wrists; or flexing the neck. The brachial plexus was the site of potential injury in 45 of these cases (65.2%). The events most often signaling impending neurologic injury were shoulder taping and the application of countertraction (n = 39; 56.5%), hyperextension of the neck (n = 19; 27.5%),

and tucking the patient's arms (n = 11; 15.9%). In all but four cases, there was complete resolution of the monitoring signals within 5 minutes of the intervention. None of the patients sustained any postoperative neurological deficit associated with a positioning injury. The researchers concluded that the results of the study demonstrated the important role of SSEP and TCeMEP monitoring in identifying altered neural function secondary to surgical positioning and allowing for prompt intervention to avoid untoward neurological sequelae.

Eager et al[208] conducted a retrospective review of 2,069 patients who underwent spine surgery with neurophysiological monitoring consisting of SSEP, TCeMEP, and electromyography. The researchers found 32 cases (1.5%) with possible intraoperative neurological events, and in 17 cases (53.1%), intraoperative neurophysiological monitoring changes affected the course of the surgery and potentially prevented postoperative neurological deficits. In four of the 17 cases (23.5%), the potential neurological injury was resolved by a change in patient positioning methods. The researchers noted the importance of multimodality intraoperative neurophysiological monitoring for spinal surgery.

8.14 **Monitor the patient's position after positioning activities and during the procedure, and take corrective actions as indicated.** *[Recommendation]*

Proactively monitoring the patient's position helps identify potential positioning problems and reduces the risk for injury.[191] Monitoring the patient's position after positioning activities verifies physiologic alignment; padding of pressure points; and clearance of fingers, toes, and genitals, and allows for necessary adjustments in the patient's position.[209] Even when correctly positioned, a patient may shift, especially during a prolonged procedure; therefore, regular intraoperative monitoring of the patient's position is necessary to detect or prevent positioning injury.[118,196]

Song et al[196] proposed conducting a second time out 3 to 4 hours after the procedure has started during robotic surgeries with extended operating times. They recommended leaving the robot arms docked and the patient draped, but turning on the room lights and examining the patient under the drapes to verify extremity placement and padding and to examine pressure points and check the tightness of safety restraints. The authors also recommended evaluating the patient's position for slippage, confirming the patient's head position and eye protection, and assessing for any changes in skin color. The authors theorized that conducting a second time out could enhance patient safety and improve the quality of care provided.

8.14.1 After positioning or repositioning the patient, verify there are no areas where devices or equipment are resting against the patient.[63,210] *[Recommendation]*

Changing the patient's position may expose or damage otherwise protected body tissue. The patient may be injured when positioning equipment is added or removed, the OR bed is adjusted, or the patient is moved on the OR bed.[210] Devices or equipment resting against the patient increase the risk for tissue or nerve damage in surgical patients.[62,210-212]

8.14.2 Scrubbed personnel should not lean against the patient.[6] *[Recommendation]*

Scrubbed personnel leaning against the patient increases the risk for tissue or nerve damage in the surgical patient.[62]

8.15 Repositioning interventions may be implemented during the procedure. *[Conditional Recommendation]*

Repositioning involves changing the patient's position for the purpose of redistributing pressure.[19] Repositioning the patient redistributes pressure from pressure points and positioning devices.[15,19,42] Simple position changes (eg, changing the degree of lateral rotation, elevating the head of the bed, moving the limbs) may be sufficient to redistribute pressure and prevent injury.[19,67]

8.15.1 Base repositioning interventions and repositioning intervals on the individual patient and the specific situation.[19] *[Recommendation]*

Repositioning options may be limited or impossible for some perioperative patients.

8.15.2 For patients undergoing robotic procedures, undock the patient from the robotic system before repositioning is initiated. *[Recommendation]*

Adjusting the OR bed or the patient's position is not possible without undocking the robot.[20,179]

9. Supine Position

9.1 Implement safe practices when positioning the patient in the supine or modifications of the supine position. *[Recommendation]*

The supine position is the most frequently used position for surgical procedures because it provides access to a number of body areas.[5,7,28,191] The supine position causes extra pressure on the skin over the occiput, scapulae, olecranon processes, sacrum, coccyx, and calcaneum.[5,36,28]

9.2 Position the patient in the supine position as described in Recommendations 8 and 9. *[Recommendation]*

Guidance for safe positioning practices is provided in Recommendation 8.

Guidance for safe practices in positioning the patient in the supine position is provided in this section (Recommendation 9).

9.3 Position the patient's arms by
- tucking them at the sides with a draw sheet,
- securing them at the sides with arm guards,
- flexing and securing them across the body, or
- extending them on arm boards.[5,143]

[Recommendation]

The position of the arms is determined by the needs of the surgical team and the physical limitations of the patient.

9.3.1 When tucking the patient's arms at the sides and securing them with a draw sheet,
- place the patient's arms in a neutral position[35,38,159] with the palms facing the body and without hyperextension of the elbows[6,36,159];
- protect the patient's elbows and hands with extra padding[36];
- pull the draw sheet up between the patient's body and arm, place it over the patient's arm, and tuck it between the patient and the OR bed mattress[36] (Figure 2);
- tuck the draw sheet snugly enough to secure the patient's arm, but not so tightly as to become a pressure source[74]; and
- extend the draw sheet from the mid-upper arm (ie, above the elbows) to the fingertips.

[Recommendation]

Neutral position is a position during which the body part distal to the joint (eg, hand is distal to wrist, forearm is distal to elbow) is not inverted or everted, adducted or abducted, flexed or extended.[213] Hyperextension of the elbow can stretch the median nerve.[7,35,156]

Padding at the elbow and hand helps redistribute pressure from the ulnar nerve and may decrease the risk for upper extremity neuropathy.[7,35,214]

Using a draw sheet that extends from the mid-upper arm to the fingertips, placing the sheet over the arm, and tucking the draw sheet between the patient's body and the OR bed mattress prevents the patient's arms from falling outside of the mattress and coming to rest on the metal portion of the OR bed.[36]

If the draw sheet is tucked too tightly, it can create a pressure or nerve injury or a compartment syndrome.[7,36,38,74,143,215]

Tucking the patient's arms may interfere with physiological monitoring (eg, blood pressure, arterial catheter) and could result in an unrecognized infiltrated IV in the tucked arm.

9.3.2 **When extending the patient's arms on arm boards,**
- **place the arms in a supinated position (ie, palms facing up),**[7,28,36,118,143]
- **pad the arm boards,**[7,36,118]
- **level the arm boards with the OR bed mattress,**[156]
- **do not abduct the arms more than 90 degrees,**[2,5-7,28,118,143]
- **do not position the arms above the head,**[11,36]
- **maintain the arms and wrists in neutral alignment**[7,36,118,191] **and do not hyperextend,**[6,12,195] **and**
- **secure the arms to the arm boards.**[28,36]

[Recommendation]

Placing the patient's palms up decreases pressure on the ulnar nerve.[35,118] When the patient's arms are pronated (ie, palms down), the ulnar nerve is more vulnerable to compression injury.[214]

The use of padded arm boards may decrease the risk for upper extremity neuropathy.[35,156]

Placement of the patient's abducted arm onto an arm board at a lower level than the OR bed mattress stretches the brachial plexus.[156]

The risk for brachial plexus injury and occlusion of the subclavian or axillary arteries is increased when the patient's arm is abducted more than 90 degrees.[11,12,36,38,68,143,156-158,191,214,216-218] The risk is further increased in patients who are thin and when both arms are extended and abducted.[68] Turning the patient's head to the side while the arms are extended on arm boards also increases stretch on the brachial plexus.[158] When the patient's arms are extended on arm boards and the patient slides caudally, excessive abduction of the arms can occur and cause a brachial neuropathy.[216] Notably, it may be difficult to ascertain the full degree of arm abduction in patients with large arms.[217]

Extreme abduction of the arm so that the hand rests above the head places considerable stretch on the brachial plexus.[11,219]

Maintaining the patient's arms and wrists in neutral alignment reduces the risk for a positioning injury.[36,220] Patients with a large muscle mass or a large amount of adipose tissue in the upper arm may be at increased risk for hyper-

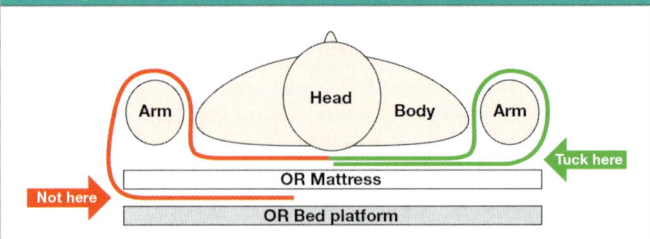

The draw sheet is pulled up between the patient's body and arm, placed over the patient's arm, and tucked between the patient and the OR bed mattress.

Illustration by Kurt Jones.

extension when the arm is extended on an arm board.[195]

In a quasi-experimental study to evaluate the effect of wrist hyperextension (as used for insertion and stabilization of intra-arterial catheters) on median nerve function, Chowet et al[221] analyzed median nerve conduction in 12 volunteer research participants. The participants were placed in the supine position with their right wrists hyperextended to 65 degrees and 85 degrees. The researchers recorded compound action potentials every 10 minutes for 2 hours. Subsequently, they released the participants' hands from hyperextension and recorded the potentials. The participants' left wrists served as the controls. The researchers concluded that wrist hyperextension for arterial line placement and stabilization was likely to result in profound impairment of median nerve function. They recommended that the patient's wrists be returned to the neutral position after arterial line placement.

Securing the arms to the arm boards reduces the risk of the patient's arms falling off the arm board.

9.4 **A pillow or pad may be placed under the patient's lumbosacral area.** *[Conditional Recommendation]*

The effects of general anesthesia may reduce or eliminate paraspinal muscle tone, leading to loss of the patient's normal lordotic curve (ie, inward curvature of the lumbar and cervical regions of the spine).[5,144] Use of a lumbosacral pad may help prevent postoperative back pain by supporting the patient's physiologic lordotic curvature.[7,41]

9.5 **Flex the patient's knees approximately 5 degrees to 10 degrees.**[222] *[Recommendation]*

Positioning the knees in slight flexion prevents popliteal vein compression and reduces the patient's risk for DVT.[19,223] Extending the patient's legs and elevating the heels may increase pressure at the sacrum and allow the knee to hyperextend, compressing the popliteal vein and increasing the risk for DVT.[137,223-226]

Huber and Huber[224] conducted an observational study to determine the incidence of popliteal vein compression in 50 patients undergoing surgery in the supine position. The researchers used duplex ultrasonography to determine the amount of popliteal vein compression when the patient's knees were flexed and extended. The researchers found that of the 90 popliteal veins studied, 39 (43%) were completely occluded and an additional 19 (21%) decreased in diameter when the patient's heels were elevated. The researchers also found that BMI was a significant factor in popliteal vein compression. Patients with a BMI > 25 kg/m² were 1.33 times more likely to have popliteal vein compression than patients with a BMI < 25 kg/m². Patients with a BMI > 30 kg/m² were 1.67 times more likely to have popliteal compression than patients with a BMI < 25 kg/m².

In a subsequent pilot study to clarify the association between popliteal vein compression and DVT, Huber et al[223] scanned the popliteal veins of 54 patients who presented to a vascular laboratory for ultrasonic scanning to determine the presence of a DVT. The researchers found that five of 18 patients with popliteal vein compression had a DVT (27.7%), and five of 36 patients without popliteal vein compression had a DVT (16.7%). This difference was statistically significant. The researchers concluded there was an association between popliteal vein compression and an increased likelihood of developing a DVT. They recommended that patients undergoing surgery in the supine position have their heels elevated and their knees slightly flexed to prevent popliteal vein compression. The researchers emphasized caution when placing anything behind the popliteal fossa, as the weight of the patient's leg could be sufficient to compress the popliteal vein. They recommended using a supportive device that redistributes the weight of the leg over a larger area.

9.5.1   **A soft pillow may be placed under the patient's knees.** *[Conditional Recommendation]*
The effects of general anesthesia relax and lengthen the hamstring, allowing the patient's knees to hyperextend.[5] Placing a pillow under the patient's knees may prevent hyperextension of the knees and help relieve pressure on the patient's lower back.[5,36,191] Using a soft pillow reduces the risk for popliteal compression[222] and provides protection for the common peroneal and tibial nerves[191] but may not be sufficient to prevent popliteal vein compression in some patients.[223]

9.6   **Place the safety strap approximately 2 inches (5 cm) above the patient's knees.**[191] *[Recommendation]*
Placing the safety strap on the patient's upper thighs or below the patient's knees does not effectively restrain the patient's legs to the OR bed. Placing the safety strap directly over the patient's knees increases the risk for nerve injury from compression of the common peroneal nerve against the head of the fibula.[191]

9.7   **Position the patient's legs parallel with the ankles uncrossed.**[2,28] *[Recommendation]*
Keeping the patient's legs parallel with ankles uncrossed reduces pressure to the occiput, scapulae, thoracic vertebrae, olecranon processes, ischial tuberosities, sacrum, coccyx, and calcaneum.[17,105]

9.8   **Elevate the patient's heels off the underlying surface.**[19,105,191] *[Recommendation]*
Offloading the supine patient's heels (ie, suspending the heels above the OR bed surface) increases perfusion and helps prevent pressure injury.[224] In a quasi-experimental study to examine heel skin temperatures in 18 adult patients during the first 3 days after hip surgery, Wong et al[227] placed temperature sensors on the plantar surfaces of each foot, close to the patient's heels. Temperature measurements were taken when the patients' heels were

- suspended above the bed surface for 20 minutes,
- on the bed surface for 15 minutes, and
- suspended again above the bed surface for 15 minutes.

The researchers found there was a trend for heel skin temperature to increase after the patients' heels were placed on the bed surface for 15 minutes, and this increase in temperature continued after the patients' heels were removed from the bed surface. The researchers recommended keeping the patients' heels off the bed surface at all times to prevent heel skin temperature changes, enhance heat dissipation, and prevent deep tissue damage.

King and Bridges[105] conducted a quasi-experimental study to determine the peak skin interface pressures of three support surfaces (ie, an OR bed mattress, a polyurethane convoluted foam overlay on the OR bed mattress, and a viscoelastic dry polymer gel pad overlay on the OR bed mattress) with participants in the supine and lateral positions. The researchers found that heel pressures were increased on all three surfaces, suggesting that elevating the patient's heels off the surface is indicated whenever possible.

In an RCT to determine the effectiveness of offloading the heels in preventing pressure injury, Donnelly et al[228] inspected the heels of 239 older patients with fractured hips each day during their admission period. The patients were randomly allocated to either the control group positioned on pressure-redistributing surfaces (n = 119) or the experimental group positioned on pressure-redistributing surfaces plus heel elevation using a commercially available heel-suspension boot (n = 120). The researchers found that 31 patients (26%) in the control group developed pressure injuries compared with eight patients (7%) in the experimental group. The researchers concluded that offloading the heels reduced the incidence of pressure injuries.

Notably, heel elevation may increase the risk for sacral pressure injury. In a prospective cohort study to identify risk factors associated with pressure injury in patients undergoing surgical procedures lasting longer than 3 hours, Primiano et al[229] collected and analyzed data on 258 patients. The researchers found that 21 patients (8.1%) developed a pressure injury, and five of those patients (23.8%) had their heels elevated during surgery. The findings of the study indicated that although heel elevation may have prevented pressure injury to the patients' heels, it may have contributed to the development of sacral pressure injury. The researchers recommended further research to investigate whether prolonged heel elevation is consistently linked to increased risk for sacral pressure injury.

9.8.1   **Redistribute pressure on the heels by**
- **using a heel-suspension device designed to elevate the heel and distribute the weight of the patient's leg along the calf**[19] **(Figure 3) or**
- **elevating and supporting the patient's calves with a pressure-redistributing surface that is wide enough to accommodate the externally rotated malleolus.**[222]

[Recommendation]

Elevating the heels in a manner that distributes the weight of the patient's leg along the calf without putting pressure on the Achilles tendon and without hyperextending the knee is the most effective way to prevent pressure injuries to the heel and sacrum.[137] Positioning devices used to reduce pressure injury to the heels are designed to work in one of three ways:
- by cradling the heel in a gel or foam surface,
- by offloading the heel by supporting the Achilles tendon, or
- by providing a surface that distributes the weight of the patient's leg along the calf.[137]

Devices designed to offload the heels by cradling the heel in a gel or foam surface or by supporting the Achilles tendon may increase pressure at the sacrum and/or Achilles tendon and allow the knee to hyperextend, compressing the popliteal vein and increasing the risk for DVT.[137,226] Offloading the heels by supporting the Achilles tendon may also increase intracompartmental pressure and lead to a compartment syndrome.[230]

Redistributing the weight of the patient's leg along the calf reduces the risk for pressure injury to the skin over the sacrum and the Achilles tendon.[222] Malkoun et al[137] investigated interface pressures at the calf, heel, Achilles tendon, and lateral malleolus using three commercially available heel positioning devices, a prototype heel-suspension device that provided heel elevation through distribution of the weight along the calf, and a standard OR bed mattress. The researchers found the interface pressures were significantly lower when devices that elevated the heel were used compared with devices designed to redistribute heel pressure. They also found that use of the prototype device resulted in significantly lower interface pressures at the Achilles tendon and the lateral malleolus than the other heel positioning devices.

Using a wide support surface helps prevent localized pressure on the lateral malleolus if the leg rotates externally.[222]

9.9   **Protect the patient's feet from hyperflexion and hyperextension.**[2] *[Recommendation]*

The patient's feet may become hyperflexed or hyperextended from the weight of blankets, drapes, or equipment (eg, the Mayo stand) resting on the patient's foot.

9.10   **When using a hyperlordotic position (ie, supine with arched spine), do not hyperextend the patient beyond a physiologic degree.**[143] *[Recommendation]*

Excessive arching of the lumbar spine (ie, beyond what is characteristic of normal functioning[231]) can stress the joints and ligaments, leading to postoperative back pain and femoral neuropathy.[144,232] Arching the spine lengthens and flattens the major vessels and can impede blood flow, leading to changes in intraspinal perfusion and causing either congestion or ischemia of the spinal canal.[144]

10. Trendelenburg Position

10.1   **Implement safe practices when positioning the patient in the Trendelenburg or modifications of the Trendelenburg position.** *[Recommendation]*

In the Trendelenburg position, the patient's feet are higher than the patient's head by 15 degrees to 30 degrees.[5] This position moves the abdominal viscera cephalad to improve surgical access to the pelvic organs.[5,233] Trendelenburg position causes a redistribution of the blood supply from the lower extremities into the central and pulmonary circulation.[69,179,234] Limb perfusion decreases.[235] Trendelenburg position also decreases venous return from the head, leading to venous pooling and increased intraocular pressure.[69,143,179,180,236-241] Swelling of the eyes, lips, tongue, and larynx can occur as a result of venous stasis.[7,179,182,242,243] Laryngeal swelling can lead to respiratory distress and the need to reintubate or delay extubation.[179,243]

Moderate-quality evidence related to the potential for cerebral desaturation in the Trendelenburg position indicates that the Trendelenburg position does not negatively affect cerebral oxygenation or autoregulation (ie, the mechanisms that maintain blood flow at physiologic levels during changes in blood pressure).[244-248] However, the Trendelenburg position does cause an elevation in cerebral blood volume and cerebrospinal fluid volume that raises intracranial pressure and may cause cerebral edema.[5,7,249] Researchers have also found that the increase in intracranial pressure associated with the Trendelenburg position may be predicted by a corresponding increase in optic nerve sheath diameter, which can be measured noninvasively using ocular sonography, allowing patients to be screened intraoperatively for increasing intracranial pressure.[250-253]

Patients who are positioned in the Trendelenburg position for prolonged periods may be at risk for postoperative vision loss.[254,255] Postoperative vision loss can be caused by an ischemic process that occurs as a result of decreased blood supply from the arteries of the optic nerve or by venous stasis that occurs as a result of decreased venous outflow.[180,242,254] Some researchers have found the increased intraocular pressure associated with the Trendelenburg position poses a risk for postoperative vision loss, particularly in patients with preexisting ocular disease.[238-241,256,257] Grosso et al[255] found that pneumoperitoneum led to mild and reversible intraocular pressure increases; however, pneumoperitoneum in combination with the Trendelenburg position led to a greater increase in intraocular pressure. Older patients who have elevated baseline intraocular pressure are at greater risk for ischemic optic neuropathy, and ophthalmology consultation may be warranted before surgery to reduce the risk for injury in these patients.[179,180,182,238,239,241,255]

The Trendelenburg position causes an increase in lower esophageal sphincter pressure.[258] To ventilate the lungs in this position, the patient's diaphragm pushes against the displaced abdominal contents, which increases the risk for the alveoli to collapse, resulting in atelectasis and hypox-

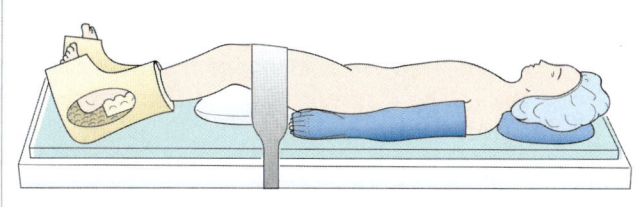

Figure 3. Redistributing Pressure on the Heels

Heel-suspension devices are designed to elevate the heel and distribute the weight of the patient's leg along the calf without placing pressure on the Achilles tendon.

Illustration by Kurt Jones.

emia.[7,69,143,234,258,259] Choi et al[259] found that the Trendelenburg position, in combination with pneumoperitoneum, enhanced atelectasis formation and decreased lung volume and lung compliance, leading to increased end-tidal carbon dioxide ($ETCO_2$) pressures. These pressures were significantly greater in older patients (ie, > 65 years) compared with middle-aged patients (ie, 45 years to 65 years).

Pulmonary functional residual capacity may be additionally impaired during laparoscopic or robotic surgery because of pneumoperitoneum.[58,179] According to Kilic et al,[260] prolonged use (ie, > 2 hours) of the steep (ie, 40-degree to 45-degree) Trendelenburg position can cause upper airway edema and reduced lung compliance. These effects may be more pronounced in patients who are obese.[260] In a retrospective review of 1,032 obese patients who underwent robotic gynecological surgery at two academic institutions, Wysham et al[261] found that only 33 patients (3%) had pulmonary complications. However, the researchers stipulated that older patients may be at increased risk for pulmonary complications when positioned in the Trendelenburg position.[261]

Evidence regarding the hemodynamic effects of the Trendelenburg position is inconclusive. Stretching of the peritoneum, either by pressure from an abdominal mass or pneumoperitoneum in combination with the Trendelenburg position, can cause bradycardia.[262] Some researchers have found that the Trendelenburg position produces negative hemodynamic effects (eg, reduced stroke volume, reduced cardiac output).[263-266] Lowenstein et al[264] suggested that women with cardiovascular disease, particularly those with arrhythmias or peripheral vascular disease, may not tolerate the hemodynamic changes associated with the steep Trendelenburg position. Other researchers have found the Trendelenburg position produces no negative hemodynamic effects[267-269] and may even improve hemodynamic function.[270,271] Further research is warranted to evaluate the hemodynamic effects of the Trendelenburg position.

Wen et al[272] conducted a retrospective review of 175,699 patients who underwent radical prostatectomy procedures during 2008 and 2009 using data extracted from the Nationwide Inpatient Sample database. The researchers found that positioning complications occurred in 0.4% of cases (n = 703). The steep (ie, 25-degree to 45-degree) Trendelenburg position was not associated with positioning complications in this sample.

10.2 | **Position the supine patient in the Trendelenburg position as described in Recommendations 8, 9, and 10.** [Recommendation]

Guidance for safe practices in positioning the supine patient is provided in Recommendations 8 and 9.

Guidance for safe practices in positioning the patient in Trendelenburg position is provided in this section (Recommendation 10).

10.3 | **Position the lithotomy patient in Trendelenburg position as described in Recommendation 8, 9, and 10.** [Recommendation]

Guidance for safe practices in positioning the patient in the lithotomy position is provided in Recommendations 8 and 9.

Guidance for safe practices in positioning the patient in Trendelenburg position is provided in this section (Recommendation 10).

10.4 | **Minimize the degree of Trendelenburg position as much as possible.**[4] [Recommendation]

There is no agreement in the literature as to the degree of Trendelenburg that constitutes "steep" or "maximum"[233,273]; however, a 30-degree to 45-degree OR bed tilt is generally considered a steep angle.[20,179,233,274] Using a more pronounced degree of Trendelenburg position places a greater physiologic strain on the patient's body and increases the potential for complications (eg, intracranial hypertension, respiratory deterioration).[233,273] The combination of pneumoperitoneum and steep degrees of Trendelenburg can lead to moderate to severe adverse hemodynamic changes (eg, reduced stroke volume, cardiac output, left ventricular end-diastolic volume[266]) and facial, ocular, and upper airway edema.[233,273,275] Retinal detachment and blindness may also result from prolonged use of the steep Trendelenburg position.[233,273]

In a study to investigate the influence of the angle of Trendelenburg position on cardiovascular and respiratory homeostasis, Kadono et al[275] found that cardiovascular and respiratory parameters were negatively affected and tended to worsen with steeper Trendelenburg. The researchers recommended completing the procedure efficiently and using the smallest degree of Trendelenburg possible.

Ghomi et al[233] conducted a descriptive study to explore the necessity of using steep (ie, 30-degree to 40-degree) Trendelenburg position in robotic gynecological surgery and to evaluate whether a lesser degree of Trendelenburg position could be used effectively. When adequate pneumoperitoneum had been achieved, the patients were placed in the degree of Trendelenburg that obtained sufficient exposure of the surgical field as determined by the primary surgeon. When the robotic portion of the procedure was completed, the degree of Trendelenburg position was measured. The surgeon and surgical team were blinded to the recorded degree of Trendelenburg. The researchers found that the median degree of Trendelenburg used was 16.4 degrees. The researchers concluded that robotic-assisted gynecological surgery could be performed using a modest degree of Trendelenburg without increasing complications or operating time.

In a quasi-experimental study to estimate the Trendelenburg angle required to perform robotic gynecological surgical procedures, Gould et al[273] measured the angle of Trendelenburg determined by the surgeons to be sufficient to perform the procedure (ie, the small bowel and sigmoid colon were displaced out of the surgical field). The researchers found the mean angle most commonly selected by the surgeons was 28.1 degrees. This difference was statistically significant when compared with the 40-degree angle the surgeons commonly used at the researchers' facility.

Raz et al[276] conducted an RCT to evaluate whether modifying the Trendelenburg position so that the patient's head and shoulders remained in a horizontal position would reduce the increase in intraocular pressure associated with the Trendelenburg position. The researchers compared intraocular pressures in 50 patients undergoing robotic-assisted laparoscopic radical prostatectomy. They found that modifying the Trendelenburg position had a significantly positive effect on patient safety by lowering intraocular pressure and accelerating its recovery to the normal range without affecting the surgery.

10.5 | **Place the patient in the Trendelenburg position for the shortest time possible.**[4,9,274,277-279] [Recommendation]

Reducing the length of time the patient is placed in Trendelenburg position decreases the potential for complications or patient injury.

The Trendelenburg position increases cephalic and intracranial pressures and can lead to otological complications,[278] cerebral edema,[249] and neurological complications (eg, stupor).[279] In a prospective cohort study, Schramm et al[274] found that steep (ie, 40-degree to 45-degree) Trendelenburg position in combination with pneumoperitoneum slowly impaired cerebrovascular autoregulation during the course of robotic-assisted prostate surgeries. The researchers recommended minimizing the length of time the patient is in the Trendelenburg position.

Patients who are positioned in the Trendelenburg position for long periods are at risk for postoperative vision loss associated with increased intraocular pressure.[180,237,242,280-282] The increase in intraocular pressure is directly correlated with the amount of time in Trendelenburg position.[242,283]

In a systematic review of the literature to identify the number and type of peripheral nerve injuries associated with laparoscopic colorectal surgery involving the Trendelenburg position, Codd et al[284] suggested that reducing procedural times or returning the OR bed to a horizontal position at specified times during the procedure could help to reduce pressure on the brachial plexus and reduce the patient's risk for nerve injury associated with the Trendelenburg position.

Patients positioned in Trendelenburg position during prolonged procedures are also at risk for developing rhabdomyolysis.[285] Mattei et al[285] conducted a prospective study of 60 consecutive patients undergoing robotic-assisted radical prostatectomy with extended pelvic lymph node dissection and found that prolonged periods (ie, 2.8 hours to 7.8 hours) in steep (ie, 30-degree) Trendelenburg position increased the patient's risk for developing rhabdomyolysis. The researchers recommended reducing the time the patient is in the Trendelenburg position.

10.6 **Reposition patients in the Trendelenburg position into the supine or reverse Trendelenburg position at established intervals during the procedure, if possible.** *[Recommendation]*

Returning the patient to the supine position, or a position in which the ocular level is above the heart, will help to reduce intraocular pressure and facilitate return to baseline levels.[182,238] Reducing intraocular pressure may reduce the risk for postoperative vision loss.[182]

In a systematic review of eight papers reporting data on ocular complications in robotic surgery on 142 patients, Gkegkes et al[254] found that the most frequent complication was increased intraocular pressure. The researchers also found that elevated intraocular pressure and ischemic damage to the optic nerve could possibly be prevented by the introduction of intervals of reverse Trendelenburg positioning.

10.6.1 **Implement repositioning interventions and repositioning intervals that are**
- **based on the individual patient and the specific situation[19] and**

- **established by the perioperative team before the beginning of the procedure, if possible.**[182]
[Recommendation]

The low-quality evidence available does not determine a time limit for the use of the Trendelenburg position or for repositioning intervals. Barr et al[249] suggested repositioning every 3 hours. Freshcoln and Diehl[182] suggested attempting a supine intervention for 5 minutes after 4 hours of steep Trendelenburg. There are numerous physiologic patient variables (eg, age, comorbidities, medications) that can affect the length of time a patient can tolerate the Trendelenburg position without injury.[255]

Current evidence also does not identify how long the patient needs to be supine or in the reverse Trendelenburg position before being repositioned back into Trendelenburg position.

10.7 **Implement measures to prevent the patient from sliding on the OR bed.**[4,20,58] *[Recommendation]*

The Trendelenburg position places the patient at risk for sliding cephalad.[9,286] Patient sliding increases the risk for skin breakdown as a result of friction and gravitational forces that pull the patient toward the head of the bed.[9,139,179] Preventing the patient from sliding on the OR bed decreases shear and reduces the potential for pressure on the brachial plexus.[4,20,179] A shift in the patient's position could place undue strain on the abdominal wall and also increase the risk for trauma to intra-abdominal structures.[179,286]

Shifting of the patient's trunk may also lead to suboptimal positioning of the extremities, increasing the risk for nerve injury from stretching or compression.[9,179,286] Preventing the patient from sliding on the OR bed is important for preventing patient injury that may occur in robotic-assisted procedures if the patient's position shifts after the device is docked.[9,32,139] If the patient slips while the robotic system is engaged, incisional tears could occur at the port sites that could cause hernias.[20] These effects may be increased in patients who are obese because they are more susceptible to downward shifting.[179]

10.7.1 **Measures to prevent patients from sliding may include using**
- **convoluted foam or viscoelastic gel overlays,**[139,179,286,287]
- **vacuum-packed positioning devices,**[139,288] **or**
- **other positioning devices designed for this purpose.**[289,290]
[Conditional Recommendation]

Evidence regarding the most effective methods and surfaces to prevent patients from sliding on the OR bed is of low quality and is inconclusive. Further research is warranted.

10.8 **After positioning in the Trendelenburg position, the anesthesia professional should check the patient's airway maintenance device and take corrective actions as indicated.**[5,144] *[Recommendation]*

When the patient is placed into the Trendelenburg position, cephalad migration of the carina causes a shortening of the trachea, allowing the airway maintenance device to migrate distally, toward the right main bronchus.[69,144,291]

An increase in airway maintenance device cuff pressure may also occur during surgery in the Trendelenburg position.[292] Wu et al[292] evaluated endotracheal cuff pressure changes before and after supine and Trendelenburg position in 70 patients undergoing laparoscopic surgery. The researchers found there was a significant increase in endotracheal tube cuff pressure after insufflation and after position changes, especially when patients were in the Trendelenburg position.

10.9 **Secure the patient's arms by**
- **tucking them at the sides with a draw sheet** (See Recommendation 9.3.1) **or**
- **securing them at the sides with arm guards.**
[Recommendation]

Tucking or securing the patient's arms at the sides reduces the potential for patient injury. Extending the patient's arms on arm boards can lead to excessive abduction of the arms and cause a brachial neuropathy when the patient slides caudally.[216]

10.10 **Do not use shoulder braces.**[9,159,277,293] *[Recommendation]*

Compression over the acromion by shoulder braces can injure the brachial plexus.[4,12,32,69,159,293] This injury is exacerbated by the muscle-relaxing, joint-mobilizing effects of general anesthesia.[4,214,293]

In a quasi-experimental study to investigate surgical positions that place the patient at risk for stretch-induced neuropathies, Coppieters et al[293] analyzed the effect of arm and neck positions in three different shoulder positions in 25 male volunteers. The tests were performed with and without fixation of the shoulder girdle to simulate the presence and absence of a shoulder brace. The researchers found that shoulder fixation resulted in a significantly reduced range of motion, even when the fixation was applied over the acromioclavicular joint. The researchers discouraged the use of shoulder braces and suggested that if they were used, it would be important to position the patient on a nonsliding surface, to monitor the pressure of the

shoulder braces regularly during the procedure, and to consider the effect of the absence of protective reflexes in an anesthetized patient.

The pressure exerted on the brachial plexus by the shoulder braces increases as the angle of Trendelenburg increases.[4,294] In a prospective descriptive study to measure the pressure placed on the shoulders and to compare the pressures during varying degrees of Trendelenburg position, Suozzi et al[294] studied three different patient positioning systems (ie, two shoulder support systems and a vacuum-packed positioning device with shoulder supports). A total of 23 volunteer participants were placed in the lithotomy position with arms tucked and tilted to 5-degree, 10-degree, 15-degree, 20-degree, 25-degree, and 30-degree Trendelenburg position. The researchers measured the pressure on the shoulders at each angle of Trendelenburg for each device.

The researchers found that as the degree of Trendelenburg increased, the shoulder pressure increased for all of the positioning systems tested. The results showed that in the 30-degree Trendelenburg position, the vacuum-packed positioning device transmitted the least amount of pressure to the shoulders and the shoulder support systems transmitted the most pressure to the shoulders. The researchers theorized this may have been caused by the larger surface area of the vacuum-packed positioning device compared with the other positioning systems. When questioned as to which positioning system was the most comfortable, 74% (n = 17) of the participants stated that they preferred the vacuum-packed positioning device.[294]

A shoulder brace that is placed proximal to the neck puts excessive pressure on the clavicle and can compress the brachial plexus as it exits the thorax between the clavicle and the first rib.[35,68,143,156,214] A shoulder brace that is placed lateral to the neck can place an upward force on the shoulder while the patient's head and neck are experiencing downward gravitational forces.[12,67,214] The opposing upward and downward forces can result in a stretching and compression injury to the brachial plexus.[12,67,156,214,293] The combination of arm abduction and shoulder braces may increase the risk for brachial plexus injury.[4,295,296]

10.11 **Do not use circumferential wrist restraints.**[277] *[Recommendation]*

Using circumferential wrist restraints to prevent patient sliding can pull the humeral head downward and cause a brachial plexus injury.[277] Shveiky et al[277] conducted a literature review to explore the anatomy, pathophysiology, diagnosis, and treatment of position-related brachial plexus injuries associated with laparoscopic- and robotic-assisted surgery. The authors reviewed 24 reported cases of brachial plexus injury and found the Trendelenburg position was used in all 24 cases, with shoulder braces used in nine cases (37.5%). Most patients recovered during the course of 1 week to 9 months; however, in one case, there was a permanent disability.

The authors found that in the Trendelenburg position, whether the patient's arms were tucked at the sides or extended on arm boards, the patient was more likely to slide down the OR bed toward the head. Circumferential wrist restraints pulled the humeral head and shoulder girdle downward, increasing the risk for brachial plexus injury. The authors recommended using the smallest degree of Trendelenburg position necessary; reducing operative times to the extent possible; avoiding lateral rotation of the patient's neck; avoiding abduction, external rotation, and extension of the upper extremities; not using shoulder braces or circumferential wrist restraints; and regularly assessing the patient's position during surgery.

10.12 **Do not use Trendelenburg position for patients who are extremely obese (ie, BMI > 40 kg/m²), if possible.**[234] *[Recommendation]*

Vaughan and Wise[297] enrolled 64 extremely obese patients (ie, 313.0 lb ± 69.2 lb [142.0 kg ± 31.4 kg]) undergoing jejunoileal bypass procedures in a quasi-experimental study to investigate the intraoperative arterial oxygenation pattern in obese patients undergoing abdominal surgeries in the Trendelenburg position. The patients were divided into two groups. Group 1 patients (n = 25) were maintained in the supine position. Group 2 patients (n = 39) were maintained in a 15-degree Trendelenburg position. The researchers found that a change from supine to 15-degree Trendelenburg position resulted in a significant reduction in mean partial pressure of oxygen in arterial blood (PaO_2).

The researchers suggested not using the Trendelenburg position for patients who are extremely obese; however, if using this position is absolutely necessary, they recommended careful monitoring of the patient's arterial blood gases. The researchers also noted that although obese, the study participants were otherwise healthy, young individuals (ie, 22.9 years to 43.7 years). Obese individuals with heart, lung, liver, or kidney disease are at increased risk for ineffective oxygenation when positioned in the Trendelenburg position.[297]

Notably, in some cases the benefits of using minimally invasive surgical approaches may exceed the potential harms of using the Trendelenburg position in patients who are extremely obese.

11. Reverse Trendelenburg Position

11.1 **Implement safe practices when positioning the patient in the reverse Trendelenburg or modifications of the reverse Trendelenburg position.** *[Recommendation]*

In the reverse Trendelenburg position, the patient's head is positioned 15 degrees to 30 degrees higher than the feet. The surgical site is elevated above the level of the heart to improve drainage of body fluids away from the surgical site, reducing intracranial pressure and decreasing bleeding in the surgical field.[7,144] Pulmonary function and hemoglobin saturation are improved.[6] Venous pooling in the lower body can result in hypotension. Venous air embolism (VAE) is a potentially lethal complication of this position.[7]

11.2 **Position the supine patient in reverse Trendelenburg position as described in Recommendations 8, 9, and 11.** *[Recommendation]*

Guidance for safe practices in positioning the supine patient is provided in **Recommendations 8 and 9**.

Guidance for safe practices in positioning the patient in the reverse Trendelenburg position is provided in this section (**Recommendation 11**).

11.3 **Use a padded foot board.**[21] *[Recommendation]*

Using a padded foot board helps prevent the patient from sliding downward on the OR bed and reduces the potential for injury to the peroneal and tibial nerves from foot and ankle flexion.[6,21]

11.3.1 **Assess and monitor the patient's feet during the procedure and implement corrective actions as indicated.** *[Recommendation]*

Assessing and monitoring the patient's feet during the procedure confirms physiologic alignment and placement against the foot board, prevents rotation and increased pressure on the ankle, and may help to prevent circulatory or nerve damage.[6]

11.4 **Patients undergoing abdominal myomectomy procedures may be positioned in the 10-degree reverse Trendelenburg position.** *[Conditional Recommendation]*

Positioning patients undergoing myomectomy procedures in the reverse Trendelenburg position may reduce the risk for VAE. An et al[298] conducted an RCT to determine the incidence and grade of VAE during abdominal myomectomy in the supine position compared with the reverse Trendelenburg position. The researchers enrolled 84 women, ASA classification I or II, who were scheduled for myomectomy under general anesthesia into the study and randomly allocated them into the supine group (n = 40) or the 10-degree Trendelenburg group (n = 44). The incidence and grade of VAE was significantly lower in the reverse Trendelenburg group than in the supine group, and the researchers recommended using the 10-degree reverse Trendelenburg position for abdominal myomectomy procedures.

12. Lithotomy Position

12.1 **Implement safe practices when positioning the patient in the lithotomy or modifications of the lithotomy position.** *[Recommendation]*

The lithotomy position provides surgical exposure for vaginal, rectal, and urological procedures.[209] Modifications of the lithotomy position include low, standard, high, hemi, and exaggerated, depending on how high the legs and pelvis are elevated for the procedure.[36,144]

- Low: The patient's hips are flexed until the angle between the posterior surface of the patient's thighs and the OR bed surface is 40 degrees to 60 degrees. The patient's lower legs are parallel with the OR bed.[144]
- Standard: The patient's hips are flexed until the angle between the posterior surface of the patient's thighs and the OR bed surface is 80 degrees to 100 degrees. The patient's lower legs are parallel with the OR bed.[144]
- Hemi: The patient's nonoperative leg is positioned in standard lithotomy. The patient's operative leg may be placed in traction.[144]
- High: The patient's hips are flexed until the angle between the posterior surface of the patient's thighs and the OR bed surface is 110 degrees to 120 degrees. The patient's lower legs are flexed.[144]
- Exaggerated: The patient's hips are flexed until the angle between the posterior surface of the patient's thighs and the OR bed surface is 130 degrees to 150 degrees. The patient's lower legs are almost vertical.[144]

Raising the patient's legs shifts the blood from the legs into the central circulation and decreases perfusion of the legs.[36,299] This results in an increase in cardiac output and venous return.[36,299] Respiratory complications can occur in the lithotomy position because the patient's abdominal organs shift when the legs are placed in leg holders.[36,209] This increases pressure on the diaphragm and can cause respiratory compromise.[7,36,69,209] In patients who are obese, there is additional chest weight and abdominal pressure, leading to an increased respiratory workload and an increased risk for aspiration.[69,209,234]

12.2 **Position the patient in lithotomy position as described in Recommendations 8, 9.3, and 12.** *[Recommendation]*

Guidance for safe practices in positioning the patient is provided in Recommendations 8 and 9.3.

Guidance for safe practices in positioning the patient in the lithotomy position is provided in this section (Recommendation 12).

12.2.1 **Protect the patient's hands and fingers from injury when the foot of the OR bed is raised, lowered, or reattached.**[5,21,36,37,143] *[Recommendation]*

If tucked at his or her sides, the patient's hands and fingers are in danger of injury when the bottom of the OR bed is raised, lowered, or reattached.[5,209]

12.3 **Place the patient in the lithotomy position for the shortest time possible.**[12,21,68,209,300-315] *[Recommendation]*

The length of time a patient may remain in the lithotomy position without risk for injury is unknown.[73,300,316] Case reports in the literature describe complications associated with prolonged time in the lithotomy position, including

- unilateral lower-leg muscle contusion after 6 hours[317];
- unilateral lower-leg compartment syndrome after 4.5 hours,[318] 5 hours,[319] 6 hours,[314,320] 10 hours,[310] and 12 hours[310];
- unilateral lower-leg compartment syndrome and thrombosis of the common iliac artery after 6 hours[321];
- bilateral lower-leg compartment syndrome after 90 minutes,[315] 4.25 hours,[313] 5 hours,[319] and 7 hours[308];
- bilateral lower-leg and left forearm compartment syndrome after 11 hours[309];
- bilateral thigh compartment syndrome, rhabdomyolysis, and acute renal failure after 6 hours[322];
- bilateral gluteal compartment syndrome after 6 hours[311]; and
- rhabdomyolysis and acute renal failure after 5.5 hours.[323]

Notably, Sadeghian et al[324] reported a bilateral femoral neuropathy in a 20-year-old man after only 30 minutes in the lithotomy position. The risk for injury is multifactorial and may be related to the patient's condition as well as the position.[73,300,302,306-308,320,323,325] The reason some patients develop an injury and others do not remains unknown.[302] The longer the patient's legs are maintained in the lithotomy position, the greater the potential for developing a neuropathy, neurovascular complication, or compartment syndrome.[32,68,73,313,320-323] The addition of Trendelenburg position to the lithotomy position increases the potential for injury because the vertical distance between the heart and the lower limbs is increased.[301,302,305,307,308,313,314]

In a review of the literature on compartment syndrome, Bauer et al[302] found that 70.6% of compartment syndrome cases (n = 10) were identified after surgery lasting longer than 5 hours. The authors concluded that time spent in the lithotomy position was the most important and potentially avoidable risk factor for development of compartment syndrome.

In a retrospective observational study to investigate the incidence and circumstances of lower extremity compartment syndrome occurring after gynecological surgery, Bauer et al[307] found that reported cases of postoperative compartment syndrome occurred after surgeries longer than 2 hours in all cases and longer than 4 hours in 76.2% of cases (n = 16).

12.3.1 **Reposition patients in the lithotomy position at established intervals during the procedure, if possible.** [Recommendation]

Low-quality evidence indicates that repositioning the patient at established intervals during the procedure may reduce the risk for compartment syndrome or other injuries associated with prolonged lithotomy position.[302,303,310,311,314,318,326]

12.3.2 **Implement repositioning interventions and repositioning intervals that are**
- **based on the individual patient and the specific situation**[19] **and**
- **established by the perioperative team before the beginning of the procedure, if possible.**[182]

[Recommendation]

The evidence regarding the most effective repositioning strategies (ie, whether it is sufficient to lower the patient's legs or whether the legs need to be completely removed from the leg holders) or repositioning intervals for the lithotomy position is of low quality and is inconclusive. Taking the patient's limbs out of lithotomy position at predetermined intervals may help to prevent position-related patient injury[73,300]; however, lowering the patient's legs while in the leg holders may be sufficient to prevent injury.

The length of time after which the patient's legs need to be repositioned is unknown and may be affected by physiologic patient variables (eg, age, comorbidities, medications).[255] The literature suggests implementing repositioning interventions at intervals ranging from 2 to 4 hours.[249,302,303,305,306,315,327-329]

Sharma and Doble[330] suggested having perioperative team members provide regular updates (ie, hourly) of the time the patient's legs have been elevated in the lithotomy position.

Current evidence does not identify how long the patient needs to be repositioned before being returned to the lithotomy position.

12.4 **Do not place the safety restraint over the patient's chest or abdomen.** [Recommendation] **P**

Correct placement of the safety restraint is difficult in the lithotomy position. The literature does not discuss best practices for placement of the safety restraint when the patient is in the lithotomy position. The perioperative RN may not be able to place the restraint low across the patient's pelvis without restricting access to the surgical site. Use of a safety restraint that is placed high or too tight across the abdomen increases the risk for pressure injury or restricting respiration. The patient's legs may seem to be secure in the leg holders with his or her arms tucked at the sides; however, there is still a risk that the patient will shift on the procedure bed, especially when being moved in and out of Trendelenburg position, which is often used in conjunction with the lithotomy position. Safe positioning practices require the patient be attended at all times by at least one surgical team member when on the OR bed[28] (See Recommendation 6.3.).

12.5 **Position the patient's buttocks even with the lower break of the procedure bed and in a manner that securely supports the sacrum on the bed surface.**[143] [Recommendation]

Supporting the patient's sacrum reduces the potential for injury.[143]

12.5.1 **When the patient is in the exaggerated lithotomy position, support the patient's sacrum.**[144] [Recommendation]

Placing a positioning support beneath the sacrum when the patient is in the exaggerated lithotomy position helps to support the patient's hips.

12.6 **Position the patient's hips in a manner that prevents excessive flexion, rotation, or abduction.**[209,304,310,331] [Recommendation]

Excessive flexion (ie, more than 80 degrees to 90 degrees) or abduction (ie, more than 30 degrees to 45 degrees) puts stress on the patient's hip joints and can cause a femoral, sciatic, obturator, or common peroneal neuropathy.[5,11,12,68,209,214,331-333] The longer the patient is in an extreme lithotomy position, the more likely an injury is to occur.[331]

When candy cane–shaped leg holders are used, the patient's hips are particularly vulnerable to excessive rotation and hyperabduction.[209,334]

Patients who are obese are at increased risk for injury to joints, muscles, nerves, and soft tissue because the difficulty in identifying anatomic landmarks can make safe levels of knee and hip flexion hard to determine.[209] Overabduction can occur because of the size and weight of the patient's thighs and the need to create sufficient space for the surgical team.[209]

Notably, in a nonexperimental study, Pannucci et al[335] found that intraoperative positioning of the lower extremities represented a modifiable risk factor for prevention of DVT. The researchers used duplex ultrasound to measure common and proximal femoral vein diameter, peak systolic velocity, and volume flow in 12 healthy patients positioned supine with knee flexion at zero degrees, 30 degrees, 60 degrees, and 90 degrees. They found that in the common femoral vein, hip flexion at 90 degrees was associated with a significant increase in mean volume flow compared with hip flexion at zero degrees. The researchers concluded that when leg holders were used, hip flexion of 90 degrees maximized venous drainage from the legs.

12.7 **Place leg holders at an even height.**[12] *[Recommendation]*

Placing the leg holders at an even height reduces the potential for injury that might occur if one leg is positioned higher than the other.[12]

12.8 **Support the patient's legs over the largest surface area of the leg possible.**[36,159,300] *[Recommendation]*

Supporting the leg over the largest surface area possible redistributes pressure and helps to prevent pressure injury.[159,300]

Boot-type leg holders support the entire leg, reducing the potential for nerve and pressure injury because pressure is evenly distributed over the leg and the foot.[159,209] Navarro-Vicente et al[336] conducted a prospective analysis of patients who underwent major colorectal abdominal surgery in a university hospital in Spain. The researchers found that eight (0.3%) of 2,304 patients developed a peripheral nerve injury. There was no association between nerve injury and patient age, sex, BMI, ASA classification, or urgent surgery; however, the use of a vacuum-packed positioning device and boot-type leg holders seemed to be protective for nerve injury in both the upper and lower limbs.

Knee-crutch leg holders support the weight of the patient's leg at the knee and may not redistribute pressure, increasing pressure on the popliteal space, which can injure the posterior and common peroneal nerves and the popliteal artery.[209,332]

Increased pressure associated with knee-crutch leg holders can obstruct or slow venous and lymphatic return, increase the risk for hypoperfusion to the lower extremities, and increase intracompartmental pressures.[325] Mizuno and Takahashi[325] investigated external pressure applied to the calf region when using knee-crutch leg holders and found that external pressure measurements were higher in men than in women, and pressure levels significantly increased with increases in height, weight, and BMI for all participants.

Patients who are placed in lithotomy with Trendelenburg position and patients with a high BMI may be at increased risk for pressure injury even when boot-type leg holders are used. Yamada et al[337] measured contact pressures of the lower extremities in 138 patients undergoing robotic-assisted radical prostatectomy procedures in the lithotomy position with 25-degree Trendelenburg. The researchers found that 33 patients (23.9%) required adjustments in leg position because of high contact pressures (ie, > 32 mmHg). Contact pressures were significantly higher when the lithotomy with 25-degree Trendelenburg position was used than when a horizontal lithotomy position was used. The researchers also found a significant correlation between increased contact pressures and higher BMI levels.

12.8.1 **When using candy cane–shaped leg holders, place additional padding around the patient's foot and ankle.**[209] *[Recommendation]* **P**

When candy cane–shaped leg holders are used, the weight of the patient's leg is supported by the foot straps.[209] Placing additional padding around the foot and ankle may help to redistribute pressure over a larger area and decrease the potential for injury to the distal sural and plantar nerves.[209]

12.9 **Place the patient's heels in the lowest position possible.**[300,306] *[Recommendation]*

Moderate-quality evidence supports using the lowest possible lithotomy position and when possible, positioning the legs at or below the level of the heart.[301,302,304,306,307,312,318,329,338] In the high and exaggerated lithotomy positions, the calf is in a more vertical position and the legs are supported at the heel, placing the heel at risk for pressure injury.[300] The risk for compartment syndrome, rhabdomyolysis, and acute renal failure may also increase as the legs are elevated.[329,338] There is a reduction in lower limb arterial pressure and an increase in venous pressure in the high and exaggerated lithotomy positions that results in an increase in compartmental pressure, reducing blood flow and leading to local ischemia.[329,338]

In a prospective study, Liu et al[339] assigned 99 patients undergoing hysterectomy procedures into three groups. Group 1 patients underwent laparoscopic-assisted hysterectomy in the low lithotomy position (n = 36), Group 2 patients underwent vaginal hysterectomy in the standard lithotomy position (n = 32), and Group 3 patients underwent abdominal hysterectomy in the supine position (n = 31). The researchers measured lower extremity venous pressures at the start of the surgery and at 5, 10, and 45 minutes. The researchers found that Group 1 patients had the highest venous pressures and Group 3 patients had the lowest. The researchers concluded that both low lithotomy position with pneumoperitoneum and standard lithotomy position without pneumoperitoneum increased lower extremity venous pressures; therefore, placing the patient's heels in a lower position represented a modifiable risk factor for prevention of DVT.

12.10 **Do not allow the patient's legs to rest against the leg holder posts.**[209,331] *[Recommendation]*

The common peroneal nerve is vulnerable to injury from the fibular neck resting against the vertical post of the leg holder when the patient is in the lithotomy position.[11,12,214,331] An injury to the common peroneal nerve can cause a paresthesia of the lateral lower leg and dorsum of the foot and result in foot drop.[209,214,331] Pressure from the lower extremities resting against leg holder posts raises compartment pressures and also increases the risk for inadequate lower-extremity perfusion.[314]

12.10.1 **Scrubbed personnel should not lean against the patient's thighs.**[214,301,331,334] *[Recommendation]*

Leaning against the patient's inner thigh increases abduction and external rotation of the thighs and can cause a femoral neuropathy.[214,331,334]

12.11 **Place the patient's legs into the leg holders slowly and simultaneously, with at least one person positioning each leg (ie, a minimum of two people).**[21,36,41] *[Recommendation]*

Slowly and simultaneously raising and lowering the patient's legs allows the patient to adjust to the sudden shift in circulatory volume.[36,209,299] Patients with pre-existing depressed cardiac function may not tolerate sudden hemodynamic changes.[299] Having a minimum of two people move the patient's legs simultaneously into the leg holders helps avoid torsional stresses at the hip joint and pelvis and prevent injury to patients and personnel.[21,41,340] In some cases, additional personnel (eg, two people per leg) may be needed to safely place the patient's legs into the leg holders.[340]

12.12 **Remove the patient's legs from the leg holders in a two-step process:**

1. **Remove the legs slowly and simultaneously from the leg holders and bring them together before the legs are lowered to the OR bed (ie, at least one person per leg for a minimum of two people).**[209]
2. **Simultaneously lower the patient's legs to the OR bed.**

[Recommendation]

Raising or lowering the patient's legs too rapidly can result in fluid volume shifts that affect blood pressure.[209] Having a minimum of two people move the patient's legs simultaneously out of the leg holders helps avoid torsional stresses at the hip joint and pelvis and prevent patient and personnel injury.[41] In some cases, additional personnel (eg, two people per leg) may be needed to safely remove the patient's legs from the leg holders.[340]

At the end of the procedure, the patient's overall circulating blood volume may be depleted when the patient's legs are lowered to the OR bed because of the blood returning quickly into the patient's peripheral circulation.[36] Simultaneously lowering the patient's legs to the OR bed may help to prevent rapid or unexpected circulatory changes.

Notably, the practice of slowly and simultaneously removing the legs from the leg holders, bringing the legs together before the legs are lowered to the OR bed, and then lowering one leg at a time to the OR bed is not incorrect and may further help to prevent rapid circulatory changes; however, there is no evidence to show this is necessary.

12.13 **Graduated compression stockings and/or intermittent pneumatic compression devices may be used on patients in the lithotomy position.** *[Conditional Recommendation]*

Evidence related to best practices for use of graduated compression stockings and intermittent pneumatic compression devices on patients in the lithotomy position is of low quality and is inconclusive. Extrinsic compression applied to the legs by graduated compression stockings or intermittent pneumatic compression devices may increase intracompartmental pressures, and this may be compounded by a prolonged lithotomy position.[309,312,314,315] It has been suggested that the combination of the lithotomy position and intermittent pneumatic compression devices impairs perfusion to muscles, which, because of the elevation of the legs in lithotomy position, are already subject to reduced perfusion.[314,341] The reperfusion of muscles caused by the cycling of the compression devices may exacerbate the potential for compartment syndrome by increasing compartmental pressures and extravasation through damaged endothelium.[315,341] For this reason it may be preferable to use other methods of venous thromboembolic prophylaxis.[312]

Rao and Jayne[304] recommended avoiding the combined use of graduated compression stockings and intermittent pneumatic compression devices, but also advised exercising the utmost of caution before omitting their combined use because the risk for DVT and pulmonary embolism is much greater than the risk for compartment syndrome. Raza et al[306] suggested that if both graduated compression stockings and pneumatic intermittent compression devices were used, it would be important to monitor the patient for potential signs of compartment syndrome, especially after a prolonged procedure.

Pfeffer et al[342] conducted a nonexperimental study to assess the effects of a pneumatic compression device on compartmental pressures in the lower leg with the leg positioned in lithotomy position. The researchers measured pressures in the tibialis anterior muscle compartment of 25 healthy volunteers with the leg supine and in the lithotomy position with and without intermittent compression. Three different leg holders were used for the lithotomy position that provided support behind the knee (knee-crutch), under the calf (boot-type), and at the ankle (candy cane–shaped).

The lithotomy position with support behind the knee or calf increased intracompartmental pressure. The addition of intermittent compression significantly decreased pressure during lithotomy and in the supine position. The researchers found that the lithotomy position with support at the ankle significantly decreased compartmental pressures. The researchers concluded that the changes in compartmental pressures in the lithotomy position were dependent on the type of leg holder used. The results of the study also showed that the use of intermittent compression significantly reduced compartmental pressures in the lower leg. The researchers cautioned that these results may not be applicable if the intermittent pneumatic compression devices are used with graduated compression stockings because of the constant pressure provided by the stockings.

Thromboembolic events are a serious and sometimes fatal event, and the risk for these events may be greater than the risk for compartment syndrome.[305,318,327] The patient's individual risk factors as well as the benefits and potential harms of not providing adequate DVT prophylaxis require careful evaluation.[303,305,318] It may be reasonable to continue the use of graduated compression stockings and intermittent pneumatic compression devices for thromboprophylaxis in patients undergoing surgical procedures in the lithotomy position.[327]

12.14 **Do not use the hemi-lithotomy position, if possible.**[12] *[Recommendation]*

Placing the patient's nonoperative leg in a hemi-lithotomy position predisposes it to the development of well-leg compartment syndrome.[12,328,343,344] In patients with an increased muscle mass, the hemi-lithotomy position can be sufficient to induce a compartment syndrome.[328] In a prospective study of 10 patients undergoing intramedullary nailing of a fractured femur in the hemi-lithotomy position, Tan et al[345] found that placement of the uninjured leg in the hemi-lithotomy position immediately increased the calf compartment pressure by more than 18 mmHg, and this pressure remained elevated until the leg was taken down. The researchers proposed that the immediate increase in compartment pressure was the direct result of mechanical compression from the leg holder. When the leg is elevated in the holder, the weight of it causes a decrease in the volume of the calf compartments pressing against the leg holder, causing the pressure within the compartments to rise. The researchers recommended avoiding the use of the hemi-lithotomy position.

Using a leg holder that allows the calf to remain free from pressure, rather than using a standard leg holder, may decrease the risk for compartment syndrome associated with the hemi-lithotomy position.[344]

13. Sitting or Semi-Sitting Position

13.1 **Implement safe practices when positioning the patient in the sitting or semi-sitting or modifications of the sitting or semi-sitting position.** *[Recommendation]*

The sitting position is also known as the Fowler position. The semi-sitting position is also known as the semi-Fowler or beach chair position. These positions are used for access to the shoulder, posterior cervical spine, or posterior or lateral head.[144]

The sitting and semi-sitting positions are variants of the supine position with the head, neck, and torso elevated 20 degrees to 90 degrees, the hips flexed 45 degrees to 60 degrees, and the knees flexed 30 degrees.[118,346-348] These positions may be accompanied by 10 degrees to 15 degrees of Trendelenburg position.[118,346]

Advantages of the sitting or semi-sitting positions include improved surgical exposure and visual alignment with critical anatomy, access to the patient's airway, ease of mechanical ventilation, reduced intracranial pressure, reduced facial swelling, improved lung excursion and diaphragmatic activity, and reduced blood pooling in the surgical field.[7,144,191,347-353]

Complications that may arise from the use of the sitting or semi-sitting positions include VAE, hemodynamic instability, pneumocephalus, quadriplegia, and compressive peripheral neuropathy.[191,348,351,352,354] A known patent foramen ovale may be a contraindication to the sitting or semi-sitting position because of the potential for a VAE to pass into the systemic arterial circulation.[348,349] There is a risk for cerebrovascular insult with these positions, and this risk is magnified when the patient is hypotensive.[353,354] There is a risk for poor venous return from the lower extremities and pooling of blood in the patient's pelvis in the sitting or semi-sitting position.[350]

The sitting or semi-sitting position may also affect bispectral index values, which are used to evaluate depth of anesthesia and prevent patient awareness during surgery.[355] Lee et al[355] found there was a significant decrease in bispectral index values associated with a change from the supine to the semi-sitting position, and this could potentially affect interpretation of the depth of anesthesia.

13.2 **Position the patient in sitting or semi-sitting position as described in** Recommendations 8 and 13. *[Recommendation]*

Guidance for safe practices in positioning the patient is provided in Recommendation 8.

Guidance for safe practices in positioning the patient in the sitting or semi-sitting position is provided in this section (Recommendation 13).

13.3 **Minimize the degree of patient head elevation as much as possible.** *[Recommendation]*

A lesser degree of patient head elevation may reduce the incidence of hypotension and the potential for subsequent cerebral desaturation.[356,357] The sitting and semi-sitting positions may cause hypotensive, bradycardic events leading to cerebral desaturation.[356,358,359] There is moderate-quality evidence to suggest a strong positive correlation between the degree of head elevation in the sitting or semi-sitting position and cerebral desaturation events.[356,358,360-365] Cerebral desaturation puts the brain at risk for ischemic injury, and the anesthetized patient is unable to express that cerebral blood flow has been reduced.[363] The consequences of cerebral desaturation include cognitive decline, organ morbidity, stroke, and death.[354,359] In the sitting and semi-sitting positions, there is a reduction in mean arterial pressure[366] and a significant decrease in cerebral artery blood flow velocity and autoregulatory response[366-368] that could lead to ischemia[368] or cognitive decline.[366]

Salazar et al[362] reviewed the literature to determine the incidence of postoperative neurocognitive deficits, number of reported complications, and incidence of postoperative cerebral desaturation events in patients who underwent arthroscopic surgery in the sitting or semi-sitting position. The authors analyzed 10 studies with a composite enrollment of 24,701 patients undergoing shoulder surgery in the sitting or semi-sitting position and found only one case of postoperative neurocognitive deficit (0.004%). The authors also identified four case reports of six patients with catastrophic neurocognitive complications after shoulder surgery in the sitting or semi-sitting position. In addition, the authors analyzed seven studies where a total of 287 patients were monitored for cerebral desaturation events. The authors found that the mean incidence of cerebral desaturation events was 41.1%.

There is also moderate-quality evidence to suggest that despite hypotension occurring in the sitting or semi-sitting position, its correlation with decreased cerebral desaturation or autoregulation has yet to be determined.[353,364,369-371] The role of hypoperfusion in cerebral infarction is unclear.[353] As well, there is a lack of evidence to define the degree and duration of cerebral desaturation required to produce a definitive and measurable neurocognitive decline.[356,372] In a blinded prospective study, Yadeau et al[369] measured cerebral oximetry levels in 99 patients undergoing ambulatory shoulder arthroscopy in the sitting position with a mean head to heart distance of 12.6 inches (32 cm). The researchers found that hypotension occurred 76% of the time with a mean duration of 71 minutes, but cerebral desaturation occurred only 0.77% of the time with a mean duration of 7 minutes. The researchers suggested that despite the presence of hypotension, adequate cerebral perfusion was maintained.

Tange et al[370] evaluated tissue oxygen index values in 30 patients undergoing shoulder surgery in the 60-degree semi-sitting position. They found that as long as the patient's blood pressure was maintained above 60 mmHg, the semi-sitting position did not alter cerebral oxygenation. To evaluate changes in cerebral tissue oxygen index values associated with the 60-degree semi-sitting position and the 90-degree sitting position, Mori et al[373] enrolled 28 healthy patients, 33 patients with one cardiovascular risk factor, and 30 patients with more than one cardiovascular risk factor (N = 91) in a prospective study. Cardiovascular risk factors included cardiac diseases, diabetes mellitus, hypertension, hypercholesterolemia, and smoking. The researchers found that the tissue oxygen index values were in the normal range of 70% before and during anesthesia in all groups.

Pin-on et al[371] conducted a comprehensive retrospective review of the records of 5,177 patients who underwent surgery in the sitting or semi-sitting position and found were no ischemic brain injuries.

13.4 **Maintain the patient's head in a neutral position without excessive flexion, extension, or rotation.**[349,374] *[Recommendation]*

Maintaining the patient's head in a neutral position when the patient is in a sitting or semi-sitting position can be challenging; however, extremes of neck flexion, extension, or rotation can result in patient injury.[346,375] Flexion of the head against the chest can lead to venous and lymphatic congestion, resulting in macroglossia.[376] Amukoa et al[374] recommended maintaining a minimum space of 1 inch (2.5 cm) between the patient's chin and chest to preserve airway patency and allow venous drainage from the face and tongue. Lindroos et al[348] also suggested that a 2-fingerbreadth distance between the patient's chin and sternum is mandatory. Hyperextension of the patient's neck could result in a spinal cord injury.[349,375] Rotation of the patient's neck while in a sitting or semi-sitting position could result in a neuropathy caused by compression and stretching of the glossopharyngeal, vagus, and hypoglossal nerves.[350]

13.4.1 **Assess and monitor the patient's head position after positioning activities and during the procedure and implement corrective actions as indicated.**[374,375] *[Recommendation]*

Assessing and monitoring the patient's head position may help prevent patient injury. Rhee and Cho[377] described two cases of hypoglossal nerve palsy after shoulder surgery. Both patients (ie, a 41-year-old man and a 71-year-old man) were positioned in a 70-degree semi-sitting position for the diagnostic shoulder arthroscopy and a 30-degree semi-sitting position for the open Bankart repair. In both cases, the procedure lasted approximately 90 minutes. In addition, in both cases, the patients' heads were immobilized by an adhesive plaster strip from the headrest across the forehead and a second adhesive plaster strip across the chin. After surgery, both patients reported difficulty pronouncing words, and they were diagnosed with a unilateral hypoglossal neuropathy that resolved within 6 weeks. The authors concluded that the most likely cause of both injuries was the change from the 70-degree to 30-degree semi-sitting position. They speculated that the change in position affected the position of the head and neck and led to unintended compression on the hypoglossal nerve.

Liang[378] opined on the duty of the perioperative team members to monitor the patient's head position during surgical procedures in describing the case of an obese woman who underwent cervical spinal surgery in the sitting position with her head flexed toward her chest. The surgeon and perioperative RN taped the patient's head to a horseshoe-shaped head positioner to prevent it from moving during the procedure but did not provide any additional padding to the patient's head or neck. When the procedure was completed, the patient was transferred to the postanesthesia care unit, where she lapsed into a coma after 20 minutes. When she emerged from the coma, the patient was only able to move one finger and to slightly move one foot. The physicians concluded that she had suffered bilateral strokes from carotid artery obstruction resulting in permanent paraplegia.

The patient sued the surgeon, anesthesiologist, and RN anesthetist. Expert physicians testifying at the trial agreed that the carotid artery obstruction resulted from the patient's chin resting on her sternum, either during the positioning process or sometime during the surgery. On cross examination, both anesthesia professionals acknowledged an obligation to inspect the patient during the procedure and ensure the patient's head is not in a position that might lead to clinical problems. If their inspections reveal a need to reposition the patient, their obligation is to inform the surgeon so that the issue can be addressed. The appeals court also observed that the only way to be assured that the patient's head remains in the correct position is through visual inspection and monitoring. Although they had attached monitors to the patient, neither of the anesthesia professionals had lifted the drapes to check the position of the patient's head. This failure to verify the patient's position was determined to be the cause of the injury to the patient.[378]

13.4.2 **Do not use a horseshoe-shaped head positioner,**[349] **if possible.** *[Recommendation]*

Using a horseshoe-shaped head positioner may cause pressure on the lesser occipital or the greater auricular nerve, resulting in a neuropathy.[349,379] The greater auricular nerve is vulnerable to injury because of its superficial location.[379,380]

13.5 **For a patient in the sitting or semi-sitting position, flex and secure the patient's arms or nonoperative arm across the body.**[21,118,144,346] *[Recommendation]*

Flexing the patient's arm(s) across the body provides surgical access and a physiologic position.

13.5.1 **The patient's operative arm may be**
- **held by the surgeon or surgical assistant or**
- **supported by an arm-positioning device designed for this purpose.**[118,347]
[Conditional Recommendation]

Using an arm-positioning device during shoulder surgery may improve visibility within the joint and provide tension on the tissues being repaired.[347] If an arm holder is not used, an assistant may be required to apply traction or joint distraction.[347]

13.5.2 **Minimize extension and external rotation of the patent's operative arm as much as possible.**[158] *[Recommendation]*

Minimizing extension and external rotation of the patient's operative arm may help to prevent injury. The available evidence is of low quality and does not define the safe limit of extension or external rotation.[158]

13.6 **Pad the patient's buttocks.**[21] *[Recommendation]*

Padding the patient's buttocks helps prevent excessive pressure on the sciatic nerve and coccyx.[191] Prolonged pressure on the buttocks during surgery in the sitting position can lead to muscle trauma and spasm of the piriformis muscle and resultant compression of the sciatic nerve.[381,382]

13.7 **Flex the patient's knees 30 degrees.**[118,346-349] *[Recommendation]*

Flexing the patient's knees reduces stretching of the sciatic nerve and may help to prevent a postoperative neuropathy.[383]

Notably, there is no evidence to specify the necessary degree of flexion required to prevent neuropathy; however, several authors have recommended 30 degrees of knee flexion in the sitting or semi-sitting position.[118,346-348]

13.8 **After the patient is moved into a sitting or semi-sitting position,**
- **prevent the patient's abdominal pannus from resting on the thighs, if possible, and**
- **verify placement and security of the safety restraint across the patient's thighs.**
[Recommendation]

Satin et al[384] described occurrences of lateral femoral cutaneous nerve palsy in four obese patients undergoing shoulder surgery in the semi-sitting position with a safety restraint applied across the thighs. The procedure times ranged from 95 minutes to 220 minutes. All patients reported severe pain and numbness in the anterolateral thighs after surgery, and in all cases, the pain and numbness resolved within 3 to 6 months. The authors noted that in patients who are obese, abdominal distention, increased visceral weight, or abundance of adipose tissue may cause the abdominal wall to bend over itself, pushing on the inguinal ligament and forcing the iliac fascia surrounding the lateral femoral cutaneous nerve to compress the underlying nerve. The authors concluded that the injuries in the reported cases were likely caused by external compression from the abdominal pannus resting on the patient's thighs. They recommended preventing the patient's abdominal pannus from resting on the thighs and reassessing the tightness of the restraint after the patient is moved into the semi-sitting position.

Notably, some methods of securing the abdominal pannus away from the thighs (eg, taping the abdomen) could lead to patient injury (eg, skin breakdown, abdominal compression); therefore, when attempting to prevent the patient's abdominal pannus from resting on the thighs, it is necessary to implement safe positioning practices and to evaluate the benefits compared with potential harms of the methods used.

A correctly placed safety restraint across the patient's thighs can tighten when the patient is moved into a sitting or semi-sitting position.[384]

13.9 **Sequential compression devices may be used when the patient is in the sitting or semi-sitting position.**[349] *[Conditional Recommendation]*

Using sequential compression devices limits venous pooling and enhances venous return from the legs.[349,374,385,386]

Kwak et al[385] conducted an RCT to investigate the effect of intermittent pneumatic sequential compression devices on the incidence of hypotension and other hemodynamic variables in the semi-sitting position. The researchers randomly assigned 50 healthy patients undergoing elective shoulder arthroscopy under general anesthesia to either the control group (n = 25) or the sequential compression devices group (n = 25). They measured hemodynamic variables before induction and at 5 minutes after the induction of anesthesia in the supine position and again at 1, 3, and 5 minutes after the patient was raised to a 70-degree semi-sitting position. The researchers found that the incidence of hypotension was significantly higher in the control group (n = 16; 64%) than in the sequential compression devices group (n = 7; 28%). The mean arterial pressure, cardiac index, and stroke volume index were also significantly higher in the sequential compression devices group than in the control group. The researchers concluded that the use of intermittent pneumatic sequential compression devices reduced the incidence of hypotension and supported venous return from the legs when patients were in the semi-sitting position.

13.10 **Do not use the sitting position for patients with ventriculoperitoneal shunts, if possible.** *[Recommendation]*

Prabhakar et al[387] reported the case of a 4-year-old girl with a ventriculoperitoneal shunt who underwent an elective midline suboccipital craniectomy in the sitting position for removal of a pineal tumor. The surgery lasted 4 hours. During a postoperative position change, the authors noted a large pneumocephalus and a right parietal hematoma. The surgeons performed a burr hole evacuation of the hematoma, and the pneumocephalus resolved without intervention. The authors concluded that the ventriculoperitoneal shunt tube led to excessive drainage of cerebrospinal fluid that resulted in intracranial hypotension and rupture of bridging veins, leading to the pneumocephalus and hematoma. They recommended not using the sitting position for patients with ventriculoperitoneal shunts.

13.11 **Be prepared to detect and implement interventions to manage VAE events.**[388-390] *[Recommendation]*

Venous air embolism can occur when air or gas is drawn into the circulation by the veins above the level of the heart and is most likely to occur during neurosurgery or open shoulder surgery in the sitting or semi-sitting position.[347-349,351,352,389-392] Rushatamukayanunt et al[391] found that the incidence of VAE was significantly higher in the sitting position (41.3%) than the horizontal positions (ie, prone and lateral; 11.0%). Venous air embolism can occur in any position in which the operative site is higher than the right atrium[388] and may also occur in the supine, reverse Trendelenburg, lateral, or prone positions.[191,388-391]

Venous air embolism can pass into the systemic arterial circulation and lead to ischemia of vital organs.[348] It can lead to cardiovascular collapse caused by obstruction of outflow from the heart with pulmonary hypertension and paradoxical air embolism.[351] The incidence of VAE is not well tolerated in patients with chronic obstructive pulmonary disease, and thus, chronic obstructive pulmonary disease may be a contraindication to using the sitting position.[352]

Successful treatment of VAE requires prompt recognition and rapid and simultaneous implementation of multiple interventions by the periopera-tive team.[351,388-391] If not diagnosed and treated immediately, VAE can be fatal.[388,391]

Notably, in addition to air, there are other potential embolic sources (eg, atherosclerotic plaque, thromboemboli, fat, bone).[349] Perelló et al[393] reported the case of a 49-year-old woman who developed a bone embolism during a craniectomy performed in the sitting position. At the end of the procedure, the patient had an episode of atrial bigeminy accompanied by an abrupt decrease in ETCO$_2$. The patient was diagnosed with a VAE, and the surgeons attempted to aspirate the air through her central venous catheter; however, rather than air, they recovered bone fragments.

13.11.1 **Manage venous air embolism by**
- **ventilating the patient with 100% oxygen**[351,374,389,390,394]**;**
- **controlling bone, dural sinus, and muscle bleeding**[348,351,394]**;**
- **filling the surgical wound with irrigation fluid or packing it with saline-soaked sponges**[348,351,374,389,394]**;**
- **placing the patient in left lateral and Trendelenburg position**[351,374,390,394]**;**
- **attempting to aspirate entrained air from a right atrial catheter**[351,374,389,390]**;**
- **initiating cardiac compressions with the patient in supine and Trendelenburg position**[374,389,390]**;**
- **administering IV fluids and vasopressors**[351,374,389,390]**;**
- **implementing transesophageal echocardiography**[394]**; and**
- **using ETCO$_2$.**[394]

[Recommendation]

The goal of air embolism management is to prevent further air entry, reduce the volume of entrained air, and provide hemodynamic support.[388-390]

Ventilating the patient with 100% oxygen maximizes patient oxygenation, aids elimination of nitrogen, and reduces embolus volume.[389,390]

Controlling bone, dural sinus, and muscle bleeding and filling the surgical wound with irrigation fluid or packing it with saline-soaked sponges helps prevent further entrainment of air.[389]

Changing the patient's position may help prevent air from traveling through the right side of the heart into the pulmonary arteries.[388,390]

Aspiration of entrained air from a central venous catheter in the right atrium may be effective; however, there are no data to support emergent catheter insertion for air aspiration during an acute VAE event.[389,390]

Initiating cardiac compressions may help to break large bubbles into smaller ones and force air out of the right ventricle into the pulmonary vessels, thus improving cardiac output.[390]

Infusion of IV fluids optimizes myocardial perfusion and may help to push the blocked airlock into the lungs where it can be absorbed.[389,390] Volume expansion increases intravascular volume and central venous pressure and may reduce further gas entry.[351,388] Administration of vasopressors increases the force and speed of ventricular contractions.[389,390]

Implementing transesophageal echocardiography may help to confirm the diagnosis of VAE.[394]

Using ETCO$_2$ can assist in assessing cardiac output and monitoring the progression and resolution of VAE.[394]

13.11.2 **Bilateral jugular compression may be used when managing VAE.**[348,374,389] *[Conditional Recommendation]*

Applying jugular compression may be effective in limiting the entry of air into the chest and right atrium from sources in the face and head by increasing venous pressure; however, increased intracranial pressure and subsequent decreased cerebral perfusion may be a direct consequence of this technique.[389,390] Additional concerns include the potential for direct carotid artery compression resulting in possible dislodgement of atheromatous plaque, venous engorgement leading to cerebral edema, and carotid sinus stimulation resulting in severe bradycardia.[389,390]

14. Lateral Position

14.1 **Implement safe practices when positioning the patient in the lateral or modifications of the lateral position.** *[Recommendation]*

In the lateral position, the patient is positioned on the nonoperative side.[5,144] In a right lateral position, the patient is lying on his or her right side.[144] This position provides exposure for a left-sided procedure.[144] In a left lateral position, the patient is lying on his or her left side. This position provides exposure for a right-sided procedure. The dependent side is the reference point for documentation.

The lateral position is used for orthopedic procedures involving the hip and, with some modification, for kidney and thoracic procedures.[5,21,36,191] The lateral position may be preferred to the prone position for patients who are obese, as the bulk of the patient's panniculus can be displaced off the abdomen.[74]

A patient in the lateral position is at risk for injury from pressure on vulnerable points on the dependent side (ie, ear, acromion process, olecranon, iliac crest, greater trochanter, lateral knee, malleolus).[21] In a retrospective review of position-related complications in 71 patients undergoing surgery in the lateral position, Furuno et al[395] found that one patient developed rhabdomyolysis and one patient developed a transient peroneal nerve palsy, but 22 patients developed Stage 1 pressure injuries (31%), and 12 patients developed Stage 2 pressure injuries (17%).

During prolonged surgery in the lateral position, the patient can experience local muscle compression with ischemia and subsequent reperfusion injury leading to compartment syndrome or rhabdomyolysis.[396] Woernle et al[396] examined serum creatinine kinase (CK) levels as markers of muscle injury in 150 patients undergoing neurosurgical procedures in the supine or prone (n = 100) or lateral (n = 50) positions. The researchers found that postoperative CK levels were significantly elevated after procedures in the lateral position. Elevated CK levels may lead to acute renal, hepatic, and respiratory complications. The researchers concluded that the elevated CK levels resulted from increased pressure associated with the lateral position.

The weight of the abdomen is shifted away from the diaphragm; however, prolonged lateral positioning can lead to vascular congestion and relative hypoventilation in the dependent lung.[7,69,234] In the lateral position, the dependent lung receives a larger blood flow and the upper lung is easier to ventilate (ie, ventilation-perfusion mismatch).[7,36] Patients with pre-existing cardiac or pulmonary disease may not be able to tolerate these physiologic changes.[36,397]

Patients with osteoporosis or other degenerative orthopedic diseases may be at risk for fracture or spinal misalignment when placed in the lateral position.[21,37,398]

In a prospective observational study of 29 consecutive patients undergoing thoracic surgery in the lateral position, Hemmerling et al[399] measured cerebral saturation to detect differences between the upper and lower hemispheres. The researchers found significantly higher saturation levels in the upper hemisphere compared with the lower hemisphere. Notably, there may be no clinical impact associated with this finding.

14.2 **Place the patient in the lateral position for the shortest time possible.**[110,400,401] *[Recommendation]*

Reducing the length of time the patient is placed in lateral position decreases the potential for rhabdomyolysis.[400,401] Dakwar et al[402] performed a retrospective review of 315 patients who underwent minimally invasive spinal surgery in the lateral position. The authors found that five patients (1.6%) developed rhabdomyolysis and acute renal failure. They concluded that the etiology of the rhabdomyolysis was likely multifactorial; however, all patients had been secured in the lateral position with safety straps and adhesive tape for the entire procedure, and all patients had operative times longer than 4 hours.

14.2.1 Patients in the lateral position may be repositioned at established intervals during the procedure. *[Conditional Recommendation]*

Moderate-quality evidence indicates that repositioning the patient at established intervals during the procedure may reduce the risk for compartment syndrome or other injury associated with prolonged lateral position.[110,400]

14.2.2 Implement repositioning interventions and repositioning intervals that are
- based on the individual patient and the specific situation[19] and
- established by the perioperative team before the beginning of the procedure, if possible.[182]

[Recommendation]

14.3 Place a head positioner or pillow under the patient's head.[21] *[Recommendation]*

Supporting the patient's head helps maintain cervical and thoracic alignment and prevent lateral flexion of the neck that could stretch the brachial plexus.[5,11,36,144] Using a head positioner may help to reduce pressure on the dependent ear.[5]

14.3.1 Assess and monitor the patient's dependent ear after positioning and during the procedure and take corrective actions as indicated.[36] *[Recommendation]*

Assessing and monitoring the patient's dependent ear verifies it is not folded.

14.3.2 Do not use a horseshoe-shaped head positioner, if possible. *[Recommendation]*

Mechanical compression from a horseshoe-shaped head positioner has been reported as a cause of postoperative facial edema and acute unilateral parotid enlargement in the lateral position.[403]

14.4 Support and secure the patient's arms on two level and parallel arm boards, with one arm on each arm board, the upper arm above the lower arm, and both arms abducted less than 90 degrees.[36,144]

- Position the lower arm on the same plane as the OR bed mattress, with the forearm and wrist in a neutral position and the palm up.[36]
- Position the upper arm on the same plane as the shoulder, with the forearm and wrist in a neutral position and the palm down.[36]

[Recommendation]

Incorrect placement of the patient's arms could cause a stretching or compression injury.[143,156]

14.4.1 The patient's operative arm may be
- held by the surgeon or surgical assistant or
- suspended by a positioning device designed for this purpose.

If the patient's arm is suspended, do not abduct more than 90 degrees.[11,118] *[Conditional Recommendation]*

The risk for brachial plexus injury and occlusion of the subclavian or axillary arteries is increased when the patient's arm is abducted more than 90 degrees.[11,12,36,38,68,143,156-158,191,214]

14.5 Place an axillary roll under the patient's dependent thorax, distal to the axillary fold, at the level of the seventh to ninth rib.[21,36,41,118,143,144,191,404] *[Recommendation]*

Using an axillary roll improves compliance of the patient's dependent hemithorax and improves cardiac output.[118,144,191] Placing the axillary roll below the axilla provides support for the rib cage, reduces pressure on the head of the dependent humerus, and avoids compression of the axillary neurovascular bundle.[5,7,11,36,118,144,191]

Notably, the term *axillary roll* is a misnomer. The word axillary implies an incorrect and potentially dangerous location for the positioning support.[144] Placing the axillary roll in the axilla can injure the long thoracic nerve,[404] cause vascular obstruction, or compromise IV infusions or intra-arterial monitors if present in the dependent arm.[144] The word *roll* may imply that the positioning support is composed of a rolled sheet or towel. Rolled sheets and towels do not redistribute pressure.

14.5.1 Use a device designed for use as an axillary support. *[Recommendation]*

Using devices designed for use as axillary supports reduces the potential for patient injury that might occur when a device is used that is not designed for this purpose (eg, an IV bag).

14.5.2 Use an axillary support that is wide enough to spread its lifting ability over the area of several contiguous ribs.[144] *[Recommendation]*

14.5.3 **Verify the patient's bilateral radial pulses after positioning in the lateral position and placement of the axillary roll, and take corrective actions as indicated.**[143,191] *[Recommendation]*

Verifying bilateral peripheral pulses confirms adequate blood flow in the dependent arm.[36,191,405]

14.6 **Maintain the patient's physiologic spinal alignment.**[5,11,36,41,144,191] *[Recommendation]*

Maintaining the patient's physiologic spinal alignment reduces the potential for injury.[11]

14.7 **Do not compress the patient's breasts and abdomen or allow them to hang over the edge of the OR bed.**[6,191] *[Recommendation]*

14.8 **Place a safety restraint across the patient's hips.**[144] *[Recommendation]*

Placing a safety restraint across the patient's hips provides stability.[144]

14.9 **Flex the patient's dependent leg at the hip and knee.**[21,143,144,191] **Position the patient's upper leg straight and support it with pillows between the legs.**[21,144,191] *[Recommendation]*

Flexing the patient's dependent leg provides a wide base of support that helps to stabilize the pelvis.[143,144] Maintaining the patient's upper leg in a straight position provides stability and also ensures that the bony prominences of the upper leg do not rest against the bony prominences of the dependent leg.[144] Placing pillows between the patient's legs facilitates venous drainage and helps to prevent pressure injury.[7,144]

14.9.1 **Pad the patient's dependent knee, ankle, and foot.**[5,21,118,143] *[Recommendation]*

The lateral position increases the risk for injury to the common peroneal nerve.[11] Using padding helps to protect the peroneal nerve on the dependent leg from being compressed between the fibula and the OR bed.[5,11,41]

14.10 **Minimize as much as possible the degree of bed flexion and the duration of kidney rest elevation used to provide additional exposure (eg, renal procedures, thoracic procedures).**[110] *[Recommendation]*

Flexing the OR bed widens the intercostal spaces.[36,110] Raising the kidney rest increases the amount of flexion and improves exposure.[36,110] However, flexing the OR bed and/or raising the kidney rest increases interface pressures, which may increase the patient's risk for pressure injury.[110]

Deane et al[110] conducted a quasi-experimental study to determine whether changes in interface pressures could be related to BMI, sex, position, or the table surface material. The researchers recruited 20 healthy volunteers (ie, 10 men, 10 women) and grouped them according to BMI (< 25 kg/m² = 5 men, 5 women; ≥ 25 kg/m² = 5 men, 5 women). The researchers placed the participants in left lateral position with the OR bed flat, half-flexed (ie, 25 degrees), fully-flexed (ie, 50 degrees), half-flexed with the kidney brace elevated, and fully-flexed with the kidney brace elevated. They recorded interface pressures for 5-minute periods in each position. The researchers found that full-bed flexion produced significantly higher pressures than both flat and half-flexed positions. Positions with the kidney rest elevated were also associated with significantly higher pressures than without the kidney rest. The researchers recommended decreasing the amount of bed flexion and limiting the duration of the elevation of the kidney rest.

14.10.1 **When using kidney braces,**
- **place the longer brace anteriorly, against the iliac crest and**
- **place the shorter brace posteriorly, against the lumbar back.**[406] *[Recommendation]*

If the kidney brace is aligned under the patient's flank rather than the iliac crest, ventilation of the dependent lung is restricted.[36]

The lateral position requires supports that do not press against the abdomen to avoid impairing venous drainage from the lower limbs.[406]

15. Prone Position

15.1 **Implement safe practices when positioning the patient in the prone or modifications of the prone position.** *[Recommendation]* **P**

The prone position provides surgical access to the dorsal aspects of the patient's body.[36] The jackknife, or Kraske, position is a variation of the prone position that provides additional exposure for sacral, rectal, or perineal areas. The knee-chest position is a modification of the prone position that provides exposure for spinal procedures and offers the advantage of reduced abdominal pressure.[191]

The prone position produces an increase in functional residual capacity and alterations in the distribution of both ventilation and perfusion throughout the lungs.[407] These changes improve ventilation/perfusion matching and consequently improve oxygenation.[407]

In a systematic review of the literature, Kwee et al[408] identified 13 potential complications associated with the prone position that included

- increased intra-abdominal pressure,
- increased bleeding,
- abdominal compartment syndrome,
- limb compartment syndrome,
- nerve injuries,
- pressure injuries,
- cardiovascular compromise,
- thrombosis and stroke,
- hepatic dysfunction,
- ocular injuries,
- oropharyngeal swelling,
- airway maintenance device dislodgement, and
- VAE.

Intra-abdominal, intrathoracic, and intraocular pressures are increased in the prone position.[407-411] Changes in intra-abdominal pressure and resultant epidural venous congestion can influence airway pressures and cause increased intraoperative blood loss.[407,409,410,412] The prone position can also cause sudden changes in inferior vena cava pressure.[407,413] These changes can be a contributing factor in the migration of an inferior vena cava filter, especially flexible retrievable filters.[413]

Patients who are obese may have increased intra-abdominal and central venous pressures in the prone position related to increased abdominal girth.[411] These physiologic changes reduce systemic venous return and cardiac output and can lead to reduced end-organ blood flow.[411] Han et al[414] studied the effect of BMI on intra-abdominal pressure and found that intra-abdominal pressures were significantly higher in obese individuals (ie, BMI 25.0 kg/m^2 to 29.9 kg/m^2) than in normal-weight individuals (ie, BMI 18.5 kg/m^2 to 22.9 kg/m^2) when in the prone position. This higher intra-abdominal pressure resulted in significantly increased intraoperative blood loss in obese individuals (495 mL ± 88 mL) compared with normal-weight individuals (435 mL ± 65 mL).

Elevated intra-abdominal pressure significantly increases the risk for abdominal compartment syndrome.[408] Patients who are obese or who have had previous abdominal surgeries are at increased risk for abdominal compartment syndrome when in the prone position.[408]

Elevated intracompartmental pressures associated with the prone position can lead to reduced limb perfusion.[408] Inadequate blood supply to the limbs can result in ischemia, which in turn leads to edema that further increases intracompartmental pressures.[408] Ischemia leads to tissue necrosis, rhabdomyolysis, and renal failure.[408] Factors such as obesity, large muscle mass, peripheral vascular dis-ease, and prolonged procedures augment the patient's risk for limb compartment syndrome.[408]

Surgery in the prone position increases the risk for neuropathic injury to the cervical spine and brachial plexus because of excessive pressure or stretch by flexion, extension, or lateral rotation.[408]

Patients who undergo procedures in the prone position are vulnerable to pressure injury on the face, breasts, lower costal margins, iliac crests, genitalia, knees, and toes.[21,36] Patients with breast implants have a theoretical risk for rupture of the implants if they are placed under direct pressure while the patient is in the prone position.[408] Respiratory function may be decreased as a result of compression on the rib cage and diaphragm.[21,36,69,144]

Hemodynamic changes associated with the prone or jack-knife position (ie, reduced cardiac output and cardiac index, increased systemic vascular resistance[407]) could increase the risk for cardiovascular compromise or collapse in patients with limited cardiovascular reserve.[408,415,416] Hemodynamic changes may be more pronounced in patients with increased thoracic and intra-abdominal pressure or with truncal obesity or when prone positioning is modified to improve surgical access (eg, exaggerated lumbar flexion).[416]

The prone position increases the patient's risk for thrombosis and stroke caused by position-related occlusion of blood flow that may lead to stasis and clotting.[408] Kinking of blood vessels related to lateral rotation of the patient's head increases the potential for intimal injury and thrombosis formation.[408]

Hepatic dysfunction can be a consequence of the increased central venous pressure associated with the prone position.[408,410] Increased central venous pressure in combination with anesthetic-induced hypotension could lead to hypoperfusion and ischemic hepatitis.[408]

General anesthesia decreases tear production and the potential for ocular injuries that include desiccation, irritation, abrasion, laceration, and subsequent inflammation or infection is increased in the prone position.[408] Ocular complications associated with the prone position include increased intraocular pressure, decreased tissue perfusion, conjunctival edema, hemorrhage, chemosis, and postoperative vision loss.[408] Patients who are predisposed to acute angle-closure glaucoma are at high risk for ocular injury even during short procedures because the prone position can shift the lens-iris diaphragm forward so it obstructs aqueous humor outflow and increases intraocular pressure.[408] Several risk factors are associated with postoperative vision loss including prolonged procedural time, high-volume infusion, intraoperative anemia, and hypotension.[417] When these risk factors are combined with a head-down position or extreme rotation of the head to one side, they may result in a loss of vision because of compromised blood flow to the optic nerve.[417]

In the prone position, gravity causes an accumulation of extravascular fluid in any dependent body part, including the hands, feet, face, and conjunctiva.[36] The longer the procedure, the more dramatic the edema.[36] This transient edema can also affect the nose, oropharynx, salivary glands, and tongue. For this reason, it may be necessary to keep the patient intubated during the immediate postoperative period.[36,408]

Both the prone and the lateral position cause dilation of the airway as a result of gravitational effects on anatomic structures. There is an increased risk for airway maintenance device displacement or dislodgement.[408]

The risk for air entrainment through the surgical wound into the venous system and the potential for VAE is greater when the surgical site is elevated above the heart or the patient is hypotensive, as may occur when the patient is in the prone position.[408]

Venous congestion associated with the prone position can lead to a rise in middle ear pressure, although the mechanism and effects of these pressure changes warrant further research.[418]

The prone position may result in impaired cerebral venous drainage with a subsequent reduction in cerebral perfusion[419]; however, evidence about the effects of the prone position on cerebral oxygenation and perfusion is inconclusive. Closhen et al[419] found a small increase in cerebral oxygen saturation of less than 5% in patients undergoing orthopedic surgery in the prone position and in awake volunteers. Babakhani et al[420] found that cerebral oxygenation could be maintained in the prone position as long as hypotension and bradycardia were prevented. Deiner et al[421] found that older patients in the prone position were more than twice as likely to experience mild cerebral desaturation as older patients in the supine position.

In a prospective observational study of 30 children ages 13 to 18 years positioned prone for scoliosis correction surgery, Brown et al[422] found there was a reduction in cardiac index and mean arterial pressure, but these changes were not significant. Further research is warranted to determine whether the effects of the prone position on cerebral oxygenation and perfusion are associated with postoperative neurological deficit.

15.2 Position patients in the prone position in 5-degree to 10-degree reverse Trendelenburg, if possible.[18,69,184,283,423-426] [Recommendation]

Positioning surgical patients with the head above the heart helps reduce venous congestion in the eye and orbit and decrease intraocular and intraorbital pressure.[118,236,425,427,428] Positioning the patient in 5-degree to 10-degree reverse Trendelenburg also decreases facial edema.[118] Emery et al[429] conducted an RCT to evaluate intraocular pressures in 63 patients undergoing lumbar spine surgery in the prone position. In 27 patients, the head was maintained in a horizontal position during the surgery. In 25 patients, the head of the OR bed was elevated to 10-degree reverse Trendelenburg position during the surgery. The researchers found that the mean intraocular pressure for the head-elevated group was significantly lower than the mean intraocular pressure for the horizontal group. The researchers concluded that this intervention could mitigate the risk for postoperative blindness associated with increased intraocular pressure.

15.2.1 Avoid using the Wilson frame,[411] if possible. [Recommendation]

The Wilson frame is sometimes used during lumbar spine surgeries to reduce lumbar lordosis and induce lumbar kyphosis; however, in doing so, the Wilson frame positions the patient's head lower than the heart, which increases orbital venous pressure and exacerbates venous congestion in the head over time.[411,424] In a case-controlled study of 80 patients with ischemic optic neuropathy compared with 315 matched control patients, the ASA Postoperative Visual Loss Study Group[411] found that Wilson frame use was an independent risk factor for postoperative vision loss. The researchers recommended reducing anesthetic time, minimizing blood loss, and not using the Wilson frame as methods for preventing postoperative vision loss associated with ischemic optic neuropathy.

15.3 Place the patient in the prone position for the shortest time possible.[283,424,430] [Recommendation]

There have been reports of subconjunctival hemorrhage,[431] subperiosteal orbital hemorrhage,[432] Horner syndrome,[433] and postoperative vision loss[423,434-437] after prolonged surgery in the prone position. Intraocular pressure increases in the anesthetized patient in the prone position, and the magnitude of this increase is related to the amount of time spent in the prone position.[236,280,438-442] Intraocular pressure can increase significantly after only a few minutes in the prone position.[283] The most dramatic increases in intraocular pressure occur when the patient is in the prone position with his or her head down (eg, jack-knife).[280,283,438]

Yoshimura et al[441] suggested that measuring intraocular pressures 1 hour after surgery in the prone position could provide an opportunity for implementing interventions to prevent additional increases in intraocular pressure (eg, head-up positioning, reducing operating time). Eddama[442] also suggested that regular measurement of intraocular pressures during prolonged surgeries provides an opportunity for implementing a change in the patient's position when critical thresholds are reached.

The length of time a patient may remain in the prone position without risk for pressure injury is unknown. Nazerali et al[443] conducted a retrospective review of the records of 10 patients who developed facial pressure injuries after neurosurgery, orthopedic surgery, or plastic surgery in the prone position. The authors found that the mean intraoperative prone time for a surgery complicated by a facial pressure injury was 8.6 hours compared with 3.2 hours for a surgery not complicated by a facial pressure injury. The authors recommended minimizing the patient's time in the prone position.

Sherman et al[444] prospectively identified position-related injuries in 17 patients undergoing 19 prone sacral procedures. The researchers found that five (29%) of the patients developed position-related injuries. One patient developed a transient ulnar nerve palsy attributed to an unrecognized shift in the arm board during the procedure. Three patients, two of whom were extremely obese, developed Stage 1 pressure injuries, and one patient developed a Stage 2 pressure injury. The researchers concluded that extreme obesity and procedural times in excess of 10 hours were risk factors for position-related complications.

Case reports describe compartment syndrome associated with prolonged time in the prone or knee-chest positions, including

- right anterior thigh compartment syndrome after 5 hours[445] and
- right lower-leg compartment syndrome with acute renal failure after 6 hours.[446]

The ASA Task Force on Perioperative Visual Loss encourages staging prone procedures that are anticipated to be lengthy.[18] Using a series of staged procedures rather than one prolonged procedure may help minimize the patient's time in the prone position; however, the risks associated with multiple surgeries (eg, infection, unstable spine) may outweigh the benefits of staged procedures.[184,423]

15.4 **Position the patient's head in a neutral position, without excessive flexion, extension, or rotation.**[18,36,184,349,374,423,430,447-452] *[Recommendation]*

Extremes of neck flexion or extension can result in patient injury.[346,375,416]

Positioning the patient's head in the midline, or neutral, position may reduce the risk for cerebral ischemia.[448,453] Maintaining a neutral head position maintains optimal cerebral blood flow and perfusion[449] and minimizes the risk of occluding the carotid or vertebral arteries.[407] Andersen et al[453] conducted a prospective controlled study of 48 patients undergoing spinal surgery in the prone position to determine whether head rotation more than 45 degrees would affect cerebral blood oxygen saturation levels. The researchers measured cerebral blood oxygen saturation levels during anesthesia with the patients' heads in neutral, rotated-left, and rotated-right positions; with the patients' heads in a face positioner; and with the patients' heads resting on a horseshoe-shaped head positioner. The researchers found that when the patients' heads were resting on the horseshoe-shaped head positioner, there was no significant decrease in cerebral blood oxygen saturation levels in the neutral, rotated-left, or rotated-right positions. When the patients' heads were in the face positioner, there was a significant decrease in cerebral oxygen saturation levels when the patients' heads were turned to the right or to the left compared with the midline or neutral position. The researchers recommended using a neutral head position for patients in the prone position.

Using a midline, or neutral, position for the head during prone positioning is also preferred because it decreases intraocular pressure, which increases perfusion of the optic nerve and reduces the potential for postoperative vision loss.[450,451,454] Using a midline position also decreases the potential for ocular compression that might occur when the patient's head is turned to the side.[450,452]

15.4.1 **When the patient's head is positioned in the midline, use a face positioner that is designed for this purpose.**[5,36,143,184,191] *[Recommendation]*

Face positioners provide protection for the patient's forehead, eyes, and chin. They allow the patient's head to remain in the midline while keeping external pressure off the eyes, providing a clear path for the airway maintenance device and allowing a clear view of the patient's face and eyes.[21,36,118,191,455,456]

Evidence related to the safest and most effective face positioner is of moderate quality and is inconclusive.[455,457,458] Further research is warranted. Nazerali et al[443] conducted a retrospective review of the records of 10 patients who developed facial pressure injuries after neurosurgery, orthopedic surgery, or plastic surgery in the prone position. The authors found the type of face positioner used contributed to facial pressure injury. After changing from a non-face-contoured positioner to a face-contoured positioner, there was a significant decrease in the occurrence of facial pressure injuries. The authors recommended using face-contoured positioners when the patient is in the prone position.

15.4.2 **Assess and monitor the position of the patient's face after positioning activities and during the procedure, and take corrective actions as indicated.**[416] *[Recommendation]*

Assessing and monitoring the position of the patient's face can help to prevent pressure injury to the eyes, nose, mouth, forehead, and chin.[416] Grover and Jangra[456] suggested positioning a mirror beneath the face positioner to allow the patient's face position to be monitored. Levan et al[459] described the case of a 66-year-old man who underwent spinal surgery in the prone position with his face positioned in a face positioner. The authors took a photograph of the patient's face in the face positioner at the beginning of the procedure and every 30 minutes during the procedure. The authors examined the pictures to assess patient positioning. They found that after 2 hours in the prone position the patient's face had progressively migrated from its initial position, and by 2.5 hours, the patient's nose was contacting the bottom of the face positioner. Perioperative team members repositioned the patient and added padding to maintain the patient's face in the face positioner. No further change in position was required during the 7-hour procedure.

15.4.3 **Do not use a horseshoe-shaped head positioner, if possible.** *[Recommendation]*

Direct compression from a horseshoe-shaped head positioner has been reported as a cause of postoperative vision loss when the patient is in the prone position.[460,461]

15.5 **Implement interventions to prevent direct pressure on the patient's eyes.**[118,404] *[Recommendation]*

There is an increased risk for direct compression on the orbit when the patient is in the prone position.[118,462] Direct pressure on the eye may increase the risk for corneal abrasion or other ocular injuries, including postoperative vision loss.[463,464]

15.5.1 **Assess and monitor the patient's eyes after positioning activities and during the procedure, and take corrective actions as indicated.**[184,416,423,456] *[Recommendation]*

Assessing and monitoring the patient's eyes verifies there is no direct pressure on the eyes and confirms the patient's position has not changed.[425,465]

In a study to explore the incidence and related risk factors for perioperative eye injuries, Yu et al[466] found that the prone and lateral positions were precipitating factors for eye injury. The researchers recommended careful positioning and intermittent assessment of the patient's eyes during the procedure.

15.6 **The anesthesia professional should assess the patient's airway maintenance device after positioning in the prone position, during the procedure, and after the patient is returned to the supine position and should implement corrective actions as indicated.**[407,467] *[Recommendation]*

Changes in the patient's position could lead to changes in airway maintenance device position or intracuff pressure.[416] Assessing the patient's airway maintenance device after positioning and during the procedure may prevent patient injury.[468] In a prospective study to determine whether the supine-to-prone position change displaced the endotracheal tube, Minonishi et al[469] measured the insertion depth of the endotracheal tube in 132 patients undergoing spinal surgery in the prone position. The researchers found that moving the patient from supine to prone position displaced the endotracheal tube in 91.7% of patients (n = 121). The endotracheal tubes had moved 0.4 inch (10 mm) or more in 47.9% of the patients (n = 58), and 86.3% of the patients (n = 104) had changes in endotracheal tube cuff pressure.

15.7 Position the patient's arms by
- tucking them at the sides with a draw sheet,[11,36,118,191]
- securing them at the sides with arm guards,
- placing them on an arm board positioned parallel to the OR bed,[11,36,118,191] or
- placing them on an arm rest with adjustment joints designed for this purpose.[36]

[Recommendation]

Placement of the arms is determined by the needs of the surgical team and the physical limitations of the patient.

15.7.1 **When tucking the patient's arms at the sides and securing them with a draw sheet,**
- place the patient's arms in a neutral position,[35,38,159] with the palms facing the body and without hyperextension of the elbows[6,36,159,191];
- pull the draw sheet up between the patient's body and arm, place it over the patient's arm, and tuck it between the patient and the OR bed mattress[36,191];
- tuck the draw sheet snugly enough to secure the patient's arm, but not so tightly as to create a pressure source[74]; and
- extend the draw sheet from the mid upper arm (ie, above the elbows) to the fingertips. *[Recommendation]*

Neutral position is a position during which the body part distal to the joint (eg, hand is distal to wrist, forearm is distal to elbow) is not inverted or everted, adducted or abducted, flexed or extended.[213] Hyperextension of the elbow can stretch the median nerve.[7,35,156]

Using a draw sheet that extends from the mid upper arm to the fingertips, placing the sheet over the arm, and tucking the draw sheet between the patient's body and the OR bed mattress prevents the patient's arms from falling outside of the mattress and coming to rest on the metal portion of the OR bed.[36]

When the draw sheet is tucked too tightly, it can create a pressure or nerve injury or a compartment syndrome.[7,36,38,74,143,215]

Notably, tucking the patient's arms may interfere with physiological monitoring (eg, blood pressure, arterial catheter) and could result in an unrecognized infiltrated IV in the tucked arm.

15.7.2 **When placing the patient's arms on arm boards or an arm rest with adjustment joints,**
- pad the arm boards or arm rest[159,191];
- place the arm boards or arm rest at a level lower than the chest[118,191];
- do not abduct the arms more than 90 degrees, with elbows flexed[5,11,67,143,161];
- do not position the arms above the patient's head[11,21,36,118,191];
- pronate the arms (ie, palms facing downward)[5,11,67,143,161];
- maintain the arms and wrists in neutral alignment[36,191]; and
- secure the arms to the arm boards.[28,36] *[Recommendation]*

The use of padded arm boards may decrease the risk for upper extremity neuropathy.[35,159]

Positioning the patient's arms at a level lower than the chest provides physiologic alignment.

The risk for brachial plexus injury and occlusion of the subclavian or axillary arteries is increased when the patient's arm is abducted more than 90 degrees.[11,12,36,38,68,143,157-159,161,191,214]

Positioning the patient's arms above the head can cause a stretch injury to the lower trunk and brachial plexus.[11,67,191]

Pronating the patient's arms and maintaining the patient's arms and wrists in neutral alignment reduces the risk for positioning injury.[36]

Securing the arms to the arm boards reduces the risk of the patient's arms falling off the arm board.

15.8 **Position the patient on two chest supports that extend from the clavicle to the iliac crest.**[5,21,118,143,191,470,471] *[Recommendation]*

Chest supports allow chest and abdominal expansion and decrease intra-abdominal pressure.[5,21,143,191]

Incorrect placement or movement of chest supports can lead to patient injury.[470] The use of the prone position with chest supports placed at the chest or pelvis can result in an acute but reversible change in hepatic blood flow and cardiac output.[472] Placing the chest supports inferior and medial to the iliac crest can result in a neuropathy associated with compression of the lateral femoral cutaneous nerve.[471]

15.8.1 **Position chest supports in a manner that permits full lung and abdominal expansion.**[5,21,118,143,191,473] *[Recommendation]*

Chest supports that do not permit full lung and abdominal expansion may increase intra-abdominal pressure. Increased intra-abdominal pressure impairs vena caval flow and can result in venous engorgement, decreased venous return to the heart, and reduced cardiac output.[7,36,234,423] Engorged epidural veins can increase bleeding at the surgical site during spinal procedures.[7,409] If the abdomen is compressed, there is a risk for mesenteric artery thrombosis and necrotic bowel.[74]

Positioning chest supports in a manner that prevents pressure on the abdomen may be difficult in a patient who is obese or pregnant and requires chest supports that are capable of supporting the patient's weight.[74]

15.9 **Position the patient's breasts, abdomen, and genitals in a manner that frees them from torsion or pressure.**[191] *[Recommendation]*

The evidence related to best practices for positioning the patient's breasts in the prone position is of low quality and is inconclusive. Some experts recommend diverting the breasts medially because lateral displacement can place traction on the vasculature and can be painful.[5,143] Another expert recommended placing a viscoelastic gel pad above the breast to support the chest and prevent neck compression from breast tissue if the patient's breasts are large and placing a viscoelastic gel pad below the patient's breasts if they are small.[191]

15.10 **Pad the patient's knees.**[5,36,143,191] *[Recommendation]*

Providing additional pressure-redistributing padding at the patient's knees helps prevent pressure injury.[5]

15.11 **Elevate the patient's toes off the bed by placing padding under the patient's shins so the shins are high enough to prevent pressure on the tips of the toes.**[5,21,143,191] *[Recommendation]*

Placing padding under the patient's shins provides greater pressure redistribution than placing padding under the dorsum of the patient's foot. Preventing pressure on the tips of the patient's toes reduces the incidence of pressure injuries and foot drop.[191]

15.12 **Assess the patient's pedal pulses after positioning in the knee-chest position and during the procedure and take corrective actions as indicated.**[191] *[Recommendation]*

A significant danger of the knee-chest position is the potential for impaired perfusion distal to the knees as a result of vascular kinking in the popliteal space.[191] Checking the patient's pedal pulses verifies adequate perfusion and allows the perioperative RN to assess color, capillary refill time, and pulses and compare them to baseline levels.[191]

15.13 **Have a gurney readily accessible when the patient is in the prone position.** *[Recommendation]*

A gurney is a height-adjustable patient transport vehicle with wheels that can be locked. A gurney may be necessary to rapidly reposition the patient from prone to supine position for CPR. Turning the patient to supine position for CPR provides superior access to the airway and chest.[407] However, turning the patient from prone to supine position causes a temporary interruption and potential disconnection of patient monitors.[416] The decision to reposition the patient may be determined by the effectiveness of cardiac compressions and defibrillation attempts in the prone position.[416] Additional considerations include the expected duration of interrupted resuscitation for repositioning, the need for access for other resuscitation procedures (eg, chest tube insertion, central venous cannulation), and the condition of the surgical wound (eg, multiple surgical instruments in place).[407,408,416]

16. Patients Who Are Pregnant

16.1 **Implement measures to reduce the risk for injuries when positioning patients who are pregnant.** *[Recommendation]*

In patients who are pregnant, venous return may be impeded because of compression from the gravid uterus on the maternal aorta and inferior vena cava.[69,474,475] Compression of the aorta reduces uterine and placental perfusion.[476] Compression of the inferior vena cava impedes venous return and decreases cardiac output.[476] At term gestation, the inferior vena cava is nearly completely compressed against the vertebral bodies by the gravid uterus.[7,477,478] Venous return occurs primarily through the collateral veins.[477]

16.2 **Position a pregnant woman undergoing obstetric surgery in a left lateral tilt by**
- **placing a 4.7-inch (12-cm) wedge-shaped positioning device under the right lumbar region above the iliac crest and below the lower costal region to achieve a 12-degree to 15-degree lateral tilt,**[479]
- **placing a wedge-shaped positioning device under the right pelvis to achieve a 12-degree to 15-degree lateral tilt,**[479] **or**
- **tilting the OR bed 15 degrees to 45 degrees to the left.**[474,476,480]

[Recommendation]

Implementing patient positions that displace the uterus to the left may help prevent supine hypotensive syndrome caused by the gravid uterus compressing the aorta and inferior vena cava.[7,474,478]

The Association of Women's Health, Obstetric and Neonatal Nurses (AWHONN)[479] recommends maintaining uterine displacement by using a wedge-shaped positioning device under the right lumbar region or under the right pelvis to achieve a 12-degree to 15-degree left lateral tilt.

A lumbar wedge may be more effective in preventing hypotension than a pelvic wedge.[478] When a pelvic wedge is used, the amount of left lateral tilt required to displace the uterus may be affected by the patient's BMI. In an observational study, Harvey et al[481] recommended tilting the OR bed or using an inflatable pelvic wedge designed for this purpose for positioning women who are obese and pregnant rather than using a pelvic wedge to displace the uterus.

Moderate-quality evidence regarding whether to use a pelvic wedge or an OR bed tilt as well as the recommended degree of OR bed tilt is inconclusive. Kinsella and Harvey[482] concluded that a right pelvic wedge and an OR bed tilt were equally effective in producing left lateral tilt sufficient to displace the uterus. Lee et al[476] concluded that aortocaval compression in patients who are pregnant could be effectively reduced by tilting the OR bed 15 degrees or greater. Higuchi et al[480] concluded that a 30-degree to 45-degree OR bed tilt was necessary to effectively reduce inferior vena cava compression in women who are pregnant. Archer et al[474] found that an OR bed tilt of 45 degrees was superior to any position with the right side down.

Saravanakumar et al[475] hypothesized that the addition of a reverse Trendelenburg tilt to a left lateral position could effectively relieve aortocaval compression. The researchers obtained magnetic resonance images of six pregnant women (32 weeks to 36 weeks pregnant; BMI 30 kg/m^2 to 35 kg/m^2) in six different positions: right lateral, left lateral, supine with a pelvic polyurethane wedge (7.9 inch; 20 cm), and 5-degree, 10-degree, and 15-degree reverse Trendelenburg. They found inferior vena cava compression was present in all participants in all positions; however, inferior vena cava dimensions were increased in the left lateral position compared to supine with a pelvic wedge. The addition of 15-degree reverse Trendelenburg position to the supine position with a pelvic wedge produced an increase in inferior vena cava diameter, but the increase was not statistically significant.

Notably, tilting the OR bed could make the surgery more difficult for the surgeon and increase the risk for injury to the mother.[483]

In a Cochrane systematic review to determine the most effective maternal position during cesarean section, Cluver et al[483] analyzed 11 RCTs representing a total of 857 women and found there was no change in hypotensive episodes with a right lumbar wedge, left OR bed tilt, right OR bed tilt, or Trendelenburg tilt compared with horizontal supine position. The researchers concluded that a left OR bed tilt might be better than a right OR bed tilt, and a lumbar wedge might be better than a left OR bed tilt. Larger studies with more robust data are needed to confirm these findings.

16.3 **Position a woman undergoing nonobstetric surgery and who is more than 18 weeks pregnant in a left lateral tilt during the operative procedure, if possible.[479] [Recommendation]**

The AWHONN[479] recommends using a left lateral tilt whenever possible for women who are more than 18 weeks pregnant.

17. Patients Who Are Obese

17.1 **Implement measures to reduce the risk for injuries when positioning patients who are obese. [Recommendation]**

According to the Centers for Disease Control and Prevention, people with a BMI of 30 kg/m^2 to < 35 kg/m^2 are classified as Class 1 obese, people with a BMI of 35 kg/m^2 to < 40 kg/m^2 are classified as Class 2 obese, and people with a BMI of 40 kg/m^2 or higher are classified as Class 3 extremely obese.[484] Obesity is associated with significant physiologic cardiovascular and pulmonary changes, and the surgical position in which the patient is placed can further alter cardiovascular and pulmonary function.[69,234] Airway and breathing mechanisms are compromised in patients who are obese because of

- excess adipose tissue leading to an increased workload for the supportive muscles[74,473,485];
- increased oxygen consumption and carbon dioxide production[74,473,485];
- decreased myocardial compliance (ie, 35% of normal)[74,473,485];
- increased breathing effort and decreased efficiency of air exchange[74,473];
- decreased resting functional residual lung capacity[74,473]; and
- increased incidence of gastroesophageal reflux, hiatal hernia, and abdominal pressure that adds to the risk for aspiration.[74,485]

In a nonexperimental study to demonstrate the relationship between BMI and regional hypoxemia in the lung, Yamane et al[486] measured the PaO$_2$ and the partial pressure of carbon dioxide from the pulmonary veins of 40 patients. The patients had normal cardiopulmonary function and were undergoing a catheter ablation for atrial fibrillation. The researchers found that the PaO$_2$ value in the inferior pulmonary veins was significantly lower than in the superior pulmonary veins in supine patients, and the extent of the hypoxemia was proportional to the patient's BMI. These findings demonstrated that even moderate obesity was associated with appreciable regional hypoxemia.

Cardiac output, pulmonary blood flow, and arterial pressure are also increased in obese patients in the supine position.[234] Excess body weight compromises the cardiovascular system by

- increasing metabolic demand and cardiac output,[74,485]
- increasing blood volume,[58,74,485]
- increasing venous return and preload,[69,157]
- increasing the work of the heart and the volume of blood pumped by the heart with each

contraction (leading to left ventricular dilation and thickening of the heart muscle),[74,485] and

- causing hypoxia and hypercapnia (leading to pulmonary vasoconstriction and right-sided heart failure).[74]

Patients who are obese may be at increased risk for postoperative rhabdomyolysis caused by traumatic compression of muscle tissue during extended procedures.[487]

17.2 The patient's head may be elevated 25 degrees. *[Conditional Recommendation]*

Use of the supine position in patients who are obese can lead to significant reductions in lung volume, increased work of breathing, and hypoxemia.[69,157,234] Patients who are obese may have difficulty breathing in a recumbent position.[24,74,485] The AWHONN[479] suggests that a head-elevated position may be indicated during positioning of women who are obese.

Airway management, ventilation, and intubation may be more difficult in patients who are obese.[69,485] Airway management may be difficult because of the patient's increased neck circumference.[58] A short, thick neck inhibits mobility and makes visualization of the larynx difficult.[24] Ventilating a patient who is obese is difficult because of the need for high pressure to overcome the weight of the chest and the abdomen when the patient is supine.[74,485] Intubation may be difficult because of the lack of landmarks and the presence of redundant tissue.[74] Large breasts may get in the way of the laryngoscope handle.[24] The weight of the patient's head may make it difficult to lift in order to visualize the larynx.[24]

Elevating the patient's head and neck helps establish a patent airway, ease intubation, decrease ventilator pressure, and prevent aspiration.[24,69,74,157] The 25-degree head-elevated position may improve visualization of anatomic structures and provide ergonomic advantages for the anesthesia professional performing the intubation.[488,489]

17.2.1 To place the patient in a head-elevated position,
- **elevate the back of the OR bed**[157,490] **or**
- **use a wedge-shaped positioning device that supports the patient's head and shoulders.**[157,491]

[Conditional Recommendation]

Wedge-shaped positioners are designed to redistribute pressure and reduce the patient's risk for pressure injury.[157] Using a wedge-shaped positioning device that supports the head and shoulders helps prevent strain on the patient's arms and brachial plexus.[69] Although potentially achieving similar results in terms of head elevation, using a stack of towels or blankets does not redistribute pressure, and may not sufficiently support the patient's arms and shoulders, increasing the risk for brachial plexus injury.[157] Using a wedge-shaped positioning device may prevent insufficient or excessive elevation of the patient's head and neck that may occur when too few or too many linens are used.[157] Excessive elevation can inhibit face mask ventilation and make the intubation process and application of cricoid pressure more difficult.[157] Likewise, using irrigation fluid bags to support the patient's head and shoulders is not recommended as these are not designed as positioning devices and may not provide the necessary stability or withstand the weight of the patient.[157] Electronically elevating and lowering the back of the OR bed is easier than manually adjusting or removing a stack of linens or a wedge-shaped positioning device and decreases the risk for personnel injury.[157,490]

17.3 A wedge-shaped positioning device may be placed under the patient's right lumbar region, or a left OR bed tilt of at least 15 degrees may be used. *[Conditional Recommendation]*

Some patients who are obese cannot tolerate recumbent positions.[234] In patients with central obesity, venous return may be impeded due to aortocaval compression similar to the effect of a gravid uterus.[69] Compression of the inferior vena cava against the vertebral bodies can lead to severe hypotension in patients who are obese.[7,234] The use of a wedge-shaped positioning device or a 15-degree left lateral OR bed tilt may offset aortocaval compression in patients in recumbent positions[69,234]; however, tilting the OR bed laterally for prolonged periods may result in sciatic nerve palsy.[157]

17.4 Padded arm guards may be used to contain the patient's arms at the sides of the body, if necessary. *[Conditional Recommendation]*

Using padded arm guards provides additional width and support and allows the patient's arms to be positioned at his or her sides.

18. Positioning Injuries

18.1 Collaborate with the perianesthesia RN to identify patient injury caused by intraoperative positioning.[21] *[Recommendation]*

Identifying patients at risk for positioning injury allows for the implementation of preventive interventions.[26] Injuries related to the patient's surgical position may be averted by effective postoperative monitoring and management.[46,492]

18.2 **The RN circulator should conduct a postoperative patient assessment to identify patient injury caused by intraoperative positioning.**[41,191] *[Recommendation]*

The RN circulator has knowledge of pressure points associated with the intraoperative position and of the locations where safety restraints, adhesives, monitoring devices, positioning equipment or devices, and other items that may present a risk for patient injury were placed during the procedure.[60]

The RN circulator also has knowledge of intraoperative factors that may increase the likelihood of a positioning injury (eg, intraoperative blood administration[493]). In a retrospective observational study of 2,695 surgical patients, O'Brien et al[493] found that intraoperative administration of blood products was significantly associated with postoperative pressure injury.

18.2.1 Use a standardized communication tool to provide information from the postoperative assessment to the perianesthesia RN, regarding
- areas of the patient's body that should be assessed and monitored for potential injury,[9]
- events during the intraoperative period that may have contributed to a position-related injury,[9,49,61,63] and
- the position of the patient during the procedure.

[Recommendation]

Communicating areas of concern may improve postoperative monitoring and management of potential position-related injuries. Using standardized communication tools helps ensure that necessary patient care information is communicated.

18.3 The perianesthesia RN should
- place the patient in a position other than the surgical position, if possible, and
- monitor areas that are at high risk for positioning injuries.[56,63]

[Recommendation]

Changing the patient's position after surgery reduces pressure on high-risk areas. Monitoring areas that are at high risk for positioning injuries assists with early recognition and treatment and allows for identification and review of positioning methods that may have contributed to or caused the injury.

18.4 **The perianesthesia RN should assess the patient for signs and symptoms of pressure injury.**[24,28,494] *[Recommendation]*

Early detection and treatment of pressure injury may help prevent skin alteration from progressing to skin loss.[26] Blanchable erythema, especially over a bony prominence, may be a normal, reactive, hyperemic response or the first clinical sign of pressure injury development after surgery.[24,26] Other early signs of pressure injury include changes in skin temperature or texture or pain sensation.[15] Pressure injuries may not appear for 1 to 4 days after surgery.[15,28,56,64] Pressure injuries that occur intraoperatively have a unique purple appearance that originates at the muscle over a bony prominence and progresses outward.[28,56,64]

Minnich et al[495] developed a postoperative skin assessment tool designed to be completed postoperatively by the RN circulator and the perianesthesia RN. Specific skin assessment processes were implemented to allow for rapid discovery and treatment. After using the assessment protocol for more than 3,000 patients over 2 years, the authors found the incidence of pressure injuries dropped from 7.1% to 3.3%.

18.5 **The perianesthesia RN should assess the patient for signs and symptoms of extremity nerve dysfunction.**[35,416,494] *[Recommendation]*

Assessment of nerve dysfunction may lead to early recognition and treatment of peripheral neuropathies.[35,65] Signs of nerve injury include a decreased range of motion, impaired limb muscle strength, numbness or tingling, or pain in the limbs or joints not associated with the procedure.[28] Symptoms of nerve damage may appear days or even weeks after the procedure because the symptoms may be confused with pain or immobility caused by the procedure.[28]

Gezginci et al[496] evaluated postoperative pain and neuromuscular complications (ie, paresthesia, numbness, weakness) associated with positioning after robotic-assisted laparoscopic radical prostatectomy in 534 patients. The researchers found that patients who had previous surgeries, comorbidities, and ASA classifications of II and III were at increased risk for neuromuscular complications.

18.6 **The perianesthesia RN should assess the patient for signs and symptoms of compartment syndrome.** *[Recommendation]*

Compartment syndrome presents as swelling; restricted movement; lack of sensation; tightness; severe pain; and, in extreme cases, no extremity pulse.[28] It is associated with significant morbidity and loss of limb function resulting from necrosis of ischemic muscle in the affected compartment as well as potential mortality from the reperfusion that occurs after surgical decompression.[492,497] Compartment syndrome is an acute medical emergency that most often requires urgent surgical treatment.[492,497] A rapid response is necessary to minimize the risk for long-term morbidity or potential mortality.[193]

Patients with compartment syndrome often present with reports of pain that are out of proportion with clinical findings and unrelieved by analgesics.[193,497] Notably, the use of a postoperative epidural can mask the initial pain associated with compartment syndrome.[497]

18.7 The perianesthesia RN should evaluate the patient for signs and symptoms of ocular injury.[18,498] *[Recommendation]*

Differences in pupillary reactivity, light sensitivity, visual field defects and patient reports of blurred, distorted, or painful vision may be indicative of ocular injury or impending postoperative vision loss.[283,498]

Patient-related risk factors for postoperative vision loss include male sex, preoperative anemia, hypertension, peripheral vascular disease, coronary artery disease, diabetes, use of tobacco, and obesity.[451] Procedure-related risk factors include spinal surgery, cardiac surgery, head-neck surgery, hip and femur surgeries, procedures longer than 6 hours, prone or Trendelenburg position, significant blood loss, and use of the Wilson frame.[451] Anesthetic related risk factors include limited intravascular fluid administration or excessive crystalloid administration.[451] Patients who are anemic before surgery or have experienced substantial blood loss during the procedure may be at increased risk for ocular injury.[451,499,500]

19. Documentation

19.1 The health care organization should maintain records of patient care related to patient positioning and organizational processes related to positioning equipment and devices. *[Recommendation]*

Documentation in the patient's medical record provides a description of the perioperative care administered, status of patient outcomes upon transfer, and information to support continuity of care.[10] Documentation provides data for identifying trends and demonstrating compliance with regulatory requirements and accreditation standards. Effective management and collection of health care information that accurately reflects the patient's care, treatment, and services is a regulatory requirement[501-504] and an accreditation standard for both hospitals[505,506] and ambulatory settings.[506-510]

19.2 The perioperative RN should document patient care and use of positioning equipment and devices on the intraoperative record. *[Recommendation]*

Accurate documentation facilitates comprehensive patient care, provides information for retrospective review and research data, and establishes a legal record.[38] Documentation provides a baseline record of the patient's condition.[9] Documentation of specific positioning actions may result in improved positioning processes by helping practitioners focus attention on relevant aspects of patient positioning and by providing information on positioning strategies that improve the quality of patient care.[28,35]

Comprehensive documentation related to patient positioning is necessary for demonstrating that the standard of care was met when defending claims that allege substandard care.[9,11,28,67,416] In an analysis of 44 cases from the AANA Foundation Closed Malpractice Claims Database, Fritzlen et al[38] found that documentation of patient positioning on the anesthesia record was judged as "adequate" in 12 (27%) of the claims studied, and documentation of padding was judged as adequate in eight claims (18%). There was a complete absence of documentation of patient positioning in 24 (55%) of the claims, and a complete absence of documentation of padding in 25 (57%) of the claims in this data set.

Rowen et al[6] suggested achieving consensus after positioning and documenting that all team members agreed that the patient was correctly and safely positioned.

19.2.1 Document the
- preoperative assessment[21];
- identification and titles of individuals participating in positioning the patient[6];
- patient's position, including the position of the patient's arms and legs, and any repositioning activities[11,28];
- type and location of positioning equipment or devices[6,43];
- type and location of safety restraints[6];
- type and location of any additional padding provided[21,28];
- specific actions taken to prevent patient injury, especially any actions taken in response to findings from the preoperative assessment[28,416]; and
- postoperative assessment.[24,88]

[Recommendation]

19.2.2 Initiate the health care organization's policies and procedures for establishing and documenting a chain of custody for jewelry or other items that are removed from the patient including
- the type and location of critical devices, superficial implants, jewelry, or other items that cannot be removed and
- any actions taken (eg, use of additional padding) to prevent patient injury from the item that cannot be removed.[21]

[Recommendation]

Establishing and documenting a chain of custody helps prevent loss or theft of jewelry and other items removed from patients. Some jewelry is easily removed; however, removal of some types of piercing jewelry requires the use of special tools.[85] The goals for nursing interventions are to prevent potential patient injuries or complications and treat actual patient problems.[511] Documenting nursing interventions promotes continuity of patient care and improves the exchange of patient care information among health care team members.[511]

19.2.3 When using photography to document injuries related to positioning, adhere to the health care organization's policies regarding medical photography and video images.[43] [Recommendation]

19.3 The health care organization should maintain records related to processes for preventive maintenance and repair of positioning equipment and devices. [Recommendation]

Records of preventive maintenance and repair of positioning equipment and devices provide a source of evidence for review during investigation of clinical issues (eg, patient injury). Records of preventive maintenance also provide evidence of maintenance, compliance with manufacturers' IFU, and information that may be useful in determining the need for repair or replacement. Records of repairs may help to identify trends in equipment and device damage and help to define practices that may reduce damage.

20. Education

20.1 Provide personnel who have responsibility for positioning patients with initial and ongoing education and competency verification activities related to patient positioning. [Recommendation]

Initial and ongoing education of perioperative personnel facilitates the development of knowledge, skills, and attitudes that affect safe patient care. It is the responsibility of the health care organization to provide initial and ongoing education and to verify the competency of its personnel[10]; however, the primary responsibility for maintaining ongoing competency remains with the individual.[512]

Competency verification activities provide a mechanism for competency documentation and help verify that personnel understand the principles and processes necessary for safe patient positioning.

Ongoing development of knowledge and skills and documentation of personnel participation is a regulatory requirement[501-504] and an accreditation standard for both hospitals[513,514] and ambulatory settings.[514-517]

20.2 The health care organization should establish education and competency verification activities for personnel and determine intervals for education and competency verification related to patient positioning. [Recommendation]

Providing education and verifying competency assists in developing knowledge and skills that may reduce the risk for errors and enhance perioperative team members' appreciation of the potential mechanisms of patient and personnel injury associated with patient positioning.[3,20,51,66,156] Education and competency verification needs and intervals are unique to the facility and to its personnel and processes.

20.2.1 Include the following in education and competency verification activities related to positioning patients:
- processes for patient assessment,[21,44,133]
- identification of factors that increase the risk for positioning injury in patients and personnel,[28,44,56,236]
- identification and effective use of pressure-redistributing support surfaces,[43,44,133]
- a description of the relevant anatomy and physiology,[28,156,214,331]
- a description of the characteristics of special populations served by the health care organization (eg, patients who are pregnant, patients who are obese, older patients, pediatric patients),[23,51]
- procedures for safe use of positioning equipment and devices,[28,416]
- implementation of safe practices for patient positioning,[21,28,236,416]
- documentation of positioning activities,[43] and
- procedures for identifying and reporting patient or personnel injury caused by patient positioning.
[Recommendation] **P**

20.3 Provide education and competency verification activities before new support surfaces or positioning equipment or devices are introduced.[28] [Recommendation]

Receiving education and completing competency verification activities before new support surfaces or equipment is introduced helps ensure correct use and promote safe positioning practices.

21. Policies and Procedures

21.1 Develop policies and procedures for positioning the patient, revise them as necessary, and make them readily available in the practice setting in which they are used. *[Recommendation]*

Policies and procedures assist in the development of patient safety, quality assessment, and performance improvement activities. Policies and procedures also serve as operational guidelines used to minimize patients' risk for injury or complications, standardize practice, and direct personnel. Policies and procedures establish authority, responsibility, and accountability within the practice setting.

Having policies and procedures that guide and support patient care, treatment, and services is a regulatory requirement[501-504] and an accreditation standard for both hospitals[518,519] and ambulatory settings.[516,519-521]

21.2 Establish a multidisciplinary team to develop perioperative policies related to positioning that are consistent with the health care organization's pressure injury prevention program.[51,133] Multidisciplinary team members may include wound specialists; wound, ostomy, and continence care RNs; infection preventionists; perioperative RNs; supply chain managers; and other involved personnel. *[Conditional Recommendation]*

The potential economic impact of pressure injury (eg, expense of treatment, lack of reimbursement) underscores the need for a multidisciplinary approach to prevention.[51]

21.3 Include the following in policies and procedures related to positioning patients:
- processes for patient assessment;
- procedures for selection, care, and maintenance of positioning equipment and devices;
- procedures for safe use of positioning equipment and devices for patients and personnel;
- identification and use of pressure-redistributing support surfaces;
- procedures for safe patient positioning;
- processes for identification and reporting of patient or personnel injury caused by patient positioning; and
- documentation of positioning activities.

[Recommendation]

21.4 Make the manufacturers' IFU for support surfaces and positioning equipment and devices readily available and monitor personnel responsible for positioning activities for adherence to the IFU. *[Recommendation]*

Instructions for use identify the validated procedures necessary for safe and effective use of support surfaces and positioning equipment and devices.

21.4.1 Review the manufacturer's IFU periodically, and review positioning procedures for compliance with the most current IFU. *[Recommendation]*

Manufacturers may make modifications to their IFU when new technology becomes available, when regulatory requirements change, or when modifications are made to a device.

22. Quality

22.1 The health care organization's quality management program should evaluate patient positioning. *[Recommendation]*

Quality assurance and performance improvement programs can facilitate the identification of problem areas and assist personnel in evaluating and improving the quality of patient care and formulating plans for corrective action. These programs provide data that may be used to determine whether an individual organization is within benchmark goals, and if not, to identify areas that may require corrective action. A quality management program provides a mechanism to evaluate effectiveness of processes, compliance with positioning policies and procedures, and function of positioning equipment and devices.

Collecting data to monitor and improve patient care, treatment, and services is a regulatory requirement[501-504] and an accreditation standard for both hospitals[522,523] and ambulatory settings.[523-527]

22.2 Include the following in the quality assurance and performance improvement program for patient positioning:
- periodic review and evaluation of positioning activities to verify compliance or to identify the need for improvement,
- identification of corrective actions directed toward improvement priorities, and
- implementation of additional actions when improvement is not achieved or sustained.

[Recommendation]

Reviewing and evaluating quality assurance and performance improvement activities may identify failure points that contribute to errors in patient positioning and help define actions for improvement and increased competency.[21,56] Taking corrective actions may improve patient safety by enhancing understanding of the principles of and compliance with best practices for patient positioning.

22.3 Participate in ongoing quality assurance and performance improvement activities related to positioning patients by identifying processes that are important for

- monitoring quality,
- developing strategies for compliance,
- establishing benchmarks to evaluate quality indicators,
- collecting data related to the levels of performance and quality indicators,
- evaluating practice based on the cumulative data collected,
- taking action to improve compliance, and
- assessing the effectiveness of the actions taken.

[Recommendation]

Participating in ongoing quality assurance and performance improvement activities is a primary responsibility of perioperative personnel engaged in practice.[10]

22.4 Checklists may be used as part of the health care organization's quality improvement program for patient positioning. [Conditional Recommendation]

Checklists are designed to prevent adverse events by promoting a team culture, standardizing practice, allowing the detection of potential errors, and improving patient safety.[192] Checklists serve as cognitive aids to improve performance.[40,528] The systematic use of checklists may help guide perioperative team members and reduce the rate of position-related injuries by improving positioning skills without dependence on long-term memory.[40,416,528] Using a checklist may direct additional attention to safe positioning requirements that might otherwise not be implemented.[67] The use of a checklist does not replace vigilant assessment, monitoring, and implementation of established safe practices when positioning patients.[528]

22.5 Report and document near misses and adverse events according to the health care organization's policy and procedure and review for potential opportunities for improvement. [Recommendation]

Near misses are unplanned events that do not result in injury. Adverse events are events that result in patient injury. Reports of near misses and adverse events can be used to identify actions that may prevent similar occurrences and reveal opportunities for improvement.

22.5.1 Submit reports regarding device malfunction that led to serious injury or death to MedWatch: The FDA Safety Information and Adverse Event Reporting Program.[121] [Recommendation]

The FDA uses medical device reports to monitor device performance, detect potential device-related safety issues, and contribute to risk-benefit assessments of suspected device-associated deaths, serious injuries, or malfunction.[121] The Manufacturer and User Facility Device Experience (MAUDE) database houses reports submitted to the FDA by mandatory reporters (ie, manufacturers, importers, device user facilities) and voluntary reporters (ie, health care professionals, patients, consumers).[529]

Mandatory reporters are required to submit reports when they become aware of information that reasonably suggests that one of their marketed devices may have caused or contributed to a death or serious injury or has malfunctioned and that the malfunction of the device would be likely to cause or contribute to a death or serious injury if the malfunction were to recur.[529] Voluntary reporters are required to submit reports when they become aware of information that reasonably suggests a device may have caused or contributed to a death or serious injury of a patient.[529]

22.5.2 Collect and analyze data on patient and health care personnel injuries related to patient positioning and use this data for performance improvement. [Recommendation]

Editor's note: Teflon is a registered trademark of the Chemours Co, Wilmington, DE.

References

1. Dybec RB. Keeping up-to-date on patient positioning. *OR Nurse.* 2013;7(2):16-17. [VC]

2. Lopes CM, Galvão CM. Surgical positioning: evidence for nursing care. *Rev Lat Am Enfermagem.* 2010;18(2):287-294. [VB]

3. Bouyer-Ferullo S. Preventing perioperative peripheral nerve injuries. *AORN J.* 2013;97(1):110-124. [VA]

4. Fleisch MC, Bremerich D, Schulte-Mattler W, et al. The prevention of positioning injuries during gynecologic operations. Guideline of DGGG (S1-Level, AWMF Registry No. 015/077, February 2015). *Geburtshilfe Frauenheilkd.* 2015;75(8):792-807. [IVB]

5. MacDonald JJ, Washington SJ. Positioning the surgical patient. *Anaesth Intensive Care Med.* 2012;13(11): 528-532. [VB]

6. Rowen L, Hunt D, Johnson KL. Managing obese patients in the OR. *OR Nurse.* 2012;6(2):26-36. [VB]

7. Washington SJ, Smurthwaite GJ. Positioning the surgical patient. *Anaesth Intensive Care Med.* 2009;10(10):476-479. [VB]

8. Sørensen EE, Kusk KH, Grønkjaer M. Operating room nurses' positioning of anesthetized surgical patients. *J Clin Nurs.* 2016;25(5-6):690-698. [IIIB]

9. Chitlik A. Safe positioning for robotic-assisted laparoscopic prostatectomy. *AORN J.* 2011;94(1):37-45. [VA]

10. Standards of perioperative nursing. In: *Guidelines for Perioperative Practice.* Denver, CO: AORN, Inc; 2015:693-732. [IVC]

11. Sawyer RJ, Richmond MN, Hickey JD, Jarratt JA. Peripheral nerve injuries associated with anaesthesia. *Anaesthesia.* 2000;55(10):980-991. [VB]

12. Kuponiyi O, Alleemudder DI, Latunde-Dada A, Eedarapalli P. Nerve injuries associated with gynaecological surgery. *Obstetrician Gynaecologist.* 2014;16(1):29-36. [VA]

13. Johnson RL, Warner ME, Staff NP, Warner MA. Neuropathies after surgery: anatomical considerations of pathologic mechanisms. *Clin Anat.* 2015;28(5):678-682. [VA]

14. Ducic I, Zakaria HM, Felder JM 3rd, Arnspiger S. Abdominoplasty-related nerve injuries: systematic review and treatment options. *Aesthet Surg J.* 2014;34(2):284-297. [IA]

15. Nilsson UG. Intraoperative positioning of patients under general anesthesia and the risk of postoperative pain and pressure ulcers. *J PeriAnesth Nurs.* 2013;28(3):137-143. [IIIB]

16. Waters T, Short M, Lloyd J, et al. AORN ergonomic tool 2: positioning and repositioning the supine patient on the OR bed. *AORN J.* 2011;93(4):445-449. [VA]

17. Lindgren M, Unosson M, Krantz AM, Ek AC. Pressure ulcer risk factors in patients undergoing surgery. *J Adv Nurs.* 2005;50(6):605-612. [IIIB]

18. Practice advisory for perioperative visual loss associated with spine surgery: an updated report by the American Society of Anesthesiologists Task Force on Perioperative Visual Loss. *Anesthesiology.* 2012;116(2):274-285. [IVA]

19. The National Pressure Ulcer Advisory Panel, European Pressure Ulcer Advisory Panel, Pan Pacific Pressure Injury Alliance. *Prevention and Treatment of Pressure Ulcers: Clinical Practice Guideline.* East Washington, DC: National Pressure Ulcer Advisory Panel; 2014. [IVA]

20. Mangham M. Positioning of the anaesthetised patient during robotically assisted laparoscopic surgery: perioperative staff experiences. *J Perioper Pract.* 2016;26(3):50-52. [VC]

21. Fletcher HC. Preventing skin injury in the OR. *OR Nurse.* 2014;8(3):29-34. [VC]

22. Jacobs A, Rose S. Assessment is more than skin deep in older adults. *OR Nurse.* 2011;5(4):29. [VC]

23. Penprase B, Johnson C. Optimizing the perioperative nursing role for the older adult surgical patient. *OR Nurse.* 2014;8(4):26-34. [VB]

24. Dybec RB. Intraoperative positioning and care of the obese patient. *Plast Surg Nurs.* 2004;24(3):118-122. [VB]

25. Schultz A. Predicting and preventing pressure ulcers in surgical patients. *AORN J.* 2005;81(5):986-1006. [IIIB]

26. Shaw LF, Chang PC, Lee JF, Kung HY, Tung TH. Incidence and predicted risk factors of pressure ulcers in surgical patients: experience at a medical center in Taipei, Taiwan. *Biomed Res Int.* 2014;2014:416896. [IIIB]

27. Tschannen D, Bates O, Talsma A, Guo Y. Patient-specific and surgical characteristics in the development of pressure ulcers. *Am J Crit Care.* 2012;21(2):116-125. [IIIB]

28. ECRI. Patient positioning. *Operating Room Risk Management.* August 2011:2. [VC]

29. Lumbley JL, Ali SA, Tchokouani LS. Retrospective review of predisposing factors for intraoperative pressure ulcer development. *J Clin Anesth.* 2014;26(5):368-374. [IIIB]

30. Armstrong D, Bortz P. An integrative review of pressure relief in surgical patients. *AORN J.* 2001;73(3):645-653. [VB]

31. Walton-Geer PS. Prevention of pressure ulcers in the surgical patient. *AORN J.* 2009;89(3):538-552. [VB]

32. Sukhu T, Krupski TL. Patient positioning and prevention of injuries in patients undergoing laparoscopic and robot-assisted urologic procedures. *Curr Urol Rep.* 2014;15(4):398. [VA]

33. Hayes RM, Spear ME, Lee SI, et al. Relationship between time in the operating room and incident pressure ulcers: a matched case-control study. *Am J Med Qual.* 2015;30(6):591-597. [IIIB]

34. Aronovitch SA. Intraoperatively acquired pressure ulcers: are there common risk factors? *Ostomy Wound Manage.* 2007;53(2):57-69. [IIIB]

35. American Society of Anesthesiologists Task Force on Prevention of Perioperative Peripheral Neuropathies. Practice advisory for the prevention of perioperative peripheral neuropathies: an updated report by the American Society of Anesthesiologists Task Force on Prevention of Perioperative Peripheral Neuropathies. *Anesthesiology.* 2011;114(4):741-754. [IVA]

36. O'Connell MP. Positioning impact on the surgical patient. *Nurs Clin North Am.* 2006;41(2):173-192. [VB]

37. Clayton JL. Special needs of older adults undergoing surgery. *AORN J.* 2008;87(3):557-574. [VB]

38. Fritzlen T, Kremer M, Biddle C. The AANA Foundation Closed Malpractice Claims Study on nerve injuries during anesthesia care. *AANA J.* 2003;71(5):347-352. [IIIB]

39. Mills JT, Burris MB, Warburton DJ, Conaway MR, Schenkman NS, Krupski TL. Positioning injuries associated with robotic assisted urological surgery. *J Urol.* 2013;190(2):580-584. [IIIB]

40. Enchev Y. Checklists in neurosurgery to decrease preventable medical errors: a review. *Balkan Med J.* 2015;32(4):337-346. [VA]

41. Adedeji R, Oragui E, Khan W, Maruthainar N. The importance of correct patient positioning in theatres and implications of mal-positioning. *J Perioper Pract.* 2010;20(4):143-147. [VB]

42. Price MC, Whitney JD, King CA, Doughty D. Wound care. Development of a risk assessment tool for intraoperative pressure ulcers. *J Wound Ostomy Continence Nurs.* 2005;32(1):19-32. [VB]

43. ECRI. Pressure ulcers. *Operating Room Risk Management.* November 2011:2. [VC]

44. Stansby G, Avital L, Jones K, Marsden G; Guideline Development Group. Prevention and management of pressure ulcers in primary and secondary care: summary of NICE guidance. *BMJ.* 2014;348:g2592. [IVA]

45. Curley MA, Razmus IS, Roberts KE, Wypij D. Predicting pressure ulcer risk in pediatric patients: the Braden Q Scale. *Nurs Res.* 2003;52(1):22-33. [IIIB]

46. Sewchuk D, Padula C, Osborne E. Prevention and early detection of pressure ulcers in patients undergoing cardiac surgery. *AORN J.* 2006;84(1):75-96. [IIIB]

47. Galvin PA, Curley MA. The Braden Q+P: a pediatric perioperative pressure ulcer risk assessment and intervention tool. *AORN J.* 2012;96(3):261-270. [VB]

48. Quigley SM, Curley MA. Skin integrity in the pediatric population: preventing and managing pressure ulcers. *J Soc Pediatr Nurs.* 1996;1(1):7-18. [VB]

49. Cherry C, Moss J. Best practices for preventing hospital-acquired pressure injuries in surgical patients. *Can Oper Room Nurs J*. 2011;29(1):6-8. [VB]

50. Centers for Medicare and Medicaid Services (CMS) HHS. Medicaid program; payment adjustment for provider-preventable conditions including health care-acquired conditions. Final rule. *Fed Regist*. 2011;76(108):32816-32838.

51. Stechmiller JK, Cowan L, Whitney JD, et al. Guidelines for the prevention of pressure ulcers. *Wound Repair Regen*. 2008;16(2):151-168. [IVA]

52. Bergstrom N, Braden BJ, Laguzza A, Holman V. The Braden Scale for Predicting Pressure Sore Risk. *Nurs Res*. 1987;36(4):205-210. [VA]

53. Cardinal Health/AORN Pressure Ulcer Prevention Project. *Instructions for the Munro Pressure Ulcer Risk Assessment Scale for Perioperative Patients for Adults*. AORN, Inc. https://www.aorn.org/-/media/aorn/guidelines/tool-kits/pressure-ulcer/instructions-for-munro-risk-assessment-scale.pdf?la=en. Accessed March 10, 2017.

54. *Munro Pressure Ulcer Risk Assessment Scale for Perioperative Patients – Adults*. AORN, Inc. https://www.aorn.org/-/media/aorn/guidelines/tool-kits/pressure-ulcer/munro-pressure-ulcer-risk-assessment-scale.xlsx?la=en. Accessed March 10, 2017.

55. Scott SM. Progress and challenges in perioperative pressure ulcer prevention. *J Wound Ostomy Continence Nurs*. 2015;42(5):480-485. [VB]

56. Giachetta-Ryan D. Perioperative pressure ulcers: how can they be prevented? *OR Nurse*. 2015;9(4):22-28. [VC]

57. He W, Liu P, Chen HL. The Braden Scale cannot be used alone for assessing pressure ulcer risk in surgical patients: a meta-analysis. *Ostomy Wound Manage*. 2012;58(2):34-40. [IIIB]

58. Owers CE, Abbas Y, Ackroyd R, Barron N, Khan M. Perioperative optimization of patients undergoing bariatric surgery. *J Obes*. 2012;2012:781546. [VB]

59. Bulfone G, Marzolil I, Wuattrin R, Fabbro C, Palese A. A longitudinal study of the incidence of pressure sores and the associated risks and strategies adopted in Italian operating theatres [corrected – published erratum appears in *J Perioper Pract*. 2012;22(4):111] [corrected – published erratum appears in *J Perioper Pract*. 2012;22(5):149]. *J Perioper Pract*. 2012;22(2):50-56. [IIIB]

60. Doerflinger DMC. Older adult surgical patients: presentation and challenges. *AORN J*. 2009;90(2):223-244. [VA]

61. Engels D, Austin M, McNichol L, Fencl J, Gupta S, Kazi H. Pressure ulcers: factors contributing to their development in the OR. *AORN J*. 2016;103(3):271-281. [VA]

62. Black J, Fawcett D, Scott S. Ten top tips: preventing pressure ulcers in the surgical patient. *Wounds Int*. 2014;54(4):14-18. [VB]

63. *Pressure Ulcer Prevention in the O.R.: Recommendations and Guidance*. St Paul, MN: Minnesota Hospital Association; 2013. https://www.mnhospitals.org/Portals/0/Documents/ptsafety/skin/OR-pressure-ulcer-recommendations.pdf. Accessed March 10, 2017. [IVC]

64. Fred C, Ford S, Wagner D, Vanbrackle L. Intraoperatively acquired pressure ulcers and perioperative normothermia: a look at relationships. *AORN J*. 2012;96(3):251-260. [IIIA]

65. Menezes S, Rodrigues R, Tranquada R, Müller S, Gama K, Manso T. Injuries resulting from positioning for surgery: incidence and risk factors. *Acta Med Port*. 2013;26(1):12-16. [IIIC]

66. Strasser LA. Improving skin integrity in the perioperative environment using an evidence-based protocol. *J Dermatol Nurses Assoc*. 2012;4(6):351-362. [VA]

67. Winfree CJ, Kline DG. Intraoperative positioning nerve injuries. *Surg Neurol*. 2005;63(1):5-18. [VB]

68. Agostini J, Goasguen N, Mosnier H. Patient positioning in laparoscopic surgery: tricks and tips. *J Visc Surg*. 2010;147(4):e227-e232. [VB]

69. Cullen A, Ferguson A. Perioperative management of the severely obese patient: a selective pathophysiological review. *Can J Anesth*. 2012;59(10):974-996. [VA]

70. Sezer SD, Küçük M, Yüksel H, Odabaşi AR, Şen S, Ogurlu M. Drop foot, an unexpected complication of vaginal hysterectomy. *Turk Jinekoloji ve Obstetrik Dernegi Dergisi*. 2012;9(1):73-76. [VC]

71. Connor T, Sledge JA, Bryant-Wiersema L, Stamm L, Potter P. Identification of pre-operative and intra-operative variables predictive of pressure ulcer development in patients undergoing urologic surgical procedures. *Urol Nurs*. 2010;30(5):289-305. [IIB]

72. Thomas DR. Does pressure cause pressure ulcers? An inquiry into the etiology of pressure ulcers. *J Am Med Dir Assoc*. 2010;11(6):397-405. [VA]

73. Anusionwu IM, Wright EJ. Compartment syndrome after positioning in lithotomy: what a urologist needs to know. *BJU Int*. 2011;108(4):477-478. [VB]

74. Bushard S. Trauma in patients who are morbidly obese. *AORN J*. 2002;76(4):585-589. [VB]

75. Mackey D. Support surfaces: beds, mattresses, overlays—oh my! *Nurs Clin North Am*. 2005;40(2):251-265. [VB]

76. Pham B, Teague L, Mahoney J, et al. Support surfaces for intraoperative prevention of pressure ulcers in patients undergoing surgery: a cost-effectiveness analysis. *Surgery*. 2011;150(1):122-132. [IIIB]

77. Silverstein JW, Matthews E, Mermelstein LE, DeWal H. Causal factors for position-related SSEP changes in spinal surgery. *Eur Spine J*. 2016;25(10):3208-3213. [IIIB]

78. Parnham A. Pressure ulcer risk assessment and prevention in children. *Nurs Child Young People*. 2012;24(2):24-29. [VA]

79. Anthony D, Willock J, Baharestani M. A comparison of Braden Q, Garvin and Glamorgan risk assessment scales in paediatrics. *J Tissue Viability*. 2010;19(3):98-105. [IIIB]

80. Willock J, Anthony D, Richardson J. Inter-rater reliability of Glamorgan Paediatric Pressure Ulcer Risk Assessment Scale. *Paediatr Nurs*. 2008;20(7):14-19. [IIIB]

81. Huffines B, Logsdon MC. The Neonatal Skin Risk Assessment Scale for predicting skin breakdown in neonates. *Issues Compr Pediatr Nurs*. 1997;20(2):103-114. [IIIB]

82. McNichol L, Lund C, Rosen T, Gray M. Medical adhesives and patient safety: state of the science: consensus statements for the assessment, prevention, and treatment of adhesive-related skin injuries. *J Wound Ostomy Continence Nurs*. 2013;40(4):365-380. [IVB]

83. Dyer A. Ten top tips: Preventing device-related pressure ulcers. *Wounds Int*. 2015;6(1):9-13. [VB]

84. Larkin BG. The ins and outs of body piercing. *AORN J*. 2004;79(2):333-342. [VA]

85. Smith FD. Caring for surgical patients with piercings. *AORN J.* 2016;103(6):583-596. [VB]

86. Ogg MJ. Preventing alternate site burns from hair accessories during electrosurgery [Clinical Issues]. *AORN J.* 2012;95(4):545-547. [VB]

87. Cho JK, Han JH, Park SW, Kim KS. Deep vein thrombosis after spine operation in prone position with subclavian venous catheterization: a case report. *Korean J of Anesthesiol.* 2014;67(1):61-65. [VA]

88. Denholm B. Caring for surgical patients who have subdermal implants [Clinical Issues]. *AORN J.* 2013;97(3):372-375. [VA]

89. Identifying and minimizing risks for surgical patients with dermal implants. *AORN J.* 2012;96(4):C5-C6. [VB]

90. Guideline for safe use of energy-generating devices. In: *Guidelines for Perioperative Practice.* Denver, CO: AORN, Inc; 2017:129-156. [IVA]

91. Haldar R, Kaushal A, Srivastava S, Singh PK. Paediatric intravenous splint: a cause of pressure injury during neurosurgery in prone position. *Pediatr Neurosurg.* 2016;51(1):55-56. [VB]

92. Weng MH. The effect of protective treatment in reducing pressure ulcers for non-invasive ventilation patients. *Intensive Crit Care Nurs.* 2008;24(5):295-299. [IIB]

93. Kuo CY, Wootten CT, Tylor DA, Werkhaven JA, Huffman KF, Goudy SL. Prevention of pressure ulcers after pediatric tracheotomy using a Mepilex Ag dressing. *Laryngoscope.* 2013;123(12):3201-3205. [IIIB]

94. Huang TT, Tseng CE, Lee TM, Yeh JY, Lai YY. Preventing pressure sores of the nasal ala after nasotracheal tube intubation: from animal model to clinical application. *J Oral Maxillofac Surg.* 2009;67(3):543-551. [IIC]

95. Gunlemez A, Isken T, Gokalp AS, Turker G, Arisoy EA. Effect of silicon gel sheeting in nasal injury associated with nasal CPAP in preterm infants. *Indian Pediatr.* 2010;47(3):265-267. [IB]

96. Ulm MA, Fleming ND, Rallapali V, et al. Position-related injury is uncommon in robotic gynecologic surgery. *Gynecol Oncol.* 2014;135(3):534-538. [IIIB]

97. Makary MA, Holzmueller CG, Thompson D, et al. Operating room briefings: working on the same page. *Jt Comm J Qual Patient Saf.* 2006;32(6):351-355. [VB]

98. Makary MA, Holzmueller CG, Sexton JB, et al. Operating room debriefings. *Jt Comm J Qual Patient Saf.* 2006;32(7):407-410, 357. [VB]

99. *AORN Position Statement: Preventing Wrong-Patient, Wrong-Site, Wrong-Procedure Events.* AORN, Inc. http://www.aorn.org/guidelines/clinical-resources/position-statements. Accessed March 10, 2017. [IVB]

100. *WHO Surgical Safety Checklist.* World Health Organization. http://www.who.int/patientsafety/safesurgery/tools_resources/SSSL_Checklist_finalJun08.pdf?ua=1. Accessed March 10, 2017.

101. UP.01.03.01: A time-out is performed before the procedure. In: *Comprehensive Accreditation and Certification Manual: Critical Access Hospitals.* July 2016 ed. Oakbrook Terrace, IL: Joint Commission Resources; 2016.

102. UP.01.03.01: A time-out is performed before the procedure. In: *Comprehensive Accreditation and Certification Manual: Ambulatory.* July 2016 ed. Oakbrook Terrace, IL: Joint Commission Resources; 2016.

103. Guideline for product selection. In: *Guidelines for Perioperative Practice.* Denver, CO: AORN, Inc; 2017:183-190. [IVB]

104. Hoshowsky VM, Schramm CA. Intraoperative pressure sore prevention: an analysis of bedding materials. *Res Nurs Health.* 1994;17(5):333-339. [IB]

105. King CA, Bridges E. Comparison of pressure relief properties of operating room surfaces. *Perioper Nurs Clin.* 2006;1(3):261-265. [IIB]

106. Reddy M. Pressure ulcers. *BMJ Clin Evid.* 2011;2011:1901 [IIIA]

107. Wu T, Wang ST, Lin PC, Liu CL, Chao YF. Effects of using a high-density foam pad versus a viscoelastic polymer pad on the incidence of pressure ulcer development during spinal surgery. *Biol Res Nurs.* 2011;13(4):419-424. [IIA]

108. McInnes E, Jammali-Blasi A, Bell-Syer SEM, Dumville JC, Middleton V, Cullum N. Support surfaces for pressure ulcer prevention. *Cochrane Database Syst Rev.* 2015;(9):CD001735. [IIB]

109. McNichol L, Watts C, Mackey D, Beitz JM, Gray M. Identifying the right surface for the right patient at the right time: generation and content validation of an algorithm for support surface selection. *J Wound Ostomy Continence Nurs.* 2015;42(1):19-37. [IVA]

110. Deane LA, Lee HJ, Box GN, et al. Third place: flank position is associated with higher skin-to-surface interface pressures in men versus women: implications for laparoscopic renal surgery and the risk of rhabdomyolysis. *J Endourol.* 2008;22(6):1147-1151. [IIB]

111. *Guidelines for Environmental Infection Control in Health-Care Facilities: Recommendations of CDC and the Healthcare Infection Control Practices Advisory Committee (HICPAC).* Atlanta, GA: Centers for Disease Control and Prevention; 2003. https://www.cdc.gov/hicpac/pdf/guidelines/eic_in_HCF_03.pdf. Accessed March 10, 2017. [IVA]

112. Ahmad R, Tham J, Naqvi SG, Butt U, Dixon J. Supports used for positioning of patients in hip arthroplasty: is there an infection risk? *Ann R Coll Surg Engl.* 2011;93(2):130-132. [IIIC]

113. Guideline for environmental cleaning. In: *Guidelines for Perioperative Practice.* Denver, CO: AORN, Inc; 2017:7-28. [IVA]

114. Neurosurgical head holders (skull clamps) and device slippage: FDA safety communication. February 25, 2016. US Food and Drug Administration. https://www.fda.gov/MedicalDevices/Safety/AlertsandNotices/ucm487665.htm. Accessed March 10, 2017. [VA]

115. Dauber MH, Roth S. Operating table failure: another hazard of spine surgery. *Anesth Analg.* 2009;108(3):904-905. [VB]

116. Ahmad FU, Madhavan K, Trombly R, Levi AD. Anterior thigh compartment syndrome and local myonecrosis after posterior spine surgery on a Jackson table. *World Neurosurg.* 2012;78(5):553.e5-553.e8. [VB]

117. Flierl MA, Stahel PF, Hak DJ, Morgan SJ, Smith WR. Traction table-related complications in orthopaedic surgery. *J Am Acad Orthop Surg.* 2010;18(11):668-675. [VA]

118. Bonnaig N, Dailey S, Archdeacon M. Proper patient positioning and complication prevention in orthopaedic surgery. *J Bone Joint Surg Am.* 2014;96(13):1135-1140. [VB]

119. Mallet R, Tricoire JL, Rischmann P, Sarramon JP, Puget J, Malavaud B. High prevalence of erectile dysfunction in young male patients after intramedullary femoral nailing. *Urology.* 2005;65(3):559-563. [IIIB]

120. Toolan BC, Koval KJ, Kummer FJ, Goldsmith ME, Zuckerman JD. Effects of supine positioning and fracture post placement on the perineal countertraction force in awake volunteers. *J Orthop Trauma.* 1995;9(2):164-170. [IIIC]

121. MedWatch: The FDA Safety Information and Adverse Event Reporting Program. US Food and Drug Administration. https://www.fda.gov/Safety/MedWatch/. Accessed March 10, 2017.

122. Poli JC, Zoia C, Lattanzi D, Balbi S. Epidural haematoma by Mayfield head-holder: case report and review of literature. *J Pediatr Sci.* 2013;5:e195. [VA]

123. Berry C, Sandberg DI, Hoh DJ, Krieger MD, McComb JG. Use of cranial fixation pins in pediatric neurosurgery. *Neurosurgery.* 2008;62(4):913-918; discussion 918-919. [IIIB]

124. Chappy S. Perioperative patient safety: a multisite qualitative analysis. *AORN J.* 2006;83(4):871-877. [IIIB]

125. Waters T, Baptiste A, Short M, Plante-Mallon L, Nelson A. AORN ergonomic tool 1: lateral transfer of a patient from a stretcher to an OR bed. *AORN J.* 2011;93(3):334-339. [VA]

126. Waters T, Lloyd JD, Hernandez E, Nelson A. AORN ergonomic tool 7: pushing, pulling, and moving equipment on wheels. *AORN J.* 2011;94(3):254-260. [VA]

127. Asiedu GB, Lowndes BR, Huddleston PM, Hallbeck S. "The Jackson Table is a pain in the...": a qualitative study of providers' perception toward a spinal surgery table. *J Patient Saf.* January 7, 2016. Epub ahead of print. [IIIB]

128. Beyea SC. Preventing patient falls in perioperative settings. *AORN J.* 2005;81(2):393-395. [VB]

129. Redman JF, McNatt SJ. Portable cushioned operating table siderails: an adjunct to pediatric surgery. *South Med J.* 2000;93(11):1081-1082. [VC]

130. Chen HL, Chen XY, Wu J. The incidence of pressure ulcers in surgical patients of the last 5 years: a systematic review. *Wounds.* 2012;24(9):234-241. [IIIB]

131. Shon YJ, Bae SK, Park JW, Kim IN, Huh J. Partial displacement of epidural catheter after patient position change: a case report. *J Clin Anesth.* 2017;37:17-20. [VB]

132. Campbell K. Pressure point measures in the operating room. *J Enterostomal Ther.* 1989;16(3):119-124. [VB]

133. Lupe L, Zambrana D, Cooper L. Prevention of hospital-acquired pressure ulcers in the operating room and beyond: a successful monitoring and intervention strategy program. *Int Anesthesiol Clin.* 2013;51(1):128-146. [VB]

134. Grous CA, Reilly NJ, Gift AG. Skin integrity in patients undergoing prolonged operations. *J Wound Ostomy Continence Nurs.* 1997;24(2):86-91. [IIIB]

135. Whitney J, Phillips L, Aslam R, et al. Guidelines for the treatment of pressure ulcers. *Wound Repair Regen.* 2006;14(6):663-679. [IVB]

136. Landis EM. Micro-injection studies of capillary blood pressure in human skin. *Heart.* 1930;15:209-228. [IIIA]

137. Malkoun M, Huber J, Huber D. A comparative assessment of interface pressures generated by four surgical theatre heel pressure ulcer prophylactics. *Int Wound J.* 2012;9(3):259-263. [IIIB]

138. Kosiak M. Etiology and pathology of ischemic ulcers. *Arch Phys Med Rehabil.* 1959;40(2):62-69. [IIIB]

139. Sutton S, Link T, Makic MB. A quality improvement project for safe and effective patient positioning during robot-assisted surgery. *AORN J.* 2013;97(4):448-456. [VB]

140. Fletcher J, Harris C, Mahoney K. A small-scale evaluation of the Dolphin Fluid Immersion Simulation® Mattress. *Wounds UK.* 2014;10(1):97-100. [VC]

141. Worsley PR, Parsons B, Bader DL. An evaluation of fluid immersion therapy for the prevention of pressure ulcers. *Clin Biomech (Bristol Avon).* 2016;40:27-32. [IIIB]

142. Kirkland-Walsh H, Teleten O, Wilson M, Raingruber B. Pressure mapping comparison of four OR surfaces. *AORN J.* 2015;102(1):61.e1-61.e9. [IIIB]

143. Akhavan A, Gainsburg DM, Stock JA. Complications associated with patient positioning in urologic surgery. *Urology.* 2010;76(6):1309-1316. [VB]

144. Martin JT, Warner MA. *Positioning in Anesthesia and Surgery.* 3rd ed. Philadelphia, PA: Saunders; 1997.

145. Stephenson LL, Webb NA, Smithers CJ, Sager SL, Seefelder C. Lateral femoral cutaneous neuropathy following lateral positioning on a bean bag. *J Clin Anesth.* 2009;21(5):383-384. [VB]

146. National Institute for Health and Care Excellence. *The Prevention and Management of Pressure Ulcers in Primary and Secondary Care. Clinical Guideline No. 179. Methods, Evidence, and Recommendations.* London, UK: National Clinical Guideline Centre; 2014:1-416. [IVA]

147. American College of Surgeons National Surgical Quality Improvement Program, American Geriatrics Society. *Optimal Perioperative Management of the Geriatric Patient.* American College of Surgeons. https://www.facs.org/~/media/files/quality%20programs/geriatric/acs%20nsqip%20geriatric%202016%20guidelines.ashx. Accessed March 10, 2017. [IVB]

148. Santamaria N, Gerdtz M, Sage S, et al. A randomised controlled trial of the effectiveness of soft silicone multi-layered foam dressings in the prevention of sacral and heel pressure ulcers in trauma and critically ill patients: the border trial. *Int Wound J.* 2015;12(3):302-308. [IB]

149. Brindle CT, Wegelin JA. Prophylactic dressing application to reduce pressure ulcer formation in cardiac surgery patients. *J Wound Ostomy Continence Nurs.* 2012;39(2):133-142. [IIB]

150. Moore ZE, Webster J. Dressings and topical agents for preventing pressure ulcers. *Cochrane Database Syst Rev.* 2013;(8):CD009362. [IB]

151. Call E, Pedersen J, Bill B, et al. Enhancing pressure ulcer prevention using wound dressings: what are the modes of action? *Int Wound J.* 2015;12(4):408-413. [IIIB]

152. Walsh NS, Blanck AW, Smith L, Cross M, Andersson L, Polito C. Use of a sacral silicone border foam dressing as one component of a pressure ulcer prevention program in an intensive care unit setting. *J Wound Ostomy Continence Nurs.* 2012;39(2):146-149. [VB]

153. Chaiken N. Reduction of sacral pressure ulcers in the intensive care unit using a silicone border foam dressing. *J Wound Ostomy Continence Nurs.* 2012;39(2):143-145. [VB]

154. Forni C, Loro L, Tremosini M, et al. Use of polyurethane foam inside plaster casts to prevent the onset of heel sores in the population at risk. A controlled clinical study. *J Clin Nurs.* 2011;20(5-6):675-680. [IIB]

155. Call E, Pedersen J, Bill B, Oberg C, Ferguson-Pell M. Microclimate impact of prophylactic dressings using in vitro body analog method. *Wounds.* 2013;25(4):94-103. [IIIB]

156. Zhang J, Moore AE, Stringer MD. Iatrogenic upper limb nerve injuries: a systematic review. *ANZ J Surg.* 2011;81(4):227-236. [VB]

157. Bale E, Berrecloth R. The obese patient. Anaesthetic issues: airway and positioning. *J Perioper Pract.* 2010;20(8):294-299. [VB]

158. Kam AW, Lam PH, Murrell GAC. Brachial plexus injuries during shoulder arthroplasty: what causes them and how to prevent them. *Tech Shoulder Elbow Surg.* 2015;15(4):109-114. [VA]

159. Colsa Gutierrez P, Viadero Cervera R, Morales-Garcia D, Ingelmo Setien A. Intraoperative peripheral nerve injury in colorectal surgery. An update. *Cir Esp.* 2016;94(3):125-136. [VA]

160. Shimizu S, Sato K, Mabuchi I, et al. Brachial plexopathy due to massive swelling of the neck associated with craniotomy in the park bench position. *Surg Neurol.* 2009;71(4):504-508. [VB]

161. Uribe JS, Kolla J, Omar H, et al. Brachial plexus injury following spinal surgery. *J Neurosurg Spine.* 2010;13(4):552-558. [VB]

162. Lin SP, Sung CS, Chan KH. Compartment syndrome and rhabdomyolysis as a positioning complication following retrosigmoid craniotomy. *Acta Anaesthesiol Taiwan.* 2013;51(4):184-186. [VB]

163. Ortega R, Suzuki S, Sekhar P, Stram JR, Rengasamy SK. Paraplegia after mastoidectomy under general anesthesia. *Am J Otolaryngol.* 2009;30(5):340-342. [VB]

164. Singha SK, Chatterjee N. Postoperative sialadenitis following retromastoid suboccipital craniectomy for posterior fossa tumor. *J Anesth.* 2009;23(4):591-593. [VB]

165. Postaci A, Aytac I, Dikmen B, Oztekin CV. Acute unilateral parotid gland swelling after lateral decubitus position under general anesthesia. *Saudi J Anaesth.* 2012;6(3):295-297. [VB]

166. Hsieh CT, Liu MY, Chen YH, Chang CF. Postoperative acute sialadenitis following posterior fossa surgery. *Neurosciences.* 2011;16(4):378-380. [VB]

167. Kim LJ, Klopfenstein JD, Feiz-Erfan I, Zubay GP, Spetzler RF. Postoperative acute sialadenitis after skull base surgery. *Skull Base.* 2008;18(2):129-133. [VB]

168. Asghar A, Karam K, Rashid S. A case of anesthesia mumps after sacral laminectomy under general anesthesia. *Saudi J Anaesth.* 2015;9(3):332-333. [VC]

169. Morrison CM, Dobryansky M, Warren RJ, Zins JE. The table tilt: preventing traction on the brachial plexus during facelift surgery. *Aesthet Surg J.* 2012;32(4):524. [VC]

170. Khokhar RS, Baaj J, Alhazmi HH, Dammas FA, Aldalati AM. Pressure-induced alopecia in pediatric patients following prolonged urological surgeries: the case reports and a review of literature. *Anesth Essays Res.* 2015;9(3):430-432. [VB]

171. Davies KE, Yesudian P. Pressure alopecia. *Int J Trichology.* 2012;4(2):64-68. [VB]

172. Gollapalli L, Papapetrou P, Gupta D, Fuleihan SF. Postoperative alopecia after robotic surgery in steep Trendelenburg position: a restated observation of pressure alopecia. *Middle East J Anesthesiol.* 2013;22(3):343-345. [VC]

173. Keidan I, Ben-Menchem E. Postoperative occipital nerve injury in a child. *Anaesth Intensive Care.* 2012;40(2):355-356. [VB]

174. Lee C, Choi PD, Scott G, Arkader A. Postoperative alopecia in children after orthopaedic surgery. *J Pediatr Orthop.* 2012;32(7):e53-e55. [VA]

175. Goodenough J, Highgate J, Shaaban H. Under pressure? Alopecia related to surgical duration. *Br J Anaesth.* 2014;113(2):306-307. [VC]

176. Matsushita K, Inoue N, Ooi K, Totsuka Y. Postoperative pressure-induced alopecia after segmental osteotomy at the upper and lower frontal edentulous areas for distraction osteogenesis. *Oral Maxillofac Surg.* 2011;15(3):161-163. [VB]

177. Bagaria M, Luck AM. Postoperative (pressure) alopecia following sacrocolpopexy. *J Robot Surg.* 2015;9(2):149-151. [VB]

178. Duimel-Peeters I, Halfens R, Berger M, Snoeckx L. The effects of massage as a method to prevent pressure ulcers. A review of the literature. *Ostomy Wound Manage.* 2005;51(4):70-80. [VB]

179. Ghomi A. Robotics in practice: new angles on safer positioning. Contemporary OB/GYN. http://contemporaryobgyn.modernmedicine.com/contemporary-obgyn/news/modernmedicine/modern-medicine-feature-articles/robotics-practice-new-angles?page=full. Published October 1, 2012. Accessed March 10, 2017. [VB]

180. Kan KM, Brown SE, Gainsburg DM. Ocular complications in robotic-assisted prostatectomy: a review of pathophysiology and prevention. *Minerva Anestesiol.* 2015;81(5):557-566. [VA]

181. Grixti A, Sadri M, Watts MT. Corneal protection during general anesthesia for nonocular surgery. *Ocul Surf.* 2013;11(2):109-118. [VB]

182. Freshcoln M, Diehl MR. Repositioning during robotic procedures to prevent postoperative visual loss. *OR Nurse.* 2014;8(4):36-41. [VC]

183. Kocatürk O, Kocatürk T, Kaan N, Dayanir V. The comparison of four different methods of perioperative eye protection under general anesthesia in prone position. *J Clin Anal Med.* 2012;3(2):163-165. [IIB]

184. Roth S. Perioperative visual loss: what do we know, what can we do? *Br J Anaesth.* 2009;103(Suppl 1):31-40. [VA]

185. Olsen GH, Krishna SG, Jatana KR, et al. Changes in intracuff pressure of cuffed endotracheal tubes while positioning for adenotonsillectomy in children. *Paediatr Anaesth.* 2016;26(5):500-503. [IIIB]

186. Anghelescu DL, Burgoyne LL, Khan RB. Multiple mechanisms of perioperative brachial plexus injury. *Anaesth Intensive Care.* 2008;36(2):276-278. [VB]

187. Truong AT, Sturgis EM, Rozner MA, Truong DT. Recurrent episodes of asystole from carotid sinus hypersensitivity triggered by positioning for head and neck surgery. *Head Neck.* 2013;35(1):E28-E30. [VB]

188. Li CC, Yie JC, Lai CH, Hung MH. Quadriplegia after off-pump coronary artery bypass surgery: look before you place the neck in an extended position. *J Cardiothorac Vasc Anesth.* 2013;27(2):e16-e17. [VB]

189. Reddy MKR, Arivazhagan A, Chandramouli BA. Intractable hypotension and bradycardia during surgical positioning in atlantoaxial dislocation. *J Neurosurg Anesthesiol.* 2008;20(1):71. [VC]

190. Addas BM. An uncommon cause of brachial plexus injury. *Neurosciences.* 2012;17(1):64-65. [VB]

191. St-Arnaud D, Paquin MJ. Safe positioning for neurosurgical patients. *AORN J.* 2008;87(6):1156-1168. [VA]

192. Ahmed K, Khan N, Khan MS, Dasgupta P. Development and content validation of a surgical safety checklist for operating theatres that use robotic technology. *BJU Int.* 2013;111(7):1161-1174. [VA]

193. Teeples TJ, Rallis DJ, Rieck KL, Viozzi CF. Lower extremity compartment syndrome associated with hypotensive general anesthesia for orthognathic surgery: a case report and review of the disease. *J Oral Maxillofac Surg.* 2010;68(5):1166-1170. [VB]

194. Judge A, Fecho K. Lateral antebrachial cutaneous neuropathy as a result of positioning while under general anesthesia. *Anesth Analg.* 2010;110(1):122-124. [VB]

195. Moore C. Intraoperative median nerve injury. *Int Student J Nurse Anesth.* 2011;10(2):11-14. [VB]

196. Song JB, Vemana G, Mobley JM, Bhayani SB. The second "time-out": a surgical safety checklist for lengthy robotic surgeries. *Patient Saf Surg.* 2013;7(1):19. [VC]

197. Drummond JC, Ciacci JD, Lee RR. Direct pressure on a pseudomeningocele resulting in intraoperative cerebral ischemia. *Can J Anaesth.* 2014;61(7):656-659. [VB]

198. Anastasian ZH, Ramnath B, Komotar RJ, et al. Evoked potential monitoring identifies possible neurological injury during positioning for craniotomy. *Anesth Analg.* 2009;109(3):817-821. [VB]

199. Jahangiri FR, Holmberg A, Vega-Bermudez F, Arlet V. Preventing position-related brachial plexus injury with intraoperative somatosensory evoked potentials and transcranial electrical motor evoked potentials during anterior cervical spine surgery. *Am J Electroneurodiagnostic Technol.* 2011;51(3):198-205. [VB]

200. Silverstein JW, Madhok R, Frendo CD, DeWal H, Lee GR. Contemporaneous evaluation of intraoperative ulnar and median nerve somatosensory evoked potentials for patient positioning: a review of four cases. *Neurodiagn J.* 2016;56(2):67-82. [VB]

201. Chung I, Glow JA, Dimopoulos V, et al. Upper-limb somatosensory evoked potential monitoring in lumbosacral spine surgery: a prognostic marker for position-related ulnar nerve injury. *Spine J.* 2009;9(4):287-295. [IIB]

202. La Neve JE, Zitney GP. Use of somatosensory evoked potentials to detect and prevent impending brachial plexus injury during surgical positioning for the treatment of supratentorial pathologies. *Neurodiagn J.* 2014;54(3):260-273. [VA]

203. Davis SF, Khalek Mohamed Abdel, Giles J, Fox C, Lirette L, Kandil E. Detection and prevention of impending brachial plexus injury secondary to arm positioning using ulnar nerve somatosensory evoked potentials during transaxillary approach for thyroid lobectomy. *Am J Electroneurodiagnostic Technol.* 2011;51(4):274-279. [VB]

204. Jellish WS, Sherazee G, Patel J, et al. Somatosensory evoked potentials help prevent positioning-related brachial plexus injury during skull base surgery. *Otolaryngol Head Neck Surg.* 2013;149(1):168-173. [IIIA]

205. Ying T, Wang X, Sun H, Tang Y, Yuan Y, Li S. Clinical usefulness of somatosensory evoked potentials for detection of peripheral nerve and brachial plexus injury secondary to malpositioning in microvascular decompression. *J Clin Neurophysiol.* 2015;32(6):512-515. [IIIA]

206. Schwartz DM, Sestokas AK, Hilibrand AS, et al. Neurophysiological identification of position-induced neurologic injury during anterior cervical spine surgery. *J Clin Monit Comput.* 2006;20(6):437-444. [IIIB]

207. Bhalodia VM, Sestokas AK, Tomak PR, Schwartz DM. Transcranial electric motor evoked potential detection of compressional peroneal nerve injury in the lateral decubitus position. *J Clin Monit Comput.* 2008;22(4):319-326. [VB]

208. Eager M, Shimer A, Jahangiri FR, Shen F, Arlet V. Intraoperative neurophysiological monitoring (IONM): lessons learned from 32 case events in 2069 spine cases. *Neurodiagn J.* 2011;51(4):247-263. [IIIA]

209. Bennicoff G. Perioperative care of the morbidly obese patient in the lithotomy position. *AORN J.* 2010;92(3):297-309. [VB]

210. Rosevear HM, Lightfoot AJ, Zahs M, Waxman SW, Winfield HN. Lessons learned from a case of calf compartment syndrome after robot-assisted laparoscopic prostatectomy. *J Endourol.* 2010;24(10):1597-1601. [VA]

211. Pandey R, Elakkumanan LB, Garg R, et al. Brachial plexus injury after robotic-assisted thoracoscopic thymectomy. *J Cardiothorac Vasc Anesth.* 2009;23(4):584-586. [VB]

212. Hobaika AB, Horiguchi CH. Radial nerve lesion after malposition and sedation by continuous target controlled infusion of propofol for extracorporeal shock wave lithotripsy. *Middle East J Anesthesiol.* 2013;22(2):235-236. [VC]

213. Neutral position of a joint. The Free Dictionary. http://medical-dictionary.thefreedictionary.com/neutral+position+of+joint. Accessed March 10, 2017.

214. Bradshaw AD, Advincula AP. Optimizing patient positioning and understanding radiofrequency energy in gynecologic surgery. *Clin Obstet Gynecol.* 2010;53(3):511-520. [VB]

215. Clark JM, Friedell ML, Gupta BR, Davenport WC, Amponsah K. Perioperative compartment syndrome of the hand. *Am Surg.* 2011;77(1):116-118. [VA]

216. Hida A, Arai T, Nakanishi K, Nagaro T. Bilateral brachial plexus injury after liver transplantation. *J Anesth.* 2008;22(3):308-311. [VB]

217. Akinbingol G, Borman H, Maral T. Bilateral brachial plexus palsy after a prolonged surgical procedure of reduction mammaplasty, abdominoplasty, and liposuction. *Ann Plast Surg.* 2002;49(2):219-220. [VC]

218. Tekin L, Akarsu S, Carli A, et al. Brachial plexus lesion due to malpositioning during thyroid surgery: a case report. *J Phys Med Rehabil Sci.* 2011;14(3-4):80-84. [VB]

219. Sabiniewicz R, Ereciński J, Zipser M. Brachial plexus injury as an unusual complication after aortic stent implantation. *Cardiol Young.* 2011;21(2):227-228. [VB]

220. Cristian DA, Grama FA, Burcos T, Poalelungi A. Brachial plexus injury after a left-side modified radical mastectomy associated with patient positioning in the operating room. *Gineco.eu.* 2013;9(3):136-137. [VB]

221. Chowet AL, Lopez JR, Brock-Utne JG, Jaffe RA. Wrist hyperextension leads to median nerve conduction block:

implications for intra-arterial catheter placement. *Anesthesiology.* 2004;100(2):287-291. [IIB]

222. Huber D. Preventing deep tissue injury of the foot and ankle in the operating theatre. *Wounds UK.* 2013;9(2):34-38. [VB]

223. Huber D, Huber J, DeYoung E. The association between popliteal vein compression and deep venous thrombosis: results of a pilot study. *Phlebology.* 2013;28(6):305-307. [IIIB]

224. Huber DE, Huber JP. Popliteal vein compression under general anaesthesia. *Eur J Vasc Endovasc Surg.* 2009;37(4):464-469. [IIIB]

225. Levine A, Huber J, Huber D. Changes in popliteal vein diameter and flow velocity with knee flexion and hyperextension. *Phlebology.* 2011;26(7):307-310. [IIIB]

226. O'Connor D, Breslin D, Barry M. Well-leg compartment syndrome following supine position surgery. *Anaesth Intensive Care.* 2010;38(3):595. [VB]

227. Wong VK, Stotts NA, Hopf HW, Dowling GA, Froelicher ES. Changes in heel skin temperature under pressure in hip surgery patients. *Adv Skin Wound Care.* 2011;24(12):562-570. [IIC]

228. Donnelly J, Winder J, Kernohan WG, Stevenson M. An RCT to determine the effect of a heel elevation device in pressure ulcer prevention post-hip fracture. *J Wound Care.* 2011;20(7):309-318. [IA]

229. Primiano M, Friend M, McClure C, et al. Pressure ulcer prevalence and risk factors during prolonged surgical procedures. *AORN J.* 2011;94(6):555-566. [IIIA]

230. O'Shea E, Power K. Well leg compartment syndrome following prolonged surgery in the supine position. *Can J Anaesth.* 2008;55(11):794-795. [VB]

231. Physiologic. The Free Dictionary. http://medical-diction ary.thefreedictionary.com/physiologic. Accessed March 10, 2017.

232. Albrecht P, Grosse J, Neukaeter W. Femoral neuropathy caused by hyperlordotic positioning. *J Anesth.* 2014;28(5):800. [VC]

233. Ghomi A, Kramer C, Askari R, Chavan NR, Einarsson JI. Trendelenburg position in gynecologic robotic-assisted surgery. *J Minim Invasive Gynecol.* 2012;19(4):485-489. [IIIC]

234. Brodsky JB. Positioning the morbidly obese patient for anesthesia. *Obes Surg.* 2002;12(6):751-758. [VB]

235. Ideno S, Miyazawa N, Yamamoto S. Muscle injury following laparoscopic appendectomy. *J Anesth.* 2014;28(5):801. [VB]

236. Kamel I, Barnette R. Positioning patients for spine surgery: avoiding uncommon position-related complications. *World J Orthop.* 2014;5(4):425-443. [VA]

237. Awad H, Santilli S, Ohr M, et al. The effects of steep Trendelenburg positioning on intraocular pressure during robotic radical prostatectomy. *Anesth Analg.* 2009;109(2):473-478. [IIB]

238. Borahay MA, Patel PR, Walsh TM, et al. Intraocular pressure and steep Trendelenburg during minimally invasive gynecologic surgery: is there a risk? *J Minim Invasive Gynecol.* 2013;20(6):819-824. [IIB]

239. Taketani Y, Mayama C, Suzuki N, et al. Transient but significant visual field defects after robot-assisted laparoscopic radical prostatectomy in deep Trendelenburg position. *Plos One.* 2015;10(4):e0123361. [IIIB]

240. Astuto M, Minardi C, Uva MG, Gullo A. Intraocular pressure during laparoscopic surgery in paediatric patients. *Br J Ophthalmol.* 2011;95(2):294-295. [IIC]

241. Mondzelewski TJ, Schmitz JW, Christman MS, et al. Intraocular pressure during robotic-assisted laparoscopic procedures utilizing steep Trendelenburg positioning. *J Glaucoma.* 2015;24(6):399-404. [IIIB]

242. Molloy BL. Implications for postoperative visual loss: steep Trendelenburg position and effects on intraocular pressure. *AANA J.* 2011;79(2):115-121. [IIIB]

243. Rewari V, Ramachandran R. Prolonged steep Trendelenburg position: risk of postoperative upper airway obstruction. *J Robot Surg.* 2013;7(4):405-406. [VB]

244. Kalmar AF, Dewaele F, Foubert L, et al. Cerebral haemodynamic physiology during steep Trendelenburg position and CO_2 pneumoperitoneum. *Br J Anaesth.* 2012;108(3):478-484. [IIIB]

245. Choi SH, Lee SJ, Rha KH, Shin SK, Oh YJ. The effect of pneumoperitoneum and Trendelenburg position on acute cerebral blood flow-carbon dioxide reactivity under sevoflurane anaesthesia. *Anaesthesia.* 2008;63(12):1314-1318. [IIA]

246. Closhen D, Treiber AH, Berres M, et al. Robotic assisted prostatic surgery in the Trendelenburg position does not impair cerebral oxygenation measured using two different monitors: a clinical observational study. *Eur J Anaesthesiol.* 2014;31(2):104-109. [IIA]

247. Park EY, Koo BN, Min KT, Nam SH. The effect of pneumoperitoneum in the steep Trendelenburg position on cerebral oxygenation. *Acta Anaesthesiol Scand.* 2009;53(7):895-899. [IIIB]

248. Lahaye L, Grasso M, Green J, Biddle CJ. Cerebral tissue O2 saturation during prolonged robotic surgery in the steep Trendelenburg position: an observational case series in a diverse surgical population. *J Robot Surg.* 2015;9(1):19-25. [IIB]

249. Barr C, Madhuri TK, Prabhu P, Butler-Manuel S, Tailor A. Cerebral oedema following robotic surgery: a rare complication. *Arch Gynecol Obstet.* 2014;290(5):1041-1044. [VB]

250. Chin JH, Seo H, Lee EH, et al. Sonographic optic nerve sheath diameter as a surrogate measure for intracranial pressure in anesthetized patients in the Trendelenburg position. *BMC Anesthesiol.* 2015;15:43. [IIB]

251. Shah SB, Bhargava AK, Choudhury I. Noninvasive intracranial pressure monitoring via optic nerve sheath diameter for robotic surgery in steep Trendelenburg position. *Saudi J Anaesth.* 2015;9(3):239-246. [IA]

252. Kim MS, Bai SJ, Lee JR, Choi YD, Kim YJ, Choi SH. Increase in intracranial pressure during carbon dioxide pneumoperitoneum with steep Trendelenburg positioning proven by ultrasonographic measurement of optic nerve sheath diameter. *J Endourol.* 2014;28(7):801-806. [IIIB]

253. Kim SH, Kim HJ, Jung KT. Position does not affect the optic nerve sheath diameter during laparoscopy. *Korean J Anesthesiol.* 2015;68(4):358-363. [IIIC]

254. Gkegkes ID, Karydis A, Tyritzis SI, Iavazzo C. Ocular complications in robotic surgery. *Int J Med Robot.* 2015;11(3):269-274. [IIIB]

255. Grosso A, Scozzari G, Bert F, Mabilia MA, Siliquini R, Morino M. Intraocular pressure variation during colorectal laparoscopic surgery: standard pneumoperitoneum leads to reversible elevation in intraocular pressure. *Surg Endosc.* 2013;27(9):3370-3376. [IIB]

256. Grosso A, Ceruti P, Morino M, Marchini G, Amisano M, Fioretto M. Comment on the paper by Mondzelewski and colleagues: "Intraocular pressure during robotic-assisted

laparoscopic procedures utilizing steep Trendelenburg positioning." *J Glaucoma.* 2015;24(6):399–404. *J Glaucoma.* August 22, 2016. Epub ahead of print. [VB]

257. Hoshikawa Y, Tsutsumi N, Ohkoshi K, et al. The effect of steep Trendelenburg positioning on intraocular pressure and visual function during robotic-assisted radical prostatectomy. *Br J Ophthalmol.* 2014;98(3):305-308. [IIB]

258. De Leon A, Thörn S-E, Ottosson J, Wattwil M. Body positions and esophageal sphincter pressures in obese patients during anesthesia. *Acta Anaesthesiol Scand.* 2010;54(4):458-463. [IIB]

259. Choi DK, Lee IG, Hwang JH. Arterial to end-tidal carbon dioxide pressure gradient increases with age in the steep Trendelenburg position with pneumoperitoneum. *Korean J Anesthesiol.* 2012;63(3):209-215. [IIA]

260. Kilic OF, Borgers A, Kohne W, Musch M, Kropfl D, Groeben H. Effects of steep Trendelenburg position for robotic-assisted prostatectomies on intra- and extrathoracic airways in patients with or without chronic obstructive pulmonary disease. *Br J Anaesth.* 2015;114(1):70-76. [IIB]

261. Wysham WZ, Kim KH, Roberts JM, et al. Obesity and perioperative pulmonary complications in robotic gynecologic surgery. *Am J Obstet Gynecol.* 2015;213(1):33.e1-33.e7. [IIIB]

262. Chin YS. Bradycardia caused by position change. *J Anesth.* 2012;26(3):475-476. [VB]

263. Darlong V, Kunhabdulla NP, Pandey R, et al. Hemodynamic changes during robotic radical prostatectomy. *Saudi J Anaesth.* 2012;6(3):213-218. [IIB]

264. Lowenstein L, Mustafa M, Burke YZ, Mustafa S, Segal D, Weissman A. Steep Trendelenburg position during robotic sacrocolpopexy and heart rate variability. *Eur J Obstet Gynecol Reprod Biol.* 2014;178:66-69. [IIIB]

265. Zorko N, Mekis D, Kamenik M. The influence of the Trendelenburg position on haemodynamics: comparison of anaesthetized patients with ischaemic heart disease and healthy volunteers. *J Int Med Res.* 2011;39(3):1084-1089. [IIC]

266. Russo A, Marana E, Viviani D, et al. Diastolic function: the influence of pneumoperitoneum and Trendelenburg positioning during laparoscopic hysterectomy. *Eur J Anaesthesiol.* 2009;26(11):923-927. [IIIB]

267. Meininger D, Westphal K, Bremerich DH, et al. Effects of posture and prolonged pneumoperitoneum on hemodynamic parameters during laparoscopy. *World J Surg.* 2008;32(7):1400-1405. [IIIB]

268. Kalmar AF, Foubert L, Hendrickx JF, et al. Influence of steep Trendelenburg position and CO(2) pneumoperitoneum on cardiovascular, cerebrovascular, and respiratory homeostasis during robotic prostatectomy. *Br J Anaesth.* 2010; 104(4):433-439. [IIIB]

269. Lestar M, Gunnarsson L, Lagerstrand L, Wiklund P, Odeberg-Wernerman S. Hemodynamic perturbations during robot-assisted laparoscopic radical prostatectomy in 45-degree Trendelenburg position. *Anesth Analg.* 2011;113(5):1069-1075. [IIIC]

270. Haas S, Haese A, Goetz AE, Kubitz JC. Haemodynamics and cardiac function during robotic-assisted laparoscopic prostatectomy in steep Trendelenburg position. *Int J Med Robot.* 2011;7(4):408-413. [IIB]

271. Mekiš D, Kamenik M. Influence of body position on hemodynamics in patients with ischemic heart disease undergoing cardiac surgery. *Wien Klin Wochenschr.* 2010;122(Suppl 2):59-62. [IIIB]

272. Wen T, Deibert CM, Siringo FS, Spencer BA. Positioning-related complications of minimally invasive radical prostatectomies. *J Endourol.* 2014;28(6):660-667. [IIIB]

273. Gould C, Cull T, Wu YX, Osmundsen B. Blinded measure of Trendelenburg angle in pelvic robotic surgery. *J Minim Invasive Gynecol.* 2012;19(4):465-468. [IIB]

274. Schramm P, Treiber AH, Berres M, et al. Time course of cerebrovascular autoregulation during extreme Trendelenburg position for robotic-assisted prostatic surgery. *Anaesthesia.* 2014;69(1):58-63. [IIIB]

275. Kadono Y, Yaegashi H, Machioka K, et al. Cardiovascular and respiratory effects of the degree of head-down angle during robot-assisted laparoscopic radical prostatectomy. *Int J Med Robot.* 2013;9(1):17-22. [IB]

276. Raz O, Boesel TW, Arianayagam M, et al. The effect of the modified Z Trendelenburg position on intraocular pressure during robotic assisted laparoscopic radical prostatectomy: a randomized, controlled study. *J Urol.* 2015;193(4):1213-1219. [IB]

277. Shveiky D, Aseff JN, Iglesia CB. Brachial plexus injury after laparoscopic and robotic surgery. *J Minim Invasive Gynecol.* 2010;17(4):414-420. [VB]

278. Addison AB, Inarra E, Watts S. Bilateral otorrhagia: a rare complication of laparoscopic abdominopelvic surgery. *BMJ Case Rep.* December 19, 2014;2014. [VB]

279. Pandey R, Garg R, Darlong V, Punj J, Chandralekha, Kumar A. Unpredicted neurological complications after robotic laparoscopic radical cystectomy and ileal conduit formation in steep Trendelenburg position: two case reports. *Acta Anaesthesiol Belg.* 2010;61(3):163-166. [VB]

280. Pinkney TD, King AJ, Walter C, Wilson TR, Maxwell-Armstrong C, Acheson AG. Raised intraocular pressure (IOP) and perioperative visual loss in laparoscopic colorectal surgery: a catastrophe waiting to happen? A systematic review of evidence from other surgical specialities. *Tech Coloproctol.* 2012;16(5):331-335. [IIIB]

281. Mizrahi H, Hugkulstone CE, Vyakarnam P, Parker MC. Bilateral ischaemic optic neuropathy following laparoscopic proctocolectomy: a case report. *Ann R Coll Surg Engl.* 2011;93(5):e53-e54. [VB]

282. Kumar G, Vyakarnam P. Postoperative vision loss after colorectal laparoscopic surgery. *Surg Laparosc Endosc Percutan Tech.* 2013;23(2):e87-88. [VB]

283. Nuzzi R, Tridico F. Ocular complications in laparoscopic surgery: review of existing literature and possible prevention and treatment. *Semin Ophthalmol.* 2016;31(6):584-592. [VB]

284. Codd RJ, Evans MD, Sagar PM, Williams GL. A systematic review of peripheral nerve injury following laparoscopic colorectal surgery. *Colorectal Dis.* 2013;15(3):278-282. [IIIB]

285. Mattei A, Di Pierro GB, Rafeld V, Konrad C, Beutler J, Danuser H. Positioning injury, rhabdomyolysis, and serum creatine kinase-concentration course in patients undergoing robot-assisted radical prostatectomy and extended pelvic lymph node dissection. *J Endourol.* 2013;27(1):45-51. [IIIB]

286. Klauschie J, Wechter ME, Jacob K, et al. Use of anti-skid material and patient-positioning to prevent patient shifting during robotic-assisted gynecologic procedures. *J Minim Invasive Gynecol.* 2010;17(4):504-507. [IIIC]

287. Wechter ME, Kho RM, Chen AH, Magrina JF, Pettit PD. Preventing slide in Trendelenburg position: Randomized trial comparing foam and gel pads. *J Robot Surg.* 2013;7(3):267-271. [IA]

288. Nakayama JM, Gerling GJ, Horst KE, Fitz VW, Cantrell LA, Modesitt SC. A simulation study of the factors influencing the risk of intraoperative slipping. *Clin Ovarian Other Gynecol Cancer.* 2014;7(1-2):24-28. [IIIB]

289. Talab SS, Elmi A, Sarma J, Barrisford GW, Tabatabaei S. Safety and effectiveness of SAF-R, a novel patient positioning device for robot-assisted pelvic surgery in Trendelenburg position. *J Endourol.* 2016;30(3):286-292. [IIIC]

290. Hewer CL. The physiology and complications of the Trendelenburg position. *Can Med Assoc J.* 1956;74(4):285-288. [VB]

291. Kalmar AF, De Wolf AM, Hendrickx JFA. Anesthetic considerations for robotic surgery in the steep Trendelenburg position. *Adv Anesth.* 2012;30(1):75-96. [VA]

292. Wu CY, Yeh YC, Wang MC, Lai CH, Fan SZ. Changes in endotracheal tube cuff pressure during laparoscopic surgery in head-up or head-down position. *BMC Anesthesiol.* 2014;14:75. [IIB]

293. Coppieters MW, Van de Velde M, Stappaerts KH. Positioning in anesthesiology: toward a better understanding of stretch-induced perioperative neuropathies. *Anesthesiology.* 2002;97(1):75-81. [IIB]

294. Suozzi BA, Brazell HD, O'Sullivan DM, Tulikangas PK. A comparison of shoulder pressure among different patient stabilization techniques. *Am J Obstet Gynecol.* 2013;209(5):478.e1-478.e5. [IIIB]

295. Devarajan J, Byrd JB, Gong MC, et al. Upper and middle trunk brachial plexopathy after robotic prostatectomy. *Anesth Analg.* 2012;115(4):867-870. [VA]

296. Eteuati J, Hiscock R, Hastie I, Hayes I, Jones I. Brachial plexopathy in laparoscopic-assisted rectal surgery: a case series. *Tech Coloproctol.* 2013;17(3):293-297. [VB]

297. Vaughan RW, Wise L. Intraoperative arterial oxygenation in obese patients. *Ann Surg.* 1976;184(1):35-42. [IIB]

298. An J, Shin SK, Kwon J-Y, Kim KJ. Incidence of venous air embolism during myomectomy: the effect of patient position. *Yonsei Med J.* 2013;54(1):209-214. [IA]

299. Ghai A, Saini S, Kiran S, Kamal K, Kad N, Bhawna. Influence of lithotomy position on the haemodynamic changes in patients with coronary artery disease. *J Anaesthesiol Clin Pharmacol.* 2008;24(3):359-360. [VB]

300. Roeder RA, Geddes LA, Corson N, Pell C, Otlewski M, Kemeny A. Heel and calf capillary-support: pressure in lithotomy positions. *AORN J.* 2005;81(4):821-830. [IIIB]

301. Wilde S. Compartment syndrome. The silent danger related to patient positioning and surgery. *Br J Perioper Nurs.* 2004;14(12):546-550. [VC]

302. Bauer EC, Koch N, Janni W, Bender HG, Fleisch MC. Compartment syndrome after gynecologic operations: evidence from case reports and reviews. *Eur J Obstet Gynecol Reprod Biol.* 2014;173:7-12. [VA]

303. Karmaniolou I, Staikou C. Compartment syndrome as a complication of the lithotomy position. *West Indian Med J.* 2010;59(6):698-701. [VA]

304. Rao MM, Jayne D. Lower limb compartment syndrome following laparoscopic colorectal surgery: a review. *Colorectal Dis.* 2011;13(5):494-499. [VB]

305. Pridgeon S, Bishop CV, Adshead J. Lower limb compartment syndrome as a complication of robot-assisted radical prostatectomy: the UK experience. *BJU Int.* 2013;112(4):485-488. [IIIB]

306. Raza A, Byrne D, Townell N. Lower limb (well leg) compartment syndrome after urological pelvic surgery. *J Urol.* 2004;171(1):5-11. [VB]

307. Bauer EC, Koch N, Erichsen CJ, et al. Survey of compartment syndrome of the lower extremity after gynecological operations. *Langenbecks Arch Surg.* 2014;399(3):343-348. [IIIB]

308. Chin KY, Hemington-Gorse SJ, Darcy CM. Bilateral well leg compartment syndrome associated with lithotomy (Lloyd Davies) position during gastrointestinal surgery: a case report and review of literature. *Eplasty.* 2009;9:e48. [VB]

309. Galyon SW, Richards KA, Pettus JA, Bodin SG. Three-limb compartment syndrome and rhabdomyolysis after robotic cystoprostatectomy. *J Clin Anesth.* 2011;23(1):75-78. [VB]

310. Awab A, El Mansoury D, Benkabbou A, et al. Acute compartment syndrome following laparoscopic colorectal surgery. *Colorectal Dis.* 2012;14(2):e76. [VC]

311. Keene R, Froelich JM, Milbrandt JC, Idusuyi OB. Bilateral gluteal compartment syndrome following robotic-assisted prostatectomy. *Orthopedics.* 2010;33(11):852. [VA]

312. Raman SR, Jamil Z. Well leg compartment syndrome after robotic prostatectomy: a word of caution. *J Robot Surg.* 2009;3(2):105-107. [VB]

313. Enomoto T, Ohara Y, Yamamoto M, Oda T, Ohkohchi N. Well leg compartment syndrome after surgery for ulcerative colitis in the lithotomy position: a case report. *Int J Surg Case Rep.* 2016;23:25-28. [VA]

314. Oman SA, Schwarz D, Muntz HG. Lower limb compartment syndrome as a complication of radical hysterectomy. *Gynecol Oncol Rep.* 2016;16:39-41. [VA]

315. Stornelli N, Wydra FB, Mitchell JJ, Stahel PF, Fabbri S. The dangers of lithotomy positioning in the operating room: case report of bilateral lower extremity compartment syndrome after a 90-minutes surgical procedure. *Patient Saf Surg.* 2016;10:18. [VA]

316. Koç G, Tazeh NN, Joudi FN, Winfield HN, Tracy CR, Brown JA. Lower extremity neuropathies after robot-assisted laparoscopic prostatectomy on a split-leg table. *J Endourol.* 2012;26(8):1026-1029. [IIIA]

317. Chikazawa K, Netsu S, Akashi K, Suzuki Y, Konno R, Motomatsu S. Delayed diagnosis of single compartment muscle contusion after radical hysterectomy in the lithotomy position: a case report. *Int J Surg Case Rep.* 2016;26:199-201. [VB]

318. Lawrenz B, Kraemer B, Wallwiener D, Witte M, Fehm T, Becker S. Lower extremity compartment syndrome after laparoscopic radical hysterectomy: brief report of an unusual complication of laparoscopic positioning requirements. *J Minim Invasive Gynecol.* 2011;18(4):531-533. [VB]

319. Boesgaard-Kjer DH, Boesgaard-Kjer D, Kjer JJ. Well-leg compartment syndrome after gynecological laparoscopic surgery. *Acta Obstet Gynecol Scand.* 2013;92(5):598-600. [VB]

320. Ulrich D, Bader AA, Zotter M, Koch H, Pristauz G, Tamussino K. Well-leg compartment syndrome after surgery for gynecologic cancer. *J Gynecol Surg.* 2010;26(4):261-262. [VC]

321. Nakamura K, Aoki H, Hirakawa T, Murata T, Kanuma T, Minegishi T. Compartment syndrome with thrombosis of common iliac artery after gynecologic surgery. *Obstet Gynecol.* 2008;112(2 Pt 2):486-488. [VB]

322. Yang RH, Chu YK, Huang CW. Compartment syndrome following robotic-assisted prostatectomy: rhabdomyolysis in bone scintigraphy. *Clin Nucl Med.* 2013;38(5):365-366. [VC]

323. Guella A, Al Oraifi I. Rhabdomyolysis and acute renal failure following prolonged surgery in the lithotomy position. *Saudi J Kidney Dis Transpl.* 2013;24(2):330-332. [VB]

324. Sadeghian H, Arasteh H, Motiei-Langroudi R. Bilateral femoral neuropathy after transurethral lithotomy in the lithotomy position: report of a case. *J Clin Neuromuscul Dis.* 2016;17(4):225-226. [VB]

325. Mizuno J, Takahashi T. Male sex, height, weight, and body mass index can increase external pressure to calf region using knee-crutch-type leg holder system in lithotomy position. *Ther Clin Risk Manag.* 2016;12:305-312. [IIIB]

326. Hsu KL, Chang CW, Lin CJ, Chang CH, Su WR, Chen SM. The dangers of hemilithotomy positioning on traction tables: case report of a well-leg drop foot after contralateral femoral nailing. *Patient Saf Surg.* 2015;9:18. [VB]

327. Sajid MS, Shakir AJ, Khatri K, Baig MK. Lithotomy-related neurovascular complications in the lower limbs after colorectal surgery. *Colorectal Dis.* 2011;13(11):1203-1213. [VB]

328. Noordin S, Allana S, Wajid. Well leg compartment syndrome: the debit side of hemilithotomy position. *J Ayub Med Coll Abbottabad.* 2009;21(1):166-168. [VA]

329. Sharma N, Doble A. A case of compartment syndrome of the thighs following urethroplasty. *Br J Med Surg Urol.* 2009;2(2):82-84. [VB]

330. Sharma N, Doble A. Response to the letter to the editor "Well leg compartment syndrome following radical cystectomy and urinary diversion in the supine position." *Br J Med Surg Urol.* 2009;2(6):260. [VB]

331. Bradshaw AD, Advincula AP. Postoperative neuropathy in gynecologic surgery. *Obstet Gynecol Clin North Am.* 2010;37(3):451-459. [VB]

332. Mizuno J, Takahashi T. Factors that increase external pressure to the fibular head region, but not medial region, during use of a knee-crutch/leg-holder system in the lithotomy position. *Ther Clin Risk Manag.* 2015;11:255-261. [IIIB]

333. Wilson M, Ramage L, Yoong W, Swinhoe J. Femoral neuropathy after vaginal surgery: a complication of the lithotomy position. *J Obstet Gynaecol.* 2011;31(1):90-91. [VB]

334. Tondare AS, Nadkarni AV, Sathe CH, Dave VB. Femoral neuropathy: a complication of lithotomy position under spinal anesthesia. *Can Anaesth Soc J.* 1983;30(1):84-86. [VB]

335. Pannucci CJ, Henke PK, Cederna PS, et al. The effect of increased hip flexion using stirrups on lower-extremity venous flow: a prospective observational study. *Am J Surg.* 2011;202(4):427-432. [IIIB]

336. Navarro-Vicente F, Garcia-Granero A, Frasson M, et al. Prospective evaluation of intraoperative peripheral nerve injury in colorectal surgery. *Colorectal Dis.* 2012;14(3):382-385. [IIIB]

337. Yamada Y, Fujimura T, Fukuhara H, et al. Measuring contact pressure of lower extremities in patients undergoing robot-assisted radical prostatectomy. *Urol Int.* 2016;96(3):268-273. [IIIB]

338. Vijay MK, Vijay P, Kundu AK. Rhabdomyolysis and myoglobinuric acute renal failure in the lithotomy/exaggerated lithotomy position of urogenital surgeries. *Urol Ann.* 2011;3(3):147-150. [VC]

339. Liu X, Wang X, Meng X, Wang H, An Z. Effects of patient position on lower extremity venous pressure during different types of hysterectomy. *J Obstet Gynaecol Res.* 2015;41(1):114-119. [IIIB]

340. Guidance statement: safe patient handling and movement in the perioperative setting. In: *Guidelines for Perioperative Practice.* Denver, CO: AORN, Inc; 2015:733-752. [IVB]

341. Pearce A. Bilateral lower limb compartment syndrome following radical cystectomy and urinary diversion in the supine position. *Br J Med Surg Urol.* 2009;2(6):258-259. [VB]

342. Pfeffer SD, Halliwill JR, Warner MA. Effects of lithotomy position and external compression on lower leg muscle compartment pressure. *Anesthesiology.* 2001;95(3):632-636. [IIIB]

343. Chung JH, Ahn KR, Park JH, et al. Lower leg compartment syndrome following prolonged orthopedic surgery in the lithotomy position—a case report. *Korean J Anesthesiol.* 2010;59(Suppl):S49-S52. [VA]

344. Meyer RS, White KK, Smith JM, Groppo ER, Mubarak SJ, Hargens AR. Intramuscular and blood pressures in legs positioned in the hemilithotomy position: clarification of risk factors for well-leg acute compartment syndrome. *J Bone Joint Surg Am.* 2002;84-A(10):1829-1835. [IIIB]

345. Tan V, Pepe MD, Glaser DL, Seldes RM, Heppenstall RB, Esterhai JL Jr. Well-leg compartment pressures during hemilithotomy position for fracture fixation. *J Orthop Trauma.* 2000;14(3):157-161. [IIIB]

346. Peruto CM, Ciccotti MG, Cohen SB. Shoulder arthroscopy positioning: lateral decubitus versus beach chair. *Arthroscopy.* 2009;25(8):891-896. [VA]

347. Li X, Eichinger JK, Hartshorn T, Zhou H, Matzkin EG, Warner JP. A comparison of the lateral decubitus and beach-chair positions for shoulder surgery: advantages and complications. *J Am Acad Orthop Surg.* 2015;23(1):18-28. [VA]

348. Lindroos AC, Niiya T, Randell T, Romani R, Hernesniemi J, Niemi T. Sitting position for removal of pineal region lesions: the Helsinki experience. *World Neurosurg.* 2010;74(4-5):505-513. [IIIB]

349. Gardner BM. The beach chair position. *S Afr Fam Pract.* 2015;57(2):S6-S9. [VA]

350. Cogan A, Boyer P, Soubeyrand M, Hamida FB, Vannier JL, Massin P. Cranial nerves neuropraxia after shoulder arthroscopy in beach chair position. *Orthop Traumatol Surg Res.* 2011;97(3):345-348. [VB]

351. Basaldella L, Ortolani V, Corbanese U, Sorbara C, Longatti P. Massive venous air embolism in the semi-sitting position during surgery for a cervical spinal cord tumor: anatomic and surgical pitfalls. *J Clin Neurosci.* 2009;16(7):972-975. [VC]

352. Dilmen OK, Akcil EF, Tureci E, et al. Neurosurgery in the sitting position: retrospective analysis of 692 adult and pediatric cases. *Turk Neurosurg.* 2011;21(4):634-640. [IIIB]

353. Friedman DJ, Parnes NZ, Zimmer Z, Higgins LD, Warner JJ. Prevalence of cerebrovascular events during shoulder surgery and association with patient position. *Orthopedics.* 2009;32(4). [IIIC]

354. Meex I, Genbrugge C, De Deyne C, Jans F. Cerebral tissue oxygen saturation during arthroscopic shoulder surgery in the beach chair and lateral decubitus position. *Acta Anaesthesiol Belg.* 2015;66(1):11-17. [VA]

355. Lee SW, Choi SE, Han JH, Park SW, Kang WJ, Choi YK. Effect of beach chair position on bispectral index values during arthroscopic shoulder surgery. *Korean J Anesthesiol.* 2014;67(4):235-239. [IIIB]

356. Pant S, Bokor DJ, Low AK. Cerebral oxygenation using near-infrared spectroscopy in the beach-chair position during shoulder arthroscopy under general anesthesia. *Arthroscopy.* 2014;30(11):1520-1527. [IIIB]

357. Mazzon D, Danelli G, Poole D, Marchini C, Bianchin C. Beach chair position, general anesthesia and deliberated hypotension during shoulder surgery: a dangerous combination! *Minerva Anestesiol.* 2009;75(5):281-282. [VB]

358. Moerman AT, De Hert SG, Jacobs TF, De Wilde LF, Wouters PF. Cerebral oxygen desaturation during beach chair position. *Eur J Anaesthesiol.* 2012;29(2):82-87. [IIIB]

359. Triplet JJ, Lonetta CM, Levy JC, Everding NG, Moor MA. Cerebral desaturation events in the beach chair position: correlation of noninvasive blood pressure and estimated temporal mean arterial pressure. *J Shoulder Elbow Surg.* 2015;24(1):133-137. [IIIB]

360. Murphy GS, Szokol JW, Marymont JH, et al. Cerebral oxygen desaturation events assessed by near-infrared spectroscopy during shoulder arthroscopy in the beach chair and lateral decubitus positions. *Anesth Analg.* 2010;111(2):496-505. [IIIB]

361. Meex I, Vundelinckx J, Buyse K, et al. Cerebral tissue oxygen saturation values in volunteers and patients in the lateral decubitus and beach chair positions: a prospective observational study. *Can J Anaesth.* 2016;63(5):537-543. [IIIB]

362. Salazar D, Hazel A, Tauchen A J, Sears BW, Marra G. Neurocognitive deficits and cerebral desaturation during shoulder arthroscopy with patient in beach-chair position: a review of the current literature. *Am J Orthop (Belle Mead NJ).* 2016;45(3):E63-E68. [IIIB]

363. Dippmann C, Winge S, Nielsen HB. Severe cerebral desaturation during shoulder arthroscopy in the beach-chair position. *Arthroscopy.* 2010;26(9 Suppl):S148-S150. [VB]

364. Salazar D, Sears B, Acosta A, et al. Effect of head and neck positioning on cerebral perfusion during shoulder arthroscopy in beach chair position. *J Surg Orthop Adv.* 2014;23(2):83-89. [IIIB]

365. Laflam A, Joshi B, Brady K, et al. Shoulder surgery in the beach chair position is associated with diminished cerebral autoregulation but no differences in postoperative cognition or brain injury biomarker levels compared with supine positioning: the anesthesia patient safety foundation beach chair study. *Anesth Analg.* 2015;120(1):176-185. [IIIB]

366. Hanouz JL, Fiant AL, Gérard JL. Middle cerebral artery blood flow velocity during beach chair position for shoulder surgery under general anesthesia. *J Clin Anesth.* 2016;33:31-36. [IIIB]

367. Buget MI, Atalar AC, Edipoglu IS, et al. Patient state index and cerebral blood flow changes during shoulder arthroscopy in beach chair position. *Braz J Anesthesiol.* 2016;66(5):470-474. [IIIB]

368. McCulloch TJ, Liyanagama K, Petchell J. Relative hypotension in the beach-chair position: effects on middle cerebral artery blood velocity. *Anaesth Intensive Care.* 2010;38(3):486-491. [IIIB]

369. Yadeau JT, Liu SS, Bang H, et al. Cerebral oximetry desaturation during shoulder surgery performed in a sitting position under regional anesthesia. *Can J Anaesth.* 2011;58(11):986-992. [IIIB]

370. Tange K, Kinoshita H, Minonishi T, et al. Cerebral oxygenation in the beach chair position before and during general anesthesia. *Minerva Anestesiol.* 2010;76(7):485-490. [IIIB]

371. Pin-on P, Schroeder D, Munis J. The hemodynamic management of 5177 neurosurgical and orthopedic patients who underwent surgery in the sitting or "beach chair" position without incidence of adverse neurologic events. *Anesth Analg.* 2013;116(6):1317-1324. [IIIA]

372. Lee JH, Min KT, Chun YM, Kim EJ, Choi SH. Effects of beach-chair position and induced hypotension on cerebral oxygen saturation in patients undergoing arthroscopic shoulder surgery. *Arthroscopy.* 2011;27(7):889-894. [IIIB]

373. Mori Y, Yamada M, Akahori T, et al. Cerebral oxygenation in the beach chair position before and during general anesthesia in patients with and without cardiovascular risk factors. *J Clin Anesth.* 2015;27(6):457-462. [IIIB]

374. Amukoa P, Reed A, Thomas JM. Use of the sitting position for pineal tumour surgery in a five-year-old child. *S Afr J Anaesth Analg.* 2011;17(6):388-392. [VB]

375. Rains DD, Rooke GA, Wahl CJ. Pathomechanisms and complications related to patient positioning and anesthesia during shoulder arthroscopy. *Arthroscopy.* 2011;27(4):532-541. [VB]

376. Vermeersch G, Menovsky T, De Ridder D, De Bodt M, Saldien V, Van de Heyning P. Life-threatening macroglossia after posterior fossa surgery: a surgical positioning problem? *B-ENT.* 2014;10(4):309-313. [VB]

377. Rhee YG, Cho NS. Isolated unilateral hypoglossal nerve palsy after shoulder surgery in beach-chair position. *J Shoulder Elbow Surg.* 2008;17(4):e28-e30. [VB]

378. Liang BA. Judgment notwithstanding the verdict: the anesthesiologist's duty to monitor head position in the perioperative period. *J Clin Anesth.* 2009;21(5):369-370. [VA]

379. Ng AK, Page RS. Greater auricular nerve neuropraxia with beach chair positioning during shoulder surgery. *Int J Shoulder Surg.* 2010;4(2):48-50. [VB]

380. LaPrade CM, Foad A. Greater auricular nerve palsy after arthroscopic anterior-inferior and posterior-inferior labral tear repair using beach-chair positioning and a standard universal headrest. *Am J Orthop (Belle Mead NJ).* 2015;44(4):188-191. [VB]

381. Wang JC, Wong TT, Chen HH, Chang PY, Yang TF. Bilateral sciatic neuropathy as a complication of craniotomy performed in the sitting position: localization of nerve injury by using magnetic resonance imaging. *Childs Nerv Syst.* 2012;28(1):159-163. [VB]

382. Kiermeir D, Banic A, Rosler K, Erni D. Sciatic neuropathy after body contouring surgery in massive weight loss patients. *J Plast Reconstr Aesthet Surg.* 2010;63(5):e454-e457. [VB]

383. Rawlani V, Lee MJ, Dumanian GA. Bilateral sciatic neurapraxia following combined abdominoplasty and mastopexy. *Plast Reconstr Surg.* 2010;125(1):31e-32e. [VC]

384. Satin AM, DePalma AA, Cuellar J, Gruson KI. Lateral femoral cutaneous nerve palsy following shoulder surgery in the beach chair position: a report of 4 cases. *Am J Orthop (Belle Mead NJ).* 2014;43(9):E206-E209. [VA]

385. Kwak HJ, Lee JS, Lee DC, Kim HS, Kim JY. The effect of a sequential compression device on hemodynamics in arthroscopic shoulder surgery using beach-chair position. *Arthroscopy.* 2010;26(6):729-733. [IA]

386. Woo KY, Kim EJ, Lee JH, Lee SG, Ban JS. Recurrent paroxysmal supraventricular tachycardia in the beach chair position for shoulder surgery under general anesthesia. *Korean J Anesthesiol.* 2014;65(6 Suppl):S75-S76. [VB]

387. Prabhakar H, Singh GP, Ali Z, Bindra A. Surgery in sitting position in patient with ventriculoperitoneal shunt in situ may be hazardous! *Childs Nerv Syst.* 2009;25(12):1531-1532. [VB]

388. Pandey V, Varghese E, Rao M, et al. Nonfatal air embolism during shoulder arthroscopy. *Am J Orthop (Belle Mead NJ).* 2013;42(6):272-274. [VB]

389. Mirski MA, Lele AV, Fitzsimmons L, Toung TJ. Diagnosis and treatment of vascular air embolism. *Anesthesiology.* 2007;106(1):164-177. [VB]

390. Natal BL. Venous air embolism treatment & management. Medscape. http://emedicine.medscape.com/article/761367-treatment. Accessed March 10, 2017. [VB]

391. Rushatamukayanunt P, Seanho P, Muangman S, Raksakietisak M. Severe venous air embolism related to positioning in posterior cranial fossa surgery in Siriraj Hospital. *J Med Assoc Thai.* 2016;99(5):511-516. [IIIB]

392. Sandwell S, Kimmell KT, Silberstein HJ, et al. 349 safety of the sitting cervical position for elective spine surgery. *Neurosurgery.* 2016;63(Suppl 1):203. [IIIC]

393. Perello L, Gracia I, Fabregas N. Bone embolism during neurosurgery in sitting position. *J Neurosurg Anesthesiol.* 2013;25(1):93. [VC]

394. Ariadne Labs, Brigham and Women's Hospital, Harvard School of Public Health. *Operating Room Crisis Checklists: Crisis Checklist Package.* 2013. http://www.projectcheck.org/uploads/1/0/9/0/1090835/or_crisis_checklists_package_10-11-13.pdf. Accessed March 10, 2017.

395. Furuno Y, Sasajima H, Goto Y, et al. Strategies to prevent positioning-related complications associated with the lateral suboccipital approach. *J Neurol Surg B Skull Base.* 2014;75(1):35-40. [IIIB]

396. Woernle CM, Sarnthein J, Foit NA, Krayenbuhl N. Enhanced serum creatine kinase after neurosurgery in lateral position and intraoperative neurophysiological monitoring. *Clin Neurol Neurosurg.* 2013;115(3):266-269. [IIB]

397. Achar SK, Paul C, Varghese E. Unilateral pulmonary edema after laparoscopic nephrectomy. *J Anaesthesiol Clin Pharmacol.* 2011;27(4):556-558. [VB]

398. Danish SF, Wilden JA, Schuster J. Iatrogenic paraplegia in 2 morbidly obese patients with ankylosing spondylitis undergoing total hip arthroplasty. *J Neurosurg Spine.* 2008;8(1):80-83. [VB]

399. Hemmerling TM, Kazan R, Bracco D. Inter-hemispheric cerebral oxygen saturation differences during thoracic surgery in lateral head positioning. *Br J Anaesth.* 2009;102(1):141-142. [IIC]

400. Kim TK, Yoon JR, Lee MH. Rhabdomyolysis after laparoscopic radical nephrectomy—a case report. *Korean J Anesthesiol.* 2010;59(Suppl):S41-S44. [VB]

401. De Tommasi C, Cusimano MD. Rhabdomyolysis after neurosurgery: a review and a framework for prevention. *Neurosurg Rev.* 2013;36(2):195-202. [VA]

402. Dakwar E, Rifkin SI, Volcan IJ, Goodrich JA, Uribe JS. Rhabdomyolysis and acute renal failure following minimally invasive spine surgery: report of 5 cases. *J Neurosurg Spine.* 2011;14(6):785-788. [VB]

403. Rowell J, Lynn AM, Filardi TZ, Celix J, Ojemann JG. Acute unilateral enlargement of the parotid gland immediately post craniotomy in a pediatric patient: a case report. *Childs Nerv Syst.* 2010;26(9):1239-1242. [VA]

404. Ameri E, Behtash H, Omidi-Kashani F. Isolated long thoracic nerve paralysis—a rare complication of anterior spinal surgery: a case report. *J Med Case Rep.* 2009;3:7366. [VB]

405. Jain V, Davies M. Axillary artery compression in park bench position during a microvascular decompression. *J Neurosurg Anesthesiol.* 2011;23(3):264. [VC]

406. Newton G, White E. Femoral artery occlusion in obese patients in the lateral position. *Anaesthesia.* 2010;65(8):863. [VC]

407. Edgcombe H, Carter K, Yarrow S. Anaesthesia in the prone position. *Br J Anaesth.* 2008;100(2):165-183. [VA]

408. Kwee MM, Ho YH, Rozen WM. The prone position during surgery and its complications: a systematic review and evidence-based guidelines. *Int Surg.* 2015;100(2):292-303. [IVA]

409. Koh JC, Lee JS, Han DW, Choi S, Chang CH. Increase in airway pressure resulting from prone position patient placing may predict intraoperative surgical blood loss. *Spine.* 2013;38(11):E678-E682. [IIIB]

410. DePasse JM, Palumbo MA, Haque M, Eberson CP, Daniels AH. Complications associated with prone positioning in elective spinal surgery. *World J Orthop.* 2015;6(3):351-359. [VA]

411. Postoperative Visual Loss Study Group. Risk factors associated with ischemic optic neuropathy after spinal fusion surgery. *Anesthesiology.* 2012;116(1):15-24. [IIIA]

412. Akinci IO, Tunali U, Kyzy AA, et al. Effects of prone and jackknife positioning on lumbar disc herniation surgery. *J Neurosurg Anesthesiol.* 2011;23(4):318-322. [IC]

413. Chalhoub V, Tohmé J, Richa F, Dagher C, Yazbeck P. Inferior vena cava filter migration during the prone position for spinal surgery: a case report. *Can J Anesth.* 2015;62(10):1114-1118. [VB]

414. Han IH, Son DW, Nam KH, Choi BK, Song GS. The effect of body mass index on intra-abdominal pressure and blood loss in lumbar spine surgery. *J Korean Neurosurg Soc.* 2012;51(2):81-85. [IIB]

415. Borodiciene J, Gudaityte J, Macas A. Lithotomy versus jack-knife position on haemodynamic parameters assessed by impedance cardiography during anorectal surgery under low

dose spinal anaesthesia: a randomized controlled trial. *BMC Anesthesiol.* 2015;15(1):1-9. [IA]

416. Chui J, Craen RA. An update on the prone position: continuing professional development. *Can J Anaesth.* 2016;63(6):737-767. [VA]

417. Shriver MF, Zeer V, Alentado VJ, Mroz TE, Benzel EC, Steinmetz MP. Lumbar spine surgery positioning complications: a systematic review. *Neurosurg Focus.* 2015;39(4):E16. [IIIB]

418. Degerli S, Acar B, Sahap M, Polat A, Horasanli E. Investigation of middle ear pressure changes during prone position under general anesthesia without using nitrous oxide. *J Craniofac Surg.* 2013;24(6):1950-1952. [IIB]

419. Closhen D, Engelhard K, Dette F, Werner C, Schramm P. Changes in cerebral oxygen saturation following prone positioning for orthopaedic surgery under general anaesthesia: a prospective observational study. *Eur J Anaesthesiol.* 2015;32(6):381-386. [IIA]

420. Babakhani B, Heroabadi A, Hosseinitabatabaei N, et al. Cerebral oxygenation under general anesthesia can be safely preserved in patients in prone position: a prospective observational study. *J Neurosurg Anesthesiol.* June 2, 2016. Epub ahead of print. [IIIB]

421. Deiner S, Chu I, Mahanian M, Lin HM, Hecht AC, Silverstein JH. Prone position is associated with mild cerebral oxygen desaturation in elderly surgical patients. *Plos One.* 2014;9(9):e106387. [IIB]

422. Brown ZE, Gorges M, Cooke E, Malherbe S, Dumont GA, Ansermino JM. Changes in cardiac index and blood pressure on positioning children prone for scoliosis surgery. *Anaesthesia.* 2013;68(7):742-746. [IIB]

423. Shifa J, Abebe W, Bekele N, Habte D. A case of bilateral visual loss after spinal cord surgery. *Pan Afr Med J.* 2016;23:119. [VA]

424. Li A, Swinney C, Veeravagu A, Bhatti I, Ratliff J. Postoperative visual loss following lumbar spine surgery: a review of risk factors by diagnosis. *World Neurosurg.* 2015;84(6):2010-2021. [VA]

425. Nickels TJ, Manlapaz MR, Farag E. Perioperative visual loss after spine surgery. *World J Orthop.* 2014;5(2):100-106. [VA]

426. Dereine T, van Pesch V, Van Boven M, Hantson P. Transient perioperative visual loss after an elective neurosurgical procedure. *Acta Anaesthesiol Belg.* 2013;64(3):109-113. [VB]

427. Grant GP, Szirth BC, Bennett HL, et al. Effects of prone and reverse Trendelenburg positioning on ocular parameters. *Anesthesiology.* 2010;112(1):57-65. [IIB]

428. Carey TW, Shaw KA, Weber ML, DeVine JG. Effect of the degree of reverse Trendelenburg position on intraocular pressure during prone spine surgery: a randomized controlled trial. *Spine J.* 2014;14(9):2118-2126. [IC]

429. Emery SE, Daffner SD, France JC, et al. Effect of head position on intraocular pressure during lumbar spine fusion: a randomized, prospective study. *J Bone Joint Surg (Am).* 2015;97(22):1817-1823. [IB]

430. Lee LA, Newman NJ, Wagner TA, Dettori JR, Dettori NJ. Postoperative ischemic optic neuropathy. *Spine.* 2010;35(9 Suppl):S105-S116. [VA]

431. Akhaddar A, Boucetta M. Subconjunctival hemorrhage as a complication of intraoperative positioning for lumbar spinal surgery. *Spine J.* 2012;12(3):274. [VC]

432. Russell DJ, Dutton JJ. Bilateral spontaneous subperiosteal orbital hemorrhages following endoscopic retrograde cholangiopancreatography. *Ophthal Plast Reconstr Surg.* 2011;27(3):e49-e50. [VC]

433. Guillaume JE, Gowreesunker P. Horner's syndrome in the prone position—a case report. *Acta Anaesthesiol Belg.* 2013;64(3):119-121. [VC]

434. Stang-Veldhouse KN, Yeu E, Rothenberg DM, Mizen TR. Unusual presentation of perioperative ischemic optic neuropathy following major spine surgery. *J Clin Anesth.* 2010;22(1):52-55. [VB]

435. Quraishi NA, Wolinsky JP, Gokaslan ZL. Transient bilateral post-operative visual loss in spinal surgery. *Eur Spine J.* 2012;21(Suppl 4):S495-S498. [VB]

436. Goni V, Tripathy SK, Goyal T, Tamuk T, Panda BB, Shashidhar BK. Cortical blindness following spinal surgery: very rare cause of perioperative vision loss. *Asian Spine J.* 2012;6(4):287-290. [VB]

437. Reddy A, Foroozan R, Edmond JC, Hinckley LK. Dilated superior ophthalmic veins and posterior ischemic optic neuropathy after prolonged spine surgery. *J Neuroophthalmol.* 2008;28(4):327-328. [VB]

438. Kendrick H. Post-operative vision loss (POVL) following surgical procedures. *J Anesth Clin Res.* 2012;3(1). [VB]

439. Agah M, Ghasemi M, Roodneshin F, Radpay B, Moradian S. Prone position in percutaneous nephrolithotomy and postoperative visual loss. *Urol J.* 2011;8(3):191-196. [IIIB]

440. Szmuk P, Steiner JW, Pop RB, et al. Intraocular pressure in pediatric patients during prone surgery. *Anesth Analg.* 2013;116(6):1309-1313. [IIIB]

441. Yoshimura K, Hayashi H, Tanaka Y, Nomura Y, Kawaguchi M. Evaluation of predictive factors associated with increased intraocular pressure during prone position spine surgery. *J Anesth.* 2015;29(2):170-174. [IIIB]

442. Eddama M. Re: Raised intraocular pressure and perioperative visual loss in laparoscopic colorectal surgery: a catastrophe waiting to happen? A systematic review of evidence from other surgical specialties. *Tech Coloproctol.* 2013;17(2):247. [VA]

443. Nazerali RS, Song KR, Wong MS. Facial pressure ulcer following prone positioning. *J Plast Reconstr Aesthet Surg.* 2010;63(4):e413-e414. [VB]

444. Sherman CE, Rose PS, Pierce LL, Yaszemski MJ, Sim FH. Prospective assessment of patient morbidity from prone sacral positioning. *J Neurosurg Spine.* 2012;16(1):51-56. [VB]

445. Dahab R, Barrett C, Pillay R, De Matas M. Anterior thigh compartment syndrome after prone positioning for lumbosacral fixation. *Eur Spine J.* 2012;21(Suppl 4):S554-S556. [VB]

446. Gupta R, Batra S, Chandra R, Sharma VK. Compartment syndrome with acute renal failure: a rare complication of spinal surgery in knee-chest position. *Spine.* 2008;33(8):E272-E273. [VB]

447. Minami K, Iida M, Iida H. Case report: central venous catheterization via internal jugular vein with associated

formation of perioperative venous thrombosis during surgery in the prone position. *J Anesth.* 2012;26(3):464-466. [VB]

448. Harman F, Yayci F, Deren S, et al. Acute cerebellar ischemia after lumbar spinal surgery: a rare clinical entity. *J Anesth.* 2012;26(6):947-948. [VC]

449. Hojlund J, Sandmand M, Sonne M, et al. Effect of head rotation on cerebral blood velocity in the prone position. *Anesthesiol Res Pract.* 2012;2012:647258. [IIB]

450. Ooi EI, Ahem A, Zahidin AZ, Bastion ML. Unilateral visual loss after spine surgery in the prone position for extradural haematoma in a healthy young man. *BMJ Case Rep.* December 13, 2013;2013. [VC]

451. Pin-On P, Boonsri S. Postoperative visual loss in orthopedic spine surgery in the prone position: a case report. *J Med Assoc Thai.* 2015;98(3):320-324. [VB]

452. Yu YH, Chen WJ, Chen LH, Chen WC. Ischemic orbital compartment syndrome after posterior spinal surgery. *Spine.* 2008;33(16):E569-E572. [VB]

453. Andersen JD, Baake G, Wiis JT, Olsen KS. Effect of head rotation during surgery in the prone position on regional cerebral oxygen saturation: a prospective controlled study. *Eur J Anaesthesiol.* 2014;31(2):98-103. [IIB]

454. Nuri Deniz M, Erakgun A, Sertoz N, Guven Yilmaz S, Ates H, Erhan E. The effect of head rotation on intraocular pressure in prone position: a randomized trial. *Rev Bras Anestesiol.* 2013;63(2):209-212. [IB]

455. Uribe AA, Baig MN, Puente EG, Viloria A, Mendel E, Bergese SD. Current intraoperative devices to reduce visual loss after spine surgery. *Neurosurgical Focus.* 2012;33(2):E14. [VB]

456. Grover VK, Jangra K. Perioperative vision loss: a complication to watch out. *J Anaesthesiol Clin Pharmacol.* 2012;28(1):11-16. [VA]

457. Grisell M, Place HM. Face tissue pressure in prone positioning: a comparison of three face pillows while in the prone position for spinal surgery. *Spine.* 2008;33(26):2938-2941. [IIB]

458. McMichael JC, Place HM. Face tissue pressures in prone positioning: a comparison of 3 pillows. *J Spinal Disord Tech.* 2008;21(7):508-513. [IIIC]

459. Levan P, O'Rourke M, Presta M, Bryam S. The use of mobile smartphone technology to enhance positioning of a prone patient for thoracic spine surgery. *Internet J Anesthesiol.* 2012;30(3):1. [VB]

460. Asok T, Aziz S, Faisal HA, Tan AK, Mallika PS. Central retinal artery occlusion and ophthalmoplegia following spinal surgery in the prone position. *Med J Malaysia.* 2009;64(4):323-324. [VB]

461. Song JS, Yim JH, Lee KB. Unilateral blindness after posterior cervical spinal surgery: a case report. *Neurosurg Q.* 2015;25(1):78-81. [VC]

462. Epstein NE. Perioperative visual loss following prone spinal surgery: a review. *Surgical Neurology International.* 2016;7(Suppl 13):S347-S360. [VB]

463. Kitthaweesin K, Moontawee K, Thanathanee O. Sudden visual loss and total ophthalmoplegia after brain surgery. *Neuroophthalmology.* 2009;33(1-2):59-61. [VB]

464. Takahashi Y, Kakizaki H, Selva D, Leibovitch I. Bilateral orbital compartment syndrome and blindness after cerebral aneurysm repair surgery. *Ophthal Plast Reconstr Surg.* 2010;26(4):299-301. [VC]

465. Woodruff C, English M, Zaouter C, Hemmerling TM. Postoperative visual loss after plastic surgery: case report and a novel continuous real-time video monitoring system for the eyes during prone surgery. *Br J Anaesth.* 2011;106(1):149-151. [VC]

466. Yu HD, Chou AH, Yang MW, Chang CJ. An analysis of perioperative eye injuries after nonocular surgery. *Acta Anaesthesiol Taiwan.* 2010;48(3):122-129. [IIIB]

467. Walker BJ, Rampersad SE. Iatrogenic endotracheal tube obstruction with foam face padding. *Paediatr Anaesth.* 2009;19(5):544-545. [VB]

468. Chae YJ, Kim JY, Yoo JY, Choi YH, Park KS. Tongue bite in a patient with tracheostomy after prone position—a case report. *Korean J Anesthesiol.* 2011;60(5):365-368. [VB]

469. Minonishi T, Kinoshita H, Hirayama M, et al. The supine-to-prone position change induces modification of endotracheal tube cuff pressure accompanied by tube displacement. *J Clin Anesth.* 2013;25(1):28-31. [IIIB]

470. Lee JA, Jeon YS, Jung HS, Kim HG, Kim YS. Acute compartment syndrome of the forearm and hand in a patient of spine surgery—a case report. *Korean J Anesthesiol.* 2010;59(1):53-55. [VB]

471. Cho KT, Lee HJ. Prone position-related meralgia paresthetica after lumbar spinal surgery: a case report and review of the literature. *J Korean Neurosurg Soc.* 2008;44(6):392-395. [VA]

472. Chikhani M, Evans DL, Blatcher AW, et al. The effect of prone positioning with surgical bolsters on liver blood flow in healthy volunteers. *Anaesthesia.* 2016;71(5):550-555. [IIIB]

473. Debbarma S, Garg S, Kumar K, Anuradha S, Dewan R. Obesity and respiratory complications. *J Int Med Sci Acad.* 2008;21(3):151-153. [VB]

474. Archer TL, Suresh P, Shapiro AE. Cardiac output measurement, by means of electrical velocimetry, may be able to determine optimum maternal position during gestation, labour and caesarean delivery, by preventing vena caval compression and maximising cardiac output and placental perfusion pressure. *Anaesth Intensive Care.* 2011;39(2):308-311. [VB]

475. Saravanakumar K, Hendrie M, Smith F, Danielian P. Influence of reverse Trendelenburg position on aortocaval compression in obese pregnant women. *Int J Obstet Anesth.* 2016;26:15-18. [IIIC]

476. Lee SW, Khaw KS, Ngan Kee WD, Leung TY, Critchley LA. Haemodynamic effects from aortocaval compression at different angles of lateral tilt in non-labouring term pregnant women. *Br J Anaesth.* 2012;109(6):950-956. [IIIB]

477. Baird EJ, Arkoosh VA. Hemodynamic effects of aortocaval compression and uterine contractions in a parturient with left ventricular outflow tract obstruction. *Anesthesiology.* 2012;117(4):879. [VC]

478. Zhou ZQ, Shao Q, Zeng Q, Song J, Yang JJ. Lumbar wedge versus pelvic wedge in preventing hypotension following combined spinal epidural anaesthesia for caesarean delivery. *Anaesth Intensive Care.* 2008;36(6):835-839. [IB]

479. Association of Women's Health, Obstetric and Neonatal Nurses. *Perioperative Care of the Pregnant Woman. Evidence-based Clinical Practice Guideline.* Washington, DC: AWHONN; 2011. [IVA]

480. Higuchi H, Takagi S, Zhang K, Furui I, Ozaki M. Effect of lateral tilt angle on the volume of the abdominal aorta and inferior vena cava in pregnant and nonpregnant women determined by magnetic resonance imaging. *Anesthesiology.* 2015;122(2):286-293. [IIIA]

481. Harvey NL, Hodgson RL, Kinsella SM. Does body mass index influence the degree of pelvic tilt produced by a Crawford wedge? *Int J Obstet Anesth.* 2013;22(2):129-132. [IIIB]

482. Kinsella SM, Harvey NL. A comparison of the pelvic angle applied using lateral table tilt or a pelvic wedge at elective caesarean section. *Anaesthesia.* 2012;67(12):1327-1331. [IIIB]

483. Cluver C, Novikova N, Hofmeyr GJ, Hall DR. Maternal position during caesarean section for preventing maternal and neonatal complications. *Cochrane Database Syst Rev.* 2013;3:007623. [IA]

484. Defining adult overweight and obesity. Centers for Disease Control and Prevention. https://www.cdc.gov/obesity/adult/defining.html. Accessed March 10, 2017.

485. Donohoe CL, Feeney C, Carey MF, Reynolds JV. Perioperative evaluation of the obese patient. *J Clin Anesth.* 2011;23(7):575-586. [VA]

486. Yamane T, Date T, Tokuda M, et al. Hypoxemia in inferior pulmonary veins in supine position is dependent on obesity. *Am J Respir Crit Care Med.* 2008;178(3):295-299. [IIIB]

487. Cheema UY, Vogler CN, Thompson J, Sattovia SL, Vallurupalli S. Protracted hypocalcemia following post-thyroidectomy lumbar rhabdomyolysis secondary to evolving hypoparathyroidism. *Ear Nose Throat J.* 2015;94(3):113-116. [VB]

488. Lee BJ, Kang JM, Kim DO. Laryngeal exposure during laryngoscopy is better in the 25 degrees back-up position than in the supine position. *Br J Anaesth.* 2007;99(4):581-586. [IIIB]

489. Collins JS, Lemmens HJ, Brodsky JB, Brock-Utne JG, Levitan RM. Laryngoscopy and morbid obesity: a comparison of the "sniff" and "ramped" positions. *Obes Surg.* 2004;14(9):1171-1175. [IB]

490. Rao SL, Kunselman AR, Schuler HG, DesHarnais S. Laryngoscopy and tracheal intubation in the head-elevated position in obese patients: a randomized, controlled, equivalence trial. *Anesth Analg.* 2008;107(6):1912-1918. [IA]

491. Cattano D, Melnikov V, Khalil Y, Sridhar S, Hagberg CA. An evaluation of the rapid airway management positioner in obese patients undergoing gastric bypass or laparoscopic gastric banding surgery. *Obes Surg.* 2010;20(10):1436-1441. [IIB]

492. Banicek J, McGarvey D. The effect of patient positioning during lengthy surgery on postoperative health. *Nurs Times.* 2010;106(3):15. [VC]

493. O'Brien DD, Shanks AM, Talsma A, Brenner PS, Ramachandran SK. Intraoperative risk factors associated with postoperative pressure ulcers in critically ill patients: a retrospective observational study. *Crit Care Med.* 2014;42(1):40-47. [IIIB]

494. American Society of PeriAnesthesia Nurses. *2017-2018 PeriAnesthesia Nursing Standards Practice Recommendations and Interpretive Statements.* Cherry Hill, NJ: ASPAN; 2017. [IVB]

495. Minnich L, Bennett J, Mercer J. Partnering for perioperative skin assessment: a time to change a practice culture. *J Perianesth Nurs.* 2014;29(5):361-366. [VA]

496. Gezginci E, Ozkaptan O, Yalcin S, Akin Y, Rassweiler J, Gozen AS. Postoperative pain and neuromuscular complications associated with patient positioning after robotic assisted laparoscopic radical prostatectomy: a retrospective non-placebo and non-randomized study. *Int Urol Nephrol.* 2015;47(10):1635-1641. [IIIB]

497. Kalin A, Hariharan V, Tudor F. Unicompartment compartment syndrome following laparascopic colonic resection. *BMJ Case Rep.* July 9, 2013;2013. [VB]

498. Hoff JM, Varhaug P, Midelfart A, Lund-Johansen M. Acute visual loss after spinal surgery. *Acta Opthalmol.* 2010;88(4):490-492. [VB]

499. Price TP, Ivashchenko A, Schurr MJ. Perioperative visual loss after excision and autografting of a thermal burn to the back. *Burns.* 2014;40(4):e31-e34. [VB]

500. Yilmaz M, Kalemci O. Visual loss after lumbar discectomy due to cortical infarction: case report. *J Neurol Sci.* 2013;30(2):422-426. [VC]

501. *State Operations Manual Appendix A—Survey Protocol, Regulations and Interpretive Guidelines for Hospitals.* Rev 151. November 20, 2015. Centers for Medicare & Medicaid Services. https://www.cms.gov/Regulations-and-Guidance/Guidance/Manuals/downloads/som107ap_a_hospitals.pdf. Accessed March 10, 2017.

502. *State Operations Manual Appendix L—Guidance for Surveyors: Ambulatory Surgical Centers.* Rev 137. April 1, 2015. Centers for Medicare & Medicaid Services. https://www.cms.gov/Regulations-and-Guidance/Guidance/Manuals/downloads/som107ap_l_ambulatory.pdf. Accessed March 10, 2017.

503. 42 CFR 482. Conditions of participation for hospitals. US Government Publishing Office. https://www.gpo.gov/fdsys/granule/CFR-2011-title42-vol5/CFR-2011-title42-vol5-part482. Accessed March 10, 2017.

504. 42 CFR 416. Ambulatory surgical services. US Government Publishing Office. https://www.gpo.gov/fdsys/granule/CFR-2011-title42-vol3/CFR-2011-title42-vol3-part416. Accessed March 10, 2017.

505. RC.01.01.01: The hospital maintains complete and accurate medical records for each individual patient. In: *Hospital Accredtation Standards.* 2016 ed. Oakbrook Terrace, IL: Joint Commission Resources; 2016.

506. MS.16: Medical record maintenance. In: *NIAHO Interpretive Guidelines and Surveyor Guidance.* Version 11 ed. Milford, OH: DNV GL - Healthcare; 2014: 37.

507. RC.01.01.01: The organization maintains complete and accurate clinical records. In: *Standards for Ambulatory Care.* Oakbrook Terrace, IL: Joint Commission Resources; 2016.

508. Clinical records and health information. In: *Accreditation Handbook for Ambulatory Health Care.* Skokie, IL: Accreditation Association for Ambulatory Health Care, Inc; 2016:51-53.

509. Medical records: operating room records. In: *Regular Standards and Checklist for Accreditation of Ambulatory Surgery Facilities.* Version 14.4 ed. Gurnee, IL: American Association for Accreditation of Ambulatory Surgery Facilities, Inc; 2016:60-63.

510. Medical records: procedure room records. In: *Procedural Standards and Checklist for Accreditation of Ambulatory Surgery Facilities.* Version 3 ed. Gurnee, IL: American Association for Accreditation of Ambulatory Surgery Facilities; 2011:64-66.

511. Guideline for patient information management. In: *Guidelines for Perioperative Practice.* Denver, CO: AORN, Inc; 2017:591-616. [IVA]

512. Jordan C, Thomas MB, Evans ML, Green A. Public policy on competency: how will nursing address this complex issue? *J Contin Educ Nurs.* 2008;39(2):86-91. [VB]

513. HR.01.05.03: Staff participate in ongoing education and training. In: *Comprehensive Accreditation Manual: CAMH for Hospitals.* 2016 ed. Oakbrook Terrace, IL: Joint Commission Resources; 2016.

514. MS.10: Continuing education. In: *NIAHO Interpretive Guidelines and Surveyor Guidance.* Version 11 ed. Milford, OH: DNV GL - Healthcare; 2014:30.

515. HR.01.05.03: Staff participate in ongoing education and training. In: Comprehensive Accreditation Manual: CAMAC for Ambulatory Care. 2016 ed. Oakbrook Terrace, IL: Joint Commission Resources; 2016.

516. Governance. In: *Accreditation Handbook for Ambulatory Health Care.* 2016 ed. Skokie, IL: Accreditation Handbook for Ambulatory Health Care, Inc; 2016:33-40.

517. Personnel: personnel records; individual personnel files. In: *Regular Standards and Checklist for Accreditation of Ambulatory Surgery Facilities.* 2016 ed. Gurnee, IL: American Association for Accreditation of Ambulatory Surgery Facilities, Inc; 2016:74-75.

518. LD.04.01.07: The hospital has policies and procedures that guide and support patient care, treatment, and services. In: *Hospital Accreditation Standards.* 2016 ed. Oakbrook Terrace, IL: Joint Commission Resources; 2016.

519. SS.1:Organization. In: *NIAHO Interpretive Guidelines and Surveyor Guidance.* Version 11 ed. Milford, OH: DNV GL - Healthcare; 2014:80-82.

520. LD.04.01.07: The organization has policies and procedures that guide and support patient care, treatment, or services. In: *Standards for Ambulatory Care.* 2016 ed. Oakbrook Terrace, IL: Joint Commission Resources; 2016.

521. Personnel: personnel records. In: *Procedural Standards and Checklist for Accreditation of Ambulatory Surgery Facilities.* Version 3 ed. Gurnee, IL: American Association for Accreditation of Ambulatory Surgery Facilities, Inc; 2011:77-79.

522. PI.03.01.01: The hospital improves performance on an ongoing basis. In: *Hospital Accreditation Standards.* 2016 ed. Oakbrook Terrace, IL: Joint Commission Resources; 2016.

523. QM.1: Quality management system. In: *NIAHO Interpretive Guidelines and Surveyor Guidance.* Version 11 ed. Milford, OH: DNV GL - Healthcare; 2014:10-17.

524. PI.03.01.01: The organization improves performance. In: *Standards for Ambulatory Care.* 2016 ed. Oakbrook Terrace, IL: Joint Commission Resources; 2016.

525. Quality management and improvement. In: *Accreditation Handbook for Ambulatory Health Care.* 2016 ed. Skokie, IL: Accreditation Association for Ambulatory Health Care, Inc; 2016:46-50.

526. Quality assessment/quality improvement: quality improvement. In: *Regular Standards and Checklist for Accreditation of Ambulatory Surgery Facilities.* Version 14.4 ed. American Association for Accreditation of Ambulatory Surgery Facilities; 2016:64.

527. Quality assessment/quality improvement: unanticipated operative sequelae. In: *Regular Standards and Checklist for Accreditation of Ambulatory Surgery Facilities.* Version 14.4 ed.

American Association for Accreditation of Ambulatory Surgery Facilities, Inc; 2016:66-69.

528. Salkind EM. A novel approach to improving the safety of patients undergoing lumbar laminectomy. *AANA J.* 2013; 81(5):389-393. [VC]

529. MAUDE—Manufacturer and User Facility Device Experience. US Food and Drug Administration. https://www .accessdata.fda.gov/scripts/cdrh/cfdocs/cfmaude/search.cfm. Accessed March 10, 2017.

Acknowledgments

Lead Author
Sharon A. Van Wicklin, MSN, RN, CNOR, CRNFA(E), CPSN-R, PLNC
Senior Perioperative Practice Specialist
AORN Nursing Department
Denver, Colorado

The author and AORN thank Marie A. Bashaw, DNP, RN, NEA-BC, CNOR, Assistant Professor, Wright State University College of Nursing and Health, Dayton, Ohio; Rodney W. Hicks, PhD, RN, FNP-BC, FAANP, FAAN, Professor, College of Graduate Nursing, Western University of Health Sciences, Pomona, California; Lynn J. Reede, DNP, MBA, CRNA, FNAP, Senior Director, Professional Practice, American Association of Nurse Anesthetists, Park Ridge, Illinois; Jay Bowers, BSN, RN, CNOR, TNCC, Clinical Educator, West Virginia University Healthcare, Morgantown; Diana L. Wadlund, MSN, ACNP-C, CRNFA, Nurse Practitioner, Paoli Hospital, Paoli, Pennsylvania; and Donna Ford, MSN, RN-BC, CNOR, CRCST, Staff Registered Nurse, Mayo Clinic, Rochester, Minnesota, for their assistance in developing this guideline.

Publication History

Originally published November 1990, *AORN Journal.*

Revised November 1995; published August 1996, *AORN Journal.*

Revised and reformatted; published January 2001, *AORN Journal.*

Revised 2007; published in *Perioperative Standards and Recommended Practices,* 2008 edition.

Minor editing revisions made to omit PNDS codes; reformatted September 2012 for publication in *Perioperative Standards and Recommended Practices,* 2013 edition.

Minor editing revisions made in November 2014 for publication as "Guideline for positioning the patient" in *Guidelines for Perioperative Practice,* 2015 edition.

Revised April 2017 for publication in *Guidelines for Perioperative Practice* online.

Evidence ratings revised and minor editorial changes made to conform to the current AORN Evidence Rating model, September 2019, for online publication in *Guidelines for Perioperative Practice.*

PRODUCT EVALUATION

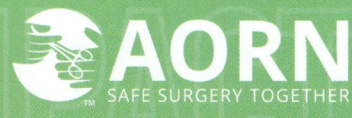
781

TABLE OF CONTENTS

MEDICAL ABBREVIATIONS & ACRONYMS

EPC – Evidence-based practice center
IDA – Innovative device assessment

RN – Registered nurse

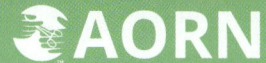
GUIDELINE FOR
MEDICAL DEVICE AND PRODUCT EVALUATION

The Guideline for Medical Device and Product Evaluation was approved by the AORN Guidelines Advisory Board and became effective November 1, 2017. It was presented as a proposed guideline for comments by members and others. The recommendations in the guideline are intended to be achievable and represent what is believed to be an optimal level of practice. Policies and procedures will reflect variations in practice settings and/or clinical situations that determine the degree to which the guideline can be implemented. AORN recognizes the many diverse settings in which perioperative nurses practice; therefore, this guideline is adaptable to all areas where operative or other invasive procedures may be performed.

Purpose

This document provides guidance to perioperative team members for developing and implementing a process for evaluating US Food and Drug Administration–cleared medical devices and products for use in the perioperative setting. The safety of patients and perioperative team members, optimal patient outcomes, and product quality are the primary concerns of perioperative registered nurses (RNs) as they participate in product review and evaluation.

The evidence regarding best practices for product evaluation in the perioperative setting is limited. The health care system is complex, with many variables that make it difficult to perform research on product selection that is generalizable to all settings. These variables include the size of the organization, financial constraints, group purchasing organization relationships, and contractual agreements.

The following subjects are outside the scope of this guideline: specific processes for cleaning, disinfection, and sterilization; management of products and devices after purchase (eg, equipment maintenance, inventory control); selection of electronic health records (eg, health information technology); processes for product waste disposal; and purchasing processes (eg, supply chain).

Evidence Review

A medical librarian conducted a systematic literature search of the databases Ovid MEDLINE®, EBSCO CINAHL®, Scopus®, and the Cochrane Database of Systematic Reviews. The search was limited to literature published in English from 2012 through April 2017. At the time of the initial search, weekly alerts were created on the topics included in the search. Results from these alerts were provided to the lead author until July 2017. The lead author requested additional articles that did not fit the original search criteria or were discovered during the appraisal process.

Search terms included *cost control, financial management, materials management, purchasing department, cost savings, value-based purchasing, surgical instruments, operating rooms, costs and cost analysis, decision-making, organizational, cost-benefit analysis, value stream mapping, financial impact analysis, product selection, quality assurance, cost effectiveness, efficiency, perioperative nursing, device approval, surgical equipment, disposable equipment,* and *equipment and supplies.* Key words and phrases included *group purchasing, surgical devices, surgical services, surgical department, consignment, vendor, committee, interdisciplinary communication, cooperative behavior, single-use devices, patient care items, par level,* and *team.*

Included were research and non-research literature in English, complete publications, and publication dates within the time restriction when available. Excluded were non–peer-reviewed publications and older evidence within the time restriction when more recent evidence was available. Editorials, news items, and brief items were excluded. Low-quality evidence was excluded when higher-quality evidence was available, and literature outside the time restriction was excluded when literature within the time restriction was available (Figure 1).

Included articles were independently evaluated and critically appraised according to the strength and quality of the evidence. Articles identified in the search were provided to the project team for evaluation. The team consisted of the lead author and one evidence appraiser. The lead author divided the search results into topics, and both members of the team reviewed and critically appraised each article using the AORN Research or Non-Research Evidence Appraisal Tools as appropriate. The literature was independently evaluated and appraised according to the strength and quality of the evidence. Each article was then assigned an appraisal score. The appraisal score is noted in brackets after each reference, as applicable.

Each recommendation rating is based on a synthesis of the collective evidence, a benefit-harm assessment, and consideration of resource use. The strength of the recommendation was determined using the AORN Evidence Rating Model and the quality and consistency of the evidence supporting a recommendation. The recommendation strength rating is noted in brackets after each recommendation.

Note: The evidence summary table is available at http://www.aorn.org/evidencetables/.

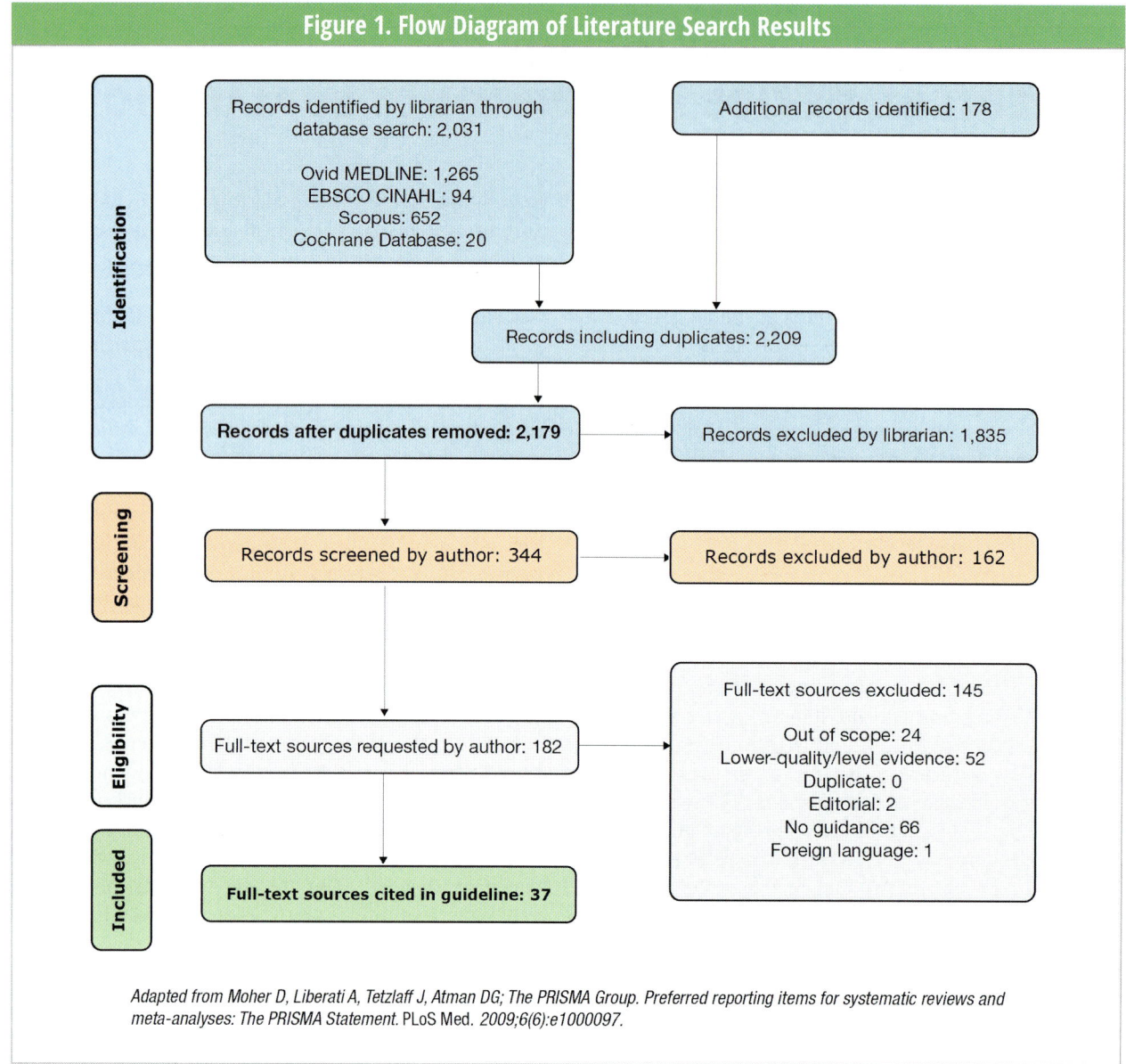

Figure 1. Flow Diagram of Literature Search Results

Adapted from Moher D, Liberati A, Tetzlaff J, Atman DG; The PRISMA Group. Preferred reporting items for systematic reviews and meta-analyses: The PRISMA Statement. PLoS Med. 2009;6(6):e1000097.

Editor's note: MEDLINE is a registered trademark of the US National Library of Medicine's Medical Literature Analysis and Retrieval System, Bethesda, MD. CINAHL, Cumulative Index to Nursing and Allied Health Literature, is a registered trademark of EBSCO Industries, Birmingham, AL. Scopus is a registered trademark of Elsevier B.V., Amsterdam, The Netherlands.

1. Interdisciplinary Team

1.1 **Establish an interdisciplinary team to be responsible for oversight of the medical device and product evaluation process.** *[Conditional Recommendation]*

Health care organizations use different titles to refer to interdisciplinary teams with responsibility for oversight of medical device and product evaluation; these titles include product selection committee, medical device and product evaluation committee, purchasing committee, and value analysis committee. Moderate-quality evidence supports an interdisciplinary team approach to the medical device and product evaluation process.[1-9]

1.2 **Perioperative RNs should have an active role in the evaluation and selection of perioperative products.**[2,3,6,7,10,11] *[Recommendation]*

Moderate-quality evidence from qualitative research studies indicates that RNs as stakeholders can provide clinical, safety, and device-user experience that may help to determine the value of a product under evaluation.

In a qualitative study conducted in five hospitals in the United Kingdom, Hinrichs et al[4] identified stakeholders with authority for making purchasing decisions and examined the challenges of promoting patient safety during the purchasing process.

The researchers identified the main stakeholders as clinical engineers, clinical end users or device users, health care industry representatives, and risk managers. The findings from the study suggest that responsibility for purchasing safe medical devices is shared among clinical end users and financial and technical stakeholders.

Grundy[2] conducted a qualitative research study of purchasing groups at four hospitals in the metropolitan area of a western US city to explore the interactions between nurses and industry representatives in clinical practice. Participants (N = 72) included RNs, supply chain professionals, administrators, and health care industry representatives. The findings indicated that RNs believed it was important for clinicians to be informed on new product developments so they would be prepared when new products were presented for evaluation. The researcher also found that involvement of nurses in hospital value analysis committees could drive quality and cost savings.

Grundy et al[3] conducted another qualitative research study of 72 participants at four acute care hospitals in a western US city to examine in depth the interactions between RNs and health care industry representatives. Data collection processes included observations of nurse-industry interactions in meetings, interviews, and focus groups. Health care industry representatives described RNs as a key audience because RNs have direct contact with patients, prescribers, and purchasers. The researchers found that RNs influenced the distribution of resources that could affect patient care.

1.3 **Include key stakeholders from within the facility on the interdisciplinary team.**[1,2,4,8,12] *[Recommendation]*

Including key stakeholders in the interdisciplinary team provides the health care organization with relevant knowledge and expertise specific to the organization's structure and patient population.

Vincent and Blandford[13] interviewed 20 purchasing committee participants in four hospitals in the United Kingdom to understand purchasing decisions, with a focus on the usability of infusion devices, purchasing practices, and the factors that shape purchasing decisions. The researchers found that a wide variety of stakeholders, including RNs, were influential in evaluating products and that having an interdisciplinary committee encouraged a holistic approach.

1.3.1 The interdisciplinary team may include
- **perioperative RNs,**[2,3,7,10,11]
- **cardiac catheterization lab/electrophysiology lab personnel,**[1]
- **interventional radiology personnel,**[1]
- **laboratory personnel,**[1]
- **materials management/supply chain personnel,**[14,15]
- **surgeons and proceduralists,**[7]
- **surgical technologists,**[7]
- **biomedical engineers,**[14,16]
- **sterile processing personnel,**[9]
- **perioperative educators,**
- **anesthesia professionals,**
- **clinical engineers,**
- **endoscopy services personnel,**
- **environmental services personnel,**
- **infection preventionists,**
- **pathology personnel,**
- **pharmacists,**
- **purchasing personnel,**
- **quality management personnel,**
- **risk managers, and**
- **others as deemed necessary.**

[Conditional Recommendation]

Including representatives from affected disciplines in the evaluation process allows input from personnel with expertise beyond clinical end users and may enhance team-work and end-user compliance with correct use of the product.

1.3.2 **Adjust the interdisciplinary team composition to include end users for specific medical devices and products under evaluation.**[4] *[Recommendation]*

Certain medical devices and products are not used in all departments, and input from key end users is needed to provide relevant and specific input.

1.3.3 **The health care organization must establish a process for selecting and evaluating sharps safety devices as part of the written blood-borne pathogens exposure control plan.**[17,18] *[Regulatory Requirement]*

2. Pre-purchase Evaluation Process

2.1 **Establish and implement a process for the pre-purchase evaluation of products.** *[Conditional Recommendation]*

A standardized medical device and product evaluation process assists in the selection of functional and reliable products that are safe, cost-effective, and environmentally friendly and that promote quality care. Moderate-quality evidence[2,6,12,19] indicates there is a need for health care organizations to be responsible for verifying that medical devices and products used within the organization are effective and safe to use. Regulatory agencies[20,21] require health care organizations to develop and promote a safe health care environment to meet the needs of patients and personnel.

2.2 **Use a decision support framework in the evaluation process.**[2,6,12,19] *[Recommendation]*

A decision support framework provides the team with a standardized tool by which to compare products equally.

Health care organizations have implemented various approaches to product evaluation and purchasing decisions. Grundy[2] developed a framework for value analysis related to medical product decision making. The framework establishes a need for the product, verifies the usability of the product, evaluates the associated costs of the product, and ends with the final decision. The researcher concluded that applying the value analysis framework might assist others in the decision-making process.

Clinical personnel at the University of Pennsylvania used an evidence-based practice center (EPC) as a mechanism for evaluating medical devices and products. The clinical personnel submitted requests to the EPC to conduct an evidence review about a device, equipment, or a supply item. The personnel at the EPC reviewed the request, conducted a rapid systematic review of the evidence, translated the evidence, and made recommendations to the purchasing committee. Jayakumar et al[6] found that the EPC process was an effective method for promoting evidence-based purchasing decisions.

Wernz et al[19] conducted a qualitative research study to identify a best practice decision-making process among hospital decision makers. The researchers conducted interviews with key stakeholders from six hospitals in five countries, including the United States. They identified a best practice approach in a US hospital that used a computer-based decision support system. The computer-based support system uses certain criteria (eg, capacity/access, financial reports, infrastructure, implementation, strategic importance, quality) and weighting of organizational goals to assist in decision-making related to the purchase of a medical device. The findings from this study suggest that use of a computer-based decision support tool may be effective for evaluation of medical devices.

Martelli et al[12] developed a criteria-based tool to assist in the analysis and evaluation of medical devices based on results of a literature review and survey that included 25 participants from 18 hospitals in France. The innovative device assessment (IDA) tool is a decision-support tool that combines multi-criteria decision analysis and a mini health technology assessment. The IDA tool consists of five weighted criteria separated into two categories:

risk and value. The risk-based criteria included the need for specific expertise and training of users, the number of patients and impact on workflow, cost per patient, additional payments for the device, and the unit cost of the device. The value-based criteria included expected risks or adverse events related to the device, expected clinical benefit for the patient, impact on quality of life, opinion concerning the device, and the quality of the evidence related to the device. The researchers applied the IDA tool at a health care system representing 38 hospitals in Paris for the evaluation of two new drug-eluting beads for transcatheter arterial chemoembolization. The IDA tool revealed that the new drug-eluting beads conferred no additional value relative to drug-eluting beads currently available. The researchers concluded that the use of the IDA tool may promote a more structured approach to health technology assessment and that it is useful as a decision-support tool.

2.3 **Perform a financial impact analysis on each medical device and product being evaluated.** *[Recommendation]*

Financial analysis is a key element in product evaluation and selection. The financial analysis assists in determining whether the product fits within the organization's overall fiscal strategy[22] and may provide data that are useful in determining global procedural costs.[23] Understanding the financial impact of a new product or device can also assist with budget development and resource utilization plans.

In some cases, a financial analysis may be required for reimbursement.[24] The Centers for Medicare & Medicaid Services[25] Hospital Value-Based Purchasing Program is an initiative that connects reimbursement with quality and patient safety. A percentage of a hospital's reimbursement is withheld until the hospital meets required quality measures. The quality measures address patient safety, patient satisfaction, and cost efficiency. The intent is to hold hospitals accountable and to improve the value of health care provided in acute health care settings.[26,27]

2.3.1 Include the following in the financial impact analysis:
- direct costs (eg, cost of the product acquisition, replacement strategy, associated equipment),
- indirect costs (eg, utilities, waste disposal, processing, personnel orientation, storage, energy use, depreciation, retrofitting of existing equipment, renovation or construction),

- reimbursement potential (eg, Centers for Medicare & Medicaid Services Value-Based Purchasing), and
- group purchasing organization contract pricing if applicable.

[Recommendation]

2.4 Include the following elements in the product evaluation:
- compliance with local, state, and regulatory requirements;
- clinical usability and cost effectiveness[5,6,13,28];
- patient and user safety[4,9];
- improved patient outcomes;
- product quality[7,29-31];
- strategic priorities[1,29,32];
- vendor contractual agreements[7,16];
- compliance with accrediting organizations;
- compatibility with existing processing methods;
- compatibility with existing disposal methods;
- patient-population needs; and
- personnel and end-user preferences.

[Recommendation]

2.5 Assess the environmental impact of a device or product. [Recommendation]

Perioperative RNs have an ethical obligation and professional responsibility to address environmental exposures and hazards for the health, welfare, and safety of all people. Perioperative RNs can help to mitigate the environmental effects of health care by supporting the selection of environmentally responsible products.[33] Serving as stewards of the environment includes implementing practices that will help preserve natural resources, reduce waste, and minimize exposure to hazardous materials.[34]

In a nonexperimental study, Kaplan et al[35] found that health care organizations are among the country's most energy-intensive facilities, accounting for a significant percentage of US greenhouse gas and carbon dioxide emissions. Health care organizations create 6,600 tons of waste per day and use large amounts of toxic chemicals.[35] Following sustainable practices that include energy-use reduction, recycling, minimization of regulated waste, reduction of landfill waste, reprocessing, reuse of single-use medical devices, and reformulation of OR custom packs may reduce waste.[36,37]

2.5.1 Use the following criteria for determining whether to purchase a single-use or reusable product:
- the useful life of the product;
- the intended use of the product;
- the ability to clean the medical device or product;

- the availability of required cleaning, disinfection, and sterilization processes;
- time required for reprocessing;
- if single-use, whether the product can be reprocessed by a US Food and Drug Administration–cleared third party reprocessor;
- if single-use, cost and requirements for disposal;
- inventory required;
- complexity of the manufacturer's instructions for use and the end user's ability to reliably follow instructions;
- competency requirements for personnel who use, maintain, and reprocess instruments, medical devices, and other equipment;
- maintenance, repair, or restoration programs for instruments and equipment; and
- storage requirements.

[Recommendation]

2.6 Obtain and review the manufacturer's technical specifications and clinical use recommendations during the product evaluation process. [Recommendation]

Health care product and device manufacturers provide clinical and technical information related to the product use and safety that is vital for product evaluation.

2.7 Develop and implement a plan to introduce new products and devices into clinical practice, including a plan for education of personnel. [Recommendation]

The development of a comprehensive plan for the introduction of a medical device or product may facilitate smooth implementation.[6]

3. Quality

3.1 Establish a quality assurance and performance improvement process for product evaluation. [Conditional Recommendation]

A quality assurance/performance improvement program provides a mechanism for verifying that new products and devices are meeting expected performance criteria and that the pre-selection evaluation process has met its objectives.

3.2 Participate in ongoing quality assurance and performance improvement activities. [Recommendation]

Participating in ongoing quality assurance and performance improvement activities is a primary responsibility of perioperative personnel engaged in practice.

3.3 **After a product or device has been introduced, develop and implement a comprehensive plan for post-purchase evaluation.** *[Conditional Recommendation]*

Glossary

Financial impact analysis: An estimate of the financial consequences associated with purchasing a new product or medical device.

References

1. Atwood D, Larose P, Uttley R. Strategies for success in purchasing medical technology. *Biomed Instrum Technol.* 2015; 49(2):93-98. [VB]

2. Grundy Q. "Whether something cool is good enough": the role of evidence, sales representatives and nurses' expertise in hospital purchasing decisions. *Soc Sci Med.* 2016;165:82-91. [IIIB]

3. Grundy Q, Bero LA, Malone RE. Marketing and the most trusted profession: the invisible interactions between registered nurses and industry. *Ann Intern Med.* 2016;164(11):733-739. [IIIB]

4. Hinrichs S, Dickerson T, Clarkson J. Stakeholder challenges in purchasing medical devices for patient safety. *J Patient Saf.* 2013;9(1):36-43. [IIIB]

5. Li CS, Vannabouathong C, Sprague S, Bhandari M. Orthopedic implant value drivers: a qualitative survey study of hospital purchasing administrators. *J Long Term Eff Med Implants.* 2015;25(3):237-244. [IIIC]

6. Jayakumar KL, Lavenberg JA, Mitchell MD, et al. Evidence synthesis activities of a hospital evidence-based practice center and impact on hospital decision making. *J Hosp Med.* 2015;11(3):185-192. [VA]

7. Plonien C, Williams M. Vendor presence in the OR. *AORN J.* 2014;100(1):81-86. [VB]

8. Sohrakoff K, Westlake C, Key E, Barth E, Antognini J, Johnson V. Optimizing the OR: a bottom-up approach. *Hosp Top.* 2014;92(2):21-27. [VB]

9. Vockley M. Choosing wisely: trends and strategies for capital planning and procurement. *Biomed Instrum Technol.* 2016;50(4):230-241. [VC]

10. Lerner DG, Pall H. Setting up the pediatric endoscopy unit. *Gastrointest Endosc Clin N Am.* 2016;26(1):1-12. [IIIB]

11. NHS Procurement & Commercial Standards. 2016. https://nhsprocurement.org.uk/files/2016-07/Standards_of_Procurement.pdf. Accessed August 23, 2017. [IVC]

12. Martelli N, Hansen P, van den Brink H, et al. Combining multi-criteria decision analysis and mini-health technology assessment: a funding decision-support tool for medical devices in a university hospital setting. *J Biomed Inform.* 2016;59:201-208. [IIIB]

13. Vincent CJ, Blandford A. How do health service professionals consider human factors when purchasing interactive medical devices? A qualitative interview study. *Appl Ergon.* 2017;59(Pt A):114-122. [IIIA]

14. Lynch PK. Do group purchasing organizations really save money on capital equipment? *Biomed Instrum Technol.* 2017;51(2):170-171. [VC]

15. Walsh SS. Suture cost savings in the OR. *AORN J.* 2012;95(5):631-634. [VB]

16. Kobernick T. How to negotiate with high-pressure vendors. *Biomed Instrum Technol.* 2013;47(1):36-37. [VC]

17. 29 CFR §1910.1030: Bloodborne pathogens. Occupational Safety and Health Administration. https://www.osha.gov/pls/oshaweb/owadisp.show_document?p_id=10051&p_table=STANDARDS. Accessed August 23, 2017.

18. Guideline for sharps safety. In: *Guidelines for Perioperative Practice.* Denver, CO: AORN, Inc; 2017: 423-446. [IVA]

19. Wernz C, Zhang H, Phusavat K. International study of technology investment decisions at hospitals. *Ind Manage Data Syst* [serial online]. 2014;114(4):568-582. [IIIC]

20. 42 CFR 482: Conditions of participation for hospitals. 2011. US Government Publishing Office. https://www.gpo.gov/fdsys/granule/CFR-2011-title42-vol5/CFR-2011-title42-vol5-part482. Accessed August 23, 2017.

21. 42 CFR 416: Ambulatory surgical services. 2011. US Government Publishing Office. https://www.gpo.gov/fdsys/granule/CFR-2011-title42-vol3/CFR-2011-title42-vol3-part416. Accessed August 23, 2017.

22. *ISO 20400:2017. Sustainable Procurement—Guidance.* Geneva, Switzerland: International Organization for Standardization; 2017.

23. Raft J, Millet F, Meistelman C. Example of cost calculations for an operating room and a post-anaesthesia care unit. *Anaesth Crit Care Pain Med.* 2015;34(4):211-215. [IIIA]

24. Sullivan SD, Mauskopf JA, Augustovski F, et al. Budget impact analysis—principles of good practice: report of the ISPOR 2012 Budget Impact Analysis Good Practice II Task Force. *Value Health.* 2014;17(1):5-14. [VA]

25. Hospital value-based purchasing. Centers for Medicare & Medicaid Services. https://www.cms.gov/Medicare/Quality-Initiatives-Patient-Assessment-Instruments/hospital-value-based-purchasing/index.html?redirect=/hospital-value-based-purchasing. Updated February 15, 2017. Accessed August 23, 2017.

26. Stacy KM. Hospital value-based purchasing: part 1, overview of the program. *AACN Adv Crit Care.* 2016;27(4):362-367. [VA]

27. Stacy KM. Hospital value-based purchasing: part 2, implications. *AACN Adv Crit Care.* 2017;28(1):16-20. [VA]

28. How healthcare executives make buying decisions. *Healthc Financ Manage.* 2012;66(6):1-7. [VC]

29. Bosko T, Dubow M, Koenig T. Understanding value-based incentive models and using performance as a strategic advantage. *J Healthc Manag.* 2016;61(1):11-14. [VB]

30. Eiferman D, Bhakta A, Khan S. Implementation of a shared-savings program for surgical supplies decreases inventory cost. *Surgery.* 2015;158(4):996-1002. [VB]

31. Farrokhi FR, Gunther M, Williams B, Blackmore CC. Application of lean methodology for improved quality and efficiency in operating room instrument availability. *J Healthc Qual.* 2015;37(5):277-286. [VB]

32. Rocchio BJ. Achieving cost reduction through data analytics. *AORN J.* 2016;104(4):320-325. [VB]

33. AORN position statement on environmental responsibility. *AORN J.* 2014;99(1):18-21. [IVB]

34. ANA's Principles of Environmental Health for Nursing Practice with Implementation Strategies. Silver Spring, MD: American Nurses Association; 2007. http://www.nursing world.org/MainMenuCategories/WorkplaceSafety/Healthy-Nurse/ANAsPrinciplesofEnvironmentalHealthforNursing Practice.pdf. Accessed August 23, 2017. [IVC]

35. Kaplan S, Sadler B, Little K, Franz C, Orris P. Can sustainable hospitals help bend the health care cost curve? *Issue Brief (Commonw Fund).* 2012;29:1-14. [IIIC]

36. Southorn T, Norrish AR, Gardner K, Baxandall R. Reducing the carbon footprint of the operating theatre: a multicentre quality improvement report. *J Perioper Pract.* 2013;23(6):144-146. [VB]

37. Wormer BA, Augenstein VA, Carpenter CL, et al. The green operating room: simple changes to reduce cost and our carbon footprint. *Am Surg.* 2013;79(7):666-671. [VA]

Acknowledgments

Lead Author

Esther M. Johnstone, DNP, RN, CNOR
Perioperative Practice Specialist
AORN Nursing Department
Denver, Colorado

Contributing Author

Ramona L. Conner, MSN, RN, CNOR, FAAN
Editor-in-Chief, Guidelines for Perioperative Practice
AORN Nursing Department
Denver, Colorado

The authors and AORN thank Marie Bashaw, DNP, RN, NEA-BC, CNOR, Assistant Professor, Wright State University, Dayton, Ohio; Barbara Nalley, MSN, RN, CRNP, CNOR, Surgical Assist RNFA Nurse Practitioner, Anne Arundel Medical Group & Chesapeake Women's Care, Crofton, Maryland; Susan Klacik, BS, CRCST, ACE, CHL, FCS,
Klacik Consulting LLC, Canfield, Ohio; Dawn Yost, MSN, BSDH, RN, RDH, CNOR, CSSM, Manager of Training & Development, Surgical Services, WVU Medicine–Ruby Memorial Hospital, Morgantown, West Virginia; James (Jay) Bowers, BSN, RN, CNOR, Clinical Educator, West Virginia Healthcare, Morgantown; Evangeline (Vangie) Dennis, BSN, RN, CNOR, CMLSO, Director of Patient Care Practice, Emory Healthcare and Ambulatory Surgery Centers, Atlanta, Georgia; Sharon Van Wicklin, MSN, RN, CNOR, CRNFA(E), CPSN-R, PLNC, Senior Perioperative Practice Specialist, AORN Nursing Department, Denver, Colorado; and Amber Wood, MSN, RN, CNOR, CIC, FAPIC, Senior Perioperative Practice Specialist, AORN Nursing Department, Denver, Colorado, for their assistance in developing this guideline.

Publication History

Originally published April 1989, *AORN Journal,* as "Recommended practices: product evaluation and selection for perioperative patient care."

Revised August 1993.

Revised November 1997; published January 1998, *AORN Journal,* as "Recommended practices for product selection in perioperative practice settings."

Reformatted July 2000.

Revised November 2003; published in *Standards, Recommended Practices, and Guidelines,* 2004 edition. Reprinted March 2004, *AORN Journal.*

Revised January 2010 for online publication in *Perioperative Standards and Recommended Practices.*

Reformatted September 2012 for publication in *Perioperative Standards and Recommended Practices,* 2013 edition.

Minor editing revisions made in November 2014 for publication as "Guideline for product selection" in *Guidelines for Perioperative Practice,* 2015 edition.

Revised November 2017 for publication in *Guidelines for Perioperative Practice* online.

Evidence ratings revised and minor editorial changes made to conform to the current AORN Evidence Rating model, September 2019, for online publication in *Guidelines for Perioperative Practice.*

AORN GUIDELINES FOR
PERIOPERATIVE PRACTICE,
2022 EDITION

RADIATION SAFETY

TABLE OF CONTENTS

A *indicates additional information is available in the Ambulatory Supplement.*

P *indicates a recommendation or evidence relevant to pediatric care.*

MEDICAL ABBREVIATIONS & ACRONYMS

AAPM – American Association of Physicists in Medicine
ACR – American College of Radiology
AK – Air kerma
ALARA – As low as reasonably achievable
BMI – Body mass index
CT – Computed tomography
DAP – Dose area product
ICRP – International Commission on Radiological Protection
FT – Fluoroscopy time
NRC – US Nuclear Regulatory Commission

OR – Operating room
PET – Positron emission tomography
RCT – Randomized controlled trial
RSO – Radiation safety officer
SPR – Society for Pediatric Radiology
TEDE – Total effective dose equivalent
TGD – Tungsten drape
UGI – Upper gastrointestinal
WSC – Water-soluable contrast

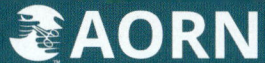
GUIDELINE FOR
RADIATION SAFETY

The Guideline for Radiation Safety was approved by the AORN Guidelines Advisory Board and became effective as of April 15, 2021. The recommendations in the guideline are intended to be achievable and represent what is believed to be an optimal level of practice. Policies and procedures will reflect variations in practice settings and/or clinical situations that determine the degree to which the guideline can be implemented. AORN recognizes the many diverse settings in which perioperative nurses practice; therefore, this guideline is adaptable to all areas where operative or other invasive procedures may be performed.

Purpose

This document provides guidance for preventing patient and health care worker injury from exposure to medical ionizing radiation during therapeutic, diagnostic, or interventional procedures performed in the perioperative environment. Guidance is included on protective measures related to the administration of **radionuclides** and **radiopharmaceuticals**; this guidance applies to patients, perioperative team members, and caregivers of patients who are treated with radionuclides or have radiopharmaceuticals circulating in their bloodstream.

Medical radiation exposure occurs

- in most perioperative specialties (eg, trauma, cardiac, neurosurgery, orthopedics, urology, vascular, podiatry)[1-3];
- in various settings (eg, operating rooms [ORs], hybrid ORs, ambulatory surgery centers, inpatient and outpatient endoscopy suites, physician offices, interventional radiology suites, cardiac catheterization laboratories)[3]; and
- in the community (eg, when a patient has **brachytherapy** implants).[4]

Studies have demonstrated that medical ionizing radiation can have adverse effects on the human body.[5-7] The adverse effects of radiation are classified as **tissue reactions** (previously known as deterministic effects) or **stochastic effects**. Tissue reactions from radiation (eg, radiation burns, radiation dermatitis, skin erythema, hair loss, cataract formation, infertility, circulatory disease) appear at various times after the exposure.[4,7-10] The reactions ranged in severity from skin rashes and epilation to necrosis of the skin and its underlying structures. These reactions may appear at any time, even years after the exposure.[4] Tissue reactions frequently appear at the radiation entrance site (eg, back, neck, buttocks, anterior of the chest).[4] Stochastic effects (eg, cancer,[11] genetic effects,[12-14] congenital anomalies[15]) can appear at any time after the exposure, but usually appear after several years.[10,16] Sto-

chastic effects occur when radiation causes a mutation within the cell or cell death. For both tissue reactions and stochastic effects, the severity and type of damage are related to the dose received (ie, the greater the dose, the greater the potential for damage).[11]

Patients and personnel may receive different amounts of radiation based on the

- modality used (eg, portable or fixed x-ray machine, brachytherapy seed or balloon implants, radiopharmaceuticals, intraoperative radiation therapy, mobile [eg, C-arm (eg, standard, mini), O-arm] or fixed fluoroscopy unit)[3,4,10,17,18];
- procedure[1,2];
- operator[19]; and
- patient-specific factors (eg, gender, body mass index [BMI], disease process).[20-26]

Farah et al[27] reviewed the radiation doses received by 319 patients undergoing a thrombectomy after a stroke. The researchers analyzed the **dose area product** (DAP), **cumulative air kerma** (AK), fluoroscopy time, and the number of images taken. They concluded that male sex, number of passages, and success of recanalization were key parameters affecting the patient dose.

The dosage is also affected by the patient's BMI. Researchers who studied patients undergoing coronary angiography,[26] fracture repairs,[23-25] fluoroscopically guided injections,[21,22] and transcatheter aortic valve replacement[20] have noted a significant increase in dosage corresponding to an increase in the patient's BMI.

Pravatà et al[28] measured the dose received by the patient and the dose received by the operator during 26 computed tomography (CT)-guided spine procedures. The researchers found that the greater the dose to the patient the greater the dose to the operator.

Although radiation doses vary by procedure and other factors, Faroux et al[29] found that for patients undergoing percutaneous coronary interventions, the DAP decreased for the same procedures between 2006 and 2016. Casella et al[19] also found a decrease in the DAP from 2010 to 2016 for 6,095 electrophysiological and 2,055 device implantation procedures. The decrease in the dosages was believed to be related to technological advances.[19,29]

Perioperative team members are exposed to radiation from three different sources independent of the modality used. These sources include

- primary radiation, which is emitted directly by the modality;
- leakage radiation, which emanates from the x-ray modality housing; and
- **scatter radiation**, which is reflected off of the patient, tabletop, and shielding material.[30]

The main source of radiation exposure for team members in the perioperative setting is scatter radiation, with different team members receiving varying doses during the same procedure.[31,32] The amount of radiation perioperative team members receive is affected by the direction of the beam,[33] the beam quality, the field size, the position of the person in relation to the position of the beam originator,[34] and the dose being administered.[28]

Limitations of the evidence include a small sample size in many of the studies, and some studies offered no recommendations for action related to minimizing exposure to radiation. Many of the studies focused on the operator, usually the physician, who stands at the sterile field close to the source of radiation; other perioperative team members in the room are frequently excluded from the study data.[35]

The following subjects are outside the scope of this document:

- management of radioactive specimens (See the AORN Guideline for Specimen Management[36]);
- safety precautions during use of magnetic resonance imaging (See the AORN Guideline for Minimally Invasive Surgery[37]);
- non-ionizing radiation (laser) precautions (See the AORN Guideline for Laser Safety[38]);
- protocols for reduction of dosage;
- safety precautions during procedures outside of the perioperative setting using gamma knife, cyber knife, or stereotactic radiosurgery;
- the informed consent process for examinations or procedures that involve radiation;
- collimation (ie, determining the size of the area of the beam);
- the principles of justification (ie, a risk-benefit assessment completed by the person requesting the radiological examination);
- precautions to be taken during positron emission tomography (PET)/CT scanning;
- selection of the C-arm orientation;
- procedural equipment selection, including use of non-radiation-emitting equipment versus radiation-emitting equipment; and
- measures to calculate or regulate the patient's radiation dose.

Evidence Review

A medical librarian with a perioperative background conducted a systematic search of the databases Ovid MEDLINE®, Ovid Embase®, EBSCO CINAHL®, and the Cochrane Database of Systematic Reviews. The search was limited to literature published in English from January 2014 through February 2020. At the time of the initial search, weekly alerts were created on the topics included in that search. Results from these alerts were provided to the lead author until April 2020. The lead author requested additional articles that either did not fit the original search criteria or were discovered during the evidence appraisal process. The lead author and the medical librarian also identified relevant guidelines from government agencies, professional organizations, and standards-setting bodies.

Search terms included *abdominal radiography, accidents (occupational), advanced imaging system, ambulatory care facility, ambulatory surgery, balloon dilatation, biplane fluoroscopy, brachytherapy, burns, catheterization, cat scan, catheterization (central venous), catheterization (peripheral), catheterization (peripheral central venous), catheterization (umbilical vessels), cleaning, conceptus, CT scan, disinfection, dose area products, dosimeter, dosimetry, equipment contamination, equipment failure, extremities, fertility, fetus, fixed advanced imaging system, fluoroscopy, glasses, goggles, gonads, hazardous waste (handling/storage/transport), heart catheterization, hybrid imaging equipment, intraoperative CT scan, intraoperative radiotherapy, interventional radiography, interventional radiology, invasive procedures, iodine radioisotopes, lead apron, lead garment, lead glasses, lead goggles, lead shield, leaded apron, leaded garment, leaded glasses, leaded goggles, leaded shield, monoplane fluoroscopy, occupational hazards, occupational accident, occupational diseases, occupational exposure, occupational health, occupational injuries, occupational radiation dose, ocular radiation injury, operating room, operating room personnel, operating suite, operating theater, operating theatre, outpatient surgery, patient injuries, patient safety, pregnancy, pregnancy outcomes, protective clothing, protective gloves, radiation, radiation burn, radiation exposure, radiation (ionizing), radiation injuries, radiation monitoring, radiation parameters, radiation protection, radiation safety officer, radiation safety precautions, radiation safety procedures, radioactive pollutants, radioactive tracers, radioactive waste (handling/storage/transport), radiography, radiography (abdominal), radiography (interventional), radioisotopes, radiometry, radiopharmaceuticals, radioprotection, radiosurgery, radiotherapy, radiotherapy (intraoperative), risk assessment, staff dose,* and *zygote.*

Included were research and non-research literature in English, complete publications, and publications with dates within the time restriction when available. Excluded were non-peer-reviewed publications and older evidence within the time restriction when more recent evidence was available. Editorials, news items, and other brief items were excluded. Low-quality evidence was excluded when higher-quality evidence was available, and literature outside the time restriction was excluded when literature within the time restriction was available (**Figure 1**).

Articles identified in the search were provided to the project team for evaluation. The team consisted of the lead author and an evidence appraiser. The lead author and the evidence appraiser reviewed and critically appraised each article using the AORN Research or Non-Research Evidence Appraisal Tools as appropriate. The literature was independently evaluated and appraised according to the strength and quality of the evidence. Each article was then assigned an appraisal score. The appraisal score is noted in brackets after each reference as applicable.

Each recommendation rating is based on a synthesis of the collective evidence, a benefit-harm assessment, and

Figure 1. Flow Diagram of Literature Search Results

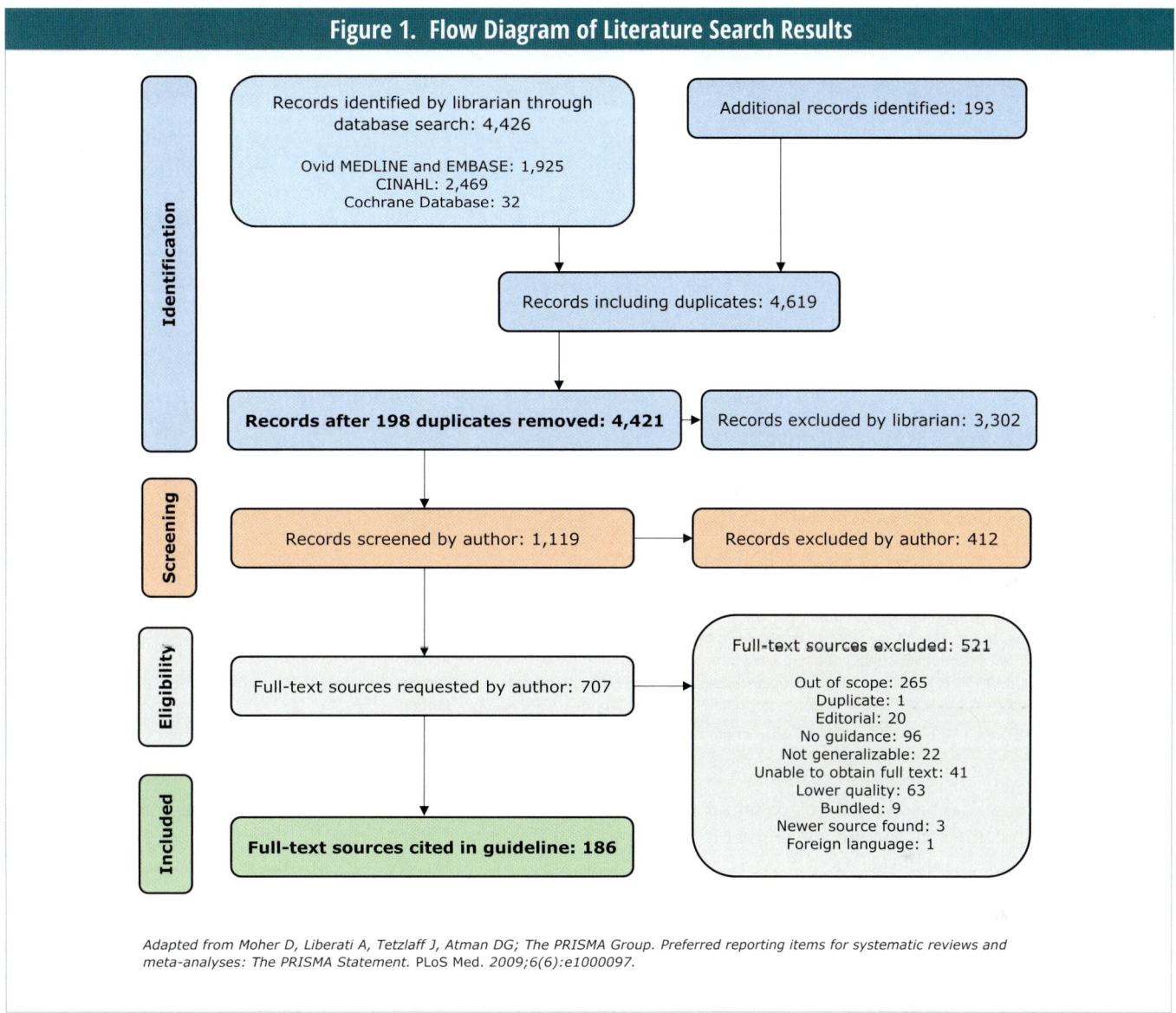

Identification

Records identified by librarian through database search: 4,426

Ovid MEDLINE and EMBASE: 1,925
CINAHL: 2,469
Cochrane Database: 32

Additional records identified: 193

Records including duplicates: 4,619

Records after 198 duplicates removed: 4,421

Records excluded by librarian: 3,302

Screening

Records screened by author: 1,119

Records excluded by author: 412

Eligibility

Full-text sources requested by author: 707

Full-text sources excluded: 521

Out of scope: 265
Duplicate: 1
Editorial: 20
No guidance: 96
Not generalizable: 22
Unable to obtain full text: 41
Lower quality: 63
Bundled: 9
Newer source found: 3
Foreign language: 1

Included

Full-text sources cited in guideline: 186

Adapted from Moher D, Liberati A, Tetzlaff J, Atman DG; The PRISMA Group. Preferred reporting items for systematic reviews and meta-analyses: The PRISMA Statement. PLoS Med. 2009;6(6):e1000097.

consideration of resource use. The strength of the recommendation was determined using the AORN Evidence Rating Model and the quality and consistency of the evidence supporting a recommendation. The recommendation strength rating is noted in brackets after each recommendation.

In the literature, various metrics were used to report the dose of radiation received; the abbreviations are listed in **Table 1**. Additional dose-related definitions are provided in the glossary.

Note: The evidence summary table is available at http://www.aorn.org/evidencetables/.

Editor's note: MEDLINE is a registered trademark of the US National Library of Medicine's Medical Literature Analysis and Retrieval System, Bethesda, MD. Embase is a registered trademark of Elsevier B.V., Amsterdam, The Netherlands. CINAHL, Cumulative Index to Nursing and Allied Health Literature, is a registered trademark of EBSCO Industries, Birmingham, AL.

Note: The use of x-ray equipment is regulated by each state and the use of radioactive materials in a medical setting is regulated by the Nuclear Regulatory Commission (NRC) or by the state in which the facility resides. The states that do not follow the NRC regulations are referred to as **Agreement States** *and many have differing regulations.[39] Before adopting the recommendations rated as regulatory requirements in this guideline, confirm with the radiation safety officer or local authority having jurisdiction whether they apply in your location.*

1. Health Care Organization

1.1 **The health care organization must establish a radiation safety program when potential for occupational radiation exposure exists.**[39-42] *[Regulatory Requirement]*

A radiation safety program manages the safety of patients and perioperative team members by

Table 1. Radiation Dosage[a] Metrics[1-3]

Term	Abbreviation	Definition
Roentgen equivalents (mammal)	rem	1 roentgen
Millirem	mrem	0.001 rem
Millirad	mrad	0.001 rad
Sievert[b]	Sv	100 rem
Millisievert	mSv	0.001 Sievert
Microsievert	μSv	0.0001 Sievert
Gray[c]	Gy	100 rad
Milligray	mGy	0.001 gray
Microgray	μGy	0.0001 gray

[a] Radiation dose is usually expressed in standard international units (SI).

[b] Effective dose or equivalent dose of radiation received is usually expressed in Sieverts. Equivalent dose may be further defined as deep-dose equivalent or shallow-dose equivalent.

[c] Absorbed dose is usually expressed in Gray.

References

1. Lakkireddy D, Nadzam G, Verma A, et al. Impact of a comprehensive safety program on radiation exposure during catheter ablation of atrial fibrillation: a prospective study. J Interv Cardiac Electrophysiol. 2009;24(2):105-112.
2. Weiss EM, Thabit O. Clinical considerations for allied professionals: radiation safety and protection in the electrophysiology lab. Heart Rhythm. 2007;4(12):1583-1587.
3. 29 CFR 1910.1096. Toxic and hazardous substances: Ionizing radiation. Occupational Safety and Health Administration. https://www.osha.gov/pls/oshaweb/owadisp.show_document?p_table=STANDARDS&p_id=10098. Accessed January 19, 2021.

providing guidance on methods to minimize exposure to ionizing radiation to a level that is as low as reasonably achievable (ALARA).[39,43]

1.2 The health care organization must appoint a radiation safety officer (RSO) and a radiation safety committee who lead and direct the radiation safety program if the facility meets the definition of a medical program as defined in the regulatory requirements.[40,42,44,45] *[Regulatory Requirement]*

These appointments are supported in a report from the NRC.[44]

1.3 The health care organization must monitor perioperative team members exposed to radiation according to local, state, and federal regulations[40,41,46] *[Regulatory Requirement]*

See Section 9 for more information on personal radiation monitoring.

1.4 The health care organization must perform an evaluation of the radiation exposure risk or concentrations of radioactive material present, to determine the need for dosimetry when there is a change in equipment (ie, purchase of a CT scanner, creation of a hybrid OR).[47] *[Regulatory Requirement]*

Federal regulations require evaluation of the levels of radiation present.[47] **See Section 9** for additional requirements for personal radiation monitoring.

1.5 The health care organization must provide radiation shielding devices (eg, aprons, rolling shields, other protective equipment) as indicated by the radiation exposure risk, for all perioperative team members.[40,41,46] *[Regulatory Requirement]*

See Sections 5 and 7 for additional requirements for shielding.

1.6 The health care organization must retain records (eg, dosimetry reports, radiology films, image records, scans, digital files) according to local, state, and federal regulatory requirements.[40,41,43] *[Regulatory Requirement]*

1.7 The health care organization must provide education to and verify competency of perioperative team members who have the potential for occupational radiation exposure, as required by state regulations and as applicable to their roles and responsibilities.[39,48] *[Regulatory Requirement]*

For more information on the educational requirements for use of radionuclides and radiopharmaceuticals, **see Recommendation 10.20.**

1.7.1 The education must be provided upon hire and annually.[42,43,49] *[Regulatory Requirement]*

1.7.2 The education should include
- radiation exposure risks,[50-55]
- biological effects of radiation exposure,[16,50,52,55,56]
- principles of radiation protection (eg, time, distance, shielding),[35,50,52,54-60]
- principles of dosimetry (eg, one versus two monitors, placement),[50,52,55,56]
- safe equipment operation,[50-52,55,59,61] and
- regulatory requirements.[55]

[Recommendation] **P**

Incorporation of the listed education content is supported by high-quality evidence[51,58,59,62] and is recommended by clinical guidelines.[50,52,54-57]

In a quasi-experimental study, Gendelberg et al[59] measured the radiation received by pediatric patients being treated for a distal radius or both-forearm bone fracture when a miniature mobile fluoroscopy unit (mini C-arm) was used for visualization of the fracture. The dose was measured before (n = 53) and after (n = 45) an education program covering radiation safety and operation of the mini C-arm was provided to residents who operated the mini C-arm. The researchers found the dose delivered for distal radius fractures was reduced from 83.1 mR before the education program to 32.6 mR after the education program. The dose delivered for combined distal radius and ulnar fractures was decreased from 90.9 mR to 30.4 mR. The researchers recommended that residents receive structured radiation safety training.

Fidalgo Domingos et al[58] performed a quasi-experimental study in which the researchers measured the average radiation dose received by the physician per procedure in one clinical setting. They obtained measurements by reading **dosimeters** located at the physicians' chest level outside of the radioprotective garments during 170 interventional vascular procedures before and 142 procedures after an education program on radiation protection. The average dose decreased from 0.4 Gy before the education program to 0.2 Gy post education, but the decrease did not reach statistical significance. The researchers concluded that education is of the utmost importance for effective radiation safety practices in the interventional vascular setting.

In a quasi-experimental study, Choi et al[51] measured the DAP for radiologists and radiographers during gastrointestinal fluoroscopic examinations before (n = 779) and after (n =

1,547) an educational program covering radiation exposure, the importance of reducing radiation exposure during fluoroscopy, and how to reduce the patient radiation dose during fluoroscopy. The examinations included colon studies with water-soluble contrast (WSC), colon studies with barium, defecography, esophagography with WSC, esophagography with barium, small bowel series with WSC, small bowel series with barium, upper gastrointestinal (UGI) series with WSC, UGI with barium, and barium swallow.

The researchers found the DAP decreased from 21.1 Gy/cm^2 before the education program to 18.2 Gy/cm^2 after the education program. They concluded that educating the radiologists and radiographers reduced radiation exposure for this population.[51]

Ghodadra et al[62] reached the same conclusion after reviewing the DAP in 1,479 diagnostic procedures (ie, UGI, voiding cystourethrograms, barium enemas) performed by nine radiologists before (n = 945) and after (n = 530) an education program.

1.8 The health care organization allows only qualified personnel to operate a radiologic device.[40,41,46,55] *[Regulatory Requirement]*

Legislation restricts the use of radiologic equipment to personnel who are either licensed to operate radiologic devices (ie, a licensed, registered radiology technologist [RT, R]), or personnel who can demonstrate successful completion of formal education and training (ie, licensed independent practitioners, physicians).[55] These regulations encompass all radiologic devices including the mini C-arm.

For more information on the responsibilities of the health care organization when radionuclides and radiopharmaceuticals are administered, **see Section 10**.

2. Radiation Safety Committee

2.1 The radiation safety committee must include
- an authorized user representing each type of use permitted by the license for administration of radioactive materials,
- the RSO,
- a representative of the nursing service, and
- a representative of management who is not an authorized user or an RSO.[42,43]

[Regulatory Requirement]

The inclusion of the listed interdisciplinary team members is required by the Centers for Medicare & Medicaid Services.[42,43]

2.1.1 The radiation safety committee also may include one or more of the following people:[42,43,49]

- a radiologist or administratively designated alternative,
- an anesthesia professional,
- a scrub person,
- environmental services personnel, and
- a medical physicist, if available.[44,63]

[Conditional Recommendation]

The interdisciplinary team members provide information in their areas of expertise (eg, a physicist provides expertise in regulatory compliance and can assist with mathematical calculations [eg, dose-specific safe distance from the radiation source], a radiologist provides expertise in optimizing protection, facility administrators provide resources to support the program). This committee makeup is supported by low-quality evidence[63] and recommended in a report from the NRC.[44]

2.1.2 Consultants or contractors may fill some of the positions on the radiation safety committee if the health care organization does not employ personnel who can fill these positions.[44,63] *[Conditional Recommendation]*

Use of consultants or contractors in the absence of employed personnel is recommended in a report from the NRC[44] and supported by low-quality evidence.[63]

2.2 The radiation safety committee is responsible for

- defining the radiation safety program,
- reviewing the licensed ALARA program,[44,64]
- establishing and verifying competency requirements for personnel,[44,63,64]
- verifying licensure of personnel,[63]
- establishing policies and procedures,
- monitoring radiation exposure,
- monitoring personnel compliance with wearing of radiation protection,[44,64]
- reviewing dosimetry records,[44,64]
- determining the unit of measure to be used for monitoring the radiation dose and the peak value for notifying the operator,
- auditing the radiation safety program annually,[44,64]
- participating in evaluation and selection of new radiology equipment,[44,64]
- registering equipment,[63] and
- providing radiation safety education for personnel not trained in radiology.[63]

[Recommendation] P

These responsibilities are recommended in a clinical guideline[65] and supported by low-quality evidence.[44,63]

For more information on the responsibilities of the radiation safety committee in facilities administering radionuclides and radiopharmaceuticals, see Recommendation 10.5.

2.2.1 Peak values should be expressed using the values recorded by the fluoroscopy unit (eg, air **kerma-area product** and AK) instead of or in addition to fluoroscopy time (FT).[55,66-68] *[Recommendation]*

Moderate-quality evidence[66-70] and clinical guidelines[55,57] support the use of air kerma-area product and AK as the reference point for comparison and documentation.

In a nonexperimental study, Kachaamy et al[66] measured the FT DAP in 463 patients undergoing endoscopic retrograde cholangiopancreatography. The researchers found the same FT produced a wide variability in DAP, and the DAP variability increased as FT increased. The researchers concluded that the FT was a poor indicator of DAP.

In a nonexperimental study, Lazarus et al[67] compared the FT and DAP for 1,011 pediatric patients undergoing procedures where fluoroscopy was used. The researchers found only limited correlation between DAP and FT and concluded that FT might be inadequate for dose monitoring.

In a nonexperimental study, Bonilha et al[68] measured the DAP radiation exposure time at various projections in 200 adults undergoing barium swallow examination. The average radiation dose expressed in $mGy\text{-}cm^2$ per second was 7 for lateral projections, 14 for upper posterior-anterior projections, 17 for middle posterior-anterior projections, and 34 for lower posterior-anterior projections. The researchers concluded the DAP did not correlate to the time of exposure.

In a nonexperimental study, Skripochnik and Loh[70] measured the AK dose during regular fluoroscopy and cinefluoroscopy, and measured the DAP in addition to the FT. The researchers found the cinefluoroscopy and fluoroscopy AK were strongly correlated to the total AK ($r = 0.95$ and 0.92, respectively); fluoroscopy DAP and cinefluoroscopy DAP also correlated strongly with total DAP ($r = 0.84$ and $r = 0.92$, respectively). Fluoroscopy time showed a poor correlation with total AK and total DAP ($r = 0.27$ and $r = 0.32$, respectively). The researchers concluded the FT was not an alternative for measuring radiation exposure. Ghelani et al[69] found similar results in a nonexperimental study in which they examined the radiation dose for 2,713 pediatric patients undergoing interventional catheterization for congenital heart disease.

2.2.2 The radiation safety committee should determine the method (eg, real time, badges) to be used for the personnel radiation dose monitoring.[50,71-78] *[Conditional Recommendation]*

Moderate-quality evidence supports the use of real-time dosimetry.[71-78] The researchers in eight different studies measured the dosage received by personnel in the room during activation of the source with (n = 1,771) and without (n = 1,860) the use of real-time dosimetry. The researchers found a decrease in the radiation dosage ranging from 7% to 60% during the use of real-time dosimetry. They concluded that the use of real-time dosimetry was beneficial.[71-78]

The use of real-time dosimetry is recommended in a clinical guideline from the International Commission on Radiological Protection (ICRP).[50]

3. Radiation Safety Officer

3.1 The RSO
- oversees the radiation safety program[43,44,55];
- assigns tasks to the assistant RSO, if one is present[43,44];
- monitors compliance with regulations put forth by the NRC and other regulatory bodies[44,55,56];
- assists in developing and implementing organizational policies and procedures[44,55];
- determines the methods that will be used in the organization for monitoring and recording occupational radiation exposure[44,55,65];
- determines which individuals require radiation monitoring devices[44,55,56];
- reviews the reports from consultants or contractors, if present[44]; and
- oversees records of personnel education.[44,55,56]

[Recommendation]

The roles and responsibilities of the RSO are described in regulatory documents,[42,43] clinical guidelines,[55,65] and low-quality literature.[44,61] **See Section 10** for more information on the RSO's responsibilities when radionuclides or radiopharmaceuticals are present.

3.2 The RSO must meet the educational requirements as listed in federal[42] or state regulations. *[Regulatory Requirement]*

3.3 The RSO oversees the quality program for radiation safety, including
- identifying radiation safety problems[42-44];
- initiating, recommending, providing, and verifying implementation of corrective actions[42-44];
- stopping unsafe practices[42-44,61]; and

- performing radiation safety audits.[44,55]

[Recommendation]

3.3.1 Include the following in the annual audits of the radiation safety program:
- patient outcomes[79];
- patient dose[44,61];
- frequency of patient-dose trigger levels requiring clinical follow-up[80];
- image quality[61];
- justification for the procedure[79];
- personal dosimeter values[44];
- use of and availability of dosimeters;
- use of and availability of radiological protection tools;
- completion of required education on radiological protection (initial and continuing);
- adherence to the radiation safety program[44]; and
- availability of personnel, such as a medical physicist.[44]

[Recommendution]

Clinical guidelines[55,65,79] and low-quality evidence[44,61] support inclusion of these criteria into the quality assurance and improvement program.

4. Radiation Safety Program

4.1 The radiation safety program should be established by a radiation safety committee. *[Recommendation]*

For more information on the radiation safety program for facilities that administer radionuclides and radiopharmaceuticals, **see Recommendation 10.4.**

4.2 The radiation safety program must include
- a list of the approved equipment operators[40,41];
- documentation and record retention requirements[40,41];
- measures, including shielding, for protecting patients and perioperative team members from unnecessary exposure to ionizing radiation[40,41];
- procedures for handling and disposing of body fluids and tissue that may be radioactive[36]; Ⓐ
- requirements for use, storage, and maintenance of radiation monitoring devices[40,41];
- a process and requirements for testing equipment for radiation hazards[40,41]; and
- methods for identifying patients who are pregnant.[40,41]

[Regulatory Requirement]

See Section 10 for additional requirements when radionuclides are being administered or implanted.

4.3 The radiation safety program should include
- methods for evaluating and selecting new equipment,
- requirements for personnel education and competency assessment,[50,55]
- a quality assurance and improvement program[54] that includes monitoring of compliance with safety precautions,[50,80,81]
- processes for radiographic testing of protective devices,[50]
- requirements for patient education, and
- provisions for acceptance testing for protective garments.[50]

[Recommendation]

Clinical guidelines recommend including this content.[50,54,55,80,81]

4.4 The radiation safety program should include annual exposure limits. The limits must not exceed those set by the NRC:
- total **effective dose** equivalent (TEDE) to radiation workers—5 rem,
- TEDE to any individual organ—50 rem,
- TEDE to an embryo or fetus of a declared pregnant woman—0.5 rem,
- dose equivalent to the eye—15 rem (0.15 Sv),
- **shallow-dose equivalent** to the skin, extremities—50 rem (0.5 Sv),
- dose to minors—10% of worker limit of 5 rem, and
- dose to members of the public—0.1 rem.[1]

[Regulatory Requirement]

4.5 The radiation safety program must be reviewed at least annually.[39] *[Regulatory Requirement]*

4.5.1 The health care organization must maintain records of changes to the radiation safety program, program audits, and individual monitoring results as prescribed by regulatory requirements.[39,43] *[Regulatory Requirement]* Ⓐ

4.5.2 The health care organization must keep records of radiation safety program changes for at least 5 years.[43] *[Regulatory Requirement]*

4.5.3 The review may include items related to equipment, processes, procedures, or staffing structures that may indicate a change is required. *[Conditional Recommendation]*

5. Patient Exposure

5.1 Consult with the RSO or the radiology professional in the room regarding the use and placement of protective shielding or garments between the patient and the source of radiation.[54,82-84] *[Recommendation]* Ⓟ

Consulting with the RSO or radiology professional can be an effective means of weighing benefits and harms that are specific to the patient and situation. The benefits of using patient shielding include protection of the patient's radiation-sensitive organs.[55,85] The harms include an increase in radiation exposure to the patient because the source automatically increases the radiation levels, or the risk of repeating the exam because of the draping falling into or being placed in the area of interest.[86]

A moderate-quality study[85] and clinical guidelines[54,55,84] support the use of shielding for patients when radiation-sensitive organs are near the source.

Use of shielding is discouraged in four high-level studies[83,86-88] and one moderate-level study[87] and in a clinical guideline authored by the American Association of Physicists in Medicine (AAPM).[89] The AAPM guideline is supported or endorsed by the American College of Radiology (ACR), Australasian College of Physical Scientists & Engineers in Medicine, Canadian Association of Radiologists, Canadian Organization of Medical Physicists, Health Physics Society, Image Gently, and Radiological Society of North America.

In a systematic review with meta-analysis, Karami et al[88] reviewed and analyzed the literature to determine the prevalence of gonad shielding and whether it is an effective method of protecting patients. The authors concluded that female gonadal shielding should be discontinued; male gonadal shielding is controversial, and its effectiveness depends on the skill of the radiographers positioning the shield. The authors also recommended that radiographers receive education on correct methods of positioning gonadal shielding.

In a quasi-experimental study, Kaplan et al[86] also challenged the use of female gonadal shielding, especially with the use of automatic exposure control sensors. The researchers measured the DAP for an adult **phantom** and a 5-year-old phantom with the automatic exposure control activated and with and without the shield in place. The researchers found the DAP increased 63% in the 5-year-old phantom and 147% in the adult phantom with the shield in place. The researchers recommended not using female gonadal shielding when the automatic exposure control is used.

In a quasi-experimental laboratory study, Phelps et al[83] measured the radiation dose received by a phantom representing a patient in-field and out-of-field at distances of 7.5 cm, 10 cm, and 12.5 cm during fluoroscopy. The dose was measured with no shield, a flat shield, and a curved shield. The flat shield was intended to block leakage radiation and the curved shield was to block scatter radiation. The researchers found the radiation dose with the flat shield decreased by an average of 1% and with the curved shield decreased by an average of 91%. Because of the minimal reduction in leakage radiation, the researchers questioned the benefit of shielding out-of-field body parts and they recommended conducting in vivo investigations.

The use of shielding is disputed in a nonexperimental study by Lee et al.[87] The researchers reviewed the radiographs of 84 boys and 84 girls randomly selected from 3,400 radiographs for orthopedic evaluation of pediatric patients. The researchers found incorrect placement of shielding for 76% of the girls and 51% of the boys. They suggested that use of the shields is ineffective.

In a nonexperimental study, Martus et al[85] measured the radiation dose received at the thyroid and gonads of 18 pediatric patients undergoing repair of supracondylar humerus fractures. The researchers placed a dosimeter under the shielding and over the thyroid and gonads. They found the dose to the thyroid was minimal and was approximately equivalent to daily radiation exposure.

5.1.1 When used, shielding should be placed
- to include, if possible, the patient's thyroid, ovaries or testes (ie, gonads), and breasts when these body parts are near the source of radiation[54,82-84];
- between the patient and the source of radiation (eg, 360 degrees around the patient for CT);
- between the source and the patient for conventional radiography; and
- beyond the edges of the path of the beam that originates from the x-ray tube.[82]

[Recommendation]

In a quasi-experimental study, Culp et al[90] used a phantom to measure the exposure to the patient when the protective shield was placed on the anterior or the posterior side of the patient with the radiation source on the anterior side. The dose received with the garment was 0.03 mrem on the anterior side and 0.37 mrem on the posterior side. The researchers concluded that the protective garment should be placed on the same side of the patient as the radiation source.

5.2 Perform a radiation safety time out before beginning the procedure.[91,92] *[Recommendation]* **P**

In a quasi-experimental study, Choi et al[91] measured the radiation dose to pediatric patients undergoing insertion of a central line in the OR. The measurements were taken before (n = 59) and after (n =

41) implementation of a radiation safety briefing and time out. After implementation of the radiation safety briefing and time-out process, the radiation dose received by the patients decreased by 79%.

Aizer et al[92] conducted a nonexperimental prospective cohort study on the radiation exposure of 1,040 patients undergoing electrophysiology procedures. They measured the DAP, reference point dose, FT, use of additional shielding, and use of alternative imaging modalities before (n = 594) and after (n = 448) the implementation of a radiation safety time out. The researchers found a significant reduction in the DAP and a significant increase in the use of additional shielding and use of alternative modalities after implementation of the time out. They concluded that use of a time out should be strongly considered.

Performance of a time-out procedure is recommended in a clinical guideline from the Environmental Protection Agency.[55]

5.2.1 The radiation safety time out may be included in the procedural time out or may be performed as a separate time out. *[Conditional Recommendation]*

5.2.2 A radiation safety time out may include the following questions:
- Is the frame rate set to the lowest acceptable rate?
- Is the patient positioned as close as safely possible to the **image intensifier**?
- Has collimation been performed?
- Is the magnification as low as possible?
- Are shields and protective drapes in place?
- Is the patient pregnant?
- Are the members of the perioperative team who are required to wear personal dosimeters wearing them?
- Will fluoroscopy images be saved rather than obtaining fluorography/cinefluoroscopy images?

[Conditional Recommendation]

5.3 During fluoroscopic procedures, keep the patient as close as possible to the image intensifier side of the fluoroscopic unit and away from the tube side of the unit **(Figure 2)**.[54,56,93] *[Recommendation]*

Positioning the patient close to the image intensifier is recommended in clinical guidelines[54,56] and a consensus document authored by the American College of Cardiology Task Force on Expert Consensus Decision Pathways developed in collaboration with Mended Hearts.[93]

Figure 2. Image Intensifier Positioned Above the Patient (A) and Below the Patient (B)

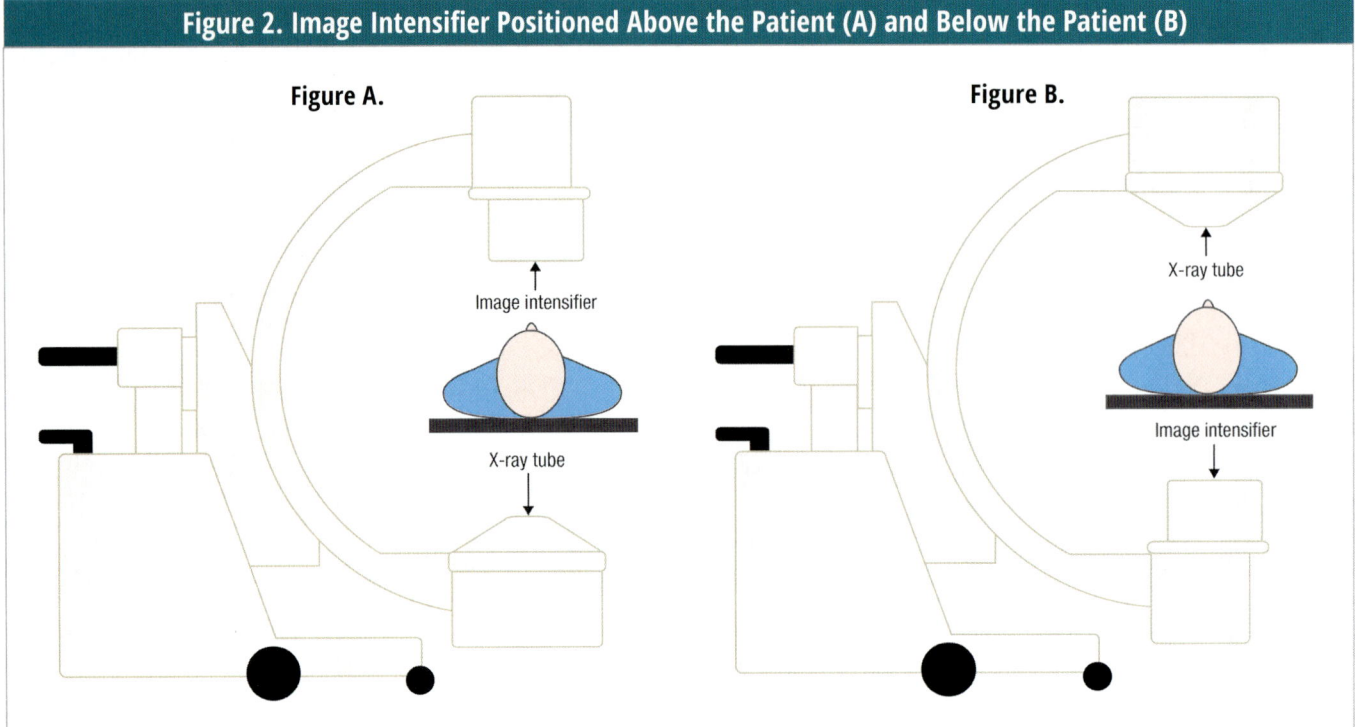

Figure A.

Image intensifier

X-ray tube

Figure B.

X-ray tube

Image intensifier

5.4 Move body parts that are not required for the study out of the path of the radiation beam.[48,54,56] [Recommendation]

Clinical guidelines recommend moving body parts that are not required for the study out of the x-ray beam.[48,54,56]

5.5 Consult with the physician regarding post-procedure education requirements and the timing of follow-up care.[4,9] [Recommendation]

Patient education is recommended in clinical guidelines[55,57,81] and in a consensus statement.[4] Follow-up care is needed to assess and, if necessary, treat the patient for complications.[4]

In a review of 2,124 patients undergoing a cardiac catheterization, Wei et al[9] found nine patients experienced radiation ulcers. The researchers recommended that high-risk patients (eg, patients who are obese, have diseases such as diabetes mellitus, or who are identified by the radiology professional as having received a large radiation dose) receive post-procedure follow-up.

5.5.1 Provide the patient with education that includes
- skin care if signs and symptoms of radiation dermatitis appear,[4,9]
- signs and symptoms of overexposure to radiation (eg, gastrointestinal symptoms, radiation burns, hair loss),[55]
- the potential time frame for appearance of signs and symptoms, and

- the importance of follow-up with the physician who performed the procedure if questions arise regarding the procedure.[55] [Recommendation]

In a review of 2,124 patients undergoing cardiac catheterization, Wei et al[9] found nine patients experienced radiation ulcers. The researchers recommended that patients receive education on post-procedure skin care to use if signs and symptoms of radiation dermatitis appear.

5.6 Create a radiation safety policy and procedure for the patient who is premenopausal that includes a
- list of procedures that require pregnancy testing,[55,94]
- method for determining pregnancy,[94]
- process for physician notification if the patient is pregnant, and
- method of protective shielding if the patient is pregnant.

[Recommendation] **P**

Assessment to determine the pregnancy status of premenopausal women undergoing certain procedures (eg, chest radiography, extremity radiography, diagnostic examination of the head or neck, mammography, CT imaging outside of the abdomen or pelvis [with the possible exception of the hip]) is supported by a clinical guideline authored by the ACR in collaboration with Society for Pediatric Radiology (SPR).[94] This document states that the risk to the fetus is uncertain but there is less risk with advanced gestational age. The goal of a screening program is to decrease unexpected exposures to patients who are pregnant, especially during vulnerable stages of gestation.[94]

Creation of a policy and procedure is recommended by a clinical guideline from the Environmental Protection Agency.[55]

For protective measures for perioperative team members who are pregnant, **see Section 8**.

5.6.1 **Determine pregnancy status according to organizational policies and procedures for patients who are undergoing a procedure on the list of pregnancy-testing-required procedures.**[56,93,94] *[Recommendation]*

Using either clinical history or pregnancy testing is supported by a clinical guideline authored by the ACR in collaboration with the SPR, which states that the clinical history may be sufficient and pregnancy testing may not be needed when the woman attests she cannot reasonably be pregnant and is between regular menstrual periods (eg, has not missed her period) or on long-term birth control, including being biologically incapable of conceiving (eg, post hysterectomy or tubal ligation), treated with ongoing oncologic therapy, or not sexually active.[94]

This guideline also states that procedures involving radiation that do not directly expose the pelvis or gravid uterus to the x-ray beam do not require verification of pregnancy status (eg, chest radiography, extremity radiography, diagnostic examination of the head or neck, mammography, CT imaging outside of the abdomen or pelvis [with the possible exception of the hip]). The clinical guideline recommends pregnancy testing for those patients undergoing interventional fluoroscopic procedures of the abdomen or pelvis, diagnostic angiography of the abdomen or pelvis, hysterosalpingography, standard-dose CT protocols of the abdomen or pelvis, and diagnostic nuclear medicine PET/CT.[94]

Other clinical guidelines[55,56] and a consensus document[93] also recommend pregnancy testing.

5.6.2 **If the patient is a minor, follow the state regulations governing pregnancy testing.**[94] *[Regulatory Requirement]*

5.6.3 **Notify the responsible physician when a patient has declared that she could be pregnant or if a woman of childbearing age or the patient's representative refuses a pregnancy test.**[56,94] *[Recommendation]*

5.6.4 **Consult with the RSO or the radiology professional in the room regarding the use and placement of protective shielding between the fetus and the source of radiation.**[94-96] *[Conditional Recommendation]*

A clinical guideline states that using lead shielding between the fetus and the source of radiation during radiation exposure to other parts of the body may support the emotional well-being of the patient but does little to reduce the scatter radiation received by the fetus.[94] The Radiological Society of North America[97] and the AAPM[89] also recommend not using lead shielding on patients who are pregnant.

In a quasi-experimental study, Chatterson et al[95] measured the radiation dose from a CT scanner to a first and third trimester gravid phantom with and without a shield. The researchers found the use of the shield decreased the radiation dose for the first trimester to below detectable levels and decreased the dose 69% for the third trimester. Moore et al[96] found similar reductions using a model representing a woman at 1 week and 12 weeks gestation.

5.7 **Document the following in the patient's health record:**
- **diagnostic and therapeutic radiation dose,**[54,80,98]
- **type and location of patient radiation protection,**[56,99]
- **preprocedural and postprocedural patient skin assessment,**[56,99] **and**
- **patient education.**

[Recommendation]

Documentation of the patient's radiation dose is supported by clinical guidelines.[54,56,57,80,81,99]

6. Perioperative Team Exposure

6.1 **Maintain the greatest distance possible from the radiation source, ideally at least 6 ft, and limit the time spent close to the radiation source.**[16,48,50,56,93,100-103] *[Recommendation]*

Maximizing the distance between the perioperative team member and the radiation source to minimize the amount of radiation exposure is supported by high-quality[102,103] and moderate-quality evidence,[100,101,104,105] and is recommended by clinical guidelines[48,50,55,56] and a consensus document.[93]

Radiation dose decreases as the square of the distance between the radiation source and the operator increases. When the distance between the person and the x-ray source is doubled, the exposure is decreased by 25%. When the distance is tripled, the dose is decreased by a factor of 9. Fluoroscopy

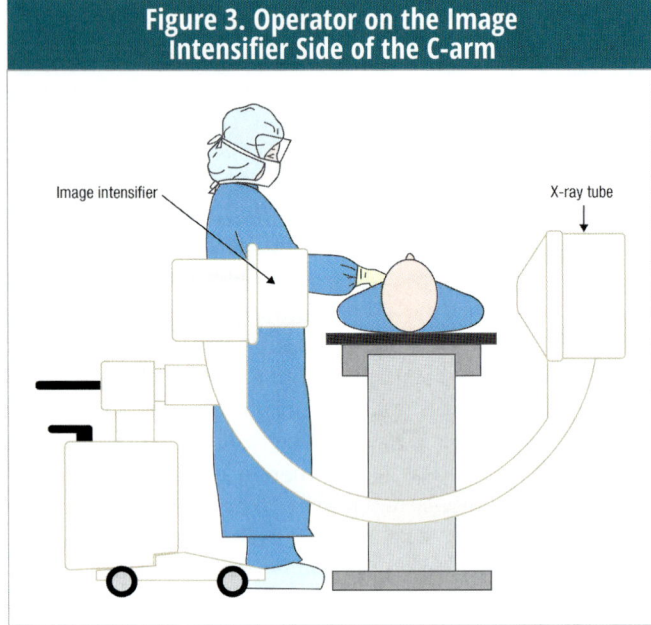

Figure 3. Operator on the Image Intensifier Side of the C-arm

Image intensifier

X-ray tube

operators and personnel can reduce their exposure accordingly by moving away from the x-ray source.[93]

In a quasi-experimental study, Sailer et al[102] measured the radiation dose to phantom operators placed near the field and one step back from the field. The researchers found the dose was decreased by a factor of 2 to 3 at the distance of one step from the field. The researchers concluded that the operator should maintain as great a distance as possible from the radiation source.

In a quasi-experimental study, Schuetze et al[103] measured the amount of scatter radiation every 0.4 m from the source to the OR wall. The researchers found a positive relationship between the distance and the amount of radiation measured (eg, the greater the distance the lower the amount of radiation). The researchers concluded that people in a hybrid OR should stay as far as possible from the source when it is activated.

6.1.1 An indication system (eg, markings on the floor) may be used to indicate areas of radiation exposure from low to high for a fixed system.[106] *[Conditional Recommendation]*

In a quasi-experimental study, Heilmaier et al[106] measured the perceptions of non-radiological personnel (N = 56) about personnel protection during CT scans. The researchers marked locations on the floor to indicate the radiation dose that may be received by a person standing at each location during a scan. The locations were labeled as lowest, intermediate, and highest radiation dose. After the participants were in the room for a scan, they were given a questionnaire that asked what effect the labels had

on their perception of personnel protection. The participants reported that the use of the system increased their radiation awareness and improved their sense of being protected from radiation.

6.2 The radiation equipment operator should alert perioperative team members in the treatment room before activating the equipment.[56] *[Recommendation]*

Alerting the perioperative team members in the room before activating the equipment allows the team members to take protective measures, such as maintaining as great a distance as possible from the source, thereby decreasing the dose of radiation received.

6.3 Stand on the image intensifier side of the fluoroscopy unit when procedural considerations allow (Figure 3).[50,54,56,100] *[Recommendation]*

Three clinical guidelines recommend standing on the image intensifier side of the fluoroscopy unit.[50,54,56]

Yu and Khan[100] performed a systematic review of literature published between January 1980 and July 2013 that examined the relationship between where the surgeon stands and the amount of radiation exposure. The authors concluded that when the surgeon stood on the side opposite the radiation source, the dose received was smaller.

6.4 Use slings, traction devices, and sandbags to maintain the patient's position during radiation exposure, and use cassette holders to secure films.[56,84] *[Recommendation]*

Clinical guidelines recommend using assistive devices, as opposed to manual positioning maintenance during radiation procedures.[56,84]

7. Perioperative Team Shielding

7.1 Wear radiation protective garments during procedures when a source of radiation is activated.[48,50,54-56,93] *[Recommendation]*

Clinical guidelines[48,50,54-56] and a consensus document[93] support wearing of protective garments (eg, apron, vest and skirt, wraparound, overlapping, thyroid shields).

Rhea et al[107] performed a systematic review of the literature to determine the amount of radiation to which anesthesia professionals were exposed during orthopedic procedures. The authors found the dose received by the anesthesia professionals at 1.5 m from the source was minimal if any. The authors concluded that wearing of lead protection by anesthesia professionals may not be necessary.

7.1.1 **Select the garment size that corresponds to the wearer's body size based on the manufacturer's sizing chart.**[50,54,56,108] *[Recommendation]*

In a quasi-experimental study, Valone et al[108] measured the amount of radiation received by a phantom representing a female orthopedic surgeon placed where an orthopedic surgeon would stand during a procedure. The phantom was first dressed in an apron that was too large, then in one that was too small, then in a proper fitting apron. The researchers measured the amount of radiation received at the upper-outer and the inner-lower quadrant of the breast. They found that the radiation doses were greater with the aprons that were too large or too small for the torso than when the apron was sized correctly. Even though the differences did not reach statistical significance, the researchers concluded that an apron that fits properly provides the greatest amount of protection, and they recommended that manufacturers should devise an apron with wings to protect the breasts.

Three clinical guidelines recommend wearing an apron of the correct size.[50,54,56]

7.1.2 **Protective garments should cover the body from the area below the chin to the knee.** *[Recommendation]*

Protective garments that cover the body from the area below the chin to the knee provide shielding from the greatest amount of scatter radiation, including that which is present under the table.

7.1.3 **Wear wraparound garments if the potential exists for exposure of the back to the radiation beam.**[50,56] *[Recommendation]*

Wearing wraparound garments can protect the wearer during clinical activities that may require turning one's back to the radiation beam.

7.1.4 **Store garments flat or hang them vertically, and do not fold them.**[50,55,56] *[Recommendation]*

Storage as described is recommended in clinical guidelines[50,55,56] because garments are susceptible to cracking when folded or creased, which can reduce the garment's effectiveness as a shielding barrier.

7.2 **Wear leaded eye protection when unable to distance from the source during activation.**[34,50,54-56,93,109-117] *[Recommendation]*

Wearing leaded glasses provides protection to the eyes, which are susceptible to radiation exposure. Wearing of leaded eye protection by personnel at the sterile field is supported by high-quality[34,112-117] and moderate-quality evidence[109-111] and is recommended by clinical guidelines[50,54-56] and a consensus document.[93]

In a quasi-experimental study, Principi et al[34] compared the radiation received to the eye in a laboratory setting with the use of radiation protective glasses with lateral shielding and small lenses, wraparound glasses, glasses with lateral shielding and large lenses, and no glasses. The researchers found that the glasses with lateral shielding and small lenses decreased the dose by one-half, and the wraparound glasses and the glasses with lateral shielding and large lenses decreased the dosage by two-thirds. The researchers concluded the use of glasses decreased the radiation dose to the eye and was specific to the type of glasses.

In a quasi-experimental study, Haga et al[117] measured the eye radiation dose in nine physicians with eye protection and three physicians without eye protection during interventional cardiology procedures (mean number of procedures 134.1 with protection, 84 without protection). The mean radiation dose was 3.1 mSv with protection and 6.3 mSv without protection. The researchers concluded that not wearing eye protection may lead to exceeding the ICRP recommended limit for eye dose (ie, 50 mSv/year).

In a quasi-experimental study, Sans Merce et al[116] measured the dose of radiation to the eyes during 32 neurointerventional procedures performed by four different physicians. The researchers measured the eye lens dose with a ceiling shield in place and with and without protective glasses. They found the dose to the eyes was decreased by a factor of 2.73 when the protective glasses were worn.

Honorio da Silva et al[115] conducted a quasi-experimental laboratory study in which they measured the amount of radiation received by the head of a phantom wearing radiation protection glasses with 0.75-mm frontal lenses or wraparound style glasses with flat frontal lenses and 0.5-mm side shielding. The researchers measured the radiation dose that reached the white matter and the hippocampus region of the brain. They found that the amount of radiation that reached the brain ranged from 10% to 17% for both styles of glasses. The researchers concluded that either style of leaded glasses contributed to shielding the brain.

In a quasi-experimental study, Hoffler and Ilyas[114] measured the radiation dose received outside and inside radiation protective glasses. They used a phantom representing a physician in a standard sitting position for hand surgery. The researchers found the dose was 66% lower inside the glasses. Even though the difference did not reach statistical significance, the researchers recommended wearing glasses because the amount of radiation exposure sufficient to increase medical risk is undefined.

In a quasi-experimental study, Ekpo et al[113] measured the exposure of the eyes of a phantom operator during a simulated CT-guided fluoroscopy. The dose to the eyes when the operator was positioned 30 degrees from the radiation source of the scanner without glasses was 10.54 µGy; the dose with glasses was 2.77 µGy. The researchers concluded that wearing the protective glasses significantly reduced the radiation dose to the eyes.

In a quasi-experimental study, Waddell et al[112] measured the radiation dose to a phantom operator using leaded glasses with and without side shields and leaded sport glasses. The researchers found a significant reduction in the radiation dose for the leaded glasses with (88.7%) and without side shields (91.4%) and the sport glasses (90.9%). They concluded that the leaded glasses without side shields and the sport glasses offered the best protection.

The need for eye protection during total hip arthroplasties was challenged in a nonexperimental study by Pomeroy et al.[118] The researchers measured the amount of eye radiation exposure to three surgeons while they performed 30 direct anterior total hip arthroplasties. The mean radiation dose per procedure for all three surgeons was 2 mGy. The researchers concluded that because of the very low exposure during this procedure, the surgeon should be able to decide when to wear eye protection. Limitations of this study are that the researchers investigated only one procedure, and the study had a small number of participants.

7.3 **Perioperative team members may wear a protective head covering if unable to distance from the beam (eg, when injecting radiation sensitive dye under fluoroscopic guidance).**[93,110,115,116,119-121] *[Conditional Recommendation]*

Wearing a protective head covering is supported by high-quality[115,119] and moderate-quality evidence[110,116,120-122] and a consensus document.[93]

In a randomized controlled trial (RCT), Alazzoni et al[119] measured the amount of scatter radiation received by the operator (N = 10) during 230 interventional coronary procedures. The dose to the operator's head was measured by placement of a dosimeter outside a cap and inside the cap in the left temporal area and with (n = 113) and without (n = 115) a protective drape. The researchers found a decrease of 2.73 µSv in dose to the operator's head for the draped group and a decrease of 7.69 µSv for the non-draped group. Both reductions were considered to be significant. The researchers concluded that the use of the cap significantly decreased the radiation dose to the operator's head.

Honorio da Silva et al[115] conducted a quasi-experimental laboratory study to compare three different protective lead head coverings: a surgical hat sized similar to a skull cap, a hood with a shielded forehead, and a hood without forehead shielding but with more shielding at the bottom of the head. The researchers measured the amount of radiation received by the head of a phantom in the hippocampus region of the brain. They found that the amount of radiation exposure depended on the model of head covering: surgical hat (11%), hood without forehead shielding (68%), and hood with forehead shielding (45%). The researchers concluded that the caps were less protective than reported in the literature found in their literature search.

7.4 **Gloves designed to protect the wearer from radiation exposure to the hands may be worn by personnel when the wearer's hands are near but not in the primary x-ray beam.**[54,56,114,123,124] *[Conditional Recommendation]*

In two moderate-quality studies, researchers measured the radiation dose inside and outside of a radiation protective glove.[114,123] The researchers concluded that wearing radiation protective gloves significantly reduced the radiation exposure that the wearer receives, by 47% to 69.8%, but these studies did not evaluate the effects of wearing gloves on patient radiation exposure. In a third, small, nonexperimental study,[124] the researchers also compared radiation exposure to the wearer with and without gloves and found that wearing gloves reduced the radiation exposure by 42.6%. This study also evaluated the effects on patient radiation exposure and found that when personnel wore gloves in the radiation beam, the patient's exposure increased by 67.6%. The researchers concluded that when worn in the direct x-ray beam, radiation protective gloves decreased the amount of scatter radiation received by personnel but increased the amount received by the patient.

Clinical guidelines recommend the use of radio-protective gloves.[50,54,56]

7.5 **Incorporate structural components (eg, walls, windows, control booths, doors, protective cubicles) into the structure of the building during construction of rooms with a fixed radiation source (eg, hybrid OR, interventional radiology room).**[55,125-127] *[Recommendation]*

Clinical guidelines recommend the use of structural components for radiation protection based on the anticipated use of the room.[55,65,125-127] Operating rooms frequently do not have these structural components unless they are designed as hybrid ORs.[55,126,127]

7.6 Use equipment-mounted and mobile shields (eg, suspended personal radiation protection systems, mobile hanging shields, under-table skirts, table-mounted side shields, rolling shields) in addition to personal shields when perioperative team members are unable to distance from the beam.[48,50,54,55,93,102,128-134]
[Recommendation]

Equipment-mounted and mobile shields can provide an added measure of protection from radiation exposure for personnel. The use of equipment-mounted shields is supported by high-quality,[102,128,129,131,132,134-137] and moderate-quality evidence[133] and is recommended in clinical guidelines[48,50,54,55] and by a consensus document.[93]

In an RCT, Muniraj et al[137] measured the radiation dose to the operator's eye and neck and the assisting nurse's neck. The dose was measured with (n = 50) and without (n = 50) a shield applied around the intensifier. The researchers found a reduction of 90%, 91%, and 93% at each area, respectively. They concluded that the shield significantly reduced the dose of radiation received by the operator and the assistant.

In an RCT, Ploux et al[136] compared the radiation dose to the operator at the thorax, back, foot, and head levels during extraction of cardiac devices with (n = 18) and without (n = 19) use of a radiation protection ceiling-suspended cabin (ie, a device with shielding on three sides that is suspended from the ceiling). The researchers found the mean dose to the head was 68 times more without the cabin and the dose to the foot was 680 times more without the cabin. They concluded that the use of the cabin offered protection to all involved.

In an RCT, Sciahbasi et al[128] compared the radiation dose to the operator at the pelvic and thorax level with (n = 102) and without (n = 103) an under-table radiation protective drape during 122 diagnostic coronary angiographies and 83 percutaneous coronary interventions with a transradial approach. The researchers found a significant decrease in the operator dose with the drape in place. The researchers concluded there was a significant reduction in radiation dose with the use of the under-table radiation protective drape.

In an RCT, Inoue et al[129] measured the radiation dose to the physician during ureteroscopy with (n = 61) and without (n = 62) radiation protective curtains placed on each side and at the foot of the table and between the operator and the source. The application of the drapes significantly decreased the mean effective doses to the operator from 0.33 µSv to 0.08 µSv. The researchers concluded that the protective curtains were effective at reducing the radiation dose to the operator at the pelvic and thorax level.

7.7 Use radiation shielding drapes as an alternative to or in addition to equipment-mounted and mobile shields when permitted by the requirements of the invasive procedure.[50,54,93,119,133,138-145]
[Recommendation]

This drape is intended to decrease the amount of scatter radiation that reaches personnel near the source and not to decrease the dose received by the patient. The drape may or may not be sterile. Use of radiation shielding drapes is supported by high-quality[31,119,138-142,144,145] and moderate-quality evidence[133,143] and recommended by clinical guidelines[50,54] and a consensus document.[93]

In an RCT, Patet et al[31] measured the radiation dose received by the operator and the nurse during 51 interventional cardiac procedures with (n = 26) and without (n = 25) a radiation protection drape. The researchers found the operator dose was 7 µSv without the drape and 1.0 µSv with the drape. The nurse dose was 2 µSv without the drape and 0 µSv with the drape. The researchers concluded the use of the drape significantly decreased radiation dose to the operator and the nurse.

In an RCT, Vlastra et al[145] measured the radiation dose to the operator during cardiac catheterizations with a radiation shield drape (n = 255), without the drape (n = 255), and with a sham drape (n = 256). The researchers found a 20% reduction in radiation dose to the operator when the shield drape was in place compared to when no shield drape was present. They also found a 44% reduction in the radiation dose received when the shield drape was present compared to the dose when the sham drape was present. Both reductions in dosage reached statistical significance. The researchers concluded the radiation shield drape reduced the radiation received by the operator.

In an RCT, Kohlbrenner et al[138] measured the radiation dose to the operator during transjugular liver biopsy with (n = 31) and without (n = 31) a lead-free radiation protective drape applied around the source. The draping consisted of square split radiation protective drape positioned around the jugular access sheath and a rectangular drape applied to the patient's shoulder and body wall, partially overlapping the drape at the access site. The researchers found the mean radiation dose for the operator decreased by 56% with the use of drapes.

In an RCT, Alazzoni et al[119] measured the amount of scatter radiation received by the operator (N = 10) during 230 interventional coronary procedures. The operator dose was measured with (n = 113) and without (n = 115) a protective drape. The researchers found a significant reduction in the operator dose (76%) when the drape was applied.

7.7.1 The radiation shielding drapes should be placed between the patient and the operator, outside of the area being imaged and not between the patient and the source. *[Recommendation]*

The drape is placed in this location to decrease the amount of scatter radiation that reaches personnel near the source. This drape is not intended to decrease the dose received by the patient, which would require positioning it between the patient and the source.

7.8 Use a combination of personal, fixed, and movable shielding devices when permitted by the requirements of the invasive procedure.[130] *[Recommendation]*

Equipment-mounted and mobile shields can provide an added measure of protection for personnel who are wearing personal protective garments during procedures that include radiation. In a quasi-experimental study, Madder et al[130] measured the radiation dose received by the RN circulator and the scrub person during cardiac interventional procedures with standard protection (n = 401) and with an additional rolling shield (n = 363). The standard radiation protection included a thyroid collar, vest, and skirt. The use of the radiation protective shield in addition to standard radiation protective garments decreased the radiation dose significantly, by 62.5% for the scrub person and 63.6% for the RN circulator.

7.9 Select shielding devices composed of lead or a lead-equivalent material (eg, tungsten antimony, bismuth-antimony).[50,55,146-149] *[Recommendation]*

High-quality evidence[146-149] and clinical guidelines[50,55] recommend that shielding devices be composed of lead or a lead-equivalent material.

In an RCT, Uthoff et al[147] measured the radiation above and under thyroid collars made from a bilayer barium sulfate-bismuth oxide composite (n = 135) and lead (n = 121). The mean radiation dose reductions for the bilayer barium sulfate-bismuth oxide composite and lead collars were 90.7% and 72.4%, respectively. The researchers concluded that the bilayer barium sulfate-bismuth oxide composite thyroid collars were more effective than the lead collars.

In a quasi-experimental study, Mayekar et al[146] measured the radiation dose received by the operator during 51 orthopedic procedures. The radiation dose was measured by dosimeters located under and above the lead apron, and one above the lead apron that was covered with a barium-bismuth fabric. The researchers found no statistically significant difference between the dose received under the lead apron and the dose under the barium and bismuth combined fabric. The lead alternative fabric apron

was 57.8% lighter than the lead apron. The researchers concluded that the alternative fabric was effective at reducing the radiation dose and could be worn safely.

In a quasi-experimental study, Kijima et al[149] measured the radiation dose at the knee, waist, chest, and eye level of a phantom operator using a lead drape compared to a tungsten drape (TGD). The radiation dose was decreased at each level (knee level 0.14% TGD versus 0.07% lead; waist level 67.8% TGD versus 64.7% lead; chest level 76.36% TGD versus 60.33% lead; eye level 70.37% TGD versus 61.8% lead). The researchers concluded that the TGD could be used instead of the lead drape.

In a quasi-experimental study, Monzen et al[148] used a phantom to measure the amount of radiation at the eye, chest, waist, and knee level of an average-height Japanese man. The radiation doses administered using the fluoroscopy mode were decreased at all levels with the addition of the various amounts of tungsten. With 10 layers of tungsten paper, the dose was decreased at the eye (4.5 mGy to 1.9 mGy), chest (14.7 mGy to 8.2 mGy), waist (33.4 mGy to 7.6 mGy), and knee (36.3 mGy to 35.4 mGy). The researchers concluded that tungsten is a potential replacement for lead in radiation protection drapes.

7.10 Visually inspect protective shielding devices for defects (eg, punctures, tears, cuts, creasing) at the time of purchase and before each use.[50,55] *[Recommendation]*

Shielding devices with defects can provide incomplete or unreliable protection for the wearer. Visual inspection to identify defects is recommended in two clinical guidelines.[50,55]

7.11 Send personal radiation protective devices to the facility-designated location for testing of shielding effectiveness
- at the time of purchase,
- at least annually for defects related to wear, and
- whenever damage is suspected.[40,41,50,56]

[Regulatory Requirement]

Testing of protective devices as described is a regulatory requirement from the Centers for Medicare & Medicaid Services[40,41] and is recommended in clinical guidelines.[50,56]

In a quasi-experimental study, Lichliter et al[150] examined the amount of radiation exposure to the operator in 16 garment models consisting of lead and non-lead equivalents and a radiation protective cabin (ie, a device with shielding on three sides). Overall, variability of operator exposures in all labeled equivalences ranged from 0.52 µSv/hour for the suspended device labeled 1.0-mm lead equivalent to 13.83 µSv/hour for a closed-back garment labeled 0.5-mm lead equivalent. The exposure for those garments labeled 0.5-mm lead equivalent ranged from 1.13 μSv/hour to 13.83 μSv/hour. The researchers recommended verification in the facility if possible.

In a quasi-experimental study, Fakhoury et al[151] measured the scatter reduction in 0.5-mm pure lead garments, non-lead blend garments, and pure barium protective garments at 60 kVp and 70 kVp. The scatter penetration was 292% greater for the non-lead blend and 258% greater for the pure barium at 60 kVp and was 214% and 233% greater at 70 kVp, respectively, when compared to the pure lead. All garments were rated by the manufacturer to have protection equivalent to 0.5-mm lead. The researchers concluded the attenuation of the lightweight aprons should be assessed before purchase.

7.11.1 **Remove devices from use that fail testing or have defects.**[55,56] *[Recommendation]*

Removing defective devices from service is supported by two clinical guidelines.[55,56]

7.11.2 **Maintain records of protective device testing in a central and accessible location.** *[Recommendation]*

7.11.3 **Notify personnel responsible for testing protective garments and shielding devices when new shielding devices are purchased.** *[Recommendation]*

Communication between the person ordering and receiving new shielding devices and the person responsible for testing the devices assists with improving testing compliance.

7.12 **Label personal shielding devices with the last test date and owner (eg, personal or department).** *[Recommendation]*

Labeling devices assists with tracking the apron and identification of the personnel or department that owns the device.[56]

7.13 **Clean and disinfect shared personal protective devices between uses and spot clean them if soiled. Clean protective garments daily if worn by only one individual.**[152-157] *[Recommendation]*

Cleaning of personal protective devices and garments is supported by high-quality[152,153] and moderate-quality evidence[154-157] and is recommended in clinical guidelines.[158,159]

In an RCT, Jain et al[153] measured the amount of bacteria present on 20 radiation protection aprons before and at zero hours and 6 hours after cleaning. Each apron was cultured in four different sites. Before cleaning, the researchers found coagulase-

negative *Staphylococcus* (n = 18), *Diphtheroids* (n = 12), *Micrococcus* species (n = 12), methicillin-resistant *Staphylococcus epidermidis* (n = 1), *Bacillus* species (n = 1), *Streptococcus viridans* (n = 1), and *Neisseria* species (n = 1). No cultures were positive at zero hours after cleaning. Six hours after cleaning, coagulase-negative *Staphylococcus* was cultured on two aprons. The researchers recommended cleaning aprons immediately before use.

In a quasi-experimental study, Lange[152] measured the contamination level of eyewear worn in the OR. The eyewear was worn during 71 surgeries in four ORs, and power tools were used in 26.7% of the procedures. For a total of 276 disposable and 39 reusable pieces of eyewear, 44.8% of all pieces and 94.9% of the reusable pieces cultured positive. The researcher concluded that eyewear could increase cross contamination and infection risk.

7.13.1 **Select cleaning methods for radiation protective garments and devices based on the garment or device manufacturer's instructions for use.** *[Recommendation]*

Some cleaning products may damage the protective garment or protective device materials. The manufacturer's instructions for use provide recommendations for cleaning solutions to be used.

8. Perioperative Team Members Who Are Pregnant

8.1 **Perioperative team members with a known or suspected pregnancy must restrict the occupational radiation dose to the levels described in local, state, and federal regulations.**[39] *[Regulatory Requirement]* **P**

Local, state, and federal regulations determine the radiation precautions to be followed by personnel who are pregnant. State guidelines are based on the regulations established by the NRC. The NRC regulations state the occupational dose to the embryo or fetus of an occupationally exposed health care worker who has declared her pregnancy must not exceed 0.5 rem during the entire gestational period and should be uniform over time (ie, the total allowed amount should not be received at one point in the gestational period).[39] The deep-dose equivalent for the worker who has declared a pregnancy is used as the dose to the embryo or fetus.[39]

For protective measures for patients who are pregnant, **see Recommendation 5.6.**

8.1.1 Perioperative team members with a known or suspected pregnancy should notify the RSO or follow other facility channels as defined in policies and procedures. *[Recommendation]*

Effective communication regarding pregnancy status initiates the organization's practices to monitor for and protect workers who are pregnant from occupational radiation exposure. Communication about pregnancy is recommended in clinical guidelines.[50,55,60]

8.2 A health care worker who is pregnant should follow standard radiation protection techniques and, in addition, may wear a maternity or double-thickness garment, a garment with ancillary shielding, or a wraparound garment that is large enough to cover the entire abdominal area.[55,60,160-163] *[Recommendation]*

Clinical guidelines[55,60] and low-quality evidence[160-162] support the use of radiation protective techniques as described.

In a nonexperimental study, Chen and Brunet[163] measured the amount of radiation received by a single female interventionalist for 10 months before she became pregnant (n = 478 cases) and 6 months after she declared her pregnancy (n = 280). During pregnancy, the interventionalist wore two lead apron skirts with a fetal dosimeter under the apron skirt in the center of the lower abdomen. She wore an additional dosimeter at the neck level outside of the apron. The mean dose outside of the apron was 105 mrem and the dose inside the apron was 0 mrem. The researchers concluded that it is safe for a woman who is pregnant to be an interventionalist if standard radiation protection precautions are taken.

8.3 Perioperative team members who are pregnant should wear radiation monitors at the waist under shielding in addition to the dosimeter worn on the collar during times of exposure to radiation.[50,56,60,93] *[Recommendation]*

Wearing radiation monitors at the waist under shielding facilitates radiation exposure monitoring to the fetus and is supported by clinical guidelines,[50,56,60] a consensus document,[93] and low-quality evidence.[161,162]

8.3.1 Dosimeters of pregnant perioperative team members should be read and reported to the individual monthly unless regulatory requirements are more stringent.[56,60] *[Recommendation]*

Timely radiation exposure monitoring of the fetus is important because it allows the mother to know if the dose received is nearing limits and, if so, helps to determine actions to be taken. Clinical guidelines recommend monthly reading of dosimeters for employees who are pregnant.[56,60]

9. Perioperative Team Radiation Monitors

9.1 Perioperative team members who may be exposed to radiation and meet the criteria defined in regulatory documents (eg, state law, 29 CFR 1910.1096) must wear radiation monitors (eg, film badges, pocket chambers, pocket dosimeters, film rings).[40,41,47] *[Regulatory Requirement]*

Regulatory agencies provide details for implementation of personnel radiation monitoring.[40,41,47]

9.2 Wear dosimeters in a consistent location on the body as determined by the RSO.[50,56] *[Recommendation]*

Clinical guidelines recommend wearing monitors consistently and in the same location on the body to achieve accurate readings.[50,56]

9.2.1 Wear a dosimeter
- on the side of the body that is closest to the radiation source when at the sterile field,
- on the center of the collar when not at the sterile field, or
- as recommended by the RSO.[164]

[Recommendation]

In a quasi-experimental study, Gerasia et al[164] measured the radiation dose received by the operator during 62 x-ray guided procedures. The dosimeters were placed outside the protective apron on the operator's anterior and posterior side. The researchers found when the operator was facing the source, the anterior dose was 11.8 μSv and the posterior dose was 0.5 μSv, but when the operator had his or her back toward the source, the anterior dose was 1.3 μSv and the posterior dose was 32.3 μSv. The researchers concluded that the dosimeter should be worn on the side of the operator that is closest to the source.

9.2.2 Wear one dosimeter outside the lead apron and one inside the lead apron or as directed by the RSO or by state regulatory bodies.[54-56] *[Recommendation]*

Clinical guidelines recommend using two dosimeters, one inside the apron and the other at the collar or left shoulder region outside the apron.[50,54-57,60]

9.2.3 Wear a finger dosimeter when working with the hands in close proximity to the primary x-ray beam, as advised by the RSO.[50,54,56] *[Recommendation]*

Four clinical guidelines recommend the use of finger dosimeters.[50,54-56]

In a nonexperimental descriptive study, Funao et al[165] measured the radiation dose on the hand, eye, thyroid, chest, and genitals of surgeons involved in 31 minimally invasive transforaminal lumbar interbody fusion procedures. The researchers found the hands, as indicated by the finger dosimeter, received the highest amount of radiation of all the areas tested (eye 0.07 mSv, thyroid 0.08 mSv, chest 0.10 mSv, genitals 0.15 mSv, finger 0.33 mSv). They concluded that the radiation exposure to the hands should be monitored.

9.2.4 An eye dosimeter may be worn when working in close proximity to the radiation source.[50,117,166] *[Conditional Recommendation]*

Use of an eye dosimeter is supported by high-quality[117] and moderate-quality[166] evidence and is recommended in two clinical guidelines.[50,57]

In a quasi-experimental study, Haga et al[117] measured the eye radiation dose in 12 physicians and 11 nurses at the eye and at the neck during interventional cardiology procedures. They found that when estimating the eye dose based on the neck dose, the eye dose tended to be overestimated for the physicians; however, the nurse's neck dose was a reasonable approximation of the eye dose. The researchers recommended the use of eye dosimeters for physicians, but said the neck dosimeter was adequate for the nurses. A limitation of the study is that the location of the nurses during the procedure was not described.

In a nonexperimental study, Betti et al[166] measured the radiation dose to the eye of 15 physician operators performing 3,117 interventional cardiology procedures. The radiation was measured using dosimeters placed on the bow of glasses. The researchers found the mean dose to the eye to be 10.8 mSv during a 12-month period of measurement. The researchers concluded that the dose received was close to the recommended maximum dose and therefore eye dosimeters should be worn.

9.2.5 Label dosimeters to indicate the location where they should be worn.[50,55] *[Recommendation]*

Identifying the location on the dosimeter (eg, inside the apron or vest, outside the apron or vest, at the chest, at the waist) helps the wearer to consistently place the dosimeter at the same location.[50,55]

9.3 Store radiation monitoring devices or dosimeters at the facility in a designated location at the end of every workday and do not remove them from the facility.[56] *[Recommendation]*

A device that is taken out of the facility may collect ionizing radiation from other sources (eg, sun, soil, airport scanners). A designated location facilitates collection of the badges for testing and can facilitate consistent wearing of the devices and timely collection and analysis of the device.[56]

9.4 The dosimetry readings must be reported to the monitored individual at least annually or more often if the individual is pregnant.[40,41,47] *[Regulatory Requirement]*

For perioperative team members who are pregnant, see Recommendation 8.3.1.

9.4.1 Dosimetry reports must be kept by the facility or health care organization and the individual for the life of the individual or as determined by regulatory requirements.[39-41] *[Regulatory Requirement]*

10. Radionuclides and Radiopharmaceuticals

10.1 The health care organization must create policies and procedures for use of radionuclides or radiopharmaceuticals, to include

- monitoring the seeds before, during, and after all uses and
- handling emergency situations, with instructions for
  - responding to a source rupture at any location,
  - retrieval of leaking or cut sources,
  - contamination control,
  - decontamination of the patient and area from a ruptured source,
  - saturation of the patient's thyroid with stable iodine in the case of an Iodine-125 source rupture,
  - restricting access to and posting warning signs at entrances to the implantation/explantation/pathology area if there is an unaccounted for or ruptured source,
  - source accountability from implantation to explantation and final disposal,
  - patient follow-up if the patient does not return for explantation,
  - waste disposal,
  - reporting to the NRC or state regulatory body, and
  - contacting the authorized users and the RSO (ie, names and telephone numbers).[49]

[Regulatory Requirement]

For more information on the responsibilities of the health care organization, see Section 1.

10.2 The health care organization must file a report with the NRC when

- an administered dose differs from prescribed dose by more than 0.05 Sv (5 rem),
- an organ or tissue receives an effective dose equivalent ≥ 0.5 Sv (50 rem),
- the skin receives a shallow-dose equivalent ≥ 0.5 Sv (50 rem),
- a wrong radioactive drug-containing by-product material or radionuclide is administered,
- the radioactive drug-containing by-product material or radionuclide is administered via the wrong route,
- the radioactive drug-containing by-product material or radionuclide is administered to the wrong individual or human research participant,
- the wrong mode of treatment is used, or
- a leak from a sealed source occurs.[42]

[Regulatory Requirement]

10.2.1 The following must be included in the report to the NRC:

- the licensee's name;
- the prescribing physician's name;
- a brief description of the event;
- the reason the event occurred;
- the effect, if any, on the individual(s) who received the medication;
- actions taken or planned to prevent recurrence; and
- certification that the licensee notified the individual or the individual's responsible relative or guardian, and if not, why not.[42]

[Regulatory Requirement]

10.3 Health care organizations in which therapeutic radionuclides (eg, brachytherapy, stereotactic radiosurgery) are administered to patients must employ an RSO, and if authorized to use two different types of by-product material, must create a radiation safety committee.[40,41,43] *[Regulatory Requirement]*

10.4 The radiation safety program must include processes for

- labeling radioactive materials, waste, and hazardous areas[40,41];
- storing radioactive materials and waste[40,41];
- safe transport of radioactive materials between locations in the hospital[40,41];
- the measures to be taken to maintain security of radioactive materials, including who may have access to radioactive materials and controlling access to radioactive materials[40,41]; and

- sterilizing radiation seeds when seed sterilization is required.

[Regulatory Requirement]

For more information on the radiation safety program, **see Section 4**.

10.5 The radiation safety committee is responsible for

- verifying radioactive waste disposal licensing requirements are met[63] and
- investigating incidents involving **licensed material**.[44]

[Recommendation]

For more information on the responsibilities of the radiation safety committee, **see Section 2**.

10.6 Radioactive materials must be used under direct supervision of the RSO or an authorized user.[42,49,167] *[Regulatory Requirement]*

10.6.1 The RSO is responsible for or delegates to a competent individual

- investigating overexposure accidents (eg, spills, losses, theft)[44,55];
- maintaining an inventory of radioactive materials[44,65];
- overseeing radioactive waste disposal[44,65];
- controlling and maintaining the surveillance program for radionuclides[42,56];
- controlling and maintaining constant surveillance of a radionuclide when it is in a controlled or unrestricted area and not in storage (eg, during sterilization or transport to the OR)[56]; and
- overseeing the security of licensed materials.[44]

[Recommendation]

For more information on the responsibilities of the RSO, **see Section 3**.

The roles and responsibilities of the RSO are described in regulatory documents,[42] clinical guidelines,[55,56,65] and an NRC report.[44]

10.7 Therapeutic radiation sources must be handled in accordance with local, state, and federal regulations.[39,43,49] *[Regulatory Requirement]*

The use of radioactive materials in a medical setting is regulated by the NRC or by the state regulatory bodies in an Agreement State, which may have differing regulations.[39]

10.7.1 Consult with the RSO to determine which of the principles listed below to follow when handling therapeutic radionuclides or radiopharmaceuticals or caring for patients who have received therapeutic radionuclides or radiopharmaceuticals:

- time (ie, spend the minimum amount of time near the source);
- distance (ie, keep as great a distance as possible from the source); and
- shielding (ie, if indicated, wear shielding when working with radionuclides and radiopharmaceuticals, or cover containers with indicated shielding devices).[50,168-171] *[Recommendation]*

Clinical guidelines recommend using indicated shielding to reduce the radiation dose to the hand.[50,171]

In a quasi-experimental study, Bruchmann et al[168] measured the amount of radiation reaching the eye of a phantom model from a syringe of nuclides. The amount of radiation reaching the eyes when radiation glasses were worn was Technetium-99 (0.28 mSv), Iodine-131 (0.79 mSv), Yttrium-90 (< 0.01 mSv), Fluorine-18 (0.86 mSv) and Gallium-68 (0.51 mSv). The researchers concluded that the need for eye protection is based on the radionuclide used.

Recommendations for protection can be found in a statement from the Occupational Safety and Health Administration and the Centers for Disease Control and Prevention.[172] Consulting with the RSO for guidance protection is recommended in two clinical guidelines.[65,169]

10.7.2 **Minimize handling of sealed radioactive sources (eg, capsules, seeds, needles, syringes) and irradiated tissues. If handling is necessary, use long forceps, tongs, or tube racks.**[50,65,169,173,174] *[Recommendation]*

Three clinical guidelines[50,65,169] and low-quality evidence[174] support use of forceps to assist with maintaining as great a distance as possible between the person and the source of radiation.

10.7.3 **Wear a covering over the scrub uniform and gloves as dictated by the procedure (eg, sterile, unsterile), and take precautions associated with the radiopharmaceutical (eg, radiation-attenuating, non-radiation-attenuating) when handling radiopharmaceuticals.** *[Recommendation]*

Wearing gloves and cover apparel (eg, lab coat, disposable gown) is recommended in a clinical guideline to protect the skin to a direct exposure in the event of a spill.[65]

10.8 **Limit the number of people in the OR to only those who are essential during all procedures for patients undergoing a radionuclide insertion, with an existing radionuclide implant, or**

with a radiopharmaceutical circulating in the bloodstream.[65] *[Recommendation]*

A clinical guideline recommends limiting the number of personnel.[65]

10.9 **Transport radiopharmaceuticals and radionuclides in a shielded container with a label indicating radioactivity unless the RSO indicates otherwise.**[65,169] *[Recommendation]*

Clinical guidelines recommend transporting radiopharmaceuticals and radionuclides in a shielded container.[65,169]

10.10 **Follow the manufacturers' written instructions for sterilizing radioactive materials.**[175] *[Recommendation]*

Sterilization instructions included in instructions for US Food and Drug Administration–cleared medical devices have been validated for effectiveness.

10.11 **Preoperatively, post a sign at all entrances stating "Radiation in Use" or an equivalent statement approved by the RSO.** *[Recommendation]*

Posting signage is recommended in a clinical guideline authored by the National Council on Radiation Protection and Measurements.[65]

10.12 **Verify the activity of sealed sources (eg, seeds) before implantation.**[49] *[Regulatory Requirement]*

10.12.1 **The following must be recorded according to the health care organization policy and procedure after verification:**
- **the radioisotope,**
- **the patient's name or identification number,**
- **the measured level of radioactivity, and**
- **the name of the individual who measured the activity.**[49]

[Regulatory Requirement]

10.13 **Personnel must account for radioactive seeds.**[42,43,49] *[Regulatory Requirement]*

The NRC mandates accounting for all seeds.[43,49] See the AORN Guideline for Prevention of Retained Surgical Items for recommendations on accounting for seeds.[176] See the AORN Guideline for Specimen Management for recommendations on accounting for seeds during radioactive seed localization procedures.[36]

10.13.1 **Maintain an inventory of all seeds removed from and returned to inventory.** *[Recommendation]*

A clinical guideline recommends maintaining an inventory (eg, a logbook).[65]

10.14 Use a standardized marking system (eg, a label on the chart, a wristband on the patient, a sign on the gurney or bed) to indicate that the patient is being treated with a radionuclide or radiopharmaceutical.[56,65] *[Recommendation]*

10.15 Prior to transferring the patient who had therapeutic radionuclides inserted, inform the personnel receiving the patient
- that the patient is radioactive and
- of the radiation source and the anatomical location.

[Recommendation]

Clinical guidelines support providing advance notification.[56,169]

10.15.1 Interventions that must be performed when transferring the patient include
- placing the patient in a private room with a private bathroom unless the patient and the roommate received the same treatment,
- posting a "Radioactive Materials" sign on the door,
- posting a sign indicating the amount of time visitors may stay in the room, and
- handling any material or waste removed from the room as radioactive unless it has been shown to be non-radioactive.[42]

[Regulatory Requirement]

10.16 After transporting the patient who has undergone a brachytherapy treatment procedure and before cleaning the OR, consult with the RSO to determine whether a radiation survey using a low-energy gamma scintillation survey instrument should be performed. *[Recommendation]*

A clinical guideline recommends completing a radiation survey of the OR to verify that no radioactive material remains in the room after the procedure.[65]

10.16.1 Use standard instrument cleaning procedures according to the manufacturer's instructions for use for instruments used during procedures involving radionuclides if the instruments were found to be nonradioactive during the postoperative survey or if instructed to do so by the RSO.[173,177] *[Recommendation]*

Use of standard instrument cleaning procedures is supported by a clinical guideline[177] and low-quality evidence.[173,177]

10.16.2 Use standard procedures for linen and surgical attire laundering that is found to be non-radioactive during the postoperative survey or if instructed to do so by the RSO.[178] *[Recommendation]*

In a quasi-experimental study, Miner et al[178] measured the amount of radioactivity present in the OR after 57 surgeries in patients receiving radiopharmaceuticals. The researchers measured the amount of radiation in the gloves, garments, sponges, linen, and OR using a swipe and meter survey. No evidence of radioactive contamination was found in the OR or in the OR waste. The researchers determined that no special waste disposal or treatment of the linen or scrubs is required after the performance of sentinel node biopsies.

10.16.3 Consult the RSO about precautions necessary if instruments or linen are found to be radioactive during the survey. *[Recommendation]*

Special handling of instruments and linen found to be radioactive is recommended in a clinical guideline authored by the National Council on Radiation Protection and Measurements.[65]

10.17 Emergency response equipment specific to the types of radioactive seeds used must be available near each surgical suite when radioactive materials are handled; this includes
- gloves (eg, sterile, nonsterile, radiation-attenuating),
- reverse action tweezers,
- shielded containers,
- a low-energy gamma scintillation survey instrument, and
- signage and labels for containers that indicate the presence of radioactive materials.[49]

[Regulatory Requirement]

According to the NRC,[49] an emergency may include loss or rupture of a seed or spill of a radiopharmaceutical.

10.17.1 In collaboration with the RSO, determine the type of gloves (eg, nonsterile, sterile, radiation-attenuating) to include in the emergency response equipment based on the types of radioactive seeds used in the facility and the risk of radiation exposure from a broken or leaking seed. *[Recommendation]*

Having emergency response equipment that will protect personnel from radioactive and biohazardous material is important. Guidance from the RSO on the risk of radiation exposure from a broken or leaking seed and the level of protection necessary will help determine the types of gloves needed in the emergency response kit.

10.18 In the event of a spill, immediately notify the RSO to determine actions to take based on the radioactive material present.[169] *[Recommendation]*

Contacting the RSO is recommended by the ICRP.[169]

10.19 Radioactive waste must be disposed of according to local, state, and federal regulations.[39,42] *[Regulatory Requirement]*

10.19.1 Use the following techniques to dispose of radioactive waste based on the levels of radioactivity:
- dilute and disperse (eg, bodily wastes with low levels of radioactivity disposed of into the sewer system using the flushing twice method)[169];
- delay and decay (eg, bodily wastes with high levels of radioactivity disposed of into the sewer system after being in a holding tank for the number of days required to decrease the radiation level to a safe level);
- concentrate and contain (used only rarely for items with a very high level of radioactivity; waste is collected into containers and then buried);
- incineration;
- return to the vendor; or
- disposal as nonregulated waste if the radioactivity of the item (eg, syringe, vial, cotton swab, tissue paper) does not exceed 1.35 microcuries.

[Conditional Recommendation]

Clinical guidelines[65,169] and low-quality evidence[179] support the use of these techniques.

10.19.2 Radioactive waste that cannot be disposed of using a dilute-and-disperse technique must be placed in a radioactive waste container in preparation for disposal.[39] *[Regulatory Requirement]*

10.19.3 A radioactive waste label must be placed on radioactive waste and should include the
- radioisotope name,
- amount of radioactivity,
- date of disposal, and
- radiation personnel or authorized user's full name and contact information.[39,180,181]

[Regulatory Requirement]

10.20 Perioperative team members (eg, RNs, scrub personnel, sterile processing personnel, environmental services personnel, anesthesia professionals) must receive education regarding handling of therapeutic radiation sources upon hire and annu-

ally as applicable to their role and responsibilities.[42,43,49] *[Regulatory Requirement]*

10.20.1 The education must include
- the size and appearance of the brachytherapy sources,[42]
- safe handling and shielding processes,[42]
- post patient death or emergency processes,[42]
- contamination control,[42]
- patient control (eg, where the patient can move within the facility);[42]
- visitor control (eg, who can visit and how many visitors are allowed),[42,43]
- waste control (eg, what waste procedures have to be followed),[42]
- dosimeter use and monitoring,[49,182] and
- emergency response to spills.[42,43,49]

[Regulatory Requirement]

10.20.2 The education and competency verification may include
- minimizing exposure to radiation (ie, ALARA),
- radiation safety procedures,[182,183]
- care of patients receiving radioactive nuclides, and
- controlling and providing security for the material (ie, constant surveillance).

[Conditional Recommendation]

This educational content is supported by clinical guidelines.[169,182,183]

10.21 Patients and caregivers must receive instructions regarding precautions to follow when a patient who has received therapeutic radionuclides is discharged.[42,43] *[Regulatory Requirement]*

10.21.1 Create individualized patient discharge instructions based on the radiation safety precautions applicable to the location of the seeds, number of seeds, and the radiation source (eg, Palladium-103, Cesium-131, Iodine-125).[65] *[Recommendation]*

Including content applicable to the location of the seeds, number of seeds, and the radiation source in patient education materials is recommended in a guideline authored by the National Council on Radiation Protection and Measurements.[65]

10.21.2 Include the following instructions for the patient:
- stay away from crowded places (eg, movie theaters);
- double flush urine and stool;
- wipe up spills of body fluids immediately;

- wear protective clothing (eg, shorts, breast shields)[184,185];
- adhere to restrictions on visitors, ambulation, and activity to maintain the integrity of the implant[65];
- cease breastfeeding[169];
- follow recommended sleeping arrangements[65]; and
- follow precautions for the specified length of time.

[Recommendation]

Including this content in education is recommended by a clinical guideline authored by the ICRP.[169]

In a nonexperimental study, Keller et al[184] calculated the amount of radiation exposure to family members of 67 female patients who had permanent breast seed implants using Palladium-103 between May 2004 and March 2007 at a single facility. The researchers measured exposure by providing the family members (ie, 39 spouses and 28 others) with dosimeters. A control badge was used to measure the atmospheric radiation, and the results of the control dosimeter were subtracted from the family-member dosimeter results. The amount of exposure to the family members was found to be below 5 mSv. The researchers recommended that the patient wear a breast shield in the presence of toddlers and women who are pregnant to provide extra protection.

10.21.3 Instruct family members, caregivers, and visitors to

- stay at least 3 ft (1 m) from the patient if possible, for a period of time equal to the half-life of the radionuclide[186] and
- follow precautions for the specified length of time.

[Recommendation]

Including this content in education is recommended by a clinical guideline authored by the ICRP.[169]

In a nonexperimental study, Yondorf et al[186] measured the radiation level at the patient's skin surface in 20 patients with Cesium-131 seeds placed in the brain. The researchers found a significant correlation between the number of seeds and the amount of radiation at the skin level. The researchers determined that increasing the distance from 14 inches (36 cm) to 40 inches (102 cm) decreased the dose by a factor of 10. The researchers concluded that the exposure to family members of patients with Cesium-131 seeds placed in the brain was below the recommended maximum dose.

10.22 Document the following in the patient's medical record:

- date and time of therapy,
- radionuclide activity level,
- any special precautions performed as indicated by the RSO, and
- patient education.[56,65]

[Recommendation]

Glossary

Absorbed dose: The energy imparted to irradiated matter by ionizing radiation to a unit mass of irradiated material at the place of interest. The special units of absorbed dose are the radiation absorbed dose or rad (ie, 0.01 joules per kg) and gray or Gy (ie, 1 joule per kg), which is equal to 100 rad.

Agreement State: Any state with which the US Nuclear Regulatory Commission or the Atomic Energy Commission has entered into a covenant under the Atomic Energy Act of 1954.

Brachytherapy: Placement of sealed radioactive sources adjacent to or in contact with a target tissue.

Cumulative air kerma: The total amount of radiation dose absorbed by air at a specific point away from the source.

Dose area product: A unit of measure used in assessing the radiation risk from diagnostic x-ray examinations and interventional procedures. It is calculated by multiplying the absorbed dose by the area irradiated.

Dosimeter: A device used to determine the external radiation dose that a person has received.

Effective dose: The sum of equivalent doses multiplied by the tissue-weighting factors of the tissue being irradiated. Describes the risks for stochastic effects when only a certain organ is irradiated.

Image intensifier: The radiation detector that produces the image in fluoroscopy.

Kerma-area product: The entire amount of radiation being delivered, measured in Gray multiplied by centimeters squared. Synonym: Dose area product.

Licensed material: Source material, special nuclear material, or by-product material received, possessed, used, transferred, or disposed of under a general or specific license issued by the US Nuclear Regulatory Commission.

Phantom: An object used as a substitute for live participants or cadavers. Frequently made to resemble human characteristics such as size and density.

Radionuclide: An unstable isotope of an element that decays or disintegrates spontaneously, resulting in radiation emission. Used on patients as seeds or as a radiopharmaceutical.

Radiopharmaceutical: A drug that emits radiation, which is administered to a patient via various routes so that the material is metabolized by the patient for distribution to various organs or tissues or the whole body for purposes of therapy.

Scatter radiation: Radiation is scattered when an x-ray beam strikes a patient's body, as it passes through the patient's body, and as it strikes surrounding structures (eg, walls, OR furniture).

Shallow-dose equivalent: The dose equivalent at a tissue depth of 0.007 cm averaged over an area of 1 cm.

Stochastic effects: The effects of the cumulative dosage of radiation, such as malignant diseases and genetic effects. The severity of the effect is not related to a threshold dose.

Tissue reactions: Localized tissue injury caused by an excessive dose of radiation. The amount of injury increases in severity as the dose is increased. Previously known as deterministic effects.

References

1. Salvo JP, Zarah J. Surgeon radiation exposure in hip arthroscopy: a prospective analysis. *Orthop J Sports Med.* 2015;3(7 Suppl 2): 2325967115S00142. [VC]

2. Sciahbasi A, Ferrante G, Fischetti D, et al. Radiation dose among different cardiac and vascular invasive procedures: the RODEO study. *Int J Cardiol.* 2017;240:92-96. [IIIA]

3. van den Haak RFF, Hamans BC, Zuurmond K, Verhoeven BAN, Koning OH. Significant radiation dose reduction in the hybrid operating room using a novel x-ray imaging technology. *Eur J Vasc Endovasc Surg.* 2015;50(4):480-486. [IIB]

4. Hirshfeld JW Jr, Ferrari VA, Bengel FM, et al. 2018 ACC/HRS/NASCI/SCAI/SCCT expert consensus document on optimal use of ionizing radiation in cardiovascular imaging—best practices for safety and effectiveness, part 1: radiation physics and radiation biology: a report of the American College of Cardiology Task Force on Expert Consensus Decision Pathways developed in collaboration with Mended Hearts. *Catheter Cardiovasc Interv.* 2018;92(2):203-221. [IVA]

5. Richardson DB, Cardis E, Daniels RD, et al. Site-specific solid cancer mortality after exposure to ionizing radiation: a cohort study of workers (INWORKS). *Epidemiology.* 2018;29(1):31-40. [IIIA]

6. Haylock RGE, Gillies M, Hunter N, Zhang W, Phillipson M. Cancer mortality and incidence following external occupational radiation exposure: an update of the 3rd analysis of the UK national registry for radiation workers. *Br J Cancer.* 2018;119(5):631-637. [IIIA]

7. Andreassi MG, Piccaluga E, Guagliumi G, Del Greco M, Gaita F, Picano E. Occupational health risks in cardiac catheterization laboratory workers. *Circ Cardiovasc Interv.* 2016;9(4):e003273. [IIIB]

8. Guesnier-Dopagne M, Boyer L, Pereira B, Guersen J, Motreff P, D'Incan M. Incidence of chronic radiodermatitis after fluoroscopically guided interventions: a retrospective study. *J Vasc Interv Radiol.* 2019;30(5):692-698. [IIIB]

9. Wei KC, Yang KC, Mar GY, et al. STROBE—radiation ulcer: an overlooked complication of fluoroscopic intervention: a cross-sectional study. *Medicine (Baltimore).* 2015;94(48):e2178. [IIIC]

10. Caird MS. Radiation safety in pediatric orthopaedics. *J Pediatr Orthop.* 2015;35(5 Suppl 1):S34-S36. [VB]

11. Preston DL, Kitahara CM, Freedman DM, et al. Breast cancer risk and protracted low-to-moderate dose occupational radiation exposure in the US radiologic technologists cohort, 1983-2008. *Br J Cancer.* 2016;115(9):1105-1112. [IIIA]

12. Ionizing radiation. Occupational Safety and Health Administration. https://www.osha.gov/SLTC/radiationionizing/healtheffects.html. Accessed January 21, 2021. [VA]

13. Basheerudeen SAS, Kanagaraj K, Jose MT, et al. Entrance surface dose and induced DNA damage in blood lymphocytes of patients exposed to low-dose and low-dose-rate X-irradiation during diagnostic and therapeutic interventional radiology procedures. *Mutat Res.* 2017;818:1-6. [IIB]

14. Kanagaraj K, Abdul Syed Basheerudeen S, Tamizh Selvan G, et al. Assessment of dose and DNA damages in individuals exposed to low dose and low dose rate ionizing radiations during computed tomography imaging. *Mutat Res Genet Toxicol Environ Mutagen.* 2015;789-790:1-6. [IIB]

15. Wiesel A, Stolz G, Queisser-Wahrendorf A. Evidence for a teratogenic risk in the offspring of health personnel exposed to ionizing radiation?! *Birth Defects Res Part A Clin Mol Teratol.* 2016;106(6):475-479. [IIIB]

16. Parikh JR, Geise RA, Bluth EI, et al. Potential radiation-related effects on radiologists. *AJR Am J Roentgenol.* 2017;208(3):595-602. [VB]

17. Kalem M, Başarir K, Kocaoğlu H, Şahin E, Kınık H. The effect of C-arm mobility and field of vision on radiation exposure in the treatment of proximal femoral fractures: a randomized clinical trial. *Biomed Res Int.* 2018;2018:6768272. [IB]

18. Georges JL, Boueri Z, Mailler B, et al. Reduction of radiation exposure associated with renewal of the radiologic systems in coronary interventions. *Ann Cardiol Angeiol (Paris).* 2018;67(5):334-338. [IIA]

19. Casella M, Dello Russo A, Russo E, et al. X-ray exposure in cardiac electrophysiology: a retrospective analysis in 8150 patients over 7 years of activity in a modern, large-volume laboratory. *J Am Heart Assoc.* 2018;7(11):e008233. [IIIA]

20. Goldsweig AM, Kennedy KF, Kolte D, et al. Predictors of patient radiation exposure during transcatheter aortic valve replacement. *Catheter Cardiovasc Interv.* 2018;92(4):768-774. [IIIA]

21. Cushman D, Mattie R, Curtis B, Flis A, McCormick ZL. The effect of body mass index on fluoroscopic time and radiation dose during lumbar transforaminal epidural steroid injections. *Spine J.* 2016;16(7):876-883. [IIIA]

22. Cushman D, Flis A, Jensen B, McCormick Z. The effect of body mass index on fluoroscopic time and radiation dose during sacroiliac joint injections. *PM R.* 2016;8(8):767-772. [IIIB]

23. Canham CD, Williams RB, Schiffman S, Weinberg EP, Giordano BD. Cumulative radiation exposure to patients undergoing arthroscopic hip preservation surgery and

occupational radiation exposure to the surgical team. *Arthroscopy.* 2015;31(7):1261-1268. [IIIB]

24. Dalgleish S, Hince A, Finlayson DF. Peri-operative radiation exposure: are overweight patients at increased risks? *Injury.* 2015;46(12):2448-2451. [IIIB]

25. Maempel JF, Stone OD, Murray AW. Quantification of radiation exposure in the operating theatre during management of common fractures of the upper extremity in children. *Ann R Coll Surg Engl.* 2016;98(7):483-487. [IIIB]

26. Madder RD, VanOosterhout S, Mulder A, et al. Patient body mass index and physician radiation dose during coronary angiography. *Circ Cardiovasc Interv.* 2019;12(1):e006823. [IIIB]

27. Farah J, Rouchaud A, Henry T, et al. Dose reference levels and clinical determinants in stroke neuroradiology interventions. *Eur Radiol.* 2019;29(2):645-653. [IIIB]

28. Pravatà E, Presilla S, Roccatagliata L, Cianfoni A. Operator radiation doses during CT-guided spine procedures. *Clin Neurol Neurosurg.* 2018;173:105-109. [IIIC]

29. Faroux L, Blanpain T, Nazeyrollas P, et al. Trends in patient exposure to radiation in percutaneous coronary interventions over a 10-year period. *Am J Cardiol.* 2017;120(6):927-930. [IIIA]

30. Rumanek J, Kudlas M. Shielding in medical imaging and radiation therapy. *Radiol Technol.* 2018;89(5):449-463. [VA]

31. Patet C, Ryckx N, Arroyo D, Cook S, Goy J. Efficacy of the SEPARPROCATH® radiation drape to reduce radiation exposure during cardiac catheterization: a pilot comparative study. *Catheter Cardiovasc Interv.* 2019;94(3):387-391. [IB]

32. Gilligan P, Lynch J, Eder H, et al. Assessment of clinical occupational dose reduction effect of a new interventional cardiology shield for radial access combined with a scatter reducing drape. *Catheter Cardiovasc Interv.* 2015;86(5):935-940. [IIB]

33. Leyton F, Nogueira MS, Gubolino LA, Pivetta MR, Ubeda C. Correlation between scatter radiation dose at height of operator's eye and dose to patient for different angiographic projections. *Appl Radiat Isot.* 2016;117:100-105. [IIIC]

34. Principi S, Farah J, Ferrari P, Carinou E, Clairand I, Ginjaume M. The influence of operator position, height and body orientation on eye lens dose in interventional radiology and cardiology: Monte Carlo simulations versus realistic clinical measurements. *Phys Med.* 2016;32(9):1111-1117. [IIB]

35. Wilson-Stewart K, Shanahan M, Fontanarosa D, Davidson R. Occupational radiation exposure to nursing staff during cardiovascular fluoroscopic procedures: a review of the literature. *J Appl Clin Med Phys.* 2018;19(6):282-297. [VA]

36. Guideline for specimen management. In: *Guidelines for Perioperative Practice.* Denver, CO: AORN, Inc; 2021:897-942. [IVA]

37. Guideline for minimally invasive surgery. In: *Guidelines for Perioperative Practice.* Denver, CO: AORN; 2021:503-534. [IVA]

38. Guideline for laser safety. In: *Guidelines for Perioperative Practice.* Denver, CO: AORN; 2021:421-442. [IVA]

39. 10 CFR 20: Standards for protection against radiation. US Nuclear Regulatory Commission. https://www.nrc. gov/reading-rm/doc-collections/cfr/part020/index.html. Accessed January 21, 2021.

40. *State Operations Manual Appendix A: Survey Protocol, Regulations and Interpretive Guidelines for Hospitals.* Rev. 200; 02-21-20. Centers for Medicare & Medicaid Services. https://www.cms. gov/Regulations-and-Guidance/Guidance/Manuals/downloads/som107ap_a_hospitals.pdf. Accessed January 21, 2021.

41. *State Operations Manual Appendix L: Guidance for Surveyors: Ambulatory Surgical Centers.* Rev. 200, 02-21-20. Centers for Medicare & Medicaid Services. https://www.cms.gov/Regulations-and-Guidance/Guidance/Manuals/downloads/som107ap_l_ambulatory.pdf. Accessed January 21, 2021.

42. 10 CFR 35: Medical use of byproduct material. US Nuclear Regulatory Commission. https://www.nrc.gov/reading-rm/doc-collections/cfr/part035/index.html. Accessed January 21, 2021.

43. 10 CFR 30.41: Transfer of byproduct material. US Nuclear Regulatory Commission. https://www.nrc.gov/reading-rm/doc-collections/cfr/part030/part030-0041.html. Accessed January 21, 2021.

44. Camper LW, Schlueter J, Woods S, et al. *Management of Radioactive Material Safety Program at Medical Facilities: Final Report [NUREG-1516].* Washington, DC: Division of Industrial and Medical Nuclear Safety, Office of Nuclear Material Safety and Safeguards, US Nuclear Regulatory Commission; 1997. [VA]

45. 42 CFR 416.49. Condition for coverage-laboratory and radiologic services. Govinfo.gov. govinfo.gov/app/details/CFR-2011-title42-vol3/CFR-2011-title42-vol3-sec416-49. Accessed January 21, 2021.

46. 42 CFR 482.26. Condition of participation: radiologic services. Govinfo.gov. https://www.govinfo.gov/app/details/CFR-2011-title42-vol5/CFR-2011-title42-vol5-sec482-26. Accessed January 21, 2021.

47. 29 CFR 1910.1096. Toxic and hazardous substances: ionizing radiation. https://www.osha.gov/laws-regs/regulations/standardnumber/1910/1910.1096. Accessed January 21, 2021.

48. Rehani MM, Ciraj-Bjelac O, Vañó E, et al. ICRP Publication 117. Radiological protection in fluoroscopically guided procedures outside the imaging department. *Ann ICRP.* 2010;40(6):1-102. [IVB]

49. Iodine-125 and Palladium-103 low dose rate brachytherapy seeds used for localization of non-palpable lesions. US Nuclear Regulatory Commission. https://www.nrc.gov/materials/miau/med-use-toolkit/seed-localization.html. Updated July 7, 2017. Accessed January 21, 2021.

50. Ortiz López P, Dauer LT, Loose R, et al. ICRP Publication 139: Occupational radiological protection in interventional procedures. *Ann ICRP.* 2018;47(2):1-118. [IVB]

51. Choi MH, Jung SE, Oh SN, Byun JY. Educational effects of radiation reduction during fluoroscopic examination of the adult gastrointestinal tract. *Acad Radiol.* 2018;25(2):202-208. [IIB]

52. Vañó E, Rosenstein M, Liniecki J, Rehani M, Martin CJ, Vetter RJ. ICRP Publication 113. Education and training in

radiological protection for diagnostic and interventional procedures. *Ann ICRP.* 2009;39(5):7-68. [IVC]

53. Jensen N, Janssen M. Quality improvement: Staff radiation exposure reduction while maintaining patient safety. *J Radiol Nurs.* 2017;36(4):242-244. [VA]

54. ICRP; Khong PL, Ringertz H, Donoghue V, et al. ICRP Publication 121: Radiological protection in paediatric diagnostic and interventional radiology. *Ann ICRP.* 2015;42(2):1-63. [IVB]

55. *Radiation Protection Guidance for Diagnostic and Interventional X-Ray Procedures* [Federal Guidance Report No. 14]. Washington, DC: Interagency Working Group on Medical Radiation; US Environmental Protection Agency; 2014. [IVB]

56. *AST Standards of Practice for Ionizing Radiation Exposure in the Perioperative Setting.* Littleton, CO; Association of Surgical Technologists; 2010. [IVC]

57. Radiation Dose Management for Fluoroscopically-Guided Interventional Medical Procedures [NCRP Report No. 168]. Bethesda, MD: National Council on Radiation Protection & Measurements; 2010. [IVB]

58. Fidalgo Domingos L, San Norberto García EM, Gutiérrez Castillo D, Flota Ruiz C, Estévez Fernández I, Vaquero Puerta C. Radioprotection measures during the learning curve with hybrid operating rooms. *Ann Vasc Surg.* 2018;50:253-258. [IIB]

59. Gendelberg D, Hennrikus W, Slough J, Armstrong D, King S. A radiation safety training program results in reduced radiation exposure for orthopaedic residents using the mini C-arm. *Clin Orthop Relat Res.* 2016;474(2):580-584. [IIB]

60. Sarkozy A, De Potter T, Heidbuchel H, et al. Occupational radiation exposure in the electrophysiology laboratory with a focus on personnel with reproductive potential and during pregnancy: A European Heart Rhythm Association (EHRA) consensus document endorsed by the Heart Rhythm Society (HRS). *Europace.* 2017;19(12):1909-1922. [IVB]

61. Sentinel Event Alert 47: Radiation risks of diagnostic imaging and fluoroscopy. The Joint Commission. https://www.jointcommission.org/resources/patient-safety-topics/sentinel-event/sentinel-event-alert-newsletters/sentinel-event-alert-issue-47-radiation-risks-of-diagnostic-imaging-and-fluoroscopy. Revised February 2019. Accessed January 21, 2021. [VB]

62. Ghodadra A, Bartoletti S. Reducing radiation dose in pediatric diagnostic fluoroscopy. *J Am Coll Radiol.* 2016;13(1):55-58. [IIB]

63. Koth J, Smith MH. Radiation safety compliance. *Radiol Technol.* 2016;87(5):511-524. [VB]

64. Guideline for medical device and product evaluation. In: *Guidelines for Perioperative Practice.* Denver, CO: AORN; 2021:719-728. [IVA]

65. *Management of Radionuclide Therapy Patients* [NCRP Report No. 155]. Bethesda, MD: National Council on Radiation Protection & Measurements; 2006. [IVC]

66. Kachaamy T, Harrison E, Pannala R, Pavlicek W, Crowell MD, Faigel DO. Measures of patient radiation exposure during endoscopic retrograde cholangiography: beyond fluoroscopy time. *World J Gastroenterol.* 2015;21(6):1900-1906. [IIIB]

67. Lazarus MS, Taragin BH, Malouf W, et al. Radiation dose monitoring in pediatric fluoroscopy: comparison of fluoroscopy time and dose-area product thresholds for identifying high-exposure cases. *Pediatr Radiol.* 2019;49(5):600-608. [IIIA]

68. Bonilha HS, Wilmskoetter J, Tipnis S, Horn J, Martin-Harris B, Huda W. Relationships between radiation exposure dose, time, and projection in videofluoroscopic swallowing studies. *Am J Speech Lang Pathol.* 2019;28(3):1053-1059. [IIIB]

69. Ghelani SJ, Glatz AC, David S, et al. Radiation dose benchmarks during cardiac catheterization for congenital heart disease in the United States. *JACC Cardiovasc Interv.* 2014;7(9):1060-1069. [IIIA]

70. Skripochnik E, Loh SA. Fluoroscopy time is not accurate as a surrogate for radiation exposure. *Vascular.* 2017;25(5):466-471. [IIIB]

71. Wilson SM, Prasan AM, Virdi A, et al. Real-time colour pictorial radiation monitoring during coronary angiography: effect on patient peak skin and total dose during coronary angiography. *EuroIntervention.* 2016;12(8):e939-e947. [IIB]

72. Baumann F, Katzen BT, Carelsen B, Diehm N, Benenati JF, Peña CS. The effect of realtime monitoring on dose exposure to staff within an interventional radiology setting. *Cardiovasc Intervent Radiol.* 2015;38(5):1105-1111. [IIB]

73. Muller MC, Welle K, Strauss A, et al. Real-time dosimetry reduces radiation exposure of orthopaedic surgeons. *Orthop Traumatol Surg Res.* 2014;100(8):947-951. [IIB]

74. Sailer AM, Vergoossen L, Paulis L, et al. Personalized feedback on staff dose in fluoroscopy-guided interventions: a new era in radiation dose monitoring. *Cardiovasc Intervent Radiol.* 2017;40(11):1756-1762. [IIB]

75. Heilmaier C, Kara L, Zuber N, Berthold C, Weishaupt D. Combined use of a patient dose monitoring system and a real-time occupational dose monitoring system for fluoroscopically guided interventions. *J Vasc Interv Radiol.* 2016;27(4):584-592. [IIB]

76. Baumgartner R, Libuit K, Ren D, et al. Reduction of radiation exposure from C-arm fluoroscopy during orthopaedic trauma operations with introduction of real-time dosimetry. *J Orthop Trauma.* 2016;30(2):e53-e58. [IIB]

77. Miller C, Kendrick D, Shevitz A, et al. Evaluating strategies for reducing scattered radiation in fixed-imaging hybrid operating suites. *J Vasc Surg.* 2018;67(4):1227-1233. [IIB]

78. Racadio J, Nachabe R, Carelsen B, et al. Effect of real-time radiation dose feedback on pediatric interventional radiology staff radiation exposure. *J Vasc Interv Radiol.* 2014;25(1):119-126. [IIB]

79. Adler DG, Lieb JG 2nd, Cohen J, et al. Quality indicators for ERCP. *Gastrointest Endosc.* 2015;81(1):54-66. [IVB]

80. Cousins C, Miller DL, Bernardi G, et al. ICRP Publication 120: Radiological protection in cardiology. *Ann ICRP.* 2013;42(1):1-125. [IVB]

81. ACR–AAPM Technical Standard for Management of the Use of Radiation in Fluoroscopic Procedures. American College of Radiology. https://www.acr.org/-/media/ACR/Files/Practice-Parameters/MgmtFluoroProc.pdf. Published 2018. Accessed January 21, 2021. [IVB]

82. Cupp SL. Radiation protection in computed tomography. *Radiol Technol.* 2016;88(2):169CT-183CT. [VA]

83. Phelps AS, Gould RG, Courtier JL, Marcovici PA, Salani C, MacKenzie JD. How much does lead shielding during fluoroscopy reduce radiation dose to out-of-field body parts? *J Med Imaging Radiat Sci.* 2016;47(2):171-177. [IIB]

84. ACR–SPR Practice Parameter for General Radiography. American College of Radiology. https://www.acr.org/-/media/ACR/Files/Practice-Parameters/RadGen.pdf. Published 2018. Accessed January 21, 2021. [IVB]

85. Martus JE, Hilmes MA, Grice JV, et al. Radiation exposure during operative fixation of pediatric supracondylar humerus fractures: is lead shielding necessary? *J Pediatr Orthop.* 2018;38(5):249-253. [IIIB]

86. Kaplan SL, Magill D, Felice MA, Xiao R, Ali S, Zhu X. Female gonadal shielding with automatic exposure control increases radiation risks. *Pediatr Radiol.* 2018;48(2):227-234. [IIB]

87. Lee MC, Lloyd J, Solomito MJ. Poor utility of gonadal shielding for pediatric pelvic radiographs. *Orthopedics.* 2017;40(4):e623-e627. [IIIB]

88. Karami V, Zabihzadeh M, Shams N, Saki Malehi A. Gonad shielding during pelvic radiography: a systematic review and meta-analysis. *Arch Iran Med.* 2017;20(2):113-123. [IIA]

89. *AAPM Position Statement on the Use of Patient Gonadal and Fetal Shielding.* American Association of Physicists in Medicine. https://www.aapm.org/org/policies/details.asp?id=468&type=PP&current=true. Published 2019. Accessed January 21, 2021. [IVC]

90. Culp MP, Barba JR, Jackowski MB. Shield placement: effect on exposure. *Radiol Technol.* 2014;85(4):369-376. [IIB]

91. Choi BH, Yaya K, Prabhu V, et al. Simple preoperative radiation safety interventions significantly lower radiation doses during central venous line placement in children. *J Pediatr Surg.* 2019;54(1):170-173. [IIB]

92. Aizer A, Qiu JK, Cheng AV, et al. Utilization of a radiation safety time-out reduces radiation exposure during electrophysiology procedures. *JACC Clin Electrophysiol.* 2019;5(5):626-634. [IIIA]

93. Hirshfeld JW Jr, Ferrari VA, Bengel FM, et al. 2018 ACC/HRS/NASCI/SCAI/SCCT expert consensus document on optimal use of ionizing radiation in cardiovascular imaging—best practices for safety and effectiveness, part 2: radiological equipment operation, dose-sparing methodologies, patient and medical personnel protection. *Catheter Cardiovasc Interv.* 2018;92(2):222-246. [IVA]

94. *ACR–SPR Practice Parameter for Imaging Pregnant or Potentially Pregnant Adolescents and Women with Ionizing Radiation.* American College of Radiology. https://www.acr.org/-/media/acr/files/practice-parameters/pregnant-pts.pdf. Published 2018. Accessed January 21, 2021. [IVB]

95. Chatterson LC, Leswick DA, Fladeland DA, Hunt MM, Webster S, Lim H. Fetal shielding combined with state of the art CT dose reduction strategies during maternal chest CT. *Eur J Radiol.* 2014;83(7):1199-1204. [IIB]

96. Moore W, Bonvento MJ, Lee D, Dunkin J, Bhattacharji P. Reduction of fetal dose in computed tomography using anterior shields. *J Comput Assist Tomogr.* 2015;39(2):298-300. [IIB]

97. *RSNA Statement on Safety of the Developing Fetus in Medical Imaging During Pregnancy.* Radiological Society of North America. https://www.rsna.org/uploadedfiles/rsna/content/role_based_pages/media/rsna-imaging-during-pregnancy-statement.pdf. Last reviewed April 3, 2018. Accessed January 21, 2021. [IVC]

98. Al Kharji S, Connell T, Bernier M, Eisenberg MJ. Ionizing radiation in interventional cardiology and electrophysiology. *Can J Cardiol.* 2019;35(4):535-538. [VB]

99. Guideline for patient information management. In: *Guidelines for Perioperative Practice.* Denver, CO: AORN; 2021:351-380. [IVA]

100. Yu E, Khan SN. Does less invasive spine surgery result in increased radiation exposure? A systematic review. *Clin Orthop Relat Res.* 2014;472(6):1738-1748. [IIIB]

101. Lee JE, Kim JH, Lee SJ, et al. Does nonexistent of your hands on the screen guarantee no radiation exposure to your body? Study on exposure of the practitioner's hands to radiation during C-arm fluoroscopy-guided injections and effectiveness of a new shielding device. *Medicine (Baltimore).* 2019;98(46):e17959. [IIIB]

102. Sailer AM, Paulis L, Vergoossen L, Wildberger JE, Jeukens CRLPN. Optimizing staff dose in fluoroscopy-guided interventions by comparing clinical data with phantom experiments. *J Vasc Interv Radiol.* 2019;30(5):701-708. [IIB]

103. Schuetze K, Kraus M, Eickhoff A, Gebhard F, Richter PH. Radiation exposure for intraoperative 3D scans in a hybrid operating room: how to reduce radiation exposure for the surgical team. *Int J Comput Assist Radiol Surg.* 2018;13(8):1291-1300. [IIB]

104. Kendrick DE, Miller CP, Moorehead PA, et al. Comparative occupational radiation exposure between fixed and mobile imaging systems. *J Vasc Surg.* 2016;63(1):190-197. [IIIB]

105. Urakov TM. Practical assessment of radiation exposure in spine surgery. *World Neurosurg.* 2018;120:e752-e754. [IIIB]

106. Heilmaier C, Mayor A, Zuber N, Fodor P, Weishaupt D. Improving radiation awareness and feeling of personal security of non-radiological medical staff by implementing a traffic light system in computed tomography. *Rofo.* 2016;188(3):280-287. [IIB]

107. Rhea EB, Rogers TH, Riehl JT. Radiation safety for anaesthesia providers in the orthopaedic operating room. *Anaesthesia.* 2016;71(4):455-461. [IIIA]

108. Valone LC, Chambers M, Lattanza L, James MA. Breast radiation exposure in female orthopaedic surgeons. *J Bone Joint Surg Am.* 2016;98(21):1808-1813. [IIB]

109. Tavares JB, Sacadura-Leite E, Matoso T, et al. The importance of protection glasses during neuroangiographies: a study on radiation exposure at the lens of the primary operator. *Interv Neuroradiol.* 2016;22(3):368-371. [IIIC]

110. Fetterly K, Schueler B, Grams M, Sturchio G, Bell M, Gulati R. Head and neck radiation dose and radiation safety for interventional physicians. *JACC Cardiovasc Interv.* 2017;10(5):520-528. [IIIB]

111. Matsubara K, Lertsuwunseri V, Srimahachota S, et al. Eye lens dosimetry and the study on radiation cataract in interventional cardiologists. *Phys Med.* 2017;44:232-235. [IIIA]

112. Waddell BS, Waddell WH, Godoy G, Zavatsky JM. Comparison of ocular radiation exposure utilizing three types of leaded glasses. *Spine (Phila Pa 1976).* 2016;41(4):E231-E236. [IIB]

113. Ekpo EU, Bakhshi S, Ryan E, Hogg P, McEntee MF. Operator eye doses during computed tomography fluoroscopic lung biopsy. *J Radiol Prot.* 2016;36(2):290-298. [IIB]

114. Hoffler CE, Ilyas AM. Fluoroscopic radiation exposure: are we protecting ourselves adequately? *J Bone Joint Surg Am.* 2015;97(9):721-725. [IIB]

115. Honorio da Silva E, Vanhavere F, Struelens L, Covens P, Buls N. Effect of protective devices on the radiation dose received by the brains of interventional cardiologists. *EuroIntervention.* 2018;13(15):e1778-e1784. [IIB]

116. Sans Merce M, Korchi AM, Kobzeva L, et al. The value of protective head cap and glasses in neurointerventional radiology. *J Neurointerv Surg.* 2016;8(7):736-740. [IIB]

117. Haga Y, Chida K, Kaga Y, Sota M, Meguro T, Zuguchi M. Occupational eye dose in interventional cardiology procedures. *Sci Rep.* 2017;7(1):569. [IIB]

118. Pomeroy CL, Mason JB, Fehring TK, Masonis JL, Curtin BM. Radiation exposure during fluoro-assisted direct anterior total hip arthroplasty. *J Arthroplasty.* 2016;31(8):1742-1745. [IIIC]

119. Alazzoni A, Gordon CL, Syed J, et al. Randomized controlled trial of radiation protection with a patient lead shield and a novel, nonlead surgical cap for operators performing coronary angiography or intervention. *Circ Cardiovasc Interv.* 2015;8(8):e002384. [IB]

120. Reeves RR, Ang L, Bahadorani J, et al. Invasive cardiologists are exposed to greater left sided cranial radiation: The BRAIN study (Brain Radiation Exposure and Attenuation During Invasive Cardiology Procedures). *JACC Cardiovasc Interv.* 2015;8(9):1197-1206. [IIIB]

121. Kirkwood ML, Arbique GM, Guild JB, et al. Radiation brain dose to vascular surgeons during fluoroscopically guided interventions is not effectively reduced by wearing lead equivalent surgical caps. *J Vasc Surg.* 2018;68(2):567-571. [IIIB]

122. Chohan MO, Sandoval D, Buchan A, Murray-Krezan C, Taylor CL. Cranial radiation exposure during cerebral catheter angiography. *J Neurointerv Surg.* 2014;6(8):633-636. [IIIB]

123. Kosaka H, Monzen H, Matsumoto K, Tamura M, Nishimura Y. Reduction of operator hand exposure in interventional radiology with a novel finger sack using tungsten-containing rubber. *Health Phys.* 2019;116(5):625-630. [IIC]

124. Kamusella P, Scheer F, Lüdtke CW, Wiggermann P, Wissgott C, Andresen R. Interventional angiography: radiation protection for the examiner by using lead-free gloves. *J Clin Diagn Res.* 2017;11(7):TC26-TC29. [IIIB]

125. ASGE Ensuring Safety in the Gastrointestinal Endoscopy Unit Task Force; Calderwood AH, Chapman FJ, Cohen J, et al. Guidelines for safety in the gastrointestinal endoscopy unit. *Gastrointest Endosc.* 2014;79(3):363-372. [IVC]

126. *Guidelines for Design and Construction of Hospitals.* St Louis, MO: Facility Guidelines Institute; 2018. [IVC]

127. *Guidelines for Design and Construction of Outpatient Facilities.* St Louis, MO: Facility Guidelines Institute; 2018. [IVC]

128. Sciahbasi A, Sarandrea A, Rigattieri S, et al. Extended protective shield under table to reduce operator radiation dose in percutaneous coronary procedures. *Circ Cardiovasc Interv.* 2019;12(2):e007586. [IA]

129. Inoue T, Komemushi A, Murota T, et al. Effect of protective lead curtains on scattered radiation exposure to the operator during ureteroscopy for stone disease: a controlled trial. *Urology.* 2017;109:60-66. [IB]

130. Madder RD, LaCombe A, VanOosterhout S, et al. Radiation exposure among scrub technologists and nurse circulators during cardiac catheterization: the impact of accessory lead shields. *JACC Cardiovasc Interv.* 2018;11(2):206-212. [IIB]

131. Crowhurst JA, Scalia GM, Whitby M, et al. Radiation exposure of operators performing transesophageal echocardiography during percutaneous structural cardiac interventions. *J Am Coll Cardiol.* 2018;71(11):1246-1254. [IIB]

132. Etzel R, König AM, Keil B, Fiebich M, Mahnken AH. Effectiveness of a new radiation protection system in the interventional radiology setting. *Eur J Radiol.* 2018;106:56-61. [IIB]

133. Sciahbasi A, Piccaluga E, Sarandrea A, et al. Operator pelvic radiation exposure during percutaneous coronary procedures. *J Invasive Cardiol.* 2018;30(2):71-74. [IIIA]

134. Hayre C, Bungay H, Jeffery C, Cobb C, Atutornu J. Can placing lead-rubber inferolateral to the light beam diaphragm limit ionising radiation to multiple radiosensitive organs? *Radiography (Lond).* 2018;24(1):15-21. [IIB]

135. Madder RD, VanOosterhout S, Mulder A, et al. Impact of robotics and a suspended lead suit on physician radiation exposure during percutaneous coronary intervention. *Cardiovasc Revasc Med.* 2017;18(3):190-196. [IIB]

136. Ploux S, Jesel L, Eschalier R, et al. Performance of a radiation protection cabin during extraction of cardiac devices. *Can J Cardiol.* 2014;30(12):1602-1606. [IB]

137. Muniraj T, Aslanian HR, Laine L, et al. A double-blind, randomized, sham-controlled trial of the effect of a radiation-attenuating drape on radiation exposure to endoscopy staff during ERCP. *Am J Gastroenterol.* 2015;110(5):690-696. [IB]

138. Kohlbrenner R, Lehrman ED, Taylor AG, et al. Operator dose reduction during transjugular liver biopsy using a radiation-attenuating drape: a prospective, randomized study. *J Vasc Interv Radiol.* 2018;29(9):1248-1253. [IB]

139. Sciahbasi A, Sarandrea A, Rigattieri S, et al. Staff radiation dose during percutaneous coronary procedures: role of adjunctive protective drapes. *Cardiovasc Revasc Med.* 2018;19(7 Pt A):755-758. [IIB]

140. Jones MA, Cocker M, Khiani R, et al. The benefits of using a bismuth-containing, radiation-absorbing drape in cardiac resynchronization implant procedures. *Pacing Clin Electrophysiol.* 2014;37(7):828-33. [IIB]

141. Arrivi A, Pucci G, Vaudo G, et al. Operators' radiation exposure reduction during cardiac catheterization using a removable shield. *Cardiovasc Interv Ther.* 2020;35(4):379-384. [IIA]

142. Dabin J, Maeremans J, Berus D, et al. Dosimetry during percutaneous coronary interventions of chronic total occlusions. *Radiat Prot Dosimetry.* 2018;181(2):120-128. [IIB]

143. Corrigan FE 3rd, Hall MJ, Iturbe JM, et al. Radioprotective strategies for interventional echocardiographers during structural heart interventions. *Catheter Cardiovasc Interv.* 2019;93(2):356-361. [IIIB]

144. Power S, Mirza M, Thakorlal A, et al. Efficacy of a radiation absorbing shield in reducing dose to the interventionalist during peripheral endovascular procedures: a single centre pilot study. *Cardiovasc Intervent Radiol.* 2015;38(3):573-578. [IIB]

145. Vlastra W, Delewi R, Sjauw KD, et al. Efficacy of the RAD-PAD protection drape in reducing operators' radiation exposure in the catheterization laboratory: a sham-controlled randomized trial. *Circ Cardiovasc Interv.* 2017;10(11):e006058. [IB]

146. Mayekar EM, Bayrak A, Shah S, Mejia A. Radiation exposure to the orthopaedic surgeon and efficacy of a novel radiation attenuation product. *J Surg Orthop Adv.* 2017;26(4):246-249. [IIB]

147. Uthoff H, Benenati MJ, Katzen BT, et al. Lightweight bilayer barium sulfate-bismuth oxide composite thyroid collars for superior radiation protection in fluoroscopy-guided interventions: a prospective randomized controlled trial. *Radiology.* 2014;270(2):601-606. [IB]

148. Monzen H, Tamura M, Shimomura K, et al. A novel radiation protection device based on tungsten functional paper for application in interventional radiology. *J Appl Clin Med Phys.* 2017;18(3):215-220. [IIB]

149. Kijima K, Krisanachinda A, Tamura M, Monzen H, Nishimura Y. Reduction of occupational exposure using a novel tungsten-containing rubber shield in interventional radiology. *Health Phys.* 2020;118(6):609-614. [IIB]

150. Lichliter A, Weir V, Heithaus RE, et al. Clinical evaluation of protective garments with respect to garment characteristics and manufacturer label information. *J Vasc Interv Radiol.* 2017;28(1):148-155. [IIB]

151. Fakhoury E, Provencher J, Subramaniam R, Finlay DJ. Not all lightweight lead aprons and thyroid shields are alike. *J Vasc Surg.* 2019;70(1):246-250. [IIB]

152. Lange VR. Eyewear contamination levels in the operating room: infection risk. *Am J Infect Control.* 2014;42(4):446-447. [IIB]

153. Jain S, Rajfer RA, Melton-Kreft R, et al. Evaluation of bacterial presence on lead X-ray aprons utilised in the operating room via IBIS and standard culture methods. *J Infect Prev.* 2019;20(4):191-196. [IC]

154. Boyle H, Strudwick RM. Do lead rubber aprons pose an infection risk? *Radiography.* 2010;16(4):297-303. [IIIC]

155. Grogan BF, Cranston WC, Lopez DM, et al. Do protective lead garments harbor harmful bacteria? *Orthopedics.* 2011;34(11):e765-e767. [IIIB]

156. La Fauci V, Riso R, Facciolà A, Merlina V, Squeri R. Surveillance of microbiological contamination and correct use of protective lead garments. *Ann Ig.* 2016;28(5):360-366. [IIIB]

157. Feierabend S, Siegel G. Potential infection risk from thyroid radiation protection. *J Orthop Trauma.* 2015;29(1):18-20. [IIIC]

158. CDC and ICAN. *Best Practices for Environmental Cleaning in Healthcare Facilities: in Resource-Limited Settings.* Version 2. Atlanta, GA: US Department of Health and Human Services, CDC; Cape Town, South Africa: Infection Control Africa Network; 2019. [IVB]

159. Guideline for environmental cleaning. In: *Guidelines for Perioperative Practice.* Denver, CO: AORN; 2021:145-176. [IVA]

160. Downes J, Rauk PN, Vanheest AE. Occupational hazards for pregnant or lactating women in the orthopaedic operating room. *J Am Acad Orthop Surg.* 2014;22(5):326-332. [VB]

161. Ghatan CE. Understanding and managing occupational radiation exposure for the pregnant interventional radiology nurse. *J Radiol Nurs.* 2020;39(1):20-23. [VA]

162. Marx MV. Baby on board: managing occupational radiation exposure during pregnancy. *Tech Vasc Interv Radiol.* 2018;21(1):32-36. [VB]

163. Chen SH, Brunet MC. Fetal radiation exposure risk in the pregnant neurointerventionalist. *J Neurointerv Surg.* 2020;12(10):1014-1017. [IIIC]

164. Gerasia R, Ligresti D, Cipolletta F, et al. Endoscopist's occupational dose evaluation related to correct wearing of dosimeter during X-ray-guided procedures. *Endosc Int Open.* 2019;7(3):E367-E371. [IIB]

165. Funao H, Ishii K, Momoshima S, et al. Surgeons' exposure to radiation in single- and multi-level minimally invasive transforaminal lumbar interbody fusion; a prospective study. *PLoS One.* 2014;9(4):e95233. [IIIB]

166. Betti M, Mazzoni LN, Belli G, et al. Surgeon eye lens dose monitoring in catheterization lab: a multi-center survey: invited for ECMP 2018 focus issue. *Phys Med.* 2019;60:127-131. [IIIA]

167. 10 CFR 20.1802. Control of material not in storage. US Nuclear Regulatory Commission. https://www.nrc.gov/reading-rm/doc-collections/cfr/part020/part020-1802.html. Accessed January 21, 2021.

168. Bruchmann I, Szermerski B, Behrens R, Geworski L. Impact of radiation protection means on the dose to the lens of the eye while handling radionuclides in nuclear medicine. *Z Med Phys.* 2016;26(4):298-303. [IIB]

169. Yonekura Y, Mattsson S, Flux G, et al. ICRP Publication 140: Radiological protection in therapy with radiopharmaceuticals. *Ann ICRP.* 2019;48(1):5-95. [IVB]

170. Kimura F, Yoshimura M, Koizumi K, et al. Radiation exposure during sentinel lymph node biopsy for breast cancer: effect on pregnant female physicians. *Breast Cancer.* 2015;22(5):469-474. [IIIB]

171. ACR-SPR Technical Standard for Diagnostic Procedures Using Radiopharmaceuticals. American College of Radiology. https://www.acr.org/-/media/ACR/Files/Practice-Parameters/

Radiopharmaceuticals.pdf. Revised 2016. Accessed January 21, 2021. [IVC]

172. Radiation emergency preparedness and response. Occupational Safety and Health Administration. https://www.osha.gov/SLTC/emergencypreparedness/radiation/radioactive_isotopes.html. Accessed January 21, 2021.

173. Michel R, Hofer C. Radiation safety precautions for sentinel lymph node procedures. *Health Phys.* 2004;86(2 Suppl):S35-S37. [VB]

174. Miller DL. Make radiation protection a habit. *Tech Vasc Interv Radiol.* 2018;21(1):37-42. [VB]

175. Guideline for sterilization. In: *Guidelines for Perioperative Practice.* Denver, CO: AORN; 2021:985-1014. [IVA]

176. Guideline for prevention of retained surgical items. In: *Guidelines for Perioperative Practice.* Denver, CO: AORN; 2021:769-820. [IVA]

177. Guideline for cleaning and care of surgical instruments. In: *Guidelines for Perioperative Practice.* Denver, CO: AORN; 2021:381-420. [IVA]

178. Miner TJ, Shriver CD, Flicek PR, et al. Guidelines for the safe use of radioactive materials during localization and resection of the sentinel lymph node. *Ann Surg Oncol.* 1999;6(1):75-82. [IIB]

179. Khan S, Syed A, Ahmad R, Rather TA, Ajaz M, Jan F. Radioactive waste management in a hospital. *Int J Health Sci (Qassim).* 2010;4(1):39-46. [VB]

180. 10 CFR 20.1905. Exemptions to labeling requirements. US Nuclear Regulatory Commission. https://www.nrc.gov/reading-rm/doc-collections/cfr/part020/part020-1905.html. Accessed January 21, 2021.

181. 10 CFR 20. Standards for protection against radiation. Subpart K: Waste disposal. US Nuclear Regulatory Commission. https://www.nrc.gov/reading-rm/doc-collections/cfr/part020/index.html. Accessed January 21, 2021.

182. *Safety Is No Accident: A Framework for Quality Radiation Oncology Care.* Arlington, VA: American Society for Radiation Oncology (ASTRO); 2019. [IVC]

183. Erickson BA, Demanes DJ, Ibbott GS, et al. American Society for Radiation Oncology (ASTRO) and American College of Radiology (ACR) practice guideline for the performance of high-dose-rate brachytherapy. *Int J Radiat Oncol Biol Phys.* 2011;79(3):641-649. [IVC]

184. Keller BM, Pignol JP, Rakovitch E, Sankreacha R, O'Brien P. A radiation badge survey for family members living with patients treated with a (103)Pd permanent breast seed implant. *Int J Radiat Oncol Biol Phys.* 2008;70(1):267-271. [IIIB]

185. Kaulich TW, Bamberg M. Radiation protection of persons living close to patients with radioactive implants. *Strahlenther Onkol.* 2010;186(2):107-112. [IIIC]

186. Yondorf MZ, Schwartz TH, Boockvar JA, et al. Radiation exposure and safety precautions following 131Cs brachytherapy in patients with brain tumors. *Health Phys.* 2017;112(4):403-408. [IIIB]

Guideline Development Group

Lead Author: Byron L. Burlingame[1], MS, BSN, RN, CNOR, Senior Perioperative Practice Specialist, AORN, Inc, Denver, Colorado

Subject Matter Experts: Stephen Balter[2], PhD, Professor of Clinical Radiology (Physics) (in Medicine) Columbia University, New York, New York; and A. Kyle Jones[3], PhD, MD Anderson Cancer Center, Associate Professor, Department of Imaging Physics, Houston, Texas

Methodologist: Erin Kyle[4], DNP, RN, CNOR, NEA-BC, Editor-in-Chief, *Guidelines for Perioperative Practice,* AORN, Inc, Denver, Colorado

Evidence Appraiser: Janice Neil[5], PhD, RN, CNE, Associate Professor, East Carolina College of Nursing, Greenville, North Carolina

Guidelines Advisory Board Member:

Linda C. Boley[6], MSN, BSN, RN, CNOR, Clinical Educator, Surgical Services, Norton Women's and Children's Hospital, Louisville, Kentucky

Guidelines Advisory Board Liaison:

Juan Sanchez[7], MD, MPA, FACS, FACHE, Associate Professor of Surgery, Johns Hopkins University School of Medicine, Baltimore, Maryland

External Review: Expert review comments were received from individual members of the American Association of Nurse Anesthetists (AANA), American College of Surgeons (ACS), Association for Professionals in Infection Control and Epidemiology (APIC), American Society of Anesthesiologists (ASA), International Association of Healthcare Central Service Materiel Management (IAHCSMM), the Society for Healthcare Epidemiology of America (SHEA), and the Surgical Infection Society (SIS). Their responses were used to further refine and enhance this guideline; however, their responses do not imply endorsement. The draft was also open for a 30-day public comment period.

Financial Disclosure and Conflicts of Interest

This guideline was developed, edited, and approved by the AORN Guidelines Advisory Board without external funding being sought or obtained. The Guidelines Advisory Board was financially supported entirely by AORN and was developed without any involvement of industry.

Potential conflicts of interest for all Guidelines Advisory Board members were reviewed before the annual meeting and each monthly conference call. None of the members of the Guideline Development Group reported a potential conflict of interest.[1-7] Had a financial conflict of interest arisen in the guideline development process, the Guideline

Advisory Board member would have recused themself from the discussion of the area of the guideline where the conflict of interest occurred.

Publication History

Originally published October 1989, *AORN Journal,* as Recommended Practices: Radiological Safety in the Practice Setting.

Published September 1993, *AORN Journal,* as Proposed Recommended Practices: Reducing Radiological Exposure in the Practice Setting.

Revised and reformatted; published January 2001, *AORN Journal,* as Recommended Practices for Reducing Radiological Exposure in the Practice Setting.

Revised November 2006; published in *Standards, Recommended Practices, and Guidelines,* 2007 edition, as Recommended Practices for Reducing Radiological Exposure in the Perioperative Practice Setting.

Minor editing revisions made to omit PNDS codes; reformatted September 2012 for publication in *Perioperative Standards and Recommended Practices,* 2013 edition.

Minor editing revisions made in November 2014 for publication in *Guidelines for Perioperative Practice,* 2015 edition, as Guideline for Reducing Radiological Exposure.

Revised June 2015 for publication in *Guidelines for Perioperative Practice* online.

Evidence ratings revised in *Guidelines for Perioperative Practice,* 2018 edition, to conform to the current AORN Evidence Rating Model.

Evidence ratings revised and minor editorial changes made to conform to the current AORN Evidence Rating model, September 2019, for online publication in *Guidelines for Perioperative Practice.*

Revised April 2021 for online publication in *Guidelines for Perioperative Practice.*

Scheduled for review in 2026.

AMBULATORY SUPPLEMENT:
RADIATION SAFETY

4. Radiation Safety Program

Ⓐ Certain hospital requirements (related to mandatory provision of radiologic services, supervision of such services by a radiologist, and practitioner signing of radiologic reports) no longer apply to ambulatory surgery centers (ASCs).

§416.49 Condition for Coverage: Laboratory and Radiologic Services

(b) Standard: Radiologic services.

(b)(1) Radiologic services may only be provided when integral to procedures offered by the ASC and must meet the requirements specified in §482.26(b), (c)(2), and (d)(2) of this chapter.

(b)(2) If radiologic services are utilized, the governing body must appoint an individual qualified in accordance with State law and ASC policies who is responsible for assuring all radiologic services are provided in accordance with the requirements of this section.[A1]

§482.26 Condition of Participation: Radiologic Services

(b)(1) Proper safety precautions must be maintained against radiation hazards. This includes adequate shielding for patients, personnel, and facilities, as well as appropriate storage, use, and disposal of radioactive materials.

(b)(2) Periodic inspection of equipment must be made and hazards identified must be promptly corrected.

(b)(3) Radiation workers must be checked periodically, by the use of exposure meters or badge tests, for amount of radiation exposure.

(b)(4) Radiologic services must be provided only on the order of practitioners with clinical privileges or, consistent with State law, of other practitioners authorized by the medical staff and the governing body to order the services.

(c)(2) Only personnel designated as qualified by the medical staff may use the radiologic equipment and administer procedures.

(d)(2) The hospital must maintain the following for at least 5 years:

(i) Copies of reports and printouts

(ii) Films, scans, and other image records, as appropriate[A2]

Ⓐ In an ASC, the individual appointed by the governing body to be the radiation safety officer is responsible for ensuring that proper radiation safety precautions are maintained. The radiation safety officer should be someone who currently works in the ASC. This individual is not required to be a radiologist but should be qualified in accordance with state law and ASC policies. As the individual responsible for oversight of the imaging services at the ASC, the radiation safety officer must maintain appropriate exposure records for each employee. In addition, this person is responsible for periodic evaluation and calibration of equipment, including testing the integrity of personal protective devices (eg, lead aprons) in compliance with federal, state, and local laws.[A3]

4.2 The radiation safety program must include
- **procedures for handling and disposing of body fluids and tissue that may be radioactive.**[A4,A5]

Ⓐ Transport personnel (couriers) may be at some risk of radiation exposure when transporting a sentinel lymph node or melanoma specimen marked with radioactive tracers if the container is improperly handled. Personnel are at risk of radiation exposure if the specimen container is held close to the body. To lessen this risk, it is advised that either the specimen itself or the specimen container be placed inside a standard bucket-type plastic specimen container, and the transport personnel should be instructed to carry the specimen container by the handle.[A6]

4.5.1 **The health care organization must maintain records of changes to the radiation safety program, program audits, and individual monitoring results as prescribed by regulatory requirements.**[A5,A7]

Ⓐ The ASC must have a policy that addresses the storage and retention of diagnostic images in accordance with federal, state, and local laws.[A5]

References

A1. Centers for Medicare and Medicaid Services. Medicare and Medicaid Programs; Regulatory Provisions to Promote Program Efficiency, Transparency, and Burden Reduction; Part II. Final rule. *Fed Regist.* 2014;79(91):27152.

A2. 42 CFR 482.26. Condition of participation: radiologic services. Govinfo.gov. http://www.govinfo.gov/app/details/

CFR-2011-title42-vol5/CFR-2011-title42-vol5-sec482-26. Accessed January 21, 2021.

A3. Diagnostic and other imaging services 13(D)(5). In: *Accreditation Handbook for Ambulatory Health Care.* Skokie, IL: Accreditation Association for Ambulatory Health Care, Inc; 2014:65.

A4. Guideline for specimen management. In: *Guidelines for Perioperative Practice.* Denver, CO: AORN, Inc; 2021:897-942.

A5. 10 CFR 20. Standards for protection against radiation. US Nuclear Regulatory Commission. https://www.nrc.gov/reading-rm/doc-collections/cfr/part020/index.html. Accessed January 21, 2021.

A6. Coventry BJ, Collins PJ, Kollias J, et al. Ensuring radiation safety to staff in lymphatic tracing and sentinel lymph node biopsy surgery—some recommendations. *J Nucl Med Radiat Ther.* 2012;S2:008.

A7. 10 CFR 30.41: transfer of byproduct material. 2014. US Nuclear Regulatory Commission. http://www.nrc.gov/reading-rm/doc-collections/cfr/part030/part030-0041.html. Accessed January 21, 2021.

Acknowledgments

Lead Author, Ambulatory Supplement
Jan Davidson, MSN, RN, CNOR, CASC
Director, Ambulatory Surgery Division
AORN, Inc
Denver, Colorado

Publication History

Originally published in *Perioperative Standards and Recommended Practices,* 2014 edition, as Ambulatory Supplement: Reducing Radiological Exposure.

Revised June 2015 for publication in *Guidelines for Perioperative Practice* online.

Minor editorial changes made to conform to revised guideline format, September 2019, for online publication in *Guidelines for Perioperative Practice.*

Revised April 2021 for online publication in *Guidelines for Perioperative Practice.*

RETAINED SURGICAL ITEMS

827

TABLE OF CONTENTS

A indicates additional information is available in the Ambulatory Supplement.

P indicates a recommendation or evidence relevant to pediatric care.

MEDICAL ABBREVIATIONS & ACRONYMS

2D – Two-dimensional
3D – Three-dimensional
ACS – American College of Surgeons
BMI – Body mass index
CT – Computed tomography
EMI – Electromagnetic interference
FDA – US Food and Drug Administration
HIPAA – Health Insurance Portability and Accountability Act
MIS – Minimally invasive surgery

MRI – Magnetic resonance imaging
OR – Operating room
QI – Quality improvement
RF – Radio frequency
RFID – Radio-frequency identification
RN – Registered nurse
RSI – Retained surgical item
UHC – University HealthSystem Consortium
WHO – World Health Organization

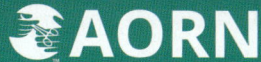
GUIDELINE FOR
PREVENTION OF UNINTENTIONALLY RETAINED SURGICAL ITEMS

The Guideline for Prevention of Unintentionally Retained Surgical Items was approved by the AORN Guidelines Advisory Board and became effective as of December 9, 2021. The recommendations in the guideline are intended to be achievable and represent what is believed to be an optimal level of practice. Policies and procedures will reflect variations in practice settings and/or clinical situations that determine the degree to which the guideline can be implemented. AORN recognizes the many diverse settings in which perioperative nurses practice; therefore, this guideline is adaptable to all areas where operative or other invasive procedures may be performed.

Purpose

This document provides guidance to perioperative team members for preventing unintentionally retained surgical items (RSIs) in patients undergoing operative and other invasive procedures. Guidance is provided for implementing a consistent interdisciplinary approach and using standardized procedures to prevent RSIs, accounting for surgical items (ie, radiopaque soft goods, sharps and miscellaneous items, instruments), preventing retention of device fragments, and reconciling count discrepancies. Guidance is also provided for use of adjunct technology during manual counting procedures.

An RSI is a rare but serious preventable error that can result in patient harm. Perioperative team members are ethically and morally obligated to protect patients by implementing measures to prevent RSIs. Prevention of RSIs requires an interdisciplinary approach that aims to reduce the risks and contributing factors associated with RSIs. In a survey conducted by Steelman et al[1] that included 3,137 responses from perioperative registered nurses (RNs), 61% of participants (n = 1,918) identified the prevention of RSIs as one of the top priorities for perioperative patient safety. The National Academy of Medicine identified avoiding injuries from care that is intended to help patients as one of six goals to achieve a better health care system.[2]

Even though unintentionally retained items continue to be one of the most common **sentinel events** reported to The Joint Commission,[3] these events are likely underreported[4-7] and underestimated.[8,9] This may be due in part to the lack of a universal definition of RSI[10] and varying reporting requirements.[11,12] The true incidence of RSIs remains unknown in part because retained items may be undetected for months or years.[7] In 2003, based on data from 1999, Gawande et al[4] esti-

mated that more than 1,500 RSIs occur annually in the United States. Since then, reports on the prevalence of RSIs have varied considerably depending on the source of the information (Table 1).

Surgical sponges are the most commonly retained items.[3,6,8,9,13-22] However, as the rates of minimally invasive procedures and the use of adjunct technologies to prevent retained soft goods increases, there could be a shift in the number and types of items that are retained compared to soft goods.[23,24] Other reported RSIs are instruments,[4,8,9,14,21,22,25,26] needles,[8,9] device fragments,[14,21,22,25,27,28] items such as guidewires,[7,8,14,21] and miscellaneous items (eg, rectal tube caps, drain bulbs).[21,22] Most counting discrepancies involve needles.[29,30]

The location of an RSI depends on the type of procedure performed. The abdomen[31] and pelvis[19,32] are reported to be the locations where RSIs are most often found,[6,10,13,15,32] and surgical sponges retained in the abdomen or pelvis can migrate into the intestine, bladder, thorax, or stomach.[31,34,35] Retained surgical items have been reported in all body cavities.[25] Other reported locations of RSIs include the brain,[4,15] face,[4,25] eye[15] and orbit,[36,37] ear,[38] mouth and airway,[15] nasal cavity,[15,39] neck,[15,31] shoulder and axilla,[15,31] thorax[4,25,40] or chest,[15] pacemaker or defibrillator pocket,[15] breast,[15,16] back,[15] spinal canal,[4] extremities,[4,15,18,25,27] inguinal hernia,[31] hip and gluteal region,[15] vagina,[4,15,25,28,40,41] scrotum,[15] and natural orifices.[13]

Retained surgical items have also been reported to occur during less-invasive procedures (eg, minimally invasive surgery [MIS], endoscopic procedures).[22,40,42,43] In a study of 308 retained object incidents that were reported to The Joint Commission between 2012 and 2018, excluding soft goods and guidewires, at least 156 incidences (50.6%) occurred during MIS.[42]

Reported methods of RSI discovery include symptoms,[25] radiological evaluation,[6,8,25,33] and physical examination.[6,25] Time to diagnosis of an RSI can vary greatly. Reports suggest that many RSIs are discovered between the time of occurrence and 2 months,[4,8,9,25,31,33,40] some have been found between 2 months and 5 years,[8,9,25,31,33] and others have been found after 5 years.[4,9,31,33] There have been reports of RSIs found after 20[44,45] to 40 years.[33,46]

Because an RSI is an event that presents significant risk for patient harm, many states require public reporting when RSI events occur.[47] Federal and state agencies, accrediting bodies, third-party payers, and professional associations consider an unintentionally retained foreign object or RSI to be a serious and largely, if not entirely, preventable event (eg, never event, health care–associated condition, sentinel event, serious reportable event).[48,49] Consequently, health care organizations and providers will not be reimbursed for additional care provided as a result of an RSI.[11,50,51]

A long-standing and evidence-based strategy for preventing RSIs is to account for all items opened or used during the operative or other invasive procedure. Health care organizations are responsible for employing standardized, transparent, verifiable, reliable practices to account for all surgical items used during a procedure. Counting radiopaque soft goods, sharps, miscellaneous items, and instruments is one method to account for all items used on the surgical field. However, there is a significant potential for inaccurate counts with the use of manual counting practices.[29,52,53] The use of adjunct technology can decrease counting discrepancies and has the potential to reduce the risk of RSIs.[8,40,54-57]

Beyond the process of counting, systems and human factors play a significant role in contributing to RSIs. Therefore, behavioral changes and education about risk-reduction strategies unique to each setting used during the adoption of systems may improve accounting for surgical items. Improving system reliability to enhance the performance of human factors (eg, compliance with policies and procedures, effective hand-over communication) may reduce the incidence of errors and improve patient safety.[23] A systems approach to preventing RSIs includes using standardized counting and reconciliation procedures, methodical wound exploration,[15] radiological confirmation, adjunct technology, team training,[58,59] and enhanced communication to promote optimal perioperative patient outcomes.[48,60-63]

The limitations of the evidence are that randomized controlled trials of RSI prevention interventions could expose patients to harm and, as such, would not be ethical.[25] Case-control studies of RSIs have been conducted and contribute valuable knowledge to the field. However, interpretation of these studies is limited by the nature of this type of research, which can only show association among study variables and cannot determine causation. Because of a lack of research on interventions to prevent RSIs, much of the available evidence is based on generally accepted practices, which were first published in the AORN "Standards for sponge, needle, and instrument procedures" in 1976.[64]

The following topics are outside the scope of this document: retrieval techniques and treatment options for RSIs, management of broken surgical drains during removal, post-procedure management of broken central line catheters, and management of retained endoscopy capsules in the gastrointestinal tract.

Evidence Review

A medical librarian with a perioperative background conducted a systematic search of the databases Ovid MEDLINE, Ovid Embase, EBSCO CINAHL, and the Cochrane Database of Systematic Reviews. The search was limited to literature published in English from January 2014 through December 2020. At the time of the initial search, weekly alerts were created on the topics included in that search. Results from these alerts were provided to the lead author until July 2021. The lead author requested additional articles that either did not fit the original search criteria or were discovered during the evidence appraisal process. The lead author and the medical librarian also identified relevant guidelines from government agencies, professional organizations, and standards-setting bodies.

Search terms included *2D matrix, 3D micro tag, adverse event, adverse health care event, anti-Semitism, awareness, attitude to obesity, bar coding, bent hypodermic needles, biliary tract surgical procedures, blood loss, blood loss estimation, blood loss (surgical), bloodless medical and surgical procedures, broken hypodermic needles, cardiac catheters, catheterization (central venous), catheterization (peripheral central venous), catheters, catheters (indwelling), catheters (vascular), central venous catheters, count board, count discrepancies, count reconciliation, count sheet, covert racism, cross-disciplinary communication, cultural bias, cultural competency, cultural diversity, cultural pluralism. delivery of health care, dentistry (operative), device fragments, difference in treatment, discrepancies in treatment, discrimination, disparities, distraction, diversity, documentation, documentation of unresolved count discrepancies, emergency surgery, emergent surgical procedures, ethnic groups, ethnicity, forceps, foreign bodies, glidewires, guidewires, gossypiboma, health care delivery, health care disparities, health care errors, health status disparities, healthcare disparities, healthcare near miss, healthcare time out, healthcare timeout, heart catheter, heart catheterization, human error, human factors, hypodermic needle defects, hypodermic needle fragments, hypodermic needles, implantable catheters, implicit bias, incorrect count, indwelling catheters, instrument breakage, instrument label defects, instrument label fragmentation, intercardiac catheter, intraoperative awareness, intraoperative imaging, intraoperative radiograph, intravascular device defects, intravascular device fragments, interdisciplinary communication, invasive procedures, Islamophobia, lengthy procedure, long procedure, malleable ribbon, medical errors, microneedles, minimally invasive procedures, minorities, minority groups, minority health, missing surgical items, morbid obesity, multiculturalism, multidisciplinary communication, nationality, near miss, near miss (healthcare), needles, never event, noise, noise pollution, nurse's role, nurse's scope of practice, nursing, nursing care, nursing role, obesity, obesity (morbid), operating room nursing, operative procedures, people of color, perioperative nursing, pocketed sponge bag system, prejudice, preventing retained surgical items, pulmonary artery catheters, race, race factors, racial disparities, racial factors, racial bias, racial discrimination, racial prejudice, racism, radio frequency, radio frequency identification, radio frequency identification device, radiopaque, reporting retained surgical items, retained foreign bodies, retained instruments, retained intravascular devices, retained surgical instruments, retained surgical items, retained surgical needle, retained surgical tool, retention, robotic surgical*

Table 1. Studies Reporting Retained Surgical Item (RSI) Incidence

RSI definition	Population			Numerator / Denominator	Incidence per 10,000*
	Dates	Location	Ages		
[1] Not provided	2007-2017	California	All	94/NR; estimated 1:300,000	0.33
[2] Not stated, but included soft goods, instruments, and sharps	2009-2016	National (Veterans)	Adults, older adults	124/2,964,472	0.42
[3] AHRQ Patient Safety Indicator 5 definition: ICD-9-CM codes 998.4, 998.7, and E891.x	2003-2007	National (Veterans)	Adults, older adults	290/2,342,690	1.20
[4] ICD-9-CM codes 998.4 and E871.0	2003	36 states participating in AHRQ Kids' Inpatient Database	Pediatric patients (< 20 years)	103/3,365,317	0.31
[5] Object unintentionally retained at time of final closure or end of procedure if no incision	2003-2006	Mayo Clinic Rochester	NR	34/191,168	1.78
[6] Retention of surgical instrument, needle, or sponge	2000-2004	A major academic health center and affiliated hospitals in New York	NR	NR; estimated 1:7,000	1.43
[7] Patients who present symptomatic and diagnosed with a retained surgical sponge	1990-2003	Ar Ramtha, Jordan (International)	NR	NR; estimated 1/5,027	1.99

Incidence bubble color legend: ● Single state; ● Veterans; ● Pediatric; ● Single medical center; ● International

NR = not reported

*Incidence rate adjusted to per 10,000 for comparison

References

1. Cohen AJ, Lui H, Zheng M, et al. Rates of serious surgical errors in California and plans to prevent recurrence. JAMA Netw Open. 2021;4(5):e217058.
2. Gunnar W, Soncrant C, Lynn MM, Neily J, Tesema Y, Nylander W. The impact of surgical count technology on retained surgical items rates in the Veterans Health Administration. J Patient Saf. 2020;16(4):255-258.
3. Chen Q, Rosen AK, Cevasco M, Shin M, Itani KM, Borzecki AM. Detecting patient safety indicators: How valid is "foreign body left during procedure" in the Veterans Health Administration? J Am Coll Surg. 2011;212(6):977-983.
4. Shah RK, Lander L. Retained foreign bodies during surgery in pediatric patients: a national perspective. J Pediatr Surg. 2009;44(4):738-742.
5. Cima RR, Kollengode A, Garnatz J, Storsveen A, Weisbrod C, Deschamps C. Incidence and characteristics of potential and actual retained foreign object events in surgical patients. J Am Coll Surg. 2008;207(1):80-87.
6. Egorova NN, Moskowitz A, Gelijns A, et al. Managing the prevention of retained surgical instruments: what is the value of counting? Ann Surg. 2008;247(1):13-18.
7. Bani-Hani KE, Gharaibeh KA, Yagha RJ. Retained surgical sponges (gossypiboma). Asian J Surg. 2005;28(2):109-115.

Figure 1. Flow Diagram of Literature Search Results

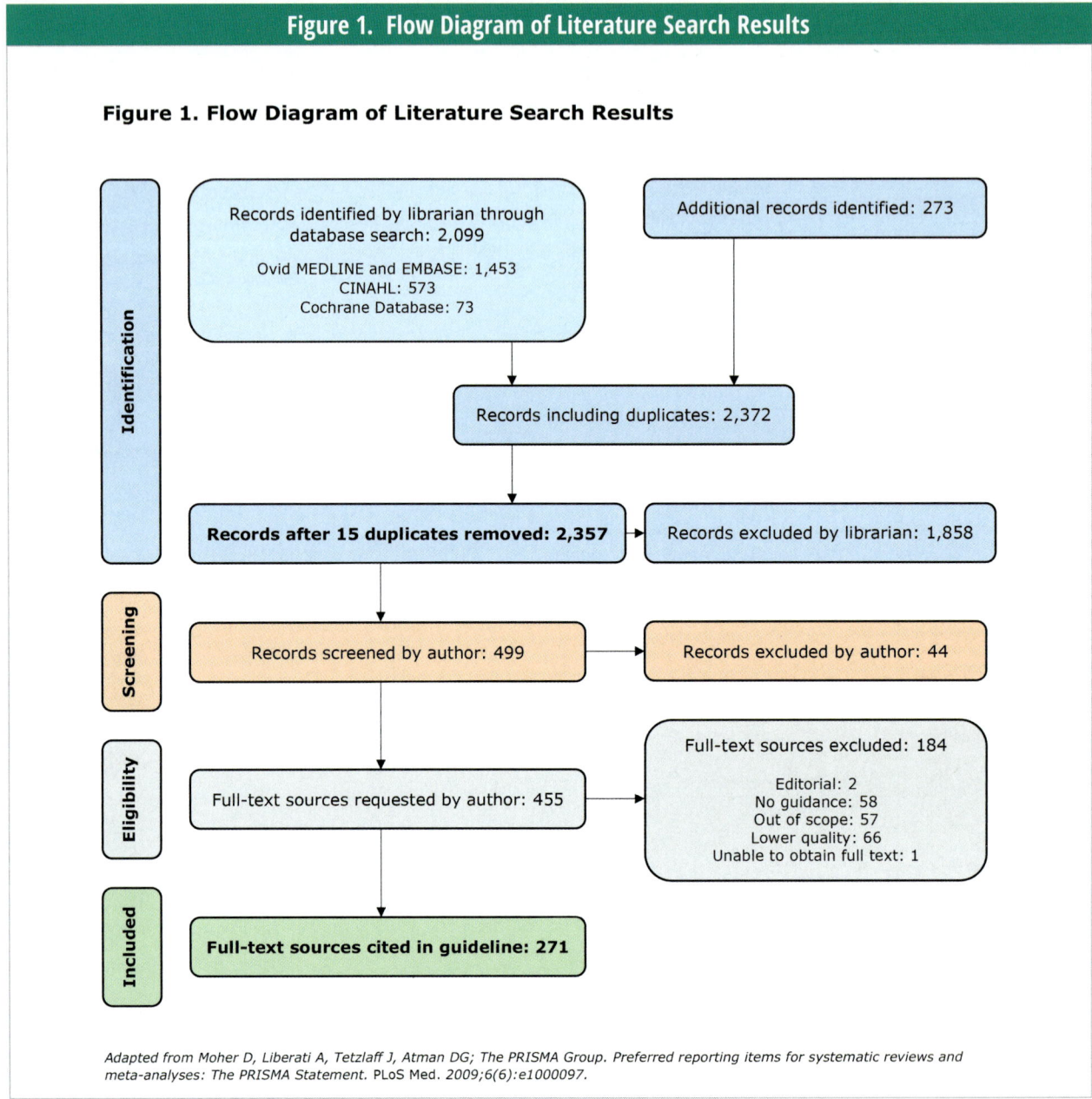

Figure 1. Flow Diagram of Literature Search Results

Adapted from Moher D, Liberati A, Tetzlaff J, Atman DG; The PRISMA Group. Preferred reporting items for systematic reviews and meta-analyses: The PRISMA Statement. PLoS Med. 2009;6(6):e1000097.

procedures, root cause analyses, root cause analysis, scope of nursing practice, sentinel event, severe obesity, shift change, shift reports, situational awareness, skin color, skin tone, small suture needles, socially responsible surgery, soft goods, speculum, surgical blood loss, surgical clamps, surgical clips, surgical count procedure, surgical count reconciliation, surgical errors, surgical hemorrhage, surgical hooks, surgical instruments, surgical nursing, surgery (operative), surgical pause, surgical plug, surgical procedures, surgical procedures (operative), surgical sponges, surgical time out, surgical timeout, surgical traumatology, surgical valves, surgical wound examination, surgical wound exploration, suture needles, tantalum clips, textiloma, therapeutic sponge packing, throat pack, time out (healthcare), trauma surgery, traumatology, trocar, underserved patients, underserved populations, unequal treatment, unretrieved device fragments,

urban population, vascular access devices, vulnerable populations, and weight bias.

Included were research and non-research literature in English, complete publications, and publications with dates within the time restriction when available. Excluded were non-peer-reviewed publications and older evidence within the time restriction when more recent evidence was available. Editorials, news items, and other brief items were excluded. Low-quality evidence was excluded when higher-quality evidence was available, and literature outside the time restriction was excluded when literature within the time restriction was available **(Figure 1)**.

Articles identified in the search were provided to the lead author for critical appraisal. The lead author distributed research articles to another evidence appraiser who independently evaluated and appraised each article using the AORN Research or Non-Research Evidence Appraisal Tools as appropriate. Each article was then assigned an appraisal score based on a consensus of the lead author and evidence appraiser. The appraisal score is noted in brackets after each reference as applicable.

Each recommendation rating is based on a synthesis of the collective evidence, a benefit-harm assessment, and consideration of resource use. The strength of the recommendation was determined using the AORN Evidence Rating Model and the quality and consistency of the evidence supporting a recommendation. The recommendation strength rating is noted in brackets after each recommendation.

Note: The evidence summary table is available at http://www.aorn.org/evidencetables/.

1. Consistent Interdisciplinary Approach

1.1 Use a consistent interdisciplinary approach for preventing RSIs during all surgical and invasive procedures. *[Recommendation]*

Moderate-quality evidence[23,58,59,62] and guidance from professional organizations[48,60,61,63,65] support that RSIs are preventable events for which the incidence can be reduced by implementing a consistent interdisciplinary approach. The approach for RSI prevention is interdisciplinary because systems that involve accounting for items used in the patient during operative or other invasive procedures are team-based activities that comprise input from multiple perioperative team members.

Establishing a system that accounts for all surgical items opened and used during a procedure constitutes a primary and proactive strategy to prevent patient harm. Reason's model of human error states that errors involve some kind of deviation from standard practice.[66] Ideal RSI prevention measures are standardized, transparent, verifiable, and reliable. Deliberate, consistent application of and adherence to standardized procedures is necessary to prevent RSIs.

In an organizational improvement initiative, Duggan et al[67] convened an interdisciplinary task force with the aim of reducing RSI events in one organization. After evaluating previous RSI events and operating room (OR) observations, the authors implemented facility-specific bundled changes. The interdisciplinary task force was successful in reducing the rate of RSIs from 1.69 per year to zero and sustaining zero RSIs for more than 1,300 days. This article demonstrates a model for improvement that organizations could emulate by engaging an interdisciplinary team for planning and implementation.

1.2 Implement measures for all perioperative team members to improve teamwork and communication as part of a collaborative interdisciplinary approach to RSI prevention. *[Recommendation]*

All perioperative team members are responsible for preventing RSIs. Professional organizations recommend engaging an interdisciplinary team as part of a systems approach to RSI prevention.[48,60-63,65] Teamwork and communication problems are common areas where failures occur in the prevention of RSIs.[15,42,66,68] Improving teamwork and communication in an effort to foster a just culture focused on patient safety is part of a systems approach to reducing surgical errors such as RSIs.[23,69]

1.2.1 The RN circulator should
- perform a room survey for open countable items from a previous procedure before conducting an initial count[70];
- verify that the count board (eg, whiteboard) and count sheets do not contain information from a previous procedure;
- initiate the count process;
- view the surgical items being counted;
- record in a visible location (eg, the count board) the counts of soft goods, sharps, miscellaneous items, and items placed in the patient[70];
- record instrument counts on preprinted count sheets;
- observe for items dropped from the sterile field;
- consult with the team about whether any supplies will be needed before initiating the closing count;
- participate in count reconciliation activities;
- report any **count discrepancy**; and
- document count activities (See Section 10).
[Recommendation]

Accurately accounting for items used during a surgical procedure is a primary responsibility of the RN circulator.[71] The RN circulator plays a leading role in implementing measures to account for surgical items. In an organizational experience study, Yang et al[72] observed 18 cardiovascular procedures for potential and actual errors to conceptualize the role that the RN circulator plays in preventing errors. Of 200 errors, 8% were attributed to counting errors. Had the RN circulator not noticed these counting errors, they might not have been resolved and could have resulted in RSIs.

Loftus et al[70] implemented the room survey as a part of count protocols in a safe surgery program. They also recommended recording the count on a whiteboard that is visible to the surgical team.

1.2.2 The scrub person should
- maintain an organized sterile field according to the health care organization's policy (there should be minimal variation in how different scrub persons organize the sterile field)[73];
- maintain awareness of the location of soft goods (eg, radiopaque sponges, towels, textiles), sharps, and instruments on the sterile field and in the patient during the course of the procedure;
- know the function configuration (eg, number of parts, assembly and disassembly methods) of all medical devices that are used during the operative or other invasive procedure;
- verify the integrity and completeness of items when they are returned from the surgical site;[73]
- consult with the surgeon about whether any supplies will be needed before performing the closing count;
- count surgical items in a manner that allows the RN circulator to see the surgical items being counted;[73]
- speak up when a discrepancy exists;[73] and
- participate in count reconciliation activities.[73]

[Recommendation]

Accurately accounting for items used during a surgical procedure is a primary responsibility of the scrub person.[73] Maintaining an organized sterile field facilitates accounting for all items during and after the procedure. Standardized sterile setups established by the health care organization's policy help reduce variation and may lessen the risk for error. Two articles from psychological journals indicated that a random arrangement of objects coupled with distracters increased counting difficulty and errors.[74,75]

1.2.3 Surgeons and surgical first assistants should actively participate in safety measures to prevent RSIs.[61] The surgeon and surgical first assistant should
- use radiopaque surgical items (eg, soft goods) in the wound;[60,61]
- maintain awareness of the location of items in the surgical wound during the course of the procedure;
- communicate placement of surgical items in the wound to the perioperative team for notation in a visible location (eg, the count board);
- acknowledge awareness of the start of the count process;

- notify the team if any supplies will be needed on the sterile field before the start of the closing count[76];
- remove unneeded counted items from the surgical field before initiation of the count process;
- perform a methodical wound exploration before closing the patient, using both visualization and touch when feasible[15,60,61];
- notify the scrub person and RN circulator about surgical items returned to the surgical field to complete the final count;
- communicate and document items left intentionally as packing[61];
- participate in count reconciliation activities;
- document actions taken to resolve count discrepancies[61]; and
- verify and document results of the final count.[48,61]

[Recommendation]

Accurately accounting for items used during a surgical procedure is a primary responsibility of the surgeon and surgical first assistant. The American College of Surgeons (ACS) recognizes patient safety as "an issue of the highest priority and strongly urges individual hospitals and health care organizations to take all reasonable measures to prevent the unintended retention of surgical items in the surgical wound."[61]

Use of radiopaque items in the surgical wound provides a mechanism to locate **misplaced items** as part of resolving count discrepancies. Not all items are manufactured with radiopaque indicators.

1.2.4 Anesthesia professionals should actively participate in safety measures to prevent RSIs. The anesthesia professional should
- plan anesthetic milestone actions (eg, emergence from anesthesia) so that these actions do not pressure the perioperative team to circumvent safe accounting practices[77];
- communicate to the perioperative team when throat packs, bite blocks, and other devices are inserted in the oropharynx, nose, or nasopharynx; and
- verify that throat packs, bite blocks, and other devices are removed from the oropharynx, nose, or nasopharynx and communicate to the perioperative team when these items are removed.[78-81]

[Recommendation]

Surgical counts and anesthetic milestones, such as emergence from anesthesia, are both critical phases of the procedure when minimizing distractions may improve patient safety.[77]

Planning and coordination will allow the perioperative team to focus on each of these critical portions of the procedure with less distraction and will potentially lessen the risk for errors.

The retention of throat packs has been reported, and moderate-quality evidence indicates that measures can be taken to prevent this type of RSI, including communication of the throat pack placement and removal.[78-81]

A case report described a piece of hydrocolloid plastic found in a patient's hypopharynx 1 year after surgery when the patient returned for a second procedure.[39] The item may have been placed between the nasal endotracheal tube and the patient's nostril to prevent a pressure injury during an oral maxillofacial procedure the year before. The authors believe that the nasal intubation before the second procedure may have pushed the item out of the nasal cavity and into the pharynx. The authors recommended accounting for these types of items.[39]

1.2.5 **Any individual who observes an item dropped from the surgical field should immediately inform the RN circulator and other members of the perioperative team.** [*Recommendation*]

1.2.6 **Verbally verify the final count as part of a checklist.** [*Recommendation*]

Moderate-quality evidence[21,42,82-86] and guidance from a professional organization[60] support using a checklist to increase communication among perioperative team members and improve surgical patient outcomes. This is important because the most common contributing factors in recent studies of retained items included problems related to human factors, ineffective leadership, and communication breakdown.[15,42,68] Although the evidence on use of checklists in surgery does not always include analysis or discussion of elements that may prevent RSIs, many checklists include a verification of the sponge, needle, and instrument count.

In a landmark study, Haynes et al[86] found that implementation of a checklist significantly reduced morbidity and mortality in patients undergoing non-cardiac surgery. Implementation of the checklist increased compliance with sponge count completion across the multicenter study.[86] However, additional research is needed to determine the influence of the organization's culture on checklist implementation[85] because successful use of a checklist for prevention of medical errors requires involvement of key perioperative stakeholders, an understanding of error occurrence, recognition of system and individual dynamics, and creation of a just culture in which there is a shared vision of patient safety.[83] Organizational support and a robust interdisciplinary process bolsters checklist effectiveness.

Steelman et al[42] recommended discussing removal of objects during a standardized postprocedural debrief. Marsh et al[87] surveyed 1,693 perioperative nurses to identify perceived missed patient care and found that 10.5% of respondents reported surgical counts were not verified as correct either occasionally, frequently, or always during closing, by either themselves or others.

1.3 **Actively participate in team training as a measure to prevent RSIs.** [*Recommendation*]

Moderate-quality evidence[21,42,58,59,88-94] and guidance from a professional organization[48] support team training as an effective intervention for improving communication and teamwork in the perioperative setting. Team training may prevent RSIs by reducing the risk for human error (eg, safety omissions) while improving team communication and attitudes. The Joint Commission recommends team training, including briefings and debriefings, to promote open communication and overcome hierarchal barriers as a measure to prevent RSIs.[48] Formal programs (ie, TeamSTEPPS,[89,92-94] Crew Resource Management,[90] Medical Team Training[91]) and their effectiveness has been studied or discussed in the literature. See the AORN Guideline for Team Communication for recommendations on team training.[95]

1.4 **Minimize distractions, noise, and unnecessary interruptions during the surgical count.** [*Recommendation*]

Moderate-quality evidence supports minimizing distractions, noise, and interruptions in the OR to create a safer environment for patients and perioperative team members.[42,69,77,96-98] See the AORN Position Statement on Managing Distractions and Noise During Perioperative Patient Care[77] for factors that contribute to distractions. See the AORN Guideline for a Safe Environment of Care[98] for recommendations to minimize distractions and noise.

In a nonexperimental study of distractions and interruptions during surgical counting processes, Bubric et al[69] found that distractions (38.5% to 46.7% of the time) and interruptions (10% to 33.3% of the time) were present during the count process and were related to the type of count (eg, initial, closing) being performed. Distractions caused attention to be taken away from the counting task. Distractions included music, nonessential conversation, personnel entering the OR, ringing telephones, multitasking, and background noise. Interruptions caused a break in performance of the count. The researchers concluded that interruptions and distractions are common and could negatively affect counting accuracy and patient safety.

Distractions and multitasking have been identified as contributing factors for RSIs.[42] Steelman and Cullen[96] conducted a health care **failure modes and effects analysis** of surgical sponge management and found that distraction was the potential cause of failures 20.8% of the time, followed closely by multitasking, which was the potential cause of failures 17.9% of the time.

In a qualitative analysis of incorrect surgical count events, Rowlands and Steeves[97] found themes of general chaos in the OR that included loud music, excessive talking, talking during critical moments of the count, fast pace, deafening noise levels, and idle chatter. In a qualitative study, Smith and Burke[99] found lack of full concentration on the scrub or circulating role, rushing for no apparent reason, and multitasking were issues identified in observational audits intended to identify compliance with the facility count policy.

The psychology literature indicates that the task of counting requires attention, and improving attention can improve count accuracy.[100-102] Ortuño et al[100] investigated the relative cerebral blood flow of 10 volunteers in Spain who were given neurocognitive tests during positron emission tomography scans. The results showed that sustained attention was required for counting tasks.[100] Camos and Barrouillet[101] investigated resource demands in 36 psychology student volunteers counting multiple arrays of dots as part of a two-series experiment. The researchers found that adult counting is a resource-demanding activity that requires switching attention between memory and counting.[101] Disruption to attention may affect count accuracy through this pathway.

In 2007, Railo et al[102] conducted a two-series laboratory-based psychology experiment in Finland with 72 and 40 adult volunteer participants, respectively. The researchers determined that even when counting small numbers of items, attentional demands increased as objects to be enumerated increased and that improving attention increased accuracy. Furthermore, they found that only the numbers one and two were counted correctly when attention was reduced, which implies that distraction affected count accuracy.

1.4.1 During the surgical count, create a no-interruption zone that prohibits nonessential conversation and activities[48,76,77] and prohibits rushing the count.[70,96,97,103] *[Recommendation]*

Clark[76] reported on a facility that successfully implemented a "Pause for the Counts" campaign to minimize interruptions during surgical counts.

As part of the interdisciplinary initiative, the RN circulator notified the team when it was time to count and asked whether any supplies would be needed on the sterile field. This communication to the team was intended to reduce interruptions from supply requests during the count.[76]

A study by Bubric et al[69] supported proactively notifying the team about the initiation of counting processes and assessing whether additional items are needed before starting, as a method to eliminate or reduce distractions and interruptions. The researchers found that most interruptions (80.4%) during counting processes were caused by the surgeon asking for an item or talking with or questioning the personnel counting. The Joint Commission supports empowering perioperative team members to call for a "closing time out" to allow for an uninterrupted closing count.[48]

Moderate-quality evidence also suggests that rushing a count is a form of interruption.[96,97,103] Butler et al[103] conducted a descriptive study in seven large ORs in Australia and found that both the RN circulator and scrub person were rushed to complete the required count procedures by the fast pace of the perioperative environment, especially when handling urgent requests of the team. The researchers also identified time pressures from the surgeon or anesthesia professional to quickly finish the surgical procedure and move to the next patient as factors that contributed to count errors.

In a qualitative study, Rowlands and Steeves[97] found that themes of chaos and feelings of being rushed contributed to safety variances and **incorrect counts**. Some participants reported that having difficulty locating equipment for a procedure caused them to rush through the initial count.[97] Steelman and Cullen[96] conducted a health care failure modes and effects analysis of surgical sponge management and found that time pressure occurred in 13.2% of potential failures. Loftus et al[70] included "no rushed counts" as part of their count protocol in a safe surgery program.

1.4.2 Do not perform counts or actions that would require a count (eg, relief of the scrub person or RN circulator) during critical phases of the procedure, including
- time-out periods,
- critical dissections,
- confirming and opening of implants,
- general anesthesia induction and emergence, and
- care and handling of specimens.[77]

[Recommendation]

2. Standard Procedure

2.1 **Use a consistent accounting methodology for all surgical counts.** *[Recommendation]*

Moderate-quality evidence[24,69,70,97,104-106] and guidance from professional organizations[48,60,61] support using a standardized, consistent accounting method to prevent RSIs. In an nonexperimental study by Rowlands and Steeves,[97] participants noted variations in counting practices between rooms and sometimes between individuals.

Variation has also been reported for the types of items counted, reconciliation procedures, and the time of counts.[104] Edel[104] reported variation in the use of tools; for example, there was inconsistency in the use of sponge bags for counting and use of needle counters. This variation was a cause for concern because of an increased risk for error when counts are recorded differently among providers.

Use of a consistent, standardized practice has been shown to reduce the reports of incorrect counts[105] and rates of overall serious reportable events that included RSIs.[70] Different measures have been implemented to reduce variability and create a consistent standardized practice, including new count procedures,[104] audits,[104] education,[105] standardization of dry-erase boards,[105] streamlining of instrument sets,[105] and updating of count sheets.[105] Using consistent count policies and increasing communication among team members has also been recommended to improve standardization.[106]

Counting protocols described in the literature are varied and are not consistently implemented across institutions in the same way. The NoThing Left Behind national surgical patient safety project is a widely referenced standardized program for RSI prevention that includes a counting protocol and is based on the principle of implementing consistent methods.[24] Additional research is needed to evaluate the effects of a count protocol on patient outcomes.

2.2 **Conduct a count of soft goods, sharps, miscellaneous items, and instruments during the phases of the procedure indicated on Table 2.** *[Recommendation]*

2.3 **Conduct a count before the procedure to establish a baseline (ie, the initial count) before the patient enters the OR or procedure room, when possible.** *[Recommendation]*

Moderate-quality evidence supports conducting the initial count before the patient enters the room as part of count protocols.[69,70,93] Bubric et al[69] reported that of 30 observed initial count processes, three (10%) were performed with only the circulator and scrub person present, eight (26.7%) were performed

while the surgical team paused for the count process, and 19 (63.3%) occurred simultaneously with other distractions (eg, conversations) or patient care being performed (eg, skin antisepsis). The researchers state that a contributing factor to distractions during the initial count process is having the patient in the room.[69]

Loftus et al[70] explained that performing the initial count before the patient is in the room allows attention to be given to the count with minimal distraction. Performing the initial count before the patient enters the room gives the perioperative team the benefit of reduced interruption from patient care distractions.

2.3.1 **When conducting the initial count before the patient enters the room is not possible, a second RN circulator may assist the primary RN circulator.** *[Conditional Recommendation]*

Loftus et al[70] also described use of a parallel process when counting before the patient enters the room is not feasible. A second RN circulator and the scrub person perform an uninterrupted baseline count while the primary team remains focused on patient care.

2.4 **An additional count may be performed at designated intervals (eg, as part of a second time out) during lengthy procedures.** *[Conditional Recommendation]*

Patients who undergo lengthy surgical procedures may be at increased risk for an RSI.[13,52] In an organizational experience article, Song et al[107] implemented a second time-out process at their facility to reduce patient complications and problems that can occur during lengthy robotic procedures. The second time-out process incorporates a standardized checklist and is intended to occur 3 to 4 hours into a lengthy robotic procedure. One of the items on the checklist is to "check if surgical counts are intact," meaning to verify surgical counts are correct during the second time-out process. The authors stated that the process received positive feedback from the perioperative team and resulted in minimal changes to the surgical procedural duration.[107] See the Guideline for Team Communication[95] for additional recommendations on second time-out processes.

2.4.1 **Collaborate with an interdisciplinary team to standardize a process for additional counts performed during lengthy procedures, including**
- **a method for identifying which procedures should have additional counts related to procedure duration,**

Table 2. Timing of Counts for Soft Goods, Sharps, Miscellaneous Items, and Instruments

	Phase of Procedure	Soft Goods	Sharps and Miscellaneous	[a] Instruments
Initial	[b] Before the procedure to establish a baseline[1-3]	×	×	×
Additional Counts	When new items are added to the field, as they are added[1-3]	Count the items added		
	[c] At the time of permanent relief of the scrub person or RN circulator[1,2]	×	×	☐
	When a discrepancy involving the type of item is suspected	Count the items in question		
	When any member of the perioperative team requests a count	Count the items in question		
	[d] At established intervals during lengthy procedures[4]	×	×	☐
Cavity	Before closure of a cavity within a cavity (eg, the uterus)[1,2]	×	×	☐
Closing	When wound closure begins[1,2]	×	×	☐
Final	[e] When skin closure begins or at the end of the procedure when counted items are no longer in use[1,2]	×	×	☐

[a] In all procedures for which the likelihood exists that an instrument could be retained (See Recommendation 5.1) and all procedures in which an open body cavity is entered (See Recommendation 5.2)
[b] Preferred to complete before the patient enters the OR or procedure room (See Recommendation 2.3)
[c] Direct visualization of all items may not be possible.
[d] Conditional Recommendation, see Recommendation 2.4 and 2.4.1.
[e] Do not consider the final count complete until all soft goods, sharps, miscellaneous items, and instruments used in closing the wound are removed and returned to the scrub person (See Recommendation 2.11)

☐ The recommendation for counting of instruments can be different depending on the procedure and types of instruments used (See Recommendation 5.2)

References

1. *Sentinel Event Alert 51: Preventing unintended retained foreign objects.* The Joint Commission. https://www.jointcommission.org/resources/patient-safety-topics/sentinel-event/sentinel-event-alert-newsletters/sentinel-event-alert-issue-51-preventing-unintended-retained-foreign-objects/. Published October 17, 2013. Accessed September 28, 2021.
2. *WHO Guidelines for Safe Surgery 2009: Safe Surgery Saves Lives.* World Health Organization. http://apps.who.int/iris/bitstream/handle/10665/44185/9789241598552_eng.pdf;jsessionid=A0223DB47B17AC150FEADA4AC1371DBF?sequence=1. Accessed September 28, 2021.
3. Loftus T, Dahl D, OHare B, et al. Implementing a standardized safe surgery program reduces serious reportable events. *J Am Coll Surg.* 2015;220(1):12-17.
4. Song JB, Vemana G, Mobley JM, Bhayani SB. The second "time-out": a surgical safety checklist for lengthy robotic surgeries. *Patient Saf Surg.* 2013;7(1):19.

- timing of the count process (eg, 3 to 4 hours into a lengthy procedure, excluding critical phases),
- items to be counted (eg, soft goods, sharps, miscellaneous items, instruments, items in use),
- communication between team members on counting results, and
- documentation.

[Recommendation]

When a facility decides to implement an additional count process as part of an RSI prevention strategy during lengthy procedures, it is important to standardize the process and clarify how it will be implemented.

2.5 Establish the standardized sequence in which the counts should be conducted in the organization. The counting sequence should have a logical progression (eg, order of standardized count board or sheet, proximal to distal from the patient). *[Recommendation]*

Moderate-quality evidence[69,70,105] and guidance from a professional organization[60] support counting in a standardized sequence. When determining the order of items to count, Loftus et al[70] followed the sequence of the standardized count board (eg, whiteboard) as part of their count protocols. Norton et al[105] implemented a count protocol that involved counting items in a manner that progressed from proximal to distal from the patient: surgical field, Mayo stand, back table, and sponge receptacle.

2.6 **Items being counted should be viewed concurrently by two individuals, one of whom should be the RN circulator, and counted audibly.** *[Recommendation]*

Moderate-quality evidence[70,105] and guidance from professional organizations[48,60] support concurrent viewing and audible counting of surgical items by two team members, including the RN circulator. Concurrent verification of counts by two individuals may lessen the risk of inaccurate counts, although additional research is needed to evaluate this theory. Loftus et al[70] and Norton et al[105] used verbal counting by two individuals as part of their count protocols. Articles in the psychology literature indicated that verbal counting resulted in fewer errors than nonverbal counting at higher numbers[108] and that suppression of count articulation increased errors.[109]

Duggan et al[67] discussed a change from having two individuals count sponges, towels, and instruments to having one individual perform the count as one element of an organizational improvement initiative for RSI prevention. After reviewing the count process, the interdisciplinary task force concluded that an element of bias or false security may occur when a count is performed by the scrub person with the RN circulator. The authors also stated that the RN circulator's focus during counts performed before the procedure may be divided because of the many tasks involved during that period.

For the initiative, the scrub person counted soft goods independently before the beginning of the procedure and notified the RN circulator of the quantities. During the procedure, counts of towels and sponges were performed by both the scrub person and the RN circulator. The reason two people counted together during the procedure was because the scrub person may be more likely to have their attention divided. Counting of sponges and towels was also performed by both the RN circulator and the scrub person at the end of the procedure. For instruments, the first count was performed by a single person in the sterile processing department during instrument tray assembly. The second instrument count took place in the OR and involved only the scrub person. The scrub person would notify the RN circulator if an error was discovered during the independent instrument count.[67]

The authors described how this process is similar to checks performed independently by personnel in the aviation industry. They reported that RSI rates were reduced from 1.69 annually to none for more than 1,300 days.[67] However, this count process was one part of an RSI prevention bundle, and use of bundled interventions prevents a clear understanding of the effect of each practice change on the outcome of the organizational improvement initiative. In addition, because this organizational improvement initiative was specific to a single institution based on internal assessments, it is not generalizable to other facilities. Additional research is needed.

2.6.1 **When possible, counts during a procedure should be performed by the same two individuals.**[53,60] *[Recommendation]*

The World Health Organization (WHO) recommends that the same two individuals conduct the counts during a procedure.[60] As part of a prospective observational study at a large academic medical center, Greenberg et al[53] found that counting activities involving a personnel change of either the RN circulator or scrub person resulted in a three-fold higher risk of a count discrepancy than in procedures with no personnel changes. The researchers noted that a limitation of the study was a small sample size.

A limitation of the evidence is a lack of studies that have examined whether multiple teams participating in a procedure may contribute to inconsistent counting methods. Although multiple teams being present during a procedure is associated with higher risk for an RSI,[13,52,53] the existing evidence has not associated multiple teams with inconsistent counting methods. Data showing multiple teams and an increased number of personnel as a risk factor for RSIs may be indicative of inconsistent counting methods, but this may be confounded by the length and complexity of the procedure (eg, transplantation), which are also risk factors for RSI.[52] However, in a systematic review with meta-analysis, Moffatt-Bruce et al[13] found that changes in nursing personnel were not significantly associated with RSI risk. Additional research is needed to determine whether the involvement of multiple teams is a risk factor for an inconsistent counting method.[53]

2.7 **The scrub person should separate**[60] **and point out**[74] **items on the sterile field while audibly counting. The RN circulator should separate**[60] **and point out**[74] **items off the sterile field while audibly counting.** *[Recommendation]*

Separating items may reduce the risk of miscounting items by omission if an item is not seen. The WHO recommends completely separating all items during counting procedures.[60]

The psychology literature supports that identifying items being counted may affect count accuracy. Individuation, or object identification, is required before enumeration can occur.[110-112] Individuation is an important part of counting that is required for tracking and counting multiple objects[113] and for counting each item only once.[114] Furthermore, Camos[74] found that a motor activity, such as pointing, facilitated verbal counting in a psychology experiment in which children and adults counted on a number line. Manual pointing may be a method of individuating objects and keeping track of items being counted.

2.8 During the initial count and when adding items to the sterile field, count packaged items according to the number in which the item is packaged. *[Recommendation]*

See Recommendation 3.3.

2.9 When introducing items to the sterile field, verify that the package contains the number of items on the product label. Packages that contain an incorrect number of items or items with a manufacturing defect (eg, missing marker, tag, or chip) should be

- excluded from the count,
- removed from the field,
- isolated from the rest of the countable items in the OR, and
- labeled.

[Recommendation]

The WHO recommends removing defective packaged items from the surgical count.[60] Incorrect numbers of items or product defects in a package can and do occur, although the prevalence has not been reported in the literature. Isolating the entire package containing an incorrect number of items can reduce the potential for error in subsequent counts.

2.9.1 When items counted before the patient enters the room are found to be defective (eg, contaminated, incorrect number in the package), these items may be removed from the room before the patient's entry.[60] *[Conditional Recommendation]*

Removing packages that contain an incorrect number of items from the room before the patient's entry can decrease confusion and the likelihood for error.

2.10 If the count is interrupted, restart the count for the type of item (eg, laparotomy sponge) that was being counted when the interruption occurred. *[Recommendation]*

The WHO recommends restarting an interrupted count to reduce the risk for a count error.[60] As part of their count protocols, Loftus et al[70] required interrupted counts to be repeated without interruption. Bubric et al[69] reported that interruptions occur most often during closing counts with at least one inter-

ruption occurring in 22 of 66 (33.3%) observed closing counts. The largest number of interruptions occurring in a single closing count process was four. Most interruptions for all counting processes were from surgeons requesting an item or questioning or speaking with personnel who were counting (See Recommendation 1.4.1).[69]

2.11 Do not consider the final count complete until all surgical soft goods, sharps, instruments, and miscellaneous items (eg, viscera retainer [ie, Fish]) used in closing the incision are removed from the patient and returned to the scrub person. *[Recommendation]*

Bubric et al[69] reported that items were still in use during 65 of 66 observed closing counts (98.5%). The researchers also observed that despite clinical practice recommendations to identify items in use during closure counts and not consider the count process finalized until they are no longer in use, 83.3% of observed closure counts did not reflect this practice.

2.11.1 For multiple procedures or sterile fields, count all items together at the final count while maintaining sterile technique. *[Conditional Recommendation]*

The evidence review for this guideline revision found no literature on the practice of counting when multiple procedures or sterile fields are being used. Multiple procedures or sterile fields increase the risk of counted items moving between setups and creating confusion during counting, which may contribute to counting errors if items are missed. Counting items across all sterile fields, while maintaining sterile technique, accounts for all surgical items in the room and validates that the items have not been retained in the patient.

The benefits of this practice include having one running count that may reduce the risk for addition or subtraction errors that could occur when supplies and instruments on each sterile field are counted separately. However, there may be instances when counting separate sterile fields together is difficult, such as when the sterile fields are associated with different surgical wound classifications (eg, clean, clean contaminated) or when isolation technique is used during wound closure. The addition of a second scrub person to help with counting processes when there are multiple sterile fields used on surgical sites of different wound classifications can reduce the risk of cross contamination. Additional research is needed on the practice of counting when multiple procedures or sterile fields are used.

2.12 A count can be requested by any perioperative team member. When any member of the perioperative team requests a count, the count should be performed. [Recommendation]

2.13 Record the count
- immediately after each type of item is counted (eg, laparotomy sponges, suture needles),[70]
- on a standardized template,[70,105]
- in a location that is visible to the surgical team (eg, count board),[21,42,70,105,115] and
- in agreement with the scrub person.[70]

[Recommendation]

Moderate-quality evidence supports recording the count in one standardized, visible location.[70,105,115] Recording of the count on a count board (eg, whiteboard) in a visible location allows all team members to view the count independently and confirm the accuracy of the counted items. Loftus et al[70] included immediate recording after counting each item in their count protocol.

The psychology literature indicates that counting requires memory to keep a running total[109] and that concurrent memory load increases counting time.[101] Immediate recording of counted items may reduce the risk of a count error by reducing reliance on memory accuracy and attentional demands that compete with counting tasks. Additional research is needed to examine the relationship between counting and memory.

2.13.1 If the RN circulator cannot immediately record the count and concurrently visualize the items being counted, the RN circulator may record the number of counted items on a standardized count sheet and then transfer the information to the count board. [Conditional Recommendation]

2.13.2 For items that are added to the field after the initial count,
- count the items immediately,
- record the item and number added on the count board in a standardized format as defined by the health care organization, and
- verify the number with the scrub person.[70]

[Recommendation]

Opening extra supplies without promptly adding them to the count board may lead to a discrepancy at the end of the procedure. Loftus et al[70] included immediate recording of added items to the count board and confirmation of the number with the scrub person as part of their count protocol. They also recommended holding the added item's package as a memory

aid until the item is written on the count board, then discarding the package.

2.13.3 Any perioperative team member (eg, anesthesia professional, float RN) who assists the surgical team by opening countable items onto the sterile field should promptly inform the RN circulator about what was added. [Recommendation]

Other team members may be asked to open supplies while the RN circulator is occupied with other patient care activities. Notifying the RN circulator of added items may reduce the risk of a count discrepancy.

2.13.4 Maintain the count running total in one location. [Recommendation]

Maintaining the running total of the count in one location can reduce the risk for errors that may occur with multiple counts. Counting using a count sheet and transferring the information is not an ideal practice, as errors in transcription can occur and multiple steps can cause confusion. However, there may be situations, depending on the room configuration for various procedures, in which immediate recording of items on the count board would not allow for the RN circulator to visualize the count. In those instances, immediate recording on the count board may not be feasible and a count sheet may need to be used as a memory aid to avoid memory lapse errors in count records.

2.14 If an item is passed or dropped from the sterile field, the RN circulator should retrieve it using standard precautions, show it to the scrub person, isolate it from the field, and include it in the final count. [Recommendation]

2.15 Do not subtract or remove items from the count. [Recommendation]

Removal or subtraction of items from the surgical count may increase the risk of a count discrepancy by introducing confusion about which items have or have not been counted. The benefits of saving time by subtracting from the count do not outweigh the risks of a count discrepancy.

2.16 Keep all counted items inside the OR or procedure room until the counts are completed and reconciled. [Recommendation]

Confining all counted items to the OR may help eliminate the possibility of a count discrepancy.

2.17 Do not remove linen and waste containers from the OR or procedure room until all counts are completed and reconciled and the patient has been transferred out of the room.[60] *[Recommendation]*

The WHO recommends keeping all counted items in the room until the final count is reconciled.[60]

2.18 Remove used or open counted items from the OR or procedure room before another procedure begins. *[Recommendation]*

Removing counted items from the room may prevent count discrepancies for the next patient. In a health care failure modes and effects analysis report, Steelman and Cullen[96] found through focus groups that leaving a sponge in the room from a previous procedure was a failure that could contribute to a **miscount**.

2.19 Perform a structured hand-over communication of accounting procedures at times of relief of the RN circulator or scrub person.[48,60,95] *[Recommendation]*

Professional organizations recommend that perioperative team members perform a structured hand over at times of relief to facilitate communication and reduce the risk of a count discrepancy or sharps injury.[48,60] As part of a quality improvement (QI) project to improve consistency in count procedures at a large city hospital, Edel[104] noted variation in numerous counting practices that caused confusion at shift change and variances in levels of communication among team members. To reduce variability in count practices and communication, Edel[104] included streamlining of hand-over communications and consistent use of count tools (eg, count board, count sheet) as part of the initiative. Greenberg et al[53] recommended additional research to standardize communication during unavoidable hand overs.

2.19.1 Perform a complete count when there is a permanent relief of the RN circulator or scrub person.[48,70] All items should be accounted for, although direct visualization of all items may not be possible. *[Recommendation]*

2.19.2 Account for counted items in use when there is relief of the RN circulator or scrub person for short durations (eg, a break). *[Recommendation]*

3. Soft Goods

3.1 Account for surgical soft goods (eg, sponges, towels, textiles) opened onto the sterile field during all procedures in which soft goods are used. *[Recommendation]*

Moderate-quality evidence suggests that the most common types of RSIs are surgical sponges.[3,6,8,9,13-15,21,22]

The abdomen[31] and pelvis[19,32] are reported to be the locations where RSIs are most often found.[6,13,15,33] However, retained surgical soft goods have also been reported in many other body locations including the brain, eye, mouth and airway, nasal cavity, neck, shoulder and axilla, chest, pacemaker or defibrillator pocket, breast, back, extremities, hip and gluteal region, vagina, and scrotum.[15]

Surgical soft goods can be retained in the smallest of incisions, including in procedures involving natural orifices,[13] such as the vagina, eye, or nose,[15] and in minimally invasive surgeries.[22,40,42,43] Surgical sponges also can be retained after a vaginal birth, therefore moderate-quality evidence[15,116-120] and guidance from a professional organization[65] support accounting for surgical items, including soft goods, before and after a vaginal delivery. Other items that could be classified as soft goods or miscellaneous items have been reported as retained, including a cotton swab and a gauze roll bite block.[42]

Reports have been published of retained surgical sponges migrating from the abdomen or pelvis to the intestine, bladder, thorax, and stomach.[31,34,35] In a laboratory animal study, Wattanasirichaigoon[121] described the stages of transmural sponge migration into the intestine:

- Stage 1 is foreign body reaction during which the sponge is encapsulated.
- Stage 2 is secondary infection during which cytolysis occurs from the cotton interacting with enzymes in the intestinal lumen.
- Stage 3 is mass formation during which a thick fibrous wall develops as part of the granuloma to prevent the infection from spreading in the abdomen and cotton filaments are released into the intestinal lumen.
- Stage 4 is remodeling during which a fibrotic scar forms after the whole surgical sponge enters the intestinal lumen.

This study demonstrated the potential for infection to occur during the process of migration and explains the mechanism of infection in the cases reported in the literature.[34,122] Although retained surgical sponges may migrate transmurally and be expelled through the rectum spontaneously, Zantvoord et al[34] reported that 93% of cases required an intervention for removal.

3.2 All soft goods used in the patient should be radiopaque and easily differentiated from non-radiopaque soft goods (eg, sponges, towels).[15,25,32,60,61,123] *[Recommendation]*

Professional organizations, including the WHO[60] and the ACS,[61] recommend using radiopaque soft goods in the surgical wound. The American College of Obstetricians and Gynecologists recommends using only radiopaque soft goods during vaginal deliveries.[65] The Society of Interventional Radiology recommends that interventional radiologists in the interventional radiology suite use only sponges with radiopaque markers to pack an incision.[124]

Radiopaque indicators facilitate locating by radiograph an item presumed lost or left in the surgical field when a count discrepancy occurs. Steelman et al[15] reported a case of retained Kerlix gauze and a non-radiopaque sponge from an anesthesia kit. There are also a number of case reports of retained non-radiopaque sponges in patients who had surgery in countries in which radiopaque sponges are not routinely used.[125-140] There has been one reported incidence of a retained radiopaque marker.[42]

3.2.1 **Before the procedure begins, isolate non-radiopaque gauze sponges used for skin antisepsis that have a similar appearance to counted radiopaque sponges to avoid possible confusion with the counted radiopaque sponges.** *[Recommendation]*

3.2.2 **If gauze sponges are used for vaginal antisepsis, the gauze sponges should be radiopaque[41] and counted.** *[Recommendation]*

In a report of a legal case, a patient experienced discomfort and required a second surgical procedure 2 months after an abdominal hysterectomy, to remove a retained sponge that was left in her vagina during preoperative vaginal antisepsis.[41] Accounting for radiopaque surgical sponges during vaginal antisepsis provides a mechanism for verifying that the sponge is not left in the patient and for detecting the sponge by radiography in the event of a discrepancy **(See Recommendation 4.8)**. See the Guideline for Preoperative Patient Skin Antisepsis[141] for more recommendations about vaginal preparation.

3.2.3 **Do not use radiopaque sponges as dressings except as therapeutic packing inside the surgical wound.** *[Recommendation]*

The use of radiopaque sponges as surface dressings may invalidate subsequent counts if the patient is returned to the OR. Radiopaque surgical sponges used as surface dressings may appear as foreign items on postoperative radiographs and falsely suggest a retained item. Williams et al[40] reported that using a surgical sponge as a dressing was a risk factor for retention. **See Recommendation 3.8** for more information about therapeutic packing.

3.2.4 **Do not use non-radiopaque towels in the surgical wound. If use of towels in the surgi-** cal wound is necessary, use towels with radiopaque markers. *[Recommendation]*

According to Steelman et al,[15] 6.9% of the retained soft goods reported to the Joint Commission between 2012 and 2017 were towels.

3.2.5 **Withhold non-radiopaque gauze dressing materials from the field until the surgical incision is closed and the final count is complete.**[32,60,70] *[Recommendation]*

One nonexperimental study[70] and the WHO[60] support withholding non-radiopaque gauze for dressings from the sterile field until the wound is closed. Separating dressing materials from counted radiopaque sponges may help prevent intermingling with the sponges used in the procedure and reduce the risk of a count discrepancy.

3.2.6 **Keep dressing sponges included in custom packs sealed and isolated on the field until the surgical incision is closed.**[70] *[Recommendation]*

3.3 **Count packaged radiopaque sponges according to the number that the item is packaged in (eg, 5, 10).** *[Recommendation]*

Counting to the number that sponges are packaged in allows perioperative team members to identify packaging errors and may serve as an indication of a miscount.

3.3.1 **Packages containing an incorrect number of sponges or that have a manufacturing defect (eg, missing marker, tag, or chip) should be**
- **excluded from the count,**
- **removed from the field,**
- **isolated from the rest of the countable items in the OR, and**
- **labeled.**

[Recommendation]

The WHO recommends removing defective packaged sponges from the surgical count.[60] Incorrect numbers of sponges or product defects inside a package occur, although the prevalence has not been reported in the literature. Isolating an entire package that contains the incorrect number of sponges may reduce the potential for error in subsequent counts.

3.3.2 **Packages containing an incorrect number of sponges or that have a manufacturing defect may be removed from the room before the patient's entry.**[60] *[Conditional Recommendation]*

Removing packages that contain an incorrect number of sponges from the room before the patient's entry may decrease confusion and the likelihood of error.

3.3.3 **If the surgical sponge package is banded, break the band and discard it before counting.** [*Recommendation*]

Leaving the package band in place may prevent the ability to completely separate and see each sponge, which may cause one or more sponges to be undetected. Removing the band may also provide a visual indicator that a count of items packaged with a band has been completed. Loftus et al[70] included removal of the surgical sponge band as part of count protocols in their safe surgery program.

3.4 **Do not cut or alter radiopaque surgical soft goods in any way.**[15,40,60] [*Recommendation*]

Altering a sponge by cutting or removing radiopaque portions invalidates counts and increases the risk of a portion being retained in the patient. The WHO recommends leaving surgical sponges in the original configuration.[60] Steelman et al[15] reported a retained portion of a Kerlix gauze that had been cut. Williams et al[40] reported that a risk factor for retained sponges was cutting the sponge.

3.5 **All radiopaque surgical soft goods placed or packed in the patient should be audibly communicated and recorded in a visible location (eg, count board) on placement and removal.**[21,32,70,115] [*Recommendation*]

The practice of verbalizing and recording placed or packed radiopaque sponges is supported in a cohort study. In the count protocol implemented by Loftus et al,[70] the surgeons were responsible for verbalizing placement and removal of placed sponges, and the RN circulators wrote the placement of sponges on a standardized count board. In an organizational experience report, Edel[115] shared a count board protocol that included the RN circulator recording the items packed in the surgical wound on a count/time-out board.

The retention of throat packs has been reported,[15] and moderate-quality evidence indicates that measures can be taken to prevent this type of RSI.[78-81] In a case report of a swallowed throat pack after maxillofacial surgery, Iwai et al[78] created a checklist for insertion and removal of the throat pack to prevent retention. At their facility, they also tied a suture to the throat pack and taped it to the patient's cheek, and the surgeon was responsible for removing the pack at the end of the procedure. Iwai et al[78] also discussed other methods of managing throat packs that they found in their literature review, such as

- having the same person place and remove the pack;
- attaching a heavy suture to the throat pack that extends outside the mouth;

- not using multiple packs;
- suturing the throat pack to the endotracheal tube; and
- placing a label in a prominent location, such as on the endotracheal tube or on the main ventilator knob.

Colbert et al[81] suggested in an expert opinion report that the anesthesia professional wear a red allergy band marked "throat pack" as a reminder to remove the throat pack. The authors alternatively suggested either placing a sticker on the patient's forehead or writing on the board that the throat pack is in place, although they discussed that these alternatives could be more prone to removal than the wristband.

In another expert opinion report, Jennings and Bhatt[79] suggested that affixing a "throat pack in situ" label on the patient's forehead was not feasible. In their experience, the head and neck surgeons placed the throat pack after draping the patient, and the forehead was not visible. As an alternative solution, the label was placed on the surgical assistant's hat and was a visible reminder to the surgeon and anesthesia professional throughout the procedure. A limitation of this expert opinion report is that the risk of the sticker becoming detached from the assistant's hat and falling into the sterile field was not addressed.

To assess variations in practice for preventing retention of throat packs, Smith et al[80] surveyed 208 members of the Neuroanaesthesia Society of Great Britain and Ireland and received 141 responses (68% response rate). Although some clinicians did not think that throat packs were indicated or that the risks outweighed the benefits of placing the throat pack (n = 69), the remaining respondents reported the following practices for pack retention:

- following formal protocols, either leaving a portion of the pack outside the mouth or attaching it to the endotracheal tube;
- using preprinted "throat pack in situ" labels;
- counting the throat pack with the sponge count; and
- documenting removal by checking a box on the anesthesia record.

3.5.1 **If feasible, leave a portion of radiopaque surgical soft goods placed in the surgical wound or cavity outside the wound so that the item remains visible.** [*Recommendation*]

Leaving a portion of a soft good item outside the wound provides a visual reminder that there is an item placed in the wound. In a case report of a retained sponge after septorhinoplasty, Cho and Jin[142] recommended using gauze packing with a thread tie left outside the nose during nasal procedures to help identify the gauze more easily.

The authors of a clinician experience article from Japan reported use of sponges with attached thread to reduce the number of missing ophthalmic sponges during trabeculectomy procedures.[143] Authors of a clinician experience article from India reported use of laparotomy sponges tied together in packs of five sponges so that no single sponge was in the surgical wound when the peritoneum was open.[144]

3.6 **The surgeon should perform a methodical wound exploration (eg, top to bottom, quadrant to quadrant) for radiopaque surgical soft goods before closing the patient, using both visualization and touch when feasible.**[15,25,60,61,123] *[Recommendation]*

Professional organizations recommend that surgeons conduct a methodical wound exploration of the cavity or surgical wound before closing, using both visualization and touch whenever possible.[60,61] The Society of Interventional Radiology recommends that interventional radiologists perform a wound exploration using visual and tactile inspection whenever sponges have been used in an incision made in the interventional radiology suite.[124] Methodical wound exploration can prevent retention of surgical sponges when counts are falsely correct and count discrepancy protocols are not implemented.

Norton et al[105] implemented a wound closure time out as part of the surgical safety checklist sign-out procedure at a large pediatric hospital. The wound closure time out included an announcement from the surgeon for a closing time out, the surgeon's statement of wound exploration completion, audible counts of surgical items, and team acknowledgment of the closing count status.[105] Methodical wound exploration is also part of the Sponge ACCOUNTing System "Pauze for the Gauze" protocol.[117]

3.6.1 **For MIS, the surgeon should perform a methodical wound exploration before camera removal.**[43] *[Recommendation]*

3.6.2 **For operative and other procedures in which the vagina is entered (eg, vaginal delivery, hysterectomy), include the vagina in postprocedure methodical wound exploration.** *[Recommendation]*

In a study of 319 retained soft goods reported to The Joint Commission between 2012 and 2017, Steelman et al[15] found that 23.9% of items were retained in the vagina and 82.2% of these items were retained after vaginal delivery. Most of the retained sponges were not discovered until 7 to 30 days after delivery. The researchers recommended a vaginal sweep for all procedures that involve the vagina.[15]

3.7 **Organize counted radiopaque surgical soft goods (ie, 4 x 4 gauze, laparotomy sponges) after use in a pocketed sponge holder with a background color that provides contrast (ie, not completely clear and colorless) or by a similar system (Figure 2).**[60,70,117] *[Recommendation]*

The WHO recommends organizing counted sponges in established multiples that are readily visible.[60] Using a pocketed holder or other system for separating used radiopaque sponges facilitates the ability to see the sponges for counting. Placement of the separated sponges in a standardized pocket holder system supports a consistent counting method.

Use of a pocketed sponge holder system is recommended as part of the Sponge ACCOUNTing System protocol.[43,117] Loftus et al[70] used a pocketed sponge system as part of the count protocol in their cohort study.

Using pocketed sponge holder systems with a contrasting background color may improve visibility of the sponges in the device. Sponges will appear white or red depending on whether they have been used. Using a pocketed sponge holder system that has a clear background can affect the ability of personnel to visually distinguish the number of sponges in each device when multiple layers of filled pocketed sponge holders are hanging on the same stand.

3.7.1 **Place used sponges in a standardized location (eg, kick bucket) until they are transferred to a pocketed holder system.**[117] **If a sponge is dropped from the sterile field, the RN circulator should retrieve it using standard precautions, show it to the scrub person, and place it in the pocketed holder system.** *[Recommendation]*

Placing the sponges in a standardized location after use may minimize the risk of miscounts that can occur by having sponges in multiple locations in the room. Placement of used sponges in kick buckets lined with clear bags is recommended in the Sponge ACCOUNTing System protocols.[117] Because the color of a red bag in the kick bucket may obscure visualization of used sponges and lead to a sponge being missed, the use of a clear bag or a bag in a color that will not obscure white or blood-soaked sponges may reduce the risk of missed sponges. The kick bucket is not the final location of surgical sponge disposal; it serves as a temporary designated location for sponge placement before transfer to a pocketed holder system.

3.7.2 Do not drape sponges over the sides of the kick bucket. *[Recommendation]*

Draping used surgical sponges over the sides of the kick bucket is discouraged because it may be difficult for all team members to see each individual sponge. Furthermore, wet used sponges may drip blood and other potentially infectious fluids onto the exterior portion of the kick bucket and the floor.

3.7.3 The RN circulator should use standard precautions to retrieve sponges, then completely open and separate each sponge before placing it in a pocketed sponge holder system. *[Recommendation]*

Separating radiopaque sponges after use minimizes errors caused by sponges sticking together.

3.7.4 Follow the manufacturer's instructions for use and facility policy and procedure for use of pocketed sponge holder systems. *[Recommendation]*

Some pocketed sponge holders have breakable perforations between horizontal sponge pockets to facilitate use of the device in different configurations (ie, 10 pockets for 4 x 4 gauze sponges, five pockets for laparotomy sponges). However, some facilities may specify in their policy and procedure how sponges are placed in the system (eg, 10 sponges per system).

3.7.5 Place only one sponge in each pocket of the pocketed sponge holder system. *[Recommendation]*

3.7.6 Place the radiopaque marker of the sponge facing forward so that it is readily visible in the pocketed holder system.[117] *[Recommendation]*

The radiopaque marker is a visual marker that distinguishes one sponge from another. Having the marker visible in the pocket may facilitate the count process. Placing sponges with the radiopaque marker facing forward is recommended in the Sponge ACCOUNTing System protocol.[117]

3.7.7 The pocketed holder system may be filled from the bottom to the top.[117] *[Conditional Recommendation]*

Filling pocketed sponge holder systems from the bottom to top, horizontally, is recommended in the Sponge ACCOUNTing System protocol.[117] Leaving open pockets at the top can provide a more-readily visible indicator of a missing sponge.

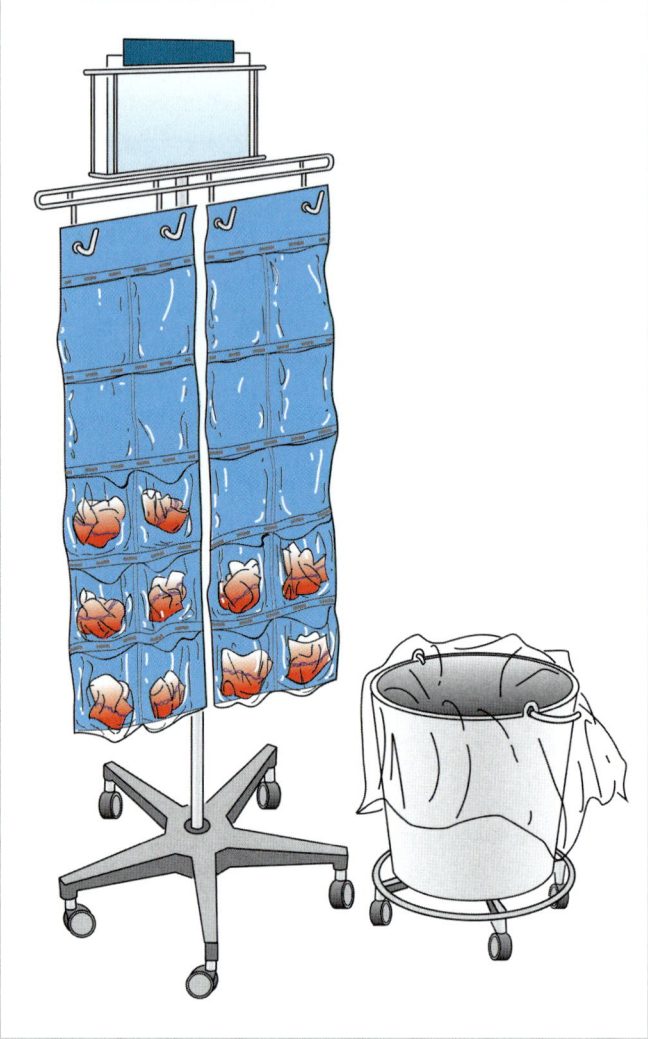

Figure 2. Pocketed Sponge Holder with Contrasting Background

3.7.8 Place the sponges in the pocketed sponge holder system with care to prevent unintended separation of horizontal pocket perforations. *[Recommendation]*

3.7.9 Discard the pocketed sponge holder if the perforations between horizontal pockets become broken unintentionally. Sponges in the pocketed sponge holder to be discarded should be placed in a new pocketed sponge system. *[Recommendation]*

Unintentional separation of the perforations between pockets could increase the risk of a counting discrepancy.

3.7.10 For the final count, unused sponges may be placed in the pocketed sponge holder system.[43,117] *[Conditional Recommendation]*

Placing unused sponges in the pocketed sponge holder system may provide a visual cue that all sponges are accounted for and are not in the patient. As part of the Sponge ACCOUNTing System, all sponges are placed in a pocketed holder system at the end of the procedure to verify that the sponges are not retained in the patient and to allow the surgeon to visualize the location of the sponges, which is called the "Show Me" step.[43,117]

3.8 Establish and implement a standardized procedure to communicate the location of packing and the plan for eventual removal of the items when radiopaque surgical soft goods are used as therapeutic packing (eg, intracavity, vaginal, oral) and the patient leaves the OR or labor and delivery room with this packing in place.[61] *[Recommendation]*

The ACS recommends communication and documentation of intentionally packed items.[61] In an organizational experience report, McIntyre et al[145] found inconsistency in documentation and changed the health care organization's policy on packed sponges to facilitate a standardized approach to communication of packing.

Steelman et al[42] reported 30 instances of retained packing placed with the intent for removal later. The material was identified as gauze or other absorbent material that were not surgical sponges. Of the retained packing, 73.3% were gauze and four instances of the gauze packing had been placed with a Bakri balloon for postpartum hemorrhage. In 17 reports, the gauze packing was located in the vagina.[42] **See Section 9** for recommendations on the use of adjunct technology for surgical soft goods.

3.8.1 When radiopaque surgical soft goods are intentionally used as therapeutic packing and the patient leaves the OR with this packing in place, document the number and types of items placed in the medical record
- **as reconciled and confirmed by the surgeon when this information is known with certainty or**
- **as incorrect if the number and type of sponges used for therapeutic packing is not known with certainty.**

[Recommendation]

When therapeutic packing is used, the number of sponges used in the wound may not be known with certainty.[40]

3.8.2 Communicate the number and types of radiopaque surgical soft goods used for therapeutic packing as part of the transfer of patient care information, and document this communication in the patient's medical record.[95,145,146] *[Recommendation]*

Steelman et al[42] recommended discussing the need for packing removal during handover processes.

3.8.3 An order for therapeutic packing removal may be added to order sets. *[Conditional Recommendation]*

Steelman et al[42] recommended providing written orders for packing removal, adding packing removal to order sets, and creating a "hard stop" to trigger packing removal in a specific time frame (eg, before discharge).

3.8.4 When the patient is returned to the OR for a subsequent procedure or to remove therapeutic packing,
- **the number and type of radiopaque soft goods to be removed should be determined based on the intraoperative record of the procedure during which the packing was placed,**
- **the number and type of radiopaque soft goods removed should be documented in the medical record,**
- **the radiopaque sponges removed should be isolated and not included in the counts for the removal procedure,**
- **the surgeon should perform a methodical wound exploration and order an intraoperative radiograph,**[145] **and**
- **the count on the removal procedure should be noted as reconciled if all radiopaque soft goods have been accounted for.**

[Recommendation]

It has been reported that the number of sponges removed in a subsequent procedure did not match the number documented during the initial procedure when therapeutic packing was used.[40]

3.8.5 The surgeon should inform the patient or patient's representative of any surgical soft goods purposely left in the wound at the end of the procedure and the plan for removing these items. *[Recommendation]*

3.8.6 Radiopaque surgical soft goods used as therapeutic packing in the surgical wound should be removed before final closure. *[Recommendation]*

Any sponge retained from use of therapeutic packing after the wound is closed is an unintentionally retained surgical item.

4. Sharps and Miscellaneous Items

4.1 **Account for sharps and other miscellaneous items that are opened onto the sterile field during all procedures in which sharps and miscellaneous items are used.** *[Recommendation]*

Professional organizations recommend accounting for sharps and miscellaneous items used in the surgical wound for prevention of RSIs in all procedures,[48,60] including vaginal deliveries.[65]

Moderate-quality evidence suggests that sharps and miscellaneous items are commonly miscounted and have been retained in patients.[8,29,52,53,62] Needles are the surgical item most likely to be miscounted,[29] although needles are retained less often than they are miscounted.[8] A possible explanation for fewer incidents of retained sharp items than surgical soft goods, despite the number of miscounts, is that sharps are often handled in a different manner than surgical sponges. Sharp items are typically exchanged one for one between the surgeon, surgical first assistant, and scrub person and are kept in designated safe locations on the sterile field.

Steelman et al[42] reported that of the 308 retained objects, excluding soft goods and guidewires, reported to The Joint Commission between 2012 and 2018, 10.7% of reports involved needles and blades, 16.9% involved catheters and drains, and 23.1% involved other items (eg, vessel loops). Cima et al[8] found in a retrospective review that needles were miscounted in 76% of the RSI cases but needles accounted for only 9% of retained items. The Pennsylvania Patient Safety Authority reported that 13% of RSIs were attributed to needles and 40.5% of RSIs were other miscellaneous items, such as guidewires.[62] In other studies of miscount events, Judson et al[52] reported needle miscounts in 48% of events and Greenberg et al[53] reported needle miscounts in 21% of events. The multitude of needles packaged in various quantities and their small size may contribute to miscounts caused by human factors.

A limitation of the evidence is that the number of retained sharp and miscellaneous items may be underreported because of the medicolegal implications of an RSI. Underdiagnosis of retained metallic items also may confound the number of reported cases because the body's immune system may not react to metal in the same way it reacts to fibrous material. Retained miscellaneous items may also be under- and misdiagnosed because these objects are often not available in radiopaque forms and may not be visible on radiographic screening.

Much like device fragments, the patient outcome from a retained sharp or miscellaneous item depends on the biocompatibility of the item's materials, location or potential migration of the item, and the patient's anatomy.[147] Outcomes may include infection, local tissue reaction, perforation or obstruction of blood vessels, and death.[147] If the retained item is metallic, the patient may be at increased risk for injury during magnetic resonance imaging (MRI) procedures because of item migration or internal tissue damage from heating of the object.[147] Additional research is needed to describe patient injury from retention of sharp items.

Retained miscellaneous surgical items (ie, guidewires, intravascular devices) in the vascular system have been reported to cause complications such as thrombosis, embolization, arrhythmia, tamponade, perforation, and death.[148-152] Authors who performed a review of 67 incidents of retained guidewires found that most events involved a physician who was inexperienced in the procedure or lack of adequate supervision (eg, the person removing the guidewire was not supervised, the supervising individual was not focused on verifying guidewire removal).[148] Twelve retained guidewires were related to the use of two catheter kits.[148] A patient's death caused by a retained pacing wire in the heart was reported in the literature.[153]

Miscellaneous items retained during minimally invasive procedures also have been reported to cause patient injury, including infection from a retained stapler anvil,[154] lung abscess from a retained specimen bag containing bowel,[155] bowel obstruction and biliary obstruction from retained free clips,[156,157] inflammatory response from a retained stapler cover,[158] urinary tract infection caused by bladder obstruction from a retained bulb syringe,[159] and vaginal abscess from a retained bulb syringe.[160]

4.1.1 **Count all suture needles, regardless of size, for all surgical procedures.** *[Recommendation]*

Accounting for all needles during a procedure, including small suture needles, reduces the risk of a needle being retained in the patient and the risk of sharps injuries to personnel. Retained small needles may cause patient injury, depending on the location of retention, such as injury during MRI procedures.[29]

Of the 33 retained needles and blades reported to The Joint Commission in a 5-year period, the majority (90.9%) of items were suture needles.[42] A barrier to the practice of counting small needles is the difficulty of reconciling a count discrepancy because needles smaller than 10 mm may be difficult to consistently locate on radiographic screening when retention is suspected.[161-164] Additional research is needed to determine more effective and consistent radiographic detection methods for small needles.[165]

4.1.2

In collaboration with an interdisciplinary team, determine which miscellaneous items should be counted. [Recommendation]

Retained miscellaneous items that have been reported in the literature include

- electrosurgery electrode tips[42];
- electrosurgery scratch pads[42];
- vessel loops[42];
- syringes[42];
- a screw cap[42];
- prep sticks[42];
- drains (eg, Penrose, close-system, bulb)[42];
- guidewires[68,148,152,166,167];
- catheters[42];
- catheter sheaths,[168] stylets, and dilators[42];
- dilator and introducer sheaths[42];
- angiocatheter glue[42];
- endostaple reload cartridges[158];
- a trocar[42];
- stapler anvils[154];
- a staple[42];
- a port sleeve[42];
- a sleeve anchor[42];
- specimen bags[42,155];
- a wound irrigator[42];
- talc straw[42];
- hemostatic sponges[42];
- Telfa[42];
- Asepto syringe bulbs (eg, for gynecological procedures)[42,159];
- a pessary guide[42];
- fetal scalp electrodes[42];
- a mouth guard[42];
- a dental guard[42];
- dental x-ray tips[42];
- an oral airway[42];
- dental retraction cords[42];
- an eye shield[42];
- Raney clips[42];
- fiducial markers (eg, navigation guide checkpoint markers)[42];
- mesh positioners[42];
- phrenic nerve pads[42]; and
- an epilepsy grid.[42]

Various types of miscellaneous items are used during procedures, and the types of items are heavily dependent on the type of procedure being performed. As such, the selection of miscellaneous items to be counted at the health care organization will depend on the types of procedures performed and the risk for retention of individual items. Items used in the surgical wound are likely to have a higher possibility for retention. A facility risk assessment can identify other items not listed above that may be at risk for retention (See Recommendation 13.3).

The evidence review for this guideline revision included several reports of miscellaneous items retained after minimally invasive procedures, including a stapler anvil, specimen bag, stapler cartridge, cervical cup, bulb syringe, and laser ablation catheter sheath.[42,154,155,158,159,168,169] Steelman et al[42] reported that catheters and drains comprised 16.9% of retained items reported to The Joint Commission in a 5-year period. The types of retained catheters or fragments described by Steelman et al[42] included cardiac, angioplasty, thrombolysis, vascular access, epidural, intrathecal, arterial line, thoracic, endotracheal guide, irrigation, paracentesis, rectal, sonogram, suction, and urinary. Of items in the drain category, Penrose drains were the most frequent, but other retained drains or drain fragments included closed-suction drains, bulb suction drains, pigtail drains, and drains that were not identified.[42] The evidence review also found many reports of RSIs from retained guidewires during placement of central line catheters before or during surgical procedures.[68,148,152,166,167] **See Section 6** on device fragments.

As part of a larger RSI prevention process, one organization described the use of a detailed list of items that were not counted or regularly accounted for.[67] The personnel used a sheet that allowed the item to be listed as "in" the surgical field or "out" when it was returned to the instrument table.[67]

4.2

The scrub person should account for and confine all sharps on the sterile field until the final count is reconciled. [Recommendation]

Unconfined sharps that remain on the sterile field may be unintentionally introduced into the incision, may be dropped on the floor, or may penetrate barriers. Confinement and containment of sharps may minimize the risk for injury to personnel as well as reduce the risk for RSIs.[60,170]

4.2.1

Confine and contain sharps in specified areas of the sterile field or inside a sharps containment device.[60,70] [Recommendation]

Sharps/needle counting devices protect scrubbed personnel during procedures by segregating sharps in one location until disposal at the end of the procedure. To prevent the accumulation of used suture needles on the sterile field, one organization limited the size of the available sterile sharps containment devices.[67] Sharps containment devices for used needles contained only 20 spaces for open procedures and 10 spaces for minimally invasive procedures.[67]

4.2.2 Sharps/needle counting devices must be
- puncture resistant,
- labeled or color coded in accordance with the Bloodborne Pathogens standard, and
- leak proof on the sides and bottom.[171]

[Regulatory Requirement]

4.2.3 When a sharps container on the sterile field is full, use an additional, new container. Include the full container in the count and do not remove it from the room until the final count reconciliation is completed. [Recommendation]

4.2.4 Securely close sharps containers before disposal. [Recommendation]

4.3 Use a **read-back method** for communicating the number of needles added to the sterile field and the number of needles recorded on the count board during the procedure. [Recommendation]

During a procedure, noise and distractions may occur. The risk of communication errors may be minimized by use of a standardized process of active listening and clear responses. Use of a read-back method for communication between the RN circulator and the scrub person was included as part of a QI process to reduce the risk of RSIs.[67] The authors describe a system that included the scrub person stating the number of needles added to the sterile field and the RN circulator stating the number of needles recorded on the count sheet.[67]

The AORN Guideline for Team Communication also recommends use of a read-back method when communicating patient information to team members.[95] Needles are commonly involved in count discrepancies[29,30] and if lost in the OR or procedure room, could increase the risk of a sharps injury to personnel entering the room.

4.4 Account for sharps and miscellaneous items used in the surgical wound in their entirety immediately on removal from the surgical site. [Recommendation]

Moderate-quality evidence[42,70] and guidance from professional organizations[48,60,147] support the practice of accounting for items used in the surgical wound in their entirety by inspecting for breakage or fragmentation immediately on removal from the surgical site. Inspection will allow for immediate detection of any device fragments and prevent the unintentional retention of fragments. Steelman et al[42] recommended verbally acknowledging removal of objects from the patient **(See Recommendation 6.3)**.

4.4.1 If a broken or separated item is returned from the surgical site, the scrub person should immediately notify the perioperative team. [Recommendation]

4.5 In the event that a needle or miscellaneous item is lost during a minimally invasive procedure, the surgeon should weigh the risks and benefits of retrieving the item.[172,173] [Recommendation]

The benefits of removing a lost needle or miscellaneous item may not outweigh the harms, depending on the clinical situation. Benefits may include reducing the risk for infection, local tissue reaction, perforation or obstruction of blood vessels, and death.[147] The risk for **adverse events** caused by an unretrieved surgical item may be affected by the biocompatibility of device materials, the location or potential migration of the item, and the patient's anatomy.[147] Magnetic fields from MRI procedures may increase the risk to the patient by causing migration of the item or internal tissue damage from heating of the object.[147]

The harms of removing the item may include additional injury to tissue and nerve damage, depending on the anatomical location of the item. Retrieving items in laparoscopic procedures may necessitate converting to an open-incision procedure,[172] which can increase the patient's risk for infection and pain and increase recovery time. In a survey of surgeons and residents, Ruscher et al[173] reported that 89.4% of respondents believed that converting to laparotomy created a greater risk than the RSI itself. However, 92.6% of the respondents also agreed that an intraperitoneally retained needle put the patient at some degree of future risk.

The evidence review for this guideline revision found reports of lost needles during minimally invasive procedures.[172,174] Small et al[175] tested the use of a laparoscopic magnet device in a porcine model and found the tool to be safe and effective for locating lost needles during porcine laparoscopic surgery. In a survey of 305 surgeons who performed MIS, use of a magnetic retriever was reported among successful needle recovery strategies. Using the survey information, Jayadevan et al[176] developed a protocol for recovering lost needles during MIS and recommended using a magnetic device, if one is available. Additional research and development is needed to establish the safety and efficacy of using a laparoscopic magnetic tip probe to locate and remove needles lost during MIS.

4.5.1 Immediately attempt to locate and retrieve the item, depending on the clinical situation. [Recommendation]

Moderate-quality evidence suggests that delay in retrieval of a lost item may cause the item to become more difficult to remove or inaccessible.[172,176] Attempting immediate retrieval may reduce the risk of the item being retained. In a protocol for retrieving lost needles based on a survey of minimally invasive surgeons, Jayadevan et al[176] recommended halting the procedure to survey for the lost needle and conduct a systematic search.

In a case report from India of a broken pediatric MIS instrument, Parelkar et al[172] emphasized the importance of retrieving broken instruments without delay. During a laparoscopic inguinal hernia repair with 2-mm instruments, a grasper blade broke but fell in the field of vision. Rather than stopping the repair or inserting another grasper to retrieve the broken instrument, the surgeon completed the hernia repair. When the surgeon attempted to retrieve the broken grasper blade, it had migrated and was no longer visible. After 20 minutes of searching, the broken grasper blade was retrieved, avoiding radiographs and possible conversion to an open procedure.

4.5.2 **Remove free clips (eg, open staples) from the abdominal cavity when possible.** *[Recommendation]*

The evidence review found reports of two patients who suffered adverse events including bowel and biliary obstructions from free clips retained in the abdomen after MIS.[156,157]

4.6 **If a sharp or miscellaneous item is passed or dropped from the sterile field, the RN circulator should**
- **retrieve it using standard precautions,**
- **handle sharp items with an instrument,**
- **show it to the scrub person,**
- **isolate it from the field,**
- **place it in a sharps/needle counting device separate from the sterile field (when applicable), and**
- **include it in the final count.**

[Recommendation]

Handling sharps with an instrument and containing the item in a sharps/needle counting device will reduce the risk of sharps injury and allow the item to be visualized in the final count.[170]

4.6.1 **Do not attach (eg, with tape) counted sharp items to the count board or sheet.** *[Recommendation]*

Using tape to attach a sharp item to the count board or sheet increases the risk of sharps injury and bloodborne pathogen exposure.

4.7 **Establish and implement a standardized procedure to communicate the location and the plan for eventual removal of the item when miscellaneous surgical items (eg, a pacing wire, a drain) are intentionally left in the surgical wound for postoperative removal.** *[Recommendation]*

Biliary stents intended for short-term (ie, 3 to 6 months) relief of biliary drainage have been reported as unintentionally retained items.[177,178] In a nonexperimental study, Kumar et al[177] found that 50% of patients did not follow the physician's instructions for removal and a third of patients thought their stent was a permanent implant. The researchers stated that they updated patient discharge paperwork to colloquial language and set up telephone services to remind patients about the presence of the stent and schedule a removal date.[177]

Steelman et al[42] reported 14 incidences of retained implants or implant fragments including ureteral and coronary stents, bariatric surgery implants (ie, lap band, gastric band), sterilization devices for occlusion of fallopian tubes, and mesh. However, it is unclear if these retained items were intended for permanent or temporary implantation.

4.7.1 **Communicate the number and types of miscellaneous surgical items intentionally placed in the patient as part of the transfer of patient care information, and document this communication in the patient's intraoperative record.**[95] *[Recommendation]*

4.7.2 **The surgeon should inform the patient or patient's representative of any miscellaneous surgical items purposely left in the wound at the end of the procedure and the plan for removing these items.** *[Recommendation]*

4.8 **Account for preparation sticks used in vaginal antisepsis.** *[Recommendation]*

Three prep sticks retained in the vagina were reported to The Joint Commission between 2012 and 2018.[42]

Vaginal antisepsis can be performed by using prepackaged preparation kits that contain prep sticks. These prep sticks are not usually radiopaque and can have a plastic handle with a foam sponge attached to one end. Use of these prep sticks can replace use of sponge sticks with gauze sponges for vaginal antisepsis **(See Recommendation 3.2.2)**, thereby reducing the risk of retained gauze sponges during vaginal antisepsis. Use of prep sticks in vaginal antisepsis may increase the risk of prep stick retention and could also increase the risk of a foam sponge detaching from the stick and being retained, although this situation was not reported in the literature reviewed for this guideline revision.

5. Instruments

5.1 **Account for instruments in all procedures for which the likelihood exists that an instrument could be retained.** [*Recommendation*]

Professional organizations recommend accounting for instruments when there is a risk for retention.[48,60] Moderate-quality evidence indicates that instruments have been retained in patients and are implicated in count discrepancies.[4,8,13,25,42,53,62] In individual retrospective reports, the prevalence of retained instruments has been reported to range from 3% to 43% of RSI cases.[4,8,21,25,42,53]

In a nonexperimental review of reports of never events to the California Department of Public Health between 2007 to 2017, Cohen et al[21] reported that clamps and retractors comprised 8.5% and 5.3% of the 94 RSIs, respectively. Steelman et al[42] reported that instruments comprised 33.1% of 308 reports of unintentionally retained foreign objects to The Joint Commission between 2012 and 2018. The study[42] did not include the 319 retained soft goods and 73 retained guidewires or guidewire fragments that were reported in other studies of The Joint Commission data completed around the same time period.[15,68]

A limitation of the evidence is that the number of retained instruments may be underreported because of the medicolegal implications of RSI. Underdiagnosis of retained metallic items also may confound the number of reported cases because the body's immune system may not react to metal in the same way it reacts to fibrous material, and the patient may be asymptomatic.

The benefits of accounting for instruments outweigh the harms. Patient harm has been associated with retained instruments.[42] Orthopedic instrumentation is the most frequently reported as retained, including instruments from joint arthroplasty procedures and arthroscopic procedures.[42] Instruments reported as retained include

- orthopedic instruments:
  - protectors,
  - k-wires,
  - pins,
  - an alignment rod,
  - a cutting jig,
  - a drill bit,
  - a humeral head shield,
  - a screw,
  - a washer,
  - a navigation guide checkpoint marker,
  - a shaver, and
  - a retractor;
- vascular instruments:
  - a bulldog clamp and
  - a micro clamp;
- retractors:
  - Balfour,
  - malleable, and
  - ribbon; and
- other instruments:
  - forceps,
  - hemostats,
  - a towel clamp,
  - a spatula,
  - a tunneler, and
  - unknown.[42]

Information from the US Food and Drug Administration (FDA) on patient outcomes from retained **unretrieved device fragments** is applicable to patient outcomes from unintentionally retained instruments. The patient outcome from a retained instrument depends on the biocompatibility of the item's materials, the location or potential migration of the item, and the patient's anatomy.[147] Outcomes may include infection, local tissue reaction, perforation or obstruction of blood vessels, and death.[147] Retained metallic items may increase the patient's risk for injury during MRI procedures because of item migration or internal tissue damage from heating of the object.[147]

5.2 **Count instruments for all procedures involving an open body cavity (ie, thorax, abdomen).** [*Recommendation*]

The WHO recommends that health care organizations determine which instruments will be counted and which procedures will have instrument counts, to include procedures involving open cavities.[60] Gawande et al[4] recommended counting instruments for every surgical procedure involving an open cavity.

5.3 **Count instruments when sets are assembled for sterilization.** [*Recommendation*]

A count of the instruments at assembly of the instrument set provides a basic inventory reference for the instrument set but is not considered the initial count before the surgical procedure.

5.4 **Do not consider the final instrument count complete until the instruments used in closing the wound (eg, malleable retractors, needle holders, scissors) are removed from the wound and returned to the scrub person.** [*Recommendation*]

Instruments used in wound closure could be retained. Malleable and ribbon retractors have been reported as retained but the circumstances of the incident were not described.[42] Researchers who surveyed Brazilian surgeons about RSIs suggested that part of the malleable retractor used during wound closure remain outside of the patient's body.[9] Steelman et al[42] recommended verbally acknowledging removal of objects from the patient.

5.5 **Account for individual pieces of assembled instruments (eg, suction tips, wing nuts, blades, sheathes) separately and record these on the count sheet.** *[Recommendation]*

Counting individual pieces of assembled instruments before and after a procedure reduces the risk of leaving a piece behind if the instrument becomes disassembled for any reason.[60] Removable instrument parts can be purposefully removed or become loose and fall into the wound or onto or off of the sterile field. The literature contains reports of both retained parts (eg, removed or loose) and fragments (eg, broken pieces) of a device or instrument.[42] It is not always clear if the retained section of the instrument or device was a part or fragment. See Section 6 for recommendations on prevention of device fragments.

Uterine manipulators may have parts that are removable and can be disassembled. Parts of uterine manipulators were the most frequently retained instrument pieces in a study of 308 retained objects reported to The Joint Commission between 2012 and 2018, excluding soft goods and guidewires.[42] The parts of the manipulator retained include Cohen manipulator tips (eg, Acorn), Koh cups or rings, and cervical caps.[42] The reason parts of these devices are retained may be attributed to the lack of visibility of the device during the laparoscopic procedure when it is inserted in the vagina and the surgeon is operating in the abdomen.[42]

5.6 **Use preprinted count sheets to record instruments as the count is conducted.**[21,60] *[Recommendation]*

Preprinted count sheets promote organization and efficiency, which are key to preventing retained surgical instruments. The WHO recommends recording counts on standardized count sheets.[18] Duggan et al[67] reported that use of the instrument list for the final count was a critical behavior to prevent RSIs.

5.6.1 **Record only the number of instruments opened for the procedure.** *[Recommendation]*

5.7 **Account for instruments used in open surgical wounds in their entirety, including any instrument labels, by inspecting for all removable parts, breakage, or fragmentation immediately on the instrument's removal from the surgical site.** *[Recommendation]*

Moderate-quality evidence[42,70,179,180] and guidance from professional organizations[48,60,147] support accounting for instruments used in the surgical wound in their entirety by inspecting instruments for breakage or fragmentation immediately on their removal from the surgical site **(See Recommendation 6.3)**.

Bansal et al[180] reported a case of a retained outflow cannula fragment found 6 years after a knee arthroscopy. The patient presented with acute pain, and radiographs showed a retained metallic object in the operative knee. The retained fragment was removed by arthroscopy and the patient subsequently developed deep vein thrombosis. The authors advised diligent inspection of instruments that have been used on a patient, even if the risk for complication is low.

Ipaktchi et al[179] reported a **near miss** event in which an instrument label fragment was discovered in the surgical wound during closing. They recommended inspecting instruments after use in their entirety, including the label, to prevent the unintentional retention of instrument label fragments.

5.8 **Keep all counted instruments inside the OR or procedure room during the procedure until all counts are completed and reconciled.** *[Recommendation]*

The WHO recommends confining all counted instruments to the room to help eliminate the possibility of a count discrepancy.[60]

5.9 **If an instrument is passed or dropped from the sterile field, the RN circulator should retrieve it using standard precautions, show it to the scrub person, isolate it from the field, and include it in the final count.** *[Recommendation]*

5.10 **Standardize instrument sets and count sheets with the minimum number and variety of instruments needed for the procedure.** *[Recommendation]*

The WHO recommends using standardized instrument sets.[60] Reducing the number and types of instruments and streamlining standardized sets increases the ease and efficiency of counting.

As part of a QI project to standardize count practices, Norton et al[105] streamlined instrument sets to remove obsolete and redundant items and updated instrument count sheets to facilitate the counting process. Instrument stringers were arranged in the same order as the count sheet, and the count sheet was updated to show a total for each instrument group (eg, scissors).[105]

5.10.1 **Remove instruments that are not routinely used in procedures from sets.** [Recommendation]

Additional or infrequently used instruments can be opened as needed and added to the count.

5.11 **Establish a policy for instrument counting.** [Recommendation]

The WHO recommends that health care organizations determine which instruments will be counted and which procedures will have instrument counts.[60]

5.11.1 **Define circumstances in which the instrument count may be waived.** [Recommendation]

Procedures in which accurate instrument counts may not be achievable or practical include

- complex procedures involving large numbers of instruments (eg, anterior-posterior spinal procedures),
- trauma procedures,[4,181,182]
- procedures that require complex instruments with numerous small parts, and
- procedures for which the width and depth of the incision is too small to retain an instrument.

5.11.2 **Define circumstances in which cavity, closing, and final instrument counts can overlap.** [Recommendation]

There may be instances when a cavity, closing, or final instrument count overlap due to the number of instruments to be counted or the time it takes to close the wound. Clarifying in the facility policy and procedure when an instrument count can include more than one type of count (eg, cavity, closing, final) is important. This provides clear, standardized information about how instrument counts are performed so that patients are protected from retained instruments but prevents personnel from rushing during closing procedures to perform a subsequent instrument count when one was just completed.

5.11.3 **Define the processes to be used to prevent retained instruments when an instrument count is waived in procedures where it would normally be performed (eg, a trauma procedure involving an unstable patient with an open abdominal cavity).** [Recommendation]

See Recommendation 8.4 on reconciling count discrepancies.

6. Device Fragments and Explants

6.1 **Take measures to prevent retention of device fragments** [Recommendation]

Serious adverse events associated with unretrieved device fragments have been reported to the FDA.[147] Fragments of devices can cause patient harm when retained and during removal. The limitations of the evidence are that few reports of device fragmentation are published in peer-reviewed literature. The harms associated with retained fragments include local tissue reaction, perforation or obstruction of blood vessels, and death.[147] Harms related to fragment removal include additional injury to tissue, increased procedure time, exposure to radiation, and conversion of laparoscopic procedures to open.[172] Additional research is needed to determine the best methods for preventing retention of device fragments.

6.2 **Take measures to prevent instrument breakage,[147] including fragmentation of instrument labels.[179]** [Recommendation]

According to the FDA, instrument fragments may cause patient harm on removal or in the event of retention.[147] Williams et al[40] found that instrument fragments were the most commonly retained item (n = 171 of 428; 40%) reported to the University HealthSystem Consortium (UHC) in 2011 and 2012. Ipaktchi et al[179] described a near miss event in which a plastic instrument label fragment was discovered in the surgical wound. The fragment was retrieved from the wound before closure. The authors recommended considering instrument labels to be part of the instrument and taking measures to prevent fragmentation.[179] See the AORN Guideline for Care and Cleaning of Surgical Instruments[183] for more information about protecting instruments from damage.

6.2.1 **Use instruments in accordance with the manufacturer's instructions for use.[147]** [Recommendation]

Using an instrument of inappropriate size or for purposes other than those intended by the manufacturer may increase the likelihood of instrument damage and fragmentation. Inappropriate use of surgical instrumentation has been reported as a major contributing factor in instrument breakage.[184] In a case report, Parelkar et al[172] reported breakage of a 2-mm grasper blade inside a pediatric patient during an inguinal hernia repair. Although the cause of breakage was not confirmed, the authors hypothesized that inserting the instrument without a trocar may have exposed the grasper tip to more force than it would have encountered through a cannula.[179]

6.2.2 **Inspect instruments, including attached labels,[179] before use to identify any defects that may increase the likelihood of fragmentation.[22,48,60,70,147] Do not use defective instruments.** [Recommendation]

Moderate-quality evidence[70] and guidance from professional organizations[48,60,147] support inspecting devices for signs of breakage or fragmentation before use. Inspection will allow for defective items to be removed from use and help prevent risks to the patient associated with a fragmented device. Identifying a broken instrument before use will also prevent the unnecessary consequences of searching for a device fragment that does not exist, such as additional injury to tissue, nerve damage, increased operative time, exposure to radiation, and conversion of a laparoscopic to an open procedure.

6.2.3 **Inspect, maintain, and service instruments, including labels,[179] in accordance with the device manufacturer's written instructions for use.[183,184]** [Recommendation]

Preventive maintenance performed according to the device manufacturer's instructions for use is necessary to maintain instruments in optimal working order.[183] In a nonexperimental study, Yasuhara et al[184] reported that 80% of all instrument breakage was identified through instrument inspections performed by personnel in the facility. A major contributing factor in instrument breakage rates was wear (eg, severe staining, cracks, discoloration, corrosion).[184]

Ipaktchi et al[179] reported a near miss event in which an instrument label fragment was discovered in the surgical wound during closing and removed. To prevent the unintentional retention of instrument label fragments, the authors recommended routine inspection and maintenance of labels.[179]

6.2.4 **Additional inspection, maintenance, and servicing of MIS instruments may be performed on a scheduled basis.[184]** [Conditional Recommendation]

Moderate-quality evidence indicates that MIS instruments have an increased risk for breakage and subsequent fragment retention.[172,184,185] Minimally invasive device fragments and instrument breakage may be difficult to identify in the OR because of the limited view of the surgical area through the camera[184,185] and the reduced lighting in the room. Therefore, identifying wear that could lead to fragmentation during instrument inspections may reduce the rate of instrument breakage that occurs intraoperatively.

Yasuhara et al[184] described a secondary monthly inspection process used for MIS instruments completed in the facility by engineering personnel contracted through the device manufacturer. Rates of MIS instrument breakage that occurred intraoperatively remained moderate (0.88%) even with the extra inspection process. However, the researchers suggested that the incidence of MIS instrument breakage could increase without it.[184]

6.3 **Account for items used in the surgical wound in their entirety by inspecting for breakage and fragmentation immediately on removal from the surgical site** (See Recommendation 4.4 and Recommendation 5.7). [Recommendation]

Moderate-quality evidence[42,172,186] and guidance from professional organizations[48,60,147] support inspecting devices for signs of breakage or fragmentation after use. Inspection will allow for immediate detection of any device fragments and reduce the risk of unintentional retention of fragments.

Steelman et al[42] stated that seven reports of retained device fragments were from orthopedic instrumentation including an arthroscopic shaver, drill bit, retractor, telescope tip, and wire tip. Steelman et al[42] also reported retained fragments of drains, gloves, uterine ablation electrodes, endobags, pacemaker wires, a laryngoscope blade, and metal fragments. In a case study of two retained dental bur fragments, the authors suggested that the fragments may have been partially caused by selection of a bur not designed for use on cortical bone and the application of force used during cutting.[186] See Recommendation 5.2.3 for information on accounting for removable instrument and device parts.

6.3.1 If a broken item is returned from the surgical site, the scrub person should immediately notify the perioperative team. [Recommendation]

6.4 If a broken instrument with a missing fragment is identified during reprocessing, sterile processing personnel should notify the perioperative team immediately.[187] When notified of a missing device fragment, the perioperative team should immediately investigate and follow established count reconciliation procedures. [Recommendation]

Notification of the perioperative team is supported in an organizational experience article. Reece et al[187] described a process for managing broken surgical instruments. If the sterile processing technician identified a damaged or fragmented instrument during the cleaning and assembly process, the technician notified the OR charge nurse. At their facility, Reece et al[187] used a bar-code system and sterile processing tracking software to allow a broken instrument with missing fragments to be traced to the patient on whom it was last used. The perioperative team then collaboratively determined whether the item was potentially retained, and a radiograph was obtained to rule out a retained device fragment if indicated.[187]

6.5 **Take measures to prevent intravascular device (ie, catheter, guidewire, sheath) fragments.** *[Recommendation]* P

Moderate-quality evidence suggests that preventive measures are needed to avoid the complications associated with removal or retention of device fragments from intravascular catheters, guidewires, and sheaths.[7,68,152,167,188] The evidence review included multiple reports of intravascular RSIs that were caused by device fragments.[149-152,167,189-192]

In a nonexperimental study of 13 retained guidewires or fragments, Moffatt-Bruce et al[167] reported that unexpected procedural factors (eg, difficult procedure, lack of familiarity with the equipment) and equipment malfunction were significantly associated with intravascular RSIs. The researchers also reported that 53.8% of intravascular RSIs were missed on the initial postprocedural imaging.[167]

In a nonexperimental study of 73 incidences of retained guidewires or fragments reported to The Joint Commission between 2012 and 2018, Steelman et al[68] reported that the majority were used with vascular catheters (eg, central line placements, peripherally inserted cardiac catheters). However, some of the retained guidewires or fragments were from nonvascular devices used during knee arthroscopy procedures, breast biopsy procedures, and placements of a biliary drain, nephrostomy tube, suprapubic catheter, and ureteral stent. Almost half of the retained guidewires or fragments migrated from the point of origin.[68]

In a review of pediatric autopsies performed on patients who underwent cardiac catheterization, heart surgery with cardiopulmonary bypass, or extracorporeal membrane oxygenation, researchers found that 33% of patients had embolic foreign material in their brain that was sometimes associated with infarction.[192] The researchers suggest that hydrophilic polymer catheter coatings can separate from the sheath or catheter and be a source of embolic material.[192]

6.5.1 Use a standardized checklist for insertion of devices with guidewires.[7,68,167] The checklist should include a two-person verbal verification that the guidewire is removed and intact.[68] *[Recommendation]*

Checklists may standardize and improve care in clinical settings by preventing the omission of important steps.[68] Two nonexperimental studies that reviewed retained guidewire and guidewire fragments recommended use of a checklist during insertion of devices with guidewires.[7,68] An important part of the checklist is a two-person check of the removal and completeness of the guidewire.[68]

Cherara et al[7] stated that checklists with a "read and verify" process allow for final verification that all steps were completed. The researchers state that a two-person process with a "challenge-response" methodology can also be used. In this process the observer reads the checklist and the individual performing the task confirms the condition of each item and states a response. For instance, the observer states, "guidewire," and the person performing the task finds the guidewire and ensures it is removed from the patient and then says, "removed." However, for a checklist to be effective, it has to be used, and success is dependent on the process the individual or team uses to implement it.[7]

6.5.2 The insertion and removal of devices with guidewires should be considered a critical phase of the procedure during which distractions are minimized. *[Recommendation]*

Distractions and interruptions may increase the likelihood of a retained guidewire or fragment.[7,68,148] See Recommendations 1.4 and 1.4.1 for more information about avoiding distractions.

6.5.3 Insert and remove intravascular devices in accordance with the manufacturer's instructions for use. *[Recommendation]*

Low-quality evidence indicates that misuse of intravascular devices leading to device fragment retention is a preventable complication and supports following the manufacturer's instructions for use, insertion, and removal.[68,149,188,190] Fischer[188] described a case of guidewire fracture in which the guidewire was weakened by manipulation into a shape for which the device was not designed.

In a review of intravascular unretrieved device fragments, Tateishi and Tomizawa[149] concluded that many preventable device-fracture complications were related to inappropriate use of intravascular devices, including use of devices for off-label purposes and reuse of single-use devices. Pillarisetti et al[190] described a specific example of failure to follow the device manufacturer's instructions in a case report of femoral vascular sheath breakage during removal. The authors emphasized the importance of following the manufacturer's instructions for use, including using an obturator or dilator when removing the sheath, to prevent adverse events associated with a retained sheath.

6.5.4 Inspect intravascular devices before use to identify any defects that may increase the likelihood of fragmentation. *[Recommendation]*

The author of an expert opinion report advised inspecting intravascular devices for breakage or manufacturing defects to minimize the risk for retained device fragments.[188] Inspection will allow for defective items to be identified and removed before use to prevent the risks to the patient associated with a fragmented device.

Identifying a broken instrument before use will also prevent unnecessary searching for a device fragment and the associated consequences, such as additional injury to tissue, nerve damage, increased operative time, and exposure to radiation. In an organizational experience article, Endicott et al[193] suggested that both the RN circulator and the scrub person inspect intravascular devices when they are opened and then the scrub person inspect them before use.

6.5.5 Do not withdraw catheters and guidewires through a needle. If the catheter or guidewire is replaced, withdraw it simultaneously with the needle. *[Recommendation]*

Low-quality evidence indicates that withdrawing a guidewire through a needle increases the risk of guidewire fracture.[152,188] Fischer[188] described catheter removal through or over a needle as an inappropriate technique that can result in unretrieved device fragments.

In a review of guidewire retention during central venous catheterizations reported to the UHC Safety Intelligence Patient Safety Organization database, Williams et al[152] advised withdrawing the guidewire together as a unit with the needle. The authors explained that withdrawing the guidewire through the needle increases the risk of damage to or shearing of the wire on the needle bevel.

6.5.6 Replace bent guidewires immediately.[152] *[Recommendation]*

Replacement of bent guidewires was supported in a review of cases of guidewire reten-

tion during central venous catheterization reported in the UHC Safety Intelligence Patient Safety Organization database.[152] Williams et al[152] found that attempts at recannulation with a bent guidewire could increase the risk of shearing the wire.

6.5.7 Account for intravascular devices in their entirety by inspecting for breakage immediately on removal from the patient. *[Recommendation]*

Low-quality evidence suggests that inspection of intravascular devices will allow for immediate detection of any breakage.[151,152,193] A review by Williams et al[152] recommended confirming removal of the guidewire and inspecting its integrity. Johnson et al[151] reported a case of a retained introducer sheath radiopaque marker. The patient underwent removal of an inferior vena cava filter, after which the filter and introducer catheters were found to be intact. On a subsequent chest radiograph, a radiopaque foreign body was found and removed from the subcutaneous tissue below the access site. Although this was a rare occurrence and related to device malfunction, the authors advised confirming the position of the radiopaque marker after its removal. Steelman et al[68] recommended documenting the verification of removal and the integrity of the guidewire.

Endicott et al[193] suggested that endovascular devices be treated differently than traditional surgical instruments because there are many products available and some may look different after use. Perioperative personnel who do not have cardiovascular education and experience and who care for patients undergoing endovascular procedures may not be able to consistently identify items that have been compromised.[193,194] Inspection of the device by the scrub person immediately after use was recommended[193] and may be aided by using a visual display of commonly used endovascular devices.[194] However, the facility interdisciplinary team involved in the QI process determined that final inspection and verification of endovascular device integrity is a responsibility of the attending surgeon or senior fellow at the end of the procedure.[193] The authors recommended that the RN circulator document during the procedural debrief that the surgeon performed a visual inspection and the surgical team document the results of the inspection in the postoperative notes.[193]

6.5.8 Develop, implement, and periodically revise policies and procedures for management of devices with guidewires. *[Recommendation]*

Inadequate policies and procedures were found to be a contributing factor related to guidewire or guidewire fragment retention.[68]

6.5.9 Provide education, training, and competency verification to perioperative team members who use guidewires.[68,167] *[Recommendation]*

Steelman et al[68] recommended education on the risks of retained guidewires, training on insertion techniques using simulation and forced-error detection, and competency assessment. The use of forced-error simulation during competency verification may help determine whether the individual can identify that the guidewire has been retained.[68,195] Pokharel et al[148] also recommended simulation in a literature review of 76 instances of guidewire retention.

6.6 Confirm removal of implants in their entirety with the surgeon. *[Recommendation]*

The literature includes cases of implants intended to be removed from the patient that were retained and caused the patient harm.[42,177,178,196,197] Steelman et al[42] reported 14 incidences of implants or parts of implants in a study of 308 retained items reported to The Joint Commission from 2012 and 2018, excluding soft goods and guidewires.

Kava and Burdick-Will[196] reported four cases of patients with retained penile prostheses that were infected. Due to the complexity of the multi-component penile prosthesis implant, the authors recommended using a removal checklist to confirm that all parts are removed. They also discussed that although complete removal of the implant is the surgeon's responsibility, implementation of an implant-specific checklist may be a rational prevention strategy to prevent unintentionally retained items from causing patient harm.

Felder et al[197] reported a case of a retained gastric band that was intended to be removed during conversion to a sleeve gastrectomy. In this case, the patient experienced recurring sharp abdominal pain and the retained implant was not identified for more than a year until the patient underwent a computed tomography (CT) scan.[197]

6.7 Take measures to prevent retention of hypodermic needle fragments. *[Recommendation]*

Low-quality evidence supports taking measures to prevent hypodermic needle fragments during inferior alveolar nerve blocks and subcutaneous injections.[198-202] The evidence review included several reports of needle fracture occurring during local anesthesia injection in dental procedures.[198-201] A case report of needle breakage during a growth hormone injection suggested similar preventive measures for needle breakage during subcutaneous injections.[202] There may be limitations to the generalizability of the evidence to other types of injections with hypodermic needles. Additional research is needed to determine the risk of hypodermic needle fracture during invasive procedures and to establish optimal prevention measures.

6.7.1 Do not use thin (ie, 30-gauge) and short (ie, 20-mm) needles unless this is clinically necessary.[198-200,203] *[Recommendation]*

The evidence review indicated that thin needles may be more prone to fracture. The harm of needle fracture from inappropriate use of a thin needle outweighs the perceived benefit of reducing patient discomfort. Use of smaller gauge needles has not been correlated with reduced patient discomfort during injection.[198-200]

The authors of two literature reviews on dental needle breakage incidence and prevention advised against using short needles and 30-gauge needles for inferior alveolar nerve blocks.[198,199] According to reports of dental needle breakage, short needles are more likely to be inserted up to the hub, which is a risk factor for needle fracture.[199,200] Augello et al[198] recommended using 25-gauge to 27-gauge and 35-mm length needles for inferior alveolar nerve blocks.

6.7.2 Inspect hypodermic needles for defects that may increase the likelihood of fragmentation before use.[198,201,202] Do not use defective hypodermic needles. *[Recommendation]*

Augello et al[198] performed a review of the literature of local anesthesia needle breakage in the oral cavity and found that hypodermic needles may have defects that could pose a risk for fracture. They recommended checking the needle before use. In a case series of four needles broken during dental anesthetic injections, Catelani et al[201] recommended that needles be inspected for manufacturing defects before use.

Inspection of hypodermic needles is also supported in a case report by Kim et al,[202] who reported a case of needle breakage during subcutaneous growth hormone injection. The authors recommended checking the needle for manufacturing defects before subcutaneous injection, checking for dull or deformed needles, and not using the needle if a defect is identified. For growth hormone injections, they also discussed that the common practice of using the same 30-gauge needle to reconstitute and inject the medication subcutaneously can lead to bending the needle tip into a hook shape that can break off and leave a needle fragment in the skin.[202]

6.7.3 **Do not bend hypodermic needles.**[198-201,203] *[Recommendation]*

Low-quality evidence found that bending of hypodermic needles before insertion of the needle for local injection is a risk factor for needle fracture.[198-201]

6.7.4 **Do not insert hypodermic needles to the hub.**[199-201,203,204] *[Recommendation]*

Low-quality evidence indicates that needle fracture is more likely to occur if the needle is inserted in the tissue up to the needle hub, which is the weakest part of the needle.[199-201,203] The literature also indicates that needle fracture retrieval is more complicated when the hub is buried in the tissue, which places the patient at increased risk for an invasive procedure to remove the fragment.[204]

Because of the risk of fracture and subsequent possible surgical intervention to locate the buried needle fragment, Malamed et al[199] advised dentists not to insert needles to the hub in soft tissue unless this is essential to the success of the injection. Augello et al[198] advised leaving at least 5 mm of the needle outside the tissue during dental local anesthesia injection to prevent insertion of the needle to the hub and needle fracture.

6.7.5 **Do not change the direction of the hypodermic needle during the injection.**[198,201,202] **If changing the needle angle is necessary, remove the needle from the tissue and reposition it.**[198] *[Recommendation]*

Low-quality evidence suggests that changing the direction of the needle during injection is a risk factor for needle fracture.[198,201,202] In a case series of four needles broken during dental anesthetic injections, Catelani et al[201] advised dentists to avoid changing the angle of the needle during injection.

In a literature review of dental needle breakage, Augello et al[198] advised taking the needle from the tissue when changing needle angulation during injection, to reduce the risk for needle fracture. Kim et al[202] also reported a case of needle breakage during subcutaneous injection and recommended not changing the direction of the needle during injection because of the risk of bending or breaking the needle.

6.7.6 **Advise patients under local anesthesia or moderate sedation about possible pain before giving an injection.**[198,202] *[Recommendation]*

A literature review[198] and a case report[203] showed that sudden or unexpected movement by the patient during injection may be a risk factor for needle breakage. Augello et al[198] recommended informing patients about possible abrupt pain and warning them of impending puncture to reduce the risk of needle breakage caused by patient movement. In their report of a broken needle from a subcutaneous growth hormone injection, Kim et al[202] also advised informing the patient about possible pain to prevent needle breakage.

6.7.7 **Do not reuse thin (ie, 30-gauge) hypodermic needles on the same patient.**[202,204] *[Recommendation]*

Low-quality evidence indicated that reuse of needles increases the risk for needle fracture.[202,204] The needle gauge size commonly associated with needle breakage was 30 gauge.

6.8 **In the event that a device fragment is retained, the surgeon should weigh the risks and benefits of retrieving the fragment.**[147] *[Recommendation]*

The FDA advises careful consideration and discussion with the patient, if possible, of the risks and benefits of retrieving versus leaving the device fragment in the patient.[147]

The benefits of removing device fragments may not outweigh the harms, depending on the clinical situation. Benefits include reducing the risk for infection, local tissue reaction, perforation or obstruction of blood vessels, and death.[147] The risk for adverse events from an unretrieved device fragment may be affected by biocompatibility of the device materials, the location or potential migration of the fragment, and the patient's anatomy.[147] Magnetic fields from MRI procedures may increase the risk to the patient by causing migration of the device fragment or internal tissue damage from heating of the object.[147]

The harms of removing device fragments may include additional injury to tissue and nerve damage, depending on the anatomical location of the fragment. Retrieving device fragments retained during laparoscopic procedures may necessitate converting to an open-incision procedure,[172] which can increase the patient's risk for infection, pain, and longer recovery time.

6.8.1 **Immediately attempt to locate and retrieve the device fragment, depending on the clinical situation.**[172,204,205] *[Recommendation]*

Low-quality evidence[172,204,205] suggests that delay in retrieval of a lost item may cause the device fragment to become more difficult to remove or inaccessible. Immediate retrieval may reduce the risk of the fragment becoming lost or retained.

In a case report from India of a broken pediatric MIS instrument, Parelkar et al[172] also emphasized the importance of retrieving broken instruments without delay. During a laparoscopic inguinal hernia repair with 2-mm instruments, a grasper blade broke but fell into the field of vision. Rather than stopping the repair or inserting another grasper to retrieve the broken instrument, the surgeon completed the hernia repair. When the surgeon attempted to retrieve the broken grasper blade, it had migrated and was no longer visible. After 20 minutes of searching, the broken grasper blade was retrieved, avoiding radiographs and possible conversion to an open procedure.

Bydon et al[205] reported a more complicated case that illustrates the practical challenges associated with immediate location of a device fragment. During a spine procedure, the surgeon noted that a rongeur tip was missing when the rongeur was withdrawn from the surgical site. An intraoperative C-arm fluoroscopic radiograph showed that the tip had migrated through a vascular injury. After consulting with the vascular team, the surgical team made the decision to complete the spine procedure given the patient's hemodynamic stability.

After surgery, the patient underwent an abdominal CT scan, chest radiograph, transthoracic echocardiogram, cardiac catheterization, and thoracic CT scan during the course of 2 days before the rongeur tip was localized to the left ventricle. The patient then underwent a sternotomy for removal of the rongeur tip and closure of a previously undiagnosed patent foramen ovale. Afterward, the patient recovered in the cardiac intensive care unit in stable condition. Although this is a rare case report of vascular injury from device fragmentation during a spine procedure, the authors emphasized the need for rapid diagnosis and collaboration to treat a potentially devastating complication from a retained device fragment.[205]

6.9 In the event that an unretrieved device fragment is left in the patient, the surgeon should inform the patient or patient's representative of the nature of the item and the risks associated with leaving it in the patient.[147] *[Recommendation]*

6.9.1 Provide the following information to the patient:
- risks and benefits of leaving the device fragment in the patient;
- material composition of the fragment (if known);
- size of the fragment (if known);
- location of the fragment;
- potential mechanisms for injury (eg, migration, infection); and
- procedures or treatments that should be avoided, such as MRI examinations in the case of metallic fragments.[147]

[Recommendation]

6.10 Unretrieved device fragments must be documented in the patient's record.[206,207] *[Regulatory Requirement]*

The Centers for Medicare and & Medicaid Services requires surgical complications to be documented in the operative report.[206,207]

6.10.1 Documentation in the patient's medical record about unretrieved device fragments, when known, should include the
- material composition of the fragment (eg, metal, plastic),
- size of the fragment,
- location,
- manufacturer,
- measures taken to recover the fragment, and
- patient notification.

[Recommendation]

When a device fragment is unintentionally retained and not retrieved, documentation that provides details on what is known about the device fragment is important to include in the patient's record.

6.11 Establish mechanisms for reporting retained device fragments.[147] *[Recommendation]*

The FDA safety communication on unretrieved device fragments advises that reportable adverse events related to unretrieved device fragments be reported through the health care organization's reporting mechanism and encourages reporting of adverse events related to device fragments that do not meet mandatory reporting requirements.[147] See the recommendations on reporting, starting with Recommendation 13.6.

6.12 Retain devices involved in fragmentation and retrieved fragments for investigation according to the health care organization's policy.[147,187] *[Recommendation]*

Retaining the device involved and retrieved fragments provides information for the health care organization to investigate the cause and to take action. The FDA safety communication on unretrieved device fragments advises retaining the device and fragment for investigation of the event by the manufacturer.[147]

In an organizational experience report, Reece et al[187] reported that at their facility, sterile processing personnel disinfected and tagged all damaged instruments and stored them for a minimum of 1 year. The retired instrument was then logged into a database that was monitored by the perioperative quality council.[187]

7. Foam Pieces

7.1 Establish and implement a standardized procedure to communicate the location and plan for eventual removal of foam pieces used in an open wound with a negative-pressure wound therapy device. *[Recommendation]*

In a nonexperimental study of reports of retained items to The Joint Commission between 2012 and 2018, Steelman et al[42] found eight incidences of retained foam pieces used in association with negative-pressure wound vacuum devices. The researchers reported that individuals removing the foam pieces may be unaware of how many pieces of foam are in the wound. Establishing a plan to standardize the care and communication regarding patients with foam dressings used in negative-pressure wound therapy is critical to prevent an RSI.[42]

7.1.1 The interdisciplinary team involved in establishing and implementing a standardized procedure for management of foam pieces used in negative-pressure wound therapy devices should include
- **physicians involved in placing, changing, or removing dressings;**
- **nurses involved in placing, changing, or removing dressings;**
- **wound care nurses;**
- **infection preventionists;**
- **quality and risk managers;**
- **materials management personnel; and**
- **other stakeholders as needed (eg, home health care nurses, manufacturer's representatives).**
[Recommendation]

Management of dressings used in negative-pressure wound therapy is a complex process that may involve interdisciplinary team members from all across the facility and in facilities to which these patients may be discharged. Involving a comprehensive interdisciplinary team supports development of a standardized process that works in all the areas in which these patients receive care, with the goal of RSI prevention.

7.2 Follow the manufacturer's instructions for use when using negative-pressure wound therapy devices including preparation of foam pieces for the dressing. *[Recommendation]*

7.3 Cut the foam only when necessary to fit it into the wound and limit the number of foam pieces used in the dressing, when possible. *[Recommendation]*

Leaving the pieces as large as possible and cutting the foam only when necessary may help provide standardization that reduces the risk of retention of foam pieces. Traditionally, foam pieces have been cut to different sizes to fit in wounds of different shapes and depths. This meant there could be unlimited combinations in the number, size, or shape of the foam pieces used. This complicates keeping track of the number of foam pieces in the wound when a dressing is changed or removed.

7.4 Document the number of the foam pieces placed in the wound in the patient's medical record. Documentation should be in an area of the patient's medical record that is accessible to all personnel involved in the placement, dressing changes, or removal of foam pieces used with negative-pressure wound therapy devices. *[Recommendation]*

Clear documentation of the number of foam pieces used in the wound may reduce the risk of an RSI by providing information to individuals changing or removing the dressing. It is unclear if foam pieces retain their size and shape after removal from the wound. Patients using negative-pressure wound therapy devices may have numerous dressing changes during which foam pieces are changed, and updating the information on the number of foam pieces in the patient's wound in the patient's medical record is important. However, many individuals in different departments of the facility and in home health agencies may be involved in wound care associated with negative-pressure wound therapy devices. Therefore, documentation that is accessible during numerous transitions of care is important.

Steelman et al[42] noted that 48.2% of retained items were identified after the patient left the hospital. The ACS recommends documenting items intentionally left as packing.[61]

7.5 Communicate the number of foam pieces used in negative-pressure wound therapy dressings as part of the transfer of patient care information, and document this communication in the patient's intraoperative record.[42,95] *[Recommendation]*

7.6 When the patient is returned to the OR for a procedure that involves removal of a negative-pressure wound therapy dressing,
- the number of foam pieces to be removed should be determined from the patient's medical record,
- the number of foam pieces removed should be documented in the patient's medical record, and
- the surgeon should perform a methodical wound examination.

[Recommendation]

7.7 The surgeon should inform the patient or patient's representative of any foam pieces purposely left in the wound at the end of the procedure as part of the dressing of the negative-pressure wound therapy device and the plan for removing these items. *[Recommendation]*

7.8 The interdisciplinary team should clarify in the facility policy and procedure what process to use when there is uncertainty about the location or retention of any foam pieces in the wound as part of a negative-pressure wound therapy dressing, including how to report the incident internally. *[Recommendation]*

Depending on the size, depth, and shape of the wound, foam pieces may be difficult to visually identify in the wound. Having a clear process to follow when there is uncertainty about removal or retention of foam pieces used in the wound may help personnel perform interventions to prevent or identify an RSI. Some facilities may have policies and procedures that provide guidance about internal reporting of incidents. **See Section 13** for more information.

7.9 No recommendation can be made for use of radiography for identification of retained foam pieces in a wound. *[No Recommendation]*

The foam pieces used in negative-pressure wound therapy dressings are not typically radiopaque. Therefore, the benefit of radiography to verify removal of all foam pieces from a wound versus exposing the patient to radiation is unclear.

7.10 Provide education to and verify competency of perioperative personnel involved in management, placement, changes, or removal of dressings; documentation; and communication. *[Recommendation]*

7.11 Monitor the processes used for prevention of retained foam pieces for quality, including the placement, changes, and removal of dressings; documentation; and communication. *[Recommendation]*

8. Reconciling Count Discrepancies

8.1 Use standardized measures for reconciling count discrepancies during the closing count and before the end of surgery. When a discrepancy in a count is identified, take actions to locate the missing item.[13,29,30,48,60] *[Recommendation]*

Professional organizations[48,60] recommend accounting for surgical items used in the wound for prevention of RSI in all procedures, including vaginal deliveries.[65] Accounting for surgical items encompasses reconciling count discrepancies.

Moderate-quality evidence indicates that count discrepancies are a risk factor for RSI.[13,29] In a meta-analysis of three case-control studies, Moffatt-Bruce et al[13] found that patients with an incorrect surgical count were at the highest risk for RSI compared with other risk factors. Egorova et al[29] were able to quantify this association, finding that retained items occurred more frequently in discrepant cases (one in 70) compared to all cases (one in 7,000).

Greenberg et al[53] conducted a prospective observational study to further investigate count discrepancy events. They categorized discrepancies as being a result of miscounts (eg, incorrect baseline count, overcount, undercount), documentation errors (eg, addition), or misplaced items (eg, retained). The most common discrepancy was from a misplaced or retained item, which occurred in 59% of cases, whereas discrepancies from human error (ie, miscount [3%], documentation [38%]) accounted for 41% of discrepancies.[53] In their study, count discrepancies occurred in one of eight cases, or one per 14 hours of operating time, and took an average of 13 minutes to resolve.[53]

Egorova et al[29] found that only 1.6% of count discrepancies led to the discovery of an item in a patient. Due to the higher frequency of count discrepancies[53] and the less-common occurrence of RSI, Stawicki et al[208] suggested that perioperative teams may be desensitized to incorrect counts to explain why they are disregarded. Human factors such as complacency and normalization of deviance may contribute to lack of follow-up on incorrect counts, although additional research is needed to confirm this.

Moderate-quality evidence indicates that risk factors for count discrepancies include personnel changes,[53,209] the number of providers,[52,209] the length of the procedure,[52] higher surgical risk,[209] procedure complexity,[209] an unplanned procedure,[209] and a low body mass index (BMI).[209] Additional research is needed to assess causal factors for count discrepancies, as the existing evidence is limited by only being able to demonstrate relationships of association.

Technological advances for identification of retained needles have been described in the literature but most are under development. Weprin et al[210] discussed the use of computer-aided detection, sharps detectors, and magnetic retrievers as methods used to identify or expedite removal of retained sharps. However, computer-aided detection and sharps detector technologies are under development or involved in clinical trials. According to the authors, magnetic retrievers are not FDA-cleared for sharps retrieval, may injure organs during the retrieval process, and have limited availability.

Ward et al[211] performed an in vivo animal study to evaluate the use of a needle coating that enhanced the visibility of 11-mm 7-0 suture needles under near infrared and ultraviolet light in the abdomen during open and laparoscopic procedures. The researchers reported that all dual dye-coated needles were located within 300 seconds compared to nine needles in the control groups that were not. The mean length of time to locate the dye-coated needles was also significantly less than for needles in the control groups.

8.2 **All perioperative team members should take immediate actions to resolve a count discrepancy (Figure 3).** *[Recommendation]*

Moderate-quality evidence[52,58,67] and guidance from a professional organization[60] support immediate notification of the team in the event of a count discrepancy and team participation in activities to reconcile the count.

8.2.1 **The RN circulator should inform the team and receive verbal acknowledgment from the surgeon, including the type and number of items missing, as soon as a discrepancy in a surgical count is identified.** *[Recommendation]*

Moderate-quality evidence[52,58,67] and guidance from a professional organization[60] support immediate notification of the team, including verbal acknowledgment, in the event of a count discrepancy. The RN circulator has a responsibility and ethical obligation to speak up promptly when a discrepancy is identified.

Marsh et al[87] conducted a nonexperimental study of missed perioperative nursing care identified from 1,693 surveys of perioperative nurses. The researchers reported that communication of count discrepancies may be missed occasionally, frequently, or always by 2.5% of

respondents. Although this communication failure was one of the least-frequent missed care opportunities,[87] it is concerning that communication of count discrepancies was missed at all.

8.2.2 **When a discrepancy in the count is identified, the RN circulator should**
- **call for assistance**[52,67]
- **search the room, including the area near the sterile field, floor, kick buckets, and linen and waste receptacles**[52,58,60]**; and**
- **recount with the scrub person.**[58,60,208]

[Recommendation]

Moderate-quality evidence[52,58] and guidance from a professional organization[60] support searching the room to locate the missing item and recounting the type of item that is involved in the count discrepancy. It is recommended that the RN circulator obtain assistance to resolve a count discrepancy.[52,67] Having assistance for roles that are needed to simultaneously continue the procedure (eg, a second RN circulator) can allow the primary team to reconcile the count without distractions.

8.2.3 **When a discrepancy in the count is identified, the scrub person should**
- **organize the sterile field**[52,97]**;**
- **search the sterile field, including drapes and tables**[60]**; and**
- **recount with the RN circulator.**[58,60,208]

[Recommendation]

Moderate-quality evidence[52,58] and guidance from a professional organization[60] support searching the sterile field to locate the missing item and recounting the type of item that is involved in the count discrepancy. Judson et al[52] and Rowlands and Steeves[97] recommended organizing the sterile field to facilitate the count process.

8.2.4 **When a discrepancy in the count is identified, the surgeon and surgical first assistant should**
- **suspend closure of the wound if the patient's condition permits,**[40,58,208]
- **perform a methodical wound examination while actively looking for the missing item,**[58,208]
- **participate in the attainment of intraoperative radiographs or other imaging modalities as indicated to find the missing item,**[58,208] **and**
- **remain in the OR until the item is found or it is determined not to be in the patient.**[208]

[Recommendation]

Figure 3. Count Reconciliation Decision Tree

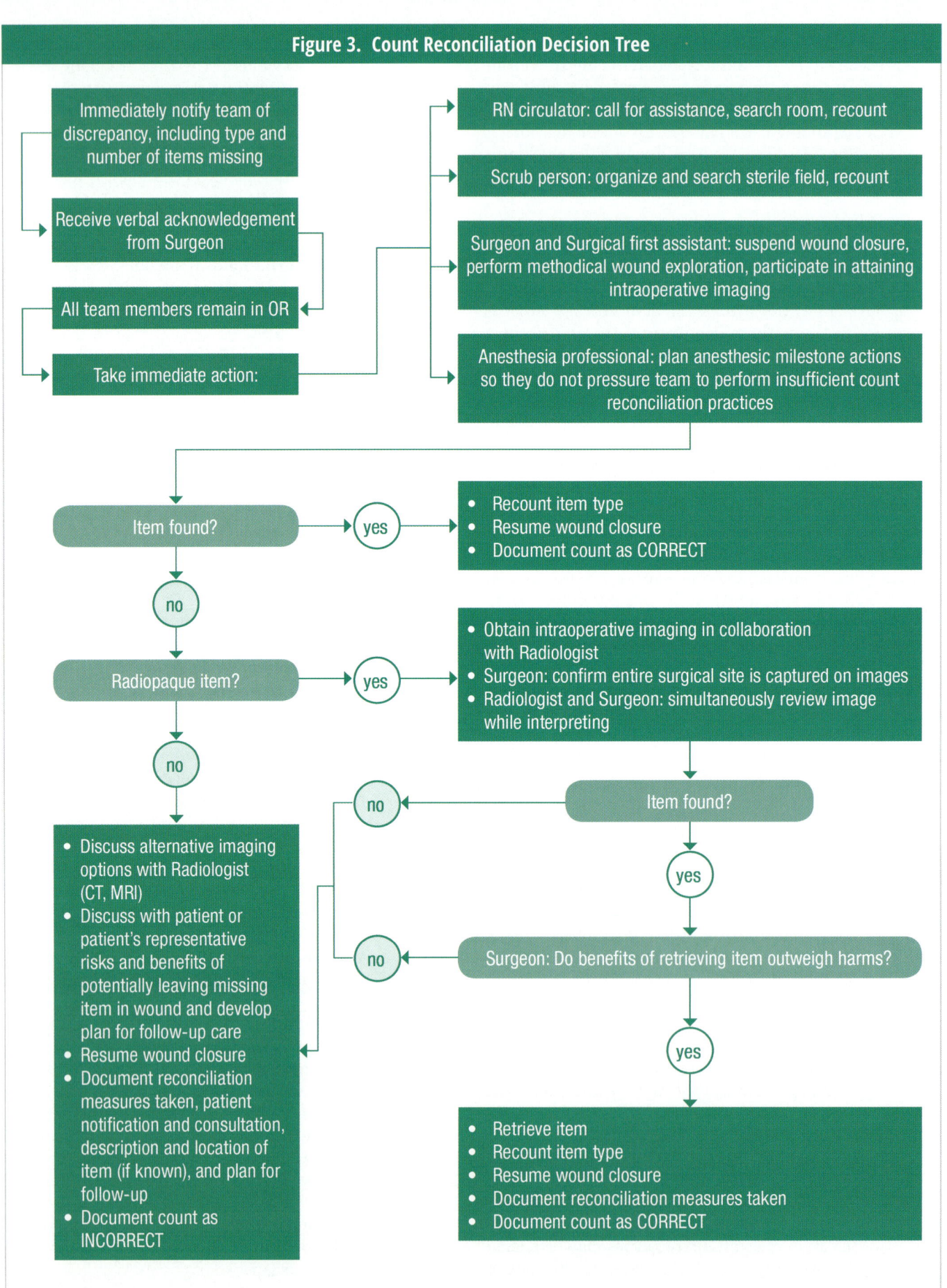

Moderate-quality evidence supports the surgeon performing a methodical wound exploration and obtaining radiographs as soon as possible when a count discrepancy is identified, if the patient's condition allows.[58,208] Stawicki et al[208] suggested that count discrepancies require a hard stop before wound closure, the patient's emergence from anesthesia, or the patient's leaving the OR, for reinspection of the surgical site and obtaining radiographic confirmation.

8.2.5 **When a discrepancy in the count is identified, the anesthesia professional should plan anesthetic milestone actions (eg, emergence from anesthesia) so that these actions do not pressure the perioperative team to perform insufficient count reconciliation practices (See Recommendation 1.2.4).**[77] *[Recommendation]*

8.2.6 **Nonessential personnel changes (eg, break, relief) should not occur until the count is resolved.** *[Recommendation]*

Judson et al[52] implemented the practice of a "No Hand-Off Zone," which defined a time when no breaks or relief of personnel were permitted until resolution of the count discrepancy.

8.2.7 **Do not use empty packages to reconcile count discrepancies.** *[Recommendation]*

Cima et al[58] recommended not reconciling counts with packages, as the number on the preprinted package may not be an accurate representation of items counted. A case report described how a third needle was found in a package of suture that was labeled as double armed.[212] The needle was found attached to the suture and was discovered when it dropped onto the table as the suture was being prepared for use. Only two suture needles were visible in the package, and that was the initial number counted.[212]

8.3 **When the missing item is found, recount the item type (eg, laparotomy sponges, suture needles).** *[Recommendation]*

Cima et al[58] recommended recounting the category of item that was missing as part of count reconciliation procedures.

8.4 **If a missing item is not recovered, perform intraoperative imaging to rule out a retained item before final closure of the wound if the patient's condition permits. If the patient's condition is**

unstable, take a radiograph as soon as possible in the next phase of care. *[Recommendation]*

Moderate-quality evidence[67,208,213] and guidance from professional organizations[60,61] support obtaining an intraoperative radiograph to find the missing item before final wound closure, if the patient's condition permits. Obtaining a radiograph when all other efforts have failed allows the surgical team to remove a potential RSI before the wound is closed completely.

8.4.1 **When accurate counting of surgical items is not possible, perform intraoperative imaging before the patient is transferred from the OR.** *[Recommendation]*

8.4.2 **If intraoperative imaging is not available, the health care organization should have a policy and procedure describing the actions and communication required between referring and receiving organizations.** *[Recommendation]* Ⓐ

8.4.3 **A radiograph to locate a possible retained item may be waived under certain circumstances as defined in the health care organization's policy and procedure.** *[Conditional Recommendation]*

There are situations in which it may be medically appropriate for the surgeon to determine that it is not in the individual patient's best interest to undergo an intraoperative radiograph to locate a potential RSI.

Researchers in one study concluded that radiography for a sponge that was 4 x 8 inches in length may be unnecessary in hand procedures when the incision is 2 cm or less in length and a misplaced sponge could be easily identified if it were in the patient.[214]

8.4.4 **Complete and detailed communication among the perioperative team, radiology technologists, and radiologists should occur during a request for radiological support to prevent an RSI. The radiology request should include standardized information about the missing surgical item, including**

- **the room in which the procedure is being performed or the patient is located,**
- **the patient's status,**
- **the type of radiograph and views needed,**
- **a description of the missing surgical item,**[42]
- **the procedure performed, and**
- **the surgical site, including involvement of any body cavities (eg, the abdomen).**

[Recommendation]

Moderate-quality evidence[52,58] and guidance from a professional organization[48] support using detailed, standardized communication with the radiologist when ordering radiographs to rule out an RSI. These activities may aid in the radiologist's ability to identify surgical items on the radiograph.

8.4.5 The radiology technologist should be called promptly and should respond expeditiously when an incorrect count occurs in the OR. [Recommendation]

8.4.6 Intraoperative imaging should provide full coverage of the surgical site and should include any views deemed necessary by the surgeon and radiologist to maximize the opportunity to identify a missing surgical item.[48] [Recommendation]

Moderate-quality evidence[8] and guidance from a professional organization[48] support imaging the entire surgical site and any involved body cavity with views deemed necessary by a collaborative decision between the surgeon and radiologist. There are reported incidents of an RSI attributed to failure to capture the full surgical site on radiographic imaging.

In a case-control study of 30 patients with RSIs, Lincourt et al[25] reported that for four patients, the imaging taken to resolve the count discrepancy did not capture the location of the retained item in the field of view. Grant-Orser et al[106] reported a case of a retained surgical sponge that was missed on imaging because the radiograph of the abdomen did not extend fully from the diaphragm to the pubis. Similarly, McIntyre et al[145] reported a case series of three patients with RSIs at the authors' institution; two of the patients had retained sponges that were missed on intraoperative imaging because of incomplete imaging of the abdomen.

As part of a radiographic screening protocol, Cima et al[8] implemented screening with high-resolution images taken with fixed radiology equipment that was located in a designated room inside the surgical suite. As part of this protocol, they identified 34 retained surgical sponges, needles, an instrument, and miscellaneous items with the high-resolution images.

Additional research is needed to determine the quality differences and effect on patient care (eg, benefits and harms, cost) of radiographs taken with fixed equipment in a radiology suite compared with images taken with portable equipment in an OR. The benefits of using portable imaging may outweigh the harms, depending on the clinical situation.

Edel[115] reported one radiology protocol for resolving count discrepancies that included obtaining an anterior and posterior film and a 20-degree view of the surgical site to provide the radiologist with two perspectives of the area.

One case report described how a metal-reinforced hair tie on the back of the patient's head resembled a retained throat pack on postoperative imaging of a patient that had bimaxillary osteotomies.[215] Details of this report show that it is important to consider objects that are in the field of the radiograph being taken.

8.4.7 Radiological techniques may include
- use of portable or fixed radiographic equipment[8];
- portable anterior and posterior and oblique views[115];
- multiple images for full coverage of the surgical site or body cavity as confirmed by the surgeon[25,106,145];
- fluoroscopy; and
- CT, which may be used postoperatively or intraoperatively (if available) when previous radiographic images are negative, and a high suspicion remains for an RSI. [Conditional Recommendation]

The evidence review found no literature to support the preference for use of a portable radiograph versus an image intensifier (ie, fluoroscopy unit). Additional research is needed to evaluate and compare the benefits and harms of various imaging techniques, such as plain portable radiograph, plain fixed radiograph, fluoroscopy (eg, C-arm),[216] CT imaging (eg, three dimensional [3D]),[165] MRI, ultrasound, and transesophageal echocardiogram[217] for intraoperative identification of radiopaque and non-radiopaque RSIs.

8.4.8 In addition to imaging of the surgical site, a sample image of an item similar to the missing object may be taken. [Conditional Recommendation]

Moderate-quality evidence suggests that a visual reference of the missing item may assist the radiologist in locating the item on the radiograph.[52,115,218] Gayer et al[219] explained various imaging presentations of RSIs and the complexity of identifying retained items amid other patient care items, such as packing, drains, and implants. Edel[115] and Judson et al[52] included imaging of a like item in their discrepancy protocols to facilitate the radiologist's review of the images. Hunter and Gimber[218] described a radiograph reference guide that was created for the radiologist reviewing radiograph screening images.

8.4.9 The radiologist and surgeon should simultaneously review and interpret intraoperative imaging for RSIs. When the radiologist is not immediately available, the surgeon should conduct a preliminary interpretation of the image. *[Recommendation]*

Judson et al[52] implemented a practice in their count discrepancy protocol, requiring that the attending surgeon speak with the attending radiologist either by telephone or in person while concurrently viewing the x-ray. Steelman et al[42] recommended a high-priority alert and a verbal report from the radiologist to the physician when an RSI is identified.

8.4.10 The health care organization's policy should define the needle size limits for which radiographs will be used to assist in identifying retained needles. *[Recommendation]*

Moderate-quality evidence is inconclusive about how effective radiographs are in detecting small suture needles. Several studies conflict regarding the ability to consistently locate 10-mm to 13-mm needles on radiographic screening when retention is suspected.[161,163,164,220]

Walter et al[30] performed a nonexperimental study of radiographs taken for surgical miscounts at a single institution. They found that the incidence of miscounts was 0.9%, and only 9% of miscounts were resolved through discovery of the item during differing times (eg, intraoperative, postoperative). The false-negative rate of the radiographs taken was 44% (four of nine). In two of three cases of missing needles, the needles were not identifiable on intraoperative radiographs. The retained needles were identified retrospectively on postoperative radiographs but were only visible in frontal and lateral views or through use of other technology such as CT. Two retained needles discovered postoperatively were not removed. The researchers stated that radiographs for small needles may be unnecessary and recommended additional study of the topic. Additional research is needed to determine the most effective and consistent radiographic detection method for small needles **(See Recommendation 4.1.1)**.

8.5 Unresolved count discrepancies must be documented in the patient's record. *[Regulatory Requirement]*

The Centers for Medicare & Medicaid Services requires surgical complications to be documented in the operative report.[206,207]

8.5.1 Documentation should include a description and the location of the item if known, all measures taken to recover the missing item, patient notification and consultation, and the plan for follow-up care. *[Recommendation]*

Moderate-quality evidence[52,58] and guidance from a professional organization[61] support documenting count reconciliation measures and consulting with the patient or patient's representative regarding the plan for follow-up, including additional imaging and possible risks of a potentially retained item. Judson et al[52] integrated their count reconciliation protocols into an electronic health record for documentation.

8.5.2 Notify environmental services personnel and the next perioperative team in the room about items reported missing in an unresolved count discrepancy. *[Recommendation]*

Having an unaccounted surgical item in the OR may affect the validity of subsequent counts. If the item missing is a sharp object, communication to other perioperative team members is important to alert them to the potential risk for a sharps injury.

9. Adjunct Technology

9.1 Use adjunct technology devices for the prevention of RSIs that are FDA-cleared or deemed exempt from premarket notification. *[Recommendation]*

The FDA uses a classification system and premarket notification process to determine the amount of regulation required for safety and effectiveness of medical devices used on humans.[221,222] Class I medical devices are generally exempt from premarket notification requirements.[222] Classification of medical devices and associated regulations are accessible in the FDA establishment registration and device listing online database.[223]

9.2 An interdisciplinary team should evaluate adjunct technologies before implementation in the health care organization. *[Recommendation]*

A thorough evaluation of any medical device is recommended before implementation into practice.[224]

9.2.1 Perioperative RNs, surgical technologists, physicians, infection preventionists, material management personnel, quality and risk managers, radiology personnel, sterile processing personnel, and other health care personnel involved in the use of the products and medical devices for prevention of RSIs should be part of the interdisciplinary product evaluation and selection committee when the health care organization is evaluating the purchase of adjunct technology.[224] [Recommendation]

The interdisciplinary team composition may differ depending on the device being evaluated. For instance, if the device selected for evaluation includes specialized instruments with **radio-frequency identification** (RFID) tags, then sterile processing personnel may provide important insights on the cleaning, disinfection, and sterilization processes.

9.2.2 Evaluate the
- manufacturer's instructions for feasibility in practice[54,55];
- process for cleaning, disinfection, and sterilization of reusable devices[183,225] (eg, instrument tags);
- process for cleaning and disinfection of equipment[226];
- preferences of perioperative personnel[55];
- associated costs[55];
- radio-frequency (RF) interference with temporary pacemakers[227,228] when applicable; and
- RFID interference with pacemakers, implantable cardioverter defibrillators, and other electronic medical devices.[229]

[Recommendation]

Evaluating adjunct technology before implementation can provide a comprehensive understanding of aspects to consider during decision-making processes and when developing an implementation plan. For a comprehensive analysis of cost, researchers have recommended including not only the cost of supplies, OR time, and radiography[230] but also costs absorbed by the facility and those that are not typically included in OR budgets, such as uncompensated patient care, state fines for retained sponges, and legal costs and settlements.[231] Several studies detailed the methods used for calculating time and costs.[40,55,230,231]

The literature search for this guideline revision identified evidence published on two different adjunct technology systems that use RF and **data-matrix-coded sponges** (eg, bar-coded sponges). Older evidence from laboratory studies on use of RFID for prevention of retained surgical sponges from a specific manufacturer is available in the literature but was not discussed because that system is not currently used in patient care.[233,234] No evidence was found on the RFID systems that are available for use with soft goods and instruments.

When evaluating the literature regarding use of adjunct technology to prevent retained sponges, it is important to note that the time to discovery of a retained sponge can vary. This is important because the follow-up period used in evidence can vary and therefore it may be possible that a retained sponge is discovered after the study has ended.

Radio-Frequency Detection
Evidence on use of RF detection adjunct technology reported either an elimination[5,54,234] or reduction[40] of retained sponges during the study period or after implementation. Inaba et al[5] reported no RSIs of any type in a 5-year period of RF use during emergency procedures. During the study, before the wound was closed, manual counting was performed, the patient was scanned with the RF system, and radiography was taken as a control. In two patients, the sponge count was reported as correct, but the RF system detected a retained sponge.[5]

In a nonexperimental study by Rupp et al,[54] the organization had previously implemented the Sponge ACCOUNTing System protocol that reduced but did not eliminate RSIs. After the organization implemented RF detection, the authors reported that no RSIs occurred with use of RF adjunct technology during a 1-year period. The researchers reported that one near miss occurred when the count was correct, but the RF device detected a sponge in the drapes. The device helped resolve 35 count discrepancies, 11 of which involved sponges found in the patient's body or surgical site.[54]

In an expert opinion article discussing the implementation of an RF detection system at a facility, Norton[234] stated that no sponges were retained in the 3 years after implementation. In an organizational experience article, Primiano et al[235] reviewed incident reports of retained sponges at a level-one trauma center before and after implementation of an RF detection system. The number of retained sponges for the 2 years before and 2 years after implementation were 56 and 18, respectively. However, a retained sponge was defined as a sponge that was not accounted for at the end of the procedure (eg, unreconciled final sponge count). No potential reasons for the 18 unaccounted sponges were discussed in the article.[235]

In a nonexperimental study, Williams et al[40] reported that use of RF detection technology at five organizations collectively reduced the rate of reported retained surgical sponges by 93% during a 6-year period. However, there was a decrease in RSI rates before the implementation of the technology, and the technology was implemented at different facilities at different times. Conversely, the reduction in the rate of reported retained surgical sponges at five organizations that did not use RF detection technology during the 6-year period was 77%. The organizations that used RF detection technology had retained sponge rates that trended down compared to a variable number of occurrences at organizations that did not use the technology.

The researchers suggested that the variability in occurrences at the organizations that did not use RF technology meant that the reduction in reported rates of retained sponges may not be sustained. They speculated that use of RF detection technology did not eliminate RSIs because there was operator error, accidental use of sponges that did not have RF detection, or because the technology was not used in all procedures.[40]

Equipment failures were described in a few reports, but the causes were unclear (eg, true equipment failure versus personnel not following the instructions for use). The researchers recommended wide adoption of the technology, consistent use, education on how to use the technology, and prevention of accidental use of non-RF sponges. The researchers stated that it is important to use RF detection technology even in areas of the body not normally identified as high risk.[40]

The use of RF detection adjunct technology is also reported to identify or reduce
- near misses[5,54,234,235];
- count discrepancies (eg, miscounted or misplaced soft goods)[5,54,235];
- time spent searching for soft goods or resolving count discrepancies[54,231,234,235];
- the number of radiographs taken,[235] associated time and costs[231] and patient exposure[40,234];
- additional procedures to remove a retained sponge[235];
- costs[234,235]; and
- the potential for contamination of personnel going through waste receptacles to find a sponge.[231]

In a nonexperimental study of retained surgical soft goods reported to The Joint Commission in a 5-year period, Steelman et al[15] stated that if RF detection technology had been used correctly, it may have prevented up to 97.2% of incidents (n = 310 of 319). Use of RF detection technology would not have prevented the retention of the nine other items reported in the study, including pledgets, Kerlix gauze, a peanut sponge, and a non-radiopaque sponge from an anesthesia kit, because those items are not available for use with this technology.[15]

Overall, the use of RF detection adjunct technology devices is reported to result in time and cost savings.[40,231,235] However, the evidence cannot be synthesized because of the differences in calculating methodologies used and may not be generalizable due to differences among facilities. Rupp et al[54] did not evaluated time in their study, but the researchers stated that time spent using the system is negligible because it was performed in tandem with other surgical processes.

In 2016, researchers in Los Angeles, California, reported that additional costs for a single RF laparotomy sponge (4 x 18) was $0.17 and a 10-pack of 4 x 8 12-ply RF gauze sponges was $0.46.[5] Authors of a 2020 QI initiative performed in Northeast Ohio estimated that the institution saved approximately $424,[292] in 1 year of routine use of RF detection technology, even with the cost of education of personnel and use of proprietary sponges, because use of the device decreased time spent resolving count discrepancies, use of radiography, and reoperations.[235]

A 2014 nonexperimental study by Williams et al[40] on data from five organizations that participated in the UHC calculated that to transition from radiology detection to RF detection technology would cost an estimated $191,352 annually or $17.09 per procedure. However, the annual costs savings from reductions in time to resolve counting discrepancies, time and use of radiography, additional hospital care of patients with retained sponges, and legal settlement fees saved from preventing two retained sponges was estimated to be $598,558. Therefore, use of RF detection technology was estimated to save $407,206 annually.[40]

In a 2019 nonexperimental study, Steelman et al[231] found implementation of a low-frequency RF identification system reduced unreconciled final counts by 71.28%, the time spent searching for sponges by 79.58% per 1,000 procedures, and the number of minutes spent obtaining radiographs by 46.31%. After implementation, the researchers reported estimated annual reductions in cost of OR time spent searching for sponges ($3,803.04 per 1,000 procedures), cost of intraoperative radiographs ($516.98 per 1,000 procedures), and cost of time spent performing the radiographs ($2,030.91 per 1,000 procedures). For facilities in which 15,000 procedures are performed per year, the total annual estimated cost savings of implementing an RF adjunct technology system on the time spent searching for sponges and performing radiography was estimated to be $95,263.95.[231]

There are some important considerations to be aware of when an RF detection system is used:

- There may be electromagnetic interference with temporary pacemakers (See Recommendation 9.3.6).
- An alert from the device indicates the presence of a sponge but not the actual location inside of the patient's body. For example, if the alarm sounded when scanning the left side of the abdomen, the sponge may be in either the left or right side of the abdomen.[56]
- Device alerts do not distinguish between the number or types of sponges in the location scanned (eg, patient, waste receptacle).[24]
- For patients with super morbid obesity (ie, BMI exceeding 50), it is recommended to use an RF wand instead of an RF mat.[57]

The presence of various types of implants, jewelry, prostheses, and other items (eg, bullets, a brace, a tracheostomy appliance) have not been found to interfere with or activate RF detection alarms.[56,57] Interference initially found with some items (eg, name badges, pagers, keys) was reported to be corrected in subsequent software updates.[56]

A survey of perioperative personnel who performed the RF detection system scan showed that the process was easy to use, did not prolong the procedure, and improved confidence in the outcome of the final count.[54] Another author reported that surveyed personnel had a high level of satisfaction specifically related to the ability of the device to locate a sponge during a count discrepancy.[234]

Data-Matrix-Coded System

There is less published evidence specific to data-matrix-coded sponge systems[55,236,237] and the evidence is too diverse to synthesize.

In a randomized controlled trial, Greenberg et al[236] compared a bar-coded sponge system (ie, two-dimensional [2D] matrix) to a traditional count protocol in 300 elective general surgery procedures and found that the bar-coding system detected significantly more counting discrepancies (eg, misplaced or miscounted sponges) than manual counting methods.[236] A misplaced sponge was found inside the patient before the patient left the OR three times when the bar-code system was used. Significantly more miscounts were identified when the bar-code system was used and four of the events included "technological saves" such as when the system alerted the individual and helped to avoid an error. Although the system helped the team identify count discrepancies, it did not decrease the time spent to resolve the discrepancy. After 60 days, a review of patient medical records did not identify any retained sponges.

The researchers reported 17 incidences of technological difficulties occurring at a rate of 2.04 per 1,000 sponges counted. Examples of technological difficulties included scanning of a sponge that was behind the sponge being actively scanned and attempting to "scan out" a sponge when the scanner was set to "scan in." The time spent counting the sponges was significantly higher when the bar-code system was used compared to the manual counting process (eg, an additional 3 minutes per procedure). However, the study was conducted in conjunction with the introduction of the system at the facility, and although no trend indicating a learning curve was identified, only 44% of personnel had used the system more than 10 times.[236]

There was no significant difference in the duration of the procedures between those in which the technology was used and those in which it was not. A survey of the personnel involved showed that most personnel felt confident that the device was tracking the sponges and that it was easy to use, but the researchers subjectively noted that some personnel struggled to use the device during the initial learning curve. The researchers concluded that by increasing detection of discrepancies, the technology has a strong potential to decrease the risk of retained sponges.[236]

In an organizational experience study, Cima et al[237] reported on implementation of a data-matrix-coded (ie, 2D matrix) sponge system at a large health care organization. They initially conducted two trials to assess the system before institution-wide implementation. In an 18-month period during which 87,404 procedures were performed, no RSIs were reported. The first trial measured time spent counting data-matrix-coded sponges (n = 365) and control sponges (n = 335) for colon and rectal procedures. Although the initial time for counting data-matrix-coded sponges was 11 seconds, the time was reduced to 5 seconds after 4 days of implementation; the average time to count control sponges was 4 seconds. Staff reported an acceptable level of satisfaction and a high degree of trust in the system. Use of the system did not cause increases in procedural duration.[237]

An organizational experience report may not be generalizable to other institutions.[237] In another organizational experience article from the same organization, Thiels et al[23] reported two retained sponges in approximately 1.5 million procedures in the 5-year period after implementation of the data-matrix-coded system.

In a study on relative cost-effectiveness, researchers predicted that use of bar-coded sponges would be cost-effective in many situations when compared with manual counting processes.[55]

9.3 Use an adjunct technology device to detect the location of surgical soft goods or to verify the outcome of manual counting procedures for surgical soft goods, when possible. *[Recommendation]*

Moderate-quality evidence[5,6,15,21,40,53,54,231,234-237] and guidance from the ACS[61] support the use of adjunct technology to verify the location or outcome of manual counting procedures for surgical soft goods. The ACS recommends the use of x-rays or adjunct technology to verify there are no unintended items in the operative field.[61] Other evidence,[8,29] literature from an accrediting body,[48] and guidance from professional organizations[60,238] support evaluating and considering the use of adjunct technology devices that become available. Use of adjunct technology does not replace manual counting processes but it may help identify counting discrepancies.

Retained sponges are the most commonly reported type of RSI[3,8,13-15] and continue to occur despite manual counting processes and use of radiography.[40,235] Manual counting of sponges continues to be important, but it can be susceptible to human error.[4,5,236] In incidences of RSIs, the count has been reported as correct (eg, **correct count**) between 62% to 88% of the time.[4,8,208] In a study specific to RSIs involving soft goods, the count was reported as correct 80.6% of the time in records that indicated a count had been performed (77.4%).[15] Other studies have also reported incidences of retained sponges when the count was reported as correct.[33,40]

The accuracy of manual counting, radiographs, and some adjunct technology devices has been reported in the literature. These data are important in evaluation of processes or technologies used to detect counting discrepancies or prevent RSIs

(Table 3).[29] The sensitivity, specificity, and positive predictive value of the manual counting processes has been reported to be 77.2%, 99.2%, and 1.6%, respectively.[29] Therefore, the ability of manual counting procedures to distinguish between a miscount, a misplaced item, or an RSI is low.[29] The researchers concluded that to reach a positive predictive value in the 50% range, manual counting processes would have to improve dramatically, and that level of improvement is unlikely to be achieved with processes that rely on manual counting alone.[29]

Cima et al[8] reported that the sensitivity of radiography in incidences of RSIs was only 67%; routine intraoperative imaging did not find six of 18 RSIs.[8] Stawicki et al[208] also reported that an RSI was missed on initial x-ray interpretation in 13 of 27 procedures (48%). In an organizational experience article, Williams et al[40] reported that two incidences of retained sponges were not identified on the x-ray taken at the end of the procedure. Conversely, in laboratory studies the overall sensitivity of an RF wand was 100%[56,57] and of an RF mat was 98.1%.[57] The sensitivity of data-matrix-coded sponge system has not been reported in the literature.

The use of an adjunct technology system to verify the outcome of the manual count may help identify count discrepancies[5,236] and increase patient safety.[56] Counting discrepancies occur in one of every eight procedures and take an average of 13 minutes to resolve.[53] When there is a count discrepancy, the odds of an RSI increase by more than 100 times.[29] Many discrepancies involve a misplaced sponge; when this occurs there is a potential risk of an RSI.[53] Other counting discrepancies include miscounting, addition errors, and documentation.[53] Therefore, use of adjunct technology could improve human performance.[53]

There are limitations to use of these devices and the supporting evidence. Adjunct technology can only be used with integrated surgical soft goods. Some surgical soft goods (eg, pledgets, peanut sponges) may not have the technology available. High-quality evidence from RCTs to identify whether use of adjunct technology significantly reduces the incidence of retained surgical sponges would require randomization of more than 100,000 patients[55] and could take years to obtain or might never become available.

Most of the evidence is also limited by a focus on one of the two different types of adjunct technology systems available: RF[5,15,40,54,56,57,230,231,234,235] or data-matrix-coded sponges (eg, bar-coded sponges).[55,236,237] The evidence specific to each system cannot be generalized to the other. Additionally, no research was identified that compared use or outcomes between the two systems. Some studies or researchers

Table 3. Reported Rates of Accuracy Related to Processes Used for Prevention of Retained Surgical Items

Type	Sensitivity[a]	Specificity[b]	Positive Predictive Value[c]
Manual Counting Processes[1]	77.2%	99.2%	1.6%
Radiography[2]	67%	NR	NR
Radio-Frequency Adjunct Technology[3,4]	Wand 100% Mat 98.1%	Wand 100% Mat 100%	Wand NR Mat 100%

NR = Not Reported

[a] **Sensitivity:** The percentage of patients with a condition in which a procedure used to identify the condition produces positive results; an assessment of the value of a process (eg, the proportion of patients who have a retained sponge correctly identified by a process).

[b] **Specificity:** The proportion of individuals who do not have a condition in whom a process used to identify the condition yields negative results; the ability of a process to exclude individuals that are free of a condition (eg, the proportion of patients correctly identified as not having a retained sponge).

[c] **Positive Predictive Value:** The probability that a positive result accurately indicated the condition is present; the percentage of times that the value (positive or negative) is the correct value.

References

1. Egorova NN, Moskowitz A, Gelijns A, et al. Managing the prevention of retained surgical instruments: what is the value of counting? Ann Surg. 2008;247(1):13-18.
2. Cima RR, Kollengode A, Garnatz J, Storsveen A, Weisbrod C, Deschamps C. Incidence and characteristics of potential and actual retained foreign object events in surgical patients. J Am Coll Surg. 2008;207(1):80-87.
3. Steelman VM. Sensitivity of detection of radiofrequency surgical sponges: a prospective, cross-over study. Am J Surg. 2011;201(2):233-237.
4. Steelman VM, Alasagheirin MH. Assessment of radiofrequency device sensitivity for the detection of retained surgical sponges in patients with morbid obesity. Arch Surg. 2012;147(10):955-960.

have been supported, at least in part, by industry,[40,53,54,57,231,236] which could be perceived as a potential conflict of interest. However, appraisals of the studies did not detect evidence of bias. Other sources did not indicate industry support,[5,234,235,237,239] and some were funded by governmental agencies.[29,55,56]

This body of evidence may also be limited by the reluctance of organizations to publish information about retained sponges[208] and susceptibility to publication bias. More research is needed, and use of standard definitions for retained sponge, near miss, count discrepancy, miscount, and misplaced item may provide clarity.

There is also conflicting evidence on the use of adjunct technology devices to reduce the rates of RSIs. Gunnar et al[239] performed a nonexperimental study of RSIs that occurred in 137 Veterans Health Administration surgical programs during a 6-year period. The purpose of the study was to compare RSI rates between programs with and without adjunct technology. The researchers found that the RSI rates for the 46 programs with adjunct technology were significantly higher than the 91 programs without it. Additionally, the researchers reported that the RSI rates before and after implementation of adjunct technology were not significantly different. However, the researchers did not report on device use (eg, if it was used, how it was used [eg, according to

manufacturer's instructions for use]). Therefore, the RSI rates before and after implementation of the device only meant that they device had been purchased by the facility. It is unclear if the device was used during procedures involving an RSI. Furthermore, the researchers did not distinguish between the types of adjunct technology used or report the rates of retained soft goods separately. The RSI rates reported in the study included soft goods, sharps, and instruments.[239] Therefore, the effect of adjunct technology on the specific soft goods with which it was used is unclear.

Time and costs associated with reconciliation of count discrepancies has been reported in the literature. According to Egorova et al[29] counting procedures occur simultaneously with other surgical tasks and therefore do not affect the duration of surgery unless there is a count discrepancy; therefore, the researchers suggested only accounting for costs attributed to counting discrepancies. Many facilities use radiology as part of the count discrepancy reconciliation process. However, selective use of radiology in high-risk procedures and counting discrepancies, although less costly than universal use (eg, after all procedures involving a cavity), is estimated to be $1 million for each retained sponge prevented.[55] It is important to note that use of radiology has additional risks and benefits not associated with adjunct technology including radiographic exposure and the potential to detect other retained items such as needles and instruments.[55]

In a 2015 nonexperimental study, Steelman et al[230] found that the total annual cost of searching for missing sponges and use of radiography was $219,056. For the 212 sponge counts that required reconciliation in a 9-month period, the time spent searching for missing sponges was between 1 and 90 minutes in each event, and the total amount was calculated to be 1,700 minutes.

In a 2009 nonexperimental study, Regenbogen et al[55] found that adjunct technology would need to almost eliminate the possibility of a retained sponge occurring and cost less than $26 per procedure to be considered cost-saving. In a systematic review using data from Regenbogen et al,[55] the authors reported that using standard counting practices is the most economical strategy compared to other technologies used to prevent retained sponges.[240]

The benefits of using adjunct technology to verify the outcome of the manual soft goods count outweighs the potential risks. Use of either system is shown to decrease count discrepancies[231,236] and may reduce the risk of retained surgical soft goods.[5,54,231,235-237] Therefore, use of adjunct technology decreases the time and costs associated with resolution of count discrepancies. When there are fewer count discrepancies, the process may be more efficient.[55] Implementation of either system will require time and education of personnel and will likely incur initial startup costs.[55] These requirements may be burdensome to smaller facilities.[55] However, the RF system[40,231,235] has been shown to reduce annual costs, and the data-matrix system[55] was predicted to be cost-effective when compared to manual counting processes.

Risk for retained soft goods still exists if the adjunct technology device is not used according to the manufacturer's instructions for use.[40,57,236] Stawicki et al[208] reported that two RSIs occurred despite use of RF tagging and cautioned that use of technology alone cannot completely prevent RSIs. An integral part of patient care is to follow safety procedures.[208] Observational audits of device use to confirm compliance with manufacturers' instructions for use have been recommended.[15] **See Recommendation 13.4** for information on monitoring for quality.

Another potential risk is detachment of the tracking device and potential RSI, which may be minimized by inspecting the product before and after use. However, no published reports of harm from manufacturing defects were found in the literature. Some benefits and risks are specific to the type of adjunct technology used and are discussed in **Section 9.2.2**.

9.3.1   **Clarify in facility policy and procedure when use of adjunct technology may be waived.** *[Conditional Recommendation]*

If use of adjunct technology may be waived in specific instances or procedures, outlining the details in facility policy and procedure can help provide clarity to personnel providing care. For instance, if surgical soft goods associated with adjunct technology are not used during an eye procedure, facility policy may specify that this procedure may be exempt from device use. Alternatively, facility personnel may believe that some procedures are extremely low risk for retained sponges, such as procedures involving small incisions performed on digits or feet. It is important to note that retained soft goods have been reported in most body locations including the eye.[15] Adjunct technology use during emergent procedures was supported in a nonexperimental study by Inaba et al.[5]

Tofte and Caldwell[214] conducted a quasi-experimental study to determine the length of a surgical sponge (ie, 4 x 8) that could fit in an incision 2 cm or less in length in the hand and the ability of physicians to visualize a sponge in the wound from different distances in the OR. The researchers found that only 3 cm of a surgical sponge could fit in a carpal tunnel incision 2 cm or less in length and that all sponges placed in a wound of this size could be visualized from 10 feet away and when the physician was standing at the table. All the simulated procedures performed in this study were in the hand specialty. Based on the study findings, the researchers concluded that use of RF detection of 4 x 8 sponges did not add benefit and can be eliminated if the sponges can be reliably visually detected.[214] However, because sponges still need to be accounted for at the end of a procedure, the location of any misplaced sponge would still need to be identified. Use of the RF system has been shown to reduce time spent reconciling count discrepancies.[231] Additionally, if a sponge is misplaced off the sterile field, the RF device may be used to locate it.[231]

9.3.2   **Use adjunct technology in accordance with the manufacturer's instructions for use.**[15,40,57] *[Recommendation]*

Using the device as intended by the manufacturer provides the highest level of assurance that the device is functioning correctly and that the data collected and reported by the device is accurate. Steelman et al[15] reported nine incidences of retained soft goods where RF detection or RFID systems were used. In most of the occurrences the technology was used after incision closure. In the remaining instances, the technology was used but the detection alarm was ignored, the scan was performed in the postanesthesia care unit, and the retained item was a Kerlix gauze that did not have the imbedded technology.

Williams et al[40] reported that incidences of retained sponges can still occur if the technology is not used in all procedures, the RF sponges necessary for the device are omitted, or the device is not used properly. For instance, using the wand of an RF system at too great of a distance from the patient's body may lead to false-negative results.[57] Some difficulties with the sponge scanning process were reported when a data-matrix-coded sponge system is used.[236] However, sponge scanning difficulties associated with data-matrix systems may be more likely when personnel are initially learning to use the technology.[236,237]

9.3.3 **Use sterile technique when using adjunct technology devices on the sterile field.** *[Recommendation]*

9.3.4 **Implement adjunct technology throughout the organization at the same time.** *[Recommendation]*

It is important to prevent simultaneous access to soft goods with and without imbedded adjunct technology. Use of both types of sponges in one organization could increase the potential for an RSI. Use of an institution-wide implementation process instead of a multiphase process (eg, different departments start device use at different times) is described in the literature.[237] Many different procedural areas may use surgical soft goods. Steelman et al[15] reported that retention of soft goods occurred in the OR, labor and delivery unit, interventional radiology lab, cardiac catheterization lab, and a urology clinic. The researchers also stated that a use of sponge counts and RF technology in labor and delivery units may decrease the risk of retained sponges and maternal morbidity.[15]

9.3.5 **Use adjunct technology even when the count is correct.** *[Recommendation]*

Retention of soft goods may still occur when the count is correct.[4,8,208] Therefore, only using the technology when there is a count discrepancy or when the count is incorrect, may prevent identification of retained sponges.

9.3.6 **Use devices that use RF and RFID technology with caution in patients with pacemakers, implantable cardioverter defibrillators, and other electronic medical devices.** *[Recommendation]*

According to the FDA, RFID transmitters may interfere with electronic medical devices.[229] No published incidents of patient harm from electromagnetic interference (EMI) from RFID devices used to prevent retained surgical sponges were found in the literature.

In an in vitro study, Seidman et al[241] tested the electromagnetic compatibility of passive RFID readers with implanted cardiac pacemakers and internal cardioverter defibrillators. The tests included 13 passive RFID readers at low-frequency (134 kHz), high-frequency (15.56 kHz), and ultra-high-frequency (915 kHz). The type of RFID readers that the researchers used for testing were not specified. The researchers found that EMI levels were different among the different frequencies, with low frequency being the most susceptible to interference, high frequency to a lesser degree, and no EMI from the ultra-high frequency RFID devices that were tested. The researchers stated that they did not believe that the current situation reveals an urgent public health risk but advised caution with increasing use of RFID into the future because of the potential for clinically significant events for patients with implanted cardiac devices.

9.3.7 **Verbally notify perioperative team members before using adjunct technology devices that use RF and RFID. Perioperative team members should verbally respond in acknowledgment of the notification.** *[Recommendation]*

Warning perioperative team members before using adjunct technology devices that use RF and RFID allows for time to take precautions to prevent EMI with medical devices in use and to prepare the sterile field for scanning.[242]

9.3.8 **Do not program pacemakers or implantable cardioverter defibrillators during active use of adjunct technology devices that use RF or RFID.**[242] *[Recommendation]*

9.3.9 **Set temporary pacemakers to asynchronous mode before using adjunct technology devices that use RF and RFID, when possible.**[15,227,228] *[Recommendation]*

Use of an asynchronous mode has been found to prevent pacemaker inhibition.[227,228] Six cases of temporary pacemaker inhibition have been reported when adjunct technology with RF was used.[227,228,242] Pacing inhibition was reported to last approximately 3 seconds[228] and lead to transient hypotension[228] and an asystolic pause.[242] Incidences of EMI occurred when a RF wand was actively used over the patient[227] and resolved when the wand was removed.[228,242] None of the patients experienced adverse outcomes, probably because of the prompt recognition and limited duration of the pacemaker inhibition.[228,242] Researchers recommend vigilant monitoring of the patient's cardiac rhythm when adjunct technology with RF is actively used near the temporary pacemaker system.[227] Inhibition has not been reported in permanent pacemaker systems[227] and this may be a result of how these systems are managed intraoperatively with the use of programing or a magnet to produce an asynchronous mode.[228]

There may be clinical situations during which the use of asynchronous mode is not optimal[228] and could contribute to cardiac complications.[242] Researchers recommend that providers weigh the risks and benefits of pacemaker inhibition for each patient individually when use of an asynchronous mode is not clinically optimal.[228]

9.3.10 **Clean and disinfect adjunct technology equipment after each use in accordance with the manufacturer's instructions for use.**[226] *[Recommendation]*

9.3.11 **Document the use of adjunct technology devices in the patients' medical record.**[234] *[Recommendation]*

9.3.12 **Additional information associated with the use of adjunct technology devices may be documented in the patients' medical record or recorded in Health Insurance Portability and Accountability Act (HIPAA)-compliant facility records.** *[Conditional Recommendation]*

When used, adjunct technology systems may provide varying levels of detailed information for each patient procedure. How information associated with adjunct technology use is documented or recorded may differ due to many variables (eg, adjunct technology system used, documentation system used). Some devices may interface directly with the patient medical record. Conversely, other systems may create HIPAA-compliant facility records.

The author of an organizational experience article described how the facility required the nurses to enter the scan identification number in the patient's medical record as a way to ver-

ify that the adjunct technology was used.[234] The authors of a second organizational experience article stated that the surgeon documented the confirmation number from the wand in the patient's operative note.[235] It is important to note that documentation of a scan identification number or a confirmation number from an adjunct technology device does not provide information on how the device was used.

9.3.13 **Facility records of information associated with use of adjunct technology devices should be retrievable by all members of the health care team that use the information (eg, perioperative nurses, wound care nurses).** *[Recommendation]*

Health care personnel outside of perioperative team members may require access to facility records involving information on use of adjunct technology. For instance, if therapeutic packing is used, wound care nurses and other members of the health care team (eg, nurses in intensive care) may need access to the records.

9.3.14 **Provide education and competency verification to perioperative personnel who use adjunct technology.**[40] *[Recommendation]*

It is important that personnel understand how the technology works and can use it according to the manufacturer's instructions for use. Without correct and consistent use of the technology, errors may still occur and could lead to retained sponges even when the technology is used.[40]

9.4 **The interdisciplinary team may evaluate RFID FDA-cleared adjunct technology for detecting retained surgical instruments as a supplement to manual count procedures.**[243-245] *[Conditional Recommendation]*

Moderate-quality evidence indicates that RFID tags used on surgical instruments is an emerging adjunct technology with potential application for prevention of retained surgical instruments.[243-245] Results from two studies with limited sample sizes showed that the technology was feasible for real-time, reliable instrument detection.[243,244] However, continuous application of electrosurgery currents[244] or placement of an instrument outside of the area detectable by the antenna may interfere with RF detection.[243] Surgical instrument tracking may also have applications for education,[244,245] usage rates, and inventory and instrument tray optimization.[243] However, additional research is needed to validate the efficacy, safety,[229] and cost-effectiveness of adjunct technology (ie, RFID tags) for surgical instrument tracking.[243-245]

9.4.1 The RFID tags for surgical instruments should be used, cleaned, and sterilized in accordance with the device and instrument manufacturer's validated and written instructions for use.[183,225] [Recommendation]

Items cannot be assumed to be clean, decontaminated, or sterile unless the manufacturer's instructions for use are derived from validation testing and the user has followed those instructions.[183] The device manufacturer has validated the cycle, identified in the instructions for use, that must be used for effective sterilization.[225]

Yamashita et al[246] evaluated the effectiveness of a washer-disinfector for cleaning surgical instruments with attached RFID tags. After fixation of simulated contaminants (sheep blood treated with heparin and 1% protamine sulfate) on the surgical instrument RFID tag, the researchers cleaned one group of instruments in a washer-disinfector and another group in an ultrasonic washer; a third group underwent no cleaning process.

Following these interventions, the residual protein was recovered and measured using cleaning appraisal guidelines from Japan and Germany. The results showed that the washer-disinfector was effective in achieving recommended residual protein amounts after cleaning of instruments with RFID tags. Although the researchers concluded that secondary infection risk from surgical instruments with RFID tags attached was low, the study was not designed to assess patient outcomes and infection risk. A major limitation of this study was that the sample size and type of instruments were not reported.[246]

9.4.2 Account for RFID tags attached to surgical instruments before and immediately after use in an operative or other invasive procedure. [Recommendation]

An RFID tag detached from a surgical instrument in the patient may become an RSI. Kranzfelder et al[244] used RFID tagged instruments in 10 laparoscopic cholecystectomies and no RFID tag failures occurred.

9.4.3 Use RFID with caution in patients with pacemakers, implantable cardioverter defibrillators, and other electronic medical devices. [Recommendation]

According to the FDA, RFID transmitters may interfere with electronic medical devices.[229] No published incidents of patient harm from electronic medical device interference or EMI were found in the evidence review. Yamashita et al[246]

found that the antenna could not detect the RFID instrument tag if there was interference from electrocautery. Kranzfelder et al[244] reported that an electromagnetic tolerance certificate was obtained to avoid interference with technology surrounding the OR.

10. Documentation

10.1 Document activities related to prevention of RSIs [Recommendation]

Documentation is a professional medicolegal standard. Documentation related to prevention of RSIs is applicable at the systems level and the patient care level. At the systems level, documentation serves as a basis for monitoring compliance and measuring performance as part of a quality assurance program. At the patient care level, documentation facilitates continuity of patient care through clear communication and supports collaboration among health care team members.

10.2 The RN circulator should document the outcome of soft good, sharp, miscellaneous item, and instrument counts on the patient's intraoperative record. [Recommendation]

Documentation of nursing activities related to the patient's perioperative care provides an account of the nursing care administered and provides a mechanism for comparing actual versus expected outcomes.[247] Such documentation is considered sound professional practice and demonstrates that all reasonable efforts were made to protect the patient's safety by preventing an RSI.

10.3 Include the following in documentation of measures taken for the prevention of RSIs:
- types of counts (eg, radiopaque sponges, sharps, miscellaneous items, instruments);
- number of counts;
- names and titles of personnel performing the counts[60,248];
- results of surgical item counts (ie, correct or incorrect)[48,60,61];
- verification of removal and integrity of objects[42];
- surgeon notification of count results[61];
- an explanation for any waived counts[60];
- number and location of any instruments intentionally remaining with the patient or radiopaque sponges intentionally retained as therapeutic packing[48,60,61];
- actions taken if count discrepancies occurred, including all measures taken to recover the

missing item or device fragment and any patient communication regarding the outcome[48,60,61];

- rationale if counts were not performed or completed as prescribed by policy[60]; and
- the outcome of actions taken. [Recommendation]

Professional organizations recommend documenting RSI prevention activities.[48,60,61] In a description of a legal RSI case in the United Kingdom, Brown and Feather[248] noted that three circulating nurses were documented as participating in the surgery but it was not clear who verified the final count. They recommended that the name of each person performing the count be clearly documented.

Extreme patient emergencies and certain individual patient considerations may necessitate waived counts to preserve a patient's life or limb. Documenting the rationale for waived counts and for variation in count procedures provides a record of the occurrence and an alert to subsequent health care providers that the patient may be at an increased risk for an RSI.

11. Policies and Procedures

11.1 Develop policies and procedures for the prevention of RSIs, review them periodically, revise them as necessary, and make them readily available in the practice setting. [Recommendation]

Policies and procedures assist in the development of patient safety, quality assessment, and performance improvement activities. Policies and procedures establish organizational authority, responsibility, and accountability. Policies and procedures also serve as operational guidelines that are used to minimize patient risk for injury or complications, standardize practice, direct perioperative personnel, and establish continuous performance improvement programs.

11.1.1 An interdisciplinary team should develop policies and procedures for preventing RSIs.[60,61,208] [Recommendation]

Developing and maintaining policies and procedures that guide patient care is a regulatory requirement for both hospitals and ambulatory settings.[206,207] Some accrediting bodies may require policies and procedures specifically for surgical counts.

In addition to regulatory and accreditation requirements, the evidence review also included recommendations for RSI prevention policies and procedures in the literature[208] and from professional organizations.[60,61] Stawicki et al[208] recommended that surgical facilities maintain and enforce a surgical safety policy for RSI prevention.

11.1.2 The interdisciplinary team should include perioperative nurses, surgeons, anesthesia professionals, sterile processing personnel, risk managers, leaders, and other stakeholders as deemed necessary. [Recommendation]

11.2 Include the following in policies and procedures for prevention of RSI:

- how noise, distractions, and unnecessary interruptions will be minimized during counting procedures;
- items to be counted;
- when counts should be performed (eg, before the patient enters the OR or procedure room, at designated intervals during lengthy procedures);
- directions for performing counts (eg, sequence, item grouping);
- waived count procedures in which baseline and/or subsequent counts may be exempt;
- interdisciplinary team actions and procedures for count discrepancy reconciliation;
- use of radiographic screening;
- use of adjunct technology; and
- documentation and reporting procedures for RSIs and near misses.

[Recommendation]

11.2.1 If intraoperative imaging is not available, the health care organization should have a policy and procedure describing actions necessary and communication required between referring and receiving organizations. [Recommendation] **A**

11.2.2 Clarify in organizational policies and procedures how adjunct technology device use will be recorded or documented. [Recommendation]

11.3 Based on risk analysis, establish policies that define when additional measures for RSI prevention should be performed or when they may be waived (eg, trauma, cystoscopy, ophthalmology). [Recommendation] **P**

Moderate-quality evidence[181,182] and guidance from professional organizations[48,60,61] indicate that there are situations in which the baseline count may need to be waived for patients in life-threatening situations, such as in trauma cases. The evidence review for this guideline revision found no other literature about criteria for waiving of count procedures, including potential differences between emergent or urgent procedures or criteria for pediatric patients. The size of a pediatric patient may dictate a correspondingly small incision that may make retention of an instrument in the surgical wound unlikely; however, RSIs can occur in the smallest of incisions.

Careful consideration is important when establishing a policy for waived counts for the pediatric patient based on age, weight, or incision size, because it is difficult to determine risk for an RSI.

Moderate-quality evidence[4,8,13,25,52,208] and guidance from professional organizations[48,60,62] support considering additional measures, such as radiographic screening of high-risk patients, as an adjunct to surgical item accounting procedures.

Lincourt et al[25] recommended routine radiographic screening for emergency procedures and when multiple major procedures are being performed because this indicates the presence of multiple surgical teams. Gawande et al[4] recommended routine intraoperative radiographic screening for select, high-risk patients (ie, patients undergoing emergency procedures, patients undergoing procedures during which unplanned changes occurred, patients with a high BMI) to detect RSIs.

Moffatt-Bruce et al[13] conducted a meta-analysis of risk factors for RSIs in three case-control studies and proposed a risk stratification system. In this system, patients were stratified by high risk and intermediate risk based on odds ratios with a cut off of three. The high-risk category includes risk factors that are associated with a more than three times greater risk for RSIs: incorrect surgical count, unexpected intraoperative factors, and more than one surgical team. The intermediate category includes risk factors with a less than three times greater risk for RSIs: surgical count not performed, more than one subprocedure, long duration of surgery, and estimated blood loss > 500 mL. The researchers recommended additional research to prospectively evaluate interventions on their effectiveness to reduce the risk for RSIs. This systematic review was limited by the retrospective nature of the review and the quality of the included studies.

Professional organizations also recommend radiographic screening of high-risk patients. The WHO recommends intraoperative imaging, when possible, when no counts were performed.[60] The Joint Commission recommends intraoperative imaging when the patient is determined to be at high risk for an RSI, even if the count was correct and a methodical wound exploration was performed.[48] The Pennsylvania Patient Safety Authority recommends intraoperative imaging for high-risk cases, including those in which there are incorrect counts, emergency procedures, procedures for patients with a high BMI, and procedures in which unplanned changes occur.[62]

Additional research is needed to evaluate the clinical application of additional measures, including intraoperative imaging, that target risk factors for RSI prevention. Additional research is also needed to determine the benefits and harms of universal imaging. Cima et al[8] recommended universal postoperative imaging surveillance for RSIs in a dedicated imaging room located in the surgical suite.

11.4 Include RSI prevention measures for organ procurement procedures in policies and procedures. [Recommendation]

Counted items that are sent with the donated organ(s) may increase the risk of count discrepancy and RSIs for the organ recipient and could create sharps injury hazards for personnel. Counted sharps and instruments that are retained in the donor may cause injury at autopsy, as reported by Burton,[249] and contribute to inventory loss.

11.5 Clarify in policies and procedures how to handle potential RSIs removed from patients (eg, send them to the pathology laboratory). [Recommendation]

Many patients with an RSI return to surgery for removal of the item.[4,8,16-20,25-27,32,41,250] Lack of clarification on how to handle a potential RSI removed from a patient may lead to disposal or questions about whether the item was an RSI.[16,250] A case report described how a specimen sent to the pathology laboratory for examination was confirmed to be a sponge after examination.[46]

11.6 Clarify in policies and procedures how to handle instruments and devices that may have contributed to an RSI or near miss. [Recommendation]

When an instrument or device is suspected of contributing to an RSI or near miss, clarifying how to handle the item (eg, sequester, report, turn in for inspection) may be important to later investigations.[27]

11.6.1 In collaboration with materials management personnel, establish a policy and procedure for reporting product packaging defects to manufacturers. [Recommendation]

12. Education

12.1 Provide education to and verify the competency of personnel who participate in RSI prevention strategies in the organization. Education topics should include

- the incidence of RSI in the organization,
- the potential consequences of an RSI event for an affected patient,
- the individual's role in
  - implementing a consistent interdisciplinary approach for RSI prevention and
  - the RSI QI program,
- how standardized counting procedures are performed,

- documentation and reporting expectations, and
- use of specialized equipment for RSI prevention (eg, adjunct technology).

[Recommendation] P

Patient injuries from RSIs described in case reports vary by the type of item retained (eg, sponge, metal), time to diagnosis, and the location of the RSI.[6,48] Many patients are reported to require reoperation for removal of an RSI.[4,6,8,16-21,23,25-27,31,32,41,250] Patient harm associated with RSIs includes pain[6,9,14,16,17,20,26-28,31-33]; nausea,[33] vomiting,[33] and digestive problems[17]; constipation;[6] infection or sepsis[4,14,18,25,31,32]; abscess[25,31-33]; purulent discharge[31]; peritonitis[9]; adhesions[14,33]; fistula[4,9,33]; obstruction[4,9,14,25,31,250]; visceral perforations[4,25]; colostomy placement[31]; gangrene and amputation[18]; partial loss of an organ[31]; delayed treatment of other medical conditions[19]; readmission or prolonged hospital stay[4]; and death.[4] Retained surgical items in the vascular system (eg, guidewires, intravascular devices, broken instruments) can cause complications such as thrombosis, embolization, arrhythmia, tamponade, perforation, or even death.[68,149-152,205] Although emotional harm has not been uniformly reported, one publication estimated the prevalence to be 1.1%.[11] There also may be an effect on the reputation of the clinicians involved and the institution.[29]

Current law does not prescribe what methods to use to prevent RSIs, who implements them, or even that they need to be used. The law does, however, require that surgical items not intended to remain in the patient be removed. The doctrine of res ipsa loquitur (ie, "the thing speaks for itself") may be applicable in RSI incidents.[146,251] In other words, the fact of an RSI alone is enough for a plaintiff patient to prove their case, and a showing of negligence on the part of the health care providers is not necessary. Furthermore, the "captain of the ship" doctrine is no longer assumed to be true, and members of the entire surgical team as well as the health care facility can be held liable in RSI litigation.[146,251,252] These cases may also be complicated by the time frame of the statute of limitations.[253] As the number of settlements increase, fewer trials for RSI cases occur.[146] Although a review of legal case findings is outside the scope of this document, the evidence review undertaken for the development of this document indicated that legal expenses and settlement payments can vary greatly, adding to the health care costs associated with RSIs.

Retained surgical items can be costly and burdensome to the health care system. The exact costs of an RSI are unknown and the published information on costs is variable. The Centers for Medicare & Medicaid Services estimated the average cost of removing an RSI to be $63,631 per hospital stay in

2007.[254] Two cost-analysis reports of RSIs in pediatric patients estimated additional hospital charges to be $35,681[255] and $42,077[256] for this complication in 2010 and 2009, respectively. In 2009, Regenbogen et al[55] stated that costs include patient care during admission for a retained item and malpractice litigation, were approximately $210,000. In 2013, Mehtsun et al[11] estimated the cost of malpractice payments for a surgical retained foreign body to range from $51 to $3,988,829, with a mean of $86,247 and median of $33,953. In 2003, Gawande et al[4] estimated malpractice claim expenses to average $52,581 per case. In 2021, Cohen et al[21] reported that when an adverse event is confirmed in a California health care facility, the state penalties may range from $75,000 for the first violation to $125,000 for the third and subsequent violations.

12.1.1 **Provide education about patient and procedural risk factors that increase the risk of an RSI occurring during**
- **surgical procedures, including**
  - **incorrect count,**[13]
  - **unexpected intraoperative factors,**[13]
  - **more than one surgical team,**[13]
  - **no count performed (due to inability or emergent situations),**[13]
  - **more than one procedure,**[13]
  - **long procedural duration,**[13]
  - **blood loss > 500 mL,**[13] **and**
  - **high BMI,**[4,208] **and**
- **intravascular procedures, including**
  - **unexpected procedural factors**[167] **and**
  - **equipment failure.**[167]

[Recommendation]

Even though many of the identified patient and procedural risk factors are nonmodifiable, providing education to perioperative personnel about these factors may improve identification of clinical practice situations that could increase the patient's risk for an RSI. Recognition of procedural or patient conditions as they are happening may help perioperative personnel focus on behaviors that may decrease risk for an RSI (eg, clear communication, calling for additional help) even when nonmodifiable situations occur.

Early RSI research focused on identifying patient and procedural risk factors that might increase the likelihood that contributing factors occur.[13,43] Moffatt-Bruce et al[13] described unexpected intraoperative factors as equipment malfunctions, an unanticipated change in the operative course, or any other complication that would not be reasonably expected during that specific procedure type. According to the researchers, a bowel resection performed during a cholecystectomy procedure and a vascular repair performed during a bowel resection procedure would be examples of an unexpected complication.[13]

Elsharydah et al[257] performed a nonexperimental study on discharge data from the Nationwide Inpatient Sample from the Healthcare Cost Utilization Project of the Agency for Healthcare Quality and Research. The study included adults who had an abdominal and pelvic procedure and were also diagnosed with an RSI or an acute reaction to a foreign substance accidentally left in the patient during a procedure between 2007 and 2011. When RSI characteristics were compared among themselves (ie, without case controls), elective procedures, procedures in teaching hospitals, and procedures on patients with morbid obesity were found to be statistically significant characteristics. These results may indicate characteristics that are higher risk among patients with an RSI.

When the 1,144 patients with an RSI were compared to similar patients without an RSI that had similar abdominal and pelvic procedures (ie, case controls), elective procedures (compared to nonelective procedures) and rural hospital locations were the characteristics that were found to be statistically significant. Elective procedures were found to be statistically significant in both analyses.[257] It is important to note that this study did not review many of the risk factors identified by Moffatt-Bruce et al[13] (eg, no count, incorrect count, procedure duration, blood loss).

12.1.2 **Provide education about contributing factors associated with RSIs, including**

- **human factors,**[15,42,68]
- **ineffective leadership,**[15,42,68]
- **communication breakdown,**[15,22,33,40,42,68]
- **operative care (eg, planning, monitoring, rushing to complete a task),**[15,42,68]
- **assessment (eg, lack of, scope, timing),**[15,42,68]
- **physical environment (eg, equipment problems, room was too small),**[15,42,68]
- **information management (eg, incomplete information, technical systems),**[15,42,68]
- **care planning/continuum of care (eg, lack of collaboration, plans lacking necessary components),**[42] **and**
- **other (eg, performance improvement issues).**[15,42,68]

[Recommendation]

More recent research has identified factors that contribute to RSIs.[15,42,68] Retained surgical items may occur more frequently during stressful situations, such as when an unexpected change in the procedure occurs, not because of the situation itself but because of the effect these conditions have on human factors (eg, teamwork, communication, mindfulness). Therefore, interdisciplinary interventions that focus on improving the system culture and addressing human factors may help decrease the risk of RSIs (See Section 1 for additional information on interdisciplinary interventions).

Focusing on modifiable interventions that target improvement of human factors or the system culture to prevent RSIs is important because many of the risk factors identified by early research were not modifiable. Thiels et al[23] found that RSIs were significantly associated with more human factors errors per event than other adverse events that occur during surgical procedures, except use of the wrong implant.

Three studies involving a review of different retained items reported to The Joint Commission between 2012 and 2018 found that the top three categories of contributing factors across all the studies were problems with human factors, ineffective leadership, and communication breakdown.[15,42,68] The individual components of the human factors category varied between studies but included inadequate orientation, education, and competency of personnel; distraction; fatigue; drift; and insufficient medical staff credentialing.[15,42]

Human factors specific to retained guidewires or guidewire fragments included inadequate supervision of personnel inserting guidewires, not following the manufacturer's instructions for use, not evaluating the guidewire on removal, distractions, lack of situational awareness, and rushing.[68]

In the leadership category, noncompliance with policies and procedures and inadequate policies and procedures were most often cited as contributing factors.[15,42,68] In the study specific to retained guidewires and guidewire fragments, inadequate policies and procedures included lack of a checklist for insertion of a guidewire and no evaluation for guidewire integrity after removal.[68]

In the communication category, barriers to communication with the physician and communication among personnel were most frequently reported.[15,42] Communication issues specific to retained guidewire and guidewire fragments included lack of communication about expectations and verification of removal and issues involving communication with the radiology department.[68] Other categories included operative care, assessment, physical environment, information management, care planning/continuum of care, and other. With regard to retained soft goods, adequacy of patient assessment was the contributing factor most reported.[15]

13. Quality and Reporting

13.1 **Participate in a variety of quality assurance and performance improvement activities that are consistent with the health care organization plan to improve understanding and compliance with the principles and processes of RSI prevention.** [Recommendation]

Quality assurance and performance improvement programs assist in evaluating and improving the quality of patient care and formulating plans for corrective action. These programs provide data that may be used to determine whether an individual organization is meeting benchmark goals and, if not, to identify areas that may require corrective action.

13.2 **Use a systems approach for quality assurance and performance improvement for prevention of RSIs. Health care organizations should value learning and respond to errors with a focus on process improvement rather than individual blame.**[23,66,67,258-261] [Recommendation]

The literature indicates that perioperative teams can better understand how adverse events like RSIs occur and learn how to redesign the system to prevent these errors when the interactions between individuals and systems are understood and the location where failure occurs is identified.[23,259,260] The perioperative setting is a highly complex system, and many factors can influence individual performance.

Butler et al[103] discussed that in addition to team performance, factors such as the type of surgery, technical complexity of the procedure, unplanned changes, and patient acuity place a high amount of pressure on the perioperative nurse to remain alert, observant, and responsive through the fatigue and stress from the physical and psychological demands of working in this setting. A systems approach targets quality interventions to address cognitive factors, team dynamics, and perceptual biases as part of a systems initiative to decrease RSIs and improve patient safety.[23]

Reason's Model of Human Error distinguishes the systems approach from individual approaches for prevention of medical errors.[66] Focusing on systems for RSI prevention, rather than blaming individuals, aims to reduce the incidence of RSIs by improving systems to prevent predictable human errors.[23,66,259]

Accountability also plays a role in systems improvement. Each perioperative team member has an ethical obligation to perform their role and responsibilities with appropriate competence and the highest level of personal integrity.[71] However, perioperative team members in a just culture are not only accountable for their own actions but are also accountable to each other in protecting patients.[261]

Riley et al[258] discussed that increasing professional accountability may improve patient safety by minimizing the effects of normalization and complacency that may occur during the repetitive task of the surgical count. However, systems improvement is beyond individual accountability and responsibility. According to Reason,[66] dealing with individual errors rather than fixing a broken system will not stop unsafe acts from occurring.

13.2.1 **Evaluate errors such that contributing factors are reviewed first and then accountability is determined in relation to actions.** [Recommendation]

Continuous quality improvement opportunities arise from documented and structured quality processes and measures that can define and resolve problems.

13.3 **Implement a multiphase, interdisciplinary process improvement program**[67] **that includes**
- **an ongoing risk assessment and review (eg, failure modes and effects analysis)**[15,67,96,262]**;**
- **a policy design and review;**
- **a review of published evidence, internal data collection, and data analysis; and**
- **plans for the ongoing monitoring and analysis of processes, near misses, and adverse events related to the prevention of RSIs.**[58,67,104,105]
[Recommendation]

A comprehensive QI program may identify opportunities for minimizing the risk of RSI events. Establishment of a quality and performance improvement program may be required by the facility's accrediting body.

Low-quality evidence supports that implementation of comprehensive process improvement programs reduced RSI events and improved count procedures in health care organizations.[58,67,104,105] As part of an organizational experience report, Cima et al[58] implemented an interdisciplinary, multiphase approach for process improvement that involved defect analysis, policy review, increasing awareness and communication among personnel, and a monitoring and control phase. After implementation of the program, the health care organization experienced a significant and sustained reduction in RSI events during a 2-year period, from an average of one RSI or near miss every 16 days to an average of one RSI or near miss every 69 days.[58]

Edel[104] reported on an organizational experience QI project that involved analysis of surgical count practice variability, policy revision, personnel education, and auditing for compliance. As a result, variability in count practices was reduced, although metrics were not reported.

In a report of an organizational experience in a pediatric teaching hospital, Norton et al[105] discussed implementation of a quality program to standardize count practices, revise policies, educate personnel, and review every reported count discrepancy. During a 1-year period, the hospital reported a 50% reduction in the number of incorrect counts and count discrepancies with sustained results.[105] Researchers in another study found that failure to adhere to facility policies and procedures and failure to enforce accountability were two of the human factors that contributed to retained guidewire or guidewire fragments.[68]

The evidence review for this guideline revision also indicated that health care failure modes and effects analysis or other QI tools may provide insight on areas of possible improvement.[15,67,96,262] In a QI article, Steelman and Cullen[96] detailed the process, results, and recommendations from a failure modes and effects analysis used to prevent retained sponges during abdominal procedures at one facility. The quality of the analysis may be dependent on the tools used, available resources, and the interdisciplinary team's experience.[262]

13.3.1 Identify the organization's RSI rate as the outcome measure for evaluating improvement. [Recommendation]

Understanding the health care organization's or facility's RSI rate provides a baseline against which to measure the outcome of performance improvement initiatives.

13.3.2 Identify and use process measures for evaluating the effects of RSI prevention improvement projects. [Recommendation]

Because RSIs are a rare event, a comparison of the health care organization's RSI rate before and after implementation of an RSI improvement process may not show a significant difference. Therefore, it may be helpful to evaluate process measures that provide information about the effects of the improvement process.

13.3.3 Process measures may include
- rates of near misses,
- rates of count discrepancies (eg, electronic medical record reports, internal variance reports)

- reports from adjunct technology devices (eg, results, reports completed compared to number of procedures in which it was intended for use),
- the number of radiographs taken for reconciling count discrepancies, and
- satisfaction of personnel involved in the process change.

[Conditional Recommendation]

The literature describes various elements that could be used to measure quality improvement processes for preventing RSIs.[5,53,234] In a nonexperimental study of time and costs associated with count discrepancies, the researchers evaluated time and costs saved from the reduction in unreconciled counts and from the decrease in radiographs taken after introduction of RF technology for the prevention of retained sponges.[231] These characteristics may provide insights about the RSI prevention improvement process; however, they may be harder to obtain or quantify.

13.4 Monitor for adherence to policies and procedures for prevention of RSI as part of quality assurance and process improvement initiatives. [Recommendation]

Moderate-quality evidence supports monitoring for adherence to policies and procedures for RSI prevention.[4,42,68,87,99,208,234] Despite best practice recommendations, some safety procedures may not be performed consistently.[87] Gawande et al[4] strongly recommended that hospitals actively monitor compliance with policies and procedures for counting, including standard sponge counting in every surgical procedure and instrument counting for every surgery involving an open cavity. Steelman et al[15] recommended monitoring that the manufacturer's instructions for use of the RF adjunct technology system are followed and providing feedback to personnel as part of the facility's quality performance measures.

In a retrospective case-control study, Stawicki et al[208] found that policy deviations identified as safety omissions/variations were significantly associated with an increased risk for RSI. The authors recommended that surgical facilities enforce a surgical safety policy for RSI prevention to foster a culture of zero tolerance for policy deviations.[208] In a QI article involving a survey and observational audits of count practices, 90% of respondents indicated that they followed the facility count policy but observational audits of clinical practice found that only 20% of personnel followed the policy.[99] The authors stated that there was a perceived lack of delegation, leadership, teaching, and coaching in the clinical setting.[99] Clinical supervision in the OR was recommended to provide reflection and motivation, encourage teamwork, and facilitate accountability.[99]

13.5 **Conduct a critical investigation of all adverse events and near misses (eg, incorrect count, incidents involving negative-pressure wound therapy foam) related to RSIs.**[15,48,105] *[Recommendation]*

Error and near miss reporting is the first step to addressing error reduction. As part of the sentinel event policy, The Joint Commission[48] requires a **root cause analysis** of all sentinel events, including unintended retention of foreign objects. There are a number of analysis methods (eg, root cause analysis, appreciative inquiry) available to health care organizations that may be used to conduct a critical investigation of adverse events.[48,105,263] Agrawal[116] reported on a root cause analysis of a retained vaginal sponge. Bell[263] reported on a critical incident analysis of a near miss where the sponge was found in the drapes during count reconciliation procedures.

As part of a multiple initiative QI project in a pediatric teaching hospital, Norton et al[105] reviewed every reported count discrepancy by root cause analysis in addition to implementing standardization of count practices, a revised policy, and personnel education. During a 1-year period, the hospital reported a 50% reduction in the number of incorrect counts and count discrepancies with sustained results.[105]

13.5.1 **Involve interdisciplinary teams in the review process and address any changes in policy that can improve patient safety.** *[Recommendation]*

13.5.2 **A human factors analysis may be used in the critical investigation of an RSI event.**[23] *[Conditional Recommendation]*

Use of human factors analysis is supported in an organizational experience report. Thiels et al[23] applied Reason's model to never events, including RSI, and identified four categories of human error: unsafe actions, preconditions for unsafe actions, oversight/supervisory factors, and organizational influences. During a 5-year period, they captured reported incidents and near misses of never events, including RSI, at a tertiary-care hospital. Human behaviors in the incident analysis were coded in subcategories of the four main categories with nano-codes. For retained foreign objects, the majority of coded behaviors (n = 221) were in the categories of unsafe actions (n = 102) and preconditions for actions (n = 94). The researchers recommended using the Human Factors Analysis and Classification System to assist in linking human factors by error type to provide targets for intervention and mitigation.[23]

Steelman et al[15] found 1,430 contributing factors associated with 319 incidents of retained soft goods, of which 79.8% were related to human factors, leadership, and communication.

13.6 **Reporting mechanisms for adverse events and near misses related to RSIs must be established.** *[Regulatory Requirement]*

Federal and state agencies, accrediting bodies, third-party payers, and professional associations consider unintentionally retained foreign objects or RSIs to be reportable events that require additional investigation.[48,264,265] Many states require public reporting when RSI events occur.[47]

13.7 **Report events that necessitate reopening a wound or creation of a new wound to retrieve an RSI in compliance with health care organizational policy, as well as local, state, and federal regulations.** *[Recommendation]*

Reopening an incision or creating a new wound can increase the risk of additional harm to the patient (eg, procedural complications, additional time under anesthesia).

13.7.1 **Facilities must report individual serious adverse events from medical devices to the FDA within 10 days of becoming aware of the event.**[147,266,267] *[Regulatory Requirement]*

Soft goods, sharps, and surgical instruments are medical devices.[268] Serious adverse events have specific criteria involving significant harm or death.[267] MedWatch is the FDA's safety information and adverse event reporting program.[269]

13.7.2 **Serious injuries related to medical devices must be reported to the device manufacturer.**[266] **If the device manufacturer cannot be identified, report the injury to the FDA.**[266] *[Regulatory Requirement]*

13.8 **Report count discrepancies and near misses internally according to the health care organization's policy and procedure.** *[Recommendation]*

Steelman et al[42] recommended encouraging reporting of near misses. Duggan et al[67] stated that robust tracking of near misses was part of the process that helped identify whether the implemented changes were working as expected.

13.9 **Promptly disclose unintentionally retained items to the patient or patient's representative according to organizational policy and procedure.** *[Recommendation]*

Both the ACS[61] and The Joint Commission[48] support disclosure of an RSI to the patient or the person responsible for making health care decisions for the patient.

In a survey of surgeons in Brazil, the authors found that 54% of patients with an RSI were not informed about the incident.[9] In the same survey, 74% of surgeons stated that they would not tell a patient about an RSI they removed that was unintentionally retained during a procedure involving a different surgeon.[9]

Theories, methods,[270] and the clinician's response[271] to disclosures of a medical error is outside the scope of this document but is examined in the literature.

Glossary

Adverse event: Any undesirable experience associated with the use of a medical product in a patient.

Correct count: No count discrepancy was identified, or a discrepancy was reconciled. This term is used for documentation purposes.

Count discrepancy: A subsequent count does not agree with the previous one.

Data-matrix-coded system: A system that identifies surgical soft goods by scanning a 2-dimensional data-matrix label.

Failure modes and effects analysis: A proactive systematic method for guiding a team in evaluating a process to determine how the process may fail, how likely the failure is to occur, and what the severity of the consequence may be for the failure. This information is used to inform improvement effort prioritization and strategies to prevent process failures.

Incorrect count: A count discrepancy that cannot be reconciled. This term is used for documentation purposes.

Miscount: A type of count discrepancy that occurs when the number of the items counted does not reflect the number of items present.

Misplaced item: A type of count discrepancy that occurs when an item is missing. Potential locations of items may include the floor, waste receptacles, drapes, or inside the patient.

Near miss: An error that is discovered and rectified before it results in harm. Identification of the error may be due to chance or to interception of the error before harm could occur. May also be referred to as a "close call" or "good catch." Definitions may vary in federal, state, and local regulations and accrediting body standards.

Radio-frequency detection: A system that locates objects with an imbedded chip using radio waves.

Radio-frequency identification: A system that locates and transmits the identity of an object (in the form of a unique serial number) wirelessly, using radio waves.

Read-back method: A dialogue in which the listener verbally repeats patient information so that the sender can confirm the accuracy of the message.

Root cause analysis: A retrospective process for identifying basic or causal factors underlying variation in performance, including the occurrence or possible occurrence of a sentinel event.

Sentinel event: An unanticipated incident involving death or serious physical or psychological injury, or the risk of serious injury or adverse outcome.

Serious adverse event: Any undesirable experience associated with the use of a medical product in a patient that involves death, hospitalization or prolonged hospitalization, disability or permanent damage, or intervention to prevent permanent impairment or damage or that is life-threatening.

Unretrieved device fragment: A fragment of a medical device that has separated and unintentionally remains in the patient after a procedure.

References

1. Steelman VM, Graling PR, Perkhounkova Y. Priority patient safety issues identified by perioperative nurses. *AORN J.* 2013;97(4):402-418. [IIIA]

2. Kohn LT, Corrigan JM, Donaldson MS, eds. *To Err Is Human: Building a Safer Health System.* Washington, DC: National Academies Press; 2000.

3. Most Commonly Reviewed Sentinel Event Types. The Joint Commission. https://www.jointcommission.org/-/media/tjc/documents/resources/patient-safety-topics/sentinel-event/most-frequently-reviewed-event-types-2020.pdf. Updated February 1, 2021. Accessed September 28, 2021. [VB]

4. Gawande AA, Studdert DM, Orav EJ, Brennan TA, Zinner MJ. Risk factors for retained instruments and sponges after surgery. *N Engl J Med.* 2003;348(3):229-235. [IIIA]

5. Inaba K, Okoye O, Aksoy H, et al. The role of radio frequency detection system embedded surgical sponges in preventing retained surgical sponges: a prospective evaluation in patients undergoing emergency surgery. *Ann Surg.* 2016;264(4):599-604. [IIIB]

6. Rabie ME, Hosni MH, Al Safty A, Al Jarallah M, Ghaleb FH. Gossypiboma revisited: a never ending issue. *Int J Surg Case Rep.* 2016;19:87-91. [VB]

7. Cherara L, Sculli GL, Paull DE, Mazzia L, Neily J, Mills PD. Retained guidewires in the Veterans Health Administration: getting to the root of the problem. *J Patient Saf.* 2018. doi: 10.1097/PTS.0000000000000475. [IIIA]

8. Cima RR, Kollengode A, Garnatz J, Storsveen A, Weisbrod C, Deschamps C. Incidence and characteristics of potential and actual retained foreign object events in surgical patients. *J Am Coll Surg.* 2008;207(1):80-87. [IIIB]

9. Birolini DV, Rasslan S, Utiyama EM. Unintentionally retained foreign bodies after surgical procedures. Analysis of 4547 cases. *Rev Col Bras Cir.* 2016;43(1):12-17. [IIIC]

10. Wallace SC. Retained surgical items: events and guidelines revisited. *Pa Patient Saf Advis.* 2017;14(1):27-35. [IVB]

11. Mehtsun WT, Ibrahim AM, Diener-West M, Pronovost PJ, Makary MA. Surgical never events in the United States. *Surgery.* 2013;153(4):465-472. [IIIB]

12. Hempel S, Maggard-Gibbons M, Nguyen DK, et al. Wrong-site surgery, retained surgical items, and surgical fires: a systematic review of surgical never events. *JAMA Surg.* 2015;150(8):796-805. [IIIB]

13. Moffatt-Bruce SD, Cook CH, Steinberg SM, Stawicki SP. Risk factors for retained surgical items: a meta-analysis and proposed risk stratification system. *J Surg Res.* 2014;190(2):429-436. [IIIA]

14. Chen Q, Rosen AK, Cevasco M, Shin M, Itani KMF, Borzecki AM. Detecting patient safety indicators: how valid is "foreign body left during procedure" in the Veterans Health Administration? *J Am Coll Surg.* 2011;212(6):977-983. [IIIB]

15. Steelman VM, Shaw C, Shine L, Hardy-Fairbanks AJ. Retained surgical sponges: a descriptive study of 319 occurrences and contributing factors from 2012 to 2017. *Patient Saf Surg.* 2018;12(1):20. [IIIA]

16. Surgeon attempts to blame nurses for sponge left in mastectomy patient. Case on point: Mitchell v. Baylor Univ. Med. Ctr., 2003 WL 21508493 S.W.3d-TX. *Nurs Law Regan Rep.* 2003;44(3):2. [VC]

17. Sponge left in pt. - Dr. settled: hospital sued for OR nurses' negligence. Savage v. Three Rivers Medical Center, C-000348-DG KYSC---S.W.3d---(10/25/2012)-KY. *Nurs Law Regan Rep.* 2012;53(7):1.

18. Sponge left in patient's leg: infection & amputation result. *Nurs Law Regan Rep.* 2006;47(7):1. [VC]

19. Sponge left in pt.: did required surgery delay treatment & cause death? *Nurs Law Regan Rep.* 2004;45(1):1. [VC]

20. Sponge left in Pt. who sued "after limitations" but right after "discovery." Case on point: Stone v. Coronado, 03-11-00243-CV TXCA3 (6/6/2012)-TX. *Nurs Law Regan Rep.* 2012;53(4):4. [VC]

21. Cohen AJ, Lui H, Zheng M, et al. Rates of serious surgical errors in California and plans to prevent recurrence. *JAMA Netw Open.* 2021;4(5):e217058. [IIIA]

22. Soncrant C, Mills PD, Neily J, Paull DE, Hemphill RR. Root cause analyses of reported adverse events occurring during gastrointestinal scope and tube placement procedures in the Veterans Health Association. *J Patient Saf.* 2020;16(1):41-46. [IIIA]

23. Thiels CA, Lal TM, Nienow JM, et al. Surgical never events and contributing human factors. *Surgery.* 2015;158(2):515-521. [IIIB]

24. Gibbs VC. Thinking in three's: changing surgical patient safety practices in the complex modern operating room. *World J Gastroenterol.* 2012;18(46):6712-6719. [VB]

25. Lincourt AE, Harrell A, Cristiano J, Sechrist C, Kercher K, Heniford BT. Retained foreign bodies after surgery. *J Surg Res.* 2007;138(2):170-174. [IIIB]

26. Foreign object left in bypass pt.: why wasn't dr. responsible? Case on pointL Breaux v. Thurston, 2003 WL 23028311 So.2d-AL. *Nurs Law Regan Rep.* 2004;44(8):4. [VC]

27. Blade left in pt.: why didn't nurses notice bladeless scalpel? Ripley v. Lanzer, WA-61952-7-1(9/14/2009)-WA. *Nurs Law Regan Rep.* 2009;50(4):1. [VC]

28. Dr. allowed to testify as expert on nursing: was this error? *Nurs Law Regan Rep.* 2008;49(4):1. [VC]

29. Egorova NN, Moskowitz A, Gelijns A, et al. Managing the prevention of retained surgical instruments: what is the value of counting? *Ann Surg.* 2008;247(1):13-18. [IIIA]

30. Walter WR, Amis ES Jr, Sprayregen S, Haramati LB. Intraoperative radiography for evaluation of surgical miscounts. *J Am Coll Radiol.* 2015;12(8):824-829. [IIIA]

31. Arikan S, Kocakusak A. Retained textile foreign bodies: experience of 27 years. *Acta Med Port.* 2015;28(4):494-500. [IIIB]

32. Gauze pad left in pt. during reversal of tubal ligation surgery. Case on point: Houserman v. Garrett, 2004 WL 2829112. *Nurs Law Regan Rep.* 2004;45(7):4. [VC]

33. Wan W, Le T, Riskin L, Macario A. Improving safety in the operating room: a systematic literature review of retained surgical sponges. *Curr Opin Anaesthesiol.* 2009;22(2):207-214. [VA]

34. Zantvoord Y, van der Weiden RMF, van Hooff MHA. Transmural migration of retained surgical sponges: a systematic review. *Obstet Gynecol Surv.* 2008;63(7):465-471. [VB]

35. Patial T, Rathore N, Thakur A, Thakur D, Sharma K. Transmigration of a retained surgical sponge: a case report. *Patient Saf Surg.* 2018;12:21. [VB]

36. Caetano FB, Duarte AF, Chahud F, Cintra MB, Cruz AAVE. Intraconal gauze mass: an unusual complication of orbital fracture repair—a case report. *Orbit.* 2018;37(2):91-93. [VC]

37. Mulay K, Sharma V, Honavar SG. Forget me not: a case of gossypiboma (textiloma) mimicking an orbital tumor. *Ophthalmic Plastic Reconstr Surg.* 2016;32(1):e5-e7. [VC]

38. Park CM, Choi KY, Heo SJ, Kim JS. Unilateral otitis media with effusion caused by retained surgical gauze as an unintended iatrogenic complication of orthognathic surgery: case report. *Br J Oral Maxillofac Surg.* 2014;52(7):e39-e40. [VC]

39. Tsukamoto M, Hirokawa J, Yokoyama T. Retained foreign body in the nasal cavity after oral maxillofacial surgery. *Anesth Prog.* 2018;65(2):111-112. [VC]

40. Williams TL, Tung DK, Steelman VM, Chang PK, Szekendi MK. Retained surgical sponges: findings from incident reports and a cost-benefit analysis of radiofrequency technology. *J Am Coll Surg.* 2014;219(3):354-364. [IIIB]

41. Nurse left sponge in pt. during preoperative procedure. Case on point: Burke v. AnMed Health, 4828 SCCA(4/27/2011)-SC. *Nurs Law Regan Rep.* 2011;52(3):4. [VC]

42. Steelman VM, Shaw C, Shine L, Hardy-Fairbanks AJ. Unintentionally retained foreign objects: a descriptive study of 308 sentinel events and contributing factors. *Jt Comm J Qual Patient Saf.* 2019;45(4):249-258. [IIIA]

43. Gibbs VC. Retained surgical items and minimally invasive surgery. *World J Surg.* 2011;35(7):1532-1539. [VA]

44. Arikan Y, Ozdemir O, Seker KG, et al. Gossypiboma: a dramatic result of human error, case report and literature review. *Prague Med Rep.* 2019;120(4):144-149. [VC]

45. Nazarinia M, Esmaeilzadeh E. Gauzoma in a scleroderma patient following open heart surgery: a case report. *Curr Rheumatol Rev.* 2019;15(1):79-81. [VC]

46. Kim DK, Hwang SK, Lee SC, et al. A 31-year-old pericardial textiloma. *Cardiovasc J Afr.* 2020;31(4):e5-e8. [VC]

47. West N, Eng T, Kirk A. Update on State Government Tracking of Health Care-Acquired Conditions and a Four-State In-Depth Review. Centers for Medicare & Medicaid Services. https://www.cms.gov/medicare/medicare-fee-for-service-payment/hospitalacqcond/downloads/phase-3-state-tracking-report.pdf. Published June 2012. Accessed September 28, 2021. [VA]

48. Sentinel Event Alert 51: Preventing unintended retained foreign objects. The Joint Commission. https://www.jointcommission.org/resources/patient-safety-topics/sentinel-event/sentinel-event-alert-newsletters/sentinel-event-alert-issue-51-preventing-unintended-retained-foreign-objects/. Published October 17, 2013. Accessed September 28, 2021. [IVB]

49. Jarrett NM, Callaham M. Evidence-Based Guidelines for Selected Hospital-Acquired Conditions. Final Report. Centers for Medicare & Medicaid Services. https://www.cms.gov/Medicare/Medicare-Fee-for-Service-Payment/HospitalAcqCond/Downloads/2016-HAC-Report.pdf. Published April 28, 2016. Accessed September 28, 2021.

50. 42 CFR 430, Subpart C—Grants; Reviews and Audits; Withholding for Failure To Comply; Deferral and Disallowance of Claims; Reduction of Federal Medicaid Payments. Electronic Code of Federal Regulations. https://www.ecfr.gov/current/title-42/chapter-IV/subchapter-C/part-430/subpart-C. Accessed September 28, 2021.

51. Ricciardi R, Baxter NN, Read TE, Marcello PW, Schoetz DJ, Roberts PL. Surgeon involvement in the care of patients deemed to have "preventable" conditions. J Am Coll Surg. 2009;209(6):707-711. [IIIB]

52. Judson TJ, Howell MD, Guglielmi C, Canacari E, Sands K. Miscount incidents: a novel approach to exploring risk factors for unintentionally retained surgical items. Jt Comm J Qual Patient Saf. 2013;39(10):468-474. [IIIA]

53. Greenberg CC, Regenbogen SE, Lipsitz SR, Diaz-Flores R, Gawande AA. The frequency and significance of discrepancies in the surgical count. Ann Surg. 2008;248(2):337-341. [IIIA]

54. Rupp CC, Kagarise MJ, Nelson SM, et al. Effectiveness of a radiofrequency detection system as an adjunct to manual counting protocols for tracking surgical sponges: a prospective trial of 2,285 patients. J Am Coll Surg. 2012;215(4):524-533. [IIIB]

55. Regenbogen SE, Greenberg CC, Resch SC, et al. Prevention of retained surgical sponges: a decision-analytic model predicting relative cost-effectiveness. Surgery. 2009;145(5):527-535. [IIIB]

56. Steelman VM. Sensitivity of detection of radiofrequency surgical sponges: a prospective, cross-over study. Am J Surg. 2011;201(2):233-237. [IIA]

57. Steelman VM, Alasagheirin MH. Assessment of radiofrequency device sensitivity for the detection of retained surgical sponges in patients with morbid obesity. Arch Surg. 2012;147(10):955-960. [IIA]

58. Cima RR, Kollengode A, Storsveen AS, et al. A multidisciplinary team approach to retained foreign objects. Jt Comm J Qual Patient Saf. 2009;35(3):123-132. [VB]

59. Stawicki SP, Cook CH, Anderson HL 3rd, et al. Natural history of retained surgical items supports the need for team training, early recognition, and prompt retrieval. Am J Surg. 2014;208(1):65-72. [VA]

60. WHO Guidelines for Safe Surgery 2009: Safe Surgery Saves Lives. World Health Organization. http://apps.who.int/iris/bitstream/handle/10665/44185/9789241598552_eng.pdf;jsessionid=A0223DB47B17AC150FEADA4AC1371DBF?sequence=1. Accessed September 28, 2021. [IVB]

61. American College of Surgeons (ACS) Committee on Perioperative Care. Revised statement on the prevention of unintentionally retained surgical items after surgery. Bull Am Coll Surg. 2016;101(10):50-51. [IVB]

62. Martindell D. Update on the prevention of retained surgical items. Pa Patient Saf Advis. 2012;9(3):106-110. [IVB]

63. ECRI. Unintentionally retained surgical items. Operating Room Risk Management. 2012;2(Surgery):1. [VC]

64. Standards for sponge, needle and instrument procedures. AORN J. 1976;23(6):971-973.

65. Committee opinion no. 464: patient safety in the surgical environment. Obstet Gynecol. 2010;116(3):786-790. [IVB]

66. Reason J. Safety in the operating theatre - Part 2: human error and organisational failure. Qual Saf Health Care. 2005;14(1):56-60. [VB]

67. Duggan EG, Fernandez J, Saulan MM, et al. 1,300 days and counting: a risk model approach to preventing retained foreign objects (RFOs). Jt Comm J Qual Patient Saf. 2018;44(5):260-269. [VB]

68. Steelman VM, Thenuwara K, Shaw C, Shine L. Unintentionally retained guidewires: a descriptive study of 73 sentinel events. Jt Comm J Qual Patient Saf. 2019;45(2):81-90. [IIIA]

69. Bubric KA, Biesbroek SL, Laberge JC, Martel JA, Litvinchuk SD. Prevalence and characteristics of interruptions and distractions during surgical counts. Jt Comm J Qual Patient Saf. 2021;47(9):556-562. [IIIA]

70. Loftus T, Dahl D, OHare B, et al. Implementing a standardized safe surgery program reduces serious reportable events. J Am Coll Surg. 2015;220(1):12-17. [IIIA]

71. Standards of perioperative nursing. AORN, Inc. https://www.aorn.org/guidelines/clinical-resources/aorn-standards. Accessed September 28, 2021. [IVB]

72. Yang YT, Henry L, Dellinger M, Yonish K, Emerson B, Seifert PC. The circulating nurse's role in error recovery in the cardiovascular OR. AORN J. 2012;95(6):755-762. [VB]

73. Recommended standard of practice for counts. Association of Surgical Technologists; https://www.ast.org/uploadedFiles/Main_Site/Content/About_Us/Standard%20Counts.pdf. Published October 27, 2006. Accessed September 28, 2021. [IVC]

74. Camos V. Coordination process in counting. Int J Psychol. 2003;38(1):24-36. [IIIB]

75. Camos V. Counting strategies from 5 years to adulthood: adaptation to structural features. Eur J Psychol Educ. 2003;18(3):251-265. [IIIA]

76. Clark GJ. Strategies for preventing distractions and interruptions in the OR. AORN J. 2013;97(6):702-707. [VB]

77. AORN Position Statement on Managing Distractions and Noise During Perioperative Patient Care. AORN, Inc. https://

www.aorn.org/guidelines/clinical-resources/position-statements. Accessed September 28, 2021. [IVB]

78. Iwai T, Goto T, Matsui Y, Tohnai I. Endoscopic removal of throat-packing gauze swallowed during general anesthesia. *J Craniofac Surg*. 2012;23(5):1547-1549. [VC]

79. Jennings A, Bhatt V. Throat packs: in your face? *Anaesthesia*. 2010;65(3):312-313. [VC]

80. Smith M, Turnbull D, Andrzejowski J. Throat packs in neuroanaesthesia. *Anaesthesia*. 2012;67(7):804-805. [IIIB]

81. Colbert S, Jackson M, Turner M, Brennan PA. Reducing the risk of retained throat packs after surgery. *Br J Oral Maxillofac Surg*. 2012;50(7):680-681. [VC]

82. Lyons VE, Popejoy LL. Meta-analysis of surgical safety checklist effects on teamwork, communication, morbidity, mortality, and safety. *West J Nurs Res*. 2014;36(2):245-261. [IIA]

83. Collins SJ, Newhouse R, Porter J, Talsma A. Effectiveness of the surgical safety checklist in correcting errors: a literature review applying Reason's Swiss Cheese Model. *AORN J*. 2014;100(1):65-79. [VB]

84. McDowell DS, McComb SA. Safety checklist briefings: a systematic review of the literature. *AORN J*. 2014;99(1):125-137. [VB]

85. Borchard A, Schwappach DLB, Barbir A, Bezzola P. A systematic review of the effectiveness, compliance, and critical factors for implementation of safety checklists in surgery. *Ann Surg*. 2012;256(6):925-933. [IIIA]

86. Haynes AB, Weiser TG, Berry WR, et al. A surgical safety checklist to reduce morbidity and mortality in a global population. *N Engl J Med*. 2009;360(5):491-499. [IIA]

87. Marsh V, Kalisch B, McLaughlin M, Nguyen L. Nurses' perceptions of the extent and type of missed perioperative nursing care. *AORN J*. 2020;112(3):237-247. [IIIA]

88. Rhee AJ, Valentin-Salgado Y, Eshak D, et al. Team training in the perioperative arena: a methodology for implementation and auditing behavior. *Am J Med Qual*. 2017;32(4):369-375. [VB]

89. Armour Forse R, Bramble JD, McQuillan R. Team training can improve operating room performance. *Surgery*. 2011;150(4):771-778. [VB]

90. Papaspyros SC, Javangula KC, Adluri RKP, O'Regan DJ. Briefing and debriefing in the cardiac operating room. Analysis of impact on theatre team attitude and patient safety. *Interact Cardiovas Thorac Surg*. 2010;10(1):43-47. [VB]

91. Young-Xu Y, Neily J, Mills PD, et al. Association between implementation of a Medical Team Training program and surgical morbidity. *Arch Surg*. 2011;146(12):1368-1373. [IIIA]

92. Weaver SJ, Rosen MA, DiazGranados D, et al. Does teamwork improve performance in the operating room? A multilevel evaluation. *Jt Comm J Qual Patient Saf*. 2010;36(3):133-142. [IIB]

93. Tibbs SM, Moss J. Promoting teamwork and surgical optimization: combining TeamSTEPPS with a specialty team protocol. *AORN J*. 2014;100(5):477-488. [VA]

94. Johnson HL, Kimsey D. Patient safety: break the silence. *AORN J*. 2012;95(5):591-601. [VB]

95. Guideline for team communication. In: Guidelines for *Perioperative Practice*. Denver, CO: AORN, Inc; 2021:1065-1096. [IVA]

96. Steelman VM, Cullen JJ. Designing a safer process to prevent retained surgical sponges: a healthcare failure mode and effect analysis. *AORN J*. 2011;94(2):132-141. [VB]

97. Rowlands A, Steeves R. Incorrect surgical counts: a qualitative analysis. *AORN J*. 2010;92(4):410-419. [IIIB]

98. Guideline for a safe environment of care. In: *Guidelines for Perioperative Practice*. Denver, CO: AORN, Inc; 2021:109-144. [IVA]

99. Smith Y, Burke L. Swab and instrument count practice: ways to enhance patient safety. *Br J Nurs*. 2014;23(11):590-593. [VB]

100. Ortuño F, Ojeda N, Arbizu J, et al. Sustained attention in a counting task: normal performance and functional neuroanatomy. *Neuroimage*. 2002;17(1):411-420. [IIIB]

101. Camos V, Barrouillet P. Adult counting is resource demanding. *Br J Psychol*. 2004;95(Pt 1):19-30. [IIIB]

102. Railo H, Koivisto M, Revonsuo A, Hannula MM. The role of attention in subitizing. *Cognition*. 2008;107(1):82-104. [IIIA]

103. Butler M, Ford R, Boxer E, Sutherland-Fraser S. Lessons from the field: an examination of count errors in the operating theatre. *ACORN*. 2010;23(3):6-16. [IIIB]

104. Edel EM. Surgical count practice variability and the potential for retained surgical items. *AORN J*. 2012;95(2):228-238. [VB]

105. Norton EK, Martin C, Micheli AJ. Patients count on it: an initiative to reduce incorrect counts and prevent retained surgical items. *AORN J*. 2012;95(1):109-121. [VB]

106. Grant-Orser A, Davies P, Singh SS. The lost sponge: patient safety in the operating room. *CMAJ*. 2012;184(11):1275-1278. [VA]

107. Song JB, Vemana G, Mobley JM, Bhayani SB. The second "time-out": a surgical safety checklist for lengthy robotic surgeries. *Patient Saf Surg*. 2013;7(1):19. [VA]

108. Boisvert MJ, Abroms BD, Roberts WA. Human nonverbal counting estimated by response production and verbal report. *Psychon Bull Rev*. 2003;10(3):683-690. [IIIB]

109. Logie RH, Baddeley AD. Cognitive processes in counting. *J Exp Psychol Learn*. 1987;13(2):310-326. [IIIB]

110. Nan Y, Knösche TR, Luo YJ. Counting in everyday life: discrimination and enumeration. *Neuropsychologia*. 2006;44(7):1103-1113. [IIIB]

111. Trick LM, Pylyshyn ZW. Why are small and large numbers enumerated differently? A limited-capacity preattentive stage in vision. *Psychol Rev*. 1994;101(1):80-102. [VA]

112. Goldfarb L, Levy S. Counting within the subitizing range: the effect of number of distractors on the perception of subset items. *PLoS One*. 2013;8(9):e74152. [IIIB]

113. Watson DG, Maylor EA, Bruce LA. The efficiency of feature-based subitization and counting. *J Exp Psychol Hum Percept Perform*. 2005;31(6):1449-1462. [IIIB]

114. Mazza V, Pagano S, Caramazza A. Multiple object individuation and exact enumeration. *J Cogn Neurosci*. 2013;25(5):697-705. [IIIB]

115. Edel EM. Increasing patient safety and surgical team communication by using a count/time out board. *AORN J*. 2010;92(4):420-424. [VB]

116. Agrawal A. Counting matters: lessons from the root cause analysis of a retained surgical item. *Jt Comm J Qual Patient Saf*. 2012;38(12):566-574. [VB]

117. Chagolla BA, Gibbs VC, Keats JP, Pelletreau B. A system-wide initiative to prevent retained vaginal sponges. *MCN Am J Matern Child Nurs.* 2011;36(5):312-317. [VB]

118. Garry DJ, Asanjarani S, Geiss DM. Policy for prevention of a retained sponge after vaginal delivery. *Case Rep Med.* 2012;2012:317856. [VB]

119. Healy P. Retained vaginal swabs: review of an adverse event in obstetrics through closed claims analysis. *Br J Midwifery.* 2012;20(9):666-669. [IIIB]

120. Lutgendorf MA, Schindler LL, Hill JB, Magann EF, O'Boyle JD. Implementation of a protocol to reduce occurrence of retained sponges after vaginal delivery. *Mil Med.* 2011;176(6):702-704. [VB]

121. Wattanasirichaigoon S. Transmural migration of a retained surgical sponge into the intestinal lumen: an experimental study. *J Med Assoc Thai.* 1996;79(7):415-422. [IIB]

122. Hyslop JW, Maull KI. Natural history of the retained surgical sponge. *South Med J.* 1982;75(6):657-660. [VB]

123. Kucuk C, Arda K, Turkkani MH, Ata N. Intrathoracic gossypiboma. *Hong Kong J Emerg Med.* 2018;25(5):290-292. [VC]

124. Statler JD, Miller DL, Dixon RG, et al. Society of Interventional Radiology position statement: prevention of unintentionally retained foreign bodies during interventional radiology procedures. *J Vasc Interv Radiol.* 2011;22(11):1561-1562. [IVC]

125. Amr AE. A submandibular gossypiboma mimicking a salivary fistula: a case report. *Cases J.* 2009;2:6413. [VB]

126. Baruah BP, Young P, Douglas-Jones A, Mansel R. Retained surgical swab following breast augmentation: a rare cause of a breast mass. *BMJ Case Rep.* 2009;2009:bcr07.2008.0519. [VB]

127. Fouelifack FY, Fouogue JT, Fouedjio JH, Sando Z. A case of abdominal textiloma following gynecologic surgery at the Yaounde Central Hospital, Cameroon. *Pan Afr Med J.* 2013;16:147. [VB]

128. Gencosmanoglu R, Inceoglu R. An unusual cause of small bowel obstruction: gossypiboma—case report. *BMC Surg.* 2003;3:6. [VB]

129. Irabor DO. Under-reporting of gossipiboma in a third-world country. a sociocultural view. *Niger J Med.* 2013;22(4):365-367. [VB]

130. Joshi MK, Jain BK, Rathi V, Agrawal V, Mohanty D. Complete enteral migration of retained surgical sponge—report of two cases. *Trop Gastroenterol.* 2011;32(3):229-232. [VC]

131. Kansakar R, Hamal BK. Cystoscopic removal of an intravesical gossypiboma mimicking a bladder mass: a case report. *J Med Case Rep.* 2011;5:579. [VC]

132. Karasaki T, Nomura Y, Nakagawa T, Tanaka N. Beware of gossypibomas. *BMJ Case Rep.* 2013;2013:brc2013010059. [VC]

133. Kim KS. Changes in computed tomography findings according to the chronicity of maxillary sinus gossypiboma. *J Craniofac Surg.* 2014;25(4):e330-e333. [VC]

134. Kohli S, Singhal A, Tiwari B, Singhal S. Gossypiboma, varied presentations: a report of two cases. *J Clin Imaging Sci.* 2013;3:11. [VC]

135. Lundin K, Allen JE, Birk-Soerensen L. Gossypiboma after breast augmentation. *Case Rep Surg.* 2013;2013:808624. [VC]

136. Naama O, Quamous O, Elasri CA, et al. Textiloma: an uncommon complication of posterior lumbar surgery. *J Neuroradiol.* 2010;37(2):131-134. [VB]

137. Ogundiran T, Ayandipo O, Adeniji-Sofoluwe A, Ogun G, Oyewole O, Ademola A. Gossypiboma: complete transmural migration of retained surgical sponge causing small bowel obstruction. *BMJ Case Rep.* 2011;2011:brc0402114073. [VC]

138. Ozkan OV, Bas G, Akcakaya A, Sahin M. Transmural migration of a retained sponge through the rectum: a case report. *Balkan Med J.* 2011;28(1):94-95. [VC]

139. Quraishi AHM. Beyond a gossypiboma. *Case Rep Surg.* 2012;2012:263841. [VB]

140. Sumer A, Carparlar MA, Uslukaya O, et al. Gossypiboma: retained surgical sponge after a gynecologic procedure. *Case Rep Med.* 2010;2010:917625. [VC]

141. Guideline for preoperative patient skin antisepsis. In: *Guidelines for Perioperative Practice.* Denver, CO: AORN, Inc; 2021:591-618. [IVA]

142. Cho SW, Jin HR. Gossypiboma in the nasal septum after septorhinoplasty: a case study. *J Oral Maxillofac Surg.* 2013;71(1):e42-e44. [VB]

143. Yuki K, Shiba D, Ota Y, Ozeki N, Murat D, Tsubota K. A new method to prevent loss of mitomycin C soaked sponges under the conjunctiva during trabeculectomy. *Br J Ophthalmol.* 2010;94(8):1111-1112. [VC]

144. Srivastava A, Kataria K, Chella VR. Prevention of gossypiboma. *Indian J Surg.* 2014;76(2):169. [VC]

145. McIntyre LK, Jurkovich GJ, Gunn ML, Maier RV. Gossypiboma: tales of lost sponges and lessons learned. *Arch Surg.* 2010;145(8):770-775. [VA]

146. Cockburn T, Davis J, Osborne S. Retained surgical items: lessons from Australian case law of items unintentionally left behind in patients after surgery. *J Law Med.* 2019;26(4):841-848. [VB]

147. FDA Public Health Notification: Unretrieved Device Fragments (archived content). US Food and Drug Administration. Published 2008. Updated 2015. Accessed December 21, 2020. [VA]

148. Pokharel K, Biswas BK, Tripathi M, Subedi A. Missed central venous guide wires: a systematic analysis of published case reports. *Crit Care Med.* 2015;43(8):1745-1756. [VA]

149. Tateishi M, Tomizawa Y. Intravascular foreign bodies: danger of unretrieved fragmented medical devices. *J Artif Organs.* 2009;12(2):80-89. [VB]

150. Al-Moghairi AM, Al-Amri HS. Management of retained intervention guide-wire: a literature review. *Curr Cardiol Rev.* 2013;9(3):260-266. [VA]

151. Johnson C, Alomari AI, Chaudry G. Detachment of introducer sheath radiopaque marker during retrieval of G2 filter. *Cardiovasc Intervent Radiol.* 2011;34(2):431-434. [VB]

152. Williams TL, Bowdle TA, Winters BD, Pavkovic SD, Szekendi MK. Guidewires unintentionally retained during central venous catheterization. *J Assoc Vasc Access.* 2014;19(1):29-34. [VA]

153. Cohen SB, Bartz PJ, Earing MG, Sheil A, Nicolosi A, Woods RK. Myocardial infarction due to a retained epicardial pacing wire. *Ann Thorac Surg.* 2012;94(5):1724-1726. [VB]

154. Kelly RJ, Whipple OC. Retained anvil after laparoscopic gastric bypass. *Surg Obes Relat Dis.* 2011;7(5):e13-e15. [VB]

155. Magalini S, Sermoneta D, Lodoli C, Vanella S, Di Grezia M, Gui D. The new retained foreign body! Case report and review of the literature on retained foreign bodies in laparoscopic bariatric surgery. *Eur Rev Med Pharmacol Sci.* 2012;16(Suppl 4):129-133. [VA]

156. Stephens M, Ruddle A, Young WT. An unusual complication of a dropped clip during laparoscopic cholecystectomy. *Surg Laparosc Endosc Percutan Tech.* 2010;20(3):e103-e104. [VC]

157. Chepla KJ, Wilhelm SM. Delayed mechanical small bowel obstruction caused by retained, free, intraperitoneal staple after laparoscopic appendectomy. *Surg Laparosc Endosc Percutan Tech.* 2011;21(1):e19-e20. [VB]

158. Ozsoy M, Celep B, Ozsan I, Bal A, Ozkececi ZT, Arikan Y. A retained plastic protective cover mimicking malignancy: case report. *Int J Surg Case Rep.* 2013;4(12):1084-1087. [VC]

159. Toubia T, Sangha R. Retained vaginal foreign body in minimally invasive gynecological surgeries. *CRSLS MIS Case Rep.* 2014:e2014.00240. [VA]

160. Sakhel K, Hines J. To forget is human: the case of the retained bulb. *J Robot Surg.* 2009;3(1):45-47. [VB]

161. Barrow CJ. Use of x-ray in the presence of an incorrect needle count. *AORN J.* 2001;74(1):80-81. [VB]

162. Macilquham MD, Riley RG, Grossberg P. Identifying lost surgical needles using radiographic techniques. *AORN J.* 2003;78(1):73-78. [VB]

163. Ponrartana S, Coakley FV, Yeh BM, et al. Accuracy of plain abdominal radiographs in the detection of retained surgical needles in the peritoneal cavity. *Ann Surg.* 2008;247(1):8-12. [VA]

164. Kieval JZ, Walsh M, Legutko PA, Daly MK. Efficacy of portable X-ray in identifying retained suture needles in ophthalmologic cases. *Eye (Lond).* 2009;23(8):1731-1734. [IIIB]

165. Hacivelioglu S, Karatag O, Gungor AC, et al. Is there an advantage of three dimensional computed tomography scanning over plain abdominal radiograph in the detection of retained needles in the abdomen? *Int J Surg.* 2013;11(3):278-281. [IIIB]

166. Horberry T, Teng YC, Ward J, Patil V, Clarkson PJ. Guidewire retention following central venous catheterisation: a human factors and safe design investigation. *Int J Risk Saf Med.* 2014;26(1):23-37. [IIIB]

167. Moffatt-Bruce SD, Ellison EC, Anderson HL 3rd, et al. Intravascular retained surgical items: a multicenter study of risk factors. *J Surg Res.* 2012;178(1):519-523. [IIIC]

168. Ren S, Liu P, Wang W, Yang Y. Retained foreign body after laser ablation. *Int Surg.* 2012;97(4):293-295. [VB]

169. Ellett L, Maher P. Forgotten surgical items: lessons for all to learn. Case report and 3-year audit of retained surgical items at a tertiary referral centre. *Gynecol Surg.* 2013;10(4):295-297. [VB]

170. Guideline for sharps safety. In: *Guidelines for Perioperative Practice.* Denver, CO: AORN, Inc; 2021:873-896. [IVA]

171. 29 CFR 1910.1030. Bloodborne pathogens. Electronic Code of Federal Regulations. https://www.ecfr.gov/current/title-29/subtitle-B/chapter-XVII/part-1910#1910.1030. Accessed September 28, 2021.

172. Parelkar SV, Sanghvi BV, Shetty SR, Athawale H, Oak SN. Needle in a haystack: Intraoperative breakage of pediatric minimal access surgery instruments. *J Postgrad Med.* 2014;60(3):324-326. [VB]

173. Ruscher KA, Modeste KA, Staff I, Papasavas PK, Tishler DS. Retained needles in laparoscopic surgery: open or observe? *Conn Med.* 2014;78(4):197-202. [IIIB]

174. Barto W, Yazbek C, Bell S. Finding a lost needle in laparoscopic surgery. *Surg Laparosc Endosc Percutan Tech.* 2011;21(4):e163-e165. [IIIB]

175. Small AC, Gainsburg DM, Mercado MA, Link RE, Hedican SP, Palese MA. Laparoscopic needle-retrieval device for improving quality of care in minimally invasive surgery. *J Am Coll Surg.* 2013;217(3):400-405. [IIIB]

176. Jayadevan R, Stensland K, Small A, Hall S, Palese M. A protocol to recover needles lost during minimally invasive surgery. *JSLS.* 2014;18(4):e2014.00165. [IIIB]

177. Kumar S, Chandra A, Kulkarni R, Maurya AP, Gupta V. Forgotten biliary stents: ignorance is not bliss. *Surg Endosc.* 2018;32(1):191-195. [IIIB]

178. Hussain Z, Malik SM, Rasool A, Mattoo S. Rare causes of foreign body in CBD: a retrospective study. *JK Science.* 2015;17(4):209-211. [VC]

179. Ipaktchi K, Kolnik A, Messina M, Banegas R, Livermore M, Price C. Current surgical instrument labeling techniques may increase the risk of unintentionally retained foreign objects: a hypothesis. *Patient Saf Surg.* 2013;7(1):31. [VC]

180. Bansal M, Heckl F, English K. Retained broken outflow cannula recovered 6 years post-knee arthroscopy. *Orthopedics.* 2011;34(12):e945-e947. [VB]

181. Teixeira PG, Inaba K, Salim A, et al. Retained foreign bodies after emergent trauma surgery: incidence after 2526 cavitary explorations. *Am Surg.* 2007;73(10):1031-1034. [IIIB]

182. Murdock D. Trauma: when there's no time to count. *AORN J.* 2008;87(2):322-328. [VB]

183. Guideline for care and cleaning of surgical instruments. In: *Guidelines for Perioperative Practice.* Denver, CO: AORN, Inc; 2021:381-420. [IVA]

184. Yasuhara H, Fukatsu K, Komatsu T, Murakoshi S, Saito Y, Uetera Y. Occult risk of broken instruments for endoscopy-assisted surgery. *World J Surg.* 2014;38(11):3015-3022. [IIIB]

185. Abe T, Murai S, Nasuhara Y, Shinohara N. Characteristics of medical adverse events/near misses associated with laparoscopic/thoracoscopic surgery: a retrospective study based on the Japanese National Database of Medical Adverse Events. *J Patient Saf.* 2019;15(4):343-351. [IIIA]

186. Matsuda S, Yoshimura H, Yoshida H, Sano K. Breakage and migration of a high-speed dental hand-piece bur during mandibular third molar extraction: two case reports. *Medicine (Baltimore).* 2020;99(7):e19177. [VB]

187. Reece M, Troeleman ND, McGowan JE, Furuno JP. Reducing the incidence of retained surgical instrument fragments. *AORN J.* 2011;94(3):301-304. [VB]

188. Fischer RA. Danger: beware of unretrieved device fragments. *Nursing.* 2007;37(11):17. [VB]

189. Omar HR, Sprenker C, Karlnoski R, Mangar D, Miller J, Camporesi EM. The incidence of retained guidewires after central venous catheterization in a tertiary care center. *Am J Emerg Med.* 2013;31(10):1528-1530. [VB]

190. Pillarisetti J, Biria M, Balda A, Reddy N, Berenbom L, Lakkireddy D. Integrity of vascular access: the story of a broken sheath! *J Vasc Nurs.* 2009;27(3):75-77. [VB]

191. DerDerian T, Ascher E, Hingorani A, Jimenez R. A rare complication of a retained wire during endovascular abdominal aortic aneurysm repair. *Ann Vasc Surg.* 2013;27(8):1183.e11-1183.e15. [VB]

192. Torre M, Lechpammer M, Paulson V, et al. Embolic foreign material in the central nervous system of pediatric autopsy patients with instrumented heart disease. *J Neuropathol Exp Neurol.* 2017;76(7):571-577. [IIIB]

193. Endicott KM, Friedrich R, Custer JW, Sarkar R, Rowen L, Anders MG. Preventing retained surgical items during endovascular procedures: bridging the gap between guidelines and practice. *AORN J.* 2020;112(6):625-633. [VB]

194. Endicott KM, Drucker CB, Orbay H, et al. Intraoperative fragmentation and retention of endovascular devices: clinical consequences and preventative strategies. *Vasc Endovascular Surg.* 2020;54(2):118-125. [VC]

195. Mariyaselvam MZA, Catchpole KR, Menon DK, Gupta AK, Young PJ. Preventing retained central venous catheter guidewires: a randomized controlled simulation study using a human factors approach. *Anesthesiology.* 2017;127(4):658-665. [IB]

196. Kava BR, Burdick-Will J. Complications associated with retained foreign bodies from infected penile implants: proposal for the use of an implant-specific checklist at the time of device removal. *J Sex Med.* 2013;10(6):1659-1666. [VA]

197. Felder SI, Liou DZ, Gangi A. Gastric adjustable band as a retained foreign object: a case report. *Bariat Surg Pract Patient Care.* 2013;8(4):166-168. [VB]

198. Augello M, von Jackowski J, Grätz KW, Jacobsen C. Needle breakage during local anesthesia in the oral cavity—a retrospective of the last 50 years with guidelines for treatment and prevention. *Clin Oral Investig.* 2011;15(1):3-8. [VB]

199. Malamed SF, Reed K, Poorsattar S. Needle breakage: incidence and prevention. *Dent Clin North Am.* 2010;54(4):745-756. [VA]

200. Pogrel MA. Broken local anesthetic needles: a case series of 16 patients, with recommendations. *J Am Dent Assoc.* 2009;140(12):1517-1522.

201. Catelani C, Valente A, Rossi A, Bertolai R. Broken anesthetic needle in the pterygomandibular space. Four case reports. *Minerva Stomatol.* 2013;62(11-12):455-463. [VB]

202. Kim SH, Huh K, Jee YS, Park MJ. Breakage of growth hormone needle in subcutaneous tissue. *J Spec Pediatr Nurs.* 2011;16(2):162-165. [VC]

203. Stein KM. Use of intraoperative navigation for minimally invasive retrieval of a broken dental needle. *J Oral Maxillofac Surg.* 2015;73(10):1911-1916. [VC]

204. Alexander G, Attia H. Oral maxillofacial surgery displacement complications. *Oral Maxillofac Surg Clin North Am.* 2011;23(3):379-386. [VA]

205. Bydon A, Xu R, Conte JV, et al. Surgical mystery: where is the missing pituitary rongeur tip? *Spine (Phila Pa 1976).* 2010;35(17):E867-E872. [VB]

206. *State Operations Manual Appendix A: Survey Protocol, Regulations and Interpretive Guidelines for Hospitals.* Rev 200 ed; 2020. Centers for Medicare & Medicaid Services. https://www.cms.gov/Regulations-and-Guidance/Guidance/Manuals/downloads/som107ap_a_hospitals.pdf. Accessed September 28, 2021.

207. *State Operations Manual Appendix L: Guidance for Surveyors: Ambulatory Surgical Centers.* Rev. 200 ed; 2020. Centers for Medicare & Medicaid Services. https://www.cms.gov/Regulations-and-Guidance/Guidance/Manuals/downloads/som107ap_l_ambulatory.pdf. Accessed September 28, 2021.

208. Stawicki SP, Moffatt-Bruce SD, Ahmed HM, et al. Retained surgical items: a problem yet to be solved. *J Am Coll Surg.* 2013;216(1):15-22. [IIIB]

209. Rowlands A. Risk factors associated with incorrect surgical counts. *AORN J.* 2012;96(3):272-284. [IIIB]

210. Weprin S, Crocerossa F, Meyer D, et al. Risk factors and preventive strategies for unintentionally retained surgical sharps: a systematic review. *Patient Saf Surg.* 2021;15(1):24.

211. Ward EP, Yang J, Delong JC, et al. Identifying lost surgical needles with visible and near infrared fluorescent light emitting microscale coating. *Surgery.* 2018;163(4):883-888.

212. Joseph M, Relano R. A typical day in cardiac theatres . . . or was it? Expect the unexpected. *J Perioper Pract.* 2014;24(9):194. [VC]

213. Hariharan D, Lobo DN. Retained surgical sponges, needles and instruments. *Ann R Coll Surg Engl.* 2013;95(2):87-92. [VB]

214. Tofte JN, Caldwell LS. Detection of retained foreign objects in upper extremity surgical procedures with incisions of two centimeters or smaller. *Iowa Orthop J.* 2017;37:189-192. [IIC]

215. Cousin G, Markose G. The incidental finding of a retained "throat pack." *Ann R Coll Surg Engl.* 2020;102(6):e125. [VC]

216. Sencimen M, Bayar GR, Gulses A. Removal of the retained suture needle under C-arm fluoroscopy: a technical note. *Dent Traumatol.* 2010;26(6):527-529. [VC]

217. Huang J, Bouvette MJ, Chari R, Vuddagiri V, Kraemer MC, Zhou J. The detection of a retained sponge in the aorta by transesophageal echocardiography. *J Cardiothorac Vasc Anesth.* 2010;24(2):314-315. [VC]

218. Hunter TB, Gimber LH. Identification of retained surgical foreign objects: policy at a university medical center. *J Am Coll Radiol.* 2010;7(9):736-738. [VB]

219. Gayer G, Lubner MG, Bhalla S, Pickhardt PJ. Imaging of abdominal and pelvic surgical and postprocedural foreign bodies. *Radiol Clin North Am.* 2014;52(5):991-1027. [VA]

220. Use of x-rays for incorrect needle counts. *PA PSRS Patient Saf Advis.* 2004;1(2):5-6. [IVC]

221. 510(k) clearances. US Food and Drug Administration. https://www.fda.gov/medical-devices/device-approvals-denials-and-clearances/510k-clearances. Accessed September 28, 2021.

222. Medical devices; exemptions from premarket notification and reserved devices; class I—FDA. Notice. *Fed Regist.* 1998;63(21):5387-5393.

223. Establishment Registration & Device Listing [Database]. US Food and Drug Administration. https://www.accessdata.fda.gov/scripts/cdrh/cfdocs/cfRL/rl.cfm. Accessed September 28, 2021.

224. Guideline for medical device and product evaluation. In: *Guidelines for Perioperative Practice.* Denver, CO: AORN, Inc; 2021:719-728. [IVA]

225. Guideline for sterilization. In: *Guidelines for Perioperative Practice*. Denver, CO: AORN, Inc; 2021:985-1014. [IVA]

226. Guideline for environmental cleaning. In: *Guidelines for Perioperative Practice*. Denver, CO: AORN, Inc; 2021:145-176. [IVA]

227. Salcedo JD, Pretorius VG, Hsu JC, et al. Compatibility of radiofrequency surgical sponge detection technology with cardiac implantable electronic devices and temporary pacemakers. *Pacing Clin Electrophysiol*. 2016;39(11):1254-1260. [IIIC]

228. Williams MR, Atkinson DB, Bezzerides VJ, et al. Pausing with the gauze: inhibition of temporary pacemakers by radiofrequency scan during cardiac surgery. *Anesth Analg*. 2016;123(5):1143-1148. [IIIB]

229. Radio frequency identification (RFID). US Food and Drug Administration. https://www.fda.gov/radiation-emitting-products/electromagnetic-compatibility-emc/radio-frequency-identification-rfid. Accessed September 28, 2021. [VA]

230. Steelman VM, Schaapveld AG, Perkhounkova Y, Storm HE, Mathias M. The hidden costs of reconciling surgical sponge counts. *AORN J*. 2015;102(5):498-506. [IIIA]

231. Steelman VM, Schaapveld AG, Storm HE, Perkhounkova Y, Shane DM. The effect of radiofrequency technology on time spent searching for surgical sponges and associated costs. *AORN J*. 2019;109(6):718-727. [IIIA]

232. Rogers A, Jones E, Oleynikov D. Radio frequency identification (RFID) applied to surgical sponges. *Surg Endosc*. 2007;21(7):1235-1237. [IIIB]

233. Macario A, Morris D, Morris S. Initial clinical evaluation of a handheld device for detecting retained surgical gauze sponges using radiofrequency identification technology. *Arch Surg*. 2006;141(7):659-662. [IIC]

234. Norton E. Using technology to prevent retained sponges. *AORN J*. 2014;99(4):C5-C6. [VC]

235. Primiano M, Sparks D, Murphy J, Glaser K, McNett M. Using radiofrequency technology to prevent retained sponges and improve patient outcomes. *AORN J*. 2020;112(4):345-352. [VC]

236. Greenberg CC, Diaz-Flores R, Lipsitz SR, et al. Bar-coding surgical sponges to improve safety: a randomized controlled trial. *Ann Surg*. 2008;247(4):612-616. [IB]

237. Cima RR, Kollengode A, Clark J, et al. Using a data-matrix-coded sponge counting system across a surgical practice: impact after 18 months. *Jt Comm J Qual Patient Saf*. 2011;37(2):51-58. [VB]

238. Retained sponges persist as a surgical complication despite manual counts. ECRI. https://www.ecri.org/search-results/member-preview/hdjournal/pages/top_10_hazards_2019_no_3_retained_sponges. Published September 26, 2018. Accessed September 28, 2021. [VC]

239. Gunnar W, Soncrant C, Lynn MM, Neily J, Tesema Y, Nylander W. The impact of surgical count technology on retained surgical items rates in the Veterans Health Administration. *J Patient Saf*. 2020;16(4):255-258. [IIIC]

240. Etchells E, Koo M, Daneman N, et al. Comparative economic analyses of patient safety improvement strategies in acute care: a systematic review. *BMJ Qual Saf*. 2012;21(6):448-456. [IIIA]

241. Seidman SJ, Brockman R, Lewis BM, et al. In vitro tests reveal sample radiofrequency identification readers inducing clinically significant electromagnetic interference to implantable pacemakers and implantable cardioverter-defibrillators. *Heart Rhythm*. 2010;7(1):99-107.

242. Plakke MJ, Maisonave Y, Daley SM. Radiofrequency scanning for retained surgical items can cause electromagnetic interference and pacing inhibition if an asynchronous pacing mode is not applied. *A A Case Rep*. 2016;6(6):143-145. [VB]

243. Yamashita K, Kusuda K, Ito Y, et al. Evaluation of surgical instruments with radiofrequency identification tags in the operating room. *Surg Innov*. 2018;25(4):374-379. [IIIC]

244. Kranzfelder M, Schneider A, Fiolka A, et al. Real-time instrument detection in minimally invasive surgery using radiofrequency identification technology. *J Surg Res*. 2013;185(2):704-710. [IIIB]

245. Neumuth T, Meissner C. Online recognition of surgical instruments by information fusion. *Int J Comput Assist Radiol Surg*. 2012;7(2):297-304. [IIIB]

246. Yamashita K, Kusuda K, Tokuda Y, et al. Validation of cleaning evaluation of surgical instruments with RFID tags attached based on cleaning appraisal judgment guidelines. *Annu Int Conf IEEE Eng Med Biol Soc*. 2013;2013:926-929. [IIC]

247. Guideline for patient information management. In: *Guidelines for Perioperative Practice*. Denver, CO: AORN, Inc; 2021:351-380. [IVA]

248. Brown J, Feather D. Surgical equipment and materials left in patients. *Br J Perioper Nurs*. 2005;15(6):259-262. [VB]

249. Burton JL. Health and safety at necropsy. *J Clin Pathol*. 2003;56(4):254-260. [VC]

250. Surgical towel left in pt.: were nurses responsible? Case on point: Hodesh v. Korlitz, 2008-Ohio-2052 (05/02/2008) -OH. *Nurs Law Regan Rep*. 2008;49(1):2. [VC]

251. Retained sponge: hospital and surgeon have independent duties to remove objects. Plymouth Meeting, PA: ECRI; 2018. [VC]

252. Murphy EK. "Captain of the ship" doctrine continues to take on water. *AORN J*. 2001;74(4):525-528. [VC]

253. Patient's discovery that clamp's presence was improper started statute-of-limitations clock. Plymouth Meeting, PA: ECRI; 2020. [VC]

254. CMS proposes additions to list of hospital-acquired conditions for fiscal year 2009. Centers for Medicare & Medicaid Services. https://www.cms.gov/newsroom/fact-sheets/cms-proposes-additions-list-hospital-acquired-conditions-fiscal-year-2009. Published April 14, 2008. Accessed September 28, 2021.

255. Camp M, Chang DC, Zhang Y, Chrouser K, Colombani PM, Abdullah F. Risk factors and outcomes for foreign body left during a procedure: analysis of 413 incidents after 1 946 831 operations in children. *Arch Surg*. 2010;145(11):1085-1090. [IIIA]

256. Shah RK, Lander L. Retained foreign bodies during surgery in pediatric patients: a national perspective. *J Pediatr Surg*. 2009;44(4):738-742. [IIIA]

257. Elsharydah A, Warmack KO, Minhajuddin A, Moffatt-Bruce SD. Retained surgical items after abdominal and pelvic surgery: incidence, trend and predictors—observational study. *Ann Med Surg (Lond)*. 2016;12:60-64. [IIIA]

258. Riley R, Manias E, Polglase A. Governing the surgical count through communication interactions: implications for patient safety. *Qual Saf Health Care*. 2006;15(5):369-374. [IIIB]

259. Karl R, Karl MC. Adverse events: root causes and latent factors. *Surg Clin North Am.* 2012;92(1):89-100. [VB]

260. Elbardissi AW, Sundt TM. Human factors and operating room safety. *Surg Clin North Am.* 2012;92(1):21-35. [VA]

261. Boysen PG 2nd. Just culture: a foundation for balanced accountability and patient safety. *Ochsner J.* 2013;13(3):400-406. [VB]

262. Chatzimichailidou MM, Ward J, Horberry T, Clarkson PJ. A comparison of the Bow-Tie and STAMP approaches to reduce the risk of surgical instrument retention. *Risk Anal.* 2018;38(5):978-990. [VB]

263. Bell R. Hide and seek, the search for a missing swab: a critical analysis. *J Perioper Pract.* 2012;22(5):151-156. [VA]

264. Hospital-acquired conditions (present on admission indicator). Centers for Medicare & Medicaid Services. https://www.cms.gov/Medicare/Medicare-Fee-for-Service-Payment/HospitalAcqCond?redirect=/hospitalacqcond/06_hospital-acquired_conditions.asp. Accessed September 28, 2021.

265. *Serious Reportable Events In Healthcare—2011 Update: A Consensus Report.* Washington, DC: National Quality Forum; 2011. [VC]

266. 21 CFR 803.10: Generally, what are the reporting requirements that apply to me? GovInfo. https://www.govinfo.gov/app/details/CFR-2006-title21-vol8/CFR-2006-title21-vol8-sec803-10/summary. Accessed September 28, 2021.

267. What is a serious adverse event? US Food and Drug Administration. https://www.fda.gov/safety/reporting-serious-problems-fda/what-serious-adverse-event. Accessed September 28, 2021. [VA]

268. Product classification [Database] US Food and Drug Administration. https://www.accessdata.fda.gov/scripts/cdrh/cfdocs/cfPCD/classification.cfm. Accessed September 28, 2021.

269. MedWatch: The FDA Safety Information and Adverse Event Reporting Program. US Food and Drug Administration. https://www.fda.gov/safety/medwatch-fda-safety-information-and-adverse-event-reporting-program. Accessed September 28, 2021.

270. Jones M, Scarduzio J, Mathews E, et al. Individual and team-based medical error disclosure: dialectical tensions among health care providers. *Qual Health Res.* 2019;29(8):1096-1108. [IIIB]

271. Swartwout E, Rodan M. The development and testing of the psychometric properties of the emotional response and disclosure of errors in clinical practice instrument. *J Nurs Meas.* 2017;25(1):184-200. [IIIA]

Guideline Development Group and Acknowledgements

Lead Author: Julie Cahn[1], DNP, RN, CNOR, RN-BC, ACNS-CP, CNS-CP, Senior Perioperative Practice Specialist, AORN, Denver, Colorado

Methodologist: Erin Kyle[2], DNP, RN, CNOR, NEA-BC, Editor-in-Chief, *Guidelines for Perioperative Practice,* AORN, Denver, Colorado

Evidence Appraisers: Lisa Spruce[3], DNP, RN, CNS-CP, CNOR, ACNS, ACNP, FAAN, Director of Evidenced-Based Perioperative Practice, AORN, Denver, Colorado

Subject Matter Expert: Victoria M. Steelman[4], PhD, RN, CNOR, FAAN, Associate Professor Emeritus, University of Iowa, Iowa City

Guidelines Advisory Board Members and Liaisons:
- Donna A. Pritchard[5], MA, BSN, RN, NE-BC, CNOR, Director of Perioperative Services, Interfaith Medical Center, Brooklyn, New York
- Brenda G. Larkin[6], MS, ACNS-BC, CNS, CNOR, Clinical Nurse Specialist, Aurora Lakeland Medical Center, Lake Geneva, Wisconsin
- Sara Reese[7], PhD, CIC, FAPIC, Association for Professionals in Infection Control and Epidemiology, Englewood, Colorado

External Review: The draft was open for a 30-day public comment period. Expert review comments were received from individual members of the American Association of Nurse Anesthesiology (AANA), American College of Surgeons (ACS), Association for Professionals in Infection Control and Epidemiology (APIC), American Society of Anesthesiologists (ASA), International Association of Healthcare Central Service Materiel Management (IAHCSMM), the Society for Healthcare Epidemiology of America (SHEA), and the Surgical Infection Society (SIS). Their responses were used to further refine and enhance this guideline; however, their responses do not imply endorsement.

Financial Disclosure and Conflicts of Interest

This guideline was developed, edited, and approved by the AORN Guidelines Advisory Board without external funding being sought or obtained. The Guidelines Advisory Board was financially supported entirely by AORN and was developed without any involvement of industry.

Potential conflicts of interest for all Guidelines Advisory Board members were reviewed before the annual meeting and each monthly conference call.

Six members of the Guideline Development Group reported no potential conflict of interest.[1-3,5-7] One member[4] disclosed potential conflict of interest (serving as a consultant in the past to a manufacturer of technology used for prevention of retained surgical items). After review and discussion of these disclosures, the Advisory Board concluded that none of the potential conflicts related to any content in this guideline.

Publication History

Originally published May 1976, *AORN Journal,* as "Standards for sponge, needle, and instrument procedures."

Format revision March 1978, July 1982.

Revised March 1984, March 1990.

Revised November 1995; published October 1996, *AORN Journal*.

Revised; published December 1999, *AORN Journal.*

Reformatted July 2000.

Revised November 2005; published as Recommended Practices for Sponge, Sharp, and Instrument Counts in *Standards, Recommended Practices, and Guidelines*, 2006 edition.

Reprinted February 2006, *AORN Journal*.

Revised July 2010 for online publication in *Perioperative Standards and Recommended Practices*.

Reformatted September 2012 for publication in *Perioperative Standards and Recommended Practices*, 2013 edition.

Minor editing revisions made in November 2014 for publication in *Guidelines for Perioperative Practice*, 2015 edition, as Guideline for Prevention of Retained Surgical Items.

Revised January 2016 for publication in *Guidelines for Perioperative Practice*, 2016 edition.

Minor editing revisions made in October 2016 for publication in *Guidelines for Perioperative Practice*, 2017 edition.

Evidence ratings revised and minor editorial changes made to conform to the current AORN Evidence Rating model, September 2019, for online publication in *Guidelines for Perioperative Practice.*

Revised December 2021 for publication in *Guidelines for Perioperative Practice*, 2022 edition.

Scheduled for review in 2026.

AMBULATORY SUPPLEMENT:
RETAINED SURGICAL ITEMS

8. Reconciling Count Discrepancies

8.4.2 **If intraoperative imaging is not available, the health care organization should have a policy and procedure describing the actions and communication required between referring and receiving organizations.**

A The ambulatory surgery facility should have a policy and procedure describing actions to take when on-site radiology services personnel are not available to perform a radiograph and interpret the result.

A A surgeon with perioperative radiologic privileges may consider using fluoroscopy to locate the retained item.[A1]

A Fluoroscopy may be used and a reading obtained by a surgeon with privileges to interpret radiographic studies.[A1]

11. Policies and Procedures

11.2.1 **If intraoperative imaging is not available, the health care organization should have a policy and procedure describing actions necessary and communication required between referring and receiving organizations.**

A Policies and procedures should include circumstances in which the patient should be transferred to the postanesthesia care unit and/ or a subsequent receiving facility for further radiologic imaging.

References

A1. *State Operations Manual Appendix L: Guidance for Surveyors: Ambulatory Surgical Centers.* Rev. 200 ed; 2020. Centers for Medicare & Medicaid Services. https://www.cms.gov/Regulations-and-Guidance/Guidance/Manuals/downloads/som107ap_l_ambulatory.pdf. Accessed September 28, 2021.

Acknowledgment

Lead Author, Ambulatory Supplement
Terri Link, MPH, BSN, CNOR, CIC, CAIP, FAPIC
Product Manager,
Guideline Implementation Tools
AORN, Inc
Denver, Colorado

Publication History

Originally published in *Perioperative Standards and Recommended Practices,* 2014 edition.

Revised January 2016 for publication in *Guidelines for Perioperative Practice,* 2016 edition.

Minor editorial changes made to conform with revised guideline format, September 2019, for online publication in *Guidelines for Perioperative Practice.*

Revised December 2021 for publication in *Guidelines for Perioperative Practice,* 2022 edition.

SAFE PATIENT HANDLING AND MOVEMENT

AORN
SAFE SURGERY TOGETHER

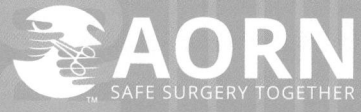

[P] *indicates a recommendation or evidence relevant to pediatric care.*

MEDICAL ABBREVIATIONS & ACRONYMS

ANA – American Nurses Association
HUDDLE – Healthcare Utilizing Deliberate Discussion Linking Events
ICU – Intensive care unit
LI – Lifting index
MIS – Minimally invasive surgery
MRKP – Multiresistant *Klebsiella pneumoniae*
MSD – Musculoskeletal disorder
N - Newton
NHANES – National Health and Nutrition Examination Survey
NIOSH – National Institute for Occupational Safety and Health

OR – Operating room
OSHA – Occupational Safety and Health Administration
PACU – Postanesthesia care unit
PHAMA – Patient handling and movement assessment
PtD – Prevention through Design
RN – Registered nurse
RNLE – Revised NIOSH Lifting Equation
ROS – Reactive oxygen species
RWL – Recommended weight limit
SPHM – Safe patient handling and movement (or mobility)
STEADI – Stopping Elderly Accidents, Deaths, and Injuries
TUG – Timed Up & Go

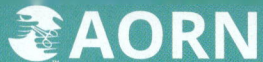

GUIDELINE FOR
SAFE PATIENT HANDLING AND MOVEMENT

The Guideline for Safe Patient Handling and Movement was approved by the AORN Guidelines Advisory Board and became effective July 1, 2018. It was presented as a proposed guideline for comments by members and others. The recommendations in the guideline are intended to be achievable and represent what is believed to be an optimal level of practice. Policies and procedures will reflect variations in practice settings and/or clinical situations that determine the degree to which the guideline can be implemented. AORN recognizes the many diverse settings in which perioperative nurses practice; therefore, this guideline is adaptable to all areas where operative or other invasive procedures may be performed.

Purpose

This document provides guidance to perioperative professionals for developing, implementing, and maintaining an effective safe patient handling and movement (SPHM) program to reduce the incidence and minimize the severity of injuries to patients and health care workers related to performance of high-risk tasks in the perioperative environment.[1] Guidance is provided for

- establishing and sustaining a culture of safety;
- establishing a formal, systemized SPHM program;
- incorporating ergonomic design principles to provide a safe environment of care;
- selecting, installing, incorporating, and maintaining safe patient handling technology in the perioperative setting;
- establishing education, training, and competency verification in safe patient handling techniques and equipment use;
- assessing the patient and the perioperative environment and developing a plan for SPHM;
- collaborating to include reasonable accommodations for post-injury return to work within the comprehensive SPHM program; and
- establishing a comprehensive quality assurance and performance improvement program to evaluate the SPHM program.

Perioperative registered nurses (RNs) and other team members are routinely faced with a wide array of occupational hazards in the perioperative setting that place them at risk for work-related **musculoskeletal disorders** (MSDs).[2,3] Work-related MSDs are disorders of the muscles, nerves, tendons, ligaments, joints, cartilage, and spinal discs.[4] The lower back, shoulder, and upper extremity are typically involved in MSDs with a gradual or chronic onset. Injuries are the result of overexertion, repetitive motion, manual lifting, and pushing and pulling.[4] When a worker's physical ability, task, workplace environment, and workplace culture are not compatible, there

is an increased risk that the worker will develop an MSD.[2] Physical stressors encountered in health care that contribute to MSDs include forceful exertions,[5] repetitive motions,[5] awkward postures,[6-9] **static postures**,[10,11] prolonged standing,[12-15] long cumulative work hours (eg, overtime, consecutive shifts),[16-20] moving or lifting patients and equipment, carrying heavy instruments and equipment, and overexertion.[2,21] Research studies have also demonstrated an association between psychosocial factors (eg, work-family conflict, workplace verbal abuse, job demands, job satisfaction) and the incidence of musculoskeletal symptoms.[22-29]

Musculoskeletal disorders are some of the most frequently occurring and costly types of occupational issues affecting nurses.[2,30-41] In 2015, RNs in the private sector reported a total of 20,360 nonfatal occupational injury and illness cases requiring days away from work, of which 8,530 (42%) were MSDs and 5,790 (28%) were back injuries.[42]

Ellapen and Narsigan[30] conducted a systematic review of 27 publications with the outcome measure of work-related MSDs among a total of 13,317 nurses. The prevalence of work-related MSDs was 71.8%. The authors concluded that nurses are vulnerable to a work-related MSDs, especially lower back pain and injury. Work-related MSDs also occur frequently in other members of the perioperative team,[20,43,47] including surgeons.[48-63] Karahan et al[43] conducted a qualitative study to describe the prevalence and high-risk factors for lower back pain among hospital workers. Of the 1,600 respondents, 65.8% reported experiencing low back pain, with 61.3% reporting an occurrence in the previous 12 months. The highest prevalence (77.1%, n = 509) was reported by nurses.

The perioperative setting poses unique challenges related to the provision of patient care and completion of procedure-related tasks. This highly technical environment is equipment intensive and necessitates the lifting and moving of heavy supplies and equipment during the perioperative team member's work shift. Many of the patients undergoing surgical or other invasive procedures are completely or partially dependent on the caregivers due to the effects of general or regional anesthesia or sedation. Patients who are unconscious cannot move, sense discomfort, or feel pain, and they must be protected from injury. This may require perioperative team members to manually lift the patient or the patient's extremities several times during a procedure.[26,64]

Nützi et al[26] conducted a correlational questionnaire study of 116 operating room (OR) nurses from eight hospitals to examine the prevalence of musculoskeletal problems in OR nurses. The frequency distribution of the sample showed that 66.1% of the OR nurses reported suffering from MSDs. The nurses reported pain in the lumbar region (52.7%), cervical region (38.4%), mid-spine region (20.5%), knees and legs

(20.5%), and hands and feet (9.8%). Many of the respondents reported more than one pain region. The authors postulated that MSD is one of the most common causes of long-term absence from work (ie, more than 2 weeks). Nurses with MSDs incur both high direct costs for treatment and high economic costs due to their absence from work and productivity loss.

A contributing factor to the incidence of musculoskeletal injuries in health care workers is the increasing prevalence of obesity in the United States.[65,66] The National Health and Nutrition Examination Survey (NHANES), a program of the National Center for Health Statistics, Centers for Disease Control and Prevention, is a cross-sectional, nationally representative health examination of the US noninstitutionalized population that includes measured weight and height. The objective of a recently published NHANES survey was to examine the obesity prevalence for 2013-2014 and trends over the decade from 2005 through 2014, adjusting for sex, age, race/Hispanic origin, smoking status, and education. The survey's main outcomes were the prevalence of obesity (body mass index ≥ 30) and class 3 obesity (body mass index ≥ 40).

The age-adjusted prevalence of obesity in 2013-2014 was 35% among men and 40.4% among women; the age-adjusted prevalence of class 3 obesity was 5.5% for men and 9.9% for women. For women, the prevalence of overall obesity and of class 3 obesity showed significant linear trends for increase from 2005 to 2014. There were no significant trends for men.[67] The relevance for the perioperative team is that more than one-third of all surgical patients cared for could be obese.

The American Nurses Association (ANA) laid the foundation for the prevention of work-related MSDs in 2003 with the release of the position statement *The Elimination of Manual Patient Handling to Prevent Work-Related Musculoskeletal Disorder*[68,69] and development of the Handle With Care® campaign.[70] In 2006, AORN developed the *Position Statement for Ergonomically Healthy Workplace Practices*.[71] The National Association of Orthopedic Nurses,[72] the Australian College of Operating Room Nurses,[73] and the Association of Occupational Health Professionals[74] have also developed safe patient handling position statements.

In 2005, AORN continued its commitment to the prevention of MSDs by forming a collaborative arrangement with the National Institute for Occupational Safety and Health (NIOSH) and the ANA to discuss, design, and advance the agenda of an ergonomically healthy workplace for perioperative professionals. The AORN Workplace Safety Task Force examined current research, literature, and patient care practices to evaluate and make recommendations to promote patient and caregiver safety in a perioperative setting.[75] While there are a number of high-risk tasks specific to perioperative nurses, the task force identified seven key activities as the starting point for developing recommendations. The result of this collaboration was the *AORN Guidance Statement: Safe Patient Handling and Movement in the Perioperative Setting*[64] developed by AORN with the assistance of a panel of experts from the Patient Safety Center of Inquiry at the James A. Haley Veterans Administration Medical Center, Tampa, Florida; the NIOSH Division of Applied

Research and Technology Human Factors and Ergonomics Research Team[76]; and the ANA.[64]

The Ergonomic Tools developed for this guidance document were based on previous work by Audrey Nelson, PhD, RN, FAAN; experts within the Veterans Administration; and nationally recognized researchers. The seven Ergonomic Tools for SPHM were developed based on professional consensus and evidence from research and were designed with the goal of eradicating job-related MSDs in perioperative nurses (See Recommendation 6).[64]

In 2013, the ANA published Safe Patient Handling and Mobility: Interprofessional National Standards Across the Care Continuum.[69] The ANA's eight core standards are:

- *Establish a Culture of Safety*
- *Implement and Sustain a Safe Patient Handling and Mobility (SPHM) Program*
- *Incorporate Ergonomic Design Principles to Provide a Safe Environment of Care*
- *Select, Install, and Maintain SPHM Technology*
- *Establish a System for Education, Training, and Maintaining Competence*
- *Integrate Patient-Centered SPHM Assessment, Plan of Care, and Use of SPHM Technology*
- *Include SPHM in Reasonable Accommodation and Post-Injury Return to Work*
- *Establish a Comprehensive Evaluation System*[69]

The ANA standards have been adapted to meet the unique needs of the perioperative patients, team members, and environment. These standards provide an important framework[77] for health care organizations to use in implementing safe patient handling practices and provide the framework for the eight recommendations in this guideline.

The benefits of implementing an SPHM program include reduced work-related MSDs,[1,78,79] reduced risk and severity of lifting and repositioning injuries,[1] increased patient safety,[1,78,79] decreased falls,[1] decreased workers' compensation costs,[1,79,80] decreased health care worker fatigue,[1] decreased employee turnover,[78] increased health care worker morale,[1,80] and increased quality of life.[1]

The following topics are outside the scope of this document:

- patient positioning (See the AORN Guideline for Positioning the Patient[81]),
- pressure injuries (See the AORN Guideline for Positioning the Patient[81]),
- patient skin antisepsis (See the AORN Guideline for Preoperative Patient Skin Antisepsis[82]), and
- mobility of postoperative patients.

Evidence Review

A medical librarian with a perioperative background conducted a systematic search of the databases Ovid MEDLINE®, EBSCO CINAHL®, Scopus®, and the Cochrane Database of Systematic Reviews. The search was limited to literature published in

Figure 1. Flow Diagram of Literature Search Results

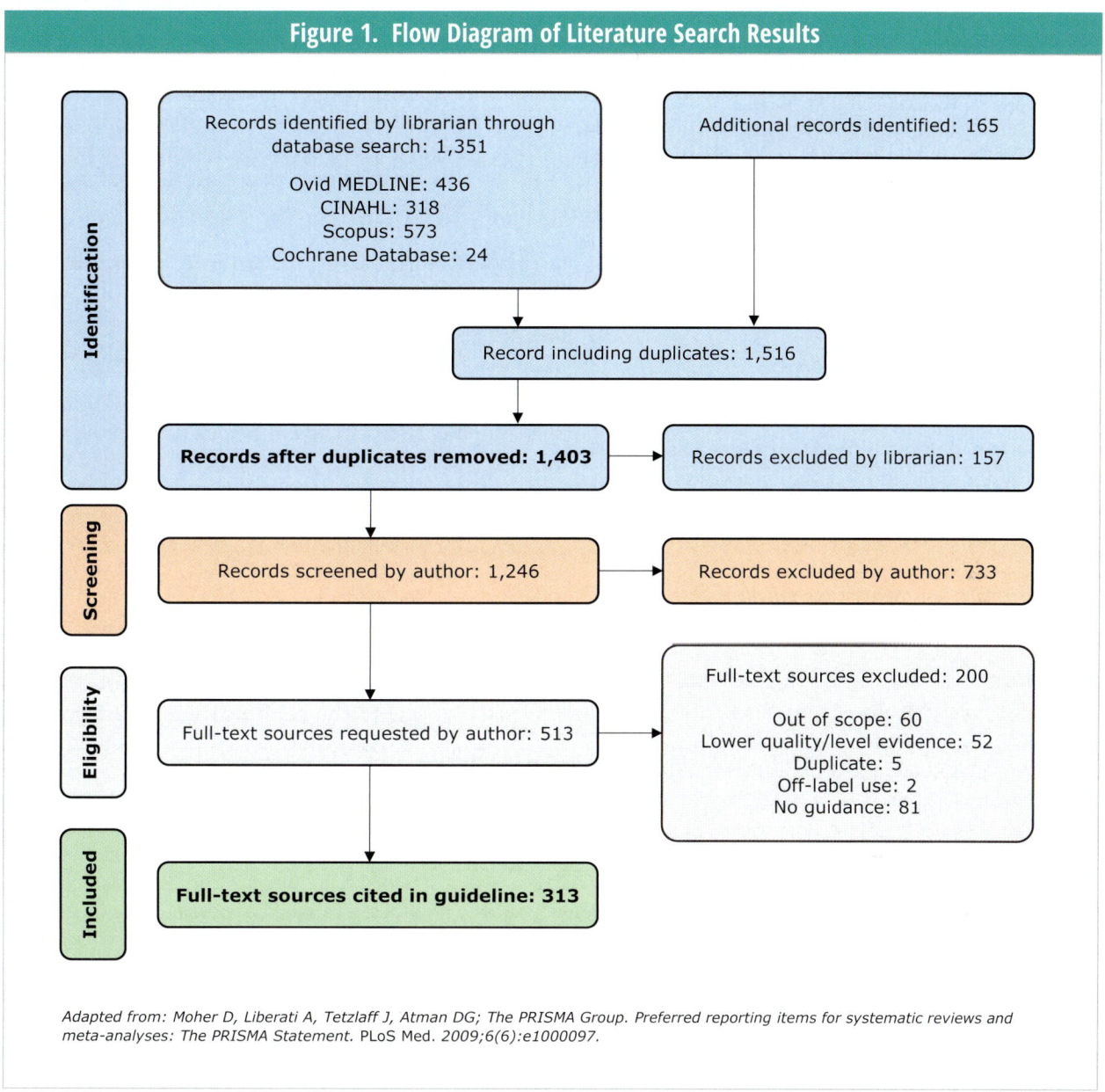

Adapted from: Moher D, Liberati A, Tetzlaff J, Atman DG; The PRISMA Group. Preferred reporting items for systematic reviews and meta-analyses: The PRISMA Statement. PLoS Med. 2009;6(6):e1000097.

English from 2005 through November 2017. At the time of the initial search, weekly alerts were created on the topics included in that search. Results from these alerts were provided to the lead author until January of 2018. The lead author requested additional articles that either did not fit the original search criteria or were discovered during the evidence appraisal process. The lead author and the medical librarian also identified relevant guidelines from government agencies, professional organizations, and standards-setting bodies. The literature review was supplemented with additional select articles following the public commenting review period.

Search terms included subject headings such as *accidental falls, accidents (occupational), allied health personnel, back injuries, biomechanics, equipment safety, ergonomics, handling and movement, health care personnel, health personnel, hoists, human engineering, lifting, lifting and transfer equipment, low back pain, muscular diseases, musculoskeletal diseases, musculoskeletal system/injuries, neck pain, nursing staff, occupational diseases, occupational exposure, occupational hazards, occupational health, occupational health services, occupational safety, occupational-related injuries, operating room personnel, patient transfer, physical complaints, posture, pull, push, risk assessment, risk management, roll board, shoulder pain, stress (physiological), surgical equipment and supplies, transfer techniques, transportation of patients, weight bearing, worker's compensation,* and *wounds and injuries/prevention and control.*

Included were research and non-research literature in English, complete publications, and publication dates within the time restriction when available. Excluded were non-peer-reviewed publications and older evidence within the time restriction when more recent evidence was available. Editorials, news items, other brief items, and publications about off-label use of devices also were excluded. Low-quality evidence was excluded when higher-quality evidence was available (Figure 1).

Articles identified in the search were provided to the project team for evaluation. The team consisted of the lead author and three evidence appraisers. The lead author divided the search results into topics, and members of the team reviewed and critically appraised each article using the AORN Research or Non-Research Evidence Appraisal Tools as appropriate. The literature was independently evaluated and appraised according to the strength and quality of the evidence. Each article was then assigned an appraisal score. The appraisal score is noted in brackets after each reference as applicable.

Each recommendation rating is based on a synthesis of the collective evidence, a benefit-harm assessment, and consideration of resource use. The strength of the recommendation was determined using the AORN Evidence Rating Model and the quality and consistency of the evidence supporting a recommendation. The recommendation strength rating is noted in brackets after each recommendation.

Note: The evidence summary table is available at http:// www.aorn.org/evidencetables/.

Editor's note: Handle With Care is a registered trademark of the American Nurses Association, Silver Spring, MD. MEDLINE is a registered trademark of the US National Library of Medicine's Medical Literature Analysis and Retrieval System, Bethesda, MD. CINAHL, Cumulative Index to Nursing and Allied Health Literature, is a registered trademark of EBSCO Industries, Birmingham, AL. Scopus is a registered trademark of Elsevier B.V., Amsterdam, The Netherlands.

1. Culture of Safety

1.1 **The health care organization and the perioperative team should collaborate to establish and sustain a culture of safety that incorporates the principles of SPHM.** *[Recommendation]*

A culture of safety incorporates the core values and behaviors resulting from a shared and sustained commitment by organizational leaders and the perioperative team to emphasize safety over competing goals.[69,78] The primary objective of the safety culture is to keep patients and perioperative team members safe.[78] Organizational leaders[83,84] and perioperative team members need to be engaged and supportive of each other to successfully implement a culture of safety.[78,85,86]

In a review of the literature of the working environment and adverse safety consequences for nurses, Geiger-Brown and Lipscomb[20] proposed improved compliance with safe work practices as the mechanism for protecting the safety and health of the workers (See the AORN Guideline for Team Communication[87]).

1.2 **Create a written statement committing to a culture of safety.**[69] *[Recommendation]*

The statement guides the health care organization's priorities, resource allocation, policies, and procedures.[69] Leadership commitment[88] is key to the development of a culture of safety within an organization.[1,89]

1.3 **Create a nonpunitive environment.**[69,89] *[Recommendation]*

A nonpunitive environment encourages team members to identify, address, and report hazards, errors, **near misses**, incidents, and accidents.[69,89] Reporting leads to a better understanding of organizational problems and can lead to improved processes and education to address patient and equipment handling incidents and injuries. The team members are held accountable for their own actions but not for system or environmental problems that are outside their control.[6]

1.3.1 **Report hazards, near misses, incidents, and accidents related to patient and equipment handling as soon as possible according to the health care organization's policy and procedure** (See Recommendation 8).[69] *[Recommendation]*

In health care organizations with a strong safety culture, errors are considered learning opportunities. Any event related to safety, particularly a human or organizational error, provides a valuable opportunity to improve safety through feedback.[89]

1.4 **The health care organization should provide the number of team members and assistive devices needed to safely move, position, or prep patients based on the algorithms in the AORN Ergonomic Tools** (See Recommendation 6).[64,69] *[Recommendation]*

Providing the number of team members and assistive devices needed to safely transfer, position, and prep a patient maintains the patient's body alignment and airway.[64]

1.5 **Implement safety huddles (ie, Healthcare Utilizing Deliberate Discussion Linking Events [HUDDLE]) to evaluate incidents and near misses related to patient and equipment handling (See the AORN Guideline for Team Communication[87]).[1]** *[Recommendation]*

Safety huddles are a means to transfer knowledge learned in one incident so it can be used the next time the perioperative team performs the same task. In the safety huddle, individuals can share their unique knowledge with the group so this knowledge can be integrated, understood by the entire team, and used when other individuals face similar circumstances.[1] Safety huddles promote a culture of safety for the patient and the perioperative team.[1]

1.5.1 Hold a brief safety huddle (eg, shorter than 15 minutes) immediately or as soon as possible after every incident or near miss.[1] *[Recommendation]*

1.5.2 Invite all perioperative team members involved in the incident or near miss to attend the safety huddle.[1] *[Recommendation]*

The input of each of the involved perioperative team member helps present a clear picture of what occurred. This information is helpful for making recommendations to prevent a similar incident in the future.[1]

1.5.3 The leader of the safety huddle should ask the team the following questions:
- *What happened to threaten patient or staff safety?*
- *What should have happened?*
- *What accounted for the differences?*
- *What corrective actions should be taken?*
- *How can the same outcome be avoided next time?*
- *What is the follow-up plan, who will take responsible for implementing the corrective actions?*[1(p88)]

[Recommendation]

1.5.4 Openly discuss the circumstances of the incident based on clear, just, and transparent processes for recognizing human and system errors and distinguishing these from unsafe, blameworthy actions.[1,87] *[Recommendation]*

The safety huddle provides opportunities for the perioperative team to make suggestions for changing their work environment based on identification of the problem and potential solutions. Safety huddles may reduce the incidence of injuries through early identification of potential problems.[1]

1.6 The health care organization should provide a mechanism for the health care worker to refuse or object to performing any patient transfer or repositioning or equipment handling that places the patient or worker at risk for injury.[69] *[Recommendation]*

The perioperative team member has a professional obligation to voice concerns about practices that may place the patient or team members at risk for injury and should be able to do so without fear of retribution.[90]

1.6.1 In the policy and procedure, describe the steps for resolving the hazard[69]; identify situations that are unsafe for the patient, team members, or both[90]; establish reporting methods[90]; and institute after-action review of a refusal to perform unsafe patient or equipment handling.[90] *[Recommendation]*

2. Safe Patient Handling and Movement (SPHM) Program

2.1 Establish a formal, systemized SPHM program. *[Recommendation]*

An SPHM program reduces the risk for patient injury and the perioperative team's risk for injuries and MSDs while improving the quality of patient care.[69]

2.2 Appoint an interdisciplinary perioperative team with the authority and responsibility to establish, evaluate, and maintain an SPHM program.[69] *[Recommendation]*

Involving key stakeholders in the development, evaluation, remediation, and maintenance of the SPHM program from the inception of the program helps to identify barriers and garners buy-in from members of the different disciplines included in the perioperative team. Staff participation in the selection of the equipment is also key to the success of the program.[91-93] In a qualitative study, Krill et al[94] concluded that it is essential to obtain information from direct-care nurses and technicians regarding the perceived barriers to safe patient handling before implementing a program.

Caspi et al[95] tested the feasibility of a multi-component intervention to improve worker safety and wellness using a pre-implementation survey (N = 374) and a post-implementation survey (N = 303) to assess changes in safety, ergonomic behaviors and practices, and social support. Three questions on the surveys assessed managerial (ie, supervisor) support. The mean reported scores of support from supervisors improved over the course of the intervention from 10.6 of 15 pre-implementation to 10.9 of 15 post-implementation. The authors concluded that managerial involvement for the planning and implementation of unit-wide changes may contribute to successful improvements in the work environment and more positive worker behaviors.

A study by Nelson et al[41] demonstrated the importance of having both the nurses' and administrators' acceptance of the **ergonomics** program. Using a pre-implementation/post-implementation design without a control group, Nelson et al[41] evaluated the effectiveness of a patient care ergonomics program on 23 high-risk units in seven facilities. The researchers compared injury rates, lost work days, modified work days, job satisfaction, staff and patient acceptance of the program, program effectiveness, and program costs and savings during two 9-month periods. They collected data prospectively through surveys, weekly process logs, injury logs, and cost logs. The six program elements includes an ergonomic assessment protocol, patient handling assessment criteria and decision algorithms, a peer leader role, state-of-the-art equipment, after-action reviews, and a no-lift policy.

Post-program implementation injury rates were significantly lower, with injury rates decreasing in 15 of the 23 units. Modified work days decreased significantly from 1,777 days pre-intervention to 539 days post-intervention. During the study, nurses self-reported the number of unsafe patient handling and lifting practices (eg, without proper equipment, without the number of staff needed) in a typical day. There was a significant decrease in the number of reported unsafe practices during the post-intervention period. Patient acceptance was moderate when the program started but increased to very high by the end of the study period. The authors concluded that the multi-faceted program resulted in an overall lower injury rate, fewer modified duty days taken per injury, and significant cost savings. The program was well accepted by patients, nursing staff members, and administrators.[41]

A random sample (n = 209) of the 825 participating nurses was invited to complete surveys before and after the interventions. The researchers surveyed six components of a nurse's work satisfaction and the number of self-reported unsafe patient handling tasks in a typical day. The overall survey score and five of the six components scores increased from the pre-intervention to the post-intervention period, indicating an increase in job satisfaction (ie, pay, professional status, task requirements, autonomy, organizational policies). Given the significant increases in two job satisfaction subscales—professional status and task requirements—an SPHM program could potentially improve nurse recruitment and retention.[41]

2.2.1 The perioperative SPHM program may be part of the health care organization's SPHM program or may be an independent perioperative program. *[Conditional Recommendation]*

Many health care organizations have implemented SPHM programs in other areas of the organization. By becoming part of the organizational SPHM, the perioperative team benefits from current best practices and lessons learned

during implementation and ongoing program maintenance.

2.2.2 Perioperative SPHM program team members may include perioperative nurses, surgeons, anesthesia professionals, surgical technologists, an industrial hygienist, perianesthesia nurses, unlicensed assistive personnel, an SPHM program coordinator, a risk manager, a materials manager, an occupational health professional, and an **ergonomist**.[1] *[Conditional Recommendation]*

2.2.3 The perioperative SPHM program team should understand the philosophy of ergonomics and ergonomic processes.[1] *[Recommendation]*

Ergonomics is the science of fitting the job to the worker. The practice of designing equipment and work tasks to conform to the capability of the worker provides a means for adjusting the work environment and work practices to prevent injuries and emphasizes work practices, **biomechanics**, work environment, and tool use.

2.3 Perform an initial comprehensive assessment[3] of SPHM needs, current patient and equipment handling technology, and **adverse events** data to determine needs, priorities, and frequency for reassessment (eg, biannually, annually) (See Recommendation 8).[69] *[Recommendation]*

2.4 Develop written goals; objectives; and a plan for ongoing evaluation, compliance, and quality improvement.[69] Include short- and long-term goals and objectives and a timeline to meet the goals and evaluation requirements.[69] *[Recommendation]*

Written short- and long-term goals and objectives and a plan for ongoing evaluation, compliance, and quality improvement are needed to evaluate the effectiveness and progress of the program.

2.4.1 The SPHM program must comply with federal, state, and local laws and regulations and should incorporate the ANA Safe Patient Handling and Mobility: Interprofessional National Standards (See the Purpose section).[69] *[Regulatory Requirement]*

Since 2005, 11 states (ie, California, Illinois, Maryland, Minnesota, Missouri, New Jersey, New York, Ohio, Rhode Island, Texas,[96,97] and Washington,[98] with a resolution from Hawaii[79,99,101]) have enacted "safe patient handling" laws, rules, or regulations. Ten states (ie, California, Illinois, Maryland, Minnesota, Missouri, New Jersey, New York, Rhode Island, Texas,[97] and Washington) require a comprehensive program in health care facilities. Common requirements in the comprehensive program include establishing a safe patient handling policy; dedicating staff to the safe patient handling program (eg, a patient handling coordinator); forming a safe patient handling committee; using lifting devices and equipment; providing education and training; reporting, tracking, and analyzing injuries; and evaluating the program.[79]

Under the General Duty Clause, Section 5(a)(1) of the Occupational Safety and Health Act of 1970, employers are required to provide their employees with a place of employment that is "free from recognizable hazards that are causing or likely to cause death or serious harm to employees."[102] A court interpretation of the Occupational Safety and Health Administration (OSHA) General Duty Clause is that the employer has a legal obligation to provide a workplace free of conditions or activities that either the employer or industry recognizes as hazardous and that cause or are likely to cause death or serious physical harm to employees when there is a feasible method to abate the hazard.[103] Recognizing the effects that ergonomic hazards have on workers,[104] OSHA has developed online resources and guidelines to help nursing homes create and implement safe patient handling assessments, policies, procedures, programs, training, and patient education.[70,105,106]

2.4.2 **Identify methods (eg, equipment, algorithms) to reduce the physical requirements of high-risk SPHM tasks (eg, positioning, transfers, static postures)** (See Recommendations 4 and 6).[69] *[Recommendation]*

Ergonomic analyses and interventions are primary preventive methods to reduce physical stressors in the workplace and may prevent work-related MSDs.[107] Use of safe patient handling equipment (eg, air-assisted transfer devices, lifts) and the AORN Ergonomic Tools can reduce the physical requirements of high-risk SPHM tasks.

2.5 **Designate individuals who will have the responsibility, authority, and accountably for implementing the plan.**[69] *[Recommendation]*

An example of an SPHM program that delineates responsibility, authority, and accountability is the Veterans Health Administration model in which a facility coordinator provides leadership and assumes continuing responsibility for the development, implementation, coordination, maintenance, and evaluation of the program at an organizational level.[1] The facility coordinator works under the direction of facility leadership.[1] The facility coordinator leads and trains SPHM peer leaders in all clinical areas. The peer leaders train their coworkers on the fundamentals of the program and assist with monitoring the program elements. A peer leader acts as a resource, coach, and team leader in his or her clinical area.[1]

2.5.1 **Establish the reporting mechanism to be used for monitoring compliance** (See Recommendation 8).[69] *[Recommendation]*

2.6 **Integrate the perioperative SPHM program across the three phases of perioperative care: preoperative, intraoperative, and postoperative.**[69] *[Recommendation]*

The evidence is limited regarding patient and equipment handling tasks in the perioperative setting. Patient and equipment handling tasks occur in all phases of perioperative care. Patient handling needs may change during the patient's perioperative stay. A patient may be fully mobile and ambulatory in the preoperative area, totally dependent in the OR during transfer from the OR bed to the stretcher, and require assistance in the postanesthesia care unit (PACU). Examples of patient handling and mobility tasks in the perioperative setting include helping an elderly patient who walks with a cane to the restroom before surgery, transferring a patient from the stretcher to the OR bed into the prone position during surgery, and repositioning a patient in the PACU.

2.7 **Identify and allocate funding to implement and sustain the program based on business-case and return-on-investment analytics.**[69] *[Recommendation]*

Health care organizations that have implemented an SPHM program have reported a return on investment within 1 to 3 years.[41,83,108,109] Overall program costs include the capital costs of the equipment, installation, maintenance, and accessories and the training costs for team members.[41,110] The return on investment can be calculated using the internal rate of return (ie, discount rate that equates the present value of the project's benefits to the project's costs). Additional costs that factor into the return on investment are the costs associated with an injury. These costs are medical treatment (eg, medical evaluation, imaging, prescriptions, therapy), workers' compensation, and lost productivity. Workers' compensation payments include continuation of payments to personnel with up to 45 lost work days (ie, short-term disability) and Department of Labor cash payments for long-term disability beyond 45 days. Lost productivity is the salary costs for the total number of lost

903

and modified work days associated with an injury. On these days, the employee is not able to perform the regular duties of his or her job.[41] The cost/benefit of the SPHM program can be attributed to lower injuries,[70,78,83,108,111-119] workers' compensation costs,[70,78,108,111,117,118,120] medical care costs,[70,112,116] and lost productivity.[41,70,83,108,112,116-118,120]

2.8 Identify the essential physical functions and provide input for the written job descriptions of personnel who perform SPHM tasks in the perioperative setting.[69] *[Recommendation]*

A written job description with identified physical functions establishes the physical requirements needed to fulfill the role. The essential physical functions in the perioperative setting were identified during the development of the *AORN Guidance Statement: Safe Patient Handling and Movement in the Perioperative Setting.*[64] The guidance statement identified seven high-risk tasks specific to perioperative nurses in the perioperative setting[64]:

- transferring a patient on and off the OR bed,[2]
- repositioning a patient in the OR bed,[2]
- lifting and holding the patient's extremities,[2]
- standing for long periods of time,[2]
- holding retractors for long periods of time,[2]
- lifting and moving equipment,[2] and
- sustaining awkward positions.

Lifting and moving patients is a frequent activity in the perioperative setting, as team members transfer patients to and from transport carts (eg, stretchers) and the OR bed many times during a typical work shift. Perioperative team members often reposition patients into a **prone**, **lateral**, or **lithotomy position** on the OR bed to provide appropriate exposure of the surgical site. This high-risk activity requires team members to physically lift and maneuver the patient or a patient's extremity while simultaneously placing a positioning device. The patient's weight may not be evenly distributed. In addition, maintaining the patient's airway and body alignment and supporting the extremities may make it difficult for team members to position themselves in an ergonomically safe position, thus exacerbating physical demands.[64]

2.8.1 Use an evidence-based process to identify the tasks that place the perioperative team members at high risk for injury.[69,121] *[Recommendation]*

2.9 Develop policies and procedures for SPHM[88] and equipment handling based on the AORN Ergonomic Tools, review them periodically, revise them as necessary, and make them readily avail-

able in the perioperative setting (See Recommendation 6). *[Recommendation]*

Safe patient handling and movement is one part of the comprehensive program to prevent team members' musculoskeletal injuries and increase patient safety.[1] Policies and procedures assist in the development of patient safety, perioperative team member safety, quality assessment, and performance improvement activities. Policies and procedures serve as operational guidelines used to minimize patients' and perioperative team members' risk for injury and standardize practice. Policies and procedures establish authority, responsibility, and accountability within the practice setting. Developing policies and procedures that guide and support patient care, treatment, and services is a regulatory requirement.[122,123]

3. Ergonomic Design

3.1 Incorporate ergonomic design principles in the planning and design of the surgical suite. *[Recommendation]*

Ergonomic design principles (eg, the Prevention through Design [PtD] initiative of NIOSH[124]) use a systemized and proactive process to prevent or reduce occupational injuries and exposures by including prevention considerations in all designs.[69] The ergonomic design of an OR is dependent on the type of procedures (eg, neurosurgery,[125,126] vascular surgery[127,128]) performed and the patient population. Koneczny[129] surveyed surgeons (N = 414) and OR nurses (N = 184) about working conditions in the OR and evaluated work plans in the ORs of five hospitals. The findings showed there was a high potential for ergonomic improvement and an increase in safety and comfort. The author concluded that the deficiencies demonstrated the need for better implementation of ergonomic design in the OR and that ORs need individualized solutions as there is not one solution that will address the needs in all ORs.

In a prospective case-controlled study, Klein et al[130] examined whether optimized ergonomic practices and technical aids within a modern OR affected psychological and physiological stress in experienced laparoscopic surgeons. Ten experienced surgeons performed laparoscopic cholecystectomies in two different ORs. In the standard OR, the equipment was on a laparoscopic cart. The monitor was positioned before surgery and not moved during the procedure. In the modern OR, two moveable flat panel monitors were fixed to the ceiling and could be moved both horizontally and vertically. One screen was in front of the surgeon and the other in front of the assistant in a neutral position. The surgeons completed a questionnaire concerning physical and psychological well-being before and after surgery. Physical parameters included pain in the right neck and shoulder, right lower arm, right hand, right side of lower back, left neck and shoulder, left lower arm, left hand, and left side of the lower back. Subjective parameters included well-being, time strain, effort, performance, frustration, and satisfaction. Preoperative to postoperative physical strain and pain measurements demonstrated a systematic difference in 14 of the 15 parameters, favoring the modern OR. Measurements for physical strain in the right neck and shoulders and pain in the right lower arm reached statistical significance. The authors concluded the physical strain on the surgeon was reduced during laparoscopic cholecystectomy performed in the modern OR compared to the standard OR.

3.2 During the planning phase of any construction or renovation of the surgical suite, integrate the assessment of ergonomic and other safety risk factors into the design.[69] *[Recommendation]*

The Facility Guidelines Institute recommends conducting a patient handling and movement assessment (PHAMA) to assist the design team in incorporating patient handling equipment into the health care environment.[110] The PHAMA consists of two phases:

- The first phase includes an assessment to identify patient handling equipment needed for each area where patient handling occurs. The needs assessment includes the projected patient population, type of high-risk tasks performed, frontline staff surveys, and appropriate equipment for high-risk tasks.
- The second phase includes defining space requirements and structural and other design considerations to accommodate integration of the safe patient handling equipment.[110]

3.3 The design team should include the perspectives and input of frontline team members and the perioperative SPHM program team[131] **at all stages and in all activities of the new construction, rebuilding, or remodeling related to ergonomic principles.**[69] *[Recommendation]*

In a qualitative study, Krill et al[94] surveyed 210 health care workers to determine the staff's perceived barriers and attitudes regarding SPHM. The staff nurses identified the lack of a "no lift" policy, adequate lifting equipment, and adequate storage space on the nursing unit as major barriers. Additionally, nurses continued to be trained to use ineffective techniques to move patients, received inadequate follow-up training for safe patient handling, and received no

safe patient handling education for increasingly complex patient care needs. The authors concluded it is essential to obtain information from frontline team members regarding perceived barriers prior to implementing a safe patient handling program, and staff participation in the selection of equipment is also key to the eventual success of the program.

3.3.1 Individualize patient handling equipment recommendations to each clinical area undergoing new construction or renovation.[110] *[Recommendation]* **P**

Patient characteristics and environmental and space characteristics vary from one clinical area to another.[110] Patient characteristics, including age (eg, pediatric[113], geriatric), size (eg, bariatric[132-136]), and procedure types (eg, spine), determine the type of equipment and design requirements needed.

3.3.2 Include process flow, evaluation of SPHM technology, and accessibility in the design of the facility (See Recommendation 4.3).[69] *[Recommendation]*

Inaccessibility,[137] inconvenient storage, and lack of storage space[138] for SPHM equipment are barriers to consistent use of the equipment.[139,140]

3.3.3 Factor storage space requirements (eg, floor space, fixed and mobile shelving) and electrical outlets needed for patient handling equipment (eg, lifts, slings, carts) into the design.[139] *[Recommendation]*

The types and amount of safe patient handling equipment determine space requirements of the storage area.[110] Shelving may be used to store slings, air-transfer mattresses, and **friction-reducing devices**. Equipment powered by rechargeable batteries needs electrical outlets for charging the batteries.[139]

3.3.4 If ceiling lifts are installed in the perioperative area, integrate the requirements for the ceiling lifts into the design process.[139,141] *[Recommendation]*

Ceiling lift installation constraints in the OR include structural capacity; boom-mounted lights and equipment towers; heating, ventilating, and air conditioning ducts; electrical conduits; and other ceiling-mounted equipment.[139] Retrofitting is costly and challenging.[142]

Thomas-Olson et al[142] surveyed 29 OR staff members after the installation of ceiling lifts in their ORs to measure the success of the project, identify barriers regarding effective use of the ceiling lifts, and determine whether there was a reduction in patient handling injuries. Three logistical barriers were identified in the survey: unavailability of slings due to supply and laundry turnaround times; an emergency pull cord that was too long and inadvertently became engaged; and the awkward location of the docking station. Two of the barriers were addressed immediately by increasing sling inventory and providing education about raising the docking station to keep it out of the way.

All of the surveyed staff members used the ceiling lift before and after surgery for **lateral transfers** and repositioning the patient and were confident in using it. The respondents believed the ceiling lifts were a practical and useful safety control and recommended them for all ORs. The slings remained with the patients postoperatively for use in other areas of the hospital with ceiling lifts, improving patient handling, patient safety, and worker safety throughout the hospital.[142]

3.3.5 **Design traverse or boom-mounted lifts to work around other ceiling-mounted equipment and to have enough coverage for lateral transfers, limb lifting, and repositioning.[139]** *[Recommendation]*

3.3.6 **Install fixed SPHM equipment according to manufacturer's specifications.[69]** *[Recommendation]*

The health care organization's engineering department is a primary resource to verify the mechanical safety of the SPHM technology and equipment, monitor the safe installation according to manufacturer's specifications, and recognize any structural concerns.[90]

4. SPHM Technology

4.1 The health care organization and the perioperative team should collaborate in the selection, installation, and maintenance of safe patient handling technology into the perioperative setting. *[Recommendation]*

Safe patient handling technology (eg, equipment, devices) facilitates SPHM, minimizing the risk for injury to the patient and health care workers.[69]

4.2 Perform an ergonomic analysis of the perioperative area.[1,69] *[Recommendation]*

The ergonomic analysis determines the type of technology, equipment, and improvements needed to decrease risk for musculoskeletal injuries.[1] The recommendations are based on a walk-through of the perioperative area, interviews with the man-

agement team and frontline perioperative team members, and a review of area-specific data.[1]

4.2.1 **Identify high-risk tasks by reviewing injury data of the perioperative area, conducting surveys, and interviewing the perioperative team.[1]** *[Recommendation]*

High-risk perioperative tasks (eg, positioning patients, transferring patients) potentially cause musculoskeletal impact and stress on the back, shoulders, neck, wrists, hands, and knees.[1,143] Examples of high-risk tasks with ergonomic hazards are tasks that require twisting,[14] bending,[14] reaching, holding patients' body parts for prolonged periods of time (ie, prepping, retracting), pushing,[144] pulling,[144] awkward postures, and repetitive motions.[1,35,64]

McCoskey[145] conducted a study to describe patient handling demands in 14 inpatient units at a military health care facility during a 24-hour period. Results of the study demonstrated the diverse nature and impact of patient-handling tasks based on the different nursing care units, patient characteristics, and available transfer equipment. A greater number of lateral transfers occurred in units in which the patients had a higher acuity level and were more dependent (eg, the intensive care unit [ICU], the OR). McCoskey concluded that the descriptions of the types of transfers performed on the nursing unit, the physical exertion required to perform the transfers, and the level of patient dependency could guide selection of the most appropriate and cost-effective equipment for specific units and patient populations.

4.2.2 **Collect information on the physical environment (eg, space, storage, structure),[1] patient characteristics (eg, age, size, procedure type), staffing, and usage and condition of existing patient handling equipment (eg, slide sheets).[1]** *[Recommendation]* **P**

Patient characteristics, including age (eg, pediatric,[113] geriatric), size (eg, bariatric[132-136]), and procedure types (eg, spine, robotics), determine the type of equipment needed.

Randall et al[146] analyzed the web-based OSHA 300 log at a 761-bed, Level I trauma center affiliated with a medical school to identify and describe the frequency, severity, and nature of bariatric versus non-bariatric patient handling injuries. Their analysis demonstrated that during a 1-year period, patients with a body mass index of ≥ 35 kg/m^2 comprised less than 10% of the patient population but accounted for 29.8% of the staff injuries related to patient handling. The narrative in the log revealed that the injured staff members were using biomechanics and not equipment to move patients. Understanding the heightened risk for injury associated with moving bariatric patients should help health care organizations identify risks and focus resources on safer patient handling solutions.

4.2.3 **Conduct a walk-through of the perioperative area.**[1] *[Recommendation]*

The walk-through evaluation serves to help identify direct and indirect factors that contribute to SPHM risks.[1] The walk-through provides a time for the SPHM team to recommend equipment and suggest changes.[1] In a qualitative study, Stucke and Menzel[147] conducted an ergonomic assessment of a critical care unit. As part of the assessment, the researchers identified several factors that contributed to unsafe SPHM practices, such as crowded hallways that made it difficult to maneuver an occupied bed through the department, broken bed wheels, and long hallways. The assessment provided objective data for recommending changes for education and training of the staff, reporting of patient handling injuries, and equipment.

4.2.4 **Generate recommendations that are achievable, accounting for constraints (eg, financial resources, administrative support, environmental factors).**[1] *[Recommendation]*

Recommendations are based on a careful review of the data, equipment availability and usage, patient population characteristics, physical environment, injury data, and high-risk tasks identified by the perioperative team.[1]

4.3 **Based on the ergonomic analysis, select types of patient handling equipment (eg, air-assisted transfer mattresses, mechanical lifting equipment) for use in the perioperative area in conjunction with the health care organization's product evaluation team, policies, and procedures.**[69,90,148] *[Recommendation]*

Before product evaluation, holding a vendor or equipment fair[1,110] is an option that allows vendors to present their products to the entire perioperative staff. The fair gives frontline employees access to different types of equipment from three to five vendors to determine the equipment that best meets their needs. The team is able to see hands-on demonstrations and evaluate ease of movement, control functions, and safety features.[1]

Lateral transfer devices help to move patients horizontally from one flat surface to another (eg, OR bed to stretcher). These devices (eg, air-assisted lateral transfer mattresses, mechanical devices, friction-reducing sheets) minimize frictional resistance and decrease the pulling forces required to move patients.[110] An **air-assisted lateral transfer device** is a mattress inflated with continuous air pressure that flows through numerous small holes in its bottom surface, thereby causing the mattress, with the patient on it, to "float" or "hover" while the health care providers guide it from one surface to the other. A mechanical device pulls the patient from one surface to another (eg, by extending a rigid surface under the patient and moving the patient). Friction-reducing devices (eg, slide sheets) are made of a slippery-type material that reduces friction.[110,149]

In a randomized controlled trial, Baptiste et al[150] assessed the performance of lateral transfer devices compared with the use of a traditional draw sheet, using the subjective feedback of 77 caregivers. Eight different types of lateral transfer devices were analyzed during 179 transfers. The devices differed in materials, transfer principle (eg, air-assisted transfer, friction-reducing), direction of force application (ie, push, pull), basic design, safety features, and cost. The elements evaluated in the survey included overall comfort, overall ease of use, effectiveness in reducing injuries, efficient use of the caregiver's time, and patient safety.

An overall performance rating was calculated as the sum of the five categories. The draw sheet performed poorly across all of the survey elements. The air-assisted transfer devices received the highest overall performance ratings. The researchers recommended that lateral transfer devices be used instead of the traditional draw sheet.[150] Studies by Lloyd and Baptiste,[151] Bartnik and Rice,[152] and Pellino et al[153] also demonstrated the benefits of using lateral transfer devices to increase patient safety and reduce the risk of health care worker injury.

Mechanical lifting equipment used with slings (eg, ceiling lifts, portable floor lifts, boom lifts) temporarily lifts the patient or suspends a body part (eg, leg, arm) during transfer, repositioning, or performance of care tasks (eg, patient skin antisepsis).[154] Slings are devices manufactured from flexible materials (eg, fabrics) that conform to the patient's body. In a single-subject study, Waters et al[155] compared the horizontal push/pull forces at the hands when using two different overhead-mounted devices and two floor-based devices. The single-subject design allowed for simple comparisons between the equipment being tested without introducing between-subject variability. The researchers focused on differences in required operating forces and estimated biomechanical loads for a typical operator. The findings demonstrated that the floor-based lifts exceeded recommended exposure limits for pushing and pulling and the overhead-mounted lifts did not. The authors recommended that overhead-mounted devices be used whenever possible.

Similarly, in a biomechanical analysis, Marras et al[156] investigated the factors associated with patient handling devices that could influence spine loads and low back pain risk. The study analyzed the three-dimensional spine forces imposed on the lumbar spines of 10 participants who manipulated ceiling-based and floor-based patient lifts through various patient handling conditions and maneuvers. The results indicated that ceiling-mounted patient lift systems imposed spine forces on the lumbar spine that would be considered safe, and the floor-based patient handling systems had the potential to increase anterior/posterior shear forces to unacceptable levels during patient handling maneuvers. The authors concluded that ceiling-based lifts are preferable to floor-based patient transfer systems.

In a cross-sectional postal survey of 361 nurses, Lee et al[157] found a significant association between lift availability and work-related low back and shoulder pain. Nurses who reported a high level of lift availability were half as likely to have work-related shoulder pain as nurses who did not have lifts available. The authors concluded that greater availability and use of lifts was associated with less musculoskeletal pain. The findings suggest that for lift interventions to be effective, the equipment must be readily available when needed and barriers against lift use must be removed.

Burdorf et al[158] conducted a systematic review of nine studies to evaluate the effect of manually lifting patients on low back pain among nurses and to estimate the effect of lifting devices on the prevention of low back pain and MSDs. Their review indicated that implementation of lifting devices and complete elimination of manual handling of patients is required to noticeably reduce low back pain and injury claims. In a qualitative study, D'Arcy et al[159] reported 41% lower odds of an injury when a lift was always available when needed.

Pompeii et al[160] retrospectively evaluated musculoskeletal injuries and disorders resulting from patient handling during a 7-year period before the implementation of mechanical lift equipment and a new minimal lift policy throughout a medical center. The authors reviewed the circumstances surrounding the injuries and tried to identify potential preventative measures. Patient handling injuries accounted for 876 (30.7%) of the 2,849 musculoskeletal injuries reported. The authors concluded that the use of mechanical lift equipment could significantly reduce the risk of some patient handling injuries and that ORs in which there are constant patient transfers would benefit from having permanent equipment (ie, ceiling lifts).

Weinel[161] described the implementation of a ceiling-mounted lift system in a new spinal cord unit. Before construction, a pilot project was initiated to compare floor-based electric lifts and a ceiling-mounted lifts. The results indicated that the nurses and the patients preferred the ceiling lift. In the next phase, the nurses were charged with identifying the ceiling lift system that would best meet the specific needs of the spinal cord unit patients and nurses. An interdisciplinary team was formed to coordinate the process of comparing the various ceiling lifts available. The team identified the basic requirements of the lifts and conducted a survey of the vendors.

A clinical evaluation of five lifts was conducted concurrently to determine patient comfort, safety, and ease of use. The lesson learned during this implementation process was that the involvement of bedside nurses during all phases of the implementation was vital and resulted in a sense of ownership. The team believed this was one of the key factors in the success of the transition. Formal and informal discussion groups, interdisciplinary teams, patient input, and field evaluations were also valuable components of the decision-making process. The discussions provided opportunities to address factors that might interfere with implementing use of the ceiling lifts.[161]

4.3.1 **Include the following in the pre-purchase evaluation of SPHM equipment:**
- **efficiency and reliability,**
- **maintenance requirements,**
- **maneuverability,**
- **storage requirements,**
- **workplace design,**
- **ease of operations,**
- **functionality and versatility, and**
- **cleaning.**[1]

[Recommendation]

4.3.2 **Determine and provide the necessary quantity of SPHM equipment to meet patient and perioperative team needs** (See Recommendation 6).[1] *[Recommendation]*

Some types of patient handling equipment can be used separately or in conjunction with other equipment.[1] Current evidence is limited on use of SPHM equipment in the OR. In developing the AORN Ergonomic Tools in 2007, the Workplace Safety Task Force determined there was a need for use of assistive devices to move,

thus, after 3 minutes, strength capability is only 29% of initial lifting strength.[64] Assistive technology is available to assist with transferring a patient into the prone position.

Asiedu et al[220] analyzed open-ended questionnaires and conducted interviews with members of the spine positioning team at a large Midwestern teaching and research hospital to identify the perceptions of the team related to patient and personnel safety during prone positioning. General challenges and themes reported in the interviews were limited staffing to position the patient, the patient's weight, and that the speed of the process creates too much movement of the patient. The participants reported that the difficulty in positioning very large patients could be a source of anxiety and stress to the positioning team. Participants also reported that the receiver role (ie, the person catching the patient during the flip from the supine position on the transport stretcher to the prone position on the OR bed) was more challenging than the sender role (ie, the person flipping the patient away from himself or herself). The difficulty of the receiver role was increased with larger patients because it took longer and required more energy.

6.5 **Before positioning or repositioning the supine patient on the OR bed, apply the algorithm described in AORN Ergonomic Tool #2: Positioning and Repositioning the Supine Patient on the OR Bed.**[64,221] *[Recommendation]*

Positioning or repositioning a patient on the OR bed requires the application of high levels of lifting, pushing, or pulling forces and therefore presents a high risk for musculoskeletal injury to the lower back and shoulders of the team member performing these tasks.[221]

6.5.1 **When positioning the patient into or from a semi-Fowler position (ie, semi-sitting position, beach chair position),**
- **if the patient's weight is less than 68 lb (30.5 kg), a minimum of three perioperative team members should be able to manually position the patient**[64,221]**;**
- **if the patient's weight exceeds 68 lb (30.5 kg), a minimum of three perioperative team members should position the patient using the automatic semi-Fowler positioning feature of the powered OR bed.**[64,221]

[Recommendation]

The mass of a patient's body from the waist up, including the head, neck, and upper extremities, equals 68.6% of the patient's total body weight.[214] Added to this is the estimated

weight of the patient positioning equipment (20 lb [9 kg]).

6.5.2 **When transferring the patient into and from the lateral position,**
- **if the patient's weight is 76 lb (34.5 kg) or less, two perioperative team members and an anesthesia professional maintaining the patient's airway should be able to position the patient**[64,221]**;**
- **if the patient's weight is between 76 lb (34.5 kg) and 115 lb (52 kg), three perioperative team members and an anesthesia professional should be able to position the patient**[64,221]**;**
- **if the patient's weight exceeds 115 lb (52 kg), a lateral positioning devices should be used. The number of team members needed to transfer the patient is dependent on the type of technology used.**[64,221]

[Recommendation]

Positioning or repositioning a patient into or out of a lateral position involves push/pull forces rather than lifting forces. Assuming that one caregiver or anesthesia professional supports the patient's head and neck during lateral positioning, the patient's remaining body mass equals 91.6% of total body mass.[214] For a pulling distance of 6.9 ft (2.1 m) or less, with a pull point (ie, starting position of the hands) between the perioperative team member's waist height and nipple line, performed no more frequently than once every 30 minutes, maximum initial force equals 57 lb (26 kg), and maximum sustained force equals 35 lb (16 kg).[64,216,221] Further research is needed to enhance technology to address this task.

6.5.3 **When positioning the patient to or from the lithotomy position,**
- **if the patient's weight is less than 141 lb (64 kg), two perioperative team members should each hold a leg with a two-handed lift to place the legs in the leg holders**[64,221]**;**
- **if the patient's weight is 141 lb (64 kg) or more, four perioperative team members (ie, two for each leg) should place the legs in the leg holders or use assistive technology**[64,221]**; or**
- **a mechanical device, such as a support sling, may be used to lift the legs to and from the lithotomy position.**

[Recommendation]

When lifting and holding body parts, the maximum load for a two-handed lift is 22 lb (10 kg). Each complete lower patient extremity,

Ergonomic Tool #2. Positioning and Repositioning the Supine Patient on the OR Bed

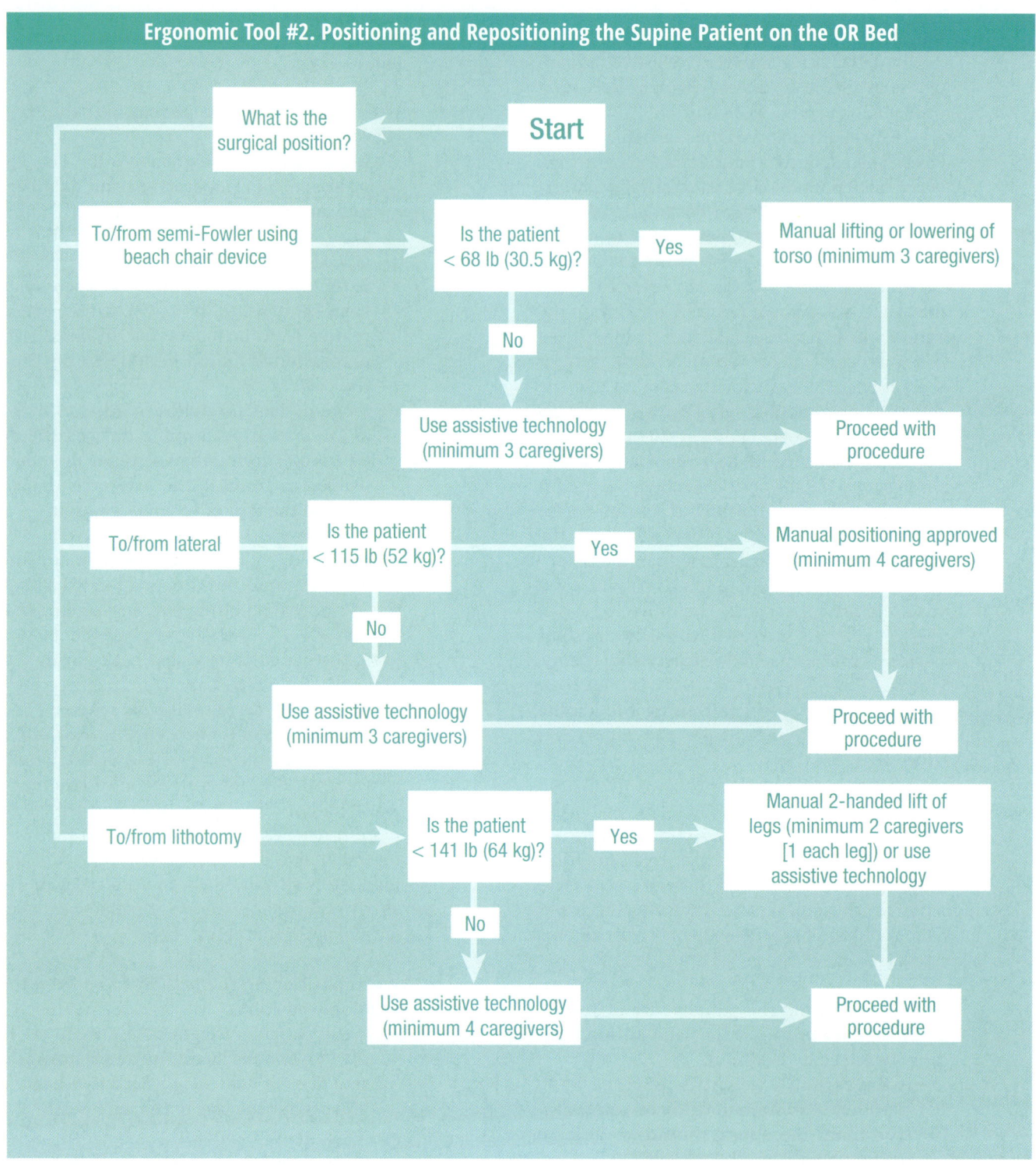

including thigh, calf, and foot, weighs 15.7% of the patient's total body mass. Two team members using two hands can safely perform this task if the patient weighs 141 lb (64 kg) or less because each leg is estimated to be less than 22 lb.[151] Patients weighing more than 141 lb (64.1 kg) require assistive technology or four team members (ie, two to lift each leg). Further

research is needed to enhance technology to address this task.[64,221]

6.6 **Before lifting and holding the patient's legs, arms, and head while prepping, apply the algorithm described in** AORN Ergonomic Tool #3: Lifting and Holding the Patient's Legs, Arms, and Head While Prepping.[64,222] *[Recommendation]*

Ergonomic Tool #3. Lifting and Holding the Patient's Legs, Arms, and Head While Prepping

Legend for action columns: □ = No shading (OK to lift and hold); ▓ = Heavy shading (Do not lift alone)

Patient Weight	Body Part	Body Part Weight		Lift 1-Hand	Lift 2-Hand	Hold 2-Hand ≤ 1 minutes	Hold 2-Hand ≤ 2 minutes	Hold 2-Hand ≤ 3 minutes
≤ 40 lb (≤ 18 kg)	Leg	< 6 lb	(< 3 kg)	□	□	□	□	□
	Arm	< 2 lb	(< 1 kg)	□	□	□	□	□
	Head	< 3 lb	(< 1 kg)	□	□	□	□	□
40-90 lb (18-41 kg)	Leg	< 14 lb	(< 6 kg)	▓	□	▓	□	□
	Arm	< 5 lb	(< 2 kg)	□	□	□	□	□
	Head	< 8 lb	(< 4 kg)	□	□	□	▓	▓
90-140 lb (41-64 kg)	Leg	< 22 lb	(< 10 kg)	▓	□	▓	▓	□
	Arm	< 7 lb	(< 3 kg)	□	□	□	□	▓
	Head	< 12 lb	(< 6 kg)	▓	□	▓	▓	▓
140-190 lb (64-86 kg)	Leg	< 30 lb	(< 14 kg)	▓	□	▓	▓	▓
	Arm	< 10 lb	(< 4 kg)	▓	□	▓	▓	▓
	Head	< 16 lb	(< 7 kg)	▓	□	▓	▓	▓
190-240 lb (86-109 kg)	Leg	< 38 lb	(< 17 kg)	▓	□	▓	▓	▓
	Arm	< 12 lb	(< 6 kg)	▓	□	▓	▓	▓
	Head	< 20 lb	(< 9 kg)	▓	▓	▓	▓	▓
240-290 lb (109-132 kg)	Leg	< 46 lb	(< 21 kg)	▓	▓	▓	▓	▓
	Arm	< 15 lb	(< 7 kg)	▓	□	▓	▓	▓
	Head	< 24 lb	(< 11 kg)	▓	▓	▓	▓	▓
290-340 lb (132-155 kg)	Leg	< 53 lb	(< 24 kg)	▓	▓	▓	▓	▓
	Arm	< 17 lb	(< 8 kg)	▓	□	▓	▓	▓
	Head	< 29 lb	(< 13 kg)	▓	▓	▓	▓	▓
340-390 lb (155-177 kg)	Leg	< 61 lb	(< 28 kg)	▓	▓	▓	▓	▓
	Arm	< 20 lb	(< 9 kg)	▓	□	▓	▓	▓
	Head	< 33 lb	(< 15 kg)	▓	▓	▓	▓	▓
390-440 lb (177-200 kg)	Leg	< 69 lb	(< 31 kg)	▓	▓	▓	▓	▓
	Arm	< 22 lb	(< 10 kg)	▓	□	▓	▓	▓
	Head	< 37 lb	(< 17 kg)	▓	▓	▓	▓	▓
> 440 lb (> 200 kg)	Leg	> 69 lb	(> 31 kg)	▓	▓	▓	▓	▓
	Arm	> 22 lb	(> 10 kg)	▓	▓	▓	▓	▓
	Head	> 37 lb	(> 17 kg)	▓	▓	▓	▓	▓

No shading: OK to lift and hold; use clinical judgment and do not hold longer than noted.
Heavy shading: Do not lift alone; use assistive device or more than 1 caregiver.

When performing preoperative patient skin antisepsis on the patient's legs, arms, and head, the body part may be raised to apply the skin antiseptic circumferentially.[82] Factors that contribute to the ability of the perioperative team member to safely perform the patient skin antisepsis and hold the limb are the size of the body part, length of holding time, posture required to hold the body part without contaminating the surgical prep, and the physical ability of the team member holding the body part. Lifting and holding limbs during skin antisepsis may be hazardous to perioperative team members because lifting and holding limbs requires arm extension that exerts strong forces on the muscles of the shoulders, arms, and back. The risk of injury is low if the muscle exertion is low and the holding time is only a few seconds. The risk of injury increases when muscle exertion exceeds acceptable levels.[214,222]

Ergonomic Tool #3 shows the calculations for average weight for an adult patient's leg, arm, and head as a function of whole body mass. Patient weight is divided into 10 categories, ranging from very light (≤ 40 lb [≤ 18 kg]) to very heavy (> 440 lb [> 200 kg]). Normalized weight for each leg, each arm, and the patient's head is calculated as a percentage of total body weight, where

- each complete lower extremity represents 15.7% of total body mass,
- each upper extremity (ie, upper arm, forearm, hand) represents 5.1% of total body mass, and
- the combination of head and neck represents 8.4% of total body mass.[214]

Maximum lift and hold loads were calculated based on 75th percentile shoulder flexion strength and endurance capabilities for the US adult female working population, where the maximum weight for a one-handed lift is 11 lb and maximum weight for a two-handed lift is 22 lb. The shaded areas of the table indicate whether it would be acceptable for one caregiver to lift the listed body parts or hold the respective body parts for zero, 1, 2, or 3 minutes using one or two hands. Adhering to these limits will minimize the risk of muscle fatigue and the potential for musculoskeletal injury.[64]

6.6.1 Assess the need for additional team member assistance or assistive devices to lift and/or hold one of these body parts according to AORN Ergonomic Tool #3[64,222] based on the amount of time required for lifting and holding and a one- or two-handed hold.[64,223]

- If the patient's weight is less than 40 lb (18 kg), one perioperative team member should be able to perform the skin antisepsis and hold the limb.
- If the patient's weight exceeds 40 lb (18 kg), one perioperative team member should perform the skin antisepsis while another team member holds the limb or the limb is suspended by a holding device.[222]

[Recommendation]

6.6.2 Assess the need for additional team member assistance or assistive devices to lift and/or hold a panniculus during skin antisepsis or the surgical procedure. [Recommendation]

While performing the abdominal patient skin antisepsis, careful attention is needed to adequately prep the skin between skin folds and under the panniculus. An extra team member or an assistive device may assist in this process.[224]

6.7 When perioperative team members (eg, scrub persons, surgeons, first assistants) are required to stand in the same position for 2 hours or longer for more than 30% of the work day or for any amount of time while wearing a lead apron, apply the algo-

rithm described in AORN Ergonomic Tool #4: Solutions for Prolonged Standing.[64,225] [Recommendation]

Prolonged standing,[226] trunk flexion, and neck flexion are all components of static load.[64] Prolonged standing at work is related to lower extremity pain or discomfort, swelling, and venous disorders.[227] Additionally, prolonged standing is associated with lower back pain, cardiovascular problems (eg, atherosclerosis), fatigue, discomfort, and pregnancy complications.[225,227,228]

In a qualitative study, Kaya et al[229] used a questionnaire to analyze problems related to ergonomic conditions during video endoscopic surgery. Medical personnel (N = 82) from eight disciplines (ie, qualified surgeons, resident surgeons, qualified orthopedists, resident orthopedists, qualified anesthesiologists, resident anesthesiologists, anesthesiology technicians, surgical nurses) answered questions related to physical, perceptive, and cognitive problems. Sixty-eight percent (n = 56) of all the medical personnel identified discomfort due to static body posture for long periods as an ergonomic problem during endoscopic surgery. Ninety-five percent (n = 19) of the surgical nurses identified static body posture as a problem.

Using a biaxial inclinometer attached with a headband to the heads of 14 surgeons and a biaxial electrogoniometer attached to their shoulder joints, Szeto et al[230] recorded real-time movement during laparoscopic and open surgeries. During laparoscopic surgeries, the surgeons held their necks in a static posture for longer periods of time. The researchers concluded that long durations of static postures in laparoscopic surgery were associated with low-level muscle tension. Muscle tension may contribute to the development of MSDs. Other studies have also identified static postures during surgery as a source musculoskeletal discomfort.[231-233]

6.7.1 Use fatigue-reducing techniques, which may include

- using anti-fatigue mats,[64,228,234,235]
- adjusting the height of the OR bed,[225,235]
- determining ergonomic monitor placement,[236,237]
- using a sit-stand stool,[64,228,238]
- wearing supportive footwear,[64,225,228] and
- alternating propping of one foot on a footstool.[225]

[Recommendation]

The interface of the foot with the floor affects body discomfort and fatigue, which may affect team performance and productivity. The type of flooring materials and characteristics (eg, elasticity, stiffness, thickness) will impact the effects of prolonged standing and comfort.

Ergonomic Tool #4. Solutions for Prolonged Standing

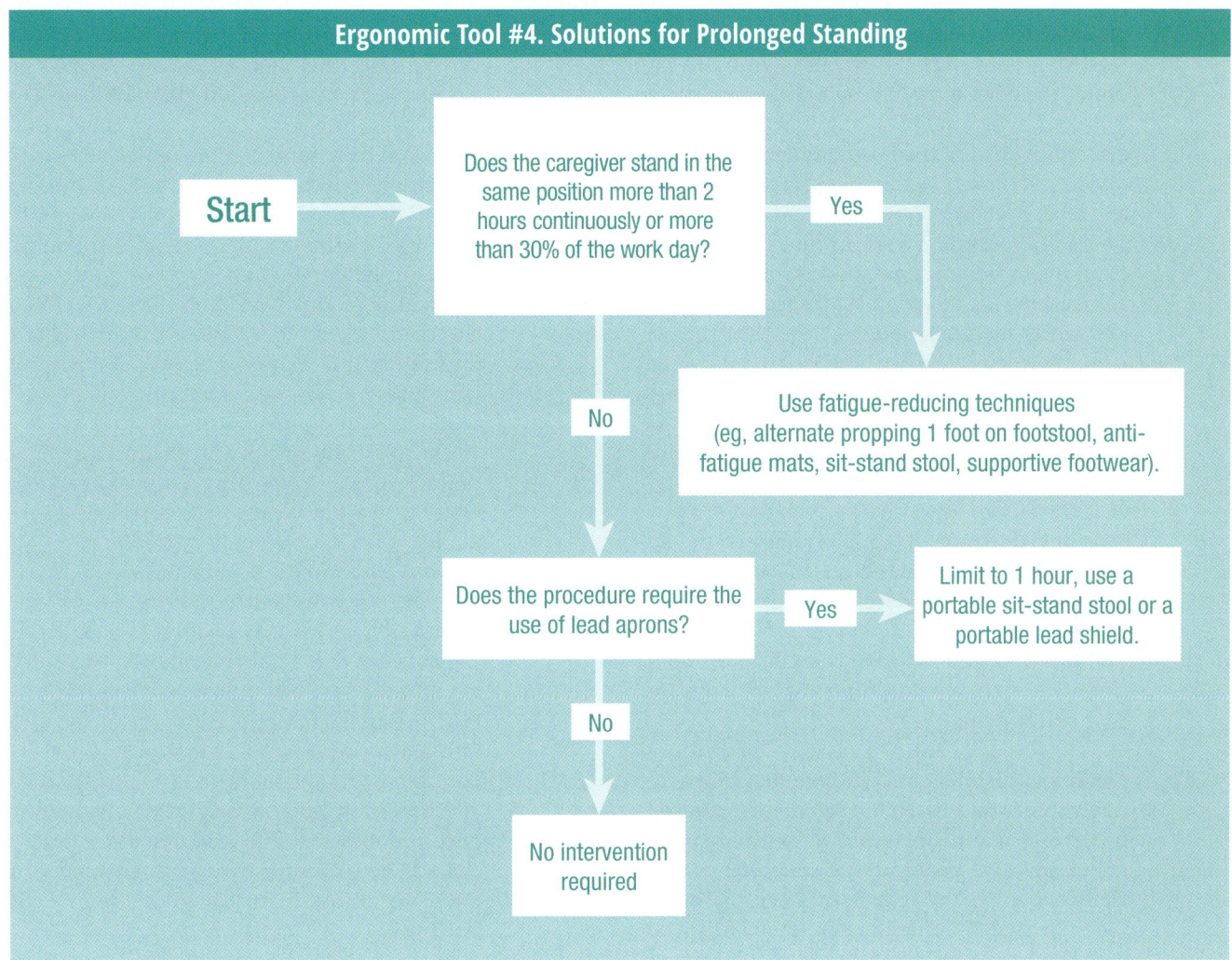

Softer floors are more comfortable for the lower back and lower extremities and less fatiguing compared to hard floors.[225] Alternating propping a foot on the footstool, using an anti-fatigue mat, wearing supportive footwear, and using a sit-stand stool decrease the effects of static posture.[225] Use of a sit-stand stool permits flexibility in body positions. The flexibility increases the number of muscles used during prolonged standing tasks and distributes the load on different body parts. The redistribution reduces the strain on individual muscles and joints that are maintaining the body in a static posture, improves blood flow, and decreases muscle fatigue.[225]

6.7.2 **Use anti-fatigue mats to cover hard flooring materials and standing stools.**[64,225] *[Recommendation]*

Flexible flooring materials (eg, wood, carpeting) are not a practicable solution to provide a safer standing surface in the perioperative environment. Wood floors and carpeting cannot be cleaned and disinfected. Anti-fatigue mats provide a softer, more elastic surface to counteract the effects of prolonged standing. The design of anti-fatigue mats cause a slight postural sway that produces a minor activation of the leg muscles, thereby improving blood flow of the lower extremities and reducing the pooling of blood.[225]

In a prospectively randomized study, Haramis et al[239] examined the comfort level of the surgical team during 100 consecutive laparoscopic renal procedures. The procedures were randomized to being performed with (n = 50) or without (n = 50) a foot gel pad. The participants were five attending physicians, six urology residents, two minimally invasive urology fellows, and five scrub nurses. The participants answered questionnaires before, immediately after, and 24 hours after the surgery.

In the preoperative period, there were no differences in the participants' comfort levels between the two groups. In the immediate postoperative evaluation, the results between the two groups were statistically significant for use of the gel pad in improving the number of times stretched, number of breaks taken, foot discomfort/pain, knee discomfort/pain, back discomfort/pain, overall amount of discomfort, and level of energy. The observed differences 24 hours after surgery were in foot discomfort/pain, overall discomfort, and level of energy. The authors introduced a simple, cost-effective, and easily maintained device (ie, the foot gel pad) into their everyday practice to reduce the discomfort of static neck and back postures associated with laparoscopic surgery. The gel pad contributed to better body posture and minimized discomfort in the knees, back, and feet.

6.7.3 **Use anti-fatigue mats that have tapered edges, anti-skid coating on the upper surface, and a slip-resistant undersurface.**[225] *[Recommendation]*

Tapered edges, anti-skid coating, and a nonslip undersurface reduce the possibility of slipping and tripping.[225]

6.7.4 **Clean and disinfect anti-fatigue mats with an Environmental Protection Agency–registered hospital-grade disinfectant after each surgical or invasive procedure if soiled or potentially soiled (eg, by splash, splatter, or spray) (See the AORN Guideline for Environmental Cleaning).**[163] *[Recommendation]*

6.7.5 **Work at an ergonomically correct height in relation to the height of the work surface.**[225,235] *[Recommendation]*

Optimal OR bed height differs depending on the team member's role (eg, surgeon, assistant, scrub person) and the individual team member's height.[237,239] The challenge is to find the ergonomically reasonable compromise for all team members, particularly when one team member is very tall[240] and another short. The optimal table height is generally at the level of the waist or elbow[241] or 5 cm above the elbow[241] but may vary depending on instrument length and design, surgery, and technique.[237]

In a quasi-experimental study, Park et al[242] studied 12 experienced spine surgeons performing a discectomy using a spine surgery simulator. They analyzed three visualization methods (ie, naked eye, loupe, out of loupe) and three operating bed heights (ie, anterior superior iliac spine, umbilicus, midpoint between the umbilicus and sternum). During the simulations conducted out of loupe and by the naked eye, the thoracic kyphosis was closer to the natural standing position when the OR bed height was at the level of the umbilicus. The researchers suggested that the optimal conditions to reduce surgeon musculoskeletal fatigue were using loupes and having the table height at the midpoint between the umbilicus and the sternum.

In a qualitative study by Kaya et al[229] of 82 medical personnel working in the OR, 70% of the respondents identified back pain due to improper table height as an ergonomic problem during endoscopic surgery. Soueid et al[243] found similar results in a qualitative study of 77 consultant surgeons who answered an anonymous survey regarding pain experienced while operating. Nearly 80% described having pain (eg, back, neck) on a regular basis. Table height was the most common cause of pain for 35% of the respondents.

Standing stools may be used to equalize the heights of the team members.[238,244,245] The height of the OR bed influences the exertion of the upper extremities of the surgeon and assistant during laparoscopic surgery.[237]

Other work surfaces that should be at an ergonomically correct height may include the decontamination sink and assembly table in the sterile processing department and computer work stations in all areas of the perioperative suite.

6.7.6 **Position video display monitors in a neutral position relative to the viewers' eyes.**[236,237] *[Recommendation]*

The position of the video display monitors affects the postures of the surgeon, assistant, and scrub person. Suboptimal placement of the video display monitors may cause static neck flexion, extension, and rotation leading to physical discomfort (eg, fatigue,[237] neck strain,[231] musculoskeletal injury[57,237]).[237]

Zehetner et al[246] evaluated the inclination and reclination angles of the cervical spines of eight surgeons using laparoscopic video towers. Three degrees to 14 degrees reclination of the cervical spine was required to view the monitors at their height on the tower. The surgeons in the study preferred a position of slight inclination to view the monitors at a lower height. The authors concluded that the monitors should be adapted to the surgeon's preferred screen height, with placement at eye level in front of the surgeon and requiring neutral or slight inclination of the cervical spine. Monitors mounted on video carts limit adjustments of height and direction. Monitors installed on ceiling-mounted booms allow for greater adjustments[237] and improved ergonomic postures for the surgeon and OR staff.[247]

Several authors[57,211,229,231,236,237,244,247-252] identified correct monitor placement (eg, 10 degrees to 25 degrees below the line of sight, in front of the viewer) as an ergonomic improvement during MIS. In a questionnaire completed by 82 medical personnel working in the OR, 72% of the respondents identified neck problems due to extension of their head when looking at a monitor as an ergonomic problem during endoscopic surgery, and 41% had perception problems due to the monitor distance.[229]

6.7.7 **During MIS, have at least two separate video display monitors to allow each team member to have an unobstructed line of vision without requiring neck torsion.**[237,238,244,253] *[Recommendation]*

One monitor is used by the surgeon. The second and additional monitors are used by the assistant and the scrub person. In a crossover trial, van Det et al[254] evaluated and compared neck posture in relation to monitor placement in a dedicated minimally invasive suite and a conventional OR. Neck flexion and rotation was assessed for 16 team members (ie, surgeons, assistants, scrub nurses) during laparoscopic cholecystectomy in the MIS and conventional OR. In the conventional OR, the laparoscopic equipment was installed on a rotating platform. The monitor was not height adjustable and was opposite the surgeon. In the MIS suite, three monitors were attached to a ceiling-mounted suspension system, allowing for versatile monitor placement around the OR bed. The dual flat panel screens were opposite the surgeon and scrub nurse. The third screen was opposite the assistant. Neck rotation was significantly reduced in the MIS suite for the surgeon and the assistant. Neck flexion was significantly reduced in the MIS suite for the surgeon and the scrub nurse. The authors concluded that the ergonomic quality of the neck posture was significantly improved in the MIS suite for the entire OR team.

6.7.8 **Do not work with the neck flexed more than 30 degrees or rotated for more than 1 minute uninterrupted.**[64,225] *[Recommendation]*

Neck flexion of more than 30 degrees or rotation for more than 1 uninterrupted minute may contribute to musculoskeletal problems of scrubbed team members.

6.7.9 **Wear supportive footwear that does not change the shape of the foot, has enough space to move toes, is closed toed, is shock-absorbing with cushioned insoles, and has a heel height that is in proportion to the shoe.**[24] *[Recommendation]*

Wearing supportive shoes with insoles that incorporate anti-fatigue properties reduces the effects of prolonged standing.[225]

6.7.10 **Perioperative team members at the sterile field may use arm supports if possible while manually retracting or performing laparoscopic surgery. Use arm rests that are large enough to allow repositioning of the arms.**[64,255] *[Conditional Recommendation]*

Arm rests may relieve hand and arm fatigue and discomfort and strain in the hands, arms, shoulders, and back. Three studies evaluated new concepts for supporting the surgeon's arms during laparoscopic surgery.[256-258]

Kim et al[256] concluded that their chair system allowed the surgeon to operate in a comfortable position with ergonomic chest, arm, and back supports. The supports minimized surgeon fatigue and discomfort during pelvic laparoscopic procedures without consequence to patient safety.

Steinhilber et al[257] researched an arm support system that reduces physical stress and is applicable to various laparoscopic interventions and OR settings. The authors concluded that the ergonomic problems (eg, increased muscle fatigue, musculoskeletal pain, injury) identified in laparoscopic surgery could be addressed by their concept of supporting the elbow from below.

6.7.11 **Team members may benefit from wearing compression stockings (eg, support hose, socks).**[64,228,235,259] *[Conditional Recommendation]*

Chronic venous insufficiency of the lower limbs is a common condition. Risk factors for chronic venous insufficiency include older age, female sex, pregnancy, family history of venous disease, obesity, and occupations requiring prolonged standing.[259]

In a quasi-experimental study, Flore et al[259] compared the venous pressure of the lower limbs and reactive oxygen species (ROS) of participants from similar working environments. The control group, who stood for less than half of their working day, included 65 outpatient department nurses and 35 laundry workers. The experimental group, who stood for the majority of their working day, included 55 theatre nurses and 23 industrial ironers. All participants were examined on two consecutive days before and after working with and without compression stockings.

Lower limb venous pressure increased significantly after work in all participants without compression stockings. Only the theatre nurses showed significantly higher mean levels of ROS. When the workers wore compression stockings, there was no significant differences in venous pressure or ROS after work between the groups. The researchers concluded that wearing compression stockings is a useful and easy preventive measure against oxidative stress in healthy workers who stand for long periods of time and cannot take rest breaks, mini breaks, or ambulate while working.[259]

6.7.12 **When using a sit-stand stool, scrubbed team members should set the level of the stool at the level of the sterile field.**[64,225] *[Recommendation]*

Alternating sitting and standing allows for flexibility in body positions. Alternating positions increases the number of muscles used during prolonged standing and better distributes the load on different parts of the body. Redistribution reduces the strain on individual muscles and joints that keep the body in a fixed standing position.[225]

Setting the height avoids changing levels during the procedure and potentially compromising the sterile field.[64] When scrubbed team members change levels, the unsterile portion of their gowns may come into contact with sterile areas (See the AORN Guideline for Sterile Technique[260]).

6.7.13 **When personal protective radiation devices are required to be worn for more than 1 hour, wear two-piece protective devices.**[64,225] *[Recommendation]*

Two-piece lead protective devices (eg, vest, skirt) reduce radiation exposure and redistribute the weight of the protective clothing from the shoulders and spine. Andreassi et al[261] examined and compared the prevalence of health problems among cardiologists, electrophysiologists, nurses, and technicians in interventional cardiology (N = 466) and cardiac electrophysiology (N = 280) with the length of occupational radiation exposure. The analysis demonstrated that workers performing fluoroscopy-guided cardiovascular procedures have significantly higher risk of several health problems compared with unexposed participants. A primary risk is an increased rate of orthopedic

illnesses (ie, cervical, hip, knee, and lumbar injuries) related to long hours of standing and a heavy lead apron.

6.8 **When perioperative team members at the sterile field are required to hold retractors or body parts for long periods of time, apply the algorithm described in** AORN Ergonomic Tool #5: Tissue Retraction in the Perioperative Setting.[64,255] *[Recommendation]*

Perioperative team members (eg, first assistants) at the sterile field may be required to hold retractors or body parts for long periods of time in addition to standing for long periods of time. **Manual retraction** to provide exposure of the operative site for the surgeon often requires first assistants to stand in an awkward posture for long periods while gripping and pulling a retractor or using their hands to retract or steady organs (eg, the heart).

The height of the surgical field in relation to the person providing retraction influences the risk for musculoskeletal injury. An optimal working height is the area between the team member's chest and waist **(See Recommendation 6.7.5).** Prolonged standing, trunk flexion, neck flexion, awkward postures,[226,262,263] and arms held higher than the optimal working height place perioperative team members at risk for a musculoskeletal injury **(See Recommendation 6.7).**[64,255]

6.8.1 **Selection of the retractor type (ie, manual, self-retaining) should be at the discretion of the surgeon.**[264] *[Recommendation]*

The type of surgery, type of tissue, and the patient's physical characteristics determine the type of retraction required.[255,264] A **self-retaining retractor** holds back the edges of the wound and tissues, providing continuous exposure of the surgical site.[255] The design (eg, size, shape) of self-retaining retractors (eg, Balfour, Weitlander) varies widely depending on type of surgery performed and anatomical structures involved.[264] The assistant is available for other tissue handling activities when a self-retaining retractor is used.[255,264]

Use of a self-retaining retractors may cause tissue damage.[264-268] In a retrospective review of a 10-year period, Noldus et al[265] analyzed operation protocols of 4,000 procedures in which a Bookwalter self-retaining retractor was used. The researchers found five cases of serious intraoperative damage to the colon and femoral nerve that were most probably attributable to the use of the Bookwalter retractor. They concluded that a table-fixed retractor was extremely useful for providing steady and reproducible

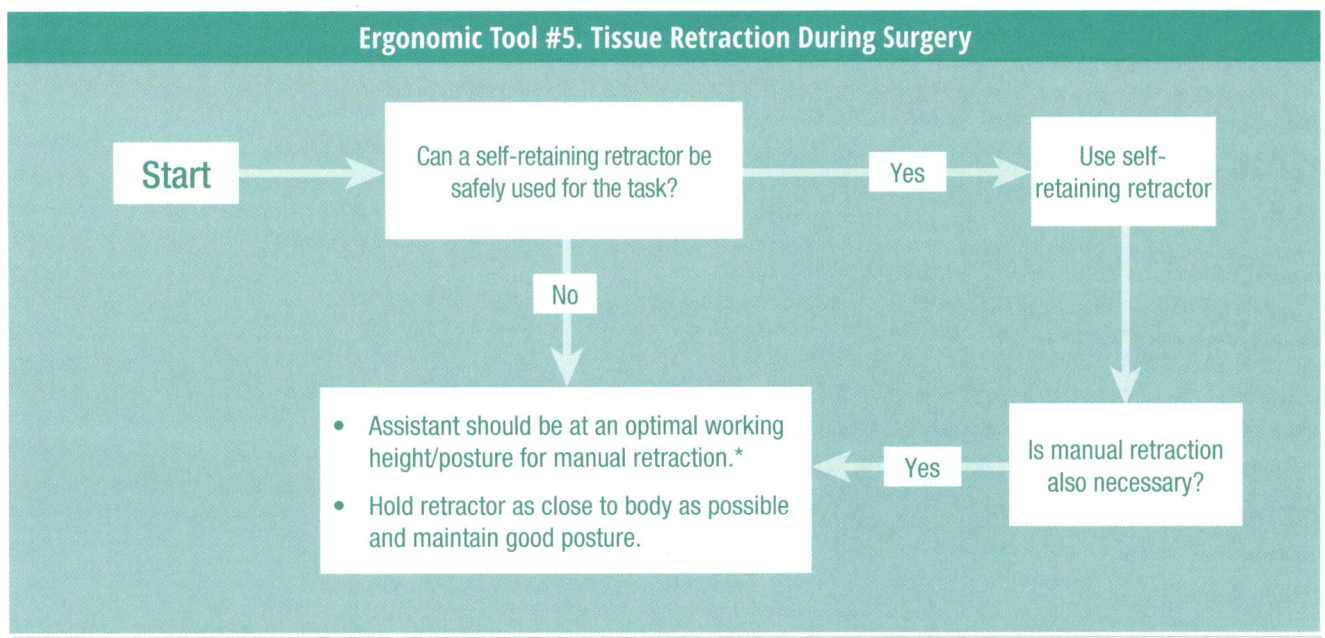

Ergonomic Tool #5. Tissue Retraction During Surgery

Start → Can a self-retaining retractor be safely used for the task?

→ **Yes** → Use self-retaining retractor

↓ **No**

- Assistant should be at an optimal working height/posture for manual retraction.*
- Hold retractor as close to body as possible and maintain good posture.

← **Yes** ← Is manual retraction also necessary?

* Optimal working height is defined as the area between the chest and the height to the operative field. Optimal posture is defined as perpendicular/straight-on to the operative field; asysmmetrical posture may be acceptable depending on load and duration; torso twisting should be avoided at all times.

exposure, although injury to secondary organs or structure is a concern as the use and variety of self-retaining retractors increases. The retractor can be applied with tension and pressure to the bowel, nerves, and other organs contrary to the use of manual retractors. The researchers' suggested recommendations to avoid self-retaining blade-related injuries included choosing the right blade for the right patient, using protective packs and padded blades, repositioning the retractor blades during prolonged procedures to prevent intraoperative damage, and using manual retractors for patients with risk factors such as immunosuppression and diverticulitis.

6.8.2 If manual retraction is necessary, the assistant should hold the retractor as close to the body as possible while maintaining good posture.[64,255] The assistant should hold the retractor with the palm facing down when retracting toward his or her body and with the palm facing up and the arm flexed at the elbow when retracting laterally.[255] *[Recommendation]*

Reaching and pulling a retractor away from or lateral to the body may cause increased muscle strain and fatigue.[255] In a qualitative study, Simonsen et al[269] evaluated the physical workload and musculoskeletal health of 99 female theatre nurses and 93 female assisting nurses. The researchers performed clinical examinations of the neck and upper extremities of the participants and assessed their physical workload using a questionnaire and technical measurements of postures, movements, and muscular load in subgroups of 12 participants in each occupation. The theatre nurses experienced prolonged and static postures while holding hooks (ie, retractors), often with raised arms. The assisting nurses experienced high physical load. Twenty-five percent of the assisting nurses and 17% of the theatre nurses reported a musculoskeletal disorder diagnosis in the neck and shoulders.

6.8.3 When using a manual retractor, the assistant should grip the retractor only as firmly as necessary for surgical exposure.[255] *[Recommendation]*

A manual retractor may or may not have a grip-shaped handle. Examples of a retractor without a handle include Army-Navy, malleable, and Deaver retractors. A single-end Richardson retractor has a handle while a double-end Richardson retractor does not. Using any hand-held retractor may cause hand and arm fatigue and discomfort and strain in the hands, arms, shoulders, and back.[255]

6.9 Before lifting and carrying supplies, instrument trays, and equipment, apply the algorithm described in AORN Ergonomic Tool #6: Lifting and Carrying Supplies and Equipment in the Perioperative Setting.[64,270] *[Recommendation]*

Perioperative team members lift and carry many different types of unsterile and sterile supplies, instrument trays, and equipment. Manual lifting and

Ergonomic Tool #6. Lifting and Carrying Supplies and Equipment in the Perioperative Setting

Lifting Task	Lifting Index	Level of Risk
3,000 mL irrigation fluid	< 0.2	
Sand bags	0.3	
Linen bags	0.4	
Lead aprons	0.4	
Custom sterile packs (eg, heart or spine)	0.5	
Garbage bags (full)	0.7	
Positioning devices off shelf or rack (eg, stirrups)	0.7	
Positioning devices off shelf or rack (eg, gel pads)	0.9	
Hand table (49 x 28 inches); largest hand table, used infrequently	1.2	
Fluoroscopy board (49 x 21 inches)	1.2	
Stirrups (2—1 in each hand)	1.4	
Wilson frame	1.4	
Irrigation containers for lithotripsy (12,000 mL)	1.5	
Instrument pans	2.0	

No shading	Minimal risk—Safe to lift
Light shading	Potential risk—Use assistive technology as available
Heavy shading	Considerable risk—1 person should not perform alone or weight should be reduced

carrying of objects is physically demanding and may place the team member at substantial risk for low back pain and back and shoulder injuries[6,64,150,189-192,237,270,271] Factors contributing to the risk for injury include the weight of the object lifted, excessive reach, location of the lifted object relative to the person lifting the object (ie, proximity of the object being lifted to the person's body), and the duration and frequency of lifting.[270] AORN Ergonomic Tool #6 is intended to assist team members in evaluating lifting and carrying tasks and taking measures to protect themselves from injury.[64]

The 2005 AORN Workplace Safety Task Force identified a series of typical OR lifting tasks and evaluated them using the Revised NIOSH Lifting Equation (RNLE). The RNLE is a tool for assessing manual lifting of objects that allows the user to calculate the **recommended weight limit** (RWL) for a specified two-handed manual lifting task. The RWL is defined for a specific set of task conditions and represents the weight of the load that nearly all healthy workers could continuously lift over a period of time (ie, 1 hour up to 8 hours) with recovery time and not increase their risk of developing lifting-related low back pain. By "healthy workers," NIOSH means workers who are free of adverse health conditions that would increase their risk of musculoskeletal injury.[64] In addition, the **lifting index** (LI) for the task can be

calculated by dividing the actual weight of the load lifted by the RWL.[64] The LI provides a relative estimate of the level of physical stress associated with a particular manual lifting task RWL.[64] The list in the tool is not all inclusive; the NIOSH equation can be used to calculate an LI value for other two-handed manual lifting tasks not on the list (Table 1).[64,199]

The concept behind the RNLE is to start with a recommended weight that is considered safe for an "ideal" lift (ie, load constant equal to 51 lb [23 kg]) and then reduce the weight as the task becomes more stressful (ie, as the task-related factors become less favorable). The fixed load constant of 51 lb (23 kg) is reduced by factors related to task geometry (ie, location of the load relative to the worker at the initial liftoff and set down points), task frequency and duration, and type of handhold on the object. The precise formulation of the revised lifting equation for calculating the RWL is based on a multiplicative model that provides a weighting (ie, multiplier) for each of six task variables. The following list briefly describes the measurements required to use the RNLE:

- **H:** horizontal distance of the load from the worker = horizontal location of hands from midpoint between the inner ankle bones. This is measured in centimeters or inches at the origin and the destination of the lift.

Table 1. Data Used to Calculate the NIOSH Lifting Index Values for Typical Items Lifted in the OR

Lifting Task	Weight	Horizontal Distance	Vertical Location-Origin	Vertical Location-Destination	Distance Carried	Lifting Index
3000 mL IV bags irrigation fluids	2.5 lb	6 inches	42 inches	30 inches	49–118 ft	< 0.2
Sand bags	10.5 lb	12 inches	30 inches	32 inches	20 ft	0.3
Linen bags	15 lb	6 inches Set = 10 inches	Floor Set = 0 inches	42 inches	140–251 ft	0.4
Lead aprons	16 lb	13 inches	36 inches	36 inches	N/A on cart	0.4
Custom sterile packs (heart or spine)	12.4 lb	18 inches	23 inches	32 inches		0.5
Garbage bags (full)	23.6 lb	6 inches Set = 10 inches	Floor Set = 0 inches	42 inches	140–251 ft	0.7
Positioning devices off shelf or rack (stirrups)	17 lb each (2 stirrups would be 34 lb)	18 inches	36 inches	36 inches		0.7
Positioning devices off shelf or rack (gel pads)	8–25 Set to 25 lb	18 inches	36 inches	36 inches	5–10 ft	0.9
Hand table (49 x 28 inches); largest hand table, used infrequently	15–27 lb Set to 27 lb	20 inches	43 inches	32 inches	49–118 ft	1.2
Fluoroscopy board (49 x 21 inches)	26 lb	20 inches	43 inches	32 inches	49–118 ft	1.2
Stirrups (2, 1 in each hand)	34 lb	18 inches	36 inches	36 inches		1.4
Wilson frame	27 lb	32 inches	31.5 inches	32 inches	49–118 ft	1.4
Irrigation containers for lithotripsy (12,000 mL)	0–50 lb Set to 50 lb	6 inches Set = 10 inches	63 inches (top shelf)	N/A Housekeeping places in bags Set to 33 inches	49–118 ft	1.5
Instrument pans	3–38 lb Set to 38 lb	19 inches	6–50 inches Set to 6 inches	Varies Set to 34 inches	5–10 ft	2.0

- V: vertical height of the lift = vertical location of the hands from the floor. This is measured in centimeters or inches at the origin and destination of the lift.
- D: vertical displacement during the lift = vertical travel distance in centimeters or inches between the origin and the destination of the lift.
- A: angle of asymmetry = angular displacement of the load from the worker's sagittal plane. This is measured in degrees at the origin and destination of the lift.
- F: frequency and duration of lifting = average frequency rate of lifting measured in lifts per minute.

Duration is defined as follows: short-duration (< 1 hour); moderate-duration (> 1 hour but < 2 hours); or long-duration (> 2 hours but < 8 hours), assuming appropriate recovery allowances (Table 2).
- C: quality of the hand-to-object coupling = quality of the interface between the worker and the load being lifted. The quality of the coupling is categorized as good, fair, or poor, depending upon the type and location of the coupling, the physical characteristics of the load, and the vertical height of the lift[64] (Table 3).

The weightings are expressed as coefficients that serve to decrease the load constant, which represents the maximum RWL to be lifted under ideal conditions. For example, as the horizontal distance between the load and the worker increases, the RWL for that task would be reduced from the ideal starting weight.[64]

The term *task variables* refers to the measurable task-related measurements that are used as input data for the formula (ie, H, V, D, A, F, C), whereas the term multipliers refers to the reduction coefficients in the equation (ie, HM, VM, DM, AM, FM, CM) (Table 4).[64]

The estimate of the level of physical stress is defined by the relationship of the weight of the load lifted and the RWL. The LI equals the load weight (weight of the object lifted) divided by the RWL. According to NIOSH, tasks with an LI value greater than 1.0 place some workers at risk for low back pain and an LI value greater than 3.0 places many workers at risk of low back pain. In a subsequent study that examined the effects of the NIOSH LI as a predictor, the risk of back pain increased when the LI exceeded 2.0.[272] Tasks with an LI value less than 1.0 can easily be performed manually. For those tasks with an LI value greater than 1.0, however, caution should be used. Alternate handling procedures may help reduce the risk of low back injury caused by lifting these objects.

The LI may be used to identify potentially hazardous lifting jobs or to compare the relative severity of two jobs for the purpose of evaluating and redesigning them. Lifting jobs should be designed to achieve an LI of 1.0 or less whenever possible. Some experts believe that worker selection criteria may be used to identify workers who can perform potentially stressful lifting tasks (ie, lifting tasks that would exceed a LI of 1.0) without significantly increasing their risk of work-related injury above the baseline level.[64] Those who endorse the use of selection criteria believe that the criteria must be based on research studies, empirical observations, or theoretical considerations that include job-related strength testing and/or aerobic capacity testing.[64]

Even these experts agree, however, that many workers will be at a significant risk for a work-related injury when performing highly stressful lifting tasks (ie, lifting tasks that would exceed an LI of 3.0). "Informal" or "natural" selection of workers may occur in many jobs that require repetitive lifting tasks. According to some experts, this may result in a unique workforce that may be able to work above an LI of 1.0, at least in theory, without substantially increasing their risk of low back injuries above the baseline rate of injury.[64]

Assessment of patient handling tasks was specifically excluded as a restriction for use of the RNLE due to limitations in the data used to derive the

Table 2. Frequencey Multipliers

Frequency lifts/minute (F)	Work Duration					
	< 1 hour		> 1 but < 2 hours		> 2 but < 8 hours	
	V < 30	V > 30	V < 30	V > 30	V < 30	V > 30
0.2	1.00	1.00	.95	.95	.85	.85
0.5	.97	.97	.92	.92	.81	.81
1	.94	.94	.88	.88	.75	.75
2	.91	.91	.84	.84	.65	.65
3	.88	.88	.79	.79	.55	.55
4	.84	.84	.72	.72	.45	.45
5	.80	.80	.60	.60	.35	.35
6	.75	.75	.50	.50	.27	.27
7	.70	.70	.42	.42	.22	.22
8	.60	.60	.35	.35	.18	.18
9	.52	.52	.30	.30	.00	.15
10	.45	.45	.26	.26	.00	.13
11	.41	.41	.00	.23	.00	.00
12	.37	.37	.00	.21	.00	.00
13	.00	.34	.00	.00	.00	.00
14	.00	.31	.00	.00	.00	.00
15	.00	.28	.00	.00	.00	.00
> 15	.00	.00	.00	.00	.00	.00

Table 3. Coupling Multiplier

	Coupling Multiplier	
	V < 30 inches (75 cm)	V > 30 inches (75 cm)
Good	1.00	1.00
Fair	0.95	1.00
Poor	0.90	0.90

Table 4. Recommended Weight Limit

	Variable		Metric	US Customary
The recommended weight limit is defined as follows: RWL = LC x HM x VM x DM x AM x FM x CM Where:	LC =	Load Constant =	23 kg	51 lb
	HM =	Horizontal Multiplier =	(25/H)	(10/H)
	VM =	Vertical Multiplier =	$1-(.003\lvert V-75\rvert)$	$1-(.0075\lvert V-30\rvert)$
	DM =	Distance Multiplier =	$.82 + (4.5/D)$	$.82 + (1.8/D)$
	AM =	Asymmetric Multiplier =	$1-(.0032A)$	$1-(.0032A)$
	FM =	Frequency Multiplier =	From Table 2	From Table 2
	CM =	Coupling Multiplier =	From Table 3	From Table 3

equation. For some patient handling tasks, however, where the person being lifted is noncombative or where there is little or no movement of the patient during the lifting task, the RNLE may be applicable, and it should be possible to determine whether the lift exceeds the RWL for those tasks. For example, the RNLE was used to derive the 35-lb weight limit for patient lifting in the AORN Ergonomic Tools.[64]

The Revised NIOSH Equation for the Design and Evaluation of Manual Lifting Tasks provides a discussion of the criteria underlying the lifting equation and of the individual multipliers[273] and identifies both the assumptions and uncertainties in the scientific studies that associate manual lifting and low back injuries. For more detailed information about how to use the RNLE, consult the *Applications Manual for the Revised NIOSH Lifting Equation*.[199]

6.9.1 **Total weight of an instrument tray should not exceed 25 lb (11.3 kg) (See the AORN Guideline for Sterilization[274]).**[274,275] *[Recommendation]*

Instrument trays weighing more than 25 lb (11.3 kg) present a risk of ergonomic injury.[274]

6.10 **Before pushing or pulling heavy equipment (eg, OR beds, patient beds) in and around the OR and between ORs, apply the algorithm described in AORN Ergonomic Tool #7: Pushing, Pulling and Moving Equipment on Wheels.[64,276]** *[Recommendation]*

Surgical procedure preparation is a combination of many activities (eg, movement of patients, supplies, and equipment in and out of the OR) that contribute to physical stress. The recommendations in Ergonomic Tool #7 include some, but not all, of the necessary activities undertaken to prepare for a surgical procedure.[216] For OR equipment not listed, the health care worker should compare physical effort to that required to push an unoccupied standard hospital bed. If greater effort is required, then additional team members and/or use of a powered transport device is recommended.[64]

The calculations used for Ergonomic Tool #7 are the push forces measured in **Newtons (N)** for each item of equipment listed (Table 5). Initial forces were measured as the peak force to initially propel the item. Sustained force was measured as the minimum force required to maintain equipment propulsion. Initial wheels turned were measured as the peak initial force where the wheels on the equipment were turned perpendicular to the desired direction of travel. The average force measured across five repeated trials for each condition and equipment item was computed and converted into US standard units.[64]

The recommendations in Ergonomic Tool #7 are based on Liberty Mutual's push force limits (Table 6).[216] The shortest acceptable push distance, considering both initial and sustained forces, was accepted. These values are based on the operator with his or her hands positioned at a middle push point of 3 ft (0.92 m) from the floor or above and performing a task no more frequently than once every 30 minutes.[64]

To measure OR equipment not listed, a measuring device can be applied to measure applicable pushing/pulling forces. Commercially available measuring instruments can be used to measure push/pull forces (eg, strain gauge, force meters, precision springs). A simple low-cost method for measuring the required forces for pushing or pulling objects, such as beds, carts, and transfer equipment, is a broom handle or other lightweight cylindrical object that can be taped to a bathroom scale and used to measure push forces. Required pull forces would be identical to the required pushing force. The scale is placed against the object to be pushed and a force is then slowly applied to the handle until the object moves. The maximum required pushing force is read off the weight scale. The scale should provide a continuous readout of applied force to obtain the maximum value. To obtain the best estimate of the actual maximum force, the measurement should be repeated several times and the average value should

Ergonomic Tool #7. Pushing, Pulling, and Moving Equipment on Wheels

OR Equipment	Pushing		Maximum Push Distance		Ergonomic Recommendation
Electrosurgery unit	8.4 lbF	(3.8 kgF)	> 200 ft	(60 m)	
Ultrasound	12.4 lbF	(5.6 kgF)	> 200 ft	(60 m)	
X-ray equipment portable	12.9 lbF	(5.9 kgF)	> 200 ft	(60 m)	
Video towers	14.1 lbF	(6.4 kgF)	> 200 ft	(60 m)	
Linen cart	16.3 lbF	(7.4 kgF)	> 200 ft	(60 m)	
X-ray equipment, C-arm	19.6 lbF	(8.9 kgF)	> 200 ft	(60 m)	
Case carts, empty	24.2 lbF	(11.0 kgF)	> 200 ft	(60 m)	
OR stretcher, unoccupied	25.1 lbF	(11.4 kgF)	> 200 ft	(60 m)	
Case carts, full	26.6 lbF	(12.1 kgF)	> 200 ft	(60 m)	
Microscopes	27.5 lbF	(12.5 kgF)	> 200 ft	(60 m)	
Hospital bed, unoccupied	29.8 lbF	(13.5 kgF)	> 200 ft	(60 m)	
Specialty equipment carts	39.3 lbF	(17.9 kgF)	> 200 ft	(60 m)	
OR stretcher, occupied, 300 lb (136 kg)	43.8 lbF	(19.9 kgF)	> 200 ft	(60 m)	
Bed, occupied, 300 lb (136 kg)	50.0 lbF	(22.7 kgF)	< 200 ft	(30 m)	Minimum 2 caregivers required
Specialty OR beds, unoccupied	69.7 lbF	(31.7 kgF)	< 100 ft	(30 m)	
OR bed, unoccupied	61.3 lbF	(27.9 kgF)	< 25 ft	(7.5 m)	Recommend powered transport device
OR bed, occupied, 300 lb (136 kg)	112.4 lbF	(51.1 kgF)	< 25 ft	(7.5 m)	
Specialty OR beds, occupied, 300 lb (136 kg)	124.2 lbF	(56.5 kgF)	< 25 ft	(7.5 m)	

No shading	Minimal risk
Light shading	Potential risk—Use assistive technology as available
Heavy shading	Considerable risk—1 person should not perform alone or weight should be reduced

* lb F: A unit of force equal to the mass of 1 lb with an acceleration equal to 1 gravitational constant (32 ft/s²). Acceleration due to gravity equals 9.8 meters per second squared (9.8 m/s²) or 32 feet per second squared (32 ft/s²).

be used for assessment. This force can then be compared to the maximum recommended push force values. For example, if the force required to push a cart was measured to be 60 lb, this task would not be acceptable for one caregiver for any distance but would be acceptable for two caregivers (assuming each pushed 26 lb) for a distance of up to 25 ft. A powered transport device would be recommended if one caregiver is performing the task.[64]

6.10.1 **Perioperative team members should push wheeled equipment.**[64,277-279] *[Recommendation]*

In a quasi-experimental study, Kao et al[277] measured electromyographic data of four muscle groups of 10 participants performing 108 experimental trials each while pushing and pulling a cart. The results showed that muscle activity was lower in the pushing task than in the pulling task.

Liberty Mutual's psychophysical limits for push forces are based on the work of Snook

and Ciriello.[216] Garg et al[280] performed a literature review of psychophysically determined maximum acceptable pushing and pulling forces. They concluded that the recommendations of Snook and Ciriello[216] for pushing and pulling forces are still valid and provide reasonable recommendations for ergonomics practitioners. In addition, they concluded that it is unclear whether pushing or pulling should be favored. The researchers concluded that epidemiological studies are needed to determine relationships between psychophysically determined maximum acceptable pushing and pulling forces and risk of musculoskeletal injuries (eg, lower back and shoulders).

6.10.2 When pushing an OR bed or an occupied standard hospital bed, a minimum of two perioperative team members should participate in the transport task or one team

member should use a powered transport device.[216] *[Recommendation]*

Patient beds and OR beds can be heavy and difficult to push, even when empty. When the bed is moved with a patient on it, the risk for injury is increased for both the patient and the perioperative team member.[276] Based on Liberty Mutual's psychophysical limits for maximum pushing distances, pushing an occupied standard hospital bed or standard or specialty OR bed, whether occupied or not, presents a moderate to high risk for injury to the team member.[64]

6.10.3 **Cart handles should be at a push height of approximately 3 ft (0.92 m) from the floor.**[216] *[Recommendation]*

Handle height influences the amount of force exerted on the cart to initiate and sustain movement, maximum voluntary strength, compressive and shear loading of spinal discs, and stresses to the shoulder joints.[280] For tasks where the push point is lower than 3 ft (0.92 m), maximum and sustained push forces will be decreased by approximately 15%.[216] For tasks performed more frequently than once every 30 minutes, maximum and sustained push forces will be decreased by approximately 6%.[216] If push force limits are exceeded, it will be necessary to reduce the weight of the load, have two or more team members complete the task together, or use a powered transport device.[64] In their review of the literature, Garg et al[280] discussed the importance of handle height in cart design, but there is inconclusive data to recommend handle heights that would result in lower strength requirements and less stress to the lower back and shoulder and minimum localized and whole body fatigue.

6.10.4 **Include equipment wheels and casters in the health care organization's routine equipment maintenance.**[64] *[Recommendation]*

Maintenance of the wheels and wheel bearings affects the amount of pushing force required to move equipment and assists in moving equipment more easily.[280] Regular maintenance (eg, cleaning, lubrication) insures that worn or broken parts are replaced in a timely and efficient manner.[278]

6.11 **Participate in their health care organization's fall reduction program**[281] **by including an evaluation of the perioperative patient's mobility and risk for falling in the preoperative assessment.** *[Recommendation]*

Identifying the patient's risk for falling is the first and most important step in preventing patient falls.[282-284] The literature search for this guideline produced only minimal evidence related to the incidence and prevention of patient falls in the perioperative environment.[284,285] Perioperative patient falls can occur in the preoperative, intraoperative, or postoperative phase[281] of care in both ambulatory and hospital settings.[284] Patients may be at increased risk for falling because of preoperative medications, anesthetic agents, lack of familiarity with the environment where care is provided, sensory-perceptual deficits related to the removal of hearing aids or glasses, and the use of elevated stretchers and OR beds.[284] The Centers for Medicare & Medicaid Services no longer pays for treatment provided for preventable complications such as falls and fall-related injuries that occur during a hospital admission.[175]

Perioperative patients may be at risk for falling when

- they are transferred to and from the stretcher or wheelchair;
- they are transferred to and from the OR bed[213];
- their extremities are lifted, held, or maneuvered into position;
- they are positioned or repositioned on the OR bed or specialty bed (eg, fracture table)[286];
- they are placed into or removed from positioning devices (eg, stirrups); or
- the position of the OR bed is changed (eg, supine to Trendelenburg[213]).[285]

Injuries from falls can result in pain, soft tissue injury, swelling, ecchymosis, lacerations, fractures, head injury,[213] functional impairment, disability, or death.[213,283,285] The physical consequences of a fall may contribute to an increased length of hospital stay, a need for rehabilitation, and increased health care costs.[283,285] Patients who have fallen may also experience emotional consequences such as anxiety, depression, or fear of falling again.[283,285] Perioperative team members caring for patients who have fallen may experience anxiety and guilt.[283]

In a systematic review of 14 controlled studies exploring the effectiveness of multifaceted interventions to prevent falls in adult hospital inpatient populations, Choi et al[287] found that the most frequently implemented approach to fall prevention was evaluation of the patient's risk for falling and modification (when possible) of fall-risk factors. The researchers found nurses' clinical assessment to be a significant and clinically meaningful predictor of the patient's risk for falling and a method to reduce hospital inpatient falls.

Table 5. Measured Push Forces for Operating Room Equipment

Equipment	Type of Force	Trial 1 (N)	Trial 2 (N)	Trial 3 (N)	Trial 4 (N)	Trial 5 (N)	Mean (N)	Mean (lbF)	Maximum Push Distance (ft)
Electrosurgical unit	initial force	30	35	35	30	30	32.0	7.2	> 200
	sustained force	10	10	10	10	10	10.0	2.2	> 200
	initial-wheels turned	40	35				37.5	8.4	> 200
OR stretcher, unoccupied	initial force	62	70	65	75		68.0	15.3	> 200
	sustained force	20	20	25	25	25	23.0	5.2	> 200
	initial-wheels turned	113	110				111.5	25.1	> 200
OR stretcher, occupied, 300 lb (136 kg)	initial force	120	120	120	115	120	119.0	26.8	> 200
	sustained force	30	35	30	40	40	35.0	7.9	> 200
	initial-wheels turned	210	180				195.0	43.8	< 50
Bed, unoccupied	initial force	115	120	125	110	105	115.0	25.9	> 200
	sustained force	30	25	30	25		27.5	6.2	> 200
	initial-wheels turned	130	135				132.5	29.8	> 200
Bed, occupied, 300 lb (136 kg)	initial force	170	160	167	135	155	157.4	35.4	> 200
	sustained force	40	50	50	40	60	48.0	10.8	> 200
	initial-wheels turned	230	215				222.5	50.0	< 25
OR bed, unoccupied	initial force	218	275	245	280	270	257.6	57.9	< 25
	sustained force	120	125	120	100	120	117.0	26.3	< 25
	initial-wheels turned	270	275				272.5	61.3	< 25
OR bed, occupied, 300 lb (136 kg)	initial force	425	432	445	405	325	406.4	91.4	< 25
	sustained force	180	180	180			180.0	40.5	< 25
	initial-wheels turned	485	515				500.0	112.4	< 25
Specialty OR beds, unoccupied	initial force	175	182	190	260	200	201.4	45.3	< 25
	sustained force	100	100	100			100.0	22.5	< 100
	initial-wheels turned	305	315				310.0	69.7	< 25
Specialty OR beds, 300-lb patient (136 kg)	initial force	365	290	320	305	305	317.0	71.3	< 25
	sustained force	140	160	140	115	115	134.0	30.1	< 25
	initial-wheels turned	560	545				552.5	124.2	< 25

6.11.1 As part of the preoperative fall risk evaluation, include an assessment of the patient's

- age,[288]
- history of previous falls,[282,283,289]
- medication use (eg, substance abuse, preoperative sedatives),[283,289,290]
- level of consciousness (eg, alert, lethargic),[282,283,288,291]
- sensory impairments (eg, vision, hearing),[289,292]
- ability to follow directions (eg, cognitive impairment, language barrier),[283,289,290,292]
- physical limitations (eg, decreased range of motion, spinal or extremity deformities),[218,290,292,293]
- level of coordination or balance,[283,288,292]
- ability to move independently (eg, limb weakness, amount of assistance required),[289,292]
- toileting needs (eg, incontinence, frequency, need for assistance),[282,283,289] and
- presence of external devices (eg, catheters, drains).[288]

[Recommendation]

Table 5 Continued. Measured Push Forces for Operating Room Equipment

Equipment	Type of Force	Trial 1 (N)	Trial 2 (N)	Trial 3 (N)	Trial 4 (N)	Trial 5 (N)	Mean (N)	Mean (lbF)	Maximum Push Distance (ft)
Microscopes	initial force	62	75	80	75	75	73.4	16.5	> 200
	sustained force	20	25	20	25	25	23.0	5.2	> 200
	initial-wheels turned	125	120				122.5	27.5	< 50
Case cart, full	initial force	62	108	75	108		88.3	19.8	> 200
	sustained force	30	40	40	40		37.5	8.4	> 200
	initial-wheels turned	122	115				118.5	26.6	> 200
Case cart, empty	initial force	60	65	65	62	65	63.4	14.3	> 200
	sustained force	40	30	35	40	35	36.0	8.1	> 200
	initial-wheels turned	120	95				107.5	24.2	> 200
X-ray equipment, C-arm	initial force	100	75	100	75	85	87.0	19.6	> 200
	sustained force	20	25	25	25	25	24.0	5.4	> 200
	initial-wheels turned	N/A	N/A				N/A	N/A	N/A
X-ray equipment, portable	initial force	60	55	55	60	58	57.6	12.9	> 200
	sustained force	25	30	30	30	30	29.0	6.5	> 200
	initial-wheels turned	N/A	N/A				N/A	N/A	N/A
Video towers	initial force	35	40	40	35	35	37.0	8.3	> 200
	sustained force	15	20	20	15	20	18.0	4.0	> 200
	initial-wheels turned	60	65				62.5	14.1	> 200
Ultrasound	initial force	35	40	45	45	40	41.0	9.2	> 200
	sustained force	20	20	25	20	20	21.0	4.7	> 200
	initial-wheels turned	55	55				55.0	12.4	> 200
Specialty equipment carts	initial force	105	90	120	125	145	117.0	26.3	> 200
	sustained force	25	30	30	25	25	27.0	6.1	> 200
	initial-wheels turned	165	185				175.0	39.3	< 200
Linen cart	initial force	50	70	55	55	65	59.0	13.3	> 200
	sustained force	20	25	20	25	20	22.0	4.9	> 200
	initial-wheels turned	75	70				72.5	16.3	> 200

The evidence review for this guideline did not reveal any research studies related to fall-risk assessments specific to the perioperative environment. The recommendation for items to be included in the perioperative fall-risk assessment has been extrapolated from research studies related to hospital falls.

In a correlational study involving a secondary analysis of data from a methodological multisite study conducted in the southeastern region of the United States, Moe et al[282] analyzed data from [281,865] falls to identify risk factors that could predict the likelihood that patients in an acute care setting might fall. The researchers found three major predictors of patient falls in the hospital setting: a previous fall within the past 6 months, patient confusion, and patient toileting issues.

Oliver et al[283] conducted a systematic review of 13 published case control or cohort studies related to hospital patient falls. The researchers found that despite the heterogeneity of the settings, populations, and risk factors studied, certain risk factors consistently emerged as significant. These factors included gait instability; lower limb weakness; urinary incontinence, frequency, or need for assisted toileting; previous fall history; agitation, confusion, or impaired judgment; and the use of certain medications, particularly sedative hypnotics. The researchers noted that some patient falls were predictable and preventable and that any successful intervention to prevent falls would likely rest on the identification and reversal of fall risk.

In a retrospective analysis of 190 postoperative falls at a Veteran's Affairs Medical Center, Church et al[288] characterized the etiology of falls as either patient related or environment related. Patient-related causes included patient delirium, disability, weakness, dizziness, loss of balance, falls that occurred during patient transfer, and patients rolling out of bed. Environment-related causes included slipping on wet or soiled floors, tripping on medical tubing, and malfunctioning assistive devices. Preoperative factors significantly associated with falls included older age, functional dependence, American Society of Anesthesiologists physical status classification of III or greater, low albumin level, anemia, and the need for emergency surgery. Intraoperative factors associated with falls included longer surgery duration and increased blood transfusion requirement.

6.11.2 **Use a standardized mobility assessment tool.**[294] [Recommendation]

A mobility assessment is an objective evaluation of a patient's mobility. A patient's mobility status determines his or her mobility, handling, and use of safe patient movement technologies. A standardized mobility assessment tool (eg, Timed Up & Go [TUG] Test[295], Banner Mobility Assessment Tool[294]) evaluates patient mobility and provides preoperative baseline information for communication to the postoperative caregiver (eg, PACU RN). If a patient is unable to stand and bear weight preoperatively, the PACU nurses need to know. The plan of care will be different to get a non-weight-bearing patient out of bed and into a chair compared to a patient capable of full weight bearing. With the mobility assessment and transfer-of-care report, the PACU nurse will not expect the patient to stand and bear weight when the patient did not do this preoperatively. Assistive devices will be needed for a non-weight-bearing patient.

The TUG assessment[295] is part of the Centers for Disease Control and Prevention's Stopping Elderly Accidents, Deaths, and Injuries (STEADI) tools and resources. The assessment provides a quick way to assess the patient's mobility. To

Table 6. Push Force Limits

Push/Pull Forces Based on 75% Acceptable for Women Design Goal					
Distance (ft)	25	50	100	150	200
Initial (lb)	51	44	42	42	37
Sustained (lb)	30	25	22	22	15

Adapted from Manual Material Handling Guidelines, http://libertymmhtables.libertymutual.com/CM_LMTablesWeb/pdf/LibertyMutualTables.pdf. Reprinted with permission from the Liberty Mutual Research Institute for Safety.

conduct the test, a stopwatch, a standard armchair, and a marked distance of 3 m (10 ft) is needed. The patient should wear their regular footwear and use a walking aid if needed.

The patient sits back in the chair. When the examiner says, "Go" the patient is to stand up, walk to the line on the floor at his or her normal pace, turn, walk back to the chair at his or her normal pace, and sit down again. The examiner uses the stopwatch to time the exercise from the word "go" until the patient sits down. The older patient who takes ≥ 12 seconds to complete the TUG is at risk for falling. The examiner should observe the patient's postural stability, gait, stride length, and sway and note a slow tentative pace, loss of balance, short strides, little or no arm swing, steadying against walls, shuffling, en bloc turning (ie, keeping the neck and trunk rigid, requiring multiple small steps to accomplish a turn), and not using an assistive device properly. These changes may signify neurological problems that require further evaluation. The TUG assessment can help with screening, assessment, and interventions to reduce patient's fall risk.

The Banner Mobility Assessment Tool[294] consists of a four-step functional task list that identifies the mobility level of the patient. Mobility level is determined on whether the patient passes or fails each assessment level. An abbreviated description of the four assessment and mobility levels follows:

- Assessment Level 1 tasks assess cognition, trunk strength, and seated balance. If the patient fails the tasks of level 1, he or she is considered to be Mobility Level 1 and requires use of a total lift with a sling, a lateral transfer device (eg, friction-reducing device), or an air-assisted device. If the patient passes the tasks of level 1, the process continues.
- Assessment Level 2 tasks assess lower extremity strength and stability. If the patient fails the tasks of level 2, he or she is considered to be Mobility Level 2 and requires use of a total

lift for the patient unable to bear weight on at least one leg and the use of a sit-to-stand lift for the patient can bear weight on at least one leg. If the patient passes the tasks of level 2, the process continues.

- Assessment Level 3 tasks assess lower extremity strength for standing. If the patient fails the tasks of level 3, he or she is considered to be Mobility Level 3 and requires the use of a non-powered raising/stand aid but defaults to the use of a powered sit-to-stand lift if no stand aid is available, use of a total lift with ambulation accessories, and use of assistive devices (eg, cane, walker, crutches). If the patient passes Assessment Level 3 but requires assistive devices to ambulate or if the cognitive assessment indicates poor safety awareness, the patient is considered to be Mobility Level 3. If the patient passes the tasks of level 3, the process continues.
- Assessment Level 4 tasks assess lower extremity strength for standing. At Assessment Level 4, the patient exhibits a steady gait, good balance, and safety awareness, and no assistance is needed. Based on the nurse's clinical judgement, supervision during ambulation may be needed. If the patient displays signs of an unsteady gait or falls, he or she is lowered to a Mobility Level 3.

6.11.3 **The perioperative RN may offer the patient the option of walking to the OR accompanied by the nurse based on the results of the mobility and falls risk assessment.**[296] *[Conditional Recommendation]*

When the patient walks to the OR, it enhances the patient's sense of independence, maintains his or her dignity, may improve the efficiency of the process, and decreases the amount of pushing and pulling of stretchers for personnel. Walking may be contraindicated if the patient is pre-medicated, had preoperative dilating ophthalmic drops, or prefers not to walk to the OR. After conducting qualitative studies, Humphrey et al,[296] Keegan-Doody,[297] and Nagraj et al[298] concluded that the patients in their studies preferred walking to the OR. In Keegan-Doody's study, the patients wore a patient gown, dressing gown (ie, robe), and socks.[297]

7. Post-Injury Return to Work

7.1 **Provide an injured employee with reasonable accommodations for post-injury return to work.** *[Recommendation]*

In a 2011 survey of 4,614 RNs conducted by the ANA, 56% of the nurses responded that they had experienced musculoskeletal pain caused or made worse by their nursing jobs, and 80% reported they frequently worked despite experiencing musculoskeletal pain.[299]

7.2 **Report to the employer any physical limitations and restrictions after an injury and provide supporting medical documentation and clearance to return to work according to the health care organization's policy.**[69] *[Recommendation]*

Medical documentation identifies any physical limitations, such as fatigue, or discomfort and identifies occupational restrictions (eg, lifting limits).[90]

7.2.1 **Monitor injuries associated with patient and equipment handling** (See Recommendation 8).[69] *[Recommendation]*

Injury monitoring establishes the frequency, severity, and cost of the perioperative team members' injuries. The data may be useful for preventing injuries in the future.[69]

7.3 **Establish, implement, and sustain a process to facilitate return to work after an injury.**[69] *[Recommendation]*

When an injured team member is able to return to work, he or she benefits by being productive and receiving a salary. The health care organization benefits by having an experienced team member back in the staffing pattern.[90] Grayson et al[107] studied 103 employees with work-related MSDs that resulted in more than 5 days away from their usual work assignments. The participants received an ergonomic evaluation consisting of an observation of usual work tasks, recommendations to minimize identified stressors, and case coordination. The researchers concluded that ergonomic risk factors are obstacles for injured workers to return to their jobs. Interventions to reduce physical stressors in the workplace may facilitate the injured worker's return to work, prevent reinjury, and decrease time away from work. The study demonstrated that introducing a limited ergonomic evaluation program early in the treatment plan for injured workers resulted in modifications of job stressors. The program was most effective when the injured worker and his or her supervisor were motivated to incorporate the recommendations of the evaluation.

In a descriptive literature review of 21 research articles, Durand et al[300] identified workplace interventions employed after a worker suffered a musculoskeletal injury. The three main objectives of workplace interventions ranged from gathering information on the work demands in a clinical setting, gradually reintroducing the worker to the demands of the work environment, and permanently reducing the demands of the job. The review elucidated the diversity of actions carried out, human resources used, and workplace environments involved. As there is confusion in the terms used to designate permanent modifications to the physical work environment (eg, modified work, work modifications, accommodations), the authors recommended future research to differentiate between temporary and permanent modifications made to the work situation.

7.3.1   **Establish a process to match the physical capabilities of the perioperative team member to the physical demands of the job.**[90] *[Recommendation]*

Depending on the severity of a musculoskeletal injury, the team member may require days away from work and a modified work assignment[70,83,108,112,116-118,120] or may potentially end his or her career in the OR. In a survey of 1,095 nurses, Fochsen et al[301] studied predictors for leaving the nursing profession. Their results showed that nurses reporting musculoskeletal problems of the neck, shoulder, and knees who had limited access to patient transfer devices were more likely to leave the profession.

Ergonomic interventions to decrease physical work load in nursing care may be a way to keep nurses in the profession longer. Injuries and disabilities are more prevalent as workers age. Reasonable accommodations[20,226] for aging workers retain talent, ability, and experience.[302] Using SPHM technology, the AORN Ergonomic Tools, and job modifications[303] are approaches to facilitating the injured employee's return to work and keeping aging team members in the workforce.[69,304]

7.3.2   **Include monitoring adherence to modified, alternative, or transitional work limits in the process.**[69] *[Recommendation]*

Modified work is a modification of the injured team member's regular work duties to accommodate work restrictions. *Alternative work* is a temporary job assignment performed when the injured team member cannot return to his or her regular work duties. *Transitional work* allows an injured team member to stay safely in his or her present workplace in a modified or alternate capacity until he or she is recovered from the injury and can return to normal work duties.[90]

7.4   **As part of a health promotion and injury prevention program, multifaceted workplace interven-**

tions (eg, physical activity,[39,305,306] cognitive behavior therapy,[307] physiotherapy,[308] participatory ergonomic sessions) may be implemented. *[Conditional Recommendation]*

Multifaceted workplace interventions may prevent or decrease low back pain.[309,310] In a randomized controlled trial, Rasmussen et al[309] analyzed 586 workers during a 3-month intervention that consisted of 12 physical training sessions, two cognitive-behavior sessions, and five participatory ergonomic sessions. The analyses of the participants' assessments demonstrated significant effects on the reduction of low back pain days, pain intensity, and bothersomeness after the intervention compared with the control group. The study established the effectiveness of this multifaceted workplace intervention to prevent low back pain.

8. Quality

8.1   **Establish a quality assurance and performance improvement program.** *[Recommendation]*

Comprehensive evaluation of the SPHM program includes perioperative team member injury incidence and severity, perioperative team member performance, and patient outcomes and injuries.[69] Quality assurance and performance improvement programs assist in evaluating and improving the quality of patient care and workplace safety and in formulating plans for corrective action. These programs provide data that may be used to determine whether an organization is within its benchmark goals and, if not, to identify areas that may require corrective action. A quality management program provides a mechanism to evaluate effectiveness of processes, compliance with patient handling and lifting and moving equipment policies and procedures, and function of equipment and devices. Collecting data to monitor and improve patient care, treatment, and services is a regulatory requirement.[122,123,175,176]

8.2   **Include the following in the quality assurance and performance improvement program for safe patient and equipment handling:**
- reviewing and evaluating patient and equipment handling activities initially and periodically (eg, biannually, annually),
- establishing benchmarks to evaluate quality indicators,
- collecting data related to the levels of performance and quality indicators,
- evaluating practice based on the cumulative data collected,
- taking action to improve compliance,

- assessing the effectiveness of the actions taken,
- verifying compliance with policies,
- identifying activities needing improvement,
- developing strategies for compliance,
- identifying corrective actions directed toward improvement priorities,
- establishing short- and long-term improvement goals,
- taking additional actions when compliance and improvement is not achieved or sustained, and
- establishing a communication plan to inform all stakeholders of the SPHM outcomes.

[Recommendation]

The plan may include one or more communication tools (eg, online summary of data, printed materials, regularly scheduled staff meetings, management meetings, organizational meetings).[69,311]

[Conditional Recommendation]

Reviewing and evaluating quality assurance and performance improvement activities may identify failure points that contribute to errors in patient handling and use of lifting and moving equipment and help define actions for improvement and increased competence. Taking corrective actions may improve patient and health care worker safety by enhancing understanding of the principles of and compliance with best practices for patient handling and lifting and moving equipment.

8.3 Participate in a variety of quality assurance and performance improvement activities consistent with the health care organization's plan to improve compliance with the principles and processes related to patient and equipment handling. [Recommendation]

Participating in ongoing quality assurance and performance improvement activities is a primary responsibility of perioperative personnel engaged in practice.[312]

8.3.1 Report and document hazards, near misses, incidents, and accidents related to SPHM according to the health care organization's policy and procedure.[69] [Recommendation]

Reports of near misses and adverse events can be used to identify actions that may prevent similar occurrences and uncover opportunities for improvement.

8.3.2 Include the following in data collection of the incident:
- a description of the event, including the
  - task being performed (eg, patient positioning),

  - action being performed (eg, turning the patient from the stretcher to the OR bed into the supine position),
  - number of team members involved in performing the task, and
  - patient factors (eg, obesity);
- whether the correct equipment was available, operable, and used according to policy and procedures;
- whether an appropriate patient assessment was performed;
- the time, shift, and date of the incident;
- the perioperative area (eg, PACU, OR); and
- the body part affected (eg, back, shoulder).[1]

[Recommendation]

8.4 After a report of an error or near miss, perform a root cause analysis and provide feedback of the results to the reporter of the incident.[89] [Recommendation]

Providing results of the analysis to the reporter of the incident demonstrates how the analysis was used to improve the system and prevent future errors.[89]

8.5 Analyze data on health care personnel and patient injuries related to patient and equipment handling and use the information for performance improvement at the start of the SPHM program and periodically.[69] Include the following in the data collection of adverse events:
- incidence of team members' MSDs;
- severity of team members' MSDs;
- medical care received as a result of the injury[1];
- number of lost work days[313];
- number of team members' light, modified, or restricted work days[313];
- amount of personal sick or vacation days taken as a result of the injury;
- total costs of team members' MSDs;
- whether an appropriate patient assessment was performed;
- staffing level;
- whether the correct equipment was available, operable, and used;
- whether the injured team member had training and competency verification on the equipment used; and
- adverse patient events (eg, falls).[90]

[Recommendation]

The data may be located in several different databases (eg, occurrence reporting, workforce management systems, employee health records, OSHA 300 log[146]), incompletely recorded, not recorded, or unavailable because of patient privacy requirements. To accurately compare incidents and results, it is important to evaluate the comparability of the data from sources and across the years.[1]

Glossary

Adverse events: Events that result in injury.

Air-assisted lateral transfer device: A mattress that is inflated with air by a portable air supply, thus facilitating a smoother lateral transfer.

Algorithm: An evidence-based clinical tool used to make health care decisions. Algorithms standardized practice based on evidence rather than requiring the health care worker to rely on his or her education and experience to make decisions.

Anti-fatigue mat: A special mat designed with friction-reducing properties for use by workers who stand for long periods of time.

Assistive devices/technology: Equipment that can be used to take all or a portion of a load, such as the weight of a body part, off of the person performing a high-risk task.

Biomechanics: The field of study that applies the laws of physics and engineering concepts to describe motion of body segments and the forces that act upon them during activity.

Ergonomics: The science of fitting the job to the worker. The practice of designing equipment and work tasks to conform to the capability of the worker, providing a means for adjusting the work environment and work practices to prevent injuries. Emphasizes work practices, biomechanics, work environment, and tool use.

Ergonomist: A practitioner in the field of ergonomics.

Fatigue-reducing technique: Any technique that will reduce fatigue experienced by the worker.

Friction-reducing devices: Low-friction (eg, slippery) material assistive aids for lateral transfer of patients and repositioning of patients.

Lateral position: Side-lying.

Lateral transfer: Movement of a patient in a supine position on a horizontal plane, such as transferring a patient from a bed to a stretcher.

Lateral transfer device: A device that is used to move a patient in a supine position from one surface to another.

Lifting index: The relative estimate of physical stress associated with a specific task. It is equal to the load weight of the object divided by the recommended weight limit.

Lithotomy position: Supine position with the hips and knees flexed and the thighs abducted and rotated externally.

Manual retraction: When a member of the perioperative sterile team (ie, scrubbed team) provides exposure of underlying anatomical parts during surgery with his or her hand or by physically holding and/or pulling with a sterile device designed to hold back the edges of tissue and organs.

Maximum sustained force: The force needed to pull or lift for a period of time.

Musculoskeletal: Relating to or involving the muscles and the skeleton.

Musculoskeletal disorder: Disorders of the muscles, nerves, tendons, ligaments, joints, cartilage, and spinal discs that result from or are worsened by work exposures.

Near misses: Unplanned events that do not result in injury but had the potential to do so.

Newton (N): A metric unit of measure for forces (1 N = 0.2248 lb).

Newton meter (Nm): A metric unit of measure for moments (ie, force × length). One Nm = 0.738 ft lb.

Optimal OR bed height: The optimal table working height is generally at the level of the waist or elbow or 5 cm above the elbow but may vary depending on instrument length and design, surgery, and technique.

Prone position: With the front (or ventral) surface of the body positioned face downward.

Recommended weight limit: The principal product of the Revised NIOSH Lifting Equation defined for a specific set of task conditions as the weight of the load that 75% of the population could perform safely.

Revised NIOSH Lifting Equation: A mathematical equation for determining the recommended weight limit and lifting index for selected two-handed manual lifting tasks.

Self-retaining retractor: A sterile device designed to mechanically hold back the edges of tissue and organs to provide exposure to underlying anatomical structures during a surgical procedure.

Semi-Fowler position: The upper half of the body raised to an incline of 30 to 45 degrees; also called the beach chair position.

Sit-stand stool: A stool that allows the worker to sit or stand while working without changing levels.

Static postures: Postures requiring a sustained position for a long period of time (eg, standing in one position during surgery).

Supine position: With the back or dorsal surface of the body positioned downward (ie, lying face up).

References

1. *Safe Patient Handling and Mobility Guidebook.* St Louis, MO: VHA Center for Engineering & Occupational Safety and Health (CEOSH); 2016. [IVB]

2. Owen BD. Preventing injuries using an ergonomic approach. *AORN J.* 2000;72(6):1031-1036. [VB]

3. Garb JR, Dockery CA. Reducing employee back injuries in the perioperative setting. *AORN J.* 1995;61(6):1046-1052. [VC]

4. Waters TR. Introduction to ergonomics for healthcare workers. *Rehabil Nurs.* 2010;35(5):185-191. [VA]

5. Gallagher S, Heberger JR. Examining the interaction of force and repetition on musculoskeletal disorder risk: a systematic literature review. *Hum Factors.* 2013;55(1):108-124. [IIIB]

6. Arvidsson I, Gremark Simonsen J, Dahlqvist C, et al. Cross-sectional associations between occupational factors and musculoskeletal pain in women teachers, nurses and sonographers. *BMC Musculoskelet Disord.* 2016;17:35. [IIIA]

7. Lee G, Lee T, Dexter D, et al. Ergonomic risk associated with assisting in minimally invasive surgery. *Surg Endosc.* 2009;23(1):182-188. [IIIC]

8. Lucas-Hernández M, Pagador JB, Pérez-Duarte FJ, Castelló P, Sánchez-Margallo F. Ergonomics problems due to the use and design of dissector and needle holder: a survey in minimally invasive surgery. *Surg Laparosc Endosc Percutan Tech.* 2014;24(5):e170-e177. [IIIB]

9. Luttmann A, Jöger M, Sökeland J. Ergonomic assessment of the posture of surgeons performing endoscopic transurethral resections in urology. *J Occup Med Toxicol.* 2009;4:26. [IIIC]

10. Yoon SH, Jung MC, Park SY. Evaluation of surgeon's muscle fatigue during thoracoscopic pulmonary lobectomy using interoperative surface electromyography. *J Thorac Dis.* 2016;8(6):1162-1169. [IIIC]

11. Welcker K, Kesieme EB, Internullo E, Kranenburg van Koppen LJ. Ergonomics in thoracoscopic surgery: results of a survey among thoracic surgeons. *Interact Cardiovasc Thorac Surg.* 2012;15(2):197-200. [IIIB]

12. Habibi E, Pourabdian S, Atabaki AK, Hoseini M. Evaluation of work-related psychosocial and ergonomics factors in relation to low back discomfort in emergency unit nurses. *Int J Prev Med.* 2012;3(8):564-568. [IIIB]

13. Adhikari S, Dhakal G. Prevalent causes of low back pain and its impact among nurses working in Sahid Gangalal National Heart Centre. *J Nepal Health Res Counc.* 2014;12(28):167-171. [IIIB]

14. Hou JY, Shiao JS. Risk factors for musculoskeletal discomfort in nurses. *J Nurs Res.* 2006;14(3):228-236. [IIIA]

15. Mohseni-Bandpei MA, Fakhri M, Bagheri-Nesami M, Ahmad-Shirvani M, Khalilian AR, Shayesteh-Azar M. Occupational back pain in Iranian nurses: an epidemiological study. *Br J Nurs.* 2006;15(17):914-917. [IIIB]

16. Hopcia K, Dennerlein JT, Hashimoto D, Orechia T, Sorensen G. Occupational injuries for consecutive and cumulative shifts among hospital registered nurses and patient care associates: a case-control study. *Workplace Health Saf.* 2012;60(10):437-444. [IIIA]

17. Dembe AE, Erickson JB, Delbos RG, Banks SM. The impact of overtime and long work hours on occupational injuries and illnesses: new evidence from the United States. *Occup Environ Med.* 2005;62(9):588-597. [IIIA]

18. Trinkoff AM, Le R, Geiger-Brown J, Lipscomb J, Lang G. Longitudinal relationship of work hours, mandatory overtime, and on-call to musculoskeletal problems in nurses. *Am J Ind Med.* 2006;49(11):964-971. [IIIA]

19. Shieh SH, Sung FC, Su CH, Tsai Y, Hsieh VC. Increased low back pain risk in nurses with high workload for patient care: a questionnaire survey. *Taiwan J Obstet Gynecol.* 2016;55(4):525-529. [IIIA]

20. Geiger-Brown J, Lipscomb J. The health care work environment and adverse health and safety consequences for nurses. *Annu Rev Nurs Res.* 2010;28:191-231. [VA]

21. Nelson A. *Safe Patient Handling and Movement: A Guide for Nurses and Other Health Care Providers.* New York, NY: Springer Publishing Co; 2006. [VA]

22. Kim SS, Okechukwu CA, Buxton OM, et al. Association between work-family conflict and musculoskeletal pain among hospital patient care workers. *Am J Ind Med.* 2013;56(4):488-495. [IIIA]

23. Simon M, Tackenberg P, Nienhaus A, Estryn-Behar M, Conway PM, Hasselhorn HM. Back or neck-pain-related disability of nursing staff in hospitals, nursing homes and home care in seven countries—results from the European NEXT-Study. *Int J Nurs Stud.* 2008;45(1):24-34. [IIIA]

24. Amin NA, Nordin R, Fatt QK, Noah RM, Oxley J. Relationship between psychosocial risk factors and work-related musculoskeletal disorders among public hospital nurses in Malaysia. *Ann Occup Environ Med.* 2014;26:23. [IIIB]

25. Schoenfisch AL, Lipscomb HJ. Job characteristics and work organization factors associated with patient-handling injury among nursing personnel. *Work.* 2009;33(1):117-128. [IIIB]

26. Nützi M, Koch P, Baur H, Elfering A. Work-family conflict, task interruptions, and influence at work predict musculoskeletal pain in operating room nurses. *Saf Health Work.* 2015;6(4):329-337. [IIIB]

27. Smedley J, Inskip H, Buckle P, Cooper C, Coggon D. Epidemiological differences between back pain of sudden and gradual onset. *J Rheumatol.* 2005;32(3):528-532. [IIIC]

28. Smedley J, Inskip H, Trevelyan F, Buckle P, Cooper C, Coggon D. Risk factors for incident neck and shoulder pain in hospital nurses. *Occup Environ Med.* 2003;60(11):864-869. [IIIB]

29. Sabbath EL, Hurtado DA, Okechukwu CA, et al. Occupational injury among hospital patient-care workers: what is the association with workplace verbal abuse? *Am J Ind Med.* 2014;57(2):222-232. [IIIB]

30. Ellapen TJ, Narsigan S. Work related musculoskeletal disorders among nurses: systematic review. *J Ergonomics.* 2014;S4:003. doi: 10.4172/2165-7556.S4-003. [IIIA]

31. Videman T, Ojajörvi A, Riihimöki H, Troup JD. Low back pain among nurses: a follow-up beginning at entry to the nursing school. *Spine (Phila Pa 1976).* 2005;30(20):2334-2341. [IIIA]

32. Lee SJ, Lee JH, Gershon RR. Musculoskeletal symptoms in nurses in the early implementation phase of California's safe patient handling legislation. *Res Nurs Health.* 2015;38(3):183-193. [IIIB]

33. Arsalani N, Fallahi-Khoshknab M, Josephson M, Lagerström M. Musculoskeletal disorders and working conditions among Iranian nursing personnel. *Int J Occup Saf Ergon.* 2014;20(4):671-680. [IIIA]

34. Chung YC, Hung CT, Li SF, et al. Risk of musculoskeletal disorder among Taiwanese nurses cohort: a nationwide population-based study. *BMC Musculoskelet Disord.* 2013;14. [IIIB]

35. Bos E, Krol B, van der Star L, Groothoff J. Risk factors and musculoskeletal complaints in non-specialized nurses, IC nurses, operation room nurses, and x-ray technologists. *Int Arch Occup Environ Health.* 2007;80(3):198-206. [IIIC]

36. de Castro AB, Cabrera SL, Gee GC, Fujishiro K, Tagalog EA. Occupational health and safety issues among nurses in the Philippines. *AAOHN J.* 2009;57(4):149-157. [IIIB]

37. Sadeghian F, Hosseinzadeh S, Aliyari R. Do psychological factors increase the risk for low back pain among nurses? A comparing according to cross-sectional and prospective analysis. *Saf Health Work.* 2014;5(1):13-16. [IIIC]

38. Naeem A, Umar M, Malik AN, ur Rehman S. Occupationally related low back pain and associated factors in nurses. *Rawal Med J.* 2015;40(2):145-147. [IIIB]

39. Letvak S. We cannot ignore nurses' health anymore: a synthesis of the literature on evidence-based strategies to improve nurse health. *Nurs Adm Q.* 2013;37(4):295-308. [IIA]

40. Serranheira F, Cotrim T, Rodrigues V, Nunes C, Sousa-Uva A. Nurses' working tasks and MSDs back symptoms: results from a national survey. *Work.* 2012;41(Suppl 1):2449-2451. [IIIA]

41. Nelson A, Matz M, Chen F, Siddharthan K, Lloyd J, Fragala G. Development and evaluation of a multifaceted ergonomics program to prevent injuries associated with patient handling tasks. *Int J Nurs Stud.* 2006;43(6):717-733. [IIA]

42. Injuries, illnesses, and fatalities. Chart 5: Rates of injuries and illnesses for selected healthcare and protective service occupations, by ownership, 2015. US Bureau of Labor Statistics. https://data.bls.gov/cgi-bin/print.pl/iif/oshwc/osh/case/chart-data-2015.htm. Updated October 20, 2017. Accessed May 10, 2018. [VA]

43. Karahan A, Kav S, Abbasoglu A, Dogan N. Low back pain: prevalence and associated risk factors among hospital staff. *J Adv Nurs.* 2009;65(3):516-524. [IIIB]

44. Dennerlein JT, Hopcia K, Sembajwe G, et al. Ergonomic practices within patient care units are associated with musculoskeletal pain and limitations. *Am J Ind Med.* 2012;55(2):107-116. [IIIA]

45. Ngan K, Drebit S, Siow S, Yu S, Keen D, Alamgir H. Risks and causes of musculoskeletal injuries among health care workers. *Occup Med (Lond).* 2010;60(5):389-394. [IIIA]

46. Moreira RF, Sato TO, Foltran FA, Silva LC, Coury HJ. Prevalence of musculoskeletal symptoms in hospital nurse technicians and licensed practical nurses: associations with demographic factors. *Braz J Phys Ther.* 2014;18(4):323-333. [IIIB]

47. Boyer J, Galizzi M, Cifuentes M, et al; Promoting Healthy Safe Employment (PHASE) in Healthcare Team. Ergonomic and socioeconomic risk factors for hospital workers' compensation injury claims. *Am J Ind Med.* 2009;52(7):551-562. [IIIB]

48. McDonald ME, Ramirez PT, Munsell MF, et al. Physician pain and discomfort during minimally invasive gynecologic cancer surgery. *Gynecol Oncol.* 2014;134(2):243-247. [IIIB]

49. Shepherd JM, Harilingam MR, Hamade A. Ergonomics in laparoscopic surgery—a survey of symptoms and contributing factors. *Surg Laparosc Endosc Percutan Tech.* 2016;26(1):72-77. [IIIB]

50. Knudsen ML, Ludewig PM, Braman JP. Musculoskeletal pain in resident orthopaedic surgeons: results of a novel survey. *Iowa Orthop J.* 2014;34:190-196. [IIIC]

51. Janki S, Mulder EEAP, IJzermans JNM, Tran TCK. Ergonomics in the operating room. *Surg Endosc.* 2017;31(6):2457-2466. [IIIB]

52. Kim-Fine S, Woolley SM, Weaver AL, Killian JM, Gebhart JB. Work-related musculoskeletal disorders among vaginal surgeons. *Int Urogynecol J.* 2013;24(7):1191-1200. [IIIB]

53. Tjiam IM, Goossens RH, Schout BM, et al. Ergonomics in endourology and laparoscopy: an overview of musculoskeletal problems in urology. *J Endourol.* 2014;28(5):605-611. [IIIB]

54. Esser AC, Koshy JG, Randle HW. Ergonomics in office-based surgery: a survey-guided observational study. *Dermatol Surg.* 2007;33(11):1304-1313; discussion 1313-1314. [IIIB]

55. Little RM, Deal AM, Zanation AM, McKinney K, Senior BA, Ebert CS Jr. Occupational hazards of endoscopic surgery. *Int Forum Allergy Rhinol.* 2012;2(3):212-216. [IIIB]

56. Vijendren A, Yung M, Sanchez J, Duffield K. Occupational musculoskeletal pain amongst ENT surgeons—are we looking at the tip of an iceberg? *J Laryngol Otol.* 2016;130(5):490-496. [IIIB]

57. Sari V, Nieboer TE, Vierhout ME, Stegeman DF, Kluivers KB. The operation room as a hostile environment for surgeons: physical complaints during and after laparoscopy. *Minim Invasive Ther Allied Technol.* 2010;19(2):105-109. [IIIB]

58. Sivak-Callcott JA, Diaz SR, Ducatman AM, Rosen CL, Nimbarte AD, Sedgeman JA. A survey study of occupational pain and injury in ophthalmic plastic surgeons. *Ophthal Plast Reconstr Surg.* 2011;27(1):28-32. [IIIB]

59. Ruitenburg MM, Frings-Dresen MH, Sluiter JK. Physical job demands and related health complaints among surgeons. *Int Arch Occup Environ Health.* 2013;86(3):271-279. [IIIB]

60. Sutton E, Irvin M, Zeigler C, Lee G, Park A. The ergonomics of women in surgery. *Surg Endosc.* 2014;28(4):1051-1055. [IIIB]

61. Godwin Y, Macdonald CR, Kaur S, Zhelin L, Baber C. The impact of cervical musculoskeletal disorders on UK consultant plastic surgeons: can we reduce morbidity with applied ergonomics? *Ann Plast Surg.* 2017;78(6):602-610. [IIIB]

62. Adams SR, Hacker MR, McKinney JL, Elkadry EA, Rosenblatt PL. Musculoskeletal pain in gynecologic surgeons. *J Minim Invasive Gynecol.* 2013;20(5):656-660. [IIIB]

63. Epstein S, Sparer EH, Tran BN, et al. Prevalence of work-related musculoskeletal disorders among surgeons and interventionalists: a systematic review and meta-analysis. *JAMA Surg.* 2018;153(2):e174947. [IIIA]

64. *AORN Guidance Statement: Safe Patient Handling and Movement in the Perioperative Setting.* Denver, CO: AORN, Inc; 2007. [IVB]

65. Ogden CL, Fakhouri TH, Carroll MD, et al. Prevalence of obesity among adults, by household income and education—United States, 2011-2014. *MMWR Morb Mortal Wkly Rep.* 2017;66(50):1369-1373. [VA]

66. Weinmeyer R. Safe patient handling laws and programs for health care workers. *AMA J Ethics.* 2016;18(4):416-421. [VA]

67. Flegal KM, Kruszon-Moran D, Carroll MD, Fryar CD, Ogden CL. Trends in obesity among adults in the United States, 2005 to 2014. *JAMA.* 2016;315(21):2284-2291. [IIIB]

68. *Position Statement on Elimination of Manual Patient Handling to Prevent Work-Related Musculoskeletal Disorders.* Silver Spring, MD: American Nurses Association; 2003. [IVB]

69. *Safe Patient Handling and Mobility: Interprofessional National Standards.* Silver Spring, MD: American Nurses Association; 2013. [IVA]

70. de Castro AB. Handle with Care: The American Nurses Association's campaign to address work-related musculoskeletal disorders. *Orthop Nurs.* 2006;25(6):356-365. [VA]

71. Ergonomically healthy workplace practices: proposed AORN position statements for consideration by House of Delegates. *AORN J.* 2006;83(1):119-122. [IVB]

72. *NAON Position Statement: Safe Patient Handling and Movement in the Orthopaedic Setting.* Chicago, IL: National Association of Orthopaedic Nurses; 2012. [IVB]

73. Position statement: safe patient and manual handling. In: *2014-2015 ACORN Standards for Perioperative Nursing: Including Nurses Roles, Guidelines, Position Statements, Competency Standards.* Lyndoch, SA, Australia: Australian College of Operating Room Nurses Ltd; 2014:143-148. [IVB]

74. *Position Statement: Safe Patient Handling. Association of Occupational Health Professionals in Healthcare.* http://aohp.org/aohp/Portals/0/Documents/ToolsForYour-Work/Position%20Statements/PositionStatements%20Jul%202017.pdf. Accessed May 10, 2018. [IVB]

75. Nelson A, Waters T, Spratt D, Peterson C, Hughes N. Development of the AORN guidance statement: safe patient handling and movement in the perioperative setting. In: *AORN Guidance Statement: Safe Patient Handling and Movement in the Perioperative Setting.* Denver, CO: AORN, Inc; 2007:5-9. [VA]

76. Waters T, Collins J, Galinsky T, Caruso C. NIOSH research efforts to prevent musculoskeletal disorders in the healthcare industry. *Orthop Nurs.* 2006;25(6):380-389. [VA]

77. Safe lifting becomes standard practice. *Hosp Case Manag.* 2013;21(2):26-28. [VA]

78. Knoblauch MD, Bethel SA. Safe patient-handling program "UPLIFTs" nurse retention. *Nursing.* 2010;40(2):67-68. [VB]

79. Dawson JM, Harrington S. Embracing safe patient handling. *Nurs Manage.* 2012;43(10):15-17. [VA]

80. Mayeda-Letourneau J. Safe patient handling and movement: a literature review. *Rehabil Nurs.* 2014;39(3):123-129. [VA]

81. Guideline for positioning the patient. In: *Guidelines for Perioperative Practice.* Denver, CO: AORN, Inc; 2018:673-744. [IVA]

82. Guideline for preoperative patient skin antisepsis. In: *Guidelines for Perioperative Practice.* Denver, CO: AORN, Inc; 2018:51-74. [IVA]

83. Cadmus E, Brigley P, Pearson M. Safe patient handling: is your facility ready for a culture change? *Nurs Manage.* 2011; 42(11):12-15. [VA]

84. Hooper J, Charney W. Creation of a safety culture: reducing workplace injuries in a rural hospital setting. *AAOHN J.* 2005;53(9):394-398. [VB]

85. Koppelaar E, Knibbe JJ, Miedema HS, Burdorf A. The influence of individual and organisational factors on nurses' behaviour to use lifting devices in healthcare. *Appl Ergon.* 2013; 44(4):532-537. [IIIB]

86. Koppelaar E, Knibbe JJ, Miedema HS, Burdorf A. Individual and organisational determinants of use of ergonomic devices in healthcare. *Occup Environ Med.* 2011;68(9):659-665. [IIIB]

87. Guideline for team communication. In: *Guidelines for Perioperative Practice.* Denver, CO: AORN, Inc; 2018:745-772. [IVA]

88. *Improving Patient and Worker Safety: Opportunities for Synergy, Collaboration and Innovation.* Oakbrook Terrace, IL: The Joint Commission; 2012. http://www.jointcommission.org/assets/1/18/TJC-improvingpatientandworkersafety-monograph.pdf. Accessed May 10, 2018. [VA]

89. Committee on the Work Environment for Nurses and Patient Safety, Institute of Medicine. Page A, ed. *Keeping Patients Safe: Transforming the Work Environment of Nurses.* Washington, DC: National Academies Press; 2004. [VA]

90. Gallagher S; American Nurses Association. *Implementation Guide to the Safe patient Handling and Mobility Interprofessional National Standards.* Silver Spring, MD: American Nurses Association; 2013. [VA]

91. Engkvist IL. Nurses' expectations, experiences and attitudes towards the intervention of a "no lifting policy." *J Occup Health.* 2007;49(4):294-304. [IIIA]

92. Hignett S, Wilson JR, Morris W. Finding ergonomic solutions—participatory approaches. *Occup Med (Lond).* 2005; 55(3):200-207. [VA]

93. Kim SL, Lee JE. Development of an intervention to prevent work-related musculoskeletal disorders among hospital nurses based on the participatory approach. *Appl Ergon.* 2010;41(3):454-460. [VA]

94. Krill C, Staffileno BA, Raven C. Empowering staff nurses to use research to change practice for safe patient handling. *Nurs Outlook.* 2012;60(3):157-162. [IIIB]

95. Caspi CE, Dennerlein JT, Kenwood C, et al. Results of a pilot intervention to improve health and safety for health care workers. *J Occup Environ Med.* 2013;55(12):1449-1455. [IIB]

96. Enos L. Texas passes first safe patient handling legislation. *Oreg Nurse.* 2005;70(3):3. [VA]

97. Hudson MA. Texas passes first law for safe patient handling in America: landmark legislation protects health-care workers and patients from injury related to manual patient lifting. *J Long-Term Eff Med Implants.* 2005;15(5):559-566. [VA]

98. Emerging issue: keeping patients and nurses safe. Nursing and musculoskeletal disorders. *N J Nurse.* 2005;35(1):12-13. [VC]

99. Hughes NL. Update on Handle with Care: the American Nurses Association's campaign to address work-related musculoskeletal disorders. *Orthop Nurs.* 2006;25(6):357. [VB]

100. Sparkman CA. Ergonomics in the workplace. *AORN J.* 2006;84(3):379-382. [VB]

101. White KM. Policy spotlight: patient care ergonomics. *Nurs Manage.* 2007;38(4):26-30. [VB]

102. OSH Act of 1970. Occupational Safety and Health Administration. https://www.osha.gov/pls/oshaweb/owadisp.show_document?p_table=OSHACT&p_id=2743. Accessed May 10, 2018.

103. OSHA general duty clause. Occupational Safety and Health Administration. https://www.osha.gov/pls/oshaweb/owadisp.show_document?p_table=OSHACT&p_id=3359. Accessed May 10, 2018.

104. Wallis L. OSHA gets serious about workplace safety for nurses. *Am J Nurs.* 2015;115(9):13. [VC]

105. de Castro AB, Hagan P, Nelson A. Prioritizing safe patient handling: the American Nurses Association's Handle with Care campaign. *J Nurs Adm.* 2006;36(7-8):363-369. [VC]

106. Safe patient handling. Safety and Health Topics: Healthcare. Occupational Safety and Health Administration. https://www.osha.gov/SLTC/healthcarefacilities/safepatienthandling.html. Accessed May 10, 2018. [VA]

107. Grayson D, Dale AM, Bohr P, Wolf L, Evanoff B. Ergonomic evaluation: part of a treatment protocol for musculoskeletal injuries. *AAOHN J.* 2005;53(10):450-457; quiz 458-459. [IIC]

108. Collins JW, Wolf L, Bell J, Evanoff B. An evaluation of a "best practices" musculoskeletal injury prevention program in nursing homes. *Inj Prev.* 2004;10(4):206-211. [IIA]

109. Enos L. Hidden costs: the case for ergonomics and safe patient handling. *Oreg Nurse.* 2010:5. [VB]

110. 2010 Health Guidelines Revision Committee. *Specialty Subcommittee on Patient Movement. Patient Handling and Movement Assessments: A White Paper.* Dallas, TX: Facility Guidelines Institute; 2010. [VA]

111. Restrepo TE, Schmid FA, Gucer PW, Shuford HL, Shyong CJ, McDiarmid MA. Safe lifting programs at long-term care facilities and their impact on workers' compensation costs. *J Occup Environ Med.* 2013;55(1):27-35. [IIIA]

112. Charney W, Simmons B, Lary M, Metz S. Zero lift programs in small rural hospitals in Washington state: reducing back injuries among health care workers. *AAOHN J.* 2006;54(8):355-358. [IIB]

113. Haglund K, Kyle J, Finkelstein M. Pediatric safe patient handling. *J Pediatr Nurs.* 2010;25(2):98-107. [IIIC]

114. Powell-Cope G, Toyinbo P, Patel N, et al. Effects of a national safe patient handling program on nursing injury incidence rates. *J Nurs Adm.* 2014;44(10):525-534. [IIA]

115. Wardell H. Reduction of injuries associated with patient handling. *AAOHN J.* 2007;55(10):407-412. [IIB]

116. Zadvinskis IM, Salsbury SL. Effects of a multifaceted minimal-lift environment for nursing staff: pilot results. *West J Nurs Res.* 2010;32(1):47-63. [IIB]

117. Nelson A, Baptiste AS. Update on evidence-based practices for safe patient handling and movement. *Orthop Nurs.* 2006;25(6):367-368. [VA]

118. Kutash M, Short M, Shea J, Martinez M. The lift team's importance to a successful safe patient handling program. *J Nurs Adm.* 2009;39(4):170-175. [VB]

119. Hunter B, Branson M, Davenport D. Saving costs, saving health care providers' backs, and creating a safe patient environment. *Nurs Econ.* 2010;28(2):130-134. [VA]

120. Meeks-Sjostrom D, Lopuszynski SA, Bairan A. The wisdom of retaining experienced nurses at the bedside: a pilot study examining a minimal lift program and its impact on reducing patient movement related injuries of bedside nurses. *Medsurg Nurs.* 2010;19(4):233-236. [IIC]

121. Vieira ER, Kumar S, Coury HJ, Narayan Y. Low back problems and possible improvements in nursing jobs. *J Adv Nurs.* 2006;55(1):79-89. [IIIB]

122. 42 CFR 482: Conditions of participation for hospitals. US Government Publishing Office. https://www.gpo.gov/fdsys/granule/CFR-2011-title42-vol5/CFR-2011-title42-vol5-part482. Accessed May 10, 2018.

123. *State Operations Manual Appendix L—Guidance for Surveyors: Ambulatory Surgical Centers.* Rev. 137; 2015. Centers for Medicare & Medicaid Services. https://www.cms.gov/Regulations-and-Guidance/Guidance/Manuals/downloads/som107ap_l_ambulatory.pdf. Accessed May 10, 2018.

124. PtD: Prevention through design. Centers for Disease Control and Prevention. https://www.cdc.gov/niosh/topics/ptd/default.html. Accessed May 10, 2018. [VB]

125. Ng I. Integrated intra-operative room design. *Acta Neurochir Suppl.* 2011;109:199-205. [VB]

126. Samii A, Gerganov VM. The dedicated endoscopic operating room. *World Neurosurg.* 2013;79(2 Suppl):S15.e19-S15.e22. [VB]

127. Sikkink CJ, Reijnen MM, Zeebregts CJ. The creation of the optimal dedicated endovascular suite. *Eur J Vasc Endovasc Surg.* 2008;35(2):198-204. [VB]

128. Hudorovi N, Rogan SA, Lovrievi I, Zovak M, Schmidt S. The vascular hybrid room—operating room of the future. *Acta Clin Croat.* 2010;49(3):289-298. [VA]

129. Koneczny S. The operating room: architectural conditions and potential hazards. *Work.* 2009;33(2):145-164. [IIIA]

130. Klein M, Andersen LP, Alamili M, Gögenur I, Rosenberg J. Psychological and physical stress in surgeons operating in a standard or modern operating room. *Surg Laparos Endosc Percutan Tech.* 2010;20(4):237-242. [IIB]

131. Anastasakis E, Protopapas A, Daskalakis G, Papadakis M, Milingos S, Antsaklis A. Transforming a conventional theatre into a gynaecological endoscopy unit. *Clin Exp Obstet Gynecol.* 2007;34(2):99-101. [VB]

132. Muir M, Heese GA, McLean D, Bodnar S, Rock BL. Handling of the bariatric patient in critical care: a case study of lessons learned. *Crit Care Nurs Clin North Am.* 2007;19(2):223-240. [VA]

133. Ginsberg GG, Pickett-Blakely O. Endoscopy unit considerations in the care of obese patients. *Gastrointest Endosc Clin N Am.* 2011;21(2):265-274. [VB]

134. *Bariatric Safe Patient Handling and Mobility Guidebook: A Resource Guide for Care of Persons of Size.* St Louis, MO: VHA Center for Engineering & Occupational Safety and Health (CEOSH); 2015. [IVB]

135. Rose MA, Drake DJ, Baker G, Watkins FR Jr, Watcrs W, Pokorny M. Caring for morbidly obese patients: safety considerations for nurse administrators. *Nurs Manage.* 2008;39(11):47-50. [VC]

136. Choi SD, Brings K. Work-related musculoskeletal risks associated with nurses and nursing assistants handling overweight and obese patients: a literature review. *Work.* 2015;53(2):439-448. [VA]

137. Schoenfisch AL, Myers DJ, Pompeii LA, Lipscomb HJ. Implementation and adoption of mechanical patient lift equipment in the hospital setting: the importance of organizational and cultural factors. *Am J Ind Med.* 2011;54(12):946-954. [IIIB]

138. de Ruiter HP, Liaschenko J. To lift or not to lift: patient-handling practices. *AAOHN J.* 2011;59(8):337-343. [IIIB]

139. *Safe Patient Handling and Mobility (SPHM) Technology—Coverage & Space Recommendations.* 2016 Revision. Washington, DC: US Department of Veterans Affairs, Veterans Health Administration; 2016. [VA]

140. Nelson A, Baptiste AS. Evidence-based practices for safe patient handling and movement. *Online J Issues Nurs.* 2004;9(3):4. [VA]

141. Guideline for a safe environment of care, part 2. In: *Guidelines for Perioperative Practice.* Denver, CO: AORN, Inc; 2018:269-294. [IVA]

142. Thomas-Olson L, Gee M, Harrison D, Helal N. Evaluating the use of ceiling lifts in the operating room. *ORNAC J.* 2015;33(1):13-16, 22-23, 26-28 passim. [IIIC]

143. Hodgson MJ, Matz MW, Nelson A. Patient handling in the Veterans Health Administration: facilitating change in the health care industry. *J Occup Environ Med.* 2013;55(10):1230-1237. [VA]

144. Waters TR, Nelson A, Proctor C. Patient handling tasks with high risk for musculoskeletal disorders in critical care. *Crit Care Nurs Clin North Am.* 2007;19(2):131-143. [VA]

145. McCoskey KL. Ergonomics and patient handling. *AAOHN J.* 2007;55(11):454-462. [IIIB]

146. Randall SB, Pories WJ, Pearson A, Drake DJ. Expanded Occupational Safety and Health Administration 300 log as metric for bariatric patient-handling staff injuries. *Surg Obes Relat Dis.* 2009;5(4):463-468. [IIIB]

147. Stucke S, Menzel NN. Ergonomic assessment of a critical care unit. *Crit Care Nurs Clin North Am.* 2007;19(2):155-165. [IIIC]

148. Guideline for medical device and product evaluation. In: *Guidelines for Perioperative Practice.* Denver, CO: AORN, Inc; 2018:183-190. [IVA]

149. Baptiste A. Technology solutions for high-risk tasks in critical care. *Crit Care Nurs Clin North Am.* 2007;19(2):177-186. [VA]

150. Baptiste A, Boda SV, Nelson AL, Lloyd JD, Lee WE 3rd. Friction-reducing devices for lateral patient transfers: a clinical evaluation. *AAOHN J.* 2006;54(4):173-180. [IB]

151. Lloyd JD, Baptiste A. Friction-reducing devices for lateral patient transfers: a biomechanical evaluation. *AAOHN J.* 2006;54(3):113-119. [IIIB]

152. Bartnik LM, Rice MS. Comparison of caregiver forces required for sliding a patient up in bed using an array of slide sheets. *Work.* 2013;61(9):393-400. [IIIB]

153. Pellino TA, Owen B, Knapp L, Noack J. The evaluation of mechanical devices for lateral transfers on perceived exertion and patient comfort. *Orthop Nurs.* 2006;25(1):4-12. [IIIB]

154. *Healthcare Recipient Sling and Lift Hanger Bar Compatibility Guidelines.* Tampa, FL: American Association for Safe Patient Handling & Movement; 2016. http://aasphm.org/wp-content/uploads/AASPHM-Sling-Hanger-Bar-Guidelines-2016.pdf. Accessed May 10, 2018. [IVB]

155. Waters TR, Dick R, Lowe B, Werren D, Parsons K. Ergonomic assessment of floor-based and overhead lifts. *Am J Safe Patient Handl Mov.* 2012;2(4):119-113. [IIIB]

156. Marras WS, Knapik GG, Ferguson S. Lumbar spine forces during manoeuvring of ceiling-based and floor-based patient transfer devices. *Ergonomics.* 2009;52(3):384-397. [IIB]

157. Lee SJ, Faucett J, Gillen M, Krause N. Musculoskeletal pain among critical-care nurses by availability and use of patient lifting equipment: an analysis of cross-sectional survey data. *Int J Nurs Stud.* 2013;50(12):1648-1657. [IIIB]

158. Burdorf A, Koppelaar E, Evanoff B. Assessment of the impact of lifting device use on low back pain and musculoskeletal injury claims among nurses. *Occup Environ Med.* 2013;70(7):491-497. [IIIA]

159. D'Arcy LP, Sasai Y, Stearns SC. Do assistive devices, training, and workload affect injury incidence? Prevention efforts by nursing homes and back injuries among nursing assistants. *J Adv Nurs.* 2012;68(4):836-845. [IIIC]

160. Pompeii LA, Lipscomb HJ, Schoenfisch AL, Dement JM. Musculoskeletal injuries resulting from patient handling tasks among hospital workers. *Am J Ind Med.* 2009;52(7):571-578. [IIIB]

161. Weinel D. Successful implementation of ceiling-mounted lift systems. *Rehabil Nurs.* 2008;33(2):63-66, 87. [VA]

162. Baptiste A, McCleerey M, Matz M, Evitt CP. Proper sling selection and application while using patient lifts. *Rehabil Nurs.* 2008;33(1):22-32. [VA]

163. Guideline for environmental cleaning. In: *Guidelines for Perioperative Practice.* Denver, CO: AORN, Inc; 2018:7-28. [IVA]

164. Guideline for a safe environment of care, part 1. In: *Guidelines for Perioperative Practice.* Denver, CO: AORN, Inc; 2018:243-268. [IVA]

165. van't Veen A, van der Zee A, Nelson J, Speelberg B, Kluytmans JA, Buiting AG. Outbreak of infection with a multiresistant *Klebsiella pneumoniae* strain associated with contaminated roll boards in operating rooms. *J Clin Microbiol.* 2005;43(10):4961-4967. [IIIB]

166. Nelson AL, Collins J, Knibbe H, Cookson K, de Castro AB, Whipple KL. Safer patient handling. *Nurs Manage.* 2007;38(3):26-32. [VA]

167. Durham CF. Safe patient handling and movement: time for a culture change. *Tar Heel Nurse.* 2007;69(4):16-18. [VB]

168. Clemes SA, Haslam CO, Haslam RA. What constitutes effective manual handling training? A systematic review. *Occup Med (Lond).* 2010;60(2):101-107. [VA]

169. Kay K, Glass N, Evans A. It's not about the hoist: a narrative literature review of manual handling in healthcare. *J Res Nurs.* 2014;19(3):226-245. [VA]

170. Sedlak CA, Doheny MO, Nelson A, Waters TR. Development of the National Association of Orthopaedic Nurses guidance statement on safe patient handling and movement in the orthopaedic setting. *Orthop Nurs.* 2009;28(2 Suppl):S2-S8. [VA]

171. Menzel NN, Hughes NL, Waters T, Shores LS, Nelson A. Preventing musculoskeletal disorders in nurses: a safe patient handling curriculum module for nursing schools. *Nurse Educ.* 2007;32(3):130-135. [VA]

172. Nelson AL, Waters TR, Menzel NN, et al. Effectiveness of an evidence-based curriculum module in nursing schools targeting safe patient handling and movement. *Int J Nurs Educ Scholarsh.* 2007;4(1):1-19. [IIA]

173. Collins JW, Bell JL, Grönqvist R. Developing evidence-based interventions to address the leading causes of workers' compensation among healthcare workers. *Rehabil Nurs.* 2010;35(6):225-261. [VA]

174. Waters TR, Nelson AL, Hughes N, Menzel N. *Safe Patient Handling Training for Schools of Nursing: Curricular Materials.* Columbus, OH: National Institute for Occupational Safety and Health; 2009. https://www.cdc.gov/niosh/docs/2009-127/pdfs/2009-127.pdf. Accessed May 10, 2018. [VA]

175. *State Operations Manual Appendix A—Survey Protocol, Regulations and Interpretive Guidelines for Hospitals.* Rev. 151; 2015. Centers for Medicare & Medicaid Services. https://www.cms

.gov/Regulations-and-Guidance/Guidance/Manuals/downloads/som107ap_a_hospitals.pdf. Accessed May 10, 2018.

176. 42 CFR 416: Ambulatory surgical services. US Government Publishing Office. https://www.gpo.gov/fdsys/granule/CFR-2011-title42-vol3/CFR-2011-title42-vol3-part416. Accessed May 10, 2018.

177. Price C, Sanderson LV, Talarek DP. Don't pay the price: utilize safe patient handling. *Nursing.* 2013;43(12):13-15. [VB]

178. Anderson MP, Carlisle S, Thomson C, et al. Safe moving and handling of patients: an interprofessional approach. *Nurs Stand.* 2014;28(46):37-41. [VA]

179. Juibari L, Sanagu A, Farrokhi N. The relationship between knowledge of ergonomic science and the occupational health among nursing staff affiliated to Golestan University of Medical Sciences. *Iran J Nurs Midwifery Res.* 2010;15(4):185-189. [IIIA]

180. Theis JL, Finkelstein MJ. Long-term effects of safe patient handling program on staff injuries. *Rehabil Nurs.* 2014;39(1):26-35. [IIB]

181. Paul A. A pilot study on awareness of ergonomics and prevalence of musculoskeletal injuries among nursing professionals. *Int J Nurs Educ.* 2012;4(1):1-4. [IIIC]

182. Lemo A, Silva AG, Tucherman M, Talerman C, Guastelli RL, e Borba CL. Risk reduction in musculoskeletal practice assistance professional nursing pilot in semi intensive care unit. *Work.* 2012;41(Suppl 1):1869-1872. [IIIC]

183. Resnick ML, Sanchez R. Reducing patient handling injuries through contextual training. *J Emerg Nurs.* 2009;35(6):504-508. [IIC]

184. Tompa E, Dolinschi R, Alamgir H, Sarnocinska-Hart A, Guzman J. A cost-benefit analysis of peer coaching for overhead lift use in the long-term care sector in Canada. *Occup Environ Med.* 2016;73(5):308-314. [IIB]

185. Knibbe HJ, Knibbe NE, Klaassen AJ. Safe patient handling program in critical care using peer leaders: lessons learned in the Netherlands. *Crit Care Nurs Clin North Am.* 2007;19(2):205-211. [IIIB]

186. Knibbe H, Knibbe NE, Klaassen A. Ergocoaches: peer leaders promoting ergonomic changes—exploring their profile and effect. *Am J Safe Patient Handl Mov.* 2012;2(3):93-99. [VA]

187. Haney LL, Wright L. Sustaining staff nurse support for a patient care ergonomics program in critical care. *Crit Care Nurs Clin North Am.* 2007;19(2):197-204. [VB]

188. Uurlu Z, Karahan A, Ünlü H, et al. The effects of workload and working conditions on operating room nurses and technicians. *Workplace Health Saf.* 2015;63(9):399-407. [IIIB]

189. Drysdale S. The incidence of upper extremity injuries in Canadian endoscopy nurses. *Gastroenterol Nurs.* 2011;34(1):26-33. [IIIB]

190. Drysdale SA. The incidence of upper extremity injuries in endoscopy nurses. *Gastroenterol Nurs.* 2007;30(3):187-192. [IIIC]

191. Drysdale SA. The incidence of upper extremity injuries in endoscopy nurses working in the United States. *Gastroenterol Nurs.* 2013;36(5):329-338. [IIIB]

192. Drysdale SA. The incidence of neck and back injuries in endoscopy nurses working in the United States of America. *Gastroenterol Nurs.* 2014;37(2):187-188. [VA]

193. Choobineh A, Movahed M, Tabatabaie SH, Kumashiro M. Perceived demands and musculoskeletal disorders in operating room nurses of Shiraz city hospitals. *Ind Health.* 2010;48(1):74-84. [IIIB]

194. Sienkiewicz Z, Paszek T, Wronska I. Strain on the spine—professional threat to nurses' health. *Adv Med Sci.* 2007;52 (Suppl 1):131-135. [IIIB]

195. Murty M. Musculoskeletal disorders in endoscopy nursing. *Gastroenterol Nurs.* 2010;33(5):354-361. [IIIC]

196. Vural F, Sutsunbuloglu E. Ergonomics: an important factor in the operating room. *J Perioper Pract.* 2016;26(7):174-178. [VA]

197. Sheikhzadeh A, Gore C, Zuckerman JD, Nordin M. Perioperating nurses and technicians' perceptions of ergonomic risk factors in the surgical environment. *Appl Ergon.* 2009; 40(5):833-839. [IIIB]

198. Waters T, Baptiste A, Short M, Plante-Mallon L, Nelson A. AORN Ergonomic Tool 1: Lateral transfer of a patient from a stretcher to an OR bed. *AORN J.* 2011;93(3):334-339. [VA]

199. Waters TR, Putz-Anderson V, Garg A. *Applications Manual for the Revised NIOSH Lifting Equation.* Cincinnati, OH: US Department of Health and Human Services, Centers for Disease Control and Prevention, National Institute for Occupational Safety and Health, Division of Biomedical and Behavioral Science; 1994. https://www.cdc.gov/niosh/docs/94-110/pdfs/94-110.pdf. Accessed May 10, 2018. [VA]

200. Waters TR. When is it safe to manually lift a patient? *Am J Nurs.* 2007;107(8):53-58. [VA]

201. Tarr ME, Brancato SJ, Cunkelman JA, Polcari A, Nutter B, Kenton K. Comparison of postural ergonomics between laparoscopic and robotic sacrocolpopexy: a pilot study. *J Minim Invasive Gynecol.* 2015;22(2):234-238. [IIIB]

202. Lawson EH, Curet MJ, Sanchez BR, Schuster R, Berguer R. Postural ergonomics during robotic and laparoscopic gastric bypass surgery: a pilot project. *J Robot Surg.* 2007;1(1):61-67. [IIA]

203. Saglam R, Muslumanoglu AY, Tokatli Z, et al. A new robot for flexible ureteroscopy: development and early clinical results (IDEAL stage 1-2b). *Eur Urol.* 2014;66(6):1092-1100. [IIIC]

204. Tung KD, Shorti RM, Downey EC, Bloswick DS, Merryweather AS. The effect of ergonomic laparoscopic tool handle design on performance and efficiency. *Surg Endosc.* 2015;29(9):2500-2505. [IIB]

205. Manukyan GA, Waseda M, Inaki N, et al. Ergonomics with the use of curved versus straight laparoscopic graspers during rectosigmoid resection: results of a multi-profile comparative study. *Surg Endosc.* 2007;21(7):1079-1089. [IIB]

206. Long JA, Tostain J, Lanchon C, et al. First clinical experience in urologic surgery with a novel robotic light-weight laparoscope holder. *J Endourol.* 2013;27(1):58-63. [IIIC]

207. Büchel D, Mårvik R, Hallabrin B, Matern U. Ergonomics of disposable handles for minimally invasive surgery. *Surg Endosc.* 2010;24(5):992-1004. [IIIB]

208. Dorion D, Darveau S. Do micropauses prevent surgeon's fatigue and loss of accuracy associated with prolonged surgery? An experimental prospective study. *Ann Surg.* 2013;257(2):256-259. [IIB]

209. Fan Y, Kong G, Meng Y, et al. Comparative assessment of surgeons' task performance and surgical ergonomics associated with conventional and modified flank positions: a simulation study. *Surg Endosc.* 2014;28(11):3249-3256. [IIB]

210. Albayrak A, Van Veelen MA, Prins JF, Snijders CJ, De Ridder H, Kazemier G. A newly designed ergonomic body support for surgeons. *Surg Endosc.* 2007;21(10):1835-1840. [IIIC]

211. van Det MJ, Meijerink WJ, Hoff C, Totté ER, Pierie JP. Optimal ergonomics for laparoscopic surgery in minimally invasive surgery suites: a review and guidelines. *Surg Endosc.* 2009;23(6):1279-1285. [VA]

212. Szeto GP, Ho P, Ting AC, Poon JT, Tsang RC, Cheng SW. A study of surgeons' postural muscle activity during open, laparoscopic, and endovascular surgery. *Surg Endosc.* 2010; 24(7):1712-1721. [IIIB]

213. Prielipp RC, Weinkauf JL, Esser TM, Thomas BJ, Warner MA. Falls from the OR or procedure table. *Anesth Analg.* 2017; 125(3):846-851. [VA]

214. Chaffin DB, Andersson GBJ, Martin BJ. Anthropometry in occupational biomechanics. In: *Occupational Biomechanics.* 3rd ed. Hoboken, NJ: Wiley; 1999:73. [VA]

215. Chaffin DB, Andersson GBJ, Martin BJ. The structure and function of the musculoskeletal system. In: *Occupational Biomechanics.* 4th ed. Hoboken, NJ: Wiley; 2006:27. [VA]

216. Snook SH, Ciriello VM. The design of manual handling tasks: revised tables of maximum acceptable weights and forces. *Ergonomics.* 1991;34(9):1197-1213. [IIIB]

217. Cherry C, Moss J. Best practices for preventing hospital-acquired pressure injuries in surgical patients. *Can Oper Room Nurs J.* 2011;29(1):6-8, 22-26. [VB]

218. Fleisch MC, Bremerich D, Schulte-Mattler W, et al. The prevention of positioning injuries during gynecologic operations. Guideline of DGGG (S1-Level, AWMF Registry No. 015/077, February 2015). *Geburtshilfe Frauenheilkd.* 2015; 75(8):792-807. [IVB]

219. Chaffin DB, Andersson GBJ, Martin BJ. Mechanical work capacity evaluation. In: *Occupational Biomechanics.* 4th ed. Hoboken, NJ: Wiley; 2006:65. [VA]

220. Asiedu GB, Lowndes BR, Huddleston PM, Hallbeck S. "The Jackson table is a pain in the...": a qualitative study of providers' perception toward a spinal surgery table. *J Patient Saf.* January 7, 2016. [Epub ahead of print]. [IIIB]

221. Waters T, Short M, Lloyd J, et al. AORN Ergonomic Tool 2: Positioning and repositioning the supine patient on the OR bed. *AORN J.* 2011;93(4):445-449. [VA]

222. Waters T, Spera P, Petersen C, Nelson A, Hernandez E, Applegarth S. AORN Ergonomic Tool 3: Lifting and holding the patient's legs, arms, and head while prepping. *AORN J.* 2011;93(5):589-592. [VA]

223. Waters TR, Sedlak CA, Howe CM, et al. Recommended weight limits for lifting and holding limbs in the orthopaedic practice setting. *Orthop Nurs.* 2009;28(2 Suppl):S28-S35. [VA]

224. Mulligan A, Young LS, Randall S, et al. Best practices for perioperative nursing care for weight loss surgery patients. *Obes Res.* 2005;13(2):267-273. [IIIB]

225. Hughes NL, Nelson A, Matz MW, Lloyd J. AORN Ergonomic Tool 4: Solutions for prolonged standing in perioperative settings. *AORN J.* 2011;93(6):767-774. [VA]

226. Abdollahzade F, Mohammadi F, Dianat I, Asghari E, Asghari-Jafarabadi M, Sokhanvar Z. Working posture and its predictors in hospital operating room nurses. *Health Promot Perspect.* 2016;6(1):17-22. [IIIA]

227. Messing K, Tissot F, Stock S. Distal lower-extremity pain and work postures in the Quebec population. *Am J Public Health.* 2008;98(4):705-713. [IIIB]

228. Waters TR, Dick RB. Evidence of health risks associated with prolonged standing at work and intervention effectiveness. *Rehabil Nurs.* 2015;40(3):148-165. [VA]

229. Kaya OI, Moran M, Ozkardes AB, Taskin EY, Seker GE, Ozmen MM. Ergonomic problems encountered by the surgical team during video endoscopic surgery. *Surg Laparosc Endosc Percutan Tech.* 2008;18(1):40-44. [IIIB]

230. Szeto GP, Cheng SW, Poon JT, Ting AC, Tsang RC, Ho P. Surgeons' static posture and movement repetitions in open and laparoscopic surgery. *J Surg Res.* 2012;172(1):e19-e31. [IIIC]

231. Supe AN, Kulkarni GV, Supe PA. Ergonomics in laparoscopic surgery. *J Minim Access Surg.* 2010;6(2):31-36. [VA]

232. Meijsen P, Knibbe HJ. Prolonged standing in the OR: A Dutch research study. *AORN J.* 2007;86(3):399-414. [IIIB]

233. Reddy PP, Reddy TP, Roig-Francoli J, et al. The impact of the Alexander technique on improving posture and surgical ergonomics during minimally invasive surgery: pilot study. *J Urol.* 2011;186(4 Suppl):1658-1662. [IIC]

234. Seagull FJ. Disparities between industrial and surgical ergonomics. *Work.* 2012;41:4669-4672. [VA]

235. Hullfish KL, Trowbridge ER, Bodine G. Ergonomics and gynecologic surgery: "Surgeon protect thyself." *J Pelvic Med Surg.* 2009;15(6):435-439. [VA]

236. Papp A, Feussner H, Seitz T, et al. Ergonomic evaluation of the scrub nurse's posture at different monitor positions during laparoscopic cholecystectomy. *Surg Laparosc Endosc Percutan Tech.* 2009;19(2):165-169. [IIIC]

237. Choi SD. A review of the ergonomic issues in the laparoscopic operating room. *J Healthc Eng.* 2012;3(4):587-603. [VA]

238. Meijsen P, Knibbe HJJ. Work-related musculoskeletal disorders of perioperative personnel in the Netherlands. *AORN J.* 2007;86(2):193-208. [IIIB]

239. Haramis G, Rosales JC, Palacios JM, et al. Prospective randomized evaluation of FOOT gel pads for operating room staff COMFORT during laparoscopic renal surgery. *Urology.* 2010;76(6):1405-1408. [IC]

240. Harper Z. It's hard work being tall. *Surg Technol.* 2013;45(2):64-65. [VC]

241. Manasnayakorn S, Cuschieri A, Hanna GB. Ergonomic assessment of optimum operating table height for hand-assisted laparoscopic surgery. *Surg Endosc.* 2009;23(4):783-789. [IIB]

242. Park JY, Kim KH, Kuh SU, Chin DK, Kim KS, Cho YE. Spine surgeon's kinematics during discectomy according to operating table height and the methods to visualize the surgical field. *Eur Spine J.* 2012;21(12):2704-2712. [IIIB]

243. Soueid A, Oudit D, Thiagarajah S, Laitung G. The pain of surgery: pain experienced by surgeons while operating. *Int J Surg*. 2010;8(2):118-120. [IIIB]

244. Marcos P, Seitz T, Bubb H, Wichert A, Feussner H. Computer simulation for ergonomic improvements in laparoscopic surgery. *Appl Ergon*. 2006;37(3):251-258. [IIIB]

245. Matern U. Ergonomic deficiencies in the operating room: examples from minimally invasive surgery. *Work*. 2009; 33(2):165-168. [VA]

246. Zehetner J, Kaltenbacher A, Wayand W, Shamiyeh A. Screen height as an ergonomic factor in laparoscopic surgery. *Surg Endosc*. 2006;20(1):139-141. [IIIC]

247. Reijnen MM, Zeebregts CJ, Meijerink WJ. Future of operating rooms. *Surg Technol Int*. 2005;14:21-27. [VB]

248. Liang B, Qi L, Yang J, et al. Ergonomic status of laparoscopic urologic surgery: survey results from 241 urologic surgeons in China. *Plos One*. 2013;8(7). [IIIB]

249. Berguer R. Surgery and ergonomics. *Arch Surg*. 1999; 134(9):1011-1016. [VA]

250. Wauben LS, van Veelen MA, Gossot D, Goossens RH. Application of ergonomic guidelines during minimally invasive surgery: a questionnaire survey of 284 surgeons. *Surg Endosc*. 2006;20(8):1268-1274. [IIIB]

251. Glickson J. Surgeons experience more ergonomic stress in the OR. *Bull Am Coll Surg*. 2012;97(4):20-26. [VB]

252. Fingerhut A, Chouillard E. Ergonomic and technical aspects of laparoscopy for trauma and nontrauma emergencies. *Eur Surg*. 2005;37(1):8-14. [VA]

253. Guideline for minimally invasive surgery. In: *Guidelines for Perioperative Practice*. Denver, CO: AORN, Inc; 2016:589-616. [IVA]

254. van Det MJ, Meijerink WJ, Hoff C, van Veelen MA, Pierie JP. Ergonomic assessment of neck posture in the minimally invasive surgery suite during laparoscopic cholecystectomy. *Surg Endosc*. 2008;22(11):2421-2427. [IIC]

255. Spera P, Lloyd JD, Hernandez E, et al. AORN Ergonomic Tool 5: Tissue retraction in the perioperative setting. *AORN J*. 2011;94(1):54-58. [VA]

256. Kim FJ, Sehrt DE, Molina WR, Huh JS, Rassweiler J, Turner C. Initial experience of a novel ergonomic surgical chair for laparoscopic pelvic surgery. *Int Braz J Urol*. 2011;37(4):455-460. [IIIC]

257. Steinhilber B, Hoffmann S, Karlovic K, et al. Development of an arm support system to improve ergonomics in laparoscopic surgery: study design and provisional results. *Surg Endosc*. 2015;29(9):2851-2858. [IIIC]

258. Galleano R, Carter F, Brown S, Frank T, Cuschieri A. Can armrests improve comfort and task performance in laparoscopic surgery? *Ann Surg*. 2006;243(3):329-333. [IC]

259. Flore R, Gerardino L, Santoliquido A, Catananti C, Pola P, Tondi P. Reduction of oxidative stress by compression stockings in standing workers. *Occup Med*. 2007;57(5):337-341. [IIA]

260. Guideline for sterile technique. In: *Guidelines for Perioperative Practice*. Denver, CO: AORN, Inc; 2018:75-104. [IVA]

261. Andreassi MG, Piccaluga E, Guagliumi G, Del Greco M, Gaita F, Picano E. Occupational health risks in cardiac catheterization laboratory workers. *Circ Cardiovasc Interv*. 2016; 9(4):e003273. [IIIB]

262. Yasobant S, Rajkumar P. Work-related musculoskeletal disorders among health care professionals: a cross-sectional assessment of risk factors in a tertiary hospital, India. *Indian J Occup Environ Med*. 2014;18(2):75-81. [IIIA]

263. Freitag S, Ellegast R, Dulon M, Nienhaus A. Quantitative measurement of stressful trunk postures in nursing professions. *Ann Occup Hyg*. 2007;51(4):385-395. [IIIC]

264. Steele PRC, Curran JF, Mountain RE. Current and future practices in surgical retraction. *Surgeon*. 2013;11(6):330-337. [VB]

265. Noldus J, Graefen M, Hartwig H. Major postoperative complications secondary to use of the Bookwalter self-retaining retractor. *Urology*. 2002;60(6):964-967. [IIIB]

266. Nozaki T, Kato T, Komiya A, Fuse H. Retraction-related acute liver failure after urological laparoscopic surgery. *Curr Urol*. 2013;7(4):199-203. [VA]

267. Lyall A, Ulaner GA. False-positive FDG PET/CT due to liver parenchymal injury caused by a surgical retractor. *Clin Nucl Med*. 2012;37(9):910-911. [VB]

268. Tamhankar A, Kelty CJ, Jacob G. Retraction-related liver lobe necrosis after laparoscopic gastric surgery. *JSLS*. 2011; 15(1):117-121. [VA]

269. Simonsen JG, Arvidsson I, Nordander C. Ergonomics in the operating room. *Work*. 2012;41(Suppl 1):5644-5646. [IIIB]

270. Waters T, Baptiste A, Short M, Plante-Mallon L, Nelson A. AORN Ergonomic Tool 6: Lifting and carrying supplies and equipment in the perioperative setting. *AORN J*. 2011;94(2):173-179. [VA]

271. Genevay S, Cedraschi C, Courvoisier DS, et al. Work related characteristics of back and neck pain among employees of a Swiss university hospital. *Joint Bone Spine*. 2011;78(4):392-397. [IIIB]

272. Waters TR, Baron SL, Piacitelli LA, et al. Evaluation of the revised NIOSH lifting equation. A cross-sectional epidemiologic study. *Spine (Phila Pa 1976)*. 1999;24(4):386-394; discussion 395. [VA]

273. Waters TR, Putz-Anderson V, Garg A, Fine LJ. Revised NIOSH equation for the design and evaluation of manual lifting tasks. *Ergonomics*. 1993;36(7):749-776. [VA]

274. Guideline for sterilization. In: *Guidelines for Perioperative Practice*. Denver, CO: AORN, Inc; 2018:957-984. [IVA]

275. *ANSI/AAMI ST79: Comprehensive Guide to Steam Sterilization and Sterility Assurance in Health Care Facilities*. Arlington, VA: Association for the Advancement of Medical Instrumentation; 2017. [IVC]

276. Waters T, Lloyd JD, Hernandez E, Nelson A. AORN Ergonomic Tool 7: Pushing, pulling, and moving equipment on wheels. *AORN J*. 2011;94(3):254-260. [VA]

277. Kao HC, Lin CJ, Lee YH, Chen SH. The effects of direction of exertion, path, and load placement in nursing cart pushing and pulling tasks: an electromyographical study. *Plos One*. 2015;10(10):e0140792. [IIIB]

278. *Using Carts in Healthcare: A Resource Guide for Reducing Musculoskeletal Injury*. Vancouver, BC, Canada: Occupational Health and Safety Agency for Healthcare (OHSAH); 2005. http://www.phsa.ca/Documents/Occupational-Health-Safety/GuideUsingCartsinHealthcareAresourceguideforreduci.pdf; http://www.ohsah.bc.ca. Accessed May 10, 2018. [VA]

279. Brace T. The dynamics of pushing and pulling in the workplace: assessing and treating the problem. *AAOHN J.* 2005;53(5):224-231. [VA]

280. Garg A, Waters T, Kapellusch J, Karwowski W. Psychophysical basis for maximum pushing and pulling forces: a review and recommendations. *Int J Ind Ergon.* 2014;44(2):281-291. [VA]

281. Diccini S, de Pinho PG, da Silva FO. Assessment of risk and incidence of falls in neurosurgical inpatients. *Rev Lat Am Enfermagem.* 2008;16(4):752-757. [IIIB]

282. Moe K, Brockopp D, McCowan D, Merritt S, Hall B. Major predictors of inpatient falls: a multisite study. *J Nurs Adm.* 2015;45(10):498-502. [IIIB]

283. Oliver D, Daly F, Martin FC, McMurdo ME. Risk factors and risk assessment tools for falls in hospital inpatients: a systematic review. *Age Ageing.* 2004;33(2):122-130. [IIB]

284. Beyea SC. Preventing patient falls in perioperative settings. *AORN J.* 2005;81(2):393-395. [VB]

285. McNamara SA. Reducing fall risk for surgical patients. *AORN J.* 2011;93(3):390-394. [VA]

286. Dauber MH, Roth S. Operating table failure: another hazard of spine surgery. *Anesth Analg.* 2009;108(3):904-905. [VB]

287. Choi YS, Lawler E, Boenecke CA, Ponatoski ER, Zimring CM. Developing a multi-systemic fall prevention model, incorporating the physical environment, the care process and technology: a systematic review. *J Adv Nurs.* 2011;67(12):2501-2524. [IIA]

288. Church S, Robinson TN, Angles EM, Tran ZV, Wallace JI. Postoperative falls in the acute hospital setting: characteristics, risk factors, and outcomes in males. *Am J Surg.* 2011;201(2):197-202. [IIIB]

289. Mohanty S, Rosenthal RA, Russell MM, Neuman MD, Ko CY, Esnaola NF. Optimal perioperative management of the geriatric patient: a best practices guideline from the American College of Surgeons NSQIP and the American Geriatrics Society. *J Am Coll Surg.* 2016;222(5):930-947. [IVB]

290. Penprase B, Johnson C. Optimizing the perioperative nursing role for the older adult surgical patient. *OR Nurse.* 2014;8(4):26-33. [VB]

291. Stansby G, Avital L, Jones K, Marsden G; Guideline Development Group. Prevention and management of pressure ulcers in primary and secondary care: summary of NICE guidance. *BMJ.* 2014;348:g2592. [IVA]

292. Doerflinger DM. Older adult surgical patients: presentation and challenges. *AORN J.* 2009;90(2):223-240; quiz 241-244. [VA]

293. Fletcher HC. Preventing skin injury in the OR. *OR Nurse.* 2014;8(3):28-34. [VC]

294. Boynton T, Kelly L, Perez A. Implementing a mobility assessment tool for nurses. *Am Nurse Today.* 2014;9(9):13-16. [VA]

295. Assessment: Timed Up & Go (TUG). Centers for Disease Control and Prevention. https://www.cdc.gov/steadi/pdf/TUG_Test-print.pdf. Accessed May 10, 2018. [VA]

296. Humphrey JA, Johnson SL, Patel S, Malik M, Willis-Owen CA, Bendall S. Patients' preferred mode of travel to the orthopaedic theatre. *World J Orthop.* 2015;6(3):360-362. [IIIC]

297. Keegan-Doody M. Walk or be driven? A study on walking patients to the operating theatre. *Can Oper Room Nurs J.* 2007;25(2):30-38. [IIIC]

298. Nagraj S, Clark CI, Talbot J, Walker S. Which patients would prefer to walk to theatre? *Ann R Coll Surg Engl.* 2006;88(2):172-173. [IIIB]

299. 2011 ANA Health and Safety Survey. American Nurses Association. https://www.nursingworld.org/practice-policy/work-environment/health-safety/health-safety-survey. Accessed May 10, 2018. [VA]

300. Durand MJ, Vézina N, Loisel P, Baril R, Richard MC, Diallo B. Workplace interventions for workers with musculoskeletal disabilities: a descriptive review of content. *J Occup Rehabil.* 2007;17(1):123-136. [IIIA]

301. Fochsen G, Josephson M, Hagberg M, Toomingas A, Lagerstrom M. Predictors of leaving nursing care: a longitudinal study among Swedish nursing personnel. *Occup Environ Med.* 2006;63(3):198-201. [IIIB]

302. Matt SB, Fleming SE, Maheady DC. Creating disability inclusive work environments for our aging nursing workforce. *J Nurs Adm.* 2015;45(6):325-330. [VA]

303. Vieira ER, Kumar S. Safety analysis of patient transfers and handling tasks. *Qual Saf Health Care.* 2009;18(5):380-384. [IIIB]

304. Hill KS. Improving quality and patient safety by retaining nursing expertise. *Online J Issues Nurs.* 2010;15(3):1. [VA]

305. Moscato U, Trinca D, Rega ML, et al. Musculoskeletal injuries among operating room nurses: results from a multicenter survey in Rome, Italy. *J Public Health.* 2010;18(5):453-459. [IIIB]

306. Warming S, Ebbehøj NE, Wiese N, Larsen LH, Duckert J, Tønnesen H. Little effect of transfer technique instruction and physical fitness training in reducing low back pain among nurses: a cluster randomised intervention study. *Ergonomics.* 2008;51(10):1530-1548. [IB]

307. Menzel NN, Lilley S, Robinson EM. Interventions to reduce back pain in rehabilitation hospital nursing staff. *Rehabil Nurs.* 2006;31(4):138-147. [IB]

308. Jaromi M, Nemeth A, Kranicz J, Laczko T, Betlehem J. Treatment and ergonomics training of work-related lower back pain and body posture problems for nurses. *J Clin Nurs.* 2012;21(11-12):1776-1784. [IB]

309. Rasmussen CD, Holtermann A, Bay H, Søgaard K, Birk Jorgensen M. A multifaceted workplace intervention for low back pain in nurses' aides: a pragmatic stepped wedge cluster randomised controlled trial. *Pain.* 2015;156(9):1786-1794. [IB]

310. Rasmussen CD, Holtermann A, Mortensen OS, Søgaard K, Jorgensen MB. Prevention of low back pain and its consequences among nurses' aides in elderly care: a stepped-wedge multi-faceted cluster-randomized controlled trial. *BMC Public Health.* 2013;13:108. [IB]

311. Morgan A, Chow S. The economic impact of implementing an ergonomic plan. *Nurs Econ.* 2007;25(3):150-156. [VB]

312. Standards of perioperative nursing. In: *Guidelines for Perioperative Practice.* Denver, CO: AORN, Inc; 2015:693-732. [IVC].

313. Schoenfisch AL, Lipscomb HJ, Pompeii LA, Myers DJ, Dement JM. Musculoskeletal injuries among hospital patient care staff before and after implementation of patient lift and transfer equipment. *Scand J Work Environ Health.* 2013;39(1):27-36. [IIIB]

Acknowledgments

Lead Author

Mary J. Ogg, MSN, RN, CNOR
Senior Perioperative Practice Specialist
AORN Nursing Department
Denver, Colorado

Contributing Authors

Sharon A. Van Wicklin, MSN, RN, CNOR, CRNFA(E), CPSN-R, PLNC, FAAN
Denver, Colorado

The authors and AORN thank Thomas R. Waters, PhD, CPE, Cincinnati, Ohio (deceased); Janice Neil, PhD, CNE, RN, Associate Professor, East Carolina College of Nursing, Greenville, North Carolina; Ramona Conner, MSN, RN, CNOR, FAAN, Editor-in-Chief, AORN, Denver, Colorado; Mary C. Fearon, MSN, RN, CNOR, Perioperative Nursing Specialist, AORN, Denver, Colorado; Megan Casey, MPH, BSN, RN, Nurse Epidemiologist, LCDR, US Public Health Service, NIOSH Respiratory Health Division Surveillance Branch, Morgantown, West Virginia; Traci Galinsky, PhD, Captain, US Public Health Service, National Institute for Occupational Safety and Helth, Cincinnati, Ohio; James Boiano, Senior Industrial Hygienist, National Institute for Occupational Safety and Health, Cincinnati, Ohio; Barbara L. Nalley, MSN, CRNP, CNOR, Manager, Anne Arundel Medical Group & Chesapeake Women's Care, Crofton, Maryland; Marie A. Bashaw, DNP, RN, NEA-BC, CNOR, Assistant Professor, Wright State University College of Nursing and Health, Dayton, Ohio; Jay Bowers, BSN, RN, CNOR, Clinical Coordinator for Trauma, General Surgery, Bariatric, Pediatric and Surgical Oncology, West Virginia University Hospitals, Morgantown; Doug Schuerer, MD, FACS, Director of Trauma, Professor of Surgery, Washington University, St Louis, Missouri; Donna A. Pritchard, MA, BSN, RN, NE-BC, CNOR, Director of Perioperative Services, Interfaith Medical Center, Brooklyn, New York; and Diana L. Wadlund, MSN, ACNP-BC, FNP-C, CRNFA, Nurse Practitioner Surgical Specialists, West Chester, Pennsylvania, for their assistance in developing this guideline.

Publication History

Originally published July 2018 in *Guidelines for Perioperative Practice* online. Supersedes the *AORN Guidance Statement: Safe Patient Handling and Movement in the Perioperative Setting;* 2007.

Evidence ratings revised and minor editorial changes made to conform to the current AORN Evidence Rating model, September 2019, for online publication in *Guidelines for Perioperative Practice.*

SHARPS SAFETY

TABLE OF CONTENTS

MEDICAL ABBREVIATIONS & ACRONYMS

ACS – American College of Surgeons
AAOS – American Academy of Orthopaedic Surgeons
AST – Association of Surgical Technologists
CDC – Centers for Disease Control and Prevention
HBV – Hepatitis B virus
HCV – Hepatitis C virus
HFT – Hands-free technique

HIV – Human immunodeficiency virus
OR – Operating room
OSHA – Occupational Safety and Health Administration
PPE – Personal protective equipment
RCT – Randomized controlled trial
SED – Safety-engineered device

SPECIMEN MANAGEMENT

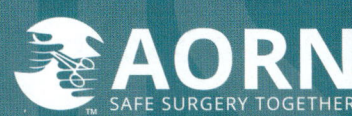
AORN
SAFE SURGERY TOGETHER

971

TABLE OF CONTENTS

MEDICAL ABBREVIATIONS & ACRONYMS

^{99m}Tc - Technetium-99M sulfur colloid
^{103}Pd - Palladium Pd-103
^{125}I - Iodine I-125
ADASP - Association of Directors of Anatomic and Surgical Pathology
ALARA - As low as reasonably achievable
ASCO - American Society of Clinical Oncology
CAP - College of American Pathologists
CBC - Complete blood count
CJD - Creutzfeldt-Jakob disease
COVID-19 - Coronavirus 2019
FDA - US Food and Drug Administration
FMEA - Failure modes and effects analysis
IFU - Instructions for use

NBF - Neutral buffered formalin
NRC - US Nuclear Regulatory Commission
OR - Operating room
OSHA - Occupational Safety and Health Administration
PPE - Personal protective equipment
RCT - Randomized controlled trial
RFID - Radio-frequency identification
RN - Registered nurse
RSL - Radioactive seed localization
RSO - Radiation safety officer
sCJD - Sporadic Creutzfeldt-Jakob disease
SLN - Sentinel lymph node
UDI - Unique device identifier
WHO - World Health Organization

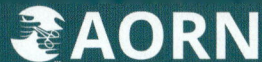
GUIDELINE FOR
SPECIMEN MANAGEMENT

The Guideline for Specimen Management was approved by the AORN Guidelines Advisory Board and became effective as of December 14, 2020. The recommendations in the guideline are intended to be achievable and represent what is believed to be an optimal level of practice. Policies and procedures will reflect variations in practice settings and/or clinical situations that determine the degree to which the guideline can be implemented. AORN recognizes the many diverse settings in which perioperative nurses practice; therefore, this guideline is adaptable to all areas where operative or other invasive procedures may be performed.

Purpose

This document provides guidance for perioperative surgical **specimen** management, including handling of specific types of specimens collected during surgical and other invasive procedures that may be sent to the pathology laboratory for examination. The specimen types included are breast cancer specimens, radioactive specimens, explanted devices, potential forensic evidence, placental tissue, highly infectious disease specimens, and prion disease specimens. Guidance is also provided for transferring specimens off the sterile field; handling, containing, labeling, preserving, and transporting specimens; temporary storage; disposal; documentation and records maintenance; policies and procedures; education; and quality.

Specimen management is a complex, interdisciplinary process that is prone to **error**.[1] Specimen errors are common, with reported rates between 0.43% and 2.9%.[2-4] Preventable errors can occur in all phases of specimen management (ie, **preanalytical**, **analytical**, **postanalytical**),[1,5-7] but most occur in the preanalytical phase. This may be due in part to the number of steps and health care personnel involved in specimen management during this phase.[3,8] The preanalytical phase of specimen management includes ordering, handling, containment, labeling, and transport.[9] An error in **specimen labeling** in the preanalytical phase may increase the likelihood that additional errors related to the same specimen will occur in the analytical phase.[10] Perioperative registered nurses (RNs) perform most of the specimen management interventions in the preanalytical phase. Therefore, perioperative RNs may significantly reduce the rate of error and the potential for patient harm by using targeted, evidenced-based nursing interventions.

Specimen errors pose a significant patient safety risk.[1-3,11,12] Steelman et al[1] conducted a nonexperimental study on specimen errors from more than 50 health care facilities during a 3-year period and found that 8% of specimen errors resulted in additional treatment or temporary or permanent patient harm. It is important to understand the type, frequency, and factors that contribute to errors in specimen management to create interventions effective in decreasing errors and reducing the potential for harm.[1,7,13]

Specimen errors in the preanalytical phase include mistakes in collection,[1-3,8,14] container labeling,[1-4,7,11,14-16] requisition completion,[1,3,7,11,14] handling (eg, contamination), storage,[1,3,7,11,14] and transport.[1,3,8,14] Factors that can contribute to errors can be categorized as poor team communication,[1,4,7,11] lack of process standardization,[1,4,11] process complexity,[1,4,7,11] and knowledge deficits.[1,7,11] However, specimen errors in the preanalytical phase have been studied less frequently than errors in other phases,[3] and study findings are not reported in a standard manner. Some researchers have categorized errors by the process step (eg, labeling or identification, collection, transport).[1,2,9,14] However, in a nonexperimental study, Bixenstine et al[3] reported preanalytical specimen errors in two categories where the errors were found: containers and requisition forms.

The following topics are outside the scope of this document:

- surgical technique used for specimen resection,
- clinical laboratory specimens (eg, complete blood count [CBC]),
- microbiology specimens (eg, culture and sensitivity),
- respiratory specimens for disease outbreaks (eg, coronavirus disease 2019 [COVID-19]),
- autologous or allograft tissue,
- traumatically amputated digits and limbs for replantation or autotransplantation;
- specimen ordering processes,
- use of florescence and methylene blue for identification,
- handling of hazardous substances (eg, formaldehyde),
- eyewash stations, and
- general radiation safety.

Refer to

- 42 CFR Part 493[17] for guidance on laboratory requirements,
- the Guideline for a Safe Environment of Care[18] for recommendations on handling of hazardous substances and eye wash stations,
- the Guideline for Autologous Tissue Management[19] for handling of autologous tissue, and
- the Guideline for Radiation Safety[20] for general radiation safety principles and safe use of radioactive seeds in brachytherapy procedures.

Figure 1. Flow Diagram of Literature Search Results

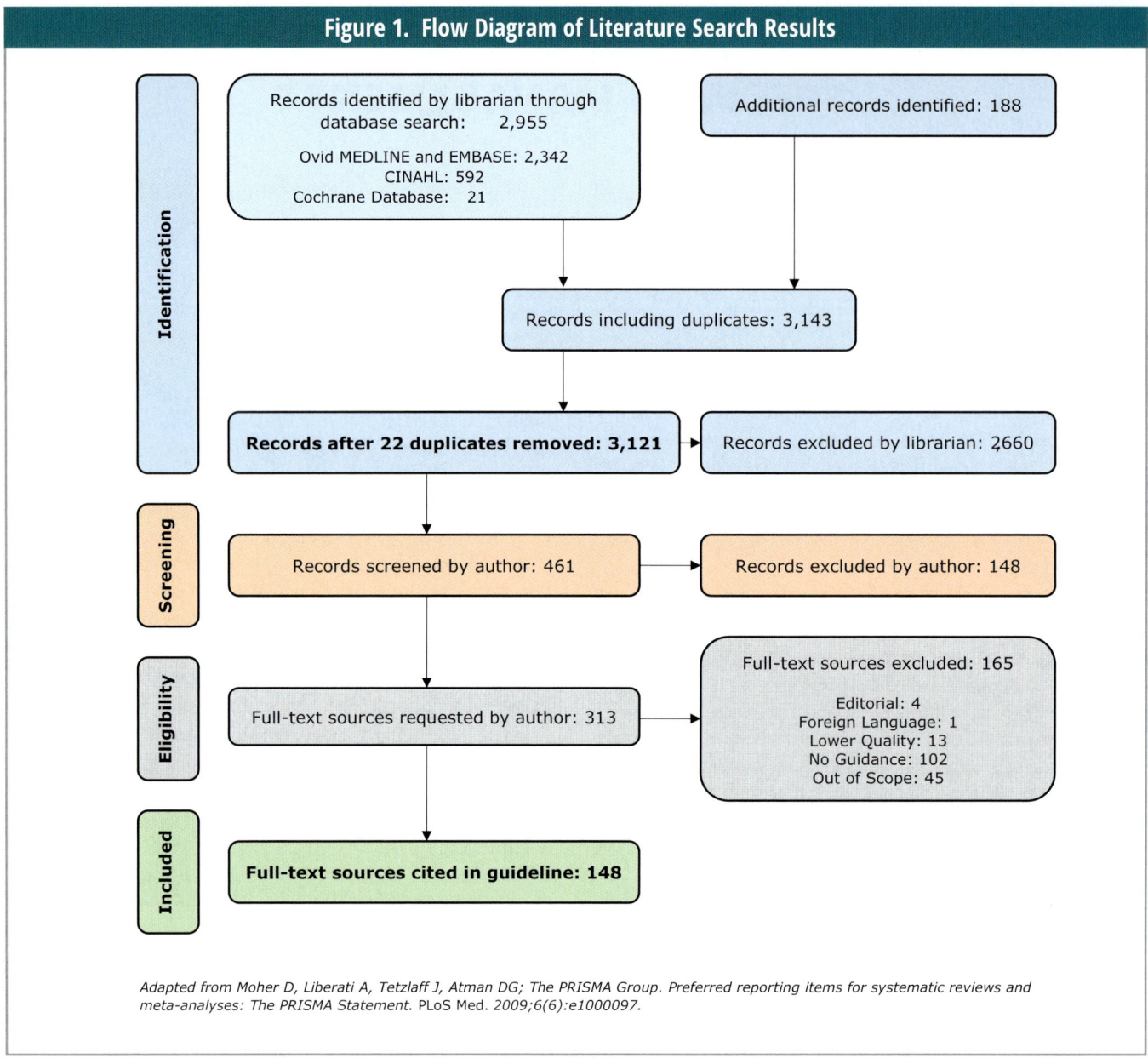

Records identified by librarian through database search: 2,955

Ovid MEDLINE and EMBASE: 2,342
CINAHL: 592
Cochrane Database: 21

Additional records identified: 188

Records including duplicates: 3,143

Records after 22 duplicates removed: 3,121

Records excluded by librarian: 2,660

Records screened by author: 461

Records excluded by author: 148

Full-text sources requested by author: 313

Full-text sources excluded: 165

Editorial: 4
Foreign Language: 1
Lower Quality: 13
No Guidance: 102
Out of Scope: 45

Full-text sources cited in guideline: 148

Identification

Screening

Eligibility

Included

Adapted from Moher D, Liberati A, Tetzlaff J, Atman DG; The PRISMA Group. Preferred reporting items for systematic reviews and meta-analyses: The PRISMA Statement. PLoS Med. 2009;6(6):e1000097.

Evidence Review

A medical librarian with a perioperative background conducted a systematic search of the databases Ovid MEDLINE®, Ovid Embase®, EBSCO CINAHL®, and the Cochrane Database of Systematic Reviews. The search was limited to literature published in English from January 2012 through November 2019. At the time of the initial search, weekly alerts were created on the topics included in that search. Results from these alerts were provided to the lead author until March 2020. The lead author requested additional articles that either did not fit the original search criteria or were discovered during the evidence appraisal process. The lead author and the medical librarian also identified relevant guidelines from government agencies, professional organizations, and standards-setting bodies.

Search terms included *accidents (occupational), amputation (traumatic), biopsy, bone nails, bone plates, bone screws, bone wires, breast neoplasms, burial practices, calculi, chain of custody, cholelithiasis, clinical information, clothing, cultural diversity, dermatologic surgical procedures, device removal, diagnostic errors, documentation, ethanol, explant, fixati*, fixation time and amount, fixatives, forensic ballistics, forensic nursing, forensic pathology, formaldehyde, formalin, fresh specimen, fresh tissue, frozen specimen, frozen tissue, funeral rites, gallstones, gross evaluation, gross examination, health care errors, honey, intraoperative care, intraoperative period, label*, lymph nodes, medical errors, mishandling, misidentification, mislabel*, normal saline, nurse's role, nursing records, occupational diseases, occupational exposure, occupational health, occupational safety, operating room nursing, operating rooms, orthopedic implants, paraffin, paraffin embedding, pathology (surgical), patient identification* systems, patient information, patient safety, perioperative care, perioperative nursing practice guidelines as topic, preoperative care, products of conception, prostheses and implants, quality assurance (health care), quality of health care, radiation effects, radiation injuries, radiation monitoring, radiation protection, radiologic health, RPMI 1640, safety, safety precautions, saline solution, specimen contaminat*, specimen defect, specimen handling, specimen storage, specimen type, surgery (operative), surgical pathology process, surgical procedures (operative), surgical site identification, surgical specimen, suture tags, tissue markers, tissue preservation, vacuum, wire localization, wounds (gunshot), and wounds (stab).

Included were research and non-research literature in English, complete publications, and publications with dates within the time restriction when available. Historical studies were also included. Excluded were non-peer-reviewed publications and older evidence within the time restriction when more recent evidence was available. Editorials, news items, and other brief items were excluded. Low-quality evidence was excluded when higher-quality evidence was available, and literature outside the time restriction was excluded when literature within the time restriction was available (Figure 1).

Articles identified in the search were provided to the project team for evaluation. The team consisted of the lead author and one evidence appraiser. The lead author and the evidence appraiser reviewed and critically appraised each article using the indicated AORN Research or Non-Research Evidence Appraisal Tools. A second appraiser was consulted in the event of a disagreement between the lead author and the primary evidence appraiser. The literature was independently evaluated and appraised according to the strength and quality of the evidence. Each article was then assigned an appraisal score. The appraisal score is noted in brackets after each reference as applicable.

Each recommendation rating is based on a systematic review and synthesis of the collective evidence, a benefit-harm assessment, and consideration of resource use. The strength of the recommendation was determined using the AORN Evidence Rating Model and the quality and consistency of the evidence supporting a recommendation. The recommendation strength rating is noted in brackets after each recommendation.

Note: The evidence summary table is available at http://www.aorn.org/evidencetables/.

Editor's note: MEDLINE is a registered trademark of the US National Library of Medicine's Medical Literature Analysis and Retrieval System, Bethesda, MD. Embase is a registered trademark of Elsevier B.V., Amsterdam, The Netherlands. CINAHL, Cumulative Index to Nursing and Allied Health Literature, is a registered trademark of EBSCO Industries, Birmingham, AL.

1. Preoperative Assessment

1.1 During the preoperative assessment, determine whether a specimen will be obtained as part of the operative procedure. [Recommendation]

1.1.1 Prepare for specimen management when the need to obtain a specimen is identified. [Recommendation]

When the items necessary for specimen management are available (eg, containers, specimen labels, forms) the process may be expedited and the risk for error related to interruptions during specimen handling may be reduced.

1.1.2 Preparation for specimen management may include
- obtaining radiographic or photographic images of the surgical site,
- notifying personnel (eg, pathology laboratory personnel for frozen section, assistive personnel for **specimen transport**),
- delivering items to the sterile field (eg, sterile containers, non-adherent pad),
- collecting containment devices (eg, containers, bags), and
- assembling required forms and labels.

[Conditional Recommendation]

1.2 Discuss **specimen collection**, **handling**, and **disposition** with the patient during the preoperative assessment. [Recommendation]

Asking the patient about preferences for specimen management before the procedure may reduce the potential for changes in the process later, potentially reducing the risk for specimen errors and increasing patient satisfaction. Patients' personal preferences for specimen management may be influenced by cultural traditions, religious beliefs, or spiritual practices (See Recommendation 15).

1.2.1 When a patient has cultural traditions, religious beliefs, or spiritual practices that result in a request for alternative methods of specimen collection, handling, and disposition, these preferences should be discussed with the surgeon and be implemented in accordance with regulatory requirements and organizational policies and procedures. [Recommendation]

1.3 Use high-quality, in-focus photographs (when available) of dermatologic lesions that clearly depict the specimen site and laterality and are labeled with the patient's identifiers[21] for surgical

site identification before Mohs procedures. *[Recommendation]*

Moderate-quality evidence supports the use of high-quality photographs for site identification of dermatologic lesions before Mohs procedures to reduce the risk for wrong site surgery.[21-24] Surgical site identification before a Mohs procedure may be difficult for both patients and physicians.[22] Lesions biopsied months before a procedure may be more difficult to identify the day of the procedure because the site may not be visible after healing.[22-24] Rates of incorrect surgical site identification before Mohs procedures have been reported as

- 5% to 29% for patients,[21-24]
- 5.9% for physicians,[23] and
- 4.4% to 12% for both the patient and physician for the same procedure.[23,24]

Therefore, reliance on the patient or surgeon for site identification may not prevent wrong site surgery.[21,22]

Factors that may increase the risk for wrong site surgery in patients undergoing Mohs procedures include

- inability of the patient to easily see the lesion[22];
- high patient volumes in dermatology practices[21,24];
- patients with multiple lesions in similar locations[24];
- limited documentation,[24] diagrams, or photographs for site reference[21,22];
- the length of time between the site biopsy and the scheduled procedure[22-24];
- the older patient population with the potential for poor eyesight or memory[24]; and
- procedures being performed by surgeons who may not have seen the patient in a preoperative consultation.[21,23]

In a nonexperimental study, McGinness and Goldstein[23] noted that surgical site identification by dermatologic surgeons necessitates the most accurate information possible. When the procedure site cannot be identified, cancelling the procedure is recommended[23] and the patient may be sent back to the referring physician.[22,24] In addition to facilitating correct surgical site identification, use of photography may reduce time, money, and potential frustration.[24] Therefore, the use of preoperative biopsy site photography is recommended as the standard of care for dermatologic site identification.[23,24]

1.3.1   **High-quality photographs of dermatologic lesions used for site identification before Mohs procedures may include**
- **a ruler to show distance,**[23]
- **a circle of the lesion with a surgical skin marker,**[23]
- **different views of the lesion (eg, one at a distance and one close),**[23] **and**

- **a view of detailed skin topography and anatomic landmarks (eg, eyebrow, nose, ear, lip).**[21]
[Conditional Recommendation]

The benefits of using high-quality dermatologic photographs for site identification before Mohs procedures include a greater level of assurance that site identification is accurate. However, there is an investment of time required to take high-quality photographs.

1.4   **Labeled photographs or radiographs of the specimen or procedure site may be displayed in the operating room (OR).** *[Conditional Recommendation]*

Personnel may help reduce the risk for wrong site surgery by displaying photographs[21-24] or radiographs of the patient's specimen or procedure site in the OR and referring to the images during the time-out process and the procedure.

2. Intraoperative Team Communication

2.1   **During the preprocedural briefing process, include a discussion of anticipated specimens.** *[Recommendation]*

A collaborative, interdisciplinary preprocedural discussion of anticipated specimens helps perioperative personnel to prepare for specimen management processes before specimen excision. Being prepared for specimen management may reduce or eliminate the potential for errors and improve efficiency.[1,25] Steelman et al[1] recommended reviewing anticipated specimens during the briefing process.

2.2   **During the hand-over process between OR personnel, use a read-back method to review specimens that are anticipated but not yet excised, and the name, type, and location of surgical specimens that are on the sterile field, in the room, or have been sent to the pathology laboratory.** *[Recommendation]*

A nonexperimental study,[1] a guideline,[25] two organization experience articles,[4,11] and two expert opinion articles[8,14] support hand-over processes for specimen management. According to Steelman et al,[1] communication failures including those that occurred during hand-over processes were among the most common factors contributing to errors in specimen management. The researchers reported that specimens were discarded, lost, or delivered to the wrong location as a result of communication failures during the hand-over process.[1] The researchers recommended that the hand-over process include verbal communication with a read-back method that reviews the specimen type, location, and other relevant information.[1] In an organizational experience article, D'Angelo and Mejabi[11] showed that institution of a consistent read-back verification process during the debriefing was an important part of the success of an improvement project. The Guideline for Team Communication[25] also recommends use of a read-back method when communicating patient information to team members.

2.3 During the procedural debriefing, confirm that
- the specimen is in the container (ie, by visual inspection)[26];
- the patient information on the label and requisition form is accurate, complete, and legible[27];
- the specimen information, including laterality on the label and requisition form, is accurate, complete, and legible[25,28,29];
- the number and type of specimens (eg, permanent, frozen section) is accurate[27];
- the indicated preservation solution was used (when applicable); and
- all pertinent information (eg, documentation of suture tags) is complete.[1,29]

[Recommendation]

Moderate-quality evidence supports having interdisciplinary specimen management discussions during procedural debriefing processes.[1,2,4,14,25,27,28] However, recommendations in the literature vary regarding what information to include in the debriefing. Some of the information supported by the evidence includes
- patient information, specimen name, and number of specimens[27];
- specimen identification and labeling[28,29];
- specimen labeling and disposition[25];
- confirmation of the pathology analysis to be performed[29];
- review of suture tag information when present[29]; and
- visual verification that the specimen is present within the container.[26]

Steelman et al[1] recommended reviewing all specimen information during the postoperative debriefing.

Martis et al[27] reported on an organizational experience in which personnel implemented a consistent process for completing the debriefing section of the World Health Organization (WHO) Safe Surgery Checklist. The sign out process included a review of the patient information, specimen description, and quantity. The authors reported a significant reduction in specimen error rates after the implementation process.[27]

2.4 Verbal communication from the pathologist related to diagnosis or specific information about the specimen (eg, results of frozen section) should be provided directly to the physician (ie, not through a third party). *[Recommendation]*

A consensus statement from the College of American Pathologists (CAP) and the Association of Directors of Anatomic and Surgical Pathology (ADASP)[30] discusses effective communication of **urgent diagnoses** and **significant, unexpected diagnoses** from surgical pathology and cytopathology. When possible, the authors recommend direct physician-to-physician communication of diagnoses.[30] The CAP[31] also recommends confirming the patient's identifiers before direct verbal communication (**See Recommendation 19.2**).

2.4.1 If direct verbal communication between the pathologist and surgeon is not possible, the perioperative RN may
- receive the communication from the pathologist,
- relay all information received from the pathologist to the surgeon using read-back verification,[25] and
- document the communication in the patient's health care record.

[Conditional Recommendation]

3. Transfer from the Sterile Field

3.1 Implement measures to minimize the risk of specimen compromise (eg, loss, contamination, crushing) on the sterile field, by
- minimizing handling,
- protecting tissue from crushing or damage,[31]
- keeping the specimen moist,[31]
- containing or covering[32] the specimen,
- labeling the specimen, and
- placing the specimen in a secure location on the sterile field.

[Recommendation]

The benefits of keeping specimens moist, covered, labeled, and secured exceed the potential harms. The benefits include preserving the integrity of the specimen by keeping it from drying out, reducing the risk of contamination from airborne sources,[32] and decreasing the risk of specimen loss. A potential harm of covering the specimen on the sterile field may be that by concealing it from view, it could be overlooked and discarded after the procedure. Steelman et al[1] reported that some specimens left on the field were accidentally discarded.

Low-quality evidence[31] supports adding a small amount of normal saline solution to tissue or wrapping solid tissue masses in saline-moistened gauze to prevent specimens from drying when they are not immediately placed in a preservative.

3.1.1 When collecting multiple specimens for patients with known or suspected infection at any surgical site, keep sterile instruments for specimen collection separate and do not use them interchangeably. *[Recommendation]*

In a quasi-experimental study, Makki et al[33] found cross contamination of biopsy specimens in patients with musculoskeletal infections. The study included nine specimens taken during the debridement procedure of each of 15 patients with foot and ankle infections. The researchers found no contamination of specimens for which new instruments were used and eight incidences of cross contamination in specimens for which instruments were reused between biopsy sites on the same patient. The researchers recommended using new instruments for each biopsy site in patients with an infection to reduce the risk of cross contamination to the specimen.[33]

The AORN Guideline for Sterile Technique[32] provides recommendations for procedures with multiple surgical sites that involve different wound classifications to assist in prevention of cross contamination.

3.2 Transfer specimens from the sterile field
- **as soon as possible after excision;**
- **using sterile technique[32];**
- **using standard precautions[34,35]; and**
- **in a manner that does not crush, twist, or compact the specimen.[31]**

[Recommendation]

The benefits of transferring the specimen as soon as possible after excision include protecting the specimen from damage, desiccation, or contamination on the sterile field and protecting the specimen from loss if overlooked later in the procedure. Collaboration with the surgeon about when the specimen may be transferred from the sterile field is important to prevent transferring a specimen before it is complete or when it might be needed later during the procedure. Using standard precautions and sterile technique can decrease risk of specimen contamination and exposure of health care personnel to bloodborne pathogens and other potentially infectious materials. A **specimen transfer** process that protects the specimen integrity can be achieved by using a method that protects it from crushing, twisting, or compacting.

Low-quality evidence supports using ideal specimen transfer methods.[1,36,37] Ideal specimen handling includes immediate transfer of fresh specimens to the pathology laboratory for prompt tissue examination and fixation.[36,37] Steelman et al[1] found that 24% of all specimen errors occurred during **specimen collection** and 15.3% of all specimen errors were delays during transport or storage. Collection errors included

- specimens not being placed in the container,
- specimen containers found to be empty,
- specimens being inadvertently discarded,
- more than one specimen in the same container,
- no preservative or solution having been used,
- use of the incorrect preservative or solution,
- solution used when none was requested, and
- use of an incorrect container.[1]

3.2.1 **Instruments used to transfer specimens into an unsterile specimen container should be considered contaminated.** *[Recommendation]*

Instruments used for specimen transfer may inadvertently contact the sides of the specimen container or come in contact with preservative agents (eg, formalin).[32] Use of contaminated instruments or instruments that come in contact with preservatives may increase the risk of surgical site infections or patient harm related to chemical exposure.[18]

3.3 **Verify patient and specimen identification on the specimen label, pathology requisition form, and patient health care record using a read-back method with the surgeon before transfer of the specimen from the sterile field.** *[Recommendation]*

Using a read-back method for specimen verification may reduce the risk for errors related to identification, labeling, and documentation. Verifying specimen and patient identifiers before transfer minimizes opportunities for error, enables immediate specimen labeling, and helps prevent misidentification of the specimen. The CAP[31] recommends verifying the patient's identity during specimen collection. The read-back method is recommended for communicating patient information to team members.[8,25]

4. Handling

4.1 **Convene an interdisciplinary team that includes a pathologist(s), a surgeon(s), a perioperative RN(s), quality and risk management personnel (when available), an infection preventionist(s), and other stakeholders identified by the organization, to establish a standardized process with embedded quality controls for handling specimens. The process should include specimen preparation for different examination methods (eg, fresh, permanent, frozen section, gross).** *[Recommendation]*

Standardizing processes to include specific methods of preparing specimens for different examination types can reduce the risk for specimen errors.

Low-quality evidence supports standardizing specimen handling.[8,11] An expert opinion article from the Pennsylvania Patient Safety Advisory[8] recommends reviewing the facility specimen handling process from the beginning of the preanalytical phase until the specimen is received by pathology personnel. The improvement process may involve going to the various departments where the work is done and discussing the process with the people involved.[8] It is important to identify parts of the process during which personnel may deviate from or circumvent standard procedures.[8]

D'Angelo and Mejabi[11] found that many nurses in their facility kept a separate running list of specimen names on note pads that were duplicated on required specimen paperwork. The authors suggested that this duplication of the specimen list was a deviation from standard processes that caused redundancy and inefficiency in the system and could increase the risk for error.[11]

4.1.1 **Quality control methods imbedded in the specimen handling process may include**
- **standardized team communication[1] and verification processes[25];**
- **pathology accession (eg, collection) processes that require review of specimen labeling and requisition forms before acceptance[10,31];**
- **clinical documentation support that alerts the user when electronic data fields are missing or incomplete[13];**
- **alarms that notify personnel of an issue that needs to be resolved (eg, a refrigerator door left open); and**
- **transport and storage logbooks with standardized fields to complete.**

[Conditional Recommendation]

Moderate-quality evidence supports imbedding methods of quality control into the specimen handling process.[1,6,8,10,38] Specimen management processes that include imbedded quality control measures may reduce the risk for specimen errors.[1,8,10]

Misidentification of specimens is most likely to occur before the specimen arrives at the pathology laboratory.[10] Steelman et al[1] found that 54% of identification and labeling errors were discovered after transport to the laboratory. Similarly, in a nonexperimental study, Nakhleh et al[10] reported that most errors were discovered one or two steps into the specimen management process, after the error had occurred. Quality checks of specimen labeling during the pathology accessioning process was significantly associated with decreased error rates.[10] Verifying congruence of the specimen and the requisition form at the point of specimen submission to pathology personnel (eg, the specimen collection area) can facilitate discovery and correction of labeling errors that

may have occurred. Discovering an error near to the time that the error is made facilitates effective correction.[1,10]

D'Angelo and Mejabi[11] implemented standard labeling for five specimen types that required special handling processes that were prone to error. The specimen types included routine pathologic examination, microbiologic examination, frozen section, lymphoma work-up, and open lung biopsy protocol.[11] The authors created standard color-coded labels that contained unique processing information for each specimen type.[11] Rolls of specimen labels were available in each OR as part of a standardized labeling station for immediate labeling and completion of requisitions. The researchers found this process was effective in expediting specimen processing.[11] An expert opinion article from the ECRI Institute[16] also supports standardizing specimen collection procedures.

In an organizational experience article, Zervakis Brent[4] discussed creation of a specimen handling process reference document. The author recommended that this document include specifics on the handling of permanent, fresh, frozen section, cytology, and tissue-banked specimens. The author also defined processes to be used during off hours (ie, after-hours, weekends, and holidays).[4]

4.2 **Reduce the number of people involved and steps required in the specimen handling process, when possible. [Recommendation]**

Low-quality evidence suggests that specimen errors that occur in the preanalytical phase may be due in part to the number of steps and people involved in the process.[6,8] Reducing the number of people and steps involved may reduce the complexity of the process and therefore reduce the risk for error.[6,8]

D'Angelo and Mejabi[11] created a triplicate layered form that served as a pathology requisition, paperwork attached to the specimen container, and a reconciliation page used during the procedural debriefing process. The reconciliation portion of the form eliminated the need for nurses to keep a separate running list of specimens on a note pad.[11]

In a nonexperimental study, Makary et al[2] reviewed specimen containers and requisition forms submitted to the pathology laboratory for 6 months. The researchers classified specimen errors as discrepancies found between the label on the specimen container and the requisition form. The researchers found 0.346% of the specimen errors occurred in the OR. As a result, they recommended standardizing requisition forms and the process for completing the forms.

4.3 Use automation technology or memory aids during specimen handling, when possible. *[Recommendation]*

Low-quality evidence indicates that specimen errors in the preanalytical phase may be due in part to little or no automation of the process.[8] Reliance on memory for complex tasks may increase the risk for error because of variability in performance.[8] When possible, increasing automation may decrease the risk of preanalytical specimen errors.[8] Examples of automation include

- use of technology (eg, software programs, paperless requisitions, vacuum containment, barcoded labels)[3,8,13,38,39] and
- memory aids (eg, checklists, procedure list, charts, logs, custom labels).[3,4,8,11,31]

D'Angelo and Mejabi[11] found that nurses did not always know how to correctly spell the specimen name and sometimes did not ask for the correct spelling. As part of the improvement project, the authors created a standardized reference listing common specimens to assist nurses with correct specimen labeling and thereby reduce errors in identification, labeling, and communication.[11]

4.4 A dedicated space for specimen management processes may be used. *[Conditional Recommendation]*

The benefits of designating a space for specimen management may exceed the harms. The benefits include having space and supplies to facilitate the procedure. Having a dedicated space may help reduce distractions, minimize the risk for error,[8] and expedite specimen handling processes.[11] Standardization of processes may be difficult if there is not a dedicated space to normalize practice. The harms may include a reduction in space for other processes or equipment and an initial set-up cost.

Low-quality evidence supports creating a dedicated space for specimen management processes.[8,11]

4.4.1 Features of the dedicated specimen management space may include
- a convenient location,
- effective lighting,[8]
- a communication device (eg, telephone),
- a counter that is clutter-free and that can be effectively cleaned and disinfected,
- supplies that support standardized processes (eg, specimen containers, gloves),[8]
- forms that support standardized processes (eg, pathology requisitions),
- memory aids that support standardized processes,[1,4]

- access to the safety data sheets of chemicals used in the space,
- contact information for collaborating personnel (eg, pathology laboratory personnel),
- temporary storage equipment (eg, refrigerator, shelving, collection bin), and
- spill kit(s) for preservatives used for **specimen preservation**.

[Conditional Recommendation]

5. Containment

5.1 Obtain containers and collection devices for specimen management before the procedure. *[Recommendation]*

Preparing for specimen management before the procedure may improve efficiency, reduce door opening,[32] and prevent damage to or loss of the specimen. Steelman et al[1] found that seven of 156 specimen collection–related errors included using the wrong container.

5.2 Specimen containers must be leak proof and puncture resistant.[40] *[Regulatory Requirement]*

Specimen containment prevents exposure of health care personnel to blood, body fluids, or other potentially infectious materials.[40]

5.2.1 Specimen containers must be placed in a second leak-proof container if the first container is compromised or leakage occurs.[40] *[Regulatory Requirement]*

5.3 When rigid specimen containers are used, they should be large enough to fully contain the specimen and preservative fluids without compressing or crushing the specimen and should allow the preservative solution (when applicable) to contact all surfaces of the specimen. *[Recommendation]*

Containing specimens in a storage device that fits may prevent leakage and personnel exposures to blood, body fluids, or other potentially infectious materials and may help preserve the integrity of the specimen for subsequent histomorphology testing.

5.3.1 Use sterile specimen collection containers for sterile specimens, when possible. *[Recommendation]*

5.3.2 Sterile or clean specimen containers may be used for unsterile specimens. *[Conditional Recommendation]*

5.3.3 **Facilities may provide specimen containers prefilled with preservative solutions (eg, formalin).** *[Conditional Recommendation]*

The benefits of providing specimen containers prefilled with preservative solutions outweigh the potential harms. The benefits include reduced risk of formaldehyde exposure from formalin fumes or splashes because perioperative personnel will not have to transfer formalin into the specimen container. The harms may include containers breaking, leaking, or spilling during storage.

5.3.4 **Two large red bags that are securely sealed may be used to contain large specimens that cannot fit in a container (eg, an amputated limb).** *[Conditional Recommendation]*

Use of two large red bags that are securely sealed (eg, knots, ties) provides containment and reduces the risk of leakage or puncture.

5.4 Contain and label the specimen immediately upon receiving it from the sterile field. *[Recommendation]*

Moderate-quality evidence supports immediate containment of specimens transferred off the sterile field.[1,8,14,26] Steelman et al[1] reported that a third of all specimen errors related to collection were attributed to specimens that were not immediately placed in containers. These errors resulted in temporary misplacement of the specimens.[1] Empty specimen containers, specimens not placed in a container, or discarded specimens accounted for 7.9% of all specimen errors in the study.[1] Similarly, in an organizational experience article, Sandbank et al[26] reported that two out of 4,400 specimens were lost as a result of not being placed in a specimen container **(See Recommendation 6.3)**.

5.5 Place the specimen container into a specimen bag when the exterior of the container is contaminated (eg, originating from the sterile field, caused by handling). *[Recommendation]*

5.6 Vacuum sealing with refrigeration at 4° C (39.2° F) may be used for containment of specimens 2 cm and larger. *[Conditional Recommendation]*

High-quality evidence from two randomized controlled trials (RCTs),[41,42] two quasi-experimental studies,[43,44] one nonexperimental study,[45] three organizational experience articles,[46-48] and three expert opinion articles[36,37,49] supports the use of vacuum sealing with refrigerated storage at 4° C (39.2° F) without formalin for specimen containment. Evidence demonstrates that specimen histomorphology and genetic markers are viable from vacuum sealing and refrigeration at 4° C (39.2° F) without the use of formalin.[42,43,45]

The Occupational Safety and Health Administration (OSHA)[50] recommend that employers select controls that emphasize hazard elimination or substitution before using other strategies described in the hierarchy of controls (ie, engineering controls, work practice controls, administrative controls, personal protective equipment [PPE]). Vacuum-sealing devices may have options for use with or without a preservative.[47] Use of vacuum sealing and cooling in place of a preservative eliminates potential formaldehyde exposures by hazard elimination. Alternatively, using vacuum-sealing devices with automatic dispensing of a preservative in an enclosed chamber may reduce the amount of preservative used and the potential for formaldehyde exposures compared to traditional methods of specimen and preservative handling through engineering controls.[41] In an RCT, Berton and Di Novi[41] found that personnel who used traditional methods of specimen handling were eight to 10 times more likely to have respiratory symptoms than personnel who used vacuum sealing and cooling without formalin for specimen containment.

It is unclear whether vacuum sealing alone is an effective method of preservation. Some literature supports the use of vacuum sealing as a method of preservation[42] although other literature questions whether it is a combination of vacuum sealing and refrigeration that affects specimen viability or refrigeration alone.[44,51] In a quasi-experimental study, Kristensen et al[44] compared the effect of vacuum sealing specimens with or without refrigeration. They found that refrigeration at 4° C (39.2° F) preserved tissue regardless of whether it was vacuum sealed. The researchers concluded that vacuum sealing alone is not an effective method of preservation and not an alternative to refrigeration at 4° C (39.2° F). Additional research is needed to clarify the source of specimen and genetic marker preservation.[42-44]

Sources that specified specimen size for vacuum containment used specimens 2 cm or larger.[37,45,46,48] Two organizational experience articles[47,48] and two expert opinion articles[36,37] reported continued use of traditional small biopsy containers (eg, 50 mL) prefilled with formalin for needle biopsy specimens or small specimens (ie, < 2 cm in size). In an organizational experience article, Zarbo[47] compared vacuum sealing of needle biopsy specimens to immediately placing needle biopsy specimens in formalin. The vacuum-sealing process for biopsy specimens included placing the tissue in a small container with holes in the lid before vacuum sealing.[47] The histological assessment scores showed a slight preference for biopsy specimens that were immediately fixed in formalin.[47]

In an organizational experience article, Di Novi et al[48] indicated that the recognized formalin penetration rate of 1 cm per 24 hours may cause faster fixation of smaller specimens. Fixation of larger specimens may occur too slowly and compromise specimen integrity.[48] In an expert opinion article, Bussolati et al[36] noted that standardization of immediate fixation of smaller specimens preserves the tissue although larger specimens require more processing steps (eg, sectioning) that affect preservation. Additional research is needed to clarify the need for, procedure for, and tissue preservation of vacuum-sealed and refrigerated specimens smaller than 2 cm.

The benefits of using vacuum sealing containment with refrigeration may include

- preservation of specimen morphology or RNA,[37,42,43,45,47,48,51]
- ability to use vacuum sealing with or without preservative,[47]
- processing that takes about 15 seconds,[37]
- ability to select the specimen-to-preservative ratio (if applicable),[46]
- automated calculation of preservative volume (if applicable),[46,47]
- automated recording of fixation time (if applicable),[36,37,48]
- ability to select the level of vacuum (eg, complete, partial),[46]
- potential for automated traceable specimen information (eg, identification, timing, temperature),[46,47]
- elimination or reduction of preservative volume used,[36,37,41,46-48]
- decreased risk of exposure to formaldehyde fumes or spills,[37,46-49]
- reduced respiratory symptoms related to workplace exposure to chemicals,[41,48]
- decreased rigid container storage space requirements,[36,37,46-48]
- specimen bags that are lighter than rigid containers, making them easier to carry,[48]
- decreased environmental waste related to less plastic used in the container,[46]
- personnel satisfaction,[36,37,46-48] and
- cost efficiency.[37,46-48]

Saliceti et al[46] conducted a comprehensive product evaluation on vacuum-sealing containment and reported no significant disadvantages related to using this device technology. Di Novi et al[48] also reported that vacuum-sealing containment was safe and reliable.

The potential risks of vacuum sealing may include

- specimen compression if the vacuum pressure is too high,
- inferior pathological examination of hollow organs,[47] and

- cross contamination to subsequent vacuum-sealed specimens if the device is not cleaned and disinfected between uses.

Saliceti et al[46] reported that some vacuum-sealing devices allowed users to select the level of vacuum, including complete air extraction, depending on the specimen type being contained.

Zarbo[47] evaluated the use of vacuum-sealing containment and refrigeration at 4° C (39.2° C) for 122 medium and large specimens from a variety of tissue types. He found only four inferior specimens during histological assessment (ie, kidney, prostate pieces, uterus, small bowel).[47] **Root cause analysis** found no cause of the inferiority in two of the specimens (ie, kidney, prostate pieces), but after analysis, the facility standardized practice to require that hollow organ specimens (eg, uterus, small bowel) be opened before vacuum sealing.[47]

Conversely, Di Novi et al[48] found that gross anatomy was preserved using vacuum-sealing containment and emphasized the importance of this finding especially when compared to the discoloration, hardening, and mucosal retraction in hollow organs (ie, stomach, colon) that is caused by formalin. More research is needed on the effect of vacuum sealing on hollow specimens.

5.6.1 **Determine a standardized process for specimen containment when vacuum sealing and refrigeration at 4° C (39.2° F) is used, including the specimen types permitted or excluded and the length of storage time before transport to the pathology laboratory.** *[Recommendation]*

Moderate-quality evidence supports standardizing processes when using vacuum-sealed specimen containment and refrigeration.[42,43,45,46] The evidence suggests that the type of tissue stored and length of storage may affect the viability of the specimen RNA or histomorphology.[42,43,45] The time frame for viability of specimen histomorphology and RNA is reported to be between 24 hours to 72 hours with use of vacuum sealing and refrigeration at 4° C (39.2° F).[42,43,45]

In an RCT, Condelli et al[42] supported the use of vacuum sealing for transport of fresh (ie, non-fixed) specimens but found that RNA stability of vacuum-sealed refrigerated specimens was dependent on the type of tissue and the length of time it was stored (eg, 24, 48, 72 hours). The researchers found that tissue morphology was intact for most specimen types with one exception: gallbladder tissue at 72 hours of storage. Viability of RNA was found to be time-dependent with increased loss of viability between 24 to 72 hours. Despite the time-dependent degradation of RNA, the researchers reported that the reduction in RNA quality was not a limitation in genetic testing. Condelli et al[42] recommended that facilities determine standardized procedures including identification of specimen types that could be used in conjunction with vacuum-sealed containment and refrigeration and the length of time specimens could be stored.

Conversely, in a quasi-experimental study, Veneroni et al[43] reported that RNA integrity was stable for up to 48 hours, and in a nonexperimental study, Annaratone et al[45] found that cells remained viable for up to 24 hours when vacuum-sealed containment and refrigeration was used. Zarbo[47] reviewed 50 pathology samples and found that 46 were viable after vacuum sealing and refrigeration at 4° C (39.2° F) and 7° C (44.6° F) using simulated transport times of 24 and 48 hours. The authors stated that simulated transport times of 72 hours produced inferior quality slides on microscopic examination.[47]

The specimen types reported in the literature to produce viable histomorphology or genetic markers when stored in vacuum-sealed containers and refrigerated for various time frames include skin, brain, tonsil, thyroid, heart, heart valve, artery, breast, lung, stomach, liver, gallbladder, spleen, fistula soft tissue, small bowel, colon, appendix, pannus tissue, lymph node, kidney, uterus, ovary, fallopian tube, placenta, hydrocele, hemorrhoid, leg, and mesenchymal tissue.[42-44,47]

5.6.2 **Follow the vacuum-sealing device manufacturer's written instructions for use (IFU) and facility policies and procedures when using vacuum-sealing containment devices and refrigeration.** *[Recommendation]*

Following the manufacturer's IFU provides the highest level of assurance that the specimen will be contained in a way that reduces the potential for exposures to preservative solutions (eg, formalin) (if applicable) and retains specimen viability for histomorphology and genetic testing (if applicable).

5.7 **Vacuum sealing with preservative solutions may be used for containment of specimens 2 cm and larger.** *[Conditional Recommendation]*

Vacuum sealing containment with preservative solution preserves the specimen for pathological examination. A benefit of this method compared to use of specimen containers prefilled with formalin is the reduced risk to personnel of formaldehyde exposure from fumes or spills because the device may add formalin in an enclosed chamber. However, because preservative solutions such as formalin are still being used, the risk, while reduced, is not eliminated as it is when vacuum-sealed containment with refrigeration is used.

A quasi-experimental study[44] and an organizational experience article[47] show that vacuum-sealing technology can be used for specimen containment alone or in combination with refrigeration and preservative solutions such as formalin.

5.8 **Establish cleaning and disinfection procedures using organization-approved disinfectants that are compatible with the vacuum-sealing containment devices, based on the vacuum-sealing device manufacturer's written IFU and facility policies and procedures.** *[Recommendation]*

Performing disinfection according to the vacuum-sealing device manufacturer's written IFU and informed by facility policies and procedures regarding available disinfection agents and practices decreases the likelihood that infectious agents will reside on device components and reduces the potential for transmission of infectious material to personnel or specimens.

6. Labeling and Requisition Forms

6.1 **Specimen containers that contain biohazardous materials must be labeled with a biohazard label.** *[Regulatory Requirement]*

Use of a fluorescent orange or orange-red biohazard label with the symbol and lettering in a contrasting color is an OSHA requirement.[40]

6.2 **Specimen containers with a chemical preservative[52] must be labeled to communicate chemical hazard.** *[Regulatory Requirement]*

For more information about chemical safety in the perioperative environment, see the AORN Guideline for a Safe Environment of Care.[18]

6.3 **Contain the specimen and label the container immediately with**
- **two patient identifiers (eg, patient name, medical record number, date of birth)[9,31];**
- **the specimen name;**
- **the specimen site including laterality, if applicable; and**
- **the date of excision.**
[Recommendation]

High-quality evidence supports specimen labeling.[1-4,9-11,14,16]

Errors in specimen labeling are consistently reported to be one of the most common types of errors in specimen management.[1-4,8-10,14] The incidence of mislabeled specimens has been reported to be between 35.8% to 49% of all surgical specimen–related errors.[1,14] Steelman et al[1] reported that 30% of the specimen labeling errors were caused by not immediately labeling the container or the requisition form. The other 70% were related to incomplete, inaccurate, or illegible information on the label or requisition.[1] The CAP[31] recommends labeling the specimen in the presence of the patient.

6.3.1   **Do not prelabel specimen containers.**[9] *[Recommendation]*

6.3.2   **Label one specimen at a time.** *[Recommendation]*
     Low-quality evidence indicates that processing more than one specimen at a time can lead to errors.[4]

6.3.3   **Use dark, indelible ink on specimen container labels and requisition forms.** *[Recommendation]*
     Using dark indelible ink may improve visibility and prevent the ink from being removed or smeared.

6.4   **Securely affix specimen identification labels to the container, not the lid.**[31,53] *[Recommendation]*
     Placing the label on the container instead of the lid may prevent specimen information loss after the lid is removed.[53]

6.4.1   **Place the label on the container in a way that prevents overlap.** *[Recommendation]*
     The CAP[31] recommends that specimen labels not overlap. This prevents patient or specimen information from being covered.[31]

6.5   **Complete the pathology requisition form according to facility policy and procedure and send it with the specimen (when applicable).** *[Recommendation]*
     Steelman et al[1] reported that some specimen labeling errors included a missing requisition form or incomplete, inaccurate, or illegible information on the requisition.[1] Eleven percent of the specimen labeling errors involved specimen labels that did not match the requisition form label.[1] The CAP[31] states that written policies and procedures on how to complete a pathology requisition form must be made available to health care personnel involved in the specimen collection and labeling process.

6.5.1   **Information recorded on a pathology requisition form should include**
- patient identifiers (eg, patient name, medical record number, date of birth),
- specimen identification (eg, name, source, tissue type, laterality [when applicable]),
- the date and time of specimen collection, and
- pathology examination required (eg, gross, frozen section).

[Recommendation]

6.5.2   **Information recorded on a pathology requisition form may include**
- the ordering physician's name and contact information,
- perioperative RN identification,
- the patient's clinical diagnosis and relevant medical history,
- additional information pertinent to the specimen (eg, location of suture tags),
- requests for special handling (eg, return of amputated limb for burial),
- **warm ischemic time** (eg, breast cancer specimens),[31]
- **cold ischemic time** (eg, breast cancer specimens),[31]
- date and time of specimen arrival in the pathology laboratory,[31] and
- nurse's or physician's signature.

[Conditional Recommendation]

6.5.3   **Protect accompanying documents (eg, pathology requisition) from contamination.** *[Recommendation]*

6.6   **Discard unused patient labels before the next patient enters the room.**[14] *[Recommendation]*
     Discarding unused patient labels before the next patient enters the room reduces the risk that the wrong patient label will be placed on a specimen container or pathology requisition form.

     Low-quality evidence supports discarding patient labels before the next patient enters the room.[4,14] During the **failure modes and effects analysis** (FMEA) process, Zervakis Brent[4] found that labeling the specimen container with a patient label that was left in the room from the previous patient was one of the potential failures in specimen management that could lead to errors. As part of the quality improvement process, patient labels were printed on 8 x 10-inch label paper that was 3-hole punched and placed in the patient chart. This reduced the risk of loose labels being left in the OR when the patient left because the labels were more likely to remain in the patient's chart that left the room with the patient.[4]

6.7 | **A point-of-care barcode system may be used for patient identification and specimen labeling.**
[Conditional Recommendation]

High-quality evidence indicates that point-of-care barcode systems may reduce the risk for patient identification and specimen labeling errors.[1,7,10,13,16,39,53-55] Snyder et al[39] conducted a systematic review and meta-analysis of observational studies on the effectiveness of barcoding technology to reduce identification errors. They concluded that barcoding is effective for reducing specimen and laboratory identification errors and recommended use of the technology as a best practice.[39]

Conversely, a survey of 136 institutions did not demonstrate a detectable benefit of reducing errors when various types of barcode technologies were used.[10] The researchers stated that the introduction of barcoding technology may improve efficiency and reduce errors, but the efficacy of the technology may be affected by the type of device involved and the consistency of its use.[10]

Although barcode technology may reduce errors, it may not eliminate them.[7] Errors may still occur when barcode technology is used, including when

- the system is not used as intended[7,10,55,56];
- the technology is not integrated into standard processes[10,55,56];
- workarounds are developed (eg, printing extra barcoded labels)[10,55,56];
- the readability of the labels is affected by printer quality or toner level[39,57];
- barcodes degrade after being worn or written on[39,57];
- the barcode scanner fails because the batteries are low[39];
- there is an incompatibility in the print size, symbol used, or scanner settings, causing a misread of the barcode[39]; and
- the small size of a pediatric wristband causes the scanner to misread the information.[39]

6.8 | **Radio-frequency identification (RFID) technology may be used for specimen management.**
[Conditional Recommendation]

The benefits of using RFID chips in specimen containers or patient wristbands may include reduced risk of specimen-related errors.[1,7,38,58] Additional benefits may include automated reading, decreased labor, greater data capacity, and increased personnel satisfaction.[58] Harms may include potential for interference with electronic medical devices[38,59] and increased cost.[58] However, the literature supporting RFID technology associated with specimen management did not report adverse effects related to electronic interference.[38,58] Implementing an RFID system for specimen management may also require an

investment of time by an interdisciplinary team to review applicable standards[60] and available systems, create or implement software and data security, and provide education for changes in clinical practice.[38,58]

Low-quality evidence supports the use of RFID technology in specimen management.[1,7,13,31,38,58] Francis et al[38] conducted a nonexperimental study in the endoscopy setting that included RFID technology on specimen bottles, paperless requisition forms, and confirmation of the site and patient for each specimen by both the endoscopy RN and the physician performing the procedure. The researchers found a significant reduction in specimen errors for all error types studied when RFID technology was used.[38] In an organizational experience article on implementation of an RFID system in the pathology laboratory, Bostwick[58] reported that 78.3% of specimens were effectively and correctly processed using RFID technology. The author stated that RFID solves most patient identification errors by linking the specimen to the patient.[58] More research is needed on the use of RFID systems during the preanalytical phase of specimen management.

7. Preservation

7.1 | **Convene an interdisciplinary team that includes a surgeon(s), a pathologist(s), a perioperative RN(s), quality management personnel, and others identified by the organization to establish, implement, and maintain standardized methods of specimen preservation, including**
- **preservative solution selection,**
- **communication about preservative solution requirements, and**
- **the volume and ratio of preservative that will effectively preserve specimens.**

[Recommendation]

The benefits of creating a standardized process for specimen preservation include preserving specimen morphology, reducing loss of molecular components into solution, preventing decomposition and **autolysis**, and minimizing contamination from microbes or fungi.[53] Unpreserved or ineffectively preserved specimens may be compromised, leading to inaccurate or incomplete diagnostic information or the need for additional procedures.

Low-quality evidence supports standardizing processes for specimen preservation.[1] Steelman et al[1] found that almost 25% of the specimen errors in their study occurred during the specimen collection phase. The errors were related to the specimen preservation solution, including not adding solution, adding the wrong solution, and adding solution when it was not indicated.[1] The CAP[31] recommends placing specimens in an effective preservative agent according to facility policy and procedure.

See the AORN Guideline for a Safe Environment of Care[18] for guidance on safe handling, storage, and monitoring related to formaldehyde and other chemical preservatives.

7.2 Confirm the use of preservatives or chemical additives for tissue preservation with the physician. [Recommendation]

Low-quality evidence supports interdisciplinary communication regarding specimen preservation solutions.[1] Steelman et al[1] found that specimen errors related to preservation included not adding the preservation solution to the specimen container, adding the wrong preservation solution, or adding a solution when it was not indicated. Specimen preservation errors occurred partly because of unclear communication about preservative solution requirements. The researchers recommended having interdisciplinary discussions regarding specimen management, enhancing communication about the specimen (eg, type, location, additional information) during the hand-over process, and educating personnel about adding solutions and preservatives to specimens.[1] The CAP[31] recommends placing specimens in preservative as soon as possible after excision except when the use of a preservative would affect the studies ordered for the specimen.

7.3 When formalin is used, fully immerse the specimen in the lowest ratio of formalin volume to specimen volume available that will effectively preserve the specimen (See Recommendation 7.1). [Recommendation]

There is no clear consensus on the ratio of formalin-to-tissue volumes for specimen preservation.[61] Preservative-to-tissue ratios reported in the literature range from 0.5:1 to 200:1.[46-48,61,62] Researchers have suggested that an "ideal ratio" of preservative volume to tissue is 10:1 or greater, including ratios between 20:1 to 50:1.[47,48,53,61] Preservative-to-tissue volume ratios of 1:20 have been advocated because most preservatives are poor buffers.[61] According to Buesa and Peshkov,[61] some literature has stated that large amounts of preservatives are needed to prevent dilution of the preservative, but this is primarily applicable to preservatives that do not contain water, which is not the case with neutral buffered formalin (NBF). The CAP[31] recommends that preservative-to-specimen volume be clarified in facility policy and procedure. The example ratio of preservative volume to tissue volume provided by the CAP[31] is between 15:1 to 20:1. The CAP recommends using 10% NBF.[31]

Buesa and Peshkov[61] conducted a quasi-experimental study on the ratio of 10% NBF to specimen volume and the timing of fixation, including ratios of 1:1, 2:1, 5:1, and 10:1. The researchers found that a 2:1 ratio of formalin-to-tissue volume was enough to result in specimen fixation after 48 hours at 20° C to 22° C (68° F to 71.6° F). However, the researchers also stated that a ratio of 2:1 at 45° C (113° F) combined with agitation and pressure may provide effective fixation in 10 hours.[61]

Vacuum-sealed containment devices may allow users to select the ratio of preservative-to-specimen weight from predetermined settings, including 1:1, 2:1, 2.5:1, 3:1, and 10:1.[46] The specimen is weighed by the device[47] and use of this feature may result in a decrease of the preservative agent required to achieve effective fixation.[46] Zarbo[47] reviewed the use of preset ratios on morphological assessments for 10 different tissue types. The author found acceptable morphologic assessments for all specimen types tested at formalin weight-to-specimen ratios of 2:1 and 1:1.[47]

The lower the formalin-to-specimen volume used, the greater the potential for reductions in formaldehyde exposure to personnel.[61] However, specimen preservation is required for subsequent testing, diagnoses, and clinical decision making. Therefore, using the lowest ratio of formalin-to-specimen volume that will effectively preserve the specimen balances the benefits with the risks.[61] Full immersion of the specimen in the formalin supports specimen fixation from formalin penetration into the tissue.[61] Preservation of specimens is dependent on tissue fixation.

7.4 No recommendation can be made for the use of alternative tissue preservation agents. [No Recommendation]

The balance of benefits versus harms of using alternative tissue preservation agents instead of formalin is unclear. The benefits include eliminating or reducing use of standard preservative agents like formalin.[41] Conversely, the risks of using formalin alternatives may include diminished tissue preservation.[63,64] Formalin is composed of 40% formaldehyde by volume, dissolved in water and 6% to 13% methanol by volume for stabilization.[65] Formaldehyde is a known carcinogen[66] and can cause skin, eye, and respiratory irritation.[65] The OSHA formaldehyde standard sets federal regulations on permissible exposure limits to reduce the risk of occupational exposures.[52] However, despite research to find a suitable alternative to formalin, nothing comparable in tissue preservation and cost has been found,[36] leading experts to suggest a focus on occupational safety by reducing instead of eliminating formalin use.[37,41,47,48,67] Substitution of formalin with alternative preservative agents does not currently seem likely[37,48,67] because an ideal preservative has not been identified; every preservative agent has positive and negative qualities.[63]

The conclusions of quasi-experimental studies[63,64,68-71] and one expert opinion article[67] conflict regarding the use of formalin alternatives. The evidence is confounded by the numerous preservative agents available, the various study methodologies used, and the difference in reported results.[63,64,67-71] Some evidence supports the use of formalin alternatives with modifications in pathology practice.[68-70] Other evidence indicates that formalin alternatives do not have the same tissue preservation properties as formalin.[63,64] Use of a new preservative agent in place of formalin may necessitate research to clarify procedures related to its use[67,69-71] and additional education for pathologists to learn how microscopic analysis associated with the new preservative may be different than with formalin.[63]

8. Transport

8.1 Convene an interdisciplinary team that includes pathology personnel, a surgeon(s), a perioperative RN(s), an infection preventionist, and personnel involved in surgical specimen transport to establish a standardized process for timely transport of specimens to the pathology laboratory. *[Recommendation]*

The benefits of a standardized process for specimen transport[8] include reduced variability and the subsequent reduced risk for specimen errors related to transport (eg, delay, loss, delivery to the wrong location).

8.2 Specimens must be transported in a manner that
- protects the integrity of the specimen[17];
- facilitates specimen identification at each point of exchange[17];
- maintains the confidentiality of protected patient information[17,72]; and
- protects health care personnel from exposure to chemicals, blood, body fluids, or other potentially infectious materials.[40,52]
[Regulatory Requirement]

8.3 Immediately transport specimens to the receiving department (when possible). *[Recommendation]*

One nonexperimental study[1] and a guideline from the CAP[31] support the immediate transport of specimens to the receiving department. Steelman et al[1] found that 38% of all specimen errors were

related to transport and temporary storage. The errors included
- delivery delays;
- specimens that were lost or not received;
- specimens that were stored in or delivered to the wrong place;
- delivery without interdepartmental communication;
- specimens that were not refrigerated when refrigeration was indicated; and
- containers that leaked, spilled, or were broken.[1]

The researchers reported that factors contributing to errors in specimen transport included interruptions, waiting to send many specimens at once, inattention, and heavy workloads.[1] Personnel may be unaware of the facility policy and procedure for specimen transport, especially during times outside of standard business hours.[1]

8.4 Confirm receipt of critical and time-sensitive information when delivering specimens to the receiving department (eg, frozen section, STAT).[1] *[Recommendation]*

8.5 Verify receipt of the specimen at the receiving department.[1] *[Recommendation]*

8.6 Devices transporting specimen containers (eg, enclosed carts) must be labeled to communicate chemical[52] and biohazard information.[40] *[Regulatory Requirement]*

When devices transporting specimen containers are used, labeling the transport device with chemical and biohazard information alerts personnel to potential hazards. Details about exceptions to the biohazard labeling process are outlined in 29 CFR 1910.1030.[40]

8.7 Minimize visibility of specimens and labels containing protected health information during transport (when possible). *[Recommendation]*

Reduced specimen visibility may help maintain patient privacy and confidentiality[72,73] and protect individuals from viewing a specimen. Reactions of patients, visitors, and other health care personnel may vary when viewing a specimen. Additionally, some specimens may be easily recognizable and of a sensitive nature (eg, amputated limbs).

8.8 No recommendation can be made for the use of pneumatic tube systems for specimen transport. *[No Recommendation]*

The balance between the benefits and harms for specimen transport in a pneumatic tube system is unclear. The benefits may include fast delivery of specimens for processing. The potential harms may include specimen loss if the specimen is sent to the wrong location[1] or stuck in the tube system or the potential for chemical or potentially infectious material to spill inside the tube system during transport. The ECRI Institute[14] recommends using caution when transporting specimens via a pneumatic tube system.

8.8.1 Follow facility policies and procedures[15] and the pneumatic tube system manufacturer's IFU when using pneumatic tube systems for specimen transport. *[Recommendation]*

8.8.2 Confirm the receipt of specimens sent through pneumatic tube systems.[1,14] *[Recommendation]*

8.9 When on-site pathology, laboratory, or courier services are not available and the need for these services is identified, services may be contracted with a third party. *[Conditional Recommendation]*

9. Temporary Storage

9.1 Specimens that will not be transported immediately to the pathology laboratory must be temporarily stored in a manner that maintains specimen integrity for examination.[17] *[Regulatory Requirement]*

9.1.1 Convene an interdisciplinary team that includes a pathologist(s), a surgeon(s), an infection preventionist(s), and a perioperative RN(s) to establish a temperature range for temporary storage of specimens in accordance with federal, state, and local regulations. *[Recommendation]*

The CAP[31] recommends refrigerated storage for specimens that cannot be immediately transported to the pathology laboratory.

9.1.2 Specimen storage logs may be compared to the available specimen container labels and requisition forms before transport to the receiving department (eg, pathology laboratory, radiology department). *[Conditional Recommendation]*

One nonexperimental study[1] recommended comparing specimen logs to the available specimen container labels and requisition forms as a quality check before transport to the receiving department. According to the CAP,[31] the log may include the

- date and time,
- patient identifiers,
- specimen identifiers,

- purpose for specimen delivery (eg, type of testing),
- name and title of the person submitting the specimen, and
- name and title of the person transporting the specimen.

10. Disposal

10.1 Specimens and chemicals used for preservation of specimens must be disposed of according to local, state, and federal regulations.[40,52,74] *[Regulatory Requirement]*

Disposal of pathology waste and chemicals is regulated by multiple entities and jurisdictions.[40,52,74] The safety data sheet states that formalin may be disposed of at an approved waste disposal plant.[75] See the Guideline for a Safe Environment of Care[18] for additional guidance on disposal of hazardous and regulated waste.

11. Breast Cancer Specimens

11.1 Convene an interdisciplinary team that includes a surgeon(s), a pathologist(s), a radiologist(s), a perioperative RN(s), perioperative leadership personnel, and other stakeholders determined by the health care organization to define and implement a standardized procedure for handling breast cancer specimens. *[Recommendation]*

Moderate-quality evidence supports creating a standard process for handling breast cancer specimens. Two nonexperimental studies,[76,77] two clinical practice guidelines,[78,79] one consensus document,[62] two organizational experience articles,[80,81] and four expert opinion articles[82-85] either describe a lack of standardization or promote standardization as necessary for handling breast cancer specimens. The 2020 American Society of Clinical Oncology (ASCO) and CAP focused guideline update[78] explained that quality control data analyzed since the previous 2010 guideline publication indicated an improvement in the quality and reproducibility of estrogen and progesterone receptor testing and that this is most likely related to improvements in standardization of different factors, including those from the preanalytical phase of specimen management.

11.1.1 Standardized processes for handling breast cancer specimens may include
- recording the time of specimen excision[62,76,78,82,83,85];
- keeping the specimen moist to prevent drying before fixation[62];

- transferring the specimen to the pathology laboratory as soon as possible[62,78,79,82-84];
- recording the time of fixation (when fixation is performed)[62,76,78,82,85];
- determining whether radiologic imaging will be used[77,80,81,83];
- determining the type of puncture-resistant, leak-proof containment device to be used[77,80,86];
- reducing the potential for sharps injuries during handling[77,80]; and
- determining whether a preservative will be used and, if so, when it will be added, the type, and the ratio of preservative-to-specimen volume (See Sections 5 and 7).[62,76,85]

[Conditional Recommendation]

Estrogen receptor **assay** test results are often used to determine the course of clinical treatment after breast-conserving procedures.[62,83,85] However, estrogen and progesterone receptors, genetic markers, and cell proliferation markers are sensitive to extended time to fixation, the length of fixation, and the type of fixation used.[76,83,87-92] The evidence conflicts, however, about the specific length of time before test results are affected.[76,83,87-92] Lack of standardization of these preanalytical variables may result in high rates of "false-negative" estrogen receptor test results or cause estrogen and progesterone receptor testing to be recorded as uninterpretable, potentially compromising patient care.[62,78,79,83] Standardizing preanalytical factors, such as the time to fixation, and recording relevant times in breast cancer specimen handling facilitates higher reliability in the test results.[76,83]

Three nonexperimental studies[77,86,93] and two organizational experience[80,81] articles indicate that there is considerable variability in the coordination of breast cancer specimens that are transferred between the OR, the radiology department, and the pathology laboratory.[77,80,81,86,93] Li and Shah[77] surveyed the members of the Society of Breast Imaging about the process used for imaging breast specimens. The survey reported that 15.3% of respondents did not have or were unaware of a facility standard for specimen processing.[77] A key finding was that 4.3% of respondents reported knowledge of needle-stick injuries that occurred during specimen handling; however, the exact cause of the injuries is unknown.[77] Breast cancer specimens may include radiopaque clips, markers, or wires.[77,81,93] Thirty-one percent of survey respondents reported that there were two or more specimen transfers during different stages in the handling process,[77] which may increase the risk for injury. The type and number of containers used throughout the process may play a role in reducing the amount of specimen handling, thereby reducing the potential for leakage or spilling of potentially infectious material and sharps injuries.[77,80]

Evidence supports using a single, rigid, leak-proof container that may include a radiopaque alphanumeric grid that may be used when specimen compression is necessary.[77,80,86] In an organizational experience article, Baltuonyte et al[80] described a reducing the number containers used during process from three to one and eliminating specimen transfers between containers, which resulted in an estimated facility savings of 27% to 28%.

Breast cancer specimens may occasionally be sent to laboratories outside of the facility for testing.[76] When this occurs, the ASCO and CAP guideline recommends that breast tissue excised in a remote location be bisected through the tumor on removal and then placed in a sufficient volume of NBF before being sent to the pathology laboratory.[78]

12. Radioactive Specimens

12.1 **Radioactive specimens must be handled according to federal, state, and local regulations.**[94,95]

[Regulatory Requirement]

The medical use of radioactive materials is regulated by the Nuclear Regulatory Commission (NRC).[94] Licensure for use of radioactive materials is obtained from the NRC or an **Agreement State**.[94] Agreement States may have differing regulations.[96] The use of radioactive seeds in localization procedures is regulated under 10 CFR 35.1000[95] "other medical uses" and the equivalent Agreement State regulations. The NRC[97] provides guidance on the safe handling of radioactive seeds during radioactive seed localization (RSL) procedures in an additional document because it is not specifically addressed in the regulations.[98]

Radiation exposure has no known safe level.[99] Therefore, a key element of the regulations regarding medical use of radioactive materials is to keep radiation exposure to individuals and the environment as low as reasonably achievable (ALARA).[94] Annual occupational ionizing radiation exposure limits are based on the **total effective dose equivalent** of radiation to which a person is exposed or the sum of the **deep-dose equivalent** and other individual exposures (eg, organ, tissue).[94] See the Guideline for Radiation Safety[20] for annual exposure limits.

Evidence for radioactive specimens is divided into two categories: sentinel lymph node (SLN) localization procedures (ie, breast, melanoma) using radioactive pharmaceuticals[100] and RSL procedures for nonpalpable breast cancer resections using radioactive brachytherapy seeds.[97]

12.1.1 Handling and management of SLN specimens during SLN localization procedures should include

- use of standard precautions,[101,102]
- minimal handling,[103]
- distance between personnel and radioactive tissue (when possible),[103]
- use of long instruments or devices when manipulating specimens,[102,103]
- containment according to the organization's standardized procedures,[101]
- recording the presence of radioactive material on the pathology requisition form,
- prompt transport of the specimen to the pathology laboratory,[101-103]
- in-person hand-over processes between personnel,[101,102]
- communication of the presence of radioactive material on delivery to the pathology laboratory,
- use of standard instrument cleaning procedures,[102]
- linen and surgical attire laundering according to standard procedures,[100] and
- waste disposal according to standard procedures.[100,103]

[Recommendation]

Moderate-quality evidence provides guidance for handling radioactive SLN specimens and management during SLN localization procedures.[99-104] Radioactive SLN specimens are not correlated with high levels of radiation exposure to personnel involved in the procedures.[100,102-104] Because low levels of radiation are found in radioactive SLN specimens, use of lead shielding is not necessary.[100] In one study, couriers transporting specimens were found to have cumulative whole-body radiation doses below the detectable limit.[103] In another study, researchers found no evidence of radioactive contamination of the OR environment, linen, garments, or waste (eg, gloves, sponges).[100]

Limiting the duration of contact and increasing the distance between personnel and radioactive tissue can reduce risk of exposure.[103] In a nonexperimental study, Coventry et al[103] found that use of instruments and surgical devices (eg, electrocautery pencils, clip devices) that are 7.8 inches (20 cm) long may reduce radiation exposure to the surgeon's hands by a factor of 30. For unscrubbed periop-

erative personnel, working 3.2 to 6.5 feet (1 to 2 m) from a radioactive source can minimize the dose received to a negligible level.[103] Excluding pregnant personnel from participating in procedures involving radiation can prevent avoidable radiation exposures.[103] Additionally, sending specimens promptly to the receiving pathology laboratory limits the time they are in the OR. Use of an in-person specimen hand-over process can reduce the risk of the specimen being left unattended.[101,102] Coventry et al[103] suggested that personnel transporting specimens carry the container away from the body.

The benefits of following evidenced-based recommendations for handling radioactive SLN specimens include maximizing safety and minimizing the risk of exposing personnel or the environment to radioactive materials.[100] Focusing on safety and reduced risk of exposure is an important part of the ALARA principle.[94]

12.1.2 Handling and management of RSL specimens containing seeds during RSL procedures should include

- communication with collaborating departments (eg, nuclear medicine, radiology, pathology) when a procedure is scheduled,[98]
- use of standard precautions,[98,105]
- minimal handling,[97]
- placement of a collection sock in the suction cannister,[96,106]
- gentle use of forceps if handling the individual seed becomes necessary,[105]
- confirmation of the seed location in the specimen with a radiation detection device before wound closure,[105-108]
- verification of the seed location in the specimen with a radiograph,[96,98,105-108]
- delay of instrument table breakdown until the seeds are accounted for,[96]
- recording the presence of a radioactive seed on the pathology requisition form,[105]
- recording intraoperative information on the **written directive** (when applicable),[96,105,106]
- prompt transport of the specimen to the pathology laboratory,
- communication about the presence of a radioactive seed on delivery to the pathology laboratory,[98]
- immediate notification to an **authorized user** when a seed is suspected to be lost,[108] and
- a radiation survey of the patient and the OR when a seed is suspected to be lost.[108]

[Recommendation]

Moderate-quality evidence is available regarding handling of specimens that contain radioactive seeds and management during RSL procedures.[96,98,105-108] Literature on the use of radioactive seeds is primarily focused on breast cancer lesions.[96,98,105,107,108] Only one nonexperimental study discussed the use of radioactive seeds for localization of nonpalpable soft tissue masses other than breast cancer lesions.[106] The locations of the 10 masses in the study included the abdomen, upper and lower back, upper arm, inguinal area, and neck.[106]

The radiation dose to personnel involved in RSL procedures or specimen handling is negligible.[98,105] Therefore, radiation monitoring for personnel, special protective equipment,[98] additional warning signs on the OR doors, and a radiographic survey of the OR are not necessary.[108]

Verifying the seed location is crucial because all seeds used must be accounted for.[96,98] Using a two-step process to verify the location of the seed in the specimen with a handheld radiation detection device followed by a specimen radiograph before wound closure may prevent the need for the patient to return to surgery for seed removal.[106,107] Intraoperative handheld radiation detection devices confirm the location of the seed(s) in the specimen and the absence of radioactivity in the patient's surgical incision before wound closure.[106-108] At least 1.1 inch (3 cm) of separation is required between seeds placed around a lesion to allow the radiation detection device to distinguish between seed locations.[96,106]

After specimen excision, radiographs are taken to verify the location of the seed(s) in the specimen[96,98,105-108] and provide evidence that the seed(s) was not lost in the OR.[98] Most specimen radiographs are taken intraoperatively on excision,[96,98,105,106] although the authors of one organizational experience article reported that specimen radiographs were taken in the radiology department before delivery of the specimen to the pathology laboratory.[108] Extruded seeds present in the wound may be caught in a vacuum and land in a suction canister.[96,106] If a seed is thought to be in a specimen collection sock, the sock may be radiographed.[96] See the Guideline for Radiation Safety[20] for recommendations on including seeds in count procedures.

Delaying the breakdown of instrument tables and Mayo stand setups in the OR until seed locations are verified is important. Adverse events may occur and identifying the location of the seed is necessary because of regulations regarding seed management and disposal. In an organizational experience article, Goudreau et al[96] recommended delaying disposal of equipment used during seed placement procedures until the seed location in the patient is confirmed. The authors described an adverse event in which a seed was inadvertently discarded in and later retrieved from a sharps disposal container.[96] In a nonexperimental study, Sung et al[107] stated that one seed placed in the axilla was lost when it fell into the axilla incision during specimen excision.[107] As a result of the proximity of the seed to nerves and vessels, it could not be safely located and removed and required a second procedure.[107] Seeds placed in the axilla may be more difficult to remove and prone to loss.

All seeds must be accounted for,[97] and the process used to trace the seed includes a written directive.[96] A written directive is required in accordance with 10 CFR 35.40(a) and (b)(6) or the equivalent state agreement.[95,97] The written directive must contain the patient's name, radionuclide, dose, treatment site, number of seeds, total source strength, and exposure time.[95] However, additional information may be included on a written directive leading to the potential for variation between facilities.[96,105,106] The intraoperative portion of the form has been reported to include the date, time, surgeon's name, location, number of seeds removed,[96] and a comment section.[105]

According to an organizational experience article by Pavlicek et al,[108] when a seed is lost, immediate notification to the nuclear technologist and the radiation safety personnel is necessary. However, different facilities may designate other personnel for notification (eg, radiation safety officer [RSO], authorized users). The authors also stated that a radiation survey of the patient and the OR may help locate the seed.[108]

The benefits of following evidenced-based recommendations for handling radioactive seeds include maximizing safety and minimizing the risk of exposing personnel or the environment to radioactive materials. Focusing on safety and reduced risk of exposure is an important part of the ALARA principle.[94]

12.1.3 **Convene an interdisciplinary team that includes the RSO, a surgeon, a perioperative RN(s), and a pathologist to establish a procedure for handling radioactive seeds separated from specimens during the procedure.** *[Recommendation]*

Establishing a procedure will help ensure that personnel are following federal and state regulations and organizational policies and procedures for containment and labeling. Specifying whether the seed will be sent to the pathology laboratory with the specimen or separately to a receiving department (eg, nuclear medicine, radiology) for disposal is important because radioactive waste disposal is regulated.[94]

12.2 **In collaboration with the RSO, establish when additional labeling of radioactive specimens is required and what should be included on the specimen label.** *[Recommendation]*

Working with the RSO provides an interdisciplinary decision-making process based on the specifics of the radioactive materials used in the facility that follows the requirements outlined in the regulations. An additional benefit may be reduced risk of radiation exposure to personnel involved in handling radioactive specimens.

Regulations for labeling licensed radioactive material and labeling exemptions are defined in sections 10 CFR 20.1904 and 10 CFR 20.1905 from the NRC.[94] When required, labeling includes a clearly visible radiation symbol and the words "caution, radioactive material." Additional information is required on the label (eg, radioactive material name, type of material [eg, seed]) to eliminate or reduce the risk of radiation exposure to personnel handling the container. However, there are many exemptions to the labeling requirement. Working with the health care organization RSO can help determine whether radioactive specimens require additional labeling or if an exemption applies.

12.3 **Determine a process for transferring radioactive specimens to an outside pathology laboratory in collaboration with the RSO, if outside transfer is required.** *[Recommendation]*

Establishing a collaborative, interdisciplinary process for transferring radioactive specimens to outside pathology laboratories will help ensure that perioperative personnel are following a process for radioactive specimen transfer that meets regulatory requirements for labeling,[94] transport,[109] and transfer[110] and is based on the specific types of radioactive material being transferred and the licensure of the receiving facility. An additional benefit is reduced risk of exposure to individuals or the environment.

12.4 **Emergency response equipment must be available near each surgical suite when radioactive seeds are handled. This includes**
- **gloves (eg, nonsterile, sterile),**
- **reverse action tweezers,**
- **shielded containers,**

- **a low-energy gamma scintillation survey instrument, and**
- **"caution, radioactive material" labels.**[97]

[Regulatory Requirement]

According to the NRC,[97] an emergency may include loss or rupture of a seed.

12.5 **Develop and maintain policies and procedures for managing radioactive specimens with an interdisciplinary team that includes the RSO, a pathologist, radiology personnel, a perioperative RN, quality and risk management personnel, and other involved perioperative team members (eg, a scrub person).** *[Recommendation]*

Collaborative development of policies and procedures can reduce the risk of exposure to radiation and keep occupational radiation doses ALARA. An additional benefit may include alignment between radiation safety policies throughout the organization.[101]

12.5.1 **Facility policies and procedures regarding emergency management of radiation exposure (eg, a broken or leaking seed) must be immediately available.**[97] *[Regulatory Requirement]*

12.6 **In collaboration with the RSO, determine the frequency, delivery method, and record keeping for education and competency verification for perioperative personnel working with radioactive specimens.** *[Recommendation]*

The benefit of a collaborative process for education and competency verification of perioperative personnel involved in SLN localization or RSL procedures is that personnel are trained in radiation safety procedures that minimize the risk of radiation exposure to individuals and the environment. An additional benefit is that personnel receive training that is consistent with the expectations of the facility radiation safety program.

Oversight of radiation safety programs including training are part of the duties assigned to the RSO of the health care organization or facility.[96]

12.6.1 **Annual training, including routine radiation monitoring and emergency procedures, must be provided for all personnel involved in RSL procedures.** *[Regulatory Requirement]*

According to the NRC,[97] all personnel involved in RSL procedures, including surgical personnel, must receive annual training that includes topics covered in 10 CFR 35.410.[95]

12.6.2 **Records of the training must be maintained according to 10 CFR 35.410**[95] **or the Agreement State regulation.**[97] *[Regulatory Requirement]*

12.7 Evaluate the ability of intraoperative radiation detection devices to distinguish among each of the specific radioactive signals to be used (eg, technetium-99m sulfur colloid [^{99m}Tc], iodine I-125 [^{125}I], palladium Pd-103 [^{103}Pd]) before starting a new program or service or before purchase of a device. [Recommendation]

Low-quality evidence indicates the need to determine whether intraoperative radiation detection equipment will distinguish between the various sources of gamma radiation that will be used in patient care.[98,108] The radioactive pharmaceutical used in SLN localization procedures is ^{99m}Tc.[98,100] Radioactive seeds contain either ^{125}I or ^{103}Pd.[97,98] Additionally, SLN localization procedures and RSL procedures may be performed simultaneously.[98,108] If equipment is not available or if devices cannot distinguish between specific radioactive signals that are being considered for patient care, new equipment may be needed. See the Guideline for Medical Device and Product Evaluation[111] for recommendations on pre-purchase decision making.

13. Explanted Medical Devices

13.1 Track and handle explanted medical devices according to federal, state, and local regulations; the device manufacturer's IFU; and facility policies and procedures. [Recommendation]

Hospitals and other health care facilities that implant medical devices are considered final distributors (ie, any person or entity that distributes a tracked device to the patient, including licensed practitioners, hospitals, and other facilities).[112] Final distributors are subject to medical device tracking requirements and are responsible for providing information to the manufacturer about explanted devices.[112,113]

Medical device tracking of class II or III devices is required by manufacturers if the US Food and Drug Administration (FDA) issues an order to the manufacturer and the device meets one of the following criteria:

- the failure of the device (ie, failure to perform or function as intended) would likely have serious adverse health consequences (ie, significant events that are life-threatening or involve permanent or long-term injury or illness);
- the device is intended to be implanted in the human body (ie, placed into a surgically or naturally formed human body cavity to continuously assist, restore, or replace the function of an organ system or structure) for more than 1 year; or
- the device is a life-sustaining or life-supporting device (ie, essential to the restoration or continuation of a bodily function) used outside of the device

user facility (ie, intended for use outside a hospital, nursing home, ambulatory surgery facility, or diagnostic or outpatient treatment facility).[112]

Explanted medical device tracking may provide information about device use, life expectancy of the device, and failure that can be used to improve devices and clinical decision making about device use. Medical device tracking, when required, benefits facilities and patients when notifications and recalls occur.

13.1.1 Explanted medical devices that require tracking must be reported to the manufacturer (Table 1).[112] Information that must be provided to the manufacturer includes the

- date the device was explanted;
- name, mailing address, and telephone number of the explanting physician; and
- date of the patient's death or the date the device was returned to the manufacturer, permanently retired from use, or otherwise disposed of permanently.[112]

[Regulatory Requirement]

13.1.2 Record the explanted device information and the process used to attempt to contact the manufacturer when the manufacturer cannot be located. [Recommendation]

13.1.3 Deaths related to an implanted medical device must be reported to both the FDA and the manufacturer.[114,115] Serious injury related to an implanted medical device must be reported to the device manufacturer.[114,115] If the medical device manufacturer cannot be identified, report the injury to the FDA.[114,115] [Regulatory Requirement]

Implanted medical device malfunctions are not required to be reported; however, the facility or health care organization may use the voluntary MedWatch program[116] to advise the FDA of potential problems with an implanted medical device.[114,115]

13.2 Follow the manufacturer's instructions and facility policies and procedures for returning, packaging, and shipping explanted devices to device manufacturers. [Recommendation]

The benefits of following the manufacturer's instructions and facility policies and procedures for returning, packaging, and shipping explanted devices include protecting the device from damage during shipping and reducing the risk of leakage of potentially hazardous or infectious materials during transport. Not all manufacturers request that explanted devices be returned.

Table 1. Medical Devices that Require Manufacturer Tracking[1]	Product Code
Aortic valve prosthesis, percutaneously delivered	NPT
Breast prosthesis, non-inflatable, internal, silicone gel filled	FTR
Defibrillator, auxiliary power supply (AC or DC) for low-energy DC defibrillator	MPD
Defibrillator, automated, external, wearable	MVK
Defibrillator, automatic, implantable, cardioverter, with cardiac resynchronization (CRT-D)	NIK
Defibrillator, DC, high energy (including paddles)	DRK
Defibrillator, DC, low energy (including paddles)	LDD
Defibrillator, implantable cardioverter (NON-CRT)	LWS
Defibrillator, implantable, dual chamber	MRM
Defibrillator, over-the-counter, automated, external	NSA
Defibrillators, automated external (AEDs) (non-wearable)	MKJ
Electrode, pacemaker, permanent	DTB
Electrode, pacing and cardioversion, temporary, epicardial	NHW
Electrodes, defibrillator, permanent	NVY
Electrodes, pacemaker, drug-eluting, permanent, right ventricular (RV) or right atrial (RA)	NVN
Endovascular graft system, aortic aneurysm treatment	MIH
Heart valve, mechanical	LWQ
Heart valve, non-allograft tissue	LWR
Heart valve, replacement	DYE
Mandibular prosthesis, condyle, temporary	NEI
Monitor, apnea, home use	NPF
Monitor, breathing frequency	BZQ
Pacemaker battery	DSZ
Pacemaker, lead adapter	DTD

13.3 The **unique device identifier** (UDI) from explanted medical devices may be documented in the patient's medical record or recorded in a facility tracking log when available.[117,118] [Conditional Recommendation]

13.4 Develop health care organization policies and procedures for handling of explanted medical devices in collaboration with an interdisciplinary team that includes perioperative leaders, legal advisors, risk management personnel, pathologists, surgeons, anesthesia professionals, infection preventionists, sterile processing personnel, and materials management personnel. [Recommendation]

13.4.1 Policies and procedures for explanted medical devices should include
- medical device tracking,[112,113]
- reporting of patient death or serious injuries,[114-116]
- returning devices to manufacturers,
- submission to the pathology laboratory if required,
- documentation of explants,[119]

- disposal of devices, and
- whether devices may be returned to the patient, including procedures for
  o communicating with personnel who perform explanted device processing,
  o decontamination processes that will be used in the facility, and
  o liability release of the facility processing the explanted device if explanted devices are returned to the patient.

[Recommendation]

The CAP[119] states that orthopedic hardware may be excluded from submission to the pathology laboratory when there is an alternative method of documenting the surgical removal of the explant. Davidovitch et al[120] conducted a nonexperimental study on submission of explanted orthopedic hardware to pathology for **gross examination** and found that the pathological examination was costly and that the resulting reports did not alter the plan of care for patients. The researchers recommended that a single radiograph of the explant site and documentation of hardware removal in the postoperative surgical report

Table 1 Continued. Medical Devices Requiring Manufacturer Tracking[1]	Product Code
Pacemaker, pulse generator (NON-CRT) implantable	LWP
Pacemaker, pulse generator, implantable	DXY
Pulmonary valve prosthesis, percutaneously delivered	NPV
Pulmonic valved conduit	MWH
Pulse generator, pacemaker, implantable, with cardiac resynchronization (CRT-P)	NKE
Pulse generator, permanent, implantable	NVZ
Pulse generator, single chamber, single	LWW
Pulse generator, dual chamber, pacemaker, external	OVJ
Pulse generator, single chamber, sensor driven, implantable	LWO
Pump, infusion or syringe, extra-luminal	FIH
Pump, infusion, implanted, programmable	LKK
Shunt, portosystemic, endoprosthesis	MIR
Stimulator, autonomic nerve, implanted (depression)	MUZ
Stimulator, cerebellar, implanted	GZA
Stimulator, diaphragmatic/phrenic nerve, implanted	GZE
Stimulator, diaphragmatic/phrenic nerve, laparoscopically implanted	OIR
Stimulator, electrical, implanted, for Parkinsonian symptoms	NHL
Temporomandibular joint, implant	LZD
Transmandibular Implant	MDL
Ventilator, continuous, home use	NOU
Ventilator, continuous, non-life-supporting	MNS
Ventilator, continuous, minimal ventilatory support, facility use	MNT
Ventilator, continuous, minimal ventilatory support, home use	NQY
Ventilator, mechanical	ONZ

Reference

1. *Medical device tracking; guidance for industry and FDA staff. US Food and Drug Administration. https://www.fda.gov/regulatory-information/search-fda-guidance-documents/medical-device-tracking. Published March 2014. Accessed September 28, 2020.*

could replace submission of explanted orthopedic hardware to the pathology laboratory.[120]

13.4.2 **No recommendation can be made for return of explanted medical devices to patients.** [*No Recommendation*]

The balance between the benefits and harms of returning explanted medical devices to the patient or patient's family is unclear. The disposition of explanted medical devices may be complicated by

- federal, state, or local regulations;
- device ownership (eg, patient, manufacturer, facility);
- verbiage in the facility's surgical informed consent form;
- whether the device is involved in a civil or criminal proceeding (eg, device failure);
- whether the device is requested for manufacturer return;
- whether the device is defined as a specimen for pathological submission;

- exposure risk to individuals from potentially infectious material on the device; and
- cleaning or decontamination of used single-use devices without instructions for reprocessing.

14. Forensic Evidence

14.1 **Convene an interdisciplinary team that includes a forensic or emergency department RN(s),**[121-123] **a surgeon, a pathologist, a perioperative RN, a surgical technologist, risk management personnel, facility security personnel, morgue personnel (if available), and a local law enforcement official to establish methods for handling, containment, documentation, chain of custody processes, and disposition of potential forensic evidence.**[122,124-126] [*Recommendation*]

The benefits of determining a process for forensic evidence management with an interdisciplinary team outweigh the harms. The benefits include having a standardized process that minimizes the handling of evidence and keeps the chain of custody intact to prevent evidence from becoming inadmissible in court.[122] An additional benefit is having a process in place for handling forensic evidence before an incident occurs. However, an investment of time is required to determine a process that may be used infrequently.

Low-quality evidence supports having an interdisciplinary team determine a process for forensic evidence management.[121-126] Preservation of potential evidence is best informed by people who collect and use evidence (eg, forensic RNs, law enforcement officials, medical examiners, state crime laboratory officials).[126] In an expert opinion article, Byrne-Dugan et al[124] discussed a collaborative effort to create a protocol for handling surgical specimens that contain forensic evidence. The interdisciplinary team included hospital personnel from three facilities, the state chief medical examiner, and a local agent from the Federal Bureau of Investigation.[124]

14.2 Use a standardized kit for collection of potential forensic evidence. *[Recommendation]*

The benefits of using a standardized evidence collection kit include reduced time needed to gather supplies, having supplies available to follow the patient to different areas of the facility (eg, emergency department, OR), and standardization of processes.[122] Additional benefits may include access to supplies that are not readily available in the OR, such as paper bags, tamper-proof tape, chain of custody forms, a camera, and body graph diagrams. There is a potential for delayed evidence collection if the kit is stored in the emergency department and is not available when needed in the OR. There is also a risk of waste if supplies kept in the kit expire before use.

14.2.1 The standardized forensic evidence collection kit may contain
- supplies for containment, including
  - specimen containers,
  - paper bags,
  - envelopes, and
  - tamper-proof tape and
- forms for documentation and reference, including
  - policies and procedures,
  - checklists,
  - chain of custody forms,
  - body graph diagrams, and
  - contact information for assistance with forensic evidence handling.[122,123,127]

[Conditional Recommendation]

Low-quality evidence supports developing an evidence collection kit and discusses items that may be included.[122,123,127,128] Forensic evidence collection kits are described as having two components: supplies for containment and forms for documentation and reference.[122,123,127] Use of checklists and policy and procedure documents may increase the standardization of processes that are performed infrequently. Facility emergency departments may have a forensic evidence collection kit available that can be used in the OR when a patient is transferred.[122]

14.3 When handling, containing, and labeling potential forensic evidence,
- collect the evidence as soon as possible[129];
- prevent the omission or disposal of potential evidence[122,125,126];
- contain the preoperative stretcher linens in a paper bag[127];
- capture photographic images before evidence removal or preoperative skin antisepsis (when possible)[124,126];
- use a measuring device or item for scale (eg, a coin) in photographed areas[125,130];
- minimize handling of the forensic evidence[122,126,127,131];
- don PPE, including gloves before handling evidence[122,123,125,127,129,131];
- change gloves after touching different body areas[129] or handling each item[122];
- use caution to prevent injuries from sharp objects (eg, needles in pockets, bullet fragments)[122,127];
- cut clothing off the patient through the seams (when necessary)[122,123,125-127,130,131];
- prevent clothes from being shaken[125] or balled up[122];
- collect and secure fabric or other debris from in or around wounds[127];
- avoid rinsing, wiping, or washing evidence[122,126];
- grasp bullets with rubber-tipped forceps[122,125-127,131];
- prevent bullets from being dropped into metal basins[122,125-127,131];
- contain fragments of the same bullet together[122,126];
- remove sharp objects without causing injury to personnel or disrupting fingerprints (when possible)[122,126,127];
- contain each piece of evidence individually[122,123,125-127,131];
- place physical evidence in a container (eg, envelope, specimen container, paper bag)[122,123,125-127,131];
- label the container with patient's identifiers, date and time of collection, and name of the person collecting the evidence[122,123,125,130,132];
- document the location on or in the patient's body where the items were obtained[122];
- seal the evidence containment device (eg, paper bags, containers) with tamper-proof tape (when available)[122,125,126] or adhesive tape[122,126,130];

- seal evidence in an envelope without licking it[122]; and
- inform law enforcement officials about items that are wet.[122,125]

[Recommendation]

Moderate-quality evidence describes processes for handling, containing, and labeling forensic evidence.[122-127,129-132] Foresman-Capuzzi,[122] in an expert opinion article, recommends keeping everything. When it is unclear if an item may be evidence (eg, soil, branches, insects, printed purchase receipts, fibers), the author recommends labeling it as "debris" and noting where it was found.[122] The linens from the preoperative stretcher may also contain physical or trace evidence.[127]

Minimizing the number of people involved in the handling of forensic evidence may reduce the risk of confusion or inconsistencies and provide a single or minimal number of contact persons for law enforcement officials.[122,124] Use of PPE reduces the risk of exposure from potentially infectious materials and may also prevent contamination of evidence.[122,127] The Faculty of Forensic and Legal Medicine[129] in the United Kingdom recommends wearing two pairs of gloves and changing the outer gloves when sampling different body areas.

The use of photography is important in evidence collection[122,126,130] but does not replace documentation.[123] Photographs can provide evidence of patient injuries.[125,126] However, some facilities may have policies and procedures that govern the use of photography.[126] Evans et al,[125] in an expert opinion article, recommended labeling printed photographs with patient information, placing the picture(s) in a sealed envelope, and following the chain of custody.

Four expert opinion articles address the packaging and containment of clothing.[122,125,130,131] One author suggests using paper bags to individually bag articles of clothing and shoes.[122] The use of separate paper bags is intended to prevent the transfer of evidence from one piece of clothing to another.[122] Authors stated that shaking out clothes can cause the loss of trace evidence[122,125] and that balling up clothes may alter stains or blood patterns.[122] However, different packaging methods were suggested to minimize the transfer of stains from one location to another on the same article of clothing. One method included placing clothing flat on pieces of paper and rolling up the clothes with paper between layers[131] and the second included wrapping clothing in a clean item (eg, clean linen) before placing it in a paper bag.[130] One author does not recommend storing wet clothing and suggests that these items be given to law enforcement officials as soon as possible.[125] The use of plastic bags for containment of wet clothes may increase the risk of mold growth that may degrade DNA.[122] Plastic bags may also contain static electricity that may remove trace evidence by lifting it off of the physical evidence.[122]

Use of metal instruments on bullets or dropping bullets into a metal container may interfere with subsequent identification of ballistic markings.[122,125-127,131] Rinsing, cleaning, or wiping evidence may remove other trace evidence.[122,126] Some authors suggest placing bullets into an envelope or nonadherent dressing and then into a specimen cup.[122,126,127,131] One author recommended wrapping the bullet in cotton and placing it in a paper-plastic pouch.[125]

Wick[126] suggests grasping objects like imbedded knives differently than how a perpetrator may have handled the item to help retain physical or trace evidence on the item.

Most literature agrees that containment devices holding forensic evidence be labeled with patient's identifiers, date and time of collection, and name of the person collecting it.[122,123,125,130,132] Some also recommends including the item name or description.[123,129] A guideline from the Faculty of Forensic and Legal Medicine[179] in the United Kingdom recommends including both the name of the collector (eg, surgeon) and the name of the person who contained the evidence (eg, perioperative RN) on evidence labels.

14.4 **Document potential informational and physical forensic evidence in the patient's medical record, including the location where physical evidence was found (eg, surgical wound) or from which it was removed (eg, pocket).** *[Recommendation]*

The benefits of documenting forensic evidence in the patient's medical record include creating a record that could be used during a civil or criminal proceeding.

Low-quality evidence supports documenting the different types of evidence with which the patient presents[122,123,125-127,131] and from where physical evidence was removed or found (Table 2).[126] Informational evidence can include odors (eg, gasoline, chemicals, alcohol) and visual clues from the patient's condition (eg, condition of clothing, visible injuries, behavior).[122,123,125-127,131] Some authors recommend that patient and family communication be documented using verbatim quotes,[123,126,131] even if slang, vulgar terms, or violent words are used.[122] The use of the words "reported" and "suspected" is advised instead of the word "alleged" that may imply disbelief or distrust.[122,123] Authors recommend describing projectile wounds by size (eg, 2 mm) and shape (eg, oval) instead of the using the words "entrance" or "exit" as a descriptor.[122,123] Documenting the location that physical evidence was removed from or found may be especially important when patients have multiple wounds.

Table 2. Types of Forensic Evidence[1]	
Informational Evidence	Stated comments, patient condition (eg, behavior, wounds), observations (eg, odors, sounds), and documented patient history
Physical Evidence	Items that can be seen, measured, and analyzed
Trace Evidence	Invisible or microscopic items

Reference
1. Foresman-Capuzzi J. CSI & U: Collection and preservation of evidence in the emergency department. J Emerg Nurs. 2014;40(3):229-236.

14.4.1 In collaboration with law enforcement officials, document patterns of blood, residue, marks, or wounds, including the shape and size[127] that are visible before preoperative skin antisepsis, when possible.[126,131] *[Conditional Recommendation]*

Evidence may be removed during preoperative patient skin antisepsis.[126,127]

14.5 Follow local, state, and federal regulations and facility policies and procedures for maintaining the chain of custody and the disposition of potential forensic evidence. *[Recommendation]*

The benefits of following a standard process for securing forensic evidence through a chain of custody include having secured, documented forensic evidence and a record of the possession and location of the evidence from the moment it is collected until it is given to a law enforcement official.[122,124] Incomplete documentation about where the evidence was or who was overseeing it may lead to questions about the evidence being left unattended that may cause the evidence to become inadmissible in court.[122] Regulations or facility policies and procedures may also outline how authorities are contacted regarding the availability of potential forensic evidence when authorities are not already present[126] and the transfer process from the facility to law enforcement personnel.

14.5.1 The process for maintaining the chain of custody for potential forensic evidence while it is within the facility may include
- keeping the number of involved personnel to a minimum,[122,126]
- transferring evidence in a secure manner,[122,124,126,127]
- identifying a secure storage location[127,130] with refrigeration (when needed) for physical forensic evidence,[124-126]
- securing digital informational forensic evidence (eg, photographs) with limited access and password protection,[124]
- recording the name and role of personnel who have contact with the evidence (eg, accessing, transporting),[122-124,126,131] and

- recording the storage location.[122,124,126] *[Conditional Recommendation]*

Low-quality evidence supports managing the chain of custody and the disposition of forensic evidence.[124-126] Reducing the number of personnel involved in the chain of custody may increase confidence in the chain of custody process by decreasing access and transfers of evidence. Having only one person involved in evidence collection and handling creates a single contact for law enforcement officials during an investigation. Personnel who collect or transport evidence may be required to testify in court.[126]

Foresman-Capuzzi[122] recommends that during the exchange of evidence from one person to another, a record of the transfer be created and signed by both individuals. One record of the transfer is kept at the facility and a copy is provided to law enforcement officials.[122]

One author suggested that physical evidence be stored in a secured area (eg, cabinet, drawer, or room) after documentation is complete.[124] Porteous[127] recommended giving evidence directly to law enforcement officials. However, when evidence cannot be given directly to law enforcement officials, facility security, or the pathology laboratory, the author recommended keeping the evidence in a locked area with limited access.[127]

14.5.2 The process for disposition of potential forensic evidence may include transferring evidence to
- law enforcement officials,[119,125,127]
- facility security personnel,[127] or
- pathology laboratory personnel.[124] *[Conditional Recommendation]*

Law enforcement officials have a legal right to obtain evidence believed to be associated with an investigation.[127] One source suggests that evidence that has been contained, labeled, and documented may be given to law enforcement officials upon patient consent, receipt of a warrant, or if the patient is under arrest.[127] When a law enforcement official is not available, the chain of custody process may include a provision to give the evidence to facility security personnel.[127] Recording the facility security officer's name and the date and time of transfer is also recommended.[127]

Disposition of forensic evidence may depend on whether the evidence is contained or imbedded in a surgical specimen. Forensic evidence that is not imbedded in a specimen may be at risk for alteration or interruptions in the chain of custody if it is sent for analysis in the pathology laboratory.[125] Byrne-Dugan et al[124] developed a protocol for pathology laboratories on handling of surgical specimens that contain forensic evidence. According to the CAP,[119] bullets and other medicolegal evidence may be given directly to law enforcement personnel. Evans et al[125] recommended that forensic evidence be collected and transferred to the authorities as soon as possible.

14.5.3 **When transferring potential forensic evidence to law enforcement officials, record the**
- **law enforcement official's name,[131]**
- **law enforcement official's badge number,[131]**
- **date and time of transfer,[127] and**
- **items transferred.[123]**
[Recommendation]

14.6 **Convene an interdisciplinary team (See Recommendation 14.1) to develop policies and procedures for forensic evidence handling, containment, labeling, documentation, chain of custody processes, and disposition.[125,131]** *[Recommendation]*

14.7 **Provide education about forensic evidence management to perioperative personnel.[125]** *[Recommendation]*

Low-quality evidence supports providing education about management of forensic evidence.[125] According to Wick,[126] it is important to understand what evidence is, its significance, and how it is processed. Educating personnel to follow a standardized checklist and policy and procedure documents that are included in a forensic evidence collection kit may increase the likelihood that personnel will perform forensic evidence collection correctly even when it is done infrequently.

15. Placental Tissue

15.1 **Convene an interdisciplinary team that includes a pathologist(s), an obstetrician(s), a perioperative RN(s), an infection preventionist(s), risk management personnel, and a legal professional(s) to develop a policy and procedure for placental tis-**

sue release when requested by the patient. *[Recommendation]*

Low-quality evidence supports having a policy and procedure in place for the release of human placental tissue to the patient or family, when allowed by federal, state, and local regulations.[119,133,134] Placental tissue may be important to patients for cultural, social, or health reasons.[133,134] Motivations for placental tissue requests include burial, consumption, or tissue banking.[133,134]

Baergen et al[133] found that the majority (61.1%) of 36 facilities participating in a survey did not allow release of the placental tissue; however, the researchers also found that the same facilities had never had a request for the tissue to be released. The researchers concluded that development of a policy and procedure for placental tissue release is important because anecdotal evidence from conversations with pathologists suggests that requests for placental tissue release to the patient or family may be increasing.[133]

15.1.1 **Incorporate federal, state, or local regulations for placental specimen management or disposal into the facility policy and procedure.** *[Recommendation]*

Regulations on managing placental tissue (eg, release, disposal, testing, education, required information to be recorded) may vary among states.[134]

15.1.2 **The policy and procedure for placental tissue management may include**
- **indications for submitting placental tissue to the pathology laboratory;**
- **requirements for placental tissue release (eg, noninfectious);**
- **state of placental tissue release (eg, fresh); and**
- **a release form that includes**
  - **patient identifiers, specimen type, signature, date, and a witness signature;**
  - **benefits of pathological examination of placental tissue (when indicated);**
  - **acknowledgment that placental release will prevent pathological examination;**
  - **disclosure that consumption of placental tissue is undertaken without endorsement or judgment from the facility; and**
  - **discussion of safe handling and disposal of tissue.[133]**
[Conditional Recommendation]

According to the CAP,[119] a placenta from an uncomplicated pregnancy may be excluded from routine submission to the pathology laboratory if the placenta appears normal at the time of delivery and the facility has not specified that pathological examination is required.

15.2 Ask the patient about preferences for placental disposition before the procedure (when applicable). *[Recommendation]*

Low-quality evidence supports asking patients about their preference for placental disposition. A nonexperimental study[133] and a qualitative study[134] found that most health care personnel view placental tissue as medical waste.[133,134] However, this assumption may not be accurate if the tissue has a cultural or religious value to the patient.[134] Engaging in cultural rituals that involve the placenta may reduce anxiety for mothers and families.[133,134]

In a qualitative study, Helsel and Mochel[134] found that many Hmong Americans believe in burying the placenta at home, but most were reluctant to ask health care personnel for the placenta. Of the 11 study participants who asked if they could take the placenta home, only five were able to do so.[134] It is important for health care personnel to be aware of how patients feel about placental disposition.[133,134] The researchers recommended that health care personnel be aware of patient beliefs and ask patients about their preferences for placental disposition (when possible).[134]

15.3 Refrigerate placentas that are not disposed of or immediately delivered to the pathology laboratory.[31] *[Recommendation]*

16. Highly Infectious Specimens

16.1 Convene an interdisciplinary team that includes an infection preventionist(s), a pathologist(s), a surgeon(s), a perioperative RN(s), and a surgical technologist(s) to develop a policy and procedure for handling surgical specimens from patients diagnosed with highly infectious diseases (eg, COVID-19, Ebola). *[Recommendation]*

Developing a standardized, interdisciplinary process for handling potentially highly infectious specimens may reduce the risk of exposure to health care personnel. However, this will require an investment of time from the interdisciplinary team to establish a process that may be used infrequently.

16.1.1 Perioperative management of highly infectious specimens may include
- identifying the potential for a highly infectious specimen during procedure scheduling,
- engaging in interdisciplinary communication about scheduled procedures when a highly infectious specimen is anticipated,
- reviewing the specimen management process during the preoperative briefing,

- alerting the pathology laboratory when the procedure has started,
- specifying the required specimen packaging and labeling,
- identifying how and when the specimen will be taken to the pathology laboratory,
- having personnel available for immediate specimen transport,
- using standard precautions during specimen transport,
- calling the pathology laboratory when the specimen is sent,
- giving the specimen directly to a receiving individual (ie, not leaving it in a collection area),
- verbally communicating the potential infectious status of the specimen during in-person **hand over**, and
- following a procedure for communication of specimen results.

[Conditional Recommendation]

16.1.2 Containment, labeling, and transfer of highly infectious specimens may include
- placing the specimen in a rigid, leak-proof specimen container;
- wiping the outside of the container with disinfectant;
- removing gloves and performing hand hygiene after specimen collection and before labeling;
- donning a clean pair of gloves before labeling the container;
- labeling the container;
- placing the container in a second container or bag;
- placing required forms in the outer pocket of the bag;
- following facility policies and procedures for labeling the outer bag or container;
- informing pathology personnel of the anticipated specimen arrival;
- transferring the specimen to personnel outside the room for transport or doffing PPE and exiting the room with the specimen;
- using standard precautions during specimen transport (eg, hand hygiene, PPE); and
- performing direct specimen hand overs and informing the individual receiving the specimen of the known or suspected disease status of the patient.

[Conditional Recommendation]

Having a standardized process for containment, labeling, and transfer of highly infectious specimens may help reduce the risk of exposure to personnel, decrease the risk of a specimen error, and maintain the integrity of the specimen.

No evidence was found to support double bagging of specimens already contained in a leak-proof specimen container. The use of additional bags may increase the risk of exposure to pathology personnel who have to reach inside the extra bag to retrieve a specimen container. The OSHA Bloodborne Pathogen standard requires secondary containment of potentially infectious material to prevent leakage when the outside of the primary container becomes contaminated.[40]

17. Prion Disease Specimens

17.1 **Convene an interdisciplinary team that includes a neuropathologist (when available) or a pathologist(s), a neurological surgeon(s), an epidemiologist (when available), an infection preventionist(s), scheduling personnel, a perioperative RN(s), and a surgical technologist(s) to establish a policy and procedure for handling specimens from patients with known or suspected prion disease.**[135-137] *[Recommendation]*

Establishing a collaborative, interdisciplinary process for handling prion disease specimens, including Creutzfeldt-Jakob disease (CJD), helps ensure that personnel are following a standardized process that meets the needs of all involved disciplines, reduces the risk of exposure to health care personnel, and decreases the risk for specimen errors.

According to the WHO,[135] there have been no confirmed cases of occupational transmission of CJD but there have been cases of CJD in health care personnel that suggest a potential for occupational exposure. Sporadic CJD (sCJD) is the most common type of CJD and the cause is unknown[137]; therefore, it is likely that the health care personnel developed sCJD spontaneously instead acquiring CJD from an occupational exposure.[138]

An extensive literature review of sCJD cases in health care personnel found that they were not at increased risk of sCJD from occupational exposure.[138] However, the authors recommended that personnel use standard precautions when in contact with high-infectivity tissue.[138] The WHO[135] also recommends following infection prevention practices to reduce the risk of exposure and transmission of prion disease to health care personnel to negligible levels. The risk of transmission and the subsequent need for special precautions is dependent on three considerations:

- the probability that a patient is known, suspected, or at risk of developing the disease;
- the level of infectivity in the tissues or fluids of a patient; and

Table 3. Categories of CJD Infectivity by Tissue Type[1]

Infectivity Category	Tissue, Blood, and Body Fluids
High Infectivity	• Brain • Spinal cord • Eye
Low Infectivity	• Cerebrospinal fluid • Kidney • Liver • Lung • Lymph nodes • Spleen • Placenta
No Detectable Infectivity	• Adipose tissue • Adrenal gland • Gingival tissue • Heart muscle • Intestine • Peripheral nerve • Prostate • Skeletal muscle • Testis • Thyroid gland • Blood* • Tears • Nasal mucous • Saliva • Sweat • Serous exudate • Milk • Semen • Urine • Feces

* Evidence on infectivity of blood conflicts. Infectivity in blood has been detected in very small amounts, but transmission of the disease by blood transfusion has not been reported.[1]

Reference

1. WHO Infection Control Guidelines for Transmissible Spongiform Encephalopathies: Report of a WHO Consultation, Geneva, Switzerland, 23-26 March 1999. *Geneva, Switzerland: World Health Organization; 2000.*

- the route of exposure to the tissue.[135]

Patients known, suspected, or at risk of developing CJD present the highest risk for disease transmission.[135] Tissue infectivity is based on the level of detectable infectivity in a specific tissue **(Table 3)**.[135] Although it is always recommended to reduce the risk of exposure of health care personnel to potential pathogens,[40] according to the WHO,[135]

- exposures of high-infectivity tissue to the intact skin or mucous membranes (except the eye) pose negligible risk, and
- exposures of high- or low-infectivity tissue to non-intact skin or mucous membranes (eg, eye splash, needlesticks, scalpel or instrument injuries) pose greater risk.

17.1.1 Use standard precautions and standard specimen handling processes for specimens from patients with known or suspected CJD. *[Recommendation]*

Two guidelines[34,135] and two expert opinion articles[136,137] indicate that standard precautions may be used for all specimens, blood, and body fluids from patients with known or suspected CJD for all levels of tissue infectivity (eg, high, low, none). Standard specimen handling was recommended for specimens from known or suspected CJD patients with high- or low-infectivity levels.[136,137] Therefore, standard specimen handling is also indicated for specimens with no infectivity levels.

17.1.2 Include the following steps when handling high- or low-infectivity specimens from patients with known or suspected CJD:

- notify the pathology laboratory when a patient with potential specimen needs is scheduled (eg, a brain biopsy procedure),[135]
- notify the pathology laboratory about impending specimen arrival,
- conduct in-person specimen hand overs to pathology personnel,
- protect patient privacy and confidentiality during hand overs,[135] and
- include the known or suspected CJD status of the patient during hand-over communication.

[Recommendation]

Two guidelines[34,135] and two expert opinion articles[136,137] address the handling of CJD specimens. Surgical specimen handling may involve different tissue types, but brain biopsy specimens are the most likely from patients known or suspected of having CJD.[135] However, it is not recommended to perform brain biopsies for the diagnosis of CJD[135] or frozen section examinations of high-infectivity tissue from patients known or suspected to have CJD.[136] The WHO[135] recommends that pathology examinations of high- or low-infectivity tissues be handled in a transmissible spongiform encephalopathy laboratory by experienced personnel. In an expert opinion article, Karasin[137] stated that trained personnel at the National Prion Disease Pathology Surveillance Center may be consulted when processing of CJD specimens is necessary. Additional considerations for processing specimens from patients with known or suspected CJD may be necessary in the pathology laboratory[34] (eg, disposable instruments, surface coverings, steel mesh gloves, decontamination and disposal procedures).[135,136] Alerting the pathology laboratory before specimen arrival may allow additional time for personnel to prepare for specimen processing (when necessary).[135]

18. Documentation

18.1 Document specimen management according to regulatory requirements, accrediting body standards, and health care organization policies and procedures. *[Recommendation]*

The benefits of documenting specimen management information include producing a legal record of care delivery (eg, specimen name, disposition), a source of information for other health care professionals in the continuum of care, and data to demonstrate the facility or health care organization's progress toward quality care outcomes.[139]

Regulatory requirements for documentation or recording of specific specimen types are described in **Recommendations 12.1.2, 13.1.1,** and **16.1.1.**

18.2 Document specimen information in the patient's health care record, including

- specimen identification (eg, name, source, tissue type, laterality [when applicable]),
- pathology examination required (eg, gross, frozen section), and
- date and time of specimen collection.

[Recommendation]

18.3 Standardized order sets for specimen management may be used. *[Conditional Recommendation]*

The benefits of developing and using standardized order sets for specimens collected in the OR outweigh the risk. The benefits may include a standard list of orders for specimens frequently collected in the OR that may reduce the risk of specimen errors. However, standardizing order sets requires an investment of time from stakeholders (eg, surgeons, pathologists, information technology personnel).

Low-quality evidence supports the development and use of order sets for specimens collected in the OR.[1,16] The CAP states that a written or electronic request for patient testing from an authorized person is necessary.[31]

18.3.1 The request for specimen testing should include

- two patient identifiers (eg, patient name, medical record number, date of birth);
- the ordering provider's name, address, and other identifiers as necessary (eg, role)
- test(s) to be performed;
- the specimen site or type; and
- the date and time of the procedure or specimen collection.[31]

[Recommendation]

Table 4. Examples of Specimens that May Be Exempt from Submission to the Pathology Laboratory[1]

- Bone donated to the bone bank
- Bone fragments removed during corrective or reconstructive orthopedic procedures (eg, rotator cuff repair), excluding large specimens (eg, femoral heads) and knee, ankle, or elbow reconstructions
- Cataracts removed by phacoemulsification
- Dental appliances
- Fat removed by liposuction
- Foreign bodies (eg, bullets) or other medicolegal evidence given directly to law enforcement personnel
- Foreskin from circumcision of a newborn
- Intrauterine contraceptive devices without attached tissue
- Medical devices (eg, catheters, gastrostomy tubes, myringotomy tubes, stents, sutures) that have not contributed to patient illness, injury, or death
- Middle ear ossicles
- Orthopedic hardware and other radiopaque medical devices, provided there is a policy for documentation of surgical removal
- Placentas from uncomplicated pregnancies that do not meet the facility or health care organization criteria for pathology examination and appear normal at the time of delivery
- Rib segments or other tissues removed for the purpose of gaining surgical access, provided the patient does not have a history of malignancy
- Saphenous vein segments harvested for coronary artery bypass
- Skin or other normal tissue removed during a cosmetic or reconstructive procedure (eg, blepharoplasty, abdominoplasty, rhytidectomy), provided it is not contiguous with a lesion and the patient does not have a history of malignancy
- Teeth with no attached tissue
- Therapeutic radioactive materials
- Toenails and fingernails that are incidentally removed

Reference

1. Appendix M. Surgical specimens to be submitted to pathology for examination. College of American Pathologists. https://webapps.cap.org/apps/docs/laboratory_accreditation/build/pdf/surgical_specimens.pdf. Revised November 2007. Accessed September 28, 2020.

18.3.2 The request for specimen testing may include the
- name and address of the individual to receive the test results (eg, surgeon, primary care physician),
- name and address of the receiving laboratory, and
- procedure performed.[31]

[Conditional Recommendation]

18.4 When documenting by hand is necessary, the handwriting should be legible. *[Recommendation]*

Illegible handwriting can increase the risk of specimen errors.

19. Policies and Procedures

19.1 Convene an interdisciplinary team that includes a pathologist(s), a surgeon(s), a perioperative RN(s), an infection preventionist(s), and other key stakeholders identified by the organization to establish and implement policies and procedures for specimen management, including
- specimens that do not require submission to the pathology laboratory (Table 4)[119];
- specimens that are exempt from microscopic examination (eg, require gross examination only) (Table 5)[119];
- personnel roles and responsibilities[6,15];

- team communication expectations (eg, briefing, hand overs, debriefing);
- selection of PPE based on anticipated exposure to both chemical and biohazardous materials[35,40,52];
- limiting exposure to potentially hazardous chemicals (eg, formaldehyde);
- prevention of specimen compromise or contamination on the sterile field;
- transfer of the specimen from the sterile field;
- containment processes;
- preservation methods (eg, type [formalin], ratio);
- labeling processes;
- requisition form requirements;
- documentation requirements;
- temporary storage methods;
- transport to the pathology laboratory, including after-hours processes;
- requirements for submission of specimens to the pathology laboratory;
- handling for different types of specimens (eg, fresh, permanent, frozen section, gross);
- documentation of removal and disposition of specimens or devices not submitted to the pathology laboratory[119];
- the process for correcting labeling discrepancies (eg, container, requisition form) found during submission to the pathology laboratory[31]; and
- nontraditional specimen management (See Section 15).

[Recommendation]

Table 5. Examples of Specimens that May Be Exempt from Microscopic Examination (eg, Require Gross Examination Only)[1]

- Accessory digits
- Bunions and hammertoes
- Extraocular muscle from corrective surgical procedures (eg, strabismus)
- Inguinal hernia sacs (with specific age requirements determined by the facility or health care organization)
- Nasal bone and cartilage from rhinoplasty or septoplasty
- Prosthetic breast implants
- Prosthetic cardiac valves without attached tissue
- Tonsils and adenoids (with specific age requirements determined by the facility or health care organization)
- Torn meniscus
- Umbilical hernia sacs (with specific age requirements determined by the facility or health care organization)
- Varicose veins

Reference

1. Appendix M. Surgical specimens to be submitted to pathology for examination. College of American Pathologists. https://webapps.cap.org/apps/docs/laboratory_accreditation/build/pdf/surgical_specimens.pdf. Revised November 2007. Accessed September 28, 2020.

A policy and procedure for specimen management developed through a collaborative, interdisciplinary process may reduce the risk for error during all phases of specimen management (eg, preanalytical, analytical, postanalytical). Policies and procedures create a standardized language and tasks that may promote consistent practice and reduce the risk for error.[8]

Moderate-quality evidence supports interdisciplinary collaboration in the development of specimen management facility policy and procedures.[8,16,119,140,141] However, there is conflicting evidence on the types of specimens that may be exempt, sent for gross examination, or routinely sent for histopathology examination.[119,140-143] Both the CAP[119] and the Royal College of Pathologists[140] have documents that discuss different specimen types and the potential level of examination (eg, histopathology, gross) or exemption. There is evidence that routinely sending specimens with a low risk of abnormal pathological examination (eg, histopathology, gross) results may be increasing health care costs.[141-143] Some researchers suggest only sending surgical specimens for pathological examination when there is a clinical suspicion to do so (eg, patient history, findings from procedures).[142,143] Researchers suggest that there is no evidence for the routine submission of all surgical specimens and that judicious use of pathological examination may result in significant savings in health care spending.[142] Conversely, submitting specimens for pathological examination may provide new information for future clinical decision making.[141]

19.2 Develop policies and procedures for communication of urgent diagnoses and significant, unexpected diagnoses. [Recommendation]

A consensus statement from the CAP and the ADASP[30] discusses effective communication of urgent diagnoses and significant, unexpected diagnoses from surgical pathology and cytopathology. The authors recommended that each institution create a policy regarding communication of urgent diagnoses and significant, unexpected diagnoses in anatomic pathology separate from other policies and procedures that discuss communication of critical results (eg, lab values) within a specific period of time (eg, less than 1 hour).[30]

The authors agreed that previous recommendations using the word "critical diagnoses" may have implied a life-threatening condition that necessitated immediate communication of results (eg, within 1 hour).[30] However, pathological examination of specimens may take as long as 24 hours to complete. Additionally, the results of pathological examination are important but do not usually represent immediately life-threatening conditions. Therefore, the results may be considered actionable and noncritical.[30] The ECRI Institute[16] also recommends using a standard process to communicate test results.

19.2.1 The policy and procedure for communication of urgent diagnoses and significant, unexpected diagnoses from the pathology laboratory may include
- the type of communication (eg, verbal, automated);
- a focus on effective and timely communication (eg, as soon as practical);
- a list of urgent diagnoses;
- examples of significant, unexpected diagnoses;
- physician-to-physician communication;
- the escalation process when the ordering physician cannot be reached;
- after-hours processes (eg, weekends);
- documentation of communication; and
- quality assurance audits of the process.[30]

[Conditional Recommendation]

A consensus statement from the CAP and the ADASP[30] states that intraoperative consultations may be excluded from the policy because of well-established expectations for this type of communication. The consensus statement also recommends written documentation of verbal or other communication when reporting urgent diagnoses and significant, unexpected diagnoses. The authors clarified that documentation may be completed in a pathology report **addendum** (eg, by the pathologist) or in an electronic or paper log[30] **(See Recommendation 2.4)**.

20. Education

20.1 Provide education and competency verification activities for perioperative personnel responsible for specimen management that include

- the prevalence and importance of reducing specimen errors (Tables 6 and Table 7);
- factors that contribute to specimen errors (Table 8);
- personnel roles and responsibilities[6,15];
- specimens that do not require submission to the pathology laboratory[119];
- specimens that are exempt from microscopic examination (eg, require gross examination only)[119];
- preoperative assessment;
- team communication expectations (eg, briefing, hand overs, debriefing);
- prevention of specimen compromise or contamination on the sterile field;
- selection and use of PPE based on anticipated exposure[35,40,52];
- transfer of specimens from the sterile field;
- handling of
  - specimens for different examination methods (eg, fresh, permanent, frozen section, gross),
  - different tissue types (eg, breast cancer, placentas),
  - radioactive specimens,
  - explanted devices,
  - forensic evidence (when applicable),
  - highly infectious specimens, and
  - prion disease specimens;
- containment processes;
- preservation methods;
- limiting exposure to potentially hazardous chemicals (eg, formaldehyde);
- labeling processes;
- requisition form requirements;
- documentation expectations;
- temporary storage methods;
- transport to the pathology laboratory, including after-hours processes;
- using a pneumatic tube system (if applicable);
- expectations for submission of specimens to the pathology laboratory;

- using specialized equipment (eg, fluorescence)[144]; and
- documentation of removal and disposition of specimens or devices not submitted to the pathology laboratory.[119]
[Recommendation]

Moderate-quality evidence supports educating personnel involved in specimen management.[1,6,8,11,15,16] Steelman et al[1] found that 38% of factors contributing to specimen management errors resulted from a lack of knowledge, training, or experience. The researchers recommended providing training during orientation, annually, and when policies and procedures are updated.[1]

D'Angelo and Mejabi[11] stated that one of the problems identified in their quality improvement project was the failure to educate and assess competency of personnel involved in specimen management. The Pennsylvania Patient Safety Advisory[8] recommends education that clarifies roles and responsibilities with observations of performance that confirm competencies are maintained.

In an organizational experience article, Meier et al[145] reviewed amended pathology reports and found a decrease in identification errors from 15.6% to 8.7% during the 4-year period of a process improvement project. One part of the project involved providing education on specimen labeling processes to personnel involved in specimen collection. However, the authors reported that the education had only a modest effect on reducing the rate of misidentification.[145] The authors stated that this finding emphasizes how misidentification errors can occur in all phases of the specimen management process.[145] Awareness and education, although important, are just one part of a multifocal process used to reduce specimen errors.

Similarly, Rees et al[15] stated that education alone was not enough to change practice. As a result of that finding, the organization in this article started a feedback process that involved the manager or director discussing with the involved personnel the circumstances of the specimen error and possible preventive measures to use in the future.[15]

20.2 Provide education to perioperative personnel who are involved in the research specimen collection process. *[Recommendation]*

The benefits of providing education for personnel on the specimen collection process for research include an understanding of the processes used for research specimen collection in the facility, a decrease in time spent during the patient assessment and specimen collection process, and assurance that specimens retain viability for research purposes.

Table 6. Negative Consequences of Specimen Management Errors

Category	Examples
Patient Harm[1-8]	• Physical or psychological injury to the patient • Increased morbidity and mortality • Extended length of stay
Diagnosis[1,5,8-10]	• Delayed diagnosis • Incomplete diagnosis • Inaccurate diagnosis
Treatment or Procedures[1-8,10,11]	• Delayed treatment • Less-than-ideal treatment • Unnecessary or inappropriate treatment • No treatment • Additional procedures
Harm to Health Care Personnel or the Facility[1-3,5-7]	• Personnel exposure to blood and other potentially infectious materials • Lengthy investigations that waste time and resources • Additional costs • Potential litigation • Community distrust

References

1. *Steelman VM, Williams TL, Szekendi MK, Halverson AL, Dintzis SM, Pavkovic S. Surgical specimen management: a descriptive study of 648 adverse events and near misses. Arch Pathol Lab Med. 2016;140(12):1390-1396.*
2. *Makary MA, Epstein J, Pronovost PJ, Millman EA, Hartmann EC, Freischlag JA. Surgical specimen identification errors: a new measure of quality in surgical care. Surgery. 2007;141(4):450-455. .*
3. *Bixenstine PJ, Zarbo RJ, Holzmueller CG, et al. Developing and pilot testing practical measures of preanalytic surgical specimen identification defects. Am J Med Qual. 2013;28(4):308-314.*
4. *Valenstein PN, Sirota RL. Identification errors in pathology and laboratory medicine. Clin Lab Med. 2004;24(4):979-996.*
5. *Lost surgical specimens, lost opportunities. PA-PSRS Patient Safety Advisory. 2005;2(3):1-5.*
6. *D'Angelo R, Mejabi O. Getting it right for patient safety: specimen collection process improvement from operating room to pathology. Am J Clin Pathol. 2016;146(1):8-17.*
7. *Dock B. Improving the accuracy of specimen labeling. Clin Lab Sci. 2005;18(4):210-212.*
8. *They Don't Make the Cut: Lost, Mislabeled, and Unsuitable Surgical Specimens. Event Reporting & Analysis – Alerts. West Conshohocken, PA: ECRI Institute; 2017.*
9. *Zervakis Brent MA. OR specimen labeling. AORN J. 2016;103(2):164-176.*
10. *Nakhleh RE, Idowu MO, Souers RJ, Meier FA, Bekeris LG. Mislabeling of cases, specimens, blocks, and slides: a College of American Pathologists study of 136 institutions. Arch Pathol Lab Med. 2011;135(8):969-974.*
11. Where Do Most Lab Errors Occur? Not the Lab. *PSO Monthly Brief. West Conshohocken, PA: ECRI Institute; 2012.*

 20.2.1 Education on the research specimen collection process may include

- the role of the perioperative RN and surgical technologist,
- how to identify patients who are enrolled in research studies,
- types of surgical specimens that are currently being collected for research,
- procedures in the organization that may involve research specimens,
- surgeons who are participating in research for which specimen collection may occur,
- additional supplies required for research specimens,
- institutional review board approval processes,
- research informed consent or assent processes,
- protection of patient confidentiality and anonymity,
- research specimen handling processes (eg, containment, timing),
- use or avoidance of preservative agents (eg, formalin),
- labeling processes for research specimens that differ from standard processes,
- forms required for the research specimen,
- institutional policies and procedures for documentation of research specimens,
- collection or transporting processes,
- contact information for personnel involved in collecting the specimens (when applicable),
- preoperative and postoperative hand-over communications when research specimens and interventions are involved, and
- facility policies and procedures related to research and research specimens.

[Conditional Recommendation]

Tissue specimens used for research may be collected during procedures. However, perioperative personnel may not be aware of the processes for research specimen collection or the related ethical considerations. Tissue collection, handling, and timing may be sensitive in research studies and affect tissue viability and study outcomes.[146]

21. Quality

21.1 **Use FMEA or other quality improvement tools to proactively identify specimen management processes with high risk for error.** *[Recommendation]*

Low-quality evidence recommends using proactive methods to identify processes prone to error to prevent errors from occurring.[1,4,9,12,16] Processes prone to risk in specimen handling include labeling, collection, preservation, transport, and reporting of test results.[1,9] In an organizational experience article, Dock[12] describes the implementation of an FMEA process for specimen handling that reduced specimen labeling errors by 75%. Zervakis Brent[4] also used an FMEA process to determine the parts of the specimen management process most prone to error. The FMEA process revealed that the facility's procedures that were most likely to lead to mislabeled specimens included

- labeling of containers,
- completing pathology requisition forms, and
- transferring the specimen off the sterile field.[4]

21.2 **Report near misses and errors in specimen management according to facility policies and procedures.** *[Recommendation]*

Moderate-quality evidence supports reporting specimen errors and near miss events.[1,2,7,15,16,26] Reporting errors and near misses helps identify contributing factors and determine the root cause.[1,26] The CAP recommends maintaining error records.[31]

21.3 **Monitor the rate, type, phase (eg, preanalytical), contributing factors, and level of harm for specimen errors and near miss events.** *[Recommendation]*

High-quality evidence supports monitoring specimen errors and near miss events.[1-4,6,7,15] Monitoring may increase attention to the problem and help decrease error rates without additional interventions.[145] Specimen error rates may be an important surgical quality indicator.[2] Specimen error rates between 0.43% and 2.9% have been reported.[2-4] Steelman et al[1] found that most specimen management errors were near miss events (43%) or involved emotional distress or inconvenience (49%).

The literature described three ways in which specimen error data were collected. The methods included incident reports,[1,4] amended pathology reports,[5,6,145,147,148] and data collected when specimens were submitted to the pathology laboratory.[2,3,11]

Pathology laboratory personnel may perform reviews of amended reports or addendums as a form of quality assurance and improvement.[145,147,148] Pathology report amendment rates have been reported between 0.47% to 0.99%.[145,147,148] **Amendments**

include misidentifications (eg, patient identifiers, tissue type, site, laterality) and other errors that are not related the preanalytical phase.[145,147,148] Additionally, misidentification rates in pathology report amendments may include identification errors that occurred in the analytical phase (eg, during accession, slide labeling, gross dictation).[145,147,148] Reported misidentification rates from pathology reports are between 13.3% to 19%.[145,147,148] A detailed discussion of the efficacy of using pathology report amendments compared to addendums is outside the scope of this document but is examined in the literature.[5,145,148]

21.3.1 **A standardized format may be used for reporting event types and levels of patient harm.** *[Conditional Recommendation]*

Low-quality evidence indicates the need for a standardized format for event reporting.[1,5,7] Steelman et al[1] used a database that incorporated the Agency for Healthcare Research and Quality common format. The common format uses a standardized taxonomy of event types and harm scales.[1]

21.4 **Evaluate data reported on specimen errors, including near miss incidents and determine root causes in collaboration with an interdisciplinary team that includes perioperative RNs, pathologists, surgeons, risk and quality management personnel, and an infection preventionist.** *[Recommendation]*

Moderate-quality evidence supports data analysis of reported specimen errors.[1-3,7,14,15,26] Reviewing the rate, type, phase, contributing factors, and level of harm for errors and near miss events may provide an in-depth understanding of the incident.[1,7] Sandbank et al[26] found that using a root cause analysis process helped to identify why specimen errors had occurred. The ECRI Institute[14] recommends monitoring incidents related to specimen errors, especially near misses, and using these reports as a patient safety measure for quality improvement projects.

Makary et al[2] collected patient errors data as part of a screening process during intake at the pathology laboratory. A quality improvement nurse was notified when specimen errors occurred and investigated the occurrence to correct the error. The researchers reported that the process was inexpensive, feasible, and provided valid measurements. Investigating errors may help facilities learn and improve.[2] The process of specimen error correction can take valuable time and resources.[3]

Table 7. Types of Specimen Errors in the Preanalytical Phase

Category	Examples
Collection[1-5]	• Not collected • No specimen in the container • Wrong container • No solution or preservative • Wrong solution • Solution should not have been added • Incorrect technique
Container or Requisition Labeling[1-3,5-10]	• Missing label • Inaccurate, incomplete, or illegible label • Missing procedure time • Missing tissue • Missing tissue site • Wrong patient (eg, label, name, number) • Missing patient identifiers • Wrong tissue or specimen • Wrong site • Wrong side • Inaccurate, incomplete, or illegible requisition form • Specimen label and requisition form do not match
Requisition Forms[1,3,5,7,8]	• Missing requisition form • Number of specimens does not match requisition form data
Storage[1,5]	• Stored in the wrong place • Wrong storage method • Not refrigerated
Transport[1,3-5]	• Delay • Not received • Not sent to the laboratory • Delivered to the wrong place • Leaking or spilled solution • Compromised or broken specimen • Pneumatic tube system delivery instead of hand delivery • Delivered without communication
Quality[1,5,10]	• Quantity not sufficient • Poor quality • Possible contamination

References

1. Steelman VM, Williams TL, Szekendi MK, Halverson AL, Dintzis SM, Pavkovic S. Surgical specimen management: a descriptive study of 648 adverse events and near misses. Arch Pathol Lab Med. 2016;140(12):1390-1396.
2. Makary MA, Epstein J, Pronovost PJ, Millman EA, Hartmann EC, Freischlag JA. Surgical specimen identification errors: a new measure of quality in surgical care. Surgery. 2007;141(4):450-455.
3. Bixenstine PJ, Zarbo RJ, Holzmueller CG, et al. Developing and pilot testing practical measures of preanalytic surgical specimen identification defects. Am J Med Qual. 2013;28(4):308-314.
4. Lost surgical specimens, lost opportunities. PA-PSRS Patient Safety Advisory. 2005;2(3):1-5.
5. They Don't Make the Cut: Lost, Mislabeled, and Unsuitable Surgical Specimens. Event Reporting & Analysis – Alerts. West Conshohocken, PA: ECRI Institute; 2017.
6. Zervakis Brent MA. OR specimen labeling. AORN J. 2016;103(2):164-176.
7. Valenstein PN, Sirota RL. Identification errors in pathology and laboratory medicine. Clin Lab Med. 2004;24(4):979-996.
8. D'Angelo R, Mejabi O. Getting it right for patient safety: specimen collection process improvement from operating room to pathology. Am J Clin Pathol. 2016;146(1):8-17.
9. Rees S, Stevens L, Mikelsons D, Quam E, Darcy T. Reducing specimen identification errors. J Nurs Care Qual. 2012;27(3):253-257.
10. Where Do Most Lab Errors Occur? Not the Lab. PSO Monthly Brief. West Conshohocken, PA: ECRI Institute; 2012.

Table 8. Factors that May Contribute to Errors in Specimen Management	
Category	**Examples**
Communication[1-4]	• Communication deficits during hand over • Communication deficits during the read-back process when transferring specimens off the sterile field • Communication deficits during the debriefing • Unclear or poor communication • Lack of communication
Lack of Standardization[1,2,4]	• Multiple methods for specimen management • Process variation or lack of standard process • Unclear or deficient policies and procedures • Practice that does not meet professional standards
Process Complexity[1-4]	• Lack of knowledge of how to spell specimen names • Failure to ask for the correct spelling of specimen names • Confusion with multiple specimens • Specimens that require special handling • Inability to label specimens immediately • Inability to fill out requisition forms immediately • Repetitive tasks • Redundant documentation • Redundant lists of specimens • Complex or time-consuming order entry or documentation • Labels from the previous patient left in the room • Distractions and interruptions • Emergency management • Inattention • Poor lighting • Staffing issues (eg, adequate number of personnel, staffing mix, float or agency personnel)
Knowledge[1,3,4]	• Lack of knowledge, training, or experience • Lack of knowledge of policies and procedures • Failure to educate and assess competency

References

1. *Steelman VM, Williams TL, Szekendi MK, Halverson AL, Dintzis SM, Pavkovic S. Surgical specimen management: a descriptive study of 648 adverse events and near misses.* Arch Pathol Lab Med. *2016;140(12):1390-1396.*
2. *Zervakis Brent MA. OR specimen labeling.* AORN J. *2016;103(2):164-176.*
3. *Valenstein PN, Sirota RL. Identification errors in pathology and laboratory medicine.* Clin Lab Med. *2004;24(4):979-996.*
4. *D'Angelo R, Mejabi O. Getting it right for patient safety: specimen collection process improvement from operating room to pathology.* Am J Clin Pathol. *2016;146(1):8-17.*

21.5 Implement changes in specimen management based on recommendations from interdisciplinary team meetings on data and root cause analysis results. *[Recommendation]*

Low-quality evidence supports implementation of changes in specimen management based on root cause analysis data.[8,26] Sandbank et al[26] implemented changes in specimen management after a root cause analysis of data on specimen errors at their institution. Even though most errors occur in the preanalytical phase, an expert opinion article from the ECRI Institute[9] recommended that strategies to reduce specimen errors include all phases and stakeholders. D'Angelo and Mejabi[11] recommended redesigning processes to simplify them; reduce variation, redundancies, and time; and create efficient,

standardized procedures that reduce the likelihood of errors.

21.6 Include perioperative and pathology personnel in patient safety and quality improvement initiatives. *[Recommendation]*

Moderate-quality evidence suggests including personnel involved in the specimen management process in improvement initiatives.[3,4,9,11-13,16] According to D'Angelo and Mejabi,[11] specimen collection procedures may be poorly designed and the individuals involved may have little control of the process. The authors recommended reviewing the whole specimen management process in the areas where the work occurs and involving personnel who do the work in the improvement process.[11]

Dock[12] also observed specimen labeling processes and interviewed personnel involved. The project resulted in increased employee and surgeon satisfaction and improved communication.[12] Extensive change often requires adjustments of personal values, attitudes, beliefs, and behaviors.[3] Therefore, collaborating with personnel about process changes may decrease the length of time it takes personnel to adopt the new procedures. Zervakis Brent[4] reported that project success is dependent on acceptance, support, and buy-in from team members involved in the process, including leaders in the involved departments.

21.6.1 | **Use a systems approach to reduce the risk of specimen errors.** [*Recommendation*]

Low-quality evidence supports using a systems approach when implementing strategies to reduce the risk of specimen errors.[6-8,11] A systems approach focuses on specimen management errors from a systems level and reduces the likelihood of viewing specimen errors as caused by specific individuals.[8] According to the Pennsylvania Patient Safety Advisory,[8] the root cause of specimen errors is more likely to be organizational processes that increase the likelihood of unintentional error by individuals. A systems approach may reveal patterns in specimen errors or near misses that highlight areas of opportunity for organizational change.[8] A focus on a systems approach may also encourage reporting and problem solving when issues arise.[8] Bixenstine et al[3] reported that efforts to reduce specimen errors require a multifaceted approach.

Glossary

Addendum: Information added to an unchanged original pathology report.

Agreement State: Any state with which the Nuclear Regulatory Commission or the Atomic Energy Commission has entered into a covenant under the Atomic Energy Act of 1954.

Amendment: A change in information on a pathology report after the report has been finalized.

Analytical phase: Processes for specimen analysis that occur within the pathology laboratory (eg, gross examination, microscopic examination).

Assay: A procedure for measuring the presence or amount of a drug or biochemical substance in a sample. The substance being measured is considered the target of the assay.

Authorized user (of radioactive materials): A physician, a person who has received special training, or a person who is credentialed to use radioactive materials and who understands radiation physics, radiobiology, radiation safety, and radiation management.

Autolysis: The destruction of cells or tissue of an organism by substances produced within the organism.

Chain of custody: A process used to maintain, secure, and document the chronological history and persons in possession of evidence that allows the evidence to be legally accepted in court.

Cold ischemic time: The period of time between removal of the specimen and placement into preservative.

Deep-dose equivalent: The dose equivalent at a tissue depth of 1 cm; applies to the external whole body exposure.

Error: An unintended act of omission (ie, failing to perform an action) or commission (ie, performing an action that results in harm).

Failure Modes and Effects Analysis: A proactive, systematic method for guiding a team in evaluating a process to determine how the process may fail, how likely the failure is to occur, and what the severity of the consequence may be for the failure. This information is used to inform improvement effort prioritization and strategies to prevent process failures.

Forensic evidence: Evidence for use in legal or criminal proceedings.

Gross examination: The inspection of surgical specimens by a pathologist using only visual examination to obtain diagnostic information.

Hand over: The transfer of patient information from one person to another during transitions of care. Synonym: hand off.

Postanalytical phase: Processes that occur after the specimen has been analyzed in the pathology laboratory (eg, recording and relaying the interpretation to the clinician).

Preanalytical phase: Processes that occur before the specimen reaches the pathology laboratory for analysis (eg, transfer of information from the physician to the perioperative RN during the procedure, labeling, containment, transport).

Radio-frequency identification: A system that transmits the identity (in the form of a unique serial number) of an object wirelessly using radio waves.

Read-back method: A dialogue in which the listener verbally repeats patient information so that the sender can confirm the accuracy of the message.

Root cause analysis: A retrospective process for identifying basic or causal factor(s) underlying variation in performance, including the occurrence or possible occurrence of a sentinel event.

Sentinel event: An unanticipated incident involving death or serious physical or psychological injury or the risk of serious injury or an adverse outcome.

Significant, unexpected diagnosis: A medical condition that is clinically unusual or unforeseen and should be addressed at some point in the patient's course.

Site identification: The act or process of positively establishing or confirming the location of tissue, foreign objects, or body substances to be removed from the patient and sent for pathology examination.

Specimen: Tissue, foreign objects, or body substances removed from a patient and sent for pathology examination.

Specimen collection: The act or process of obtaining a biopsy or resecting a specimen.

Specimen containment: The act or process of securing a specimen by placing it in a container used for storage or transport.

Specimen disposition: The act of positioning or distributing tissue, foreign bodies, explanted items, or body fluids removed from a patient for pathology examination.

Specimen handling: The act or process of holding, securing, moving, or manipulating a specimen.

Specimen labeling: The process of affixing information to a container that establishes or indicates the specifications or characteristics of the enclosed sample.

Specimen preservation: The act or process of protecting a specimen to maintain morphology, reduce the loss of molecular components, prevent decomposition and autolysis, and prevent microbial growth.

Specimen transfer: The process of moving a specimen from the sterile field to the containment device.

Specimen transport: The act of carrying or conveying a specimen from one location to another.

Total effective dose equivalent: The sum of deep-dose equivalent (ie, external exposures) and the committed effective dose equivalent (ie, internal exposures) of radiation.

Unique device identifier: A unique alphanumeric or numeric code consisting of a device identifier (DI) and product information (PI).

Urgent diagnosis: A medical condition that, in most cases, should be addressed as soon as possible.

Warm ischemic time: The time required for arterial ligation and removal of a specimen.

Written directive: A written order from an authorized user for the administration of by-product material or radiation from by-product material to a specific patient, as specified in 10 CFR 35.40(a) and (b)(6) or the equivalent state agreement.

References

1. Steelman VM, Williams TL, Szekendi MK, Halverson AL, Dintzis SM, Pavkovic S. Surgical specimen management: a descriptive study of 648 adverse events and near misses. *Arch Pathol Lab Med.* 2016;140(12):1390-1396. [IIIA]

2. Makary MA, Epstein J, Pronovost PJ, Millman EA, Hartmann EC, Freischlag JA. Surgical specimen identification errors: a new measure of quality in surgical care. *Surgery.* 2007;141(4):450-455. [IIIA]

3. Bixenstine PJ, Zarbo RJ, Holzmueller CG, et al. Developing and pilot testing practical measures of preanalytic surgical specimen identification defects. *Am J Med Qual.* 2013;28(4):308-314. [IIIB]

4. Zervakis Brent MA. OR specimen labeling. *AORN J.* 2016;103(2):164-176. [VB]

5. Cooper K. Errors and error rates in surgical pathology: an Association of Directors of Anatomic and Surgical Pathology survey. *Arch Pathol Lab Med.* 2006;130(5):607-609. [IIIC]

6. Novis DA. Detecting and preventing the occurrence of errors in the practices of laboratory medicine and anatomic pathology: 15 years' experience with the College of American Pathologists' Q-PROBES and Q-TRACKS programs. *Clin Lab Med.* 2004;24(4):965-978. [VB]

7. Valenstein PN, Sirota RL. Identification errors in pathology and laboratory medicine. *Clin Lab Med.* 2004;24(4):979-996. [VA]

8. Lost surgical specimens, lost opportunities. *PA-PSRS Patient Safety Advisory.* 2005;2(3):1-4. [VA]

9. Ask HRC: Best practices for specimen handling. ECRI Institute. https://www.ecri.org/components/HRC/Pages/AskHRC072417.aspx. Published July 24, 2017. Accessed September 28, 2020. [VA]

10. Nakhleh RE, Idowu MO, Souers RJ, Meier FA, Bekeris LG. Mislabeling of cases, specimens, blocks, and slides: a College of American Pathologists study of 136 institutions. *Arch Pathol Lab Med.* 2011;135(8):969-974. [IIIB]

11. D'Angelo R, Mejabi O. Getting it right for patient safety: specimen collection process improvement from operating room to pathology. *Am J Clin Pathol.* 2016;146(1):8-17. [VA]

12. Dock B. Improving the accuracy of specimen labeling. *Clin Lab Sci.* 2005;18(4):210-212. [VB]

13. *Patient Identification Errors.* Health Technology Assessment Information Service: Special Report. West Conshohocken, PA: ECRI Institute; 2016. [VA]

14. *They Don't Make the Cut: Lost, Mislabeled, and Unsuitable Surgical Specimens.* Event Reporting & Analysis – Alerts. West Conshohocken, PA: ECRI Institute; 2017. [VA]

15. Rees S, Stevens L, Mikelsons D, Quam E, Darcy T. Reducing specimen identification errors. *J Nurs Care Qual.* 2012;27(3):253-257. [VB]

16. *Where Do Most Lab Errors Occur? Not the Lab.* PSO Monthly Brief. West Conshohocken, PA: ECRI Institute; 2012. [VB]

17. 42 CFR 493: Laboratory requirements. Electronic Code of Federal Regulations. https://www.ecfr.gov/cgi-bin/text-idx?node=pt42.5.493&rgn=div5. Accessed September 28, 2020.

18. Guideline for a safe environment of care. In: *Guidelines for Perioperative Practice.* Denver, CO: AORN, Inc; 2020:115-150. [IVA].

19. Guideline for autologous tissue management. In: *Guidelines for Perioperative Practice.* Denver, CO: AORN, Inc; 2020:1-34. [IVA]

20. Guideline for radiation safety. In: *Guidelines for Perioperative Practice.* Denver, CO: AORN, Inc; 2020:715-754. [IVA]

21. Nemeth SA, Lawrence N. Site identification challenges in dermatologic surgery: a physician survey. *J Am Acad Dermatol.* 2012;67(2):262-268. [IIIB]

22. Rossy KM, Lawrence N. Difficulty with surgical site identification: what role does it play in dermatology? *J Am Acad Dermatol.* 2012;67(2):257-261. [IIIB]

23. McGinness JL, Goldstein G. The value of preoperative biopsy-site photography for identifying cutaneous lesions. *Dermatol Surg.* 2010;36(2):194-197. [IIIB]

24. Ke M, Moul D, Camouse M, et al. Where is it? The utility of biopsy-site photography. *Dermatol Surg.* 2010;36(2):198-202. [IIIC]

25. Guideline for team communication. In: *Guidelines for Perioperative Practice.* Denver, CO: AORN, Inc; 2020:1039-1070. [IVA]

26. Sandbank S, Klein D, Westreich M, Shalom A. The loss of pathological specimens: incidence and causes. *Dermatol Surg.* 2010;36(7):1084-1086. [VB]

27. Martis WR, Hannam JA, Lee T, Merry AF, Mitchell SJ. Improved compliance with the World Health Organization Surgical Safety Checklist is associated with reduced surgical specimen labelling errors. *N Z Med J.* 2016;129(1441):63-67. [VA]

28. *Implementation Manual WHO Surgical Safety Checklist 2009: Safe Surgery Saves Lives.* Geneva, Switzerland: World Health Organization; 2009. [IVA]

29. Makary MA, Holzmueller CG, Sexton JB, et al. Operating room debriefings. *Jt Comm J Qual Patient Saf.* 2006;32(7):407-410, 357. [VB]

30. Nakhleh RE, Myers JL, Allen TC, et al. Consensus statement on effective communication of urgent diagnoses and significant, unexpected diagnoses in surgical pathology and cytopathology from the College of American Pathologists and Association of Directors of Anatomic and Surgical Pathology. *Arch Pathol Lab Med.* 2012;136(2):148-154. [IVA]

31. Lott R, Tunnicliffe J, Sheppard E, et al. *Pre-Microscopic Examination Specimen Handling Guidelines in the Surgical Pathology Laboratory.* 8.0th ed. Northfield, IL: College of American Pathologists; 2018. [IVB]

32. Guideline for sterile technique. In: *Guidelines for Perioperative Practice.* Denver, CO: AORN, Inc; 2020:917-958. [IVA]

33. Makki D, Abdalla S, El Gamal TA, Harvey D, Jackson G, Platt S. Is it necessary to change instruments between sampling sites when taking multiple tissue specimens in musculoskeletal infections? *Ann R Coll Surg Engl.* 2018;100(7):563-565. [IIC]

34. Siegel JD, Rhinehart E, Jackson M, Chiarello L; Healthcare Infection Control Practices Advisory Committee, eds. *2007 Guidelines for Isolation Precautions: Preventing Transmission of Infectious Agents In Healthcare Settings.* Updated July 2019. Atlanta, GA: Centers for Disease Control and Prevention: Healthcare Infection Control Practices Advisory Committee; 2019. [IVA]

35. Guideline for transmission-based precautions. In: *Guidelines for Perioperative Practice.* Denver, CO: AORN, Inc; 2020:1071-1100. [IVA]

36. Bussolati G, Annaratone L, Maletta F. The pre-analytical phase in surgical pathology. *Recent Results Cancer Res.* 2015;199:1-13. [VB]

37. Comanescu M, Annaratone L, D'Armento G, Cardos G, Sapino A, Bussolati G. Critical steps in tissue processing in histopathology. *Recent Pat DNA Gene Seq.* 2012;6(1):22-32. [VB]

38. Francis DL, Prabhakar S, Sanderson SO. A quality initiative to decrease pathology specimen-labeling errors using radiofrequency identification in a high-volume endoscopy center. *Am J Gastroenterol.* 2009;104(4):972-975. [IIIB]

39. Snyder SR, Favoretto AM, Derzon JH, et al. Effectiveness of barcoding for reducing patient specimen and laboratory testing identification errors: a Laboratory Medicine Best Practices systematic review and meta-analysis. *Clin Biochem.* 2012;45(13-14):988-998. [IIIB]

40. 29 CFR 1910.1030: Bloodborne pathogens. Occupational Safety and Health Administration. https://www.osha.gov/pls/oshaweb/owadisp.show_document?p_id=10051&p_table=STANDARDS. Accessed September 28, 2020.

41. Berton F, Di Novi C. Occupational hazards of hospital personnel: assessment of a safe alternative to formaldehyde. *J Occup Health.* 2012;54(1):74-78. [IB]

42. Condelli V, Lettini G, Patitucci G, et al. Validation of vacuum-based refrigerated system for biobanking tissue preservation: analysis of cellular morphology, protein stability, and RNA quality. *Biopreserv Biobank.* 2014;12(1):35-45. [IB]

43. Veneroni S, Dugo M, Daidone MG, et al. Applicability of under vacuum fresh tissue sealing and cooling to omics analysis of tumor tissues. *Biopreserv Biobank.* 2016;14(6):480-490. [IIB]

44. Kristensen T, Engvad B, Nielsen O, Pless T, Walter S, Bak M. Vacuum sealing and cooling as methods to preserve surgical specimens. *Appl Immunohistochem Mol Morphol.* 2011;19(5):460-469. [IIB]

45. Annaratone L, Marchiò C, Russo R, et al. A collection of primary tissue cultures of tumors from vacuum packed and cooled surgical specimens: a feasibility study. *PLoS One.* 2013;8(9):e75193. [IIIB]

46. Saliceti R, Nicodemo E, Giannini A, Cortese A. Health Technology Assessment: introducing a vacuum-based preservation system for biological materials in the anatomic pathology workflow. *Pathologica.* 2016;108(1):20-27. [VA]

47. Zarbo RJ. Histologic validation of vacuum sealed, formalin-free tissue preservation, and transport system. *Recent Results Cancer Res.* 2015;199:15-26. [VA]

48. Di Novi C, Minniti D, Barbaro S, Zampirolo MG, Cimino A, Bussolati G. Vacuum-based preservation of surgical specimens: an environmentally-safe step towards a formalin-free hospital. *Sci Total Environ.* 2010;408(16):3092-3095. [VB]

49. Dämmrich ME, Kreipe HH. Standardized processing of native tissue in breast pathology. *Recent Results Cancer Res.* 2015;199:45-53. [VC]

50. *Recommended Practices for Safety and Health Programs.* Washington, DC: Occupational Safety and Health Administration; 2016. [IVA]

51. Zeugner S, Mayr T, Zietz C, Aust DE, Baretton GB. RNA quality in fresh-frozen gastrointestinal tumor specimens—experiences from the tumor and healthy tissue bank TU Dresden. *Recent Results Cancer Res.* 2015;199:85-93. [IB]

52. 29 CFR 1910.1048: Formaldehyde. Occupational Safety and Health Administration. https://www.osha.gov/pls/oshaweb/owadisp.show_document?p_id=10075&p_table=STANDARDS. Accessed September 28, 2020.

53. Bell WC, Young ES, Billings PE, Grizzle WE. The efficient operation of the surgical pathology gross room. *Biotechnic & Histochemistry.* 2008;83(2):71-82. [VB]

54. Trask L, Tournas E. Barcode specimen collection improves patient safety. *MLO Med Lab Obs.* 2012;44(4):42, 44-45. [VB]

55. Granata J. Getting a handle on specimen mislabeling. *J Emerg Nurs.* 2011;37(2):167-168. [VC]

56. Hill PM, Mareiniss D, Murphy P, et al. Significant reduction of laboratory specimen labeling errors by implementation of an electronic ordering system paired with a bar-code specimen labeling process. *Ann Emerg Med.* 2010;56(6):630-636. [IIIB]

57. Colard D. Reduction of patient identification errors using technology. *Point Care.* 2005;4(1):61-63. [VB]

58. Bostwick DG. Radiofrequency identification specimen tracking in anatomical pathology: pilot study of 1067 consecutive prostate biopsies. *Ann Diagn Pathol.* 2013;17(5):391-402. [VA]

59. Radio frequency identification (RFID). US Food and Drug Administration. https://www.fda.gov/radiation-emitting-products/electromagnetic-compatibility-emc/radio-frequency-identification-rfid. Accessed September 28, 2020. [VA]

60. *ANSI/HIBC 4.0: The Health Industry Supplier Standard for RFID Product Identification.* Phoenix, AZ: Health Industry Business Communications Council; 2009. [IVB]

61. Buesa RJ, Peshkov MV. How much formalin is enough to fix tissues? *Ann Diagn Pathol.* 2012;16(3):202-209. [IIB]

62. Yaziji H, Taylor CR, Goldstein NS, et al. Consensus recommendations on estrogen receptor testing in breast cancer by immunohistochemistry. *Appl Immunohistochem Mol Morphol.* 2008;16(6):513-520. [IVB]

63. Titford ME, Horenstein MG. Histomorphologic assessment of formalin substitute fixatives for diagnostic surgical pathology. *Arch Pathol Lab Med.* 2005;129(4):502-506. [IIB]

64. Prentø P, Lyon H. Commercial formalin substitutes for histopathology. *Biotech Histochem.* 1997;72(5):273-282. [IIB]

65. OSHA fact sheet: Formaldehyde. https://www.osha.gov/OshDoc/data_General_Facts/formaldehyde-factsheet.html. Accessed September 28, 2020.

66. *Formaldehyde, 2-Butoxyethanol and 1-tert-Butoxypropan-2-ol.* IARC Monographs on the Evaluation of Carcinogenic Risks to Humans; No. 88. Lyon, France: World Health Organization: International Agency for Research on Cancer; 2006. [IVA]

67. Buesa RJ. Histology without formalin? *Ann Diagn Pathol.* 2008;12(6):387-396. [VA]

68. van Essen HF, Verdaasdonk MAM, Elshof SM, de Weger RA, van Diest PJ. Alcohol based tissue fixation as an alternative for formaldehyde: influence on immunohistochemistry. *J Clin Pathol.* 2010;63(12):1090-1094. [IIB]

69. Gillespie JW, Best CJ, Bichsel VE, et al. Evaluation of nonformalin tissue fixation for molecular profiling studies. *Am J Pathol.* 2002;160(2):449-457. [IIB]

70. Ozkan N, Salva E, Cakalağaoğlu F, Tüzüner B. Honey as a substitute for formalin? *Biotech Histochem.* 2012;87(2):148-153. [IIC]

71. Al-Maaini R, Bryant P. The effectiveness of honey as a substitute for formalin in the histological fixation of tissue. *J Histotechnol.* 2006;29:173-176. [IIC]

72. Modifications to the HIPAA Privacy, Security, Enforcement, and Breach Notification rules under the Health Information Technology for Economic and Clinical Health Act and the Genetic Information Nondiscrimination Act; other modifications to the HIPAA rules. *Fed Regist.* 2013;78(17):5565-5702.

73. *Standards of Perioperative Nursing.* AORN, Inc. https://www.aorn.org/guidelines/clinical-resources/aorn-standards. Last published 2015. Accessed September 28, 2020. [IVB]

74. 40 CFR 260: Hazardous waste management system: general. Electronic Code of Federal Regulations. https://www.ecfr.gov/cgi-bin/text-idx?SID=e890c50a0ff246a8e05409a398695337&mc=true&node=pt40.26.260&rgn=div5. Accessed September 28, 2020.

75. *Safety Data Sheet: Formalin, Buffered, 10%.* Creation Date May 12, 2011. Revision Date April 13, 2018. Fair Lawn, NJ; Thermo Scientific; 2018. [VA]

76. Nkoy FL, Hammond MEH, Rees W, et al. Variable specimen handling affects hormone receptor test results in women with breast cancer: a large multihospital retrospective study. *Arch Pathol Lab Med.* 2010;134(4):606-612. [IIIB]

77. Li JK, Shah BA. Survey on imaging management and handling of breast surgical specimens by radiologists. *J Am Coll Radiol.* 2014;11(9):890-893. [IIIB]

78. Allison KH, Hammond MEH, Dowsett M, et al. Estrogen and progesterone receptor testing in breast cancer: ASCO/CAP guideline update. *J Clin Oncol.* 2020;38(12):1346-1366. [IVB]

79. Wolff AC, Hammond MEH, Allison KH, et al. Human epidermal growth factor receptor 2 testing in breast cancer: American Society of Clinical Oncology/College of American Pathologists clinical practice guideline focused update. *Arch Pathol Lab Med.* 2018;142(11):1364-1382. [IVB]

80. Baltuonyte A, Ruparelia V, Shah BA. In the clinic. Surgical breast tissue specimen handling and transportation in radiology. *Radiol Technol.* 2016;87(5):564-568. [VB]

81. Kallen ME, Sim MS, Radosavcev BL, Humphries RM, Ward DC, Apple SK. A quality initiative of postoperative radiographic imaging performed on mastectomy specimens to reduce histology cost and pathology report turnaround time. *Ann Diagn Pathol.* 2015;19(5):353-358. [VB]

82. Hicks DG, Boyce BF. The challenge and importance of standardizing pre-analytical variables in surgical pathology specimens for clinical care and translational research. *Biotech Histochem.* 2012;87(1):14-17. [VB]

83. Hicks DG, Kushner L, McCarthy K. Breast cancer predictive factor testing: the challenges and importance of standardizing tissue handling. *J Natl Cancer Inst Monogr.* 2011;2011(42):43-45. [VB]

84. Balch CM. Reexamining our routines of handing surgical tissue in the operating room. *J Natl Cancer Inst Monogr.* 2011;2011(42):39-40. [VB]

85. Hewitt SM, Lewis FA, Cao Y, et al. Tissue handling and specimen preparation in surgical pathology: issues concerning the recovery of nucleic acids from formalin-fixed, paraffin-embedded tissue. *Arch Pathol Lab Med.* 2008;132(12):1929-1935. [VB]

86. Graham RA, Homer MJ, Katz J, Rothschild J, Safaii H, Supran S. The pancake phenomenon contributes to the inaccuracy of margin assessment in patients with breast cancer. *Am J Surg.* 2002;184(2):89-93. [IIIB]

87. Khoury T, Sait S, Hwang H, et al. Delay to formalin fixation effect on breast biomarkers. *Mod Pathol.* 2009;22(11):1457-1467. [IIB]

88. Portier BP, Wang Z, Downs-Kelly E, et al. Delay to formalin fixation "cold ischemia time": effect on ERBB2 detection by in-situ hybridization and immunohistochemistry. *Mod Pathol.* 2013;26(1):1-9. [IIIB]

89. Moatamed NA, Nanjangud G, Pucci R, et al. Effect of ischemic time, fixation time, and fixative type on HER2/neu

immunohistochemical and fluorescence in situ hybridization results in breast cancer. *Am J Clin Pathol.* 2011;136(5):754-761. [IIB]

90. Arima N, Nishimura R, Osako T, et al. The importance of tissue handling of surgically removed breast cancer for an accurate assessment of the Ki-67 index. *J Clin Pathol.* 2016;69(3):255-259. [IIIB]

91. Li X, Deavers MT, Guo M, et al. The effect of prolonged cold ischemia time on estrogen receptor immunohistochemistry in breast cancer. *Mod Pathol.* 2013;26(1):71-78. [IIIIB]

92. Arber DA. Effect of prolonged formalin fixation on the immunohistochemical reactivity of breast markers. *Appl Immunohistochem Mol Morphol.* 2002;10(2):183-186. [IIIB]

93. Tevis SE, Neuman HB, Mittendorf EA, et al. Multidisciplinary intraoperative assessment of breast specimens reduces number of positive margins. *Ann Surg Oncol.* 2018;25(10):2932-2938. [IIIB]

94. 10 CFR 20: Standards for protection against radiation. US Nuclear Regulatory Commission. https://www.nrc.gov/reading-rm/doc-collections/cfr/part020/. Accessed September 28, 2020.

95. 10 CFR 35: Medical use of byproduct material. US Nuclear Regulatory Commission. https://www.nrc.gov/reading-rm/doc-collections/cfr/part035/. Accessed September 28, 2020.

96. Goudreau SH, Joseph JP, Seiler SJ. Preoperative radioactive seed localization for nonpalpable breast lesions: technique, pitfalls, and solutions. *Radiographics.* 2015;35(5):1319-1334. [VB]

97. Iodine-125 and Palladium-103 low dose rate brachytherapy seeds used for localization of non-palpable lesions. US Nuclear Regulatory Commission. http://www.nrc.gov/materials/miau/med-use-toolkit/seed-localization.html. Updated July 7, 2017. Accessed September 28, 2020.

98. Graham RP, Jakub JW, Brunette JJ, Reynolds C. Handling of radioactive seed localization breast specimens in the pathology laboratory. *Am J Surg Pathol.* 2012;36(11):1718-1723. [VB]

99. Renshaw AA, Kish R, Gould EW. Increasing radiation from sentinel node specimens in pathology over time. *Am J Clin Pathol.* 2010;134(2):299-302. [IIIB]

100. Miner TJ, Shriver CD, Flicek PR, et al. Guidelines for the safe use of radioactive materials during localization and resection of the sentinel lymph node. *Ann Surg Oncol.* 1999;6(1):75-82. [IIB]

101. Fitzgibbons PL, LiVolsi VA. Recommendations for handling radioactive specimens obtained by sentinel lymphadenectomy. Surgical Pathology Committee of the College of American Pathologists, and the Association of Directors of Anatomic and Surgical Pathology. *Am J Surg Pathol.* 2000;24(11):1549-1551. [IVB]

102. Michel R, Hofer C. Radiation safety precautions for sentinel lymph node procedures. *Health Phys.* 2004;86(2 Suppl):S35-S37. [VB]

103. Coventry BJ, Collins PJ, Kollias J, et al. Ensuring radiation safety to staff in lymphatic tracing and sentinel lymph node biopsy surgery—some recommendations. *J Nucl Med Radiat Ther.* 2012;(S2:008):1-5. [IIIC]

104. Law M, Chow LW, Kwong A, Lam CK. Sentinel lymph node technique for breast cancer: radiation safety issues. *Semin Oncol.* 2004;31(3):298-303. [VB]

105. Dessauvagie BF, Frost FA, Sterrett GF, et al. Handling of radioactive seed localisation breast specimens in the histopathology laboratory: the Western Australian experience. *Pathology.* 2015;47(1):21-26. [VB]

106. Garner HW, Bestic JM, Peterson JJ, Attia S, Wessell DE. Preoperative radioactive seed localization of nonpalpable soft tissue masses: an established localization technique with a new application. *Skeletal Radiol.* 2017;46(2):209-216. [IIIC]

107. Sung JS, King V, Thornton CM, et al. Safety and efficacy of radioactive seed localization with I-125 prior to lumpectomy and/or excisional biopsy. *Eur J Radiol.* 2013;82(9):1453-1457. [IIIB]

108. Pavlicek W, Walton HA, Karstaedt PJ, Gray RJ. Radiation safety with use of I-125 seeds for localization of nonpalpable breast lesions. *Acad Radiol.* 2006;13(7):909-915. [VB]

109. 10 CFR 71.5: Transportation of licensed material. US Nuclear Regulatory Commission. https://www.nrc.gov/reading-rm/doc-collections/cfr/part071/part071-0005.html. Accessed September 28, 2020.

110. 10 CFR 30.41: Transfer of byproduct material. US Nuclear Regulatory Committee. https://www.nrc.gov/reading-rm/doc-collections/cfr/part030/part030-0041.html. Accessed September 28, 2020.

111. Guideline for medical device and product evaluation. In: *Guidelines for Perioperative Practice.* Denver, CO: AORN, Inc; 2020:705-714. [IVA]

112. 21 CFR 821: Medical device tracking requirements. Electronic Code of Federal Regulations. https://www.ecfr.gov/cgi-bin/text-idx?SID=3ecf60fc34260612326bbc9d5a87fd1c&mc=true&node=pt21.8.821&rgn=div5. Accessed September 28, 2020.

113. Medical device tracking; guidance for industry and FDA staff. US Food and Drug Administration. https://www.fda.gov/regulatory-information/search-fda-guidance-documents/medical-device-tracking. Published March 2014. Accessed September 28, 2020. [VA]

114. 21 CFR 803 subpart C: User facility reporting requirements. Electronic Code of Federal Regulations. https://www.ecfr.gov/cgi-bin/text-idx?SID=56a92292f48628d7687166c5765d8b74&mc=true&node=sp21.8.803.c&rgn=div6. Accessed September 28, 2020.

115. Medical device reporting (MDR): how to report medical device problems. US Food and Drug Administration. https://www.fda.gov/medical-devices/medical-device-safety/medical-device-reporting-mdr-how-report-medical-device-problems. Accessed September 28, 2020. [VA]

116. MedWatch: the FDA safety information and adverse event reporting program. https://www.fda.gov/safety/medwatch-fda-safety-information-and-adverse-event-reporting-program. Accessed September 28, 2020. [VA]

117. Unique device identification system. Final rule. *Fed Regist.* 2013;78(185):58785-58828.

118. Burlingame BL, Maxwell-Downing D. Clinical issues-November 2015. *AORN J.* 2015;102(5):536-544. [VA]

119. Appendix M. Surgical specimens to be submitted to pathology for examination. College of American Pathologists. https://webapps.cap.org/apps/docs/laboratory_accreditation/build/pdf/surgical_specimens.pdf. Revised November 2007. Accessed September 28, 2020. [IVB]

120. Davidovitch RI, Temkin S, Weinstein BS, Singh JR, Egol KA. Utility of pathologic evaluation following removal of

explanted orthopaedic internal fixation hardware. *Bull NYU Hosp Jt Dis.* 2010;68(1):18-21. [IIIC]

121. Bush K. *Position Statement: Forensic Evidence Collection in the Emergency Care Setting.* Schaumburg, IL: Emergency Nurses Association; 2018. [IVB]

122. Foresman-Capuzzi J. CSI & U: Collection and preservation of evidence in the emergency department. *J Emerg Nurs.* 2014;40(3):229-236. [VA]

123. Peel M. Opportunities to preserve forensic evidence in emergency departments. *Emerg Nurse.* 2016;24(7):20-26. [VC]

124. Byrne-Dugan CJ, Cederroth TA, Deshpande A, Remick DG. The processing of surgical specimens with forensic evidence: lessons learned from the Boston Marathon bombings. *Arch Pathol Lab Med.* 2015;139(8):1024-1027. [VA]

125. Evans MM, Stagner PA, Rooms R. Maintaining the chain of custody—evidence handling in forensic cases. *AORN J.* 2003;78(4):563-569. [VA]

126. Wick JM. "Don't destroy the evidence!" *AORN J.* 2000;72(5):807-827. [VB]

127. Porteous J. Don't tip the scales! Care for patients involved in a police investigation. *Can Oper Room Nurs J.* 2005;23(3):12-14, 16. [VA]

128. Recommended equipment for obtaining forensic samples from complainants and suspects. Faculty of Forensic & Legal Medicine. https://fflm.ac.uk/wp-content/uploads/2020/06/Recommended-equipment-for-obtaining-forensic-samples-Dr-M-Stark-July-2020.pdf. Published July 2020. Accessed September 28, 2020. [IVB]

129. Recommendations for the collection of forensic specimens from complainants and suspects. Faculty of Forensic & Legal Medicine. https://fflm.ac.uk/wp-content/uploads/2020/06/Recommendations-for-the-collection-of-forensic-specimens-FSSC-July-2020.pdf. Published July 2020. Accessed September 28, 2020. [IVB]

130. Koehler SA. Firearm evidence and the roles of the ER nurse and forensic nurse. *J Forensic Nurs.* 2009;5(1):46-48. [VC]

131. Carrigan M, Collington P, Tyndall J. Forensic perioperative nursing. Advocates for justice. *Can Oper Room Nurs J.* 2000;18(4):12-16. [VA]

132. Labelling forensic samples. Faculty of Forensic & Legal Medicine. https://fflm.ac.uk/wp-content/uploads/2019/01/Labelling-Forensic-Samples-Jan-2019.pdf. Published January 2019. Accessed September 28, 2020. [IVB]

133. Baergen RN, Thaker HM, Heller DS. Placental release or disposal? Experiences of perinatal pathologists. *Pediatr Dev Pathol.* 2013;16(5):327-330. [IIIC]

134. Helsel DG, Mochel M. Afterbirths in the afterlife: cultural meaning of placental disposal in a Hmong American community. *J Transcult Nurs.* 2002;13(4):282-286. [IIIB]

135. *WHO Infection Control Guidelines for Transmissible Spongiform Encephalopathies: Report of a WHO Consultation, Geneva, Switzerland, 23-26 March 1999.* Geneva, Switzerland: World Health Organization; 2000. [IVA]

136. Pizzella N, Kurec A. The proper handling of CJD-infected patient samples in the pathology laboratory. *MLO Med Lab Obs.* 2018;50(5):40-42. [VA]

137. Karasin M. Special needs populations: perioperative care of the patient with Creutzfeldt-Jakob disease. *AORN J.* 2014;100(4):390-410. [VA]

138. Alcalde-Cabero E, Almazán-Isla J, Brandel JP, et al. Health professions and risk of sporadic Creutzfeldt-Jakob disease, 1965 to 2010. *Euro Surveill.* 2012;17(15):20144. [VA]

139. Guideline for patient information management. In: *Guidelines for Perioperative Practice.* Denver, CO: AORN, Inc; 2020:357-386. [IVA]

140. Liebmann R, Varma M, eds. *Best Practice Recommendations: Histopathology and Cytopathology of Limited or No Clinical Value.* 3rd ed. London, United Kingdom: Royal College of Pathologists; 2019. [IVB]

141. Damjanov I, Vranic S, Skenderi F. Does everything a surgeon takes out have to be seen by a pathologist? A review of the current pathology practice. *Virchows Arch.* 2016;468(1):69-74. [VB]

142. Fisher M, Alba B, Bhuiya T, Kasabian AK, Thorne CH, Tanna N. Routine pathologic evaluation of plastic surgery specimens: are we wasting time and money? *Plast Reconstr Surg.* 2018;141(3):812-816. [IIIA]

143. Bizzell JG, Richter GT, Bower CM, Woods GL, Nolder AR. Routine pathologic examination of tonsillectomy specimens: a 10-year experience at a tertiary care children's hospital. *Int J Pediatr Otorhinolaryngol.* 2017;102:86-89. [IIIA]

144. Teraphongphom N, Kong CS, Warram JM, Rosenthal EL. Specimen mapping in head and neck cancer using fluorescence imaging. *Laryngoscope Investig Otolaryngol.* 2017;2(6):447-452. [VA]

145. Meier FA, Varney RC, Zarbo RJ. Study of amended reports to evaluate and improve surgical pathology processes. *Adv Anat Pathol.* 2011;18(5):406-413. [VA]

146. Gillio-Meina C, Zielke HR, Fraser DD. Translational research in pediatrics IV: solid tissue collection and processing. *Pediatrics.* 2016;137(1). [VB]

147. Harrison BT, Dillon DA, Richardson AL, Brock JE, Guidi AJ, Lester SC. Quality assurance in breast pathology: lessons learned from a review of amended reports. *Arch Pathol Lab Med.* 2017;141(2):260-266. [IIIA]

148. Volmar KE, Idowu MO, Hunt JL, Souers RJ, Meier FA, Nakhleh RE. Surgical pathology report defects: a College of American Pathologists Q-Probes study of 73 institutions. *Arch Pathol Lab Med.* 2014;138(5):602-612. [IIIA]

Guideline Development Group

Lead Author: Julie Cahn[1], DNP, RN, CNOR, RN-BC, ACNS-BC, CNS-CP, Perioperative Practice Specialist, AORN, Denver, Colorado

Methodologist: Erin Kyle[2], DNP, RN, CNOR, NEA-BC, Editor-in-Chief, *Guidelines for Perioperative Practice*, AORN, Denver, Colorado

Evidence Appraisers: Julie Cahn[1]; Marie A. Bashaw[3], DNP, RN, NEA-BC, CNOR, Assistant Professor, Wright State University College of Nursing and Health, Dayton, Ohio; Janice Neil[4], PhD, CNE, RN, Associate Professor, East Carolina College of Nursing, Greenville, North Carolina; and Erin Kyle[2]

Guidelines Advisory Board Members:

- Donna A. Pritchard[5], MA, BSN, RN, NE-BC, CNOR, Director of Perioperative Services, Interfaith Medical Center, Brooklyn, New York
- Susan Lynch[6], PhD, RN, CSSM, CNOR, Associate Director, Surgical Services, Chester County Hospital, West Chester, Pennsylvania
- Linda C. Boley[7], MSN, BSN, RN, CNOR, Clinical Educator, Surgical Services, Norton Women's and Children's Hospital, Louisville, Kentucky
- Brenda G. Larkin[8], MS, CNS-CP, CNOR, CSSM Clinical Nurse Specialist, Aurora Lakeland Medical

Guidelines Advisory Board Liaisons:

- Craig S. Atkins[9], DNP, CRNA, Chief Nurse Anesthetist, Belmar Ambulatory Surgical Center, Lakewood, Colorado
- Shandra R. Day[10], MD, Assistant Professor, Infectious Disease, The Ohio State University Wexner Medical Center, Columbus, Ohio
- Cassie Dietrich[11], MD, Anesthesiologist, Anesthesia Associates of Kansas City, Overland Park, Kansas
- Jared Huston[12], MD, Director, Trauma Research, Northwell Health, Manhasset, New York
- Susan G. Klacik[13], BS, CRCST, FCS, Clinical Educator, International Association of Healthcare Central Service Materiel Management (IAHCSMM), Chicago, Illinois
- Sara Reese[14], PhD, CIC, FAPIC, Association for Professionals in Infection Control and Epidemiology, Englewood, Colorado
- Juan Sanchez[15], MD, Associate Professor of Surgery, Johns Hopkins University School of Medicine, Baltimore, Maryland.

External Review: Expert review comments were received from individual members of the American Association of Nurse Anesthetists (AANA), American College of Surgeons (ACS), Association for Professionals in Infection Control and Epidemiology (APIC), American Society of Anesthesiologists (ASA), International Association of Healthcare Central Service Materiel Management (IAHCSMM), the Society for Healthcare Epidemiology of America (SHEA), and the Surgical Infection Society (SIS). Subject matter expert comments were also received from Victoria M. Steelman[16], PhD, RN, CNOR, FAAN, Associate Professor Emeritus, University of Iowa, Iowa City; and Joyce Foresman-Capuzzi[17], MSN, APRN, CCNS, CEN, CCRN, TCRN, CTRN, CPN, CPEN, SANE-A, AFN-BC, EMT-P, FAEN, Clinical Nurse Educator, Lankenau Medical Center, Wynnewood, Pennsylvania. Their responses were used to further refine and enhance this guideline; however, their responses do not imply endorsement. The draft was also open for a 30-day public comment period.

Financial Disclosure and Conflicts of Interest

This guideline was developed, edited, and approved by the AORN Guidelines Advisory Board without external funding being sought or obtained. The Guidelines Advisory Board was financially supported entirely by AORN and was developed without any involvement of industry.

Potential conflicts of interest for all Guidelines Advisory Board members were reviewed before the annual meeting and each monthly conference call. None of the members of the Guideline Development Group reported a potential conflict of interest.[1-17]

Publication History

Originally approved November 2005, AORN Board of Directors. Published in *Standards, Recommended Practices, and Guidelines*, 2006 edition.

Reprinted March 2006, *AORN Journal*.

Minor editing revisions made to omit PNDS codes; reformatted September 2012 for publication in *Perioperative Standards and Recommended Practices*, 2013 edition.

Revised May 2014 for online publication in *Perioperative Standards and Recommended Practices*.

Minor editing revisions made in November 2014 for publication in *Guidelines for Perioperative Practice*, 2015 edition.

Evidence ratings revised in *Guidelines for Perioperative Practice*, 2018 edition, to conform to the current AORN Evidence Rating Model.

Evidence ratings revised and minor editorial changes made to conform to the current AORN Evidence Rating model, September 2019, for online publication in *Guidelines for Perioperative Practice*.

Revised December 2020 for online publication in the *Guidelines for Perioperative Practice*.

Scheduled for review in 2025.

STERILE TECHNIQUE

1017

TABLE OF CONTENTS

MEDICAL ABBREVIATIONS & ACRONYMS

AAMI – Association for the Advancement of
    Medical Instrumentation
CDC – Centers for Disease Control and Prevention
CFU – Colony-forming unit
CVC – Central venous catheter
FDA – US Food and Drug Administration
IFU – Instructions for use

OR – Operating room
PAPR – Powered air-purifying respirator
PICC – Peripherally inserted central catheter
PPE – Personal protective equipment
RCT – Randomized controlled trial
SSI – Surgical site infection
WHO – World Health Organization

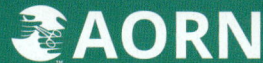
GUIDELINE FOR
STERILE TECHNIQUE

The Guideline for Sterile Technique was approved by the AORN Guidelines Advisory Board and became effective November 1, 2018. It was presented as a proposed guideline for comments by members and others. The recommendations in the guideline are intended to be achievable and represent what is believed to be an optimal level of practice. Policies and procedures will reflect variations in practice settings and/or clinical situations that determine the degree to which the guideline can be implemented. AORN recognizes the many diverse settings in which perioperative nurses practice; therefore, this guideline is adaptable to all areas where operative or other invasive procedures may be performed.

Purpose

This document provides guidance on the principles and processes of **sterile technique**. Sterile technique involves the use of specific actions and activities to maintain sterility and prevent contamination of the **sterile field** and sterile items during operative and other invasive procedures. Thoughtful and diligent implementation of sterile technique is a cornerstone of perioperative nursing practice and a key strategy in the prevention of surgical site infections (SSIs).

All individuals who are involved in operative or other invasive procedures have a responsibility to provide a safe environment for patient care.[1] Perioperative team members must be vigilant in preventing contamination of the sterile field and ensuring that the principles and processes of sterile technique are implemented. Perioperative leaders have a duty to promote a culture of safety by creating an environment in which perioperative personnel are encouraged to identify, question, or stop practices believed to be unsafe without fear of repercussions.[2]

Adhering to the principles and processes of sterile technique is a matter of ethical obligation, individual conscience, and patient advocacy that applies to all members of the perioperative team.[1,3] Surgical patients are vulnerable; thus, perioperative team members are required to mindfully practice the principles of sterile technique to ensure the sterile field is maintained. Perioperative nurses have a long-standing reputation of advocating for patients and working with members of the interdisciplinary health care team to provide a safe perioperative environment.[2]

Although these recommendations include references to other AORN Guidelines, the focus of this document is sterile technique. Surgical attire, hand hygiene, product evaluation, and the effects of forced-air warming equipment are outside the scope of these recommendations. Refer to the AORN Guideline for Surgical Attire,[4] Guideline for Hand Hygiene,[5] Guideline for Medical Device and Product Evaluation,[6] and Guideline for Prevention of Unplanned Patient Hypothermia[7] for additional guidance.

Evidence Review

A medical librarian with a perioperative background conducted a systematic search of the databases Ovid MEDLINE®, EBSCO CINAHL®, Scopus®, and the Cochrane Database of Systematic Reviews. The search was limited to literature published in English from 2012 through 2017. At the time of the initial search, weekly alerts were created on the topics included in that search. Results from these alerts were provided to the lead author until April 2018. The lead author requested additional articles that either did not fit the original search criteria or were discovered during the evidence appraisal process. The lead author and the medical librarian also identified relevant guidelines from government agencies, professional organizations, and standards-setting bodies.

Search terms included subject headings such as *abdominal and perineal surgery, aerosolization, asepsis, aseptic practice, aseptic technique, assembled instruments, assisted gloving, barrier precautions, blocked vents, blood, body exhaust suits, bone and bones, bone cements, bowel isolation technique, bowel surgery, bowel technique, break in sterile technique, C-arm, case classifications, cerebrospinal fluid shunts, cesarean birth, cesarean section, changing levels, chemical indicator, chemical integrator, chewing gum, clamped instruments, clean closure technique, clean to dirty case, closed gloving, closing instruments, closing trays, colorectal surgery, complex procedure, contamination, conversations, corrective actions, cough, cover equipment, cover implants, cover instrument trays, critical zone, cuffing, cystoscopic surgery, cystoscopy, debris, delivery of sterile items, delivery to sterile field, dispensing sterile items, doffing, donning, door openings, double gloving, dual sterile fields, education, endovascular procedures, endovascular surgery, event-related sterility, extended cuffs, facing back to back, facing front to front, fluid and fat absorption, fluid warmers, fluoroscopy, gastrointestinal tract, glove compromise, glove expansion and fluid, glove gown interface, glove inspection, glove integrity, glove perforation, gloves (surgical), gowns, grease, hair, hand hygiene, handling sterile items, health physics, heavy items, human factors, hybrid operating room, hybrid procedure room, hybrid surgical suites, immediate action, increased activity, indicator systems, indicators and reagents, individual interventions, inspection of sterile supplies, instrument inspection, instrument set removal, instrument trays, instrument wrap, interoperative MRI, intraoperative MRI, introduction of sterile supplies, Ioban, iodine impregnated drape, isolation technique, Kimguard, lead apron, lead garment, leaning over, level of the sterile field, maintain*

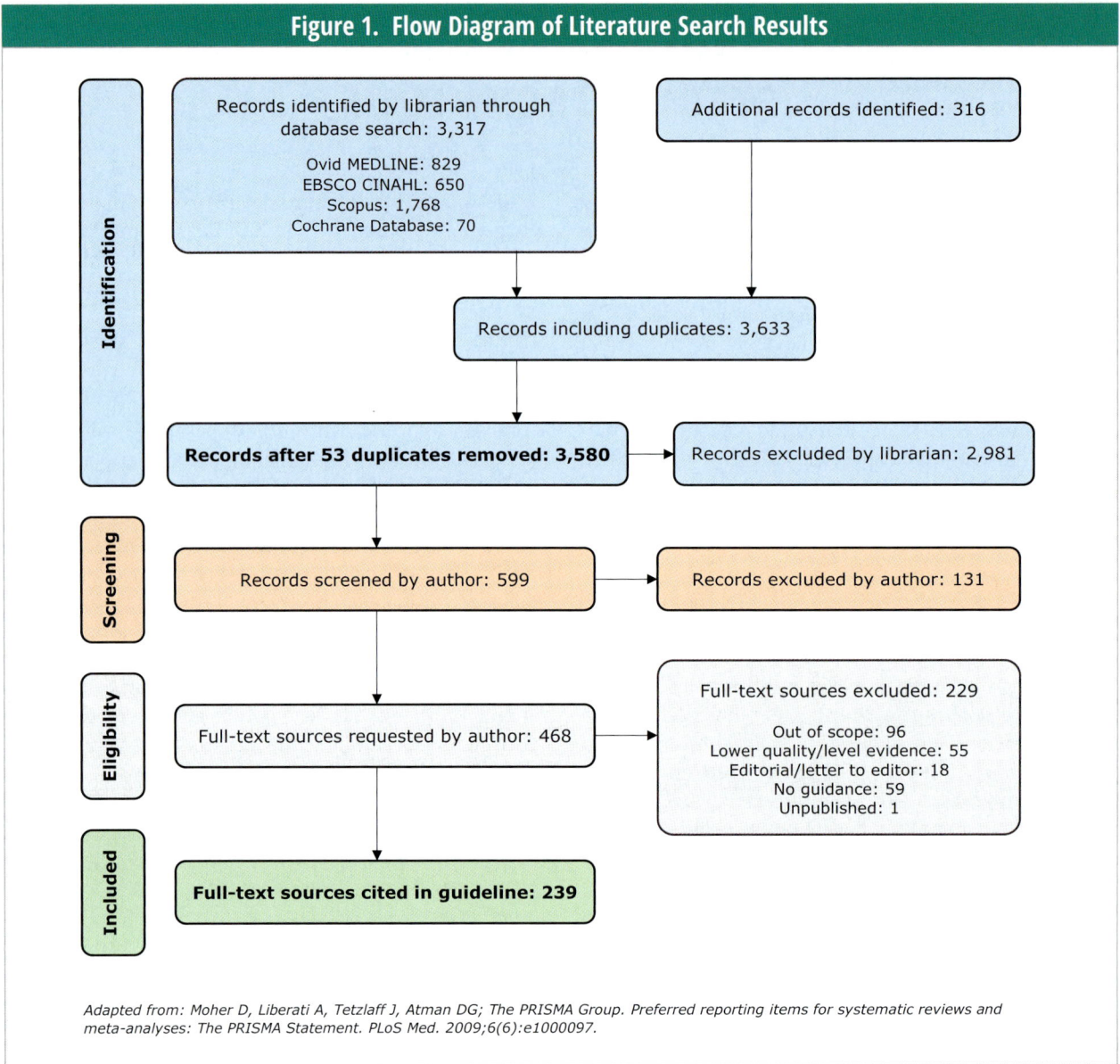

Figure 1. Flow Diagram of Literature Search Results

Records identified by librarian through database search: 3,317

Ovid MEDLINE: 829
EBSCO CINAHL: 650
Scopus: 1,768
Cochrane Database: 70

Additional records identified: 316

Records including duplicates: 3,633

Records after 53 duplicates removed: 3,580

Records excluded by librarian: 2,981

Records screened by author: 599

Records excluded by author: 131

Full-text sources requested by author: 468

Full-text sources excluded: 229

Out of scope: 96
Lower quality/level evidence: 55
Editorial/letter to editor: 18
No guidance: 59
Unpublished: 1

Full-text sources cited in guideline: 239

Identification
Screening
Eligibility
Included

Adapted from: Moher D, Liberati A, Tetzlaff J, Atman DG; The PRISMA Group. Preferred reporting items for systematic reviews and meta-analyses: The PRISMA Statement. PLoS Med. 2009;6(6):e1000097.

integrity, major break, Maxair, medications, metastatic tumors, methyl methacrylate, microscope eyepiece, microscopes, minimally invasive, minimally invasive procedures, minimally invasive surgical procedures, minimize handling, minor break, monitoring sterile field, movement of personnel, multiple sterile fields, multiple surgical specialties, neoplasm metastasis, non-penetrating clamps, opening sterile items, opening sterile items in a rigid container, operative microscope, organic material, orthopedic hoods, otolaryngology, package integrity, packaging, pharmaceutical preparations, plastic adhesive incise drape, plastic bandages to cover holes, polymethyl methacrylate, procedural drapes, product evaluation, product packaging, product selection, protective clothing, radiologic exposure, retrieve sterilizer items, robotic surgery, robotic surgical procedures, seated procedures, securement, sharp items, simulation, slush machines, sneezing, solutions, space suits, Spaulding classification, speech, sterile areas or sections, sterile barrier, sterile drapes, sterile field, sterile field preparation, sterile part of gown, sterile practices, sterile surgical gloves, sterile surgical gown, sterile technique, sterility, strikethrough, sub-sterile, surgery (digestive system), surgical air systems, surgical conscience, surgical doors shut, surgical drapes, surgical draping, surgical equipment and supplies, surgical gown, surgical gown cuffs, surgical gown seams, surgical gown strikethrough, surgical helmet system, surgical hood, surgical instruments, surgical site infection bundle, surgical wound, table covering, talking, tape doors, team interventions, time-related sterility, tissue, traffic patterns, training, unanticipated delay, ventriculoperitoneal shunts, visible defect, waist level, wound classification, and wrapped items.

Included were research and non-research literature in English, complete publications, and publications with dates within the time restriction when available. Excluded were non-peer-reviewed publications and older evidence within the time restriction when more recent evidence was available. Editorials, news items, and other brief items were excluded. Low-quality evidence was excluded when higher-quality evidence was available **(Figure 1)**.

Articles identified by the search were provided to the project team for evaluation. The team consisted of the lead author and two evidence appraisers. The lead author divided the search results into topics and assigned members of the team to review and critically appraise each article using the AORN Research or Non-Research Evidence Appraisal Tools as appropriate. The literature was independently evaluated and appraised according to the strength and quality of the evidence. Each article was then assigned an appraisal score agreed upon by consensus of the team. The appraisal score is noted in brackets after each reference as applicable.

Each recommendation rating is based on a synthesis of the collective evidence, a benefit-harm assessment, and consideration of resource use. The strength of the recommendation was determined using the AORN Evidence Rating Model and the quality and consistency of the evidence supporting a recommendation. The recommendation strength rating is noted in brackets after each recommendation.

Note: The evidence summary table is available at http://www.aorn.org/evidencetables/.

Editor's note: MEDLINE is a registered trademark of the US National Library of Medicine's Medical Literature Analysis and Retrieval System, Bethesda, MD. CINAHL, Cumulative Index to Nursing and Allied Health Literature, is a registered trademark of EBSCO Industries, Birmingham, AL. Scopus is a registered trademark of Elsevier B.V., Amsterdam, The Netherlands. Ioban is a registered trademark of 3M Company, St Paul, MN. Kimguard is a registered trademark of Kimberly-Clark Worldwide, Inc, Neenah, WI. Maxair is a registered trademark of Maxair Manufacturing Ltd, Port Coquitlam, British Columbia, Canada.

1. Before Preparing the Sterile Field

1.1 **Before preparing a sterile field, implement practices to prevent contamination of the sterile field.** *[Recommendation]*

The perioperative setting is a controlled environment that is designed to minimize the risk of infection during operative and other invasive procedures. In addition to environmental controls, the work practices of perioperative personnel are essential for preventing contamination of the sterile field. Wearing clean surgical attire that has been laundered by a health care–accredited laundry facility, wearing a clean surgical mask, and performing hand hygiene are all work practices that may prevent contamination of the sterile field.

1.2 **Wear clean surgical attire and a surgical head covering when entering an operating room (OR) or invasive procedure room for any reason (eg,** stocking supplies, delivering equipment, transporting specimens).[8] *[Recommendation]*

Surgical attire helps contain bacterial shedding and promotes environmental cleanliness.[4] Clean surgical attire supports patient safety and helps preserve the integrity of the sterile field. Covering all hair with a clean surgical head covering minimizes the risk of hair and scalp skin contaminating the sterile field.[4] Specific guidance regarding surgical attire is provided in the AORN Guideline for Surgical Attire.[4]

1.3 **When open sterile supplies are present, wear a clean surgical mask that covers the mouth and nose and is secured in a manner that prevents venting at the sides of the mask.**[8] *[Recommendation]*

The Centers for Disease Control and Prevention (CDC) 2017 Guideline for the Prevention of Surgical Site Infection[8] recommends that a surgical mask that fully covers the mouth and nose be worn when a surgical procedure is beginning or in progress or when sterile surgical instruments are open. The CDC and various professional organizations recommend mask use in specific procedures, including

- placement of central venous catheters (CVCs), placement of peripherally inserted central catheters (PICCs), and guidewire exchange[9-11];
- high-risk spinal canal procedures (eg, myelogram, lumbar puncture, spinal anesthesia)[10,12,13]; and
- interventional radiology procedures.[14]

There is conflicting evidence on the benefits of wearing masks for prevention of SSI. The findings from seven studies indicate that the use of a clean surgical mask may help protect the sterile field from oropharyngeal and nasopharyngeal microbial contamination, which may reduce the patient's risk for SSI.[15-21] Although there is consensus on the use of masks for preventing personnel exposure to potentially infectious materials,[22] there is conflicting evidence on mask use for prevention of microbial contamination of the sterile field or the effectiveness of mask use for prevention of SSI, and the evidence is dated.[23-30] The research on surgical masks is further limited by

- the availability of a variety of mask types,[31]
- a wide range of facial types and different methods of securing mask fit,
- a lack of consistency in the study methodology (eg, outcomes tested, sampling types),
- the lack of reporting of mask type and facial fit of the mask in the research,
- the varied environments (eg, OR, procedure room, cardiac catheterization lab)[20-22,26] and air delivery systems where surgical masks are used,[23]
- the focus on limited surgical specialties[15,16,18,19,21,26-28] or the exclusion of certain surgical specialties

or procedure types (eg, orthopedic procedures, emergencies),[27,28] and

- the multicausal nature of SSIs.

The research on mask effectiveness cannot be synthesized into one generalizable statement because of the various complications inherent to the prevention of SSI. The authors of a systematic review on the use of disposable surgical masks for the prevention of SSI in clean surgery also concluded that their findings were not generalizable.[32] More research is needed on the correlation between SSI and the use of surgical masks, especially for surgical wounds classified as clean.[31,32]

One factor that determines mask effectiveness is the fit of the mask on the face. Wearing a clean surgical mask according to manufacturer's instructions for use (IFU) may limit venting at the sides of the mask and therefore potentially reduce the chance of oropharyngeal or nasopharyngeal droplet dispersal.[4] Mask use is also required by the Occupational Safety and Health Administration[22] when there is a reasonable anticipation of exposure to potentially infectious material. The AORN Guideline for Prevention of Transmission-Based Precautions[33] and Guideline for Surgical Smoke Safety[34] provide additional information on the use of masks in the perioperative setting.

1.4 **An interdisciplinary team that includes an infection preventionist and an occupational health professional should determine whether powered air-purifying respirators (PAPRs) may be used for respiratory protection in the perioperative environment when a sterile field is present.** *[Conditional Recommendation]*

The use of PAPRs in the health care setting may be indicated for respiratory protection of personnel from certain diseases transmissible by the airborne route, although the use of PAPRs in the perioperative setting may contaminate the sterile field. The CDC does not recommend the use of a PAPR with exhalation valves during invasive procedures in the presence of a sterile field.[35,36] The battery-powered blower in the PAPR filters the air intake for the person wearing the device, but it does not filter the wearer's exhaled air. The unfiltered air exhausted from the PAPR may contribute to increased levels of OR air contamination and potentially increase the patient's risk for SSI.[37] In addition, the CDC states that the external belt-mounted blower and tubing is designed to be worn on the outside of the gown.[38] Depending on the PAPR manufacturer's IFU, wearing the blower and tubing externally may allow for proper airflow into the PAPR unit, but wearing the blower outside of a sterile gown would contaminate the gown.[38] The AORN Guideline for

Transmission-Based Precautions[33] provides additional information on this topic.

1.4.1 **If PAPR use is allowed, create a standardized procedure for perioperative PAPR use and protection of the sterile field from contamination (eg, portions of the sterile field to be covered; direction of the blower exhaust; type of PAPR allowed, such as loose-fitting, full face piece, hood style).** *[Recommendation]*

A standardized procedure for PAPR use allows the health care organization to evaluate specific patient and organizational needs.[39]

1.5 **Perform hand hygiene before opening sterile supplies.**[5] *[Recommendation]*

Hand hygiene helps reduce the potential for transmission of potentially infectious material to patients and health care personnel.[33] Hand hygiene is not only effective, but also cost efficient for infection prevention (See the AORN Guideline for Hand Hygiene).[5]

2. Donning Gowns and Gloves

2.1 **Select the surgical gown by task and anticipated degree of exposure to blood, body fluids, or other potentially infectious materials, as determined by the following factors:**

- **team member's role,**
- **type of procedure (eg, minimally invasive versus open, superficial incision versus deep body cavity incision),**
- **procedure duration,**
- **anticipated blood loss,**
- **anticipated volume of irrigation fluid,**
- **possibility of handling hazardous medications,**[40] **and**
- **anticipated patient contact (eg, splash, soaking, leaning).**[41]

[Recommendation]

The Occupational Safety and Health Administration requires personnel to wear personal protective equipment (PPE) based on anticipated risk for exposure to blood, body fluids, and other potentially infectious materials.[22] In an expert guidance document for selection and use of protective apparel, the Association for Advancement of Medical Instrumentation (AAMI) recommends assessing risk for exposure based on the presence of liquid, the pressure and type of contact, the duration of the procedure, the type of procedure, and the role of each surgical team member.[41]

The AORN Guideline for Medication Safety[40] includes information about gown and glove selection for handling of hazardous medications (eg, chemotherapy medications).

2.1.1 Select the surgical gown needed for the procedure according to the barrier performance class as stated on the product label (Table 1).[41,42] [Recommendation]

Surgical gowns are labeled with the barrier properties of the gown's **critical zone**. The US Food and Drug Administration (FDA) requires gown manufacturers to test and validate liquid barrier claims for surgical gowns and recognizes the ANSI/AAMI PB70 barrier performance levels as the preferred method for assessing gown liquid barrier protection.[42,43] The size and configuration of the critical zone varies by each design and is specified by the manufacturer on the product label (See the AORN Guideline for Transmission-Based Precautions).[33]

2.1.2 Select and wear surgical gowns that wrap around the body and completely cover the wearer's back. The gown sleeves should

- conform to the shape of the wearer's arms,[42,44]
- be of sufficient length to allow gloves to completely cover the cuffs,[42,45] and
- be of sufficient length to prevent the gown cuffs from being exposed when the wearer's arms are extended.[42,45]

[Recommendation]

When a gown is of insufficient size or has insufficient sleeve length to cover the perioperative team member's body, it may restrict movement, increase the potential for the scrubbed team member's unsterile skin or clothing to contact the sterile field, or fail to provide adequate coverage to protect the scrubbed team member from exposure to blood, body fluids, or other potentially infectious materials. Sterile gowns that are too large or sleeves that are too long may brush against unsterile objects or surfaces. The gown manufacturer's IFU may provide size dimensions for gown fit.

In a quasi-experimental study to evaluate various combinations of surgical attire, Ritter et al[46] found that the addition of a wrap-around gown reduced environmental microbial contamination by 51% compared to surgical attire worn without a gown.

2.1.3 Scrubbed personnel may wear a **surgical helmet system** when splashes, spray, splatter, or droplets of blood or other potentially infectious materials may be generated and

Table 1. Gown Liquid Barrier Performance Class

Barrier Level[1]	Anticipated Risk of Exposure (eg, fluid amount, splash risk, pressure on the gown)[2]
Level 1	Minimal
Level 2	Low
Level 3	Moderate
Level 4	High

References
1. ANSI/AAMI PB70:2012. Liquid Barrier Performance and Classification of Protective Apparel and Drapes Intended for Use in Health Care Facilities. *Arlington, VA: Association for the Advancement of Medical Instrumentation; 2012.*
2. AAMI TIR11:2005. Selection and Use of Protective Apparel and Surgical Drapes in Health Care Facilities. *Arlington, VA: Association for the Advancement of Medical Instrumentation; 2005.*

facial contamination can be reasonably anticipated. [Conditional Recommendation]

Surgical helmet systems provide more protective coverage to scrubbed personnel than a surgical gown does.[47-49] Personal protective equipment is critical in orthopedic and trauma procedures that present a higher risk for exposure to bloodborne pathogens and other potentially infectious materials.[22,47,50-52] Two studies of surgical helmet systems showed that these systems are significantly more protective against splatter and spray than traditional goggles, visors,[48] or masks with a face shield.[47] The authors of a nonexperimental study on personnel contamination from hydrosurgical debridement devices also recommended the use of surgical helmet systems during procedures involving these devices.[49]

2.2 Perform surgical hand antisepsis before donning a sterile gown and gloves.[5] [Recommendation]

Surgical hand antisepsis decreases transient and resident microorganisms on the skin, which may reduce the incidence of health care–associated infections. Healthy hand skin and nail condition, no jewelry on hands or wrists, hand hygiene, and surgical hand antisepsis are the most effective ways to prevent and control infections and represent the least expensive means of achieving both (See the AORN Guideline for Hand Hygiene).[5]

2.3 Use sterile technique when donning and wearing a sterile gown. [Recommendation]

2.3.1 When donning the sterile gown without assistance, prevent contamination of the sterile field by

- following the manufacturer's instructions for donning, if available;

- opening and donning the sterile gown and gloves away from the sterile field[53];
- not opening sterile gloves directly on top of the open sterile gown[54];
- completely drying hands and arms prior to donning the gown;
- only touching the inside of the sterile gown when picking it up for donning; and
- not touching the sterile glove wrapper or gloves until the sterile gown has been donned.[54]

[Recommendation]

Donning a gown and gloves in an area separate from any sterile fields may reduce the risk for contamination from potential contact with the unprotected skin and clothing. In addition, in a nonexperimental study, Noguchi et al[53] found that the activities of unfolding a sterile surgical gown and donning the gown had a high rate of airborne particle dispersal, and the researchers recommended that gowns be unfolded and donned away from the sterile field. Although the particles dispersed from a sterile gown are sterile, the researchers noted that the airborne particles could potentially become a vector for transmission of pathogens if they came in contact with nonsterile areas.[53]

Donning a gown and gloves in a separate area also may prevent droplets of water or used antiseptic solution from contaminating instrument tables. When the gown is retrieved, droplets of water or used antiseptic solution from the scrubbed team member's wet hands may drip onto the glove wrapper and contaminate the sterile gloves.[54] In a nonexperimental study, Heal et al[54] studied water droplets from surgeons' arms after a standard 5-minute mechanical surgical scrub and tap water rinse. Water droplets were collected from the surgeons' arms and cultured. Pathogenic and environmental bacteria were recovered from the water droplets.

The researchers also reviewed the paper wrappers from two different brands of gloves for permeability and bacterial penetration. The paper was found to be permeable. The researchers concluded that the pathogenic bacteria could be transferred from the surgeons' arms to the gloves by water dropped on the glove packaging during the gowning and gloving process and that this represented a theoretical source of wound contamination.[54]

Touching only the inside of the gown when picking it up prevents the scrubbed team member's hands from contaminating the exterior of the gown. After the sterile gown is donned, the scrubbed team member's hands are covered by the gown sleeves, which prevents the scrubbed team member's unprotected hands from contaminating the glove wrapper and gloves.[54]

2.3.2 Consider the following parts of the gown to be sterile:
- the front of a sterile gown from the chest to the level of the sterile field and
- the gowns sleeves from the cuff to 2 inches above the elbow, circumferentially.

[Recommendation]

In a quasi-experimental study, Bible et al[55] evaluated the most sterile areas of surgical gowns. The researchers found that the contamination rates were lowest between the wearer's chest and the operative field. Bacterial growth from the gowns was highest in areas above the chest level and below the OR bed. The researchers theorized that the increased levels of bacterial growth in the areas above the chest were likely related to microbial shedding from the scrubbed team member's head or mask, whereas the portion below the OR bed was likely contaminated by direct contact with unsterile objects below the level of the operative field.[55] The area 2 inches below the elbow to the cuff of the gown is adjacent to the area of the front of the gown that is considered sterile.[55]

2.3.3 Consider the following parts of the surgical gown to be contaminated or unsterile:
- the neckline, shoulders, and axillary regions[55];
- the gown back; and
- the sleeve cuffs after the scrubbed team member's hands pass through and beyond the cuff.

[Recommendation]

The neckline, shoulders, and axillary regions are areas of friction and may not provide effective microbial barriers; these regions have been shown to have higher levels of bacterial growth.[55] The back of the gown cannot be constantly monitored. Sleeve cuffs are not impervious[42,44] and could allow for microbial transfer from the scrubbed team member's hands.[45,56]

2.3.4 When a gown sleeve is contaminated by an unsterile object, use clinical judgment to determine whether a sterile sleeve should be worn to cover the area of contamination or if the gown should be removed, surgical hand antisepsis performed, and a sterile gown and gloves donned. Base the decision on a risk assessment of the following variables:
- the part of the gown that was contaminated;

- the degree of contamination;
- the risk of exposing the patient or other perioperative personnel to blood, body fluids, or other potentially infectious materials; and
- the length of time remaining in the procedure.

[Recommendation]

Gown-sleeve contamination may vary depending on the situation, which requires perioperative personnel to make a decision based on their clinical judgement of the situation. The evidence review for this guideline found no evidence as to whether using sterile surgical gown sleeves to cover gown sleeves contaminated by unsterile objects would compromise sterile technique.

2.4 Use sterile technique when donning, wearing, and changing sterile gloves. *[Recommendation]*

2.4.1 Perform gloving without assistance by touching only the inside of the glove. *[Recommendation]*

2.4.2 Perform initial gowning and gloving with assistance in the following order:
1. The team member being gloved should don a surgical gown with the gown cuffs remaining at or beyond the finger tips.
2. A scrubbed team member should hold open the glove to be donned.
3. The person donning the glove should insert his or her hand into the glove with the gown cuff touching only the inside of the glove (Figure 2).

[Recommendation]

The risk for glove contamination may be reduced when the hand has not passed through the gown cuff. In a randomized controlled trial (RCT), Jones et al[57] compared contamination of the inside of the glove cuff during open (ie, gown cuff at the wrist) and closed (ie, gown cuff at the fingertips) **assisted gloving**. As part of the study, two surgeons were gloved 20 times after covering their fingers and hands with a fluorescent powder. One surgeon was gloved by the closed assisted method and the other by the open assisted method. The results showed that **open assisted gloving** led to significantly greater glove cuff contamination than **closed assisted gloving**.

2.4.3 When the gown cuff is at the wrist level, perform gloving with assistance in the following order:

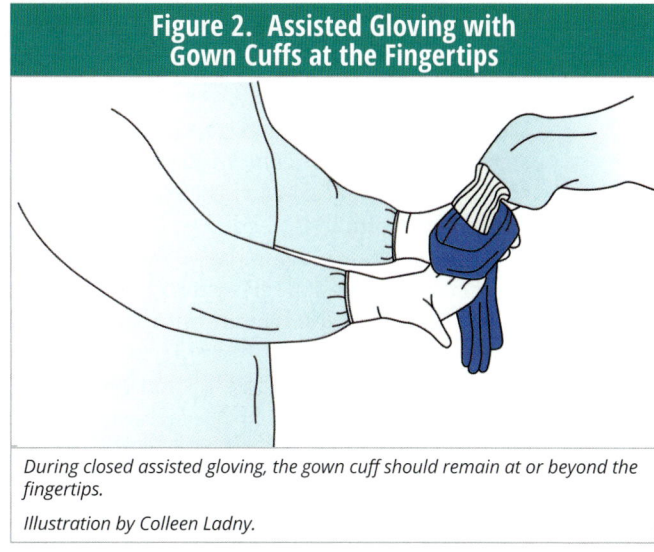

Figure 2. Assisted Gloving with Gown Cuffs at the Fingertips

During closed assisted gloving, the gown cuff should remain at or beyond the fingertips.

Illustration by Colleen Ladny.

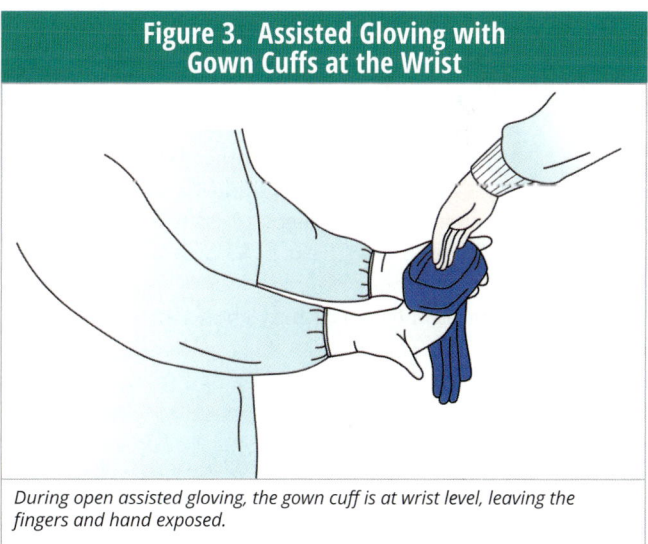

Figure 3. Assisted Gloving with Gown Cuffs at the Wrist

During open assisted gloving, the gown cuff is at wrist level, leaving the fingers and hand exposed.

Illustration by Colleen Ladny.

1. The team member being gloved should leave the gown cuff at wrist level, leaving the fingers and hand exposed.
2. A scrubbed team member should hold open the glove to be donned.
3. The person donning the glove should insert his or her hand into the glove with the gown cuff touching only the inside of the glove (Figure 3).

[Recommendation]

2.4.4 Scrubbed team members should wear two pairs of sterile surgical gloves (ie, double glove), and use a **perforation indicator system**. *[Recommendation]*

Moderate-quality evidence indicates that double gloving provides a more protective sterile barrier for the prevention of microbial transfer from the surgical team member to the patient or transfer of potentially infectious materials from the patient to the surgical team member.[33,58-62] A systematic review of 12 RCTs showed that the addition of a second pair of surgical gloves significantly reduced glove perforations.[58] The researchers stated that no additional research is needed to determine the efficacy of double gloving.

The American College of Surgeons recommends "the universal adoption of the double gloving (or underglove) technique to reduce exposure to body fluids resulting from glove tears and sharps injuries. In certain delicate operations, and in situations where it may compromise the safe conduct of the operation or safety of the patient, the surgeon may decide to forgo this safety measure."[63(p1)] The American Academy of Orthopaedic Surgeons also supports double gloving during invasive surgical procedures.[50] A nonexperimental study on double gloving during oral and maxillofacial surgery conducted by Kuroyanagi et al[61] also supported double gloving. However, the 2016 World Health Organization (WHO) *Global Guidelines for the Prevention of Surgical Site Infection*[64] concluded that insufficient evidence existed about whether double gloving during surgery is more effective and thus did not make a recommendation.

Han et al[65] found that conventional outer gloves were not more prone to perforations than thick outer gloves. Their study also revealed reduced tactile sensitivity when thick outer gloves were worn as part of a double-gloving method.

Perforation indicator systems enable personnel to detect more glove perforations **(Figure 4)**.[33,58-60,62,66] A meta-analysis of five RCTs showed that scrubbed team members only identified 21% of perforations when wearing two pairs of standard color double gloves.[66] Scrubbed team members wearing perforation indicator systems detected 77% of perforations.[66]

2.4.5 **Completely cover the gown cuffs with the gloves.** *[Recommendation]*

Maintaining coverage of the gown cuff by the glove is important to protect the wearer from exposure at the wrist to blood, body fluids, and other potentially infectious materials. The interface between the gown and the glove can be an area of contamination and transfer for potentially infectious materials.[44,45,67,68] Excess material at the gown sleeves may pleat when sterile gloves are applied over the sleeves.[44] Choosing a gown of the right size may reduce pleating at the interface between the gown and the glove.

Surgical gown cuffs are made of knit material, which is permeable and may allow for microbial transfer to the patient. Fraser et al[45] found that all of the gown-glove interfaces had varying degrees of simulated contamination leak from inside the gown out onto the area surrounding the junction.

2.4.6 **Surgical gloves with extended cuffs may be worn to maintain coverage of the gown cuffs.** *[Conditional Recommendation]*

When worn in combination with a gown, the glove cuff may not be long enough to cover the gown cuff during use, depending on the task being performed. Gloves with extended cuffs may provide additional protection to prevent wrist exposure during use. The authors of two studies and one expert opinion article discussed how the interface between the gown and the glove may be the part of the surgical gown-glove barrier system that is most prone to leakage of potentially infectious materials onto the person wearing the PPE.[44,67,68] In a nonexperimental study of OR exposures to potentially infectious materials, Panlilio et al[52] found that 15% of exposures involved skin contact through soaked clothing on the arms. The majority of skin contacts were reported by surgeons.[52]

2.5 **Inspect all gloves for integrity after donning, before contact with the sterile field, throughout use, and when an outer glove perforation is discovered and outer gloves are changed.** *[Recommendation]*

Holes or defects in surgical gloves may allow for passage of microorganisms, particulates, and fluids between sterile and unsterile areas. Careful inspection of glove integrity after donning and before contact with the sterile field may reveal holes or defects that have occurred during the manufacturing or donning process. Inspecting glove integrity throughout the procedure may prevent unnoticed glove perforation. Kojima and Ohashi[69] found that the incidence of unnoticed glove damage during thoracoscopic procedures was 25% for surgeons and 12% for all the gloves used during the procedures studied.

2.5.1 **Change surgical gloves worn during invasive surgical procedures**
- **after each patient procedure**[10,70];
- **every 90 to 150 minutes**[50,59,69,71-73];
- **when a visible defect or perforation is noted or when a suspected or actual perforation**

from a needle, suture, bone, or other object occurs[22,71];

- immediately after direct contact with methyl methacrylate[40,74-77];
- after touching optic eye pieces on the operative microscope[78];
- after touching a fluoroscopy machine[79];
- after touching a surgical helmet system hood or visor[80-82]; and
- when suspected or actual contamination occurs.

[Recommendation]

Failure to change gloves after each patient procedure may lead to transmission of microorganisms from one patient to another.[70] Three studies on glove perforations showed that the frequency of glove perforations was directly correlated to the length of time the gloves were worn.[71-73] All three studies recommended changing gloves every 90 minutes based on the rate of glove perforations after 90 minutes.[71-73] In two of the studies, some bacterial migration occurred through the perforations.[71,72] Researchers who conducted a nonexperimental study on double gloving during oral and maxillofacial surgery also suggested glove changes but did not define the interval duration.[61] The American Academy of Orthopaedic Surgeons recommends changing the outer pair of gloves at least every 2 hours.[50]

Surgical helmet systems may become contaminated during surgery.[80,82] One nonexperimental study showed that 22% of surgical helmet systems were contaminated immediately after donning.[81] Consequently, sterile glove changes are recommended after a surgical helmet system has been touched.[80-82] These findings were also supported by a nonexperimental study by Young et al,[82] in which results showed potential for contamination on the outside of the surgical helmet system hood.

The AORN Guideline for Sharps Safety[62] includes recommendations for prevention of occupational exposures to bloodborne pathogens. The AORN Guideline for Medication Safety[40] includes information about glove use during handling of hazardous medications. The AORN Guideline for a Safe Environment of Care[74] includes recommendations about handling methyl methacrylate.

2.5.2 Surgical gloves worn during invasive surgical procedures may be changed
- after draping is complete[50,83-85];
- after handling of heavy, coarse, or sharp instrumentation[61,84,86];

Figure 4. Perforation Indicator Systems

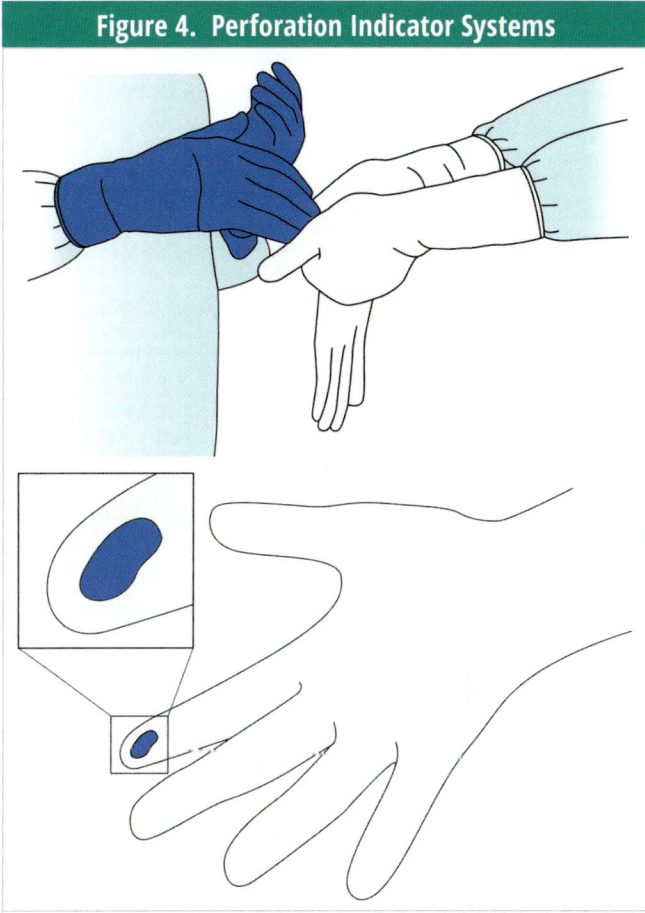

The use of perforation indicator systems may increase safety and reduce the potential for exposure to blood, body fluids, or other potentially infectious materials. When glove perforation occurs, the site of perforation can be more easily seen because of the colored gloves worn beneath the standard gloves.

Illustration by Colleen Ladny.

- after manipulation of rough edges of bone[61,83,84,86]; and
- before handling of implants.[83,84,87]

[Conditional Recommendation]

Moderate-quality evidence suggests that glove changes may be warranted after certain events during a procedure because of the likelihood of glove contamination or perforation.[61,83,84,86,87] However, the evidence may not be generalizable to procedures that do not involve handling bone tissue because four of the five studies were performed in orthopedic populations[83,84,86,87] and one was performed in oral and maxillofacial surgery.[61]

Glove contamination may occur during draping because there is potential for contact with the patient's skin, which has been shown to be a potential source of staphylococci.[85]

The rough edges of bone may perforate gloves. Changing gloves may prevent contamination of the sterile field or of implants in the event that the glove perforation is not identified. In a nonexperimental study, Carter et al[83] evaluated glove perforations during total joint arthroplasty procedures and found that 79.6% of all glove perforations occurred in the time between incision and the placement of implants. The researchers found that 40% of the glove perforations occurred between the time of incision and bone resection but before final implant placement.

In another nonexperimental study, Ward et al[87] recommended changing gloves prior to handling implants. The researchers reviewed glove contamination rates at 1 hour and at 1 hour and 15 minutes. The researchers found that the group of surgeons who did not change their outer gloves at 1 hour were 2.5 times more likely to be contaminated at the 1 hour and 15 minute mark. This study was performed during orthopedic procedures, and the 1 hour time point for glove changes was chosen to represent the approximate time of implant handling.

2.5.3 **When a perforation occurs in the outer pair of double gloves, change the outer gloves and inspect the inner gloves.** [Recommendation]

When the outer glove is perforated, the inner glove may also have a perforation. In a quasi-experimental study, Harnoss et al[71] found that almost 50% of outer glove perforations were associated with inner glove perforations. In a nonexperimental study, Carter et al[83] found that personnel who double gloved and had perforations in both the inner and outer gloves always noticed the outer glove perforation but only identified the inner glove perforation 19% of the time.

2.5.4 **When a glove change is indicated, use clinical judgment to determine whether the individual glove should be changed or if the gown and gloves should be removed, surgical hand antisepsis performed, and a sterile gown and gloves donned. Base the decision on a risk assessment of the following variables:**
- **the part of the glove that was contaminated;**
- **the degree of contamination;**
- **the risk of exposing the patient or other perioperative personnel to blood, body fluids, or other potentially infectious materials; and**
- **the length of time remaining in the procedure.**

[Recommendation]

Glove contamination may vary depending on the situation, which requires perioperative personnel to make a decision based on their clinical judgement in the situation. The evi-

dence review for this guideline found no evidence to indicate whether changing a contaminated glove without performing surgical hand antisepsis and donning another sterile gown would compromise sterile technique.

2.5.5 **Change gloves in a location away from the sterile field.** [Recommendation]

Noguchi et al[53] found that glove removal dispersed a large number of particles into the air. The researchers thought the particles could be glove powders, skin squames, and lint from textiles (eg, drapes). Based on their findings, the researchers concluded that gloves should not be removed in close proximity to the surgical site or sterile instruments.

2.5.6 **To change a sterile glove during a procedure, perform gloving with assistance in the following order:**
1. **An unscrubbed team member should remove the glove to be changed without altering the position of the gown cuff (ie, not pulling the cuff down over the scrubbed team member's hand).**
2. **A scrubbed team member should hold open the glove to be donned.**
3. **The person donning the glove should insert his or her hand into the glove with the gown cuff touching only the inside of the glove.**

[Recommendation]

2.6 **Use sterile technique in accordance with the manufacturer's IFU when donning and wearing a surgical helmet system.** [Recommendation]

Surgical helmet systems may become contaminated during the donning process, which may increase the risk for SSI. The CDC does not make a recommendation for or against surgical helmet system use for SSI prevention due to lack of evidence to guide practice.[8] In a systematic review with meta-analysis, Young et al[88] found that surgical helmet systems do not reduce the risk for deep SSIs during arthroplasty procedures.

2.6.1 **Don the unsterile helmet and a surgical mask before performing surgical hand antisepsis.** [Recommendation]

Wearing a mask during surgical hand antisepsis reduces the risk for contamination of the hands.[5]

2.6.2 **Don the sterile visor hood or toga that covers the unsterile helmet before donning the sterile gown and gloves.** [Recommendation]

2.6.3 The mask may be removed in accordance with the manufacturer's IFU during donning of the sterile visor hood or toga. [*Conditional Recommendation*]

2.6.4 Turn the fan in the unsterile helmet on after gowning is completed. [*Recommendation*]

In a nonexperimental study, Hanselman et al[89] found that the fan located within the helmet may increase OR environmental contamination.

3. Preparing the Sterile Field

3.1 Prepare a sterile field for patients undergoing operative or other invasive procedures. [*Recommendation*]

Preparing a sterile field for patients undergoing operative or other invasive procedures reduces the risk of microbial contamination and is a cornerstone of infection prevention. The prevention of SSIs is crucial, and adherence to sterile technique during an invasive procedure can reduce the patient's risk for infection.[8,64]

3.2 Perform surgical hand antisepsis and don a sterile gown and gloves before preparing or using a sterile field. [*Recommendation*]

Surgical hand antisepsis reduces transient and resident microorganisms on the skin, which may prevent SSIs.[5,8,90] Sterile surgical gowns and gloves help maintain the sterile field and decrease the risk of transmitting potentially infectious materials to patients or perioperative personnel.[64] Wearing a sterile surgical gown and gloves may minimize microbial dissemination in the form of shedding skin squames.[46] Wearing a sterile gown during sterile field set up also provides some level of assurance that the surgical attire of the person performing the set up did not contaminate the sterile field. The CDC recommends maximal barrier precautions, including a gown, during placement of CVCs, placement of PICCs, and guidewire exchanges.[9] Wearing sterile gowns is also recommended during interventional radiology procedures.[14]

3.3 Prepare the sterile field as close as possible to the time of use.[91-96] [*Recommendation*]

Preparing a sterile field as close as possible to the time of use reduces the risk for particulate matter and potentially infectious materials to settle on opened sterile fields. High-quality evidence suggests that contamination of the sterile field increases over time.[91-96]

3.4 Open the sterile field for only one patient at a time. [*Recommendation*]

Opening sterile supplies onto the sterile field for multiple patients in a single OR or procedure room increases the risk for cross contamination. There may be an increased risk for errors to occur when sterile supplies are opened for more than one patient at a time, due to confusion and distraction in a complex environment.[97]

3.5 One patient at a time should occupy the OR or procedure room.[10] [*Recommendation*]

The presence of multiple patients in the same OR or procedure room may expose patients to unnecessary hazards and an increased risk for SSI. Infectious diseases may be transmitted by contact, droplet, or airborne methods.[10] The risk for disease transmission or cross contamination may be increased when multiple sterile fields and surgical teams are confined to a single OR or procedure room.

3.6 Prepare the sterile field in the OR or procedure room where it will be used and do not move to another room.[98,99] [*Recommendation*]

Moving the sterile field from one location to another increases the potential for contamination. A nonexperimental study of sterile instrument table contamination levels based on set-up location demonstrated a 24-fold reduction in bacteria colony-forming units (CFU) on sterile tables prepared in ORs with laminar airflow versus those prepared in an instrument preparation room with conventional ventilation.[98] Another nonexperimental study showed that preparation rooms had higher levels of bacteria than an OR with laminar airflow when air samples were taken.[99] This evidence suggests that preparing the sterile field in an OR with laminar airflow may be preferred because preparation rooms may not have the same quality of ventilation systems as the OR.[99]

3.7 Only sterile items should come into contact with the sterile field.[64,100] [*Recommendation*]

Using only sterile items during invasive procedures minimizes the risk for infection and provides the highest level of assurance that the sterile field is free of microorganisms.[64,100]

3.8 For procedures that involve different wound classifications (ie, clean, clean-contaminated, contaminated, dirty), keep sterile fields and instrumentation separate and do not use them interchangeably on the cleaner wound. [*Recommendation*]

Separating sterile fields and instrumentation for incision sites of varying levels of wound classification may reduce the patient's risk for infection by preventing contamination of the cleaner wound.

3.9 Use **isolation technique** during
- **bowel surgery and**
- **procedures involving resection of metastatic tumors.**

[Recommendation]

Isolation technique, also known as bowel or contamination technique or clean closure, is intended to prevent the transfer of bacteria, microorganisms, or cancerous cells from one location to another, thereby reducing the risk of SSI or the potential for cancerous cells to re-seed.[101-103]

There are large numbers of bacteria and anaerobic microorganisms in the large bowel.[104-106] The proximal small intestine has smaller populations of bacteria due to the destructive action of gastric acid and bile, digestion by proteolytic enzymes, and bacterial clearance by intestinal peristalsis.[104-106] However, some gastrointestinal disorders that require surgical repair in the upper gastrointestinal tract (eg, obstruction, diverticula, fistula) may be associated with an increased number of bacteria and may warrant the implementation of isolation technique.[104-106]

The evidence of bacterial and microorganism loads in the various parts of the digestive tract is consistent with the results of a study that assessed the risk factors for SSI during gastrointestinal surgery. Watanabe et al[107] found that the incidence of SSIs after gastric surgery was 8%, while the incidence of SSIs after small bowel, colorectal, appendectomy, and stoma surgeries was as high as 20% to 30%. The overall infection rate was 15.5%. The researchers concluded that strict adherence to sterile technique and minimal blood loss were associated with a lower incidence of SSI.[107]

Several studies have evaluated surgical instrument contamination during bowel surgery. Porteous et al[103] found that surgical instruments used in large bowel resections were more heavily contaminated than instruments used in small bowel resections. Saito et al[108] found that forceps used throughout the procedure on digestive tissue in elective laparotomies were significantly correlated with higher rates of positive cultures than forceps used during wound closure. The contamination rate for all forceps was 31.4%. The researchers concluded that while perioperative personnel generally practice under the assumption that sterile instruments remain sterile, instrument contamination is considerably high even without obvious contamination, and sterile technique is crucial in decreasing the patient's risk for SSI.

Saito et al[108] found that adenosine triphosphate assays completed on the forceps could not be statis-

tically correlated to microbial contamination. This led the researchers to conclude that adenosine triphosphate assays could not be reliably used to test for surgical instrument microbial contamination.

Hashimoto et al[109] found that sterile forceps and drapes used only during abdominal wound closure significantly lowered the rates of incisional SSIs in open pancreatic procedures, specifically pancreatic duodenectomies. This finding is important because patients with pancreatic tumors may also have diabetes mellitus, which may contribute to increased risk for SSI.[109] Four of six wound cultures from incisional SSIs indicated enteric bacteria (ie, from the gastrointestinal tract).[109] Instrument microbial load may lead to contamination of the peritoneal cavity and abdominal wall if the instruments are not isolated.[103,108,109] The *WHO Global Guidelines for the Prevention of Surgical Site Infection*[64] does not make a recommendation on isolation technique. However, the WHO stated that instrument changes prior to wound closure may be a common practice and that it may be logical in contaminated procedures, especially in colorectal surgery or for patients with diffuse peritonitis.[64]

In a study on using closing technique as part of a bundle approach, Johnson et al[110] found that the overall SSI rate dropped from 6.0% to 1.1%. The study involved ovarian cancer procedures with and without bowel resections and open uterine cancer procedures. The bundle elements included a sterile closing tray with glove changes for fascial and skin closure, dressing removal 1 to 2 days after surgery, discharge with 4% chlorhexidine gluconate, and nursing follow-up telephone calls.[110] A limitation of bundled studies is the inability to determine the effect of a single intervention among multiple study elements.

The use of isolation technique is a precaution to prevent the potential spread of cancer cells. There have been reports of local and distant implantation of tumor cells associated with instrumentation used for both resection and subsequent closure or reconstruction.[111-116] In three cases, the authors reported that seeding from a primary tumor site to a secondary site was the result of instruments contaminated with cancerous cells from tumor excision that were then used during graft harvest, reconstruction, or closure.[111-113] Two of the cases resulted in the patient's death.[111,112] The authors of one case report recommended removing resection instrumentation before closure and irrigating the surgical site.[111]

3.9.1 **Develop and implement a standardized procedure for isolation technique.** *[Conditional Recommendation]*

A standard procedure for isolation technique that follows the same patterns and processes each time may assist perioperative personnel in

Table 2. Isolation Technique for Single and Dual Sterile Fields	
Single Sterile Field	**Dual Sterile Fields**
Prepare 1 sterile field for the procedure and closure.	Prepare 1 sterile field for the procedure. Prepare and cover a 2nd sterile field for the closure.
Before transection of the bowel or metastatic tumor excision, place a wound protector or clean sterile towels around the surgical site.	
Segregate all contaminated instruments and other items that have contacted the bowel lumen or metastatic tumor to a designated area (eg, Mayo stand, basin).	Not applicable
Refrain from touching the sterile back table while the bowel is open or metastatic tumor excision is in progress.	Not applicable
When the anastomosis/resection is complete, remove the contaminated instruments, wound protector, towel drapes, and any other potentially contaminated items (eg, electrosurgical pencil, suction, light handles) from the surgical site and place them in a separate area of the sterile field that will not be touched during closing.	When the anastomosis/resection is complete, remove the contaminated instruments, wound protector, towel drapes, and any other potentially contaminated items (eg, electrosurgical pencil, suction, light handles) from the surgical site and place them on the sterile field used during the procedure that will not be touched during closing.
Irrigate the wound and initiate accounting procedures.	
Announce the change to clean closure.	
Have one scrubbed team member remain at the sterile field while all other team members change gloves. Gowns may also be changed. The scrubbed team member who remained at the sterile field should remove the moist counted sponges or towels, then change gloves when the other team members are back at the sterile field.	
Apply sterile light handles.	
Apply sterile drapes to cover the existing drapes, which may be soiled with bowel contents or may have been in contact with the metastatic tumor tissue.	
Secure a sterile electrosurgical pencil and suction to the field.	
Proceed with wound closure using only sterile instrumentation and items.	Proceed with wound closure using only sterile instrumentation and items from the sterile field for the closure.

achieving accuracy, efficiency, and continuity among perioperative team members.[97] Studies of human error have shown that many errors involve a deviation from routine practice.[97] Creation of a facility-specific standard procedure allows health care organizations to determine best practices that meet the needs of their patient population.

3.9.2   Include the following in isolation technique procedures:
- organizing the sterile field in a manner that minimizes the risk of sterile field exposure to intestinal tract bacteria[101-107] or cancerous cells from metastatic tumor excisions,[102,111-116]
- initiating isolation technique immediately before resection of the bowel[101,103] or metastatic tumor and concluding when the resection or anastomosis is complete,
- no longer using instruments or items that had contact with the inside of the bowel lumen after it has been closed[101-103,107] or that were used for metastatic tumor excision,[111]

- removing contaminated instruments and items from the sterile field or placing them in a separate area that will not be touched by members of the sterile team,[101-103,111]
- changing surgical gloves[101,102,109,110,117] and changing the surgical gown when soiled,[110,117]
- covering existing sterile drapes with new sterile drapes,[109,117] and
- using clean instruments to close the wound after anastomosis or resection.[101-103,111,112] *[Recommendation]*

3.9.3   Isolation technique may be implemented using either a single sterile field or a dual sterile field (Table 2). *[Conditional Recommendation]*

3.10   Use a **wound protector** according to the manufacturer's IFU for procedures that enter the gastrointestinal or biliary tract. *[Recommendation]*

A wound protector may reduce the risk for surgical wound contamination from the gastrointestinal or biliary tract, which may decrease the risk for SSI. The WHO recommends wound protector use for reducing SSI rates in abdominal procedures with wound classes of clean-contaminated, contaminated, and dirty.[64] However, the WHO guideline recommends exercising caution during placement of wound protectors for patients who have adhesions.[64]

The Society for Healthcare Epidemiology of America and the Infectious Diseases Society of America[90] also recommended the use of wound protectors based on the results of a meta-analysis that showed a 45% reduction in SSIs with their use. No difference was found between the dual- or single-ring versions of the device.[90]

In an RCT, Bressan et al[118] found that dual ring wound protectors provided an absolute risk reduction of 23% and a relative risk reduction of 52% in pancreaticoduodenectomy patients after preoperative insertion of an intrabiliary stent. In a nonexperimental study, Papaconstantinou et al[119] also found significant decreases in overall and enteric bacteria with the use of a wound protector that irrigates and suctions around the wound edge.

4. Sterile Drapes

4.1 Use sterile drapes to establish a sterile field. *[Recommendation]*

Sterile drapes provide a barrier that minimizes the passage of microorganisms from unsterile to sterile areas and reduces the risk of health care–associated infections.[42] The WHO states that the use of drapes is good clinical practice in surgery.[64] The CDC recommends maximal sterile barrier precautions, including the use of a full body drape, during the placement of CVCs, placement of PICCs, and guidewire exchanges.[9] A bundle program that included the use of maximal sterile barriers during CVC insertion in 103 intensive care units in Michigan resulted in a 66% decrease in infection rates.[120]

4.2 Place sterile drapes on the patient, furniture, and equipment in the sterile field in a manner that prevents contamination of the sterile field. *[Recommendation]*

4.2.1 Handle sterile drapes as little as possible and in a controlled manner that prevents contamination.[53] *[Recommendation]*

Rapid movement of draping materials creates air currents that can cause dust, lint, and other particles to migrate.[53]

4.2.2 Place sterile drapes in a manner that does not require the scrubbed team members to lean across an unsterile area and that prevents the sterile gowns from contacting an unsterile surface. *[Recommendation]*

4.2.3 During draping, shield gloved hands by cuffing the interior portion of the drape material over the sterile gloves.[42,84,85] *[Recommendation]*

Cuffing gloved hands beneath the draping material may protect gloves from contact with unsterile items or areas. Two nonexperimental studies indicated that gloves may become contaminated during draping.[84,85]

4.2.4 Place sterile drapes first at the surgical site then outward toward the peripheral areas. *[Recommendation]*

4.2.5 Cover unsterile equipment (eg, the Mayo stand) on the top, bottom, and sides with a sterile drape before introducing to or bringing over a sterile field. Cover unsterile equipment that will be positioned immediately adjacent to the sterile field with a sterile drape. *[Recommendation]*

4.2.6 Drape large equipment (eg, microscopes, robotic arms, C-arm fluoroscopy unit) as close as possible to the time of use and in accordance with the drape manufacturer's IFU.[78,79,121,122] *[Recommendation]*

When available, manufacturer's instructions for draping equipment may help with proper drape placement and potentially limit overheating caused by covering equipment ventilation areas.

4.3 Do not move the portion of the sterile drape that establishes the sterile field after initial positioning. *[Recommendation]*

4.4 Secure surgical equipment (eg, tubing, cables) on the sterile field to the sterile field with nonperforating devices. *[Recommendation]*

Perforation of barrier materials may provide portals of entry and exit for microorganisms, blood, and other potentially infectious materials.[42]

4.5 Consider only the top surface of the sterile drape to be sterile. Consider items that fall below the level of the sterile field to be contaminated.[42,123] *[Recommendation]*

Items that are below the level of the sterile field (eg, sterile trash bags, suture tails) have a higher risk of becoming contaminated since those items are not as easily monitored for contact with unsterile surfaces.[42,123] A nonexperimental study of C-arm draping methods also demonstrated increased levels of contamination below the level of the sterile field.[123]

4.6 When a C-arm is moved into lateral position,
- consider the upper portion of a C-arm drape to be contaminated[79,122] and
- do not bring the sterile drape that is below the level of the OR bed up into the sterile field.[79,123]

[Recommendation]

Several studies have evaluated the sterility of C-arm drapes and draping methods for lateral positioning. One study showed that the area of greatest contamination was at the top of the C-arm.[122] When the C-arm is rotated into lateral position, the top portion of the draped C-arm machine has an increased risk of becoming contaminated. This led the researchers to recommend that the top portion of the C-arm drape be considered unsterile and that personnel avoid contact with this area **(Figure 5)**.[122] Peters et al[79] studied contamination of C-arm drapes and found that 17% of drapes were contaminated from the time of draping and 80% of all C-arm drapes were contaminated at 80 minutes. There was a significant positive correlation between lateral C-arm position changes and time to drape contamination. The researchers recommended that the surgeon not touch the C-arm drape.[79]

Gershkovich et al[123] reviewed three different methods of lateral C-arm receiver draping and measured contamination in distance. The traditional three-quarter sheet draping method was compared with a three-quarter clip draping method and a commercially available C-arm draping product. When all three draping methods were compared, the distance between the contamination areas for the different methods was statistically significant. The traditional three-quarter sheet drape was contaminated at a level that was within the sterile field when the receiver was brought into a lateral position.[123] The traditional method of three-quarter sheet draping also contaminated the surgeon's gown and gloves while the other two methods did not.[123]

4.7 Do not use adhesive incise drapes without antimicrobial properties. *[Recommendation]*

Iodophor-impregnated adhesive incise drapes may be used in accordance with the manufacturer's IFU, unless contraindicated by a patient's allergy to iodine. *[Conditional Recommendation]*

High-quality evidence regarding the benefits of using adhesive incise drapes for prevention of SSI conflicts. The evidence indicates that use of plain adhesive incise drapes without antimicrobial properties is correlated with an increase in SSI rates.[124] A systematic review found that use of an iodophor-impregnated drape has no effect on SSI rates,[124] and a more recent study found that use of an iodophor-impregnated drape may reduce SSI rates.[125] Recent evidence also indicates that the adhesiveness of the

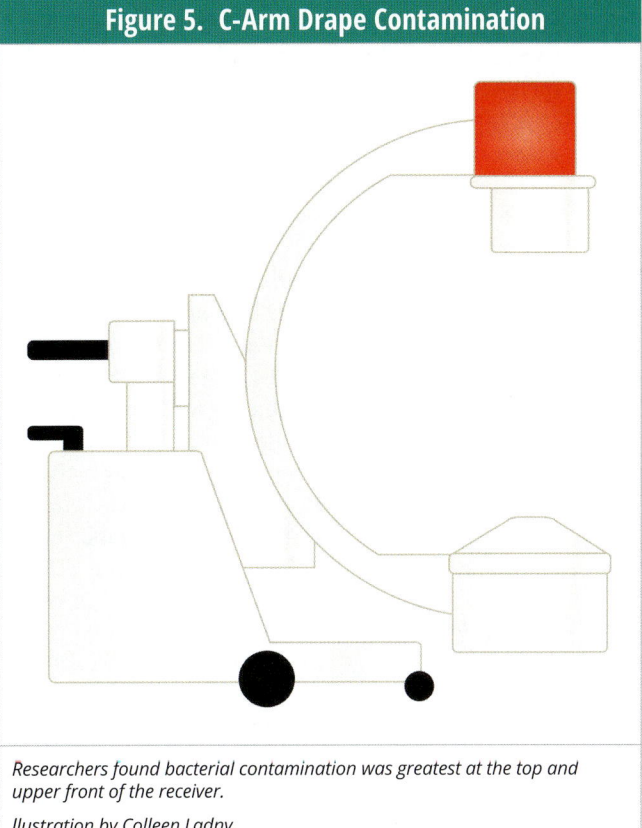

Figure 5. C-Arm Drape Contamination

Researchers found bacterial contamination was greatest at the top and upper front of the receiver.

Ilustration by Colleen Ladny.

incise drape to the skin may improve the effectiveness of the product and that iodophor-impregnated drapes may be useful for maintaining sterile technique by securing sterile drapes without increasing the risk for SSI.[125,126]

Surgical site infection guidelines also give conflicting recommendations for use of adhesive incise drapes. The WHO, CDC, Society for Healthcare Epidemiology of America, and Infectious Diseases Society of America do not recommend the use of adhesive incise drapes for prevention of SSI.[8,64,90] However, more recent guidelines from organizations in other countries support the use of iodophor-impregnated adhesive incise drapes (unless the patient has an iodine allergy) but do not recommend use of noniodophor-impregnated adhesive incise drapes.[127-129]

In a systematic review of seven RCTs involving 4,195 patients, Webster and Alghamdi[124] concluded there was no evidence to support the use of nonantimicrobial plastic adhesive incise drapes as a method for reducing infection and that there was some evidence that infection rates may be increased when adhesive incise drapes are used. A meta-analysis of five studies included in the review, which included 3,082 participants, compared plain plastic adhesive incise drapes with no drape and showed a significantly higher number of patients developed an SSI when the adhesive incise drape was used. There was no effect on SSI rates according to a meta-analysis of two additional studies in the systematic review that included 1,113 participants and compared iodine-impregnated plastic adhesive incise drapes with no drape.

The researchers theorized that the patient's skin is not likely to be a primary cause of SSI if it is properly disinfected, and they concluded that attempting to isolate the skin from the surgical wound is of no benefit and may create increased moisture and bacterial growth under adhesive drapes.[124] It is important to note that this systematic review did not compare non-iodine-impregnated plastic adhesive incise drapes with iodine-impregnated plastic adhesive incise drapes because no research that fit the inclusion criteria was available.

Since this systematic review[124] was published in 2015, new evidence has been generated on the use of plastic adhesive incise drapes that conflicts with the systematic review findings.[125,126,130,131] Two of the studies suggest that the adhesiveness of the drape, including how it is applied initially and how the adhesiveness is maintained throughout the surgery may be a factor affecting SSI rates when these drapes are used.[125,126] The manufacturer's IFU can provide information on the correct drape application technique for maximum product effectiveness. More research is needed in the form of large RCTs comparing the use of iodine-impregnated plastic adhesive incise drapes and non-iodine-impregnated plastic adhesive incise drapes on SSI rates in multiple specialties. Researchers should also report the skin preparation process, including the preoperative bathing and intraoperative skin antiseptic product used and the adhesiveness of the drape initially and throughout the procedure.

In a quasi-experimental study, Bejko et al[125] prospectively collected data for 5,100 patients undergoing cardiac surgery. For outcome analysis, the researchers matched 1,616 cardiac surgery patients to study the difference in SSI rates for the iodine-impregnated plastic adhesive drape group (n = 808) and the non-iodine-impregnated plastic adhesive drape group (n = 808). They found that both the overall SSI rate and the superficial SSI rate were significantly lower in the iodine-impregnated plastic adhesive drape group. In addition, the iodine-impregnated plastic adhesive incise drape group needed significantly fewer vacuum-assisted closures. Notably, the authors also reported that only 57.9% of the patients with the non-iodine-impregnated drape had complete adherence of the drape to the skin at the end of the procedure versus 95% of the patients with the iodine-impregnated drape. The researchers concluded that the higher rate of adhesiveness in the iodine-impregnated plastic adhesive drape group

may have been a variable contributing to the lower superficial SSI rate.[125]

In a single center, single surgeon RCT, Rezapoor et al[126] studied the use of iodine-impregnated plastic adhesive incise drapes in patients undergoing hip procedures (N = 101). In this study, 50 participants were randomly assigned to the intervention group and had iodine-impregnated plastic adhesive incise drapes used on the operative hip. The participants not assigned to the intervention group (N = 51) had no plastic adhesive incise drapes used. The researchers took a total of five swabs from the skin or drape of each participant

- prior to skin preparation,
- after skin preparation,
- immediately after skin incision,
- after closure of the capsule and tensor fasciae latae, and
- immediately after the skin was closed and the iodine-impregnated plastic adhesive drape was removed if used.

The researchers ended the study early because they found a significant decrease in bacterial colonization after skin closure, with only 12% positive cultures for the iodine-impregnated plastic adhesive drapes group and 27.5% for the group with no plastic adhesive drapes. No SSIs were identified in either group. Six of the 50 patients in the iodine-impregnated plastic adhesive drape group had some gaps between the skin and the drape. Interestingly, there was a non-statistically significant increase in bacterial contamination rates when the iodine-impregnated plastic adhesive incise drape was separated and lifted off of the skin.[126]

In an RCT with a small sample size (N = 40) in a simulated surgery setting, Milandt et al[130] found no statistical difference in bacterial recolonization rates of the knee (ie, the simulated surgical site) when an iodine-impregnated plastic adhesive incise drape was used or when the knee was only exposed to air. Therefore, the researchers concluded that iodine-impregnated plastic adhesive drapes do not increase bacterial colonization and can be used for at least 75 minutes in uncomplicated total knee arthroplasty procedures without the risk of potential recolonization. The researchers also stated that the results might lead to questioning the need for these drapes because there was no difference in the colonization rates and stated that they might be used in clinical practice for other reasons, such as securing other drape material.[130]

In an ex vivo laboratory study, Casey et al[131] studied the effect of iodine-impregnated plastic adhesive incise drapes and nonantimicrobial drapes on donor skin inoculated with methicillin-resistant *Staphylococcus aureus* and the permeation of iodine into the skin from drape use. Overall, the researchers found that the iodine-impregnated drape had significant antimicrobial properties compared with the nonantimicrobial plastic adhesive incise drape. The researchers also found skin permeation of iodine down to the deeper skin layers, up to 1,500 μm below the skin.[131]

5. Opening Sterile Items

5.1 **Open, dispense, and transfer sterile items to the sterile field by methods that maintain the sterility and integrity of the item and the sterile field.** *[Recommendation]*

5.2 **Introduce sterile items to the sterile field as close as possible to the time of use.** *[Recommendation]*

High-quality evidence indicates that sterile items will remain sterile with the passage of time when correctly wrapped or packaged and sterilized.[92,132-135] However, sterile items that have been opened have an increased chance of becoming contaminated.[91-96,98] To reduce the risk of contamination, it is best to have the item conveniently available and ready to open when it is needed rather than to open the item (eg, implant, medication, non-emergent suture, dressing) hours before use.[91] Additional benefits of opening sterile items as close as possible to the time of use include reducing waste and the financial impact of opening items that are not used.

Leaving implants in sterile packaging until as close to the moment of implantation as possible reduces the risk of contamination through exposure to the OR environment and increased handling. In a quasi-experimental study, Menekse et al[93] found that uncovered implant trays were significantly more contaminated during a 2-hour period compared to implant trays covered with a sterile towel. Patient receiving implants, especially those undergoing an implant replacement, may be at greater risk for infection. The CDC has stated that implants can be susceptible to formation of biofilm with microorganisms that have a higher chance of being resistant to antibiotics.[90] A typical pathogen associated with infected implants is *Staphylococcus epidermidis,* which has demonstrated antimicrobial resistance.[136] However, studies on current methodologies to prevent implant contamination and reduce biofilm formation are limited.

5.3 **Immediately before presenting items to the sterile field, inspect sterile items for**
- **sterility of the contents, as noted on the packaging;**
- **the expiration date, when applicable;**

- **package integrity;**
- **product integrity (eg, discoloration or particulate formation in medications and solutions); and**
- **verification that the external chemical indicators have changed to the correct color, indicating that the parameters for sterilization have been met.**[100,137]

[Recommendation]

Inspecting items before they are presented to the sterile field helps verify that conditions required for sterility have been met. Inspection also prevents microbial contamination of the sterile field that may occur if the integrity of the container has been breached and the item is placed on the sterile field. Implants may have additional elements that require inspection, such as sizing and factors specific to that item.

High-quality evidence shows that correctly wrapped or packaged and sterilized items will remain sterile with the passage of time.[92,132-135] However, the sterility of a packaged item may be affected by particular events (eg, amount of handling) or environmental conditions (eg, humidity).[137,138] Therefore, the sterility of packages is event-related and depends on maintenance of the integrity of the package.[100,132,138]

Items that have an expiration date should not be used after the date has passed. Manufacturers will not typically guarantee that a product meets expected parameters after the expiration date, and the product could have reduced effectiveness.

5.3.1 **Have an interdisciplinary team, including the surgeon and an infection preventionist, perform a risk/cost/benefit analysis to determine whether items that are not labeled as sterile (eg, antiseptic solution) or not packaged for sterile delivery to the sterile field (eg, vancomycin powder) may be used on the sterile field. Isolate items that have been approved for use on the sterile field by an interdisciplinary team from other items on the sterile field.** *[Conditional Recommendation]*

As part of the Code of Federal Regulations, the FDA requires that items have specific labeling and adequate directions for use.[139,140] The directions for use guide personnel in using the item safely within parameters set for the intended purpose of the product.[140]

In 2012, the FDA raised awareness about microbial contamination of antiseptic drug products intended for use as preoperative skin preparation agents.[141] One of the intended outcomes was to alert clinicians that not all skin antiseptic agents are sterile and therefore could be a potential source of infection.[141] The FDA does not require skin antiseptic agents to be sterile but has requested that manufacturers voluntarily clarify on their label the sterility status (ie, sterile, nonsterile). As part of this recommendation, there was further emphasis that the products should be used according to the manufacturer's IFU. Since the FDA does not currently require skin antisepsis products to be manufactured as sterile, it is crucial that products be used according to the directions provided. When sterility, labeling, packaging, or directions for use are unclear or unavailable, additional consideration by an interdisciplinary team is needed to evaluate risks and benefits to the patient. When antimicrobial products are being evaluated, the risk for antimicrobial resistance may also be considered a potential patient or population harm.[142]

Items not packaged for sterile delivery to the sterile field may increase the risk of contamination. Removal of a medication stopper that is not designed to be removed may expose the contents to contamination when the contents are transferred over the unsterile lip of the container. The AORN Guideline for Medication Safety[40] includes more information on sterile delivery of medications to the sterile field.

5.4 **Deliver items to the sterile field in a manner that prevents unsterile objects or unscrubbed team members from leaning or reaching over the sterile field.** [Recommendation]

Microorganisms are shed from the skin of perioperative personnel.[64,96] Maintaining distance from the sterile field decreases the potential for contamination when items are passed from unsterile to sterile areas.[143,144]

5.5 **Present sterile items directly to the scrubbed team member or placed securely on the sterile field.** [Recommendation]

Items tossed onto a sterile field may roll off the edge, create a hole in the sterile drape, or cause other items to be displaced, leading to contamination of the sterile field.

5.5.1 **Present heavy or sharp items directly to a scrubbed team member or opened them on a separate clean, dry surface.** [Recommendation]

5.6 **Open items packaged in sterile barrier systems according to the manufacturers' IFU, if available.** [Recommendation]

5.6.1 **Inspect rigid sterilization containers for intact external locks, secured latch filters, valves, and tamper-evident devices, and for the correct color change to external chemical indicators before they are opened onto a clean, flat, and dry surface.**[137] **Open the rigid sterilization container in the following order:**

1. **An unscrubbed person should lift the lid up and toward himself or herself while moving the lid away from the container.**
2. **The unscrubbed person should inspect the integrity of the lid filter or valve and consider the contents to be contaminated if the filter is dislodged, damp, or not intact (eg, holes, tears, punctures).**
3. **A scrubbed team member should lift the inner basket(s) out of and above the container without contacting the unsterile surfaces of the table or container.**
4. **Before the instruments are placed on the sterile field, the scrub person should examine the internal chemical indicator for the correct color change and inspect the inside surface of the container for debris, moisture, contamination, or damage.**[137]
5. **If there are any filters in the bottom of the container, an unscrubbed person should inspect the integrity of the filters.**

[Recommendation]

Opening rigid sterilization containers on a clean, flat, and dry surface facilitates removal of sterile items from their containers without contaminating the items or the sterile field. Checking that container locks, latch filters, valves, and tamper-evidence devices are intact helps to verify there has not been a breach of the container seal. Opening the container according to the manufacturer's written IFU facilitates aseptic removal of the contents. Lifting the lid up and away from the container and toward oneself helps to prevent potential contamination from contact between the unsterile lid and the sterile inner rim, contents, and inside of the container system and also helps to prevent the unscrubbed person from leaning over the sterile contents of the container. Inspection of filters by unscrubbed personnel prevents contamination of the scrub person's sterile gloves by the portion of the filter that was exposed to the external side of the packaging.

5.6.2 Inspect wrapped sterile packages for intact tape and the correct color change for external chemical indicators before they are opened. An unscrubbed person should open the wrapped sterile package by

1. opening the farthest wrapper flap and securing the flap in the hand that is holding the item;
2. opening each of the side flaps, one at a time, and securing the flaps in the hand that is holding the item;
3. opening the nearest wrapper flap and presenting the item to the scrubbed team member; and
4. visually inspecting the entire wrapper for integrity (eg, no holes, tears, punctures) and presence of moisture before the sterile item is placed onto the sterile field. *[Recommendation]*

Opening the wrapper flap that is farthest away first prevents contamination that might occur from passing an unsterile arm over sterile items. Wrapper edges are considered contaminated. Securing the loose edges helps prevent them from contaminating sterile areas or items.

Instrument tray wrappers used in accordance with the manufacturer's IFU provide a barrier against contamination of the contents. Holes or tears in instrument wrappers interrupt the barrier properties of the wrapper, calling into question the sterility of the contents.[137]

In a nonexperimental study, Mobley and Jackson[145] evaluated staff member identification of varying sized holes and tears in disposable instrument wrappers and found that personnel trained to detect holes and tears correctly identified them only 56.1% of the time. The staff members followed the standard practice of holding the wrapper up to overhead lights in the OR to identify holes and tears. It was easier for staff members to recognize an intact or torn wrapper than it was to identify a punctured wrapper. The researchers did not find that the data were correlated to role or experience level. They concluded that the current method of wrapper hole and tear identification is not adequate. The study results suggest that facilities should evaluate the use of wrappers versus other methods of packaging as a measure to limit the potential for holes and tears in wrappers. Additional research on methods for hole and tear identification in instrument wrappers is needed.

5.6.3 Inspect paper-plastic pouches (ie, peel pouches) for intact seals and for the correct color change of external chemical indicators. Present the pouch to the scrubbed team member or opened onto the sterile field by pulling back the flaps without touching the inside of the package, allowing the contents to slide over the unsterile edges of the package, or tearing the package. *[Recommendation]*

Touching the inside of the peel pouch packaging or allowing the contents to slide over the unsterile edges may contaminate the contents of the package. In a nonexperimental study, Trier et al[146] showed that items in large peel pouches had significantly greater contamination on opening than those in small peel pouches. The researchers did not correlate contamination with levels of personnel experience or job role.

5.7 When transferring medications and sterile solutions (eg, normal saline) to the sterile field,
- transfer as close to the time of use as possible[40];
- transfer in a slow, controlled manner using a sterile transfer device (eg, sterile vial spike, filter straw, plastic catheter)[40] unless the item is packaged for sterile delivery to the sterile field;
- transfer into a receptacle that is placed near the sterile table's edge or is held by a scrubbed team member; and
- verify and label the medication or solution immediately after transfer.[40,147-150]

[Recommendation]

Transferring and handling medications and solutions on the sterile field poses increased risks for contamination of the medication, solution, sterile field, and surgical site because medications and solutions are removed from their original containers, stored on the sterile field, and passed from a scrubbed team member to a licensed practitioner for administration.[40] Using transfer devices designed to reduce the potential for contamination by minimizing splashing, spilling, or the need to reach over the sterile field enables personnel to comply with principles of sterile technique. Pouring the entire contents of the container slowly prevents splashing. Splashing may cause strikethrough and splashback from unsterile surfaces to the sterile field. Placing the solution receptacle near the edge of the sterile table or having the scrubbed team member hold the receptacle reduces the potential for contamination of the sterile table and allows the unscrubbed team member to pour fluids without leaning over the sterile field.

5.7.1 Do not remove medication vial stoppers from vials for the purpose of pouring medications unless they are specifically designed for removal and pouring by the manufacturer. *[Recommendation]*

1037

5.7.2 **Pour medications or sterile solutions from the container only once, and do not replace the cap. Discard any remaining fluids in the opened container at the end of the procedure.** *[Recommendation]*

The sterility of the contents of opened medication or solution containers cannot be maintained if the cap is replaced. In addition, reuse of open containers may contaminate sterile solutions from drops that contact unsterile areas and then run back over the container opening. Irrigation and IV solutions and supplies are considered to be for single use. Using surplus volume from any irrigation or IV solution container or using the same supplies for more than one patient increases the risk of cross contamination.

6. Maintaining the Sterile Field

6.1 **Continually maintain the sterile field.** *[Recommendation]*

The sterile field is subject to contamination by personnel, breaks in sterile technique, vectors (eg, insects), and exposure to air.

6.2 **Monitor for contamination of the sterile field and potential breaks in sterile technique and correct them immediately.** *[Recommendation]*

Continual observation for breaks in sterile technique may prevent microbial contamination. Breaks in sterile technique may expose the patient to increased microbial contamination. Microbial contamination can increase the risk for infection.[138,151-153]

6.2.1 **When a break in sterile technique occurs, take corrective action immediately unless the patient's safety is at risk. When a break in technique cannot be corrected immediately, take corrective action as soon as it is safe for the patient.** *[Recommendation]*

The longer the contamination remains uncorrected, the more complex and difficult containment can be, and it becomes more likely that full containment may not be possible.[154]

6.2.2 **Consider instruments contaminated when they are found**
- assembled or clamped closed,[100]
- with organic material (eg, blood, hair, tissue, bone fragments) on or in the instrument,[155] or
- with other debris (eg, bone cement, grease, mineral deposits) on or in the instrument.

[Recommendation]

Sterilization or high-level disinfection can only be achieved if all surfaces of an instru-

ment have contacted the sterilizing or disinfecting agent under appropriate conditions and for the appropriate amount of time.[100,137,138] If an instrument has not been correctly dissembled or is clamped closed before sterilization or high-level disinfection, there is no way to ensure that the sterilant or high-level disinfectant made contact with all surfaces of the item; therefore, sterility or high-level disinfection may not have been achieved.

Organic and inorganic material that remains on a surgical instruments after the sterilization process is not considered sterile[155] and may increase the risk for SSI.[151-153] Organic materials and other debris may act as barriers that interfere with sterilization[155] or high-level disinfection or may combine with and deactivate the sterilant or disinfectant.[100,137,138] If organic material or other debris is found on an instrument that has been through a sterilization or high-level disinfection cycle, there is no way to ensure that the sterilant or high-level disinfectant made contact with all surfaces of the item; therefore, sterility or high-level disinfection may not have been achieved. More information on sterilization is available in the AORN Guideline for Sterilization.[100]

6.2.3 **When contaminated instruments are found in an instrument set, consider the entire set contaminated.** *[Recommendation]*

If one instrument within an instrument set was clamped closed, was assembled, or had organic or other debris present during the sterilization or high-level disinfection process, there is no way to confirm that the sterilant or high-level disinfectant made contact with all surfaces of the item and with the other items in the set. Sterility or high-level disinfection may not have been achieved[100,137,138]; therefore, the sterility of the entire set is in question.

6.2.4 **When an item or items are found to be contaminated, take the following corrective actions, at a minimum:**
- remove the contaminated item(s),
- remove any other items that may have come in contact with the contaminated item(s),
- change the gloves of any team member who may have touched the contaminated item(s), and
- take any additional corrective actions required after thoughtful assessment and informed decision making based on the specific factors associated with the individual event.

[Recommendation]

Taking immediate corrective action when breaks in sterile technique occur may minimize the amount of contamination and reduce the subsequent risk for SSI.

6.3 **Cover the sterile field if it will not be used immediately (eg, procedural delay, sterile field for closure, multiple tables) or during periods of increased activity (eg, pre-incision, repositioning).** [Recommendation]

If the sterile field is in use, the portion of the sterile field that will not be immediately used (eg, implants, instruments not in use) may be covered. [Conditional Recommendation]

Exposure to air may affect the **event-related sterility** of open sterile items and sterile fields. Moderate-quality evidence suggests that covering the sterile field reduces contamination over time.[91,93,95,98] Although opening instruments and sterile supplies as close to the time of use is the primary strategy to reduce exposure to potential air contamination,[91] covering the sterile field may be used as a secondary strategy to reduce the potential for contamination from exposure to the OR environment.[91,93,98,156] The OR environment is not sterile, and potentially infectious organisms may be present in the air.[91,93,95,98] Therefore, covering the sterile field or even portions of the sterile field that are not actively being used, especially implants and instruments, may be crucial in minimizing potential air contamination of the sterile field.[157,158]

In a nonexperimental study, Markel et al[156] compared covered and uncovered tables in static and dynamic (ie, active) environments. The researchers found that covering sterile tables significantly reduced the bacterial contamination under the sterile drape when reviewed at the 4- and 8-hour time periods. However, no differences in contamination rates were found above or below the sterile covers at the 24-hour period.[156] Based on the findings of their study, the researchers also suggested that covering implants or portions of the instrument table during the active procedure might significantly reduce the risk for contamination.

Moderate-quality evidence on environmental (eg, air particle, bacterial) contamination indicates that the OR environment may be progressively contaminated over time, especially with increased numbers of personnel and increased activity (eg, movement, door openings).[25,99,144,159-166] Conversely, there is some conflicting evidence[162,167] demonstrating that increased surgical duration or numbers of people do not increase OR environmental contamination.

Three nonexperimental studies demonstrated higher levels of environmental bacteria during the pre-incision time frame correlated to periods of increased activity that increases the risk of sterile field contamination.[98,164,168] These findings are also supported by Lynch et al[169] and Darnley et al[170] who both found higher rates of traffic during the pre-incision time frame.

Chosky et al[98] found that all bacterial contamination occurred during instrument setup. The researchers also found that instruments that were set up and covered in an OR with ultraclean air had a 28-fold decrease in contamination. This led the researchers to conclude that instruments should be set up and covered until the patient is transferred to the OR bed. This finding was also supported by Hansen et al[164] who found a significant number of CFU prior to incision, leading the researchers to conclude that there was a period of increased activity prior to the procedure start.

Radcliff et al[168] also found that risk to patients was increased in the pre-incision time frame. The researchers studied surgical delays from the time the patient entered the OR until the time of incision in patients undergoing spinal procedures. They found that in-room delays of more than 1 hour in length prior to incision were significantly correlated to an increase in SSI risk,[168] supporting table covering during this period when possible. The researchers theorized that this finding was due to additional exposure of the sterile field to airborne contaminants, traffic, and direct contact.[168]

Two studies found that strategic covering of implant trays may reduce the potential for contamination.[93,95] Bible et al[95] evaluated implant tray covering in an RCT of 105 spinal procedures by one surgeon. In the control procedures, the spinal implant trays were not covered; in the intervention procedures, the spinal implant trays were covered with a sterile towel upon opening. Swabs of the top layer of the implant trays were taken after the implantation phase of the procedure was complete. The implant trays that were covered had only a 2.0% contamination rate while the uncovered spinal implant trays had a 16.7% contamination rate.

Menekse et al[93] also studied covered and uncovered spinal implant trays for contamination during a 2-hour period. The researchers found that after 30 minutes, there was a significant difference in contamination rates between the covered and uncovered trays. In addition, the uncovered trays progressively became more contaminated than the trays covered with a sterile towel. At the 2-hour point, the contamination rates were 18.2% and 55% for covered and uncovered trays, respectively. The implant contamination levels were not linked to SSI rates.[93]

It should be noted that both studies used sterile surgical towels as the covering method, which may explain the presence of contamination on covered implant trays in both studies. Sterile surgical towels do not meet the same standards as a sterile drape, which is required to resist strikethrough of liquids or microorganisms carried in liquids.[42] Further research is needed to compare the effectiveness of using a sterile drape to using a sterile surgical towel to protect the sterile field from contamination.

6.3.1 **Cover the sterile field with a sterile drape in a manner that allows the cover to be removed without compromising the sterility of the table (eg, bringing a portion of the table cover up and over the field from below the level of the table surface,[123] cutting the drape down the middle). The sterile field may be covered with a sterile drape designed for this purpose or by the sterile two-"cuffed"-drape method described as follows:**

- **Place the first drape horizontally over the table or other area to be covered, with the cuff at or just beyond the halfway point. Place the second drape from the opposite side of the table with the cuff positioned so that it completely covers the cuff of the first drape (Figure 6).**
- **Remove the drapes by placing the hands within the cuff of the top drape and lifting the drape up and away from the table and toward the person removing the drape. Remove the second drape from the opposite side in the same manner.**

[Recommendation]

Removing the cover from the sterile field may result in a part of the cover that was below the sterile field being drawn above the sterile field, which may allow air currents to draw microorganisms and other contaminants (eg, dust, debris) from an unsterile area (eg, the floor) and deposit them in sterile areas.[96,123]

6.3.2 **Have an interdisciplinary team that includes an infection preventionist develop and implement measures to minimize risk of contamination to covered sterile fields. Measures may include**

- **posting a sign notifying personnel that a covered sterile field is in the room,**
- **limiting traffic in the OR or procedure room with covered sterile field, or**
- **directly observing the covered sterile field.**

[Conditional Recommendation]

The evidence review for this guideline found no evidence to support that the presence of a person directly observing a covered sterile table during a procedural delay prevents contamination of the sterile field. The presence of person-

nel may increase the level of particle or bacterial contamination in the OR[25,94,144,159,160,166] or the risk for SSI,[163,171] whereas bacterial contamination in an empty OR is comparatively low.[25,164,172] There is conflicting evidence on whether the presence of personnel affects OR contamination[162,167,173] and whether instruments always become contaminated over time.[174]

There is also conflicting evidence regarding the length of time a sterile field may remain covered. In an RCT, Dalstrom et al[91] found that covered sterile instruments had no contamination after 4 hours. This study was limited because the trays were covered and left in a locked OR without traffic and the study only tested the instrument trays for contamination up to 4 hours. In a nonexperimental study comparing table covering methods and levels of contamination, Markel et al[156] found significantly reduced contamination of covered sterile tables for 8 hours. However, there was no differences in contamination rates above or below the sterile table cover at the 24-hour period. A nonexperimental study by Campbell et al[175] found 2% contamination on the third day of testing of covered sterile tables that were repeatedly covered and uncovered by a rolled method. The second part of the study found only a 7.5% contamination rate of sterile covered tables after 7 days. Based on their findings, the researchers suggested that covering tables for up to 24 hours reduces contamination, presents minimal patient risk, and may be clinically relevant to certain surgical specialties where patient emergencies are time sensitive.[175]

Further research is needed to determine what measures should be taken to prevent contamination of a covered sterile field. Facility design and practices may affect the risk of contamination of a covered sterile field.

6.3.3 **Develop a standardized procedure to delineate the specific circumstances under which the sterile field should be covered and to clarify the length of time a sterile field may be covered.** *[Recommendation]*

Standard procedures (ie, following the same patterns and processes each time) assist in achieving accuracy, efficiency, and continuity among perioperative team members. Studies of human error have shown that many errors involve a deviation from routine practice.[97] Creating a facility-specific standardized practice allows facilities to review procedures or situations specific to their organization that might necessitate table covering, such as during intraoperative magnetic resonance imaging procedures when the patient is being scanned.

6.4 **When a <u>unidirectional ultraclean air delivery system</u> (eg, laminar airflow) is in use, position the surgical site and instrument tables within the air curtain of the system, if possible.** *[Recommendation]*

A unidirectional ultraclean air delivery system provides a steady stream of high-efficiency particulate air filtration within the air curtain (ie, impact area of the air delivery system).[161,167,176-178] The stream of clean air theoretically reduces the risk of bacterial contamination at the surgical site by constantly moving clean air across the area.[161,167] Unidirectional ultraclean air delivery systems may also decrease contamination of the instrument tables in the sterile field when the tables are positioned within the airflow curtain.[174,179]

In a systematic review of methods for SSI prevention, Barr et al[180] found that the evidence supported the use of a unidirectional ultraclean air delivery system for reducing sterile field contamination. In a nonexperimental study, Markel et al[156] found that the air velocity at the approximate site of the surgical incision was significantly higher than the air velocity at the instrument table. These findings were negatively correlated to a significant increase in contamination at the instrument table compared to the approximate site of the surgical incision. The researchers concluded that the instruments should be placed in the unidirectional ultraclean air delivery system air curtain.[156]

In another nonexperimental study, Diab-Elschahawi et al[167] compared the effects of unidirectional ultraclean air delivery systems of different sizes on air contamination levels. The researchers found that ORs without a unidirectional ultraclean air delivery system and ORs with a small unidirectional ultraclean air delivery system had a significant increase in CFU on the instrument table.[167] The researchers stated that smaller unidirectional ultraclean air delivery systems cause air turbulence from insufficient airflow in the areas on the very edge of the stream of air, such as the area including the instrument table.[167] In a nonexperimental study, Friberg et al[181] also found high amounts of air contamination at the instrument table, which was similar to contamination in turbulent airflow systems.

Smith et al[161] conducted a quasi-experimental study on passive contamination rates of culture plates both inside and outside the air curtain of a vertical unidirectional ultraclean air delivery sys-

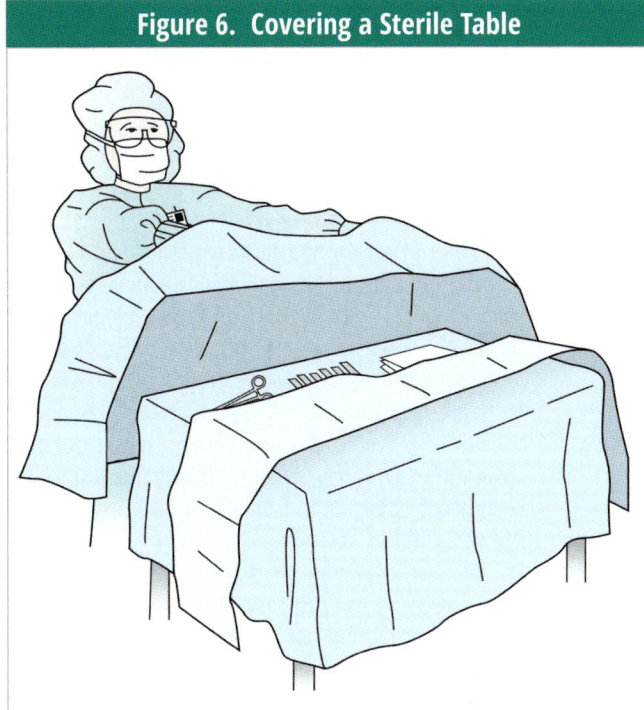

Figure 6. Covering a Sterile Table

The first drape is placed with the cuff at the halfway point. The second drape is placed from the opposite side and completely covers the cuff of the first drape

Illustration by Colleen Ladny and Kurt Jones.

tem. The researchers found consistently lower levels of contamination within the air curtain area than outside of it. The researchers discussed that minimizing obstacles within the air curtain (eg, staff, lights, microscopes) may reduce air turbulence, thereby making the system more effective against the spread of airborne contaminants.

In a small simulated study, Cao et al[182] found that thermal plumes within the unidirectional ultraclean air delivery system air curtain affected the velocity of the air distribution in that space. The researchers also found that the position of the moveable overhead surgical lights affected the air velocity distribution within the unidirectional ultraclean air delivery system air curtain. The researchers recommended that clinicians carefully consider the position of moveable overhead surgical lights to minimize blocking the air curtain from the surgical site.

The effectiveness of the air handling systems may depend on many factors. Perez et al[179] found that increased numbers of scrubbed personnel was positively associated with increased levels of bacterial contamination inside the unidirectional ultraclean air delivery system air curtain. The researchers also observed that increased numbers of scrubbed personnel was associated with an increased risk that the instrument table would be moved out of the unidirectional ultraclean air delivery system air curtain.

6.4.1

The unidirectional ultraclean air delivery system impact area may be visually identified on the OR floor. *[Conditional Recommendation]*

In a mixed methods study, De Korne et al[183] found that placing visual markers of the unidirectional ultraclean air delivery system impact area on the OR floor led to more consistent placement of the patient, Mayo stand, and sterile back table into the air curtain. During the 2-year period following the study, the SSI rate was lower than in the 4 years prior to the study.[183] However, since the previous rate of SSIs was low to begin with and the surgical volume had been increasing, the finding was not statistically significant.[183] The researchers found the following insightful comments from the qualitative interviews included in their study:

- The unidirectional ultraclean air delivery system air curtain may be too small to adequately provide enough space to both move sufficiently and position the Mayo stand and instrument table within the impact area.
- The open corneal implants were being kept outside of the air curtain.
- The unidirectional ultraclean air delivery system air curtain space above the patient may be compromised when both the overhead lights and microscope are inside of it.
- It was difficult for personnel to visually estimate the air curtain area above the patient since it was not visually marked like the OR floor.
- It was easier for unsterile visitors to understand where they could not stand when the impact area was marked on the floor.[183]

6.4.2

When a horizontal unidirectional ultraclean air delivery system is in use, do not stand or walk between the airflow curtain and the sterile field or surgical wound. *[Recommendation]*

Salvati et al[171] retrospectively reviewed data from 3,175 primary single total hip arthroplasty and total knee arthroplasty procedures for a period of 8 years at a single center specializing in these procedures. The researchers found that the infection rate for total hip arthroplasty decreased from 1.4% to 0.9% when the procedure was performed in the horizontal unidirectional ultraclean air delivery system room. However, the infection rate for total knee arthroplasty increased from 1.4% to 3.9% when the surgery was completed in a horizontal unidirectional ultraclean air delivery system room. The researchers concluded that during the total knee arthroplasty procedures, the scrubbed personnel were occasionally positioned between the horizontal airflow source and the patient's surgical incision site, whereas the horizontal airflow was not blocked by personnel during total hip arthroplasty procedures.

6.4.3

When a fixed unidirectional ultraclean air delivery system is not available or is not large enough to cover the entire sterile field, a portable unidirectional ultraclean air delivery system may be used at the instrument table or delivered to the surgical incision site in a sterile manner in accordance with the manufacturer's IFU. *[Conditional Recommendation]*

High-quality evidence supports the use of portable unidirectional ultraclean air delivery systems at the surgical site, instrument table, or both.[177,184-189] Two RCTs showed that the use of a sterile hose to deliver unidirectional ultraclean airflow over the surgical wound decreased bacterial contamination.[177,184] Darouiche et al[184] also found that the amount of bacterial contamination at the incision site significantly correlated with implant infections. A total of four implant infections all occurred in the control group participants, who underwent procedures without the use of the portable ultraclean air delivery system.[184]

Fixed ceiling- or wall-mounted unidirectional ultraclean air delivery systems may

- not always be functioning,
- not be available in the area where an operative[187,188] or other invasive procedure is planned,[185]
- be too small to accommodate all the items included in the sterile field,[186] and
- be affected by the position of scrubbed perioperative team members[171] and moveable overhead lights.[182]

In a laboratory smoke test, Nilsson et al[186] found that a portable unidirectional ultraclean air delivery system mounted to an instrument table outside of the ceiling-mounted unidirectional ultraclean air delivery system did not affect the air curtain of the ceiling-mounted system. Lapid-Gortzak et al[185] found that positioning a portable unidirectional air delivery system toward a simulated surgical site for intravitreal injection and the associated instrument table significantly reduced the particle counts in both areas. The researchers concluded that the use of a portable unidirectional ultraclean air delivery system may aid in reducing contamination in procedures not completed in locations with fixed unidirectional ultraclean air delivery systems.[185]

Clear identification of the target area for potential contaminant reduction, strategic positioning of the unit, and an unobstructed air curtain are important during the use of portable unidirectional ultraclean air delivery systems.[189] Following the manufacturer's IFU may aid in decision making to promote optimal product efficiency.

6.5 **Position heater-cooler devices away from the sterile field, and direct the airflow exhaust of the equipment away from the sterile field.** [Recommendation]

When heater-cooler devices are used in an OR with a unidirectional ultraclean air delivery system, positioning equipment outside of the air curtain and away from the sterile field may help decrease ventilation disruptions and turbulent airflow. Awareness of where the equipment exhaust fan is directed is crucial because there is the possibility for the fan's exhaust to blow into the surgical field.[190] In a nonexperimental study, Sommerstein et al[157] demonstrated that a heater-cooler device directed at the surgical site was more likely to cause the airflow exhaust to flow into the vertical unidirectional ultraclean air delivery system air curtain coming down toward the surgical site. The ability to maintain cleanliness of the air intake and internal exhaust systems of heater-cooler devices has recently been called into question.[191] The difficulty in ensuring cleanliness of the air intake and internal exhaust systems of the heater-cooler device makes it crucial to mitigate the effect of exhaust on the OR environment.

6.6 **When using intraoperative debridement devices with irrigation (ie, hydrosurgery, pulse lavage, low-frequency ultrasonic debridement) on open, infected wounds, implement interventions to minimize personnel exposure to potentially infectious materials and reduce contamination of the sterile field. Interventions may include**
- **wearing PPE**[33,49,192-197];
- **wearing a surgical helmet system**[47-49];
- **training personnel on correct use of the device**[49,192,196];
- **using manufacturer's recommendations for power, irrigation, and suction settings that limit mist, splatter, or spray, if patient care allows**[193,194,196,198]**; and**
- **covering the active hand piece with a clear sterile drape.**[49,192,197,199,200]

[Recommendation]

Moderate-quality evidence suggests that certain types of debridement devices (ie, hydrosurgery,[49,192-195] pulse lavage,[196,197,199,200] and low-frequency ultrasonic debridement[195,198]) may lead to dispersion of bacteria when used on open and infected wounds. The result-

ing mist, spray, or splatter may increase the risk of transmission of potentially infectious material to perioperative personnel and may contaminate the sterile field and OR environment.[49,192-198]

Moderate-quality evidence indicates that dispersion contamination may be reduced by either limiting[193,194,196,198] or containing[49,192,197,199,200] the device mist, spray, or splatter. The manufacturer's IFU may provide guidance on specific power, irrigation, and suction settings to reduce the amount of mist, splatter, or spray produced during use.[193,194,196,198] Covering the active hand piece with a clear sterile drape,[42] if not contraindicated by the manufacturer's IFU, may limit the number of particulates expelled on personnel or into the OR environment.[49,192,197,199,200]

Michailidis et al[198] studied the potential for dispersion contamination of aerosolized mist from a low-frequency ultrasonic debridement device. The researchers compared how different device settings, flow rates of saline irrigation, use of suction, and procedure locations affected the potential for increased CFU. Higher microbial counts were found with lower device settings, lower irrigation settings, no suction use, and a large wound area. There was no correlation of CFU to where the procedure was performed, whether the wound was infected, the type of hand piece used, or the duration of treatment. These findings led the researchers to conclude that contamination dispersal could be reduced with the use of higher device settings, higher irrigation flow rates, and suction. This was consistent with the device manual, which stated that higher settings result in a finer mist. There was a significant difference between CFU found before use of the device and when the device was used. The active air-sampling results showed that even in a clinic or patient room setting, there was a return to baseline levels of aerosolized microbes after 30 minutes. Wearing full PPE, including an impervious gown, a mask, a face shield with a plastic visor, and gloves was strongly recommended during use of low-frequency ultrasonic debridement devices.[198]

In a laboratory study, Sönnergren et al[193] studied the risk for bacterial transmission from three debridement methods including steel curette, plasma-mediated bipolar radio-frequency ablation, and hydrosurgery. Twelve porcine joint specimens were inoculated with *Staphylococcus aureus* and divided among treatment groups. Aerosolized bacteria was captured by active and passive sampling methods both during and after debridement. The researchers found that debridement by hydrosurgery caused significant aerosolization of bacteria at both default and maximum settings. However, aerosolization was not correlated to use of the curette or plasma-mediated bipolar radio-frequency ablation at the default or maximum settings. Although the bacterial counts for hydrosurgery were consistently higher than both curette and plasma-mediated bipolar radio-frequency ablation throughout the study, bacterial counts for hydrosurgery did decrease at the 15-, 30-, and 60-minute intervals. Plasma-mediated bipolar radio-frequency ablation was also able to significantly reduce the bacterial load in the wound.[193] The results of this study were confirmed in a second study by the same lead researcher.[194]

Angobaldo et al[197] studied dispersion of bacteria with pulse lavage use. The pulse lavage was used either with a sterile irrigation bag made for the purpose of containing splatter and spray or without a cover bag. Five culture plates were set at 1, 2, and 3 ft for each of the 10 participants. The rate of contamination when the bag was used during pulse lavage was 0.24%; when no bag was used, the contamination rate was 30.1%. A significant difference in contamination rates between groups was found at all distances measured. The researchers recommended the use of additional protective measures such as a bag to minimize the dissemination of potentially infectious material to personnel and the immediate vicinity.[197]

In another nonexperimental study, Putzer et al[49] tested whether use of a disposable draping device over the hydrosurgery device had an effect on contamination of personnel and the environment. The researchers found saline irrigation fluid purposefully contaminated with bacteria to simulate an infected wound on all OR personnel and in the OR environment when high-pressure hydrosurgery was used. Significant reductions in bacterial contamination were found on personnel and in the OR environment when a drape with a window was used over the high-powered hydrosurgical device. Notably, the surgeon and the surgical assistant had the largest reduction in dispersion contamination, emphasizing the protection that additional draping provided. However, the use of the drape only reduced contamination but did not completely eliminate dispersion contamination from either personnel or the OR environment.[49]

7. Moving Around a Sterile Field

7.1 **Move within or around a sterile field in a manner that prevents contamination of the sterile field.**
[Recommendation]

Airborne contaminants and microbial levels in the surgical environment are directly proportional to the amount of movement and the number of people in the OR or other procedure room.[24,25,96,143,144,169,172,201,202]

7.2 Scrubbed team members should
- remain close to the sterile field and touch only sterile areas or items;
- keep their hands and arms above waist level at all times[55,123];
- not fold their arms with their hands positioned in the axillary area[42];
- avoid changing levels, and be seated only when the entire procedure will be performed at that level[123];
- not turn their backs on the sterile field[42];
- turn back to back or face to face while maintaining distance from each other, the sterile field, and unsterile areas during position changes;
- not be positioned between the horizontal unidirectional ultraclean air delivery system air curtain and the surgical site[171];
- not leave the sterile field to retrieve items from the sterilizer; and
- use shielding devices (eg, lead aprons, mobile shields) that reduce radiological exposure in order to stay near the sterile field when radiology equipment is used.[203]

[Recommendation]

Keeping the hands and arms above waist level allows constant monitoring by the perioperative team member. Contamination may occur when a perioperative team member moves his or her hand or arms below waist level.[55,123]

The axillary area has the potential to become contaminated by perspiration, allowing for strikethrough of the gown and potential contamination of the gloved hands. The axillary area of the gown is an area of friction and is not considered an effective microbial barrier.[42]

When scrubbed team members change levels, the unsterile portion of their gowns may come into contact with sterile areas.[55,123]

Contamination of sterile gowns and gloves and the sterile field may be prevented when scrubbed team members maintain distance from each other and the sterile field when changing position and by establishing patterns of movement that reduce the risk of contact with unsterile areas.

Walking outside the periphery of the sterile field or leaving and then returning to the OR or other procedure room in sterile attire increases the potential for contamination.

7.3 Unscrubbed team members should
- face the sterile field on approach,
- not walk between sterile fields or scrubbed persons,
- not reach over an uncovered sterile field,
- stay as far back from the sterile field[143,144] and scrubbed persons as possible,

- remain outside of a vertical unidirectional ultra-clean air delivery system air curtain,[144] and
- not walk between the horizontal unidirectional ultraclean air delivery system air curtain and the sterile field.[171]

[Recommendation]

Facing the sterile field on approach allows perioperative personnel to observe their proximity to sterile areas and monitor for potential contamination of the sterile field. Walking between sterile fields or scrubbed personnel may increase the risk for contamination because both sides of a person cannot be monitored at the same time. Reaching over a sterile field increases the potential for contamination from unsterile items above it.

When possible, non-scrubbed personnel may reduce the potential for contamination by staying away from the sterile field[143,144] and out of unidirectional ultraclean air delivery system air curtains. Two studies have demonstrated that traffic or the presence of personnel in a specific space are correlated to increased particles[144] or bacteria.[143] The same studies demonstrated lower particle[144] or microbial[143] counts in areas of less movement or fewer personnel. One of the studies also found that increasing numbers of people within a unidirectional ultraclean air delivery system air curtain caused rising heat thermals that disrupted the airflow in that area.[144]

7.4 | **Limit nonessential conversations in the presence of a sterile field.** *[Recommendation]*

Conversations that are irrelevant to the patient or surgical process may be a barrier to effective communication[2] and may add unnecessary noise and distractions to the OR or other invasive procedure room.[74] In addition, microorganisms are transported on airborne particles, including respiratory droplets.[96] Letts and Doermer[172] studied the role of conversation in the OR by using small spherical particles of human albumin ranging in size from 10 μm to 35 μm in diameter to simulate particles that carry bacteria. Approximately 300,000 albumin particles were sprayed on the faces of the study participants and in their nostrils beneath the surgical masks.

The participants read aloud continuously for periods of 5, 10, 20, 30, 40, 50, and 60 minutes from a position 30 cm above a water bath simulating a surgical wound. The researchers collected particles from the water bath and processed them after each reading session. The results of the study showed that the longer the period of conversation, the greater the number of particles in the simulated wound. The effect of both time and conversation were found to be significant. The researchers concluded that conversation contributes to airborne contamination of surgical wounds.[172] Conversely, Hansen et al[164] did not find a correlation between particle counts and the amount of conversation during surgical procedures.

7.5 | **Keep doors to the operative or invasive procedure room closed as much as possible except during the entry and exit of patients, required personnel, and necessary equipment.** *[Recommendation]*

Moderate-quality evidence on door openings indicates that perioperative personnel contribute significantly to door openings, which may increase OR environmental contamination and subsequent patient risk for SSIs.[94,169,179,201,202,204] Door openings affect the OR positive pressure[162,169,205-208] and may interrupt the laminar airflow, possibly leading to more environmental contamination and greater risk for infection.[160,201,202,209-212] The authors of a systematic review found that the evidence supported limiting door openings.[180] One nonexperimental study significantly correlated an increased number of door openings with increased bacterial counts in the OR environment.[166]

Smith et al[161] studied door openings and the effect on contamination rates inside and outside of the vertical unidirectional ultraclean air curtain. The researchers found that the use of unidirectional airflow reduced but did not completely negate the contamination rates associated with door openings. For example, the researchers found that if the doors were opened just once, even with the use of unidirectional airflow, the contamination rates on culture plates increased by 63.9%. The researchers recommended using unidirectional airflow systems, limiting door openings, and restricting access to personnel.

Villafruela et al[213] studied the direction and magnitude of air velocity during door openings and closures, with personnel entering and exiting an OR that had vertical unidirectional airflow. The researchers found that the OR maintained a steady rate of positive pressure with no door openings. Another finding was that more air enters the OR from the adjacent corridor when a person enters the OR than when a person exits. This researchers also demonstrated that during door opening in an OR with functional unidirectional airflow, the air moves into the OR at the top of the doorway and out of the OR at the bottom of the doorway. The researchers concluded that this was most likely due to the fact that vertical unidirectional airflow causes movement of air from the ceiling down, which subsequently causes the air by the walls and door to flow upward. When personnel entered the OR, the air volume was found to be greater on the side of the doorway closest to where the person walked. This led the researchers to conclude that personnel should not walk close to either door frame when entering an OR, in order to minimize air volumes entering the OR.[213]

Conversely, some literature has not correlated OR door opening to higher microbial counts[143] or SSIs in procedures involving clean surgical wounds.[214] Wanta et al[214] found that SSIs were significantly correlated to a patient history of diabetes mellitus and operative duration. In a study on the effect of door opening on OR positive pressure rates, Weiser et al[208] found that OR positive pressure was only affected when two OR doors were opened simultaneously.

7.5.1 **Have an interdisciplinary team of key stakeholders develop and implement interventions to decrease door openings. Interventions may include**
- **preplanning and consolidating supply and equipment retrieval,**[160-162,169,202,207,211,212]
- **keeping the surgeons' preference cards current,**[169,207,209,212,215,216]
- **confirming that all instruments and supplies are present before the incision is made,**[212]
- **posting a sign on the door to restrict traffic while a procedure is in progress,**[204,207,210,216,217]
- **using means of communication that do not involve opening the door during procedures (eg, intercom systems, video monitoring systems, mobile communication devices),**[162,169,201,204,207,209,210,212,216,217]
- **assessing the phase of the procedure before relieving for breaks,**[94,169,207,209,211,212]
- **evaluating the culture in the perioperative environment,**[162,217]
- **having the surgeon state a preference for limited door openings,**[216,218]
- **storing frequently needed supplies in the OR,**[94,161,169,207,209,210,212,215,216]
- **using pass-through windows or compartments,**[207,210]
- **installing automatic door opening counters,**[169,204,207,210,212,216,217,219]
- **installing door alarms,**[169,219]
- **installing viewing windows,**[210,216] **and**
- **providing education about the effects of opening the doors.**[94,160-162,204,207,212,216,217,220]

[Conditional Recommendation]

Moderate-quality evidence contains various evidenced-based interventions that may help reduce door openings. The facilities that have introduced some of these measures have seen a decrease in door openings, and some have noted a decrease in the number of SSIs.[210,215] Two studies showed that door opening is multifactorial and concluded that having an interdisciplinary

team develop interventions to decrease door openings may be effective.[204,215] Education of OR personnel may be particularly important.

Understanding the reasons for door openings may facilitate the selection of interventions to reduce door openings. Moderate-quality evidence shows a large inconsistency in the range of door openings (ie, 35 to 259) during similar types of procedures, with nursing personnel responsible for the majority of door openings during procedures.[94,169,201,204,209,212,217] The most common reasons for door openings were information retrieval and supply gathering.[162,169,204,207,209,215] The researchers of one blinded study reported that 47% of door openings had no clear cause, leading the researchers to question whether these door openings were necessary.[94] Andersson et al[160] found that nearly 30% of all door openings may be unnecessary. The evidence has led researchers to conclude that door openings can be significantly reduced through interventions targeting modifiable behaviors.[162,169,201,204,207,209,212,215,220]

7.5.2 **Establish a quality assurance process to monitor door openings that occur while sterile supplies are open.** *[Recommendation]*

A quality assurance program to monitor numbers of door openings can help facilities understand whether there is a high rate of door openings overall or in certain specialties.[94,162,169,201,204,207,209,212,215,217] A quality monitoring program that tracks reasons for door openings may find potentially modifiable behaviors that can be targeted for change.[162,169,201,204,207,209,212,215,220] In a small study at a single institution, no change in behavior was found when a traffic surveillance monitoring program was implemented.[207] However, the researchers still recommended monitoring and including perioperative personnel in the development of monitoring protocols. The researchers concluded that while monitoring is important, other interventions or incentives might be essential.[207]

7.6 **Keep the number and movement of individuals in an operative or invasive procedure room to a minimum.** *[Recommendation]*

Moderate-quality evidence supports limiting the number of personnel during procedures.[24,159,166,169,179,180,207,221-223] Bacterial shedding increases with additional people[179] and levels of activity.[25] Air currents can pick up contaminated particles shed from patients, personnel, and drapes and distribute them to sterile areas.[25,96,224] One study found that an increased number of people in an OR was significantly correlated to increased bacterial counts in the OR environment.[166] Lynch et al[169] found an exponential relationship between door openings and the maximum number of people in a procedure room at any time point. In a simulated study, Sadrizadeh et al[144] found that increasing numbers of people around the sterile field may create greater potential for rising thermal air, which may interfere with air currents above the OR bed. In a small simulated study, Cao et al[182] also found that heat from personnel within the vertical unidirectional ultraclean air delivery system may decrease air velocity. Perez et al[179] found that increased numbers of scrubbed personnel increased bacterial contamination within the unidirectional ultraclean air delivery system air curtain, but associated the increase with bacterial shedding from personnel in that area.

Despite the evidence to support limiting personnel in ORs and procedure rooms, there is limited evidence clarifying what the number of individuals should be. Sadrizadeh et al[144] stated that critical procedures with the potential for high rates of SSIs should not have more than five or six personnel in order to keep the airborne bacterial counts below 10 CFU/m³. Castella et al[225] found that the average number of personnel was six to seven but that this number was sometimes higher in teaching facilities or in hospitals where complex surgeries are performed.

In a nonexperimental study to evaluate whether the behaviors and number of OR personnel can predict the density of airborne bacteria at the surgical site, Stocks et al[159] measured the number of airborne particulates and viable bacteria during 22 joint arthroplasty procedures with a range of five to 12 team members in the OR. The results indicated a relationship between the number and activity of team members present in the periphery of the OR and the number of particulates and CFU at the surgical site. The researchers recommended minimizing the number of team members who are present during the procedure.[159]

Conversely, in a retrospective case control study, Wanta et al,[214] found no significant correlation between numbers of people in an OR and rates of SSI in procedures classified as clean.

8. Quality

8.1 **Participate in quality assurance and performance improvement activities that are consistent with the health care organization's plan to improve understanding of and compliance with the principles and processes of sterile technique.** *[Recommendation]*

Quality assurance and performance improvement programs assist in evaluating and improving the quality of patient care and formulating plans for corrective action. These programs provide data that may be used to determine whether an individual organization is within benchmark goals and, if not, to identify areas that may require corrective actions.

8.2 **If a patient develops an SSI, have an interdisciplinary team that includes an infection preventionist evaluate sterile technique practices that may have contributed to the development of the infection, including**
- **intraoperative delays[168];**
- **adherence to surgical attire policies or procedures;**
- **performance of hand hygiene and surgical hand antisepsis;**
- **the use of a PAPR;**
- **use of surgical helmet systems;**
- **performance of routine glove changes per facility policy;**
- **use of isolation technique;**
- **use of a wound protector;**
- **use of medications and solutions on the sterile field[40,191];**
- **use of items that are not sterile, not labeled as sterile, or not packaged for sterile delivery to the sterile field;**
- **number of door openings and associated reasons;**
- **number of personnel and their roles during the procedure;**
- **movement of personnel around and within the sterile field;**
- **use and maintenance of heater-cooler devices;**
- **use of debridement devices on open, infected wounds; and**
- **use of table covering.**
[Recommendation]

Lack of evidence on the clinical application of sterile technique principles may create a gap in understanding potential contributing factors when a patient develops an SSI.[90,191] Evidence reviewed as part of the evaluation may include clinical documentation or data collected through a quality monitoring process.[226] Not all applications of sterile technique practices may be appropriate for inclusion into the patient's medical record, which serves as the legal record of care delivery. Documentation of nursing activities is dictated by health care organization policy and regulatory and accrediting agency requirements.[227-230]

Radcliff et al[168] found that delays longer than 60 minutes from when the patient came into the OR to the time of incision were predictive of a patient's risk for SSI. Procedural delays from in-room time to incision time also may correspond to periods of

Figure 7. Surgical Wound Classification Decision Tree

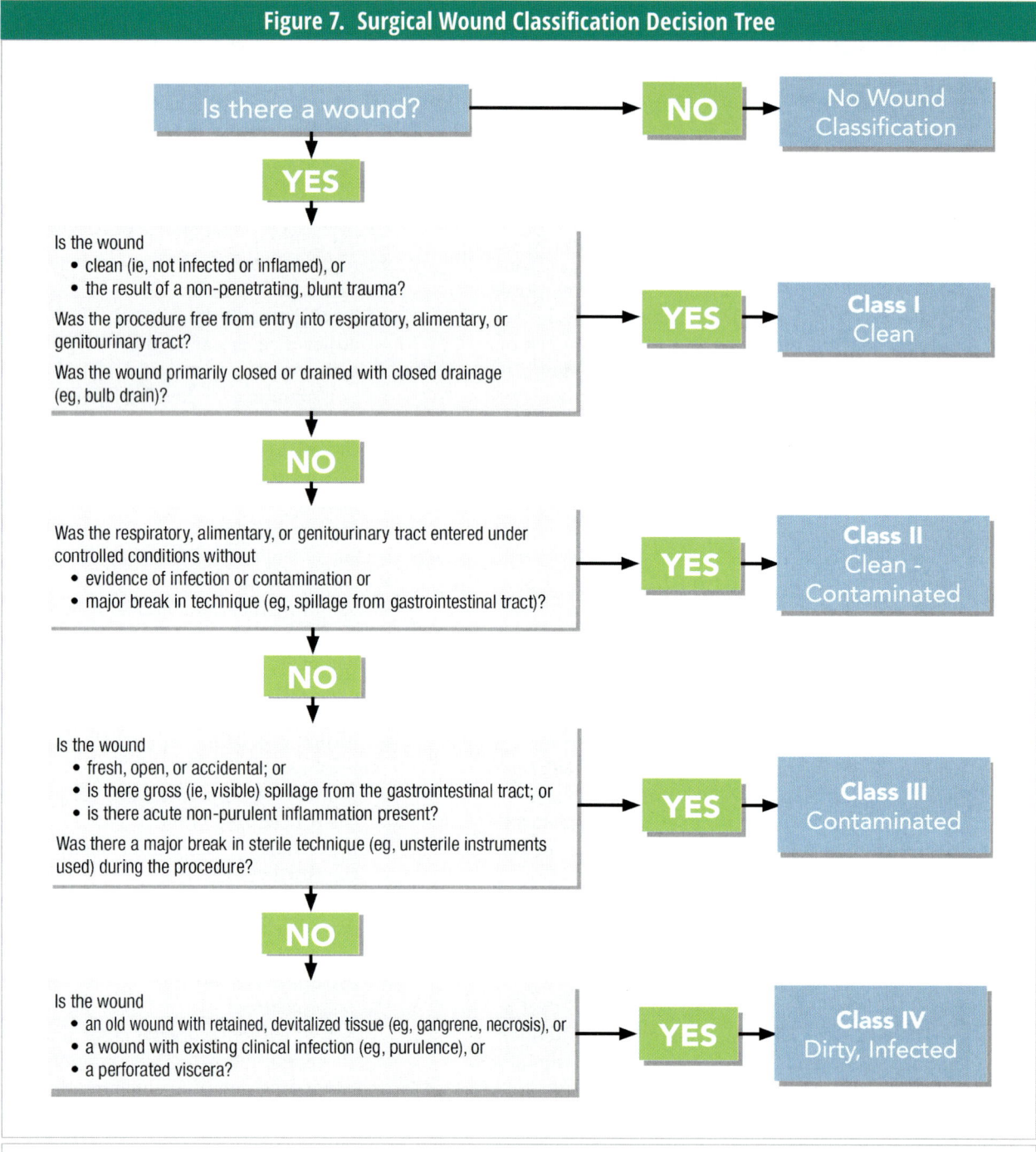

References

1. Mangram AJ, Horan TC, Pearson ML; Hospital Infection Control Practices Advisory Committee. Guidelines for prevention of surgical site infection, 1999. Am J Infect Control. 1999;27(2):97-132.
2. Surgical site infection (SSI) event. January 2017. Centers for Disease Control and Prevention. National Healthcare Safety Network. http://www.cdc.gov/nhsn/pdfs/pcssmanual/9pcssicurrent.pdf. Accessed June 20, 2017.

increased activity found to increase the potential for environmental contamination and traffic prior to incision.[98,164,169]

8.3 **Document significant or major breaks in sterile technique that are not immediately corrected or report these per organizational policy. [Recommendation]**

Effective management and collection of health care information that accurately reflects the patient's care, treatment, and services is a regulatory and accreditation requirement for both hospitals and ambulatory settings.[227-238] Clear and concise perioperative documentation is essential for the continuity of outcome-focused nursing care and for effective comparison of realized versus anticipated patient outcomes (eg, SSIs).

8.3.1 **Have an interdisciplinary team that includes perioperative nurses, an infection preventionist, quality personnel, risk managers, surgeons, and others key stakeholders determine what types of breaks in sterile technique necessitate documentation of a change in the surgical wound classification.** [Recommendation]

There is limited evidence on what constitutes a major or minor break in sterile technique. The AORN Surgical Wound Classification Decision Tree (Figure 7) classifies wounds as contaminated if there was a major break in sterile technique, such as the use of unsterile instruments during the procedure or spillage from the gastrointestinal tract. The CDC[239] states that a wound should be classified as contaminated if there is a major break in technique, such as open cardiac massage. In an expert opinion article, Hopper and Moss[154] described categories of breaks in sterile technique based on the length of time until recognition that the break has occurred.

Glossary

Assisted gloving: A method by which a gowned and gloved person assists another gowned person to don sterile gloves.

Closed assisted gloving: A technique used for donning sterile gloves during which the gown cuff of the team member being gloved remains at or beyond the fingertips. The glove to be donned is held open by a scrubbed person, while the team member being gloved inserts his or her hand into the glove with the gown cuff touching only the inside of the glove.

Critical zone: The area of protective apparel or surgical drape where direct contact with blood, body fluids, or other potentially infectious materials is most likely to occur.

Event-related sterility: Sterility maintenance that is not based on expiration dating but rather factors such as the quality of packaging material, the storage conditions, the methods and conditions of transport, the amount and conditions of handling, or environmental conditions (eg, humidity, exposure to airborne contaminants).

Isolation technique: Instruments and equipment that have contacted the inside of the bowel or the bowel lumen are no longer used after the lumen has been closed. Clean instruments are used to close the wound. The contaminated instruments and equipment are either removed from the sterile field or placed in a separate area that will not be touched by members of the sterile team. Synonyms: bowel technique, contamination technique.

Open assisted gloving: A technique for donning sterile gloves during which the gown sleeve of the team member being gloved is pulled up so that the gown cuff is at the wrist level, leaving the fingers and hand exposed. The glove to be donned is held open by a scrubbed team member, while the team member being gloved inserts his or her hand into the glove without touching the outside of the glove.

Perforation indicator system: A double-gloving system comprising a colored pair of surgical gloves worn beneath a standard pair of surgical gloves. When a glove perforation occurs, the inner, colored glove showing through the perforation allows the site of the perforation to be more easily seen.

Powered air-purifying respirator: A respirator that uses a battery-powered blower to move the airflow through the filters.

Sterile barrier system: A package that prevents ingress of microorganisms and allows aseptic presentation of the product at the point of use.

Sterile field: The area surrounding the site of the incision or perforation into tissue, or the site of introduction of an instrument into a body orifice that has been prepared for an invasive procedure. The area includes all working areas, furniture, and equipment covered with sterile drapes and drape accessories and all personnel in sterile attire.

Sterile technique: The use of specific actions and activities to prevent contamination and maintain sterility of identified areas during operative or other invasive procedures.

Surgical helmet system: A nonsterile, reusable helmet with a built-in ventilation fan covered with a single-use, disposable sterile visor mask hood or toga (ie, hood and gown combination); often referred to as a "space suit."

Unidirectional ultraclean air delivery system: An air delivery system that delivers particle-free air that moves over the sterile field at a uniform velocity of 0.3 to 0.5 µm/second. Unidirectional airflow is recirculated air that is filtered through a high-efficiency particulate air filter and can be either vertical or horizontal; often referred to as "laminar airflow."

Wound protector: A double ring, self-retaining circumferential device that is designed to protect the incision site during surgical manipulation.

References

1. Standards of perioperative nursing. In: *Guidelines for Perioperative Practice.* Denver, CO: AORN, Inc; 2015:693-732. [IVB]

2. Guideline for team communication. In: *Guidelines for Perioperative Practice.* Denver, CO: AORN, Inc; 2018:745-772. [IVA]

3. *AORN's Perioperative Explications for the ANA Code of Ethics for Nurses with Interpretive Statements.* AORN, Inc. https://www.aorn.org/guidelines/clinical-resources/code-of-ethics. Updated 2017. Accessed September 10, 2018. [IVB]

4. Guideline for surgical attire. In: *Guidelines for Perioperative Practice.* Denver, CO: AORN, Inc; 2018:105-128. [IVA]

5. Guideline for hand hygiene. In: *Guidelines for Perioperative Practice.* Denver, CO: AORN, Inc; 2018:29-50. [IVA]

6. Guideline for medical device and product evaluation. In: *Guidelines for Perioperative Practice.* Denver, CO: AORN, Inc; 2018:183-190. [IVA]

7. Guideline for prevention of unplanned patient hypothermia. In: *Guidelines for Perioperative Practice.* Denver, CO: AORN, Inc; 2018:549-572. [IVA]

8. Berrios-Torres SI, Umscheid CA, Bratzler DW, et al. Centers for Disease Control and Prevention guideline for the prevention of surgical site infection, 2017. *JAMA Surg.* 2017;152(8):784-791. [IVA]

9. O'Grady NP, Alexander M, Burns LA, et al. Guidelines for the prevention of intravascular catheter-related infections. *Am J Infect Control.* 2011;39(4 Suppl 1):S1-S34. [IVA]

10. Siegel JD, Rhinehart E, Jackson M, Chiarello L; Health Care Infection Control Practices Advisory Committee. 2007 guideline for isolation precautions: preventing transmission of infectious agents in health care settings. *Am J Infect Control.* 2007;35(10 Suppl 2):S65-S164. [IVA]

11. Weber DJ, Rutala WA. Central line-associated bloodstream infections: prevention and management. *Infect Dis Clin North Am.* 2011;25(1):77-102. [IVB]

12. Centers for Disease Control and Prevention(CDC). Bacterial meningitis after intrapartum spinal anesthesia—New York and Ohio, 2008-2009. *MMWR Morb Mortal Wkly Rep.* 2010;59(3):65-69. [VA]

13. Hebl JR. The importance and implications of aseptic techniques during regional anesthesia. *Reg Anesth Pain Med.* 2006;31(4):311-323. [IVB]

14. Chan D, Downing D, Keough CE, et al. Joint practice guideline for sterile technique during vascular and interventional radiology procedures: from the Society of Interventional Radiology, Association of periOperative Registered Nurses, and Association for Radiologic and Imaging Nursing, for the Society of Interventional Radiology (Wael Saad, MD, Chair), Standards of Practice Committee, and Endorsed by the Cardiovascular Interventional Radiological Society of Europe and the Canadian Interventional Radiology Association. *J Radiol Nurs.* 2012;31(4):130-143. [IVB]

15. Berger SA, Kramer M, Nagar H, Finkelstein A, Frimmerman A, Miller HI. Effect of surgical mask position on bacterial contamination of the operative field. *J Hosp Infect.* 1993;23(1):51-54. [IB]

16. Edmiston CE Jr, Seabrook GR, Cambria RA, et al. Molecular epidemiology of microbial contamination in the operating room environment: is there a risk for infection? *Surgery.* 2005;138(4):573-582. [IIIB]

17. McLure HA, Talboys CA, Yentis SM, Azadian BS. Surgical face masks and downward dispersal of bacteria. *Anaesthesia.* 1998;53(7):624-626. [IIB]

18. Ha'eri G, Wiley AM. The efficacy of standard surgical face masks: an investigation using "tracer particles." *Clin Orthop Relat Res.* 1980;148 160-162. [IIIB]

19. Chamberlain GV, Houang E. Trial of the use of masks in the gynaecological operating theatre. *Ann R Coll Surg Engl.* 1984;66(6):432-433. [IC]

20. Philips BJ, Fergusson S, Armstrong P, Anderson FM, Wildsmith JA. Surgical face masks are effective in reducing bacterial contamination caused by dispersal from the upper airway. *Br J Anaesth.* 1992;69(4):407-408. [IIC]

21. Alwitry A, Jackson E, Chen H, Holden R. The use of surgical facemasks during cataract surgery: is it necessary? *Br J Ophthalmol.* 2002;86(9):975-977. [IB]

22. 29 CFR 1910.1030: Bloodborne pathogens. Occupational Safety and Health Administration. https://www.osha.gov/pls/oshaweb/owadisp.show_document?p_id=10051&p_table=STANDARDS. Accessed September 11, 2018.

23. Mitchell NJ, Hunt S. Surgical face masks in modern operating rooms—a costly and unnecessary ritual? *J Hosp Infect.* 1991;18(3):239-242. [IIIB]

24. Ritter MA. Operating room environment. *Clin Orthop Relat Res.* 1999;369:103-109. [IIB]

25. Ritter MA, Eitzen H, French ML, Hart JB. The operating room environment as affected by people and the surgical face mask. *Clin Orthop Relat Res.* 1975;111:147-150. [IIIC]

26. Laslett LJ, Sabin A. Wearing of caps and masks not necessary during cardiac catheterization. *Cathet Cardiovasc Diagn.* 1989;17(3):158-160. [IIIB]

27. Orr NW. Is a mask necessary in the operating theatre? *Ann R Coll Surg Engl.* 1981;63(6):390-392. [IIIC]

28. Tunevall TG. Postoperative wound infections and surgical face masks: a controlled study. *World J Surg.* 1991;15(3):383-387; discussion 387-388. [IB]

29. Webster J, Croger S, Lister C, Doidge M, Terry MJ, Jones I. Use of face masks by non-scrubbed operating room staff: a randomized controlled trial. *ANZ J Surg.* 2010;80(3):169-173. [IA]

30. Schweizer RT. Mask wiggling as a potential cause of wound contamination. *Lancet.* 1976;2(7995):1129-1130. [IIIB]

31. Romney MG. Surgical face masks in the operating theatre: re-examining the evidence. *J Hosp Infect.* 2001;47(4):251-256. [VB]

32. Vincent M, Edwards P. Disposable surgical face masks for preventing surgical wound infection in clean surgery. *Cochrane Database Syst Rev.* 2016;4:CD002929. [IIA]

33. Guideline for transmission-based precautions. In: *Guidelines for Perioperative Practice.* Denver, CO: AORN, Inc; 2018. [IVA]

34. Guideline for surgical smoke safety. In: *Guidelines for Perioperative Practice.* Denver, CO: AORN, Inc; 2018:469-498. [IVA]

35. Jensen PA, Lambert LA, Iademarco MF, Ridzon RCDC. Guidelines for preventing the transmission of *Mycobacterium tuberculosis* in health-care settings, 2005. *MMWR Recomm Rep.* 2005;54(RR-17):1-141. [IVA]

36. *Hospital Respiratory Protection Program Toolkit Resources for Respirator Program Administrators.* Washington, DC: Occupational Safety and Health Administration; Department of Health and Human Services (NIOSH); 2015. [VA]

37. *Implementing Respiratory Protection Programs in Hospitals: A Guide for Respirator Program Administrators.* Richmond, CA: Occupational Health Branch: California Department of Public Health; 2015. [VA]

38. Guidance on personal protective equipment (PPE) to be used by healthcare workers during management of patients with confirmed Ebola or persons under investigation (PUIs) for

Ebola who are clinically unstable or have bleeding, vomiting, or diarrhea in US hospitals, including procedures for donning and doffing PPE. Centers for Disease Control and Prevention. https://www.cdc.gov/vhf/ebola/healthcare-us/ppe/guidance.html. Updated August 27, 2015. Accessed September 11, 2018. [VA]

39. Roberts V. To PAPR or not to PAPR? *Can J Respir Ther.* 2014;50(3):87-90. [VB]

40. Guideline for medication safety. In: *Guidelines for Perioperative Practice.* Denver, CO: AORN, Inc; 2018:295-330. [IVA]

41. *AAMI TIR11:2005. Selection and Use of Protective Apparel and Surgical Drapes in Health Care Facilities.* Arlington, VA: Association for the Advancement of Medical Instrumentation; 2005. [VC]

42. *ANSI/AAMI PB70:2012. Liquid Barrier Performance and Classification of Protective Apparel and Drapes Intended for Use in Health Care Facilities.* Arlington, VA: Association for the Advancement of Medical Instrumentation; 2012. [IVC]

43. *Infection Control Devices Branch Division of General and Restorative Devices. Guidance on Premarket Notification [510(k)] Submissions for Surgical Gowns and Surgical Drapes.* US Food and Drug Administration. https://www.fda.gov/downloads/medicaldevices/deviceregulationandguidance/guidancedocuments/ucm081305.pdf. Published 1993. Accessed September 11, 2018.

44. Meyer KK, Beck WC. Gown-glove interface: a possible solution to the danger zone. *Infect Control Hosp Epidemiol.* 1995;16(8):488-490. [IIIB]

45. Fraser JF, Young SW, Valentine KA, Probst NE, Spangehl MJ. The gown-glove interface is a source of contamination: a comparative study. *Clin Orthop Relat Res.* 2015;473(7):2291-2297. [IIIB]

46. Ritter MA, Eitzen IIE, Hart JB, French ML. The surgeon's garb. *Clin Orthop Relat Res.* 1980;153:204-209. [IIB]

47. Wendlandt R, Thomas M, Kienast B, Schulz AP. In-vitro evaluation of surgical helmet systems for protecting surgeons from droplets generated during orthopaedic procedures. *J Hosp Infect.* 2016;94(1):75-79. [IIB]

48. Hirpara KM, O'Halloran E, O'Sullivan M. A quantitative assessment of facial protection systems in elective hip arthroplasty. *Acta Orthop Belg.* 2011;77(3):375-380. [IIIB]

49. Putzer D, Lechner R, CoracaHuber D, Mayr A, Nogler M, Thaler M. The extent of environmental and body contamination through aerosols by hydro-surgical debridement in the lumbar spine. *Arch Orthop Trauma Surg.* 2017;137(6):743-747. [IIB]

50. Information statement: preventing the transmission of bloodborne pathogens. American Association of Orthopaedic Surgeons. https://www.aaos.org/uploadedFiles/PreProduction/About/Opinion_Statements/advistmt/1018%20Preventing%20the%20Transmission%20of%20Bloodborne%20Pathogens.pdf. Updated 2008. Accessed September 11, 2018. [IVB]

51. Tokars JI, Chamberland ME, Schable CA, et al. A survey of occupational blood contact and HIV infection among orthopedic surgeons. The American Academy of Orthopaedic Surgeons Serosurvey Study Committee. *JAMA.* 1992;268(4):489-494. [IIIB]

52. Panlilio AL, Foy DR, Edwards JR, et al. Blood contacts during surgical procedures. *JAMA.* 1991;265(12):1533-1537. [IIIB]

53. Noguchi C, Koseki H, Horiuchi H, et al. Factors contributing to airborne particle dispersal in the operating room. *BMC Surg.* 2017;17(1):78 [IIIB]

54. Heal JS, Blom AW, Titcomb D, Taylor A, Bowker K, Hardy JR. Bacterial contamination of surgical gloves by water droplets spilt after scrubbing. *J Hosp Infect.* 2003;53(2):136-139. [IIIC]

55. Bible JE, Biswas D, Whang PG, Simpson AK, Grauer JN. Which regions of the operating gown should be considered most sterile? *Clin Orthop Relat Res.* 2009;467(3):825-830. [IIC]

56. Laufman H, Eudy WW, Vandernoot AM, Harris CA, Liu D. Strike-through of moist contamination by woven and nonwoven surgical materials. *Ann Surg.* 1975;181(6):857-862. [IIIC]

57. Jones C, Brooker B, Genon M. Comparison of open and closed staff-assisted glove donning on the nature of surgical glove cuff contamination. *ANZ J Surg.* 2010;80(3):174-177. [IB]

58. Mischke C, Verbeek JH, Saarto A, Lavoie MC, Pahwa M, Ijaz S. Gloves, extra gloves or special types of gloves for preventing percutaneous exposure injuries in healthcare personnel. *Cochrane Database Syst Rev.* 2014(3):CD009573. [IA]

59. de Oliveira AC, Gama CS. Evaluation of surgical glove integrity during surgery in a Brazilian teaching hospital. *Am J Infect Control.* 2014;42(10):1093-1096. [IIIB]

60. Korniewicz D, El-Masri M. Exploring the benefits of double gloving during surgery. *AORN J.* 2012;95(3):328-336. [IIIA]

61. Kuroyanagi N, Nagao T, Sakuma H, et al. Risk of surgical glove perforation in oral and maxillofacial surgery. *Int J Oral Maxillofac Surg.* 2012;41(8):1014-1019. [IIIB]

62. Guideline for sharps safety. In: *Guidelines for Perioperative Practice.* Denver, CO: AORN, Inc; 2018:415-438. [IVA]

63. Revised statement on sharps safety. American College of Surgeons. https://www.facs.org/about-acs/statements/94-sharps-safety. Updated October 1, 2016. Accessed September 11, 2018. [IVB]

64. *Global Guidelines for the Prevention of Surgical Site Infection.* Geneva, Switzerland: World Health Organization; 2016. [IVA]

65. Han CD, Kim J, Moon SH, Lee BH, Kwon HM, Park KK. A randomized prospective study of glove perforation in orthopaedic surgery: is a thick glove more effective? *J Arthroplasty.* 2013;28(10):1878-1881. [IIIA]

66. Tanner J, Parkinson H. Double gloving to reduce surgical cross-infection. *Cochrane Database Syst Rev.* 2006;3:CD003087. [IA]

67. Edlich RF, Wind TC, Hill LG, Thacker JG. Creating another barrier to the transmission of bloodborne operative infections with a new glove gauntlet. *J Long Term Eff Med Implants.* 2003;13(2):97-101. [IIIB]

68. Fernandez M, Del Castillo JL, Nieto MJ. Surgical gown's cuff modification to prevent surgical contamination. *J Maxillofac Oral Surg.* 2015;14(2):474-475. [VB]

69. Kojima Y, Ohashi M. Unnoticed glove perforation during thoracoscopic and open thoracic surgery. *Ann Thorac Surg.* 2005;80(3):1078-1080. [IIIB]

70. Boyce JM, Pittet D; Healthcare Infection Control Practices Advisory Committee, HICPAC/SHEA/APIC/IDSA Hand Hygiene Task Force. Guideline for hand hygiene in healthcare settings. Recommendations of the Healthcare Infection Control Practices Advisory Committee and the HICPAC/SHEA/

APIC/IDSA Hand Hygiene Task Force. Society for Healthcare Epidemiology of America/Association for Professionals in Infection Control/Infectious Diseases Society of America. *MMWR Recomm Rep.* 2002;51(RR-16):1-45; quiz CE1-CE4. [IVA]

71. Harnoss JC, Partecke LI, Heidecke CD, Hubner NO, Kramer A, Assadian O. Concentration of bacteria passing through puncture holes in surgical gloves. *Am J Infect Control.* 2010;38(2):154-158. [IIA]

72. Hubner NO, Goerdt AM, Stanislawski N, et al. Bacterial migration through punctured surgical gloves under real surgical conditions. *BMC Infect Dis.* 2010;10:192. [IIIB]

73. Partecke LI, Goerdt AM, Langner I, et al. Incidence of microperforation for surgical gloves depends on duration of wear. *Infect Control Hosp Epidemiol.* 2009;30(5):409-414. [IA]

74. Guideline for a safe environment of care. In: *Guidelines for Perioperative Practice.* Denver, CO: AORN, Inc; 2018:e103-e132. [IVA]

75. Thomas S, Padmanabhan TV. Methyl methacrylate permeability of dental and industrial gloves. *N Y State Dent J.* 2009;75(4):40-42. [IIIB]

76. Waegemaekers TH, Seutter E, den Arend JA, Malten KE. Permeability of surgeons' gloves to methyl methacrylate. *Acta Orthop Scand.* 1983;54(6):790-795. [IIIB]

77. Edwards TB, Habetz S, D'Ambrosia RD. The effect of polymethyl methacrylate on latex-free surgical gloves. *J Arthroplasty.* 2001;16(4):541-542. [IIIC]

78. Bible JE, O'Neill KR, Crosby CG, Schoenecker JG, McGirt MJ, Devin CJ. Microscope sterility during spine surgery. *Spine (Phila Pa 1976).* 2012;37(7):623-627. [IIIB]

79. Peters PG, Laughlin RT, Markert RJ, Nelles DB, Randall KL, Prayson MJ. Timing of C-arm drape contamination. *Surg Infect (Larchmt).* 2012;13(2):110-113. [IIIB]

80. Singh VK, Hussain S, Javed S, Singh I, Mulla R, Kalairajah Y. Sterile surgical helmet system in elective total hip and knee arthroplasty. *J Orthop Surg (Hong Kong).* 2011;19(2):234-237. [IIB]

81. Kearns KA, Witmer D, Makda J, Parvizi J, Jungkind D. Sterility of the personal protection system in total joint arthroplasty. *Clin Orthop Relat Res.* 2011;469(11):3065-3069. [IIIC]

82. Young S, Chisholm C, Zhu M. Intraoperative contamination and space suits: a potential mechanism. *Eur J Orthop Surg Traumatol.* 2014;24(3):409-413. [IIIB]

83. Carter AH, Casper DS, Parvizi J, Austin MS. A prospective analysis of glove perforation in primary and revision total hip and total knee arthroplasty. *J Arthroplasty.* 2012;27(7):1271-1275. [IIIB]

84. Beldame J, Lagrave B, Lievain L, Lefebvre B, Frebourg N, Dujardin F. Surgical glove bacterial contamination and perforation during total hip arthroplasty implantation: when gloves should be changed. *Orthop Traumatol Surg Res.* 2012;98(4):432-440. [IIIB]

85. Mazurek MJ, Rysz M, Jaworowski J, et al. Contamination of the surgical field in head and neck oncologic surgery. *Head Neck.* 2014;36(10):1408-1412. [IIIB]

86. X Li, Li M, Li J, et al. Glove perforation and contamination in fracture fixation surgeries. *Am J Infect Control.* 2017;45(4):458-460. [IIIC]

87. Ward WG, Cooper JM, Lippert D, Kablawi RO, Neiberg RH, Sherertz RJ. Glove and gown effects on intraoperative bacterial contamination. *Ann Surg.* 2014;259(3):591-597. [IIIB]

88. Young SW, Zhu M, Shirley OC, Wu Q, Spangehl MJ. Do "surgical helmet systems" or "body exhaust suits" affect contamination and deep infection rates in arthroplasty? A systematic review. *J Arthroplasty.* 2016;31(1):225-233. [IIIB]

89. Hanselman AE, Montague MD, Murphy TR, Dietz MJ. Contamination relative to the activation timing of filtered-exhaust helmets. *J Arthroplasty.* 2016;31(4):776-780. [IIIB]

90. Anderson DJ, Podgorny K, Berrios-Torres SI, et al. Strategies to prevent surgical site infections in acute care hospitals: 2014 update. *Infect Control Hosp Epidemiol.* 2014;35(Suppl 2):S66-S88. [IVA]

91. Dalstrom DJ, Venkatarayappa I, Manternach AL, Palcic MS, Heyse BA, Prayson MJ. Time-dependent contamination of opened sterile operating-room trays. *J Bone Joint Surg Am.* 2008;90(5):1022-1025. [IC]

92. de Araujo Moriya GA, de Souza RQ, Gomes Pinto FM, Graziano KU. Periodic sterility assessment of materials stored for up to 6 months at continuous microbial contamination risk: laboratory study. *Am J Infect Control.* 2012;40(10):1013-1015. [IB]

93. Menekse G, Kuscu F, Suntur BM, et al. Evaluation of the time-dependent contamination of spinal implants: prospective randomized trial. *Spine.* 2015;40(16):1247-1251. [IIA]

94. Panahi P, Stroh M, Casper DS, Parvizi J, Austin MS. Operating room traffic is a major concern during total joint arthroplasty. *Clin Orthop Relat Res.* 2012;470(10):2690-2694. [IIIB]

95. Bible JE, O'Neill KR, Crosby CG, Schoenecker JG, McGirt MJ, Devin CJ. Implant contamination during spine surgery. *Spine J.* 2013;13(6):637-640. [IB]

96. Edmiston CE Jr, Sinski S, Seabrook GR, Simons D, Goheen MP. Airborne particulates in the OR environment. *AORN J.* 1999;69(6):1169-1179. [IIB]

97. Reason J. Safety in the operating theatre—part 2: human error and organisational failure. *Qual Saf Health Care.* 2005;14(1):56-60. [VA]

98. Chosky SA, Modha D, Taylor GJS. Optimisation of ultra-clean air. The role of instrument preparation. *J Bone Joint Surg Br.* 1996;78(5):835-837. [IIIB]

99. Andersson AE, Petzold M, Bergh I, Karlsson J, Eriksson BI, Nilsson K. Comparison between mixed and laminar airflow systems in operating rooms and the influence of human factors: experiences from a Swedish orthopedic center. *Am J Infect Control.* 2014;42(6):665-669. [IIIA]

100. Guideline for sterilization. In: *Guidelines for Perioperative Practice.* Denver, CO: AORN, Inc; 2018:e76-e101. [IVA]

101. Zach J. A review of the literature on bowel technique. *ACORN.* 2004;17(4):14-19. [VB]

102. Bruen E. Clean/dirty scrub technique: is it worth the effort? *Br J Perioper Nurs.* 2001;11(12):532-537. [VA]

103. Porteous J, Gembey D, Dieter M. Bowel technique in the OR: is it really necessary? *Can Oper Room Nurs J.* 1996;14(1):11-14. [IIA]

104. Hao WL, Lee YK. Microflora of the gastrointestinal tract: a review. *Methods Mol Biol.* 2004;268:491-502. [VA]

105. Bures J, Cyrany J, Kohoutova D, et al. Small intestinal bacterial overgrowth syndrome. *World J Gastroenterol.* 2010;16(24):2978-2990. [VA]

106. Husebye E. The pathogenesis of gastrointestinal bacterial overgrowth. *Chemotherapy.* 2005;51 (Suppl 1):1-22. [VA]

107. Watanabe A, Kohnoe S, Shimabukuro R, et al. Risk factors associated with surgical site infection in upper and lower gastrointestinal surgery. *Surg Today.* 2008;38(5):404-412. [IIIB]

108. Saito Y, Kobayashi H, Uetera Y, Yasuhara H, Kajiura T, Okubo T. Microbial contamination of surgical instruments used for laparotomy. *Am J Infect Control.* 2014;42(1):43-47. [IIIB]

109. Hashimoto D, Chikamoto A, Arima K, et al. Unused sterile instruments for closure prevent wound surgical site infection after pancreatic surgery. *J Surg Res.* 2016;205(1):38-42. [IIB]

110. Johnson MP, Kim SJ, Langstraat CL, et al. Using bundled interventions to reduce surgical site infection after major gynecologic cancer surgery. *Obstet Gynecol.* 2016;127(6):1135-1144. [IIB]

111. Bekar A, Kahveci R, Tolunay S, Kahraman A, Kuytu T. Metastatic gliosarcoma mass extension to a donor fascia lata graft harvest site by tumor cell contamination. *World Neurosurg.* 2010;73(6):719-721. [VA]

112. Zemmoura I, Ben Ismail M, Travers N, Jan M, Francois P. Maxillary surgical seeding of a clival chordoma. *Br J Neurosurg.* 2012;26(1):102-103. [VB]

113. McLemore MS, Bruner JM, Curry JL, Prieto VG, Torres-Cabala CA. Anaplastic oligodendroglioma involving the subcutaneous tissue of the scalp: report of an exceptional case and review of the literature. *Am J Dermatopathol.* 2012;34(2):214-219. [VA]

114. Chang H, Ding Y, Wang P, Wang Q, Lin Y, Li B. Cutaneous metastases of the glioma. *J Craniofac Surg.* 2018;29(1):e94-e96. [VB]

115. Vogin G, Calugaru V, Bolle S, et al. Investigation of ectopic recurrent skull base and cervical chordomas: the Institut Curie's proton therapy center experience. *Head Neck.* 2016;38(Suppl 1):E1238-E1246. [IIIC]

116. Iloreta AMC, Nyquist GG, Friedel M, Farrell C, Rosen MR, Evans JJ. Surgical pathway seeding of clivo-cervical chordomas. *J Neurol Surg Rep.* 2014;75(2):e246-e250. [VB]

117. Ortiz H, Armendariz P, Kreisler E, et al. Influence of rescrubbing before laparotomy closure on abdominal wound infection after colorectal cancer surgery: results of a multicenter randomized clinical trial. *Arch Surg.* 2012;147(7):614-620. [IA]

118. Bressan AK, Aubin JM, Martel G, et al. Efficacy of a dual-ring wound protector for prevention of surgical site infections after pancreaticoduodenectomy in patients with intrabiliary stents: a randomized clinical trial. *Ann Surg.* 2018;268(1):35-40. [IB]

119. Papaconstantinou HT, Ricciardi R, Margolin DA, et al. A novel wound retractor combining continuous irrigation and barrier protection reduces incisional contamination in colorectal surgery. *World J Surg.* 2018;42(9):3000-3007. [IIIA]

120. Pronovost P, Needham D, Berenholtz S, et al. An intervention to decrease catheter-related bloodstream infections in the ICU. *N Engl J Med.* 2006;355(26):2725-2732. [IIIB]

121. Barnes S. Infection prevention: the surgical care continuum. *AORN J.* 2015;101(5):512-518. [VB]

122. Biswas D, Bible JE, Whang PG, Simpson AK, Grauer JN. Sterility of C-arm fluoroscopy during spinal surgery. *Spine (Phila Pa 1976).* 2008;33(17):1913-1917. [IIB]

123. Gershkovich GE, Tiedeken NC, Hampton D, Budacki R, Samuel SPDE, Saing M. A comparison of three C-arm draping techniques to minimize contamination of the surgical field. *J Orthop Trauma.* 2016;30(10):e351-e356. [IIIB]

124. Webster J, Alghamdi A. Use of plastic adhesive drapes during surgery for preventing surgical site infection. *Cochrane Database Syst Rev.* 2015;(4):CD006353. [IA]

125. Bejko J, Tarzia V, Carrozzini M, et al. Comparison of efficacy and cost of iodine impregnated drape vs. standard drape in cardiac surgery: study in 5100 patients. *J Cardiovasc Transl Res.* 2015;8(7):431-437. [IIA]

126. Rezapoor M, Tan TL, Maltenfort MG, Parvizi J. Incise draping reduces the rate of contamination of the surgical site during hip surgery: a prospective, randomized trial. *J Arthroplasty.* 2018;33(6):1891-1895. [IA]

127. *The APSIC Guidelines for the Prevention of Surgical Site Infections.* Asian Pacific Society of Infection Control. http://apsic-apac.org/wp-content/uploads/2018/05/APSIC-SSI-Prevention-guideline-March-2018.pdf. Accessed September 11, 2018. [IVB]

128. Surgical site infections: prevention and treatment. Clinical guideline [CG74]. National Institute for Health and Care Excellence. https://www.nice.org.uk/guidance/cg74. Updated February 2017. Accessed September 11, 2018. [IVC]

129. Prävention postoperativer Wundinfektionen: Empfehlung der Kommission für Krankenhaushygiene und Infektionsprävention (KRINKO) beim Robert Koch-Institut [Article in German]. *Bundesgesundheitsblatt Gesundheitsforschung Gesundheitsschutz.* 2018;61(4):448-473. [IVC]

130. Milandt N, Nymark T, Kolmos Hjø, Emmeluth C, Overgaard S. Iodine-impregnated incision drape and bacterial recolonization in simulated total knee arthroplasty. *Acta Orthop.* 2016;87(4):380-385. [IA]

131. Casey AL, Karpanen TJ, Nightingale P, Conway BR, Elliott TS. Antimicrobial activity and skin permeation of iodine present in an iodine-impregnated surgical incise drape. *J Antimicrob Chemother.* 2015;70(8):2255-2260. [IIB]

132. Lakhan P, Faoagali J, Steinhardt R, Olesen D. Shelf life of sterilized packaged items stored in acute care hospital settings: factors for consideration. *Healthc Infect.* 2013;18(3):121-129. [VB]

133. Barker CS, Soro V, Dymock D, Fulford M, Sandy JR, Ireland AJ. Time-dependent recontamination rates of sterilised dental instruments. *Br Dent J.* 2011;211(8):E17. [IIB]

134. Butt WE, Bradley DV Jr, Mayhew RB, Schwartz RS. Evaluation of the shelf life of sterile instrument packs. *Oral Surg Oral Med Oral Pathol.* 1991;72(6):650-654. [IA]

135. Webster J, Lloyd W, Ho P, Burridge C, George N. Rethinking sterilization practices: evidence for event-related outdating. *Infect Control Hosp Epidemiol.* 2003;24(8):622-624. [IIB]

136. McCann MT, Gilmore BF, Gorman SP. *Staphylococcus epidermidis* device-related infections: pathogenesis and clinical management. *J Pharm Pharmacol.* 2008;60(12):1551-1571. [VB]

137. *ANSI/AAMI ST79: Comprehensive Guide to Steam Sterilization and Sterility Assurance in Health Care Facilities.* Arlington, VA:

Association for the Advancement of Medical Instrumentation (AAMI); 2017. [IVC]

138. Rutala WA, Weber DJ; Healthcare Infection Control Practices Advisory Committee (HICPAC). Guideline for disinfection and sterilization in healthcare facilities, 2008 Centers for Disease Control and Prevention. https://www.cdc.gov/infection-control/pdf/guidelines/disinfection-guidelines.pdf. Accessed September 12, 2018. [IVA]

139. 21 CFR 801: Labeling. US Government Publishing Office. https://www.gpo.gov/fdsys/granule/CFR-2011-title21-vol8/CFR-2011-title21-vol8-part801. Accessed September 12, 2018

140. 21 CFR 801.5: Medical devices; adequate directions for use. US Government Publishing Office. https://www.gpo.gov/fdsys/granule/CFR-2012-title21-vol8/CFR-2012-title21-vol8-sec801-5. Accessed September 12, 2018.

141. Chang CY, Furlong LA. Microbial stowaways in topical antiseptic products. N Engl J Med. 2012;367(23):2170-2173. [VB]

142. Edmiston CE Jr, Leaper D, Spencer M, et al. Considering a new domain for antimicrobial stewardship: topical antibiotics in the open surgical wound. Am J Infect Control. 2017;45(11):1259-1266. [VB]

143. Taaffe K, Lee B, Ferrand Y, et al. The influence of traffic, area location, and other factors on operating room microbial load. Infect Control Hosp Epidemiol. 2018;39(4):391-397. [IIIC]

144. Sadrizadeh S, Tammelin A, Ekolind P, Holmberg S. Influence of staff number and internal constellation on surgical site infection in an operating room. Particuology. 2014;1342-51. [IIIA]

145. Mobley KS, Jackson JB 3rd. A prospective analysis of clinical detection of defective wrapping by operating room staff. Am J Infect Control. 2018;46(7):837-839. [IIIB]

146. Trier T, Bello N, Bush TR, Bix L. The role of packaging size on contamination rates during simulated presentation to a sterile field. Plos One. 2014;9(7):e100414. [IIIB]

147. National Patient Safety Goals effective January 2018 hospital accreditation program. In: The Joint Commission Comprehensive Accreditation and Certification Manual. E-dition. Oakbrook. Terrace, IL: The Joint Commission; 2017. https://www.jointcommission.org/hap_2017_npsgs/. Accessed September 12, 2018.

148. National Patient Safety Goals effective January 2018 critical access hospital accreditation program. In: The Joint Commission Comprehensive Accreditation and Certification Manual. E-dition. Oakbrook Terrace, IL: The Joint Commission; 2017. https://www.jointcommission.org/cah_2017_npsgs/. Accessed September 12, 2018.

149. National Patient Safety Goals effective January 2018 ambulatory health care accreditation program. In: The Joint Commission Comprehensive Accreditation and Certification Manual. E-dition. Oakbrook Terrace, IL: The Joint Commission; 2017. https://www.jointcommission.org/ahc_2017_npsgs/. Accessed September 12, 2018.

150. National Patient Safety Goals effective January 2018 office-based surgery accreditation program. In: The Joint Commission Comprehensive Accreditation and Certification Manual. E-dition Oakbrook Terrace, IL: The Joint Commission; 2017. https://www.jointcommission.org/obs_2017_npsgs/. Accessed September 12, 2018.

151. Tosh PK, Disbot M, Duffy JM, et al. Outbreak of Pseudomonas aeruginosa surgical site infections after arthroscopic procedures: Texas, 2009. Infect Control Hosp Epidemiol. 2011;32(12):1179-1186. [VB]

152. Parada SA, Grassbaugh JA, DeVine JG, Arrington ED. Instrumentation-specific infection after anterior cruciate ligament reconstruction. Sports Health. 2009;1(6):481-485. [VB]

153. Blevins FT, Salgado J, Wascher DC, Koster F. Septic arthritis following arthroscopic meniscus repair: a cluster of three cases. Arthroscopy. 1999;15(1):35-40. [VB]

154. Hopper WR, Moss R. Common breaks in sterile technique: clinical perspectives and perioperative implications. AORN J. 2010;91(3):350-364. [VB]

155. Smith K, Araoye I, Gilbert S, et al. Is retained bone debris in cannulated orthopedic instruments sterile after autoclaving? Am J Infect Control. 2018;46(9):1009-1013. [IIB]

156. Markel TA, Gormley T, Greeley D, Ostojic J, Wagner J. Covering the instrument table decreases bacterial bioburden: an evaluation of environmental quality indicators. Am J Infect Control. 2018. 10.1016/j.ajic.2018.02.032. [IIIB]

157. Sommerstein R, Ruegg C, Kohler P, Bloemberg G, Kuster SP, Sax H. Transmission of Mycobacterium chimaera from heater-cooler units during cardiac surgery despite an ultra-clean air ventilation system. Emerg Infect Dis. 2016;22(6):1008-1013. [IIIC]

158. Schreiber PW, Kuster SP, Hasse B, et al. Reemergence of Mycobacterium chimaera in heater-cooler units despite intensified cleaning and disinfection protocol. Emerg Infect Dis. 2016;22(10):1830-1833. [IIIC]

159. Stocks GW, Self SD, Thompson B, Adame XA, O'Connor DP. Predicting bacterial populations based on airborne particulates: a study performed in nonlaminar flow operating rooms during joint arthroplasty surgery. Am J Infect Control. 2010;38(3):199-204. [IIIB]

160. Andersson AE, Bergh I, Karlsson J, Eriksson BI, Nilsson K. Traffic flow in the operating room: an explorative and descriptive study on air quality during orthopedic trauma implant surgery. Am J Infect Control. 2012;40(8):750-755. [IIIB]

161. Smith EB, Raphael IJ, Maltenfort MG, Honsawek S, Dolan K, Younkins EA. The effect of laminar air flow and door openings on operating room contamination. J Arthroplasty. 2013;28(9):1482-1485. [IIB]

162. Teter J, Guajardo I, Al Rammah T, Rosson G, Perl TM, Manahan M. Assessment of operating room airflow using air particle counts and direct observation of door openings. Am J Infect Control. 2017;45(5):477-482. [IIIA]

163. Alfonso-Sanchez JL, Martinez IM, Martin-Moreno JM, Gonzalez RS, Botia F. Analyzing the risk factors influencing surgical site infections: the site of environmental factors. Can J Surg. 2017;60(3):155-161. [IIIB]

164. Hansen D, Krabs C, Benner D, Brauksiepe A, Popp W. Laminar air flow provides high air quality in the operating field even during real operating conditions, but personal protection seems to be necessary in operations with tissue combustion. Int J Hyg Environ Health. 2005;208(6):455-460. [IIIB]

165. Namba RS, Inacio MC, Paxton EW. Risk factors associated with deep surgical site infections after primary total knee arthroplasty: an analysis of 56,216 knees. *J Bone Joint Surg Am.* 2013;95(9):775-782. [IIIA]

166. Agodi A, Auxilia F, Barchitta M, et al. Italian Study Group of Hospital Hygiene. Operating theatre ventilation systems and microbial air contamination in total joint replacement surgery: results of the GISIO-ISChIA study. *J Hosp Infect.* 2015;90(3):213-219. [IIIB]

167. Diab-Elschahawi M, Berger J, Blacky A, et al. Impact of different-sized laminar air flow versus no laminar air flow on bacterial counts in the operating room during orthopedic surgery. *Am J Infect Control.* 2011;39(7):e25-e29. [IIIB]

168. Radcliff KE, Rasouli MR, Neusner AK, Christopher K, et al. Preoperative delay of more than 1 hour increases the risk of surgical site infection. *Spine.* 2013;38(15):1318-1323. [IIIB]

169. Lynch RJ, Englesbe MJ, Sturm L, et al. Measurement of foot traffic in the operating room: implications for infection control. *Am J Med Qual.* 2009;24(1):45-52. [IIIB]

170. Darnley J, Denham Z, Phieffer LS, et al. Cracking the case: should orthopaedic case carts be subjected to more stringent regulations? *Curr Orthop Pract.* 2017;28(5):453-458. [VB]

171. Salvati EA, Robinson RP, Zeno SM, Koslin BL, Brause BD, Wilson PDJ. Infection rates after 3175 total hip and total knee replacements performed with and without a horizontal unidirectional filtered air-flow system. *J Bone Joint Surg Am.* 1982;64(4):525-535. [IIIB]

172. Letts RM, Doermer E. Conversation in the operating theater as a cause of airborne bacterial contamination. *J Bone Joint Surg Am.* 1983;65(3):357-362. [IIB]

173. Mathijssen NMC, Hannink G, Sturm PDJ, et al. The effect of door openings on numbers of colony forming units in the operating room during hip revision surgery. *Surg Infect (Larchmt).* 2016;17(5):535-540. [IIIB]

174. Ritter MA, Eitzen HE, French ML, Hart JB. The effect that time, touch and environment have upon bacterial contamination of instruments during surgery. *Ann Surg.* 1976;184(5):642-644. [IIB]

175. Campbell BA, Manos J, Stubbs TM, Flynt NC. Pre-preparation of the sterile instrument table for emergency cesarean section. *Surg Gynecol Obstet.* 1993;176(1):30-32. [IIIC]

176. Dharan S, Pittet D. Environmental controls in operating theatres. *J Hosp Infect.* 2002;51(2):79-84. [VB]

177. Stocks GW, O'Connor DP, Self SD, Marcek GA, Thompson BL. Directed air flow to reduce airborne particulate and bacterial contamination in the surgical field during total hip arthroplasty. *J Arthroplasty.* 2011;26(5):771-776. [IB]

178. Fischer S, Thieves M, Hirsch T, et al. Reduction of airborne bacterial burden in the OR by installation of unidirectional displacement airflow (UDF) systems. *Med Sci Monit.* 2015;212367-2374. [IIA]

179. Perez P, Holloway J, Ehrenfeld L, et al. Door openings in the operating room are associated with increased environmental contamination. *Am J Infect Control.* 2018;46(8):954-956. [IIIB]

180. Barr SP, Topps AR, Barnes NL, et al. Infection prevention in breast implant surgery—a review of the surgical evidence, guidelines and a checklist. *Eur J Surg Oncol.* 2016;42(5):591-603. [IIIB]

181. Friberg B, Friberg S, Burman LG. Inconsistent correlation between aerobic bacterial surface and air counts in operating rooms with ultra clean laminar air flows: proposal of a new bacteriological standard for surface contamination. *J Hosp Infect.* 1999;42(4):287-293. [IIIB]

182. Cao G, Storås MCA, Aganovic A, Stenstad L, Skogås JG. Do surgeons and surgical facilities disturb the clean air distribution close to a surgical patient in an orthopedic operating room with laminar airflow? *Am J Infect Control.* 2018. 10.1016/j.ajic.2018.03.019. [IIIB]

183. De Korne DF, Van Wijngaarden JDH, Van Rooij J, Wauben LSGL, Hiddema UF, Klazinga NS. Safety by design: effects of operating room floor marking on the position of surgical devices to promote clean air flow compliance and minimise infection risks. *BMJ Qual Saf.* 2012;21(9):746-752. [IIIB]

184. Darouiche RO, Green DM, Harrington MA, et al. Association of airborne microorganisms in the operating room with implant infections: a randomized controlled trial. *Infect Control Hosp Epidemiol.* 2017;38(1):3-10. [IB]

185. Lapid-Gortzak R, Traversari R, van der Linden JW, Lesnik Oberstein SY, Lapid O, Schlingemann RO. Mobile ultra-clean unidirectional airflow screen reduces air contamination in a simulated setting for intravitreal injection. *Int Ophthalmol.* 2017;37(1):131-137. [IIB]

186. Nilsson K, Lundholm R, Friberg S. Assessment of horizontal laminar air flow instrument table for additional ultraclean space during surgery. *J Hosp Infect.* 2010;76(3):243-246. [IIC]

187. Ferretti S, Pasquarella C, Fornia S, et al. Effect of mobile unidirectional air flow unit on microbial contamination of air in standard urologic procedures. *Surg Infect (Larchmt).* 2009;10(6):511-516. [IIB]

188. Sossai D, Dagnino G, Sanguineti F, Franchin F. Mobile laminar air flow screen for additional operating room ventilation: reduction of intraoperative bacterial contamination during total knee arthroplasty. *J Orthop Traumatol.* 2011;12(4):207-211. [IIB]

189. Thore M, Burman LG. Further bacteriological evaluation of the TOUL mobile system delivering ultra-clean air over surgical patients and instruments. *J Hosp Infect.* 2006;63(2):185-192. [IIIB]

190. Information for health care providers and staff at health care facilities. US Food and Drug Administration. https://www.fda.gov/MedicalDevices/ProductsandMedicalProcedures/CardiovascularDevices/Heater-CoolerDevices/ucm492583.htm. Accessed September 11, 2018. [VA]

191. Nagpal A, Wentink JE, Berbari EF, et al. A cluster of *Mycobacterium wolinskyi* surgical site infections at an academic medical center. *Infect Control Hosp Epidemiol.* 2014;35(9):1169-1175. [IIIB]

192. Bowling FL, Stickings DS, Edwards-Jones V, Armstrong DG, Boulton AJM. Hydrodebridement of wounds: effectiveness in reducing wound bacterial contamination and potential for air bacterial contamination. *J Foot Ankle Res.* 2009;2(1):1-8. [IIIB]

193. Sönnergren HH, Strombeck L, Aldenborg F, Faergemann J. Aerosolized spread of bacteria and reduction of bacterial

wound contamination with three different methods of surgical wound debridement: a pilot study. *J Hosp Infect.* 2013; 85(2):112-117. [IIIB]

194. Sönnergren HH, Polesie S, Strombeck L, Aldenborg F, Johansson BR, Faergemann J. Bacteria aerosol spread and wound bacteria reduction with different methods for wound debridement in an animal model. *Acta Derm Venereol.* 2015;95(3):272-277. [IIIB]

195. Granick M, Rubinsky L, Parthiban C, Shanmugam M, Ramasubbu N. Dispersion risk associated with surgical debridement devices. *Wounds.* 2017;29(10):E88-E91. [IIIB]

196. Maragakis LL, Cosgrove SE, Song X, et al. An outbreak of multidrug-resistant *Acinetobacter baumannii* associated with pulsatile lavage wound treatment. *JAMA.* 2004;292(24):3006-3011. [VB]

197. Angobaldo J, Marks M, Sanger C. Prevention of projectile and aerosol contamination during pulsatile lavage irrigation using a wound irrigation bag. *Wounds.* 2008;20(6):167-170. [IB]

198. Michailidis L, Kotsanas D, Orr E, et al. Does the new low-frequency ultrasonic debridement technology pose an infection control risk for clinicians, patients, and the clinic environment? *Am J Infect Control.* 2016;44(12):1656-1659. [IIIB]

199. Tobias AM, Chang B. Pulsed irrigation of extremity wounds: a simple technique for splashback reduction. *Ann Plast Surg.* 2002;48(4):443-444. [VC]

200. Greene DL, Akelman E. A technique for reducing splash exposure during pulsatile lavage. *J Orthop Trauma.* 2004;18(1):41-42. [VC]

201. Bedard M, Pelletier-Roy R, Angers-Goulet M, Leblanc PA, Pelet S. Traffic in the operating room during joint replacement is a multidisciplinary problem. *Can J Surg.* 2015;58(4):232-236. [IIIB]

202. Scaltriti S, Cencetti S, Rovesti S, Marchesi I, Bargellini A, Borella P. Risk factors for particulate and microbial contamination of air in operating theatres. *J Hosp Infect.* 2007; 66(4):320-326. [IIIB]

203. Guideline for radiation safety. In: *Guidelines for Perioperative Practice.* Denver, CO: AORN, Inc; 2018:331-366. [IVA]

204. DiBartola AC, Patel PG, Scharschmidt TJ, et al. Operating room team member role affects room traffic in orthopaedic surgery: a prospective observational study. *Curr Orthop Pract.* 2017;28(3):281-286. [IIIA]

205. Mears SC, Blanding R, Belkoff SM. Door opening affects operating room pressure during joint arthroplasty. *Orthopedics.* 2015;38(11):e991-e994. [IIIB]

206. Allo MD, Tedesco M. Operating room management: operative suite considerations, infection control. *Surg Clin North Am.* 2005;85(6):1291-1297; xii. [VC]

207. Parikh SN, Grice SS, Schnell BM, Salisbury SR. Operating room traffic: is there any role of monitoring it? *J Pediatr Orthop.* 2010;30(6):617-623. [IIC]

208. Weiser MC, Shemesh S, Chen DD, Bronson MJ, Moucha CS. The effect of door opening on positive pressure and airflow in operating rooms. *J Am Acad Orthop Surg.* 2018;26(5): e105-e113. [IIIB]

209. Sturm L, Sturm LK, Jackson J, Murphy S, Chenoweth C. Measurement and analysis of foot traffic in a university hospital operating room. *Am J Infect Control.* 2012;40(5):e124-e125. [IIIB]

210. Barbara D. Looking forward—infection prevention in 2017. *AORN J.* 2016;104(6):531-535. [VB]

211. Crolla RM, van der Laan L, Veen EJ, Hendriks Y, van Schendel C, Kluytmans J. Reduction of surgical site infections after implementation of a bundle of care. *Plos One.* 2012;7(9):e44599. [IIB]

212. Young RS, O'Regan DJ. Cardiac surgical theatre traffic: time for traffic calming measures? *Interact Cardiovasc Thorac Surg.* 2010;10(4):526-529. [IIIC]

213. Villafruela JM, San José JF, Castro F, Zarzuelo A. Airflow patterns through a sliding door during opening and foot traffic in operating rooms. *Build Environ.* 2016;109:190-198. [IIIA]

214. Wanta BT, Glasgow AE, Habermann EB, et al. Operating room traffic as a modifiable risk factor for surgical site infection. *Surg Infect (Larchmt).* 2016;17(6):755-760. [IIIB]

215. Elliott S, Parker S, Mills J, et al. STOP: can we minimize OR traffic? *AORN J.* 2015;102(4):409.e1-409.e7. [VB]

216. Rovaldi CJ, King PJ. The effect of an interdisciplinary QI project to reduce OR foot traffic. *AORN J.* 2015;101(6):666-681. [VB]

217. Esser JMN, Shrinski K, Cady R, Belew J. Reducing OR traffic using education, policy development, and communication technology. *AORN J.* 2016;103(1):82-88. [VA]

218. Pulido RW, Kester BS, Ran. Effects of intervention and team culture on operating room traffic. *Qual Manag Health Care.* 2017;26(2):103-107. [IIIB]

219. Eskildsen SM, Moskal PT, Laux J, Del Gaizo DJ. The effect of a door alarm on operating room traffic during total joint arthroplasty. *Orthopedics.* 2017;40(6):e1081-e1085. [IIIA]

220. Hamilton WG, Balkam CB, Purcell RL, Parks NL, Holdsworth JE. Operating room traffic in total joint arthroplasty: identifying patterns and training the team to keep the door shut. *Am J Infect Control.* 2018;46(6):633-636. [IIIB]

221. Liu Z, Dumville JC, Norman G, et al. Intraoperative interventions for preventing surgical site infection: an overview of Cochrane Reviews. *Cochrane Database Syst Rev.* 2018;2:CD012653. [IB]

222. Ahn DK, Park HS, Kim TW, et al. The degree of bacterial contamination while performing spine surgery. *Asian Spine J.* 2013;7(1):8-13. [IIIB]

223. Chauveaux D. Preventing surgical-site infections: measures other than antibiotics. *Orthop Traumatol Surg Res.* 2015; 101(Suppl 1):S77-S83. [VB]

224. Howard JL, Hanssen AD. Principles of a clean operating room environment. *J Arthroplasty.* 2007;22(7 Suppl 3):6-11. [VB]

225. Castella A, Charrier L, Di Legami V, et al. Surgical site infection surveillance: analysis of adherence to recommendations for routine infection control practices. *Infect Control Hosp Epidemiol.* 2006;27(8):835-840. [IIIB]

226. Quality improvement/quality assessment: quality improvement. In: *Procedural Standards and Checklist for Accreditation of Ambulatory Surgery Facilities.* Version 31. Gurnee, IL: American Association for Accreditation of Ambulatory Surgery Facilities; 2018:65.

227. 06: Clinical records and health information. In: *2017 Accreditation Handbook for Ambulatory Health Care*. Skokie, IL: Accreditation Association for Ambulatory Health Care; 2017:51-53.

228. Medical records: general. In: *Regular Standards and Checklist for Accreditation of Ambulatory Surgery Facilities*. Version 145. Gurnee, IL: American Association for Accreditation of Ambulatory Surgery Facilities; 2017:57-59.

229. Medical records: pre-operative medical record. In: *Regular Standards and Checklist for Accreditation of Ambulatory Surgery Facilities*. Version 145. Gurnee, IL: American Association for Accreditation of Ambulatory Surgery Facilities; 2017:58-59.

230. Medical records: operating room records. In: *Regular Standards and Checklist for Accreditation of Ambulatory Surgery Facilities*. Version 145. Gurnee, IL: American Association for Accreditation of Ambulatory Surgery Facilities; 2017:60-63.

231. *State Operations Manual Appendix A—Survey Protocol, Regulations and Interpretive Guidelines for Hospitals*. Rev 176. 2017. Centers for Medicare & Medicaid Services. https://www.cms.gov/Regulations-and-Guidance/Guidance/Manuals/downloads/som107ap_a_hospitals.pdf. Accessed September 12, 2018.

232. *State Operations Manual Appendix L—Guidance for Surveyors: Ambulatory Surgical Centers*. Rev 137. 2015. Centers for Medicare & Medicaid Services. https://www.cms.gov/Regulations-and-Guidance/Guidance/Manuals/Downloads/som107ap_l_ambulatory.pdf. Accessed September 12, 2018.

233. Medical records: general. In: *Procedural Standards and Checklist for Accreditation of Ambulatory Surgery Facilities*. Version 31. Gurnee, IL: American Association for Accreditation of Ambulatory Surgery Facilities; 2018:58-59.

234. Medical records: procedure room records. In: *Procedural Standards and Checklist for Accreditation of Ambulatory Surgery Facilities*. Version 31. Gurnee, IL: American Association for Accreditation of Ambulatory Surgery Facilities; 2018:63-65.

235. Critical access hospital. Record of care, treatment, and services. RC.01.01.01: The critical access hospital maintains complete and accurate medical records for each individual patient. In: *Comprehensive Accreditation Manual*. E-dition. Oakbrook Terrace, IL: The Joint Commission; 2018.

236. Hospital. Record of care, treatment, and services. RC.01.01.01: The hospital has policies and procedures that guide and support patient care, treatment, and services. In: *Comprehensive Accreditation Manual*. E-dition. Oakbrook Terrace, IL: The Joint Commission; 2018.

237. Ambulatory. Record of care, treatment, and services. RC.01.01.01: The organization maintains complete and accurate clinical records. In: *Comprehensive Accreditation Manual*. E-dition. Oakbrook Terrace, IL: The Joint Commission; 2018.

238. Office based surgery. Record of care, treatment, and services. RC.01.01.01: The practice maintains complete and accurate clinical records. In: *Comprehensive Accreditation Manual*. E-dition. Oakbrook Terrace, IL: The Joint Commission; 2018.

239. Surgical site infection (SSI) event. In: *National Healthcare Safety Network (NHSN) Patient Safety Component Manual*. Atlanta GA: National Healthcare Safety Network, Centers for Disease Control and Prevention; 2018:9-1–9-24.

Acknowledgments

Lead Author
Julie A. Cahn, DNP, RN, CNOR, RN-BC, ACNS-BC, CNS-CP
Perioperative Practice Specialist
AORN Nursing Department
Denver, Colorado

Contributing Author
Amber Wood, MSN, RN, CNOR, CIC, FAPIC
Editor-in-Chief, Guidelines for Perioperative Practice
AORN Nursing Department
Denver, Colorado

The authors and AORN thank Donna A. Pritchard, MA, BSN, RN, NE-BC, CNOR, Director of Perioperative Services, Interfaith Medical Center, Brooklyn, New York; Bernard C. Camins, MD, MSc, Associate Professor of Medicine, University of Alabama at Birmingham; Heather A. Hohenberger, MSN, RN, CIC, CNOR, CPHQ, Administrative Director Surgical Services, IU Health Arnett Hospital, Lebanon, Indiana; Jennifer Butterfield, MBA, RN, CNOR, CASC, Administrator/COE, Lakes Surgery Center, West Bloomfield, Michigan; Gerald McDonnell, PhD, BSc, Johnson & Johnson Family of Companies, Raritan, New Jersey; Kate McGee, BSN, RN, CNOR, Staff Nurse, Aurora West Allis Medical Center, East Troy, Wisconsin; Mary Anderson, MS, RN, CNOR, OR RN - II, Parkland Health & Hospital System, Dallas, Texas; Mary Fearon, MSN, RN, CNOR, Service Line Director Neuroscience, Overlake Medical Center, Sammamish, Washington; Jennifer Hanrahan, DO, Medical Director of Infection Prevention, Metrohealth Medical Center, Cleveland, Ohio; Susan Ruwe, MSN, RN, CPHQ, CIC, Senior Infection Preventionist, Carle Foundation Hospital, Argenta, Illinois; Doug Schuerer, MD, FACS, FCCM, Professor of Surgery, Trauma Director, Washington University School of Medicine, St Louis, Missouri; Brenda G. Larkin, MS, ACNS-BC, CNS, CNOR, Clinical Nurse Specialist, Aurora Lakeland Medical Center, Lake Geneva, Wisconsin; Jay Bowers, BSN, RN, CNOR, Clinical Coordinator for Trauma, General Surgery, Bariatric, Pediatric and Surgical Oncology, West Virginia University Hospitals, Morgantown; Marisa (Missi) Merlino, MHA, RN-BC, CNOR, CSSM, Scott & White Medical Center-Temple, Staff Nurse II, Temple, Texas; Elizabeth (Lizz) Pincus, MSN, RN, CNS-CP, CNOR, Clinical Nurse Specialist, St Francis Hospital, Roslyn, NY; and Marie A. Bashaw, DNP, RN, NEA-BC, CNOR, Assistant Professor, Wright State University College of Nursing and Health, Dayton, Ohio, for their assistance in developing this guideline.

Publication History

Originally published as "AORN Standards—OR wearing apparel, draping and gowning materials," March 1975, *AORN Journal*.

Revised; published as "Standards of technical and aseptic practice: OR," March 1978, *AORN Standards of Practice*.

Revised October 1985; published as "Recommended practices: basic aseptic technique," March 1987, *AORN Journal.*

Revised February 1991; published as "Recommended practices: aseptic technique," October 1991, *AORN Journal.*

Revised January 1996; published as "Recommended practices for maintaining a sterile field," November 1996, *AORN Journal.*

Revised; published February 2001, *AORN Journal.*

Revised November 2005; published in *Standards, Recommended Practices, and Guidelines,* 2006 edition. Reprinted February 2006, *AORN Journal.*

Revised December 2012; published as "Recommended practices for sterile technique," *Perioperative Standards and Recommended Practices,* 2013 edition.

Evidence ratings revised 2013 to conform to the AORN Evidence Rating Model.

Minor editing revisions November 2014; published as "Guideline for sterile technique" in *Guidelines for Perioperative Practice,* 2015 edition.

Evidence rating revised to conform to the current AORN Evidence Rating Model in *Guidelines for Perioperative Practice,* 2018 edition.

Revised November 2018 for publication in *Guidelines for Perioperative Practice* online.

Evidence ratings revised and minor editorial changes made to conform to the current AORN Evidence Rating model, September 2019, for online publication in *Guidelines for Perioperative Practice.*

STERILIZATION

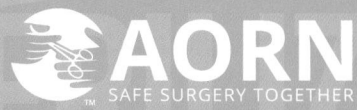

TABLE OF CONTENTS

MEDICAL ABBREVIATIONS & ACRONYMS

AAMI – Association for the Advancement of Medical Instrumentation
ACGIH – American Conference of Governmental Industrial Hygienists
BI – Biological indicator
CDC – Centers for Disease Control and Prevention
CI – Chemical indicator
EO – Ethylene oxide
EPA – Environmental Protection Agency
EPCRA – Emergency Planning and Community Right-To-Know Act

FDA – US Food and Drug Administration
IARC – International Agency for Research on Cancer
IFU – Instructions for use
IUSS – Immediate use steam sterilization
OSHA – Occupational Safety and Health Administration
PCD – Process challenge device
PPE – Personal protective equipment
ppm – Parts per million
SDS – Safety data sheet
SSI – Surgical site infection
TLV – Threshold limit value

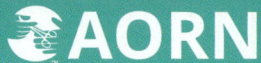
GUIDELINE FOR
STERILIZATION

The Guideline for Sterilization was approved by the AORN Guidelines Advisory Board and became effective September 1, 2018. It was presented as a proposed guideline for comments by members and others. The recommendations in the guideline are intended to be achievable and represent what is believed to be an optimal level of practice. Policies and procedures will reflect variations in practice settings and/or clinical situations that determine the degree to which the guideline can be implemented. AORN recognizes the many diverse settings in which perioperative nurses practice; therefore, this guideline is adaptable to all areas where operative or other invasive procedures may be performed.

Purpose

This document provides guidance for sterilizing reusable medical devices to be used in perioperative and procedural settings. Items that enter sterile tissue, including the vascular system, are categorized as critical using the Spaulding classification and should be sterile when used.[1] An important factor in preventing surgical site infections (SSIs) is the use of only sterile instruments and medical devices for operative and other invasive procedures. Surgical site infections are among the most common health care–associated infections, comprising 31% of all health care–associated infections among hospitalized patients.[2] Between 2006 and 2009, SSIs complicated an estimated 1.9% of surgical procedures in the United States.[3] The Centers for Disease Control and Prevention (CDC) health care–associated infection prevalence survey found there were an estimated 157,500 SSIs associated with inpatient surgeries in 2011.[2]

Surgical site infections may cause serious injury or death at enormous cost to patients, their families, and the health care organization. A systematic review of the literature on SSI from 1998 to 2014 found the estimated average cost of an SSI ranged between $10,433 (2005 dollars) and $25,546 (2002 dollars),[3] which equates to approximately $13,300 to $35,400 in 2018 dollars. Costs can exceed $90,000 per infection when the SSI involves a prosthetic joint implant or an antimicrobial-resistant organism.[3]

Sterility is accomplished through a multistep process. This process begins immediately after instrument use with the removal of gross soil, followed by further cleaning, decontamination, inspection, packaging, and finally sterilization. Each step is critical in producing sterile items and maintaining sterility until the item is opened and delivered to the sterile field for use. Effective sterilization cannot take place without effective cleaning, decontamination, and

packaging. Substances such as bioburden, biofilm, plaques, soils, and oils inhibit sterilization. The degree to which sterilization is inhibited is correlated with the amount, number, type, and inherent resistance of these substances. Any of these substances may shield microorganisms on items from contact with the sterilant or combine with and inactivate the sterilant. Sterile barrier packaging increases the probability that sterility will be achieved and maintained until the package is opened at the point of use.

Sterility may be achieved by a variety of physical or chemical processes. The selection of the sterilization method is dependent on a number of factors including device design, material, packaging, compatibility with the sterilant, load limitations, safety requirements, and organization-specific considerations. The most common sterilization methods used in health care in the United States are addressed in this guideline. New sterilization technologies are being developed and may become commercially available in the future but are not yet cleared by the US Food and Drug Administration (FDA) for use in the United States. This document provides guidance only for sterilization processes commonly used in health care and currently cleared by the FDA.

The guideline addresses

- saturated steam under pressure;
- ethylene oxide;
- low-temperature hydrogen peroxide gas plasma;
- low-temperature hydrogen peroxide vapor;
- ozone combined with hydrogen peroxide;
- dry heat;
- liquid chemical sterilization using peracetic acid;
- loading the sterilizer and load configuration;
- transport of sterile items;
- quality control measures; and
- installation, care, and maintenance of sterilization equipment.

Guidance for the following topics is outside of the scope of this document:

- specific guidance for reprocessing of medical devices labeled as single use, criteria for evaluating the services of a third-party reprocessor, and identifying single-use items for reprocessing;
- cleaning and decontamination of surgical instruments;
- high-level disinfection;
- packaging;
- loaned instruments;
- facility design;
- sterilization processes not cleared by the FDA for use in health care facilities (eg, gamma or electron beam radiation, chlorine dioxide, nitrogen dioxide);

Figure 1. Flow Diagram of Literature Search Results

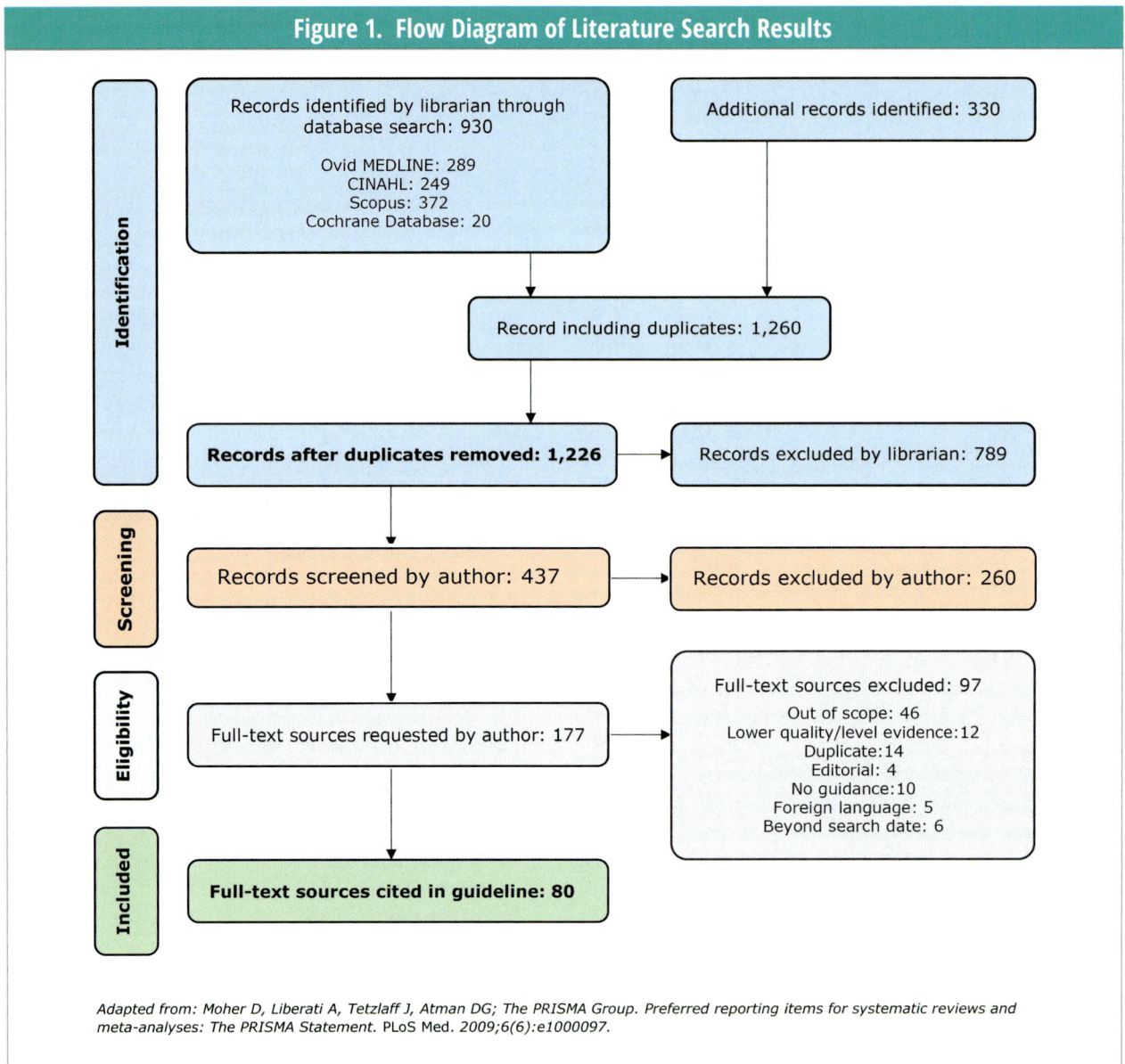

Adapted from: Moher D, Liberati A, Tetzlaff J, Atman DG; The PRISMA Group. Preferred reporting items for systematic reviews and meta-analyses: The PRISMA Statement. PLoS Med. 2009;6(6):e1000097.

- processing of medical devices that have been or potentially have been exposed to prions; and
- cost comparison and analysis of various methodologies.

Refer to the AORN Guideline for Cleaning and Care of Surgical Instruments,[4] Guideline for Manual Chemical High-Level Disinfection,[5] Guideline for Flexible Endoscopes,[6] Guideline for Selection and Use of Packaging Systems for Sterilization,[7] and Guideline for Design and Maintenance of the Surgical Suite[8] for guidance on these important topics related to the sterilization process.

Evidence Review

A medical librarian conducted a systematic search of the databases Ovid MEDLINE®, EBSCO CINAHL®, Scopus®, and the Cochrane Database of Systematic Reviews. The search was limited to literature published in English from January 2012 through December 2017. At the time of the initial search, weekly alerts were created on the topics included in that search. Results from these alerts were provided to the lead author until February 2018. The lead author requested additional articles that either did not fit the original search criteria or were discovered during the evidence appraisal process. The lead author and the medical librarian also identified relevant guidelines from government agencies, professional organizations, and standards-setting bodies.

Search terms included *autoclave, biofilms, biological indicators, biomaterial, burns, central services department, chemical indicators, clinical quality measures, disinfectant agent, dry heat, dynamic air cycles, ethylene oxide, flash sterilization, gravity displacement, hydrogen peroxide, hydrogen peroxide gas, hydrogen peroxide gas plasma, immediate use, immediate use flash sterilization, immediate use steam sterilization, indicators and reagents, **installation qualification**, instrument* processing, instrument sterilization, IUSS, liquid chemical sterilants, load release, loading sterilizer, Medivators, mixed loads, moist heat, *operational qualification*, ozone, peracetic acid, *performance qualification*, prevacuum, process challenge, quality assurance testing, reagent strips, satellite processing, steam, steam flush pressure pulse, sterile processing department, sterility assurance levels, sterilization, sterilization and disinfection, sterilization cycles, sterilization efficacy, sterilization modalities, sterilization monitoring, sterilization parameters, sterilization quality, sterilizer load configuration, sterilizer load weight limit, Steris, Sterrad, surgical equipment, surgical instruments/microbiology, tabletop sterilizer, user validation, vacuum sterilizer, vaporized hydrogen peroxide, wet heat, and wet instrument trays.

Included were research and non-research literature in English, complete publications, and publications with dates within the time restriction when available. Excluded were non-peer-reviewed publications and older evidence within the time restriction when more recent evidence was available. Editorials, news items, and other brief items were excluded. Low-quality evidence was excluded when higher-quality evidence was available, and literature outside the time restriction was excluded when literature within the time restriction was available (Figure 1).

Articles identified in the search were provided to the project team for evaluation. The team consisted of the lead author, a coauthor, and two evidence appraisers. The lead author divided the search results into topics and assigned members of the team to review and critically appraise each article using the AORN Research or Non-Research Evidence Appraisal Tools as appropriate. The literature was independently evaluated and appraised according to the strength and quality of the evidence. Each article was then assigned an appraisal score. The appraisal score is noted in brackets after each reference as applicable.

Each recommendation rating is based on a synthesis of the collective evidence, a benefit-harm assessment, and consideration of resource use. The strength of the recommendation was determined using the AORN Evidence Rating Model and the quality and consistency of the evidence supporting a recommendation. The recommendation strength rating is noted in brackets after each recommendation.

Note: The evidence summary table is available at http://www.aorn.org/evidencetables/.

Editor's note: MEDLINE is a registered trademark of the US National Library of Medicine's Medical Literature Analysis and Retrieval System, Bethesda, MD. CINAHL, Cumulative Index to Nursing and Allied Health Literature, is a registered trademark of EBSCO Industries, Birmingham, AL. Scopus is a registered trademark of Elsevier B.V., Amsterdam, The Netherlands. Sterrad is a registered trademark of Johnson & Johnson, New Brunswick, NJ.

1. Process Based on Intended Use

1.1 **Process reusable medical devices based on the intended use of the item.** *[Recommendation]*

1.2 **Items that enter sterile tissue, including the vascular system, should be sterile when used.**[1,9-11] *[Recommendation]*

Medical devices that contact sterile body tissues or fluids are considered critical items.[1] The CDC recommends that these items be sterile when used because any microbial contamination could result in disease transmission. Sterilization provides the highest level of assurance that surgical items are free of viable microbes.[1]

1.3 **Sterilize reusable semicritical items that are manufacturer-validated for sterilization if possible.**[10,12-14] *[Recommendation]*

Reusable semicritical items processed by high-level disinfection present a greater risk of disease transmission than items processed by sterilization.[12] The Spaulding classification has been a reliable and useful tool for determining needed levels of disinfection since 1957. However, there is a growing scientific debate on practices and expectations of disinfection.[14] This debate is fueled by two concepts. First, the Spaulding classification, at its inception, considered high-level disinfection to be effective against most pathogens known at that time.[14] It is now known that pathogens resistant to high-level disinfection exist, including but not limited to small non-enveloped viruses (eg, parvoviruses, coxsackieviruses, other enteroviruses, hepatitis A, norovirus) and resistant bacteria (eg, the mycobacteria *M tuberculosis*, *M avium* and *M abscessus*, *M fortuitum*, *M chimaera*).[14] Second, studies in many countries have documented a lack of compliance with sterilization and disinfection guidelines that have led to numerous infectious outbreaks.[15,16] A large number of these have been related to items classically identified as semicritical (eg, endoscopes).

McDonnell and Burke[14] suggested that although much of the Spaulding classification scheme remains relevant, some devices, such as flexible endoscopes, currently categorized as semicritical may no longer fit into the semicritical classification. It is now known that various types of viruses, bacterial strains, and protozoa survive high-level disinfection. Infectious outbreaks have been associated with the use of some high-level disinfected semicritical devices (eg, flexible duodenoscopes). Respiratory therapy and anesthesia equipment, gastrointestinal endoscopes, bronchoscopes, laryngoscopes, esophageal manometry probes, anorectal manometry catheters, endocavity probes, prostate biopsy probes, infrared coagulation devices, nasopharyngoscopes, cystoscopes, and diaphragm fitting rings are included in the category of semicritical devices. Intact mucous membranes, such as those of the lungs or the gastrointestinal tract, generally are resistant to infection by common bacterial spores but are susceptible to other organisms such as bacteria, mycobacteria, and viruses.[14]

1.4 **Sterilize reusable medical devices according to the manufacturers' instructions for use (IFU) for the specific device, packaging, and sterilizer equipment.**[17-21] *[Recommendation]*

Manufacturers of FDA-cleared reusable medical devices, packaging systems, and sterilization equipment provide validated instructions on how to sterilize devices and operate sterilization equipment.[17-21] Items cannot be assumed to be clean, decontaminated, or sterile unless the manufacturers' IFU have been followed.

1.4.1 **Make manufacturers' written IFU accessible to personnel who perform sterile processing.**[21-23] *[Recommendation]*

1.4.2 **Reconcile the sterilization method and cycle parameters recommended by the device manufacturer and the packaging manufacturer with the sterilizer manufacturer's written instructions for the specific sterilization cycle and load configuration.**[22-24] *[Recommendation]*

The parameters required to achieve sterilization are determined by the design of the device, the characteristics of the load, the sterilizer capabilities, and the packaging.[23] The increasingly complex design of instruments, the configuration of instrument trays, and the variety of packaging materials have resulted in the need for complicated and specific processing recommendations from instrument manufacturers.[22] Device manufacturers' instructions are sometimes unclear, incomplete, or require processes or cycles that are not available in the health care facility.[22]

Certain complex instruments (eg, some pneumatically powered instruments, orthopedic sets, robotic instruments) and implants may require prolonged exposure times or drying times. These sterilization cycle parameters may not have been validated by the sterilizer manufacturer.

1.4.3 **When the device, sterilizer, and packaging manufacturers' IFU conflict, follow the device manufacturer's IFU.**[23,25] *[Recommendation]*

The device manufacturer's instructions are not always compatible with the sterilizer instructions or the instructions for the type of packaging used. The device manufacturer performs validation studies to determine the sterilization parameters required to achieve sterility of the specific device.[17,26] The sterilizer and packaging manufacturers may have performed validation studies on specific devices. However, sterilizing the device in a package or sterilizer that is not validated by the device manufacturer may not be supported by the device manufacturer.

1.5 **Devices labeled for single use must not be reprocessed unless the FDA guidelines for reprocessing of single-use devices can be met.**[27] *[Regulatory Requirement]*

In 2000, the FDA issued a guidance document for reprocessing of single-use devices.[27] This document details the requirements that a reprocessor must meet. These requirements are the same requirements that the original device manufacturer must meet.[27] They include

- registering as a reprocessing firm and listing all products that are reprocessed;
- submitting reports of associated adverse events to the FDA;
- tracking devices that, in the event of failure, could lead to serious adverse outcomes;
- correcting or removing from the market unsafe devices; and
- meeting manufacturing and labeling requirements.[26]

Third-party and hospital reprocessors of single-use devices are subject to all the regulatory requirements currently applicable to original equipment manufacturers, including premarket submission requirements (Section 513 and 515 of the FDA Act[27]; 21 CFR Parts 807[28] and 814[29]).

1.5.1 **Health care organizations that are considering reprocessing single-use devices should identify devices labeled as for single use that they would like to reprocess; review the FDA guidance document[27]; and, based on the requirements in the document, make a determination as to the feasibility of reprocessing those devices within the facility or contracting with a third-party reprocessor.** *[Recommendation]*

Meeting these requirements is beyond the capabilities of most health care organizations.

1.5.2 **If it is determined that inhouse reprocessing of single-use devices is feasible, form an interdisciplinary team to develop a program for reprocessing single-use devices that**

meets the FDA requirements[27] and includes policies, procedures, competencies, and educational requirements for personnel. *[Conditional Recommendation]*

2. Area for Sterilization Processes

2.1 Perform sterilization in an area intended, designed, and equipped for sterilization processes.[30] *[Recommendation]*

The requirements for processing reusable medical devices do not vary by location. Equivalent competent personnel, environments, procedures, supplies, equipment, and quality assurance measures are needed in all locations where processing is performed.

2.2 Perform sterilization processes in an area equipped and designed to be functionally equivalent to central sterile processing areas (ie, a satellite sterile processing area).[30] Do not perform sterilization processes in an OR or procedure room. *[Recommendation]*

Physical separation of patient care areas from areas where sterilization processes are performed minimizes the risk of cross contamination.

2.3 Place sterilizers in a clean work area or room with restricted access (eg, the semi-restricted area of the perioperative suite), with physical separation from high-traffic hallways or other potential sources of contamination, such as scrub sinks, clinical sinks or hoppers, wash sinks, or containers for the disposal of linen and trash.[23] *[Recommendation]*

2.4 Sterile processing areas, including satellite sterile processing areas should have

- cleaning and decontamination spaces, which may be rooms or areas, that are separated by one of three methods:
  - a wall with a door or pass-through,
  - a partial wall or partition that is at least 4-ft high and at least the width of the counter, or
  - a distance of 4 ft between the instrument-washing sink and the area where the instruments are prepared for sterilization;
- provisions for sterilization equipment and storage of related supplies in the clean area;
- separate sinks for washing instruments and washing hands;
- decontamination equipment (eg, automated washer, ultrasonic cleaner); and
- storage space for personal protective equipment (PPE) and cleaning supplies in the decontamination area.[23,30]

[Recommendation]

2.5 Establish traffic patterns that define requirements for access, movement of personnel, and attire.[8,23] *[Recommendation]*

Control of traffic patterns is intended to protect personnel, equipment, supplies, and instrumentation from sources of potential contamination.

2.5.1 Establish functional workflow patterns to create and maintain physical separation between the decontamination and sterilization areas. Establish functional workflow patterns from areas with high contamination potential to clean areas in the following order:
1. cleaning and decontamination area,
2. preparation and packaging,
3. sterilization processing, and
4. sterile storage or the point of use.[23]

[Recommendation]

A workflow pattern that begins in the decontamination area and flows to the storage area or the point of use can help prevent clean or sterile items from reentering a contaminated area where they may become recontaminated.[23]

3. Transport of Sterile Items

3.1 Protect sterile items from contamination, damage, or tampering during transport to a designated storage area or to the point of use. *[Recommendation]*

Sterility is event-related and is dependent on the amount of handling, the conditions during transport and storage, the quality of the packaging material, and adherence to the packaging material manufacturer's IFU.[1] Controlled transport and storage conditions reduce the risk of contamination and damage. Mishandling or tampering with sterile packages can damage the integrity of the package and the contents.

3.2 Contain sterile items in a **sterile barrier system** for transport to the point of use or storage.[1,7,23,24,31-35] *[Recommendation]*

Sterile barrier systems are designed and validated to protect the contents of the package from contamination until the enclosed item is used.

Sterile barrier systems are defined by the FDA in 21 CFR 880.6850 as "devices intended to be used to enclose another medical device that is to be sterilized by a health care provider. It is intended to allow sterilization of the enclosed medical device and also to maintain sterility of the enclosed device until used."[35]

3.2.1 When transport carts or bins are used, select carts that are either covered or enclosed and have solid bottom shelves.[23,24] *[Recommendation]*

Covered or enclosed carts and bins protect sterile items from exposure to environmental contaminants during transport. Solid bottom shelves protect the packages on the cart from contaminants on the floor.

3.2.2 Sterile items transported in an elevator designated for clean and sterile supply transport may be transported on uncovered carts.[23,24] [Conditional Recommendation]

3.2.3 When an elevator is used to transport both sterile and contaminated supplies, use covered or enclosed transport carts.[23,24] [Recommendation]

3.2.4 Segregate sterile items from contaminated items, trash, and food during transport.[23,24] [Recommendation]

Physical separation minimizes potential contamination of sterile items.

3.2.5 Use fluid-resistant transport carts, containers, and reusable covers and clean and disinfect them after each use.[23] [Recommendation]

3.3 Establish and implement standardized sterile processing procedures and measures for oversight of all aspects of processing and transport, including when all instruments are processed at one facility, requiring transport of packaged sterilized items between facilities. [Conditional Recommendation]

Some multisite organizations centralize sterile processing functions at one site and distribute sterilized items to other locations owned and operated by the same organization. Coordination of the process through standardization and oversight facilitates a consistent standard of care across the organization.

4. Storage of Sterile Items

4.1 Store sterile items in a controlled environment.[23] [Recommendation]

Limiting exposure to moisture, dust, direct sunlight, handling, and temperature and humidity extremes decreases the potential for contamination and degradation of sterilized items.[23] Factors that contribute to contamination include handling,[23,24] air movement, humidity, temperature, location of storage, dust, presence of vermin, whether shelving is open or closed, and properties of the sterile barrier system.[1]

4.2 Establish a process for determining the **shelf life** of sterilized items. The shelf life should be event-related unless otherwise specified by the packaging system manufacturer's labeled expiration date. Events that may compromise the sterility of a package include

- **multiple instances of handling that leads to seal breakage or loss of package integrity,**
- **moisture penetration, and**
- **exposure to airborne contaminants.**[23,36,37]

[Recommendation]

Shelf life is dependent on packaging material, storage conditions, transport, and handling (See the AORN Guideline for Selection and Use of Packaging Systems for Sterilization).[7]

4.3 Store sterile items under controlled conditions.[23] [Recommendation]

Controlled conditions reduce the risk of contaminating sterile items (See the AORN Guideline for Design and Maintenance of the Surgical Suite).[8]

4.3.1 Limit access to sterile supply areas to authorized personnel.[1,23,24] [Recommendation]

4.3.2 **Sterile storage rooms** may contain closed or open shelves, racks, and cabinets. [Conditional Recommendation]

4.3.3 Sterile items outside a designated sterile storage room should be stored in closed cabinets or covered carts.[23,24] [Recommendation]

4.3.4 The bottom shelf of an open shelving unit should be solid.[23,24] [Recommendation]

4.3.5 Keep racks, bins, and containers clean and dry on shelving that allows air circulation and ease of environmental cleaning (See the AORN Guideline for Environmental Cleaning).[23,24,38] [Recommendation]

4.3.6 Store sterile items in a manner that protects the integrity of the sterile barrier system.[1,23,24] [Recommendation]

4.3.7 Do not store sterile items under sinks or in other locations where they can become wet.[1,23,24] [Recommendation]

4.3.8 If a variance occurs in the parameters of the heating, ventilation, and air conditioning system in the sterile storage areas, have an interdisciplinary team perform a risk assessment (See the AORN Guideline for Design & Maintenance of the Surgical Suite).[8] [Recommendation]

4.4 Remove supplies and equipment from external shipping containers and open-edged corrugated cardboard boxes before transfer to the sterile storage area or point of use.[23] [*Recommendation*]

External shipping containers and open-edged cardboard boxes may collect dust, debris, and insects during shipment and may carry contaminants into the surgical suite.[23,36,37]

5. Steam Sterilization

5.1 **Use saturated steam under pressure to sterilize heat- and moisture-stable items unless otherwise indicated by the device manufacturer.** [*Recommendation*]

Saturated steam under pressure is the preferred sterilization method for items validated for this sterilization method.[1] It has a large margin of safety because of its reliability, consistency, and effectiveness. It is an inexpensive and relatively rapid sterilization method for most porous and nonporous materials.[1,39]

5.2 **Follow the manufacturers' written IFU for operating specific steam sterilizers, including**
- **gravity-displacement steam sterilizers that permit only gravity-displacement cycles,**
- **dynamic air-removal steam sterilizers (eg, prevacuum, steam-flush pressure-pulse) that permit only dynamic air-removal cycles, and**
- **sterilizers that permit either gravity-displacement or dynamic air-removal cycles.**[1,19,23]
[*Recommendation*]

Steam sterilizers vary in size, design, and performance characteristics. Steam sterilizers may be large capacity (ie, greater than 2 cu ft) or small capacity table-top models and may differ in how they generate steam.[23]

Air removal is critical to successful steam sterilization.[23] Medical device manufacturers, in their written IFU, may recommend a specific type of steam sterilization cycle or specify the achievement of certain cycle parameters based on validation of a specific method of air removal.[23]

5.3 **Packages containing phacoemulsification hand pieces may be sterilized in an upright (ie, vertical) position and held in a manner that allows for free drainage of the channel during steam sterilization.**[40-42] [*Conditional Recommendation*]

The device manufacturers' IFU may specify device position for sterilization. Van Doornmalen Gomez Hoyos et al[40] investigated the influence of the position of phacoemulsification hand pieces on the required conditions for steam sterilization. In this quasi-experimental study, three brands of phacoemulsification hand pieces were packaged individu-

ally in sterilization pouches. The packaged hand pieces were placed in a hospital steam sterilizer and oriented in three different ways: vertical with free drainage of the open end, horizontal, and vertical without free drainage of the open end. The hand pieces were sterilized for 4 minutes at 134° C (273° F). During the sterilization process, the temperature and pressure in the middle of the phacoemulsification hand piece channels were measured. The researchers found that horizontally oriented hand pieces or vertically oriented hand pieces with a blocked distal end preventing gravity drainage may not achieve sterilization conditions in the channel. They concluded that for effective and reproducible steam sterilization of phacoemulsification hand pieces, the hand pieces should be oriented vertically with no obstruction of the end of the channel. This research may be applicable to other channeled instruments, and further research is warranted.

van Wezel et al[42] conducted a quasi-experimental study as a follow-up to the study by van Doornmalen Gomez Hoyos et al.[40] In this study, three brands of phacoemulsification hand pieces were individually wrapped with regular and heavy duty wrapping material instead of a sterilization pouch and placed in a basket. The phacoemulsification hand pieces were fixed in five different angles (ie, zero, 30, 45, 60, and 90 degrees). During the sterilization process, the researchers measured the temperature and pressure in the middle of the phacoemulsification hand piece channels. The results of this study were similar to the findings of the previous study.[40] Sterilization conditions ($\geq 134°$ C [$\geq 273°$ F] for at least 3 minutes) were reached in 16 of the 43 studied cycles (37%). Failure rates varied among the different brands of hand pieces and were higher for hand pieces placed at zero degrees and 30 degrees than those placed at larger angles. The authors concluded that it is more likely for sterilization conditions to be met when hand pieces are vertically oriented.

5.4 **After steam sterilization, remove the sterilization rack containing sterilized items from the chamber and do not touch it until the items are cooled.**[23] [*Recommendation*]

The Association for the Advancement of Medical Instrumentation (AAMI) recommends that "terminally sterilized items should be allowed to cool to room temperature before handling."[23(p64)] However, the temperature is not specified. There is a lack of scientific evidence supporting precisely the amount of time needed for cooling or the temperature at which the items are safe to touch. A period of 30 minutes to more than 2 hours may be necessary for the cooldown. Cooling time will vary according to how hot items are at the end of the cycle; the density and composition of the materials contained within the load; the packaging material; heating, ventilation, and air conditioning in the cooling area; and the temperature and humidity of the ambient environment.[23] Containers made from plastic may require an extended cooling period to ensure moisture is removed from the container. High-density items retain heat and may require extended cooling times.

At the end of a steam sterilization cycle, a package may contain moisture that migrates out of the package as a gas (ie, water vapor) during the drying and cooling period. Depending on the type of packaging, if touched, a moist area may be created that can act as a wick and draw bacteria from hands before the package is cooled and dry.

5.4.1 Do not place warm or hot items on cool or cold surfaces. When the sterilizer has a sterilization rack, allow items to cool on the rack.[23] *[Recommendation]*

When hot and cold surfaces are brought together, moisture may condense from both inside and outside the package. Moisture may compromise the integrity of woven and nonwoven packaging materials and the sterility of the contents. Moisture may indicate problems with the packaging or sterilization process.[23]

5.4.2 When items are moved from the cooling rack for transport to storage or to the point of use, inspect the package for integrity, moisture, and change of the external **chemical indicator**.[23] If there is any question of sterility, resterilize the item(s). *[Recommendation]*

5.4.3 Before handling, the temperature of the sterilized item may be measured with a calibrated infrared thermometer or similar device.[23] *[Conditional Recommendation]*

5.4.4 Cool sterilized items before use to prevent thermal injury to the patient.[43-45] *[Recommendation]*

Injuries have occurred when warm or hot items were used in the surgical wound or for positioning. In addition to the temperature of the item, the use, pressure exerted on tissue, and contact time contribute to the risk of a thermal injury to the patient. Rutala et al[45] reported two incidents of patient burn injuries. One patient who underwent an anterior cruciate ligament reconstruction received a partial thickness burn to her thigh when a hot shaver that had been "flash" sterilized (ie, processed by **immediate use steam sterilization**) was placed on her leg. Attempts had been made

to cool the instrument and the scrub person was able to hold the instrument, although it felt warm. The second patient suffered a full-thickness burn from a "flash" sterilized self-retaining retractor weight.

Another incident of a patient injury occurred when a warm positioning device was used to position a patient's arm during hand surgery. Following the surgery, a third-degree burn was discovered on the patient's upper arm and a portion of the patient's lower back.[44] During a dental procedure, a 20-year-old patient sustained a superficial burn from a "recently sterilized instrument."[43(p689)]

5.5 Perform immediate use steam sterilization (IUSS) only when all of the following conditions are met:
- the device and sterilizer manufacturer's written IFU include instructions for IUSS;
- the device manufacturer's written instructions for cleaning, cycle type, exposure times, temperature settings, and drying times (if recommended) are readily available and followed;
- items are placed in a containment device that has been validated for IUSS and cleared by the FDA for this purpose and in a manner that allows steam to contact all instrument surfaces;
- the rigid sterilization container manufacturer's written IFU are followed; and
- measures are taken to prevent contamination during removal from the sterilizer and transfer to the sterile field.[23]

[Recommendation]

A multi-organization position paper published in 2011[25] and endorsed by AORN; the Association for Professionals in Infection Control and Epidemiology; the International Association of Healthcare Central Service Materiel Management; the Accreditation Association of Ambulatory Healthcare; the Association of Surgical Technologists; and the ASC Quality Collaboration, which represents the ambulatory surgery center industry, recommended that the same critical processing steps (ie, cleaning, decontaminating, and transporting sterilized items) be followed regardless of the specific sterilization cycle employed. The paper states that "a safe process does not include short-cuts or work-arounds."[25(p1)]

Time constraints and lack of equipment and supplies may result in pressure on OR personnel to eliminate or modify one or more steps in the cleaning and sterilization process. In a report of an organizational experience from a hospital in Ohio, Sheffer[46] noted that when performing IUSS in the OR, personnel did not have the same tools for complete cleaning and sterilization or access to specific device manufacturer's IFU as were available in the sterile processing area. When the organization implemented measures that reduced the incidence of IUSS (from 330 to 25 in a 28-day period), practices improved and efficiency was maximized.

5.5.1 Subject items to be steam sterilized for immediate use to the decontamination processes described in the AORN Guideline for Cleaning and Care of Surgical Instruments.[4,25] *[Recommendation]*

As with **terminal sterilization**, decontamination is essential for removing bioburden, debris, and biofilm, thus preparing an item for IUSS. Abbreviated processing steps (eg, inadequate decontamination) place patients at increased risk for SSI or other complications.[1]

5.5.2 Contain devices processed using IUSS in a rigid sterilization container and transport them to the point of use in a manner that minimizes the risk of contamination of the item and thermal injury to patients or personnel.[23] *[Recommendation]*

Items sterilized by IUSS may be vulnerable to contamination by exposure to the environment and handling by personnel transporting the sterile devices to the point of use. It is important that sterilization processing be carried out in a clean environment and that IUSS devices be transferred to the point of use in a manner that prevents contamination.[23]

Because drying may not be required as part of a preprogrammed IUSS cycle, the items processed may be wet at the conclusion of the cycle and will be hot when removed from the sterilizer chamber immediately after the cycle.

5.5.3 Use items processed by IUSS immediately and do not store them for future use or hold them from one procedure to the next.[23,25] *[Recommendation]*

5.5.4 Do not use immediate use steam sterilization for implantable devices except in cases of defined emergency when no other option is available.[1,23] *[Recommendation]*

Implants are foreign bodies, and they increase the risk of SSI.[47] Careful planning, packaging, and inventory management in cooperation with suppliers can minimize the need for IUSS of implantable medical devices.

5.5.5 When IUSS of an implant is unavoidable, determine cycle selection by the device manufacturer's written IFU, and run a **biological indicator** (BI) and a type 5 chemical integrating indicator

with the load. For dynamic air-removal cycles, a preassembled process challenge device may be used. When an implant is used before the BI results are known and the BI is later determined to have a positive result, notify the surgeon and infection preventionist(s) as soon as the results are known. *[Recommendation]*

5.5.6 Maintain documentation of IUSS cycle information and monitoring results.[23] *[Recommendation]*

Documentation of cycle information provides a means for tracking items that are processed using IUSS to individual patients and for quality monitoring.

5.6 Investigate wet loads or **wet packs** in a terminal sterilization cycle and take corrective measures.[23] *[Recommendation]*

Loads or packages found to be wet after a complete terminal sterilization cycle that includes drying may indicate a problem with the steam supply, sterilizer function, or load configuration.

In a 2015, peer-reviewed, expert opinion article, Sandle[48] described three possible scenarios for a wet load: visible moisture on the outside of the pack, moisture inside the pack (eg, a moist towel), and visible water inside the tray. The author also discussed potential causes of wet loads. First, steam supply could be problematic. Poor **steam quality** (eg, insufficient dryness) can lead to excessive condensate formation within the sterilizer. Excessive demands on the steam supply can lead to wet steam. Steam supply infrastructure issues can also lead to problems with steam, including pipework with dead ends, improperly trapped or insulated piping, or inadequate maintenance of steam traps. The farther the steam line is from the heating source, the more likely condensate is to form. If the steam generator does not have sufficient capacity for the autoclave, a pressure drop may occur at times of peak demand and residual water (condensate) may enter the sterilizer. Malfunctioning or improperly sized steam traps can cause excessive water formation that might overwhelm the sterilizer.

Second, overloaded and densely packed loads can cause excessive condensation and pose a challenge for steam circulation and evacuation during the sterilization cycle. Additional load considerations include type of packaging materials, metal density in each set, and loading technique (eg, rigid containers should be spaced and not stacked unless this is allowed by the container manufacturer's IFU). Less common contributing factors may include

- a temperature differential between the sterilizer jacket, sterilizer door, and chamber;

- a stainless steel carriage, which creates more condensate than an aluminum carriage;
- an inadequate preheating process;
- items touching the sterilizer wall;
- items loaded when wet;
- a load configuration that traps water;
- blocked condensate drains;
- buildup of condensate in the steam supply pipework (especially when it has not been used for a few days); and
- an open drain valve (leading to drain water being returned).[48]

Basu[49] reviewed potential causes for wet packs and loads, which are the same as those noted by Sandle.[48] The author offered a simplified list of preventive measures, including

- performing periodic maintenance and calibration of steam sterilizers;
- avoiding sterilizer overload;
- ensuring adequate dry time per the manufacturer's IFU;
- allowing adequate cool time inside the sterilizer to acclimate with room temperature;
- avoiding instrument tip protectors, which can hold moisture;
- using good quality wrapping material;
- ensuring set packing is performed per the manufacturer's IFU;
- choosing the correct size of wrappers and containers;
- checking gaskets and drain valves to ensure good working order for all rigid containers;
- maintaining environmental temperature and humidity in the sterile processing department per guidelines; and
- implementing corrective measures in the sterile processing department in response to deviations from temperature and humidity guidelines.

Two laboratory quasi-experimental studies challenged the notion that wet packs are unsuitable for use. These studies analyzed sterility of packaged items after terminal steam sterilization where the drying phase was intentionally interrupted. In one small study, Fayard et al[50] assessed the effect of residual moisture on microbial contamination of surgical instruments. The authors tested two types of packaging: rigid sterilization containers with disposable filter papers and double-layer nonwoven sterilization wrap. The containers were tested in batches of six tests where each batch was sterilized at 135° C [275° F] for 18 minutes with a 1-minute drying phase and then stored for different durations (zero, 1, 3, 7, and 14 days) to equal 30 tests per packaging type.

Positive controls for rigid containers after zero, 3, and 7 days were found to be contaminated; however, positive controls for double-wrapped packages were culture-negative. Rigid containers were found to have no residual water after 3 days of storage; double-wrapped packages contained no residual water after 7 days. Culture samples from the study groups were negative for all rigid and wrapped containers for each storage duration. The researchers acknowledged study limitations in some important areas. First, some control packages cultured microbial contaminants on porcelain test carriers yet yielded sterile water on analysis. Second, some of the positive controls expected to show positive culture were negative. Additionally, the researchers suggested that the study was conducted in "real world" simulation; however, the strict environmental controls present in the study may not be as tightly controlled in all locations where steam sterilization occurs.[50]

In another study, Moriya and Graziano[51] conducted a laboratory experiment after considering how to respond to situations in which stored sterile items needed for an emergency procedure were found to be in wet packs. The study was conducted in Brazil using packaging practices that are specific to that country, which included surgical perforated boxes without lids, single wrapped with nonwoven cloth covering. Forty surgical boxes (ie, 20 in the control and 20 in study sample) were sterilized in a pre-vacuum cycle at 134° C (273° F) for 4 minutes, with the study group's dry cycle interrupted in "the early drying stage." After sterilization, the external faces of all packages were deliberately contaminated with *Serratia marcescens* and then stored for 30 days.

The researchers found no microbial growth when the surgical boxes were opened after 30 days in either the experimental or the control groups. The researchers made no mention of the presence or absence of residual moisture in the experimental group. The researchers did not intend to contradict recommendations that items should be dried after completing the sterilization process; their intent was to present scientific evidence to support decision making in emergent situations, such as when a patient is anesthetized and wet packs are discovered with no alternative surgical instruments available.[51]

Seavey[52] described a practical approach to investigating causes of wet loads. Potential causes listed in this expert opinion article are quality of steam supply to the sterilizer, performance of the sterilizer itself, and human processing errors. The author suggested that approximately 60% of wet packs can be attributed to steam supply. She recommended the use of the moisture assessment investigation tools found in Annex O of ANSI/AAMI ST79.[23]

5.6.1 Include the following in the investigation:
- date and time of the load in question;
- load configuration;
- number and description of trays reported as wet;
- cycle parameters;
- type of sterile barrier system used (eg, rigid sterilization container system, paper-plastic pouch);
- identification of the personnel who packaged the items;
- tray contents, configuration, and weight; and
- sterilizer performance.[23]

[Recommendation]

6. Low-Temperature Hydrogen Peroxide

6.1 Use low-temperature hydrogen peroxide sterilization methods (eg, vapor, gas plasma combination, ozone combination) to sterilize moisture- and heat-sensitive items when indicated by the device manufacturer. [Recommendation]

Manufacturers of medical devices that may be damaged by exposure to the high temperature of steam sterilization provide instructions for sterilization by low-temperature methods that rely on chemical effects to achieve sterility.[24] New and innovative surgical instrumentation made with heat-sensitive materials often requires low-temperature sterilization. Sterilizers that employ exposure to hydrogen peroxide gas plasma, vapor, or a combination of ozone and hydrogen peroxide are cleared by the FDA and are available to meet the need for safe and effective low-temperature sterilization methods.[53] However, hydrogen peroxide is listed as an extremely hazardous substance on the Environmental Protection Agency (EPA) Consolidated List of Chemicals Subject to Emergency Planning and Community Right-To-Know Act (EPCRA) and in Section 112(r) of the Clean Air Act of 1990.[54]

Hydrogen peroxide exposure has potential acute and chronic health effects, including the following:
- Hydrogen peroxide is corrosive to skin, eyes, and mucous membranes at high concentration (> 10%).
- Eye contact may result in ulceration or perforation of the cornea.
- Skin contact can cause irritation and temporary bleaching of the skin and hair and may cause severe skin burns with blisters.
- Vapors, mists, or aerosols of hydrogen peroxide can cause upper airway irritation, inflammation of the nose, hoarseness, shortness of breath, and a sensation of burning or tightness in the chest.
- Inhalation exposure to high concentrations can result in severe mucosal congestion of the trachea and bronchi and delayed accumulation of fluid in the lungs.
- Survivors of severe inhalation injury may sustain permanent lung damage.[55,56]

The World Health Organization International Agency for Research on Cancer (IARC) has determined that hydrogen peroxide is not classifiable as carcinogenic to humans[56]; but it is classified as carcinogenic to animals by the American Conference of Governmental Industrial Hygienists (ACGIH).[57]

The Occupational Safety and Health Administration (OSHA) sets a limit of 1 part of hydrogen peroxide in 1 million parts of air (1 ppm) in the workplace for an 8-hour work shift in a 40-hour work week.[58]

Ozone in combination with hydrogen peroxide has entered the marketplace as a sterilant. Ozone is listed as an extremely hazardous substance and toxic chemical on the EPA Consolidated List of Chemicals Subject to EPCRA.[54] The IARC does not provide a monograph for ozone cancer risk. The ACGIH has determined that ozone is not classifiable as a human carcinogen.[59] Numerous studies detailed in the ACGIH **Threshold Limit Value** (TLV®) profile[59] have demonstrated that the primary site of acute injury after ozone exposure in both experimental animals and humans exposed to ozone is the lung, with relatively low concentrations for short periods producing pulmonary congestion, edema, and hemorrhage. Exposure to ozone at increased workload potentiates greater effects on the lungs.[59] In humans, ozone concentrations of 1.5 parts per million and lower result in
- headaches,
- dryness of the throat and mucous membranes of the nose and eyes, and
- reduced pulmonary function values.[59]

Permissible limits for exposure to ozone, as established by OSHA, are 0.1 parts of ozone in 1 million parts of air (0.1 ppm) in the workplace for an 8-hour work shift in a 40-hour work week.[58] The ACGIH TLV exposure recommendations are workload-dependent. Heavy work limits are 0.05 ppm, moderate work limits are 0.08 ppm, and light work limits are 0.1 ppm.[59]

Items processed using low-temperature hydrogen peroxide do not require additional **aeration** because the residuals and by-products are oxygen and water, and these by-products are typically nontoxic.[24]

6.2 Follow the sterilizer manufacturer's written instructions for operation, monitoring, and maintenance of the sterilizer.[24] [Recommendation]

There are several manufacturers and models of hydrogen peroxide sterilizers with differing chamber sizes and FDA-cleared cycles available to US health care facilities. Each sterilizer has specific operating instructions and limitations on the type of items that may be sterilized (eg, non-lumened, lumen diameter and length, device material, packaging material, weight, number of channels).[53,60] Failure to follow the sterilizer manufacturer's IFU may damage the sterilizer or medical device, fail to result in sterility, or accidentally expose personnel to the chemical sterilant.

6.2.1 **Obtain written documentation of the acceptability of low-temperature hydrogen peroxide sterilization for specific devices from the device and sterilizer manufacturers.**[24] *[Recommendation]*

6.2.2 **Evaluate devices with lumens to determine whether the lumen diameter and length are within the sterilizer manufacturer's acceptable dimensions as specified in the sterilizer manufacturer's IFU.**[24] *[Recommendation]*

Complexity of some devices makes sterilization more challenging. Complex aspects of these devices (eg, endoscopes) include materials of construction, length, diameter, and number of lumens.[24] These can affect the ability of the sterilant to effectively contact all surfaces.[24]

6.3 **Clean and thoroughly dry items to be sterilized using low-temperature hydrogen peroxide sterilization before packaging in sterilization wraps, pouches, trays, or containers cleared by the FDA for use in hydrogen peroxide sterilizers.**[7,24,61] *[Recommendation]*

Liquids, powders, and cellulose based (ie, paper based) packaging materials or products are not suitable for low-temperature hydrogen peroxide gas plasma sterilization.[24] Excess moisture can also impact the effectiveness of some gaseous chemical sterilants because the system may rely on the absence or control of moisture.[24] In some sterilizers, excess moisture can cause cycle cancellation.[24]

6.3.1 **Place items in the sterilizer chamber as specified by the sterilizer and device manufacturers' IFU.**[24] *[Recommendation]*

Correct placement and configuration of items within the chamber facilitate contact of the sterilant with the items to be sterilized. Sterilant contact is essential for sterilization.

7. Peracetic Acid

7.1 **Liquid chemical sterilant instrument processing systems that use peracetic acid may be used for devices that can be immersed, are approved for this process by the device manufacturer, and**

cannot be sterilized using terminal sterilization methods.[1,24,62] *[Conditional Recommendation]*

Peracetic acid is an oxidizing agent that is an effective biocide at low temperatures and, in FDA-cleared formulated products, is effective in the presence of organic matter.[1] Peracetic acid is listed as an extremely hazardous substance, toxic chemical, and hazardous air pollutant on the EPA Consolidated List of Chemicals Subject to EPCRA and in Section 112(r) of the Clean Air Act of 1990.[54] The IARC does not provide a monograph for peracetic acid cancer risk. According to the ACGIH, peracetic acid is not classifiable as a human carcinogen, but peracetic acid has been found to be carcinogenic to animals.[63] In some animal studies with repeated dermal application at high concentrations, the authors concluded that peracetic acid is a strong promoter of skin tumors.[63]

Peracetic acid exposure has potential acute and chronic health effects, including the following:

- skin inflammation characterized by itching, scaling, reddening, and occasionally blistering;
- burns and ulcerations from prolonged skin exposure;
- lacrimation and extreme discomfort and irritation of nasal membranes at levels as low as 2 parts per million;
- red, watering, and itching eyes;
- toxic effects to blood, kidneys, lungs, liver, mucous membranes, heart, cardiovascular system, upper respiratory tract, skin, eyes, the central nervous system, and teeth; and
- general deterioration of health by accumulation in one or many human organs caused by repeated or prolonged exposure.[63]

The ACGIH recommends a limit of 0.4 parts of peracetic acid in 1 million parts of air (0.4 ppm) in the workplace for an 8-hour work shift in a 40-hour work week.[63]

7.2 **When using liquid chemical sterilant processing systems, follow the manufacturer's written instructions for operation, monitoring, and maintenance.**[24] *[Recommendation]*

Items processed in a liquid peracetic acid sterilant processing system that are not validated for these systems may not be compatible with the sterilant or the process, which could result in damage or an ineffective process. Processing devices that are not compatible with liquid chemical sterilant processing systems can shorten the life of the devices.

7.3 **When using liquid chemical sterilant processing systems, verify the correct selection of adapters and connect the device to the adapters as recommended by the manufacturers of both the device** and the liquid chemical sterilant processing system.[24] *[Recommendation]*

Failure to do so may result in failure of the liquid chemical sterilant to contact the lumen of the item.

7.4 **Transport items processed in liquid chemical sterilant systems to the point of use immediately and do not store for later use or hold from one procedure to another.**[24] *[Recommendation]*

Items processed in a liquid chemical sterilant processing system are wet, and the cassette or container in which they are processed is not sealed to prevent contamination, thereby increasing the risk for contamination from delivery to the sterile field and if not used immediately.[9] Processing trays used in liquid chemical sterilant systems are not intended for storage of processed items.

8. Ethylene Oxide

8.1 **Ethylene oxide sterilization may be used to sterilize moisture- and heat-sensitive surgical items when indicated by the device manufacturer.**[36] *[Conditional Recommendation]*

Ethylene oxide (EO) has a long history of use in sterilization applications in health care. Ethylene oxide–based sterilization processes are effective and reliable sterilization modes for moisture- and heat-sensitive critical surgical items when used according to device and sterilizer manufacturers' written IFU. Ethylene oxide is a known carcinogen in humans and animals.[64] Because inhalation risk is at its highest when the chamber has not been aerated, effective March 1, 2010, the EPA requires hospitals and health care facilities to use a single-chamber process for EO, which combines sterilization and aeration in a single unit.[65]

Ethylene oxide is listed as an extremely hazardous substance, toxic chemical, and hazardous air pollutant on the EPA Consolidated List of Chemicals Subject to EPCRA and in Section 112(r) of the Clean Air Act of 1990.[54] In December 2016, the EPA updated its EO inhalation risk to be based on human studies rather than animal studies. Formerly categorized as a reproductive hazard and probable carcinogen, the 2016 update concluded that EO is carcinogenic to humans, in agreement with the IARC, which classifies EO as "Group 1 - carcinogenic to humans."[64] Human studies illustrate that sufficient exposure to EO may result in lymphoid cancer and breast cancer in women.[66,67] In addition to cancer risk, EO carries other health and safety hazards, including the following[64,67]:

- Inhaling EO at high concentrations can cause nausea, vomiting, and neurological disorders.
- In solution, EO can severely irritate and burn the skin, eyes, and lungs.
- Ethylene oxide may damage the central nervous system, liver, and kidneys or cause cataracts.
- Ethylene oxide is extremely reactive and flammable, increasing risk of chemical accidents when used. Even static electricity can cause EO to ignite.[67]
- Ethylene oxide emissions in the atmosphere can cause community exposure (the EO half-life is 69 to 149 days).[67]

Permissible limits for exposure to EO, as established by OSHA, are 1 part ethylene oxide in 1 million parts of air (1 ppm) in the workplace for an 8-hour work shift in a 40-hour work week.[58] The ACGIH TLV exposure recommendations are also 1 ppm for ethylene oxide.[68]

8.2 **Be aware of and comply with federal, state, and local regulations for EO sterilizers.** *[Recommendation]*

Mixtures of EO with inert diluent gases are no longer commercially available, as EPA regulations have dictated a phase-out of these mixtures. Only 100% EO is commercially available in the United States.

8.3 **Items must be sterilized and aerated in a single-chamber EO sterilizer.**[65] *[Regulatory Requirement]*

The purpose of aeration is to reduce EO vapors and residue to a safe level. Some manufacturers' IFU require extended aeration times. Ethylene oxide is a known human carcinogen and a chemical that has the potential to cause adverse reproductive effects in humans.[64] If not aerated, EO residue absorbed into sterilized items represents a hazard to patients and personnel. Items that are not sufficiently aerated may cause injury (eg, chemical burns). Mechanical aeration is the only safe and effective way to remove residual EO. The EPA does not permit transfer of EO-sterilized loads to a separate aerator.[65]

8.3.1 **Do not open the EO sterilizer chamber or handle load contents until aeration is complete.**[36,65] *[Recommendation]*

Safety measures are necessary to prevent health care personnel from coming in contact with EO residues.

8.4 **The health care organization must establish a program for monitoring occupational exposure to EO in compliance with OSHA requirements.**[69] *[Regulatory Requirement]*

Compliance with regulations promotes a safe work environment that is within federal and state mandated limits for EO exposure. General environmental monitoring is not required, although it may provide an indicator of problems with the ventilation or EO system.

Permissible limits for exposure to EO, as established by OSHA, are 1 part per million (ppm) of airborne EO expressed as a time-weighted average for an 8-hour work shift in a 40-hour work week or 5 ppm for short-term exposure. Monitoring of short-term exposures during a 15-minute period is required while sterilization and aeration activities are being performed.[69]

8.4.1 **Personnel who have the potential for exposure should wear EO-monitoring badges that meet the National Institute for Occupational Safety and Health standards for accuracy.**[68,69] *[Recommendation]*

8.4.2 **Documentation of employee monitoring must be maintained in employees' health records for the duration of employment plus 30 years after termination of employment.**[69] *[Regulatory Requirement]*

Regulations from OSHA require that documentation of monitoring of the employee breathing zone (ie, 2 ft surrounding the employee's head) must be maintained. Health and safety procedures must be developed for health care personnel who are at risk for exposure to EO.[69,70]

Established procedures help to identify, eliminate, or minimize risk from exposure to hazards as well as facilitate timely responses to accidental exposure and emergencies.

8.4.3 **To communicate the potential environmental hazards of EO, signage with the following information must be posted at the doors of the rooms where the EO is located: "Ethylene oxide, Cancer hazard and reproductive hazard, Authorized personnel only, Respirators and protective clothing may be required to be worn in this area."**[68] *[Regulatory Requirement]*

8.4.4 **Personnel must be educated about the health effects and potential hazards associated with exposure to EO before assignment to an area where there is potential for exposure to EO.**[69] *[Regulatory Requirement]*

8.4.5 **Ethylene oxide safety procedure competency must be verified and documented at the time of assignment to an area where EO is used and at least annually thereafter.**[68,69] *[Regulatory Requirement]*

8.4.6 **Periodic employee and environmental physical assessment and testing must be carried out and documented according to current OSHA regulations.**[68,69] *[Regulatory Requirement]*

8.4.7 **Personnel must be familiar with the organization's emergency EO exposure plan.**[69] *[Regulatory Requirement]*

8.4.8 **Personnel must be aware of safety procedures to implement following exposure to EO.**[67] **The safety data sheet (SDS) for the type of EO used should be consulted for specific first-aid measures after exposure.**[67,68] *[Regulatory Requirement]*

8.4.9 **People who have inhaled concentrated EO gas should seek fresh air and medical attention immediately.**[68,69] *[Recommendation]*

8.5 **Review the device manufacturer's written instructions to determine whether the device is compatible with EO.**[36] *[Recommendation]*

8.6 **Select EO sterilizer cycle parameters in accordance with the sterilizer and device manufacturers' written IFU. Variables influencing cycle parameters in the device manufacturer's IFU include**
- **item composition and size,**
- **item preparation and packaging,**
- **density of the load,**
- **type of EO sterilizer/aerator used, and**
- **the device and sterilizer manufacturers' written IFU.**[36]

[Recommendation]

8.7 **Clean and dry items, including all lumens, before packaging for EO sterilization.**[36] *[Recommendation]*

Soils, including biofilm, inhibit sterilization, and residual moisture may produce toxic by-products. Ethylene oxide is reactive with water and can result in the formation of ethylene glycol, a form of antifreeze.[36]

8.8 **Follow the sterilizer manufacturers' written instructions for EO sterilization load configuration.**[36] *[Recommendation]*

Ethylene oxide sterilizers differ in design and operating characteristics. This information is found in the manufacturer's written IFU.

8.8.1 **Place items in EO sterilizers in baskets or on loading carts in a manner that allows free circulation and penetration of the EO and moisture vapor.**[36] *[Recommendation]*

9. Dry-Heat Sterilization

9.1 Use dry-heat sterilization only for materials that are impenetrable to moist heat.[1] When indicated by the device manufacturer, dry heat may be used to sterilize anhydrous (ie, waterless) items that can withstand high temperatures. *[Conditional Recommendation]*

Items that can withstand the high temperatures generated by dry-heat sterilization may be sterilized using this method. Dry heat is an oxidation or slow-burning process that causes the coagulation of proteins in microbial cells. Sterilization is accomplished through the transfer of heat energy to objects on contact. There is no moisture present in a dry-heat process, so microorganisms are destroyed by a very slow process of heat absorption.

Presterilized oils and powders are commercially available and may eliminate the need for a dry-heat sterilizer.

9.2 When using dry-heat sterilizers, follow the manufacturer's written instructions for operation, monitoring, and maintenance.[37] *[Recommendation]*

Dry-heat sterilizers may vary in design and performance characteristics.

9.3 Only use packaging and container materials designed and validated by the packaging manufacturer to withstand the high temperature of dry-heat sterilization.[37] *[Recommendation]*

If packaging is not formulated for dry-heat sterilization, pouches may char, compromising the package integrity of sterilized items.

9.3.1 Use closed containers or cassettes based on the manufacturer's instructions and BI monitoring results.[37] *[Recommendation]*

Closed containers or cassettes may extend the time needed to achieve sterilization.

9.3.2 Consult packaging manufacturers to confirm the compatibility of the packaging material with sterilizer temperatures before selecting packaging materials for dry-heat sterilization.[37] *[Recommendation]*

Most types of tape are not designed to withstand the high temperatures of dry-heat sterilization. Tape adhesive can melt when subjected to dry-heat sterilization, which may result in loss of tape adhesion and may leave a sticky residue on sterilized packages that degrades, leaving baked-on tape residue on the items.

9.3.3 When possible, use small containers for items to be dry-heat sterilized, and keep package density as low as possible.[37] *[Recommendation]*

9.4 Place items within the sterilizer chamber according to the sterilizer manufacturer's IFU.[37] *[Recommendation]*

Correct placement and configuration of items within the chamber facilitates contact of the sterilant with the items to be sterilized. Sterilant contact is essential for sterilization.

9.5 Be aware of the hazards associated with dry-heat sterilization and use the necessary PPE (eg, insulated gloves, transfer handles).[37] *[Recommendation]*

Burns are the most common safety hazard associated with dry-heat sterilization.

9.5.1 On completion of a dry-heat sterilization cycle, both the sterilizer chamber and the items in the chamber are very hot and should not be touched.[37] *[Recommendation]*

9.5.2 Cool packages before being handled or removed from the dry-heat sterilizer.[37] *[Recommendation]*

10. Quality

10.1 Establish a quality assurance and performance improvement program to evaluate and monitor sterilization processes in all areas of the facility where sterilization processes are performed. *[Recommendation]*

Quality assurance and performance improvement programs can facilitate the identification of problem areas and assist personnel in evaluating and improving the quality of patient care and formulating plans for corrective action. These programs provide data that may be used to determine whether an individual organization is within benchmark goals, and if not, to identify areas that may require corrective action. A quality management program provides a mechanism to evaluate effectiveness of processes, compliance with manufacturer's IFU, sterilization policies and procedures, and function of equipment.

10.2 Appoint an interdisciplinary team with responsibility and authority to establish and implement a quality assurance and performance improvement program for sterilization processes. *[Recommendation]*

Seavey[71] described a collaborative interdisciplinary approach to improvement efforts in an expert opinion article. The author describes potential causes of conflict between operating room and sterile processing personnel, including ineffective communication, hierarchical and autocratic cultures, rapidly changing technology pressures, intimidating management styles, inconsistent policies and procedures, worker fatigue, multitasking, time pressures, staffing shortages, a blaming culture, unclear expectations, and insufficient orientation and training. She recommended activities to promote a culture of safety, including building trust among team members, disseminating information to personnel at all levels, developing and sustaining a proactive approach, and establishing safety as the first priority at all levels within the team. These activities can help reduce errors; facilitate understanding of teamwork and human factors as vital elements of a safety culture; and foster interdisciplinary trust, conflict resolution, team commitment to a safety culture, accountability, a focus on results and outcomes, and improvements in team communication. To further foster interdepartmental collaboration, the author recommended combining team activities, including assignment of an interdepartmental liaison and hosting shared celebrations and educational opportunities.

10.3 **Use chemical, physical, and biological indicators to monitor sterilization processes.**[23] *[Recommendation]*

Sterilization process monitoring is a critical component of quality assurance. Deviation from recommended practices and recommendations can compromise the quality of sterilization processes.

10.4 **Use external and internal chemical indicators (CIs) specific for the sterilization method with each package.** *[Recommendation]*

Chemical indicators are used to immediately verify that one or more of the conditions necessary for sterilization has been achieved within each package.[23] The purpose of the external CI is to differentiate between processed and unprocessed items.[72] Chemical indicators do not establish whether the item is sterile, but they do demonstrate that the contents were exposed to the sterilant.[72] Although CIs do not verify sterility, they help detect procedural errors and equipment malfunctions.

10.4.1 Place a **type 1 CI (ie, process indicator)** on the outside of every package unless the internal indicator is visible through the packaging material.[23] *[Recommendation]*

10.4.2 Place a **type 5 CI (ie, integrating indicator)** or **type 6 CI (ie, emulating indicator)** inside every package.[23] *[Recommendation]*

10.4.3 A **type 3 CI** or **type 4 CI** may be used within a package to meet requirements for internal monitoring.[23] *[Conditional Recommendation]*

10.4.4 Read and interpret (eg, color, migration, other change) the internal CI before the tray or items are placed on the sterile field. If a pass result has not been achieved, do not place trays or items on the sterile field. *[Recommendation]*

10.4.5 If the interpretation of the external or internal process indicators suggests inadequate or questionable processing, do not use the items. *[Recommendation]*

10.5 Review **physical monitors** (eg, time, temperature, pressure, humidity, sterilant concentration) at the end of each cycle. Verify that all sterilization parameters were met for every cycle and every sterilization method.[72] *[Recommendation]*

Physical monitoring provides real-time assessments of cycle conditions as well as historic records by means of printouts, digital readings, graphs, or gauges. Reviewing data from physical monitoring can readily identify sterilizer malfunctions and expedite corrective actions.

10.6 Label each package with load control numbers.[23] *[Recommendation]*

Load control numbers allow items to be identified or retrieved in the event of a sterilizer failure or malfunction.

10.6.1 Record the following information for each load:
- identification of the sterilizer (eg, "sterilizer #1"),
- type of sterilizer and cycle used,
- load control number,
- load contents (eg, set names, individually packaged instrument names),
- critical parameters for the specific sterilization method (eg, exposure time, temperature for steam sterilization),
- operators' identification, and
- results of sterilization process monitoring (ie, chemical, physical, biological).[23]

[Recommendation]

10.6.2 An electronic instrument tracking system may be used.[23] *[Conditional Recommendation]*

Electronic instrument tracking systems provide a mechanism for labeling packages with each of the load identification elements (See Recommendation 10.6.1) in the form of a barcode or unique device identifier. This information may be used for the purpose of item identification and retrieval in the event of a sterilizer failure or malfunction.

10.7 Use biological indicators (BIs) specific to each sterilization method and exposure time.[23] *[Recommendation]*

Biological indicators are used to monitor sterilizer efficacy. Sterilizer efficacy monitoring reduces the possibility that items will be processed under suboptimal conditions. Biological indicators are intended to demonstrate whether the conditions were adequate within the sterilizer, specific to the sterilization method, to be lethal to resistant spores.

10.7.1 Determine the frequency of sterilizer quality assurance testing. Perform biological indicator testing at least weekly, but preferably each day the sterilizer is used, for steam and dry-heat sterilizers and more frequently for low-temperature sterilization processes.[1,23,24,36] *[Recommendation]*

The CDC recommends routine sterilizer efficacy monitoring with a BI at least weekly; and if a sterilizer is used frequently (eg, several loads per day), daily use of BIs allows earlier discovery of equipment malfunctions or errors and thus minimizes the extent of patient surveillance and product recall necessary in the event of a positive BI result.[1] ANSI/AAMI ST79[23] recommends routine sterilizer efficacy monitoring using a **process challenge device** (PCD) containing a BI weekly, but preferably each day the sterilizer is used. ANSI/AAMI ST41[36] recommends that a BI within a PCD be used in each sterilization cycle unless the BI challenge test pack is part of the load. ANSI/AAMI ST58[24] recommends that a PCD with a BI be used at least each day the sterilizer is used, but preferably in every sterilization cycle.

10.7.2 Place a positive control in each incubator each day a test vial is run and incubated. Use a test vial that is from the same lot as the control vial.[23] *[Recommendation]*

10.7.3 Run loads containing implants with a BI, and quarantine the implants until BI results are known.[23,36] *[Recommendation]*

10.7.4 Report positive BI results immediately and take corrective actions (See Recommendation 10.14).[23] *[Recommendation]*

10.8 Perform process monitoring specific to steam sterilizers.[23] *[Recommendation]*

10.8.1 Use *Geobacillus stearothermophilus* spore BIs for sterilizer **qualification testing** and routine sterilizer efficacy monitoring. *Geobacillus stearothermophilus* spore BIs may also be used for routine load release.[23] *[Recommendation]*

10.8.2 Include the following in quality assurance testing for steam sterilizers:
- using a PCD[73] containing a BI,
- testing for each cycle used if a steam sterilizer is intended to be used for multiple types of cycles (eg, **gravity displacement**, **dynamic air removal**),
- testing of the shortest (ie, the most challenging) exposure time if one temperature is used with different exposure times,
- testing in a fully loaded chamber for **table-top sterilizers** and for sterilizers larger than 2 cu ft,
- placing the biological monitor in the most challenging location within the sterilizer chamber and within the rigid sterilization container as indicated by the sterilizer and container manufacturers, and
- PCD monitoring (containing a BI and a type 5 CI) for each load containing an implantable device.[23,73]

[Recommendation]

10.8.3 For dynamic air-removal steam sterilizer cycles, perform a Bowie-Dick air-removal test (**type 2 indicator**) each day the sterilizer is used by
- running the test in an empty chamber,
- performing the test before the first load of the day but after a warm-up cycle is run, and
- running the test in accordance with the **Bowie-Dick test** manufacturer's IFU.[23]

[Recommendation]

The air-removal test is designed to detect residual air in the sterilizer chamber. A warm-up cycle enables the Bowie-Dick testing to be performed under the conditions in which the sterilizer will be used.

10.8.4 Perform qualification testing after installation, relocation, malfunction, major repair, or sterilizer process failure and include
- one Bowie-Dick air-removal test run in three consecutive cycles in an empty chamber for dynamic air-removal steam sterilizer cycles;
- one BI PCD[73] run in three consecutive cycles in an empty chamber for each cycle type (eg, gravity displacement, dynamic air removal);

- qualification testing of sterilizers larger than 2 cu ft and for IUSS cycles in an empty chamber; and
- qualification testing of table-top sterilizers in a fully loaded chamber.[23]

[Recommendation]

10.9 Perform process monitoring specific to EO sterilizers.[36] *[Recommendation]*

10.9.1 Use *Bacillus atrophaeus* spore BIs for routine load release, routine sterilizer efficacy monitoring, and sterilizer qualification testing.[36] *[Recommendation]*

10.9.2 Run a PCD containing a BI with every load.[36,73] *[Recommendation]*

10.9.3 Perform qualification testing in accordance with the sterilizer manufacturer's IFU after installation, relocation, malfunction, major repair, or sterilization process failure.[36] *[Recommendation]*

10.10 Perform process monitoring specific to low-temperature hydrogen peroxide sterilizers (eg, vapor, gas plasma combination, ozone combination).[24] *[Recommendation]*

10.10.1 Use *Geobacillus stearothermophilus* spore BIs for routine load release, routine sterilizer efficacy monitoring, and sterilizer qualification testing. *[Recommendation]*

10.10.2 Perform routine sterilizer efficacy monitoring every day the sterilizer is used for each cycle type (eg, standard, advanced, lumen, non-lumen), preferably with each load. Use the BI-containing quality monitoring product according the BI manufacturer's IFU.[24] *[Recommendation]*

10.10.3 Perform qualification testing in accordance with sterilizer manufacturer's IFU after installation, relocation, malfunction, major repair, or sterilization process failure.[24] Test each sterilization cycle type that is used for three consecutive cycles in an empty chamber.[24] *[Recommendation]*

10.11 Perform process monitoring specific to peracetic acid sterilant systems.[24] *[Recommendation]*

10.11.1 Use *Geobacillus stearothermophilus* spore BIs for routine load release, routine sterilizer efficacy monitoring, and sterilizer qualification testing. *[Recommendation]*

10.11.2 Perform routine sterilizer efficacy monitoring each day the sterilizer is used.[24] Run a diagnostic cycle in accordance with the sterilizer manufacturer's IFU.[24] *[Recommendation]*

10.11.3 Perform qualification testing in accordance with the sterilizer manufacturer's IFU after installation, relocation, malfunction, major repair, or sterilization process failure.[24] *[Recommendation]*

10.12 Perform process monitoring specific to dry-heat sterilizers.[37] *[Recommendation]*

10.12.1 Use *Bacillus atrophaeus* spore BIs for routine load release, routine sterilizer efficacy monitoring, sterilizer qualification testing, and periodic product quality assurance testing.[37] *[Recommendation]*

10.12.2 Perform routine sterilizer efficacy monitoring in an empty sterilizer at least weekly, but preferably each day the sterilizer is used.[37] *[Recommendation]*

10.12.3 Perform qualification testing in accordance with the sterilizer manufacturer's IFU after installation, relocation, malfunction, major repair, or sterilization process failure.[37] Perform testing for three consecutive cycles in an empty chamber.[37] *[Recommendation]*

10.13 All chemical, physical, and biological monitoring results, including results from controls, should be interpreted by qualified personnel. Interpret the results in the time frame specified by the manufacturer of the monitor and include the results in the sterilization records.[19,23,24,36,37] *[Recommendation]*

10.14 All sterilizer failures (eg, wet packs or loads; failed CI, physical indicator, or BI results) should be investigated, documented, and reported to the affected department (eg, operating room, cardiac catheterization lab, emergency department), an infection preventionist, the quality assurance or risk management department, and through the organizational chain of command. Take immediate corrective actions in the event of a sterilization failure.[23,24,37,74] *[Recommendation]*

10.14.1 Investigate sterilization process failure(s) in a standardized, systematic manner.[23,24,37] *[Recommendation]*

10.14.2 The investigation may include the following steps:

1. immediately quarantining any potentially affected items;
2. removing the affected sterilizer from use until function is restored and qualification testing is completed;
3. confirming the process failure (eg, that a CI or BI result is not a false positive);
4. informing key stakeholders (eg, leaders, infection preventionist[s], affected service area);
5. conducting a complete and thorough investigation of the cause of the failure;
6. preparing a list of potentially exposed patients;
7. assessing whether the failure increases patients' risk for infection;
8. informing additional stakeholders of the sterilization issue per the organizational chain of command;
9. developing a hypothesis for failure and initiating corrective action;
10. developing a method to further assess potential adverse patient events;
11. when required, notifying regulatory agencies (eg, the health department, the FDA);
12. determining whether patient notification is warranted;
13. if patients are notified, determining whether these patients require medical evaluation for possible postexposure therapy and followup to detect infection;
14. developing a detailed plan to prevent similar failures in the future; and
15. completing an after-action report.[15]

[Conditional Recommendation]

Weber and Rutala[15] proposed a standardized approach to sterilization process failures using these 15 steps, recognizing that failure events are often unique.

10.14.3 Check the sterilizer's physical cycle monitors. If the cycle parameters were not met, remove the sterilizer from service, quarantine the load, and investigate the cause of the failure.[23,24,37] *[Recommendation]*

10.14.4 If the cause of the failure is immediately identified (eg, not a result of mechanical issues with the sterilizer) or the failure is confined to a single item within the load, correct the cause, return the sterilizer to service, and reprocess the load.[23,24,37] *[Recommendation]*

10.14.5 If the cause of the failure is not immediately identified, quarantine the load and take the sterilizer out of service. Investigate the cause and only return the sterilizer to service when the cause is identified and rectified and qualification testing is complete.[23,24,37] *[Recommendation]*

10.14.6 When possible, recall items that were processed in the suspect sterilizer (ie, back to the last known negative BI test) and reprocess the items before use.[23,24,37] *[Recommendation]*

10.15 Preventive maintenance and repairs should be performed by qualified personnel as specified in the sterilizer manufacturer's written IFU.[19,23,24,36,37] *[Recommendation]*

Periodic inspections, maintenance, and replacement of components that are subject to wear (eg, recording devices, steam traps, filters, valves, drain pipes, gaskets) help maintain optimal sterilizer performance.[23,24,37]

10.15.1 Maintain the maintenance records for each sterilizer and include the

- date of service;
- sterilizer model and serial number;
- sterilizer location;
- description of any malfunction;
- name of the person who is performing the maintenance and the name of his or her company;
- description of the type of service and any parts that are replaced;
- results of BI testing, if performed;
- results of process-specific CI testing (eg, Bowie-Dick), if performed;
- name of the person requesting the service; and
- signature and title of the person acknowledging the completed work.[19,23,24,36,37]

[Recommendation]

Accurate and complete records are required for sterilization process verification.

10.15.2 Perform sterilizer inspection and routine maintenance including cleaning as specified in the manufacturer's written IFU.[19,23,24,36,37] *[Recommendation]*

Inspection and maintenance minimizes sterilizer downtime and helps prevent sterilizer malfunctions.

10.16 Facility engineering personnel should monitor and control the steam supply system to steam sterilizers that have a volume greater than 56.63 L (2 cu ft).[23,75] *[Recommendation]*

Table-top steam sterilizers typically have a water reservoir that injects a set volume of water to create steam during the cycle. Because they are not dependent on a utility system to generate steam, steam quality monitoring by a facility engineer is not necessary, although water quality is important.[23,75]

10.16.1 **Treat major repairs of or changes to the steam supply system as major repairs to the sterilizer, and perform sterilizer qualification testing before use.**[23] *[Recommendation]*

Significant changes to the utilities connected to the sterilizer (eg, installation of new boilers, annual boiler maintenance, changes necessitated by water-main breaks, or additional equipment loads) could affect sterilizer performance.[23,75]

10.16.2 **Conduct steam quality evaluation on installation of steam-consuming equipment or steam supply, after repairs to steam-consuming equipment or steam supply, after modification of steam routing infrastructure, and during investigation of steam sterilization cycle failures.**[19,23] *[Recommendation]*

The performance of the sterilizer is dependent on the quality of the steam supply.[19] Steam that is too dry can contribute to **superheating** and, consequently, to suboptimal steam sterilization conditions. Steam that is too wet can lead to wet packs after sterilization and can compromise sterility.[23]

10.17 **Facility engineering personnel should monitor and control the water supply system to steam sterilizers that have a volume less than 56.63 L (2 cu ft).**[76] *[Recommendation]*

Quality of the water supply is an important factor influencing steam quality in table-top steam sterilizers.

11. Environmental Impact

11.1 **Assess the environmental impact of sterilization processes and equipment.** *[Recommendation]*

Nurses have an ethical and professional responsibility to advocate for patients' health. Because human health is dependent on the environment, by extension, it is important that nurses work to actively protect the environment by promoting and participating in initiatives that mitigate negative environmental impact.[77]

11.2 **The health care organization may establish a strategy for shutting down idle steam sterilizers.**[78] *[Conditional Recommendation]*

McGain et al[78] evaluated the energy and cost savings potential of shutting down idle steam sterilizers in one hospital in Australia with 24-hour operations. The authors looked at the number of hours that the hospital's four steam sterilizers were idle and could be turned off until needed. They found that the sterilizers were active 38% of the time, off 14%, and idle 48%. A policy of switching the sterilizers off instead of to idle when no loads were waiting was implemented. The difference in electrical and water use resulted in savings of 65,662 kWh and 1,003,509 L of water per year for each sterilizer. The authors estimated that the sterilizers used 40% of their electricity and 21% of their water while idle. Turning off the sterilizers when not in use would reduce the annual cost of electricity by $9,855 AUD ($7,745.91 US) and the annual cost of water by $1,824 AUD ($1,433.64 US) and reduce carbon emissions by approximately 78.7 tons. Although the authors recognized that their strategy for reducing energy consumption of the steam sterilizers may not be practical for all practice settings, their results suggest that other health care organizations may find other opportunities and strategies to switch off idle steam sterilizers and benefit from financial efficiencies while reducing the environmental impact of steam sterilization.

11.2.1 Perform a risk/cost/benefit analysis to determine that
- sterilizer performance would not be adversely affected by frequent shut downs,
- the sterilizer manufacturer's IFU for turning off and restarting the sterilizer can accommodate frequent restarts,
- steam quality would not be adversely affected by frequent interruption of the steam supply system,
- there would not be a buildup of residual water in the steam lines that could flush through the system on re-start, and
- there would not be delays or interruptions of sterilization services that could affect patient care.[78]
[Recommendation]

11.3 **Evaluate environmentally safe and responsible strategies for sterilization (eg, energy consumption, harmful emissions, toxicity, cost reduction) when making sterilization purchase and usage decisions.** *[Recommendation]*

Energy conservation, emission reduction, and resource stewardship are important elements in health care delivery. Human toxicity and environmental effects are important considerations in selecting and utilizing sterilization methods. Sterilization practices evolve over time within an organization to meet service line needs. Each time changes occur in service lines or new technology is acquired, opportunities arise to evaluate and make improvements in existing sterilization processes (See the *AORN Position Statement on Environmental Responsibility*).[77]

12. Leadership

12.1 Assign responsibility and authority for leadership of the sterile processing team to qualified personnel. *[Recommendation]*

Personnel who are qualified to lead the sterile processing team are knowledgeable in sterilization fundamentals, quality monitoring, sterilization safety issues, regulatory compliance, sterilization equipment, and facility design related to sterilization. The complexity of sterilization tasks coupled with ever-changing technologies in surgical and procedural instrumentation demand a high degree of expertise among sterile processing leaders.

12.2 Leaders should be knowledgeable about sterilization processes.[23,24,36] *[Recommendation]*

Managers who supervise the work of others maintain extensive knowledge of the techniques and equipment used by personnel to perform their work. Technical knowledge is necessary to plan and organize work operations; to direct and train personnel in specialized activities; and to monitor quality of work, evaluate performance, and coordinate improvement efforts. Technical expertise prepares leaders for dealing with disruptions in the work due to equipment failures, quality defects, accidents, insufficient materials, and coordination problems.

12.3 Leaders should maintain departmental quality programs that meet regulatory requirements and industry guidelines.[74] *[Recommendation]*

Effective quality programs require committed leaders to organize plans to establish priorities, manage data, and conduct improvement activities and to empower personnel to implement improved processes.

12.3.1 Leaders should prioritize quality improvement efforts in accordance with regulatory requirements, industry guidelines, and concerns specific to the health care organization.[23,24,36,74] *[Recommendation]*

12.3.2 Leaders should provide oversight for systematic data collection and surveillance to inform quality improvement efforts.[74] *[Recommendation]*

12.3.3 Leaders should champion collaboration between sterile processing, infection prevention, and perioperative teams in quality improvement initiatives.[74] *[Recommendation]*

12.3.4 Leaders should organize the work for improvement initiatives and provide performance evaluation feedback to the team.[74] *[Recommendation]*

12.4 Leaders should maintain safe working conditions for those performing sterilization duties.[23,24,36,74] *[Recommendation]*

12.5 Leaders should monitor adherence to professional standards and regulatory compliance related to sterilization.[23,24,36,69,74] *[Recommendation]*

12.6 Leaders should oversee procurement of equipment and materials for sterilization processes. *[Recommendation]*

Maintaining supplies (eg, CIs and BIs, packaging materials, sterilant solutions) that support the demand for sterilization services is crucial for safe and effective sterilization processes.

Capital equipment and medical device procurement are collaborative processes that require clinical, business, financial, and legal acumen. Strategic planning for procuring major sterilization equipment is an important leadership function.

12.7 Leaders should maintain a staffing plan for sterilization personnel.[74] *[Recommendation]*

12.8 Leaders should participate in planning of facility design for sterilization.[8] *[Recommendation]*

13. Education

13.1 Provide initial and ongoing education and competency verification activities related to sterilization processes for personnel who perform sterilization. *[Recommendation]*

Initial and ongoing education of perioperative personnel on sterilization processes facilitates the development of knowledge, skills, and attitudes that affect safe patient care. It is the responsibility of the health care organization to provide initial and ongoing education and to verify the competency of its personnel; however, the primary responsibility for maintaining ongoing competency remains with the individual. Competency verification provides a mechanism for documentation and helps verify that perioperative personnel understand the principles and processes necessary for safe and effective sterilization.

13.2 **Sterilization activities should be performed only by personnel whose competence in such activities has been verified and documented.**[23,24,79] *[Recommendation]*

Sterilization involves complex processes that should be performed by educated and competent personnel.

13.3 **Include the following in education and competency verification activities related to sterilization processes:**
- sterilization equipment operation and maintenance according to the manufacturers' IFU[23,24,36];
- sterilization of items according to the device, container, and sterilizer manufacturers' IFU[23,24,36];
- use and interpretation of CIs according to the manufacturer's IFU[23,24,36];
- use and interpretation of BIs according to the manufacturer's IFU[23,24,36];
- interpretation of sterilizer physical monitor results[23,24,36,74];
- requirements for maintaining records of sterilization[23,24,36,74];
- requirements for employee exposure monitoring[24,36];
- location and use of
  - SDS,
  - eyewash stations,
  - chemical spill kits, and
  - PPE[23,24,36];
- quality assurance measures for sterilization[23,24,36,74];
- team communication and a patient safety culture; and
- processes for reporting adverse events and occupational exposure incidents.[24,36]
[Recommendation]

13.4 **Determine intervals for education and competency verification related to sterilization.** *[Recommendation]*

Education and competency verification needs and intervals are unique to the facility and to its personnel and processes.

13.5 **The health care organization must provide education about the written hazard communication program for personnel who use, handle, or may be exposed to sterilants.**[69] *[Regulatory Requirement]*

Personnel who have received education and completed competency verification activities related to the plan may have a greater understanding of how to reduce potential adverse effects associated with exposure to hazardous chemicals.[80]

13.5.1 **Education related to the hazard communication program must include**
- an explanation of the SDS and chemical labeling system and how to obtain and use this hazard information;
- methods and observations that may be used to detect the presence or release of all chemicals used in the workplace;
- the physical and health hazards of all chemicals used in the workplace; and
- the measures personnel can take to protect themselves, including specific procedures the organization has implemented to protect personnel from exposure to chemicals used in the workplace (eg, emergency procedures, PPE).[69]
[Regulatory Requirement]

14. Records

14.1 **Maintain records of sterilization processes.** *[Recommendation]*

Records provide data for the identification of quality improvement opportunities and demonstrate compliance with regulatory requirements and accreditation agency standards.

14.2 **Maintain sterilization records for a time period specified by the health care organization and in compliance with regulatory and accreditation requirements.**[23,24,36] *[Recommendation]*

14.3 **Record every sterilization cycle including the**
- contents of each load,
- load identification,
- exposure parameters,
- operators' identification,
- results of physical monitors, and
- results of CIs and BIs.[23,24,36]
[Recommendation]

14.4 **Maintain documentation detailing sterilization process failures and corrective action for a time period specified by the health care organization and in compliance with regulatory and accreditation requirements.**[23,24,36] *[Recommendation]*

14.5 **Maintain documentation detailing preventive maintenance and equipment repairs for a time**

period specified by the health care organization and in compliance with regulatory and accreditation requirements.[23,24,36] *[Recommendation]*

Editor's note: Threshold Limit Value (TLV) is a registered trademark of the American Conference of Governmental Industrial Hygienists (ACGIH), Cincinnati, OH.

Glossary

Aeration: A method by which absorbed ethylene oxide is removed from ethylene oxide–sterilized items by circulation of warm air in an enclosed cabinet specifically designed for this purpose.

Biofilm: A coating containing biologically active organisms that have the ability to develop in water, water solutions, or in vivo, which coat the surface of structures (eg, teeth, inner surfaces of catheters, tubes, implanted or indwelling devices, instruments, other medical devices). Biofilms contain viable and nonviable microorganisms that adhere to surfaces and become trapped within a matrix of organic matter (eg, proteins, glycoproteins, carbohydrates), which prevents antimicrobial agents from reaching the cells.

Biological indicator: A sterilization process-monitoring device commercially prepared with a known population of highly resistant spores that tests the effectiveness of the method of sterilization being used. The indicator is used to demonstrate that conditions necessary to achieve sterilization were met during the sterilizer cycle being monitored.

Bowie-Dick test: A test designed to detect air leaks, ineffective air removal, and presence of noncondensable gases in dynamic air-removal steam sterilizers. See Chemical indicators, Type 2.

Chemical indicator: A sterilization-monitoring device used to monitor the attainment of one or more critical parameters required for sterilization. A characteristic color or other visual change indicates a defined level of exposure based on the classification of the chemical indicator used.

- **Type 1 CI (process indicator):** A chemical indicator intended for use with an individual package to indicate that the item has been exposed to the sterilization process and to distinguish between processed and unprocessed units.

- **Type 2 CI:** A chemical indicator that is used for a specific test procedure, such as the dynamic air-removal test (eg, Bowie-Dick test).

- **Type 3 CI:** A chemical indicator designed to react to one of the critical parameters of sterilization to indicate exposure to a sterilization process at a stated value of the chosen parameter.

- **Type 4 CI:** A chemical indicator designed to react to two or more of the critical parameters of sterilization to indicate exposure to a sterilization process at stated values of the chosen parameters.

- **Type 5 CI (integrating indicator):** A chemical indicator designed to react to all critical parameters over a specified range of sterilization cycles and whose performance has been correlated to the performance of the stated test organism under the labeled conditions of use.

- **Type 6 CI (emulating indicator):** A chemical indicator designed to react to all critical parameters of specified sterilization cycles, with the stated values having been generated from the critical variables of the specific sterilization process. This type of indicator is also referred to as a cycle verification indicator.

Decontamination: Any physical or chemical process that removes or reduces the number of microorganisms or infectious agents and renders reusable medical products safe for handling or disposal. The process by which contaminants are removed, either by manual cleaning or mechanical means, using specific solutions capable of rendering blood and debris harmless and removing them from the surface of an object or instrument.

Dynamic air removal: Mechanically assisted air removal from the sterilization chamber, including in prevacuum and steam-flush pressure-pulse steam sterilizers.

Gravity displacement: Type of sterilization cycle during which incoming steam replaces residual air through a port or drain near the bottom of the sterilizer chamber.

Immediate use steam sterilization: A sterilization method that involves the shortest possible time between a sterilized item's removal from the sterilizer and its aseptic transfer to the sterile field. Immediacy implies that a sterilized item is used during the procedure for which it was sterilized and in a manner that minimizes its exposure to air and other environmental contaminants. A sterilized item intended for immediate use is not stored for future use nor held from one surgical procedure to another. Immediacy, rather than being defined according to a specific time frame, is established through the critical analysis and expert collaboration of the health care team.

Physical monitors: Automated devices (eg, printouts, digital readings, graphs, gauges) that monitor sterilization parameters for the sterilization method in use.

Process challenge device (PCD): A device designed to represent a defined challenge or resistance to a sterilization process. A commercially prepared PCD may contain a biological indicator, a chemical indicator, or both. A PCD is used to test the efficacy of the sterilization process.

Qualification testing: Sterilizer testing performed after installation, relocation, malfunction, major repair, or sterilizer process failure to verify that the sterilizer equipment performs within predetermined limits when used in accordance with the manufacturer's instructions for use.

- **Installation qualification:** Process of obtaining and documenting evidence that equipment has been provided and installed in accordance with the sterilizer's specifications.

- **Operational qualification:** Process of obtaining and documenting evidence that installed equipment operates within predetermined limits when used in accordance with the sterilizer's operational procedures.

- **Performance qualification:** Process of obtaining and documenting evidence that the equipment, as installed and operated in accordance with operational procedures, consistently performs in accordance with predetermined criteria and thereby yields product meeting the sterilizer's specification.

Shelf life: The period of time during which a stored product remains effective, useful, or suitable for use.

Steam quality: Steam characteristic reflecting the dryness fraction (ie, weight of dry steam present in a mixture of dry saturated steam and entrained water) and the level of noncondensable gas (ie, air or other gas that will not condense under the conditions and temperature and pressure used during the sterilization process).

Sterile barrier system: A package that prevents ingress of microorganisms and allows aseptic presentation of the product at the point of use.

Sterile storage room: A room with four walls and at least one door where sterile items are stored.

Superheating: Condition that occurs in steam sterilization when the temperature of the steam is higher than the temperature of the saturated steam, thereby creating a dry or superheated steam effect and adversely affecting the steam sterilization process.

Table-top sterilizer: A compact steam sterilizer that has a chamber volume of less than or equal to 2 cu ft and that generates its own steam when distilled or deionized water is added.

Terminal sterilization: A process by which the product is sterilized within a sterile barrier that permits storage for use at a later time.

Threshold Limit Value: Refers to airborne concentrations of chemical substances and represents conditions to which it is believed that nearly all workers may be repeatedly exposed, day after day, over a working lifetime, without adverse health effects.

Wet pack: A sterilized package with surface or internal moisture in the form of dampness, droplets, or puddles of liquid (eg, water) on or within the package after a completed sterilization cycle, drying, and cooldown period. Wet packs are generally associated with steam; however, they can also occur with ethylene oxide and hydrogen peroxide gas sterilization systems.

References

1. Rutala WA, Weber DJ; Healthcare Infection Control Practices Advisory Committee. *Guideline for Disinfection and Sterilization in Healthcare Facilities, 2008.* Atlanta, GA: Centers for Disease Control and Prevention; 2008. [IVA]

2. *Procedure-Associated Module: Surgical Site infection (SSI) Event.* Atlanta, GA: Centers for Disease Control and Prevention; 2017.

3. Berrios-Torres SI, Umscheid CA, Bratzler DW, et al. Centers for Disease Control and Prevention guideline for the prevention of surgical site infection, 2017. *JAMA Surg.* 2017;152(8):784-791. [IVA]

4. Guideline for cleaning and care of surgical instruments. In: *Guidelines for Perioperative Practice.* Denver, CO: AORN, Inc; 2018:907-942. [IVA]

5. Guideline for manual chemical high level disinfection. In: *Guidelines for Perioperative Practice.* Denver, CO: AORN, Inc; 2018:883-906. [IVA]

6. Guideline for processing flexible endoscopes. In: *Guidelines for Perioperative Practice.* Denver, CO: AORN, Inc; 2018:799-882. [IVA]

7. Guideline for selection and use of packaging systems for sterilization. In: *Guidelines for Perioperative Practice.* Denver, CO: AORN, Inc; 2018:943-956. [IVA]

8. Design and maintenance of the surgical suite. In: *Guidelines for Perioperative Practice.* Denver, CO: AORN, Inc; 2018:e49-e75. [IVA]

9. Rutala WA, Weber DJ. Sterilization, high-level disinfection, and environmental cleaning. *Infect Dis Clin North Am.* 2011;25(1):45-76. [VA]

10. *High-Level Disinfection (HLD) and Sterilization BoosterPak.* The Joint Commission. https://www.jointcommission.org/standards_booster_paks/. Accessed July 13, 2018.

11. Rutala WA, Weber DJ. Disinfection and sterilization: an overview. *Am J Infect Control.* 2013;41(5 Suppl):S2-S5. [VA]

12. Rutala WA, Weber DJ. Reprocessing semicritical items: current issues and new technologies. *Am J Infect Control.* 2016;44(5 Suppl):e53-e62. [VA]

13. Rutala WA, Weber DJ. New developments in reprocessing semicritical items. *Am J Infect Control.* 2013;41(5 Suppl):S60-S66. [VA]

14. McDonnell G, Burke P. Disinfection: is it time to reconsider Spaulding? *J Hosp Infect.* 2011;78(3):163-170. [VA]

15. Weber DJ, Rutala WA. Assessing the risk of disease transmission to patients when there is a failure to follow recommended disinfection and sterilization guidelines. *Am J Infect Control.* 2013;41(5 Suppl):S67-S71. [VA]

16. Weber DJ, Rutala WA. Lessons learned from outbreaks and pseudo-outbreaks associated with bronchoscopy. Infect Control Hosp Epidemiol. 2012;33(3):230-234. [VA]

17. *AAMI TIR12:2010: Designing, Testing, and Labeling Reusable Medical Devices for Reprocessing in Health Care Facilities: A Guide for Medical Device Manufacturers.* Arlington, VA: Association for the Advancement of Medical Instrumentation; 2010. [IVC]

18. *AAMI TIR30:2011: A Compendium of Processes, Materials, Test Methods, and Acceptance Criteria for Cleaning Reusable Medical Devices.* Arlington, VA: Association for the Advancement of Medical Instrumentation; 2011. [IVC]

19. *ANSI/AAMI ST8:2013: Hospital Steam Sterilizers.* Arlington, VA: Association for the Advancement of Medical Instrumentation; 2013:33. [IVC]

20. *ANSI/AAMI/ISO 17664: Processing of Health Care Products—Information to be Provided by the Medical Device Manufacturer for the Processing of Medical Devices.* Arlington, VA: Association for the Advancement of Medical Instrumentation; 2017. [IVB]

21. Duro M. Manufacturer's written instructions for use: a critical component. *AORN J.* 2013;97(6):C7-C8. [VC]

22. Seavey R. High-level disinfection, sterilization, and antisepsis: current issues in reprocessing medical and surgical instruments. *Am J Infect Control.* 2013;41(5 Suppl):S111-S117. [VA]

23. *ANSI/AAMI ST79: Comprehensive Guide to Steam Sterilization and Sterility Assurance in Health Care Facilities.* Arlington, VA: Association for the Advancement of Medical Instrumentation; 2017. [IVC]

24. *ANSI/AAMI ST58:2013. Chemical Sterilization and High-Level Disinfection in Health Care Facilities.* Arlington, VA: Association for the Advancement of Medical Instrumentation; 2013. [IVC]

25. AAMI; Accreditation Association for Ambulatory Health Care, Inc; AORN, Inc; et al. Immediate-use steam sterilization. 2011. http://s3.amazonaws.com/rdcms-aami/files/production/public/FileDownloads/Products/ST79_Immediate_Use_Statement.pdf. Accessed July 18, 2018. [IVC]

26. US Department of Health and Human Services, US Food and Drug Administration, Center for Devices and Radiological Health, Center for Biologics Evaluation and Research. *Reprocessing Medical Devices in Health Care Settings: Validation Methods and Labeling. Guidance for Industry and Food and Drug Administration Staff.* 2015. US Food and Drug Administration. https://www.fda.gov/downloads/medicaldevices/deviceregulationandguidance/guidancedocuments/ucm253010.pdf. Accessed July 18, 2018.

27. US Department of Health and Human Services; US Food and Drug Administration, Center for Devices and Radiological Health. *Enforcement Priorities for Single-Use Devices Reprocessed by Third Parties and Hospitals.* 2000. US Food and Drug Administration. https://www.fda.gov/downloads/Medical Devices/DeviceRegulationandGuidance/GuidanceDocuments/ucm107172.pdf. Accessed July 18, 2018.

28. 21 CFR 807: Establishment registration and device Listing for manufacturers and initial importers of devices. Electronic Code of Federal Regulations. https://www.ecfr.gov/cgi-bin/text-idx?SID=3efdf3cc98a571f1c17fdeaa6807d423&mc=true&tpl=/ecfrbrowse/Title21/21cfr807_main_02.tpl. Accessed July 18, 2018.

29. 21 CFR 814: Premarket approval of medical devices. Electronic Code of Federal Regulations. https://www.ecfr.gov/cgi-bin/text-idx?SID=76317c63bf257feaa77b460e5d4ef182&mc=true&node=pt21.8.814&rgn=div5. Accessed July 18, 2018.

30. The Facility Guidelines Institute. *Guidelines for Design and Construction of Health Care Facilities.* Chicago, IL: American Society for Healthcare Engineering of the American Hospital Association; 2010. [IVB]

31. Dunkelberg H, Schmelz U. Determination of the efficacy of sterile barrier systems against microbial challenges during transport and storage. *Infect Control Hosp Epidemiol.* 2009;30(2):179-183. [IIIA]

32. Wagner T, Scholla MH. Sterile barrier systems: managing changes and revalidations. *J Validation Technol.* 2013;19(3):1-8. [VB]

33. Moriya GA, Souza RQ, Pinto FM, Graziano KU. Periodic sterility assessment of materials stored for up to 6 months at continuous microbial contamination risk: laboratory study. *Am J Infect Control.* 2012;40(10):1013-1015. [IIB]

34. Shaffer HL, Harnish DA, McDonald M, Vernon RA, Heimbuch BK. Sterility maintenance study: dynamic evaluation of sterilized rigid containers and wrapped instrument trays to prevent bacterial ingress. *Am J Infect Control.* 2015;43(12):1336-1341. [IIA]

35. 21 CFR 880.6850: Sterilization wrap. US Food and Drug Administration. https://www.accessdata.fda.gov/scripts/cdrh/cfdocs/cfcfr/CFRSearch.cfm?fr=880.6850. Accessed July 18, 2018.

36. *ANSI/AAMI ST41:2008/(R)2012: Ethylene Oxide Sterilization in Health Care Facilities: Safety and Effectiveness.* Arlington, VA: Association for the Advancement of Medical Instrumentation; 2012. [IVC]

37. *ANSI/AAMI ST40:2004/(R)2010: Table-Top Dry Heat (Heated Air) Sterilization and Sterility Assurance in Health Care Facilities.* Arlington, VA: Association for the Advancement of Medical Instrumentation; 2010. [IVC]

38. Guideline for environmental cleaning. In: *Guidelines for Perioperative Practice.* Denver, CO: AORN, Inc; 2018:7-28. [IVA]

39. Yoon JH, Yoon BC, Lee HL, et al. Comparison of sterilization of reusable endoscopic biopsy forceps by autoclaving and ethylene oxide gas. *Dig Dis Sci.* 2012;57(2):405-412. [IIIC]

40. van Doornmalen Gomez Hoyos JPCM, van Wezel RAC, van Doornmalen HWJM. Case study on the orientation of phaco hand pieces during steam sterilization processes. *J Hosp Infect.* 2015;90(1):52-58. [IIB]

41. van Doornmalen JPCM, Verschueren M, Kopinga K. Penetration of water vapour into narrow channels during steam sterilization processes. *J Phys D Appl Phys.* 2013;46(6):065201. [IIA]

42. van Wezel RAC, van Doornmalen HWJM, de Geus J, Rutten S, van Doornmalen GH. Second case study on the orientation of phaco hand pieces during steam sterilization. *J Hosp Infect.* 2016;94(2):194-197. [IIB]

43. Zadik Y. Iatrogenic lip and facial burns caused by an overheated surgical instrument. *J Calif Dent Assoc.* 2008;36(9):689-691. [VB]

44. Nurse "flash" sterilized surgical equipment: pt. burned. Case on point: Ford v. Stringfellow Memorial Hospital, 2080567 (10/23/2009)-AL. *Nurs Law Regan Rep.* 2009;50(7):2. [VC]

45. Rutala WA, Weber DJ, Chappell KJ. Patient injury from flash-sterilized instruments. *Infect Control Hosp Epidemiol.* 1999;20(7):458. [VB]

46. Sheffer J. Bright ideas: hospital takes hard look at immediate-use steam sterilization. *Biomed Instrum Technol.* 2015;49(4):273-276. [VB]

47. Mangram AJ, Horan TC, Pearson ML, Silver LC, Jarvis WR. Guideline for prevention of surgical site infection, 1999. Hospital Infection Control Practices Advisory Committee. *Infect Control Hosp Epidemiol.* 1999;20(4):250-278; quiz 279-280. [IVA]

48. Sandle T. Ensuring sterility: autoclaves, wet loads, and sterility failures. *J GXP Compliance.* 2015;19(2):9. [VC]

49. Basu D. Reason behind wet pack after steam sterilization and its consequences: an overview from central sterile supply department of a cancer center in eastern India. *J Infect Public Health.* 2017;10(2):235-239. [VC]

50. Fayard C, Lambert C, Guimier-Pingault C, Levast M, Germi R. Assessment of residual moisture and maintenance of sterility in surgical instrument sets after sterilization. *Infect Control Hosp Epidemiol.* 2015;36(8):990-992. [IIB]

51. Moriya GA, Graziano KU. Sterility maintenance assessment of moist/wet material after steam sterilization and 30-day storage. *Rev Lat Am.* 2010;18(4):786-791. [IIC]

52. Seavey R. Troubleshooting failed sterilization loads: process failures and wet packs/loads. *Am J Infect Control.* 2016;44(5 Suppl):e29-e34. [VA]

53. Wallace CA. New developments in disinfection and sterilization. *Am J Infect Control.* 2016;44(5 Suppl):e23-e27. [VB]

54. Consolidated List of Chemicals Subject to the Emergency Planning and Community Right-To-Know Act (EPCRA), Comprehensive Environmental Response, Compensation and Liability Act (CERCLA) and Section 112(r) of the Clean Air Act. 2015. United States Environmental Protection Agency, Office of Solid Waste and Emergency Response. https://www.epa.gov/sites/production/files/2015-03/documents/list_of_lists.pdf. Accessed July 18, 2018.

55. Medical management guidelines for hydrogen peroxide (H2O2). Agency for Toxic Substances and Disease Registry. https://www.atsdr.cdc.gov/MMG/MMG.asp?id=304&tid=55. Accessed July 18, 2018. [VA]

56. *Re-evaluation of Some Organic Chemicals, Hydrazine and Hydrogen Peroxide.* IARC Monographs on the Evaluation of Carcinogenic Risks to Humans; No. 71. Lyon, France: World Health Organization International Agency for Research on Cancer; 1999. https://monographs.iarc.fr/wp-content/uploads/2018/06/mono71.pdf. Accessed July 18, 2018. [VA]

57. Hydrogen peroxide. In: *Documentation of the Threshold Limit Values & Biological Exposure Indices.* 7th ed. Cincinnati, OH: American Conference of Governmental Industrial Hygienists; 2001. [VA]

58. OSHA standards and exposure limits. OSHA Occupational Chemical Database. https://www.osha.gov/chemicaldata/. Updated 2018. Accessed July 18, 2018.

59. Ozone. In: *Documentation of the Threshold Limit Values & Biological Exposure Indices.* 7th ed. Cincinnati, OH: American Conference of Governmental Industrial Hygienists; 2001. [VA]

60. Dufresne S, Richards T. The first dual-sterilant low-temperature sterilization system. *Can J Infect Control.* 2016;31(3):169-174. [VB]

61. *ANSI/AAMI/ISO 11607-1:2006/(R)2015: Packaging for Terminally Sterilized Medical Devices—Part 1: Requirements for Materials, Sterile Barrier Systems, and Packaging Systems.* Arlington, VA: Association for the Advancement of Medical Instrumentation; 2015. [IVB]

62. *Summary for System 1E Liquid Chemical Sterilant Processing.* 2010. US Food and Drug Administration. https://www.accessdata.fda.gov/cdrh_docs/pdf9/k090036.pdf. Accessed July 18, 2018.

63. Peracetic acid. In: *Documentation of the Threshold Limit Values & Biological Exposure Indices.* 7th ed. 2014 Suppl. Cincinnati, OH: American Conference of Governmental Industrial Hygienists; 2014. [VA]

64. *1,3-Butadiene, Ethylene Oxide and Vinyl Halides (Vinyl Fluoride, Vinyl Chloride and Vinyl Bromide).* IARC Monographs on the Evaluation of Carcinogenic Risks to Humans; No. 97. Lyon, France: World Health Organization: International Agency for Research on Cancer; 2008. https://monographs.iarc.fr/wp-content/uploads/2018/06/mono97.pdf. Accessed July 18, 2018. [VA]

65. Ethylene oxide (ETO): hospitals and healthcare facilities must use a single chamber when sterilizing medical equipment with ETO. 2010. US Environmental Protection Agency. https://archive.epa.gov/pesticides/reregistration/web/html/ethylene_oxide_fs.html. Accessed July 18, 2018.

66. Ethylene oxide (EtO): evidence of carcinogenicity. The National Institute for Occupational Safety and Health. https://www.cdc.gov/niosh/docs/81-130/default.html. Published 1981. Updated 2014. Accessed July 18, 2018. [VA]

67. Environmental Protection Agency. Reducing ethylene oxide use. 2018. Great Lakes Regional Pollution Prevention Roundtable. http://www.glrppr.org/docs/r5-eto-factsheet-revised-feb2018.pdf. Accessed July 18, 2018. [VA]

68. Ethylene oxide. In: *Documentation of the Threshold Limit Values & Biological Exposure Indices.* 7th ed. Cincinnati, OH: American Conference of Governmental Industrial Hygienists; 2001. [VA]

69. 29 CFR 1910.1047: Ethylene oxide. Occupational Safety and Health Administration. https://www.osha.gov/pls/oshaweb/owadisp.show_document?p_table=standards&p_id=10070. Accessed July 18, 2018.

70. Supporting statement for the information-collection requirements of the ethylene oxide (EtO) standard (29 CFR 1910.1047). 2000. Occupational Safety and Health Administration. https://www.osha.gov/Reduction_Act/1218-eto.html. Accessed July 18, 2018.

71. Seavey RE. Collaboration between perioperative nurses and sterile processing department personnel. *AORN J.* 2010;91(4):454-462. [VA]

72. *ANSI/AAMI/ISO 15882 2008/(R)2013: Sterilization of Health Care Products—Chemical Indicators—Guidance for Selection, Use, and Interpretation of Results.* Arlington, VA: Association for the Advancement of Medical Instrumentation; 2013. [IVB]

73. *AAMI TIR31:2008: Process Challenge Devices/Test Packs for Use in Health Care Facilities.* Arlington, VA: Association for the Advancement of Medical Instrumentation; 2008. [IVC]

74. *ANSI/AAMI ST90: Processing of Health Care Products—Quality Management Systems for Processing in Health Care Facilities.* Arlington, VA: Association for the Advancement of Medical Instrumentation; 2017. [IVC]

75. *ANSI/AAMI ST8: Hospital Steam Sterilizers.* Arlington, VA: Association for the Advancement of Medical Instrumentation; 2008. [IVB]

76. *ANSI/AAMI ST55:2016: Table-Top Steam Sterilizers.* Arlington, VA: Association for the Advancement of Medical Instrumentation; 2016. [IVC]

77. *AORN Position Statement on Environmental Responsibility.* AORN, Inc. https://www.aorn.org/guidelines/clinical-resources/position-statements. Published 2014. Accessed July 18, 2018. [IVB]

78. McGain F, Moore G, Black J. Hospital steam sterilizer usage: could we switch off to save electricity and water? *J Health Serv Res Policy.* 2016;21(3):166-171. [VB]

79. Passut J, Duro M, Berg DS, Seavey R, Swenson D. A roundtable discussion: the many challenges of sterile processing. *Biomed Instrum Technol.* 2015;49(4):261-267. [VC]

80. Ethylene oxide (EtO): understanding OSHA's exposure monitoring requirements. Occupational Safety and Health Administration. https://www.osha.gov/Publications/ethylene_oxide.html. Published 2007. Accessed July 18, 2018. [VA]

Acknowledgments

Lead Author
Ramona Conner, MSN, RN, CNOR, FAAN
Editor-in-Chief, Guidelines for Perioperative Practice
AORN Nursing Department
Denver, Colorado

Co-Author
Erin Kyle, DNP, RN, CNOR, NEA-BC
Perioperative Practice Specialist
AORN Nursing Department
Denver, Colorado

Contributing Author
Amber Wood, MSN, RN, CNOR, CIC, FAPIC
Senior Perioperative Practice Specialist
AORN Nursing Department
Denver, Colorado

The authors and AORN thank Mary A. Anderson, MS, RN, CNOR, OR RN – II, Parkland Health & Hospital System, Dallas, Texas; Marie A. Bashaw, DNP, RN, NEA-BC, CNOR, Assistant Professor, Wright State University College of Nursing and Health, Dayton, Ohio; Bernard C. Camins, MD, MSc, Associate Professor of Medicine, University of Alabama at Birmingham; Vangie Dennis, BSN, RN, CNOR, CMLSO, Director of Patient Care Practice, Emory Healthcare and Ambulatory Surgery Centers, Atlanta, Georgia; Judith L. Goldberg, DBA, MSN, RN, CNOR, CSSM, CHL, CRCST, Director Perioperative and Procedural Services, Lawrence & Memorial Hospital, Waterford, Connecticut; Heather A. Hohenberger, MSN, RN, CIC, CNOR, CPHQ, Administrative Director Surgical Services, IU Health Arnett Hospital, Lebanon, Indiana; Brenda G. Larkin, MS, ACNS-BC, CNS, CNOR, Clinical Nurse Specialist, Aurora Lakeland Medical Center, Lake Geneva, Wisconsin; Gerald McDonnell, PhD, BSc, Johnson & Johnson Family of Companies, Raritan, New Jersey; Donna A. Pritchard, MA, BSN, RN, NE-BC, CNOR, Director of Perioperative Services, Interfaith Medical Center, Brooklyn, New York; Sue G. Klacik, BS, CRCST, FCS, President Klacik Consulting, Canfield, Ohio; and Susan Ruwe, MSN, RN, CPHQ, CIC, Senior Infection Preventionist, Carle Foundation Hospital, Argenta, Illinois, for their assistance in developing this guideline.

Publication History

Originally published August 1980, *AORN Journal.* Format revision July 1982.

Revised February 1987, October 1992. Published as proposed recommended practices in July 1994.

Revised; published August 1999, *AORN Journal.* Reformatted July 2000.

Revised November 2005; published March 2006, *AORN Journal.*

Revised 2007; published in *Perioperative Standards and Recommended Practices,* 2008 edition.

Minor editing revisions made in November 2010 for publication in *Perioperative Standards and Recommended Practices,* 2011 edition.

Revised June 2012 for online publication in *Perioperative Standards and Recommended Practices.*

Reformatted September 2012 for publication in *Perioperative Standards and Recommended Practices,* 2013 edition.

Evidence ratings revised 2013 to conform to the AORN Evidence Rating Model.

Minor editing revisions made in November 2014 for publication in *Guidelines for Perioperative Practice,* 2015 edition.

Evidence ratings revised in *Guidelines for Perioperative Practice,* 2018 edition, to conform to the current AORN Evidence Rating Model.

Revised September 2018 for publication in *Guidelines for Perioperative Practice* online.

Evidence ratings revised and minor editorial changes made to conform to the current AORN Evidence Rating model, September 2019, for online publication in *Guidelines for Perioperative Practice.*

AORN GUIDELINES FOR
PERIOPERATIVE PRACTICE,
2022 EDITION

SURGICAL ATTIRE

AORN
SAFE SURGERY TOGETHER

1089

TABLE OF CONTENTS

MEDICAL ABBREVIATIONS & ACRONYMS

CFU – Colony-forming units
HAI – Health care–associated infection
MRSA – Methicillin-resistant *Staphylococcus aureus*

OR – Operating room
PPE – Personal protective equipment
RCT – Randomized controlled trial

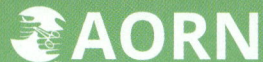
GUIDELINE FOR
SURGICAL ATTIRE

The Guideline for Surgical Attire was approved by the AORN Guidelines Advisory Board and became effective as of July 1, 2019. The recommendations in the guideline are intended to be achievable and represent what is believed to be an optimal level of practice. Policies and procedures will reflect variations in practice settings and/or clinical situations that determine the degree to which the guideline can be implemented. AORN recognizes the many diverse settings in which perioperative nurses practice; therefore, this guideline is adaptable to all areas where operative or other invasive procedures may be performed.

Purpose

This document provides guidance to perioperative team members for laundering **surgical attire**; wearing long sleeves, cover apparel, head coverings, and shoes in **semi-restricted** and **restricted areas**; and cleaning identification badges, stethoscopes, and personal items such as backpacks, briefcases, cell phones, and electronic tablets.

Surgical attire and personal protective equipment (PPE) are worn to provide a high level of cleanliness and hygiene within the perioperative environment and to promote patient and worker safety. Reducing the patient's exposure to microorganisms that are shed from the skin and hair of perioperative personnel may reduce the patient's risk for surgical site infection (SSI).

This document does not address patient clothing or linens used in health care facilities. The use of masks as PPE and the use of masks at the sterile field are outside the scope of this document; the reader should refer to the AORN Guideline for Sterile Technique[1] and the Guideline for Transmission-Based Precautions[2] for additional information. The wearing of rings, bracelets, watches, nail polish, artificial nails, or other nail enhancements is outside the scope of this document; the reader should refer to the AORN Guideline for Hand Hygiene[3] for additional information.

Evidence Review

A medical librarian with a perioperative background conducted a systematic search of the databases Ovid MEDLINE®, Ovid Embase®, EBSCO CINAHL®, and the Cochrane Database of Systematic Reviews. The search was limited to literature published in English from January 2014 through February 2018. At the time of the initial search, weekly alerts were created on the topics included in that search. Results from these alerts were provided to the lead author until August 2018. The lead author requested additional articles that either did not fit the original search criteria or were discovered during the evidence appraisal process. The lead author and the medical librarian also identified relevant guidelines from government agencies, professional organizations, and standards-setting bodies.

Search terms included *armpit, axilla, backpack, bacterial load, badge, beard, bedding and linens, bouffant, briefcase, bunny suit, cell phone, cellular phone, clean room, clothing, colonization, computers, computers (handheld/hand-held/portable), computers and computerization, coveralls, cross infection, dandruff, dermatitis (exfoliative/seborrheic), desquamate, desquamation, disease transmission, disposable hats, dust, ear, environment (controlled), epithelial cells, epithelium, equipment contamination, eyelashes, facial hair, fanny pack, fleece,* **fomites**, *fungi, groin, hair, head covering, hoods, infection control, infectious disease transmission, iPad, iPhone, jewelry, jumpsuit, lanyard, laundering, laundering scrubs, laundering service (hospital), mobile communication device, mobile phone, mold, nosocomial, pollen, protective clothing, purse, scalp, scrubs, seborrhea, seborrheic dermatitis, shed, shedding, skin, skullcaps, smartphone, squames, stethoscopes, surgical attire, surgical cap, surgical wound infection, tablet computer, textiles, tie, uniforms,* and *washing machine.*

Included were research and non-research literature in English, complete publications, and publications with dates within the time restriction when available. Excluded were non-peer-reviewed publications and older evidence within the time restriction when more recent evidence was available. Editorials, news items, and other brief items were excluded. Low-quality evidence was excluded when higher-quality evidence was available, and literature outside the time restriction was excluded when literature within the time restriction was available (Figure 1).

Articles identified in the search were provided to the project team for evaluation. The team consisted of the lead author and one evidence appraiser. The lead author and the evidence appraiser reviewed and critically appraised each article using the AORN Research or Non-Research Evidence Appraisal Tools as appropriate. A second appraiser was consulted if there was a disagreement between the lead author and the primary evidence appraiser. The literature was independently evaluated and appraised according to the strength and quality of the evidence. Each article was then assigned an appraisal score. The appraisal score is noted in brackets after each reference as applicable.

Each recommendation rating is based on a synthesis of the collective evidence, a benefit-harm assessment, and consideration of resource use. The strength of the recommendation was determined using the AORN Evidence Rating Model and the quality and consistency of the evidence supporting a

Figure 1. Flow Diagram of Literature Search Results

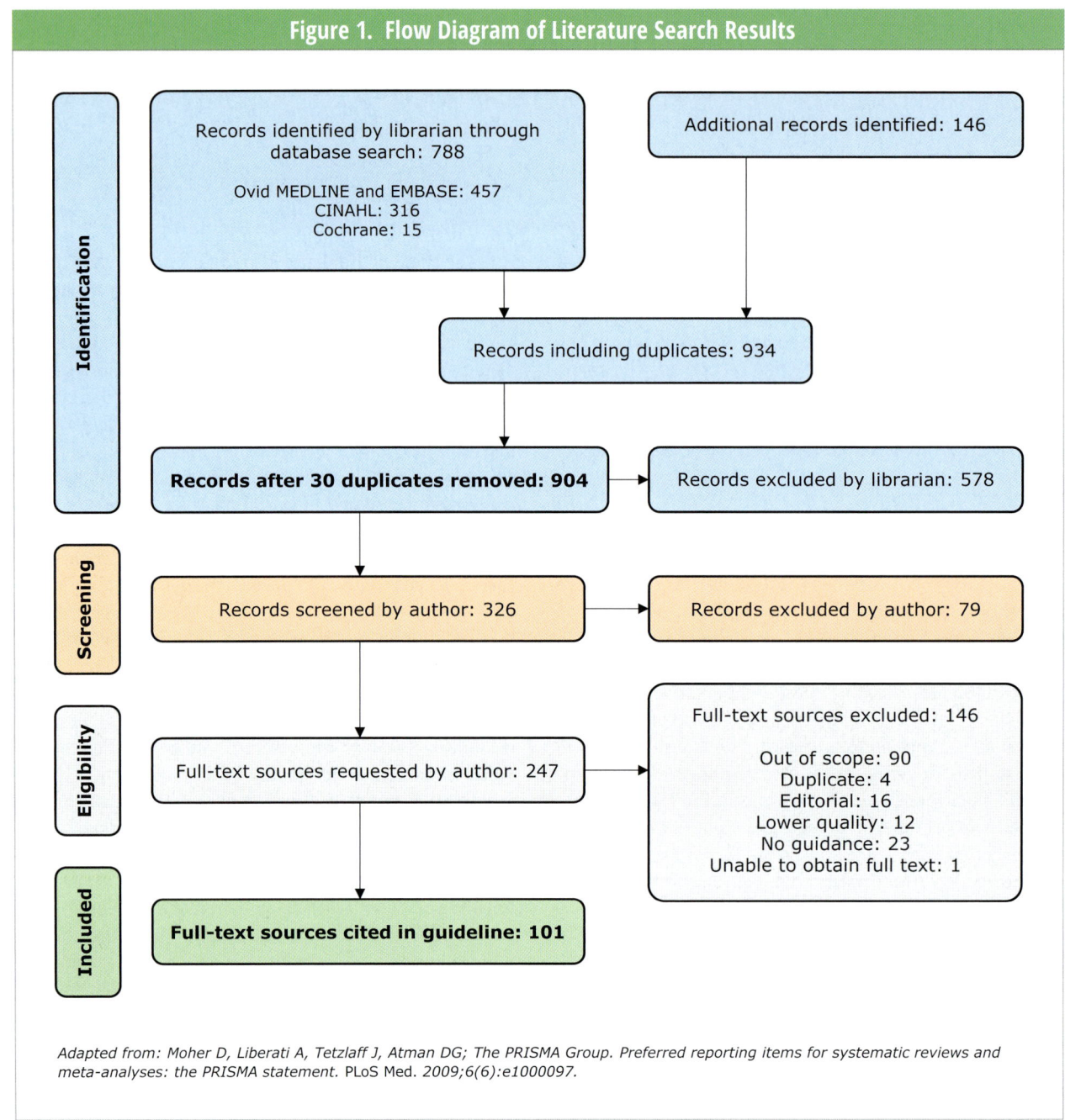

Adapted from: Moher D, Liberati A, Tetzlaff J, Atman DG; The PRISMA Group. Preferred reporting items for systematic reviews and meta-analyses: the PRISMA statement. PLoS Med. 2009;6(6):e1000097.

recommendation. The recommendation strength rating is noted in brackets after each recommendation.

Note: The evidence summary table is available at http://www.aorn.org/evidencetables/.

Editor's note: MEDLINE is a registered trademark of the US National Library of Medicine's Medical Literature Analysis and Retrieval System, Bethesda, MD. Embase is a registered trademark of Elsevier B.V., Amsterdam, The Netherlands. CINAHL, Cumulative Index to Nursing and Allied Health Literature, is a registered trademark of EBSCO Industries, Birmingham, AL. iPad and iPhone are registered trademarks of Apple, Inc; Cupertino, CA.

1. Laundering

1.1 Wear clean surgical attire when entering the semi-restricted and restricted areas. *[Recommendation]*

Wearing **clean** surgical attire may protect patients from exposure to microorganisms that could contribute to an SSI.

1.2 After each daily use, launder **scrub attire** at
- a **health care–accredited laundry facility**,
- the health care organization according to state regulatory requirements, or

- the health care organization according to Centers for Disease Control and Prevention recommendations for laundering[4] in the absence of state requirements.

[Recommendation]

Wearing attire that is laundered at a health care–accredited laundry facility or at the health care organization in accordance with state regulatory requirements provides control of the laundering process and helps ensure that effective laundering standards have been met.

Home laundering is not monitored for quality, consistency, or safety. Home washing machines may not have the adjustable parameters or controls required to achieve the necessary thermal measures (eg, water temperature); mechanical measures (eg, agitation); or chemical measures (eg, capacity for additives to neutralize the alkalinity of the water, soap, or detergent) to reduce microbial levels in soiled scrub attire.

Moderate-quality evidence demonstrates that scrubs become contaminated with bacteria during the workday, including potentially pathogenic organisms that can be transmitted to other people or the environment.[5-15] Several studies have found that microorganisms can survive the home laundering process due to low water temperature and household detergents and can be transferred to other garments.[16-19] Biofilm may form in home washing machines, which can be transferred to other clothing and textiles washed in the same machine.[18,20]

After performing a systematic review, Goyal et al[15] concluded that provider attire is a potential source of pathogenic bacterial transmission in health care settings. There is limited data to link provider attire and health care–associated infections (HAIs). This review gave some guidance on strategies to reduce the spread of bacterial pathogens, including multidrug-resistant organisms that have the potential to cause HAIs. The authors recommended that facilities determine where scrubs will be laundered and, when required, provide laundering instructions for home laundering, such as to use hot water and bleach.

Wright et al[21] reported three cases of postoperative *Gordonia bronchialis* sternal infections after coronary artery bypass grafting surgery. *G bronchialis* was isolated from the scrub attire, axilla, hands, and purse of a nurse anesthetist and was implicated as the cause of the SSIs. Cultures taken from her roommate, who was also a nurse, showed the same microorganism. After notification of the culture results, the nurse anesthetist discarded her front-loading washing machine. During the next year, the nurse anesthetist's and her roommate's scrub attire, hands, nares, and scalps tested negative for

G bronchialis. The authors concluded that the home washing machine was the likely bacterial reservoir. Home laundering may not reliably kill all pathogens, and the pathogens may survive in the form of biofilm within the washing machine. Biofilms have been implicated in malodor emitting from washing machines. The authors recommended that hospital laundering of scrub attire be implemented as a measure to reduce patients' risk of developing an SSI. Further research is needed to demonstrate a causal relationship between home laundering and human disease.

In a nonexperimental study of OR surgical attire conducted as the result of an increase in multidrug-resistant organisms and HAIs, Nordstrom et al[17] took swatches from unwashed, hospital-laundered, home-laundered, new cloth, and disposable scrub attire and tested them for the presence of microorganisms. The researchers found that the home-laundered scrub attire had a significantly higher total bacterial count than the facility-laundered attire, and they found no significant difference in bacterial counts between hospital-laundered, unused, or disposable scrub attire. The researchers concluded that although it is not known how contaminated scrub attire contributes to the spread of HAIs, hospital administrators and infection preventionists need to consider the potential for transmission of infection versus cost savings to the facility if home laundering is allowed. The researchers advised that health care workers be made aware of the risks of home laundering and be provided with instructions for best methods for home laundering in order to reduce the risk of infection.

Mitchell et al[10] conducted a literature review on the role of health care apparel and other textiles in the transmission of pathogens and determined that laundering scrubs at home may not be safe. Due to child safety laws to prevent scalding and burns, typical home washing machine temperatures do not exceed 110° F (43° C) and cannot reach the recommended water temperature of 160° F (71° C) required to remove significant quantities of microorganisms. However, the authors also discussed that industrial post-laundering practices may recontaminate attire.

Some evidence supports home laundering within specific parameters. Lakdawala et al[22] conducted a nonexperimental investigation of the effect of low-temperature washing cycles (140° F [60° C]) by assessing the amount of bioburden on health care workers' uniforms before and after laundering. The researchers concluded that a washing cycle of 140° F (60° C) for 10 minutes was sufficient to decontaminate hospital uniforms and decrease the bacterial load by at least a 7-log reduction. The uniforms could become recontaminated after laundering, but the organisms could be easily removed by ironing.

Patel et al[23] conducted a study to determine the effectiveness of home laundering in removing *Staphylococcus aureus* from scrub attire. The researchers cut hospital-laundered scrub attire into squares, inoculated them with *S aureus,* and washed them at a typical household laundry temperature of 104° F (40° C) and a higher temperature of 140° F (60° C). The researchers concluded that the lower temperature did not remove *S aureus;* however, adding sequential tumble drying or ironing reduced the number of bacteria to an undetectable level. Washing at 140° F (60° C) produced a greater reduction in total viable organisms compared with washing at 104° F (40° C). The researchers concluded that scrub attire can be safely washed at 104° F (40° C) if tumble dried for 30 minutes or ironed.

Al-Benna[24] conducted a literature review to explore home laundering of scrub attire and found there was little scientific evidence that facility laundering was better than home laundering.

1.3 Prevent contamination of laundered surgical attire during transport to the health care facility.[25] *[Recommendation]*

Preventing clean surgical attire from contamination during transport from the laundry facility to the health care facility helps prevent physical damage to the surgical attire and minimizes the potential for contamination from the external environment.[25]

1.3.1 Transport laundered surgical attire in enclosed carts or containers and in vehicles that are cleaned and disinfected regularly.[25] *[Recommendation]*

Carts, containers, and vehicles can be a source of contamination.

1.4 Store laundered surgical attire in enclosed carts, cabinets, or dispensing machines that are cleaned and disinfected regularly.[25] *[Recommendation]*

Storing laundered surgical attire in clean enclosed carts, cabinets, or dispensing machines helps prevent contamination. Storing clean attire in a facility locker with personal items from outside of the facility may contaminate the clean scrub attire.

1.5 Scrub attire that has been penetrated by blood, body fluids, or other potentially infectious materials must be removed immediately or as soon as possible, and replaced with clean attire.[26,27] *[Regulatory Requirement]*

Changing contaminated, soiled, or wet attire may reduce the potential for contamination and protect personnel from exposure to potentially pathogenic microorganisms.

1.5.1 Scrub attire contaminated with visible blood or body fluids must remain at the health care facility for laundering.[26] *[Regulatory Requirement]*

1.5.2 Contaminated scrub attire must be bagged or containerized at the location where it was used and not be rinsed or sorted.[26] *[Regulatory Requirement]*

Rinsing or sorting contaminated reusable attire may expose the health care worker to blood, body fluids, or other potentially infectious materials.

1.6 Remove surgical attire before leaving the health care facility. *[Recommendation]*

The benefits of removing surgical attire before leaving the facility outweigh the harms. Moderate-quality evidence supports changing out of surgical attire into street clothes when leaving the building to reduce the potential for health care workers to transport pathogenic microorganisms from the facility or health care organization into the home or community.

In a systematic review, Goyal et al[15] concluded that provider attire is a potential source of pathogenic bacterial transmission in health care settings. There is limited data to link provider attire and HAIs. The authors recommended that providers wear clean scrub clothes when exiting and returning to the facility.

Sanon and Watkins[12] conducted a study to investigate the pathogens that nurses potentially take into a public setting outside the work environment. The 10 nurses who participated in the study were given sterilized scrub attire to wear prior to the beginning of their shift, and the scrubs were collected at the end of the shift. Microbial assessment of the scrubs showed that the average bacteria colony growth per square inch was 1,246 for the day shift and 5,795 for the night shift. After 48 hours, methicillin-resistant *Staphylococcus aureus* (MRSA) was present on four of the scrubs worn during the day shift and three of the scrubs worn during the night shift. Other bacteria present were *Bacillus* species, *Micrococcus luteus, Staphylococcus aureus, Staphylococcus epidermidis,* and *Micrococcus roseus.* In light of public health concerns about antibiotic resistance, the researchers recommended that facilities consider implementing policy regarding the wearing of scrub attire outside of the work environment.

1.7 No recommendation can be made regarding personal clothing worn under scrub attire. *[No Recommendation]*

No evidence was found to evaluate the benefits and harms of wearing personal clothing under scrub attire.

1.7.1 Establish and implement a process for managing personal clothing that may be worn under scrub attire, including
- the type of fabrics (eg, nonlinting) that may be worn under scrub attire,
- the amount of fabric that may extend beyond the scrub attire (eg, a crew neck collar under V-neck scrub attire),
- laundering frequency (eg, daily), and
- laundering method (eg, facility laundering, home laundering).

[Conditional Recommendation]

1.7.2 Personal clothing contaminated with blood, body fluids, or other potentially infectious materials must remain at the health care facility for laundering.[26] *[Regulatory Requirement]*

2. Fabric

2.1 Select fabrics for scrub attire that are tightly woven and low linting. *[Recommendation]*

Moderate-quality evidence supports wearing tightly woven scrub attire. One quasi-experimental[28] and four nonexperimental[29-32] studies compared airborne bacterial contamination levels when perioperative team members wore various types of scrub attire. The results of four of the studies indicated that tightly woven scrub attire was superior to other types of scrub attire in decreasing bacterial contamination of the air.[28-31] Tammelin et al[28] defined conventional scrub attire as 50% cotton/50% polyester woven with 270 × 230 threads/10 cm and defined tightly woven scrub attire as 50% cotton/50% polyester woven with 560 × 395 threads/10 cm. However, there was no common definition of "tightly woven fabric" used in the collective evidence.

Wearing scrub attire that is low linting may help prevent lint particles from being disseminated into the environment where bacteria may attach to the lint and settle in surgical sites and wounds and increase the potential for postoperative patient complications.[33]

2.2 No recommendation can be made for wearing surgical attire made of antimicrobial fabric. *[No Recommendation]*

Although the evidence regarding the use of antimicrobial scrub attire is of high quality, there is a wide range of variability in study results and several studies were performed in the laboratory setting. Six studies support its use as a means to decrease bacterial contamination of scrubs,[34-39] and four studies found no difference between standard scrubs and antimicrobial scrubs.[40-43]

Bearman et al[39] conducted a randomized controlled trial (RCT) to determine the effectiveness of antimicrobial fabric for reducing the bacterial burden on the hands and scrub attire of health care workers in an intensive care unit setting of an academic medical center. All study participants (N = 30) were randomly assigned to wear either traditional scrub attire or scrub attire made of antimicrobial fabric during a clinical shift for a 4-week period. Each health care worker underwent unannounced weekly garment and hand cultures. Cultures taken at the beginning and end of the shifts included garment cultures taken from the abdominal and leg pockets of the scrub attire. The researchers did not specify the length of the clinical shifts. The antimicrobial scrubs were associated with a 4 to 7 mean log reduction in MRSA but not in vancomycin-resistant *Enterococcus* or gram-negative rod bacteria.

Boutin and colleagues[40] conducted a randomized crossover trial to determine bacterial contamination of antimicrobial scrubs (chitosan/DMDM hydantoin) at the end of a typical 12-hour hospital shift. Standard untreated scrubs served as the control. A total of 110 health care workers participated in the study, and 720 samples were taken. Samples were taken at 4 and 12 hours. The researchers concluded that there was no difference in bacterial contamination between the antimicrobial scrubs and untreated scrubs and more research is needed before facilities invest in antimicrobial scrubs.

Anderson et al[43] conducted a three-arm RCT to test the efficacy of antimicrobial impregnated scrubs compared to standard scrubs. Two antimicrobial scrub types were compared with standard cotton/polyester scrubs. Forty nurses were enrolled in the study, and each completed three shifts in the scrub type that they were randomly assigned to wear. The researchers found that the antimicrobial fabric was not effective in reducing microbial contamination of the scrubs; however, the environment was an important source of contamination of the scrubs.

Further research is needed to determine the potential harms to the wearer of wearing surgical attire made from antimicrobial fabric.

2.2.1 Follow the health care organization's process for the pre-purchase evaluation of products when considering the purchase of antimicrobial surgical attire. *[Conditional Recommendation]*

3. Long Sleeves

3.1 **Arms may be covered during performance of pre-operative patient skin antisepsis.** [*Conditional Recommendation*]

Although the benefits of wearing long sleeves during performance of preoperative patient skin antisepsis are likely to exceed the harms, further research is needed to confirm the risk-benefit assessment and the effect on SSI outcomes.

Markel at al[44] conducted an experimental study to compare air contamination during intraoperative patient skin prep with and without arm coverage of the person performing the prep. A mock patient skin prep was performed in three hospitals with a total of 12 experiments, six with bare arms and six with arms covered. The researchers used particle counters to measure airborne particulate contamination. Active and passive microbial assessment was measured using air samplers and settle plate analysis. In one operating room (OR), there was a decrease in 5.0 μm-sized particles when the arms were covered. In the other two ORs, there was a decrease in total microbes when the arms were covered. Wearing long sleeves specifically appeared to decrease the amount of *Micrococcus* in the environment. The researchers recommended wearing attire with long sleeves when performing the intraoperative patient skin prep.

Contamination of the prep by loose-fitting sleeves is a potential harm of wearing long sleeves during preoperative patient skin antisepsis. This risk may be reduced by wearing a tight-fitting sleeve, avoiding reaching over the prep area, or wearing a sterile sleeve, which may reduce the potential for introducing pathogens to the prep area. Research is needed to evaluate this potential harm and risk-reduction interventions.

3.2 **No recommendation can be made for wearing long sleeves in the semi-restricted and restricted areas other than during performance of preoperative patient skin antisepsis.** [*No Recommendation*]

No evidence was found to evaluate the benefits and harms of wearing long sleeves in the semi-restricted and restricted areas during any activities other than preoperative patient skin antisepsis.

In an organizational report, Chow et al[45] adopted a policy requiring all personnel to wear cover jackets in perioperative areas. They compared SSI data from before and after implementation and did not find any statistically significant differences in SSI outcomes. The authors noted that laundry costs increased approximately $1,000 per month.

In an independent cost analysis, Elmously et al[46] described implementation of disposable long-sleeve jackets at two facilities in the same hospital system. The added cost of implementing use of disposable jackets was $1,128,078 annually.

4. Cover Apparel

4.1 **If worn, cover apparel (eg, lab coats) should be clean.** [*Recommendation*]

Moderate-quality evidence shows that lab coats worn as cover apparel can be contaminated with large numbers of pathogenic microorganisms.[47-53] Researchers have found that cover apparel is not always discarded daily after use or laundered on a frequent basis.[47,48]

In a systematic review, Haun et al[52] examined bacterial contamination of health care personnel attire and other devices. The researchers found 72 studies that assessed contamination of a variety of items including white coats. Pathogens recovered from these items included *Staphylococcus aureus*, gram-negative rods, and *Enterococcus*.

In another systematic review, Goyal et al[15] concluded that provider attire is a potential source of pathogenic bacterial transmission in health care settings. There is limited data to link provider attire and HAIs. The authors recommended increasing the frequency of laundering of white coats to at least weekly and when visibly soiled; providing multiple white coats to allow for laundering; and providing guidance for laundering at home when required, including the use of hot water, bleach, and heated drying.

In a nonexperimental study, Munoz-Price et al[48] investigated the laundering practices of 160 health care providers related to scrub attire and lab coats. Overall, lab coats were washed every 12.4 days and scrub attire every 1.7 days. Ninety percent of respondents laundered their lab coats only once per month, and four people washed their lab coats only once every 90 days to 12 months. Water temperature used by health care providers to launder their lab coats included cold (11%), warm (21%), and hot (52%); 11% did not know the temperature used; and 6% dry-cleaned their lab coats. Ninety percent of respondents acknowledged that their lab coats were potentially contaminated with hospital pathogens. The researchers recommended that lab coats be laundered regularly (ie, at least once or twice per week) and whenever dirty or soiled with body fluids. The researchers also recommended that the lab coats be laundered in hot water with bleach to reduce or eliminate potential pathogens.

In a nonexperimental study of contamination levels of health care practitioners' cover apparel, Treakle et al[47] found that cover apparel in inpatient and outpatient areas, intensive care units, administrative areas, and the OR was contaminated with *Staphylococcus aureus,* including MRSA. Two-thirds of the health care practitioners perceived their cover apparel to be dirty because it had not been washed in more than 1 week. Notably, health care personnel with contaminated cover apparel were more likely to have home laundered their cover apparel.

5. Head Coverings

5.1 **Cover the scalp and hair when entering the semi-restricted and restricted areas.** *[Recommendation]*

Wearing a head covering may contain hair and bacteria that is shed by perioperative team members, which may prevent contamination of the sterile field and reduce the patient's risk for SSI.[54-57] Although there is a potential benefit to the patient, research has not demonstrated that covering the hair affects the multifactorial outcome of SSI rates.[55,58-60] Case studies have demonstrated, however, that human-to-human transmission of bacteria shed from the scalp and hair of perioperative team members can occur and has been directly attributed to SSI outbreaks.[61-64]

Hair and skin can harbor bacteria that may be dispersed into the perioperative environment. Moderate-quality evidence suggests that hair is a reservoir for bacteria.[7,54,61,65,66]

Mase et al[66] conducted a laboratory study to determine whether staphylococci that were present on the hair could be removed by shampooing. The results of the study showed that staphylococci become firmly attached to the human hair surface and the edge of hair cuticles. Extensive treatment with neutral detergents did not remove the organism, suggesting that conventional shampooing has little effect on removing staphylococci from hair. Moreover, these neutral detergents had little bactericidal activity on staphylococci. These results suggest that hair falling into the sterile field could be a source of multidrug-resistant staphylococci in SSIs.

5.2 **Cover a beard when entering the restricted areas and while preparing and packaging items in the clean assembly section of the sterile processing area.** *[Recommendation]*

Several studies have demonstrated that beards can be a source of bacterial organisms.[67-69]

In a nonexperimental study, McLure et al[68] examined dispersal of bacteria by men with and without beards and by women. The results of the study showed that there was significantly more bacterial shedding by bearded men than by clean-shaven men or by women even when a mask was worn. The researchers suggested that beards may act as a reservoir for bacteria and dead organic material.

Wakeam et al[69] compared facial bacterial colonization rates among 408 male health care workers with and without facial hair. The results of this study demonstrated that male hospital workers with facial hair did not harbor more potentially concerning bacteria than clean shaven workers. Clean shaven workers were significantly more likely to be colonized with *Staphylococcus aureus,* including MRSA. Both groups shed bacteria at high rates. The researchers suggested standard infection prevention practices be followed to prevent contamination during the performance of sterile procedures.

Parry et al[67] conducted a study to determine whether nonsterile surgical hoods reduce the risk of bacterial shedding by bearded men. Ten bearded and 10 clean-shaven surgeons completed three sets of standardized facial motions, each lasting 90 seconds while unmasked, masked, and masked and hooded. The addition of surgical hoods did not decrease the total number of bacteria as measured in colony-forming units (CFU). The unmasked men shed a significantly higher number of CFU than the masked men. The researchers concluded that the bearded surgeons did not appear to have an increased likelihood of bacterial shedding compared to the non-bearded surgeons while wearing surgical masks, and the addition of surgical hoods did not decrease the amount of shedding

5.3 **No recommendation can be made for the type of head covers worn in the semi-restricted and restricted areas.** *[No Recommendation]*

The evidence does not demonstrate any association between the type of surgical head covering material or extent of hair coverage and the outcome of SSI rates.

Markel et al[70] compared disposable bouffant style caps and skull caps to newly home-laundered cloth hats to determine permeability, particle transmission, and pore size. All three types of hats were evaluated twice at two different institutions for a total of four 1-hour-long mock surgeries for each hat. All hat types underwent permeability and porosity testing. The researchers found that disposable bouffant hats were more permeable to bacteria compared to the disposable skull caps and cloth caps. The researchers acknowledged that cloth hats are not always laundered daily, and a dirty, unwashed cloth hat could possibly lead to airborne contamination and transmission of bacteria.

Kothari et al[59] conducted a nonexperimental study to compare SSI rates of patients whose attending surgeon's preferred cap style was either bouffant or skullcap. The data for this study came from a previously published, prospective RCT on the impact of hair clipping on SSI. A total of 1,543 patients were included in the trial, and the prevalence of diabetes and tobacco use were similar among both groups. Thirty-nine percent of the surgeons preferred wearing bouffant caps and 61% preferred wearing skullcaps. Surgical site infections occurred in 8% of patients whose surgeons preferred a bouffant cap and 5% of the patients whose surgeons preferred a skullcap. When adjusting for the type of surgery, there was no significant difference in SSI rates for skullcaps compared to bouffant caps. A limitation of this study design is that it was a retrospective review of a previous clinical trial and the head coverings of other team members were not documented. The researchers concluded that type of cap worn did not significantly affect SSI rates after accounting for surgical procedure type.

Haskins et al[58] conducted a nonexperimental study to investigate the incidence of postoperative wound infections following ventral hernia repair and the type of surgical hat worn, using data from the Americas Hernia Society Quality Collaborative database. Surgeons were sent a survey asking them what type of surgical hair covering they wear in the OR. The association of the type of hat worn, operative factors, and patient variables was compared with 30-day wound infections using multivariate logistic regression. A total of 68 surgeons responded, resulting in 6,210 cases analyzed. The researchers concluded that the type of surgical hat worn was not associated with an increased risk of 30-day SSIs or surgical site occurrences requiring procedural intervention. A limitation of this study design is that the survey may have introduced response bias. Furthermore, the survey did not capture the types of surgical hats worn by other team members in the OR and may have overgeneralized the type of surgical hat worn.

5.3.1 An interdisciplinary team, including members of the surgical team and infection preventionists, may determine the type of head covers that will be worn at the health care organization. [*Conditional Recommendation*]

5.3.2 Religious head coverings (eg, head scarves [hijabs], veils, turbans, bonnets) that are clean, constructed of tightly-woven and low-linting material, are without adornments, and fit securely with loose ends tucked in the scrub top may be worn to cover the hair and scalp in the semi-restricted and restricted area. [*Conditional Recommendation*]

Some religious traditions include the practice of wearing specific head coverings. Some of these head coverings are configured in a way that covers the hair and scalp and others also cover portions of the wearer's neck and chest.

Policy restrictions or policies that do not address the use of religious head coverings in perioperative settings can be a barrier for members of some religious groups who currently work or aspire to work in procedural areas. In a survey, Malik[71] explored the experiences of female Muslim health care professionals who wore a headscarf in the surgical setting and their view on "bare below the elbows" policies. Most of the professionals (94%) agreed that wearing a headscarf was important to them because of their religious beliefs, yet more than half (51.5%) experienced problems trying to wear a headscarf in the perioperative setting; some women reported feeling embarrassed (23.4%), anxious (37.1%), or bullied (36.5%). The researchers concluded that policies can be at odds with an individual's personal beliefs, which may contribute to a decrease in workplace diversity and fewer opportunities for certain groups.

See **Section 1 Laundering** and **Section 2 Fabric** for more information.

5.3.3 Religious head coverings that cover only a portion of the hair and scalp (eg, kippahs, yarmulkes) may be worn under another head covering. [*Conditional Recommendation*]

5.3.4 Establish and implement a process for managing reusable head coverings (eg, cloth personal head coverings, religious head coverings), including

- the type of fabrics (eg, nonlinting) that may be worn,
- laundering frequency (eg, daily), and
- laundering method (eg, facility laundering, home laundering) when reusable head coverings are worn in the facility.

[*Conditional Recommendation*]

5.4 No recommendation can be made for covering the ears in the semi-restricted and restricted areas. [*No Recommendation*]

Moderate-quality evidence suggests that ears are a potential reservoir for pathogens, although research has not demonstrated any association between covering the ears and SSI rates.

Kanayama Katsuse et al[72] conducted a nonexperimental study of the earlobes and fingers of 200 nurses working at a university hospital to determine whether cross transmission could occur between bacteria-colonized pierced earring holes and fingers. *Staphylococcus aureus* was recovered from the earlobes of 24 nurses (19%) with pierced ears (n = 128) and seven nurses (10%) without pierced ears (n = 72). Of the nurses who were positive for *S aureus* (n = 31), 15 also had *S aureus* on their fingers, which included 12 from the pierced-ear group and three from the unpierced-ear group. With the exception of one nurse, the susceptibility patterns and genotypes of *S aureus* were identical for the earring hole and fingers. The researchers concluded that pierced earlobes can be a source of HAIs due to cross contamination from earring holes to fingers.

Covering ears may also prevent earrings worn by scrubbed team members from falling into the sterile field, which increases the patient's risk for SSI and a retained item. However, covering the ears may have potential harms such as impairing hearing and potentially impeding team communication, interfering with use of a stethoscope, and hindering the fit of protective eyewear or loupes.

5.5   **Remove head coverings at the end of the shift or when they are contaminated.** *[Recommendation]*

5.5.1   **Reusable head coverings contaminated with blood, body fluids, or other potentially infectious materials must remain at the health care facility for laundering.**[26] *[Regulatory Requirement]*

6. Shoes

6.1   **Wear clean shoes when entering the semirestricted or restricted areas.** *[Recommendation]*

In a systematic review, Rashid et al[73] found that shoes have the ability to transfer infectious organisms to the floor and contribute to floor contamination.

In a nonexperimental study, Amirfeyz et al[74] examined shoes worn outdoors and shoes worn only in the surgical suite (N = 120). The results of the study demonstrated that 98% of the outdoor shoes were contaminated with coagulase-negative staphylococci, coliform, and *Bacillus* species compared with 56% of the shoes worn only in the surgical suite. Bacteria on the perioperative floor may contribute up to 15% of CFU dispersed into the air by walking. The researchers concluded that shoes worn only in the perioperative area may help to reduce contamination of the perioperative environment.

6.2   **Wear protective footwear that meets the health care organization's safety requirements.** *[Recommendation]*

The OSHA regulations for foot protection[75] require the use of protective footwear that meets ASTM F2414 standards[76] in areas where there is a danger of foot injuries from falling or rolling objects or objects piercing the sole. The employer is responsible for determining whether foot injury hazards exist and what, if any, protective footwear is required. The OSHA regulations mandate that employers perform a workplace hazard risk assessment and ensure that employees wear footwear that provides protection from identified potential hazards (eg, needlesticks, scalpel cuts, splashing from blood or other potentially infectious materials).[75] The National Institute for Occupational Safety and Health recommends wearing slip-resistant shoes for prevention of slips, trips, and falls.[77]

In a laboratory study, Barr and Siegel[78] examined 15 different types of shoes and tested them with an apparatus that measured resistance to penetration by scalpels. The materials of the shoes included leather, suede, rubber, and canvas. Sixty percent of the shoes sustained scalpel penetration through the shoe into a simulated foot. Only six materials prevented complete penetration. These materials included sneaker suede, suede with inner mesh lining, leather with inner canvas lining, nonpliable leather, rubber with inner leather lining, and rubber. Wearing shoes made of these materials could potentially prevent harm to the perioperative team member.

6.3   **Fluid-resistant shoe covers or boots must be worn in instances when gross contamination can reasonably be anticipated.**[75] *[Regulatory Requirement]*

6.4   **Shoe covers worn as PPE must be removed immediately after use. After removal, discard the shoe covers and perform hand hygiene.**[75] *[Regulatory Requirement]*

7. Identification Badges

7.1   **Clean identification badges with a low-level disinfectant when the badge becomes soiled with blood, body fluids, or other potentially infectious materials.** *[Recommendation]*

Moderate-quality evidence supports that identification badges may be contaminated with pathogens.

In a prospective cross-sectional study, Caldwell at al[79] cultured employee common access cards and identification badges in a burn unit. The overall contamination rate was 75%. There was an 86% bacterial contamination rate on the access cards and a 65% bacterial contamination rate on the identification badges. When the badges and cards were cleaned weekly, the contamination rate dropped to 50%, which indicated that even weekly cleaning appeared to have an effect on the contamination rate.

7.1.1 **Determine the frequency for routine badge disinfection (eg, daily, weekly).** [*Conditional Recommendation*]

7.2 **Clean lanyards with a low-level disinfectant when the lanyard becomes soiled with blood, body fluids, or other potentially infectious materials.** [*Recommendation*]

Moderate-quality evidence supports that lanyards may be contaminated with pathogens.

In a cross-sectional study, Kotsanas et al[80] examined the pathogenic contamination of identification badges and lanyards and found that the median bacterial load was tenfold more for lanyards (3.1 CFU/cm²) than for identification badges (0.3 CFU/cm²). The microorganisms recovered from lanyards and identification badges were methicillin-sensitive *Staphylococcus aureus*, MRSA, *Enterococcus* species, and *Enterobacteriaceae*. The researchers concluded that identification badges should be clipped on and disinfected regularly and that lanyards should be changed frequently or should not be worn.

8. Stethoscopes

8.1 **Clean stethoscopes before each patient use according to the manufacturer's instructions for use.** [*Recommendation*]

Moderate-quality evidence supports that hand hygiene and stethoscope cleaning by health care personnel decreases the risk of transmitting pathogens to patients and environmental surfaces.[52,81-91] Stethoscopes come in direct contact with patients' skin and could be a mechanism for transmission of pathogens from patient to patient, from patient to health care worker, or from health care worker to patient.

In a systematic review, Haun et al[52] examined bacterial contamination of health care personnel attire and other personal devices. The review found 72 studies that assessed contamination of a variety of items including stethoscopes. Pathogens recovered from these items included *Staphylococcus aureus*, MRSA, gram-negative rods, and *Enterococcus* species.

In a comparative study, Denholm et al[92] examined the microbial contamination levels of the stethoscopes of 155 physicians and medical students and compared personal stethoscopes with facility-owned stethoscopes. The researchers isolated significantly more organisms from personal stethoscopes than from facility-owned stethoscopes; however, there was no significant relationship between the frequency of stethoscope cleaning and the degree of contamination. The researchers concluded that even regular cleaning of stethoscopes may be insufficient to prevent colonization with pathogenic organisms and that stethoscopes used for patients at high risk for HAIs should be restricted to single-patient use.

In a nonexperimental cross-sectional study, Campos-Murguía et al[90] examined the number of potentially pathogenic organisms present on stethoscopes by analyzing 112 stethoscopes from 12 hospital departments. Forty-eight stethoscopes (43%) had microorganisms that were potentially pathogenic. The results of this study showed that stethoscopes could be significant contributors to MRSA infections and that they should be routinely cleaned and disinfected before and after each patient use.

9. Personal Items

9.1 **Establish a process to prevent contamination of the semi-restricted and restricted areas from personal items (eg, briefcases, backpacks). The process may include cleaning or containing the item or placing the item in a designated location.** [*Conditional Recommendation*]

Items brought into the semi-restricted and restricted areas, such as briefcases, backpacks, and other personal items, may be difficult to clean and may harbor pathogens, dust, and bacteria. Cleaning these items may help to decrease the transmission of potentially pathogenic microorganisms from external surfaces to perioperative surfaces and from perioperative surfaces to external surfaces.

9.2 **Clean cell phones, tablets, and other personal communication or hand-held electronic equipment according to the device manufacturer's instructions for use before these items are brought into the OR, and perform hand hygiene.** [*Recommendation*]

Moderate-quality evidence[52,93-101] demonstrates that cell phones, tablets, and other personal hand-held devices are highly contaminated with microorganisms, some potentially pathogenic. Researchers recommended regular cleaning of these devices and implementing hand hygiene before and after use. Reducing the numbers of microorganisms present on the devices may protect patients from the risk of HAIs resulting from the transfer of microorganisms from the devices or hands of health care workers to patients.

Datta et al[93] conducted a nonexperimental study to investigate the rate of bacterial contamination of the mobile phones of health care workers employed in a tertiary health care teaching hospital. Of the 200 health care workers' mobile phones sampled, 144 (72%) were contaminated with bacteria, and 18% of those bacteria were MRSA. The researchers concluded that simple measures such as regular cleaning of cell phones and other hand-held electronic devices and improving hand hygiene may decrease patients' risk of acquiring HAIs from pathogens carried on personal mobile devices.

9.3 No recommendation can be made for whether a necklace may be worn in the semi-restricted and restricted areas. [No Recommendation]

No evidence was found to evaluate the benefits and harms of wearing a necklace in the semi-restricted and restricted areas. Wearing a necklace while scrubbed poses a risk that the necklace could fall into the sterile field and result in a retained foreign body.

10. Visitor Attire

10.1 Visitors entering the semi-restricted or restricted areas of the surgical suite (eg, law enforcement officers, parents, biomedical engineers) should don either clean surgical attire or a single-use jumpsuit (eg, coveralls, bunny suit) designed to completely cover personal apparel. [Recommendation]

The benefits of wearing clean attire in the semi-restricted and restricted areas of the surgical suite for non-emergent situations may outweigh the harms. Donning clean scrub attire or single-use jumpsuits before entry into the semi-restricted and restricted areas may help to maintain a clean environment and decrease the possibility of transferring microorganisms from external areas and personal attire to perioperative surfaces and patients.

Glossary

Clean: The absence of visible dust, soil, debris, or blood.

Fomite: An inanimate object that, when contaminated with a viable pathogen (eg, bacterium, virus), can transfer the pathogen to a host.

Health care–accredited laundry facility: An organization that processes health care linens and has successfully passed an inspection of its facility, policies and procedures, training programs, and relationships with customers.

Low-level disinfectant: An agent that destroys all vegetative bacteria, some fungi, and some viruses but not all bacterial spores.

Restricted area: Includes the OR and is accessible only from a semi-restricted area.

Scrub attire: Nonsterile apparel designed for the perioperative practice setting that includes two-piece pantsuits and scrub dresses.

Semi-restricted area: Includes the peripheral support areas of the surgical suite and has storage areas for sterile and clean supplies, work areas for storage and processing of instruments, and corridors leading to the restricted areas of the surgical suite.

Surgical attire: Nonsterile apparel designated for the perioperative practice setting that includes scrub attire (eg, two-piece pantsuits, scrub dresses), scrub jackets, and head coverings.

References

1. Guideline for sterile technique. In: *Guidelines for Perioperative Practice.* Denver, CO: AORN, Inc; 2019:931-972. [IVA]

2. Guideline for transmission-based precautions. In: *Guidelines for Perioperative Practice.* Denver, CO: AORN, Inc; 2019:1093-1120. [IVA]

3. Guideline for hand hygiene. In: *Guidelines for Perioperative Practice.* Denver, CO: AORN, Inc; 2019:289-314. [IVA]

4. Background G. Laundry and bedding. In: *Guidelines for Environmental Infection Control in Health-Care Facilities (2003).* Centers for Disease Control and Prevention. https://www.cdc.gov/infectioncontrol/guidelines/environmental/background/laundry.html. Updated November 5, 2015. Accessed April 3, 2019. [IVA]

5. Abu Radwan M, Ahmad M. The microorganisms on nurses' and health care workers' uniforms in the intensive care units. *Clin Nurs Res.* 2019;28(1):94-106. [IIIB]

6. Colclasure VJ, Soderquist TJ, Lynch T, et al. Coliform bacteria, fabrics, and the environment. *Am J Infect Control.* 2015;43(2):154-158. [IIB]

7. Davidson T, Lewandowski E, Smerecki M, et al. Taking your work home with you: potential risks of contaminated clothing and hair in the dental clinic and attitudes about infection control. *Can J Infect Control.* 2017;32(3):137-142. [IIB]

8. Gupta P, Bairagi N, Priyadarshini R, Singh A, Chauhan D, Gupta D. Bacterial contamination of nurses' white coats after first and second shift. *Am J Infect Control.* 2017;45(1):86-88. [IIC]

9. Gupta P, Bairagi N, Priyadarshini R, Singh A, Chauhan D, Gupta D. Bacterial contamination of nurses' white coats made from polyester and polyester cotton blend fabrics. *J Hosp Infect.* 2016;94(1):92-94. [IIC]

10. Mitchell A, Spencer M, Edmiston Jr C, Edmiston CJ. Role of healthcare apparel and other healthcare textiles in the transmission of pathogens: a review of the literature. *J Hosp Infect.* 2015;90(4):285-292. [VA]

11. Thom KA, Escobar D, Boutin MA, Zhan M, Harris AD, Johnson JK. Frequent contamination of nursing scrubs is associated with specific care activities. *Am J Infect Control.* 2018;46(5):503-506. [IIA]

12. Sanon MA, Watkins S. Nurses' uniforms: how many bacteria do they carry after one shift? *J Public Health Epidemiol.* 2012;4(10):311-315. [IIC]

13. Halliwell C. Nurses' uniforms: off the radar. A review of guidelines and laundering practices. *Healthc Infect.* 2012;17(1):18-24. [VA]

14. Perry C, Marshall R, Jones E. Bacterial contamination of uniforms. *J Hosp Infect.* 2001;48(3):238-241. [IIIB]

15. Goyal S, Khot SC, Ramachandran V, Shah KP, Musher DM. Bacterial contamination of medical providers' white coats and surgical scrubs: a systematic review. *Am J Infect Control.* 2019. doi: 10.1016/j.ajic.2019.01.012. [IIIA]

16. Munk S, Johansen C, Stahnke LH, Adler-Nissen J. Microbial survival and odor in laundry. *J Surfact Deterg.* 2001:4(4)385-394. [IIB]

17. Nordstrom JM, Reynolds KA, Gerba CP. Comparison of bacteria on new, disposable, laundered, and unlaundered hospital scrubs. *Am J Infect Control.* 2012;40(6):539-543. [IIIA]

18. Callewaert C, Van Nevel S, Kerckhof FM, Granitsiotis MS, Boon N. Bacterial exchange in household washing machines. *Front Microbiol.* 2015;6:1381. [IIIC]

19. Gerba CP, Kennedy D. Enteric virus survival during household laundering and impact of disinfection with sodium hypochlorite. *Appl Environ Microbiol.* 2007;73(14):4425-4428. [IIB]

20. Gattlen J, Amberg C, Zinn M, Mauclaire L. Biofilms isolated from washing machines from three continents and their tolerance to a standard detergent. *Biofouling.* 2010;26(8):873-882. [IIIB]

21. Wright SN, Gerry JS, Busowski MT, et al. *Gordonia bronchialis* sternal wound infection in 3 patients following open heart surgery: intraoperative transmission from a healthcare worker. *Infect Control Hosp Epidemiol.* 2012;33(12):1238-1241. [VA]

22. Lakdawala N, Pham J, Shah M, Holton J. Effectiveness of low temperature domestic laundry on the decontamination of healthcare workers' uniforms. *Infect Control Hosp Epidemiol.* 2011;32(11):1103-1108. [IIIA]

23. Patel SN, Murray-Leonard J, Wilson AP. Laundering of hospital staff uniforms at home. *J Hosp Infect.* 2006;62(1):89-93. [IIA]

24. Al-Benna S. Laundering of theatre scrubs at home. *J Perioper Pract.* 2010;20(11):392-396. [VA]

25. *ANSI/AAMI ST65:2008/(R)2013: Processing of Reusable Surgical Textiles for Use in Health Care Facilities.* Arlington, VA: Association for the Advancement of Medical Instrumentation; 2013. [IVC]

26. 29 CFR 1910.1030: Bloodborne pathogens. Occupational Safety and Health Administration. https://www.osha.gov/pls/oshaweb/owadisp.show_document?p_id=10051&p_table=STANDARDS. Accessed April 3, 2019.

27. 29 CFR 1910.132: General requirements. Occupational Safety and Health Administration. https://www.osha.gov/laws-regs/regulations/standardnumber/1910/1910.132. Accessed April 3, 2019.

28. Tammelin A, Domicel P, Hambraeus A, Stahle E. Dispersal of methicillin-resistant *Staphylococcus epidermidis* by staff in an operating suite for thoracic and cardiovascular surgery: relation to skin carriage and clothing. *J Hosp Infect.* 2000;44(2):119-126. [IIC]

29. Tammelin A, Hambraeus A, Stahle E. Source and route of methicillin-resistant *Staphylococcus epidermidis* transmitted to the surgical wound during cardio-thoracic surgery. Possibility of preventing wound contamination by use of special scrub suits. *J Hosp Infect.* 2001;47(4):266-276. [IIIC]

30. Andersen BM, Solheim N. Occlusive scrub suits in operating theaters during cataract surgery: effect on airborne contamination. *Infect Control Hosp Epidemiol.* 2002;23(4):218-220. [IIIC]

31. Tammelin A, Ljungqvist B, Reinmüller B. Comparison of three distinct surgical clothing systems for protection from air-borne bacteria: a prospective observational study. *Patient Saf Surg.* 2012;6(1):23. [IIIC]

32. Tammelin A, Ljungqvist B, Reinmüller B. Single-use surgical clothing system for reduction of airborne bacteria in the operating room. *J Hosp Infect.* 2013;84(3):245-247. [IIIC]

33. Lidwell OM, Lowbury EJL, Whyte W, Blowers R, Stanley SJ, Lowe D. Airborne contamination of wounds in joint replacement operations: the relationship to sepsis rates. *J Hosp Infect.* 1983;4(2):111-131. [IIIB]

34. Mariscal A, Lopez-Gigosos RM, Carnero-Varo M, Fernandez-Crehuet J. Antimicrobial effect of medical textiles containing bioactive fibres. *Eur J Clin Microbiol Infect Dis.* 2011;30(2):227-232. [IIB]

35. Chen-Yu JH, Eberhardt DM, Kincade DH. Antibacterial and laundering properties of AMS and PHMB as finishing agents on fabric for health care workers' uniforms. *Clothing and Textiles Research Journal.* 2007;25(3):258-272. [IIA]

36. Kasuga E, Kawakami Y, Matsumoto T, et al. Bactericidal activities of woven cotton and nonwoven polypropylene fabrics coated with hydroxyapatite-binding silver/titanium dioxide ceramic nanocomposite "Earth-plus." *Int J Nanomedicine.* 2011;6:1937-1943. [IIB]

37. Sun G, Qian L, Xu X. Antimicrobial and medical-use textiles. *Textile Asia.* 2001;32(9):33-35. [IIIB]

38. Gerba CP, Sifuentes LY, Lopez GU, Abd-Elmaksoud S, Calabrese J, Tanner B. Wide-spectrum activity of a silver-impregnated fabric. *Am J Infect Control.* 2016;44(6):689-690. [IIC]

39. Bearman GM, Rosato A, Elam K, et al. A crossover trial of antimicrobial scrubs to reduce methicillin-resistant *Staphylococcus aureus* burden on healthcare worker apparel. *Infect Control Hosp Epidemiol.* 2012;33(3):268-275. [IA]

40. Boutin MA, Thom KA, Zhan M, Johnson JK. A randomized crossover trial to decrease bacterial contamination on hospital scrubs. *Infect Control Hosp Epidemiol.* 2014;35(11):1411-1413. [IA]

41. Burden M, Keniston A, Frank MG, et al. Bacterial contamination of healthcare workers' uniforms: a randomized controlled trial of antimicrobial scrubs. *J Hosp Med.* 2013;8(7):380-385. [IA]

42. Condo C, Messi P, Anacarso I, et al. Antimicrobial activity of silver doped fabrics for the production of hospital uniforms. *New Microbiol.* 2015;38(4):551-558. [IIA]

43. Anderson DJ, Addison R, Lokhnygina Y, et al. The Antimicrobial Scrub Contamination and Transmission (ASCOT) trial: a three-arm, blinded, randomized controlled trial with crossover design to determine the efficacy of antimicrobial-impregnated

scrubs in preventing healthcare provider contamination. *Infect Control Hosp Epidemiol.* 2017;38(10):1147-1154. [IA]

44. Markel TA, Gormley T, Greeley D, Ostojic J, Wagner J. Wearing long sleeves while prepping a patient in the operating room decreases airborne contaminants. *Am J Infect Control.* 2018;46(4):369-374. [IIB]

45. Chow CJ, Hayes LM, Saltzman DA. The impact of perioperative warm-up jackets on surgical site infection: cost without benefit? *Am J Surg.* 2016;212(5):863-865. [VC]

46. Elmously A, Gray KD, Michelassi F, et al. Operating room attire policy and healthcare cost: favoring evidence over action for prevention of surgical site infections. *J Am Coll Surg.* 2019;228(1):98-106. [VB]

47. Treakle AM, Thom KA, Furuno JP, Strauss SM, Harris AD, Perencevich EN. Bacterial contamination of health care workers' white coats. *Am J Infect Control.* 2009;37(2):101-105. [IIIB]

48. Munoz-Price LS, Arheart KL, Lubarsky DA, Birnbach DJ. Differential laundering practices of white coats and scrubs among health care professionals. *Am J Infect Control.* 2013;41(6):565-567. [IIIA]

49. Munoz-Price LS, Arheart KL, Mills JP, et al. Associations between bacterial contamination of health care workers' hands and contamination of white coats and scrubs. *Am J Infect Control.* 2012;40(9):e245-e248. [VA]

50. Kaplan C, Mendiola R, Ndjatou V, Chapnick E, Minkoff H. The role of covering gowns in reducing rates of bacterial contamination of scrub suits. *Am J Obstet Gynecol.* 2003;188(5):1154-1155. [IIC]

51. Loh W, Ng VV, Holton J. Bacterial flora on the white coats of medical students. *J Hosp Infect.* 2000;45(1):65-68. [IIIB]

52. Haun N, Hooper-Lane C, Safdar N. Healthcare personnel attire and devices as fomites: a systematic review. *Infect Control Hosp Epidemiol.* 2016;37(11):1367-1373. [IIIA]

53. Du ZY, Zhang MX, Shi MH, Zhou HQ, Yu Y. Bacterial contamination of medical uniforms: a cross-sectional study from Suzhou City, China. *J Pak Med Assoc.* 2017;67(11):1740-1742. [IIIB]

54. Summers MM, Lynch PF, Black T. Hair as a reservoir of staphylococci. *J Clin Pathol.* 1965;18:13-15. [IIIB]

55. Spruce L. Surgical head coverings: a literature review. *AORN J.* 2017;106(4):306-316. [VA]

56. Boyce JM. Evidence in support of covering the hair of OR personnel. *AORN J.* 2014;99(1):4-8. [VA]

57. Berrios-Torres SI, Umscheid CA, Bratzler DW, et al; Healthcare Infection Control Practices Advisory Committee. *Centers for Disease Control and Prevention guideline for the prevention of surgical site infection, 2017* (Supplement). https://jamanetwork.com/journals/jamasurgery/fullarticle/2623725. Accessed April 4, 2019. [IVA]

58. Haskins IN, Prabhu AS, Krpata DM, et al. Is there an association between surgeon hat type and 30-day wound events following ventral hernia repair? *Hernia.* 2017;21(4):495-503. [IIIC]

59. Kothari SN, Anderson MJ, Borgert AJ, Kallies KJ, Kowalski TJ. Bouffant vs skull cap and impact on surgical site infection: does operating room headwear really matter? *J Am Coll Surg.* 2018;227(2):198-202. [IIIA]

60. Rios-Diaz AJ, Chevrollier G, Witmer H, et al. The art and science of surgery: do the data support the banning of surgical skull caps? *Surgery.* 2018;164(5):921-925. [VB]

61. Mastro TDMD, Farley TAMD, Elliott JAPD, et al. An outbreak of surgical-wound infections due to group A streptococcus carried on the scalp. *N Engl J Med.* 1990;323(14):968-972. [VA]

62. Rahav G, Pitlik S, Amitai Z, et al. An outbreak of Mycobacterium jacuzzii infection following insertion of breast implants. *Clin Infect Dis.* 2006;43(7):823-830. [VA]

63. Richet HM, Craven PC, Brown JM, et al. A cluster of *Rhodococcus (Gordona) bronchialis* sternal-wound infections after coronary-artery bypass surgery. *N Engl J Med.* 1991;324(2):104-109. [VB]

64. Scheflan M, Wixtrom RN. Over troubled water: an outbreak of infection due to a new species of *Mycobacterium* following implant-based breast surgery. *Plast Reconstr Surg.* 2016;137(1):97-105. [VA]

65. Dineen P, Drusin L. Epidemics of postoperative wound infections associated with hair carriers. *Lancet.* 1973;302(7839):1157-1159. [VA]

66. Mase K, Hasegawa T, Horii T, et al. Firm adherence of *Staphylococcus aureus* and *Staphylococcus epidermidis* to human hair and effect of detergent treatment. *Microbiol Immunol.* 2000;44(8):653-656. [IIC]

67. Parry JA, Karau MJ, Aho JM, Taunton M, Patel R. To beard or not to beard? Bacterial shedding among surgeons. *Orthopedics.* 2016;39(2):e290-e294. [IIA]

68. McLure HA, Mannam M, Talboys CA, Azadian BS, Yentis SM. The effect of facial hair and sex on the dispersal of bacteria below a masked subject. *Anaesthesia.* 2000;55(2):173-176. [IIC]

69. Wakeam E, Hernandez RA, Rivera Morales D, Finlayson SRG, Klompas M, Zinner MJ. Bacterial ecology of hospital workers' facial hair: a cross-sectional study. *J Hosp Infect.* 2014;87(1):63-67. [IIIA]

70. Markel TA, Gormley T, Greeley D, et al. Hats off: a study of different operating room headgear assessed by environmental quality indicators. *J Am Coll Surg.* 2017;225(5):573-581. [IIC]

71. Malik A, Qureshi H, Abdul-Razaq H, et al. "I decided not to go into surgery due to dress code": a cross-sectional study within the UK investigating experiences of female Muslim medical health professionals on bare below the elbows (BBE) policy and wearing headscarves (hijabs) in theatre. *BMJ Open.* 2019;9(3):e019954. [IIIB].

72. Kanayama Katsuse A, Takishima M, Nagano M, et al. Cross-contamination of bacteria-colonized pierced earring holes and fingers in nurses is a potential source of health care-associated infections. *Am J Infect Control.* 2019;47(1):78-81. [IIIB]

73. Rashid T, Vonville H, Hasan I, Garey KW. Mechanisms for floor surfaces or environmental ground contamination to cause human infection: a systematic review. *Epidemiol Infect.* 2017;145(1):347-357. [IIIA]

74. Amirfeyz R, Tasker A, Ali S, Bowker K, Blom A. Theatre shoes—a link in the common pathway of postoperative wound infection? *Ann R Coll Surg Engl.* 2007;89(6):605-608. [IIB]

75. 29 CFR 1910.136. Personal protective equipment: foot protection. Occupational Safety and Health Administration. https://

www.osha.gov/pls/oshaweb/owadisp.show_document?p_table=standards&p_id=9786. Accessed April 3, 2019.

76. *ASTM F2412-18a. Standard Test Methods for Foot Protection.* West Conshohocken, PA: ASTM International; 2018. [IVC]

77. Bell J, Collins JW, Dalsey E, Sublet V. *Slip, Trip, and Fall Prevention for Healthcare Workers* (DHHS [NIOSH] Publication Number 2011-123). Washington, DC: National Institute for Occupational Safety and Health; 2010. [IVB]

78. Barr J, Siegel D. Dangers of dermatologic surgery: protect your feet. *Dermatol Surg.* 2004;30(12 Pt 1):1495-1497. [IIIB]

79. Caldwell NW, Guymon CH, Aden JK, Akers KS, Mann-Salinas E. Bacterial contamination of burn unit employee identity cards. *J Burn Care Res.* 2016;37(5):e470-e475. [IIIA]

80. Kotsanas D, Scott C, Gillespie EE, Korman TM, Stuart RL. What's hanging around your neck? Pathogenic bacteria on identity badges and lanyards. *Med J Aust.* 2008;188(1):5-8. [IIIA]

81. Fafliora E, Bampalis VG, Lazarou N, et al. Bacterial contamination of medical devices in a Greek emergency department: impact of physicians' cleaning habits. *Am J Infect Control.* 2014;42(7):807-809. [IIIB]

82. Rao DA, Aman A, Muhammad Mubeen S, Shah A. Bacterial contamination and stethoscope disinfection practices: a cross-sectional survey of healthcare workers in Karachi, Pakistan. *Trop Doct.* 2017;47(3):226-230. [IIIB]

83. Wood MW, Lund RC, Stevenson KB. Bacterial contamination of stethoscopes with antimicrobial diaphragm covers. *Am J Infect Control.* 2007;35(4):263-266. [IIIB]

84. Bernard L, Kereveur A, Durand D, et al. Bacterial contamination of hospital physicians' stethoscopes. *Infect Control Hosp Epidemiol.* 1999;20(9):626-628. [IIIB]

85. Uneke CJ, Ogbonna A, Oyibo PG, Onu CM. Bacterial contamination of stethoscopes used by health workers: public health implications. *J Infection Dev Ctries.* 2010;4(7):436-441. [IIIA]

86. Russell A, Secrest J, Schreeder C. Stethoscopes as a source of hospital-acquired methicillin-resistant *Staphylococcus aureus. J Perianesth Nurs.* 2012;27(2):82-87. [IIA]

87. Mehta AK, Halvosa JS, Gould CV, Steinberg JP. Efficacy of alcohol-based hand rubs in the disinfection of stethoscopes. *Infect Control Hosp Epidemiol.* 2010;31(8):870-872. [IIIB]

88. Uneke CJ, Ogbonna A, Oyibo PG, Ekuma U. Bacteriological assessment of stethoscopes used by medical students in Nigeria: implications for nosocomial infection control. *Healthc Q.* 2009;12(3):132-138. [IIIB]

89. Bhatta DR, Gokhale S, Ansari MT, et al. Stethoscopes: a possible mode for transmission of nosocomial pathogens. *J Clin Diagn Res.* 2012;5(6):1173-1176. [IIIB]

90. Campos-Murguía A, León-Lara X, Muñoz JM, Macías AE, Álvarez JA. Stethoscopes as potential intrahospital carriers of pathogenic microorganisms. *Am J Infect Control.* 2014;42(1):82-83. [IIIB]

91. Worster A, Tang PH, Srigley JA, Main CL. Examination of staphylococcal stethoscope contamination in the emergency department (pilot) study (EXSSCITED pilot study). *Can J Emerg Med.* 2011;13(4):239-244. [IIIB]

92. Denholm JT, Levine A, Kerridge IH, Ashhurst-Smith C, Ferguson J, D'Este C. A microbiological survey of stethoscopes in Australian teaching hospitals: potential for nosocomial infection? *Aust Infect Control.* 2005;10(3):79. [IIIA]

93. Datta P, Rani H, Chander J, Gupta V. Bacterial contamination of mobile phones of health care workers. *Indian J Med Microbiol.* 2009;27(3):279-281. [IB]

94. Byrns G, Foong YC, Green M, et al. Mobile phones as a potential vehicle of infection in a hospital setting. *J Occup Environ Hyg.* 2015;12(10):D232-D235. [IIIB]

95. Chang C, Chen S, Lu J, Chang C, Chang Y, Hsieh P. Nasal colonization and bacterial contamination of mobile phones carried by medical staff in the operating room. *Plos One.* 2017;12(5):e0175811. [IIIB]

96. Khan A, Rao A, Reyes-Sacin C, et al. Use of portable electronic devices in a hospital setting and their potential for bacterial colonization. *Am J Infect Control.* 2015;43(3):286-288. [IIIB]

97. Kirkby S, Biggs C. Cell phones in the neonatal intensive care unit: How to eliminate unwanted germs. *Adv Neonatal Care.* 2016;16(6):404-409. [VA]

98. Lee YJ, Yoo CG, Lee CT, et al. Contamination rates between smart cell phones and non-smart cell phones of healthcare workers. *J Hosp Med.* 2013;8(3):144-147. [IIIB]

99. Martínez-Gonzáles NE, Solorzano-Ibarra F, Cabrera-Díaz E, et al. Microbial contamination on cell phones used by undergraduate students. *Can J Infect Control.* 2017;32(4):211-216. [IIIB]

100. Murgier J, Coste JF, Cavaignac E, et al. Microbial flora on cell-phones in an orthopedic surgery room before and after decontamination. *Orthop Traumatol Surg Res.* 2016;102(8):1093-1096. [IIIB]

101. Shakir IA, Patel NH, Chamberland RR, Kaar SG. Investigation of cell phones as a potential source of bacterial contamination in the operating room. *J Bone Joint Surg (Am).* 2015;97(3):225-231. [IIB]

Guideline Development Group

Lead Author: Lisa Spruce[1], DNP, RN, CNS-CP, CNOR, ACNS, ACNP, FAAN, Director of Evidence-Based Perioperative Practice, AORN, Denver, Colorado

Methodologist: Amber Wood[2], MSN, RN, CNOR, CIC, FAPIC, Editor-in-Chief, Guidelines for Perioperative Practice, AORN, Denver, Colorado

Evidence Appraisers: Lisa Spruce[1]; Janice Neil[3], PhD, CNE, RN, Associate Professor, East Carolina College of Nursing, Greenville, North Carolina; and Amber Wood[2]

Guidelines Advisory Board Members:
- Donna A. Pritchard[4], MA, BSN, RN, NE-BC, CNOR, Director of Perioperative Services, Interfaith Medical Center, Brooklyn, New York
- Bernard C. Camins[5], MD, MSc, Medical Director, Infection Prevention, Mount Sinai Health System, New York, New York
- Heather A. Hohenberger[6], MSN, RN, CIC, CNOR, CPHQ, Administrative Director Surgical Services, IU Health Arnett Hospital, Lebanon, Indiana

- Mary Fearon[7], MSN, RN, CNOR, Service Line Director Neuroscience, Overlake Medical Center, Sammamish, Washington
- Jennifer Butterfield[8], MBA, RN, CNOR, CASC, Administrator, Lakes Surgery Center, West Bloomfield, Michigan
- Kate McGee[9], BSN, RN, CNOR, Staff Nurse, Aurora West Allis Medical Center, East Troy, Wisconsin
- Mary Anderson[10], MS, RN, CNOR, OR RN–II, Parkland Health & Hospital System, Dallas, Texas
- Gerald McDonnell[11], PhD, BSc, Senior Director, Sterility Assurance, DePuy Synthes, Johnson & Johnson Family of Companies, Raritan, New Jersey
- Judith L. Goldberg[12], DBA, MSN, RN, CNOR, CSSM, CHL, CRCST, Director Nursing Excellence & Professional Development, Yale New Haven Health, Lawrence + Memorial Hospital, New London, Connecticut
- Brenda G. Larkin[13], MS, ACNS-BC, CNS, CNOR, Clinical Nurse Specialist, Aurora Lakeland Medical Center, Lake Geneva, Wisconsin
- Jay Bowers[14], BSN, RN, CNOR, Clinical Coordinator for Trauma, General Surgery, Bariatric, Pediatric and Surgical Oncology, West Virginia University Hospitals, Morgantown
- Elizabeth (Lizz) Pincus[15], MSN, RN, CNS-CP, CNOR, Clinical Nurse Specialist, St Francis Hospital, Roslyn, New York

Guidelines Advisory Board Liaisons:
- Doug Schuerer[16], MD, FACS, FCCM, Professor of Surgery, Trauma Director, Washington University School of Medicine, St Louis, Missouri
- Cassie Dietrich[17], MD, Anesthesiologist, Anesthesia Associates of Kansas City, Overland Park, Kansas
- Leslie Jeter[18], MSNA, RN, CRNA, Staff CRNA, Ambulatory Anesthesia of Atlanta, Georgia
- Jennifer Hanrahan[19], DO, Medical Director of Infection Prevention, Metrohealth Medical Center, Cleveland, Ohio
- Susan Ruwe[20], MSN, RN, CPHQ, CIC, Senior Infection Preventionist, Carle Foundation Hospital, Argenta, Illinois
- Susan G. Klacik[21], BS, CRCST, FCS, Clinical Educator, International Association of Healthcare Central Service Materiel Management (IAHCSMM), Chicago, Illinois
- Julie K. Moyle[22], MSN, RN, Member Engagement Manager, Centura – Avista Adventist Hospital, Golden, Colorado

External Review: Expert review comments were received from individual members of the American Association of Nurse Anesthetists (AANA), American College of Surgeons (ACS), Association for Professionals in Infection Control and Epidemiology (APIC), American Society of Anesthesiologists (ASA), International Association of Healthcare Central Service Materiel Management (IAHCSMM), Practice Greenhealth, and the Society for Healthcare Epidemiology of America (SHEA). Their responses were used to further refine and enhance this guideline; however, their responses do not imply endorsement. The draft was also open for a 52-day public comment period.

Financial Disclosure and Conflicts of Interest

This guideline was developed, edited, and approved by the AORN Guidelines Advisory Board without external funding being sought or obtained. The Guidelines Advisory Board was financially supported entirely by AORN and was developed without any involvement of industry.

Potential conflicts of interest for all Guidelines Advisory Board members were reviewed before the annual meeting and each monthly conference call. Nineteen members of the Guideline Development Group reported no potential conflict of interest.[1-5,7-10,12-18,20-22] Three members[6,11,19] disclosed potential conflicts of interest. After review and discussion of these disclosures, the Advisory Board concluded that none of the potential conflicts related to any content in this guideline.

Publication History

Originally published March 1975, *AORN Journal,* as AORN "Standards for proper OR wearing apparel."

Format revision March 1978, July 1982.

Revised March 1984, March 1990. Published as proposed recommended practices, August 1994.

Revised November 1998; published December 1998. Reformatted July 2000.

Revised November 2004; published in *Standards, Recommended Practices, and Guidelines,* 2005 edition. Reprinted February 2005, *AORN Journal.*

Revised October 2010 for online publication in *Perioperative Standards and Recommended Practices.*

Reformatted September 2012 for publication in *Perioperative Standards and Recommended Practices,* 2013 edition.

Revised September 2014 for online publication in *Perioperative Standards and Recommended Practices.*

Minor editing revisions made in November 2014 for publication in *Guidelines for Perioperative Practice,* 2015 edition.

Revised 2019 for online publication in *Guidelines for Perioperative Practice.*

Minor revisions in May 2021, addition to Section 5 Head Coverings (5.3.2, 5.3.3), for online publication in *Guidelines for Perioperative Practice.*

Scheduled for review in 2024.

SURGICAL SMOKE SAFETY

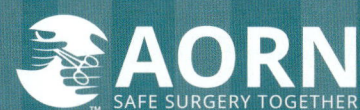

AORN
SAFE SURGERY TOGETHER

MEDICAL ABBREVIATIONS & ACRONYMS

AQI – Air quality index
BPV – Bovine papillomavirus
CAE – Continuous aerosol evacuation
CDC – Centers for Disease Control and Prevention
CO₂ – Carbon dioxide
dBA – A-weighted decibels
EAP – Electrostatic aerosol precipitation
ESP – Electrostatic precipitation
ESU – Electrosurgical unit
FDA – US Food and Drug Administration
HBsAg – Hepatitis B surface antigen
HBV – Hepatitis B virus
HEPA – High-efficiency particulate air
HIV – Human immunodeficiency virus
HPV – Human papillomavirus
HVAC – Heating, ventilation, and air conditioning
LASIK – Laser in-situ keratomileusis

LEEP - Loop electrosurgery excision procedure
MPPS – Most penetrating particulate size
NIOSH – National Institute for Occupational
  Safety and Health
OR – Operating room
OSHA – Occupational Safety and Health Administration
PAH – Polycyclic aromatic hydrocarbon
PCR – Polymerase chain reaction
PM – Particulate matter
PPE – Personal protective equipment
REL – Recommended exposure limits
RRP – Recurrent respiratory papillomatosis
SAEC – Small airway epithelial cells
SWPF – Simulated workplace protection factor
TVOC – Total volatile organic compound
ULPA – Ultra-low particulate air
VOC – Volatile organic compound

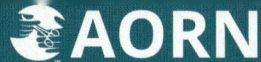

GUIDELINE FOR
SURGICAL SMOKE SAFETY

The Guideline for Surgical Smoke Safety was approved by the AORN Guidelines Advisory Board and became effective as of October 14, 2021. The recommendations in the guideline are intended to be achievable and represent what is believed to be an optimal level of practice. Policies and procedures will reflect variations in practice settings and/or clinical situations that determine the degree to which the guideline can be implemented. AORN recognizes the many diverse settings in which perioperative nurses practice; therefore, this guideline is adaptable to all areas where operative or other invasive procedures may be performed.

Purpose

This document provides guidance on **surgical smoke** safety precautions to support the perioperative team in establishing a safe environment for both surgical patients and team members through consistent use of control measures.

Surgical smoke is the vaporous and gaseous by-product of the use of surgical energy devices (eg, electrosurgical units [ESUs], lasers, ultrasonic devices, high-speed powered instruments).[1,2] When surgical energy devices raise intracellular temperatures to 100° C (212° F) or higher, the tissue vaporizes, producing surgical smoke.[3]

Electrosurgical devices use radio-frequency current to cut and coagulate; radio-frequency current passing through body tissues generates heat, which causes cell walls to rupture, releasing the cellular fluid as steam and the cell contents into the air. Lasers produce an intense, coherent, directional beam of light and also produce high heat, which raises the temperature within the cell, vaporizing the contents and releasing steam and cell contents.[1] Ultrasonic scalpel devices apply mechanical movement of 55.5 kHz frequency at the tip of the device; mechanisms of cavitation, protein denaturation, and heat generation of 50° C to 100° C (122° F to 212° F) cause temperature and pressure fluctuations within the cells, releasing vapor.[4] Ultrasonic aspirators produce a fine mist from interaction of the high-speed hollow tip on tissue and the irrigation fluid.[1] High-speed electrical devices (eg, bone saws, drills) cut, dissect, and resect tissue; the mechanical action of the saw or drill combined with the irrigation fluid used to cool the device produces aerosols.[5]

Surgical smoke is visible and malodorous.[2] The contents of surgical smoke have been widely studied. Researchers began analyzing the contents of surgical smoke as early as 1976.[6] In a 1981 study, Tomita et al[7] found that the contents of surgical **smoke** were similar to the contents of cigarette smoke, with known and suspected carcinogens and mutagens. This finding is supported by a recent concept analysis.[2]

Surgical smoke is reported to contain toxic compounds (eg, **hydrogen cyanide**, toluene, benzene), bio-aerosols, viruses (eg, hepatitis B virus [HBV],[8] human papillomavirus [HPV],[9] human immunodeficiency virus [HIV]),[10] viable cancer cells,[11-13] particles (ie, lung-damaging dust of 5.0 μm and smaller),[14] blood fragments, and bacteria.[15] **Ultrafine particles** of 0.1 μm (ie, 100 nm) and smaller can comprise 70% or more of surgical smoke and concentrations vary based on the type of tissue treated.[16,17] The water vapor content of surgical smoke from laser and vessel-sealing devices ranges from 1% to 11%,[18,19] and experts report that surgical smoke may have a water content of up to 95%.[1]

The Occupational Safety and Health Administration (OSHA) acknowledges the hazards of surgical smoke and recognizes that many health care workers are exposed to surgical smoke, including surgeons, nurses, anesthesia professionals, and surgical technologists.[20] Acute and chronic exposure to ambient concentrations of fine and ultrafine particulate matter have been associated with cardiovascular and pulmonary health effects.[21] Occupational exposure to **volatile organic compounds** (VOCs) in surgical smoke remains a concern because of the potential risk of long-term health effects[22] and possible reproductive effects.[23]

Perioperative nurses report twice the incidence of many respiratory problems (eg, allergies, sinus infections/problems, asthma, bronchitis) compared to the general population.[24] Case reports have established a link between inhalation of surgical smoke during excision of anogenital condylomata procedures and transmission of HPV to health care providers.[25-27] For example, a laser surgeon developed laryngeal papillomatosis of the same virus genotype as his patient,[27] and experts at a virological institute confirmed a high probability of occupational exposure in a gynecologic perioperative nurse who developed recurrent and histologically proven laryngeal papillomatosis.[26]

Surgical smoke exposure can also be hazardous to patients. Although exposure to surgical smoke might be brief, potential risks to patients include reduced visibility of the surgical field during minimally invasive procedures[28-31] with potential to delay the procedure,[32] possible port site metastasis,[12,33] exposure to carbon monoxide,[34-36] and increased levels of carboxyhemoglobin.[34,35]

AORN, the National Institute for Occupational Safety and Health (NIOSH),[37] and other professional organizations[38-41] have recommended surgical smoke evacuation for more than 25 years. However, perioperative team members continue to demonstrate a lack of knowledge of the hazards of surgical smoke[42,43] and a lack of compliance in evacuating surgical smoke and adhering to surgical smoke safety practices.[24,42-51] Even though smoke generated by electrosurgery is more hazardous than laser-generated surgical smoke,[7] there is greater compliance with smoke evacuation for laser procedures.[50,51]

The COVID-19 pandemic required the health care community to implement transmission-based precautions. As a result, a renewed interest developed in protecting health care workers from the potential for viral transmission from surgical smoke during operative or other invasive procedures. Researchers who performed a systematic scoping review through June 2020 to assess the risk of viral transmission from surgical smoke during intraabdominal surgery found no evidence to support the presence of respiratory viruses in peritoneal fluid.[52] In a subsequent prospective pilot study conducted in Italy to evaluate the presence of the SARS-CoV-2 virus in surgical smoke, the researchers concluded that theoretically, SARS-CoV-2 might be transmitted through surgical smoke and aerosolized from fluid in the abdominal cavity.[53]

Because the presence, viability, and transmission potential of the SARS-CoV-2 virus in surgical smoke remain unknown,[54] authors of professional society consensus documents,[55,56] literature reviews,[54,57-62] and expert opinion articles[63-65] recommend adhering to surgical smoke safety practices to guide safe perioperative care while protecting health care workers from possible exposure to the novel coronavirus that causes COVID-19. For further guidance on transmission-based precautions, such as respiratory protection recommendations for aerosol-generating procedures, refer to the AORN Guideline for Transmission-Based Precautions.[66] Specific guidance on infection control practices related to SARS-CoV-2 is available from the Centers for Disease Control and Prevention (CDC).[67]

Surgical smoke is often referred to as surgical plume, smoke plume, bio-aerosols, **laser-generated airborne contaminants**, and **lung-damaging dust**. For the purpose of this document, the term *surgical smoke* will be used unless another term has been specifically used in a reference source.

Evidence Review

This systematic review is an update to the Guideline for Surgical Smoke Safety, which was published December 16, 2016. A medical librarian with a perioperative background conducted a systematic search of the databases Ovid MEDLINE, Ovid Embase, EBSCO CINAHL, and the Cochrane Database of Systematic Reviews. The search was limited to literature published in English from January 2015 through June 2020. At the time of the initial search, weekly alerts were created on the topics included in that search. Results from these alerts were provided to the lead author until April 2021. The lead author requested addi-

tional articles that either did not fit the original search criteria or were discovered during the evidence appraisal process. The lead author and the medical librarian also identified relevant guidelines from government agencies, professional organizations, and standards-setting bodies.

Search terms included (*active or passive*) [*close to*] *filtration, aerosol generating procedures, aerosol generating procedures and (surg* or device or instrument), air pollutants (occupational), bacterial aerosols, bioaerosol*, cautery and (surg* or device or instrument), cautery smoke, coronavirus infections, COVID-19, diathermy, diathermy and (surg* or device or instrument), diathermy fume, diathermy mist, diathermy plume, diathermy smoke, diathermy (surgical) and (surg* or device or instrument), dissection, dissection and (surg* or device or instrument), (electrosurg* or laser or ultrasonic) and (surg* or device or instrument), electrocautery, electrocautery and (surg* or device or instrument), electrocautery exhaust, electrocautery fume, electrocautery mist, electrocautery plume, electrocautery smoke, electrocoagulation, electrocoagulation and (surg* or device or instrument), electrostatic precipitation, electrosurg*, electrosurg* and (surg* or device or instrument), electrosurg* exhaust, electrosurg* fume, electrosurg* mist, electrosurg* plume, electrosurg* smoke, HIV, human immunodeficiency virus, human papillomavirus, laparoscopy, laparoscopy and (surg* or device or instrument), laser exhaust, laser fume, laser mist, laser plume, laser smoke, laser surgery, laser surgery and (device or instrument), laser therapy smoke, lasers, lasers and (surg* or device or instrument), local exhaust ventilation, occupational air pollutants, occupational hazards, operative procedures, operative procedures and (surg* or device or instrument), Papillomaviridae, particulate matter, (smoke or aerosol) [close to] evacuation, (surgery, operative+) and smoke, smoke extract*, smoke inhalation injury, surg* fume, surg* mist, surg* plume, surg* smoke, surgical procedures (operative) and smoke, surgical smoke precipitator, tissue ablation, tissue ablation and (surg* or device or instrument), (ultrastatic or ultrafine) [close to] particulate, viral aerosols,* and *virus aerosols.*

Included were research and non-research literature in English, complete publications, and publications with dates within the time restriction when available. Excluded were non-peer-reviewed publications and older evidence within the time restriction when more recent evidence was available. Editorials, news items, and other brief items were excluded. Low-quality evidence was excluded when higher-quality evidence was available, and literature outside the time restriction was excluded when literature within the time restriction was available. Citations from the original guideline were retained when newer research was not available or the citations remained relevant in explaining the rationale for a practice recommendation **(Figure 1)**.

Articles identified in the search were provided to the project team for evaluation. The team consisted of the lead author and three evidence appraisers. The lead author divided the search results into topics and assigned members of the team to review and critically appraise each article

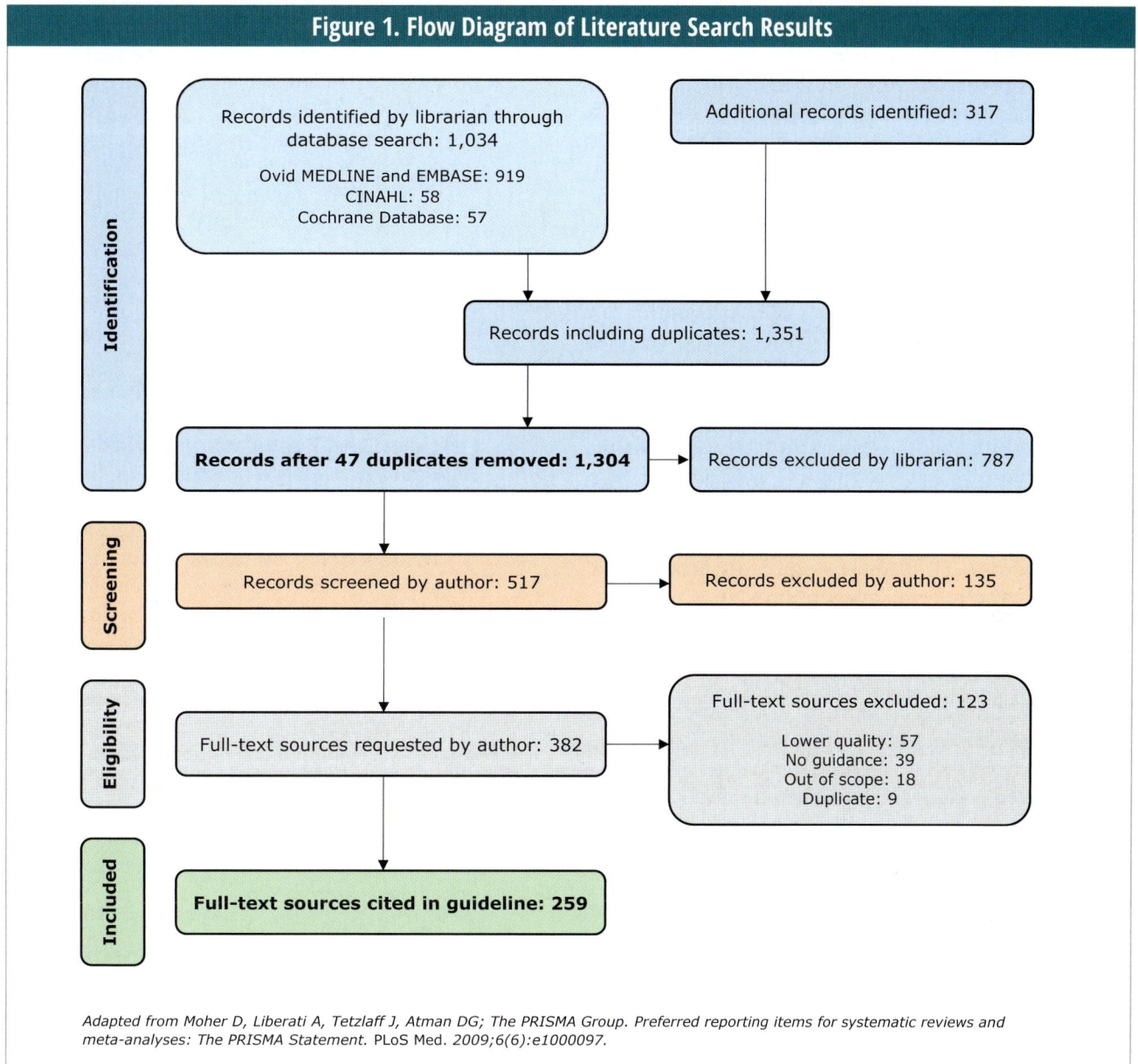

Figure 1. Flow Diagram of Literature Search Results

Records identified by librarian through database search: 1,034

Ovid MEDLINE and EMBASE: 919
CINAHL: 58
Cochrane Database: 57

Additional records identified: 317

Records including duplicates: 1,351

Records after 47 duplicates removed: 1,304

Records excluded by librarian: 787

Records screened by author: 517

Records excluded by author: 135

Full-text sources requested by author: 382

Full-text sources excluded: 123

Lower quality: 57
No guidance: 39
Out of scope: 18
Duplicate: 9

Full-text sources cited in guideline: 259

Identification

Screening

Eligibility

Included

Adapted from Moher D, Liberati A, Tetzlaff J, Atman DG; The PRISMA Group. Preferred reporting items for systematic reviews and meta-analyses: The PRISMA Statement. PLoS Med. 2009;6(6):e1000097.

using the AORN Research or Non-Research Evidence Appraisal Tools as appropriate. The literature was independently evaluated and appraised according to the strength and quality of the evidence. Each article was then assigned an appraisal score. The appraisal score is noted in brackets after each reference, as applicable.

Each recommendation rating is based on a synthesis of the collective evidence, a benefit-harm assessment, and consideration of resource use. The strength of the recommendation was determined using the AORN Evidence Rating Model and the quality and consistency of the evidence supporting a recommendation. The recommendation strength rating is noted in brackets after each recommendation.

Note: The evidence summary table is available at http:// www.aorn.org/evidencetables/.

1. Smoke-Free Environment

1.1 **The health care organization should provide a surgical smoke–free work environment.** *[Recommendation]*

The hazards related to surgical smoke are explicitly acknowledged by OSHA[20]; however, no OSHA regulatory standards specifically address protection from smoke generated from surgical energy devices used in the operating room (OR) or procedural setting. Related standards, as interpreted by OSHA, include the OSHA General Duty Clause and OSHA general industry standards (29 CFR 1910).[68]

The General Duty Clause, Section 5(a)(1) of the Occupational Safety and Health Act of 1970, is used when no other specific standards address the particular hazard. Under the General Duty Clause, an employer is required to provide employees with a place of employment that is "free from recognized hazards that are causing or are likely to cause death or serious physical harm to his employees."[68,69] A 2016 OSHA interpretation of the OSHA General Duty Clause reinforces the employer requirements related to worker protection from surgical smoke hazards.[70] An employer may be found in violation for failure to provide reasonable prevention or abatement for an existing recognized serious hazard.

The interpretation further outlines the OSHA general industry standards relevant to surgical smoke, including OSHA Standard 29 CFR 1910.132, Personal Protective Equipment,[71] which requires employers to provide personal protective equipment (PPE) to minimize exposure to hazards; OSHA Standard 29 CFR 1910.134, Respiratory Protection,[72] which requires employers to provide appropriate respiratory protection to control respiratory hazards; and OSHA Standard 29 CFR 1910.1000, Air Contaminants,[73] which requires employers to control exposure to air contaminants at or below permissible exposure limits.[70]

Many states and territories have federal OSHA-approved occupational health and safety programs in place. These state standards are required to be at least as effective as the federal OSHA equivalent.[74]

1.2 **The health care organization should evaluate the perioperative team's risk of exposure to surgical smoke.** *[Recommendation]*

Surgical smoke contains many components that are recognized health hazards. High-quality evidence describes the particulate and chemical contents of surgical smoke and demonstrates the exposure risks and hazards to the perioperative team. Evidence of varying quality levels describes the potential presence of biohazardous materials in surgical smoke. Moderate-quality evidence suggests that HPV can be present in surgical smoke from HPV lesions,[9] and there is evidence of occupational transmission of HPV among clinicians who participate in smoke-generating procedures involving HPV lesions. Limited evidence suggests the potential presence of HBV in surgical smoke from infected patients, but there is no evidence of occupational transmission.[8] Surgical smoke can contain

- particles (eg, fine particulate matter [$PM_{2.5}$] and ultrafine particulate matter [$PM_{0.1}$])[14,17,75-86];
- chemicals, including
  - **aromatic hydrocarbons** (eg, benzene,[75,87-90] toluene,[75,88,90-99] xylenes [75,76,90,92,96,98-100]),
  - VOCs[22,87-90,100-102] (eg, acetone[90,101], aldehydes[89] [acetaldehyde,[101,103] formaldehyde][101]),
  - polycyclic aromatic hydrocarbons (PAHs)[79,87,104-106] (eg, naphthalene,[75,79,104] phenanthrene,[75,79,104] benzo[a]pyrene,[79] anthracene[79]),
  - hydrogen cyanide,[88]
  - **inorganic gases** (eg, carbon monoxide[75,107,108]),
  - **nitriles** (eg, acetonitrile,[76,100] acrylonitrile[92,93,109]); and
- biohazardous materials, including
  - viruses[59,61,110-113] (eg, HPV,[9,114-117] HIV[5,10], HBV[8]),
  - bacteria,[118,119]
  - blood,[120-124] and
  - potentially viable cancer cells.[11-13]

Particles and Respiratory Hazards

High-quality evidence indicates that the particles in surgical smoke generated by surgical energy devices (eg, monopolar and bipolar electrosurgery, ultrasonic scalpels, lasers) are within the respirable range.[17,75,77,80-86] The size (ie, aerodynamic diameter) of the particles in the surgical smoke directly influences the type of adverse respiratory health effects experienced by the perioperative team.[14,82,83,119,125-127] Particle size depends on the type of device generating the surgical smoke.[1,126,128] Electrosurgery generates the smallest aerodynamic size particles (< 0.07 μm to 0.1 μm); laser tissue ablation creates larger particles (~ 0.31 μm); and ultrasonic scalpels create the largest particles (0.35 μm to 6.5 μm).[1] Particulate composition may include chemicals,[79] viruses, bacteria, or cellular material.[14,125]

Particle size affects how far the particle can travel in the respiratory system.[14,126] Particles that are 5 μm or larger settle in the walls of the nose and pharynx; particles 3 μm to 5 μm settle in the trachea; particles 1 μm to 3 μm settle in the bronchus and bronchioles; and particles smaller than 1 μm can penetrate to the alveoli **(Figure 2)**.[125,129,130] Particles smaller than 5 μm are categorized as lung-damaging dust[14] because they can penetrate to the deepest areas of the lung and obstruct gas exchange.[14,126,127] The effects of concentration of ultrafine particles on health is unclear; however, the health effects of exposure to ultrafine particles is thought to be cumulative.[85]

High-quality evidence suggests that fine particle and ultrafine particle concentrations[77,78] are associated with the type of tissue treated and with the degree of personal exposure.[17,78,83] Liver tissue has been found to consistently produce the highest concentrations of total particles and ultrafine particles.[77,78]

Tan et al[77] quantified fine particle concentrations in surgical smoke produced from various tissues during surgery on hemihepatectomy patients (n = 50) and compared fine particle concentrations in surgical smoke during ultrasonic scalpel use and

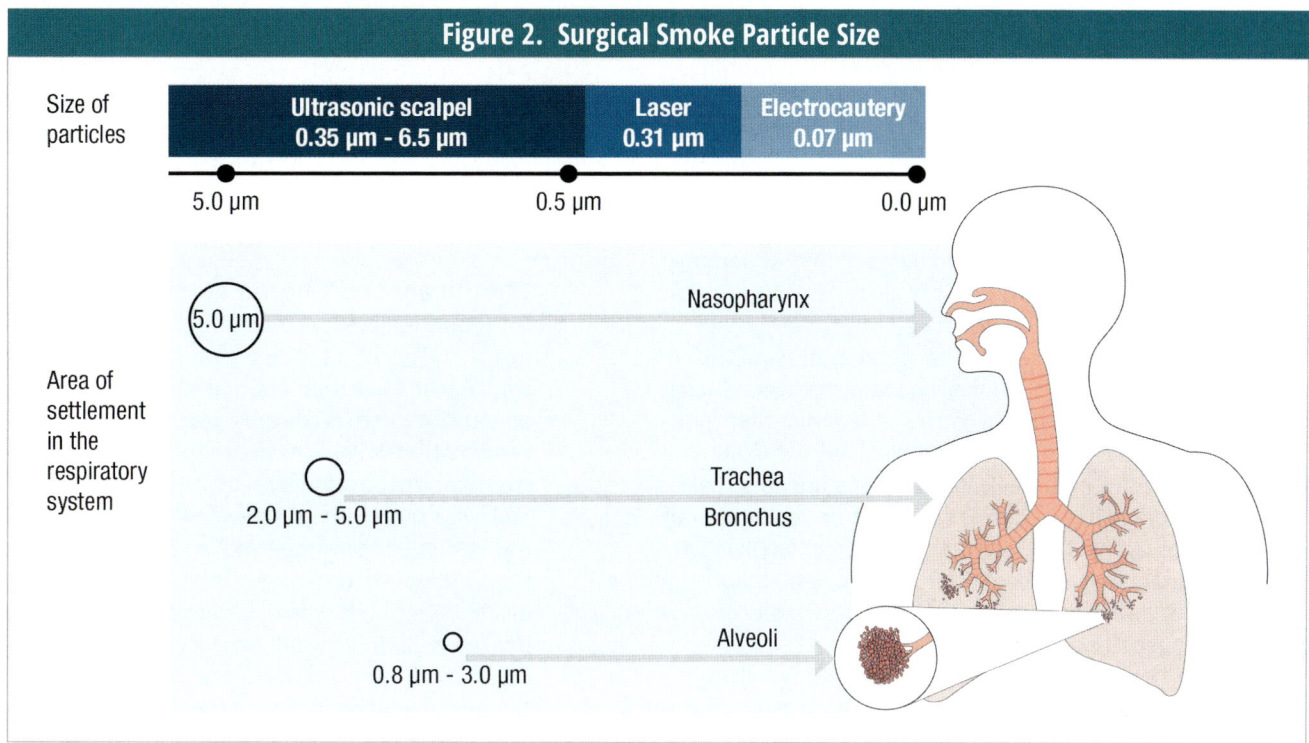

Figure 2. Surgical Smoke Particle Size

Size of particles

| Ultrasonic scalpel 0.35 µm - 6.5 µm | Laser 0.31 µm | Electrocautery 0.07 µm |

5.0 µm   0.5 µm   0.0 µm

Area of settlement in the respiratory system

5.0 µm — Nasopharynx

2.0 µm - 5.0 µm — Trachea / Bronchus

0.8 µm - 3.0 µm — Alveoli

electrosurgical knife use on liver tissue (n = 20). Fine particle concentrations were collected at the head height of the surgeon during electrosurgical knife use on different tissues including adipose, muscle, and liver tissues, and blood vessels. Of the different tissues, liver tissue produced the highest fine particle concentration in surgical smoke (303.10 +/- 108.95 µg/m³), significantly higher than in surgical smoke from other tissue (muscle = 110.07 +/- 50.47 µg/m³, adipose = 46.89 +/- 20.39 µg/m³, blood vessel = 8.35 +/- 6.87 µg/m³). The results demonstrated that when used on liver tissue, the ultrasonic scalpel produced a significantly higher average concentration of fine particles, reaching 531.28 +/- 71.58 µg/m³, compared to the average concentration of fine particles produced by the electrosurgical knife (279.88 +/- 69.51 µg/m³).[77]

Karjalainen et al[78] evaluated particulate matter characteristics of electrosurgical smoke produced from 10 porcine tissue samples of different types (ie, skeletal muscle, liver, subcutaneous fat, renal pelvis, renal cortex, lung, bronchus, cerebral matter [gray and white], and skin) all from the same animal. Concentrations and aerodynamic size distribution of particles were measured in 10 samples from each tissue type. The researchers also estimated health implications for OR personnel by calculating the airway deposition fractions for the upper airways, bronchial tube, and the alveoli from the measured aerosol particle mass distributions. Liver tissue was found to have the highest concentration of particulate matter (PM_{10} = 9,100 mg/m³,

$PM_{2.5}$ = 1,100 mg/m³, $PM_{1.0}$ = 470 mg/m³) with the greatest overall calculated mass that could be deposited to the alveoli of OR personnel. The researchers concluded that tissue types could be separated into three distinct groups related to the particulate matter and potential risk of exposure to the surgical team: high-PM tissues with high exposure risk (ie, liver), medium-PM tissues with moderate risk (ie, renal cortex, renal pelvis, muscle), and low-PM tissues with low risk (ie, skin, cerebral matter, bronchus, subcutaneous fat).

Ragde et al[17] conducted an observational study to assess exposure of surgical personnel to ultrafine particles, to identify the predictors of exposure to ultrafine particles, and to characterize the particle size distribution of surgical smoke in five different procedures (ie, nephrectomy, breast reduction, abdominoplasty, hip replacement, transurethral resection of the prostate). The researchers measured personal exposures for the surgeon, assistant, scrub person, and anesthesia professional throughout each of the five procedures and used spectrometry to characterize the particle distribution and assess the exposure to ultrafine particles. Possible predictors of exposure were investigated using linear mixed effects models. The researchers found that exposure to ultrafine particles was highest during abdominoplasty and lowest during hip replacement surgeries.

Among the studied procedures, 70% or more of the measured particles were in the ultrafine range. The use of electrosurgery resulted in short-term exposure at a high level, with a maximum peak exposure of 272,000 ultrafine particles/cm³ during a breast reduction surgery. The peaks corresponded to the use of the ESU. Nephrectomy, transurethral resection of the prostate, and hip replacement surgeries produced the smallest size particles (9 nm) and also had the highest percentages of ultrafine particles. Breast reduction surgery and abdominoplasty produced larger sized particles (70 nm and 81 nm, respectively) and had a lower percentage of ultrafine particles. There were no significant differences in exposure among the team members during any of the studied procedures. The researchers concluded that the use of electrosurgery resulted in short-term, high-peak exposures to ultrafine particles, and they recommended the correct use of smoke evacuators, the use of a built-in smoke evacuator tubing on the electrosurgery pencil, and the use of two smoke evacuators when two electrosurgery pencils are required.[17]

Wang et al[83] conducted a prospective study to analyze fine particles in surgical smoke by time and distance during open urology procedures, laparoscopic partial nephrectomy, and transurethral resection of bladder tumors. Three subtypes of the open surgery group, according to surgery depth, were inguinal lymph node dissection for penile cancer (superficial), partial nephrectomy (abdominal), and radical prostatectomy (pelvic). There were five participants in each of the five procedure groups (N = 25). All procedures were performed in the same laminar airflow OR. The researchers measured particle counts at 40 cm, 60 cm, and 120 cm from the surgical smoke source during open and laparoscopic surgeries to simulate the positions of the surgeon, assistant, and scrub person and at 40 cm during the transurethral surgeries. During the open procedures, fine particles were measured with and without wall suction used for smoke evacuation. To evaluate the air quality, the researchers used the Air Quality Index (AQI) – the National Ambient Air Quality Standards for Particle Pollution revised by the US Environmental Protection Agency.

Background particle measurements in the OR before the surgeries were nearly 5 μg/m³. The AQI of the air 40 cm from the open surgery incisions turned to unhealthy (ie, 55.5 μg/m³ to 150.4 μg/m³) and very unhealthy (ie, 150.5 μg/m³ to 250.4 μg/m³) in 3 to 6 seconds. In laparoscopic surgeries, the AQI 40 cm from the trocar reached hazardous levels within 3 seconds after the trocar valve was opened, releasing the surgical smoke. In the transurethral surgeries, the AQI was moderate 40 cm from the resectoscope. Use of wall suction decreased the inhalation dose of fine particles 48% in superficial surgeries and 52% in abdominal surgeries. The

researchers found that the concentration of fine particles of a single smoke plume could become very unhealthy for the surgeon. They concluded that increasing the distance to the incision site decreased the concentration and inhalation of fine particles and that using smoke evacuation can reduce the concentration of fine particles.[83]

Chemicals and Chemical Hazards

High-quality evidence establishes the presence of potentially hazardous chemicals in surgical smoke,[37,131,132] with an estimated 150 chemical compounds[89,133] discovered using gas chromatography,[104] a combination of gas chromatography and mass spectrometry/spectrography,[22,75,76,87,89,90,92,93,100-102,105,106,109,134-136] and laser spectroscopy[18,19,91,94,137] (Table 1). The chemical content of surgical smoke varies by the type of tissue treated (eg, liver, muscle, adipose, skin, hair),[75,76,89,98,102,125,138] type of surgical energy device used (eg, laser, ESU, ultrasonic energy, argon beam),[95,103,139] duration of the procedure,[105] and the amount of time the surgical energy device was in use.[91,94,98]

Cheng et al[22] conducted an observational study to compare VOC exposure during laparotomic/laparoscopic, mastectomy, and orthopedic procedures (N = 10) performed using electrocautery and pulsed electron avalanche knife energy devices. Breath samples (N = 24) were obtained from operating personnel including surgeons, surgeon assistants, scrubbed persons, and registered nurse (RN) circulators immediately before and after surgery. Area samples were also collected in the ORs and in a control area outside the OR (ie, the nursing station). Volatile organic compounds found in OR air samples that were thought to be associated with electrocautery included significantly high levels of benzene (96 ppb), toluene (17.3 ppb), ethylbenzene (62.3 ppb), and m/p-xylene (199.8 ppb). The researchers also found 18 VOCs in breath samples, including benzene, hexamethyldisiloxane, toluene, ethylbenzene, m/p-xylene, and 1,3,5-trimethylbenzene, although these remained at a similar level or decreased after the procedure compared to the before-surgery breath sample mean values.

Van Gestel et al[87] conducted a 5-day study to identify exposure to VOCs and PAHs from electrosurgical smoke by analyzing the environment and personal biomarkers for the purpose of comparing internal to external exposure. The researchers collected room air samples and personal air samples of surgeons, scrub assistants, and circulating RNs (N = 15) involved in general surgery procedures performed using electrosurgery in the same OR. Urine samples were also collected pre-shift, mid-shift, and end of shift from each participant. Volatile organic compounds including styrene, ethyl benzene, benzene, and toluene and the PAH naphthalene were detected in air samples. Although o-creosol urine levels increased, an association between VOCs and PAHs present in surgical smoke and urine metabolites was unclear.

Markowska et al[89] sought to identify surgical smoke chemical composition during procedures involving previously burned tissue. The study participants were 10 patients with full-thickness burn injuries undergoing escharotomy (n = 6) or necrotomy (n = 4) procedures with monopolar and bipolar electrocautery. Four surgical smoke samples collected using solid-phase microextraction sampling fibers were obtained during each surgery (N = 40). The morning after the study was conducted, background air samples were obtained from clean, empty ORs to serve as controls.

Analysis revealed a total of 432 compounds with 153 VOCs identified in the surgical smoke after background compounds, including those present in disinfectants, were removed. Volatile organic compounds included aldehydes and ketones (5.16%), alkanes (14.28%), alcohols (4.06%), benzene and benzene derivatives (25.73%), cyclic compounds (22.55%), esters (4.30%), and other compounds (10.14%). Benzene, a known carcinogen, constituted 17.65% of the total compounds found. Ethylbenzene was present at 5.23%. The analysis revealed a significant difference between the compounds found and the type of surgery performed, though benzene was found in large amounts in all samples. The researchers concluded that further research is needed to examine and quantify surgical smoke released during burn procedures and that surgical teams should include surgical smoke safety during the planning phase of surgery.[89]

Hollman et al[140] conducted an assay of surgical smoke generated during a reduction mammoplasty procedure. Monopolar electrocautery was used for dissection and resection, which resulted in intense smoke production. The researchers collected smoke samples (N = 25) whenever the electrocautery was in use. Laser spectroscopy was used to determine the gas components and corresponding concentration in the smoke samples collected. The researchers identified and quantified 11 gases (ie, 1-ethenyl-3-methyl-benzene; 1,3-butadiene; propanenitrile; toluene; thiocyanic acid, methyl ester; 1-heptene; ethylene; ammonia; 1-decene; 2-furancarbox aldehyde; methylpropene). They concluded that surgical smoke generated by electrocautery is a potential health danger to the OR team, although the degree of the threat is unclear.

Sagar et al[141] collected samples of surgical smoke generated by electrocautery during colorectal surgery to determine the chemical composition of surgical smoke. The sampling tube was attached near the end of the electrocautery pencil or held in the plume above the pencil. The researchers analyzed the collected smoke samples for PAHs, nitrosamines, nitrates, nitrites, and VOCs by using high-performance liquid chromatography, gas chromatography with a thermal energy analyzer, ion chromatography, and mass spectrometry. The electrocautery smoke contained significant levels of benzene, ethyl benzene, styrene, carbon disulphide, and toluene. Benzene, a known carcinogen, was detected in significant quantities (71 µg/m³). The substances detected can cause eye irritation, dermatitis, central nervous system effects, and hepatic and renal toxicity. The researchers concluded that additional studies are needed to determine the extent of exposure to the entire OR team and to develop methods to reduce the health risks.

Petrus et al[137] used laser photoacoustic spectroscopy to quantitatively analyze the trace gas concentrations in surgical smoke produced in vitro in nitrogen or synthetic air atmospheres. The researchers used a carbon dioxide (CO_2) laser to generate surgical smoke by irradiating fresh animal tissue and then measured the levels of ethylene, benzene, ammonia, and methanol. Benzene was detected in high concentrations in all smoke samples at a level hundreds of times higher than the recommended exposure limit established by OSHA and NIOSH. Ammonia also exceeded the exposure limit. Methanol and ethylene were detected in the smoke but were within recommended exposure limits. The researchers concluded that additional factors to consider are the cumulative effect of all VOCs released during laser surgery and the harmful effects to the surgical team of continuous exposure by surgical smoke inhalation.

In a subsequent study, Petrus et al[91] quantitatively analyzed surgical smoke produced in vitro by vaporization of fresh animal tissue with a CO_2 laser in a closed nitrogen atmosphere. The concentrations of acetonitrile, acrolein, ammonia, benzene, ethylene, and toluene in surgical smoke were determined with laser photoacoustic spectroscopy. The researchers investigated different types of tissue (ie, pig kidney, muscle, skin, heart) at a laser vaporization power of 10 W and 15 W with exposure times of 5 seconds and 15 seconds. The researchers collected several smoke samples and measured the average gas concentrations. The concentrations of the six gases measured were acetonitrile 190 ppm, acrolein 35 ppm, ammonia 25 ppm, benzene 20 ppm, ethylene 0.410 ppm, and toluene 45 ppm. The researchers concluded that the concentrations of all six gases increased depending on the laser power, exposure time, and type of tissue and that

Table 1. Chemical Contents, Exposure Limits, and Health Effects of Surgical Smoke[1-6]

Chemical	Exposure Limits[1]	IDLH[a] Values[2]	Symptoms[1]
1,2-Dichloroethane	ENIOSH REL[b]: **Ca**[c] TWA[d] 1 ppm (4 mg/m³) ST[e] 2 ppm (8 mg/m³) OSHA PEL[f]: TWA 50 ppm 200 ppm [5-minute maximum peak in any 3 hours]	50 ppm	Irritation of the eyes, corneal opacity; central nervous system depression; nausea, vomiting; dermatitis; liver, kidney, cardiovascular system damage; **potential occupational carcinogen**
2-Propanol	ENIOSH REL: TWA 400 ppm (980 mg/m³) OSHA PEL: TWA 400 ppm (980 mg/m³)	2,000 ppm	Irritation of the eyes, nose, throat; drowsiness, dizziness, headache; dry cracking skin
Acetonitrile	NIOSH REL: TWA 20 ppm (34 mg/m³) OSHA PEL: TWA 40 ppm (70 mg/m³)	137 ppm	Irritation of the nose, throat; asphyxia; nausea, vomiting; chest pain; lassitude (weakness, exhaustion); stupor; convulsions
Acetaldehyde	NIOSH REL: **Ca** OSHA PEL: TWA 200 ppm (360 mg/m³)	2,000 ppm	Irritation of the eyes, nose, throat; eye, skin burns; dermatitis; conjunctivitis; cough; central nervous system depression; delayed pulmonary edema; **potential carcinogenic effects**
Acetonitrile	NIOSH REL: TWA 20 ppm (34 mg/m³) OSHA PEL: TWA 40 ppm (70 mg/m³)	137 ppm	Irritation of the nose, throat; asphyxia; nausea, vomiting; chest pain; lassitude; stupor; convulsions
Acetone	NIOSH REL: TWA 250 ppm (590 mg/m³) OSHA PEL: TWA 1000 ppm (2,400 mg/m³)	2,500 ppm	Irritation of the eyes, nose, throat; headache, dizziness; central nervous system depression; dermatitis
Acetylene	NIOSH REL: Cg 2,500 ppm (2,662 mg/m³)		Headache, dizziness, asphyxia
Acrolein	NIOSH REL: TWA 0.1 ppm (0.25 mg/m³) ST 0.3 ppm (0.8 mg/m³) OSHA PEL: TWA 0.1 ppm (0.25 mg/m³)	2 ppm	Irritation of the eyes, skin, mucous membranes; decreased pulmonary function; delayed pulmonary edema; chronic respiratory disease
Acrylonitrile	NIOSH REL: **Ca** TWA 1 ppm C 10 ppm [15-minute] [skin] OSHA PEL: [1910.1045] TWA 2 ppm C 10 ppm [15-minute] [skin]	60 ppm	Irritation of the eyes, skin; asphyxia; headache; sneezing; nausea, vomiting; lassitude; dizziness; skin vesiculation, scaling dermatitis; **potential carcinogenic effects (brain tumors, lung and bowel cancer)**
Benzene	NIOSH REL: **Ca** TWA 0.1 ppm ST 1 ppm OSHA PEL: [1910.1028] TWA 1 ppm ST 5 ppm	500 ppm	Irritation of the eyes, skin, nose, respiratory system; dizziness; headache; nausea; staggered gait; anorexia; lassitude; dermatitis; bone marrow depression; **potential occupational carcinogen (leukemia)**
Butadiene	NIOSH REL: **Ca** OSHA PEL: [1910.1051] TWA 1 ppm ST 5 ppm	2,000 ppm	Irritation of the eyes, nose, throat; drowsiness; dizziness; **potential occupational carcinogen (blood cancer)**
Carbon monoxide	NIOSH REL: TWA 35 ppm (40 mg/m³) C 200 ppm (229 mg/m³) OSHA PEL: TWA 50 ppm (55 mg/m³)	1,200 ppm	Headache, tachypnea, nausea, lassitude, dizziness, confusion, hallucinations, cyanosis, depressed S-T segment of electrocardiogram, angina, syncope
Creosol (o-, m-, p- isomers)	NIOSH REL: TWA 2.3 ppm (10 mg/m³) OSHA PEL: TWA 5 ppm (22 mg/m³) [skin]	250 ppm	Irritation of the eyes, skin, mucous membranes; central nervous system effects: confusion, depression, respiratory failure; dyspnea (breathing difficulty), irregular rapid respirations, weak pulse; eye, skin burns; dermatitis; lung, liver, kidney, pancreas damage
Cyclohexanone	NIOSH REL: TWA 25 ppm (100 mg/m³) [skin] OSHA PEL: TWA 50 ppm (200 mg/m³)	700 ppm	Irritation of the eyes, skin, mucous membranes; headache; narcosis, coma; dermatitis
Ethanol	NIOSH REL: TWA 1,000 ppm (1,900 mg/m³) OSHA PEL: TWA 1,000 ppm (1,900 mg/m³)	3,300 ppm	Irritation of the eyes, skin, nose; headache; drows-iness, lassitude, narcosis; cough; liver damage; anemia; reproductive, teratogenic effects

Table 1. Continued. Chemical Contents, Exposure Limits, and Health Effects of Surgical Smoke[1-6]

Chemical	Exposure Limits[1]	IDLH[a] Values[2]	Symptoms[1]
Ethyl benzene	NIOSH REL: TWA 100 ppm (435 mg/m³) ST 125 ppm (545 mg/m³) OSHA PEL: TWA 100 ppm (435 mg/m³)	800 ppm	Irritation of the eyes, skin, mucous membranes; headache; dermatitis; narcosis, coma
Formaldehyde	NIOSH REL: **Ca** TWA 0.016 ppm C 0.1 ppm [15-minute] OSHA PEL: [1910.1048] TWA 0.75 ppm ST 2 ppm	20 ppm	Irritation of the eyes, nose, throat, respiratory system; lacrimation (discharge of tears); cough; wheezing; dermatitis; **[potential occupational carcinogen] (nasal cancer)**
Furfural	NIOSH: no established REL OSHA PEL: TWA 5 ppm (20 mg/m³) [skin]	100 ppm	Irritation of the eyes, skin, upper respiratory system; headache; dermatitis
Hydrogen cyanide	NIOSH REL: ST 4.7 ppm (5 mg/m³) [skin] OSHA PEL: TWA 10 ppm (11 mg/m³) [skin]	50 ppm	Asphyxia; lassitude, headache, confusion; nausea, vomiting; increased rate and depth of respiration or slow and gasping respiration; thyroid, blood changes
Phenol	NIOSH REL: TWA 5 ppm (19 mg/m³) C 15.6 ppm (60 mg/m³) [15-minute] [skin] OSHA PEL: TWA 5 ppm (19 mg/m³) [skin]	250 ppm	Irritation of the eyes, nose, throat; anorexia, weight loss; lassitude, muscle ache, pain; dark urine; cyanosis; liver, kidney damage; skin burns; dermatitis; ochronosis; tremor, convulsions, twitching
Pyridine	NIOSH REL: TWA 5 ppm (15 mg/m³) OSHA PEL: TWA 5 ppm (15 mg/m³)	1,000 ppm	Irritation of the eyes; headache, anxiety, dizziness, insomnia; nausea, anorexia; dermatitis; liver, kidney damage
Styrene	NIOSH REL: TWA 50 ppm (215 mg/m³) ST 100 ppm (425 mg/m³) OSHA PEL: TWA 100 ppm C 200 ppm 600 ppm (5-minute maximum peak in any 3 hours)	700 ppm	Irritation of the eyes, nose, respiratory system; headache, lassitude, dizziness, confusion, malaise (vague feeling of discomfort), drowsiness, unsteady gait; narcosis; defatting dermatitis; possible liver injury; reproductive effects
Toluene	NIOSH REL: TWA 100 ppm (375 mg/m³) ST 150 ppm (560 mg/m³) OSHA PEL: TWA 200 ppm C 300 ppm 500 ppm (10-minute maximum peak)	500 ppm	Irritation of the eyes, nose; lassitude, confusion, euphoria, dizziness, headache; dilated pupils, lacrimation (discharge of tears); anxiety, muscle fatigue, insomnia; paresthesia; dermatitis; liver, kidney damage
Xylene (o-, m-, p- isomers)	NIOSH REL: TWA 100 ppm (435 mg/m³) ST 150 ppm (655 mg/m³) OSHA PEL: TWA 100 ppm (435 mg/m³)	900 ppm	Irritation of the eyes, skin, nose, throat; dizziness, excitement, drowsiness; incoordination, staggering gait; corneal vacuolization; anorexia, nausea, vomiting, abdominal pain; dermatitis

[a] IDLH: Immediately dangerous to life or health

[b] NIOSH REL: National Institute for Occupational Safety and Health recommended exposure limits

[c] **Ca**: A potential occupational carcinogen, per NIOSH

[d] TWA: Time-weighted average; the employee's average exposure in any 10-hour work shift during a 40-hour work week, which shall not be exceeded

[e] ST: Short-term exposure limit

[f] OSHA PEL: Occupational Safety and Health Administration permissible exposure limits

[g] C: Ceiling value; the ceiling value should not be exceeded at any time

References

1. NIOSH Pocket Guide to Chemical Hazards. *3rd ed. Washington, DC: US Department of Health and Human Services; 2007.*
2. *Immediately dangerous to life or health (IDLH) values. The National Institute for Occupational Safety and Health. Centers for Disease Control and Prevention. https://www.cdc.gov/niosh/idlh/intridl4.html. Reviewed October I, 2019. Accessed August 31, 2021.*
3. *Barrett WL, Garber SM. Surgical smoke: a review of the literature. Is this just a lot of hot air? Surg Endosc. 2003;17(6):979-987.*
4. *Pierce JS, Lacey SE, Lippert JF, Lopez R, Franke JE, Colvard MD. An assessment of the occupational hazards related to medical lasers. J Occup Environ Med. 2011;53(11):1302-1309.*
5. *Okoshi K, Kobayashi K, Kinoshita K, Tomizawa Y, Hasegawa S, Sakai Y. Health risks associated with exposure to surgical smoke for surgeons and operation room personnel. Surg Today. 2015;45(8):957-965.*
6. *Choi SH, Choi DH, Kang DH, et al. Activated carbon fiber filters could reduce the risk of surgical smoke exposure during laparoscopic surgery: application of volatile organic compounds. Surg Endosc. 2018;32(10):4290-4298.*

Table 2. US Environmental Protection Agency Priority Pollutants Polycyclic Aromatic Hydrocarbons[1]

- Benzo[a]anthracene
- Benzo[a]pyrene
- Benzo[b]fluoranthene
- Benzo[k]fluoranthene
- Chrysene/triphenylene
- Dibenzo[a,h]anthracene
- Indenol[1,2,3-cd]pyrene
- Acenaphthene
- Acenaphthylene
- Anthracene
- Benzo[ghi]perylene
- Phenanthrene
- Fluoranthene
- Fluorene
- Naphthalene
- Pyrene

Reference

1. Näslund Andréasson S, Mahteme H, Sahlberg B, Anundi H. Polycyclic aromatic hydrocarbons in electrocautery smoke during peritonectomy procedures. J Environ Public Health. 2012;2012:929053.

the laser photoacoustic spectroscopy system was efficient in analyzing a multicomponent gas mixture.

Näslund Andréasson et al[106] collected personal and stationary samplings of PAHs in electrocautery smoke during 40 peritonectomy procedures for pseudomyxoma peritonei (n = 22), colorectal cancer (n = 11), appendiceal cancer (n = 5), and ovarian cancer (n = 2). All but three patients received hyperthermic intraperitoneal chemotherapy (n = 37) as part of the procedure. The primary aim of the study was to identify and quantify the US Environmental Protection Agency's 16 priority pollutant PAHs (Table 2) present in the OR during the procedure. Personal samplings were collected using a 40-mm absorbent filter cassette fixed near the surgeon's breathing zone to absorb organic compounds. The stationary samplings were collected with a 20-mm smoke evacuator hose connected to a smoke evacuator system. The absorbent filter cassette tubing was inserted in a small slit 5 cm from the tip of the electrocautery device.

All 16 PAHs were detected in personal and stationary samples. Naphthalene, a possible human carcinogen, was the most abundant PAH and was found in all but one of the samples (97.5%). In addition to naphthalene, phenanthrene (93%), fluorene (63.3%), acenaphthene (40%), and acenaphthylene (36.7%) were detected in the personal samplings. Acenaphthylene (93.3%), phenanthrene (90%), acenaphthene (90%), and fluorene (83.3%) were detected in the stationary samplings. The researchers postulated that long-term exposure to PAHs could lead to high cumulative levels of PAHs in perioperative team members, and consideration should be given to the possibility that simultaneous exposure to particles, PAHs, and VOCs may have synergistic and additive effects.[106]

Carcinogenic Hazards

The evidence is inconclusive as to whether exposure to surgical smoke places perioperative team members or patients at increased risk of developing cancer due to the presence of potentially viable malignant cells[11-13] or exposure to carcinogenic compounds.[88,90,96,102,105,129,138]

Tseng et al[105] investigated particle number concentrations, size distribution, and gaseous and particle phase PAHs as the tracers of surgical smoke in the OR. Through their investigation of PAH concentrations for different surgical personnel, the potential cancer risk can be estimated for OR team members exposed to electrosurgery smoke. The researchers chose mastectomy procedures because of procedure length and high electrocautery use. During 14 mastectomy procedures, samples from the breathing zones of the surgeon and anesthesia provider were collected at 5-minute intervals. The majority of the airborne particles (70%) were 0.3 μm in size.

The researchers found that the downward flow of air (ie, positive pressure) from the OR ceiling distributed the smoke into the surrounding environment, exposing all personnel in the room instantaneously. The particle and gaseous PAH concentrations for the surgeon and anesthesia provider increased 40 to 100 times over the initial baseline measurements. The surgeon was exposed to the highest level of PAHs, approximately 1.5 times higher than the anesthesia provider. Although the anesthesia provider's levels were lower than the surgeon's, longer hours working in the OR increased the risk. The researchers concluded that the submicron particles in the smoke contained carcinogenic chemicals that could threaten the health of the OR team through respiration of the particles. Using the toxicity equivalency factor, the average cancer risk in a 70-year lifetime for the surgeons and the anesthesia providers was calculated to be 117×10^{-6} and 270×10^{-6}, respectively, which is significantly higher than the safety level adopted by the US Army for deployed personnel (1×10^{-4}).[105,142]

In et al[11] conducted a two-part experiment to determine whether viable cells were present in surgical smoke. If viable tumor cells were found in the in vitro portion of the study, the researchers evaluated their carcinogenicity in the in vivo study portion. Viable cells were identified in the smoke at 5 cm from the ultrasonic scalpel. No viable cells were detected in the smoke from the ESU or radio-frequency ablation device. The viable cells were injected on both sides of the lower back of 20 mice. After 2 weeks, there was tumor growth in 16 of the 40 injection sites. Biopsies for morphological assessment showed highly mitotic cells, including irregularly shaped nuclei consistent with malignant tumors. The researchers concluded that smoke from an ultrasonic scalpel may contain viable tumor cells, and there is a theoretical risk of transfer of the viable tumor cells to anyone close to the surgical procedure.

Mowbray et al[129] conducted a systematic review of the literature to evaluate the properties of surgical smoke and the evidence of the harmful effects to the OR team. The authors reviewed 20 studies that met the inclusion criteria for documentation of the contents of surgical smoke during human surgical procedures, methods to analyze the smoke, implication of smoke exposure, and type of energy device. The authors concluded that their review confirmed surgical smoke contains potentially carcinogenic compounds small enough to be respirable and reach the lower airways.

Mutagenic Hazards

Moderate-quality evidence supports that surgical smoke is potentially mutagenic.[7,96,143-145]

Gatti et al[143] collected multiple air samples in the OR during reduction mammoplasty procedures in which electrocautery was used for dissection and excision of the breast tissue. The OR samples were collected approximately 2.5 ft to 3 ft above the surgical field. Control air samples were taken in a separate room. All of the samples were tested for mutagenic activity in standard tester strains TA98 and TA100 of Salmonella typhimurium using the Salmonella microsomal microsuspension test. The results showed the air samples were mutagenic to the TA98 strain of Salmonella typhimurium. The TA100 strain of Salmonella typhimurium did not appear to be significantly altered by the smoke. The researchers concluded from this preliminary study that the smoke produced by the electrocautery during reduction mammoplasty is mutagenic. Mutagenic potential may vary among patients. Safe levels of ambient mutagens have not been determined.

To test the mutagenic activity of surgical smoke condensates, Tomita et al[7] used a CO_2 laser to irradiate and an ESU to cauterize excised canine tongue. The researchers tested the generated smoke with the microbial strains TA98 and TA100 of Salmonella typhimurium. The laser condensates showed mutagenicity on TA98 in the presence of S9 mix. The S9 mix contained 50 µmoles sodium phosphate buffer, 4 µmoles magnesium chloride, 16.5 µmoles potassium chloride, 2.5 µmoles glucose-6 phosphate, 2 µmoles nicotinamide adenine dinucleotide phosphate, and 150 µL of S9 fraction (prepared from rat liver pretreated with polychlorobiphenyl) in a total volume of 0.5 mL. The ESU condensates exhibited mutagenic activity on both strains in the presence of S9 mix. The mutagenic ability of laser condensates was one-half that of the ESU condensates for the microbial strain TA98. The microbial strain TA98 of Salmonella typhimurium was 10 times more sensitive than microbial strain TA100 of Salmonella typhimurium to the condensates.

The researchers found that the mutagenic potency of the condensates was comparable to that of cigarette smoke. The researchers collected about 40 mg of laser and ESU condensates from 1 g of vaporized or cauterized tissue. This amount of laser condensate was equivalent to that from three cigarettes, and this amount of ESU condensate was equivalent to that from six cigarettes. The researchers concluded that more research is needed to evaluate the hazards of laser and ESU smoke on human health and, unless proven otherwise, there is a potential health risk to surgeons, anesthesia providers, nurses, and patients.[7]

Hill et al[146] studied six human and 78 porcine tissue samples to find the mass of tissue ablated during 5 minutes of monopolar ESU use. They also recorded electronically the total daily duration of ESU use in a plastic surgery OR during a 2-month period. An initial pilot study compared a human tissue sample with the animal model. No difference was found between the two tissue types. Porcine tissue is the most physiologically similar tissue to human tissue. For the human tissue, the mass of the ESU tissue ablation after 5 minutes of continuous cutting ablation was 2.4 g and the mass after coagulation ablation was 1.6 g. For the porcine tissue, the mass of the ESU tissue ablation after 5 minutes of continuous cutting ablation was 2.4 g and the mass after coagulation ablation was 1.5 g. The mean daily ESU activation time was 12 minutes, 43 seconds. Using Tomita's results that 1 g of tissue equals six unfiltered cigarettes,[7] the researchers quantified the environmental OR air pollution. They concluded that the equivalent of 27 to 30 unfiltered cigarettes would need to be smoked in the OR on a daily basis to generate a passive air pollution with an equivalent mutagenicity.

Cytotoxic Hazards

There is limited evidence regarding the cytotoxic effects of surgical smoke.[76,145,147-149]

Sisler et al[76] investigated the induced cytotoxicity of surgical smoke produced from using electrocautery on breast tissue. To quantify the airborne and dissolved chemical composition, the researchers sampled and analyzed surgical smoke ultrafine particle concentrations and VOCs in headspace and canister samples during six separate sampling sessions. Acetaldehyde, acetone, acetonitrile, benzene, ethanol, ethylbenzene, isopropyl alcohol, m/p-xylene, and toluene were found in both canister and headspace analysis. To measure induced cytotoxicity in vitro, the researchers exposed human small airway epithelial cells (SAEC) and RAW 264.7 mouse macrophages to the surgical smoke (N = 62). After 24 hours, the cultures were assayed for cell viability, superoxide production, and lactate dehydrogenase. Results indicated that surgical smoke from human breast tissue induced cytotoxicity, as demonstrated by lactate dehydrogenase increases in both SAEC and RAW samples. Induced superoxide production was not observed. The researchers concluded that surgical smoke in vitro is cytotoxic and therefore could be considered an occupational hazard.

Hensman et al[147] exposed cultured cells for a short period of time to smoke produced in a confined space in vitro to determine whether significant toxicity can occur. The smoke was produced in helium, CO_2, and air-saturated environments. The toxic, infective, and mutagenic risks of surgical smoke during open surgeries are known. In minimally invasive surgery, it is unknown whether the smoke produced in a CO_2-saturated environment may have a different composition. The chemical contents identified in the smoke produced in helium, CO_2, and air were similar in composition. The researchers concluded the ESU smoke generated in a closed environment produced several toxic chemicals. The effect of the toxic chemicals on cell viability, macrophage, and endothelial cell activation is unknown.

Viral Presence and Viral Hazards

HPV

Human papillomavirus has been detected in the surgical smoke generated by lasers and ESUs during treatment of cervical lesions,[116,117,150] genital infections,[151-154] verrucae,[155,156] laryngeal papillomas,[157] and bovine papillomavirus–induced cutaneous fibropapillomas.[111] However, some studies have found no detectable HPV in laser plume generated during treatment of laryngeal papillomas.[158-160]

Although the evidence regarding the presence and infectivity of HPV in surgical smoke from treated HPV-related lesions conflicts, recent moderate-quality evidence demonstrates that HPV DNA in electrosurgical smoke can contaminate the nasal epithelia of surgeons.[117] Due to this uncertainty, experts recommend wearing respiratory protection (eg, a surgical N95 filtering facepiece respirator) in addition to evacuating surgical smoke when treating HPV-infected tissue with electrosurgery or laser (**See Recommendation 3.3**).[9,114,115,161]

Zhou et al[117] sought to explore the presence of HPV DNA in electrosurgical smoke from loop electrosurgery excision procedures (LEEP) and its possible effects on those performing the procedure. The participants were patients with persistent HPV infection undergoing outpatient LEEP for cervical intraepithelial neoplasia (N = 134). Surgeons employed surgical smoke evacuation within 2 cm to 10 cm of the surgical site, wearing either an N95 respirator (n = 41) or a surgical mask (n = 93).

The researchers sampled surgical smoke from the LEEP, collected exfoliated cervical cells from the patients, and obtained nasopharyngeal swabs from surgeons before the procedure and at 3, 6, 12, 18, and 24 months. Human papillomavirus DNA analysis was performed using fluorescence in situ hybridization and polymerase chain reaction (PCR). The researchers found that 40 of the 134 smoke samples tested positive for HPV DNA, including HPV-16, HPV-58, HPV-52, HPV-33, HPV-31, and HPV-18 subtypes that were consistent with the patients' cervical cell HPV subtypes. They found a significant association between HPV-positive exfoliated cervical cells and HPV-positive surgical smoke.[117]

All preoperative nasal epithelial swab samples were negative. Two of the postoperative samples from surgeons wearing surgical masks were positive, one for HPV-16 and one for HPV-58. Neither surgeon's positive results persisted beyond 6 months. None of the surgeons wearing an N95 respirator had positive results. The researchers concluded that HPV DNA is present in LEEP surgical smoke and is potentially infectious. They recommended use of an N95 respirator and smoke evacuation during these procedures.[117]

Neumann et al[116] conducted a study to determine whether high-risk HPV is present in surgical plume from routine LEEP for high-grade squamous intraepithelial lesions. Surgical smoke was collected during LEEP (N = 24). Additionally, resected cervical tissue was analyzed to determine HPV subtype. Human papillomavirus was found in four of 24 samples, with all positive surgical smoke samples matching the cervical tissue HPV subtype (ie, one with HPV-16, one with HPV-39, two with HPV-53). The researchers acknowledged that infectivity remains unclear, but they recommended that smoke evacuation and respiratory protection be employed for LEEP. They also suggested that HPV vaccination may be useful for health care professionals who perform LEEP (See Recommendation 3.6).

In contrast, moderate-quality evidence[154,162-166] has demonstrated a low risk of HPV transmission and subsequent infection.

Kofoed et al[162] investigated the prevalence of mucosal HPV types in medical personnel employed in the gynecology and dermato-venereology departments of multiple Danish hospitals in relation to occupational exposure to HPV. The participants (N = 287) completed a questionnaire with demographic data, their previous and current work-related HPV exposure, and history of HPV-related disease. The researchers collected oral and nasal mucosa samples from the participants and analyzed the samples using HPV genotyping. In relation to exposure, a mucosal HPV type was found in

- 5.8% of participants with experience in treating genital warts with a laser compared to 1.7% of the participants who did not have this experience,
- 6.5% of participants with experience in treating genital warts with electrosurgery compared to 2.8% of the participants who did not have this experience, and
- 4.7% of participants with experience in treating genital warts with LEEP compared to 4.6% of the participants who did not have this experience.

Physician and non-physician laser personnel who had treated patients with genital warts for at least 5 years had a significantly higher prevalence of mucosal HPV types than personnel who had less than 5 years of experience or no experience treating genital warts with a laser. The researchers found that participating in CO_2 laser or electrosurgical evaporation of genital warts or loop electrode excision of cervical dysplasia did not significantly increase the prevalence of nasal or oral HPV. Mucosal HPV types are infrequent in the oral and nasal cavities of health care personnel.[162]

Despite the low risk of transmission and subsequent infection with HPV, there have been reported cases of occupational transmission of HPV.[25-27] In 1991, Hallmo and Naess[27] reported the case of a 44-year-old laser surgeon who presented with a large, confluent papillomatous mass in the anterior commissure and along the right vocal cord and four smaller, discrete, smooth papillomas on the left vocal cord. Biopsies of the laryngeal lesions showed squamous papillomas with moderate focal dysplasia. Types HPV-6 and HPV-11 DNA were identified in groups of tumor cells. The surgeon had no known source of infection other than that he had used the Nd:YAG laser for therapeutic procedures involving anogenital condyloma acuminata. Anogenital condylomas harbor HPV types 6 and 11. The authors concluded that any of the surgeon's patients with anogenital warts could have been the source of the surgeon's HPV infection, and there is a similar risk for laser procedure team members.

Calero and Brusis[26] reported the case of a 28-year-old OR nurse who developed recurrent and histologically proven laryngeal papillomatosis. The nurse's occupational history included assisting on electrosurgical and laser surgical excisions of anogenital condylomas. After a virological institute confirmed the high probability of correlation between the occupational exposure and laryngeal papillomatosis, the nurse's condition was accepted as an occupational disease. Hallmo and Naess[27] and Calero and Brusis[26] concluded that the occupational transmission risk of HPV is low when recommended protective measures (eg, smoke evacuation) are employed.

Rioux et al[25] described the cases of HPV-16–positive oropharyngeal squamous cell carcinomas in two surgeons with long-term histories of occupational laser plume exposure to HPV. A 53-year-old gynecologist sought consultation for a lesion on his right tonsil and a lump in the right side of his neck. The biopsy of the right tonsil confirmed invasive squamous cell carcinoma of moderate to poor differentiation. The lesion was positive for HPV-16 by hybrid capture assay. The patient was a non-smoker who consumed alcohol occasionally, was in a monogamous relationship, and whose partner tested negative for HPV. The only identifiable risk factor for oropharyngeal cancer and HPV was occupational exposure to HPV-positive laser plume. The surgeon had performed more than 3,000 laser ablations and LEEP surgeries for dysplastic cervical and vulvar lesions over 20 years.

The second case was a 62-year-old gynecologist who sought consultation for a foreign body sensation in his throat. A biopsy of the base of his tongue was positive for squamous cell carcinoma and HPV-16. The surgeon was a non-smoker who consumed alcohol occasionally and had been married twice. The surgeon's occupational history consisted of performing weekly laser ablations with a CO_2 laser for 15 years and performing LEEP for 15 years. The authors suggested prophylactic HPV vaccination against oncogenic HPV strains to prevent infection and reduce the risk of oropharyngeal cancer.[25]

Garden et al[111] investigated whether laser-generated plume from infected animal tissue (ie, bovine papillomavirus [BPV]-induced cutaneous fibropapilloma) can reproduce disease. The researchers evaluated three laser settings, suctioned and collected the laser plume at each setting, and re-inoculated the laser plume onto the skin of three calves. All of the laser plume samples at the three laser settings contained BPV DNA. Two calves developed marked lesions at the sites of BPV inoculum, and the third calf developed minimal growth. The histological evaluation of the excised laser plume–induced lesions was typical of BPV fibropapillomas. The DNA extracts from each of the three induced tumors contained high levels of BPV DNA, thus confirming that the lesions resulted from the BPV infection. The researchers found the lesions induced by the laser plume were identical to the original lesions based on the histopathological and viral typing.

Kashima et al[157] conducted a prospective study to determine whether HPV DNA was in the smoke plume after CO_2 laser treatment of recurrent respiratory papillomatosis (RRP). Twenty-two patients with diagnoses of adult-onset RRP (n = 7), juvenile-onset RRP (n = 12), laryngeal carcinoma (n = 2), and nonspecific laryngitis (n = 1) participated in the study. The researchers collected 30 paired tissue and smoke samples during microlaryngoscopy with CO_2 laser excision under general anesthesia. To avoid contamination, the samples were processed separately with a PCR assay for amplification of HPV-6 and HPV-11 sequences. Seventeen of the 30 smoke samples were positive for HPV DNA; three of the samples were identified as HPV-6, and 14 samples were identified as HPV-11. Only the RRP specimens were HPV positive. The DNA types HPV-6 and HPV-11 are recognized as etiological agents in RRP. The researchers concluded that the consequences of HPV in smoke plume are unknown. To reduce the risk of potential infection to the patient and perioperative team members, they recommended using PPE (eg, masks, gowns, gloves) and a gas-scavenging system whenever viral-infected lesions are treated with a CO_2 laser.

In a prospective study, Hughes and Hughes[159] collected and evaluated the laser plume of erbium:YAG laser-treated human warts to determine the presence or absence of HPV DNA in the plume. The researchers excised half of five patients' verrucae vulgaris and submitted the specimens for histopathological diagnosis and HPV DNA detection (HPV-1 and HPV-2) with in situ hybridization for HPV. The remaining half of the verrucae vulgaris were ablated with the erbium:YAG laser. A smoke evacuator collected the plume for evaluation of HPV DNA by PCR with consensus primers for the HPV previously detected in the verruca vulgaris specimens. The histopathological diagnosis of all five specimens was verruca vulgaris. All of the specimens with in situ hybridization contained HPV-2 DNA. Using PCR with

consensus primers for HPV-2, the researchers did not detect HPV-2 in the laser plume of the same specimens. They concluded that the negative HPV plume results with the erbium:YAG laser were contradictory to the positive HPV plume findings in two other studies[155,156] in which CO_2 laser and electrosurgical excision and CO_2 laser excision were used. Hughes and Hughes postulated that the negative results could be a result of the radical explosive ejection of the erbium:YAG laser disrupting the HPV and rendering it undetectable.

HIV

Low-quality evidence suggests that HIV-1 may be present in cool aerosols produced from HIV-1–positive cultures in a laboratory setting.[5] No evidence exists to demonstrate HIV-1 presence in surgical smoke from high-temperature devices and no evidence exists of occupational transmission of HIV-1 from surgical smoke.

Johnson and Robinson[5] conducted an experimental laboratory-based study to determine whether infectious HIV-1 could be isolated from aerosols generated from human blood containing HIV-1 during orthopedic and other surgical procedures that generate aerosols. The researchers prepared a mixture of human packed red blood cells negative for cytomegalovirus and HIV antibodies, a culture medium, and a culture medium containing a 105 tissue culture infectious dose of HIV-1. Individually, samples of the mixture were subjected to electrocautery in the coagulation and cutting modes, a high-speed bone cutting router, an oscillating bone saw, and a wound irrigation syringe jet. The cool aerosol or smoke plume generated by the procedures was suctioned and cultured. The cultures positive for HIV-1 developed from the cool aerosols generated by the effects of the high-speed router tip and the oscillating bone saw on the blood mixture containing HIV-1. Cultures negative for HIV-1 developed from the cool aerosols generated by the wound irrigation syringe jet. Negative culture results were also obtained from six experiments of cutting and six experiments of coagulation with the electrocautery. The researchers concluded that infectious HIV-1 could be isolated from cool aerosols created from HIV-1–positive blood exposed to orthopedic routers and oscillating saws but that the high temperature of the electrocautery may inactivate HIV-1.[5]

HBV

Low-quality evidence suggests that HBV may be present in surgical smoke from patients with HBV infection[8]; however, there is no evidence of occupational transmission of HBV from surgical smoke.

Kwak et al[8] conducted an observational study to detect whether HBV was present in aerosolized gas of surgical smoke. The researchers sampled and analyzed surgical smoke of patients (N = 11) with positive hepatitis B surface antigen (HBsAg). Preoperative HBV DNA blood levels ranged from undetectable to 1.7×10^8 IU/mL. All patients underwent laparoscopic surgery or robotic abdominal surgery. Surgical smoke was analyzed using nested PCR methodology with previously identified HBV primers. Hepatitis B virus DNA was detected in 10 of the 11 samples of surgical smoke. The researchers concluded that HBV may be present in the surgical smoke generated from patients with HBV infection.

Other Viruses

No evidence exists to support the presence of the SARS-CoV-2 virus in surgical smoke; however, researchers agree that there is a theoretical potential for transmission from surgical smoke.[52,53]

Bogani et al[53] performed a prospective observational pilot study in Italy during the COVID-19 pandemic to investigate the presence of the SARS-CoV-2 virus in surgical smoke generated during laparoscopy and the potential for virus transmission. The participants were women with suspected or documented gynecologic cancer (N = 17) undergoing laparoscopic procedures. All patients were tested and negative for COVID-19 prior to surgery. At the end of surgery, swabs of both the endotracheal tube and trocar valve filter were obtained and reverse-transcription PCR testing was performed. One patient's swab results both showed amplification on the N gene in reverse-transcription PCR testing. In another patient, positive amplification on the N gene was noted for the filter swab test. Amplification on the N gene is not specific for SARS-CoV-2 and may be positive for any coronavirus infection. No results showed amplification for the ORF1ab test, which is specific to the SARS-CoV-2 virus. The researchers concluded that there is a theoretical potential for transmission of the SARS-CoV-2 virus from surgical smoke generated during laparoscopic surgery.

The evidence conflicts as to whether pathogenic virus transfer occurs during excimer laser treatment of corneal tissue.[112,167,168] Hagen et al[167] developed a model system to test the possibility of virus transmission during excimer laser treatment through airborne excimer laser debris. The researchers used an excimer laser to ablate a culture plate infected with pseudorabies virus (ie, a porcine enveloped herpes virus similar in structure and lifecycle to HIV and the herpes simplex virus). In vitro transfer of viable pseudorabies virus by excimer laser plume did not appear to occur. The researchers concluded that the surgeon and team members are at low risk of infection from enveloped viruses (eg, HIV, herpes simplex) transmitted by the excimer laser plume.

In 1997, Taravella et al[168] used an excimer laser to ablate fibroblasts infected with attenuated varicella-zoster virus. The researchers collected the laser plume for PCR analysis and viral cultures. Their results suggested that viral DNA fragments remain intact after ablation but the virus particles capable of causing infection in the fibroblast culture do not. They concluded that attenuated varicella-zoster virus does not seem to survive excimer laser ablation, and further research is needed to determine whether other viruses could remain infectious after exposure to excimer laser radiation.

In a subsequent experimental study in 1999, Taravella et al[112] used an excimer laser to ablate fibroblasts infected with oral polio vaccine virus. The researchers collected the laser plume for viral cultures. The cultures were positive for the virus. The researchers also analyzed the role of virus size and its ability to remain infectious after excimer laser ablation. The oral polio virus is approximately 30 nm in size compared with 200 nm for the herpes virus family. The results suggested that smaller viruses might be able to escape ablation, whereas larger viruses may not. The researchers concluded that the oral polio virus can survive excimer laser ablation and that whether other viruses, such as HIV, can withstand ablation and remain infectious needs to be determined.

Bacterial Hazards

Capizzi et al[169] conducted a prospective study to analyze the potential bacterial and viral exposure to OR personnel from the laser smoke plume generated by CO_2 laser resurfacing. During 13 consecutive laser resurfacing procedures, the researchers captured the smoke plume using a smoke evacuator with a **high-efficiency particulate air (HEPA) filter**. Before the resurfacing procedures, the room air was filtered with the smoke evacuator. The HEPA filter served as the control. Two bacterial and two viral cultures were collected per filter. The bacterial cultures were incubated for 14 days if the results were negative, and the viral cultures were incubated for 28 days if the results were negative.

There was no growth from any of the viral cultures. Five patients had a bacterial culture that grew +1 coagulase-negative *Staphylococcus*. Two of these five cultures also had a concomitant bacterial growth of either *Corynebacterium* or *Neisseria*. The researchers concluded that viable bacteria exist within the smoke plume generated during laser resurfacing and additional research is needed to define the exposure risk associated with patients who have hepatitis, HIV, and antibiotic-resistant bacteria.[169]

Blood

Jewett et al[123] conducted a study to characterize the hemoglobin content by particle size of blood-containing aerosols generated by surgical power tools. Part of this study extends the work of Johnson and Robinson[5] described earlier. The researchers used two different protocols to generate aerosols. In a laboratory simulation of an OR, an oscillating bone saw, a high-speed air-driven drill, and a high-speed irrigating drill were used to "operate" on bone, and an ESU was used to cut and coagulate tendons. To simulate the blood present during surgery, blood was dripped onto the working area.

The researchers collected a sampling from each test condition in addition to a control sampling using distilled water instead of blood. The second protocol was the same as that described by Johnson and Robinson,[5] except the blood was not infected with HIV. All the instrumentation tested produced blood-containing aerosol particles in the respirable size range (< 5 μm). The researchers concluded that hemoglobin is an adequate marker of blood and therefore of bloodborne pathogens. The results suggest there is potential for breathing-zone exposure to respirable blood-containing particles during surgery performed with similar instrumentation. Additional research is needed in clinical settings.[123]

In a prospective, single-center trial, Ishihama et al[121] investigated whether blood-contaminated aerosols were present in a room where oral surgery procedures (N = 100) were performed with a high-speed drill. The sampling results were 76% positive in blood presumptive tests at 20 cm (7.9 inches) from the surgical site and 57% positive at 100 cm (39.4 inches) from the surgical site. The researchers concluded that these results suggest a risk for floating blood particles with the potential to cause airborne infection during use of high-speed instruments in oral surgery procedures.

In a subsequent study, Ishihama et al[122] used two protocols to investigate the presence of blood-contaminated aerosols in ORs during oral surgery procedures. For both protocols, the exhaust ducts of the central air-conditioning system were covered with a filter to collect the atmospheric samples. In the accumulation protocol, the researchers left the filters in place for 1, 2, and 4 weeks in one OR. In the second protocol, to analyze contributing factors, the test filters were changed after each surgical procedure. A leucomalachite green presumptive test for blood was used to test each filter. The researchers also collected additional data, including the type of procedure, the use of a high-speed rotating instrument or electric coagulator device, blood loss volume, and length of the procedure. In the accumulation protocol, the sites positive for blood increased from 26 after 1 week to 92 and 143 after 2 and 4 weeks, respectively.

There were sites positive for blood in 21 of 33 individual procedures. Factors contributing to a positive result for blood included use of a high-speed instrument (nine of 10 surgeries), use of an electric coagulator (16 of 17 surgeries), and use of a high-speed instrument or electric coagulator (20 of 21 surgeries). Factors contributing to a negative result for blood included use of no device (11 of 12 surgeries). The researchers discussed the lack of evidence of infection risk from inhalation of floating infectious materials. Most health care workers who contract an occupational infection cannot pinpoint a causative injury such as a mucous membrane exposure. The researchers recommended using caution, especially for personnel who remain in the OR for long periods (eg, anesthesia providers, surgical assistants).[122]

1.2.1 Determine the hazard exposure to the perioperative team according to the
- job descriptions and job tasks that place team members at risk,[17,170]
- types of procedures where surgical smoke is generated,[17]
- types of tissue involved in production of surgical smoke,[77,78]
- duration of surgical energy applied to tissues,[21,146]
- type of surgical energy devices used,[28,95,103,139]
- number of surgical energy devices used during a procedure,[17]
- availability of smoke management systems (eg, surgical smoke evacuation and filtration systems),[171] and
- availability of smoke evacuation disposable supplies (ie, smoke evacuator tubing, smoke evacuator filters, in-line filters, laparoscopic filters).[171]

[Recommendation]

1.3 Use the OSHA-endorsed CDC/NIOSH hierarchy of controls[170,172] to reduce the perioperative team's exposure to surgical smoke and establish safe practices, including
- eliminating the hazard (eg, avoiding use of smoke-generating surgical devices),[170]
- substituting the hazard (eg, using alternative devices),[170]
- using engineering controls (eg, surgical smoke evacuation and filtration, room ventilation of 20 total air exchanges per hour,[173] work practices),[37,170]
- using administrative controls (eg, policies and procedures, education and training),[170] and
- wearing PPE (ie, respiratory protection).[66,170,172]

[Recommendation]

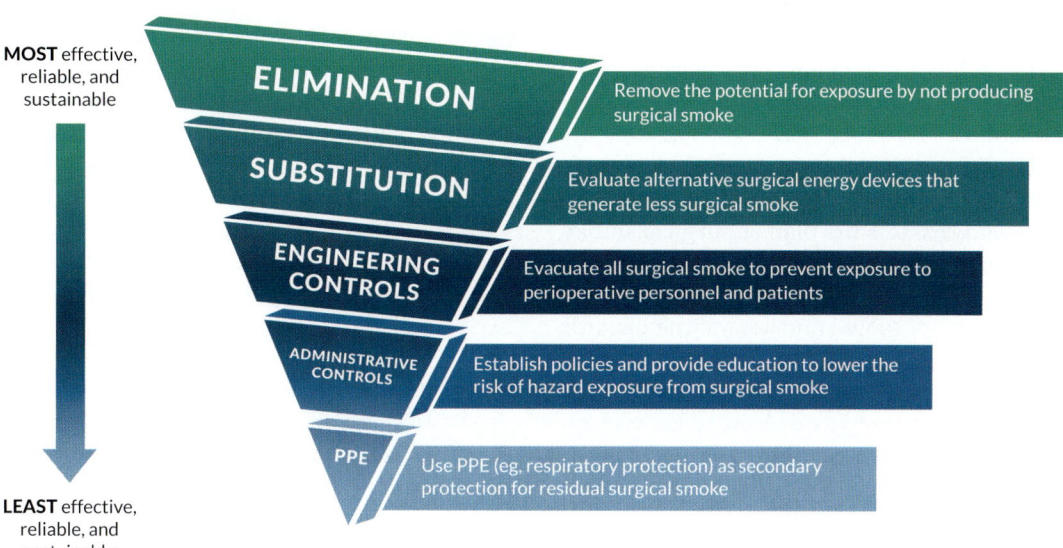

Figure 3. Surgical Smoke Hierarchy of Controls[1]

MOST effective, reliable, and sustainable

ELIMINATION — Remove the potential for exposure by not producing surgical smoke

SUBSTITUTION — Evaluate alternative surgical energy devices that generate less surgical smoke

ENGINEERING CONTROLS — Evacuate all surgical smoke to prevent exposure to perioperative personnel and patients

ADMINISTRATIVE CONTROLS — Establish policies and provide education to lower the risk of hazard exposure from surgical smoke

PPE — Use PPE (eg, respiratory protection) as secondary protection for residual surgical smoke

LEAST effective, reliable, and sustainable

Reference

1. Hierarchy of controls. The National Institute for Occupational Safety and Health. https://www.cdc.gov/niosh/topics/hierarchy/. Reviewed January 13, 2015. Accessed August 30, 2021.

Controlling exposures to hazards and toxic substances is the fundamental method of protecting workers. A hierarchy of controls is used as a means of determining how to implement feasible and effective controls. The CDC/NIOSH hierarchy of controls[172] is a systematic approach that can be used to identify the most effective method of risk reduction.[170] Where possible, elimination or substitution is the most effective, reliable, and sustainable approach followed by use of engineering controls **(Figure 3)**. Engineering controls are physical changes to the work environment that will minimize the health care worker's exposure to the hazard. Engineering controls include surgical smoke evacuation and filtration. Operating rooms require a minimum of 20 air exchanges per hour.[173] Administrative controls (eg, policies and procedures) are used in conjunction with the other controls that more directly reduce exposure to the hazard. The last line of defense is the use of PPE. Both OSHA and NIOSH identify PPE as likely the least effective, reliable, and sustainable method to control hazards. Personal protective equipment reduces exposure to the risks and is the last line of defense against exposure to surgical smoke when exposure cannot be managed through a higher level of control.

1.3.1 **When possible, use the highest level of control.[170] If the hazard (eg, surgical smoke) cannot be eliminated, employ the next level in the hierarchy.** [*Recommendation*]

1.3.2 **Use smoke evacuation and filtration (ie, local exhaust ventilation) in addition to room ventilation.** [*Recommendation*]

Because general room ventilation is insufficient to capture the contaminants, NIOSH recommends using a combination of ventilation techniques to control the airborne contaminants of surgical smoke.[37] Supporting evidence demonstrates that despite efficient room ventilation, surgical smoke ultrafine particles accumulated and peaked at > 100,000 particles/cm^3 within minutes.[85] Additionally, Romano et al[174] found that ventilation design may affect ultrafine particle air contamination; ORs equipped with downward unidirectional ventilation have greater removal of air contaminants than ORs with upward displacement ventilation, though ventilation alone cannot remove ultrafine particle air contamination.

In a subsequent study, Romano et al[175] further identified that downward unidirectional airflow with peripheral mixing systems (ie, hybrid ventilation) was more effective than upward displacement ventilation in reducing airborne contamination during various stages of surgery, although ESU use increased ultrafine particle concentrations regardless of the type of ventilation. The researchers concluded that local exhaust ventilation (eg, surgical smoke evacuation) should be used to reduce surgical smoke diffusion.

Seipp et al[176] found that surgical smoke evacuation efficiency in particle reduction is maximized when high unidirectional displacement flow is present. See the AORN Guideline for Sterile Technique for more information about unidirectional displacement airflow.[177]

1.4 In collaboration with the perioperative team, determine a surgical smoke safety plan before the procedure and reassess the plan as surgical smoke management needs change.[178] [Recommendation]

When surgical smoke is anticipated, all members of the surgical team should understand the plan for surgical smoke management and have the opportunity to provide input into the smoke safety plan and the need for possible respiratory protection prior to the start of the procedure.

1.4.1 The decision to evacuate or not evacuate surgical smoke should be a team decision and not be made at the discretion of an individual practitioner.[42] [Recommendation]

Moderate-quality evidence demonstrates that the patient and other perioperative team members are continually exposed to the hazards of surgical smoke. In a 5-day exposure study, Van Gestel et al[87] found that circulating RNs and scrub assistants may have more exposure to surgical smoke than surgeons, as evidenced by increased levels of VOCs in personal air samples and urine analysis.

In a workplace survey of nurses, anesthesia professionals, surgical technologists, and surgical assistants, 47% of 4,533 respondents reported that local exhaust ventilation (eg, smoke evacuation) was always used during laser surgery and only 14% reported that local exhaust ventilation was always used during electrosurgical procedures. Many reported that they felt they had no control over whether a smoke evacuator was used. The researchers concluded that smoke evacuation use should be a team decision since all members of the surgical team experience exposure to surgical smoke.[42]

1.5 Select and use smoke evacuation and filtration devices and accessories based on the type of procedure and amount of surgical smoke anticipated. [Recommendation]

1.5.1 A smoke evacuation decision tool may be used. [Conditional Recommendation]

A decision tool (**Figure 4**) for surgical smoke evacuation can assist with initial assessment and intraoperative reassessment of surgical smoke evacuation and filtration needs based on the type of procedure and anticipated amount of surgical smoke.[179]

1.6 An interdisciplinary team that includes one or more perioperative RNs, surgeons, anesthesia professionals, and scrub personnel should select surgical smoke safety equipment to be used in the perioperative setting. Additional team members may include an infection preventionist, engineers (eg, biomedical; heating, ventilation, and air conditioning [HVAC] systems), and a materials manager. [Recommendation]

Involvement of an interdisciplinary committee allows input from all departments in which the product will be used and from personnel with expertise beyond clinical end users (eg, infection preventionists, materials management personnel). The perioperative RN has a professional responsibility to consider "factors related to safety, effectiveness, efficiency, and the environment, as well as the cost in planning, delivering, and evaluating patient care."[180] Perioperative RNs play a crucial role in providing practical insight and expertise in the use and evaluation of surgical products.

1.6.1 In collaboration with the perioperative team, the surgical specialty physicians (eg, generalist, otorhinolaryngologist, plastic surgeon, urologist) should evaluate alternative surgical energy devices or techniques that generate less surgical smoke.[181] [Recommendation]

High-quality evidence indicates that bipolar instruments,[29,182,183] ultrasonic instruments,[28,29,95,184-186] vessel-sealing devices,[182] certain surgical techniques,[187,188] and use of lower energy settings[80,189,190] generate low amounts of surgical smoke.

High-quality evidence supports that ultrasonic devices produce less surgical smoke than electrosurgery. Choi et al[28] conducted a randomized controlled trial to compare surgical smoke and lateral thermal damage from two electrosurgical devices in patients undergoing laparoscopic hysterectomy. Patients were randomly assigned to either the ultrasonic device group (n = 20) or the monopolar electrosurgery group (n = 20). Via videorecording, two blinded gynecologic surgeons used a 5-point Likert scale (ie, 1 = very clear to 5 = extremely smoky) to independently measure surgical smoke by degree of visual obstruction. Lateral thermal damage from tissue samples was measured under a light microscope. A significant difference in lateral thermal damage was found between the monopolar electrosurgery group (1,500 μm) and the ultrasonic device group (950 μm). Additionally, the ultrasonic device group had a significantly lower

Figure 4. Smoke Evacuation and Filtration Decision Tool

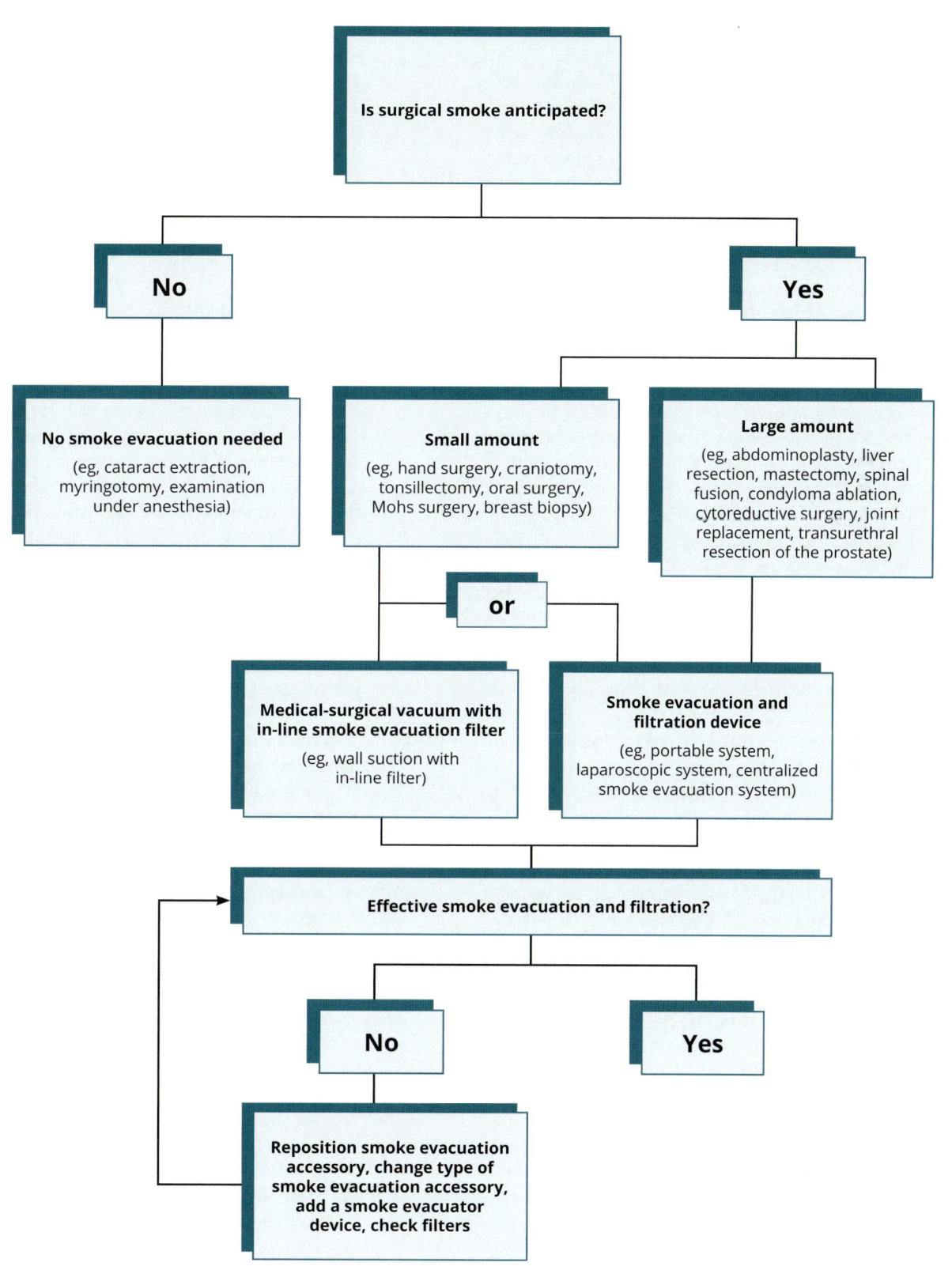

degree of visual obstruction from surgical smoke compared to the monopolar electrosurgery group. The researchers concluded that ultrasonic devices created less thermal tissue damage and less visible surgical smoke.

However, Tan et al[77] found that the concentration of fine particles was significantly higher in surgical smoke from ultrasonic scalpel use (531.28 +/- 71.58 µg/m³) compared to electrosurgical knife use (279.88 +/- 69.51 µg/m³) on liver tissue.

Moderate-quality evidence supports using lower energy settings to generate lower amounts of surgical smoke. Carr et al[189] conducted a cross-sectional study to examine the relationship between monopolar electrocautery settings and the use of surgical smoke evacuation via wall suction on surgical smoke particulate concentration during tonsillectomy procedures for pediatric patients (N = 36). Air samples were obtained from particle counters worn by the surgeons during four experimental conditions: electrocautery at 12 W with a smoke evacuation system, electrocautery at 20 W with a smoke evacuation system, electrocautery at 12 W without a smoke evacuation system, and electrocautery at 20 W without a smoke evacuation system (n = 9 patients in each group).

Analysis of variance revealed a significant difference in particle concentrations among the four groups. The mean particle concentration was highest at the 20 W energy setting without a smoke evacuation system (78,506 particles/cm³) compared to the 12 W energy setting without a smoke evacuation system (8,208 particles/cm³), the 20 W energy setting with a smoke evacuation system (5,515 particles/cm³), and the 12 W energy setting with a smoke evacuation system (1,661 particles/cm³). The mean electrocautery time ranged from 3.6 to 8.4 minutes and was not controlled for during the study. The researchers concluded that lower monopolar electrocautery energy settings and the use of smoke evacuation minimized the concentration of surgical smoke.[189]

Moderate-quality evidence demonstrates that despite the use of effective smoke evacuation and filtration, some chemicals from surgical smoke may remain above OSHA-established permissible exposure limits and NIOSH recommended exposure limits (REL). In an observational study, Ha et al[134] found that concentrations of formaldehyde remained above REL after filtration using built-in trocar filters. In a study using porcine tissue, Kocher et al[88] found that butadiene and benzene levels were decreased but remained above REL after use of a smoke evacua-

tor. Further, in an experimental simulated animal modeling study to measure the health effects of surgical smoke exposure to surgeons, Hui and Yan[107] demonstrated that use of smoke evacuators in a laminar flow ventilation OR decreased the height of the smoke plume, although standing in the area on both sides of the middle portion of the OR bed with exposure for 5 consecutive days significantly affected blood pH, oxygen saturation, and oxygen content with increased mean carboxyhemoglobin levels of 11.61% +/- 1.12%.

High-quality evidence conflicts on the use of nonstick electrocautery blades. In a high-quality experimental study, Kisch et al[187] found that Teflon-coated blades used during electrocautery created significantly less surgical smoke compared to stainless steel blades. Further, the use of both feedback electrocautery mode and Teflon-coated blades was associated with decreased amounts of surgical smoke. However, in a high-quality observational study, Cheng et al[22] found elevated average concentrations of hexamethyldisiloxane, the chemical used to coat nonstick electrosurgical tips, in breath samples (21.9 +/- 59.7 ppb) and in area samples (9.1 +/- 12.2 ppb) after occupational exposure to electrosurgical smoke during laparotomy/laparoscopy procedures. It was unclear whether the laparotomy/laparoscopy procedures involved coated blades.

1.6.2 **Evaluate surgical smoke evacuators and filters before purchase and use.**[191] *[Recommendation]*

Manufacturers use various technological approaches for surgical smoke management.

1.6.3 **Items to evaluate may include the**
- **equipment effectiveness and efficiency,**[171,191-193]
- **portability (eg, stationary, mobile),**[171]
- **type of filters (eg, prefilter, ultra-low particulate air [ULPA], activated carbon),**[171]
- **capture characteristics (eg, variable flow rate, capture velocity),**[171]
- **type of filtration method (eg, active, passive),**[171]
- **vacuum pressure (ie, less than 150 mm Hg),**[171]
- **noise level (ie, less than 60 A-weighted decibels [dBA]),**[171]
- **type of activation (eg, automatic, foot switch/foot pedal, hand switch),**[171]
- **type of filter monitoring system,**
- **type of equipment alarms and alerts (eg, audible, visual),**[171]
- **compatibility of products,**
- **dimensions of equipment,**

- adherence to industry standards,[191,194] and
- cost of equipment (eg, installation, operating cost) and disposable accessories (eg, tubing, filters).[171]

[Conditional Recommendation]

Combination filters offer many benefits.[64] A prefilter captures small amounts of liquid or tissue to protect the filter from debris or moisture damage.[191] A wet filter may lose effectiveness. The prefilter may be made of sponge or wire materials or may include a container, fluid drop out, or suction catheter.[191] The ULPA filter captures particles in surgical smoke with an overall particulate efficiency of not less than 99.999%.[194] The activated carbon filter adsorbs the gases (ie, VOCs) and odors in surgical smoke. Some manufacturers may include specialized filters that adsorb specific gases.[192]

The ECRI Institute[192] and NIOSH[37] recommend a minimum capture velocity of 100 ft to 150 ft per minute at the nozzle inlet, but the vacuum pressure should not exceed 150 mmHg. High vacuum pressures can cause damage to tissue.

A noise level of 60 dBA or louder can interrupt effective team communication during the procedure.[171] Seipp et al[176] tested efficiency and noise levels of five commercially available portable smoke evacuation systems. Sound levels ranged from 51 to 69 dBA during medium and maximum suction capacities.

Manufacturers determine the replacement method for filters. This may be based on the length of time the filter is used to filter surgical smoke or may be determined by a device to measure filter resistance.[192]

The AORN Guideline for Medical Device and Product Evaluation provides further guidance on developing and implementing a process for product evaluation and selection.[195]

1.6.4 **Medical devices that are intended to clear the visual field (eg, a surgical smoke precipitator) should be evaluated by the perioperative team before purchase and use.**[181] *[Recommendation]*

The surgical smoke precipitator utilizes electrostatic precipitation (ESP) technology to clear the visual field by negatively charging suspended smoke particles during laparoscopic surgery.[32,196] The device precipitates the charged particles onto the inner surface of the patient's peritoneum.[32,196] It is categorized by the US Food and Drug Administration (FDA) as a surgical smoke precipitator.[197]

The balance between the benefits and any potential harms of using surgical smoke precipitators for surgical smoke filtration remains unclear.

The benefits of ESP use during laparoscopic surgery can include clearing of the visual field,[32] reducing delays related to camera cleaning,[32] reducing bioaerosol concentrations in the abdominal cavity,[198] and facilitating lower-pressure surgery by maintaining insufflation pressure.[196] Researchers have noted that the use of electrostatic precipitation technology results in the retention of surgical smoke particulates inside the patient's abdominal cavity, although no adverse events were observed.[196,199] Experts highlight the usefulness of ESP technology as an adjunct to surgical smoke evacuation and filtration.[181,199]

High-quality evidence demonstrates the benefits of using ESP for visual clearing during laparoscopic surgery.[32,196,198] Ansell et al[32] performed a prospective double-blinded randomized controlled pilot study to evaluate the effectiveness of electrostatic precipitation in clearing the visual field during laparoscopic cholecystectomy. Thirty patients were randomly assigned to either the experimental condition of "device on" or the control of "device off." Operating surgeons and independent blinded reviewers rated visibility using a 5-point scale (ie, 1 = excellent to 5 = bad). The operating surgeons rated the mean visibility for the active device as 2.2 and 3.2 for controls. Independent blinded reviewers rated the mean visibility for the active device as 2.3 and 3.2 for controls. Effective visibility was 89.2% when the device was on and 71.2% when the device was off. Camera cleaning was not required in 85% of active cases and 35% of control cases. The researchers concluded that ESP improves visibility and reduces surgical delays related to camera cleaning and smoke clearing.

Buggisch et al[198] performed a laboratory study using porcine gallbladders and a simulated abdominal trainer to compare the efficacy of electrostatic aerosol precipitation (EAP) and continuous aerosol evacuation (CAE) in bioaerosol elimination during laparoscopic surgery. Bioaerosols were generated using monopolar and ultrasonic cutting energies. The researchers found a reduction in bioaerosol concentration with the use of EAP compared to CAE during the simulated surgery. The authors concluded that EAP is an efficient means to eliminate bioaerosols during laparoscopic surgery.

Levine et al[196] conducted a prospective blinded randomized controlled trial in women undergoing low pressure laparoscopic hysterectomy to evaluate the feasibility of using ESP to clear the visual field and reduce interruptions. Participants (N = 35) were randomly assigned to the experimental group (ESP) or the control group (no ESP). An additional third study group of five nonrandomized patients underwent myomectomy surgery with ESP. The investigator surgeon, who was blinded to group allocation, rated visibility from 1 (ie, excellent) to 5 (ie, bad). The investigator also rated the proportion of effective visibility during the surgery from 1 to 100. The researchers found a 42% improvement in visibility when ESP was used. Fewer procedural pauses were noted in the ESP group (ie, 1.5 per case) than in the no ESP group (3.7 per case). Low-pressure surgery was carried out in 87% of procedures with ESP compared to 53% without ESP. The researchers concluded that ESP can facilitate low-pressure laparoscopic hysterectomy by reducing procedural pauses and clearing the visual field.

Further research is needed to evaluate any potential harms of using ESP technology, including the possible ozone by-product levels when using surgical smoke precipitators,[181] efficiency of ESP in eliminating surgical smoke hazards (eg, viruses, chemicals), size characterization of eliminated particles during ESP use,[198] and patient effects when ESP technology is used (ie, whether precipitated chemical components of surgical smoke are absorbed by the patient) during laparoscopic procedures.

2. Smoke Evacuation and Filtration

2.1 Evacuate and filter all surgical smoke. *[Recommendation]*

High-quality evidence[11,17,42,44,75,77,79,96,101,118,189,200-202]; standards[203,204]; and guidance from NIOSH,[37] the Healthcare Infection Control Practices Advisory Committee,[205] accreditation agencies,[206] and professional organizations[38-41,207] indicate that evacuating and filtering surgical smoke protects patients and health care workers from the hazards of surgical smoke **(See Recommendation 1.2).**

Benson et al[75] observed levels of VOCs, PAHs, and ultrafine particles during live surgery with full-shift personal and area air sampling (n = 6) compared to background samples (n = 2) during a 3-day period. All surgeons used electrocautery surgical energy devices with combinations of local exhaust ventilation (ie, none, wall suction, smoke evacuator). The researchers detected 17 analytes in personal sampling; the most commonly occurring chemicals were 2-propanol, acetone, dichlorodifluoromethane, ethanol, fluorene, propene, and toluene. During breast reduction surgery, ultrafine particle concentrations when no smoke evacuator was used reached a full-shift average of 2,257 particles/cm^3 with 15-minute

maximums reaching 17,554 particles/cm^3 and 1-minute maximums reaching 21,951 particles/cm^3. When a smoke evacuator was used during a different breast reduction surgery, ultrafine particle concentrations reached a full-shift average of 773 particles/cm^3 with 15-minute maximums reaching 4,643 particles/cm^3 and 1-minute maximums reaching 7,011 particles/cm^3. The researchers found that smoke evacuator use was associated with decreased airborne ultrafine particle concentrations from electrocautery surgical smoke.

2.2 Use a smoke evacuation system (eg, portable smoke evacuator with filtration, medical-surgical vacuum with an in-line filter, centralized stationary smoke evacuation system) to evacuate and filter all surgical smoke. *[Recommendation]*

Using smoke evacuation systems to reduce potential acute and chronic health risks to health care personnel and patients is recommended by NIOSH.[37] The hazards of surgical smoke exposure to the perioperative team are respiratory, chemical, biologic (eg, blood, virus, bacteria), carcinogenic, mutagenic, and cytotoxic. Repeated exposure to the contents of surgical smoke may be cumulative,[24,126] which could increase the possibility of adverse effects.[96] Although exposure to surgical smoke may be brief, surgical smoke exposure risks to patients during minimally invasive procedures can include reduced visibility in the surgical field[28-31] with potential to delay the procedure,[32] possible port site metastasis,[12,33] exposure to carbon monoxide,[34-36] and increased levels of carboxyhemoglobin.[34,35] Risks to the patient during open procedures include potential respiratory inflammation[208] and postoperative refractive errors.[209]

Tokuda et al[101] conducted a prospective randomized study in Japan to investigate the effectiveness of surgical smoke evacuation in reducing nurses' and surgeons' occupational exposure to VOCs found in surgical smoke. The researchers measured environmental conditions (ie, total volatile organic compound [TVOC] levels, formaldehyde levels) at two locations within the OR (ie, near the OR bed, away from the OR bed) and personal exposure levels of OR personnel (ie, surgeons, surgical assistants, scrub nurses, circulating nurses, anesthetists) during breast surgery procedures performed with (n = 30) and without (n = 31) the use of surgical smoke evacuation, determined randomly. The analysis demonstrated that surgical smoke evacuation significantly lowered TVOC and formaldehyde concentrations at both locations. A multiple regression analysis revealed that the surgical smoke evacuator was a factor that significantly reduced personal exposure to formaldehyde and acetaldehyde for the entire team. The researchers concluded that surgical smoke evacuators are effective in reducing personal exposure to the hazards of surgical smoke.

Seipp et al[176] sought to evaluate efficiencies and noise levels of surgical smoke evacuation systems. They tested five commercially available smoke evacuation systems with corresponding electrosurgical pencils under various experimental conditions, including different electrocautery cutting angles (ie, 45 degrees, 90 degrees), device suction capacities (ie, minimum, medium, maximum), and room ventilation unidirectional displacement flow rates (ie, 7,500 m³/hour; 9,000 m³/hour; 10,500 m³/hour). A cutting angle of 45 degrees was found to have the most efficient particle reduction. The researchers found that maximum suction capacity was most efficient but had the highest sound pressure level (ie, 69 dBA).

Dobrogowski et al[96] conducted a study to identify and quantitatively measure selected chemical substances in surgical smoke and to assess the risk of the chemicals to medical personnel. The researchers collected air samples in the OR during laparoscopic cholecystectomy procedures. A complete qualitative and quantitative analysis of the samples showed the presence of aldehydes, benzene, toluene, ethylbenzene, xylene, ozone, and dioxins in concentrations lower than the hygienic standards used in the European Union. The researchers noted that the synergistic and antagonistic interactions of these substances have not been studied and are difficult to predict, and they concluded that surgical smoke should be evacuated to protect the OR team from the toxic and possibly carcinogenic, mutagenic, and genotoxic effects.

Moot et al[210] used selected ion flow tube mass spectrometry to analyze the composition of VOCs in diathermy plume produced during abdominal surgery. The researchers identified hydrogen cyanide, acetylene, and 1,3-butadiene in the plume. They concluded that although there is no evidence of adverse health effects from VOCs in surgical smoke plume, there is no evidence to indicate that it is safe to breathe smoke plume; thus, they recommended using smoke evacuators.

Hassan et al[211] conducted a prospective study to quantify the exposure of the surgeon and the patient to known chemical toxins in electrocautery smoke, and to determine whether there were qualitative or quantitative differences in exposure during laparoscopic or open ileal loop pouch anastomosis. The researchers measured the surgeon's exposure to benzene, toluene, xylene, acetone, and styrene. They tested the patient's blood preoperatively within 6 hours of surgery and at the end of the procedure for benzene, ethyl benzene, toluene, xylene, carboxyhemoglobin, and cyanide. During the laparoscopic procedures, a smoke filter was used to maintain visibility,

and during the open procedures, the electrocautery smoke was suctioned by the first assistant.

The samplings of the surgeon's exposure were all negative. The patients' preoperative and postoperative levels of cyanide, carbon monoxide, benzene, ethyl benzene, toluene, and xylene were below standard detectable levels in the laparoscopic and open procedures. The researchers concluded that the methods (ie, suction devices) used to remove smoke from the surgical field and the OR air exchanges of the HVAC system were effective and minimized exposure of the health care team and the patient to the chemicals in surgical smoke. The researchers further concluded that additional qualitative and quantitative studies of the contents of electrocautery smoke are needed as well as technology that more efficiently and effectively evacuates surgical smoke from the surgical site and the OR environment.[211]

Patient Health Effects

Moderate-quality evidence shows potential hazardous effects to patients from laser smoke exposure related to visual acuity during LASIK procedures and possible bronchial inflammation.[208,209]

Charles[209] retrospectively studied the effects of laser plume evacuation on laser in-situ keratomileusis (LASIK) outcomes in 199 patients (n = 82 with no evacuation, n = 117 with plume evacuation). There were no statistical differences in the frequency of corneal abrasion or flap slippage or the level of postoperative debris. A significant difference was noted in postoperative residual refractive error and uncorrected visual acuity. In the group with no plume evacuation, 90% had uncorrected visual acuity of 20/40 or better, 68% saw 20/25 or better, and 59% saw 20/20 or better. In the plume evacuation group, 96% had uncorrected visual acuity of 20/40 or better, 89% saw 20/25 or better, and 74% saw 20/20 or better. Charles concluded that using plume evacuation for LASIK procedures improved refractive and uncorrected visual acuity outcomes.

Freitag et al[208] investigated the harmful effects of surgical smoke inhalation for the patient and the OR team in an animal study. To simulate a single patient exposure of the respiratory system during a procedure, the researchers measured the effects of one 10-minute exposure on airway resistance, gas exchange, and mucociliary clearance rate in the trachea. To simulate the repetitive exposures of surgical smoke inhalation by the OR team, the researchers measured the effects of three separate 10-minute exposures on airway resistance, gas exchange, and mucociliary clearance rate in the trachea. They found a decrease in arterial partial pressure of oxygen after smoke inhalation. Tracheal mucous velocity was significantly depressed in a dose-dependent manner with increasing smoke exposure. Results of bronchoalveolar lavage showed smoke inhalation induced a severe inflammation with increases in inflammatory cells. The researchers concluded that the surgeons should be informed that inhalation of laser-generated smoke may cause transient hypoxia, depression of lung defense mechanisms, and delayed airway inflammation.

Patient Experience

High-quality evidence describes the effect of surgical smoke evacuation on the patient experience.[212,213]

Golda et al[212] conducted a single-blinded randomized controlled trial that included 160 adult patients undergoing Mohs micrographic surgery to compare smoke evacuation to no smoke evacuation on the patient experience. Patients were asked about their experience related to lights, smoke, and noise during surgery. The researchers found that patients in the smoke evacuation group noticed the smoke smell significantly less frequently than those in the control group. Further, patients in the smoke evacuation group were significantly less bothered by the smoke smell than patients for whom no smoke evacuator was used. They concluded that patients undergoing dermatologic procedures notice and are bothered by the surgical smoke smell and that the use of smoke evacuation may improve the patient experience.

In a comparative pilot study, Yonan and Ochoa[213] surveyed patients (N = 36) about their perception of electrosurgery smoke after undergoing Mohs surgery where smoke evacuation by wall suction was used during closure but not during Mohs staging. All patients (100%) reported perceiving a burning odor when smoke removal was not employed during Mohs staging compared to 40% who perceived a burning odor during closure. Moreover, 66.6% reported that the odor during Mohs staging was unpleasant. Only 16.6% of patients reported an unpleasant odor during closure when smoke was evacuated. The researchers concluded that smoke evacuation can create a more pleasant patient experience during Mohs surgery.

2.2.1 Use a smoke evacuator system that contains an ULPA filter with an activated carbon filter when surgical smoke is anticipated.[38,40,41,191,192,203] [Recommendation]

Electrosurgery generates the smallest aerodynamic size particles (< 0.07 μm to 0.1 μm); laser tissue ablation creates larger particles (~ 0.31 μm); and ultrasonic scalpels create the largest particles (0.35 μm to 6.5 μm).[1]

An ULPA filter demonstrates an efficiency of no less than 99.999% at a **most penetrating particle size** (MPPS) (eg, 0.12 μm).[192,194] Capture efficiency (%) and MPPS diameter (μm) of a filter are functions of straining, diffusion, inertial impaction, and interception. These mechanisms allow greater filter efficiencies for particles larger and smaller than the MPPS.[194,214]

Surgical energy devices applied to tissue produce by-products of toxic gaseous chemicals and vapors.[37,171,181,203,215,216] An activated carbon filter acts to adsorb odors and gases (eg, VOCs) in surgical smoke.[191,192,203]

2.2.2 When using a medical-surgical vacuum system, place an in-line ULPA filter with an activated carbon filter between the suction wall connection and the suction cannister.[40,41,192,203] [Recommendation]

An in-line ULPA filter captures airborne contaminants in surgical smoke.[192] Placement between the suction cannister and the wall connection prevents moisture from reaching the filter media. Surgical energy devices applied to tissue produce by-products of toxic gaseous chemicals and vapors.[37,171,181,203,215,216] An activated carbon filter acts to adsorb odors and gases (eg, VOCs) in surgical smoke.[191,192,203]

2.2.3 A medical-surgical vacuum system (ie, wall suction) with an in-line ULPA filter may be used to evacuate small amounts[192] of surgical smoke as defined by the health care organization's policy and procedures. [Conditional Recommendation]

Low suction flow rates associated with medical-surgical vacuum systems limit their efficiency in evacuating surgical smoke, making them suitable only for the evacuation of small amounts of smoke.[37,179,192,217]

2.2.4 An additional suction device may be needed to remove large amounts of fluid from the surgical field when a dual function system is being used (eg, a medical-surgical vacuum system with an in-line filter). [Conditional Recommendation]

2.3 Use smoke management equipment and accessories according to manufacturers' written instructions.[37,192,203] [Recommendation]

Manufacturers of medical devices provide specific instructions for use. This information includes safety information, device settings, applications for which the device is intended, filter change information, and the recommended distance of the capture device from the generation of surgical smoke.

2.4 **Position the smoke capture device (eg, wand, tubing) of a smoke evacuation system as close to the surgical site as necessary to maximize surgical smoke capture.** [Recommendation]

Standards[191,203] and guidance from NIOSH[37] and professional organizations[38-41] recommend that the surgical smoke capture device be kept as close as possible to the surgical site; NIOSH[37,218] recommends that the device be kept within 2 inches (5 cm) of the surgical site. Capture performance is affected by the smoke evacuator flow rate, distance of the evacuator nozzle to the surgical site, tubing size, and amount of smoke generated.[192] The ECRI Institute[192] and NIOSH[37] recommend a minimum capture velocity of 100 ft to 150 ft per minute at the nozzle inlet, but the vacuum pressure should not exceed 150 mmHg. High vacuum pressures can cause damage to tissue.

The choice of smoke evacuator capture device and its positioning related to the source of surgical smoke production can influence surgical smoke evacuation effectiveness. Liu et al[219] conducted a prospective study to compare two types of surgical smoke evacuator accessory capture devices (ie, a surgical smoke evacuation pencil and a para incisional capture device). Participants in both the surgical smoke evacuator group (n = 26) and the para incisional evacuator group (n = 25) underwent posterior spine surgery with electrocautery. The researchers measured the concentration of ultrafine particles including the average smoke level and the peak smoke level during surgery with and without smoke evacuator use. The average smoke reduction rate for both evacuator types was similar, although the peak smoke reduction rate was significantly greater for the para incisional evacuator (95.9%, range 57.9% to 98.7%) compared to the smoke evacuation pencil (75.3%, range 14.7% to 87.9%). The authors concluded that using surgical smoke evacuation that is optimized for the procedure, such as using a para incisional capture device for spine procedures, can significantly decrease the concentration of ultrafine particles.

In a randomized controlled trial, Pillinger et al[202] investigated whether a suction clearance device would reduce the amount of smoke reaching the surgeon's mask. All of the patients underwent either thyroid or parathyroid surgery with a standard anterior cervical collar incision and division of the strap muscles. The amount of smoke reaching the level of the surgeon's mask was measured with an aerosol monitor. Smoke evacuation was used for the patients in the experimental group (n = 15), and no smoke evacuation was used for the patients in the control group (n = 15). Baseline measurements were taken before the patients entered the OR, con-

tinuously during surgery, and postoperatively after the patients left the OR. Use of smoke extraction resulted in a significant reduction in the mean amount of smoke detected at the level of the surgeon's mask (control group 137 µg/m³; experimental group 12 µg/m³) and the maximum amount of smoke detected at the level of the surgeon's mask (control group 2,411 µg/m³; experimental group 255 µg/m³). Clearing the smoke improved visibility of the surgical field and reduced the characteristic diathermy smell. The researchers concluded that evacuation of surgical smoke is advisable.[202]

2.4.1 **If there is a detectable odor when a smoke evacuation system is in use, evaluate the smoke evacuation system to verify that**

- **smoke is being captured at the site where it is being generated,**
- **there is efficient air movement through the suction device,**
- **an activated charcoal filter is present, and**
- **the filter is within its useful life.**[191,192]

[Recommendation]

2.4.2 **If intraoperative smoke evacuation is ineffective or equipment is malfunctioning, adjustments for smoke evacuation and filtration may include**

- **repositioning the smoke evacuation accessory,**
- **changing the type of smoke evacuation accessory,**
- **switching from wall-suction with an in-line ULPA filter to a smoke evacuator device,**
- **adding an activated charcoal filter,**
- **replacing the filter, or**
- **adding a smoke evacuator device.**

[Conditional Recommendation]

2.4.3 **Activate the smoke evacuation system (eg, surgical smoke evacuator with ULPA filtration, medical-surgical vacuum with an in-line ULPA filter) at all times while surgical smoke is being generated.**[37,83,161] [Recommendation]

Surgical smoke concentration of fine particles accumulates to unhealthy levels within the first few seconds after surgical smoke production starts, and individuals closest to the site of surgical smoke generation are at the highest risk of exposure.[83] However, exposure to surgical smoke has been demonstrated for all members of the surgical team.[87]

2.5 **Use a surgical smoke management system during minimally invasive procedures.** *[Recommendation]*

In addition to possible perioperative staff risk of exposure to surgical smoke **(See Recommendation 1.2)**, high-quality evidence demonstrates that the risks of surgical smoke exposure to the patient during minimally invasive procedures may include

- reduced visibility of the surgical site during the procedure,[28-31]
- potential delays during the procedure,[32]
- absorption and excretion of smoke by-products (eg, carbon monoxide,[34-36] benzene,[220,221] carboxyhemoglobin[34,35]), and
- possible port site metastasis.[12,33]

Dobrogowski et al[221] assessed patients' exposure to organic substances identified in surgical smoke generated during laparoscopic cholecystectomy procedures. The researchers collected urine samples from 69 patients undergoing laparoscopic cholecystectomy procedures both before and after surgery and analyzed them for benzene, toluene, ethylbenzene, and xylene. Samples of the gases in the abdominal cavity were obtained from the trocar during the procedure for identification of the main chemical compounds. The researchers identified about 40 substances, such as aldehydes, unsaturated and saturated hydrocarbons, aromatic hydrocarbons, and dioxins. The concentrations of benzene and toluene were significantly higher in the urine samples after surgery compared with preoperative levels, indicating that the compounds were produced intraoperatively and absorbed into the blood. The postoperative levels of benzene, a known human carcinogen, were three times higher than before surgery (0.28 ± 0.045 versus 0.867 ± 0.143). The researchers concluded that the concentrations of the compounds in the urine were only a small percentage of the total absorbed dose. The mixture of the toxic compounds in the urine can significantly increase the overall toxicity potential caused by the interaction of the compounds. There is also a potential threat from carcinogenic compounds (eg, benzene) despite a short exposure time and low concentrations.

Takahashi et al[222] used an industrial smoke-detection device to evaluate the efficacy of an automatic smoke evacuator in eliminating surgical smoke in a laboratory-based animal study that included experimental surgery on six pigs. Smoke was generated with either a high-frequency ESU or laparoscopic coagulating shears. Ten laparoscopic surgeons independently and subjectively evaluated the laparoscopic field of view. The composition of the smoke was analyzed by mass spectrometry and more than 40 chemical compounds were identified in the smoke. The surgeons reported a superior field of view in the evacuation group compared with the control group at 15 seconds after activation of the ESU. The estimated volume of residual intraabdominal smoke after activation of the ESU was significantly lower in the smoke evacuation group. The researchers concluded that the use of an automatic smoke evacuator enhanced the field of view and reduced smoke exposure in experimental laparoscopic surgery.

The evidence is unclear about whether elevated blood[34,35,108,223,224] or intraperitoneal[35,108,223] levels of carbon monoxide absorbed by the patient pose a health risk. However, researchers agree that the use of smoke evacuation lowers the patient's exposure to carbon monoxide produced by surgical smoke during minimally invasive surgery.

In a prospective study, Nezhat et al[224] analyzed the blood samples of patients undergoing laparoscopic procedures with accompanying laser and bipolar ESU smoke generation. Carboxyhemoglobin concentrations were measured with gas chromatography. Preoperatively, the mean carboxyhemoglobin levels were 0.70 ± 0.15%, and postoperatively, the levels were 0.58 ± 0.20%. The decrease was statistically significant. The researchers concluded that carbon monoxide poisoning is not associated with laparoscopic procedures. They attributed the results to aggressive smoke evacuation that minimized the patients' exposure to carbon monoxide and to active elimination by ventilation with high oxygen concentrations.

To determine the absorption of carbon monoxide from the peritoneal cavity, Ott[34] measured patients' preoperative, intraoperative, and postoperative levels of carboxyhemoglobin. For the control group (n = 25), no lasers or smoke-generating devices were used during the laparoscopic procedure. For the experimental group (n = 25), lasers were used during the laparoscopic procedures. Patients were screened preoperatively for environmental or occupational sources of elevated carbon monoxide. The patients were evaluated for carbon monoxide levels before induction of anesthesia, periodically during the procedure, and postoperatively at 2, 3, 6, 12, and 24 hours.

The control group showed no statistical change between preoperative, intraoperative, and postoperative levels of carboxyhemoglobin. Significant elevation of carboxyhemoglobin was found in all 25 of the experimental group members at 10 minutes. The carboxyhemoglobin levels ranged from 2.8% to 18.5% saturation of whole blood and were elevated for as long as 16 hours after the end of the procedure. The patients with the highest postoperative levels had symptoms of carbon monoxide poisoning (eg, dizziness, nausea, headache, weakness).

Ott concluded that patients having laparoscopic procedures with a CO_2 laser were exposed to high levels of carbon monoxide and that smoke evacuation reduces the hazards of carbon monoxide absorption, decreases carboxyhemoglobin formation, and reduces the consequences of acute iatrogenic surgical carbon monoxide exposure resulting from laser-generated smoke during laparoscopic surgery.[34]

2.5.1 **Minimally invasive surgical smoke evacuation equipment may include trocars, tubing, or accessories with ULPA and activated carbon filtration.** *[Conditional Recommendation]*

Activated carbon filters in laparoscopic surgical smoke evacuation equipment reduce the levels of VOCs released during surgery. Moderate-quality evidence supports the effectiveness of built-in trocar filters.[90,134,225] Choi et al[90] studied the effectiveness of activated carbon fiber filters on volatile organic gas elimination during transperitoneal laparoscopic nephrectomy cases (n = 20). The researchers found the total elimination rate for VOCs was 86.49 +/- 2.83% with the activated carbon fiber filter, reducing calculated cancer risk for benzene, ethylbenzene, and styrene to negligible levels. In a small prospective study, Ha et al[134] found that built-in filter ports significantly reduced concentrations of xylene; benzene, toluene, ethyl benzene, and styrene; and butyraldehyde and isovaleraldehyde. Hahn et al[225] found significant removal rates of benzene, toluene, and butyraldehyde with the use of built-in filter trocars compared to use of nonfiltered trocars during laparoscopic rectal surgery.

2.5.2 **Do not release unfiltered surgical smoke into the OR during minimally invasive procedures.** *[Recommendation]*

2.5.3 **Before removal of trocars, the insufflation gas may be filtered using a mechanical exsufflation or a passive filtration method.**[55,56] *[Conditional Recommendation]*

Surgical smoke may contain potentially hazardous material, including viruses (eg, HBV,[8] HPV,[9] HIV[10]), viable cancer cells,[11-13] particles (ie, lung damaging dust of 5.0 µm and smaller),[14] blood fragments,[37] and bacteria.[15] Although no evidence exists that demonstrates the presence of SARS-CoV-2 in surgical smoke, experts agree that surgical teams should practice caution to minimize potential exposure.[55,56] Filtering insufflation gas before removal of trocars prevents possible perioperative team member exposure to surgical smoke contaminants.

2.6 **Used smoke evacuator filters, tubing, and wands must be handled using standard precautions, and disposed of as biohazardous waste.**[37,226] *[Regulatory Requirement]*

Surgical smoke contains potentially hazardous material, which can include viruses (eg, HBV,[8] HPV,[9] HIV),[10] potentially viable cancer cells,[11-13] particles (ie, lung damaging dust of 5.0 µm and smaller),[14] blood fragments,[37] and bacteria.[15]

3. Respiratory Protection

3.1 **Personal protective equipment used for respiratory protection should not be considered a replacement for effective surgical smoke evacuation and filtration.** *[Recommendation]*

According to the CDC/NIOSH hierarchy of controls, PPE is the least effective method for controlling exposures to occupational hazards such as surgical smoke.[172] Personal protective equipment is employed only after methods to remove or replace the hazard (eg, elimination and substitution) or practices to isolate the hazard with engineering controls (eg, surgical smoke evacuation and filtration) have been evaluated and implemented.[172] In addition, N95 filtering facepiece respirators do not provide protection against gases or vapors.[170]

3.2 **Wear PPE (ie, respiratory protection) as secondary protection against residual surgical smoke.** *[Recommendation]*

Standards,[203] regulations,[170] and guidance from professional organizations[38-41,207] recommend using PPE (eg, a fit-tested surgical N95 filtering facepiece respirator[170]) as secondary protection against the inhalation of residual surgical smoke. After considering removal of or substitution for the hazard of surgical smoke, general room ventilation and smoke evacuation (ie, local exhaust ventilation) are the next lines of protection against the hazards of surgical smoke.[37] When respiratory protection is required, the minimum respiratory protection device is a filtering facepiece respirator (eg, surgical N95 facepiece respirator).[66,170]

A fit-tested surgical N95 filtering facepiece respirator is a personal protective device that is worn on the face, covers the nose and mouth, and is used to reduce the wearer's risk of inhaling hazardous airborne particles including infectious agents.[14] The NIOSH respirator approval regulation defines the term *N95* as a filter class that removes at least 95% of airborne particles during "worse case" testing using a "most-penetrating" sized particle.[227] Filters meeting the criteria are given a 95 rating. Many filtering facepiece respirators have an N95 class filter, and those meeting this filtration performance are often referred to simply as "N95 respirators."[227] A surgical N95 filtering facepiece respirator is fluid resistant on the outside to protect the wearer from splashes or sprays of body fluids.[170]

3.2.1 **A surgical mask must not be considered respiratory protection.**[170] *[Regulatory Requirement]*

A surgical mask is a loose-fitting face mask intended to prevent the release of potential contaminants from the user into their immediate environment and does not meet the requirements to be classified as respiratory protection.[14,170] A surgical mask is fluid resistant, providing protection from large droplets, sprays, and splashes of body fluids[14] but does not give the wearer a reliable level of protection against inhaling small airborne particles.[170,228] Additionally, surgical masks do not effectively filter VOCs found in surgical smoke, such as 1,3-butadiene, benzene, and furfural.[88] A high-filtration surgical face mask is designed to filter particulate matter that is 0.1 µm in size and larger. Similar to a surgical mask, a high-filtration mask does not create a seal between the face and the mask and may allow dangerous contaminants to enter the health care worker's breathing zone.[14,229]

High-quality evidence demonstrates that there is measurable superiority in protection provided by a surgical N95 respirator compared with high-filtration and surgical masks.[228,230-234]

Gao et al[228] investigated the performance of two surgical masks and two surgical N95 respirators during exposure to surgical smoke. Ten participants were fit tested for the N95 respirators before the experiment. The participants performed surgical dissections on animal tissue in a simulated OR with an electrocautery device to generate surgical smoke. Each of the participants wore each of the four types of masks or respirators in random order. The generated surgical smoke was sampled in the breathing zone directly outside the mask or respirator to represent the inhalation exposure of an unprotected individual and inside the mask or respirator to represent the inhalation exposure of a protected wearer.

The aerosol concentrations and particle size distribution of the inside- and outside-sampled aerosols were measured for 12 minutes each with a particle size spectrometer in combination with an optical particle counter. The simulated workplace protection factor (SWPF) was calculated for the masks and respirators. The SWPF values for both surgical masks were close to 1, indicating essentially no protection. The SWPF values for both N95 respirators exceeded 100, the OSHA fit-test passing level. The results suggest that surgical masks cannot protect health care workers against surgical smoke but that N95 NIOSH-certified respiratory protection devices can.[228]

High-quality evidence demonstrates that surgical masks have inadequate filter performance for aerosols[235,236] and submicron particles.[228,229]

Rengasamy et al[229] investigated the filtration performance of surgical masks for a wide size range of submicron particles, including the size of many viruses. Masks cleared by the FDA can be categorized into three barrier types: high, moderate, and low. High and moderate barrier masks are cleared with > 98% bacterial filtration efficiency and particle filtration efficiency. Low barrier masks require > 95% for bacterial filtration efficiency only. The researchers tested five models of FDA-cleared surgical masks (n = 1 high barrier type, n = 2 moderate barrier type, and n = 2 low barrier type) for room air particle penetrations under constant and cyclic flow conditions. The following tests were performed:

- room air particle penetration at constant flow condition,
- room air particle penetration as a function of particle size,
- particle penetration measurement at cyclic flow conditions,
- polydisperse sodium chloride aerosol penetration measurement,
- monodisperse aerosol test method, and
- effect of isopropanol treatment on monodisperse aerosol penetrations.

Results of this study showed a wide variation in filtration performance. The researchers concluded that the wide variation in penetration levels for room air particles, which included particles in the viruses size range, confirms that surgical masks should not be used as respiratory protection.[229]

Oberg and Brosseau[237] evaluated nine types of surgical masks for filtration performance and facial fit. The types included surgical, laser, and procedure masks that were cupped, flat, and duckbilled with ties and ear loops. The masks' filter efficiency varied from very low to high. Facial fit was evaluated quantitatively and qualitatively. When filter performance and facial fit were evaluated, none of the surgical masks met the qualifications of respiratory protection devices.

See the AORN Guideline for Transmission-Based Precautions for guidance on respiratory protection during aerosol-generating procedures and procedures on patients with known or suspected aerosol transmissible infections (eg, tuberculosis, varicella, rubeola, SARS-CoV-2).[66]

3.3 **Wear respiratory protection (eg, a surgical N95 filtering facepiece respirator) in conjunction with smoke evacuation and filtration when participating in procedures using smoke-generating surgical devices on tissue containing HPV.[161]**
[Recommendation]

High-quality evidence supports that surgical smoke from HPV lesions treated with lasers[9,114,115] or electrosurgery[9,115] may have the potential for transmission during exposure. Observational studies identified the presence of HPV DNA in surgical smoke from cervical LEEP surgery.[116,117] Possible cases of HPV transmission through surgical smoke have been reported, resulting in laryngeal and oropharyngeal squamous cell carcinoma.[25-27]

Some researchers have not detected HPV DNA in surgical smoke,[238] indicating that further research is needed to examine the transmissibility of HPV in surgical smoke. However, experts agree that HPV transmission remains plausible and that smoke evacuation and respiratory protection should be employed during high-risk procedures.[9,114,115,161]

3.4 **For open smoke-generating procedures involving the liver, respiratory protection (eg, a surgical N95 filtering facepiece respirator) may be worn in conjunction with smoke evacuation and filtration.**
[Conditional Recommendation]

High-quality evidence supports that concentrations of fine and ultrafine particulate matter in surgical smoke from liver tissue are high compared to other tissue.[77,78]

Tan et al[77] quantified fine particle concentrations in surgical smoke produced during surgery on hemihepatectomy patients (n = 50) and tested various mask filtering capabilities. Fine particle concentrations were collected at the head height of the surgeon during electrosurgical knife use on different tissues including adipose, muscle, and liver tissues and blood vessels. Also tested during surgical smoke production was the filtering effectiveness of three types of masks: a single-layer medical mask, a double-layer medical mask, and a surgical particulate respirator (ie, an N95 filtering facepiece respirator). Additionally, the researchers measured and compared fine particle concentrations in surgical smoke during ultrasonic scalpel use and electrosurgical knife use on liver tissue in an additional sample of hemihepatectomy patients (n = 20).

Of the different tissues studied, liver tissue produced the highest fine particle concentration in surgical smoke, significantly higher than surgical smoke from other tissues **(Table 3).** The N95 respirator demon-

Table 3. Fine Particle Concentration in Surgical Smoke in Different Types of Tissue

Tissue Type	Fine Particle[a] Concentration (µg/m³)
Liver	303.10 +/- 108.95
Muscle	110.07 +/- 50.47
Adipose	46.89 +/- 20.39
Blood vessel	8.35 +/- 6.87

[a] Fine particle (PM2.5) = particles 2.5 µm and smaller

Reference
1. Tan W, Zhu H, Zhang N, et al. Characterization of the PM2.5 concentration in surgical smoke in different tissues during hemihepatectomy and protective measures. *Environ Toxicol Pharmacol.* 2019;72:103248.

strated the best protection capacity, reducing fine particle concentration by about 75%. Finally, the results demonstrated that when used on liver tissue, the ultrasonic scalpel produced a significantly higher average concentration of fine particles, reaching 531.28 +/- 71.58 µg/m³, compared to the electrosurgical knife concentration of 279.88 +/- 69.51 µg/m³. The researchers concluded that medical masks do not provide protection, and that use of surgical smoke evacuators and surgical particulate respirators should be considered.[77]

Karjalainen et al[78] evaluated particulate matter characteristics of electrosurgical smoke produced from porcine tissue samples (N = 10) of different types (ie, skeletal muscle, liver, subcutaneous fat, renal pelvis, renal cortex, lung, bronchus, cerebral matter [gray and white], and skin), all of which were taken from the same animal. The researchers then estimated health implications for OR personnel by calculating the airway deposition fractions for the upper airways, bronchial tube, and the alveoli from the measured aerosol particle mass distributions. Concentrations and aerodynamic size distribution of particles were measured in 10 samples from each tissue type. Liver tissue was found to have the highest concentration of particulate matter (PM_{10} = 9,100 mg/m³, $PM_{2.5}$ = 1,100 mg/m³, $PM_{1.0}$ = 470 mg/m³) with the greatest overall calculated mass that could be deposited to the alveoli among OR personnel **(Table 4).** The researchers concluded that tissue types could be separated into three distinct groups related to the particulate matter and potential risk of exposure to the surgical team:
- high-PM tissues with high exposure risk (ie, liver),
- medium-PM tissues with moderate risk (ie, renal cortex, renal pelvis, muscle), and
- low-PM tissues with low risk (ie, skin, cerebral matter, bronchus, subcutaneous fat).

Table 4: Concentration and Type of Particulate Matter in Different Types of Tissue

Tissue Type	Total PM$_{10}$ Particles[a] (mg/m³)	PM$_{2.5}$ Particles[b] (mg/m³)	PM$_1$ Particles[c] (mg/m³)
Liver	9,100	1,100	470
Muscle	3,000	370	150
Renal cortex	2,500	330	140
Renal pelvis	2,400	300	130
Grey matter	760	100	47
Bronchus	720	100	52
Skin	370	61	34
White matter	370	52	25
Lung	210	29	14
Adipose	210	28	12

[a] particles 10 µm and smaller (PM$_{10}$)

[b] particles 2.5 µm and smaller (PM$_{2.5}$)

[c] particles 1 µm and smaller (PM$_1$)

Reference

1. Karjalainen M, Kontunen A, Saari S, et al. The characterization of surgical smoke from various tissues and its implications for occupational safety. PLoS One. 2018;13(4):e0195274.

Statistical modeling extrapolation revealed that medium-PM and high-PM tissue particle concentration 1-hour exposure without smoke removal remained in the "very high" air quality index, ranging from 110 µg/m³ to 1,700 µg/m³. They concluded that assuming general purpose surgical suction could decrease particulate exposure by 50% and a smoke evacuator could decrease exposure by up to 88%, estimated air quality indices remained "very high" in high-PM tissue even with smoke evacuation. The researchers recommended the use of surgical smoke evacuation and particulate filtration masks for surgery on high-PM and medium-PM tissue, especially for personnel at the surgical field.[78]

3.5 Notify OR team members that respiratory protection is being used as secondary protection from surgical smoke during an operative or other invasive procedure (eg, post signs at the OR entrance).[239] [Recommendation]

Surgical smoke has the potential to reach all areas of the OR.[107] Notifying team members that respiratory protection is being used supports effective team communication and allows team members to don appropriate PPE prior to entering the OR.

3.6 No recommendation can be made regarding occupational HPV vaccination for personnel who participate in surgical smoke-generating procedures involving tissue containing oncogenic HPV (eg, HPV-16, HPV-18). [No Recommendation]

No evidence exists as to whether occupational HPV vaccination would provide protection for OR personnel who participate in surgical smoke–generating procedures involving tissue containing oncogenic HPV types (eg, HPV-16, HPV-18). The CDC currently does not provide HPV vaccination recommendations for health care workers,[240] although clinical trials are underway.[241] Further research is needed to determine the benefits and harms of HPV vaccination for health care workers.

Refer to the AORN Guideline for Transmission-Based Precautions for guidance on health care worker vaccination for the perioperative area.[66]

4. Education

4.1 **Provide initial and ongoing education to and verify competency of perioperative team members for surgical smoke safety.** [Recommendation]

Initial and ongoing education of perioperative team members facilitates the development of knowledge, skills, and attitudes that affect safe patient care and workplace safety. The health care organization is responsible for providing initial and ongoing education and verifying the competency of its personnel; however, the primary responsibility for maintaining ongoing competency remains with the individual.[180]

Competency verification activities provide a mechanism for competency documentation and help verify that perioperative team members understand the hazards of surgical smoke, evacuation methods, proper equipment usage, and disposal of used tubing and filters.

High-quality evidence from observational studies,[42,44-47,242] literature reviews,[15,149,216,243] expert opinion articles,[55,244,245] and organizational experience reports[246-249] supports interdisciplinary education for surgical smoke safety.

4.1.1 **Establish intervals for education and competency verification related to surgical smoke safety practices.** [Recommendation]

4.2 **Include the following in interdisciplinary education and competency verification related to surgical smoke safety:**
- **the health effects of surgical smoke exposure on health care workers and patients;**
- **the definition of surgical smoke (ie, vaporous and gaseous by-product of the use of surgical energy devices);**
- **critical factors for managing surgical smoke for all procedures that generate surgical smoke;**
- **sources of surgical smoke (eg, lasers, ESUs, ultrasonic devices, high-speed drills, burrs, saws);**
- **the effect of particle size on the speed and distance smoke travels;.**
- **selecting smoke management systems and supplies (eg, ESU pencils with incorporated evacuation tubing, trocars with built-in filters, in-line ULPA filters, smoke evacuator units)** in accordance with the procedure being performed (eg, by using a decision tool);
- **applying the CDC/NIOSH hierarchy of controls to surgical smoke safety, including**
  - **elimination (physically removing the hazard),**
  - **substitution (replacing the hazard),**
  - **engineering controls (isolating people from the hazard),**
  - **administrative controls (changing the way people work), and**
  - **PPE (protecting the worker with protective equipment);**
- **testing smoke management equipment before the procedure;**
- **connecting equipment according to the manufacturer's instructions for use;**
- **using smoke evacuation equipment according to the manufacturer's instructions for use;**
- **using standard precautions to handle used smoke evacuation supplies and discarding biohazardous waste;**
- **policies and procedures related to smoke evacuation; and**
- **participation in quality improvement programs related to the management of surgical smoke as assigned.**

[Recommendation]

The evidence indicates there is a lack of knowledge among perioperative team members regarding surgical smoke. Steege et al[42] conducted a web-based survey of members of professional organizations representing health care occupations in which there is routine contact with selected chemical agents, including surgical smoke. Laser surgery and electrosurgery were addressed in separate submodules of the survey. Eligible respondents (N = 4,533) worked within 5 ft of surgical smoke generation during electrosurgery (99%) or laser surgery (31%). The respondents were nurse anesthetists (33%), perioperative nurses (19%), physician anesthesiologists (21%), surgical technologists (16%), and others (11%). In response to questions about training, 49% of the respondents to the survey laser submodule and 44% of the respondents to the electrosurgery submodule reported that they had never received training on the hazards of surgical smoke.

4.3 **Provide education to and verify competency of perioperative team members before new smoke management systems and accessories are introduced.**[191] [Recommendation]

Receiving education and completing competency verification activities in advance of a change helps ensure safe practice and adherence to surgical smoke management practices.

5. Policies and Procedures

5.1 Develop policies and procedures for surgical smoke safety, review them periodically, revise them as necessary, and make them readily available in the practice setting in which they are used. *[Recommendation]*

Policies and procedures regarding surgical smoke safety provide guidance to perioperative team members for creating an environment that reduces the exposure of patients and the perioperative team to surgical smoke. Policies and procedures assist in the development of patient safety, workplace safety, quality assessment, and performance improvement activities. Policies and procedures also serve as operational guidelines used to minimize patients' and perioperative team members' risk for injury or complications, standardize practice, direct personnel, and establish continuous performance improvement programs. Policies and procedures establish authority, responsibility, and accountability within the practice setting. Having policies and procedures in place that guide and support patient care, treatment, and services is a regulatory requirement.[250-253]

5.2 Include the following in policies and procedures for surgical smoke safety:

- evacuating all surgical smoke generated by surgical energy devices (eg, ESUs, lasers, ultrasonic scalpels/dissectors) during operative or other invasive procedures;
- selecting a smoke management system and supplies (eg, ESU pencils with smoke evacuator tubing, in-line ULPA filters, smoke evacuator units, minimally invasive filtering equipment) based on the procedure being performed;
- using a smoke evacuator with a 99.999% efficient filter (eg, an ULPA filter) and activated carbon filter or a medical-surgical vacuum system with an in-line ULPA filter and activated carbon filter in place between the suction wall connection and the suction canister to evacuate small amounts of surgical smoke;
- positioning the smoke capture device (eg, wand, tubing) as close to the surgical site as necessary to effectively collect surgical smoke;
- activating the smoke evacuator at all times when surgical smoke is produced during surgical procedures;
- using a smoke management system during minimally invasive procedures;
- handling used smoke evacuator filters, tubing, and wands as potentially infectious waste by using standard precautions and disposing of these items as biohazardous waste;
- wearing respiratory protective equipment as secondary protection against residual surgical smoke;
- knowing the criteria (eg, procedure type) for use of a suction tubing with an in-line ULPA filter to evacuate a small amount of surgical smoke and the indications to convert to using a smoke evacuator with larger tubing and suction capacity; and
- defining education and competency verification requirements.

[Recommendation]

5.3 Include procedures for reporting instances of health problems associated with surgical smoke exposure (eg, reporting to the occupational health department) in the policy. *[Recommendation]*

The potential hazards of surgical smoke exposure to the perioperative team are respiratory, biologic (eg, blood, virus, bacteria), carcinogenic, chemical, cytotoxic, and mutagenic. Repeated exposure to the contents of surgical smoke increases the possibility of developing adverse effects (Table 5).

At the request of several health care organizations,[254-258] the Hazard Evaluation and Technical Assistance Branch of NIOSH conducted field investigations of possible health hazards associated with surgical smoke in the workplace. At the Laser Institute at the University of Utah Health Sciences Center in Salt Lake City[255]; Inova Fairfax Hospital in Falls Church, Virginia[256]; Morton Plant Hospital in Dunedin, Florida[257]; and Carolinas Medical Center in Charlotte, North Carolina,[258] NIOSH tested the air for chemicals commonly found in surgical smoke and surveyed employees about heath symptoms associated with surgical smoke exposure. At Inova Fairfax Hospital, Morton Plant Hospital, and the Carolinas Medical Center, formaldehyde, acetaldehyde, and toluene were present in the air. The levels of the compounds were below the relevant criteria for occupational exposure.

Of the employees surveyed at the hospitals, the range of at least one symptom associated with surgical smoke exposure was 36% to 52%. In the hospitals tested, 33% to 46% of the employees described eye and upper respiratory irritation. The NIOSH investigators recommended that the health care organization's management team implement engineering controls during smoke-producing procedures and that the employees report instances of health symptoms associated with surgical smoke exposure to the organization's occupational health personnel. At the Laser Institute at the University of Utah Health Sciences Center, the investigators found detectable levels of ethanol, isopropanol, anthracene, formaldehyde, cyanide, and airborne mutagenic substances. They recommended the use of smoke evacuators to minimize the potential for health effects and improve visualization of the surgical field.[254-258]

Ball[24] conducted a web-based survey in a sample of 777 perioperative RN participants to understand the association between key indicators and compliance with recommendations for smoke evacuation. Reported respiratory problems included

- nasal congestion (32.8%),
- increased coughing (24.7%),
- allergies (24.2%),
- sinus infection or problems (22.9%),
- asthma (10.9%), and
- bronchitis (9%).

The prevalence results indicated that perioperative RNs reported twice the incidence of some respiratory problems compared to the general population.[24]

Asdornwised et al[44] surveyed 377 OR nurses in Thailand to assess practices regarding smoke evacuation. Results demonstrated a lack of adherence to recommended surgical smoke evacuation practices and a lack of consistent training, although respondents reported having knowledge about the hazards of surgical smoke. The researchers also surveyed participants on perceived health effects. Headache was reported most frequently followed by sore throat, coughing/sneezing, weakness, and eye irritation. Also reported were nausea/dizziness, chronic bronchitis, and asthma with low severity scores (< 3 on a scale of 1 to 7). Only 11.9% of the respondents stated that they "always" complied with guidelines for surgical smoke protection.

Ilce et al[45] conducted a descriptive study in Turkey to investigate symptoms of surgical smoke exposure reported by nurses (n = 45) and physicians (n = 36). Both physicians and nurses reported headache, watering eyes, cough, throat burning, nausea, drowsiness, dizziness, and sneezing. Nurses reported headache (48.9%) and cough (48.9%) most frequently; physicians reported headache (58.3%) most frequently, with 50% reporting "other" symptoms including irritability, respiratory tract infection, weakness, myalgia, dermatitis, conjunctivitis, anemia, cardiovascular disease, nasopharyngeal lesion, abdominal pain, or vomiting. Though study participants had knowledge of smoke evacuation, only 13.3% of nurses and no physicians reported using smoke evacuation.

5.4 Include procedures for reporting injuries or failures with smoke evacuator devices that potentially affect patient or staff safety. [*Recommendation*]

Table 5. Health Effects of Surgical Smoke Exposure

- Acute and chronic inflammatory respiratory changes (eg, emphysema, asthma, chronic bronchitis)
- Anemia
- Anxiety
- Carcinoma
- Cardiovascular dysfunction
- Colic
- Dermatitis
- Eye irritation
- Headache
- Hepatitis
- Hypoxia or dizziness
- Lacrimation
- Leukemia
- Lightheadedness
- Nasopharyngeal lesions
- Nausea or vomiting
- Sneezing
- Throat irritation
- Weakness

Reference

1. Alp E, Bijl D, Bleichrodt RP, Hansson B, Voss A. Surgical smoke and infection control. J Hosp Infect. 2006;62(1):1-5.

From Ulmer BC. The hazards of surgical smoke. AORN J. 2008;87(4): 721-734. *Adapted with permission.*

5.4.1 The health care organization must report any suspected device-related serious injury or death to the FDA and the manufacturer, or only to the FDA if the manufacturer is unknown.[259] [*Regulatory Requirement*]

The FDA provides specific guidance for device mandatory reporting.[259]

5.4.1 The health care organization may report device malfunction to the FDA.[259] [*Conditional Recommendation*]

The FDA provides specific guidance for voluntary reporting for near miss events and other device concerns.[259]

6. Quality

6.1 Participate in a variety of quality assurance and performance improvement activities that are consistent with the health care organization's plan to improve understanding and compliance with the principles and processes of surgical smoke evacuation. *[Recommendation]*

Quality assurance and performance improvement programs assist in evaluating and improving the quality of patient care and workplace safety and in formulating plans for corrective action. These programs provide data that may be used to determine whether an organization is within its benchmark goals and, if not, to identify areas that may require corrective action.

6.2 Include assessment of compliance with surgical smoke evacuation in the quality assurance and performance improvement program for surgical smoke safety. Compliance indicators include

- surgical smoke is evacuated with a smoke evacuation system, a laparoscopic filter, or suction with an in-line filter during all smoke-generating procedures;
- the smoke evacuation capture device is positioned as close as possible to the generation of surgical smoke to effectively collect all traces of the smoke;
- smoke evacuation filters are used according to manufacturer's instructions for use (eg, single use, all day);
- perioperative team members wear PPE (eg, gloves) when disposing of contaminated filters and smoke supplies; and
- perioperative team members adhere to policies and procedures for smoke evacuation.

[Recommendation]

Moderate-quality evidence indicates there is a lack of compliance with surgical smoke evacuation and respiratory protection.[24,42-51] Steege et al[42] conducted a web-based survey of members of professional organizations representing health care occupations in which there is routine contact with selected chemical agents including surgical smoke. Laser surgery and electrosurgery were addressed in separate submodules of the survey. Eligible respondents (N = 4,533) worked within 5 ft of surgical smoke generation during electrosurgery (99%) or laser surgery (31%). The respondents were nurse anesthetists (33%), perioperative nurses (19%), anesthesiologists (21%), surgical technologists (16%), and others (11%). Only 47% of the respondents reported always using local exhaust ventilation during laser procedures and 14% reported always using local exhaust ventilation during electrosurgery.

Reasons reported for not using local exhaust ventilation included that it was not provided by the employer, the smoke exposure was minimal, and use of local exhaust ventilation was not part of the facility's protocol. Respondents also wrote in answers in the "other" category, and the majority responded that they did not know why local exhaust ventilation was not used and that they had no control over the decision to use local exhaust ventilation. The authors concluded that the decision to use local exhaust ventilation should not be made at the discretion of an individual practitioner when others (eg, anesthesia personnel, nurses) will be exposed to surgical smoke. The survey results provide a valuable snapshot of existing practices and can be used to raise awareness of surgical smoke controls.[42]

6.2.1 Measure smoke evacuation practices by direct observation. *[Recommendation]*

6.2.2 Other measures to evaluate smoke evacuation practices when direct observation is not feasible may include product usage or documentation of smoke evacuation in the perioperative patient record. *[Conditional Recommendation]*

6.3 Identify barriers to implementing surgical smoke evacuation and filtration in the perioperative setting and address them through interventions to improve smoke safety practices. *[Recommendation]*

Barriers to implementing smoke evacuation can include

- unreliable or inefficient smoke evacuator equipment,[24]
- unavailability of smoke evacuator equipment or supplies,[24]
- lack of support to evacuate surgical smoke,[24]
- noisy smoke evacuator equipment,[24]
- equipment that is difficult to use (eg, bulky, uncomfortable,[42] inconvenient[24]),
- cost of smoke evacuator equipment,[24]
- knowledge gaps,[24,42] and
- competency deficits (eg, equipment use).[24,42]

Identifying barriers to smoke safety practices allows the health care organization to develop relevant interventions to improve surgical smoke evacuation.

6.4 Identify barriers to wearing recommended PPE (ie, respiratory protection) in the perioperative setting when indicated as secondary protection against residual surgical smoke, and address them through interventions to improve compliance. *[Recommendation]*

Barriers to wearing recommended respiratory protection can include

- no respiratory protection indications in the smoke evacuation policy,
- perception of low exposure potential,
- unavailability of appropriate PPE,
- discomfort or difficulty during use, and
- competency deficits.[47]

Addressing barriers to wearing appropriate PPE (ie, respiratory protection) supports a safe work environment.

6.5 When performing preventive maintenance for a centralized stationary smoke evacuation system, inspect and clean the smoke evacuator lines according to the manufacturer's instructions.[191] *[Recommendation]*

A centralized stationary smoke evacuation system is permanently installed in mechanical spaces and provides evacuation to several points of use. The filtered air is exhausted outside of the building. Regular maintenance and inspection of the smoke evacuator lines prevents particulate matter buildup or contamination of the suction line.[191]

Glossary

Adsorb: To collect molecules (eg, volatile organic compounds) in a thin layer on the surface of another substance. An example is the activated carbon filter that adsorbs and neutralizes odors and gases in surgical smoke.

Aldehydes: Organic compounds containing the hydridooxidocarbon (CHO) radical. Examples are acetaldehyde and formaldehyde.

Aromatic hydrocarbon: Any of a class of hydrocarbon molecules that have multiple carbon rings and that include carcinogenic substances and environmental pollutants.

High-efficiency particulate air (HEPA) filter: A filter that demonstrates an overall particulate efficiency of not less than 99.99%. Manufacturers report filtering efficiencies based on standardized validation and testing procedures; therefore, reported filtering qualities (ie, particulate efficiency, most penetrating particle size) may vary slightly.

Hydrogen cyanide: A poisonous, usually gaseous compound, also known as hydrocyanic acid (HCN), that has the odor of bitter almonds and boils at 25.6° C (78.1° F).

Inorganic gases: Gases that do not contain carbon and hydrogen as the principle elements (eg, carbon monoxide, carbon dioxide, sulphur dioxide, nitrous oxide, nitrogen dioxide).

Laser-generated airborne contaminants: Particles, toxins, and steam produced by vaporization of target tissues.

Lung-damaging dust: Categorization of particles smaller than 5 µm that can penetrate to the deepest areas of the lung and obstruct gas exchange.

Most penetrating particle size: The particle diameter that allows maximum penetration through the filter medium.

Nitriles: Organic compounds that contain a cyanide group – cyanide bound to an alkyl group.

Smoke: The visible vapors and gases given off by a burning or smoldering substance, especially of organic origin, made visible by the presence of small particles of carbon.

Surgical smoke: The vaporous and gaseous by-product of burning organic material created as a result of the destruction of tissue by lasers, electrosurgical units, ultrasonic devices, powered instruments, and other heat-producing surgical tools. Surgical smoke can contain toxic gases and vapors such as benzene, hydrogen cyanide, formaldehyde, bioaerosols, dead and live cellular material including blood fragments, and viruses. At high concentrations, surgical smoke causes ocular and upper respiratory tract irritation in health care workers and creates obstructive visual problems for the surgeon. Surgical smoke has unpleasant odors and has been shown to have mutagenic potential. Synonyms: surgical plume, laser-generated airborne contaminants.

Surgical smoke precipitator: A class II medical device intended to clear the visual field by electrostatic precipitation of surgical smoke and other aerosolized particulate matter created during laparoscopic surgery.

Ultrafine particles: Airborne particles measuring ≤ 0.1 µm in aerodynamic diameter. Other terms include nanoparticles or $PM_{0.1}$. Concentration is measured in particles/cm³.

Ultra-low particulate air (ULPA) filter: A filter that demonstrates an overall particulate efficiency of not less than 99.999%. Manufacturers report filtering efficiencies based on standardized validation and testing procedures; therefore reported filtering qualities (ie, particulate efficiency, most penetrating particle size) may vary slightly. Synonym: ultra-low penetration air filter.

Volatile organic compounds: Carbon-based chemicals that evaporate easily.

References

1. Ulmer BC. The hazards of surgical smoke. *AORN J.* 2008;87(4):721-734. [VB]

2. Vortman R, McPherson S, Cecilia Wendler M. State of the science: a concept analysis of surgical smoke. *AORN J.* 2021;113(1):41-51. [VA]

3. Ott DE. Proposal for a standard for laser plume filter technology. *J Laser Appl.* 1994;6(2):108-110. [VB]

4. Mayo-Yánez M, Calvo-Henríquez C, Lechien JR, Fakhry N, Ayad T, Chiesa-Estomba CM. Is the ultrasonic scalpel recommended in head and neck surgery during the COVID-19 pandemic? State-of-the-art review. *Head Neck.* 2020;42(7):1657-1663. [VB]

5. Johnson GK, Robinson WS. Human immunodeficiency virus-1 (HIV-1) in the vapors of surgical power instruments. *J Med Virol.* 1991;33(1):47-50. [IIA]

6. Mihashi S, Jako GJ, Incze J, Strong MS, Vaughan CW. Laser surgery in otolaryngology: interaction of CO_2 laser and soft tissue. *Ann N Y Acad Sci.* 1976;267(1):263-294. [IIIC]

7. Tomita Y, Mihashi S, Nagata K, et al. Mutagenicity of smoke condensates induced by CO_2-laser irradiation and electrocauterization. *Mutat Res.* 1981;89(2):145-149. [IIB]

8. Kwak HD, Kim SH, Seo YS, Song K-J. Detecting hepatitis B virus in surgical smoke emitted during laparoscopic surgery. *Occup Environ Med.* 2016;73(12):857-863. [IIIC]

9. Fox-Lewis A, Allum C, Vokes D, Roberts S. Human papillomavirus and surgical smoke: a systematic review. *Occup Environ Med.* 2020;77(12):809-817. [IIIB]

10. Baggish MS, Poiesz BJ, Joret D, Williamson P, Refai A. Presence of human immunodeficiency virus DNA in laser smoke. *Lasers Surg Med.* 1991;11(3):197-203. [IIA]

11. In SM, Park DY, Sohn IK, et al. Experimental study of the potential hazards of surgical smoke from powered instruments. *Br J Surg.* 2015;102(12):1581-1586. [IIA]

12. Fletcher JN, Mew D, Descôteaux JG. Dissemination of melanoma cells within electrocautery plume. *Am J Surg.* 1999;178(1):57-59. [IIB]

13. Nahhas WA. A potential hazard of the use of the surgical ultrasonic aspirator in tumor reductive surgery. *Gynecol Oncol.* 1991;40(1):81-83. [VB]

14. Benson SM, Novak DA, Ogg MJ. Proper use of surgical N95 respirators and surgical masks in the OR. *AORN J.* 2013;97(4):457-470. [VA]

15. Addley S, Quinn D. Surgical smoke—what are the risks? *Obstet Gynaecol.* 2019;21(2):102-106. [VB]

16. Schultz L. An analysis of surgical smoke plume components, capture, and evacuation. *AORN J.* 2014;99(2):289-298. [VB]

17. Ragde SF, Jørgensen RB, Føreland S. Characterisation of exposure to ultrafine particles from surgical smoke by use of a fast mobility particle sizer. *Ann Occup Hyg.* 2016;60(7):860-874. [IIB]

18. Bratu AM, Petrus M, Patachia M, Dumitras DC. Carbon dioxide and water vapors detection from surgical smoke by laser photoacoustic spectroscopy. *UPB Sci Bull Series A.* 2013;75(2):139-146. [IIB]

19. Gianella M, Hahnloser D, Rey JM, Sigrist MW. Quantitative chemical analysis of surgical smoke generated during laparoscopic surgery with a vessel-sealing device. *Surg Innov.* 2014;21(2):170-179. [IIB]

20. Laser/electrosurgery plume. Occupational Safety and Health Administration. https://www.osha.gov/laser-electro-surgery-plume. Accessed August 30, 2021. [VA]

21. Eshleman EJ, LeBlanc M, Rokoff LB, et al. Occupational exposures and determinants of ultrafine particle concentrations during laser hair removal procedures. *Environ Health.* 2017;16(1):30. [IIC]

22. Cheng NY, Chuang HC, Shie RH, Liao WH, Hwang YH. Pilot studies of VOC exposure profiles during surgical operations. *Ann Work Expo Health.* 2019;63(2):173-183. [IIIB]

23. Anderson M, Goldman RH. Occupational reproductive hazards for female surgeons in the operating room: a review. *JAMA Surg.* 2020;155(3):243-249. [VA]

24. Ball K. Surgical smoke evacuation guidelines: compliance among perioperative nurses. *AORN J.* 2010;92(2):e1-e23. [IIIB]

25. Rioux M, Garland A, Webster D, Reardon E. HPV positive tonsillar cancer in two laser surgeons: case reports. *J Otolaryngol Head Neck Surg.* 2013;42(1):54. [VB]

26. Calero L, Brusis T. Laryngeal papillomatosis—first recognition in Germany as an occupational disease in an operating room nurse [Article in German]. *Laryngorhinootologie.* 2003;82(11):790-793. [VB]

27. Hallmo P, Naess O. Laryngeal papillomatosis with human papillomavirus DNA contracted by a laser surgeon. *Eur Arch Otorhinolaryngol.* 1991;248(7):425-427. [VB]

28. Choi C, Do IG, Song T. Ultrasonic versus monopolar energy-based surgical devices in terms of surgical smoke and lateral thermal damage (ULMOST): a randomized controlled trial. *Surg Endosc.* 2018;32(11):4415-4421. [IB]

29. Weld KJ, Dryer S, Ames CD, et al. Analysis of surgical smoke produced by various energy-based instruments and effect on laparoscopic visibility. *J Endourol.* 2007;21(3):347-351. [IIB]

30. Khoder WY, Stief CG, Fiedler S, et al. In-vitro investigations on laser-induced smoke generation mimicking the laparoscopic laser surgery purposes. *J Biophotonics.* 2015;8(9):714-722. [IIA]

31. Loukas C, Georgiou E. Smoke detection in endoscopic surgery videos: a first step towards retrieval of semantic events. *Int J Med Robot.* 2015;11(1):80-94. [IIIB]

32. Ansell J, Warren N, Wall P, et al. Electrostatic precipitation is a novel way of maintaining visual field clarity during laparoscopic surgery: a prospective double-blind randomized controlled pilot study. *Surg Endosc.* 2014;28(7):2057-2065. [IB]

33. Nduka CC, Monson JR, Menzies-Gow N, Darzi A. Abdominal wall metastases following laparoscopy. *Br J Surg.* 1994;81(5):648-652. [VC]

34. Ott DE. Carboxyhemoglobinemia due to peritoneal smoke absorption from laser tissue combustion at laparoscopy. *J Clin Laser Med Surg.* 1998;16(6):309-315. [IIB]

35. Wu JS, Luttmann DR, Meininger TA, Soper NJ. Production and systemic absorption of toxic byproducts of tissue combustion during laparoscopic surgery. *Surg Endosc.* 1997;11(11):1075-1079. [IIB]

36. Esper E, Russell TE, Coy B, Duke BE 3rd, Max MH, Coil JA. Transperitoneal absorption of thermocautery-induced carbon monoxide formation during laparoscopic cholecystectomy. *Surg Laparosc Endosc.* 1994;4(5):333-335. [IIB]

37. Control of smoke from laser/electric surgical procedures (DHHS [NIOSH] Publication No 96-128). The National Institute for Occupational Safety and Health. 1996. Accessed August 30, 2021. [IVB]

38. IFPN guideline for surgical plume (IFPN statement 1012). International Federation of Perioperative Nurses. https://www.ifpn.world/resources/education-tools. Accessed August 30, 2021. [IVB]

39. Standard: surgical plume. In: Murphy C, ed. Standards for *Perioperative Nursing in Australia: Clinical Standards.* Vol 1. 16th ed. Adelaide, South Australia: Australian College of Operating Room Nurses; 2020. [IVB]

40. AST standards of practice for use of electrosurgery. 2012. Association of Surgical Technologists. https://www.ast.org/uploadedfiles/main_site/content/about_us/standard%20electrosurgery.pdf. Accessed August 30, 2021. [IVB]

41. AST guidelines for best practices in laser safety. 2019. Association of Surgical Technologists. https://www.ast.org/uploadedFiles/Main_Site/Content/About_Us/Standard%20Laser%20Safety.pdf. Accessed August 30, 2021. [IVB]

42. Steege AL, Boiano JM, Sweeney MH. Secondhand smoke in the operating room? Precautionary practices lacking for surgical smoke. *Am J Ind Med.* 2016;59(11):1020-1031. [IIIA]

43. Steege AL, Boiano JM, Sweeney MH. NIOSH health and safety practices survey of healthcare workers: training and awareness of employer safety procedures. *Am J Ind Med.* 2014;57(6):640-652. [IIIB]

44. Asdornwised U, Pipatkulchai D, Damnin S, Chiswangwatanakul V, Boonsripitayanon M, Tonklai S. Recommended practices for the management of surgical smoke and bio-aerosols for perioperative nurses in Thailand. *J Perioper Nurs.* 2018;31(1):33-41. [IIIA]

45. Ilce A, Yuzden GE, Yavuz van Giersbergen M. The examination of problems experienced by nurses and doctors associated with exposure to surgical smoke and the necessary precautions. *J Clin Nurs.* 2017;26(11-12):1555-1561. [IIIB]

46. Michaelis M, Hofmann FM, Nienhaus A, Eickmann U. Surgical smoke-hazard perceptions and protective measures in German operating rooms. *Int J Environ Res Public Health.* 2020;17(2):515. [IIIB]

47. Wizner K, Nasarwanji M, Fisher E, Steege AL, Boiano JM. Exploring respiratory protection practices for prominent hazards in healthcare settings. *J Occup Environ Hyg.* 2018;15(8):588-597. [IIIB]

48. Oganesyan G, Eimpunth S, Kim SS, Jiang SI. Surgical smoke in dermatologic surgery. *Dermatol Surg.* 2014;40(12):1373-1377. [IIIB]

49. Spearman J, Tsavellas G, Nichols P. Current attitudes and practices towards diathermy smoke. *Ann R Coll Surg Engl.* 2007;89(2):162-165. [IIIB]

50. Edwards BE, Reiman RE. Comparison of current and past surgical smoke control practices. *AORN J.* 2012;95(3):337-350. [IIIB]

51. Edwards BE, Reiman RE. Results of a survey on current surgical smoke control practices. *AORN J.* 2008;87(4):739-749. [IIIB]

52. Gavin DJ, Wilkie BD, Tay J, Loveday BPT, Furlong T, Thomson BNJ. Assessing the risk of viral infection from gases and plumes during intra-abdominal surgery: a systematic scoping review. *ANZ J Surg.* 2020;90(10):1857-1862. [VB]

53. Bogani G, Ditto A, De Cecco L, et al. Transmission of SARS-CoV-2 in surgical smoke during laparoscopy: a prospective, proof-of-concept study. *J Minim Invasive Gynecol.* 2021;28(8):1519-1525. [IIIB]

54. Moletta L, Pierobon ES, Capovilla G, et al. International guidelines and recommendations for surgery during COVID-19 pandemic: a systematic review. *Int J Surg.* 2020;79:180-188. [VA]

55. Francis N, Dort J, Cho E, et al. SAGES and EAES recommendations for minimally invasive surgery during COVID-19 pandemic. *Surg Endosc.* 2020;34(6):2327-2331. [IVA]

56. Porter J, Blau E, Gharagozloo F, et al. Society of Robotic Surgery review: recommendations regarding the risk of COVID-19 transmission during minimally invasive surgery. *BJU Int.* 2020;126(2):225-234. [IVA]

57. Alqadi GO, Saxena AK. Smoke and particulate filters in endoscopic surgery reviewed during COVID 19 pandemic. *J Ped Endo Surg.* 2020;2(2):61-67. [VA]

58. Mintz Y, Arezzo A, Boni L, et al. The risk of COVID-19 transmission by laparoscopic smoke may be lower than for laparotomy: a narrative review. *Surg Endosc.* 2020;34(8):3298-3305. [VA]

59. Pavan N, Crestani A, Abrate A, et al. Risk of virus contamination through surgical smoke during minimally invasive surgery: a systematic review of the literature on a neglected issue revived in the COVID-19 pandemic era. *Eur Urol Focus.* 2020;6(5):1058-1069. [VA]

60. Pini Prato A, Conforti A, Almstrom M, et al. Management of COVID-19-positive pediatric patients undergoing minimally invasive surgical procedures: systematic review and recommendations of the Board of European Society of Pediatric Endoscopic Surgeons. *Front Pediatr.* 2020;8:259. [VA]

61. Vourtzoumis P, Alkhamesi N, Elnahas A, Hawel JE, Schlachta C. Operating during COVID-19: is there a risk of viral transmission from surgical smoke during surgery? *Can J Surg.* 2020;63(3):E299-E301. [VA]

62. Zakka K, Erridge S, Chidambaram S, et al; PanSurg Collaborative Group. Electrocautery, diathermy, and surgical energy devices: are surgical teams at risk during the COVID-19 pandemic? *Ann Surg.* 2020;272(3):e257-e262. [VB]

63. [COVID-19] Considerations for smoke evacuation during non-deferrable surgery [ECRI exclusive hazard report]. Health Devices Alerts. ECRI. https://www.ecri.org/Components/Alerts/Pages/TrackingUser/AlertDisplay.aspx?AId=1643206&entryID=2&Page=AlertDisplay. Published May 18, 2020. Accessed August 30, 2021. [VA]

64. Mowbray NG, Ansell J, Horwood J, et al. Safe management of surgical smoke in the age of COVID-19. *Br J Surg.* 2020;107(11):1406-1413. [VA]

65. Van den Eynde J, De Groote S, Van Lerberghe R, Van den Eynde R, Oosterlinck W. Cardiothoracic robotic assisted

surgery in times of COVID-19. *J Robot Surg.* 2020;14(5):795-797. [VB]

66. Guideline for transmission-based precautions. In: *Guidelines for Perioperative Practice.* Denver, CO: AORN, Inc; 2021:1097-1126. [IVA]

67. Interim infection prevention and control recommendations for healthcare personnel during the coronavirus disease 2019 (COVID-19) pandemic. Centers for Disease Control and Prevention. https://www.cdc.gov/coronavirus/2019-ncov/hcp/infection-control-recommendations.html. Updated February 23, 2021. Accessed August 30, 2021. [IVA]

68. OSHA General Duty Clause. Occupational Safety and Health Administration.. https://www.osha.gov/laws-regs/oshact/section5-duties. Accessed August 30, 2021.

69. Occupational Safety and Health Act of 1970. Occupational Safety and Health Administration. https://www.osha.gov/laws-regs/oshact/completeoshact. Accessed August 30, 2021.

70. Galassi T. OSHA requirements for smoke plume generated from laser and electrosurgical instruments in dental offices and hospital operating rooms [Standards interpretations]. October 7, 2016. Accessed August 30, 2021. [VB]

71. 29 CFR 1910.132. General requirements. Electronic Code of Federal Regulations. https://www.ecfr.gov/cgi-bin/retrieveECFR?gp=1&SID=22f04ddbddca6fe30d5f2073f85ab334&ty=HTML&h=L&mc=true&n=pt29.5.1910&r=PART#se29.5.1910_1132. Accessed August 30, 2021.

72. 29 CFR 1910.134. Respiratory protection. Electronic Code of Federal Regulations. https://www.ecfr.gov/cgi-bin/retrieveECFR?gp=1&SID=22f04ddbddca6fe30d5f2073f85ab334&ty=HTML&h=L&mc=true&n=pt29.5.1910&r=PART#se29.5.1910_1134. Accessed August 30, 2021.

73. 29 CFR 1910.1000 Air contaminants. Electronic Code of Federal Regulations. https://www.ecfr.gov/cgi-bin/retrieveECFR?gp=1&SID=22f04ddbddca6fe30d5f2073f85ab334&ty=HTML&h=L&mc=true&r=SECTION&n=se29.6.1910_11000. Accessed August 30, 2021.

74. State plans. Occupational Safety and Health Administration. https://www.osha.gov/stateplans. Accessed August 30, 2021.

75. Benson SM, Maskrey JR, Nembhard MD, Unice KM, Shirley MA, Panko JM. Evaluation of personal exposure to surgical smoke generated from electrocautery instruments: a pilot study. *Ann Work Expo Health.* 2019;63(9):990-1003. [IIB]

76. Sisler JD, Shaffer J, Soo JC, et al. In vitro toxicological evaluation of surgical smoke from human tissue. *J Occup Med Toxicol.* 2018;13(1):12. [IIIB]

77. Tan W, Zhu H, Zhang N, et al. Characterization of the PM2.5 concentration in surgical smoke in different tissues during hemihepatectomy and protective measures. *Environ Toxicol Pharmacol.* 2019;72:103248. [IIA]

78. Karjalainen M, Kontunen A, Saari S, et al. The characterization of surgical smoke from various tissues and its implications for occupational safety. *PLoS One.* 2018;13(4):e0195274. [IIIB]

79. Li CI, Pai JY, Chen CH. Characterization of smoke generated during the use of surgical knife in laparotomy surgeries. *J Air Waste Manag Assoc.* 2020;70(3):324-332. [IIIB]

80. Andréasson SN, Anundi H, Sahlberg B, et al. Peritonectomy with high voltage electrocautery generates higher levels of ultrafine smoke particles. *Eur J Surg Oncol.* 2009;35(7):780-784. [IIB]

81. Taravella MJ, Viega J, Luiszer F, et al. Respirable particles in the excimer laser plume. *J Cataract Refract Surg.* 2001;27(4):604-607. [IIB]

82. Pierce JS, Lacey SE, Lippert JF, Lopez R, Franke JE. Laser-generated air contaminants from medical laser applications: a state-of-the-science review of exposure characterization, health effects, and control. *J Occup Environ Hyg.* 2011;8(7):447-466. [VB]

83. Wang HK, Mo F, Ma CG, et al. Evaluation of fine particles in surgical smoke from an urologist's operating room by time and by distance. *Int Urol Nephrol.* 2015;47(10):1671-1678. [IIB]

84. Farrugia M, Hussain SY, Perrett D. Particulate matter generated during monopolar and bipolar hysteroscopic human uterine tissue vaporization. *J Minim Invasive Gynecol.* 2009;16(4):458-464. [IIA]

85. Brüske-Hohlfeld I, Preissler G, Jauch KW, et al. Surgical smoke and ultrafine particles. *J Occup Med Toxicol.* 2008;3:31. [IIB]

86. DesCoteaux JG, Picard P, Poulin EC, Baril M. Preliminary study of electrocautery smoke particles produced in vitro and during laparoscopic procedures. *Surg Endosc.* 1996;10(2):152-158. [IIB]

87. Van Gestel EAF, Linssen ES, Creta M, et al. Assessment of the absorbed dose after exposure to surgical smoke in an operating room. *Toxicol Lett.* 2020;328:45-51. [IIIB]

88. Kocher GJ, Sesia SB, Lopez-Hilfiker F, Schmid RA. Surgical smoke: still an underestimated health hazard in the operating theatre. *Eur J Cardiothorac Surg.* 2019;55(4):626-631. [IIB]

89. Markowska M, Krajewski A, Maciejewska D, Jeleń H, Kaczmarek M, Stachowska E. Qualitative analysis of surgical smoke produced during burn operations. *Burns.* 2020;46(6):1356-1364. [IIB]

90. Choi SH, Choi DH, Kang DH, et al. Activated carbon fiber filters could reduce the risk of surgical smoke exposure during laparoscopic surgery: application of volatile organic compounds. *Surg Endosc.* 2018;32(10):4290-4298. [IIB]

91. Petrus M, Bratu AM, Patachia M, Dumitras DC. Spectroscopic analysis of surgical smoke produced in vitro by laser vaporization of animal tissues in a closed gaseous environment. *Rom Rep Phys.* 2015;67(3):954-965. [IIA]

92. Weston R, Stephenson RN, Kutarski PW, Parr NJ. Chemical composition of gases surgeons are exposed to during endoscopic urological resections. *Urology.* 2009;74(5):1152-1154. [IIB]

93. Zhao C, Kim MK, Kim HJ, Lee SK, Chung YJ, Park JK. Comparative safety analysis of surgical smoke from transurethral resection of the bladder tumors and transurethral resection of the prostate. *Urology.* 2013;82(3):744.e9-744.e14. [IIB]

94. Bratu AM, Petrus M, Patachia M, et al. Quantitative analysis of laser surgical smoke: targeted study on six toxic compounds. *Rom J Phys.* 2015;60(1-2):215-227. [IIA]

95. Fitzgerald JEF, Malik M, Ahmed I. A single-blind controlled study of electrocautery and ultrasonic scalpel smoke plumes in laparoscopic surgery. *Surg Endosc.* 2012;26(2):337-342. [IIA]

96. Dobrogowski M, Wesolowski W, Kucharska M, et al. Health risk to medical personnel of surgical smoke produced during laparoscopic surgery. *Int J Occup Med Environ Health.* 2015;28(5):831-840. [IIIB]

97. Lin YW, Fan SZ, Chang KH, Huang CS, Tang CS. A novel inspection protocol to detect volatile compounds in breast surgery electrocautery smoke. *J Formos Med Assoc.* 2010;109(7):511-516. [IIIB]

98. Wu YC, Tang CS, Huang HY, et al. Chemical production in electrocautery smoke by a novel predictive model. *Eur Surg Res.* 2011;46(2):102-107. [IIB]

99. Al Sahaf OS, Vega-Carrascal I, Cunningham FO, McGrath JP, Bloomfield FJ. Chemical composition of smoke produced by high-frequency electrosurgery. *Ir J Med Sci.* 2007;176(3):229-232. [IIB]

100. Lee T, Soo JC, LeBouf RF, et al. Surgical smoke control with local exhaust ventilation: experimental study. *J Occup Environ Hyg.* 2018;15(4):341-350. [IIC]

101. Tokuda Y, Okamura T, Maruta M, et al. Prospective randomized study evaluating the usefulness of a surgical smoke evacuation system in operating rooms for breast surgery. *J Occup Med Toxicol.* 2020;15:13. [IB]

102. Yeganeh A, Hajializade M, Sabagh AP, Athari B, Jamshidi M, Moghtadaei M. Analysis of electrocautery smoke released from the tissues frequently cut in orthopedic surgeries. *World J Orthop.* 2020;11(3):177-183. [IIIC]

103. Krones CJ, Conze J, Hoelzl F, et al. Chemical composition of surgical smoke produced by electrocautery, harmonic scalpel and argon beaming—a short study. *Eur Surg.* 2007;39(2):118-121. [IIA]

104. Claudio CV, Ribeiro RP, Martins JT, Marziale MHP, Solci MC, Dalmas JC. Polycyclic aromatic hydrocarbons produced by electrocautery smoke and the use of personal protective equipment 1. *Rev Lat Am Enfermagem.* 2017;25:e2853. [IIIC]

105. Tseng HS, Liu SP, Uang SN, et al. Cancer risk of incremental exposure to polycyclic aromatic hydrocarbons in electrocautery smoke for mastectomy personnel. *World J Surg Oncol.* 2014;12:31. [IIB]

106. Näslund Andréasson S, Mahteme H, Sahlberg B, Anundi H. Polycyclic aromatic hydrocarbons in electrocautery smoke during peritonectomy procedures. *J Environ Public Health.* 2012;2012:929053. [IIA]

107. Hui Y, Yan J. Effect of electrosurgery in the operating room on surgeons' blood indices: a simulation model and experiment on rabbits. *J Int Med Res.* 2018;46(12):5245-5256. [IB]

108. Beebe DS, Swica H, Carlson N, Palahniuk RJ, Goodale RL. High levels of carbon monoxide are produced by electrocautery of tissue during laparoscopic cholecystectomy. *Anesth Analg.* 1993;77(2):338-341. [IIB]

109. Chung YJ, Lee SK, Han SH, et al. Harmful gases including carcinogens produced during transurethral resection of the prostate and vaporization. *Int J Urol.* 2010;17(11):944-949. [IIB]

110. Stephenson DJ, Allcott DA, Koch M. The presence of P22 bacteriophage in electrocautery aerosols. In: *Proceedings of the National Occupational Research Agenda Symposium.* Salt Lake City, UT; 2004. [IIB]

111. Garden JM, Kerry O'Banion M, Bakus AD, Olson C. Viral disease transmitted by laser-generated plume (aerosol). *Arch Dermatol.* 2002;138(10):1303-1307. [IIB]

112. Taravella MJ, Weinberg A, May M, Stepp P. Live virus survives excimer laser ablation. *Ophthalmology.* 1999;106(8):1498-1499. [IIB]

113. Ziegler BL, Thomas CA, Meier T, Müller R, Fliedner TM, Weber L. Generation of infectious retrovirus aerosol through medical laser irradiation. *Lasers Surg Med.* 1998;22(1):37-41. [IIB]

114. Cox SV, Dobry AS, Zachary CB, Cohen JL. Laser plume from human papillomavirus-infected tissue: a systematic review. *Dermatol Surg.* 2020;46(12):1676-1682. [VA]

115. Palma S, Gnambs T, Crevenna R, Jordakieva G. Airborne human papillomavirus (HPV) transmission risk during ablation procedures: a systematic review and meta-analysis. *Environ Res.* 2021;192:110437. [VA]

116. Neumann K, Cavalar M, Rody A, Friemert L, Beyer DA. Is surgical plume developing during routine LEEPs contaminated with high-risk HPV? A pilot series of experiments. *Arch Gynecol Obstet.* 2018;297(2):421-424. [IIIB]

117. Zhou Q, Hu X, Zhou J, Zhao M, Zhu X, Zhu X. Human papillomavirus DNA in surgical smoke during cervical loop electrosurgical excision procedures and its impact on the surgeon. *Cancer Manage Res.* 2019;11:3643-3654. [IIIB]

118. Schultz L. Can efficient smoke evacuation limit aerosolization of bacteria? *AORN J.* 2015;102(1):7-14. [IIB]

119. Cukier J, Price MF, Gentry LO. Suction lipoplasty: biohazardous aerosols and exhaust mist—the clouded issue. *Plast Reconstr Surg.* 1989;83(3):494-499. [IIB]

120. Nogler M, Lass-Flörl C, Wimmer C, Mayr E, Bach C, Ogon M. Contamination during removal of cement in revision hip arthroplasty. A cadaver study using ultrasound and high-speed cutters. *J Bone Joint Surg Br.* 2003;85(3):436-439. [IIA]

121. Ishihama K, Koizumi H, Wada T, et al. Evidence of aerosolised floating blood mist during oral surgery. *J Hosp Infect.* 2009;71(4):359-364. [IIB]

122. Ishihama K, Sumioka S, Sakurada K, Kogo M. Floating aerial blood mists in the operating room. *J Hazard Mater.* 2010;181(1-3):1179-1181. [IIC]

123. Jewett DL, Heinsohn P, Bennett C, Rosen A, Neuilly C. Blood-containing aerosols generated by surgical techniques: a possible infectious hazard. *Am Ind Hyg Assoc J.* 1992;53(4):228-231. [IIB]

124. Collins D, Rice J, Nicholson P, Barry K. Quantification of facial contamination with blood during orthopaedic procedures. *J Hosp Infect.* 2000;45(1):73-75. [IIC]

125. Okoshi K, Kobayashi K, Kinoshita K, Tomizawa Y, Hasegawa S, Sakai Y. Health risks associated with exposure to surgical

smoke for surgeons and operation room personnel. *Surg Today.* 2015;45(8):957-965. [VB]

126. Alp E, Bijl D, Bleichrodt RP, Hansson B, Voss A. Surgical smoke and infection control. *J Hosp Infect.* 2006;62(1):1-5. [VB]

127. Born H, Ivey C. How should we safely handle surgical smoke? *Laryngoscope.* 2014;124(10):2213-2215. [VB]

128. Barrett WL, Garber SM. Surgical smoke: a review of the literature. Is this just a lot of hot air? *Surg Endosc.* 2003;17(6):979-987. [VA]

129. Mowbray N, Ansell J, Warren N, Wall P, Torkington J. Is surgical smoke harmful to theater staff? A systematic review. *Surg Endosc.* 2013;27(9):3100-3107. [IIIA]

130. Kunachak S, Sobhon P. The potential alveolar hazard of carbon dioxide laser–induced smoke. *J Med Assoc Thai.* 1998;81(4):278-282. [IIB]

131. *NIOSH Pocket Guide to Chemical Hazards.* 3rd ed. Washington, DC: US Department of Health and Human Services; 2007. [IVA]

132. Immediately dangerous to life or health (IDLH) values. The National Institute for Occupational Safety and Health. Centers for Disease Control and Prevention. https://www.cdc.gov/niosh/idlh/intridl4.html. Reviewed October I, 2019. Accessed August 31, 2021. [IVA]

133. Pierce JS, Lacey SE, Lippert JF, Lopez R, Franke JE, Colvard MD. An assessment of the occupational hazards related to medical lasers. *J Occup Environ Med.* 2011;53(11):1302-1309. [VB]

134. Ha HI, Choi MC, Jung SG, et al. Chemicals in surgical smoke and the efficiency of built-in-filter ports. *JSLS.* 2019;23(4):e2019.00037. [IIC]

135. Choi SH, Kwon TG, Chung SK, Kim TH. Surgical smoke may be a biohazard to surgeons performing laparoscopic surgery. *Surg Endosc.* 2014;28(8):2374-2380. [IIB]

136. Park SC, Lee SK, Han SH, Chung YJ, Park JK. Comparison of harmful gases produced during GreenLight High-Performance System laser prostatectomy and transurethral resection of the prostate. *Urology.* 2012;79(5):1118-1124. [IIB]

137. Petrus M, Matei C, Patachia M, Dumitras DC. Quantitative in vitro analysis of surgical smoke by laser photocoustic spectroscopy. *Journal of Optoelectronics and Advanced Materials.* 2012;14(7-8):664-670. [IIA]

138. Chuang GS, Farinelli W, Christiani DC, Herrick RF, Lee NCY, Avram MM. Gaseous and particulate content of laser hair removal plume. *JAMA Dermatol.* 2016;152(12):1320-1326. [IIC]

139. Lippert JF, Lacey SE, Jones RM. Modeled occupational exposures to gas-phase medical laser-generated air contaminants. *J Occup Environ Hyg.* 2014;11(11):722-727. [IIIB]

140. Hollmann R, Hort CE, Kammer E, Naegele M, Sigrist MW, Meuli-Simmen C. Smoke in the operating theater: an unregarded source of danger. *Plast Reconstr Surg.* 2004;114(2):458-463. [IIB]

141. Sagar PM, Meagher A, Sobczak S, Wolff BG. Chemical composition and potential hazards of electrocautery smoke. *Br J Surg.* 1996;83(12):1792. [IIB]

142. National Research Council. Review of the *Army's Technical Guides on Assessing and Managing Chemical Hazards to Deployed Personnel.* Washington, DC: The National Academies Press; 2004. [VA]

143. Gatti JE, Bryant CJ, Noone RB, Murphy JB. The mutagenicity of electrocautery smoke. *Plast Reconstr Surg.* 1992;89(5):781-784. [IIB]

144. Stocker B, Meier T, Fliedner TM, Plappert U. Laser pyrolysis products: sampling procedures, cytotoxic and genotoxic effects. *Mutat Res.* 1998;412(2):145-154. [IIA]

145. Plappert UG, Stocker B, Helbig R, Fliedner TM, Seidel HJ. Laser pyrolysis products—genotoxic, clastogenic and mutagenic effects of the particulate aerosol fractions. *Mutat Res.* 1999;441(1):29-41. [IIA]

146. Hill DS, O'Neill JK, Powell RJ, Oliver DW. Surgical smoke—a health hazard in the operating theatre: a study to quantify exposure and a survey of the use of smoke extractor systems in UK plastic surgery units. *J Plast Reconstr Aesthet Surg.* 2012;65(7):911-916. [IIB]

147. Hensman C, Baty D, Willis RG, Cuschieri A. Chemical composition of smoke produced by high-frequency electrosurgery in a closed gaseous environment. An in vitro study. *Surg Endosc.* 1998;12(8):1017-1019. [IIB]

148. Hensman C, Newman EL, Shimi SM, Cuschieri A. Cytotoxicity of electro-surgical smoke produced in an anoxic environment. *Am J Surg.* 1998;175(3):240-241. [IIB]

149. Bhatt A, Mittal S, Gopinath KS. Safety considerations for health care workers involved in cytoreductive surgery and perioperative chemotherapy. *Indian J Surg Oncol.* 2016;7(2):249-257. [VB]

150. Sood AK, Bahrani-Mostafavi Z, Stoerker J, Stone IK. Human papillomavirus DNA in LEEP plume. *Infect Dis Obstet Gynecol.* 1994;2(4):167-170. [IIB]

151. Andre P, Orth G, Evenou P, Guillaume JC, Avril MF. Risk of papillomavirus infection in carbon dioxide laser treatment of genital lesions. *J Am Acad Dermatol.* 1990;22(1):131-132. [IIB]

152. Ferenczy A, Bergeron C, Richart RM. Human papillomavirus DNA in CO2 laser-generated plume of smoke and its consequences to the surgeon. *Obstet Gynecol.* 1990;75(1):114-118. [IIB]

153. Ferenczy A, Bergeron C, Richart RM. Carbon dioxide laser energy disperses human papillomavirus deoxyribonucleic acid onto treatment fields. *Am J Obstet Gynecol.* 1990;163(4 Pt 1):1271-1274. [IIB]

154. Weyandt GH, Tollmann F, Kristen P, Weissbrich B. Low risk of contamination with human papilloma virus during treatment of condylomata acuminata with multilayer argon plasma coagulation and CO_2 laser ablation. *Arch Dermatol Res.* 2011;303(2):141-144. [IIB]

155. Sawchuk WS, Weber PJ, Lowy DR, Dzubow LM. Infectious papillomavirus in the vapor of warts treated with carbon dioxide laser or electrocoagulation: detection and protection. *J Am Acad Dermatol.* 1989;21(1):41-49. [IIB]

156. Garden JM, O'Banion MK, Shelnitz LS, et al. Papillomavirus in the vapor of carbon dioxide laser–treated verrucae. *JAMA.* 1988;259(8):1199-1202. [IIB]

157. Kashima HK, Kessis T, Mounts P, Shah K. Polymerase chain reaction identification of human papillomavirus DNA in CO2 laser plume from recurrent respiratory papillomatosis. *Otolaryngol Head Neck Surg.* 1991;104(2):191-195. [IIB]

158. Abramson AL, DiLorenzo TP, Steinberg BM. Is papillomavirus detectable in the plume of laser-treated laryngeal papilloma? *Arch Otolaryngol Head Neck Surg.* 1990;116(5):604-607. [IIB]

159. Hughes PS, Hughes AP. Absence of human papillomavirus DNA in the plume of erbium:YAG laser-treated warts. *J Am Acad Dermatol.* 1998;38(3):426-428. [IIB]

160. Kunachak S, Sithisarn P, Kulapaditharom B. Are laryngeal papilloma virus–infected cells viable in the plume derived from a continuous mode carbon dioxide laser, and are they infectious? A preliminary report on one laser mode. *J Laryngol Otol.* 1996;110(11):1031-1033. [IIB]

161. Health and safety practices survey of healthcare workers. The National Institute for Occupational Safety and Health. https://www.cdc.gov/niosh/topics/healthcarehsps/smoke.html. Updated March 30, 2017. Accessed August 30, 2021. [VA]

162. Kofoed K, Norrbom C, Forslund O, et al. Low prevalence of oral and nasal human papillomavirus in employees performing CO2-laser evaporation of genital warts or loop electrode excision procedure of cervical dysplasia. *Acta Derm Venereol.* 2015;95(2):173-176. [IIIB]

163. Manson LT, Damrose EJ. Does exposure to laser plume place the surgeon at high risk for acquiring clinical human papillomavirus infection? *Laryngoscope.* 2013;123(6):1319-1320. [VB]

164. Ilmarinen T, Auvinen E, Hiltunen-Back E, Ranki A, Aaltonen LM, Pitkäranta A. Transmission of human papillomavirus DNA from patient to surgical masks, gloves and oral mucosa of medical personnel during treatment of laryngeal papillomas and genital warts. *Eur Arch Otorhinolaryngol.* 2012;269(11):2367-2371. [IIB]

165. Wisniewski PM, Warhol MJ, Rando RF, Sedlacek TV, Kemp JE, Fisher JC. Studies on the transmission of viral disease via the CO2 laser plume and ejecta. *J Reprod Med.* 1990;35(12):1117-1123. [IIB]

166. Gloster HM Jr, Roenigk RK. Risk of acquiring human papillomavirus from the plume produced by the carbon dioxide laser in the treatment of warts. *J Am Acad Dermatol.* 1995;32(3):436-441. [IIIB]

167. Hagen KB, Kettering JD, Aprecio RM, Beltran F, Maloney RK. Lack of virus transmission by the excimer laser plume. *Am J Ophthalmol.* 1997;124(2):206-211. [IIB]

168. Taravella MJ, Weinberg A, Blackburn P, May M. Do intact viral particles survive excimer laser ablation? *Arch Ophthalmol.* 1997;115(8):1028-1030. [IIB]

169. Capizzi PJ, Clay RP, Battey MJ. Microbiologic activity in laser resurfacing plume and debris. *Lasers Surg Med.* 1998;23(3):172-174. [IIC]

170. Hospital Respiratory Protection Program Toolkit: Resources for Respirator Program Administrators (DHHS [NIOSH] Publication Number 2015-117). The National Institute of Occupational Safety and Health. https://www.cdc.gov/niosh/docs/2015-117/default.html. Accessed August 30, 2021. [VA]

171. Surgical smoke evacuation. Health System Risk Management. ECRI. https://www.ecri.org/search-results/member-preview/hrc/pages/surgan17_1. Published May 16, 2018. Accessed August 30, 2021. [VB]

172. Hierarchy of controls. The National Institute for Occupational Safety and Health. https://www.cdc.gov/niosh/topics/hierarchy/. Reviewed January 13, 2015. Accessed August 30, 2021. [VA]

173. Guideline for design and maintenance of the surgical suite. In: *Guidelines for Perioperative Practice.* Denver, CO: AORN, Inc; 2021:51-82. [IVA]

174. Romano F, Gustén J, De Antonellis S, Joppolo CM. Electrosurgical smoke: ultrafine particle measurements and work environment quality in different operating theatres. *Int J Environ Res Public Health.* 2017;14(2):137. [IIB]

175. Romano F, Milani S, Gustén J, Joppolo CM. Surgical smoke and airborne microbial contamination in operating theatres: influence of ventilation and surgical phases. *Int J Environ Res Public Health.* 2020;17(15):5395. [IIIB]

176. Seipp HM, Steffens T, Weigold J, et al. Efficiencies and noise levels of portable surgical smoke evacuation systems. *J Occup Environ Hyg.* 2018;15(11):773-781. [IIB]

177. Guideline for sterile technique. In: *Guidelines for Perioperative Practice.* Denver, CO: AORN, Inc; 2021:943-984. [IVA]

178. Guideline for team communication. In: *Guidelines for Perioperative Practice.* Denver, CO: AORN, Inc; 2021:1065-1096. [IVA]

179. Ogg MJ, Johnstone EM. Clinical Issues–June 2017. *AORN J.* 2017;105(6):619-627. [VA]

180. Standards of perioperative nursing practice. AORN, Inc. https://aorn.org/guidelines/clinical-resources/aorn-standards. Accessed August 30, 2021. [IVB]

181. Limchantra IV, Fong Y, Melstrom KA. Surgical smoke exposure in operating room personnel: a review. *JAMA Surg.* 2019;154(10):960-967. [VB]

182. Hubner M, Sigrist MW, Demartines N, Gianella M, Clavien PA, Hahnloser D. Gas emission during laparoscopic colorectal surgery using a bipolar vessel sealing device: a pilot study on four patients. *Patient Saf Surg.* 2008;2:22. [IIB]

183. Edelman DS, Unger SW. Bipolar versus monopolar cautery scissors for laparoscopic cholecystectomy: a randomized, prospective study. *Surg Laparosc Endosc.* 1995;5(6):459-462. [IB]

184. Kim FJ, Sehrt D, Pompeo A, Molina WR. Laminar and turbulent surgical plume characteristics generated from curved- and straight-blade laparoscopic ultrasonic dissectors. *Surg Endosc.* 2014;28(5):1674-1677. [IIB]

185. Schneider A, Doundoulakis E, Can S, Fiolka A, Wilhelm D, Feussner H. Evaluation of mist production and tissue dissection efficiency using different types of ultrasound shears. *Surg Endosc.* 2009;23(12):2822-2826. [IIB]

186. Ott DE, Moss E, Martinez K. Aerosol exposure from an ultrasonically activated (Harmonic) device. *J Am Assoc Gynecol Laparosc.* 1998;5(1):29-32. [IIB]

187. Kisch T, Liodaki E, Kraemer R, et al. Electrocautery devices with feedback mode and Teflon-coated blades create less surgical smoke for a quality improvement in the operating theater. *Medicine (Baltimore)*. 2015;94(27):e1104. [IIB]

188. Bui MH, Breda A, Gui D, Said J, Schulam P. Less smoke and minimal tissue carbonization using a thulium laser for laparoscopic partial nephrectomy without hilar clamping in a porcine model. *J Endourol*. 2007;21(9):1107-1111. [IIB]

189. Carr MM, Patel VA, Soo JC, Friend S, Lee EG. Effect of electrocautery settings on particulate concentrations in surgical plume during tonsillectomy. *Otolaryngol Head Neck Surg*. 2020;162(6):867-872. [IIB]

190. Lopez R, Lacey SE, Lippert JF, Liu LC, Esmen NA, Conroy LM. Characterization of size-specific particulate matter emission rates for a simulated medical laser procedure—a pilot study. *Ann Occup Hyg*. 2015;59(4):514-524. [IIB]

191. ISO 16571:2014(en): Systems for evacuation of plume generated by medical devices. International Organization for Standardization; 2014. https://www.iso.org/obp/ui/#iso:std:iso:16571:ed-1:v1:en. Accessed August 30, 2021. [IVA]

192. Smoke evacuation systems, surgical. Device Overviews & Specifications - Comparative Data. https://www.ecri.org/components/HPCS/Pages/Smoke-Evacuation-Systems,-Surgical.aspx [subscription required]. Published 1/1/2020. Accessed August 31, 2021. [VB]

193. CSA Z305.13:13 (R2020). Plume scavenging in surgical, diagnostic, therapeutic, and aesthetic settings. 2013. Canadian Standards Association. https://www.csagroup.org/store/product/Z305.13-13/. Accessed August 31, 2021. [IVB]

194. ISO 29463-1:2017(en): High efficiency filters and filter media for removing particles from air—Part 1: classification, performance, testing and marking. International Organization for Standardization; 2017. https://www.iso.org/obp/ui/#iso:std:iso:29463:-1:ed-2:v1:en. Accessed August 30, 2021. [IVA]

195. Guideline for medical device and product evaluation. In: *Guidelines for Perioperative Practice*. Denver, CO: AORN, Inc; 2021:719-728. [IVA]

196. Levine D, Petroski GF, Haertling T, Beaudoin T. Electrostatic precipitation in low pressure laparoscopic hysterectomy and myomectomy. *JSLS*. 2020;24(4):e2020.00051. [IB]

197. 21 CFR 878.5050: Surgical smoke precipitator. Electronic Code of Federal Regulations. https://www.ecfr.gov/cgi-bin/retrieveECFR?gp=1&SID=5eb8ca1702aa639c15a7186f80efad89&ty=HTML&h=L&mc=true&r=SECTION&n=se21.8.878_15050. Accessed August 30, 2021.

198. Buggisch JR, Göhler D, Le Pape A, et al. Experimental model to test electrostatic precipitation technology in the COVID-19 era: a pilot study. *J Am Coll Surg*. 2020;231(6):704-712. [IIB]

199. Wexner SD, Cortés-Guiral D, Gilshtein H, Kent I, Reymond MA. COVID-19: impact on colorectal surgery. *Colorectal Dis*. 2020;22(6):635-640. [VB]

200. O'Brien DC, Lee EG, Soo JC, Friend S, Callaham S, Carr MM. Surgical team exposure to cautery smoke and its mitigation during tonsillectomy. *Otolaryngol Head Neck Surg*. 2020;163(3):508-516. [IIB]

201. Mattes D, Silajdzic E, Mayer M, et al. Surgical smoke management for minimally invasive (micro)endoscopy: an experimental study. *Surg Endosc*. 2010;24(10):2492-2501. [IIB]

202. Pillinger SH, Delbridge L, Lewis DR. Randomized clinical trial of suction versus standard clearance of the diathermy plume. *Br J Surg*. 2003;90(9):1068-1071. [IB]

203. 7.4 laser generated airborne contaminants (LGAC); plume and airborne contaminants (PAC). In: *ANSI Z136.3: Safe Use of Lasers in Health Care*. Orlando, FL.: Laser Institute of America; 2018:36-37. [IVB]

204. American Association of Physics in Medicine; American College of Medical Physics. *Medical Lasers: Quality Control, Safety Standards, and Regulations*. Joint Report Task Group No. 6. Madison, WI: Medical Physics Publishing; 2001. [IVB]

205. *Guidelines for Environmental Infection Control in Health-Care Facilities. Recommendations of CDC and the Healthcare Infection Control Practices Advisory Committee (HICPAC)*. Atlanta GA: Centers for Disease Control and Prevention; 2003. https://www.cdc.gov/infectioncontrol/pdf/guidelines/environmental-guidelines-P.pdf. Updated 2019. Accessed August 31, 2021. [IVA]

206. EC.02.02.01: The hospital manages risks related to hazardous materials and waste. Element of performance 9. In: *Comprehensive Accreditation Manual for Hospitals*. Oakbrook Terrace, IL: The Joint Commission; 2021.

207. Surgical smoke evacuation. In: *Standards, Guidelines, and Position Statements for Perioperative Registered Nursing Practice*. 12th ed. Bath, Ontario, Canada: Operating Room Nurses' Association of Canada (ORNAC); 2015:229-231. [IVC]

208. Freitag L, Chapman GA, Sielczak M, Ahmed A, Russin D. Laser smoke effect on the bronchial system. *Lasers Surg Med*. 1987;7(3):283-288. [IIB]

209. Charles K. Effects of laser plume evacuation on laser in situ keratomileusis outcomes. *J Refract Surg*. 2002;18(3 Suppl):S340-S342. [IIIB]

210. Moot AR, Ledingham KM, Wilson PF, et al. Composition of volatile organic compounds in diathermy plume as detected by selected ion flow tube mass spectrometry. *ANZ J Surg*. 2007;77(1-2):20-23. [IIB]

211. Hassan I, Drelichman ER, Wolff BG, Ruiz C, Sobczak SC, Larson DW. Exposure to electrocautery toxins: understanding a potential occupational hazard. *Prof Saf*. 2006;4:38-41. [IIB]

212. Golda N, Huber A, Gole H. Determining the impact of intraoperative smoke evacuation on the patient experience during outpatient surgery: a randomized controlled trial. *J Am Acad Dermatol*. 2018;78(5):1007-1009. [IC]

213. Yonan Y, Ochoa S. Impact of smoke evacuation on patient experience during Mohs surgery. *Dermatol Surg*. 2017;43(11):1363-1366. [IIIB]

214. Perry J, Agui J, Vijayakumar R, eds. *Submicron and Nanoparticulate Matter Removal by HEPA-Rated Media Filters and Packed Beds of Granular Materials*. No. NASA/TM—2016–218224. Washington, DC: National Aeronautics and Space Administration; 2016. [VA]

215. Tramontini CC, Galvão CM, Vieira Claudio C, Perfeito Ribeiro R, Trevisan Martins J. Composition of the electrocautery

smoke: integrative literature review [Article in Portuguese]. *Rev Esc Enferm USP*. 2016;50(1):144-157. [VB]

216. Georgesen C, Lipner SR. Surgical smoke: risk assessment and mitigation strategies. *J Am Acad Dermatol*. 2018;79(4):746-755. [VB]

217. Ball K. Protecting patients from surgical smoke. *AORN J*. 2018;108(6):680-684. [VA]

218. Control of smoke from laser/electrical surgical procedures. Engineering Controls Database. The National Institute for Occupational Safety and Health. https://www.cdc.gov/niosh/engcontrols/ecd/detail193.html. Reviewed November 16, 2018. Accessed August 31, 2021. [VA]

219. Liu N, Filipp N, Wood KB. The utility of local smoke evacuation in reducing surgical smoke exposure in spine surgery: a prospective self-controlled study. *Spine J*. 2020;20(2):166-173. [IIB]

220. Ott D. Smoke production and smoke reduction in endoscopic surgery: preliminary report. *Endosc Surg Allied Technol*. 1993;1(4):230-232. [IIB]

221. Dobrogowski M, Wesolowski W, Kucharska M, Sapota A, Pomorski LS. Chemical composition of surgical smoke formed in the abdominal cavity during laparoscopic cholecystectomy—assessment of the risk to the patient. *Int J Occup Med Environ Health*. 2014;27(2).314-325. [IIIB]

222. Takahashi H, Yamasaki M, Hirota M, et al. Automatic smoke evacuation in laparoscopic surgery: a simplified method for objective evaluation. *Surg Endosc*. 2013;27(8):2980-2987. [IIB]

223. Wu JS, Monk T, Luttmann DR, Meininger TA, Soper NJ. Production and systemic absorption of toxic byproducts of tissue combustion during laparoscopic cholecystectomy. *J Gastrointest Surg*. 1998;2(5):399-405. [IIB]

224. Nezhat C, Seidman DS, Vreman HJ, Stevenson DK, Nezhat F, Nezhat C. The risk of carbon monoxide poisoning after prolonged laparoscopic surgery. *Obstet Gynecol*. 1996;88(5):771-774. [IIB]

225. Hahn KY, Kang DW, Azman ZAM, Kim SY, Kim SH. Removal of hazardous surgical smoke using a built-in-filter trocar: a study in laparoscopic rectal resection. *Surg Laparosc Endosc Percutan Tech*. 2017;27(5):341-345. [IIC]

226. 29 CFR 1910.1030. Bloodborne pathogens. Occupational Safety and Health Administration. https://www.osha.gov/laws-regs/regulations/standardnumber/1910/1910.1030. Accessed August 31, 2021.

227. Respirator trusted-source information. The National Personal Protective Technology Laboratory. Centers for Disease Control and Prevention. http://www.cdc.gov/niosh/npptl/topics/respirators/disp_part/RespSource.html. Accessed August 31, 2021. [IVB]

228. Gao S, Koehler RH, Yermakov M, Grinshpun SA. Performance of facepiece respirators and surgical masks against surgical smoke: simulated workplace protection factor study. *Ann Occup Hyg*. 2016;60(5):608-618. [IIB]

229. Rengasamy S, Miller A, Eimer BC, Shaffer RE. Filtration performance of FDA-cleared surgical masks. *J Int Soc Respir Prot*. 2009;26(3):54-70. [IIB]

230. Elmashae Y, Koehler RH, Yermakov M, Reponen T, Grinshpun SA. Surgical smoke simulation study: physical characterization and respiratory protection. *Aerosol Sci Technol*. 2018;52(1):38-45. [IIB]

231. Davidson C, Green CF, Panlilio AL, et al. Method for evaluating the relative efficiency of selected N95 respirators and surgical masks to prevent the inhalation of airborne vegetative cells by healthcare personnel. *Indoor Built Environ*. 2011;20(2):265-277. [IIB]

232. Derrick JL, Li PT, Tang SP, Gomersall CD. Protecting staff against airborne viral particles: in vivo efficiency of laser masks. *J Hosp Infect*. 2006;64(3):278-281. [IIA]

233. Eninger RM, Honda T, Adhikari A, Heinonen-Tanski H, Reponen T, Grinshpun SA. Filter performance of N99 and N95 facepiece respirators against viruses and ultrafine particles. *Ann Occup Hyg*. 2008;52(5):385-396. [IIB]

234. Redmayne AC, Wake D, Brown RC, Crook B. Measurement of the degree of protection afforded by respiratory protective equipment against microbiological aerosols. *Ann Occup Hyg*. 1997;41(Suppl 1):636-640. [IIB]

235. Chen CC, Willeke K. Aerosol penetration through surgical masks. *Am J Infect Control*. 1992;20(4):177-184. [IIB]

236. Weber A, Willeke K, Marchioni R, et al. Aerosol penetration and leakage characteristics of masks used in the health care industry. *Am J Infect Control*. 1993;21(4):167-173. [IIB]

237. Oberg T, Brosseau LM. Surgical mask filter and fit performance. *Am J Infect Control*. 2008;36(4):276-282. [IIB]

238. Subbarayan RS, Shew M, Enders J, Bur AM, Thomas SM. Occupational exposure of oropharyngeal human papillomavirus amongst otolaryngologists. *Laryngoscope*. 2020;130(10):2366-2371. [IIIC]

239. Engelman DT, Lother S, George I, et al. Adult cardiac surgery and the COVID-19 pandemic: aggressive infection mitigation strategies are necessary in the operating room and surgical recovery. *Ann Thorac Surg*. 2020;110(2):707-711. [IVB]

240. Advisory Committee on Immunization Practices; Centers for Disease Control and Prevention (CDC). Immunization of health-care personnel: recommendations of the Advisory Committee on Immunization Practices (ACIP). *MMWR Recomm Rep*. 2011;60(RR-7):1-45. [IVA]

241. Derkay C. Occupational exposure to human papilloma virus (HPV) and prophylactic vaccination. US National Library of Medicine. ClinicalTrials.gov. https://clinicaltrials.gov/ct2/show/NCT03350698?term=occupational&cond=HPV&draw=2&rank=1. Published November 22, 2017. Updated August 19, 2021. Accessed August 30, 2021.

242. Golda N, Merrill B, Neill B. Intraoperative electrosurgical smoke during outpatient surgery: a survey of dermatologic surgeon and staff preferences. *Cutis*. 2019;104(2):120-124. [IIIB]

243. Bree K, Barnhill S, Rundell W. The dangers of electrosurgical smoke to operating room personnel: a review. *Workplace Health Saf*. 2017;65(11):517-526. [VA]

244. Swerdlow BN. Surgical smoke and the anesthesia provider. *J Anesth*. 2020;34(4):575-584. [VA]

245. ECRI. Clearing the air around surgical smoke: know the risks. Health Devices. https://www.ecri.org/components/HDJournal/Pages/Clearing-the-Air-around-Surgical-Smoke.aspx#. Published July 24, 2019. Accessed August 24, 2021. [VB]

246. Chavis S, Wagner V, Becker M, Bowerman MI, Jamias MS. Clearing the air about surgical smoke: an education program. *AORN J.* 2016;103(3):289-296. [VB]

247. Dobbie MK, Fezza M, Kent M, Lu J, Saraceni ML, Titone S. Operation clean air: implementing a surgical smoke evacuation program. *AORN J.* 2017;106(6):502-512. [VB]

248. Tagle M. Reduction of surgical smoke in the operating room: application of the evidence. *J Pediatr Surg Nurs.* 2020;9(2):49-51. [VC]

249. York K, Autry M. Surgical smoke: putting the pieces together to become smoke-free. *AORN J.* 2018;107(6):692-703. [VB]

250. 42 CFR 482. Conditions of participation for hospitals. Electronic Code of Federal Regulations. https://www.ecfr.gov/cgi-bin/retrieveECFR?gp=1&SID=5eb8ca1702aa639c15a7186f80efad89&ty=HTML&h=L&mc=true&r=PART&n=pt42.5.482. Accessed August 30, 2021.

251. 42 CFR 416: Ambulatory surgical services. Electronic Code of Federal Regulations. https://www.ecfr.gov/cgi-bin/retrieveECFR?gp=1&SID=5eb8ca1702aa639c15a7186f80efad89&ty=HTML&h=L&mc=true&r=PART&n=pt42.3.416. Accessed August 30, 2021.

252. *State Operations Manual Appendix A: Survey Protocol, Regulations and Interpretive Guidelines for Hospitals.* Rev. 200; 02-21-20. Centers for Medicare & Medicaid Services. https://www.cms.gov/Regulations-and-Guidance/Guidance/Manuals/downloads/som107ap_a_hospitals.pdf. Accessed August 31, 2021.

253. *State Operations Manual Appendix L: Guidance for Surveyors: Ambulatory Surgical Centers.* Rev. 200, 02-21-20. Centers for Medicare & Medicaid Services. https://www.cms.gov/Regulations-and-Guidance/Guidance/Manuals/downloads/som107ap_l_ambulatory.pdf. Accessed August 31, 2021.

254. Bryant CJ, Gorman R, Stewart J, Whong Z. Health hazard evaluation report: HETA-85-126-1932, Bryn Mawr Hospital, Bryn Mawr, Pennsylvania. The National Institute for Occupational Safety and Health. https://www.cdc.gov/niosh/hhe/reports/pdfs/85-126-1932.pdf. Published September 1988. Accessed August 30, 2021. [VA]

255. Moss CE, Bryant CJ, Whong Z, Stewart J. Health hazard evaluation report: HETA-88-101-2008, University of Utah Health Sciences Center, Salt Lake City, Utah. The National Institute for Occupational Safety and Health. https://www.cdc.gov/niosh/hhe/reports/pdfs/1988-0101-2008.pdf?id=10.26616/NIOSHHETA881012008. Published February 1990. Accessed August 30, 2021. [VA]

256. King B, McCullough J. Health hazard evaluation report: HETA-2000-0402-3021, Inova Fairfax Hospital, Falls Church, Virginia. The National Institute for Occupational Safety and Health. https://www.cdc.gov/niosh/hhe/reports/pdfs/2000-0402-3021.pdf?id=10.26616/NIOSHHETA200004023021. Published November 2006. Accessed August 30, 2021. [VA]

257. King B, McCullough J. Health hazard evaluation report: HETA-2001-0066-3019, Morton Plant Hospital, Dunedin, Florida. The National Institute for Occupational Safety and Health. https://www.cdc.gov/niosh/hhe/reports/pdfs/2001-0066-3019.pdf?id=10.26616/NIOSHHETA200100663019. Published October 2006. Accessed August 30, 2021. [VA]

258. King B, McCullough J. Health hazard evaluation report: HETA-2001-0030-3020, Carolinas Medical Center, Charlotte, North Carolina. The National Institute for Occupational Safety and Health. https://www.cdc.gov/niosh/hhe/reports/pdfs/2001-0030-3020.pdf. Published November 2006. Accessed August 30, 2021. [VA]

259. Medical device reporting (MDR): How to report medical device problems. US Food and Drug Administration. https://www.fda.gov/medical-devices/medical-device-safety/medical-device-reporting-mdr-how-report-medical-device-problems#overview. Updated October 2, 2020. Accessed August 30, 2021.

Guideline Development Group

Lead Author: Emily Jones[1], MSN, RN, CNOR, NPD-BC, Perioperative Practice Specialist, AORN, Denver, Colorado

Methodologist: Erin Kyle[2], DNP, RN, CNOR, NEA-BC, Editor-in-Chief, Guidelines for Perioperative Practice, AORN, Denver, Colorado

Evidence Appraisers: Mary Ogg[3], MSN, RN, CNOR; Amber Wood[4], MSN, RN, CNOR, CIC, FAPIC, Perioperative Practice Specialist, AORN, Denver, Colorado; Julie Cahn[5], DNP, RN, CNOR, RN-BC, ACNS-BC, CNS-CP, Perioperative Practice Specialist, AORN, Denver, Colorado

Guidelines Advisory Board Members:

- Susan Lynch[6], PhD, RN, CSSM, CNOR, Associate Director/Surgical Services, Penn Medicine-Chester County Hospital
- Mary Fearon[7], MSN, RN, CNOR, Retired, Sammamish, Washington.
- Crystal A. Bricker[8], MSN, RN, CNOR, Clinical Practice Partner, Perioperative Services, Advocate Health Care, Bloomington, Illinois
- Michele J. Brunges[9], RN, MSN, Director, Perioperative Services, University of Florida Health Shands Hospital, Gainesville, Florida
- Craig S. Atkins[10], DNP, CRNA, Chief Nurse Anesthetist, Belmar Ambulatory Surgical Center, Lakewood, Colorado
- Shandra R. Day[11], MD, Assistant Professor, Infectious Disease, Ohio State University Wexner Medical Center, Columbus, Ohio
- Cassie Dietrich[12], MD, Anesthesiologist, Anesthesia Associates of Kansas City, Overland Park, Kansas
- Jared M. Huston[13], MD, Director, Trauma Research, Northwell Health, Manhasset, New York

- Susan G. Klacik[14], BS, CRCST, FCS, Clinical Educator, International Association of Healthcare Central Service Materiel Management (IAHCSMM), Chicago, Illinois
- Sara Reese[15], PhD, MPH, CIC, System Director of Infection Prevention, SCL Health, Englewood, Colorado
- Juan Sanchez[16], MD, MPA, FACS, FACHE, Associate Professor of Surgery, Johns Hopkins University School of Medicine, Baltimore, Maryland
- Valerie M. Deloney[17], MBA, Guidelines Consultant, Society for Healthcare Epidemiology of America, Arlington, Virginia
- Brenda G. Larkin[18], MS, ACNS-BC, CNS, CNOR, Clinical Nurse Specialist, Aurora Lakeland Medical Center, Lake Geneva, Wisconsin
- Brandy L. Miller[19], MHA, MSN, RN, CNOR, Director, Southwest Surgical Suites, Fort Wayne, Indiana

External Review: Expert review comments were received from members of the Guidelines Advisory Board during the guideline development process. Additional expert review comments were received from individual members of the American Association of Nurse Anesthetists (AANA), American College of Surgeons (ACS), Association for Professionals in Infection Control and Epidemiology (APIC), American Society of Anesthesiologists (ASA), International Association of Healthcare Central Service Materiel Management (IAHCSMM), the Society for Healthcare Epidemiology of America (SHEA), and the Surgical Infection Society (SIS). Their responses were used to further refine and enhance this guideline; however, their responses do not imply endorsement. The draft was also open for a 30-day public comment period.

Financial Disclosure and Conflicts of Interest

This guideline was developed, edited, and approved by the AORN Guidelines Advisory Board without external funding being sought or obtained. The Guidelines Advisory Board was financially supported entirely by AORN, Inc.

Potential conflicts of interest for all Guidelines Advisory Board members were reviewed before the annual meeting and each monthly conference call. None of the members of the Guideline Development Group reported a potential conflict of interest.[1-19]

Publication History

Originally published December 2016 in *Guidelines for Perioperative Practice* online.

Evidence ratings revised and minor editorial changes made to conform to the current AORN Evidence Rating model, September 2019, for online publication in *Guidelines for Perioperative Practice.*

Revised in October 2021 for online publication in Guidelines for Perioperative Practice.

Scheduled for review in 2026.

AORN GUIDELINES FOR
PERIOPERATIVE PRACTICE,
2022 EDITION

TEAM COMMUNICATION

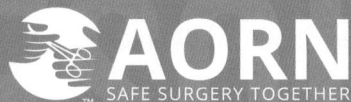

TABLE OF CONTENTS

MEDICAL ABBREVIATIONS & ACRONYMS

CMS – Centers for Medicare & Medicaid Services
HUDDLE – Healthcare Utilizing Deliberate
    Discussion Linking Events
I PASS the BATON – Introduction, Patient, Assessment,
    Situation, Safety Concerns, (the)
    Background, Actions, Timing,
    Ownership, Next
ICU – Intensive care unit
IHI – Institute for Healthcare Improvement
NOTSS – Nontechnical Skills for Surgeons

QI – Quality improvement
RN – Registered nurse
SBAR – Situation, Background, Assessment,
    Recommendation
SOP – Standard operating procedure
SURPASS – SURgical PAtient Safety System
SWITCH – Surgical Procedure, Wet, Instruments, Tissue,
    Counts, Have You Any Questions
WHO – World Health Organization

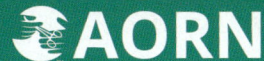
GUIDELINE FOR
TEAM COMMUNICATION

The Guideline for Team Communication was approved by the AORN Guidelines Advisory Board and became effective January 15, 2018. It was presented as a proposed guideline for comments by members and others. The recommendations in the guideline are intended to be achievable and represent what is believed to be an optimal level of practice. Policies and procedures will reflect variations in practice settings and/or clinical situations that determine the degree to which the guideline can be implemented. AORN recognizes the many diverse settings in which perioperative nurses practice; therefore, this guideline is adaptable to all areas where operative or other invasive procedures may be performed.

Purpose

This document provides guidance for improving perioperative team communication through a culture of safety that incorporates team training, simulation training, standardized transfer of patient information (commonly referred to as **hand overs** or hand offs), **briefings**, **time outs**, surgical safety checklists, and **debriefings**. In 1999, the Institute of Medicine report To Err Is Human: Building a Safer Health System stated that between 44,000 and 98,000 hospital patients die annually as a result of medical **errors** in the United States.[1] Subsequent studies have estimated the incidence to be as high as 180,000 to 400,000 deaths annually.[2] Since this landmark report, the health care industry has embraced the need for change. Numerous organizations have written position statements on the importance of team communication and the use of a safe surgery checklist to reduce the incidence of medical errors.[3-9]

The collective evidence[10-13] demonstrates that communication breakdowns in the perioperative setting are a factor in events that adversely affect patients. Seventy percent of adverse events in the surgical environment are caused by breakdowns in communication among health care providers.[14,15] The perioperative environment is stressful, and perioperative team members are under increasing pressure from numerous demands and complex functions that lend themselves to error. Despite these pressures, patient safety is a top priority for perioperative RNs and cannot be sacrificed for efficiency. Communication tools and team training programs provide a foundation to improve the chances that communication is conveyed effectively and received accurately. The surgical safety checklist is one tool that the literature supports as improving communication in the perioperative environment.[16-62] The use of checklists in hand overs, briefings, and debriefings provides a defense against adverse events.[46,63,64]

Successful perioperative team communication requires a **high-reliability team** with a shared goal. According to Wahr et al,[50] high-reliability teams have six elements in common: communication, coordination, cooperation, cognition, conflict resolution, and coaching. An understanding by each team member of his or her role and responsibilities is necessary to achieve a successful surgical outcome for the patient. Beginning with the patient's decision to consent to the procedure, valuable information is collected and handed over to multiple personnel during the patient's surgical encounter. Effective communication among team members is important for understanding the surgical plan for each individual patient. A **shared mental model** increases the effectiveness of communication between team members because each team member is knowledgeable about his or her own role, other team members' roles, and how these roles interrelate. As the surgery progresses, a shared mental model facilitates timely communication and response by each team member to changes in the surgical plan.[50]

Communication is a process that consists of sending and receiving messages; however, a variety of **distractions** can impede the ability to send or receive the message accurately. Distractions can be internal or external. Internal distractions are related to the individual's nontechnical skills and individual **resilience** to human factors (eg, hunger, thirst, anxiety, anger, fatigue) when communicating within the team.[65] External or environmental distractions can be divided into two types: essential and nonessential. Essential distractions come from components necessary for patient care, such as equipment alarms, telephones, pagers, and equipment **noise**. Nonessential distractions occur in the environment but are not necessary for patient care, such as irrelevant conversations, music, and **interruptions** from personnel not essential to the procedure. Hierarchical and personal relationships among the individuals on the team can be barriers to effective communication. Other individual barriers include educational background, language preference, culture, race, and gender.[63]

Interprofessional team members send and receive multiple messages throughout a patient's surgical experience. Mohorek and Webb[66] described the Linear Model of Communication as a conceptual framework for hand overs between physicians and described different reasons for errors during the hand-over process. Viewing the flow of communication in a linear model may be beneficial for mapping out the critical messages that are covered in each team conversation and for preventing repetition of information that is not critical.

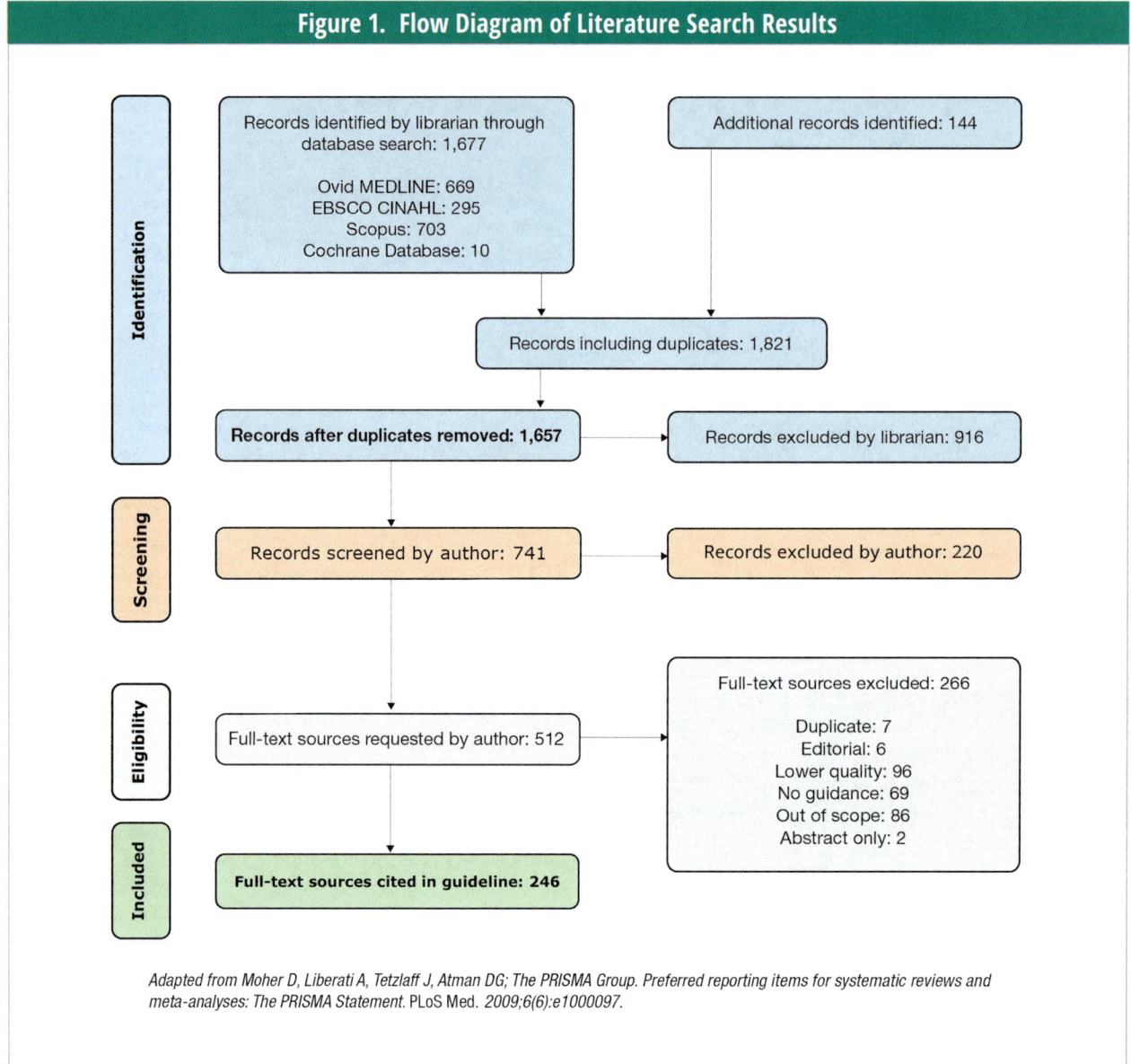

Figure 1. Flow Diagram of Literature Search Results

Records identified by librarian through database search: 1,677

Ovid MEDLINE: 669
EBSCO CINAHL: 295
Scopus: 703
Cochrane Database: 10

Additional records identified: 144

Records including duplicates: 1,821

Records after duplicates removed: 1,657

Records excluded by librarian: 916

Records screened by author: 741

Records excluded by author: 220

Full-text sources requested by author: 512

Full-text sources excluded: 266

Duplicate: 7
Editorial: 6
Lower quality: 96
No guidance: 69
Out of scope: 86
Abstract only: 2

Full-text sources cited in guideline: 246

Identification

Screening

Eligibility

Included

Adapted from Moher D, Liberati A, Tetzlaff J, Atman DG; The PRISMA Group. Preferred reporting items for systematic reviews and meta-analyses: The PRISMA Statement. PLoS Med. 2009;6(6):e1000097.

Nontechnical skills, including situational awareness, decision making, leadership, communication, and teamwork, may affect team communications. Nontechnical skills have been extensively studied in aviation and have been added to training programs for pilots. Although tools for observing nontechnical skills have been validated for other professional roles in the perioperative setting, a standardized tool has not been developed for observing nontechnical skills in the perioperative registered nurse (RN) role. Validated tools for observing nontechnical skills in the perioperative environment include Observational Teamwork Assessment for Surgery (OATS),[67,68] Anesthetist Non-Technical Skills (ANTS),[69] Nontechnical Skills for Surgeons (NOTSS),[14,70-72] and Scrub Practitioners' List of Intraoperative Nontechnical Skills (SPLINTS).[69]

The following topics are outside the scope of this document: workplace violence, bullying, incivility, and workplace safety. Although disruptive behavior is mentioned in the description of the literature, guidance for addressing disruptive behavior is also outside the scope of this document.

Evidence Review

A medical librarian conducted a systematic search of the databases Ovid MEDLINE®, EBSCO CINAHL®, Scopus®, and the Cochrane Database of Systematic Reviews. The search was limited to literature published in English from 2011 through April 2017. At the time of the initial search, weekly alerts were created on the topics included in that search. Results from these alerts were provided to the lead author until July 2017. The lead author requested additional articles that either did not fit the original search criteria or were discovered during the evidence appraisal process. The lead author and the medical librarian also identified relevant guidelines from government agencies, professional organizations, and standards-setting bodies.

Search terms included subject headings such as *operating rooms, communication, patient handoff, clinical protocols, intraoperative complications, interdisciplinary communication, hand off (patient safety),* and *Universal Protocol.* Additional keywords and phrases included *time-out, briefings, debriefings, passive, assertive, sentinel event, never event, TeamSTEPPS, system reliability, misinformation, miscommunication,* and *process improvement.*

Included were research and non-research literature in English, complete publications, and publications with dates within the time restriction. Excluded were non-peer-reviewed publications and older evidence within the time restriction when more recent evidence was available. Editorials, news items, and other brief items were excluded. Low-quality evidence was excluded when higher-quality evidence was available (**Figure 1**).

Articles identified in the search were provided to the project team for evaluation. The team consisted of the lead author, a coauthor, and one evidence appraiser. The lead author divided the search results into topics and assigned the members of the team to review and critically appraise each article using the AORN Research or Non-Research Evidence Appraisal Tools as appropriate. The literature was independently evaluated and appraised according to the strength and quality of the evidence. Each article was then assigned an appraisal score. The appraisal score is noted in brackets after each reference as applicable.

Each recommendation rating is based on a synthesis of the collective evidence, a benefit-harm assessment, and consideration of resource use. The strength of the recommendation was determined using the AORN Evidence Rating Model and the quality and consistency of the evidence supporting a recommendation. The recommendation strength rating is noted in brackets after each recommendation.

Note: The evidence summary table is available at http:// www.aorn.org/evidencetables/.

Editor's note: MEDLINE is a registered trademark of the US National Library of Medicine's Medical Literature Analysis and Retrieval System, Bethesda, MD. CINAHL, Cumulative Index to Nursing and Allied Health Literature, is a registered trademark of EBSCO Industries, Birmingham, AL. Scopus is a registered trademark of Elsevier B.V., Amsterdam, The Netherlands.

1. Patient Safety Culture

1.1 **Establish administrative processes to create a patient safety culture and encourage individual team members to actively engage in and support the culture.** *[Recommendation]*

Commitment to a patient safety culture in the perioperative setting improves patient care, teamwork, and communication, which reduces the patient's risk for adverse events.[73,74] In a patient safety culture, perioperative team members reduce risk by communicating safety concerns. Team members adapt and modify their behavior by learning from mistakes or by receiving rewards for use of safety behaviors.[75] The pillars of a patient safety culture—trust, report, and improve—provide a foundation for health care organizations to achieve high levels of patient safety.[76]

Establishing a patient safety culture is a system-level intervention to improve patient safety. Investigations in the aviation, nuclear power, and oil and gas industries have found that major factors in accidents were system failures.[75,77]

1.2 **The health care organization should promote respect among team members by**
- **encouraging honesty;**
- **fostering learning;**
- **encouraging collaborative practice;**
- **encouraging team members to speak up;**
- **holding team members accountable for their behavior;**
- **maintaining adequate staffing systems;**
- **providing expert, credible, and visible leadership;**
- **providing opportunities for shared decision making at all levels; and**
- **recognizing the value of each team member's contributions.**[1,76,78]

[Recommendation]

Promoting respectful behaviors among team members facilitates effective communication and teamwork and encourages individuals to speak up when a variance may lead to an unsafe outcome. Effective teamwork, a systems approach, and blameless communication are the best strategies for building a patient safety culture.[79-82] A nonexperimental study conducted by Kolbe et al[82] provides evidence that team communication is improved when there is a positive relationship between speaking-up behavior and technical team performance. The researchers defined speaking up as "explicitly communicating task-relevant observations, requesting clarification, or explicitly challenging or correcting a task-relevant decision or a procedure."[82(p1100)] They found that speaking up during the briefing was associated with speaking up later when a situation became more critical.

In the Silence Kills study, a nonexperimental study conducted by VitalSmarts, AORN, and the American Association of Critical-Care Nurses, the researchers surveyed RNs (N = 4,235) about three concerns identified in an earlier study: dangerous shortcuts, incompetence, and disrespect.[83] The survey responses indicated that 82% (n = 3,472) of the respondents worked with people who demonstrated disrespectful behaviors such as condescending responses, insults, rude comments, yelling, shouting, swearing, or name calling. Forty-six percent of the RN respondents (n = 1,948) identified that disrespect prevented them from communicating effectively and undermined their professional credibility. Forty-nine percent (n = 2,075) stated that they spoke to their managers about the person who was being disrespectful, and 16% (n = 678) spoke to the person who was demonstrating disrespectful behaviors. The researchers concluded that health care organizations that created an environment where RNs were personally, socially, and structurally supported to speak up increased the incidence of respectful behavior.

Adequate staffing systems in a healthy perioperative practice environment respects the needs of perioperative team members.[78]

1.3 **The health care organization should hold the executives and managers at all levels accountable for promoting a patient safety culture.** [Recommendation]

Moderate-quality evidence[22,80,82,84-97] supports the need for leaders to promote factors that shape the sense of safety for the perioperative team. An expert panel convened by the National Patient Safety Foundation advised that leaders should consistently prioritize safety and the well-being and safety of the health care workforce through the use of standardized definitions of safety terms and measurement of safety outcomes.[98]

A nonexperimental study conducted by Vital-Smarts, AORN, and the American Association of Critical-Care Nurses[83] found that only 41% (n = 341) of perioperative RN managers (N = 832) followed up on reported deviations from safety protocols that could have caused patient harm.

1.3.1 **Health care organization leaders should encourage the reporting of errors, unsafe conditions, and intimidating behaviors.**[50,81,99,100] [Recommendation]

Health care organization leaders provide the foundation for building a patient safety culture. A patient safety culture reflects actions that provide safe care in the health care organization.[84] Disruptive behavior has an adverse effect on staff relationships, communication flow, and patient care. Moderate-quality evidence[50,81,99-103] identifies that disruptive behavior can cause increased workplace stress, contribute to dysfunctional teams, reduce the quality of care for patients and their family members, and increase the risk of litigation. Leaders of high-reliability teams foster a patient safety culture by discour-

aging disruptive team member behaviors and encouraging behaviors that promote reporting of safety concerns.

1.4 **Use human factor analysis in the development of processes for establishing a patient safety culture.** [Recommendation]

A patient safety culture incorporates human factor analysis to decrease adverse events or errors. Moderate-quality evidence[82,83,104-108] demonstrates that the use of standardization, checklists, and protocols mitigates the human factor risk. The perioperative team should be constantly adapting to mitigate human factor risk and promote resilience in the environment. Maxfield et al[83] reported that 85% (n = 2,020) of RN survey respondents had used tools that minimize human factor errors, such as checklists, hand-over tools, and drug interaction warning systems. These tools identify problems that may have been missed, to assist in prevention of unintentional slips and errors.

1.5 **Establish an environment that promotes resilience in individual team members.** [Recommendation]

Low-quality evidence[50,90,109] supports the relationship between human error and personal factors, such as fatigue, nutritional state, emotional states including anger and stress, multitasking, and loss of awareness of what is happening. Brennan et al[90] describes using the mnemonic HALT (Hungry, Anxious or angry, Late or lonely, and Tired) to assess team members' abilities to perform their roles. The researchers concluded that a team member can use the mnemonic to stop himself or herself from potentially creating an error or to inform and help if they observe any of these factors in another team member.

1.6 **Establish patient safety goals.** [Recommendation]

Establishing patient safety goals guides the team in working toward a patient safety culture.

1.7 **Implement clear, just, and transparent processes for recognizing human and system errors and distinguishing these from unsafe, blameworthy actions.** [Recommendation]

Errors are frequently the consequence of system failures.[110-112] Reason defined errors as "all those occasions in which a planned sequence of mental or physical activities fails to achieve its intended outcome, and when these failures cannot be attributed to the intervention of some chance agency."[111(p9)] These errors can be slips, lapses, or mistakes in memory or actions when executing the action or plan.

In a **just culture**, determination of individual and system errors is balanced with personal accountability and system improvement. People are encouraged to provide essential safety-related information but are also clear about where the line must be drawn between acceptable and unacceptable behavior. Blaming an individual for an error may be more immediate than taking the time to investigate and correct the system issue that was the **root cause**. However, blaming does not help personnel or the health care organization understand how mistakes occur, fix a broken system, or help an individual improve his or her performance, and it will not stop unsafe acts from occurring.[110-112]

1.7.1 When an error is caused by a system failure, take steps to improve the system.[28,111,113] [*Recommendation*]

1.7.2 When an error is caused by the action of an individual, provide the individual with counseling, coaching, or other corrective action.[95,114-116] [*Recommendation*]

1.8 Establish a process for conflict resolution. [*Recommendation*]

Moderate-quality evidence[101-103,117-119] indicates that conflicts are inevitable in the high-volume, complex, and constantly changing perioperative environment. Providing a process to resolve conflict in a constructive manner may decrease frustration and stress in the workplace. In a quasi-experimental study, Saxton[118] conducted a survey of 17 perioperative nurses before and after they attended a two-day Crucial Conversations® workshop. In the post-workshop survey, 71% of the participants (n = 12) reported having more confidence in their ability to address disruptive physician behavior.

1.9 Establish an interdisciplinary team with authority and responsibility to provide oversight for the patient safety culture. [*Recommendation*]

Establishing an interdisciplinary team of key stakeholders who oversee the implementation of team training and system design provides a forum for discussion of barriers to the patient safety culture.[50,53,120] The National Surgical Patient Safety Summit[3] recommends having a centralized and coordinated oversight committee to monitor the patient safety culture.

1.9.1 Include the following representatives on the interdisciplinary team:
- nurses,
- support personnel,
- surgeons,
- anesthesia professionals,
- perioperative services executives,
- quality management personnel, and
- risk management personnel.[50,53,120]
[*Recommendation*]

1.9.2 The interdisciplinary team should
- oversee the implementation of the culture of safety and team training;
- develop and implement the communication tools that will be used for briefing, time out, debriefing, and hand overs;
- review the safety measures and identify actions to be taken to sustain safety measures; and
- report safety data to the perioperative executive team.[50,53,120]
[*Recommendation*]

1.10 Identify perioperative team leaders who will provide leadership by
- organizing the team,
- identifying and articulating clear goals,
- assigning tasks and responsibilities,
- monitoring and modifying the plan,
- reviewing the team's performance,
- managing and allocating resources,
- facilitating information sharing,
- encouraging team members to assist one another,
- facilitating conflict resolution in the learning environment, and
- modeling effective teamwork.
[*Recommendation*]

Low-quality evidence[50,96,113,121-123] supports the need for strong leadership in teams. Henrickson Parker et al[96] conducted a literature review on surgeon leadership skills. The review revealed two common categories for leadership: task focus and team focus. A team supported by a leader who can focus on both the task and the team can work well together and accomplish goals. Although the authors found many studies on leadership theory and leadership in the workplace, only one study was conducted in the perioperative setting. The authors found that the perception of teamwork differed among surgeons and nursing personnel. Nurses viewed good leadership as good collaboration where their input is respected, whereas surgeons defined collaboration as having a team that can anticipate needs and follow instructions.

Further research is needed to determine ideal intraoperative leadership behaviors for safe surgical practice and whether the surgeon should lead the team or maintain focus on the task of performing surgery.

1.11 Reduce barriers to effective communication, including

- facility design barriers,[124-127]
- irrelevant conversations,[127,128]
- noise levels,[126,129,130]
- social setting barriers (eg, status, hierarchy),[101]
- distractions,[124,131] and
- interruptions.[126,127,131,132]

[Recommendation]

Moderate-quality evidence[124-127,130-132] supports that distractions lead to miscommunication and adverse events.

Jothiraj et al[131] conducted a qualitative study in which they observed anesthesiologists in 32 separate procedures during which distractions were recorded by two trained medical student observers. Distractions caused by another anesthesiologist were frequent, and in one-third of those events, the distraction had an observable effect on the anesthesiologist caring for the patient. The authors suggested that the anesthesiologists needed to address themselves as causes of distractions and the potential impact on patient safety.

In an observational study, Keller et al[129] compared peak noise levels on the influence of communication in the surgical setting. The results showed that high noise peaks reduced the frequency of patient-related communication, and communication was impaired because the noise was distracting. The researcher recommended interventions to reduce the noise level in the OR.

Weigl et al[132] conducted an observational study that compared the effect of intraoperative interruptions on surgeons' perceived workload in orthopedic surgery. The researchers observed 56 elective procedures and determined that intraoperative interruptions occurred an average of 9.78 times per hour. The interruptions that occurred most often included people entering or exiting the OR (30.6%) and telephone- or pager-related disruptions (23.6%). The researchers determined that interruptions contributed to the deterioration of the surgeon's mental focus.

1.11.1 Refrain from nonessential activities to minimize distractions during important tasks (ie, the **sterile cockpit** rule) or during critical communication phases of the procedure (eg, briefing, time out, debriefing, induction of or emergence from anesthesia, count process, specimen handling).[113,131-134] *[Recommendation]*

Moderate-quality evidence[113,131-133] supports that mental fatigue and stress can be reduced when a hand over is performed in a private, quiet setting with minimal interruptions and distractions where the participants can focus their attention on the information being provided.

1.11.2 Implement strategies to decrease distractions or interruptions. Strategies may include

- identifying sources of noise that can be reduced,[113,134]
- leaving cell phones and pagers outside of the OR or procedure room,[134]
- prioritizing conversations during critical phases of care,
- muting cell phones,[134,135]
- limiting nonessential conversation,[135]
- controlling voice level and tone,[134]
- setting equipment alarms and alerts to the lowest audible level,[135]
- limiting the number of people in the OR,[134]
- limiting overhead paging,[134]
- displaying "quiet please" posters,[113,134] and
- providing education on the importance of minimizing interruptions.[113]

[Recommendation]

1.11.3 When a distraction or interruption occurs that could affect patient safety, a safety pause should be implemented by any perioperative team member. A safety pause may consist of

- identifying a safety event,
- calling for a safety pause and communicating the concern,
- resolving the event with a team response to the concern, and
- discussing the event during the debriefing process and identifying ways to improve patient care.[100,132]

[Recommendation]

A safety pause provides an opportunity for any perioperative team member to pause patient care when he or she perceives that a distraction or interruption is causing potentially unsafe conditions.[108,134]

In an organizational experience described by Meginniss et al,[108] personnel used a standardized communication technique called "Time-out for patient safety." This technique provided a critical language for safety situations and empowered the team members to speak up when they had a safety concern.

1.12 Perioperative team members should collaborate and support each other by

- crosschecking and monitoring;
- asking a question, making a request, or voicing a concern;
- using the chain of command;
- giving timely and specific feedback for peer coaching;
- questioning attitudes; and

- reading back and verifying the receipt of critical patient information.[95,114-116]

[*Recommendation*]

Moderate-quality evidence[95,114-116] supports collaboration among team members that improves accurate communication. When individuals ask for more information at the hand over, the hand over is perceived as more accurate. Boyd et al[116] found that read-back techniques increased the transfer of critical patient information between team members.

1.13 Speak up and address behavior that may lead to patient harm by

- collecting the facts;
- assuming the best intent of each team member;
- helping the team member as well as the patient;
- making the conversation safe to prevent defensiveness;
- using facts and data as much as possible;
- avoiding telling negative stories or making accusations; and
- diffusing or deflecting the person's anger and emotion.[83]

[*Recommendation*]

A perioperative team member's willingness to speak up is dependent on whether he or she perceives it is safe to do so, that there is opportunity to do so, that doing so will be effective, and that he or she has credibility with other members of the team.[105] Nembhard et al[105] conducted a qualitative study in which they interviewed 99 surgeons, anesthesia professionals, and nursing personnel at 12 randomly selected hospitals in the United States about their willingness to speak up. They found that factors such as tenure, work configuration, culture, benchmarking, and external environment influenced the health professionals' sense of safety, efficacy, opportunity, or legitimacy, all of which affected their belief about the risk and benefit of speaking up and willingness to speak up. They also found the team members would speak up for three purposes: to learn for themselves, to inform others, and to protect patients. The researchers concluded that leaders can influence or elicit a willingness to voice concerns by attending to these factors.

Raemer et al[107] conducted a randomized controlled trial in which they concluded that an educational intervention alone was ineffective in improving the speaking-up behaviors of practicing non-trainee anesthesiologists. The anesthesiologists (N = 337) completed a survey after participating in a simulation course designed to observe speaking-up behavior in different simulated scenarios. The five most frequently mentioned hurdles to speaking up were uncertainty about the issue, stereotypes about others on the team, unfamiliarity with the individual they were speaking to, respect for other's experience, and the repercussion expected. The five most frequently mentioned strategies to increase speaking up were realizing the speaking-up problem, having a speaking-up rubric, certainty about the consequences of speaking up, familiarity with the individual they were speaking to, and getting a second opinion or getting help.[107]

2. Hand-Over Process

2.1 Establish and implement a standardized hand-over process for the transfer of patient information between individuals and teams. [*Recommendation*]

High-quality evidence[136-150] suggests that communication failure and incomplete or missing patient information are the most common causes of sentinel events and pose a significant threat to patient safety. Communication failures during transfer of information are common in the perioperative setting and can compromise patient safety and contribute to inefficiency.[138] A standardized hand-over process may improve patient safety by promoting optimal communication by all perioperative team members during the transfer of patient information, which is a critical phase in a patient's perioperative experience.

2.2 Establish an interdisciplinary team at the facility level to develop a standardized hand-over process. [*Recommendation*]

A standardized hand-over process helps to identify risks during the perioperative phases so the team can take action to minimize threats to patient safety. In a systematic review of nonexperimental studies, Møller et al[151] recognized that patient hand over is an ever-changing and complex process designed to analyze and address the challenges in the local setting. The author recommended that the hand-over process be designed to fit the context in which it will take place.

2.2.1 Include the following representatives on the interdisciplinary team:

- perioperative RNs,
- perianesthesia RNs,
- RNs from receiving patient care units,
- surgeons,
- anesthesia professionals,
- **licensed independent practitioners**,
- allied health care providers, and
- support personnel.

[*Recommendation*]

2.3 The hand-over process should include

- assigning the roles and responsibilities of team members,
- individualizing the hand over for the specific patient population (eg, child, adult) and level of acuity (eg, severity of symptoms, complexity of surgery, comorbid conditions),
- notifying the receiving team member that the patient is being transferred and of the potential equipment needs before the patient's arrival,
- completing urgent tasks before starting the hand-over communication,
- limiting the hand-over conversation to only patient-specific discussions,
- allowing only one person to speak at a time,
- keeping distractions and interruptions (eg, personal conversations) to a minimum with only urgent clinical interruptions allowed,
- using supporting documentation (eg, lab test results), and
- providing an opportunity for participants to voice concerns and ask questions.[151]

[Recommendation]

A structured hand-over process that includes strategies for safe patient care helps to identify and mitigate risks to patient safety.[151]

In a systematic review of quasi-experimental and nonexperimental studies, Segall et al[152] identified recommendations for hand-over structure and information transfer. The researchers found an association between poor quality hand-over processes and adverse patient safety events.

2.3.1 The interdisciplinary team should assign team member roles and responsibilities for the hand-over process.[153,154] *[Recommendation]*

Ambiguous roles and responsibilities can cause confusion during the hand-over process and can contribute to potential patient harm. In a nonexperimental study, McElroy et al[153] identified that team member participation was important to the development of a high-quality hand-over process. The physical presence of all team members was clearly identified as key to conveying all of the patient care issues that need to be addressed between transferring and receiving team members.

In a qualitative study, McElroy et al[154] found that clarifying team member roles and expectations decreased ambiguity and the risk of patient harm. The researchers determined that there were varying degrees of team member participation in the hand-over process, and roles within a team determined the team members' perspectives of the hand-over process.

2.4 Use the **read-back method** when communicating patient information to other team members. *[Recommendation]*

The read-back method improves communication during hand overs. In a nonexperimental study conducted by Boyd et al,[116] postanesthesia care unit nurses and anesthesia assistants participated in 88 simulated scenarios involving a clinical crisis. Participants used either a read-back method, verbal acknowledgement without read-back, or no verbal reply to respond to patient information. Participants who used the read-back method were 8.27 times more likely to correctly recall information and those that responded verbally were 3.16 times more likely to correctly recall information compared to participants who gave no verbal response.

2.5 Use standardized hand-over tools, checklists, or protocols. *[Recommendation]*

High-quality evidence[46,64,143,155-163] demonstrates that the use of standardized tools, protocols, and checklists improves the quality of information transfer and decreases communication breakdowns during hand overs.

In a systematic review of quasi-experimental and nonexperimental studies, Pucher et al[46] found that using a checklist or standardized process may improve transfers of patient information.

In a randomized controlled trial, Salzwedel et al[64] implemented use of a written checklist in a university hospital. The researchers observed 40 hand overs before the checklist implementation and 80 hand overs after implementation. They determined that the percentage of overall items included in the hand over were significantly increased with use of the checklist. The researchers concluded that the quality of patient hand overs was improved because of the additional patient information relayed with the use of a written checklist.

In a quality improvement (QI) project, Petrovic et al[164] implemented use of a perioperative hand-over tool to improve postprocedural patient transfers. The tool established a mandate that all members of the hand-over team be present at the bedside and provided a series of structured steps that guided the hand over. The authors found that implementation of the tool resulted in improved information sharing, increased team satisfaction, and decreased distractions during the hand over.

2.5.1 The perioperative team may use evidence-based tools during the hand over, such as

- SBAR: situation, background, assessment, recommendation[157,160];
- I PASS the BATON: introduction, patient, assessment, situation, safety concerns, (the) background, actions, timing, ownership, next[165];
- SWITCH: surgical procedure, wet, instruments, tissue, counts, have you any questions[158]; and
- SURgical PAtient Safety System (SURPASS).[56]

[Conditional Recommendation]

In a prospective intervention study, Randmaa et al[160] implemented the SBAR communication tool in anesthetic clinics in two hospitals. The researchers used preassessment and postassessment data to determine the number of incident reports generated because of communication errors. In the intervention group using the SBAR tool, there was a significant improvement in communication accuracy, and the number of incident reports resulting from communication errors decreased from 31% of all incident reports in the year before the tool implementation to 11% of all incident reports in the year after the implementation.

Eberhardt[157] reported on an organizational experience in which a team comprised of medical/surgical and perioperative RNs implemented the SBAR hand-over tool to standardize the hand-over process between the medical-surgical unit and the OR. The team implemented a pilot test and refined the tool based on the feedback from the perioperative and medical-surgical RNs. The team then implemented the process throughout the facility and received positive responses from all the RNs who used it in the hand-over process.

As part of TeamSTEPPS®, the mnemonic I PASS THE BATON was created to structure the critical communication elements that need to be conveyed during a hand over or patient care transition.[165]

Johnson et al[158] developed the SWITCH intraoperative tool in response to identified inconsistencies in communication of essential information during the transfer of patient care from one perioperative care provider to another. The tool enabled the perioperative team to have a standardized reporting process, address communication barriers, and maintain focus on patient care during critical moments, such as shift changes, thereby improving patient safety.

The SURPASS checklist was developed as a multidisciplinary checklist designed to follow the patient from admission to discharge, and it can be used for the hand-over process. In a quasi-experimental study, deVries et al[56] compared rates of complication in patients before (n = 3,760) and after (n = 3,820) implementation of the SURPASS checklist. The researchers found that the total number of complications per 100 patients decreased from 27.3 to 16.7.

2.6 Include all phases and locations of patient care in a standardized hand-over process design. Phases of care include

- scheduling,
- preadmission,
- preoperative,
- intraoperative, and
- postoperative.

Locations of care may include the

- primary care provider's office,
- surgeon's office,
- scheduling department,
- preanesthesia testing unit,
- presurgical testing unit,
- preoperative holding area,
- OR or procedure room,
- postanesthesia care unit, and
- other areas where postoperative care is provided (eg, medical/surgical ward, intensive care unit).

[Recommendation]

Moderate-quality evidence[143,146,152] indicates that poor standardization, incomplete transfer of information, incomplete team involvement, and absence of clinical task execution are barriers to effective postoperative hand overs. Hand overs can be inconsistent, and items deemed important may vary by team member, patient population, patient acuity, and facility.

2.6.1 When performing a hand-over from scheduling to the preoperative phase, verify

- the correct patient and procedure including site and side;
- completion of the history and physical;
- completion of required consultations;
- informed consent;
- preoperative orders;
- an anesthesia consult as needed;
- implant, instrumentation, and equipment needs; and
- the identification of the patient's caregiver who will be present at the preoperative visit.[56,166]

[Recommendation]

In a nonexperimental study, Wu and Aufses[167] reviewed scheduling errors reported in one institution's adverse event reporting system and identified that in 17,606 surgeries, there were 151 errors in scheduling. The most common scheduling errors were wrong-side booking (eg, left, right), incomplete booking (eg, additional procedures added after booking, bilateral cases scheduled for one side), and wrong approach (eg, laparoscopic versus open). The incomplete booking and wrong approach scheduling errors resulted in delays and increased cost to the health care organization. The researchers concluded that scheduling errors were infrequent but caused disruptions in OR team dynamics, delays, and substantial costs.

In a literature review, Zahiri et al[166] found that the first encounter with the patient is crucial for ensuring that the correct and compete medical record is available to prevent wrong site surgery. The authors recommended that the surgeon perform a thorough history and physical and that this information be entered meticulously into the patient's medical record; that the consent be completed with the patient and immediately placed in the patient's medical record; and that a standardized, efficient scheduling process be instituted in the surgeon's office to decrease risk to the patient as a result of scheduling errors.

2.6.2 The hand-over process for the preoperative to the intraoperative phase may include information on
- the correct patient and procedure;
- the correct operative side/site;
- the history and physical;
- the patient's allergies;
- the patient's current medications and adjustments if needed (eg, anticoagulants, antibiotics);
- significant diagnostic test results;
- medications given or prescribed;
- anticoagulation prophylaxis, if applicable;
- patient mobility issues;
- blood products available, if ordered; and
- a plan for communicating with the patient's significant other.[56]

[Conditional Recommendation]

2.6.3 The hand-over process during the intraoperative phase for personnel change may include information on
- the correct patient and procedure,
- the correct operative side/site,
- special considerations or precautions,

- intraoperative imaging,
- the type of incision and dressing needed,
- the postoperative plan of care,
- medications or other solutions on the sterile field,
- blood products given or available,
- current blood loss,
- urine output,
- the presence of drains,
- implants needed,
- instruments needed and the location of the instruments,
- specimen management,
- grafts (eg, type, location),
- the status of counts (eg, sponges, needles, instruments) and the location of counted items (eg, body cavities, off the sterile field),
- the status of documentation, and
- a plan for communicating with the patient's significant other.[146,158]

[Conditional Recommendation]

2.6.4 The hand-over process for the intraoperative to postoperative phase may include information on
- the patient's circulation, airway, and breathing[133,143];
- the patient's name, age, weight, vital signs[143,152];
- the patient's allergies[143,146,152];
- the patient's diagnosis and pertinent medical history[146,152];
- the procedure performed[143,146,152];
- surgical complications and corrective interventions[146,152];
- time in the OR[146];
- the patient's current condition (eg, hemodynamic status)[143,152];
- the patient's skin condition[143];
- the pressure injury risk assessment;
- the patient's hypothermia status[146];
- the type of anesthesia[146,152];
- complications from the anesthesia[152];
- intraoperative medications administered, including dose and time[146,152];
- IV fluids and lines present[146,152];
- drains and tubes present[143];
- wound packing (eg, type, location)[143];
- blood products used, including type and amount[152];
- estimated blood loss[146,152];
- any intraoperative testing performed (eg, radiograph, echocardiogram)[152];
- surgical site information (eg, dressings, tubes, drains, packing)[152];

- the postoperative management plan and orders,[152] including
  - anticipated recovery concerns[152];
  - the monitoring plan and the acceptable range of physiological variables[152];
  - the plan for pain management[152];
  - the plan for IV fluids, medications, antibiotics, and venous thromboembolism prophylaxis[146,152];
  - the plan for feeding and oral hydration[143,146,152];
  - disposition of the patient (eg, discharge or admission)[143]; and
  - the receiving patient care unit, if applicable[143];
- special considerations or precautions; and
- a plan for communicating with the patient's significant other.

[Conditional Recommendation]

2.6.5 The hand-over process for patients being transferred directly from the OR to an intensive care unit (ICU) should include activities before and upon arrival.

The perioperative RN should prepare for the hand over before arrival at the ICU, by

- notifying the ICU before leaving the OR or at predetermined notification time frames established by the interdisciplinary team[145,168,169];
- notifying the ICU of ventilator settings, if applicable[145,168,169];
- verifying that all transport equipment is available and functioning correctly[168];
- creating a written or digital OR summary data sheet for the ICU team[168];
- notifying the ICU if the patient will need isolation precautions and what type[143];
- notifying the ICU to prepare monitors, drains, IV fluids, and medications before the patient's arrival[133,169]; and
- disentangling patient device tubing and lines before leaving the OR.[143,169]

On arrival at the ICU, the hand-over process should include completion of patient care tasks and communication of patient information, including

- a call for a safety pause at the start of the hand over[169];
- a review of hand-over elements from the intraoperative to postoperative phases (See Recommendation 2.6.4);
- connection of the breathing circuit to the ICU ventilator[143];

- a check of oxygenation and ventilation status (eg, breath sounds, chest expansion, oxygen saturation)[148,169];
- connection of the patient to monitoring equipment[169];
- connection of chest tubes to suction[169];
- communication of the anesthesia details by the anesthesia professional (eg, type of induction, central line, arterial lines placed, complications)[144,145,148,169];
- communication of the surgery details by the surgeon (eg, surgery performed, cardiopulmonary bypass time, cross clamp time, transesophageal echocardiogram results)[144,145,148,169];
- discussion by the team of postoperative details (eg, blood loss, blood products administered, blood products currently available, pacemaker, vital signs, intracardiac pressures, medications administered, fluid volume, sedatives, laboratory test results, tubes, drains)[144,145,148,169];
- confirmation that medications and IV drips are correctly labeled[144,145,148,169];
- discussion of the expected postoperative course, potential complications or risks, and anticipatory guidance[145,168,169]; and
- discussion of specific concerns for the patient.[144,145,147,148,168,169]

[Recommendation]

High-quality evidence[133,143-145,147,148,153,168,169] suggests that hand overs to an intensive care setting can be difficult because of the acuity of the patient; the numerous drains, lines, and tubes present; distractions and noise; and the lack of all team members being present during the hand-over process, all of which can increase a patient's risk for harm.

Developing protocols and checklists for use in hand overs between the OR and the ICU increases team-member involvement, reduces errors, and may improve efficiencies during the hand-over process.[133,143-145,147,148,153,168,169]

In a qualitative study, McElroy et al[168] assessed systems and processes involved in the hand over between the OR and the ICU. Using a failure modes, effects, and criticality analysis, the researchers identified 37 individual steps in the hand-over process. The researchers found 81 process failures, 22 of which were in critical processes. The processes with the greatest risk to cause harm were lack of preliminary OR to ICU communication, team members being absent during the hand over, and equipment malfunctioning during transport.

Chen et al[133] conducted an observational, cross-sectional study of hand-over communications between the OR and the pediatric cardiac ICU in one facility. The team used a protocol that included the "sterile cockpit" environment where all hand-over team participants refrained from nonessential activities to decrease distractions during the hand-over process. The researchers concluded that the hand-over process in a sterile cockpit environment decreased distraction and improved discussion about the anticipated patient course.

3. Briefing

3.1 Establish and implement a standardized briefing process before the surgical procedure. [Recommendation]

Moderate-quality evidence[114,120,170-178] supports the use of briefings to improve teamwork and team communication and improve the quality of patient care by increasing efficiency, decreasing interruptions and delays, and improving patient outcomes. Briefing improves team communication by allowing teams to develop a shared mental model.[179]

Thanapongsathorn et al[172] reported on an organizational experience in which a project team implemented a preoperative briefing that included the entire perioperative team. The perioperative team met before each procedure, and the briefing lasted no longer than 10 minutes. The project team collected team satisfaction data and found that the briefings increased the level of satisfaction for teamwork and decreased operative time because preventable delays were identified before the start of the surgery.

Although evidence supports the performance of the time out just before the incision, further research is needed to determine the ideal timing for the briefing.[50,63,66,180]

3.2 The interdisciplinary team should create a standardized briefing process with input from perioperative team members representing individual service lines (eg, cardiac, orthopedic, neurosurgical, obstetric). [Recommendation]

Johnston et al[171] reported on an organizational experience in which they developed an auditing tool to determine how preoperative briefings were conducted at an academic medical center. They found a high degree of variability in participation among team members and across service lines and highlighted the need for service-specific customization of the briefing process.

3.2.1 The briefing process should include
- introduction of the team members[175,181];
- the patient's name and identifiers (the patient may participate)[171,173,175];
- the consent signed[171];
- the planned procedure and side[171,173];
- the goals of the procedure[175];
- the estimated length of the procedure[173];
- a review of laboratory results and radiographs[171,172,175];
- the planned intraoperative patient position[171,173,175];
- the pressure injury risk assessment;
- the planned patient skin antisepsis[171];
- that the needed equipment is available,[175];
- that the needed instruments are available[172];
- the patient's known allergies or sensitivities[171];
- special considerations or precautions[173,175];
- a fire risk assessment[182]; and
- questions, safety concerns, and equipment concerns.[173,175]

[Recommendation]

3.2.2 The briefing process may include information about
- venous thromboembolism prophylaxis[171,175];
- difficult airway or risk of aspiration[171];
- antibiotic administration[170,171,175];
- anticipated antibiotic redosing[171,175];
- the need for glucose management[171,175];
- the plan for regional, neuraxial, or local anesthesia[173];
- anticipated blood loss[171,173,175];
- planned pneumatic tourniquet use[173];
- the availability of blood and blood products[171,172,175];
- the availability of implants[175];
- the intraoperative imaging needed[171]; and
- the postoperative plan of care.[173]

[Conditional Recommendation]

3.3 The briefing may be guided by the use of a checklist.[170] [Conditional Recommendation]

In a quasi-experimental study, Lingard et al[170] assessed the effect of a checklist-driven preoperative team briefing on the timing of the administration of prophylactic antibiotics. The percentage of patients who received on-time administration of antibiotics improved from 77.6% in the pre-intervention phase to 87.6% in the post-intervention phase.

3.4 Stop all unnecessary activities and conversations when the briefing is initiated.[120,134,183,184] [Recommendation]

Distractions and interruptions during critical conversations and phases of perioperative care can contribute to surgical errors.

4. Site Marking

4.1 The patient's identity, procedure, and procedural site including laterality must be verified and the site marked.[185] *[Regulatory Requirement]*

Identifying the correct site on the patient's body where the procedure or surgery is to be performed helps to decrease the risk for wrong site surgery.[120,185,186] **Site marking** is required by the Centers for Medicare & Medicaid Services (CMS).[185] All accrediting agencies with CMS deemed status require site marking.

The Universal Protocol was developed by The Joint Commission to provide guidance for prevention of wrong site, wrong procedure, and wrong person surgery.[186] The protocol consists of three steps: preprocedure verification, patient site marking, and a time out. The World Health Organization also recommends site marking for cases involving laterality or multiple structures or levels.[120]

4.2 The site marking process must be consistent throughout the health care organization and not open to interpretation.[185,186] *[Regulatory Requirement]*

Consistent site marking processes applied throughout the health care organization decrease confusion and risk for wrong site surgery.

4.2.1 Identify procedures that will require site marking.[120,186] *[Recommendation]*

4.2.2 At a minimum, perform site marking when there is more than one possible location for the surgery to occur.[186] *[Recommendation]*

4.3 The procedure site must be marked before the procedure begins.[120,185,186] *[Regulatory Requirement]*

Marking the site before the procedure helps to promote patient involvement and minimize the risk for wrong site surgery.

4.3.1 Involve the patient or the patient's representative in the marking of the site if possible.[186] *[Recommendation]*

4.3.2 The procedure site must be marked by a licensed independent practitioner who is accountable and will be present when the procedure is performed.[185,186] *[Regulatory Requirement]*

4.3.3 Site marking may be delegated to another individual as defined in health care organization policy, which may include

- a postgraduate medical student who is being supervised by the licensed independent practitioner performing the procedure, is familiar with the patient, and will be present when the surgery or procedure is performed or

- a person who has a collaborative or supervisory agreement with the licensed independent practitioner performing the procedure, is familiar with the patient, and will be present when the procedure or surgery is performed (an advanced practice RN or physician assistant).[186]

[Conditional Recommendation]

4.3.4 The mark should be made at or near the procedure site and be visible after surgical skin antisepsis and draping.[186] *[Recommendation]*

4.3.5 Create an alternative marking process for patients who refuse site marking or for cases when it is anatomically or technically impossible (eg, mucosal surfaces, the perineum, teeth) or impractical (eg, minimal access procedures that involve a lateralized internal organ, whether through a natural orifice or percutaneous access; procedures on premature infants for whom marking may cause a permanent tattoo).[186] *[Recommendation]*

4.3.6 For spinal procedures, in addition to skin marking, use intraoperative imaging techniques to determine the exact vertebral level.[120,186,187] *[Recommendation]*

5. Time Out

5.1 The perioperative team must perform a time out before an operative or invasive procedure begins.[185] *[Regulatory Requirement]*

The collective evidence[26,50,120,166,183-185,188,189] supports the time out as a tool to prevent wrong site surgeries. The purpose of the time out is to conduct a final check that the correct patient, correct site, and correct procedure are identified. During a time out, all activities are stopped so that the perioperative team can focus on the factors that contribute to a wrong person, wrong site, and wrong procedure surgery and other risks to patient safety.[120,184,189] A time out provides an opportunity for all perioperative team members to speak up and address any concerns or problems that would affect the safety of the patient.

5.2 **The time out should be a standardized process as defined by the facility.** [Recommendation]

A standardized process is most effective when it is conducted consistently throughout the facility.

5.2.1 **A designated perioperative team member should call for the time out to begin.**[183] [Recommendation]

5.2.2 **The time out should involve all members of the perioperative team. The participating team members must include the individual performing the procedure, the anesthesia professional, the RN circulator, the scrub person, and any other team members who will be participating in the procedure from the beginning.**[120,189] [Recommendation]

5.2.3 **If two or more procedures are being performed on the same patient and the person performing the procedure is different, conduct a time out before each procedure.**[120,189] [Recommendation]

5.2.4 **During the time-out process, the team must confirm, at a minimum, the correct patient, site, and procedure to be performed.**[120,185,189] [Regulatory Requirement]

5.2.5 **Stop all unnecessary activities and conversations in the OR when the time out is called.**[120,183,184] [Recommendation]

5.2.6 **If perioperative team members have not introduced themselves, each person should state his or her name and role on the team.**[188] [Recommendation]

5.2.7 **Discuss any patient safety concerns or concerns about the procedure during the time out.**[120,188] [Recommendation]

5.2.8 **Document the time out as completed in accordance with facility policy (amount and type of documentation).**[189] [Recommendation]

5.3 **Perform a time out before regional anesthesia procedures.**[21] [Recommendation]

Barrington et al[21] conducted a literature review to describe the phenomenon of wrong site regional anesthetic blocks and to identify preventive strategies. The authors found that the incidence of wrong regional block procedures may be as frequent as 7.5

per 10,000 procedures. They identified factors that contribute to wrong regional blocks, including scheduling changes, poor communication, incomplete documentation, patient position change, physician distraction, lack of surgical consent, inadequate supervision of residents, lack of situational awareness, fatigue, site marking not visible, cognitive overload, and failure to perform a time out. The authors recommended performing a time out immediately before all regional anesthesia procedures and repeating the time out with any patient position change or procedures performed by a different team.

5.4 **Identify when a subsequent or second time out may be performed for a lengthy procedure.** [Recommendation]

Patients who are undergoing lengthy surgical procedures are at increased risk for positioning and nerve injuries and other complications. In an organizational experience, Song et al[190] implemented a second time out in their facility that was aimed at reducing patient complications and addressing problems encountered during lengthy robotic surgeries. The authors developed a standardized surgical checklist to address potential problems and improve patient safety. The second time out provided an opportunity for members of the perioperative team to discuss concerns for patient safety and address issues unique to robotic surgery. The implementation of the second time out received positive feedback from the perioperative team, and there was minimal intrusion into the surgical procedure time.

5.5 **Use a standardized surgical safety checklist during the time-out process.** [Recommendation]

High-quality evidence[16-62] supports the use of a standardized safe surgery checklist during the time-out process to improve communication, reduce the potential for error, reduce patient complications, improve adherence to critical processes and safety measures, and decrease surgical mortality. A surgical safety checklist is designed to enhance communication and teamwork and helps create an environment in which perioperative team members' input is solicited and welcomed and information sharing is encouraged.[53]

In a systematic review of quasi-experimental and nonexperimental studies, Treadwell et al[16] found that the use of a safe surgery checklist, such as the World Health Organization (WHO) Surgical Safety Checklist or the SURPASS checklist, could potentially decrease patient morbidity and mortality in surgery. Safe surgery checklists were associated with fewer complications, improved communication, improvements in facility safety culture, and increased detection of potential safety issues.

Thomassen et al[17] also conducted a systematic review of quasi-experimental and nonexperimental studies and found that safe surgery checklists could be used in all clinical settings to increase compliance with national guidelines, reduce the number of safety events, decrease morbidity and mortality, and mitigate errors attributable to human factors. The researchers did not find evidence that the safe surgery checklists had negative effects on patient safety or quality of care.

In another systematic review, Russ et al[18] found that patient outcomes could be improved when perioperative teams used a safe surgery checklist because the use of the checklist improved teamwork and communication.

Lyons and Popejoy[19] conducted a systematic review with meta-analysis on the effects of the use of a safe surgery checklist on teamwork, communication, morbidity, mortality, and safety. The researchers found that using a checklist improved team communication and teamwork, reduced morbidity and mortality, and improved compliance with safety measures.

Bock et al[25] conducted a quasi-experimental retrospective comparative analysis of administrative outcome data before and after implementation of a surgical safety checklist in one large hospital in Italy. The researchers collected data 3 months before and 3 months after checklist implementation (N = 10,741 procedures). Thirty- and 90-day all-cause mortality were the outcomes for this study. The introduction of the surgical safety checklist was associated with a significant reduction in 90-day all-cause mortality (2.4% [n = 129] compared with 2.2% [n = 118] after the surgical safety checklist implementation). The implementation of the safe surgery checklist was not associated with a reduction of 30-day all-cause mortality.

The evidence conflicts about the actual rate of improved surgical mortality with checklist use. Urbach et al[191] surveyed 101 hospitals in Canada in a nonexperimental study to determine operative mortality, rates of surgical complications, lengths of hospital stay, and rates of hospital readmission and emergency department visits within 30 days after discharge among patients undergoing a variety of surgical procedures before and after adoption of a safe surgery checklist. The researchers found no significant reduction in operative mortality after checklist implementation. In addition, there were no reductions in risk of surgical complications, hospital readmissions, or emergency department visits after the safe surgery checklist implementation. The researchers noted that a greater effect from the use

of the safe surgery checklist may occur with intensive team training or increased monitoring for compliance. The researchers also acknowledged that the safe surgery checklist may be beneficial in improving teamwork and communication.

In a prospective study, Sewell et al[192] evaluated the outcomes of mortality, early complications, and personnel perceptions of the WHO Surgical Safety Checklist after an educational program was instituted to increase use of a safe surgery checklist in one facility. The researchers reviewed 480 patient procedures before the educational program and 485 after the educational program. They determined that the use of the checklist for emergency and elective orthopedic patients at their facility was not associated with a significant reduction in early major complications or mortality. The educational program significantly increased the accurate use of the checklist and improved personnel perceptions of the WHO Surgical Safety Checklist.

Standardized checklist formats include the WHO Surgical Safety Checklist,[120] the SURPASS Checklist,[93] and AORN's Comprehensive Surgical Checklist.

5.6 **Adapt the safe surgery checklist to the patient population served.** [Recommendation]

High-quality evidence[20,27,32,35,36,47,52-55,59,193-196] supports the customization of checklists based on specialized surgical procedures and unique characteristics of patients, with input from all members of the perioperative team.

5.6.1 **Develop the checklist with input from perioperative team members representing individual service lines.** [Recommendation]

Input from individual team members helps to identify care relevant to specific patient populations, provide meaning to the safe surgery checklist, and decrease variability.

Fargen et al[32] reported on the experience of one organization that implemented a three-part, 20-item checklist specific to the neurointerventional service line. Nurses, physicians, and radiology technologists were surveyed after each neurointerventional procedure 4 weeks before and 4 weeks after checklist implementation. Seventy-one procedures were performed before checklist implementation and 60 after implementation. Post-checklist surveys indicated that communication improved and the number of adverse events was significantly lower after checklist use (ie, decreased from 25 to six adverse events).

5.7 Use memory aid tools such as whiteboards, electronic whiteboards, or other tools to guide safe surgery checklist use. *[Recommendation]*

Using tools as a memory aid helps to increase compliance with the safe surgery checklist. In a quasi-experimental study, Mainthia et al[39] implemented an electronic checklist system in all ORs in one institution. They performed direct observations of 80 cases 1 month before and 1 month and 9 months after implementation of the electronic tool (N = 240). The researchers found that the core elements of the time out were performed approximately 50% of the time before implementation and approximately 80% at both 1 month and 9 months postintervention. The researchers concluded that implementing an electronic whiteboard for checklist use dramatically increased compliance with performing preprocedural time outs.

6. Debriefing

6.1 Establish and implement a standardized debriefing process. *[Recommendation]*

Moderate-quality evidence[23,50,53,59,114,174-176,179,192] supports the use of debriefings to improve teamwork and team communication, foster continuous team learning, and improve the quality of patient care by identifying defects or system barriers in care and allowing teams to learn from those defects.

The debriefing process is an active process with engagement from all members of the perioperative team focusing on specific events and applying what they learned to their practice. Debriefings allow the perioperative team to identify opportunities to improve efficiency and patient safety, identify any defects in care, and discuss the plan for the transition of patient care from the OR to another team.[50,53,175]

In an organizational experience report, Van Herzeele et al[179] identified that the debriefing process fosters team learning because members of the perioperative team can discuss what went well and what needs improvement in individual patient cases, allowing them to improve team performance.

Although evidence supports the performance of the time out just before the incision, further research is needed to determine the ideal timing for the debriefing.[50,63,66,180]

6.2 Create a standardized debriefing process with input from perioperative team members representing individual service lines. *[Recommendation]*

Input from individual team members helps to identify care relevant to specific patient populations, which provides meaning to the debriefing process. Hicks et al[175] implemented a standardized debriefing

process for patients undergoing colorectal surgery and structured the process to include focused questions relevant to colorectal surgery. They recognized that although it can be labor intensive to engage frontline providers, a debriefing process relevant to individual service lines may prove to be more sustainable and acceptable than one created with a top-down approach.

6.2.1 The debriefing process may include a discussion of
- counts performed and confirmed[175];
- the procedure performed[176];
- labeling and disposition of specimen containers[175];
- equipment and instrumentation issues[175];
- missing supplies[176];
- blood loss[175];
- glycemic control[175];
- pain management[175];
- venous thromboembolism prophylaxis[175];
- the wound classification[176];
- team members' concerns regarding the recovery and management of the patient[192]; and
- safety concerns and questions.[176]

[Conditional Recommendation]

6.3 Stop all unnecessary activities and conversations in the OR or procedure room when the debriefing is called.[120,183,184] *[Recommendation]*

6.4 The debriefing may be guided by the use of a checklist. *[Conditional Recommendation]*

7. Quality

7.1 The health care organization's quality management program should evaluate and monitor team communication and the culture of safety. *[Recommendation]*

Quality assurance and performance improvement programs can facilitate the identification of problem areas and assist personnel in evaluating and improving the quality of patient care and formulating plans for corrective action. These programs provide data that may be used to determine whether an individual organization is within benchmark goals, and if not, to identify areas that may require corrective action. A quality management program provides a mechanism to evaluate effectiveness of processes and compliance with team communication policies and procedures.

Collecting data to monitor and improve patient care, treatment, and services is a regulatory requirement[197-200] and an accreditation standard for both hospitals[201,202] and ambulatory settings.[203,204]

Sustaining a change in culture requires an organization to commit to high reliability and monitoring of quality initiatives. Health care organizations can be distracted by new initiatives and lose track of improvements that were gained in QI initiatives, like team training, effective communication, and a culture of safety.[205] A white paper published by the Institute for Healthcare Improvement (IHI)[206] described systems for sustaining improvement developed by 10 outstanding health care systems. The IHI framework outlines key factors for implementing a high-performing medical system. This framework defines primary drivers of high-performing systems as quality control, QI, and establishing a culture of high-performance management. Creating positive trust relationships encourages and sustains frontline personnel engagement in quality control and QI. The IHI framework further defined 13 secondary drivers: standardization, accountability, visual management, problem solving, escalation, integration, prioritization, assimilation, implementation, policy, feedback, transparency, and trust.

7.2 **Review patterns of error causality to develop QI projects.** *[Recommendation]*

Moderate-quality evidence[92,97,110,188,207-212] supports increased error reporting to assist with improving health care systems. The use of reporting to analyze system failures and develop QI initiatives helps decrease the potential for human error.

In a nonexperimental study, Rogers et al[213] reviewed alleged surgical errors that resulted in patient injury in 258 of the 444 (58%) malpractice claims reported from four malpractice liability insurers. Surgeon reviewers looked at each case to determine the factors that led to a surgical error. The reviewers found that most of the 258 cases involved more than one clinician and one-third involved chains of events contributing to patient harm, such as communication breakdowns, lack of supervision, technology failures, and patient-related factors. The researchers concluded that malpractice claims can be a source for surgical error analysis.

Reason[111] developed the Swiss Cheese Model, which illustrates how a chain of errors can "slip through the holes" as a result of failures in system defenses, barriers, and safeguards. High-reliability organizations develop strong systems and provide individual support to keep the "holes" from aligning and leading to an adverse event. Failure in the defense developed to decrease error can be attributed to two reasons: **active failure** and **latent failure**. Reason described resilient high-reliability

systems with error management programs that use a system approach by reviewing all factors such as the person, the team, the task, the workplace, and the institution as a whole.

7.3 **The health care organization may implement a huddle to discuss safety concerns.** *[Conditional Recommendation]*

Low-quality evidence[214-216] supports the use of Healthcare Utilizing Deliberate Discussion Linking Events (HUDDLE) as a QI tool for managers to check in on safety issues on a daily basis and escalate concerns quickly to resolve potential safety concerns in the system.

Morrison and Sanders[216] reported on an organizational experience in which huddles were used to improve communication and teamwork on a unit. The huddle was performed 15 minutes after change-of-shift reports. All personnel were expected to attend, and a huddle champion (ie, charge nurse) summarized key points at the end of the huddle to refocus on the safety issues identified. Each member was given an opportunity to speak and share ideas.

7.4 **Develop patient safety indicators that measure the patient safety culture.** *[Recommendation]*

High-quality evidence[16-33,35-38,40,42-45,48,49,51,53] supports the reporting of morbidity, mortality, and adverse event data to measure patient safety. Adverse event reporting has been reported to increase when a just culture is established. Providing information on improvements in patient safety keeps the team members engaged in high-reliability teams. Two expert opinions challenge this reporting mechanism because there are so many factors involved in morbidity and mortality of patients.[191,192]

7.4.1 **Develop dashboards of patient safety indicators and make them available for the perioperative team.** *[Recommendation]*

Dashboards provide personnel with visual information on progress in improving safety and sustaining safety measures.[217]

7.4.2 **Review patient safety indicators with perioperative team members.** *[Recommendation]*

8. Education

8.1 **Provide initial and ongoing education and competency verification activities related to team communication and a patient safety culture.** *[Recommendation]*

Initial and ongoing education of perioperative personnel facilitates the development of knowledge, skills, and attitudes that affect safe patient care. It is the responsibility of the health care organization to provide initial and ongoing education and to verify the competency of its personnel[53,218]; however, the primary responsibility for maintaining ongoing competency remains with the individual.

Competency verification activities provide a mechanism for competency documentation and help verify that personnel understand the principles and processes necessary for safe patient care.

Ongoing development of knowledge and skills and documentation of personnel participation is a regulatory requirement[198-200] and an accreditation standard for both hospitals and ambulatory settings.

8.2 **Establish education and competency verification activities for its personnel and determine intervals for education and competency verification related to a patient safety culture and team communication.** *[Recommendation]*

Education and competency verification needs and intervals are unique to the facility and to its personnel and processes. Formal didactic instruction and competency verification is implemented to relay the importance of team communication for patient safety, strategies for safe and effective team communication, and expectations regarding team communication processes.[218]

8.3 **The health care organization should provide perioperative team training.** *[Recommendation]*

Moderate-quality evidence and guidance from professional organizations[3,5,6,50,179,219,220] support team training as an effective intervention for improving communication and teamwork in the perioperative setting. Team training may reduce the risk for human error (eg, safety omissions) while improving team communication and attitudes.

Moderate-quality evidence[14,69-72,96,221-225] indicates that approximately half of all adverse events could have been prevented and that the underlying causes are often attributable to human factors and nontechnical skills of personnel rather than to a lack of technical training or expertise. Generic nontechnical skills such as communication, teamwork, leadership, situational awareness, and decision making have been found to be critical for safety in most high-risk occupations.

Teamwork is dependent on individual performance and the performance of the team collectively through communication, cooperation, coordination, cognition, conflict resolution, and leadership. Improving communication in the perioperative environment requires an environment in which open communication is encouraged and the removal of hierarchical barriers.[50,63]

8.3.1 **Incorporate principles of human factor analysis in perioperative team training.** *[Recommendation]*

Human factors, including repetition, stress, and fatigue, can impede team performance.[75,84,90]

In an organizational experience report, Hu et al[84] investigated the etiology and resolution of unanticipated events in the OR during 10 high-acuity surgical procedures. The researchers developed a tool to track deviations caused by human factors and classified the deviations as either delays or safety compromises. Delays were defined as complete halts in forward progress for the entire team lasting more than 2 minutes. Safety compromises were defined as episodes of increased risk of harm to the patient. The researchers found there were multiple deviations per procedure (ie, one every 79.5 minutes). The researchers developed a conceptual model that illustrates the occurrence of the safety compromises in the OR. Communication and organizational structure was frequently identified as the root causes in both types of deviations. Strategies to resolve deviations were categorized as vigilance, communication, coordination, cooperation, and leadership.[84]

8.3.2 **Incorporate the safe surgery checklist in perioperative team training.** *[Recommendation]*

Providing team training on checklist use fosters team communication and team building, which are necessary components to have in place before checklist implementation.[53] High-quality evidence[16,22-24,29,31,34,38,42,44,45,49,54,57,59,61-63,192,226-231] supports team training with the implementation of a safe surgery checklist to foster mutual understanding among team members, improve communication, flatten the surgical hierarchy, promote team responsibility and accountability, and build toward high reliability in perioperative teams. Using a safe surgery checklist without training is little more than a tick-box exercise that has no real meaning to perioperative teams. Training and input from all perioperative team members is essential to achieving a significant commitment to a patient safety culture.

Rydenfalt[226] conducted an observational study to examine the actual usage of each component of safe surgery checklists in 24 surgical procedures. Overall, the safe surgery checklist was used 96% of the time; however, all of the individual items on the checklist were only completed 54% of the time. The researchers determined that the time-out process could be improved by educating and training perioperative team members on how the safe surgery checklist affects patient safety and by designing safe surgery checklists with input from the perioperative teams that will use them.

Pugel et al[62] conducted a literature review to examine how the safe surgery checklist could be used as a communication tool with a focus on team attitudes and behaviors in the OR. The authors determined that implementation strategy is important, and perioperative leaders need to assess the patient safety climate at the facility to make the surgical safety checklist relevant to those who will be using it rather than a challenge to team use. In addition, customizing the safe surgery checklist allows teams to have a feeling of ownership and increases compliance with use of the safe surgery checklist.

Ariadne labs created a safe surgery checklist implementation guide for hospitals and ambulatory surgery centers that can be used as a resource for team leaders to design their own safe surgery checklist, support implementation efforts, avoid common problems, and improve team buy in.[53]

8.4 Perioperative team training should include all team members. *[Recommendation]*

Team training reduces professional silos during perioperative team interactions. Paige et al[223] reported on an organizational experience of implementing interprofessional simulation-based training. The authors defined interprofessional education as bringing together two or more students from different health care professions to learn with, from, and about each other. Core interprofessional competencies were categorized into four major domains: values and ethics for interprofessional practice, roles and responsibilities, interprofessional communication, and teamwork.[223] The authors noted the value of interprofessional education in the OR where team dynamics continue to be less than ideal. The OR environment has been described as a silo where the interaction among team members is more multiprofessional than interprofessional. Communication between team members with differing roles (eg, physician to nurse, nurse to technician) is a challenge because of educational level, cultural background, and hierarchical barriers. The silo mentality is perpetuated and fosters a less than ideal OR culture. The authors list several problems caused by silos of professional practice, such as lack of communication, role confusion, heightened tension, and ineffective teamwork.

8.4.1 Perioperative team members should actively participate in team training. *[Recommendation]*

High-quality evidence[16-62] indicates that team training is effective for improving team communication and reducing patient morbidity. A statement from the American Heart Association[50] reported that poor teamwork contributes to errors and that team training reduces the incidence of errors. Therefore, the American Heart Association recommends that all cardiac OR team members participate in team training to improve communication, leadership, and situational awareness.

Crew Resource Management is a team training program widely used in health care. In a quasi-experimental study that took place in five hospitals in the United Kingdom, McCulloch et al[232] compared the effectiveness of Crew Resource Management team training, standard operating procedures (SOPs), and Lean thinking for promoting compliance with completion of the WHO Surgical Safety Checklist. Using the Oxford Nontechnical Skills Assessment (NOTECHS) II, the researchers compared the effectiveness of each intervention independently, a combination of team training with SOPs, and a combination of team training with Lean thinking. The researchers found that the group using team training combined with SOPs improved compliance with nontechnical skills and technical team performance when completing the WHO checklist. The researchers asserted that the use of SOPs and Lean thinking empowered the team to make changes to the process for completing the WHO checklist and improve their work environment.

Low-quality evidence[121,233,234] indicates that implementing TeamSTEPPS® in the perioperative setting may improve teamwork as part of QI processes. Tibbs and Moss[233] conducted a QI program implementing TeamSTEPPS and recommended that perioperative team members participate in team training to improve communication and team relationships.

Medical Team Training is a program developed by the Veterans Health Administration that emphasizes communication and teamwork with the use of checklist-driven operative briefings and debriefings.[235] One difference in the Medical Team Training Program compared to other Crew Resource Management-based programs is that the training faculty members work with an implementation team, including surgical personnel, for a 2-month planning and preparation phase before implementation.[235] In a retrospective cohort study of 119,383 procedures in Veterans Health Administration facilities, Young-Xu et al[235] found that facilities participating in the Medical Team Training program (n = 42) had a significantly lower surgical morbidity rate than facilities that were not participating in the program (n = 32). This study demonstrated an important link between improvement of teamwork in the OR and improvement of a measurable patient outcome, surgical morbidity.

8.5 **Include simulation scenarios that incorporate the health care organization's standardized communication tools for briefing, time out, debriefing, and hand overs in perioperative team training.** *[Recommendation]*

High-quality evidence[16,22-24,29,31,34,38,42,44,45,49,54,57,59,61-63, 192,226-231,235,236] supports the use of simulation with interprofessional groups for improving communication and decreasing adverse outcomes from lack of communication in critical patient care moments, such as the time out and hand overs.

In addition, moderate-quality evidence[93,123,237-240] suggests that interprofessional training with simulation-based scenarios is effective in improving nontechnical skills and teamwork. Moderate-quality evidence also supports using either video recordings or observational scenarios to assess team skills and improve communication.[93,237,239,241-245]

8.5.1 **Include simulation training with all perioperative team members in perioperative team training.[150,163,246]** *[Recommendation]*

Simulation training for the hand-over process helps to improve interprofessional communication. In an organizational experience report, Weinger et al[246] used formal education and simulation training to train perioperative team members in the hand-over process. They concluded that this education and training process significantly improved interprofessional communication.

Pukenas et al[163] evaluated the percentage of hand-over omissions plus errors by surgical residents before and after simulation training using a hand-over checklist in a qualitative study. The researchers found that the communication failure rate (incorrect and omitted items) decreased from 29.7% to 16.8% after initial training and additionally decreased to 13.2% 1 year after the simulation training was completed.

8.5.2 **Perioperative team training observers should provide feedback to participants on nontechnical skills.** *[Recommendation]*

Moderate-quality evidence[68-72,222,244] supports the use of observational tools to assess non-

technical skills, such as situational awareness, decision making, leadership, communication, and teamwork. Further research is needed to validate a tool for observation of nontechnical skills in the perioperative RN.

In a quasi-experimental study, Dedy et al[72] trained 11 surgical residents on nontechnical skills and used the NOTSS rating system to score observed behaviors in four categories: situational awareness, decision making, communication and teamwork, and leadership. The residents were observed and given baseline scores and individual feedback based on the observations. Then, each resident and the educator developed a plan to change target behaviors identified for improvement or to maintain performance. Scores on nontechnical skills improved significantly after the training. Participants reported that the intervention was useful and they believed it was important to incorporate debriefing and feedback on nontechnical skills into surgical training.

Editor's note: Crucial Conversations is a registered trademark of VitalSmarts, Provo, UT. TeamSTEPPS is a registered trademark of the US Department of Health and Human Services, Washington, DC, and the US Department of Defense, Washington, DC.

Glossary

Active failure: An error that is the result of an individual's failure and occurs at the point of contact between a human and an aspect of a larger system.

Briefing: A short dialogue for planning before the start of an operative or invasive procedure to discuss team formation, assign essential team roles, establish expectations and climate, and anticipate outcomes.

Debriefing: A short dialogue conducted after the procedure has concluded that is designed to improve team performance and effectiveness.

Distraction: An event that causes a diversion of attention or concentration during performance of a task.

Error: An act of commission (doing something wrong) or omission (failing to do what is right) that leads to an undesirable outcome or significant potential for such an outcome. These can be slips, lapses, or mistakes in memory or actions when executing the action or plan.

Hand over: The transfer of patient information from one person to another during transitions of care. Synonym: hand off.

High-reliability team: A team that is organized to anticipate and detect defects, maintain stable operations, and respond to abnormalities.

Interruption: An unplanned or unexpected event causing discontinuation of a task.

Just culture: A culture that balances personal accountability and system improvement.

Latent failure: An error that is a result of organizational system or design failure that allows active errors to occur and cause harm.

Licensed independent practitioner: A physician, dentist, nurse practitioner, nurse midwife, or any other individual permitted by law and the organization to provide care and services without direction or supervision, within the scope of the individual's license and consistent with individually granted clinical privileges.

Noise: Any sound that interferes with normal hearing and is undesired.

Patient safety culture: A culture in which every perioperative team member places value on safety and commits to personal responsibility for patient safety.

Read-back method: A dialogue in which the listener verbally repeats patient information so that the sender can confirm the correctness of the message.

Resilience: Human adaptation to an imperfect system.

Root cause: Basic or causal factor(s) underlying variation in performance, including the occurrence or possible occurrence of a sentinel event.

Shared mental model: The perception of, understanding of, or knowledge of a situation or process that is shared among team members through communication.

Site marking: The act of identifying the correct site on the patient's body where the operative or invasive procedure is to be performed.

Sterile cockpit: An environment in which personnel refrain from nonessential activities to minimize distractions during important tasks.

Time out: The pause in patient care activity taken by the surgical team immediately before the start of the procedure to conduct a final assessment that the correct patient, site, positioning, and procedure are identified and that, as applicable, all relevant documents, related information, and necessary equipment are available.

References

1. Institute of Medicine. Kohn LT, Corrigan JM, Donaldson MS, eds. *To Err Is Human: Building a Safer Health System.* Washington, DC: National Academy Press; 2000.

2. Makary MA, Daniel M. Medical error—the third leading cause of death in the US. *BMJ.* 2016;353:i2139. [VB]

3. *Information Statement: Surgical Patient Safety.* American Academy of Orthopaedic Surgeons. https://www.aaos.org/uploadedFiles/PreProduction/About/Opinion_Statements/advistmt/ 1049%20Surgical%20Patient%20Safety.pdf. Published 2016. Accessed September 28, 2017. [VA]

4. *Information Statement: Surgical Site and Procedure Confirmation.* American Academy of Orthopaedic Surgeons. https://www.aaos.org/uploadedFiles/PreProduction/About/Opinion_Statements/advistmt/1043%20Surgical%20Site%20and%20Procedure%20Confirmation.pdf. Published March 2015. Accessed September 28, 2017. [VA]

5. *Information Statement: Consistency for Safety in Orthopaedic Surgery.* American Academy of Orthopaedic Surgeons. https://www.aaos.org/uploadedFiles/PreProduction/About/Opinion_Statements/advistmt/ 1042%20Consistency%20for%20Safety%20in%20Orthopaedic%20Surgery.pdf. Published March 2015. Accessed September 28, 2017. [VA]

6. *Information Statement: Surgeon and Surgical Team Concentration.* American Academy of Orthopaedic Surgeons. https://www.aaos.org/uploadedFiles/PreProduction/About/Opinion_Statements/advistmt/1041%20Sur-geon%20and%20Surgical%20Team%20Concentration.pdf. Published December 2014. Accessed September 28, 2017. [VA]

7. American College of Surgeons (ACS) Committee on Perioperative Care. Revised statement on safe surgery checklists, and ensuring correct patient, correct site, and correct procedure surgery. *Bull Am Coll Surg.* 2016;101(10):52. [VA]

8. American College of Surgeons (ACS) Committee on Perioperative Care. Statement on distractions in the operating room. *Bull Am Coll Surg.* 2016;101(10):42-44. [VA]

9. American College of Surgeons (ACS); American Society of Anesthesiologists. Statement on physician-led team-based surgical care. *Bull Am Coll Surg.* 2016;101(8):50. [VA]

10. Ajlan AM, Harsh GR 4th. The human factor and safety attitudes in neurosurgical operating rooms. *World Neurosurg.* 2015;83(1):46-48. [VA]

11. Arriaga AF, Elbardissi AW, Regenbogen SE, et al. A policy-based intervention for the reduction of communication breakdowns in inpatient surgical care: results from a Harvard surgical safety collaborative. *Ann Surg.* 2011;253(5):849-854. [IIA]

12. Barzallo Salazar MJ, Minkoff H, Bayya J, et al. Influence of surgeon behavior on trainee willingness to speak up: a randomized controlled trial. *J Am Coll Surg.* 2014;219(5):1001-1007. [IA]

13. Braaf S, Manias E, Finch S, Riley R, Munro F. Healthcare service provider perceptions of organisational communication across the perioperative pathway: a questionnaire survey. *J Clin Nurs.* 2013;22(1-2):180-191. [IIIA]

14. Michinov E, Jamet E, Dodeler V, Haegelen C, Jannin P. Assessing neurosurgical non-technical skills: an exploratory study of a new behavioural marker system. *J Eval Clin Pract.* 2014;20(5):582-588. [IIIB]

15. Update: sentinel event statistics. *Jt Comm Perspect.* 2006; 26(10):14-15.

16. Treadwell JR, Lucas S, Tsou AY. Surgical checklists: a systematic review of impacts and implementation. *BMJ Qual Saf.* 2014;23(4):299-318. [IIIA]

17. Thomassen Ø, Storesund A, Søfteland E, Brattebø G. The effects of safety checklists in medicine: a systematic review. *Acta Anaesthesiol Scand.* 2014;58(1):5-18. [IIIA]

18. Russ S, Rout S, Sevdalis N, Moorthy K, Darzi A, Vincent C. Do safety checklists improve teamwork and communication in the operating room? A systematic review. *Ann Surg.* 2013;258(6):856-871. [IIIA]

19. Lyons VE, Popejoy LL. Meta-analysis of surgical safety checklist effects on teamwork, communication, morbidity, mortality, and safety. *West J Nurs Res.* 2014;36(2):245-261. [IA]

20. Arriaga AF, Bader AM, Wong JM, et al. Simulation-based trial of surgical-crisis checklists. *N Engl J Med.* 2013;368(3):246-253. [IIA]

21. Barrington MJ, Uda Y, Pattullo SJ, Sites BD. Wrong-site regional anesthesia: review and recommendations for prevention? *Curr Opin Anaesthesiol.* 2015;28(6):670-684. [VA]

22. Bergs J, Lambrechts F, Simons P, et al. Barriers and facilitators related to the implementation of surgical safety checklists: a systematic review of the qualitative evidence. *BMJ Qual Saf.* 2015;24(12):776-786. [IB]

23. Berrisford RG, Wilson IH, Davidge M, Sanders D. Surgical time out checklist with debriefing and multidisciplinary feedback improves venous thromboembolism prophylaxis in thoracic surgery: a prospective audit. *Eur J Cardiothorac Surg.* 2012;41(6):1326-1329. [IIIB]

24. Bliss LA, Ross-Richardson CB, Sanzari LJ, et al. Thirty-day outcomes support implementation of a surgical safety checklist. *J Am Coll Surg.* 2012;215(6):766-776. [IIA]

25. Bock M, Fanolla A, Segur-Cabanac I, et al. A comparative effectiveness analysis of the implementation of surgical safety checklists in a tertiary care hospital. *JAMA Surg.* 2016;151(7):639-646. [IIA]

26. Starling J 3rd, Coldiron BM. Outcome of 6 years of protocol use for preventing wrong site office surgery. *J Am Acad Dermatol.* 2011;65(4):807-810. [VB]

27. Calland JF, Turrentine FE, Guerlain S, et al. The surgical safety checklist: lessons learned during implementation. *Am Surg.* 2011;77(9):1131-1137. [IB]

28. Collins SJ, Newhouse R, Porter J, Talsma A. Effectiveness of the surgical safety checklist in correcting errors: a literature review applying Reason's Swiss Cheese Model. *AORN J.* 2014;100(1):65-79. [VA]

29. Conley DM, Singer SJ, Edmondson L, Berry WR, Gawande AA. Effective surgical safety checklist implementation. *J Am Coll Surg.* 2011;212(5):873-879. [VB]

30. Cullati S, Le Du S, Rae AC, et al. Is the surgical safety checklist successfully conducted? An observational study of social interactions in the operating rooms of a tertiary hospital. *BMJ Qual Saf.* 2013;22(8):639-646. [IIIB]

31. Cullati S, Licker M, Francis P, et al. Implementation of the surgical safety checklist in Switzerland and perceptions of its benefits: cross-sectional survey. *Plos One.* 2014;9(7):e101915. [IIIB]

32. Fargen KM, Velat GJ, Lawson MF, Firment CS, Mocco J, Hoh BL. Enhanced staff communication and reduced near-miss errors with a neurointerventional procedural checklist. *J Neurointerv Surg.* 2013;5(5):497-500. [VB]

33. Gordon BM, Lam TS, Bahjri K, Hashmi A, Kuhn MA. Utility of preprocedure checklists in the congenital cardiac catheterization laboratory. *Congenit Heart Dis.* 2014;9(2):131-137. [IIB]

34. Graling PR. Designing an applied model of perioperative patient safety. *Clin Scholars Rev.* 2011;4(2):104-114. [VA]

35. Hawranek M, Gasior PM, Buchta P, et al. Periprocedural checklist in the catheterisation laboratory is associated with decreased rate of treatment complications. *Kardiol Pol.* 2015;73(7):511-519. [IIB]

36. Helmiö P, Blomgren K, Takala A, Pauniaho SL, Takala RS, Ikonen TS. Towards better patient safety: WHO Surgical Safety Checklist in otorhinolaryngology. *Clin Otolaryngol.* 2011;36(3):242-247. [IIB]

37. Hullfish KL, Miller T, Pastore LM, et al. A checklist for timeout on labor and delivery: a pilot study to improve communication and safety. *J Reprod Med.* 2014;59(11-12):579-584. [VA]

38. Jones S. Your life in WHO's hands: The World Health Organization Surgical Safety Checklist: a critical review of the literature. *J Perioper Pract.* 2011;21(8):271-274. [VA]

39. Mainthia R, Lockney T, Zotov A, et al. Novel use of electronic whiteboard in the operating room increases surgical team compliance with pre-incision safety practices. *Surgery.* 2012;151(5):660-666. [IIA]

40. Nissan J, Campos V, Delgado H, Matadial C, Spector S. The automated operating room: a team approach to patient safety and communication. *JAMA Surg.* 2014;149(11):1209-1210. [IIIC]

41. Norton EK, Singer SJ, Sparks W, Ozonoff Al, Baxter J, Rangel S. Operating room clinicians' attitudes and perceptions of a pediatric surgical safety checklist at 1 institution. *J Patient Saf.* 2016;12(1):44-50. [IIIA]

42. Nugent E, Hseino H, Ryan K, Traynor O, Neary P, Keane FBV. The surgical safety checklist survey: a national perspective on patient safety. *Ir J Med Sci.* 2013;182(2):171-176. [IIIA]

43. Oak SN, Dave NM, Garasia MB, Parelkar SV. Surgical checklist application and its impact on patient safety in pediatric surgery. *J Postgrad Med.* 2015;61(2):92-94. [IIC]

44. Papaconstantinou HT, Jo CH, Reznik SI, Smythe WR, Wehbe-Janek H. Implementation of a surgical safety checklist: impact on surgical team perspectives. *Ochsner J.* 2013;13(3):299-309. [IIA]

45. Porter AJ, Narimasu JY, Mulroy MF, Koehler RP. Sustainable, effective implementation of a surgical preprocedural checklist: an "attestation" format for all operating team members. *Jt Comm J Qual Patient Saf.* 2014;40(1):3-9. [IIIC]

46. Pucher PH, Johnston MJ, Aggarwal R, Arora S, Darzi A. Effectiveness of interventions to improve patient handover in surgery: a systematic review. *Surgery.* 2015;158(1):85-95. [IIIA]

47. Raman J, Leveson N, Samost AL, et al. When a checklist is not enough: how to improve them and what else is needed. *J Thorac Cardiovasc Surg.* 2016;152(2):585-592. [VA]

48. Silva Araújo MP, de Oliveira AC. "Safe surgery saves lives" program contributions in surgical patient care: integrative review. *Rev Enferm UFPE.* 2015;9(4):7448-7457. [VA]

49. Takala RS, Pauniaho SL, Kotkansalo A, et al. A pilot study of the implementation of WHO surgical checklist in Finland: improvements in activities and communication. *Acta Anaesthesiol Scand.* 2011;55(10):1206-1214. [IIIB]

50. Wahr JA, Prager RL, Abernathy JH, et al. Patient safety in the cardiac operating room: human factors and teamwork: a scientific statement from the American Heart Association. *Circulation.* 2013;128(10):1139-1169. [IVA]

51. Walker IA, Reshamwalla S, Wilson IH. Surgical safety checklists: do they improve outcomes? *Br J Anaesth.* 2012; 109(1):47-54. [VB]

52. Zeeni C, Carabini L, Gould RW, et al. The implementation and efficacy of the Northwestern High Risk Spine Protocol. *World Neurosurg.* 2014;82(6):e815-e823. [VA]

53. *Safe Surgery Checklist Implementation Guide.* Boston MA: Ariadne Labs; 2015. Safe Surgery 2015. http://www.safesurgery2015.org/uploads/1/0/9/0/1090835/safe_surgery_implementation _guide__092515.012216_.pdf. Accessed September 28, 2017. [VA]

54. Berlinger N, Dietz E. Time-out: the professional and organizational ethics of speaking up in the OR. *AMA J Ethics.* 2016;18(9):925-932. [VB]

55. Dagey D. Using simulation to implement an OR cardiac arrest crisis checklist. *AORN J.* 2017;105(1):67-72. [VA]

56. de Vries EN, Prins HA, Crolla RM, et al. Effect of a comprehensive surgical safety system on patient outcomes. *N Engl J Med.* 2010;363(20):1928-1937. [IIA]

57. Haynes AB, Weiser TG, Berry WR, et al. Changes in safety attitude and relationship to decreased postoperative morbidity and mortality following implementation of a checklist-based surgical safety intervention. *BMJ Qual Saf.* 2011;20(1): 102-107. [IIA]

58. Safe surgery saves lives: surgical safety checklist. In: *The ORNAC Standards for Perioperative Registered Nursing Practice.* 12th ed. Kingston, Ontario: Operating Room Nurses Association of Canada (ORNAC); 2015:34-35. [IVB]

59. Russ S, Rout S, Caris J, et al. Measuring variation in use of the WHO Surgical Safety Checklist in the operating room: a multicenter prospective cross-sectional study. *J Am Coll Surg.* 2015;220(1):1-11. [IIIA]

60. Position statement: surgical safety. In: *2014-2015 ACORN Standards for Perioperative Nursing.* Adelaide, South Australia: The Australian College of Operating Room Nurses; 2014:154-156. [IVB]

61. Michael R, Della P, Zhou H. The effectiveness of the Surgical Safety Checklist as a means of communication in the operating room. *ACORN.* 2013;26(2):48-52. [IIIA]

62. Pugel AE, Simianu VV, Flum DR, Dellinger EP. Use of the surgical safety checklist to improve communication and reduce complications. *J Infect Public Health.* 2015;8(3):219-225. [VB]

63. Gillespie BM, Withers TK, Lavin J, Gardiner T, Marshall AP. Factors that drive team participation in surgical safety checks: a prospective study. *Patient Saf Surg.* 2016;10(1):3. [IIIA]

64. Salzwedel C, Bartz HJ, Kühnelt I, et al. The effect of a checklist on the quality of post-anaesthesia patient handover: a randomized controlled trial. *Int J Qual Health Care.* 2013;25(2):176-81. [IA]

65. Sexton JB, Schwartz SP, Chadwick WA, et al. The associations between work-life balance behaviours, team-work climate and safety climate: cross-sectional survey introducing the work-life climate scale, psychometric properties, benchmarking data and future directions. *BMJ Qual Saf.* 2017;26(8):632-640. [IIIA]

66. Mohorek M, Webb TP. Establishing a conceptual framework for handoffs using communication theory. *J Surg Educ.* 2015;72(3):402-409. [VB]

67. Hull L, Arora S, Kassab E, Kneebone R, Sevdalis N. Observational teamwork assessment for surgery: content validation and tool refinement. *J Am Coll Surg.* 2011;212(2):234-243.e1-e5. [IIIB]

68. Sharma B, Mishra A, Aggarwal R, Grantcharov TP. Non-technical skills assessment in surgery. *Surg Oncol.* 2011;20(3):169-177. [IIIB]

69. Mitchell L, Mitchell J. "Pass the buzzy thing, please." Recognising and understanding information: an essential non-technical skill element for the efficient scrub practitioner. *J Perioper Pract.* 2011;21(6):203-205. [IIC]

70. Spanager L, Beier-Holgersen R, Dieckmann P, Konge L, Rosenberg J, Oestergaard D. Reliable assessment of general surgeons' non-technical skills based on video-recordings of patient simulated scenarios. *Am J Surg.* 2013;206(5):810-817. [IIB]

71. Geraghty AM, McIlhenny C. Human factor skills in the surgical environment. *Br J Hosp Med (Lond).* 2016;77(1):14-16. [VC]

72. Dedy NJ, Fecso AB, Szasz P, Bonrath EM, Grantcharov TP. Implementation of an effective strategy for teaching nontechnical skills in the operating room: a single-blinded nonrandomized trial. *Ann Surg.* 2016;263(5):937-941. [IIA]

73. Han SJ, Rolston JD, Lau CY, Berger MS. Improving patient safety in neurologic surgery. *Neurosurg Clin North Am.* 2015;26(2):143-147. [VB]

74. Hemingway MW, O'Malley C, Silvestri S. Safety culture and care: a program to prevent surgical errors. *AORN J.* 2015;101(4):404-415. [VA]

75. El Bardissi AW, Sundt TM. Human factors and operating room safety. *Surg Clin North Am.* 2012;92(1):21-35. [VA]

76. *Leading a Culture of Safety: A Blueprint for Success.* Boston, MA: National Patient Safety Foundation; 2017.

77. Espin S, Lingard L, Baker GR, Regehr G. Persistence of unsafe practice in everyday work: an exploration of organizational and psychological factors constraining safety in the operating room. *Qual Saf Health Care.* 2006;15(3):165-170. [IIIB]

78. *AORN Position Statement on a Healthy Perioperative Practice Environment.* AORN, Inc. https://www.aorn.org/guidelines/clinical-resources/position-statements. Updated 2015. Accessed September 29, 2017. [IVB]

79. Lipira LE, Gallagher TH. Disclosure of adverse events and errors in surgical care: challenges and strategies for improvement. *World J Surg.* 2014;38(7):1614-1621. [VB]

80. Merry AF, Weller J, Mitchell SJ. Improving the quality and safety of patient care in cardiac anesthesia. *J Cardiothorac Vasc Anesth.* 2014;28(5):1341-1351. [VA]

81. Tsao K, Browne M. Culture of safety: a foundation for patient care. *Semin Pediatr Surg.* 2015;24(6):283-287. [VA]

82. Kolbe M, Burtscher MJ, Wacker J, et al. Speaking up is related to better team performance in simulated anesthesia inductions: an observational study. *Anesth Analg.* 2012;115(5):1099-1108. [IIIB]

83. Maxfield D, Grenny J, Lavandero R, Groah L. *The Silent Treatment: Why Safety Tools and Checklists Aren't Enough to Save Lives.* Provo, UT: VitalSmarts; 2011. [IIIA]

84. Hu YY, Arriaga AF, Roth EM, et al. Protecting patients from an unsafe system: the etiology and recovery of intraoperative deviations in care. *Ann Surg.* 2012;256(2):203-210. [VA]

85. Hickson GB, Pichert JW, Webb LE, Gabbe SG. A complementary approach to promoting professionalism: identifying, measuring, and addressing unprofessional behaviors. *Acad Med.* 2007;82(11):1040-1048. [VA]

86. Reiter CE, Pichert JW, Hickson GB. Addressing behavior and performance issues that threaten quality and patient safety: what your attorneys want you to know. *Prog Pediatr Cardiol.* 2012;33(1):37-45. [VA]

87. Lane-Fall MB, Brooks AK, Wilkins SA, Davis JJ, Riesenberg LA. Addressing the mandate for hand-off education: a focused review and recommendations for anesthesia resident curriculum development and evaluation. *Anesthesiology.* 2014;120(1):218-229. [VA]

88. Prati G, Pietrantoni L. Attitudes to teamwork and safety among Italian surgeons and operating room nurses. *Work.* 2014;49(4):669-677. [IIIA]

89. Vannucci A, Kras JF. Decision making, situation awareness, and communication skills in the operating room. *Int Anesthesiol Clin.* 2013;51(1):105-127. [VA]

90. Brennan PA, Mitchell DA, Holmes S, Plint S, Parry D. Good people who try their best can have problems: recognition of human factors and how to minimise error. *Br J Oral Maxillofac Surg.* 2016;54(1):3-7. [VA]

91. Kirschbaum KA, Rask JP, Brennan M, Phelan S, Fortner SA. Improved climate, culture, and communication through multidisciplinary training and instruction. *Am J Obstet Gynecol.* 2012;207(3):200.e1-200.e7. [VB]

92. Singer SJ, Rivard PE, Hayes JE, Shokeen P, Gaba D, Rosen A. Improving patient care through leadership engagement with frontline staff: a Department of Veterans Affairs case study. *Jt Comm J Qual Patient Saf.* 2013;39(8):349-360. [VA]

93. Bearman M, O'Brien R, Anthony A, et al. Learning surgical communication, leadership and teamwork through simulation. *J Surg Educ.* 2012;69(2):201-207. [IIIB]

94. The Joint Commission. The essential role of leadership in developing a safety culture. *Sentinel Event Alert.* 2017;57. https://www.jointcommission.org/assets/1/18/SEA_57_Safety_Culture_Leadership_0317.pdf. Accessed September 29, 2017. [VA]

95. Huang LC, Conley D, Lipsitz S, et al. The surgical safety checklist and teamwork coaching tools: a study of inter-rater reliability. *BMJ Qual Saf.* 2014;23(8):639-650. [IIIA]

96. Henrickson Parker S, Yule S, Flin R, McKinley A. Towards a model of surgeons' leadership in the operating room. *BMJ Qual Saf.* 2011;20(7):570-579. [VA]

97. Taylor AM, Chuo J, Figueroa-Altmann A, Di Taranto S, Shaw KN. Using four-phased unit-based patient safety walkrounds to uncover correctable system flaws. *Jt Comm J Qual Patient Saf.* 2013;39(9):396-403. [VA]

98. *Free from Harm: Accelerating Patient Safety Improvement Fifteen Years After To Err is Human.* Boston, MA: National Patient Safety Foundation; 2015. http://c.ymcdn.com/sites/www.npsf.org/resource/resmgr/PDF/Free_from_Harm.pdf. Accessed September 29, 2017. [VA]

99. Figueroa MI, Sepanski R, Goldberg SP, Shah S. Improving teamwork, confidence, and collaboration among members of a pediatric cardiovascular intensive care unit multidisciplinary team using simulation-based team training. *Pediatr Cardiol.* 2013;34(3):612-619. [VB]

100. Gillespie BM, Gwinner K, Chaboyer W, Fairweather N. Team communications in surgery—creating a culture of safety. *J Interprof Care.* 2013;27(5):387-393. [IIIA]

101. Rosenstein A. Managing disruptive behaviors in the health care setting: focus on obstetrics services. *Am J Obstet Gynecol.* 2011;204(3):187-182. [VB]

102. Walrath JM, Dang D, Nyberg D. An organizational assessment of disruptive clinician behavior: findings and implications. *J Nurs Care Qual.* 2013;28(2):110-121. [VA]

103. Swiggart WH, Dewey CM, Hickson GB, Finlayson AJ, Spickard WA Jr. A plan for identification, treatment, and remediation of disruptive behaviors in physicians. *Front Health Serv Manage.* 2009;25(4):3-11. [VA]

104. Hu YY, Arriaga AF, Peyre SE, Corso KA, Roth EM, Greenberg CC. Deconstructing intraoperative communication failures. *J Surg Res.* 2012;177(1):37-42. [VB]

105. Nembhard IM, Labao I, Savage S. Breaking the silence: determinants of voice for quality improvement in hospitals. *Health Care Manage Rev.* 2015;40(3):225-236. [IIIA]

106. Reid J, Bromiley M. Clinical human factors: the need to speak up to improve patient safety. *Nurs Stand.* 2012;26(35):35-40. [VA]

107. Raemer DB, Kolbe M, Minehart RD, Rudolph JW, Pian-Smith MC. Improving anesthesiologists' ability to speak up in the operating room: a randomized controlled experiment of a simulation-based intervention and a qualitative analysis of hurdles and enablers. *Acad Med.* 2016;91(4):530-539. [IA]

108. Meginniss A, Damian F, Falvo F. Time out for patient safety. *J Emerg Nurs.* 2012;38(1):51-53. [VB]

109. Sexton JB, Thomas EJ, Helmreich RL. Error, stress, and teamwork in medicine and aviation: cross sectional surveys. *BMJ.* 2000;320(7237):745-749. [IIIA]

110. Stein JE, Heiss K. The Swiss Cheese Model of adverse event occurrence—closing the holes. *Semin Pediatr Surg.* 2015;24(6):278-282. [VA]

111. Reason J. *Human Error.* New York, NY: Cambridge University Press; 1990:302. [VA]

112. Herzer KR, Mirrer M, Xie Y, et al. Patient safety reporting systems: sustained quality improvement using a multidisciplinary team and "good catch" awards. *Jt Comm J Qual Patient Saf.* 2012;38(8):399-347. [VA]

113. Pape TM. The role of distractions and interruptions in operating room safety. *Perioper Nurs Clin.* 2011;6(2):101-111. [VA]

114. Kleiner C, Link T, Maynard MT, Halverson Carpenter K. Coaching to improve the quality of communication during briefings and debriefings. *AORN J.* 2014;100(4):358-368. [VA]

115. McCulloch P, Mishra A, Handa A, Dale T, Hirst G, Catchpole K. The effects of aviation-style non-technical skills training on

technical performance and outcome in the operating theatre. *Qual Saf Health Care.* 2009;18(2):109-115. [VB]

116. Boyd M, Cumin D, Lombard B, Torrie J, Civil N, Weller J. Read-back improves information transfer in simulated clinical crises. *BMJ Qual Saf.* 2014;23(12):989-993. [IIIB]

117. Patel B, Johnston M, Cookson N, King D, Arora S, Darzi A. Interprofessional communication of clinicians using a mobile phone app: a randomized crossover trial using simulated patients. *J Med Internet Res.* 2016;18(4):e79. [IB]

118. Saxton R. Communication skills training to address disruptive physician behavior. *AORN J.* 2012;95(5):602-611. [IIA]

119. Simmons A. "Territorial games" aim to help curb disruptive behavior in the OR. *OR Manager.* 2014;30(1):24-26. [VC]

120. *Implementation Manual WHO Surgical Safety Checklist 2009: Safe Surgery Saves Lives.* Geneva, Switzerland: World Health Organization; 2009. http://apps.who.int/iris/bitstream/10665/44186/1/9789241598590_eng.pdf. Accessed September 29, 2017. [IVA]

121. Plonien C, Williams M. Stepping up teamwork via TeamSTEPPS. *AORN J.* 2015;101(4):465-470. [VB]

122. Sentinel events (SE). In: *Comprehensive Accreditation Manual.* E-dition. Oakbrook Terrace, IL: The Joint Commission; 2017:SE-1–SE-20.

123. Klipfel JM, Carolan BJ, Brytowski N, Mitchell CA, Gettman MT, Jacobson TM. Patient safety improvement through in situ simulation interdisciplinary team training. *Urol Nurs.* 2014;34(1):39-46. [VA]

124. Al-Hakim LG, Xiao Y. On the day of surgery: how long does preventable disruption prolong the patient journey? *Int J Health Care Qual Assur.* 2012;25(4):322-342. [IIIB]

125. Steeples LR, Hingorani M, Flanagan D, Kelly SP. Wrong intraocular lens events—what lessons have we learned? A review of incidents reported to the national reporting and learning system: 2010-2014 versus 2003-2010. *Eye.* 2016;30(8):1049-1055. [IIIA]

126. Campbell G, Arfanis K, Smith AF. Distraction and interruption in anaesthetic practice. *Br J Anaesth.* 2012;109(5):707-715. [IIIA]

127. Stewart DE, Tlusty SM, Taylor KH, et al. Trends and patterns in reporting of patient safety situations in transplantation. *Am J Transplant.* 2015;15(12):3123-3133. [IIIA]

128. Wheelock A, Suliman A, Wharton R, et al. The impact of operating room distractions on stress, workload, and teamwork. *Ann Surg.* 2015;261(6):1079-1084. [IIIA]

129. Keller S, Tschan F, Beldi G, Kurmann A, Candinas D, Semmer NK. Noise peaks influence communication in the operating room. an observational study. *Ergonomics.* 2016;59(12):1541-1552. [IIIB]

130. Way TJ, Long A, Weihing J, et al. Effect of noise on auditory processing in the operating room. *J Am Coll Surg.* 2013;216(5):933-938. [IIA]

131. Jothiraj H, Howland-Harris J, Evley R, Moppett IK. Distractions and the anaesthetist: a qualitative study of context and direction of distraction. *Br J Anaesth.* 2013;111(3):477-482. [IIIB]

132. Weigl M, Antoniadis S, Chiapponi C, Bruns C, Sevdalis N. The impact of intra-operative interruptions on surgeons'

perceived workload: an observational study in elective general and orthopedic surgery. *Surg Endosc.* 2015;29(1):145-153. [IIIB]

133. Chen JG, Wright MC, Smith PB, Jaggers J, Mistry KP. Adaptation of a postoperative handoff communication process for children with heart disease: a quantitative study. *Am J Med Qual.* 2011;26(5):380-386. [VB]

134. *AORN Position Statement on Managing Distractions and Noise During Perioperative Patient Care.* https://www.aorn.org/guidelines/clinical-resources/position-statements. Updated 2014. Accessed September 29, 2017. [IVB]

135. Wright MI. Implementing no interruption zones in the perioperative environment. *AORN J.* 2016;104(6):536-540. [VA]

136. Saleem AM, Paulus JK, Vassiliou MC, Parsons SK. Initial assessment of patient handoff in accredited general surgery residency programs in the United States and Canada: a cross-sectional survey. *Can J Surg.* 2015;58(4):269-277. [IIIA]

137. Nagpal K, Abboudi M, Manchanda C, et al. Improving postoperative handover: a prospective observational study. *Am J Surg.* 2013;206(4):494-501. [IIA]

138. Nagpal K, Arora S, Vats A, et al. Failures in communication and information transfer across the surgical care pathway: interview study. *BMJ Qual Saf.* 2012;21(10):843-849. [IIIB]

139. Manser T, Foster S. Effective handover communication: an overview of research and improvement efforts. *Best Pract Res Clin Anaesthesiol.* 2011;25(2):181-191. [VA]

140. Grover A, Duggan E. Chinese whispers in the post anaesthesia care unit (PACU). *Ir Med J.* 2013;106(8):241-243. [VB]

141. Evanina EY, Monceaux NL. Anesthesia handoff: a root cause analysis based on a near-miss scenario. *Clin Scholars Rev.* 2012;5(2):132-136. [VB]

142. Chard R, Makary MA. Transfer-of-care communication: nursing best practices. *AORN J.* 2015;102(4):329-342. [VA]

143. Petrovic MA, Aboumatar H, Scholl AT, et al. The perioperative handoff protocol: evaluating impacts on handoff defects and provider satisfaction in adult perianesthesia care units. *J Clin Anesth.* 2015;27(2):111-119. [IIA]

144. Agarwal HS, Saville BR, Slayton JM, et al. Standardized postoperative handover process improves outcomes in the intensive care unit: a model for operational sustainability and improved team performance. *Crit Care Med.* 2012;40(7):2109-2115. [VA]

145. Breuer RK, Taicher B, Turner DA, Cheifetz IM, Rehder KJ. Standardizing postoperative PICU handovers improves handover metrics and patient outcomes. *Pediatr Crit Care Med.* 2015;16(3):256-263. [IIA]

146. Siddiqui N, Arzola C, Iqbal M, et al. Deficits in information transfer between anaesthesiologist and post-anaesthesia care unit staff: an analysis of patient handover. *Eur J Anaesthesiol.* 2012;29(9):438-445. [IIIB]

147. Craig R, Moxey L, Young D, Spenceley NS, Davidson MG. Strengthening handover communication in pediatric cardiac intensive care. *Paediatr Anaesth.* 2012;22(4):393-399. [IIA]

148. Joy BF, Elliott E, Hardy C, Sullivan C, Backer CL, Kane JM. Standardized multidisciplinary protocol improves handover of cardiac surgery patients to the intensive care unit. *Pediatr Crit Care Med.* 2011;12(3):304-308. [IIB]

149. Raiten JM, Lane-Fall M, Gutsche JT, et al. Transition of care in the cardiothoracic intensive care unit: a review of hand-offs in perioperative cardiothoracic and vascular practice. *J Cardiothorac Vasc Anesth.* 2015;29(4):1089-1095. [VB]

150. Johner AM, Merchant S, Aslani N, et al. Acute general surgery in Canada: a survey of current handover practices. *Can J Surg.* 2013;56(3):E24-E28. [IIIB]

151. Møller TP, Madsen MD, Fuhrmann L, Østergaard D. Postoperative handover: characteristics and considerations on improvement: a systematic review. *Eur J Anaesthesiol.* 2013; 30(5):229-242. [IIIA]

152. Segall N, Bonifacio AS, Schroeder RA, et al; Durham VA Patient Safety Center of Inquiry. Can we make postoperative patient handovers safer? A systematic review of the literature. *Anesth Analg.* 2012;115(1):102-115. [IIIA]

153. McElroy LM, Daud A, Lapin B, et al. Detection of medical errors in kidney transplantation: a pilot study comparing proactive clinician debriefings to a hospital-wide incident reporting system. *Surgery.* 2014;156(5):1106-1115. [IIIA]

154. McElroy LM, Macapagal KR, Collins KM et al. Clinician perceptions of operating room to intensive care unit handoffs and implications for patient safety: a qualitative study. *Am J Surg.* 2015;210(4):629-635. [IIIB]

155. Agarwala AV, Firth PG, Albrecht MA, Warren L, Musch G. An electronic checklist improves transfer and retention of critical information at intraoperative handoff of care. *Anesth Analg.* 2015;120(1):96-104. [VA]

156. Schuster KM, Jenq GY, Thung SF, et al. Electronic hand-off instruments: a truly multidisciplinary tool? *J Am Med Inform Assoc.* 2014;21(e2):e352-e357. [VB]

157. Eberhardt S. Improve handoff communication with SBAR. *Nursing.* 2014;44(11):17-20. [VC]

158. Johnson F, Logsdon P, Fournier K, Fisher S. SWITCH for safety: perioperative hand-off tools. *AORN J.* 2013;98(5):494-507. [VA]

159. Morris AM, Hoke N. Communication is key in the continuum of care. *OR Nurse.* 2015;9(5):14-19. [VC]

160. Randmaa M, Mårtensson G, Swenne CL, Engström M. SBAR improves communication and safety climate and decreases incident reports due to communication errors in an anaesthetic clinic: a prospective intervention study. *BMJ Open.* 2014;4(1):e004268. [IIA]

161. Ryan S, O'Riordan JM, Tierney S, Conlon KC, Ridgway PF. Impact of a new electronic handover system in surgery. *Int J Surg.* 2011;9(3):217-220. [IIIB]

162. Weiss MJ, Bhanji F, Fontela PS, Razack SI. A preliminary study of the impact of a handover cognitive aid on clinical reasoning and information transfer. *Med Educ.* 2013;47(8):832-841. [VA]

163. Pukenas EW, Dodson G, Deal ER, Gratz I, Allen E, Burden AR. Simulation-based education with deliberate practice may improve intraoperative handoff skills: a pilot study. *J Clin Anesth.* 2014;26(7):530-538. [IIIA]

164. Petrovic MA, Martinez EA, Aboumatar H. Implementing a perioperative handoff tool to improve postprocedural patient transfers. *Jt Comm J Qual Patient Saf.* 2012;38(3):135-142. [VA]

165. Department of Defense Patient Safety Program. *Healthcare Communications Toolkit to Improve Transitions in Care.* Falls Church, VA: TRICARE Management Activity; 2005. https://www.oumedicine.com/docs/ad-obgyn-workfiles/handofftoolkit.pdf?sfvrsn=2. Accessed September 29, 2017. [IVA]

166. Zahiri HR, Stromberg J, Skupsky H, et al. Prevention of 3 "never events" in the operating room: fires, gossypiboma, and wrong-site surgery. *Surg Innov.* 2011;18(1):55-60. [VA]

167. Wu RL, Aufses A Jr. Characteristics and costs of surgical scheduling errors. *Am J Surg.* 2012;204(4):468-473. [IIIA]

168. McElroy LM, Collins KM, Koller FL, et al. Operating room to intensive care unit handoffs and the risks of patient harm. *Surgery.* 2015;158(3):588-594. [IIB]

169. Fabila TS, Hee HI, Sultana R, Assam PN, Kiew A, Chan YH. Improving postoperative handover from anaesthetists to non-anaesthetists in a children's intensive care unit: the receiver's perception. *Singapore Med J.* 2016;57(5):242-253. [VA]

170. Lingard L, Regehr G, Cartmill C, et al. Evaluation of a preoperative team briefing: a new communication routine results in improved clinical practice. *BMJ Qual Saf.* 2011;20(6):475-482. [IIB]

171. Johnston FM, Tergas AI, Bennett JL, et al. Measuring briefing and checklist compliance in surgery: a tool for quality improvement. *Am J Med Qual.* 2014;29(6):491-498. [VA]

172. Thanapongsathorn W, Jitsopa J, Wongviriyakorn O. Interprofessional preoperative briefing enhances surgical teamwork satisfaction and decrease operative time: a comparative study in abdominal operation. *J Med Assoc Thai.* 2012;95(Suppl 12):S8-S14. [VA]

173. Jain AL, Jones KC, Simon J, Patterson MD. The impact of a daily pre-operative surgical huddle on interruptions, delays, and surgeon satisfaction in an orthopedic operating room: a prospective study. *Patient Saf Surg.* 2015;9(1):8. [VA]

174. Bethune R, Sasirekha G, Sahu A, Cawthorn S, Pullyblank A. Use of briefings and debriefings as a tool in improving team work, efficiency, and communication in the operating theatre. *Postgrad Med J.* 2011;87(1027):331-334. [VA]

175. Hicks CW, Rosen M, Hobson DB, Ko C, Wick EC. Improving safety and quality of care with enhanced teamwork through operating room briefings. *JAMA Surg.* 2014;149(8):863-868. [VA]

176. Bandari J, Schumacher K, Simon M, et al. Surfacing safety hazards using standardized operating room briefings and debriefings at a large regional medical center. *Jt Comm J Qual Patient Saf.* 2012;38(4):154-160. [VA]

177. Symons NRA, Wong HWL, Manser T, Sevdalis N, Vincent CA, Moorthy K. An observational study of team-work skills in shift handover. *Int J Surg.* 2012;10(7):355-359. [VA]

178. Einav Y, Gopher D, Kara I, et al. Preoperative briefing in the operating room: shared cognition, teamwork, and patient safety. *Chest.* 2010;137(2):443-449. [IIA]

179. Van Herzeele I, Sevdalis N, Lachat M, Desender L, Rudarakanchana N, Rancic Z. Team training in ruptured EVAR. *J Cardiovasc Surg.* 2014;55(2):193-206. [VA]

180. Gillespie BM, Gwinner K, Fairweather N, Chaboyer W. Building shared situational awareness in surgery through distributed dialog. *J Multidiscip Healthc.* 2013;6:109-118. [IIIA]

181. Birnbach DJ, Rosen LF, Fitzpatrick M, Paige JT, Arheart KL. Introductions during time-outs: do surgical team members know one another's names? *Jt Comm J Qual Patient Saf.* 2017;43(6):284-288. [IIIB]

182. Guideline for a safe environment of care, part 1. In: *Guidelines for Perioperative Practice.* Denver, CO: AORN, Inc; 2017:243-268. [IVA]

183. Clarke JR, Waddell L, Wolff DD Jr. Quarterly update on wrong-site surgery: how to do an effective time-out in the dark. *Penn Patient Saf Advis.* 2014;11(2):88-92. [VA]

184. Weiser TG, Berry WR. Review article: perioperative checklist methodologies. *Can J Anesth.* 2013;60(2):136-142. [VB]

185. Revised guidance related to new & revised regulations for hospitals, ambulatory surgical centers (ASCs), rural health clinics (RHCs) and federally qualified health centers (FQHCs). 2015. Centers for Medicare & Medicaid Services. https://www.cms.gov/Medicare/Provider-Enrollment-and-Certification/SurveyCertificationGenInfo/Downloads/Survey-and-Cert-Letter-15-22.pdf. Accessed September 29, 2017.

186. UP.01.02.01: Mark the procedure site. In: *Comprehensive Accreditation Manual.* E-dition. Oakbrook Terrace, IL: The Joint Commission; 2017.

187. Mayer JE, Dang RP, Duarte Prieto GF, Cho SK, Qureshi SA, Hecht AC. Analysis of the techniques for thoracic- and lumbar-level localization during posterior spine surgery and the occurrence of wrong-level surgery: results from a national survey. *Spine J.* 2014;14(5):741-748. [IIIB]

188. Yoon RS, Alaia MJ, Hutzler LH, Bosco JA 3rd. Using "near misses" analysis to prevent wrong-site surgery. *J Healthc Qual.* 2015;37(2):126-132. [VA]

189. A time-out is performed before the procedure. In: *Comprehensive Accreditation Manual.* E-dition. Oakbrook Terrace, IL: The Joint Commission; 2017.

190. Song JB, Vemana G, Mobley JM, Bhayani SB. The second "time-out": a surgical safety checklist for lengthy robotic surgeries. *Patient Saf Surg.* 2013;7(1):19. [VA]

191. Urbach DR, Govindarajan A, Saskin R, Wilton AS, Baxter NN. Introduction of surgical safety checklists in Ontario, Canada. *N Engl J Med.* 2014;370(11):1029-1038. [IIIA]

192. Sewell M, Adebibe M, Jayakumar P, et al. Use of the WHO Surgical Safety Checklist in trauma and orthopaedic patients. *Int Orthop.* 2011;35(6):897-901. [VA]

193. Fourcade A, Blache JL, Grenier C, Bourgain JL, Minvielle E. Barriers to staff adoption of a surgical safety checklist. *BMJ Qual Saf.* 2012;21(3):191-197. [IIB]

194. Lyons VE, Popejoy LL. Time-out and checklists: a survey of rural and urban operating room personnel. *J Nurs Care Qual.* 2017;32(1):E3-E10. [IIIB]

195. Cima R, Dankbar E, Lovely J, et al. Colorectal surgery surgical site infection reduction program: a National Surgical Quality Improvement Program-driven multidisciplinary single-institution experience. *J Am Coll Surg.* 2013;216(1):23-33. [VB]

196. Maniar RL, Sytnik P, Wirtzfeld DA, et al. Synoptic operative reports enhance documentation of best practices for rectal cancer. *J Surg Oncol.* 2015;112(5):555-560. [IIIA]

197. *State Operations Manual Appendix A—Survey Protocol, Regulations and Interpretive Guidelines for Hospitals.* Rev 151; 2015. Centers for Medicare & Medicaid Services. https://www.cms.gov/Regulations-and-Guidance/Guidance/Manuals/downloads/som107ap_a_hospitals.pdf. Accessed September 29, 2017.

198. *State Operations Manual Appendix L—Guidance for Surveyors: Ambulatory Surgical Centers.* Rev. 137; 2015. Centers for Medicare & Medicaid Services. https://www.cms.gov/Regulations-and-Guidance/Guidance/Manuals/downloads/som107ap_l_ambulatory.pdf. Accessed September 29, 2017.

199. 42 CFR 482. Conditions of participation for hospitals. 2011. Government Publishing Office. https://www.gpo.gov/fdsys/granule/CFR-2011-title42-vol5/CFR-2011-title42-vol5-part482. Accessed September 29, 2017.

200. 42 CFR 416. Ambulatory surgical services. 2011. Government Publishing Office. https://www.gpo.gov/fdsys/granule/CFR-2011-title42-vol3/CFR-2011-title42-vol3-part416. Accessed September 29, 2017.

201. Patient safety systems for hospitals. In: *Comprehensive Accreditation Manual for Hospitals.* Oakbrook Terrace, IL: The Joint Commission; 2017:PS-1–PS-50. https://www.jointcommission.org/assets/1/18/CAMH_04a_PS.pdf. Accessed September 29, 2017. [VA]

202. NIAHO: National Integrated Accreditation for Healthcare Organizations. Surgical services (SS). In: *Interpretive Guidelines and Surveyor Guidance.* Version 11. Milford, OH: DNV GL Healthcare USA, Inc; 2014:80-91.

203. Quality assessment/quality improvement: quality improvement. In: *Regular Standards and Checklist for Accreditation of Ambulatory Surgery Facilities.* Version 14.5. Gurnee, IL: American Association for Accreditation of Ambulatory Surgery Facilities, Inc; 2017:64.

204. Quality assessment/quality improvement: unanticipated operative sequelae. In: *Regular Standards and Checklist for Accreditation of Ambulatory Surgery Facilities.* Version 14.5. American Association for Accreditation of Ambulatory Surgery Facilities, Inc; 2017:66-69.

205. Cassin BR, Barach PR. Making sense of root cause analysis investigations of surgery-related adverse events. *Surg Clin North Am.* 2012;92(1):101-115. [VA]

206. Scoville R, Little K, Rakover J, Luther K, Mate K. *Sustaining Improvement.* IHI White Paper. Cambridge, MA: Institute for Healthcare Improvement; 2016. http://www.ihi.org/resources/Pages/IHIWhitePapers/Sustaining-Improvement.aspx. Accessed September 29, 2017. [VA]

207. Blackmore CC, Bishop R, Luker S, Williams BL. Applying lean methods to improve quality and safety in surgical sterile instrument processing. *Jt Comm J Qual Patient Saf.* 2013;39(3):99-105. [VB]

208. Wakeam E, Hyder JA, Ashley SW, Weissman JS. Barriers and strategies for effective patient rescue: a qualitative study of outliers. *Jt Comm J Qual Patient Saf.* 2014;40(11):503-513. [IIIB]

209. Johnson M, Sanchez P, Suominen H, et al. Comparing nursing handover and documentation: forming one set of patient information. *Int Nurs Rev.* 2014;61(1):73-81. [IIIB]

210. Pronovost PJ, Armstrong CM, Demski R, et al. Creating a high-reliability health care system: improving performance on core processes of care at Johns Hopkins Medicine. *Acad Med.* 2015;90(2):165-172. [VA]

211. Chassin MR, Loeb JM. High-reliability health care: getting there from here. *Milbank Q.* 2013;91(3):459-490. [VA]

212. Lin M, Heisler S, Fahey L, McGinnis J, Whiffen TL. Nurse knowledge exchange plus: human-centered implementation for spread and sustainability. *Jt Comm J Qual Patient Saf.* 2015;41(7):303-312. [VA]

213. Rogers SO Jr, Gawande AA, Kwaan M, et al. Analysis of surgical errors in closed malpractice claims at 4 liability insurers. *Surgery.* 2006;140(1):25-33. [IIIA]

214. Glymph DC, Olenick M, Barbera S, Brown EL, Prestianni L, Miller C. Healthcare utilizing deliberate discussion linking events (HUDDLE): a systematic review. *AANA J.* 2015;83(3):183-188. [VA]

215. Krenzischek DA, Xie Y, Petrovic M, et al. The perioperative handoff protocol: application of a multidisciplinary model to promote teamwork and reduce perioperative miscommunication. *J Perianesth Nurs.* 2011;26(3):188-189. [VC]

216. Morrison D, Sanders C. Huddling for optimal care outcomes. *Nursing.* 2011;41(12):22-24. [VB]

217. Park KW, Smaltz D, McFadden D, Souba W. The operating room dashboard. *J Surg Res.* 2010;164(2):294-300. [VB]

218. Johnson JK, Arora VM, Bacha EA, Barach PR. Improving communication and reliability of patient handovers in pediatric cardiac care. *Prog Pediatr Cardiol.* 2011;32(2):135-139. [VB]

219. HR.01.05.03: Staff participate in ongoing education and training. In: *Comprehensive Accreditation and Certification Manual.* E-dition. Oakbrook Terrace, IL: The Joint Commission; 2016.

220. Committee on Development of High Performance Teamwork; American College of Surgeons. Statement on high-performance teams. *Bull Am Coll Surg.* 2010;95(2):23-24. [IVC]

221. Larsson J, Holmström IK. How excellent anaesthetists perform in the operating theatre: a qualitative study on non-technical skills. *Br J Anaesth.* 2013;110(1):115-121. [IIIB]

222. McClelland G. Assessing scrub practitioner nontechnical skills: a literature review. *J Perioper Pract.* 2015;25(1-2):12-18. [VA]

223. Paige JT, Garbee DD, Brown KM, Rojas JD. Using simulation in interprofessional education. *Surg Clin North Am.* 2015;95(4):751-766. [VA]

224. Rudarakanchana N, Van Herzeele I, Desender L, Cheshire NJW. Virtual reality simulation for the optimization of endovascular procedures: current perspectives. *Vasc Health Risk Manag.* 2015;11:195-202. [VB]

225. Willems A, Waxman B, Bacon AK, Smith J, Peller J, Kitto S. Interprofessional non-technical skills for surgeons in disaster response: a qualitative study of the Australian perspective. *J Interprof Care.* 2013;27(2):177-183. [IIIA]

226. Rydenfält C, Johansson G, Odenrick P, Akerman K, Larsson PA. Compliance with the WHO Surgical Safety Checklist: deviations and possible improvements. *Int J Qual Health Care.* 2013;25(2):182-187. [VB]

227. Nurok M, Sundt TM 3rd, Frankel A. Teamwork and communication in the operating room: relationship to discrete outcomes and research challenges. *Anesthesiol Clin.* 2011;29(1):1-11. [IIIB]

228. Marshall MB, Emerson D. Patient safety in the surgical setting. *Thorac Surg Clin.* 2012;22(4):545-550. [VA]

229. Bohmer AB, Kindermann P, Schwanke U, et al. Long-term effects of a perioperative safety checklist from the viewpoint of personnel. *Acta Anaesthesiol Scand.* 2013;57(2):150-157. [IIIA]

230. Braaf S, Manias E, Riley R. The "time-out" procedure: an institutional ethnography of how it is conducted in actual clinical practice. *BMJ Qual Saf.* 2013;22(8):647-655. [IIIB]

231. Weiser TG, Porter MP, Maier RV. Safety in the operating theatre—a transition to systems-based care. *Nat Rev Urol.* 2013;10(3):161-173. [VA]

232. McCulloch P, Morgan L, New S, et al. Combining systems and teamwork approaches to enhance the effectiveness of safety improvement interventions in surgery: the safer delivery of surgical services (S3) program. *Ann Surg.* 2017;265(1):90-96. [IIA]

233. Tibbs SM, Moss J. Promoting teamwork and surgical optimization: combining TeamSTEPPS with a specialty team protocol. *AORN J.* 2014;100(5):477-488. [VA]

234. Li Y. Evidence summary. TeamSTEPPS. The Joanna Briggs Institute EBP Database, JBI@Ovid. 2017;JBI5271. [IVA]

235. Young-Xu Y, Neily J, Mills PD, et al. Association between implementation of a medical team training program and surgical morbidity. *Arch Surg.* 2011;146(12):1368-1373. [IIA]

236. Nurok M, Evans LA, Lipsitz S, Satwicz P, Kelly A, Frankel A. The relationship of the emotional climate of work and threat to patient outcome in a high-volume thoracic surgery operating room team. *BMJ Qual Saf.* 2011;20(3):237-242. [IB]

237. Brown LL, Overly FL. Simulation-based interprofessional team training. *Clin Pediatr Emerg Med.* 2016;17(3):179-184. [VB]

238. Burke C, Grobman W, Miller D. Interdisciplinary collaboration to maintain a culture of safety in a labor and delivery setting. *J Perinat Neonatal Nurs.* 2013;27(2):113-123. [IIIB]

239. Cumin D, Boyd MJ, Webster CS, Weller JM. A systematic review of simulation for multidisciplinary team training in operating rooms. *Simul Healthc.* 2013;8(3):171-179. [IIIA]

240. Gardner AK, Scott DJ. Concepts for developing expert surgical teams using simulation. *Surg Clin North Am.* 2015;95(4):717-728. [VB]

241. Andrew B, Plachta S, Salud L, Pugh CM. Development and evaluation of a decision-based simulation for assessment of team skills. *Surgery.* 2012;152(2):152-157. [IIIB]

242. Arain NA, Hogg DC, Gala RB, et al. Construct and face validity of the American College of Surgeons/Association of Program Directors in Surgery laparoscopic troubleshooting team training exercise. *Am J Surg.* 2012;203(1):54-62. [IIIA]

243. Bilotta FF, Werner SM, Bergese SD, Rosa G. Impact and implementation of simulation-based training for safety. *Sci World J.* 2013;2013:652956. [VA]

244. Pena G, Altree M, Field J, et al. Nontechnical skills training for the operating room: a prospective study using simulation and didactic workshop. *Surgery.* 2015;158(1):300-309. [IIIB]

245. Nicksa GA, Anderson C, Fidler R, Stewart L. Innovative approach using interprofessional simulation to educate

surgical residents in technical and nontechnical skills in high-risk clinical scenarios. *JAMA Surg.* 2015;150(3):201-207. [IIIB]

246. Weinger MB, Slagle JM, Kuntz AH, et al. A multimodal intervention improves postanesthesia care unit handovers. *Anesth Analg.* 2015;121(4):957-971. [VA]

Acknowledgments

Lead Author

Mary C. Fearon, MSN, RN, CNOR
Perioperative Practice Specialist
AORN Nursing Department
Denver, Colorado

Co-Author

Lisa Spruce, DNP, RN, CNS-CP, CNOR, ACNS, ACNP, FAAN
Director, Evidence-Based Perioperative Practice
AORN Nursing Department
Denver, Colorado

Contributing Authors

Ramona L. Conner, MSN, RN, CNOR, FAAN
Editor-in-Chief, Guidelines for Perioperative Practice
AORN Nursing Department
Denver, Colorado

Amber Wood, MSN, RN, CNOR, CIC, FAPIC
Senior Perioperative Practice Specialist
AORN Nursing Department
Denver, Colorado

The authors and AORN thank Janice Neil, PhD, CNE, RN, Associate Professor, East Carolina College of Nursing, Greenville, North Carolina; Barbara L. Nalley, MSN, CRNP, CNOR, Manager, Jackson Surgical Assistants, Crofton, Maryland; David R. Urbach, MD, Clinical Epidemiology MSc, University Health Network, Toronto, Canada; Marie A. Bashaw, DNP, RN, NEA-BC, CNOR, Assistant Professor, Wright State University College of Nursing and Health, Dayton, Ohio; Jennifer Butterfield, MBA, RN, CNOR, CASC, Administrator/ CEO, Lakes Surgery Center, Northville, Michigan; Susan Ruwe, MSN, RN, CPHQ, CIC, Senior Infection Preventionist, Carle Foundation Hospital, Argenta, Illinois; Donna A. Pritchard, MA, BSN, RN, NE-BC, CNOR, Director of Perioperative Services, Interfaith Medical Center, Brooklyn, New York; Juan A. Sanchez, MD, MPA, Associate Professor of Surgery, Johns Hopkins University School of Medicine, Chair of Surgery, Saint Agnes Hospital, Baltimore, MD; Marisa Merlino, MHA, RN-BC, CNOR, CSSM, Staff Nurse II, Scott & White Memorial Hospital, Temple, Texas; and Vangie Dennis, BSN, RN, CNOR, CMLSO, Director of Patient Care Practice, Emory Clinic Ambulatory Surgery Center, Duluth, Georgia, for their assistance in developing this guideline.

Publication History

Originally published January 2018 in *Guidelines for Perioperative Practice*. Supersedes the "Guideline for transfer of patient care information."

Evidence ratings revised and minor editorial changes made to conform to the current AORN Evidence Rating model, September 2019, for online publication in *Guidelines for Perioperative Practice*.

TRANSMISSION-BASED PRECAUTIONS

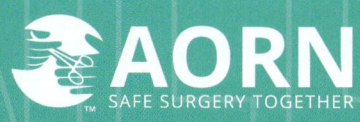

AORN
SAFE SURGERY TOGETHER

1187

TABLE OF CONTENTS

Ⓐ *indicates additional information is available in the Ambulatory Supplement.*

Ⓟ *indicates a recommendation or evidence relevant to pediatric care.*

MEDICAL ABBREVIATIONS & ACRONYMS

AIIR – Airborne infection isolation room
ASC – Ambulatory surgery center
CDC – Centers for Disease Control and Prevention
CMS – Centers for Medicare & Medicaid Services
CPR – Cardiopulmonary resuscitation
FDA – US Food and Drug Administration
HEPA – High-efficiency particulate air
HIV – Human immunodeficiency virus
IFU – Instructions for use
MAUDE – Manufacturer and User Facility Device Experience
MDRO – Multidrug-resistant organism
NIOSH – National Institute for Occupational Safety and Health

OR – Operating room
OSHA – Occupational Safety and Health Administration
PAPR – Powered air-purifying respirator
PAS – Portable anteroom system
PPE – Personal protective equipment
RN – Registered nurse
SARS – Severe acute respiratory syndrome
SHEA – Society for Healthcare Epidemiology of America
TB – Tuberculosis
TDAP – Tetanus toxoid, reduced diphtheria toxoid, and acellular pertussis
UVGI – Ultraviolet germicidal irradiation

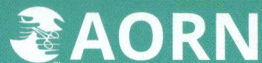
GUIDELINE FOR
TRANSMISSION-BASED PRECAUTIONS

The Guideline for Transmission-Based Precautions was approved by the AORN Guidelines Advisory Board and became effective December 1, 2018. It was presented as a proposed guideline for comments by members and others. The recommendations in the guideline are intended to be achievable and represent what is believed to be an optimal level of practice. Policies and procedures will reflect variations in practice settings and/or clinical situations that determine the degree to which the guideline can be implemented. AORN recognizes the many diverse settings in which perioperative nurses practice; therefore, this guideline is adaptable to all areas where operative or other invasive procedures may be performed.

Purpose

The rapidly changing health care environment presents perioperative personnel with continual challenges in the form of newly recognized pathogens and well-known microorganisms that have become more resistant to today's therapeutic modalities. Protecting patients and personnel from transmission of potentially infectious agents continues to be a primary focus for perioperative registered nurses (RNs). The prevention and control of multidrug-resistant organisms requires that all health care organizations implement, evaluate, and adjust efforts to decrease the risk of transmission.

Three principal elements are required for an infection to occur:
- a source or reservoir,
- a susceptible host with a portal of entry to receive the infectious agent, and
- a method of transmission.[1]

This document provides guidance to perioperative RNs for implementing **standard precautions** and **transmission-based precautions** (ie, contact, droplet, airborne) to prevent pathogen transmission in the perioperative practice setting. Additional guidance is provided for personal protective equipment (PPE); bloodborne pathogens; immunization; and activities of health care workers with infections, exudative lesions, and nonintact skin. Refer to the Centers for Disease Control and Prevention (CDC) when seeking the most current information for pathogen-specific guidance, especially during an outbreak when guidance for PPE use and transmission-based precautions may change rapidly. Guidance for prevention of surgical site infections, catheter-associated urinary tract infections, intravascular catheter-related infections, and ventilator-associated events is outside the scope of this document.

Prevention of pathogen transmission is a priority in the perioperative environment and includes considerations for hand hygiene, environmental cleaning, sharps safety, safe injection practices, surgical attire, sterile technique, and surgical smoke safety. These topics are addressed in other AORN guidelines, and although they are mentioned briefly where applicable (eg, standard precautions), the broader discussions are outside the scope of this document.

Evidence Review

A medical librarian with a perioperative nursing background conducted a systematic search of the databases Ovid MEDLINE®, EBSCO CINAHL®, Scopus®, and the Cochrane Database of Systematic Reviews. The search was limited to literature published in English from 2012 through 2018. At the time of the initial search, weekly alerts were created on the topics included in that search. Results from these alerts were provided to the lead author until April 2018. The lead author requested additional articles that either did not fit the original search criteria or were discovered during the evidence appraisal process. The lead author and the medical librarian also identified relevant guidelines from government agencies, professional organizations, and standards-setting bodies.

Search terms included *airborne precautions, biological warfare, biological warfare agents, bioterrorism, blood-borne pathogens, chemical terrorism, chemical warfare, Clostridium difficile, communicable diseases, disaster planning, disease outbreaks, disease transmission (horizontal, infectious, patient-to-professional, professional-to-patient), doffing, donning, droplet precautions, drug resistance (microbial), Ebola, Ebola virus, Ebolavirus, emergency preparedness, extensively drug-resistant tuberculosis, gram-negative bacteria, gram-negative bacterial infections, gram-positive bacteria, hemorrhagic fever (Ebola, viral) HEPA filter, hepatitis C, hepatitis (viral, human), herpesvirus, HIV infections, HIV-infected patients, infectious disease transmission, infectious skin diseases, isolation precautions, latent tuberculosis, meningitis (viral), methicillin resistance, methicillin-resistant Staphylococcus aureus, microbial drug resistance, multidrug resistant organism, needle stick injuries, needlestick injuries, negative pressure environment, patient isolation, personal protective equipment, quarantine, skin diseases (infectious, viral), staging wound closure, standard precautions, Staphylococcus aureus, TB precautions in tissue, transmissible infections, tuberculosis, tuberculosis (central nervous system, cutaneous, gastrointestinal, meningeal, multidrug-resistant, ocular, pulmonary), tuberculosis cutaneous precautions, tuberculosis precautions, tuberculosis tissue precautions, universal*

Figure 1. Flow Diagram of Literature Search Results

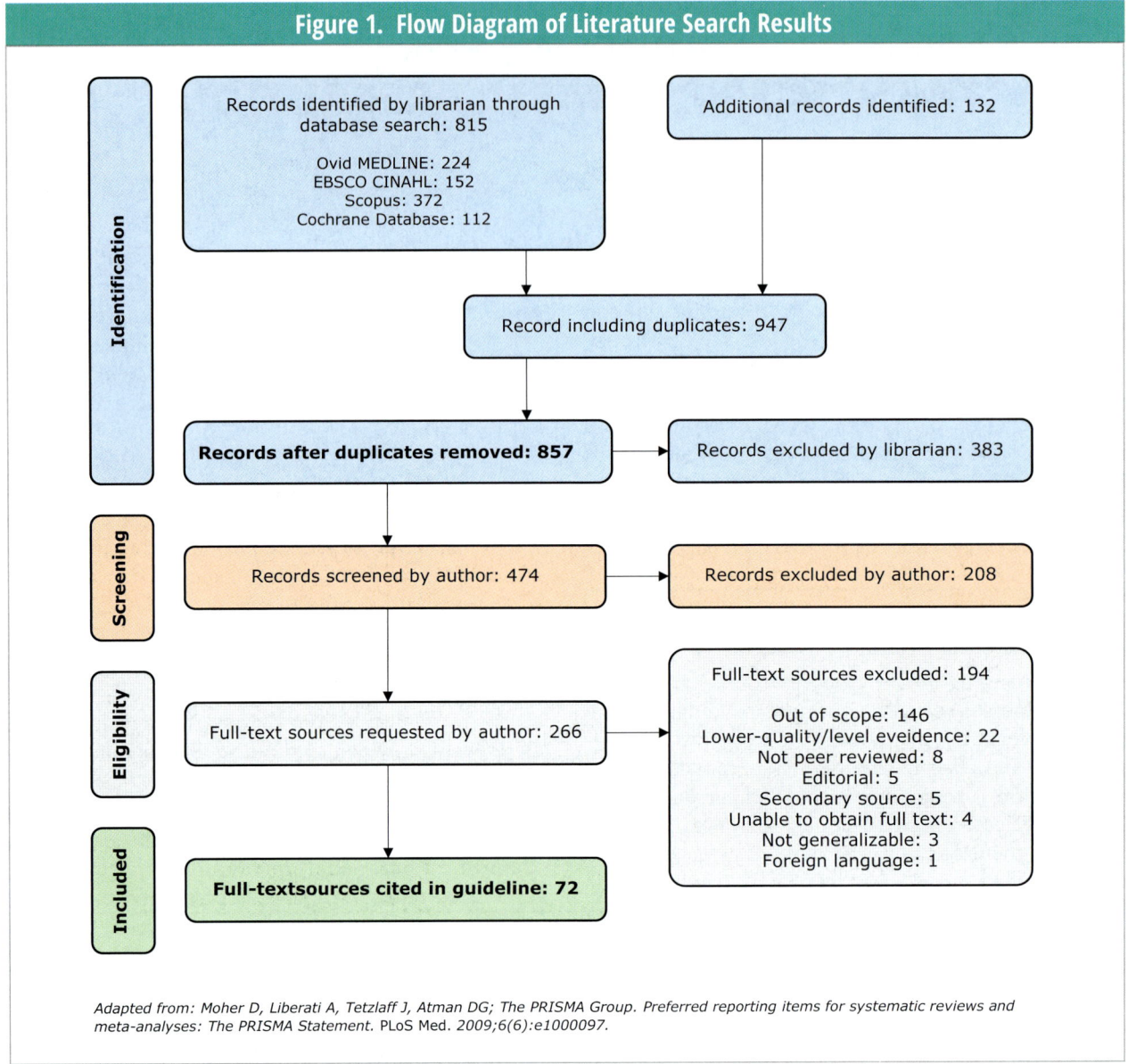

Adapted from: Moher D, Liberati A, Tetzlaff J, Atman DG; The PRISMA Group. Preferred reporting items for systematic reviews and meta-analyses: The PRISMA Statement. PLoS Med. 2009;6(6):e1000097.

precautions, vancomycin resistance, vancomycin-resistant Enterococci, viral hepatitis, viral meningitis, and *viral skin diseases.*

Included were research and non-research literature in English, complete publications, and publication dates within the time restriction when available. Excluded were non-peer-reviewed publications and older evidence within the time restriction when more recent evidence was available. Editorials, news items, and other brief items were excluded. Low-quality evidence was excluded when higher-quality evidence was available, and literature outside the time restriction was excluded when literature within the time restriction was available (Figure 1).

Articles identified in the search were provided to the project team for evaluation. The team consisted of the lead author and one evidence appraiser. The lead author divided the search results into topics. The members of the team reviewed and critically appraised each article using the AORN Research or Non-Research Evidence Appraisal Tools

as appropriate. The literature was independently evaluated and appraised according to the strength and quality of the evidence. Each article was then assigned an appraisal score. The appraisal score is noted in brackets after each reference as applicable.

Each recommendation rating is based on a synthesis of the collective evidence, a benefit-harm assessment, and consideration of resource use. The strength of the recommendation was determined using the AORN Evidence Rating Model and the quality and consistency of the evidence supporting a recommendation. The recommendation strength rating is noted in brackets after each recommendation.

Note: The evidence summary table is available at http://www.aorn.org/evidencetables/.

Editor's note: *MEDLINE is a registered trademark of the US National Library of Medicine's Medical Literature Analysis and*

Retrieval System, Bethesda, MD. CINAHL, Cumulative Index to Nursing and Allied Health Literature, is a registered trademark of EBSCO Industries, Birmingham, AL. Scopus is a registered trademark of Elsevier B.V., Amsterdam, The Netherlands.

1. Standard Precautions

1.1 **Use standard precautions when caring for all patients.**[1,2] *[Recommendation]*

Standard precautions are the foundation for preventing transmission of infectious diseases. They apply to all patients across all health care settings (eg, hospitals, ambulatory surgery centers, free-standing specialty care sites, interventional sites) and to the handling of any blood, body fluids, or other potentially infectious materials.[1] These practices protect perioperative personnel and prevent transmission of pathogens to patients.[2]

1.2 **All personnel in the health care organization should follow established hand hygiene practices (See the AORN Guideline for Hand Hygiene**[3]**).**[1-5] *[Recommendation]*

Hand hygiene is one of the most effective ways to prevent disease transmission and control infections in health care settings.[5]

1.3 **Provide the patient with a clean, safe environment (See the AORN Guideline for Environmental Cleaning**[6]**).**[2,6-9] *[Recommendation]*

Establishing a clean environment decreases the risk for cross contamination from environmental reservoirs and decreases the risk for disease transmission to the patient.[6]

1.4 **Perioperative personnel must wear PPE whenever the possibility exists for exposure to blood, body fluids, or other potentially infectious materials.**[1,2,10] *[Regulatory Requirement]*

The use of PPE protects the wearer's mucous membranes, airway, skin, and clothing from contact with blood, body fluids, and other potentially infectious materials (See Recommendation 2).[1,10]

1.4.1 **Use mouth pieces, resuscitation bags, or other ventilation devices during resuscitation.**[1] *[Recommendation]*

Respiratory droplets are generated during cardiopulmonary resuscitation (CPR). If CPR is given to a patient with a transmissible infection, disease transmission is possible. Mouth pieces, resuscitation bags, pocket masks with one-way valves, and other ventilation devices allow caregivers to perform CPR without exposing their mouths and noses to oral and respiratory fluids.[1]

1.5 **All people who enter the health care facility should practice respiratory hygiene and cough etiquette.**[1,2] *[Recommendation]*

Respiratory hygiene and cough etiquette may minimize potential exposures by reducing the transmission of respiratory infections within the facility.[2]

1.5.1 **Separate patients with respiratory symptoms from others as soon as possible (eg, during triage, at entry into the facility).**[1,2] *[Recommendation]*

1.5.2 **Establish and implement policies and procedures to screen visitors who have signs or symptoms of a communicable infection and limit patient visitation.**[1] *[Recommendation]*

1.5.3 **Promote respiratory hygiene and cough etiquette by**
- **posting signs that provide instructions for respiratory hygiene and cough etiquette at entrances and in strategic places within ambulatory and inpatient settings in all languages that are applicable to the population served,**
- **providing resources (eg, alcohol-based hand rub dispensers, handwashing supplies) and instructions in convenient locations and near waiting areas on how to perform hand hygiene,**
- **providing tissues and no-touch waste receptacles for disposal of tissues, and**
- **providing masks for patients who exhibit signs of respiratory infection.**[1]

[Recommendation]

1.5.4 **Promote compliance with respiratory hygiene and cough etiquette by educating perioperative personnel, patients, and visitors to**
- **cover their mouth and nose with a tissue or a sleeve rather than the hand when coughing or sneezing;**
- **quickly dispose of used tissues into waste receptacles;**
- **perform hand hygiene after coming into contact with respiratory secretions;**
- **wear a mask if exhibiting signs of respiratory infection; and**
- **stay at least 3 ft away from others in common areas if exhibiting signs of respiratory symptoms.**[1]

[Recommendation]

1.6 Use safe injection practices (eg, aseptic technique, single-use syringe and needle, single-dose vials, sharps safety) when administering medication (See the AORN Guideline for Medication Safety[11] and the AORN Guideline for Sharps Safety[12]).[1,2,10-12] *[Recommendation]*

Using syringes, needles, and vials more than once increases the risk for disease transmission and infection, and unsafe medication injection practices have been implicated in outbreaks of hepatitis B and hepatitis C.[1] Safe injection practices also protect health care workers by decreasing the risk for bloodborne pathogen transmission through sharps injuries and are required by Occupational Safety and Health Administration (OSHA) regulations.[10,12]

1.7 Clean reusable medical equipment (eg, blood glucose meters, blood pressure cuffs, pulse oximeter probes, surgical instruments, endoscopes) that has been used for one patient and disinfect or sterilize equipment in accordance with the manufacturer's written instructions for use (IFU) before use for another patient and when soiled.[1,2,8] *[Recommendation]*

Cleaning and disinfection or sterilization of soiled reusable medical equipment decreases the risk for cross contamination and disease transmission to the patient.

2. Personal Protective Equipment

2.1 Perioperative personnel must wear PPE when exposure to blood, body fluids, or other potentially infectious materials is anticipated.[10] *[Regulatory Requirement]*

Personal protective equipment protects the wearer's skin, clothing, mucous membranes, and respiratory tract from contact with blood, body fluids, and other potentially infectious materials. Blood and body fluids may contain bloodborne pathogens, such as hepatitis B, hepatitis C, and human immunodeficiency virus (HIV), that can infect perioperative personnel if exposure occurs. The selection of PPE is based on the mode of transmission (eg, contact, droplet, airborne) and the nature of the patient interaction.[1]

2.2 The health care organization must provide PPE to personnel at no cost.[10] *[Regulatory Requirement]*

The OSHA Bloodborne Pathogens standard requires employers to provide PPE to personnel at no cost to reduce the risk of skin and mucous membrane exposure to blood, body fluids, and other potentially infectious materials.[10] It is also the employer's responsibility to ensure that PPE is available and readily accessible, that alternatives are available for employees with allergies, and that personnel wear the appropriate PPE for the task being performed. Personal protective equipment includes gloves, gowns, eye protection, masks, and respirators.

2.3 Perioperative personnel must wear gloves when contact of the hands with blood, body fluids, or other potentially infectious materials can be reasonably anticipated, including when
- touching mucous membranes or nonintact skin,
- performing vascular access procedures, and
- touching contaminated patient care items or environmental surfaces.[10]

[Regulatory Requirement]

Gloves protect the wearer's hands from contamination by contact with blood, body fluids, and other potentially infectious materials.

2.3.1 Wear gloves during care of a patient who requires **contact precautions** or for coming into contact with potentially contaminated surfaces in the patient's environment (See Recommendation 3).[1] *[Recommendation]*

2.3.2 Wear low-protein, powder-free natural rubber latex gloves or gloves labeled as "not made with natural rubber latex."[13] *[Recommendation]*

The use of low-protein, powder-free natural rubber latex gloves or synthetic rubber gloves may minimize latex exposure and the risk of reactions in both health care personnel and patients.[13] Although natural rubber latex gloves pose an allergy risk, they may be more protective to the wearer in the event of a glove breach.

In a laboratory study, Bardorf et al[14] compared glove elasticity and bacterial passage through nine different types of medical gloves and two types of surgical gloves. The glove materials included nitrile, latex, neoprene, and thermoplastic elastomer. The researchers found that bacterial passage through glove punctures decreased when the glove material was more elastic, such as natural rubber latex, which may protect the wearer in the event of a glove breach. Medical examination gloves made of nitrile and neoprene had 10-fold higher bacterial passage through the glove puncture than latex gloves, although all the surgical gloves had less bacterial passage than the examination gloves. Because of the risk for latex allergy in patients and health care personnel, the researchers recommended conducting a risk-benefit assessment to balance the risk of allergy with the degree of protection required in the event of a glove puncture.

Patient examination gloves and surgical gloves are regulated as medical devices by the US Food and Drug Administration (FDA).[15] In 2016, the FDA determined that powdered gloves present an unreasonable and substantial risk of causing illness or injury and therefore banned powdered patient examination gloves and powdered surgeon's gloves.[16] As part of this rule, gloves may not include more than trace amounts of residual powder from manufacturing processes, not to exceed 2 mg per glove. See the AORN Guideline for a Safe Environment of Care[13] for additional information.

2.3.3 Scrubbed team members should wear two pairs of sterile surgical gloves (ie, double glove). When wearing two pairs of gloves, use a perforation indicator system. (See the AORN Guideline for Sterile Technique[17] and the AORN Guideline for Sharps Safety[12]). *[Recommendation]*

2.3.4 Limit the use of polyvinyl chloride or vinyl examination gloves to situations in which exposure risk is low. *[Recommendation]*

Research has shown that vinyl and polyvinyl gloves have a higher failure rate in use than nitrile or latex gloves.[18-21] In a quasi-experimental study of 137 procedures, the researchers noted higher microbial contamination of the hands of health care personnel and a higher frequency of leaks in vinyl gloves compared to latex gloves.[18] Similarly, another quasi-experimental study of 886 examination gloves showed vinyl gloves were much more likely to leak than latex gloves (51.3% versus 19.7%) as demonstrated by a standardized clinical protocol designed to mimic patient care activities.[19] Research also has indicated that polyvinyl chloride gloves fail to protect against virus exposure 22% of the time.[22]

Comparisons of different glove types have supported the lesser durability of vinyl and polyvinyl chloride gloves. Rego and Roley[21] evaluated 2,000 gloves (ie, 800 latex, 800 vinyl, 400 nitrile) by testing them immediately out of the box and after manipulations designed to simulate in-use conditions. Vinyl gloves failed 12% to 61% of the time, whereas latex and nitrile gloves had failure rates of 0% to 4% and 1% to 3%, respectively.

Another comparison involving 5,510 medical examination gloves (ie, 1,464 nitrile, 1,052 latex, 1,006 copolymer, 1,988 vinyl) showed that vinyl and copolymer (ie, polyvinyl chloride) gloves were less-effective barriers than latex and nitrile gloves.[20] Results showed 8.2% failure rates for the vinyl and copolymer gloves compared to 1.3% for nitrile gloves and 2.2% for latex gloves.

2.3.5 When handling hazardous medications, wear two pairs of chemotherapy gloves or other gloves as described in the manufacturer's IFU (See the AORN Guideline for Medication Safety).[11] *[Recommendation]*

2.3.6 Perform hand hygiene before donning gloves for patient contact or performing a clean or sterile task.[4,5] *[Recommendation]*

The use of gloves does not replace the need for hand hygiene.[4,5] Glove boxes may be contaminated by the hands of perioperative personnel retrieving gloves, which may be an indication for performing hand hygiene before donning gloves or for the need for a solution to reduce box contamination during glove dispensing.[3] See the AORN Guideline for Hand Hygiene[3] for additional information.

2.3.7 Visually inspect gloves for perforations and tears upon donning and during use. If a glove defect is identified, remove the gloves. *[Recommendation]*

Gloves may have perforations or tears that occur in the manufacturing process, as gloves are donned, or during use.

2.3.8 When hand hygiene is indicated, remove gloves to perform hand hygiene.[4,5] *[Recommendation]*

The use of gloves does not replace the need for hand hygiene.[4,5] Loveday et al[23] conducted a nonexperimental study at a single academic center in the United Kingdom by auditing glove use and interviewing health care personnel (N = 125) about clinical glove use. The researchers found that gloves were worn as an alternative to hand hygiene. In 37% of episodes of inappropriate glove use, there was a risk for cross contamination due to failure to remove gloves or perform hand hygiene after use. See the AORN Guideline for Hand Hygiene[3] for additional information.

2.3.9 Gloves may be removed in the following order (Figure 2):
1. With a gloved hand, grasp the palm area of the other glove; peel the glove away from the hand, allowing the glove to turn inside out; and hold the removed glove.
2. With the ungloved hand, slide a finger under the glove cuff and remove the second glove by peeling it off the hand.
3. Discard the removed gloves into a waste receptacle and perform hand hygiene.[5,24]

[Conditional Recommendation]

Figure 2. Glove Removal Sequence[1]

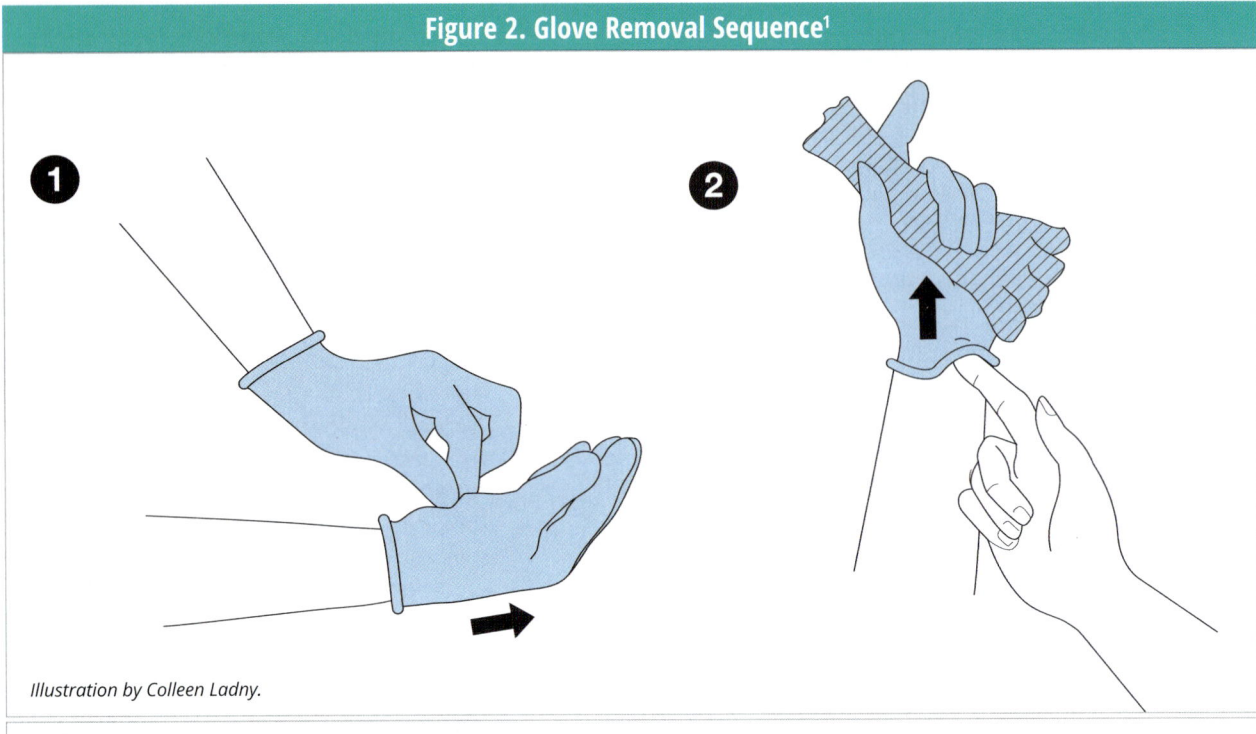

Illustration by Colleen Ladny.

Reference

1. *How to safely remove personal protective equipment (PPE). Centers for Disease Control and Prevention. https://www.cdc.gov/hai/pdfs/ppe/PPE-Sequence.pdf. Accessed October 15, 2018.*

The outer surface of the gloves may contaminate the hands during removal if touched.

2.3.10 Submit reports of glove malfunction that leads to serious injury or death to MedWatch: The FDA Safety Information and Adverse Event Reporting Program. *[Recommendation]*

The FDA classifies medical and surgical gloves as medical devices. The FDA uses medical device reports to monitor device performance, detect potential device-related failures or safety issues, and contribute to risk-benefit assessments of suspected device-associated deaths, serious injuries, or malfunction. The Manufacturer and User Facility Device Experience (MAUDE) database houses reports submitted to the FDA by mandatory reporters (ie, manufacturers, importers, device user facilities) and voluntary reporters (ie, health care professionals, patients, consumers).

Mandatory reporters are required to submit reports when they become aware of information that reasonably suggests that one of their marketed devices may have caused or contributed to a death or serious injury or has malfunctioned and that the malfunction of the device would be likely to cause or contribute to a death or serious injury if the malfunction were to recur. Voluntary reporters are required to sub-

mit reports when they become aware of information that reasonably suggests a device may have caused or contributed to a death or serious injury to a patient.

2.4 Perioperative personnel must wear gowns when contact of the arms or clothing with blood, body fluids, or other potentially infectious materials can be reasonably anticipated.[2,10] *[Regulatory Requirement]*

A gown protects the wearer's skin and clothing from contamination by contact with blood, body fluids, and other potentially infectious materials.

2.4.1 Wear a gown during care of a patient who requires contact precautions or for coming into contact with potentially contaminated surfaces or equipment in the patient's environment (See Recommendation 3).[1] *[Recommendation]*

2.4.2 Determine the type of gown needed (eg, isolation, surgical) by the task and degree of exposure anticipated.[2,10,25-27] *[Recommendation]*

2.4.3 Select the type of isolation or surgical gown needed for the procedure according to the barrier performance class as stated on the product label.[26,27] *[Recommendation]*

The level of protection provided by the gown may be stated on the product label, with

Table 1. Gown Liquid Barrier Performance Class*		
Barrier Level[1]	**Test Methods[1]**	**Anticipated Risk of Exposure (eg, fluid amount, splash risk, pressure on the gown)[2]**
Level 1	AATCC 42	Minimal
Level 2	AATCC 42 AATCC 127 (≥ 20 cm)	Low
Level 3	AATCC 42 AATCC 127 (≥ 50 cm)	Moderate
Level 4	AATCC F1671	High

*The barrier performance class may be stated on the label as the barrier level or test method.

AATCC = American Association of Textile Chemists and Colorists

References

1. AAMI PB70: Liquid Barrier Performance and Classification of Protective Apparel and Drapes Intended for Use in Health Care Facilities. *Arlington, VA: Association for the Advancement of Medical Instrumentation; 2012.*
2. AAMI TIR11:2005. Selection and Use of Protective Apparel and Surgical Drapes in Health Care Facilities. *Arlington, VA: Association for the Advancement of Medical Instrumentation; 2005.*

higher barrier levels providing more protection to the wearer (Table 1). The FDA requires gown manufacturers to test and validate liquid barrier claims for surgical gowns and isolation gowns that provide moderate (ie, Level 3) and high (ie, Level 4) levels of protection.[28] The FDA recognizes the ANSI/AAMI PB70 barrier performance levels and associated test methods as the preferred methods for assessing gown liquid barrier protection.[28]

Surgical gowns are labeled with the barrier properties of the gown's critical zone. The size and configuration of the critical zone varies by each design and is specified by the manufacturer on the product label. See the AORN Guideline for Sterile Technique[17] for additional information. Isolation gowns may be labeled with either the barrier level or the associated test method.

2.4.4 **Select a gown that fully covers the wearer's torso from the neck to the knees and the wearer's arms to the end of wrists and wraps around the back.**[24-26] *[Recommendation]*

A gown that is of an insufficient size may expose the wearer's clothing or restrict the wearer's movement.

2.4.5 **Secure the gown at the neck and waist.**[24] *[Recommendation]*

A gown that is not secured at the neck and waist may expose the wearer's skin and clothing to blood, body fluids, and other potentially infectious materials.

2.4.6 **Completely cover the gown cuffs with the gloves.**[24]

- **A gown with a thumb loop may be worn under the gloves to secure the gown sleeve.**[25]

- **Gloves with extended cuffs may be worn to maintain coverage of the gown cuffs.** *[Recommendation]*

Maintaining coverage of the gown cuff by the glove is important to protect the wearer from exposure at the wrist to blood, body fluids, and other potentially infectious materials.[25] A gown with a thumb loop may be used to secure the gown sleeve and cuff under the gloves to keep the cuff from moving up the forearm. When worn in combination with a gown, the glove cuff may not be long enough to cover the gown cuff during use, depending on the task being performed. Gloves with extended cuffs may provide additional protection to prevent wrist exposure during use.

2.4.7 **Remove the gown and gloves in the following order (Figure 3):**

1. **Grasp the front of the gown with gloved hands.**
2. **Pull the gown away from the body so that the attachments break.**
3. **While removing the gown, roll the gown inside out into a bundle, touching only the outside of the gown with gloved hands.**
4. **Peel off the gloves as the gown is being removed, touching only the inside of the gloves and gown with bare hands.**
5. **Discard the gown and gloves into a waste container or soiled linen bin and perform hand hygiene.**[24]

[Recommendation]

The outside of the gown may be contaminated. Rolling the gown into a bundle with the most contaminated part on the inside may reduce environmental contamination when discarding the gown. Removing the gloves

Figure 3. Gown and Gloves Removal Sequence[1]

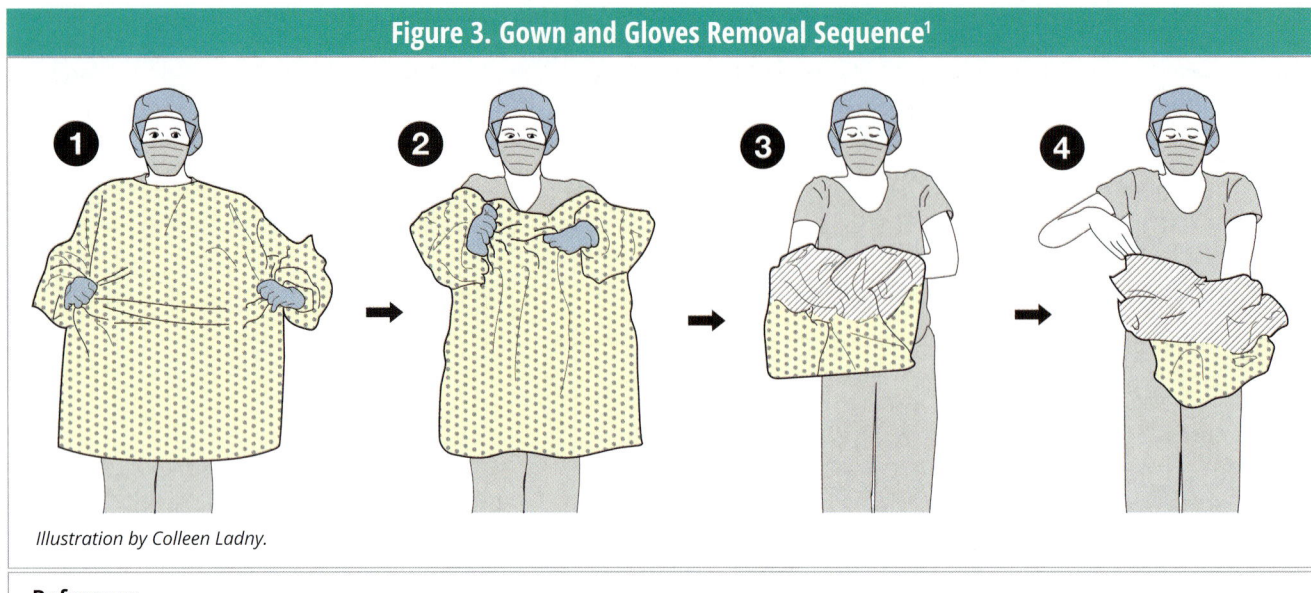

Illustration by Colleen Ladny.

Reference

1. *How to safely remove personal protective equipment (PPE). Centers for Disease Control and Prevention. https://www.cdc.gov/hai/pdfs/ppe/PPE-Sequence.pdf. Accessed October 15, 2018.*

simultaneously with the gown may prevent hand contamination during the gown removal process.

2.4.8 When the wearer is unable to break the gown ties and there is no assistant available to untie the gown, remove the gloves and perform hand hygiene (See Recommendation 2.3.9). The gown may be removed in the following order (Figure 4):

1. Unfasten gown ties; when reaching for the ties, take care that the sleeves do not contact the body.
2. Touching only the inside of the gown, pull the gown away from the body while rolling the gown inside out.
3. Place the gown in a waste container or soiled linen bin and perform hand hygiene.[24]

[Recommendation]

2.5 Perioperative personnel must wear eye protection when splashes, spray, spatter, or droplets of blood or other potentially infectious materials may be generated and eye contamination can be reasonably anticipated.[1,2,10] *[Regulatory Requirement]*

Eye protective devices,[10] such as goggles, glasses with solid side shields, a surgical mask with an attached eye shield, or a chin-length face shield may protect the wearer's eyes from contamination by contact with blood, body fluids, and other potentially infectious materials. Personal eyeglasses do not provide the same level of protection as eye protective devices and may not have protection at the sides. Prescription eyeglasses with side protection are available but may not protect against splashes or droplets as well as goggles do.[29]

2.5.1 Wear eye protection during aerosol-generating procedures, including bronchoscopy, endotracheal intubation, and open suctioning of the respiratory tract.[1] *[Recommendation]*

The performance of procedures that can generate small particle aerosols (ie, aerosol-generating procedures) has been associated with transmission of infectious agents to health care personnel.[1]

2.5.2 Determine the type of eye protection needed by the task, degree of exposure anticipated, and personal vision needs.[1,29] *[Recommendation]*

2.5.3 Select goggles that fit snugly, especially at the corners of the eyes and across the brow, are indirectly vented, and have anti-fog properties.[29] *[Recommendation]*

Fitted, indirectly vented goggles with a manufacturer's anti-fog coating are the most reliable and practical means of protecting the wearer's eyes from splashes, sprays, and respiratory droplets.[29]

2.5.4 Use a face shield when more coverage is needed to protect the face and eyes outside the area covered by the mask and goggles.[1,29] *[Recommendation]*

Face shields provide protection to the eyes and other areas of the face.[1,29,30] Face shields that have crown and chin protection and wrap around the face to the point of the ear protect the eyes and sides of the face from splashes and sprays.

2.5.5 **After use, remove the protective eyewear with ungloved hands by handling only the ear or head pieces without touching the front, and perform hand hygiene.**[1,29] *[Recommendation]*

Protective eyewear may be contaminated with blood, body fluid, or other potentially infectious materials during use, especially the front of the goggles or face shield.[1,29] Handling the eyewear by the cleaner part may reduce hand contamination during removal.

2.5.6 **Discard disposable eyewear and disinfect reusable eyewear after each use.**[1,29] *[Recommendation]*

Reusable eyewear may be a reservoir for pathogens in the perioperative setting. In a nonexperimental study conducted at one facility, Lange[31] cultured disposable and reusable eyewear and found that 37.7% of disposable and 94.9% of reusable eyewear was contaminated after use. After disinfection, 74.4% of reusable eyewear remained contaminated.

2.6 **Perioperative personnel must wear masks when splashes, spray, spatter, or droplets of blood or other potentially infectious materials may be generated and nose or mouth contamination can be reasonably anticipated.**[1,2,10] *[Regulatory Requirement]*

A mask protects the wearer's nose, mouth, and face from contamination by contact with blood, body fluids, and other potentially infectious materials. Masks also are worn as part of sterile technique to protect patients from exposure to pathogens that may be carried in the mouths or noses of perioperative personnel. See the AORN Guideline for Sterile Technique[17] for additional information.

In a nonexperimental study, Lakhani et al[32] found that 54% of the masks worn by scrubbed personnel during otolaryngology procedures were contaminated with blood splashes. For tonsillectomy procedures, the most common surgical procedure, 76.9% of the masks were contaminated with blood splashes.

2.6.1 **Wear a mask during aerosol-generating procedures, including bronchoscopy, endotracheal intubation, and open suctioning of the respiratory tract.**[1] *[Recommendation]*

The performance of procedures that can generate small particle aerosols (ie, aerosol-generating procedures) has been associated with transmission of infectious agents to health care personnel.[1]

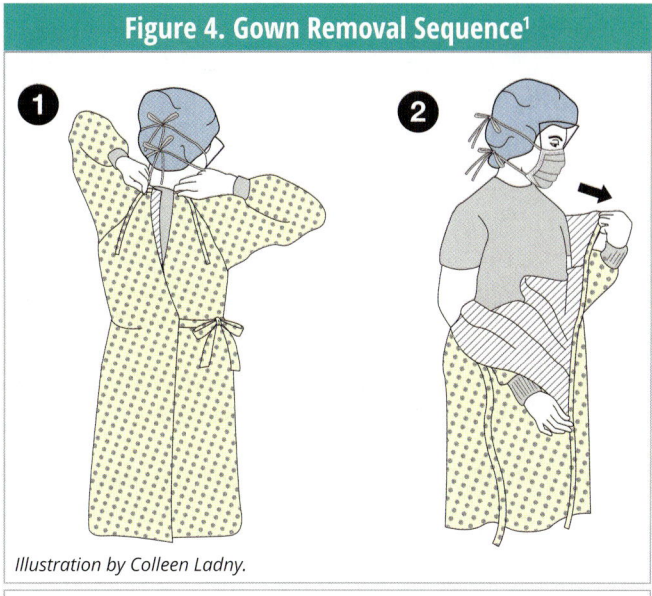

Figure 4. Gown Removal Sequence[1]

Illustration by Colleen Ladny.

Reference

1. *How to safely remove personal protective equipment (PPE). Centers for Disease Control and Prevention. https://www.cdc.gov/hai/pdfs/ppe/PPE-Sequence.pdf. Accessed October 15, 2018.*

2.6.2 **Wear a mask during care of a patient who requires droplet precautions (See Recommendation 4).**[1] *[Recommendation]*

2.6.3 **Determine the type of mask needed by the task and degree of exposure anticipated.**[2,10] *[Recommendation]*

2.6.4 **Select the type of surgical mask needed for the procedure according to the barrier level as stated on the product label.** *[Recommendation]*

The level of protection provided by the mask may be determined by the ASTM barrier level as stated on the product label, with higher barrier levels providing more protection to the wearer.[33] The FDA recommends that mask manufacturers test the masks for risks to the health of the wearer, including the risk for inadequate fluid resistance, inadequate barrier for bacteria (ie, particulate filtration efficiency, bacterial filtration efficiency), inadequate air exchange (ie, differential pressure), and flammability.[34] The label "surgical mask" on a product does not necessarily indicate that the product underwent the FDA-recommended fluid-resistance testing.

2.6.5 **The mask should completely cover the mouth, nose, and chin and fit snugly in a manner that prevents gaps at the sides of the mask.** *[Recommendation]*

A mask that conforms to the wearer's face decreases the risk that the health care worker will transmit nasopharyngeal and respiratory microorganisms to the patient or the sterile field.

2.6.6 Select the mask attachment that provides the best facial fit for the individual (eg, ties, ear loop, elastic). [Recommendation]

The wearer's facial shape will determine which mask attachment provides the best fit. Ear loop attachments may not provide a secure facial fit that prevents venting at the sides of the mask.

2.6.7 Don clean masks before the performing or assisting with each new procedure. [Recommendation]

2.6.8 Replace the mask and discard it whenever it becomes wet or soiled. [Recommendation]

The filtering capacity of a surgical mask may become compromised when it is wet or soiled.

2.6.9 Remove the mask last when worn in combination with other PPE, including a gown, gloves, or eye protection.[24] [Recommendation]

2.6.10 Remove the mask by touching only the ties without touching the front of the mask. Discard it in a waste receptacle and perform hand hygiene.[24] [Recommendation]

2.6.11 Do not wear used masks hanging around the neck. [Recommendation]

The filter portion of a surgical mask harbors bacteria collected from the nasopharyngeal airway. The contaminated mask may cross contaminate the attire when the mask is worn hanging around the neck.

2.7 When respiratory protection is needed, wear a National Institute for Occupational Safety and Health (NIOSH)-approved, fit-tested, surgical N95 respirator or higher level respirator in accordance with the facility's respiratory protection program.[1,35,36] [Recommendation]

Respiratory protection of personnel is regulated by OSHA[37] as part of an employer's respiratory protection program, which includes the provision and use of respirators, medical clearance of personnel to wear respirators, fit testing of respirators, education on respirator use, and evaluation of the respiratory protection program.

Respirators used in health care settings are certified by NIOSH.[1,38] The NIOSH-approval process verifies that the N95 filtering face piece respirator performs as intended by removing at least 95% of airborne particles during "worst case" testing with particles that are most likely to penetrate the respirator.[39] The respirator's NIOSH-approval status may

be identified by the "TC number" on the product label and confirmed by looking up the respirator on the NIOSH Certified Equipment List.[39]

The FDA requires surgical N95 manufacturers to meet several conditions, including having NIOSH approval, conducting flammability testing, and conducting testing to demonstrate the ability to resist penetration by blood and body fluids at a velocity consistent with the intended use of the device.[40] The FDA-recommended test for fluid-resistance of surgical masks is ASTM F1862, which demonstrates resistance to penetration by synthetic blood at a minimum velocity (80 mmHg, 120 mmHg, or 160 mmHg), with the higher velocity indicating a higher level of fluid-resistance (Table 2).[34] The level of fluid resistance may be stated on the surgical N95 product label as either the ASTM barrier level (ie, Level 1, Level 2, Level 3) or the ASTM F1862 test results (ie, 80 mmHg, 120 mmHg, 160 mmHg).

A surgical mask is not considered respiratory protection.[36] A surgical mask is a loose-fitting face mask intended to prevent the release of potential contaminants from the wearer into his or her immediate environment.[36,38] A surgical mask does not give the wearer a reliable level of protection from inhaling small airborne particles.[36]

The CDC recommends that health care personnel wear fit-tested N95 respirators or higher-level respirators as respiratory protection when caring for patients with airborne transmissible infections.[1] However, there is conflicting evidence on the benefits of wearing an N95 respirator for prevention of acute respiratory infection, such as pandemic influenza. Smith et al[41] conducted a systematic review with meta-analysis and found there was insufficient evidence in the clinical setting to determine whether N95 respirators are superior to surgical masks for protecting health care personnel from infection with acute respiratory pathogens. In a quasi-experimental study performed in Hong Kong, Suen et al[42] found that the body movements during nursing procedures may increase the risk for respirator face-seal leakage. The researchers recommended further research and product development to improve respirator fit during clinical use.

2.7.1 Wear respiratory protection before entering the room of a patient who is under airborne precautions (See Recommendation 5).[1,35] [Recommendation]

2.7.2 Wear respiratory protection during aerosol-generating procedures (eg, bronchoscopy, endotracheal intubation, open suctioning of the respiratory tract) for patients under droplet

Table 2. Medical Face Mask Barrier Levels[1]

Barrier Level[1]	Anticipated Risk of Exposure	Fluid Resistance*	Filtration**	Air Exchange†	Flammability‡
Level 1	Low	80 mmHg	≥ 95%	< 4.0	Class 1
Level 2	Moderate	120 mmHg	≥ 98%	< 5.0	Class 1
Level 3	High	160 mmHg	≥ 98%	< 5.0	Class 1

*Resistance to penetration by synthetic blood as tested by ASTM F1862 minimum pressure for pass result.
**Bacterial filtration efficiency to the wearer and sub-micron particulate filtration efficiency at 0.1 µm.
†Differential pressure in mm H_2O/cm^2
‡Flame spread

Reference
1. ASTM F2100-11(2018): Standard Specification for Performance of Materials Used in Medical Face Masks. *West Conshohocken, PA: ASTM International; 2018.*

precautions with suspected or proven infections transmitted by respiratory aerosols (eg, severe acute respiratory syndrome [SARS], avian influenza, seasonal influenza, pandemic influenza, viral hemorrhagic fevers) (See Recommendation 4).[1] *[Recommendation]*

2.7.3 Wear respiratory protection as secondary protection against surgical smoke that is not evacuated or is incompletely evacuated. *[Recommendation]*

Respiratory protection does not replace the need to use a smoke evacuation system as the first line of protection against the hazards of surgical smoke. See the AORN Guideline for Surgical Smoke Safety[43] for additional information.

2.7.4 Don respirators in accordance with the manufacturers' IFU and perform a **user seal check** (ie, fit check) for each use.[1,38] *[Recommendation]*

2.7.5 Facial hair should not cross under the seal of a fit-tested N95 respirator.[36] *[Recommendation]*

Facial hair of any length may compromise the seal of the respirator, and alternative respiratory protection may be needed.

2.7.6 Remove the respirator after leaving the patient's room and closing the door.[24] *[Recommendation]*

2.7.7 Remove the respirator last when worn in combination with other PPE (eg, gown, gloves, eye protection).[24] *[Recommendation]*

2.7.8 Remove the surgical N95 respirator in accordance with the manufacturer's written IFU by touching only the ties and without touching the front of the respirator. Discard it in a waste receptacle and perform hand hygiene.[24] *[Recommendation]*

2.7.9 Have an interdisciplinary team determine whether **powered air-purifying respirators** (PAPRs) may be used for respiratory protection in accordance with state and federal regulations and the PAPR manufacturer's written IFU when a sterile field is present. The interdisciplinary team should include an infection preventionist and an occupational health professional. *[Conditional Recommendation]*

The use of PAPRs in the health care setting may be indicated for respiratory protection of personnel from certain diseases transmissible by the airborne route, although the use of PAPRs in the perioperative setting may contaminate the sterile field. The CDC does not recommend the use of a PAPR with exhalation valves during invasive procedures in the presence of a sterile field.[35] The battery-powered blower in the PAPR filters the air intake for the person wearing the device, but it does not filter the wearer's exhaled air. The unfiltered exhausted air from the PAPR may contribute to increased levels of operating room (OR) air contamination and potentially increase the patient's risk for surgical site infection.[36,44] See the AORN Guideline for Sterile Technique[17] for additional information.

2.8 Perioperative personnel must wear fluid-resistant surgical hoods when gross contamination can reasonably be anticipated (eg, during orthopedic surgery).[10] *[Regulatory Requirement]*

2.9 Perioperative personnel must wear fluid-resistant shoe covers or boots when gross contamination can reasonably be anticipated (eg, during orthopedic surgery).[10] *[Regulatory Requirement]*

2.10 Perioperative personnel must remove PPE and clothing as soon as possible after exposure to blood, body fluids, or other potentially infectious materials.[10] *[Regulatory Requirement]*

Talbot et al[45] reported that after surgical debridement of a patient with group A *Streptococcus* necrotizing fasciitis, two surgeons acquired group A *Streptococcus* infections, one of whom developed necrotizing fasciitis with associated toxic shock syndrome. Both surgeons had gross contamination through their surgical gowns and continued to wear contaminated clothing after the procedure had ended. The surgeon who developed necrotizing fasciitis in the right leg also noted soaking of his socks with blood and body fluid. The authors recommended adherence to standard precautions, including the removal of contaminated clothing as soon as possible after exposure and cleaning of contaminated skin. The authors also suggested that the health care organization should design systems that enhance access to replacement scrubs and shower facilities.

2.11 Perioperative personnel must remove all PPE before leaving the work area and must place used PPE in a designated area or closed container for storage, washing, decontamination, or disposal.[10] *[Regulatory Requirement]*

2.11.1 Perform hand hygiene after removing PPE.[1,3-5,10] *[Recommendation]*

2.12 Identify barriers to PPE use in the perioperative setting and implement interventions to improve PPE compliance. *[Recommendation]*

Identifying barriers to PPE use allows the health care organization to develop relevant interventions to improve compliance. The collective evidence indicates that health care personnel frequently fail to use PPE correctly, especially during PPE removal, which may lead to self-contamination with potential pathogens.[46-54]

In a nonexperimental study, Kang et al[50] found that PPE contamination occurred during PPE removal in 79.2% of simulations. The health care personnel in the study reported that PPE use was time consuming and cumbersome and reported concerns about PPE effectiveness. Herlihey et al[53] used a mixed methods approach to evaluate PPE usability testing and recommended that health care organizations use human factor methods to identify risk and failure points with PPE use and implement modifications based on iterative evaluations of end-user feedback.

The culture of the health care organization may also be a barrier to PPE compliance. Neo et al[55] conducted a review of qualitative literature regarding nursing noncompliance with wearing PPE. The authors recommended the promotion of an environment that fosters teamwork and PPE use, commitment from managers to ensure availability and access to PPE, and the provision of sustainable education related to PPE and standard precautions. In a quasi-experimental study, Moore et al[56] implemented an education program and found that team support and leadership was essential to enhancing PPE compliance in the perioperative setting.

2.13 Deliver education on PPE use and removal procedures to perioperative personnel in an active training format (eg, face-to-face instruction, fluorescent marker simulation).[57] *[Recommendation]*

In a systematic review, Verbeek et al[57] found that active training (eg, spoken instruction, computer simulation) in PPE use may reduce PPE doffing errors more than passive training (eg, videos, files), although further research is needed to confirm these findings. In a quasi-experimental study, Tomas et al[48] found that educational interventions that include practice with immediate visual feedback by use of a fluorescent marker on skin and clothing contamination can significantly reduce the risk of contamination during removal of PPE. Tomas et al[58] also studied a novel reflective marker with flash photography to simulate contamination during PPE doffing procedures and recommended this as a useful tool for visualizing personnel contamination during PPE removal. Drew et al[59] recommended use of an ultraviolet tracer to assess the effectiveness of personnel education on correct PPE donning and doffing procedures.

3. Contact Precautions

3.1 Use contact precautions when providing care to patients who are known or suspected to be infected or colonized with pathogens that are transmitted by direct or indirect contact.[1,60] *[Recommendation]* Ⓐ

In addition to standard precautions, the CDC recommends using contact precautions to minimize the risk of transmission of microorganisms (eg, multidrug-resistant organisms [MDROs], *Clostridium difficile*) that are transmitted by **direct contact** or **indirect contact**.[1,60] Contact precautions that may be implemented after consultation with an infection preventionist include the use of PPE (eg, gloves, gowns), interventions during patient transport, considerations for patient placement to minimize contact with other patients, and **enhanced environmental cleaning** (Table 3).

3.2 Wear gloves and a gown when coming into contact with a patient who is known to be colonized or infected with pathogens transmitted by contact (eg, MDROs, *C difficile*) or potentially contaminated equipment and environmental surfaces in close proximity to the patient.[1] *[Recommendation]*

Table 3. Guide for Perioperative Personnel Caring for Patients Under Transmission-Based Precautions[1]

Type of Precaution	Type of Organism/Disease	Transport	Protection for Unscrubbed Personnel*	Preoperative Area	Environmental Measures
Contact	• Draining abscess • Infectious wounds • *Clostridium difficile* • Acute viral infection • Methicillin-resistant *Staphylococcus aureus* (MRSA) • Vancomycin-resistant *Enterococci* (VRE) • Vancomycin-intermediate/resistant *S aureus* (VISA/VRSA) • Extended-spectrum beta-lactamase (ESBL) • Multidrug-resistant organism	• Cover or contain the infected or colonized areas of the patient's body. • Remove and dispose of contaminated personal protective equipment (PPE) and perform hand hygiene before transporting the patient. • Don clean PPE to handle the patient at the transport destination.	• Use standard precautions. • Wear gloves whenever touching the patient's skin or items that are in close proximity to the patient. • Wear a gown when it can be anticipated that clothing will come into contact with the patient or contaminated environmental surfaces. • Don a gown upon entry into the room. Remove the gown and perform hand hygiene before exlting.	• Hold the patient in a single-patient room if possible; otherwise keep ≥ 3 ft separation between patients.	• Clean the room immediately after patient use. Focus on frequently touched surfaces.
Droplet	• Diphtheria • Haemophilus influenzae type b • Seasonal influenza • Pandemic influenza • Meningococcal disease • Mumps • Mycoplasma pneumonia • Group A streptococcus • Pertussis • Adenovirus • Rubella	• Instruct the patient to wear a mask and follow respiratory hygiene and cough etiquette. • The transporter is not required to wear a mask.	• Use standard precautions. • Wear a mask upon entry into the room.	• Hold the patient in a single-patient room if possible; otherwise keep ≥ 3 ft separation between patients. • Draw a privacy curtain between beds to minimize the opportunity for close contact.	• Routine
Airborne	• *Mycobacterium tuberculosis* • Disseminated herpes zoster • Rubeola Monkeypox • Smallpox • Varicella zoster • Chicken pox	• Instruct the patient to wear a mask and follow respiratory hygiene and cough etiquette. • Cover and contain affected skin lesions. • The transporter is not required to wear a mask.	• Use standard precautions. • Wear a fit-tested N95 or higher level respirator that is approved by the National Institute for Occupational Safety and Health.	• Place the patient in an airborne infection isolation room (AIIR), if possible. • Provide at least 6 (existing facility) or 12 new construction/renovation) air changes per hour.	• Consult an infection preventionist before patient placement to determine the safety of an alternative room that does not meet AIIR requirements. • If an AIIR is not available, the OR should remain vacant postoperatively for sufficient time to allow for a full exchange of air, generally 1 hour.

*"Unscrubbed personnel" include anesthesia professionals, the circulating RN, and preoperative and postanesthesthia care personnel.
This table should be adapted according to local conditions and special patient considerations.

Reference

1. Siegel JD, Rhinehart E, Jackson M, Chiarello L; the Healthcare Infection Control Practices Advisory Committee. *2007 Guideline for Isolation Precautions: Preventing Transmission of Infectious Agents in Health Care Settings.* Am J Infect Control. 2007;35(10 Suppl 2):S65-S164.

3.2.1 Don the gown and gloves upon room entry and discard them upon exiting the room (See Recommendation 2.3).[1] *[Recommendation]*

3.3 When patient transport is necessary, take precautions to reduce the opportunity for transmission of pathogens to other patients, personnel, and visitors and to reduce contamination of the environment.[1] *[Recommendation]*

3.3.1 Before transporting the patient,
- notify the receiving team members that the patient is coming and what precautions should be taken,
- perform hand hygiene,
- don a gown and gloves,
- contain and cover the infected or colonized areas of the patient's body,
- remove and dispose of contaminated PPE, and
- perform hand hygiene.[1]

[Recommendation]

3.3.2 Don gloves to clean and disinfect the bed rails and controls that will be touched by personnel during patient transport. *[Recommendation]*

3.3.3 Wear PPE during transport according to organizational policy and when direct contact with the patient is necessary during transport (eg, an intubated patient). Do not touch doors, elevator buttons, identification badges, or environmental surfaces with contaminated PPE (ie, gloves, gowns) during transport. *[Recommendation]* **P**

3.3.4 At the transport destination, don a gown and gloves before coming into contact with the patient.[1] *[Recommendation]*

3.4 Place a patient who requires contact precautions in a single-patient room before and after surgery when one is available.[1] *[Recommendation]*

Single-patient placement may help to prevent the inadvertent sharing of patient care items that could transmit pathogens to other patients.[1]

3.4.1 When single-patient placement is not possible, consult with an infection preventionist to establish optimal preoperative and postoperative placement for a patient who requires contact precautions.[1] *[Recommendation]*

The infection preventionist can help assess and mitigate the risks associated with non-isolation placement options (eg, cohorting, keeping the patient with an existing room-

mate) to minimize the potential for cross contamination.[1]

3.4.2 Place patients who require contact precautions at least 3 ft away from other patients.[1] *[Recommendation]*

3.5 Implement enhanced environmental cleaning, in consultation with an infection preventionist, for cleaning following the care of patients who are known to be infected or colonized with MDROs.[1,60] *[Recommendation]*

Decreasing environmental contaminants on high-touch surfaces may decrease the risk of MDRO transmission. See the AORN Guideline for Environmental Cleaning[6] for additional information.

3.5.1 Use an Environmental Protection Agency–registered disinfectant that is effective against *C difficile* spores during cleaning following the care of patients diagnosed with or suspected to have a *C difficile* infection.[6-8] *[Recommendation]*

Thorough cleaning of environmental surfaces and equipment using a disinfectant that effectively kills *C difficile* spores is a foundational requirement for preventing the transmission of *C difficile* infection and colonization. See the AORN Guideline for Environmental Cleaning[6] for additional information.

3.6 Have an interdisciplinary team, including an infection preventionist, identify the preferred method for hand hygiene (ie, soap and water, alcohol-based hand rub) to use when caring for patients under contact precautions for *C difficile* infection in the perioperative setting.
- Perform hand hygiene with soap and water after direct contact with feces or body areas where fecal contamination is likely (eg, the perineum).[61]
- Hand hygiene may be performed with an alcohol-based hand rub in a non-outbreak setting.[61]

[Conditional Recommendation]

Soap and water may remove *C difficile* spores from the hands more effectively than an alcohol-based hand rub (See the AORN Guideline for Hand Hygiene[3]). In an outbreak setting, hand hygiene with soap and water may be indicated to prevent *C difficile* spore transmission.[61] However, sinks are not readily accessible in the perioperative setting and hand hygiene with an alcohol-based hand rub during patient care may improve hand hygiene compliance and reduce the patient's risk for acquiring a health care–associated infection.

3.7 Clean and disinfect all noncritical equipment (eg, commodes, IV pumps, ventilators, computers, personal electronic devices) between uses for patient care and handle them in a manner to prevent personnel exposure or environmental contact with potentially infectious materials.[1] *[Recommendation]*

3.7.1 Dedicated noncritical equipment such as stethoscopes, blood pressure cuffs, and electronic thermometers may be used.[1,60] *[Conditional Recommendation]*

The CDC recommends using dedicated noncritical equipment for patients who require contact precautions.[1,60] In a nonexperimental study, Grewal et al[62] found high bacterial colonization rates on blood pressure cuffs from three hospital departments, including the OR, although methicillin-resistant *Staphylococcus aureus* and vancomycin-resistant enterococci were not frequently found. The researchers identified the need for improving disinfection and infection prevention and control protocols because of the high number of microorganisms found on the inner surfaces of the blood pressure cuffs.

John et al[63] cultured electronic thermometers in a nonexperimental study and found that 8% of the thermometer handles in three hospitals were contaminated with one or more potential pathogen. In this study, a DNA marker inoculated onto the handles of electronic thermometers in hospital and long-term care facility settings spread to surfaces in patient rooms, to other types of portable equipment, and to patients' hands. The researchers identified the need for effective strategies to reduce the risk for pathogen transmission by electronic thermometers.

3.8 Assess the patient for any adverse effects (eg, anxiety, depression, perceptions of stigma, reduced contact with perioperative personnel) caused by using contact precautions and implement interventions (eg, social contact, patient education, increased communication) to address the adverse effects.[1] *[Recommendation]*

Patients who require transmission-based precautions may experience increased anxiety and depression and decreased levels of satisfaction.[1] Two systematic literature reviews[64,65] found that patients under contact precautions may experience adverse outcomes, including

- less patient-to-health care provider contact;
- changes to systems of care that produce delays and more noninfectious adverse events;

- increased symptoms of depression, anxiety, and anger; and
- decreased satisfaction with care.

However, more recent quasi-experimental research found that placement under contact precautions did not affect the anxiety and depression levels of the patients.[66,67] Rather, the personal attributes of the patient were associated with the development of depression.[66]

Perioperative RNs are in a position to assess patients for negative feelings, improve social contact, and provide education and frequent communication to the patient. By educating a patient who requires contact precautions and his or her family members,[64] the perioperative RN may minimize feelings of isolation, depression, and anxiety and may increase patient satisfaction.

3.9 Instruct a patient's visitors to wear gowns and gloves in the patient's room and to perform hand hygiene upon entering and exiting the room.[68] *[Recommendation]*

The Society for Healthcare Epidemiology of America (SHEA)[68] states that visitors to patients with an MDRO infection or colonization who are interacting with multiple patients may increase the risk for transmission of these organisms. In the perioperative setting, patients' visitors have a high number of contacts with other visitors and patients in common waiting areas, depending on the layout and flow of patients through perioperative phases of care. As such, a perioperative patient's visitors may reduce the risk for transmission of pathogens to other patients in common waiting areas by following contact precautions and performing hand hygiene when entering and exiting the patient's room or treatment bay. Extended-stay visitors to inpatients may have been exempted from following contact precautions in the inpatient unit because of the impracticality of this practice, and explaining the rationale for the difference in the perioperative setting may facilitate visitor participation.

4. Droplet Precautions

4.1 Use droplet precautions when providing care to patients who are known or suspected to be infected with pathogens transmitted by respiratory droplets (ie, large particle droplets > 5 μm in size) that are generated by a patient who is coughing, sneezing, or talking.[1] *[Recommendation]* **A**

In addition to standard precautions, the CDC recommends droplet precautions to reduce the risk of transmitting pathogens (eg, adenovirus, group A *Streptococcus*, influenza, *Neisseria meningitides*, *Bordetella pertussis*, rhinovirus) that spread through close respiratory or mucous membrane contact.[1] Droplet precautions include the use of PPE (eg, a surgical mask), placing a mask on the patient during transport, and considering the patient's placement to minimize contact with other patients.

4.2 **Don masks upon entering the room or cubicle of a patient who requires droplet precautions (See Recommendation 2.6).**[1] *[Recommendation]*

Masks prevent the transmission of large droplets (ie, greater than 5 μm) and, worn correctly, protect perioperative personnel who are within close proximity of a patient who requires droplet precautions.[1]

4.2.1 Don NIOSH-approved, fit-tested, surgical N95 respirators or higher-level respirators in accordance with the facility's respiratory protection program before performing aerosol-generating procedures (eg, bronchoscopy, endotracheal intubation, open suctioning of the respiratory tract) on patients under droplet precautions with suspected or proven infections transmitted by respiratory aerosols (eg, SARS, avian influenza, pandemic influenza, viral hemorrhagic fevers) (See Recommendation 2.7).[1] *[Recommendation]*

4.3 **When patient transport is necessary, take precautions to reduce the opportunity for transmission of pathogens to other patients, personnel, and visitors and to reduce contamination of the environment.**[1] *[Recommendation]*

4.3.1 Before transporting the patient, notify the receiving team members that the patient is coming and to follow droplet precautions.[1] *[Recommendation]*

4.3.2 If possible, have the patient wear a mask and follow respiratory hygiene and cough etiquette during transport (See Recommendation 1.5).[1] *[Recommendation]*

4.3.3 Perioperative personnel should not wear masks during patient transport.[1] *[Recommendation]*

4.4 **Place a patient who requires droplet precautions in a single-patient room before and after surgery.**[1] *[Recommendation]*

Single-patient placement helps prevent the spread of infection from patient to patient.[1] Special air handling and ventilation are not required as a part of droplet precautions.[1]

4.4.1 When single-patient placement is not possible, consult with an infection preventionist to establish optimal preoperative and postoperative placement for a patient who requires droplet precautions.[1] *[Recommendation]*

The infection preventionist can help assess and mitigate the risks associated with non-isolation placement options (eg, cohorting, keeping the patient with an existing roommate) to minimize the potential for cross contamination.[1]

4.4.2 Place patients who require droplet precautions at least 3 ft away from other patients.[1] *[Recommendation]*

The defined risk area (ie, > 3 ft) around the patient is based on epidemiologic and simulated infection studies.[1]

4.4.3 When possible, close the door or curtain to the patient's room.[1] *[Recommendation]*

Curtains and doors help to separate patients and reduce transmission of infectious organisms.

4.5 **Instruct a patient's visitors to wear masks in the patient's room and to perform hand hygiene upon entering and exiting the room.**[68] *[Recommendation]*

The SHEA recommends that visitors to patients who require droplet precautions wear masks, although visitors may be exempted if they have significant documented exposure (eg, household contact) to the symptomatic patient and are not ill themselves.[68]

5. Airborne Precautions

5.1 **Use airborne precautions when providing care to patients who are known or suspected to be infected with pathogens that are transmitted by the airborne route (ie, small particles or droplet nuclei < 5 μm in size).**[1,35] *[Recommendation]*

In addition to standard precautions, the CDC recommends airborne precautions to minimize transfer of pathogens that are spread by the airborne route (eg, *Mycobacterium tuberculosis*, rubeola virus [measles], varicella-zoster virus [chickenpox], disseminated herpes zoster).[1,35] Airborne precautions include the use of PPE (eg, respiratory protection), placing a mask on the patient during transport, environmental controls, and administrative controls.

5.2 **Don a NIOSH-approved, fit-tested, surgical N95 respirator or higher-level respirator in accordance with the facility's respiratory protection program before entering the room of a patient who requires airborne precautions (See Recommendation 2.7).**[1] *[Recommendation]*

5.3 When patient transport is necessary, take precautions to reduce the opportunity for transmission of pathogens to other patients, personnel, and visitors and to reduce contamination of the environment.[1] [Recommendation]

5.3.1 Before transporting the patient, notify the receiving team members that the patient is coming and to follow airborne precautions.[1] [Recommendation]

5.3.2 For patients with skin lesions associated with varicella or smallpox or draining skin lesions caused by *M tuberculosis,* cover the affected areas before patient transport.[1] [Recommendation]

5.3.3 If possible, have the patient wear a mask and follow respiratory hygiene and cough etiquette during transport (See Recommendation 1.5).[1] [Recommendation]

5.3.4 Transport the patient who is in an **airborne infection isolation room** (AIIR) directly to the OR, bypassing the preoperative area. At the end of the procedure, transfer the patient directly to an AIIR in the postanesthesia care unit or other inpatient unit. [Recommendation]

5.3.5 Perioperative personnel should not wear a mask or respiratory protection during patient transport if the patient is wearing a mask.[1] [Recommendation]

5.4 Elective surgery should be postponed for a patient who has a suspected or confirmed airborne-transmissible disease (eg, tuberculosis [TB]) until the patient is determined to be noninfectious. If surgery cannot be postponed, the surgery should be scheduled when a minimum number of perioperative personnel are present and at the end of the day when possible.[7,35] [Recommendation] Ⓐ

Scheduling the surgery as the last procedure of the day may reduce the likelihood for personnel exposure and maximizes the time available for removal of airborne contamination.

5.5 Place a patient who requires airborne precautions in an AIIR if one is available, including during surgery and postoperative recovery.[1,35] [Recommendation]

The CDC recommends use of special air handling and ventilation systems such as an AIIR to help prevent the spread of airborne pathogens, particularly *M tuberculosis.*[1,35]

5.5.1 Keep the doors to the AIIR or OR closed, and minimize traffic into and out of the room.[35] [Recommendation]

5.6 If an AIIR is not available, consult with an infection preventionist to determine whether supplemental air-cleaning technologies (eg, portable high-efficiency particulate air [HEPA] filtration, ultraviolet germicidal irradiation [UVGI]) are necessary.[35] [Recommendation]

5.6.1 If intubation or extubation is performed in the OR, a portable HEPA filter may be used to supplement air cleaning in accordance with the manufacturers' written IFU and in the following manner:
- position the unit near the patient's breathing zone,
- obtain engineering consultation to determine the correct placement, and
- switch the portable unit off during the surgical procedure.[7]
[Conditional Recommendation]

Switching the unit off during the procedure is recommended because after the patient is intubated, the airway is circulating in a closed system; therefore, the portable units do not serve any purpose while the patient is intubated.

5.6.2 A portable anteroom system (PAS)-HEPA combination unit may be used. [Conditional Recommendation]

In a pilot study, Olmstead[69] compared freestanding portable HEPA filter units placed inside the OR to a novel PAS-HEPA combination unit that was placed outside the OR and found that the PAS-HEPA unit was more effective in removing potentially contaminated air from the room. The PAS-HEPA unit achieved a downward evacuation of plume, away from the sterile field and toward the main entry door. Comparatively, the portable freestanding HEPA unit inside the OR moved the plume vertically upward and directly into the breathing zone where the surgical team would be during a procedure. A limitation of this pilot study is that it was performed in a single OR during a 2-day period and may not be generalizable to other settings.

5.7 Place a single-use, disposable bacterial filter on the patient's endotracheal tube or exhalation breathing circuit.[7,35] [Recommendation]

Placing a bacterial filter on the patient's endotracheal tube or exhalation breathing circuit prevents contamination of the anesthesia equipment and release of tubercle bacilli into the room.[35] The preferred filter will filter particles 0.3 μm or larger in size in both loaded and unloaded states and will have a filter efficiency of 95% (ie, filter penetration of < 5%) at the maximum design flow rates of the ventilator for the service life of the filter.[35]

5.8 After cough-inducing procedures (eg, intubation, extubation, bronchoscopy) are performed in the OR on a patient who requires airborne precautions, restrict room access until 99% of airborne particles have been removed from the air (eg, 15 air exchanges per hour for 28 minutes to remove 99.9% of airborne contaminants).[7,35] *[Recommendation]*

Performing cough-inducing procedures increases the likelihood that droplet nuclei will be expelled into the air.[35] The length of time required to expel more than 99% of airborne contaminants varies by the efficiency of the ventilation or filtration system. By waiting to place another patient in the room, the risk of airborne transmission is reduced.

5.8.1 When entering the room before 99% of airborne contaminants are removed, wear respiratory protection.[7,35] *[Recommendation]*

5.9 Establish administrative controls to reduce the risk of TB exposure to patients and personnel, including
- implementing work practices for managing patients with suspected or confirmed TB;
- ensuring that potentially contaminated equipment (eg, bronchoscopes, laryngoscopes, endoscopes) is cleaned and sterilized or processed by high-level disinfection in accordance with the manufacturers' IFU;
- educating perioperative personnel about TB prevention, transmission, and symptoms;
- establishing a TB screening program to evaluate perioperative personnel who are at risk for TB or who might be exposed to *M tuberculosis;* and
- implementing a respiratory protection program for personnel that requires fit testing and certification to use an N95 respirator.[35]
[Recommendation]

5.10 Instruct visitors to wear masks while in the patient's room and to perform hand hygiene upon entering and exiting the room.[68] *[Recommendation]*

The SHEA recommends that visitors to patients who require airborne precautions wear masks.[68] Although the visitor may wear an N95 respirator, the respirator is most effective when the mask is fit tested and the wearer is trained in respirator use. Visitors may be exempted if they have significant documented exposure (eg, household contact) to the symptomatic patient and are not ill themselves.

6. OSHA Bloodborne Pathogens Standard

6.1 Perioperative personnel must follow the OSHA Bloodborne Pathogens standard when there is a risk of exposure to blood, body fluids, and other potentially infectious materials.[10] *[Regulatory Requirement]*

The OSHA Bloodborne Pathogens standard mandates practices to reduce health care worker exposure to blood, body fluids, and other potentially infectious materials. Methods for preventing bloodborne pathogen exposure include a hierarchy of controls: eliminating the hazard, implementing engineering and work practice controls, implementing administrative controls, establishing and following an exposure control plan, and using PPE.[10]

6.2 Perioperative personnel must use engineering controls (eg, safety-engineered devices) and work practice controls (eg, neutral zone, hands-free technique).[10] *[Regulatory Requirement]*

Engineering controls isolate or remove the risk of exposure, and work practice controls reduce the likelihood of exposure by changing the method of performing a task.[10] See the AORN Guideline for Sharps Safety[12] for additional information.

6.3 The health care organization must establish a written exposure control plan, make it accessible to employees, and review and update it at least annually.[10] *[Regulatory Requirement]*

A written exposure control plan that is consistent with federal, state, and local rules and regulations and that governs occupational exposure to bloodborne pathogens, is reviewed periodically, and is readily available in the practice setting promotes safe practices with medical devices and blood and body fluids.[10]

6.4 Perioperative personnel must wear PPE when exposure to blood, body fluids, or other potentially infectious materials is anticipated (See Recommendation 2).[10] *[Regulatory Requirement]*

6.5 Perioperative personnel must wash their hands and skin with soap and water or flush their mucous membranes with water immediately or as soon as possible after coming into direct contact with blood, body fluids, or other potentially infectious materials.[10] *[Regulatory Requirement]*

6.6 Food and drink must not be taken into the semi-restricted or restricted areas of the perioperative suite. Food and drink must not be kept in refrigerators, freezers, or cabinets or on shelves, countertops, or work spaces where blood or other potentially infectious materials are present.[10] *[Regulatory Requirement]*

6.7 Cosmetics and lip balm must not be applied and contact lenses must not be handled in the semi-restricted or restricted areas of the perioperative suite.[10] *[Regulatory Requirement]*

6.8 Perioperative personnel must receive training before assignment to tasks where occupational exposure to blood, body fluids, and other potentially infectious materials may occur; at least annually thereafter; and when changes to procedures or tasks affect occupational exposure.[10] *[Regulatory Requirement]*

Employers are responsible for providing training on the bloodborne pathogens standard during working hours at no cost to employees. Employers are also responsible for ensuring employees participate in the training program and for offering materials in appropriate languages and at appropriate literacy levels.[10]

Providing the basis for the prevention of bloodborne pathogen exposure may instill an understanding of the processes that need to be followed and thereby prevent disease transmission. Education and training efforts are equally important in promoting awareness of hazards and acceptance of safe work and material-handling procedures in the workplace. Educating employees on safe work practices (eg, using PPE) can help protect personnel, their family members, and the community from take-home transmissions.

6.8.1 Employee education must include
- an explanation of the modes of transmission of bloodborne pathogens and an explanation of the employer's exposure control plan;
- an explanation of the use and limitations of methods for reducing exposure (eg, engineering controls, work practices, PPE); and
- information on the hepatitis B vaccine, its efficacy and safety, the method of administration, and the benefits of vaccination.[10]

[Regulatory Requirement]

6.8.2 Employers must maintain training records related to bloodborne pathogens for 3 years.[10] The records must include
- training dates,
- content or a summary of the training,
- names and qualifications of trainer(s), and
- names and job titles of trainees.

[Regulatory Requirement]

7. Personnel with Infections

7.1 Restrict the activities of perioperative personnel who have infections, exudative lesions, and nonintact skin when these activities pose a risk of transmission of infection to patients and other personnel.[70] *[Recommendation]*

Restricting activities of personnel who have transmissible infections reduces transmission between providers and patients depending on the mode of transmission and epidemiology of the disease.[70] Work restrictions for perioperative personnel with bloodborne infections who provide direct patient care may depend on several factors, including circulating viral burden and category of clinical activities. Danzmann et al[71] conducted a systematic review and found that outbreaks caused by health care workers are rare, although awareness of personnel carrier status may significantly decrease the risk of causing large outbreaks.

7.2 An employee health nurse, infection preventionist, or physician should assess perioperative personnel who have infections, exudative lesions, or nonintact skin before they are allowed to return to work providing direct patient care or handling medical devices that are used in operative or other invasive procedures.[70] *[Recommendation]*

Medical clearance is necessary before perioperative personnel who have infections, exudative lesions, or nonintact skin can return to work with patients or other personnel.[70] Infections that may require restrictions from providing direct patient care, entering the patient's environment, or handling instruments or devices that may be used during operative or invasive procedures include
- viral respiratory infections (eg, influenza, respiratory syncytial virus infections);
- keratoconjunctivitis or purulent conjunctivitis;
- acute gastrointestinal illnesses (ie, vomiting or diarrhea with or without nausea, fever, or abdominal pain);
- diphtheria (ie, identification as an asymptomatic carrier);
- pertussis (ie, whooping cough);
- exudative lesions that cannot be contained (eg, eczema, impetigo, smallpox);
- herpes simplex infections of the fingers or hands (ie, herpetic whitlow);
- pediculosis (eg, head lice, body lice);
- scabies;
- hand, foot, and mouth disease; and
- meningococcal infection (ie, until 24 hours after the start of effective therapy).[70]

7.2.1 Follow state, federal, and professional guidelines to determine the need for work restrictions for perioperative personnel with blood-borne infections. *[Recommendation]*

7.3 Report exposures as soon as they occur and infections as soon as the disease process is noted.[70] *[Recommendation]*

Early self-reporting of exposures and infections helps prevent transmission to patients and other personnel.

7.4 All exposure incidents (eg, needlesticks, blood exposures) must be reported according to health care organization policy and based on the OSHA Bloodborne Pathogens standard.[10] *[Regulatory Requirement]*

7.4.1 All incidents of occupational exposure to blood, body fluids, or other potentially infectious materials must be documented.[10] Documentation must include
- the route of exposure;
- the circumstances associated with the exposure;
- the source individual's serological status, if known;
- the employee's name and social security number;
- the employee's hepatitis B vaccination status and other relevant medical information for both the employee and source, including vaccination dates and any medical records related to the employee's ability to receive vaccinations;
- results of all related examinations, medical tests, and postexposure evaluation and follow-up procedures;
- a licensed health care professional's written opinion; and
- a copy of the information provided to the employee.

[Regulatory Requirement]

Documenting each exposure incident provides a record of the incident, what follow-through was taken, and the current status of the incident.

7.4.2 Employers must maintain a sharps injury log to document all percutaneous injuries from contaminated sharps and must maintain the log in such a way that an injured employee's identification remains confidential.[10] At a minimum, a sharps injury log must include
- the type and brand of device involved in the incident,

- the department or work area where the exposure incident occurred, and
- an explanation of how the incident occurred.

[Regulatory Requirement]

Some health care employers may be exempt from maintaining a sharps injury log. The requirement to establish and maintain a sharps injury log applies to any employer who is required to maintain a log of occupational injuries and illnesses under 29 CFR §1904.4.

7.4.3 Documentation related to exposure incidents must be maintained for the employee's duration of employment plus 30 years.[10] *[Regulatory Requirement]*

Documenting all exposure incidents provides the employer with feedback regarding the circumstances of employee exposures. This information can be used to focus efforts on decreasing or eliminating specific circumstances or routes of exposure.

7.5 All perioperative personnel should receive baseline TB screening upon hire. Follow-up testing should be performed in the case of exposure to TB.[35] *[Recommendation]*

7.5.1 Maintain records and results of TB screening for each employee in the employee's health record. If an employee has symptoms of TB, record the symptoms in the employee health record or medical record.[35] *[Recommendation]*

7.6 Have a written policy regarding perioperative personnel who have potentially transmissible infections that establishes responsibility for reporting the condition, work restrictions, and guidelines for clearing the employee for work after an illness that required a restriction.[70] *[Recommendation]*

7.6.1 Design the policy to prevent judgement or penalty (eg, loss of wages, benefits, job status) for self-reporting of exposures or infections.[70] *[Recommendation]*

Policies that are designed to prevent judgment or penalty may encourage self-reporting of exposures or infections.[70]

8. Personnel Immunization

8.1 Perioperative personnel should be immunized against vaccine-preventable diseases. *[Recommendation]* Ⓐ

The CDC Advisory Committee for Immunization Practices[72] recommends that health care personnel receive immunizations if they come into contact with patients or infectious material from patients that may put them at risk for exposure and possible transmission of vaccine-preventable disease (ie, hepatitis B, seasonal influenza, measles, mumps, rubella, pertussis, varicella). Including vaccinations as part of an organizational infection prevention and control program reduces the risk of occupationally acquired infections and, therefore, harm to patients from vaccine-preventable diseases.[72]

8.2 **Employers must make the hepatitis B vaccination series available to all perioperative employees whose work involves a reasonable risk of exposure to blood, body fluids, or other potentially infectious materials and must provide postexposure evaluation and follow-up to all employees who have an exposure incident.[10,72]** *[Regulatory Requirement]*

Hepatitis B is highly contagious and is transmitted via percutaneous exposure (eg, needlestick injury) or mucosal exposure to infected blood or body fluids. The risk of acquiring hepatitis B infection from occupational exposure depends on the frequency of percutaneous and mucosal exposure to blood or body fluids that contain the virus.[72]

8.2.1 **Repeat serologic testing after hepatitis B vaccination for perioperative personnel who are at "high risk" of occupational percutaneous or mucosal exposure to blood or body fluids. If antibody levels are too low (< 10 mIU/mL), revaccinate personnel and test again after completing the series.[72]** *[Recommendation]*

Performing serologic testing 1 to 2 months after the last dose of the vaccine helps determine whether there is a need for revaccination and guides postexposure prophylaxis in the event of an exposure incident.[72]

8.2.2 **In the event of blood or body fluid exposure (ie, percutaneous, ocular, mucous membrane, nonintact skin), evaluate the need for postexposure prophylaxis immediately based on the hepatitis B surface antigen status of the source and the employee's vaccination history and vaccine-response status.[72]** *[Recommendation]*

8.3 **All perioperative personnel should receive annual influenza vaccinations, unless contraindicated.[72]** *[Recommendation]*

Perioperative personnel are exposed to patients who have influenza and are therefore at risk for occupationally acquired influenza and transmitting the disease to patients and other providers.[72]

8.3.1 **Establish and implement strategies to improve influenza vaccination rates among perioperative personnel, including**
- **establishing evidence-based educational and promotional programs to communicate about the disease and the vaccine,**
- **running a campaign that emphasizes the benefits of vaccination for personnel and patients,**
- **implementing a vaccine declination policy,**
- **encouraging senior medical staff members or opinion leaders to get vaccinated,**
- **removing administrative barriers (eg, costs),**
- **providing incentives for getting vaccinated,**
- **providing the vaccine in locations and at times that are easily accessible to health care providers, and**
- **monitoring and reporting provider vaccination rates.[72]**

[Recommendation]

8.4 **Perioperative personnel should have evidence of immunity to measles, mumps, and rubella, and this information should be documented and readily available in the health care setting.[72]** *[Recommendation]*

Presumptive evidence includes written documentation of vaccination with two doses of measles-mumps-rubella vaccine administered at least 28 days apart, laboratory evidence of immunity, laboratory confirmation of disease, or birth before 1957.

Measles and mumps are highly contagious and can have serious consequences. Rubella was declared eliminated from the United States in 2004, but there is a risk of resurgence from importation.[72]

Exposure to measles, mumps, or rubella in the health care setting can be expensive and disruptive because of containment measures, necessary personnel furloughs or reassignments, and potential facility closures.[72]

8.4.1 **When caring for a patient who is suspected to have a measles infection, use respiratory protection regardless of immunity status.[72]** *[Recommendation]*

Measles vaccination can fail and is ineffective for preventing measles about 1% of the time. Measles is highly contagious and transmission can occur anywhere from 4 days before presentation of a rash to 4 days after the rash resolves.[72]

8.4.2 **Only allow perioperative personnel with evidence of immunity to care for a patient who is suspected of having mumps or rubella.[72]** *[Recommendation]*

8.5 Perioperative personnel should receive a single dose of tetanus toxoid, reduced diphtheria toxoid, and acellular pertussis (Tdap) as soon as feasible upon hire if they have not been vaccinated previously.[72] *[Recommendation]*

Pertussis (ie, whooping cough) is a highly contagious bacterial infection and is transmitted via contact and droplet routes.[72] The Tdap vaccine protects against pertussis and reduces the risk of transmission to patients, other health care personnel, family members, and the community.[72]

8.5.1 Only allow perioperative personnel with evidence of immunity to care for a patient who is suspected to have pertussis.[72] *[Recommendation]*

8.5.2 Perioperative personnel should receive a booster vaccination against tetanus and diphtheria every 10 years.[72] *[Recommendation]*

8.5.3 Establish programs to increase Tdap vaccination among personnel, including providing convenient access to the vaccination, giving the vaccination free of charge, and educating perioperative personnel about the benefits of vaccination.[72] *[Recommendation]*

8.6 Verify that all perioperative personnel have evidence of immunity to varicella, and that personnel who have no evidence of immunity receive the varicella vaccine. This information should be documented and readily available in the health care setting.[72] *[Recommendation]*

Varicella is highly infectious and is transmitted via contact, droplet, and airborne routes. Primary infection usually results in lifetime immunity, and the US vaccination program that began in 1995 has led to greater than 85% declines in varicella incidence, hospitalizations, and deaths.[72]

Despite the reduced incidence, health care–associated transmission is still a risk, and the disease can be fatal. Varicella is more likely to spread in hospital settings and long-term care facilities.[72] Varicella exposure among patients and health care personnel can disrupt patient care and cost the facility in terms of identifying susceptible patients and staff members, managing those who are exposed, and mandating furloughs for exposed staff members.

8.6.1 When a patient with a confirmed or suspected varicella infection enters the health care facility, implement and follow airborne and contact precautions, and allow only perioperative personnel who have evidence of immunity provide care to the patient.[72] *[Recommendation]*

8.7 Establish and implement a comprehensive vaccination policy for all perioperative personnel,[72] including a method to validate that
- all perioperative personnel are up to date with recommended vaccines,
- perioperative personnel vaccination and immunity status is reviewed at the time of hire and at least annually thereafter, and
- necessary vaccines are offered to employees in conjunction with routine annual disease prevention measures (eg, influenza vaccination, TB testing).[72]

[Recommendation]

8.8 Maintain vaccination records for each employee. Include the following in the records of any vaccinations administered during employment:
- the type of vaccine given;
- the date on which the vaccine is given;
- the name of the vaccine manufacturer and the lot number;
- any documented episodes of adverse reactions to a vaccination;
- the name, address, and title of the person who administered the vaccination; and
- the edition and distribution date of the language-appropriate vaccine information statement provided to the employee at the time of vaccination.[72]

[Recommendation]

Accurate vaccination records make it possible to quickly identify health care personnel who are susceptible to infection during an outbreak and can reduce costs and disruptions to health care operations.[72]

8.8.1 Record the employee's immunity status for vaccine-preventable diseases, including documented disease, vaccination history, and serology results, in the employee's record.[72] *[Recommendation]*

8.8.2 Use a secure computerized system to manage vaccination records for perioperative personnel.[72] *[Recommendation]*

Computerized systems allow records to be retrieved easily and as needed.[72]

Glossary

Airborne infection isolation room: A single-patient room that supplies negative air pressure relative to the surrounding area, has a minimum of 12 air exchanges per hour, and exhausts air directly to the outside or recirculates air through high-efficiency particulate air filtration before return.

Airborne precautions: Precautions that reduce the risk of an airborne transmission of infectious airborne droplet nuclei (ie, particle residue 5 μm or smaller).

Contact precautions: Precautions designed to reduce the risk of transmission of epidemiologically important microorganisms by direct or indirect contact.

Direct contact: Person-to-person contact resulting in physical transfer of infectious microorganisms between an infected or colonized person and a susceptible host.

Droplet precautions: Precautions that reduce the risk of large particle droplet transmission of infectious agents (ie, 5 μm or larger).

Enhanced environmental cleaning: Environmental cleaning practices implemented to prevent the spread of infections or outbreaks that promote consistent and standardized cleaning procedures beyond routine cleaning.

Indirect contact: Contact of a susceptible host with a contaminated object (eg, instruments, hands).

Powered air-purifying respirator: A respirator that uses a battery-powered blower to move the air flow through the filters.

Standard precautions: Precautions used for care of all patients regardless of their diagnosis or presumed infectious status.

Transmission-based precautions: Precautions designed to be used with patients known or suspected of being infected or colonized with highly transmissible or epidemiologically important pathogens for which additional precautions are needed to prevent transmission in the practice setting.

User seal check: An action conducted by the respirator user to determine whether the respirator is properly seated to the face.

References

1. Siegel JD, Rhinehart E, Jackson M, Chiarello L; Health Care Infection Control Practices Advisory Committee. 2007 guideline for isolation precautions: preventing transmission of infectious agents in health care settings. *Am J Infect Control.* 2007; 35 (10 Suppl 2):S65-S164. [IVA]

2. *Core Infection Prevention and Control Practices for Safe Healthcare Delivery in All Settings—Recommendations of the Health-care Infection Control Practices Advisory Committee (HICPAC).* Atlanta, GA: Centers for Disease Control and Prevention, Healthcare Infection Control Practices Advisory Committee; 2017. [IVA]

3. Guideline for hand hygiene. In: *Guidelines for Perioperative Practice.* Denver, CO: AORN, Inc; 2018:29-50. [IVA]

4. Centers for Disease Control and Prevention. Guideline for hand hygiene in health-care settings. recommendations of the Healthcare Infection Control Practices Advisory Committee and the HICPAC/SHEA/APIC/IDSA Hand Hygiene Task Force. Society for Healthcare Epidemiology of America/Association for Professionals in Infection Control/Infectious Diseases Society of America. *MMWR Recomm Rep.* 2002;51(RR-16):1-45. [IVA]

5. WHO Guidelines on Hand Hygiene in Health Care. *First Global Patient Safety Challenge, Clean Care Is Safer Care.* Geneva, Switzerland: World Health Organization; 2009. [IVA]

6. Guideline for environmental cleaning. In: *Guidelines for Perioperative Practice.* Denver, CO: AORN, Inc; 2018:7-28. [IVA]

7. Sehulster L, Chinn RY. Guidelines for environmental infection control in health-care facilities. Recommendations of CDC and the Healthcare Infection Control Practices Advisory Committee (HICPAC) [published correction appears in *MMWR Morb Mortal Wkly Rep.* 52(42);1025-1026] *MMWR Recomm Rep.* 2003; 52 (RR-10):1-42. [IVA]

8. Rutala WA, Weber DJ; Healthcare Infection Control Practices Advisory Committee (HICPAC), eds. *Guideline for Disinfection and Sterilization In Healthcare Facilities 2008.* Atlanta, GA: Centers for Disease Control and Prevention. 2008. [IVA]

9. *Practice Guidance for Healthcare Environmental Cleaning.* 2nd ed. Chicago, IL: American Society for Healthcare Environmental Services; 2012. [IVC]

10. 29 CFR §1910.1030: Bloodborne pathogens. Electronic Code of Federal Regulations. https://www.ecfr.gov/cgi-bin/text-idx?SID=71a8c4b5ed8145f7559e5a72e9f008df&mc=true&node=se29.6.1910_11030&rgn=div8. Accessed October 10, 2018.

11. Guideline for medication safety. In: *Guidelines for Perioperative Practice.* Denver, CO: AORN, Inc; 2018:295-330. [IVA]

12. Guideline for sharps safety. In: *Guidelines for Perioperative Practice.* Denver, CO: AORN, Inc; 2018:415-438. [IVA]

13. Guideline for a safe environment of care. In: *Guidelines for Perioperative Practice.* Denver, CO: AORN, Inc; 2018:243-268. [IVA]

14. Bardorf MH, Jäger B, Boeckmans E, Kramer A, Assadian O. Influence of material properties on gloves' bacterial barrier efficacy in the presence of microperforation. *Am J Infect Control.* 2016;44(12):1645-1649. [IIIB]

15. *Guidance for Industry and FDA Staff: Medical Glove Guidance Manual; 2008.* US Department of Health and Human Services; Food and Drug Administration; Center for Devices and Radiological Health; Office of Device Evaluation; Division of Anesthesiology, General Hospital, Infection Control, and Dental Devices; Infection Control Devices Branch. https://www.fda.gov/downloads/medicaldevices/deviceregulationandguidance/guidancedocuments/ucm428191.pdf. Accessed October 15, 2018. [VA]

16. Banned devices; powdered surgeon's gloves, powdered patient examination gloves, and absorbable powder for lubricating a surgeon's glove. Final rule. *Fed Regist.* 2016;81(243):91722-91731.

17. Guideline for sterile technique. In: *Guidelines for Perioperative Practice.* Denver, CO: AORN, Inc; 2018:75-104 [IVA]

18. Olsen RJ, Lynch P, Coyle MB, Cummings J, Bokete T, Stamm WE. Examination gloves as barriers to hand contamination in clinical practice. *JAMA.* 1993;270(3):350-353. [IIB]

19. Korniewicz DM, Kirwin M, Cresci K, et al. Barrier protection with examination gloves: double versus single. *Am J Infect Control.* 1994;22(1):12-15. [IIB]

20. Korniewicz DM, ElMasri M, Broyles JM, Martin CD, O'Connell KP. Performance of latex and nonlatex medical examination gloves during simulated use. *Am J Infect Control.* 2002;30(2):133-138. [IIB]

21. Rego A, Roley L. In-use barrier integrity of gloves: latex and nitrile superior to vinyl. *Am J Infect Control.* 1999;27(5):405-410. [IIB]

22. Klein RC, Party E, Gershey EL. Virus penetration of examination gloves. *Biotechniques.* 1990;9(2):196-199. [IIB]

23. Loveday HP, Lynam S, Singleton J, Wilson J. Clinical glove use: healthcare workers' actions and perceptions. *J Hosp Infect.* 2014;86(2):110-116. [IIIB]

24. *Guidance for the Selection and Use of Personal Protective Equipment in Healthcare Settings.* Atlanta, GA: Centers for Disease Control and Prevention, National Center for Emerging and Zoonotic Infectious Diseases (NCEZID), Division of Healthcare Quality Promotion (DHQP); 2010. [VA]

25. Kilinc FS. A review of isolation gowns in healthcare: fabric and gown properties. *J Eng Fiber Fabr.* 2015;10(3):180-190. [VA]

26. *AAMI PB70: Liquid Barrier Performance and Classification of Protective Apparel and Drapes Intended for Use in Health Care Facilities.* Arlington, VA: Association for the Advancement of Medical Instrumentation; 2012. [IVC]

27. *AAMI TIR11:2005. Selection and Use of Protective Apparel and Surgical Drapes in Health Care Facilities.* Arlington, VA: Association for the Advancement of Medical Instrumentation; 2005. [VB]

28. *Premarket Notification Requirements Concerning Gowns Intended for Use in Health Care Settings. Guidance for Industry and Food and Drug Administration Staff; 2015.* US Department of Health and Human Services; Food and Drug Administration; Center for Devices and Radiological Health; Office of Device Evaluation; Division of Anesthesiology, General Hospital, Respiratory, Infection Control, and Dental Devices. https://www.fda.gov/downloads/medicaldevices/deviceregulation-andguidance/guidancedocuments/ucm452804.pdf. Accessed October 15, 2018. [VA]

29. Eye safety. Centers for Disease Control and Prevention. https://www.cdc.gov/niosh/topics/eye/eye-infectious.html. Updated July 29, 2013. Accessed October 10, 2018. [VA]

30. Roberge RJ. Face shields for infection control: a review. *J Occup Environ Hyg.* 2016;13(4):235-242. [VB]

31. Lange VR. Eyewear contamination levels in the operating room: infection risk. *Am J Infect Control.* 2014;42(4):446-447. [IIIB]

32. Lakhani R, Loh Y, Zhang TT, Kothari P. A prospective study of blood splatter in ENT. *Eur Arch Otorhinolaryngol.* 2015;272(7):1809-1812. [IIIB]

33. *ASTM F2100-11(2018): Standard Specification for Performance of Materials Used in Medical Face Masks.* West Conshohocken, PA: ASTM International; 2018. [IVC]

34. *Guidance for Industry and FDA Staff: Surgical Masks—Premarket Notification [510(K)] Submissions; Guidance for Industry and FDA; 2004.* US Department of Health and Human Services; Food and Drug Administration; Center for Devices and Radiological Health; Division of Anesthesiology, General Hospital, Infection Control, and Dental Devices; Office of Device Evaluation. https://www.fda.gov/RegulatoryInformation/Guidances/ucm072549.htm. Accessed October 15, 2018. [VA]

35. Centers for Disease Control and Prevention (CDC). Guidelines for preventing the transmission of *Mycobacterium tuberculosis* in health-care settings, 2005. *MMWR Morb Mortal Wkly Rep.* 2005;54(RR-17):1-140. [IVA]

36. *Hospital Respiratory Protection Program Toolkit: Resources for Respirator Program Administrators; 2015.* DHHS (NIOSH) Publication Number 2015-117, OSHA Publication Number 3767-05 2015. https://www.osha.gov/Publications/OSHA3767.pdf. Accessed October 15, 2018. [VA]

37. 29 CFR 1910.134: Respiratory protection. Occupational Safety and Health Administration. https://www.osha.gov/pls/oshaweb/owadisp.show_document?p_id=12716&p_table=standards. Accessed October 15, 2018.

38. Benson SM, Novak DA, Ogg MJ. Proper use of surgical N95 respirators and surgical masks in the OR. *AORN J.* 2013;97(4):457-470. [VA]

39. Respirator trusted-source information. Centers for Disease Control and Prevention. http://www.cdc.gov/niosh/npptl/topics/respirators/disp_part/RespSource.html. Accessed October 15, 2018. [VA]

40. Medical Devices; Exemption from Premarket Notification: Class II Devices; Surgical Apparel. Final Order. *Fed Regist.* 2018;83(96):22846-22848.

41. Smith JD, MacDougall CC, Johnstone J, Copes RA, Schwartz B, Garber GE. Effectiveness of N95 respirators versus surgical masks in protecting health care workers from acute respiratory infection: a systematic review and meta-analysis. *CMAJ.* 2016;188(8):567-574. [IIIA]

42. Suen LKP, Yang L, Ho SSK, et al. Reliability of N95 respirators for respiratory protection before, during, and after nursing procedures. *Am J Infect Control.* 2017;45(9):974-978. [IIB]

43. Guideline for surgical smoke safety. In: *Guidelines for Perioperative Practice.* Denver, CO: AORN, Inc; 2018:469-498. [IVA]

44. *Implementing Respiratory Protection Programs in Hospitals: A Guide for Respirator Program Administrators.* Richmond, CA: Occupational Health Branch: California Department of Public Health; 2015.

45. Talbot TR, May AK, Obremskey WT, Wright PW, Daniels TL. Intraoperative patient-to-healthcare-worker transmission of invasive group A streptococcal infection. *Infect Control Hosp Epidemiol.* 2011;32(9):924-926. [VB]

46. Krein SL, Mayer J, Harrod M, et al. Identification and characterization of failures in infectious agent transmission precaution practices in hospitals: a qualitative study. *JAMA Intern Med.* 2018;178(8):1051-1057. [IIIA]

47. Zellmer C, Van Hoof S, Safdar N. Variation in health care worker removal of personal protective equipment. *Am J Infect Control.* 2015;43(7):750-751. [IIIC]

48. Tomas ME, Kundrapu S, Thota P, et al. Contamination of health care personnel during removal of personal protective equipment. *JAMA Intern Med.* 2015;175(12):1904-1910. [IIA]

49. Mitchell R, Roth V, Gravel D, et al. Are health care workers protected? An observational study of selection and removal of personal protective equipment in Canadian acute care hospitals. *Am J Infect Control.* 2013;41(3):240-244. [IIIB]

50. Kang J, O'Donnell JM, Colaianne B, Bircher N, Ren D, Smith KJ. Use of personal protective equipment among health care personnel: results of clinical observations and simulations. *Am J Infect Control.* 2017;45(1):17-23. [IIIB]

51. Kwon JH, Burnham CD, Reske KA, et al. Assessment of healthcare worker protocol deviations and self-contamination during personal protective equipment donning and doffing. *Infect Control Hosp Epidemiol.* 2017;38(9):1077-1083. [IIB]

52. Honda H, Iwata K. Personal protective equipment and improving compliance among healthcare workers in high-risk settings. *Curr Opin Infect Dis.* 2016;29(4):400-406. [VA]

53. Herlihey TA, Gelmi S, Flewwelling CJ, et al. Personal protective equipment for infectious disease preparedness: a human factors evaluation. *Infect Control Hosp Epidemiol.* 2016;37(9):1022-1028. [IIIB]

54. Doll M, Feldman M, Hartigan S, et al. Acceptability and necessity of training for optimal personal protective equipment use. *Infect Control Hosp Epidemiol.* 2017;38(2):226-229. [IIIB]

55. Neo F, Edward K, Mills C. Current evidence regarding non-compliance with personal protective equipment—an integrative review to illuminate implications for nursing practice. *ACORN.* 2012;25(4):22-30. [VB]

56. Moore C, Edward KL, King K, Giandinoto JA. Using the team to reduce risk of blood and body fluid exposure in the perioperative setting. *ORNAC J.* 2015;33(4):37-46, 28-36. [IIC]

57. Verbeek JH, Ijaz S, Mischke C, et al. Personal protective equipment for preventing highly infectious diseases due to exposure to contaminated body fluids in healthcare staff. *Cochrane Database Syst Rev.* 2016;4:CD011621. [IIA]

58. Tomas ME, Cadnum JL, Mana TSC, et al. Utility of a novel reflective marker visualized by flash photography for assessment of personnel contamination during removal of personal protective equipment. *Infect Control Hosp Epidemiol.* 2016;37(6):711-713. [IIC]

59. Drew JL, Turner J, Mugele J, et al. Beating the spread: developing a simulation analog for contagious body fluids. *Simul Healthc.* 2016;11(2):100-105. [IIB]

60. Siegel JD, Rhinehart E, Jackson M, Chiarello L; Health-care Infection Control Practices Advisory Committee, eds. *Management of Multidrug-Resistant Organisms in Healthcare Settings, 2006.* Atlanta, GA: Centers for Disease Control and Prevention; 2006. [IVA]

61. McDonald LC, Gerding DN, Johnson S, et al. Clinical practice guidelines for *Clostridium difficile* infection in adults and children: 2017 update by the Infectious Diseases Society of America (IDSA) and Society for Healthcare Epidemiology of America (SHEA). *Clin Infect Dis.* 2018;66(7):e1-e48. [IVA]

62. Grewal H, Varshney K, Thomas LC, Kok J, Shetty A. Blood pressure cuffs as a vector for transmission of multi-resistant organisms: colonisation rates and effects of disinfection. *Emerg Med Australas.* 2013;25(3):222-226. [IIIB]

63. John AR, Alhmidi H, Cadnum JL, Jencson AL, Gestrich S, Donskey CJ. Evaluation of the potential for electronic thermometers to contribute to spread of healthcare-associated pathogens. *Am J Infect Control.* 2018;46(6):708-710. [IIIB]

64. Abad C, Fearday A, Safdar N. Adverse effects of isolation in hospitalised patients: a systematic review. *J Hosp Infect.* 2010;76(2):97-102. [IIIB]

65. Morgan DJ, Diekema DJ, Sepkowitz K, Perencevich EN. Adverse outcomes associated with contact precautions: a review of the literature. *Am J Infect Control.* 2009;37(2):85-93. [VA]

66. Findik UY, Ozbaş Ayfer, Ikbal C, Tulay E, Topcu SY. Effects of the contact isolation application on anxiety and depression levels of the patients. *Int J Nurs Pract.* 2012;18(4):340-346. [IIC]

67. Day HR, Perencevich EN, Harris AD, et al. Depression, anxiety, and moods of hospitalized patients under contact precautions. *Infect Control Hosp Epidemiol.* 2013;34(3):251-258. [IIA]

68. Munoz-Price LS, Banach DB, Bearman G, et al. Isolation precautions for visitors. *Infect Control Hosp Epidemiol.* 2015;36(7):747-758. [VA]

69. Olmsted RN. Pilot study of directional airflow and containment of airborne particles in the size of *Mycobacterium tuberculosis* in an operating room. *Am J Infect Control.* 2008;36(4):260-267. [IIC]

70. Bolyard EA, Tablan OC, Williams WW, Pearson ML, Shapiro CN, Deitchman SD. Guideline for infection control in health care personnel, 1998. *Am J Infect Control.* 1998;26(3):289-354. [IVA]

71. Danzmann L, Gastmeier P, Schwab F, Vonberg RP. Health care workers causing large nosocomial outbreaks: a systematic review. *BMC Infect Dis.* 2013;13:98. [IIIA]

72. Advisory Committee on Immunization Practices, Centers for Disease Control and Prevention (CDC). Immunization of health-care personnel: recommendations of the Advisory Committee on Immunization Practices (ACIP). *MMWR Recomm Rep.* 2011;60(RR-7):1-45. [IVA]

Acknowledgments

Lead Author
Amber Wood, MSN, RN, CNOR, CIC, FAPIC
Editor-in-Chief
Guidelines for Perioperative Practice
AORN Nursing Department
Denver, Colorado

The author and AORN thank Donna A. Pritchard, MA, BSN, RN, NE-BC, CNOR, Director of Perioperative Services, Interfaith Medical Center, Brooklyn, New York; Gerald McDonnell, PhD, BSc, Johnson & Johnson Family of Companies, Raritan, New Jersey; Bernard C. Camins, MD, MSc, Associate Professor of Medicine, University of Alabama at Birmingham; Heather A. Hohenberger, MSN, RN, CIC, CNOR, CPHQ, Administrative Director Surgical Services, IU Health Arnett Hospital, Lebanon, Indiana; Jennifer Hanrahan, DO, Medical Director of Infection Prevention, Metrohealth Medical Center, Cleveland, Ohio; Susan Ruwe, MSN, RN, CPHQ, CIC, Senior Infection Preventionist, Carle Foundation Hospital, Argenta, Illinois; Leslie Jeter, MSNA, RN, CRNA, Staff CRNA, Ambulatory Anesthesia of Atlanta, Georgia; Mary J. Ogg, MSN,

RN, CNOR, Senior Perioperative Practice Specialist, AORN, Denver, Colorado; Janice Neil, PhD, CNE, RN, Associate Professor, East Carolina College of Nursing, Greenville, North Carolina; Brenda G. Larkin, MS, ACNS-BC, CNS, CNOR, Clinical Nurse Specialist, Aurora Lakeland Medical Center, Lake Geneva, Wisconsin; Jay Bowers, BSN, RN, CNOR, Clinical Coordinator for Trauma, General Surgery, Bariatric, Pediatric and Surgical Oncology, West Virginia University Hospitals, Morgantown; and Vangie Dennis, BSN, RN, CNOR, CMLSO, Director of Patient Care Practice, Emory Healthcare and Ambulatory Surgery Centers, Atlanta, Georgia, for their assistance in developing this guideline.

Publication History

Originally published February 1993, *AORN Journal,* as "Recommended practices for universal precautions in the perioperative practice setting."

Revised November 1998 as "Recommended practices for standard and transmission-based precautions in the perioperative practice setting"; published February 1999, *AORN Journal.* Reformatted July 2000.

Approved June 2006, AORN Board of Directors, as "Recommended practices for prevention of transmissible infections in perioperative practice settings." Published in *Standards, Recommended Practices, and Guidelines,* 2007 edition.

Revised and reformatted December 2012 for online publication in *Perioperative Standards and Recommended Practices.*

Evidence ratings revised 2013 to conform to the AORN Evidence Rating Model.

Minor editing revisions made in November 2014 for publication in *Guidelines for Perioperative Practice,* 2015 edition.

Revised December 2018 for publication in *Guidelines for Perioperative Practice* online.

Evidence ratings revised and minor editorial changes made to conform to the current AORN Evidence Rating model, September 2019, for online publication in *Guidelines for Perioperative Practice.*

AMBULATORY SUPPLEMENT:
TRANSMISSION-BASED PRECAUTIONS

3. Contact Precautions

Ⓐ The facility should screen individuals for infectious agents (eg, MDROs) transmitted by contact.[A1] Identification of infected individuals before their admission to the ambulatory surgery center (ASC) may prevent infection transmission.[A1]

4. Droplet Precautions

Ⓐ The facility should screen individuals for infectious agents (eg, influenza, pertussis) transmitted by droplets.[A1] Identification of infected individuals before their admission to the ASC may prevent infection transmission.[A1]

5. Airborne Precautions

5.4 Elective surgery should be postponed for a patient who has a suspected or confirmed airborne-transmissible disease (eg, tuberculosis [TB]) until the patient is determined to be noninfectious. If surgery cannot be postponed, the surgery should be scheduled when a minimum number of perioperative personnel are present and at the end of the day when possible.

Ⓐ Personnel in an ASC in which care is provided to patients with confirmed or suspected TB should follow **Recommendation 5**.

Ⓐ Unless the facility has the capability to establish a negative pressure room, patients with suspected or confirmed cases of TB should be transferred to or rescheduled at a facility with a negative pressure room. An airborne infection isolation room and a respiratory protection program are needed for airborne precautions. Airborne precautions are required for any patient with suspected or confirmed active pulmonary TB.[A1,A2]

8. Personnel Immunization

Ⓐ A facility participating in the Centers for Medicare & Medicaid Services (CMS) Ambulatory Surgical Quality Reporting Program must report influenza vaccination data for the following categories of health care professionals: employees, licensed independent practitioners, students, and volunteers.[A3]

Ambulatory Recommendations

Perioperative personnel should receive initial and ongoing education and competency validation of their understanding of the principles of infection prevention and the performance of standard, contact, droplet, and airborne precautions for prevention of transmissible infections and MDROs.

Ⓐ An ASC that is certified by the CMS must have a licensed health care professional qualified through training in infection control and designated to direct the ASC's infection prevention program.[A4]

> *Interpretive Guidelines: §416.51(b)(1): The ASC must designate in writing, a qualified licensed health care professional who will lead the facility's infection control program. The ASC must determine that the individual has had training in the principles and methods of infection control.*[A5]

Ⓐ Ambulatory surgery center personnel should receive infection prevention education. Personnel include
- medical personnel,
- nursing personnel,
- other staff providing direct patient care,
- personnel responsible for on-site sterilization/high-level disinfection processes, and
- environmental services personnel.[A4]

Ⓐ Infection prevention education should be conducted
- upon hire,
- annually, and
- periodically as needed.[A4]

Ⓐ Infection prevention education records should be maintained for all personnel.[A4]

Documentation should reflect activities related to infection prevention and control.

Ⓐ A CMS-certified facility's infection prevention program must document the consideration, selection, and implementation of a nationally recognized infection control guideline,[A4] such as the AORN Guidelines for Perioperative Practice.

Policies and procedures for the prevention and control of transmissible infections and MDROs should be developed, reviewed periodically, revised as necessary, and readily available within the practice setting.

Ⓐ The infection prevention policy and procedure must comply with the state's reporting requirements for notifiable diseases.[A4]

Perioperative team members should participate in a variety of quality assurance and performance improvement activities to monitor and improve the prevention of infections and MDROs.

Ⓐ A risk assessment should be conducted as part of the infection prevention plan. There are diverse floor plans and environmental controls in ASCs that may present challenges to supporting current infection prevention practices.

Ⓐ The patient population and community served should be part of the risk assessment.

Ⓐ The ASC must have a program to control and investigate infectious and communicable diseases.[A6]

References

A1. Siegel JD, Rhinehart E, Jackson M, Chiarello L; Health Care Infection Control Practices Advisory Committee. 2007 guideline for isolation precautions: preventing transmission of infectious agents in health care settings. *Am J Infect Control.* 2007;35(10 Suppl 2):S65-S164.

A2. Jensen PA, Lambert LA, Iademarco MF, Ridzon R; CDC. Guidelines for preventing the transmission of *Mycobacterium tuberculosis* in healthcare settings, 2005. *MMWR Recomm Rep.* 2005;54(RR17):1-141

A3. Influenza Vaccination Coverage Among Healthcare Personnel Centers for Medicare & Medicaid Services. https://cmit.cms.gov/CMIT_public/ReportMeasure?measureId=854. Accessed October 15, 2018.

A4. Exhibit 351: Ambulatory Surgical Center (ASC) Infection Control Surveyor Worksheet (Rev 142, Issued: 07-17-15, Effective: 07-07-15, Implementation: 07-07-15). Centers for Medicare & Medicaid Services. https://www.cms.gov/Regulations-and-Guidance/Guidance/Manuals/downloads/som107_exhibit_351.pdf. Accessed October 15, 2018.

A5. §416.51(b)(1). In: *State Operations Manual Appendix L—Guidance for Surveyors: Ambulatory Surgical Centers.* Rev. 137; 2015. Centers for Medicare & Medicaid Services. https://www.cms.gov/Regulations-and-Guidance/Guidance/Manuals/downloads/som107ap_l_ambulatory.pdf. Accessed October 15, 2018.

A6. §416.51(b)(3). In: *State Operations Manual Appendix L—Guidance for Surveyors: Ambulatory Surgical Centers.* Rev. 137; 2015. Centers for Medicare & Medicaid Services. https://www.cms.gov/Regulations-and-Guidance/Guidance/Manuals/downloads/som107ap_l_ambulatory.pdf. Accessed October 15, 2018.

Acknowledgments

Lead Author, Ambulatory Supplement
Jan Davidson, MSN, RN, CNOR, CASC
Director, Ambulatory Surgery Division
AORN, Inc
Denver, Colorado

Publication History

Originally published as Ambulatory Supplement: Transmissible Infections in *Perioperative Standards and Recommended Practices,* 2014 edition.

Revised December 2018 for publication in *Guidelines for Perioperative Practice* online.

Minor editorial changes made to conform to revised guideline format, September 2019, for online publication in *Guidelines for Perioperative Practice.*

VENOUS THROMBOEMBOLISM

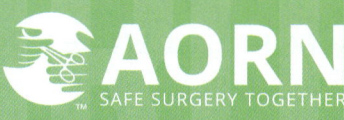

TABLE OF CONTENTS

[P] *indicates a recommendation or evidence relevant to pediatric care.*

MEDICAL ABBREVIATIONS & ACRONYMS

ACCP – American College of Chest Physicians
ACFAS – American College of Foot and Ankle Surgeons
ACOG – American Congress of Obstetricians and Gynecologists
ASMBS – American Society for Metabolic Bariatric Surgery
DVT – Deep vein thrombosis
ERAS – Enhanced Recovery After Surgery

MRI – Magnetic resonance imaging
NICE – National Institute for Health and Care Excellence
PE – Pulmonary embolism
RCT – Randomized controlled trial
RN – Registered nurse
VTE – Venous thromboembolism

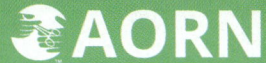
GUIDELINE FOR
PREVENTION OF VENOUS THROMBOEMBOLISM

The Guideline for Prevention of Venous Thromboembolism was approved by the AORN Guidelines Advisory Board and became effective November 1, 2017. It was presented as a proposed guideline for comments by members and others. The recommendations in the guideline are intended to be achievable and represent what is believed to be an optimal level of practice. Policies and procedures will reflect variations in practice settings and/or clinical situations that determine the degree to which the guideline can be implemented. AORN recognizes the many diverse settings in which perioperative nurses practice; therefore, this guideline is adaptable to all areas where operative or other invasive procedures may be performed.

Purpose

This document provides guidance to perioperative team members for developing and implementing a protocol for prevention of venous thromboembolism (VTE), including prevention of deep vein thrombosis (DVT) by mechanical and pharmacologic prophylaxis and prevention of pulmonary embolism (PE) as a complication of DVT.

According to the Centers for Disease Control and Prevention,[1] approximately 900,000 people in the United States experience VTE each year. Approximately 33% of patient deaths related to VTE in the United States occur following a surgical procedure.[2] Among people who develop VTE,

- 50% have long-term complications (eg, swelling, pain, discoloration, scaling in the affected limb) as part of a condition called post-thrombotic syndrome,[1]
- 33% have a recurrence within 10 years,[1,3]
- 10% to 30% die within 1 month of diagnosis,[1]
- 25% with PE experience sudden death as the first symptom,[1,3] and
- 4% who survive PE develop chronic thromboembolic pulmonary hypertension.[4]

Treatment for VTE involves therapeutic anticoagulation, often for a minimum of 3 months; this treatment is associated with minor bruising and hematoma as well as major bleeding events that can be fatal.[4] Patients who have survived VTE have experienced anxiety, adverse effects from anticoagulant treatment, financial burden, loss of function, and fear of recurrence.[4]

Hospital-associated VTE, including DVT and PE, has been identified as a major public health concern.[1,4] Although as many as 70% of hospital-associated VTE cases could be prevented, fewer than half of hospitalized patients receive preventive measures according to the standard of care.[1] The gap between evidence-based practice and actual clinical practice for VTE prevention is concerning and presents a major opportunity for improvement in patient care.[4]

Prevention of VTE is also important for reducing economic burden,[5,6] as costs attributed to VTE in surgical patients have been found to be 1.5 times greater than costs for care of patients without VTE, and the expenses may persist for up to 5 years.[3,7] Although the prevention of VTE should be a priority for the entire health care organization, the particular risks facing surgical patients makes it critical that perioperative registered nurses (RNs) take an active role in VTE prevention.[8-12]

All perioperative patients, including children, may be at risk for VTE because of immobility, vessel injury, compression of tissue caused by retraction, and patient positioning requirements. As such, recommendations for prevention of VTE are applicable to all perioperative patients, including children. The patient may have one or more of the three primary causative factors of venous thrombus formation, which is commonly referred to as Virchow's triad (ie, venous stasis, vessel wall injury, hypercoagulability). Although DVT usually occurs in the lower extremities, it also may occur in the upper extremities.[13-20] **P**

Pulmonary embolism may result as a complication of DVT, although PE may occur independently from DVT.[21] Further research is needed to determine the ideal means to prevent PE and whether a reduction in DVT will lead to a reduction in the incidence of PE.[21]

The selection of VTE prophylaxis, including inferior vena cava filter use, is a medical decision and is outside the scope of this document. The following topics are also outside the scope of this document:

- diagnosis of VTE,
- treatment of VTE and complications (eg, post-thrombotic syndrome, venous stasis ulcers, chronic thromboembolic pulmonary hypertension),
- arterial thrombosis,
- superficial vein thrombosis,
- thrombosis at the surgical site (eg, flap, brain, portal vein thrombosis),
- use of regional anesthesia with DVT prophylaxis,
- laboratory testing of D-dimer levels to assess VTE risk,
- conditions that were studied as potential risk factors and found not to be associated with VTE (eg, use of cement, preoperative travel, Asian ethnicity, hemophilia, arthroscopy, laparoscopic cholecystectomy, shoulder procedures, non-oncologic otorhinolaryngology procedures),
- thromboprophylaxis for a patient with an implanted stent,
- anticoagulation for cardiac bypass,
- medication administration, and
- recommendations for bridging anticoagulant therapy.

Figure 1. Flow Diagram of Literature Search Results

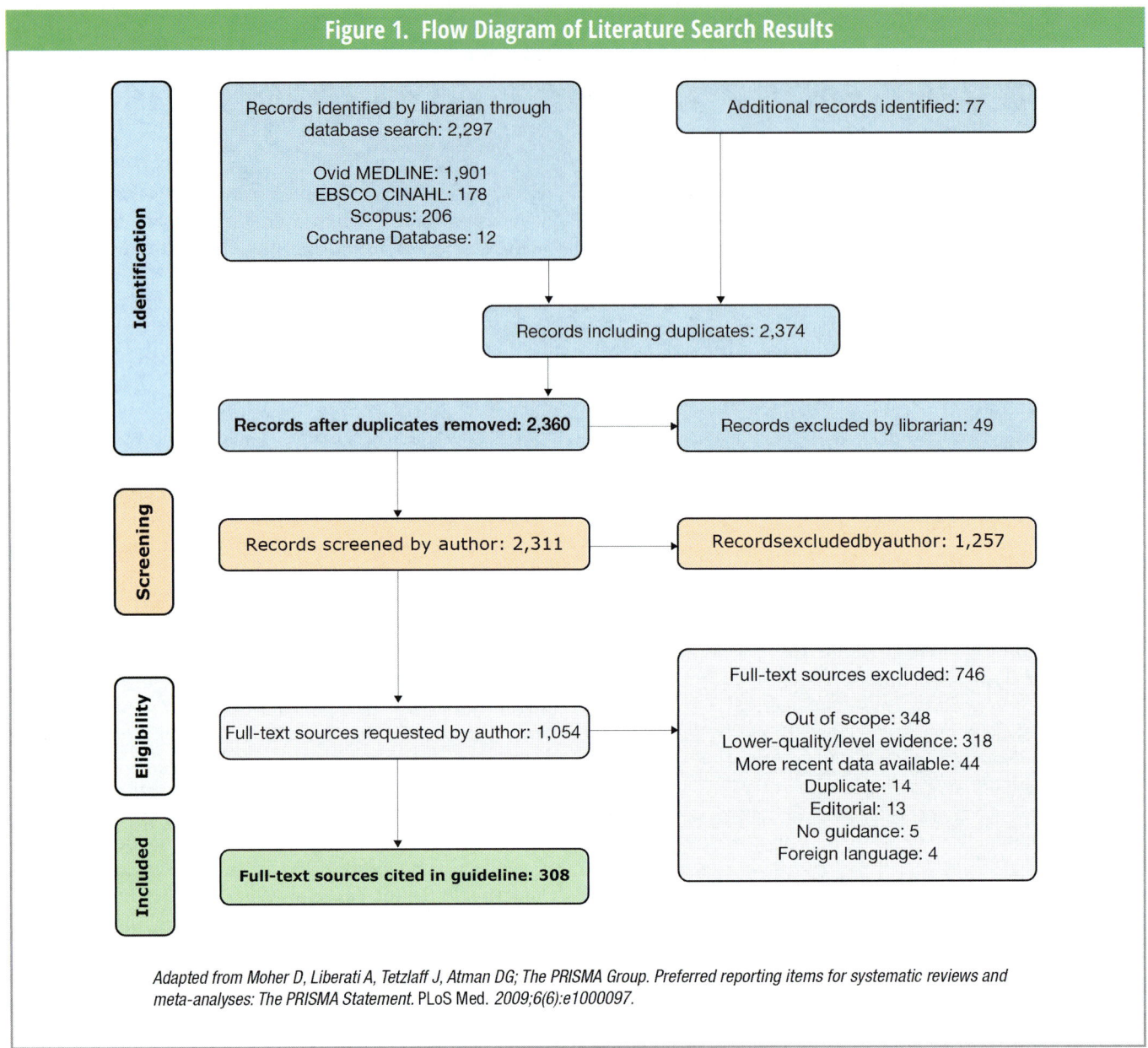

Adapted from Moher D, Liberati A, Tetzlaff J, Atman DG; The PRISMA Group. Preferred reporting items for systematic reviews and meta-analyses: The PRISMA Statement. PLoS Med. *2009;6(6):e1000097.*

Evidence Review

A medical librarian conducted a systematic search of the databases Ovid MEDLINE®, EBSCO CINAHL®, Scopus®, and the Cochrane Database of Systematic Reviews. The search was limited to literature published in English from 2011 through April 2016. A second search of the same databases was performed using the same topics as in the initial search for literature published from 2016 to March 2017. The lead author requested additional articles that either did not fit the original search criteria or were discovered during the evidence appraisal process. The lead author and the medical librarian also identified relevant guidelines from government agencies, professional organizations, and standards-setting bodies.

Search terms included subject headings such as *operating rooms, venous thrombosis, thromboembolism, compression garments, intermittent pneumatic compression, risk factors, Caprini, prophylaxis, foot inflation device,* and *thromboprophylaxis.* Additional keywords and phrases included the names of relevant pharmaceuticals.

Included were research and non-research literature in English, complete publications, and publication dates within the time restriction when available. Excluded were non-peer-reviewed publications, older evidence within the time restriction when more recent evidence was available, research conducted in nonsurgical patient populations (eg, stroke, critical care), and research on mechanical prophylaxis for indications other than prevention of VTE (eg, pain control, lymphedema, ischemia). Editorials, news items, and other brief items were excluded. Lower-level and lower-quality evidence was excluded when higher-quality evidence was available, and literature outside the time restriction was excluded when literature within the time restriction was available. In total, 1,054 research and non-research sources of evidence were identified for possible inclusion, and of these, 308 are cited in the guideline (Figure 1).

Articles identified in the search were provided to the project team for evaluation. The team consisted of the lead author and two evidence appraisers. The lead author divided the search results into topics and assigned members of the team to review and critically appraise each article using the AORN Research or Non-Research Evidence Appraisal Tools as appropriate. The literature was independently evaluated and appraised according to the strength and quality of the evidence. Each article was then assigned an appraisal score. The appraisal score is noted in brackets after each reference as applicable.

Each recommendation rating is based on a synthesis of the collective evidence, a benefit-harm assessment, and consideration of resource use. The strength of the recommendation was determined using the AORN Evidence Rating Model and the quality and consistency of the evidence supporting a recommendation. The recommendation strength rating is noted in brackets after each recommendation.

Note: The evidence summary table is available at http://www.aorn.org/evidencetables/.

Editor's note: MEDLINE is a registered trademark of the US National Library of Medicine's Medical Literature Analysis and Retrieval System, Bethesda, MD. CINAHL, Cumulative Index to Nursing and Allied Health Literature, is a registered trademark of EBSCO Industries, Birmingham, AL. Scopus is a registered trademark of Elsevier B.V., Amsterdam, The Netherlands.

1. Venous Thromboembolism Protocol

1.1 **Establish and implement a protocol for the prevention of VTE.** [*Recommendation*]

Using an organization-wide protocol that is developed using evidence-based, professional guidelines and that includes clinical decision support for prophylactic choices prompts health care providers to give consistent and effective care for the prevention of VTE.[4]

1.2 **The VTE protocol should be developed by an interdisciplinary team, including**
- **a clinical team leader;**
- **a quality improvement facilitator;**
- **process owners, including frontline personnel from each discipline (eg, pharmacists, RNs, surgeons, anesthesia professionals);**
- **information technology and health information system experts; and**
- **patient representatives.**[4]

[*Recommendation*]

The Agency for Healthcare Research and Quality recommends assembling an effective, interdisciplinary team that is empowered and supported by the health care organization's leaders to facilitate achieving meaningful improvement in VTE prevention.[4]

1.3 **The VTE protocol should**
- **be evidence-based;**
- **standardize assessment of VTE and bleeding risk;**
- **provide clinical decision support for evidence-based prophylaxis based on level of risk for VTE and bleeding at critical phases of care (eg, admission, transfer of care, post surgery); and**
- **be easy to use in clinical practice.**[4]

[*Recommendation*]

Protocols for VTE prevention establish best practice at the local level.[4]

1.3.1 **Include a standardized VTE risk assessment model.**[4] [*Recommendation*]

The Agency for Healthcare Research and Quality recommends using a standardized VTE risk assessment model to improve the reliability of the VTE protocol.[4] Qualitative and quantitative VTE risk assessment models have been validated in various perioperative patient populations.[4,22-44] A limitation of the evidence is that there is no consensus regarding a preferred VTE risk assessment tool.[4]

1.3.2 **Include a standardized bleeding risk assessment model.**[4] [*Recommendation*]

The Agency for Healthcare Research and Quality recommends using a standardized bleeding risk assessment model to improve the reliability of the VTE protocol.[4] Bleeding risk is evaluated concurrently with the VTE risk assessment and may be influenced by patient- or procedure-specific factors.[4]

1.3.3 **Include a start time (eg, upon admission, before surgery, after surgery) for all types of prophylaxis based on the clinical condition of the patient.** [*Recommendation*]

The risk for VTE formation begins with preoperative immobility and administration of anesthesia and continues throughout the postoperative phase of care until the patient regains mobility.[45] Some prophylactic measures, such as pharmacologic methods, may be contraindicated because of the increased risk for bleeding and may need to be started postoperatively when the risk for bleeding decreases.[2]

1.3.4 The VTE protocol may include specialty- or procedure-specific (eg, orthopedic, cardiac) clinical decision support for prophylaxis. *[Conditional Recommendation]*

1.4 Use a clinical decision support system with alerts to notify clinicians of a potential lapse in prophylaxis according to the VTE protocol. *[Recommendation]*

High-quality evidence[4,46,47] indicates that clinical decision support systems and alerts can improve compliance with the VTE protocol and reduce the patient's risk for VTE. Borab et al[46] conducted a systematic review with meta-analysis of 11 nonexperimental studies in which computerized clinical decision support systems were implemented for VTE prevention in surgical patients. The researchers found that these systems significantly increased compliance with recommended prophylaxis and significantly reduced the risk for VTE events.

In a systematic review with meta-analysis of 54 randomized controlled trials (RCTs) and quasi-experimental studies, Kahn et al[47] found that use of alerts significantly improved prescription of prophylaxis, especially as part of a multifaceted intervention to improve compliance. However, this systematic review did not find a significant benefit for reduction of VTE.

When alerts are used as a strategy to improve compliance with the VTE protocol, notifying the clinician of only critical events indicating a lapse in care, rather than all screening events, may reduce the risk of alert fatigue from unnecessary alerts.[4]

2. VTE Risk Factors

2.1 Assess the patient preoperatively to determine VTE risk factors. *[Recommendation]* **P**

The preoperative assessment provides information necessary to determine the individual patient's risk for VTE and identify prophylaxis measures recommended by the health care organization's VTE protocol.

2.2 Assess the patient for the following VTE risk factors that contribute to venous stasis, vessel wall injury, and hypercoagulability:
- age greater than 40 years[2,48];
- cancer (ie, active or occult) or cancer treatment[48-50];
- obesity[33,48,51-66];
- previous history of VTE or stroke[2,48,67-70];
- prolonged bed rest (> 3 days) or immobilization [2,48];
- varicose veins[48,71-74];
- presence of a central venous catheter[2,75-77];
- trauma[2,48,78-80];
- spinal cord injury[2,48,81,82];

- inherited or acquired **thrombophilia**[48,67,83,84];
- estrogen therapy (ie, oral contraceptive, hormone replacement therapy)[48,67,85-89];
- critical care admission[48];
- dehydration[48];
- comorbidities, including
  - heart disease[90-92] (eg, congestive heart failure,[93-96] hypertension,[71,97] pacemaker[98]),
  - metabolic or endocrine disease (eg, Cushing's disease[99,100]),
  - respiratory disease[95,101] (eg, chronic obstructive pulmonary disease[33,94]),
  - acute infectious disease[33,102-104] (eg, sepsis[2,27,105,106]), and
  - inflammatory conditions[107] (eg, inflammatory bowel disease,[54,108-112] rheumatoid arthritis,[113] psoriasis[114])[48];
- pregnancy and the postpartum period[67,115-117];
- smoking[54,58,118-120];
- steroid therapy[121-124];
- American Society of Anesthesiologists physical status classification of 3 or higher[27,30,64,90,92,111,125,126];
- recent surgery (ie, within 30 days)[27,58,122];
- preoperative hospitalization[122];
- blood transfusion[127-131];
- known non-O blood type[128,132];
- obstructive sleep apnea[120]; and
- asplenia.[133]

[Recommendation]

Clinical practice guidelines and moderate-quality evidence indicate that patients with any of these risk factors exhibit a greater potential for developing VTE.

2.2.1 Assess the patient for procedure-related VTE risk factors, including
- duration of surgery (ie, surgery and general anesthesia time longer than 90 minutes or longer than 60 minutes for procedures involving the lower limb or pelvis[48])[27,48,55,58,64,65,71,131,134-140];
- the intraoperative patient position (eg, excessive hip flexion, hyperextension of the knee, reverse Trendelenburg)[141];
- use of a pneumatic tourniquet, especially during prolonged periods of inflation[142];
- major orthopedic surgery (eg, hip arthroplasty, knee arthroplasty, hip fracture surgery)[48,143-147];
- bariatric surgery[48,51,53,55,56,60-63,138,148];
- cardiothoracic surgery[2,48,149,150];
- vascular surgery[48,151-153];
- general surgery involving the abdomen or pelvis (eg, hepatic resection[131,154-156])[2,27,48,157,158];
- urologic surgery involving the abdomen or pelvis (eg, nephrectomy)[2,48,159-161];

- neurosurgery[2,48,124,162-165];
- spine surgery[2,35,48,64,96,166-172];
- immobilizing cast of a lower limb[48];
- open procedure[60,61,95,111,173-178];
- emergency procedure[125,157];
- concurrent procedures[27,101,125,179-181];
- transplant surgery[182-192];
- cesarean delivery[115-117];
- major foot and ankle surgery (eg, Achilles tendon rupture, total ankle arthroplasty, ankle fracture)[193-200];
- major hand, wrist, or elbow surgery (eg, elbow arthroplasty)[201];
- procedures involving hardware placement[202]; and
- major plastic surgery (eg, body contouring, abdominoplasty, breast reconstruction).[31,66,181,203]

[Recommendation]

2.3 Consult and collaborate with perioperative team members regarding the need for and selection of prophylaxis based on the organizational protocol and the individual patient's VTE risk factor assessment. [Recommendation]

The perioperative RN has a professional responsibility to advocate for the patient regarding the need for and selection of VTE prophylaxis by consulting and collaborating with other professional colleagues regarding patient care.

3. Mechanical VTE Prophylaxis

3.1 Implement mechanical VTE prophylaxis in a safe and effective manner as prescribed. [Recommendation]

Mechanical prophylaxis is used for prevention of VTE in patients undergoing operative and invasive procedures. Nursing interventions are necessary to decrease the potential for complications associated with mechanical VTE prophylaxis. Mechanical prophylaxis includes the use of intermittent pneumatic compression devices, use of graduated compression stockings, early ambulation, and foot and ankle exercises.

The benefit of using mechanical prophylaxis modalities is reduction of VTE risk without increasing the risk for bleeding.[45] Mechanical prophylaxis is often used in combination with pharmacologic prophylaxis. Unless a patient is at low risk for VTE or is at high risk for bleeding complications, mechanical prophylaxis alone is not recommended for effective VTE prevention.[49,50,204]

The American College of Chest Physicians (ACCP)[2] recommends mechanical prophylaxis for all surgical patients, including early ambulation for patients at very low risk for VTE and intermittent pneumatic compression devices for patients at low, moderate, or high risk for VTE. The American Society for Metabolic and Bariatric Surgery (ASMBS)[51] recommends mechanical prophylaxis and early ambulation for all patients who undergo bariatric surgery. The American College of Foot and Ankle Surgeons (ACFAS)[193] recommends a multimodal approach for preventing VTE in high-risk patients undergoing foot and ankle surgery, which includes early mobilization and use of intermittent pneumatic compression devices and graduated compression stockings. The ERAS® (Enhanced Recovery After Surgery) guidelines[205-207] also recommend mechanical prophylaxis (ie, intermittent pneumatic compression devices and graduated compression stockings) as part of a multimodal approach.

3.2 When prescribed, verify that intermittent pneumatic compression devices are functioning and graduated compression stockings are applied before the administration of regional or general anesthesia.[48] [Recommendation]

Regional or general anesthesia dilates the calf veins due to the loss of leg muscle tone. According to Caprini,[45] the best theoretical approach to prophylaxis is to minimize venous stasis and dilation, starting before the anticipated confinement of surgery and continuing throughout the entire period of risk. The National Institute for Clinical Excellence (NICE)[48] guidelines recommend starting mechanical prophylaxis for surgical patients at admission.

3.3 Perform interventions for safe and effective use of intermittent pneumatic compression devices. [Recommendation]

Low-quality evidence indicates that patients may be harmed by wearing intermittent pneumatic compression devices for prevention of VTE.[208,209] The harms caused by intermittent pneumatic compression devices may include pressure injury[208] and hypothermia.[209] Another potential harm associated with intermittent pneumatic compression devices may be a fall when the patient ambulates. However, Boelig et al[210] found that patient falls were rarely associated with sequential compression device use in one health care organization database (0.45% of total patient falls). The harms may be mitigated by interventions implemented by the perioperative RN to facilitate the patient's wearing of intermittent pneumatic compression devices in accordance with the manufacturer's instructions for use, prevent pressure injury, and prevent unplanned hypothermia.

The benefits of intermittent pneumatic compression include a reduction in VTE rates similar to those for pharmacologic prophylaxis methods while also reducing the risk for major bleeding in surgical patients.[211-214] Research has demonstrated that the addition of intermittent pneumatic compression to pharmacologic prophylaxis significantly reduces the risk for VTE compared to either modality alone.[212,215-219] Although the exact mechanism of VTE prevention by intermittent pneumatic compression devices is unknown, evidence suggests that intermittent pneumatic compression devices reduce venous stasis, improve venous return from the lower extremities, and cause flow-induced endothelial reactions that increase fibrinolytic activity.[45,213,220,221] Foot inflation devices reduce venous stasis by simulating natural walking and providing compression to the plantar venous plexus.

For mechanical prophylaxis, the ACCP[2,143] recommends the use of intermittent pneumatic compression devices in preference to graduated compression stockings because of the risk for skin complications associated with the stockings. The American Congress of Obstetricians and Gynecologists (ACOG)[115,222,223] also preferentially recommends intermittent pneumatic compression for all patients undergoing gynecologic surgical procedures or cesarean delivery. In an RCT involving 108 high-risk patients undergoing gynecological pelvic surgery, Gao et al[224] found that a combination of intermittent pneumatic compression and graduated compression stockings significantly reduced VTE rates compared with use of graduated compression stockings alone. Further research is needed to determine whether graduated compression stockings limit the hemodynamic performance of intermittent pneumatic compression devices by preventing filling of veins.[225]

Morris and Woodcock[225] conducted a systematic review to compare intermittent pneumatic compression and graduated compression stockings and found weak and potentially biased nonexperimental evidence indicating that intermittent pneumatic compression was superior in effectiveness to graduated compression stockings for VTE prevention. The researchers urged caution in interpreting the results, and warned that insufficient evidence that one is more effective does not imply strong evidence of equivalency.

The limitations of the evidence are that optimal compression techniques (eg, sequential, simultaneous, cycle method), area of compression (eg, foot, calf, entire leg), and time of inflation are unknown. Several intermittent pneumatic compression devices have been cleared by the US Food and Drug Administration with a wide variety of design features that provide inflation on the foot, calf, or entire leg. In subgroup analysis of a systematic review, Pavon et al[212] did not find any significant differences in effectiveness based on intermittent pneumatic compression device mode of inflation or device location. Only one study in the systematic review compared various lengths of pneumatic compression devices; this study found that calf-length pneumatic compression was more effective than plantar compression for reduction of thigh swelling, although no cases of DVT or PE were reported.[226] Several studies have found that venous foot pump devices are safe and effective for prevention of VTE,[227-229] although one study did not find a difference in VTE rates with foot pump use.[230]

3.3.1 **Assess the patient for potential contraindications related to use of the intermittent pneumatic compression device, including**
- **any leg condition (eg, dermatitis, recent skin graft, gangrene) that pneumatic compression may exacerbate,[2,48]**
- **known allergy or sensitivity to the sleeve or tubing material,[48]**
- **cardiac failure or pulmonary edema from congestive heart failure,[48,220]**
- **any factor that prevents correct fitting of sleeves (eg, exceeding the size limit, severe leg edema, deformity),[48,231]**
- **pre-existing DVT, and**
- **severe arteriosclerosis or other ischemic vascular disease.**

[Recommendation]

In a nonexperimental study, Hou et al[232] found that application of intermittent pneumatic compression in patients with pre-existing DVT was safe. The International Compression Club[220] has stated that further research is needed in this area.

3.3.2 **Notify the prescriber and anesthesia professional of any identified contraindications related to use of the intermittent pneumatic compression device.** *[Recommendation]*

3.3.3 **Apply sleeves for intermittent pneumatic compression devices according to the manufacturer's instructions for use.** *[Recommendation]*

3.3.4 **When the manufacturer's instructions for use require the use of stockinet, graduated compression stockings, or other material under the sleeves, verify that the material is wrinkle-free when applied to the skin.** *[Recommendation]*

Some manufacturers may recommend stockinet, graduated compression stockings, or other materials for skin protection under the sleeves. Smooth, wrinkle-free undersleeve material may reduce the risk of skin injury.

3.3.5 During application of the sleeve, place the tubing on the external surface of the sleeve facing away from the patient's skin and away from locations that may create a pressure injury. *[Recommendation]*

Placement of the tubing between the patient's skin and the sleeve may lead to a pressure injury. Tubing may also cause pressure injury depending on the patient's position.

3.3.6 Verify that the sleeves for intermittent pneumatic compression devices are applied correctly, connected to the device pump, and operating and that the tubing is away from locations that may create a pressure injury after the patient is transferred to the OR bed or repositioned. *[Recommendation]*

3.3.7 When intermittent pneumatic compression is used, implement interventions to prevent unplanned hypothermia as recommended in the AORN Guideline for Prevention of Unplanned Patient Hypothermia.[209,233] *[Recommendation]*

Use of intermittent pneumatic compression may increase the patient's risk for hypothermia. In an RCT, Huh et al[209] found that temperatures dropped significantly for patients wearing calf- or thigh-length sequential compression devices compared with patients not wearing the devices. The researchers recommended temperature monitoring and active warming methods because of the core temperature drop noted in the group wearing the sequential compression devices.

3.3.8 Sleeves for intermittent pneumatic compression devices used on the sterile field should be sterile (See the AORN Guideline for Sterile Technique).[234] *[Recommendation]*

Failure to adhere to aseptic practices during invasive procedures has been associated with surgical site infections.[234]

Intermittent pneumatic compression devices are used on the sterile field. Research has shown that patients undergoing bilateral total knee arthroplasty are twice as likely to develop VTE as patients undergoing unilateral arthroplasty.[235] In a retrospective study of a single clinician's experience,[236] sterile intermittent pneumatic compression devices were applied to 157 patients undergoing bilateral total knee arthroplasty when the tourniquet was not

inflated, as part of a multimodal approach for VTE prevention.

3.3.9 Intermittent pneumatic compression devices used during procedures with intraoperative magnetic resonance imaging (MRI) should be MRI safe (ie, non-ferromagnetic).[237] *[Recommendation]*

Intermittent pneumatic compression devices that are not MRI safe can become lethal projectiles, causing harm to personnel and patients or damage to the scanner.[237] Two nonexperimental studies showed that use of intermittent pneumatic compression devices during intraoperative MRI significantly reduced the risk of DVT.[238,239] Maybody et al[239] found that the sleeves and tubing of an intermittent compression device were MRI safe, although the control unit was not MRI safe. To comply with MRI safety requirements, the control unit was placed in the MRI control room and connected to the sleeves using extended tubing. Use of the extended tubing did not cause device failure or interfere with the procedure.

3.3.10 The intermittent pneumatic compression device should remain on for a minimum of 18 hours daily during the intraoperative and immediate postoperative period unless removal is necessitated by patient care needs.[2,48,143] *[Recommendation]*

The ACCP and NICE guidelines[2,48,143] recommend that patients wear intermittent pneumatic compression devices for as much time as possible to obtain the optimal benefit for VTE prevention. In a nonexperimental study of patients undergoing urologic surgery (N = 100), Ritsema et al[240] found that noncompliance with wearing sequential compression devices was more likely to be caused by hospital factors, such as availability of equipment and timely restarting of the devices by nursing personnel, than by patient factors.

3.3.11 The intermittent pneumatic compression device should be portable. *[Recommendation]*

High-quality evidence and clinical practice guidelines[2,143,235,241-246] support that mobile compression devices are safe and effective for prevention of VTE in surgical patients. In an RCT, Obi et al[241] investigated patient compliance (N = 67) with intermittent pneumatic compression device use for battery-powered devices (n = 35) compared to stationary devices that must remain plugged into the electrical outlet (n = 32). The researchers found that use of portable, battery-operated intermittent pneumatic compression devices significantly increased patient compliance compared to use of stationary devices.

3.3.12 | **The intermittent pneumatic compression device should be capable of recording wear time.** [Recommendation]

High-quality evidence and clinical practice guidelines[2,143,235,241-246] support use of intermittent pneumatic compression devices that record wear time as a mechanism to monitor patient adherence. In a systematic review with meta-analysis of eight nonexperimental studies, Craigie et al[247] found that as many as 25% of hospitalized surgical patients were not compliant with wearing mechanical prophylaxis.

3.4 | **Perform interventions for safe and effective use of graduated compression stockings.** [Recommendation]

Moderate-quality evidence and clinical practice guidelines[2,48,248-252] indicate that patients may be harmed by wearing graduated compression stockings for prevention of VTE when graduated compression stockings are incorrectly worn or sized. The harms may include skin injury[2,48]; nerve injury[248,249]; compartment syndrome[250]; and tourniquet effect, which increases the risk for VTE.[251,252] The harms may be mitigated by interventions implemented by the perioperative RN to facilitate the patient's wearing of graduated compression stockings in accordance with the manufacturer's instructions for use.

Although the exact mechanism of graduated compression stockings function is unknown, evidence suggests that exerting graded pressure distally to proximally in combination with muscular contraction displaces blood from the superficial to deep venous system of the leg. This displacement of blood increases the velocity and volume of blood flow in the deep system, thereby potentially preventing VTE.[253] Sachdeva et al[253] conducted a systematic review with meta-analysis and found that graduated compression stockings were effective in reducing the risk for VTE in hospitalized surgical patients, although the included research was conducted primarily with patients undergoing general and orthopedic surgery. In another systematic review, Mandavia et al[254] did not find a clear benefit of graduated compression stockings in addition to pharmaceutical prophylaxis in surgical inpatients when compared to patients receiving only pharmaceutical prophylaxis.

A limitation of the evidence is that the effect of graduated compression stockings alone for prevention of VTE is not clear because stockings are often used in combination with other interventions, including intermittent pneumatic compression devices and pharmaceutical prophylaxis.

3.4.1 | **Assess the patient for potential contraindications related to the use of graduated compression stockings, including**
- **any skin conditions (eg, dermatitis, recent skin graft, leg ulcer) that stockings may exacerbate,**[2,48]
- **any vascular conditions (eg, peripheral vascular disease, peripheral arterial bypass grafting, severe arteriosclerosis) that stockings may exacerbate,**[2,48,231]
- **severe peripheral neuropathy or other sensory impairment,**[48]
- **gangrene,**[48]
- **known allergy or sensitivity to stocking material,**[48]
- **cardiac failure or pulmonary edema from congestive heart failure,**[48] **and**
- **any factor that prevents correct fitting of stockings (eg, exceeding the size limit, severe leg edema, deformity).**[48,231]

[Recommendation]

3.4.2 | **Notify the prescriber and anesthesia professional of any identified contraindications related to the use of the graduated compression stockings.** [Recommendation]

3.4.3 | **Assess the patient's ability to wear thigh-length graduated compression stockings in accordance with the manufacturer's instructions for use and the patient's preference for length (ie, thigh or knee length). When thigh-length graduated compression stockings are contraindicated based on the patient assessment, collaborate with the prescriber to determine whether knee-length graduated compression stockings may be substituted for thigh-length stockings.** [Recommendation]

The evidence regarding the ideal length for graduated compression stockings conflicts. The ACCP[2] recommends that surgical patients wear thigh-length graduated compression stockings instead of knee length, citing evidence showing greater benefit for prevention of VTE in stroke patients who wore thigh-length stockings. For hospitalized surgical patients, three systematic reviews with meta-analysis[255-258] found insufficient high-quality evidence to determine a statistical difference in effectiveness between thigh- and knee-length graduated compression stockings. Because of this conflicting evidence and the theory that prevention of VTE with graduated compression stockings is unlikely to be effective when patient compliance is low,[259] the authors of one systematic review[256] suggested a pragmatic approach of providing thigh-length graduated compression stockings only to patients who can consistently use the stockings according to the manufacturer's instructions.

An RCT conducted with Turkish patients undergoing abdominal-pelvic surgeries (N = 219) directly compared patient satisfaction with thigh- and knee-length graduated compression stockings. Ayhan et al[260] found that patients who wore low-pressure (ie, 15 mmHg to 18 mmHg), knee-length stockings (n = 73) were more satisfied and had fewer problems than those who wore low-pressure, thigh-length stockings (n = 73) or moderate-pressure (20 mmHg to 30 mmHg), knee-length stockings (n = 73). The researchers monitored the patients 5 to 7 days after surgery using duplex ultrasonography and found no patients in the study had experienced DVT.

Another study recommended considering patient preference based on evidence showing similar hemodynamic performance between thigh- and knee-length graduated compression stockings. In this quasi-experimental study, Lattimer et al[261] found that graduated compression stockings significantly improved all hemodynamic performance tests, including venous filling index, venous volume, and time to fill 90% of venous volume, regardless of length (ie, thigh- or knee-length) or compression class (18 mmHg to 21 mmHg versus 23 mmHg to 32 mmHg). The majority of patients in the study (62%, n = 21) preferred knee-length graduated compression stockings. The authors recommended basing stocking selection on patient preference because of a lack of significance in hemodynamic performance by length or compression class.

Further research is needed to determine the most effective graduated compression stocking length for prevention of VTE in surgical patients, patient adherence,[259] and cost.

3.4.4 **Fit graduated compression stockings to the individual patient. Measure the patient's legs separately and according to the manufacturer's instructions.**[2,48] *[Recommendation]*

Incorrect sizing of graduated compression stockings may cause injury to the patient or reduce the effectiveness for VTE prevention. The ACCP[2] recommends that the stockings be fitted to ensure efficacy, with pressure at the ankle between 18 mmHg and 23 mmHg. Measuring each of the patient's legs is necessary because there may be enough variability in length and circumference to require a different stocking size for each leg.

An insufficient range of stocking sizes may contribute to the use of an incorrectly sized stocking. In a nonexperimental study, Bowling et al[252] found that one facility had only three of six sizes of stockings available. Only 14% of stockings showed gradation in accordance with the manufacturers' intended compression, and 23% of stockings exerted more pressure at the calf than the ankle, thereby creating a tourniquet effect, which increases the risk for VTE. The authors discussed that a wide variety of sizes was necessary to achieve individual patient fit, although available products in larger sizes increased in length but not girth at the calf. In addition to the lack of all available sizes of stockings, patients were not universally remeasured for size 24 hours after surgery in accordance with facility policy, which may have contributed to the poor fit.

In a nonexperimental study, Thompson et al[251] implemented a protocol for sizing knee-length stockings in patients undergoing total hip and knee replacements (N = 57). The standardized protocol significantly improved correct sizing of stockings, reduced the proportion of patients with **proximal indentation** from stockings, reduced the number of patients with **reverse gradients**, and improved patient compliance with wearing stockings.

Compartment syndrome has been reported as a result of incorrect stocking size. Hinderland et al[250] reported a case of lateral leg compartment syndrome after ankle surgery in a patient's nonoperative extremity. The authors attributed the compartment syndrome to a graduated compression stocking that was a size too small. The patient complained of severe pain when he awoke from surgery. Removal of the stocking and intermittent pneumatic compression device provided minimal relief of the patient's pain. No defect was found with the pneumatic compression device. The patient was assessed for compartment syndrome; however, the compartment pressures were initially normal. The patient returned 2 days later with severe, increasing pain and underwent surgical decompression fasciotomy of the lateral leg compartment, split-thickness skin graft, and 3 weeks of non-weight bearing of bilateral extremities. The patient was able to return to full activity 4 months after surgery with no muscle deficits, although he was treated for mild neuropraxia of the foot.

3.4.5 Apply graduated compression stockings according to the manufacturer's written instructions. After application, verify that the

- stockings are not rolled up the foot or down the leg,
- stockings are smooth when fitted,
- toe holes lie underneath the toes,
- heel patches are in the correct position, and
- thigh gussets are positioned on the patient's inner thighs.

[Recommendation]

3.4.6 Verify that the graduated compression stockings have not rolled up the foot or down the leg during transfer to and from the OR bed or during procedural positioning. [Recommendation]

3.4.7 If the patient develops postoperative leg edema, remove the stockings, remeasure the patient's legs, and refit the stockings.[48,252] [Recommendation]

Postoperative leg edema may alter the fit of the graduated compression stockings, which may reduce the pressure exerted at the ankle and reduce the effectiveness of the stockings.[252] The NICE[48] guidelines recommend remeasurement and refitting of graduated compression stockings for patients with postoperative leg edema or swelling.

At a single facility that required stocking remeasurement at 24 hours after surgery, Bowling et al[252] found that the remeasurement was not taking place according to recommendations from NICE. Only 14% of stockings worn by patients had gradation in accordance with the manufacturers' intended compression, and 23% of stockings exerted more pressure at the calf than the ankle, which increases the risk for VTE.

In a nonexperimental study, Thompson et al[251] implemented a protocol for refitting knee-length graduated compression stockings 48 hours after surgery for patients undergoing total hip and knee replacements. The standardized protocol significantly improved correct sizing of stockings, reduced the proportion of patients with proximal indentation from stockings, reduced the number of patients with reverse gradients, and improved patient compliance with wearing the stockings.

3.4.8 Do not use elastic bandages as a replacement for graduated compression stockings. [Recommendation]

Potential harms of using elastic bandages include risk for skin, pressure, and nerve injury. Elastic bandages may not provide a protective effect for VTE due to variability in pressure exerted and inability to control for tourniquet effect. Inconsistent bandaging technique may be associated with poor patient outcomes.[220] Further research is needed to determine the safety and efficacy of using elastic bandages for VTE prevention.

3.5 Graduated compression stockings and intermittent pneumatic compression devices may be used on patients in the lithotomy position (See the AORN Guideline for Positioning the Patient).[141] [Conditional Recommendation]

The risk for VTE may be greater than the risk for compartment syndrome when mechanical prophylaxis is used for a patient in the lithotomy position, and it may be reasonable to continue the use of graduated compression stockings and intermittent pneumatic compression devices for thromboprophylaxis in patients undergoing surgical procedures in the lithotomy position.[141]

3.6 Assess the patient for adverse effects related to the use of mechanical VTE prophylaxis, including

- skin injury[2,48,208];
- hypothermia from the use of intermittent pneumatic compression devices[209];
- numbness, tingling, discomfort, or pain[248-250];
- proximal indentation from knee-length graduated compression stockings[251]; and
- ischemia.

[Recommendation]

Skin injury,[2,48,208] nerve injury,[248,249] compartment syndrome,[250] and vascular compromise (eg, ischemia) are potential complications related to use of mechanical VTE prophylaxis.

In a nonexperimental study, Thompson et al[251] identified proximal indentation on the calves of patients wearing knee-length graduated compression stockings and found that patients with proximal indentation were significantly more likely to have reverse gradients (41%) than patients without proximal indentation (8%). The researchers implemented a protocol for refitting knee-length stockings 48 hours after surgery and found that the standardized protocol significantly reduced the proportion of patients with proximal indentation from stockings (53% to 19%).

3.6.1 Specify in the VTE protocol when mechanical VTE prophylaxis (ie, intermittent pneumatic compression device, graduated compression stockings) should be removed for patient assessment and patient care activities (eg, ambulation, before discharge, transfer of care). [Recommendation]

3.6.2 When evidence of complications related to the use of mechanical VTE prophylaxis is present,

- remove the stocking and compression device,[48]
- notify the physician and anesthesia professional, and
- document actions taken.

[Recommendation]

3.6.3 When patient injury or equipment failure occur during the use of intermittent pneumatic compression devices,

- remove the intermittent pneumatic compression device from service;
- retain all sleeve and tubing accessories if possible; and
- report the adverse event details, including device identification and maintenance and service information, according to the health care organization's policy and procedures.

[Recommendation]

Retaining the intermittent pneumatic compression device, sleeves, and tubing accessories facilitates the incident investigation.

3.7 The patient should ambulate as soon as possible after surgery. *[Recommendation]*

Ambulation decreases venous stasis by creating natural compression of the venous system through muscle contraction and compression of the venous foot pump. Several guidelines[2,48,51,85,144,193] recommend early ambulation or mobilization as a postoperative intervention to prevent VTE. The NICE[48] guidelines recommend encouraging mobilization as soon as possible after surgery for all surgical patients. Other guidelines recommend early ambulation for a specific surgical procedure, VTE risk level, or patient population. For example, the ACCP[2] recommends early ambulation as the only method of VTE prophylaxis for patients undergoing general and abdominal-pelvic surgery who are at very low risk for VTE. Similarly, the ACOG[85] recommends early ambulation for low-risk patients undergoing gynecologic surgery who do not require other mechanical or pharmaceutical prophylaxis. The American Academy of Orthopaedic Surgeons[144] recommends early mobilization after elective hip and knee arthroplasty, in addition to mechanical and pharmaceutical prophylaxis. The ACFAS[193] recommends a multimodal approach that includes early mobilization and weight bearing for preventing VTE in high-risk patients undergoing foot and ankle surgery. The ASMBS[51] recommends early ambulation for all patients who have undergone bariatric surgery in addition to mechanical and

pharmaceutical prophylaxis based on the patient's risk assessment.

Early mobilization is also included in multimodal protocols for improving recovery of surgical patients, including ERAS[205-207,262] and fast-track[263-267] protocols. The ERAS guidelines for elective rectal/pelvic surgery recommend a care plan that supports patient independence and mobilization, with patients out of bed for 2 hours on the day of surgery and 6 hours on postoperative days thereafter.[207] The ERAS guidelines for gynecologic/oncology surgery recommend encouraging the patient to mobilize within 24 hours after surgery.[206] Fast-track protocols for patients undergoing hip and knee arthroplasty include mobilization as soon as 2 to 4 hours[263,264] or 3 to 5 hours[267] after surgery.

Further research is needed to compare multimodal protocols with early mobilization to a protocol without early mobilization to determine the specific benefits of early mobilization.[264]

The benefits of early postoperative ambulation outweigh the harms. Benefits of ambulation include reduced VTE complications, reduced pulmonary complications, reduced muscle atrophy, reduced hospital length of stay, and counteracting insulin resistance from immobilization.[205,206] Postoperative ambulation is a low-cost intervention for VTE prevention.[144] Benefits of early mobilization may include a reduced need for prolonged pharmaceutical prophylaxis, although further research is needed.[263-265] The harms may include patient falls.

3.7.1 Assess the patient's risk for falls and implement measures to prevent falls during postoperative ambulation. *[Recommendation]*

3.7.2 Collaborate with the perioperative team to minimize barriers to postoperative ambulation, including

- inadequate pain control,[205,206,264]
- pain management techniques that reduce patient mobility (eg, regional anesthesia),
- an indwelling urinary catheter,[205,206]
- IV infusion,[205,206] and
- lack of patient motivation (eg, sedation).[205]

[Recommendation]

Moderate-quality evidence and clinical practice guidelines support that barriers to early postoperative ambulation include inadequate pain control,[264] IV fluid infusion, an indwelling urinary catheter, lack of patient motivation, and pre-existing comorbidities.[205,206] Compliance with a multimodal ERAS protocol may minimize these barriers.[206] Pain management techniques that limit the patient's mobility, such as regional anesthesia, may also be a barrier to postoperative ambulation.

3.8 Instruct the patient to perform postoperative foot and ankle exercises. *[Recommendation]*

Foot and ankle exercises decrease venous stasis by creating natural compression of the venous system through muscle contraction. The ACFAS[193] recommends early rehabilitation and mobilization of the operative limb, including ankle exercises, to reengage the calf muscle pump as part of a multimodal approach for VTE prevention in high-risk patients. Wang et al[268] found that patients in an RCT who were selected to perform active ankle movements postoperatively for 7 days (n = 96) had fewer occurrences of thrombosis and DVT, less swelling of the thigh and calf, and improved maximum venous outflow and capacity, which may prevent formation of DVT, than patients who did not perform ankle movements (n = 78). The active ankle movements included a range of movement to 20-degree dorsal flexion, 30-degree varus and valgus, and 40-degree plantar flexion at a frequency of 30 times per minute, 20 times per day.

Shimizu et al[269] found that a novel leg apparatus to facilitate active ankle movement improved venous flow in the femoral veins of eight healthy volunteers after 1 minute of exercise compared to application of intermittent pneumatic compression for 10 minutes. The novel leg apparatus enabled movement from the supine position to 30-degree dorsiflexion, 60-degree plantar flexion, combined flexion and rotation of the ankle, flexion and extension of the knee and hip, and combined leg motion.

The limitations of the evidence are that research has not confirmed the effect of foot and ankle exercises on VTE development. Further research is needed to determine the optimal method, sequence, and frequency of foot and ankle exercises.

The benefits of the patient performing foot and ankle exercises outweigh the harms. Benefits include improvement of blood flow in the lower extremities, which may prevent VTE.[268,269] The effect of benefits may be limited by the patient's ability to perform foot and ankle exercises in the full range of motion (eg, because of a rigid cast[193] or contractures) or to contract muscles in the lower extremities (eg, because of paralysis).

4. Pharmacologic VTE Prophylaxis

4.1 Implement pharmacologic VTE prophylaxis in a safe and effective manner as prescribed. *[Recommendation]*

Nursing interventions are necessary to decrease the risk of potential complications from pharmacologic prophylaxis that may be used throughout the perioperative period. Pharmacologic prophylaxis consists of administering anticoagulant medications that inhibit blood clotting. The pharmacologic regimen may include medications such as low molecular weight heparin, low-dose unfractionated heparin, warfarin, factor Xa inhibitors (ie, fondaparinux, rivaroxaban, apixaban), dabigatran, vitamin K antagonists, or aspirin.

4.2 Assess the patient for potential contraindications related to use of pharmacologic VTE prophylaxis, including

- **active bleeding**[2,48,270];
- **previous major bleeding**[2,143,270,271];
- **known, untreated bleeding disorder**[2,48,270];
- **severe renal or hepatic failure**[2,48,143,270,271];
- **thrombocytopenia**[2,48,270,271];
- **acute stroke**[2,48];
- **uncontrolled systemic hypertension**[2,48,270,271];
- **lumbar puncture or epidural or spinal anesthesia within the previous 4 hours or planned within the next 12 hours**[2,48,270-272];
- **concomitant use of anticoagulants, antiplatelet therapy, or thrombolytic drugs**[2,48,143,270,271];
- **procedures in which bleeding complications may have especially severe consequences (eg, craniotomy, spinal surgery, spinal trauma, reconstructive procedures involving a free flap)**[2,270];
- **bacterial endocarditis**[270,271];
- **allergy to medication**[271];
- **pregnancy**[270];
- **ophthalmic surgery**[270]; **and**
- **prosthetic heart valve.**[270]

[Recommendation]

4.2.1 Notify the prescriber of any identified contraindications. *[Recommendation]*

4.3 Assess the patient for adverse effects related to the use of pharmacologic VTE prophylaxis, including

- **bleeding**[2,270,271];
- **hematoma formation**[2,270];
- **thrombocytopenia**[2,270,271];
- **osteoporosis and osteopenia**[271];
- **skin necrosis**[270,273];
- **calciphylaxis**[270];
- **atheroembolism**[270]; **and**
- **injection site irritation, pain, bruising, bleeding, or itching.**[270]

[Recommendation]

4.3.1 Notify the prescriber and anesthesia professional of any identified adverse effects. *[Recommendation]*

5. Patient Education

5.1 Provide the patient and the patient's designated caregiver(s) with instructions regarding prevention of VTE and prescribed prophylactic measures. *[Recommendation]*

Education related to VTE prevention may reduce the patient's risk for developing VTE by increasing the patient's awareness and, potentially, compliance with prophylaxis.[274]

5.2 Provide the patient and the patient's designated caregiver(s) with verbal and written instructions on the prevention of VTE,[48,274,275] including

- common signs and symptoms of DVT or PE (eg, leg pain, swelling, unexplained shortness of breath, wheezing, chest pain, palpitations, anxiety, sweating, coughing up blood)[48];
- the importance of seeking medical help and who to contact if the patient suspects DVT, PE, or an adverse effect[48];
- the importance of adhering to the entire duration of prescribed VTE prophylaxis[48];
- who to contact if the patient has any problems using the prescribed VTE prophylaxis[48];
- the importance of mobilization, including ambulation and foot and ankle exercises[48];
- maintaining adequate hydration[48,276];
- preventive measures to use when travelling long distances after surgery, including frequent ambulation, calf muscle exercise, and wearing fitted, knee-length graduated compression stockings[277];
- elevating the legs[276];
- avoiding clothing that constricts the lower extremities;
- avoiding sitting with knees bent or legs crossed for long periods of time; and
- avoiding sitting or standing for long periods of time.

[Recommendation]

Venous thromboembolism frequently develops or becomes evident after the patient is discharged. One analysis of the National Surgical Quality Improvement Program database found that 30% of patients with VTE were diagnosed after hospital discharge.[111] Education provides the patient with the signs and symptoms of VTE, an awareness of VTE prevention measures, and information about when to seek medical help. Three audits of patients' preoperative knowledge found that patients lacked awareness of risk for VTE and methods of prevention.[274,275,278] One quasi-experimental study found that implementation of targeted patient education on VTE risk and prevention significantly improved patient awareness.[274]

5.3 Provide the patient receiving mechanical prophylaxis and the patient's designated caregiver(s) with preoperative and postoperative instructions, including

- the benefits of mechanical prophylaxis[48];
- the importance of compliance[2,48,143,247,259];
- the importance of wearing sized, graduated compression stockings in accordance with the manufacturer's instructions for use[2,48];
- instructions for removal, laundering, and reapplication of graduated compression stockings[48,249];
- instructions for removal and reapplication of the intermittent compression device immediately after ambulation[2,143];
- the importance of postoperative ambulation[48];
- potential complications, including
  ○ skin injury (eg, marking, blistering),[2,48,208]
  ○ ischemia (eg, discoloration), and
  ○ numbness, tingling, discomfort, or pain[248-250]; and
- who to contact if the patient has any problems using the prescribed mechanical prophylaxis.[48]

[Recommendation]

Education helps the patient understand the potential complications of mechanical prophylaxis as well as the importance of compliance with its correct use.

5.3.1 Assess the patient's ability to remove and replace intermittent pneumatic compression devices and graduated compression stockings or the availability of someone to help the patient.[48] *[Recommendation]*

5.3.2 Monitor the patient's use of intermittent pneumatic compression devices and graduated compression stockings and compliance with the manufacturer's instructions for use. If these are not being used correctly, assist the patient and provide reeducation.[48] *[Recommendation]*

5.3.3 Provide the patient prescribed an alternative mechanical prophylaxis device (ie, continuous passive motion,[279] electrical calf muscle stimulation[280]) and the patient's designated caregiver(s) with preoperative and postoperative instructions for use of the device. *[Recommendation]*

5.4 Provide the patient receiving pharmacologic VTE prophylaxis and the patient's designated caregiver(s) with preoperative and postoperative instructions, including

- the importance of following through with medication-related laboratory tests[270];
- the importance of continuing medication post discharge as prescribed[270];
- who to contact if the patient has any problems self-administering the prescribed pharmacologic prophylaxis[48];
- the importance of not stopping medication or of not starting a new medication, including over-the-counter medications (eg, aspirin, ibuprofen), without consulting the physician[270];
- potential adverse effects and when to seek medical attention[281];
- interactions with herbal and other over-the-counter preparations (eg, ginger, ginkgo biloba, ginseng, garlic, chamomile)[270,282];
- reporting signs of bleeding, including
  - unusual bruising,
  - pink or brown urine,
  - red or black tarry stools,
  - coughing up blood,
  - vomiting blood or vomit that looks like coffee grounds,
  - pain, swelling, or discomfort in a joint,
  - recurring nose bleeds,
  - unusual bleeding from gums, or
  - cuts that do not stop bleeding[270,282];
- reporting signs of epidural hematoma if the patient underwent any spine procedures, including
  - back pain,
  - tingling or numbness,
  - muscle weakness, or
  - incontinence[270];
- avoiding eating large amounts of food high in vitamin K such as green, leafy vegetables;
- avoiding certain activities (eg, contact sports)[282];
- using an electric razor when shaving[282];
- using a soft toothbrush and waxed dental floss gently[282];
- informing health care workers about pharmacologic prophylaxis before undergoing any procedures (eg, dental work, laboratory tests)[270,282];
- carrying or wearing medical identification to let health care providers know that the patient takes anticoagulation therapy[282]; and
- informing the physician if the patient is breastfeeding.[270]

[Recommendation]

Education assists the patient in understanding the potential complications of pharmacologic prophylaxis, as well as the importance of compliance as prescribed.

6. Documentation

6.1 Document activities taken for prevention of VTE. *[Recommendation]*

Documentation in the patient's medical record provides a description of the perioperative care administered, status of patient outcomes upon transfer, and information to support continuity of care.[283] Documentation provides data for identifying trends and demonstrating compliance with regulatory requirements and accreditation standards. Effective management and collection of health care information that accurately reflects the patient's care, treatment, and services is a regulatory requirement[284-287] and an accreditation standard for both hospitals[288,289] and ambulatory settings.[289-293]

6.2 Document in a manner consistent with the health care organization's policies and procedures and include

- pharmacologic prophylaxis administration (eg, medication, dose, time, route),[281]
- presence of VTE risk factors,[294]
- contraindications to mechanical or pharmacologic prophylaxis and actions taken,[294]
- adverse effects from mechanical or pharmacologic prophylaxis and actions taken,[294]
- patient education provided,[221,294]
- the reason for any variance from the VTE protocol,[4]
- the type and size of the intermittent pneumatic compression sleeve and graduated compression stockings applied,[294]
- results of a fall risk assessment and measures taken to prevent patient falls during postoperative ambulation,
- application and removal times for all mechanical prophylactic measures,
- intermittent pneumatic compression device identification (eg, serial or biomedical number) and settings, and
- results of a patient skin assessment for mechanical prophylactic measures.

[Recommendation]

Miller[294] conducted an audit of graduated compression use in surgical patients (N = 80) at a teaching hospital in Australia. Limb measurement, stocking size, and patient education were not documented for any patient. Assessment for DVT risk factors was documented for 17.5% of patients and daily skin assessment was recorded for 29% of patients. The author recommended using a documentation tool to ensure consistency of VTE risk assessment, assessment for contraindications to graduated compression stockings, patient education, and monitoring of patients wearing stockings for complications and compliance.

7. Education

7.1 Provide initial and ongoing education and competency verification activities related to VTE prevention. *[Recommendation]*

Initial and ongoing education of perioperative personnel facilitates the development of knowledge, skills, and attitudes that affect safe patient care. It is the responsibility of the health care organization to provide initial and ongoing education and to verify the competency of its personnel[283]; however, the primary responsibility for maintaining ongoing competency remains with the individual.[295]

Competency verification activities provide a mechanism for competency documentation and help verify that personnel understand the principles and processes necessary for safe patient care.

Ongoing development of knowledge and skills and documentation of personnel participation is a regulatory requirement[284-287] and an accreditation standard for both hospitals[296,297] and ambulatory settings.[297-300]

7.2 Establish education and competency verification activities for personnel and determine intervals for education and competency verification related to VTE prevention.[47] *[Recommendation]*

Providing education and verifying competency assists in developing knowledge and skills that may improve compliance with the VTE protocol and thus may reduce the patient's risk for VTE. In a systematic review with meta-analysis, Kahn et al[47] found that educational interventions to improve use of VTE prophylaxis significantly improved the quality of prophylaxis, especially when combined with other interventions as part of a multifaceted systems approach.

Education and competency verification needs and intervals are unique to the facility or health care organization and to its personnel and processes.

7.2.1 Include the following in education and competency verification activities related to VTE prevention:
- the pathophysiology of VTE formation;
- VTE protocol and updates;
- assessment for VTE risk factors, including patient- and procedure-specific risk factors;
- manufacturers' instructions for use and sizing of graduated compression stockings;
- manufacturers' instructions for use and sizing of intermittent pneumatic compression devices;
- contraindications and adverse effects of mechanical prophylaxis;
- the importance of compliance with mechanical prophylaxis;
- contraindications and adverse effects of pharmacologic prophylaxis; and
- the importance of patient education on prevention of VTE and prescribed prophylactic measures.

[Recommendation]

8. Quality

8.1 The health care organization's quality management program should evaluate the outcomes of VTE prophylaxis and protocol compliance. *[Recommendation]*

Quality assurance and performance improvement programs can facilitate the identification of problem areas and assist personnel in evaluating and improving the quality of patient care and formulating plans for corrective action. These programs provide data that may be used to determine whether an individual organization is within benchmark goals, and if not, to identify areas that may require corrective action. A quality management program provides a mechanism to evaluate effectiveness of processes, including processes in the VTE prevention protocol.

Collecting data to monitor and improve patient care, treatment, and services is a regulatory requirement[284-287] and an accreditation standard for both hospitals[301,302] and ambulatory settings.[302-306]

8.2 Include the following in the quality assurance and performance improvement program for VTE prevention:
- monitoring the rate of perioperative venous thromboembolism, including DVT and PE[4,307,308];
- assessing compliance with prophylaxis according to the health care organization's VTE prevention protocol[4];
- addressing barriers to compliance with prophylaxis, including complications from prophylaxis use[4];
- identifying common failure modes in VTE prevention processes[4]; and
- providing ongoing evaluation, feedback to perioperative team members, and refinement of the VTE protocol as needed.[4]

[Recommendation]

Editor's note: ERAS (Enhanced Recovery After Surgery) is a registered trademark of the ERAS Society, Stockholm, Sweden.

Glossary

Atheroembolism: A cholesterol embolism, with or without calcified matter, originating from an atheroma of the aorta or other diseased artery.

Calciphylaxis: A condition of induced systemic hypersensitivity in which tissues respond to challenging agents with local calcification.

Proximal indentation: An indentation of the proximal calf from graduated compression stockings, creating a reverse gradient.

Reverse gradient: A condition in which proximal pressures from graduated compression stockings are higher than distal pressures, causing the advantageous pressure gradient for venous thromboembolism to reverse, which compromises venous return and increases the risk for venous thromboembolism. Synonym: tourniquet effect.

Thrombophilia: A condition in which the blood coagulates faster than normal.

References

1. Venous thromboembolism (blood clots). Centers for Disease Control and Prevention. https://www.cdc.gov/ncbddd/dvt/index.html. Accessed August 24, 2017. [VA]

2. Gould MK, Garcia DA, Wren SM, et al. Prevention of VTE in nonorthopedic surgical patients: Antithrombotic Therapy and Prevention of Thrombosis, 9th ed: American College of Chest Physicians Evidence-Based Clinical Practice Guidelines. *Chest.* 2012;141(2 Suppl):e227S-e277S. [IVA]

3. Heit JA. Epidemiology of venous thromboembolism. *Nat Rev Cardiol.* 2015;12(8):464-474. [VB]

4. Maynard G. *Preventing Hospital-Associated Venous Thromboembolism: A Guide for Effective Quality Improvement.* 2nd ed. [AHRQ Publication No. 16-0001-EF]. Rockville, MD: Agency for Healthcare Research and Quality; 2016. https://www.ahrq.gov/sites/default/files/publications/files/vteguide.pdf. Accessed August 24, 2017. [VA]

5. Vekeman F, LaMori JC, Laliberté F, et al. Risks and cost burden of venous thromboembolism and bleeding for patients undergoing total hip or knee replacement in a managed-care population. *J Med Econ.* 2011;14(3):324-334. [IIIA]

6. Baser O, Supina D, Sengupta N, Wang L, Kwong L. Clinical and cost outcomes of venous thromboembolism in Medicare patients undergoing total hip replacement or total knee replacement surgery. *Curr Med Res Opin.* 2011;27(2):423-429. [IIIA]

7. Cohoon KP, Leibson CL, Ransom JE, et al. Direct medical costs attributable to venous thromboembolism among persons hospitalized for major operation: a population-based longitudinal study. *Surgery.* 2015;157(3):423-431. [IIIA]

8. Adams A. Proactivity in VTE prevention: a concept analysis. *Br J Nurs.* 2015;24(1):20-25. [VA]

9. Findlay J, Keogh M, Cooper L. Venous thromboembolism prophylaxis: the role of the nurse. *Br J Nurs.* 2010;19(16):1028-1032. [VB]

10. Frostick S. Pharmacological thromboprophylaxis and total hip or knee replacement. *Br J Nurs.* 2016;25(1):45-53. [VB]

11. McNamara SA. Prevention of venous thromboembolism. *AORN J.* 2014;99(5):642-647. [VB]

12. Collins R, MacLellan L, Gibbs H, MacLellan D, Fletcher J. Venous thromboembolism prophylaxis: the role of the nurse in changing practice and saving lives. *Aust J Adv Nurs.* 2010;27(3):83-89. [VA]

13. Smith T, Daniell H, Hing C. Upper extremity deep vein thrombosis in orthopaedic and trauma surgery: a systematic review. *Eur J Orthop Surg Traumatol.* 2011;21(2):79-85. [IIIB]

14. Desai K, Dinh TP, Chung S, Pierpont YN, Naidu DK, Payne WG. Upper extremity deep vein thrombosis with tourniquet use. *Int J Surg Case Rep.* 2015;6C:55-57. [VB]

15. Durant TJS, Swanson BT, Cote MP, Allen DA, Arciero RA, Mazzocca AD. Upper extremity deep venous thromboembolism following arthroscopic labral repair of the shoulder and biceps tenodesis: a case report. *Int J Sports Phys Ther.* 2014;9(3):377-382. [VB]

16. Garofalo R, Notarnicola A, Moretti L, Moretti B, Marini S, Castagna A. Deep vein thromboembolism after arthroscopy of the shoulder: two case reports and a review of the literature. *BMC Musculoskelet Disord.* 2010;11:65. [VB]

17. Oofuvong M, Oearsakul T, Chittithavorn V, Viboonjuntra P. Upper extremity deep vein thrombosis related to fatal massive pulmonary embolism after spinal surgery. *J Med Assoc Thai.* 2012;95(2):279-281. [VB]

18. Saleh H, Pennings A, Elmaraghy A. Venous thromboembolism after shoulder arthroplasty: a report of three cases. *Acta Orthop Traumatol Turc.* 2015;49(2):220-223. [VB]

19. Wood J, Halen JV, Samant S. Upper extremity deep vein thrombosis and pulmonary embolus after radial forearm free flap: a case report and literature review. *J Reconstr Microsurg.* 2014;30(4):275-278. [VB]

20. Yamamoto T, Tamai K, Akutsu M, Tomizawa K, Sukegawa T, Nohara Y. Pulmonary embolism after arthroscopic rotator cuff repair: a case report. *Case Rep Orthop.* 2013;2013:801752. [VB]

21. Parvizi J, Parmar R, Raphael IJ, Restrepo C, Rothman RH. Proximal deep venous thrombosis and pulmonary embolus following total joint arthroplasty. *J Arthroplasty.* 2014;29(9):1846-1848. [IIIA]

22. Bikdeli B, Sharif-Kashani B, Shahabi P, et al. Comparison of three risk assessment methods for venous thromboembolism prophylaxis. *Blood Coagul Fibrinolysis.* 2013;24(2):157-163. [IIIB]

23. Hewes PD, Hachey KJ, Zhang XW, et al. Evaluation of the Caprini model for venothromboembolism in esophagectomy patients. *Ann Thorac Surg.* 2015;100(6):2072-2078. [IIIB]

24. Lobastov K, Barinov V, Schastlivtsev I, Laberko L, Rodoman G, Boyarintsev V. Validation of the Caprini risk assessment model for venous thromboembolism in high-risk surgical patients in the background of standard prophylaxis. *J Vasc Surg.* 2016;4(2):153-160. [IIIB]

25. Pannucci CJ, Bailey SH, Dreszer G, et al. Validation of the Caprini risk assessment model in plastic and reconstructive surgery patients. *J Am Coll Surg.* 2011;212(1):105-112. [IIIB]

26. Pannucci CJ, Barta RJ, Portschy PR, et al. Assessment of postoperative venous thromboembolism risk in plastic surgery patients using the 2005 and 2010 Caprini risk score. *Plast Reconstr Surg.* 2012;130(2):343-353. [IIIB]

27. Pannucci CJ, Basta MN, Fischer JP, Kovach SJ. Creation and validation of a condition-specific venous thromboembolism risk assessment tool for ventral hernia repair. *Surgery.* 2015;158(5):1304-1313. [IIIA]

28. Pannucci CJ, Laird S, Dimick JB, Campbell DA, Henke PK. A validated risk model to predict 90-day VTE events in postsurgical patients. *Chest.* 2014;145(3):567-573. [IIIA]

29. Nam D, Nunley RM, Johnson SR, Keeney JA, Clohisy JC, Barrack RL. The effectiveness of a risk stratification protocol for thromboembolism prophylaxis after hip and knee arthroplasty. *J Arthroplasty.* 2016;31(6):1299-1306. [IIIA]

30. Shaikh M, Jeong HS, Mastro A, Davis K, Lysikowski J, Kenkel JM. Analysis of the American Society of Anesthesiologists physical status classification system and Caprini risk assessment model in predicting venous thromboembolic outcomes in plastic surgery patients. *Aesthet Surg J.* 2016;36(4):497-505. [IIIB]

31. Iorio ML, Venturi ML, Davison SP. Practical guidelines for venous thromboembolism chemoprophylaxis in elective plastic surgery. *Plast Reconstr Surg.* 2015;135(2):413-423. [IVC]

32. Cassidy MR, Rosenkranz P, McAneny D. Reducing postoperative venous thromboembolism complications with a standardized risk-stratified prophylaxis protocol and mobilization program. *J Am Coll Surg.* 2014;218(6):1095-1104. [VA]

33. Shah DR, Wang H, Bold RJ, et al. Nomograms to predict risk of in-hospital and post-discharge venous thromboembolism after abdominal and thoracic surgery: an American College of Surgeons National Surgical Quality Improvement Program analysis. *J Surg Res.* 2013;183(1):462-471. [IIIA]

34. Stroud W, Whitworth JM, Miklic M, et al. Validation of a venous thromboembolism risk assessment model in gynecologic oncology. *Gynecol Oncol.* 2014;134(1):160-163. [IIIB]

35. Goz V, McCarthy I, Weinreb JH, et al. Venous thromboembolic events after spinal fusion: which patients are at high risk? *J Bone Joint Surg Am.* 2014;96(11):936-942. [IIIA]

36. Cavazza S, Rainaldi MP, Adduci A, Palareti G. Thromboprophylaxis following cesarean delivery: one site prospective pilot study to evaluate the application of a risk score model. *Thromb Res.* 2012;129(1):28-31. [IIB]

37. Shuman AG, Hu HM, Pannucci CJ, Jackson CR, Bradford CR, Bahl V. Stratifying the risk of venous thromboembolism in otolaryngology. *Otolaryngol Head Neck Surg.* 2012;146(5):719-724. [IIIB]

38. Janus E, Bassi A, Jackson D, Nandurkar H, Yates M. Thromboprophylaxis use in medical and surgical inpatients and the impact of an electronic risk assessment tool as part of a multi-factorial intervention. A report on behalf of the elVis study investigators. *J Thromb Thrombolysis.* 2011;32(3):279-287. [IIIA]

39. Novis SJ, Havelka GE, Ostrowski D, et al. Prevention of thromboembolic events in surgical patients through the creation and implementation of a computerized risk assessment program. *J Vasc Surg.* 2010;51(3):648-654. [IIA]

40. Bahl V, Hu HM, Henke PK, Wakefield TW, Campbell DAJ, Caprini JA. A validation study of a retrospective venous thromboembolism risk scoring method. *Ann Surg.* 2010;251(2):344-350. [IIIA]

41. Connelly CR, Laird A, Barton JS, et al. A clinical tool for the prediction of venous thromboembolism in pediatric trauma patients. *JAMA Surg.* 2016;151(1):50-57. [IIIA]

42. Atchison CM, Arlikar S, Amankwah E, et al. Development of a new risk score for hospital-associated venous thromboembolism in noncritically ill children: findings from a large single-institutional case-control study. *J Pediatr.* 2014;165(4):793-798. [IIIA]

43. Prentiss AS. Early recognition of pediatric venous thromboembolism: a risk-assessment tool. *Am J Crit Care.* 2012;21(3):178-183. [IIIC]

44. Caprini JA. Identification of patient venous thromboembolism risk across the continuum of care. *Clin Appl Thromb Hemost.* 2011;17(6):590-599. [VA]

45. Caprini JA. Mechanical methods for thrombosis prophylaxis. *Clin Appl Thromb Hemost.* 2010;16(6):668-673. [VA]

46. Borab ZM, Lanni MA, Tecce MG, Pannucci CJ, Fischer JP. Use of computerized clinical decision support systems to prevent venous thromboembolism in surgical patients: a systematic review and meta-analysis. *JAMA Surg.* 2017;152(7):638-645. [IIIC]

47. Kahn SR, Morrison DR, Cohen JM, et al. Interventions for implementation of thromboprophylaxis in hospitalized medical and surgical patients at risk for venous thromboembolism. *Cochrane Database Syst Rev.* 2013;(7):CD008201. [IIA]

48. Venous thromboembolism: reducing the risk for patients in hospital. Clinical guideline. NICE: National Institute for Health and Care Excellence. http://www.nice.org.uk/guidance/cg92. Published January 2010. Updated June 2015. Accessed August 24, 2017. [IVA]

49. Farge D, Debourdeau P, Beckers M, et al. International clinical practice guidelines for the treatment and prophylaxis of venous thromboembolism in patients with cancer. *J Thromb Haemost.* 2013;11(1):56-70. [IVA]

50. Lyman GH, Bohlke K, Khorana AA, et al. Venous thromboembolism prophylaxis and treatment in patients with cancer: American Society of Clinical Oncology clinical practice guideline update 2014. *J Clin Oncol.* 2015;33(6):654-656. [IVA]

51. American Society for Metabolic and Bariatric Surgery Clinical Issues Committee. ASMBS updated position statement on prophylactic measures to reduce the risk of venous thromboembolism in bariatric surgery patients. *Surg Obes Relat Dis.* 2013;9(4):493-497. [IVC]

52. Hoefnagel D, Kwee LE, van Putten EHP, Kros JM, Dirven CMF, Dammers R. The incidence of postoperative thromboembolic complications following surgical resection of intracranial meningioma. A retrospective study of a large single center patient cohort. *Clin Neurol Neurosurg.* 2014;123:150-154. [IIIB]

53. Agarwal R, Hecht TEH, Lazo MC, Umscheid CA. Venous thromboembolism prophylaxis for patients undergoing bariatric surgery: a systematic review. *Surg Obes Relat Dis.* 2010; 6(2):213-220. [IIIB]

54. Pellino G, Sciaudone G, Candilio G, De Fatico GS, Canonico S, Selvaggi F. Predictors of venous thromboembolism after colorectal surgery in a single unit. *Acta Chir Belg.* 2015; 115(4):288-292. [IIIB]

55. Finks JF, English WJ, Carlin AM, et al. Predicting risk for venous thromboembolism with bariatric surgery: results from the Michigan Bariatric Surgery Collaborative. *Ann Surg.* 2012;255(6):1100-1104. [IIIA]

56. Stein PD, Matta F. Pulmonary embolism and deep venous thrombosis following bariatric surgery. *Obes Surg.* 2013;23(5):663-668. [IIIA]

57. Wang L, Pryor AD, Altieri MS, et al. Perioperative rates of deep vein thrombosis and pulmonary embolism in normal weight vs obese and morbidly obese surgical patients in the era post venous thromboembolism prophylaxis guidelines. *Am J Surg.* 2015;210(5):859-863. [IIIA]

58. Nwaogu I, Yan Y, Margenthaler JA, Myckatyn TM. Venous thromboembolism after breast reconstruction in patients undergoing breast surgery: an American College of Surgeons NSQIP analysis. *J Am Coll Surg.* 2015;220(5):886-893. [IIIA]

59. Parkin L, Sweetland S, Balkwill A, et al. Body mass index, surgery, and risk of venous thromboembolism in middle-aged women: a cohort study. *Circulation.* 2012;125(15):1897-1904. [IIIA]

60. Jamal MH, Corcelles R, Shimizu H, et al. Thromboembolic events in bariatric surgery: a large multi-institutional referral center experience. *Surg Endosc.* 2015;29(2):376-380. [IIIA]

61. Winegar DA, Sherif B, Pate V, DeMaria EJ. Venous thromboembolism after bariatric surgery performed by bariatric surgery center of excellence participants: analysis of the bariatric outcomes longitudinal database. *Surg Obes Relat Dis.* 2011; 7(2):181-188. [IIIA]

62. Becattini C, Agnelli G, Manina G, Noya G, Rondelli F. Venous thromboembolism after laparoscopic bariatric surgery for morbid obesity: clinical burden and prevention. *Surg Obes Relat Dis.* 2012;8(1):108-115. [IIIA]

63. Bartlett MA, Mauck KF, Daniels PR. Prevention of venous thromboembolism in patients undergoing bariatric surgery. *Vasc Health Risk Manag.* 2015;11:461-477. [IIIA]

64. Schoenfeld AJ, Herzog JP, Dunn JC, Bader JO, Belmont PJ Jr. Patient-based and surgical characteristics associated with the acute development of deep venous thrombosis and pulmonary embolism after spine surgery. *Spine.* 2013;38(21):1892-1898. [IIIA]

65. Swenson CW, Berger MB, Kamdar NS, Campbell DAJ, Morgan DM. Risk factors for venous thromboembolism after hysterectomy. *Obstet Gynecol.* 2015;125(5):1139-1144. [IIIA]

66. Wes AM, Wink JD, Kovach SJ, Fischer JP. Venous thromboembolism in body contouring: an analysis of 17,774 patients from the National Surgical Quality Improvement databases. *Plast Reconstr Surg.* 2015;135(6):972e-980e. [IIIA]

67. Anderson JAM, Weitz JI. Hypercoagulable states. *Crit Care Clin.* 2011;27(4):933-952. [VA]

68. Allen D, Sale G. Lower limb joint replacement in patients with a history of venous thromboembolism. *Bone Joint J.* 2014; 96-B(11):1515-1519. [IIIB]

69. Liem TK, Huynh TM, Moseley SE, et al. Symptomatic perioperative venous thromboembolism is a frequent complication in patients with a history of deep vein thrombosis. *J Vasc Surg.* 2010;52(3):651-657. [IIIB]

70. Pedersen AB, Sorensen HT, Mehnert F, Overgaard S, Johnsen SP. Risk factors for venous thromboembolism in patients undergoing total hip replacement and receiving routine thromboprophylaxis. *J Bone Joint Surg Am.* 2010;92(12):2156-2164. [IIIA]

71. Qu H, Li Z, Zhai Z, et al. Predicting of venous thromboembolism for patients undergoing gynecological surgery. *Medicine.* 2015;94(39):e1653. [IIIB]

72. Testroote MJG, Wittens CHA. Prevention of venous thromboembolism in patients undergoing surgical treatment of varicose veins. *Phlebology.* 2013;28(Suppl 1):86-90. [IIIB]

73. Sutton PA, El-Dhuwaib Y, El-Duhwaib Y, Dyer J, Guy AJ. The incidence of post operative venous thromboembolism in patients undergoing varicose vein surgery recorded in hospital episode statistics. *Ann R Coll Surg Engl.* 2012;94(7):481-483. [IIIB]

74. Chen K, Yu GF, Huang JY, et al. Incidence and risk factors of early deep venous thrombosis after varicose vein surgery with routine use of a tourniquet. *Thromb Res.* 2015;135(6):1052-1056. [IIIA]

75. Minami K, Iida M, Iida H. Case report: central venous catheterization via internal jugular vein with associated formation of perioperative venous thrombosis during surgery in the prone position. *J Anesth.* 2012;26(3):464-466. [VB]

76. Smith BR, Diniz S, Stamos M, Nguyen NT. Deep venous thrombosis after general surgical operations at a university hospital: two-year data from the ACS NSQIP. *Arch Surg.* 2011;146(12):1424-1427. [IIIB]

77. Wang TF, Wong CA, Milligan PE, Thoelke MS, Woeltje KF, Gage BF. Risk factors for inpatient venous thromboembolism despite thromboprophylaxis. *Thromb Res.* 2014;133(1):25-29. [IIIB]

78. Holley AB, Petteys S, Mitchell JD, et al. Venous thromboembolism prophylaxis for patients receiving regional anesthesia following injury in Iraq and Afghanistan. *J Trauma Acute Care Surg.* 2014;76(1):152-159. [IIIB]

79. Dahl OE, Harenberg J, Wexels F, Preissner KT. Arterial and venous thrombosis following trauma and major orthopedic surgery: molecular mechanisms and strategies for intervention. *Semin Thromb Hemost.* 2015;41(2):141-145. [VA]

80. Allen CJ, Murray CR, Meizoso JP, et al. Risk factors for venous thromboembolism after pediatric trauma. *J Pediatr Surg.* 2016;51(1):168-171. [IIIA]

81. Matsumoto S, Suda K, Iimoto S, et al. Prospective study of deep vein thrombosis in patients with spinal cord injury not receiving anticoagulant therapy. *Spinal Cord.* 2015; 53(4):306-309. [IIIB]

82. Giorgi Pierfranceschi M, Donadini MP, Dentali F, et al. The short- and long-term risk of venous thromboembolism

in patients with acute spinal cord injury: a prospective cohort study. *Thromb Haemost.* 2013;109(1):34-38. [IIB]

83. Hunt BJ. Venous thromboembolism and thrombophilia testing. *Medicine (United Kingdom).* 2013;41(4):234-237. [VB]

84. Banks-Gonzales V, Ruppert SD. Thrombophilia and hypercoagulation: risk assessment and screening. *J Nurse Pract.* 2012;8(8):649-655. [VA]

85. Committee on Practice Bulletins—Gynecology, American College of Obstetricians and Gynecologists. ACOG Practice Bulletin No. 84: Prevention of deep vein thrombosis and pulmonary embolism. *Obstet Gynecol.* 2007;110(2 Pt 1):429-440. [IVC]

86. Amar S, Van Boven M, Rooijakkers H, Momeni M. Massive postoperative pulmonary embolism in a young woman using oral contraceptives: the value of a preoperative anesthetic consult. *Acta Anaesthesiol Belg.* 2014;65(2):73-75. [VA]

87. Barsoum MK, Heit JA, Ashrani AA, Leibson CL, Petterson TM, Bailey KR. Is progestin an independent risk factor for incident venous thromboembolism? A population-based case-control study. *Thromb Res.* 2010;126(5):373-378. [IIIA]

88. Paresi RJ Jr, Myers RS, Matarasso A. Contraceptive vaginal rings: do they pose an increased risk of venous thromboembolism in aesthetic surgery? *Aesthet Surg J.* 2015;35(6):721-727. [VB]

89. Alaia MJ, Zuskov A, Davidovitch RI. Contralateral deep venous thrombosis after hip arthroscopy. *Orthopedics.* 2011; 34(10):e674-e677. [VB]

90. Zeng Y, Shen B, Yang J, Zhou Z, Kang P, Pei F. Preoperative comorbidities as potential risk factors for venous thromboembolism after joint arthroplasty: a systematic review and meta-analysis of cohort and case-control studies. *J Arthroplasty.* 2014;29(12):2430-2438. [IIIA]

91. Markovic-Denic L, Zivkovic K, Lesic A, Bumbasirevic V, Dubljanin-Raspopovic E, Bumbasirevic M. Risk factors and distribution of symptomatic venous thromboembolism in total hip and knee replacements: prospective study. *Int Orthop.* 2012;36(6):1299-1305. [IIIB]

92. Singh JA, Jensen MR, Harmsen WS, Gabriel SE, Lewallen DG. Cardiac and thromboembolic complications and mortality in patients undergoing total hip and total knee arthroplasty. *Ann Rheum Dis.* 2011;70(12):2082-2088. [IIIB]

93. Haskins IN, Amdur R, Sarani B, Vaziri K. Congestive heart failure is a risk factor for venous thromboembolism in bariatric surgery. *Surg Obes Relat Dis.* 2015;11(5):1140-1145. [IIIA]

94. Kapoor A, Labonte AJ, Winter MR, et al. Risk of venous thromboembolism after total hip and knee replacement in older adults with comorbidity and co-occurring comorbidities in the Nationwide Inpatient Sample (2003-2006). *BMC Geriatrics.* 2010;10:63. [IIIB]

95. Masoomi H, Buchberg B, Reavis KM, Mills SD, Stamos M, Nguyen NT. Factors predictive of venous thromboembolism in bariatric surgery. *Am Surg.* 2011;77(10):1403-1406. [IIIB]

96. Gephart MGH, Zygourakis CC, Arrigo RT, Kalanithi PSA, Lad SP, Boakye M. Venous thromboembolism after thoracic/thoracolumbar spinal fusion. *World Neurosurg.* 2012;78(5):545-552. [IIIA]

97. Huang L, Li J, Jiang Y. Association between hypertension and deep vein thrombosis after orthopedic surgery: a meta-analysis. *Eur J Med Res.* 2016;21(1):13. [IIIC]

98. Delos D, Rodeo SA. Venous thrombosis after arthroscopic shoulder surgery: pacemaker leads as a possible cause: pacemaker leads as a possible cause. *HSS J.* 2011;7(3):282-285. [VB]

99. Barbot M, Daidone V, Zilio M, et al. Perioperative thromboprophylaxis in Cushing's disease: what we did and what we are doing? *Pituitary.* 2015;18(4):487-493. [IIIA]

100. Manetti L, Bogazzi F, Giovannetti C, et al. Changes in coagulation indexes and occurrence of venous thromboembolism in patients with Cushing's syndrome: results from a prospective study before and after surgery. *Eur J Endocrinol.* 2010;163(5):783-791. [IIIB]

101. Masoomi H, Paydar KZ, Wirth GA, Aly A, Kobayashi MR, Evans GRD. Predictive risk factors of venous thromboembolism in autologous breast reconstruction surgery. *Ann Plast Surg.* 2014;72(1):30-33. [IIIA]

102. Monn MF, Hui X, Lau BD, et al. Infection and venous thromboembolism in patients undergoing colorectal surgery: what is the relationship? *Dis Colon Rectum.* 2014;57(4):497-505. [IIIA]

103. Baker D, Sherrod B, McGwin GJ, Ponce B, Gilbert S. Complications and 30-day outcomes associated with venous thromboembolism in the pediatric orthopaedic surgical population. *J Am Acad Orthop Surg.* 2016;24(3):196-206. [IIIA]

104. Barmparas G, Fierro N, Lamb AW, et al. Clostridium difficile increases the risk for venous thromboembolism. *Am J Surg.* 2014;208(5):703-709. [IIIA]

105. Donze JD, Ridker PM, Finlayson SRG, Bates DW. Impact of sepsis on risk of postoperative arterial and venous thromboses: large prospective cohort study. *BMJ.* 2014;349:g5334. [IIIA]

106. Hatch Q, Nelson D, Martin M, et al. Can sepsis predict deep venous thrombosis in colorectal surgery? *Am J Surg.* 2016;211(1):53-58. [IIIA]

107. Albayati MA, Grover SP, Saha P, Lwaleed BA, Modarai B, Smith A. Postsurgical inflammation as a causative mechanism of venous thromboembolism. *Semin Thromb Hemostas.* 2015;41(6):615-620. [VA]

108. Wilson MZ, Connelly TM, Tinsley A, Hollenbeak CS, Koltun WA, Messaris E. Ulcerative colitis is associated with an increased risk of venous thromboembolism in the postoperative period: the results of a matched cohort analysis. *Ann Surg.* 2015;261(6):1160-1166. [IIIA]

109. Kaplan GG, Lim A, Seow CH, et al. Colectomy is a risk factor for venous thromboembolism in ulcerative colitis. *World J Gastroenterol.* 2015;21(4):1251-1260. [IIIB]

110. Merrill A, Millham F. Increased risk of postoperative deep vein thrombosis and pulmonary embolism in patients with inflammatory bowel disease: a study of National Surgical Quality Improvement Program patients. *Arch Surg.* 2012;147(2):120-124. [IIIA]

111. Moghadamyeghaneh Z, Hanna MH, Carmichael JC, Nguyen NT, Stamos MJ. A nationwide analysis of postoperative deep vein thrombosis and pulmonary embolism in colon and rectal surgery. *J Gastrointest Surg.* 2014;18(12):2169-2177. [IIIA]

112. Colorectal Writing Group for Surgical Care and Outcomes Assessment Program-Comparative Effectiveness

Research Translation Network (SCOAP-CERTAIN) Collaborative; Nelson DW, Simianu VV, et al. Thromboembolic complications and prophylaxis patterns in colorectal surgery. *JAMA Surg.* 2015;150(8):712-720. [IIIA]

113. Mameli A, Marongiu F. Thromboembolic disease in patients with rheumatoid arthritis undergoing joint arthroplasty: update on prophylaxes. *World J Orthop.* 2014;5(5):645-652. [IIIB]

114. Ahlehoff O, Gislason GH, Lindhardsen J, et al. Psoriasis carries an increased risk of venous thromboembolism: a Danish nationwide cohort study. *Plos One.* 2011;6(3):e18125. [IIIA]

115. James A; Committee on Practice Bulletins—Obstetrics. Practice Bulletin No. 123: Thromboembolism in pregnancy. *Obstet Gynecol.* 2011;118(3):718-729. [IVB]

116. D'Alton ME, Friedman AM, Smiley RM, et al. National partnership for maternal safety: consensus bundle on venous thromboembolism. *Obstet Gynecol.* 2016;128(4):688-698. [IVB]

117. Tepper NK, Boulet SL, Whiteman MK, et al. Postpartum venous thromboembolism: incidence and risk factors. *Obstet Gynecol.* 2014;123(5):987-996. [IIIA]

118. Musallam KM, Rosendaal FR, Zaatari G, et al. Smoking and the risk of mortality and vascular and respiratory events in patients undergoing major surgery. *JAMA Surg.* 2013;148(8):755-762. [IIIA]

119. Sweetland S, Parkin L, Balkwill A, et al. Smoking, surgery, and venous thromboembolism risk in women: United Kingdom cohort study. *Circulation.* 2013;127(12):1276-1282. [IIIA]

120. Deflandre E, Degey S, Opsomer N, Brichant J, Joris J. Obstructive sleep apnea and smoking as a risk factor for venous thromboembolism events: review of the literature on the common pathophysiological mechanisms. *Obes Surg.* 2016;26(3):640-648. [VB]

121. Kantar RS, Haddad AG, Tamim H, Jamali F, Taher AT. Venous thromboembolism and preoperative steroid use: analysis of the NSQIP database to evaluate risk in surgical patients. *Eur J Intern Med.* 2015;26(7):528-533. [IIIA]

122. Greaves SW, Holubar SD. Preoperative hospitalization is independently associated with increased risk for venous thromboembolism in patients undergoing colorectal surgery: a National Surgical Quality Improvement Program database study. *Dis Colon Rectum.* 2015;58(8):782-791. [IIIA]

123. Lieber BA, Han J, Appelboom G, et al. Association of steroid use with deep venous thrombosis and pulmonary embolism in neurosurgical patients: a national database analysis. *World Neurosurg.* 2016;89:126-132. [IIIA]

124. Rolston JD, Han SJ, Bloch O, Parsa AT. What clinical factors predict the incidence of deep venous thrombosis and pulmonary embolism in neurosurgical patients? *J Neurosurg.* 2014;121(4):908-918. [IIIA]

125. Mueller MG, Pilecki MA, Catanzarite T, Jain U, Kim JYS, Kenton K. Venous thromboembolism in reconstructive pelvic surgery. *Am J Obstet Gynecol.* 2014;211(5):552.e1-552.e6. [IIIA]

126. Miller TJ, Jeong HS, Davis K, et al. Evaluation of the American Society of Anesthesiologists physical status classification system in risk assessment for plastic and reconstructive surgery patients. *Aesthet Surg J.* 2014;34(3):448-456. [IIIB]

127. Ghazi L, Schwann TA, Engoren MC, Habib RH. Role of blood transfusion product type and amount in deep vein thrombosis after cardiac surgery. *Thromb Res.* 2015;136(6):1204-1210. [IIIB]

128. Tollefson MK, Karnes RJ, Rangel L, Carlson R, Boorjian SA. Blood type, lymphadenectomy and blood transfusion predict venous thromboembolic events following radical prostatectomy with pelvic lymphadenectomy. *J Urol.* 2014;191(3):646-651. [IIIA]

129. Xenos ES, Vargas HD, Davenport DL. Association of blood transfusion and venous thromboembolism after colorectal cancer resection. *Thromb Res.* 2012;129(5):568-572. [IIIA]

130. Yang S, Ding W, Yang D, et al. Prevalence and risk factors of deep vein thrombosis in patients undergoing lumbar interbody fusion surgery: a single-center cross-sectional study. *Medicine.* 2015;94(48):e2205. [IIIB]

131. Turley RS, Reddy SK, Shortell CK, Clary BM, Scarborough JE. Venous thromboembolism after hepatic resection: analysis of 5,706 patients. *J Gastrointest Surg.* 2012;16(9):1705-1714. [IIIA]

132. Wang JK, Boorjian SA, Frank I, et al. Non-O blood type is associated with an increased risk of venous thromboembolism after radical cystectomy. *Urology.* 2014;83(1):140-145. [IIIB]

133. Ha LP, Arrendondo M. Fatal venous thromboembolism after splenectomy: pathogenesis and management. *J Am Osteopath Assoc.* 2012;112(5):291-300. [VB]

134. Abel EJ, Wong K, Sado M, et al. Surgical operative time increases the risk of deep venous thrombosis and pulmonary embolism in robotic prostatectomy. *JSLS.* 2014;18(2):282-287. [IIIA]

135. Kim JYS, Khavanin N, Rambachan A, et al. Surgical duration and risk of venous thromboembolism. *JAMA Surg.* 2015;150(2):110-117. [IIIA]

136. Kimmell KT, Walter KA. Risk factors for venous thromboembolism in patients undergoing craniotomy for neoplastic disease. *J Neurooncol.* 2014;120(3):567-573. [IIIA]

137. Kim BD, Hsu WK, De Oliveira GSJ, Saha S, Kim JYS. Operative duration as an independent risk factor for postoperative complications in single-level lumbar fusion: an analysis of 4588 surgical cases. *Spine.* 2014;39(6):510-520. [IIIA]

138. Chan MM, Hamza N, Ammori BJ. Duration of surgery independently influences risk of venous thromboembolism after laparoscopic bariatric surgery. *Surg Obes Relat Dis.* 2013;9(1):88-93. [IIIA]

139. Montoya TI, Leclaire EL, Oakley SH, et al. Venous thromboembolism in women undergoing pelvic reconstructive surgery with mechanical prophylaxis alone. *Int Urogynecol J.* 2014;25(7):921-926. [IIIA]

140. Leung ASM, Fok MWM, Fung BKK. Fatal bilateral lower-limb deep vein thrombosis and pulmonary embolism following single digit replantation. *Hong Kong Med J.* 2015;21(3):283-285. [VB]

141. Guideline for positioning the patient. In: *Guidelines for Perioperative Practice.* Denver, CO: AORN, Inc; 2017:e1-e72. [IVA]

142. Guideline for care of patients undergoing pneumatic tourniquet-assisted procedures. In: *Guidelines for Perioperative Practice.* Denver, CO: AORN, Inc; 2017:157-182. [IVA]

143. Falck-Ytter Y, Francis CW, Johanson NA, et al. Prevention of VTE in orthopedic surgery patients: antithrombotic therapy and prevention of thrombosis, 9th ed: American College of Chest Physicians Evidence-Based Clinical Practice Guidelines. *Chest.* 2012;141(2 Suppl):e278S-e325S. [IVA]

144. Mont MA, Jacobs JJ, Boggio LN, et al. Preventing venous thromboembolic disease in patients undergoing elective hip and knee arthroplasty. *J Am Acad Orthop Surg.* 2011;19(12):768-776. [IVA]

145. Januel J, Chen G, Ruffieux C, et al. Symptomatic in-hospital deep vein thrombosis and pulmonary embolism following hip and knee arthroplasty among patients receiving recommended prophylaxis: a systematic review. *JAMA.* 2012;307(3):294-303. [IIIA]

146. Zhang J, Chen Z, Zheng J, Breusch SJ, Tian J. Risk factors for venous thromboembolism after total hip and total knee arthroplasty: a meta-analysis. *Arch Orthop Trauma Surg.* 2015;135(6):759-772. [IIIA]

147. Lewis CG, Inneh IA, Schutzer SF, Grady-Benson J. Evaluation of the first-generation AAOS clinical guidelines on the prophylaxis of venous thromboembolic events in patients undergoing total joint arthroplasty: experience with 3289 patients from a single institution. *J Bone Joint Surg Am.* 2014;96(16):1327-1332. [IIB]

148. Steele KE, Schweitzer MA, Prokopowicz G, et al. The long-term risk of venous thromboembolism following bariatric surgery. *Obes Surg.* 2011;21(9):1371-1376. [IIIA]

149. Di Nisio M, Peinemann F, Porreca E, Rutjes AWS. Primary prophylaxis for venous thromboembolism in patients undergoing cardiac or thoracic surgery. *Cochrane Database Syst Rev.* 2015;(6):CD009658. [IB]

150. Ho KM, Bham E, Pavey W. Incidence of venous thromboembolism and benefits and risks of thromboprophylaxis after cardiac surgery: a systematic review and meta-analysis. *J Am Heart Assoc.* 2015;4(10):e002652. [IIIA]

151. Aziz F, Patel M, Ortenzi G, Reed AB. Incidence of postoperative deep venous thrombosis is higher among cardiac and vascular surgery patients as compared with general surgery patients. *Ann Vasc Surg.* 2015;29(4):661-669. [IIIA]

152. Ramanan B, Gupta PK, Sundaram A, et al. In-hospital and postdischarge venous thromboembolism after vascular surgery. *J Vasc Surg.* 2013;57(6):1589-1596. [IIIA]

153. Scarborough JE, Cox MW, Mureebe L, Pappas TN, Shortell CK. A novel scoring system for predicting postoperative venous thromboembolic complications in patients after open aortic surgery. *J Am Coll Surg.* 2012;214(4):620-626. [IIIA]

154. Aloia TA, Geerts WH, Clary BM, et al. Venous thromboembolism prophylaxis in liver surgery. *J Gastrointest Surg.* 2016;20(1):221-229. [IVC]

155. Ejaz A, Spolverato G, Kim Y, et al. Defining incidence and risk factors of venous thromboembolism after hepatectomy. *J Gastrointest Surg.* 2014;18(6):1116-1124. [IIIA]

156. Newhook TE, Lapar DJ, Walters DM, et al. Impact of postoperative venous thromboembolism on postoperative morbidity, mortality, and resource utilization after hepatectomy. *Am Surg.* 2015;81(12):1216-1223. [IIIB]

157. Bouras G, Burns EM, Howell A, Bottle A, Athanasiou T, Darzi A. Risk of post-discharge venous thromboembolism and associated mortality in general surgery: a population-based cohort study using linked hospital and primary care data in England. *Plos One.* 2015;10(12):e0145759. [IIIA]

158. Humes DJ, Walker AJ, Hunt BJ, Sultan AA, Ludvigsson JF, West J. Risk of symptomatic venous thromboembolism following emergency appendicectomy in adults. *Br J Surg.* 2016;103(4):443-450. [IIIA]

159. Violette PD, Cartwright R, Briel M, Tikkinen KAO, Guyatt GH. Guideline of guidelines: thromboprophylaxis for urological surgery. *BJU Int.* 2016;118(3):351-358. [VA]

160. Tikkinen KAO, Agarwal A, Craigie S, et al. Systematic reviews of observational studies of risk of thrombosis and bleeding in urological surgery (ROTBUS): introduction and methodology. *Syst Rev.* 2014;3:150. [IIIB]

161. Tyson MD, Castle EP, Humphreys MR, Andrews PE. Venous thromboembolism after urological surgery. *J Urol.* 2014;192(3):793-797. [IIIA]

162. Salmaggi A, Simonetti G, Trevisan E, et al. Perioperative thromboprophylaxis in patients with craniotomy for brain tumours: a systematic review. *J Neurooncol.* 2013;113(2):293-303. [IB]

163. Harris DA, Lam S. Venous thromboembolism in the setting of pediatric traumatic brain injury. *J Neurosurg Pediatr.* 2014;13(4):448-455. [IIIA]

164. Algattas H, Kimmell KT, Vates GE, Jahromi BS. Analysis of venous thromboembolism risk in patients undergoing craniotomy. *World Neurosurg.* 2015;84(5):1372-1379. [IIIA]

165. Kimmell KT, Jahromi BS. Clinical factors associated with venous thromboembolism risk in patients undergoing craniotomy. *J Neurosurg.* 2015;122(5):1004-1011. [IIIA]

166. Sansone JM, del Rio AM, Anderson PA. The prevalence of and specific risk factors for venous thromboembolic disease following elective spine surgery. *J Bone Joint Surg Am.* 2010;92(2):304-313. [IIIA]

167. Oglesby M, Fineberg SJ, Patel AA, Pelton MA, Singh K. The incidence and mortality of thromboembolic events in cervical spine surgery. *Spine.* 2013;38(9):E521-E527. [IIIA]

168. Fineberg SJ, Oglesby M, Patel AA, Pelton MA, Singh K. The incidence and mortality of thromboembolic events in lumbar spine surgery. *Spine.* 2013;38(13):1154-1159. [IIIA]

169. Schairer WW, Pedtke AC, Hu SS. Venous thromboembolism after spine surgery. *Spine.* 2014;39(11):911-918. [IIIA]

170. Hohl JB, Lee JY, Rayappa SP, et al. Prevalence of venous thromboembolic events after elective major thoracolumbar degenerative spine surgery. *J Spinal Disord Tech.* 2015;28(5):E310-E315. [IIIA]

171. Cox JB, Weaver KJ, Neal DW, Jacob RP, Hoh DJ. Decreased incidence of venous thromboembolism after spine surgery with early multimodal prophylaxis: clinical article. *J Neurosurg Spine.* 2014;21(4):677-684. [IIIA]

172. Jain A, Karas DJ, Skolasky RL, Sponseller PD. Thromboembolic complications in children after spinal fusion surgery. *Spine.* 2014;39(16):1325-1329. [IIIA]

173. Barber EL, Neubauer NL, Gossett DR. Risk of venous thromboembolism in abdominal versus minimally invasive hysterectomy for benign conditions. *Am J Obstet Gynecol.* 2015;212(5):609.e1-609.e7. [IIIA]

174. Buchberg B, Masoomi H, Lusby K, et al. Incidence and risk factors of venous thromboembolism in colorectal surgery: does laparoscopy impart an advantage? *Arch Surg.* 2011;146(6):739-743. [IIIA]

175. Shapiro R, Vogel JD, Kiran RP. Risk of postoperative venous thromboembolism after laparoscopic and open colorectal surgery: an additional benefit of the minimally invasive approach? *Dis Colon Rectum.* 2011;54(12):1496-1502. [IIIA]

176. Cui G, Wang X, Yao W, Li H. Incidence of postoperative venous thromboembolism after laparoscopic versus open colorectal cancer surgery: a meta-analysis. *Surg Laparosc Endosc Percutan Tech.* 2013;23(2):128-134. [IA]

177. Xie YZ, Fang K, Ma WL, Shi ZH, Ren XQ. Risk of postoperative deep venous thrombosis in patients with colorectal cancer treated with open or laparoscopic colorectal surgery: a meta-analysis. *Indian J Cancer.* 2015;51(Suppl 2):e42-e44. [IB]

178. Autorino R, Zargar H, Butler S, Laydner H, Kaouk JH. Incidence and risk factors for 30-day readmission in patients undergoing nephrectomy procedures: a contemporary analysis of 5276 cases from the national surgical quality improvement program database. *Urology.* 2015;85(4):843-849. [IIIA]

179. Saad AN, Parina R, Chang D, Gosman AA. Risk of adverse outcomes when plastic surgery procedures are combined. *Plast Reconstr Surg.* 2014;134(6):1415-1422. [IIIA]

180. Fischer JP, Wes AM, Tuggle CT, Wu LC. Venous thromboembolism risk in mastectomy and immediate breast reconstruction: analysis of the 2005 to 2011 American College of Surgeons National Surgical Quality Improvement Program data sets. *Plast Reconstr Surg.* 2014;133(3):263e-273e. [IIIA]

181. Tran BH, Nguyen TJ, Hwang BH, et al. Risk factors associated with venous thromboembolism in 49,028 mastectomy patients. *Breast.* 2013;22(4):444-448. [IIIA]

182. Elboudwarej O, Patel JK, Liou F, et al. Risk of deep vein thrombosis and pulmonary embolism after heart transplantation: clinical outcomes comparing upper extremity deep vein thrombosis and lower extremity deep vein thrombosis. *Clin Transplant.* 2015;29(7):629-635. [IIIA]

183. Annamalai A, Kim I, Sundaram V, Klein A. Incidence and risk factors of deep vein thrombosis after liver transplantation. *Transplant Proc.* 2014;46(10):3564-3569. [IIIA]

184. Cherian TP, Chiu K, Gunson B, et al. Pulmonary thromboembolism in liver transplantation: a retrospective review of the first 25 years. *Transplant Int.* 2010;23(11):1113-1119. [IIIA]

185. Emuakhagbon V, Philips P, Agopian V, Kaldas FM, Jones CM. Incidence and risk factors for deep venous thrombosis and pulmonary embolus after liver transplantation. *Am J Surg.* 2016;211(4):768-771. [IIIA]

186. Alvarez-Alvarez RJ, Barge-Caballero E, Chavez-Leal SA, et al. Venous thromboembolism in heart transplant recipients: incidence, recurrence and predisposing factors. *J Heart Lung Transplant.* 2015;34(2):167-174. [IIIA]

187. Abualhassan N, Aljiffry M, Thalib L, Coussa R, Metrakos P, Hassanain M. Post-transplant venous thromboembolic events and their effect on graft survival. *Saudi J Kidney Dis Transpl.* 2015;26(1):1-5. [IIIB]

188. Salami A, Qureshi W, Kuriakose P, Moonka D, Yoshida A, Abouljoud M. Frequency and predictors of venous thromboembolism in orthotopic liver transplant recipients: a single-center retrospective review. *Transplant Proc.* 2013;45(1):315-319. [IIIB]

189. Verhave JC, Tagalakis V, Suissa S, Madore F, Hebert M, Cardinal H. The risk of thromboembolic events in kidney transplant patients. *Kidney Int.* 2014;85(6):1454-1460. [IIIB]

190. Ooi CY, Brandao LR, Zolpys L, et al. Thrombotic events after pediatric liver transplantation. *Pediatr Transplant.* 2010;14(4):476-482. [IIIB]

191. Saez-Gimenez B, Berastegui C, Loor K, et al. Deep vein thrombosis and pulmonary embolism after solid organ transplantation: an unresolved problem. *Transplant Rev.* 2015;29(2):85-92. [VB]

192. Arshad F, Lisman T, Porte RJ. Hypercoagulability as a contributor to thrombotic complications in the liver transplant recipient. *Liver Int.* 2013;33(6):820-827. [VB]

193. Fleischer AE, Abicht BP, Baker JR, Boffeli TJ, Jupiter DC, Schade VL. American College of Foot and Ankle Surgeons' clinical consensus statement: risk, prevention, and diagnosis of venous thromboembolism disease in foot and ankle surgery and injuries requiring immobilization. *J Foot Ankle Surg.* 2015;54(3):497-507. [IVB]

194. Calder JDF, Freeman R, Domeij-Arverud E, van Dijk CN, Ackermann PW. Meta-analysis and suggested guidelines for prevention of venous thromboembolism (VTE) in foot and ankle surgery. *Knee Surg Sports Traumatol Arthrosc.* 2016;24(4):1409-1420. [IIIA]

195. Mangwani J, Sheikh N, Cichero M, Williamson D. What is the evidence for chemical thromboprophylaxis in foot and ankle surgery? Systematic review of the English literature. *Foot.* 2015;25(3):173-178. [IIIB]

196. Barg A, Henninger HB, Hintermann B. Risk factors for symptomatic deep-vein thrombosis in patients after total ankle replacement who received routine chemical thromboprophylaxis. *J Bone Joint Surg Br.* 2011;93(7):921-927. [IIIA]

197. Basques BA, Miller CP, Golinvaux NS, Bohl DD, Grauer JN. Risk factors for thromboembolic events after surgery for ankle fractures. *Am J Orthop (Belle Mead NJ).* 2015;44(7):E220-E224. [IIIA]

198. Altintas F, Ozler T, Guven M, Ozkut AT, Ulucay C. Deep venous thrombosis and pulmonary embolism as rare complications after hallux valgus surgery: case report and literature review. *J Am Podiatr Med Assoc.* 2013;103(2):145-148. [VB]

199. Kadous A, Abdelgawad AA, Kanlic E. Deep venous thrombosis and pulmonary embolism after surgical treatment of ankle fractures: a case report and review of literature. *J Foot Ankle Surg.* 2012;51(4):457-463. [VB]

200. Makhdom AM, Garceau S, Dimentberg R. Fatal pulmonary embolism following Achilles tendon repair: a case report and a review of the literature. *Case Rep Orthop.* 2013;2013:401968. [VB]

201. Roberts DC, Warwick DJ. Venous thromboembolism following elbow, wrist and hand surgery: a review of the literature and prophylaxis guidelines. *J Hand Surg Br.* 2014;39(3):306-312. [VA]

202. Mathur M, Shafi I, Alkhouli M, Bashir R. Surgical hardware-related iatrogenic venous compression syndrome. *Vasc Med.* 2015;20(2):162-167. [VA]

203. Pannucci CJ, MacDonald JK, Ariyan S, et al. Benefits and risks of prophylaxis for deep venous thrombosis and pulmonary embolus in plastic surgery: a systematic review and meta-analysis of controlled trials and consensus conference. *Plast Reconstr Surg.* 2016;137(2):709-730. [IIIA]

204. Zareba P, Wu C, Agzarian J, Rodriguez D, Kearon C. Meta-analysis of randomized trials comparing combined compression and anticoagulation with either modality alone for prevention of venous thromboembolism after surgery. *Br J Surg.* 2014;101(9):1053-1062. [IA]

205. Gustafsson UO, Scott MJ, Schwenk W, et al. Guidelines for perioperative care in elective colonic surgery: Enhanced Recovery After Surgery (ERAS®) Society recommendations. *Clin Nutr.* 2012;31(6):783-800. [IVA]

206. Nelson G, Altman AD, Nick A, et al. Guidelines for postoperative care in gynecologic/oncology surgery: Enhanced Recovery After Surgery (ERAS®) Society recommendations—part II. *Gynecol Oncol.* 2016;140(2):323-332. [IVA]

207. Nygren J, Thacker J, Carli F, et al. Guidelines for perioperative care in elective rectal/pelvic surgery: Enhanced Recovery After Surgery (ERAS®) Society recommendations. *Clin Nutr.* 2012;31(6):801-816. [IVA]

208. Skillman J, Thomas S. An audit of pressure sores caused by intermittent compression devices used to prevent venous thromboembolism. *J Perioper Pract.* 2011;21(12):418-420. [VB]

209. Huh J, Cho YB, Yang MK, Yoo YK, Kim DK. What influence does intermittent pneumatic compression of the lower limbs intraoperatively have on core hypothermia? *Surg Endosc.* 2013;27(6):2087-2093. [IC]

210. Boelig MM, Streiff MB, Hobson DB, Kraus PS, Pronovost PJ, Haut ER. Are sequential compression devices commonly associated with in-hospital falls? A myth-busters review using the patient safety net database. *J Patient Saf.* 2011;7(2):77-79. [IIIA]

211. Eppsteiner RW, Shin JJ, Johnson J, van Dam RM. Mechanical compression versus subcutaneous heparin therapy in postoperative and posttrauma patients: a systematic review and meta-analysis. *World J Surg.* 2010;34(1):10-19. [IB]

212. Pavon JM, Adam SS, Razouki ZA, et al. Effectiveness of intermittent pneumatic compression devices for venous thromboembolism prophylaxis in high-risk surgical patients: a systematic review. *J Arthroplasty.* 2016;31(2):524-532. [IIIA]

213. Arverud E, Azevedo J, Labruto F, Ackermann PW. Adjuvant compression therapy in orthopaedic surgery-an evidence-based review. *Eur Orthop Traumatol.* 2013;4(1):49-57. [VB]

214. Feng JP, Xiong YT, Fan ZQ, Yan LJ, Wang JY, Gu ZJ. Efficacy of intermittent pneumatic compression for venous thromboembolism prophylaxis in patients undergoing gynecologic surgery: a systematic review and meta-analysis. *Oncotarget.* 2017;8(12):20371-20379. [IIIB]

215. O'Connell S, Bashar K, Broderick BJ, et al. The use of intermittent pneumatic compression in orthopedic and neurosurgical postoperative patients. A systematic review and meta-analysis. *Ann Surg.* 2016;263(5):888-899. [IIIA]

216. Sadaghianloo N, Dardik A. The efficacy of intermittent pneumatic compression in the prevention of lower extremity deep venous thrombosis. *J Vasc Surg.* 2016;4(2):248-256. [IIIB]

217. Kakkos SK, Warwick D, Nicolaides AN, Stansby GP, Tsolakis IA. Combined (mechanical and pharmacological) modalities for the prevention of venous thromboembolism in joint replacement surgery. *J Bone Joint Surg Br.* 2012;94(6):729-734. [IIB]

218. Sobieraj DM, Coleman CI, Tongbram V, et al. Comparative effectiveness of combined pharmacologic and mechanical thromboprophylaxis versus either method alone in major orthopedic surgery: a systematic review and meta-analysis. *Pharmacotherapy.* 2013;33(3):275-283. [IIB]

219. Parry K, Sadeghi A, van der Horst S, Westerink J, Ruurda JP, van Hillegersberg R. Intermittent pneumatic compression in combination with low-molecular weight heparin in the prevention of venous thromboembolic events in esophageal cancer surgery. *J Surg Oncol.* 2017;115(2):181-185. [IIIB]

220. Delos Reyes AP, Partsch H, Mosti G, Obi A, Lurie F. Report from the 2013 meeting of the international compression club on advances and challenges of compression therapy. *J Vasc Surg Venous Lymphat Disord.* 2014;2(4):469-476. [VA]

221. Larkin BG, Mitchell KM, Petrie K. Translating evidence to practice for mechanical venous thromboembolism prophylaxis. *AORN J.* 2012;96(5):513-527. [VB]

222. Committee opinion no 610: chronic antithrombotic therapy and gynecologic surgery. *Obstet Gynecol.* 2014;124(4):856-862. [IVC]

223. Rahn DD, Mamik MM, Sanses TVD, et al. Venous thromboembolism prophylaxis in gynecologic surgery: a systematic review. *Obstet Gynecol.* 2011;118(5):1111-1125. [IIIA]

224. Gao J, Zhang Z, Li Z, et al. Two mechanical methods for thromboembolism prophylaxis after gynaecological pelvic surgery: a prospective, randomised study. *Chin Med J (Engl).* 2012;125(23):4259-4263. [IB]

225. Morris RJ, Woodcock JP. Intermittent pneumatic compression or graduated compression stockings for deep vein thrombosis prophylaxis? A systematic review of direct clinical comparisons. *Ann Surg.* 2010;251(3):393-396. [IIIB]

226. Zhao JM, He ML, Xiao ZM, Li TS, Wu H, Jiang H. Different types of intermittent pneumatic compression devices for preventing venous thromboembolism in patients after total hip replacement. *Cochrane Database Syst Rev.* 2012;11:CD009543. [IIC]

227. Pour AE, Keshavarzi NR, Purtill JJ, Sharkey PF, Parvizi J. Is venous foot pump effective in prevention of thromboembolic disease after joint arthroplasty: a meta-analysis. *J Arthroplasty.* 2013;28(3):410-417. [IIA]

228. Dohm M, Williams KM, Novotny T. Micro-mobile foot compression device compared with pneumatic compression device. *Clin Orthop Relat Res.* 2011;469(6):1692-1700. [IB]

229. Pitto RP, Koh CK. Flowtron foot-pumps for prevention of venous thromboembolism in total hip and knee replacement. *J Orthop.* 2015;12(1):35-38. [IIIA]

230. Sakai T, Izumi M, Kumagai K, et al. Effects of a foot pump on the incidence of deep vein thrombosis after total knee arthroplasty in patients given edoxaban: a randomized controlled study. *Medicine.* 2016;95(1):e2247. [IB]

231. Wickham N, Gallus AS, Walters BNJ, Wilson A; NHMRC VTE Prevention Guideline Adaptation Committee. Prevention of venous thromboembolism in patients admitted to Australian hospitals: summary of National Health and Medical Research Council clinical practice guideline. *Intern Med J.* 2012;42(6):698-708. [IVA]

232. Hou H, Yao Y, Zheng K, et al. Does intermittent pneumatic compression increase the risk of pulmonary embolism in deep venous thrombosis after joint surgery? *Blood Coagul Fibrinolysis.* 2016;27(3):246-251. [IIIB]

233. Guideline for prevention of unplanned patient hypothermia. In: *Guidelines for Perioperative Practice.* Denver, CO: AORN, Inc; 2017:567-590. [IVA]

234. Guideline for sterile technique. In: *Guidelines for Perioperative Practice.* Denver, CO: AORN, Inc; 2017:75-104. [IVA]

235. Levy YD, Hardwick ME, Copp SN, Rosen AS, Colwell CWJ. Thrombosis incidence in unilateral vs simultaneous bilateral total knee arthroplasty with compression device prophylaxis. *J Arthroplasty.* 2013;28(3):474-478. [IIIB]

236. Morris JK, Fincham BM. Intermittent pneumatic compression for venous thromboembolism prophylaxis in total knee arthroplasty. *Orthopedics.* 2012;35(12):e1716-e1721. [IIB]

237. Guideline for minimally invasive surgery. In: *Guidelines for Perioperative Practice.* Denver, CO: AORN, Inc; 2017:629-658. [IVA]

238. Frisius J, Ebeling M, Karst M, et al. Prevention of venous thromboembolic complications with and without intermittent pneumatic compression in neurosurgical cranial procedures using intraoperative magnetic resonance imaging. A retrospective analysis. *Clin Neurol Neurosurg.* 2015;133:46-54. [IIIB]

239. Maybody M, Taslakian B, Durack JC, et al. Feasibility of intermittent pneumatic compression for venous thromboembolism prophylaxis during magnetic resonance imaging-guided interventions. *Eur J Radiol.* 2015;84(4):668-670. [IIIB]

240. Ritsema DF, Watson JM, Stiteler AP, Nguyen MM. Sequential compression devices in postoperative urologic patients: an observational trial and survey study on the influence of patient and hospital factors on compliance. *BMC Urol.* 2013;13:20. [IIIB]

241. Obi AT, Alvarez R, Reames BN, et al. A prospective evaluation of standard versus battery-powered sequential compression devices in postsurgical patients. *Am J Surg.* 2015;209(4):675-681. [IB]

242. Sobieraj-Teague M, Hirsh J, Yip G, et al. Randomized controlled trial of a new portable calf compression device (Venowave) for prevention of venous thrombosis in high-risk neurosurgical patients. *J Thromb Haemost.* 2012;10(2):229-235. [IB]

243. Colwell CWJ, Froimson MI, Anseth SD, et al. A mobile compression device for thrombosis prevention in hip and knee arthroplasty. *J Bone Joint Surg Am.* 2014;96(3):177-183. [IIA]

244. Haynes J, Barrack RL, Nam D. Mobile pump deep vein thrombosis prophylaxis: just say no to drugs. *Bone Joint J.* 2017;99-B(1 Suppl A):8-13. [IIIB]

245. Nam D, Nunley RM, Johnson SR, Keeney JA, Barrack RL. Mobile compression devices and aspirin for VTE prophylaxis following simultaneous bilateral total knee arthroplasty. *J Arthroplasty.* 2015;30(3):447-450. [IIIB]

246. Hardwick ME, Pulido PA, Colwell CWJ. A mobile compression device compared with low-molecular-weight heparin for prevention of venous thromboembolism in total hip arthroplasty. *Orthop Nurs.* 2011;30(5):312-316. [IA]

247. Craigie S, Tsui JF, Agarwal A, Sandset PM, Guyatt GH, Tikkinen KAO. Adherence to mechanical thromboprophylaxis after surgery: a systematic review and meta-analysis. *Thromb Res.* 2015;136(4):723-726. [IIIA]

248. Kim JH, Kim WI, Kim JY, Choe WJ. Peroneal nerve palsy after compression stockings application. *Saudi J Anaesth.* 2016;10(4):462-464. [VB]

249. Guzelkucuk U, Skempes D, Kumnerddee W. Common peroneal nerve palsy caused by compression stockings after surgery. *Am J Phys Med Rehabil.* 2014;93(7):609-611. [VB]

250. Hinderland MD, Ng A, Paden MH, Stone PA. Lateral leg compartment syndrome caused by ill-fitting compression stocking placed for deep vein thrombosis prophylaxis during surgery: a case report. *J Foot Ankle Surg.* 2011;50(5):616-619. [VB]

251. Thompson A, Walter S, Brunton LR, et al. Antiembolism stockings and proximal indentation. *Br J Nurs.* 2011;20(22):1426-1430. [IIIB]

252. Bowling K, Ratcliffe C, Townsend J, Kirkpatrick U. Clinical thromboembolic deterrent stockings application: Are thromboembolic deterrent stockings in practice matching manufacturers application guidelines. *Phlebology.* 2015;30(3):200-203. [IIIB]

253. Sachdeva A, Dalton M, Amaragiri SV, Lees T. Graduated compression stockings for prevention of deep vein thrombosis. *Cochrane Database Syst Rev.* 2014;(12):CD001484. [IA]

254. Mandavia R, Shalhoub J, Head K, Davies AH. The additional benefit of graduated compression stockings to pharmacologic thromboprophylaxis in the prevention of venous thromboembolism in surgical inpatients. *J Vasc Surg Venous Lymphat Disord.* 2015;3(4):447-455.e1. [IB]

255. Sajid MS, Desai M, Morris RW, Hamilton G. Knee length versus thigh length graduated compression stockings for prevention of deep vein thrombosis in postoperative surgical patients. *Cochrane Database Syst Rev.* 2012;(5):CD007162. [IB]

256. Wade R, Paton F, Rice S, et al. Thigh length versus knee length antiembolism stockings for the prevention of deep vein thrombosis in postoperative surgical patients; a systematic review and network meta-analysis. *BMJ Open.* 2016;6(2):e009456. [IA]

257. Wade R, Sideris E, Paton F, et al. Graduated compression stockings for the prevention of deep-vein thrombosis in postoperative surgical patients: a systematic review and economic model with a value of information analysis. *Health Technol Assess.* 2015;19(98):1-220. [IA]

258. Loomba RS, Arora RR, Chandrasekar S, Shah PH. Thigh-length versus knee-length compression stockings for deep vein thrombosis prophylaxis in the inpatient setting. *Blood Coagul Fibrinolysis.* 2012;23(2):168-171. [IIB]

259. Feist WR, Andrade D, Nass L. Problems with measuring compression device performance in preventing deep vein thrombosis. *Thromb Res.* 2011;128(3):207-209. [VB]

260. Ayhan H, Iyigun E, Ince S, Can MF, Hatipoglu S, Saglam M. A randomised clinical trial comparing the patient comfort and efficacy of three different graduated compression stockings in the prevention of postoperative deep vein thrombosis. *J Clin Nurs.* 2015;24(15-16):2247-2257. [IB]

261. Lattimer CR, Azzam M, Kalodiki E, Makris GC, Geroulakos G. Compression stockings significantly improve hemodynamic performance in post-thrombotic syndrome irrespective of class or length. *J Vasc Surg.* 2013;58(1):158-165. [IIB]

262. Bell BR, Bastien PE, Douketis JD; Thrombosis Canada. Prevention of venous thromboembolism in the Enhanced Recovery After Surgery (ERAS) setting: an evidence-based review. *Can J Anaesth.* 2015;62(2):194-202. [VB]

263. Glassou EN, Pedersen AB, Hansen TB. Risk of readmission, reoperation, and mortality within 90 days of total hip and knee arthroplasty in fast-track departments in Denmark from 2005 to 2011. *Acta Orthop.* 2014;85(5):493-500. [IIIA]

264. Husted H, Otte KS, Kristensen BB, Orsnes T, Wong C, Kehlet H. Low risk of thromboembolic complications after fast-track hip and knee arthroplasty. *Acta Orthop.* 2010;81(5):599-605. [IIIB]

265. Jorgensen CC, Jacobsen MK, Soeballe K, et al. Thromboprophylaxis only during hospitalisation in fast-track hip and knee arthroplasty, a prospective cohort study. *BMJ Open.* 2013;3(12):e003965. [IIIA]

266. Jorgensen CC, Kehlet H; Lundbeck Foundation Centre for Fast-track Hip and Knee Replacement Collaborative Group. Early thromboembolic events. *Thromb Res.* 2016;138:37-42. [IIIB]

267. Khan SK, Malviya A, Muller SD, et al. Reduced short-term complications and mortality following enhanced recovery primary hip and knee arthroplasty: results from 6,000 consecutive procedures. *Acta Orthop.* 2014;85(1):26-31. [IIIB]

268. Wang Z, Chen Q, Ye M, Shi G, Zhang B. Active ankle movement may prevent deep vein thrombosis in patients undergoing lower limb surgery. *Ann Vasc Surg.* 2016;32:65-72. [IB]

269. Shimizu Y, Kamada H, Sakane M, et al. A novel apparatus for active leg exercise improves venous flow in the lower extremity. *J Sports Med Phys Fitness.* 2016;56(12):1592-1597. [IIC]

270. DailyMed. US National Library of Medicine. https://dailymed.nlm.nih.gov/dailymed/. Accessed August 28 , 2017.

271. Mahan CE, Spyropoulos AC. ASHP therapeutic position statement on the role of pharmacotherapy in preventing venous thromboembolism in hospitalized patients. *Am J Health Syst Pharm.* 2012;69(24):2174-2190. [IVB]

272. Horlocker TT, Wedel DJ, Rowlingson JC, et al. Regional anesthesia in the patient receiving antithrombotic or thrombolytic therapy: American Society of Regional Anesthesia and Pain Medicine Evidence-Based Guidelines (Third Edition). *Reg Anesth Pain Med.* 2010;35(1):64-101. [IVA]

273. Karuppiah SV, Johnstone AJ. Skin necrosis associated with thromboprophylaxis after total knee replacement. *Case Rep Orthop.* 2014;2014:139218. [VB]

274. Sadideen H, O'Callaghan JM, Navidi M, Sayegh M. Educating surgical patients to reduce the risk of venous thromboembolism: an audit of an effective strategy. *JRSM Short Rep.* 2011;2(12):97. [IIB]

275. Haymes A. Venous thromboembolism: patient awareness and education in the pre-operative assessment clinic. *J Thromb Thrombolysis.* 2016;41(3):459-463. [IIIB]

276. Keiter JE, Johns D, Rockwell WB. Importance of postoperative hydration and lower extremity elevation in preventing deep venous thrombosis in full abdominoplasty: a report on 450 consecutive cases over a 37-year period. *Aesthet Surg J.* 2015;35(7):839-841. [IIIB]

277. Guyatt GH, Akl EA, Crowther M, Gutterman DD, Schünemann HJ. Executive summary: Antithrombotic Therapy and Prevention of Thrombosis, 9th ed: American College of Chest Physicians Evidence-Based Clinical Practice Guidelines. *Chest.* 2012;141(2 Suppl):7S-47S. [IVA]

278. Alzoubi KH, Khassawneh BY, Obeidat B, Asfoor SS, Alazzam SI. Awareness of patients who undergo cesarean section about venous thromboembolism prophylaxis. *J Vasc Nurs.* 2013;31(1):15-20. [IIIA]

279. He ML, Xiao ZM, Lei M, Li TS, Wu H, Liao J. Continuous passive motion for preventing venous thromboembolism after total knee arthroplasty. *Cochrane Database Syst Rev.* 2012;1:CD008207. [IA]

280. Lobastov K, Barinov V, Laberko L, Obolensky V, Boyarintsev V, Rodoman G. Electrical calf muscle stimulation with Veinoplus device in postoperative venous thromboembolism prevention. *Int Angiol.* 2014;33(1):42-49. [IIB]

281. Guideline for Medication Safety. In: *Guidelines for Perioperative Practice.* Denver, CO: AORN, Inc; 2017:295-333. [IVB]

282. Eisenstein DH. Anticoagulation management in the ambulatory surgical setting. *AORN J.* 2012;95(4):510-521. [VB]

283. Standards of perioperative nursing. In: *Guidelines for Perioperative Practice.* Denver, CO: AORN, Inc; 2015:693-732. https://www.aorn.org/aorn-org/guidelines/clinical-resources/aorn-standards. Accessed August 24, 2017. [IVC]

284. *State Operations Manual Appendix A—Survey Protocol, Regulations and Interpretive Guidelines for Hospitals.* Rev 151; 2015 Centers for Medicare & Medicaid Services. https://www.cms.gov/Regulations-and-Guidance/Guidance/Manuals/downloads/som107ap_a_hospitals.pdf. Accessed August 24, 2017.

285. *State Operations Manual Appendix L—Guidance for Surveyors: Ambulatory Surgical Centers.* Rev. 137; 2015. Centers for Medicare & Medicaid Services. https://www.cms.gov/Regulations-and-Guidance/Guidance/Manuals/downloads/som107ap_l_ambulatory.pdf. Accessed August 24, 2017.

286. 42 CFR 482. Conditions of participation for hospitals. 2011. Government Publishing Office. https://www.gpo.gov/fdsys/granule/CFR-2011-title42-vol5/CFR-2011-title42-vol5-part482. Accessed August 24, 2017.

287. 42 CFR 416. Ambulatory surgical services. 2011. Government Publishing Office. https://www.gpo.gov/fdsys/granule/CFR-2011-title42-vol3/CFR-2011-title42-vol3-part416. Accessed August 24, 2017.

288. RC.01.01.01: The hospital maintains complete and accurate medical records for each individual patient. In: *The Joint Commission Comprehensive Accreditation and Certification Manual.* E-dition. Oakbrook Terrace, IL: The Joint Commission; 2016.

289. MS.16: Medical record maintenance. In: *National Integrated Accreditation for Healthcare Organizations (NIAHO): Interpretive Guidelines and Surveyor Guidance.* Version 11. Milford, OH: DNV-GL Healthcare; 2014:37. http://cms.ipressroom.com.s3.amazonaws.com/107/files/20146/DNVGL+Healthcare+-+NIAHO+Accreditation+Requirements+and+Interpretive+Guidelines+-+Rev+11.pdf. Accessed August 24, 2017.

290. RC.01.01.01: The organization maintains complete and accurate clinical records. In: *The Joint Commission Comprehensive Accreditation and Certification Manual.* E-dition. Oakbrook Terrace, IL: The Joint Commission; 2016.

291. Clinical records and health information. In: *Accreditation Handbook for Ambulatory Health Care.* Skokie, IL: Accreditation Association for Ambulatory Health Care, Inc; 2016:51-53. https://www.aaahc.org/Global/Handbooks/2016/HB16_FNL-interactive_v2.pdf. Accessed August 24, 2017.

292. Medical records: operating room records. In: *Regular Standards and Checklist for Accreditation of Ambulatory Surgery Facilities.* Version 14.4. Gurnee, IL: American Association for Accreditation of Ambulatory Surgery Facilities, Inc; 2016:60-63.

293. Medical records: procedure room records. In: *Regular Standards and Checklist for Accreditation of Ambulatory Surgery Facilities.* 3rd ed. Gurnee, IL: American Association for Accreditation of Ambulatory Surgery Facilities, Inc; 2011:64-66. https://www.aaaasf.org/docs/default-source/accreditation/standards/standards-manual-and-checklist-v3-(obp).pdf?sfvrsn=5. Accessed August 24, 2017.

294. Miller JA. Use and wear of anti-embolism stockings: a clinical audit of surgical patients. *Int Wound J.* 2011;8(1):74-83. [IIIB]

295. Jordan C, Thomas MB, Evans ML, Green A. Public policy on competency: how will nursing address this complex issue? *J Contin Educ Nurs.* 2008;39(2):86-91. [VB]

296. HR.01.05.03: Staff participate in ongoing education and training. In: *The Joint Commission Comprehensive Accreditation and Certification Manual.* E-dition. Oakbrook Terrace, IL: The Joint Commission; 2016.

297. MS.10: Continuing education. In: *National Integrated Accreditation for Healthcare Organizations (NIAHO): Interpretive Guidelines and Surveyor Guidance.* Version 11. Milford, OH: DNV-GL Healthcare; 2014:30. http://cms.ipressroom.com.s3.amazonaws.com/107/files/20146/NVGL+Healthcare+ -+NIAHO+Accreditation+Requirements+and+Interpretive+Guidelines+-+Rev+11.pdf. Accessed August 24, 2017.

298. HR.01.05.03: Staff participate in ongoing education and training. In: *The Joint Commission Comprehensive Accreditation and Certification Manual.* E-dition. Oakbrook Terrace, IL: The Joint Commission; 2016.

299. Governance. In: *Accreditation Handbook for Ambulatory Health Care.* Skokie, IL: Accreditation Association for Ambulatory Health Care, Inc; 2016:33-40. https://www.aaahc.org/Global/Handbooks/2016/HB16_FNL-interactive_v2.pdf. Accessed August 24, 2017.

300. Personnel: Personnel records; individual personnel files. In: *Regular Standards and Checklist for Accreditation of Ambulatory Surgery Facilities.* Version 14.4. Gurnee, IL: American Association for Accreditation of Ambulatory Surgery Facilities, Inc; 2016:74-75.

301. PI.03.01.01: The hospital improves performance on an ongoing basis. In: *The Joint Commission Comprehensive Accreditation and Certification Manual.* E-dition. Oakbrook Terrace, IL: The Joint Commission; 2016.

302. QM.1: Quality management system. In: *National Integrated Accreditation for Healthcare Organizations (NIAHO): Interpretive Guidelines and Surveyor Guidance.* Version 11. Milford, OH: DNV-GL Healthcare; 2014:10-17. http://cms.ipressroom.com.s3.amazonaws.com/107/files/20146/DNVGL+Healthcare+-+NIAHO+Accreditation+Requirements+and+Interpretive+Guidelines+-+Rev+11.pdf. Accessed August 24, 2017.

303. PI.03.01.01: The organization improves performance. In: *The Joint Commission Comprehensive Accreditation and Certification Manual.* E-dition. Oakbrook Terrace, IL: The Joint Commission; 2016.

304. Quality management and improvement. In: *Accreditation Handbook for Ambulatory Health Care.* Skokie, IL: Accreditation Association for Ambulatory Health Care, Inc; 2016:46-50. https://www.aaahc.org/Global/Handbooks/2016/HB16_FNL-interactive_v2.pdf. Accessed August 24, 2017.

305. Quality assessment/quality improvement: Quality improvement. In: *Regular Standards and Checklist for Accreditation of Ambulatory Surgery Facilities.* Version 14.4. Gurnee, IL: American Association for Accreditation of Ambulatory Surgery Facilities, Inc; 2016:64.

306. Quality assessment/quality improvement: unanticipated operative sequelae In: *Regular Standards and Checklist for Accreditation of Ambulatory Surgery Facilities.* Version 14.4. Gurnee, IL: American Association for Accreditation of Ambulatory Surgery Facilities, Inc; 2016:66-69.

307. *PSI 90: Patient Safety for Selected Indicators. Technical Specifications.* Rockville, MD: Agency for Healthcare Research and Quality; 2015.

308. Venous thromboembolism national hospital inpatient quality measures. In: *Specifications Manual for National Hospital Inpatient Quality Measures.* Version 5.2a. Oakbrook Terrace, IL: The Joint Commission; 2016:VTE-1. https://www.jointcommission.org/assets/1/6/HIQR_SpecsManual_v52a.zip. Accessed August 24, 2017.

Acknowledgments

Lead Author
Amber Wood, MSN, RN, CNOR, CIC, FAPIC
Senior Perioperative Practice Specialist
AORN Nursing Department
Denver, Colorado

Contributing Author
Ramona L. Conner, MSN, RN, CNOR, FAAN
Editor-in-Chief, Guidelines for Perioperative Practice
AORN Nursing Department
Denver, Colorado

The authors and AORN thank Heather A. Hohenberger, MSN, RN, CIC, CNOR, CPHQ, FAPIC, System Perioperative Quality Improvement Consultant, Indiana University Health, Indianapolis; Jocelyn M. Chalquist, BSN, RN, CNOR, Surgical Services Educator, Aurora Medical Center-Kenosha, Kenosha, Wisconsin; Barbara L. Nalley, MSN, CRNP, CNOR, Manager, Anne Arundel Medical Group, Annapolis, Maryland; Marie A. Bashaw, DNP, RN, NEA-BC, CNOR, Assistant Professor, Wright State University College of Nursing and Health, Dayton, Ohio; Janice Neil, PhD, RN, CNE, Associate Professor, College of Nursing, East Carolina University, Greenville, North Carolina; Diana L. Wadlund, MSN, ACNP-C, CRNFA, Nurse Practitioner, Paoli Hospital, Paoli, Pennsylvania; Lynn Reed, DNP, MBA, CRNA, FNAP, Senior Director, Professional Practice, American Association of Nurse Anesthetists, Des Plaines, Illinois; David Urbach, MD, MSc, Clinical Epidemiology, University Health Network, Toronto, Ontario, Canada; Dawn Yost, MSN, RN, CNOR, CSSM, Manager of Training & Development, Surgical Services, West Virginia University Medicine-Ruby Memorial Hospital, Morgantown; Carrie Simpson, BSN, BA, RN-BC, CNOR, Owner& Principal Consultant, CS Perioperative Education Solution, New Orleans, Louisiana; Vangie Dennis, BSN, RN, CNOR, CMLSO, Director of Patient Care Practice, Emory Healthcare and Ambulatory Surgery Centers, Atlanta, Georgia; Jay Bowers, BSN, RN, CNOR, TNCC, Clinical Educator, West Virginia University Healthcare, Morgantown; and Esther Johnstone, DNP, RN, CNOR, Perioperative Practice Specialist, AORN Nursing Department, Denver, Colorado, for their assistance in developing this guideline.

Publication History

Originally published March 2011 as "Recommended practices for prevention of deep vein thrombosis" in *Perioperative Standards and Recommended Practices* online.

Reformatted September 2012 for publication in *Perioperative Standards and Recommended Practices*, 2013 edition.

Minor editing revisions made in November 2014 for publication as "Guideline for prevention of deep vein thrombosis" in *Guidelines for Perioperative Practice*, 2015 edition.

Revised November 2017 for publication in *Guidelines for Perioperative Practice* online.

Evidence ratings revised and minor editorial changes made to conform to the current AORN Evidence Rating model, September 2019, for online publication in *Guidelines for Perioperative Practice*.

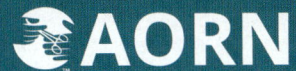

INDEX TO THE *GUIDELINES FOR PERIOPERATIVE PRACTICE* 2022 EDITION